A PRACTICAL TOOL FOR LEARNING CRITICAL AND APPLYING INFORMATION TO NEW SITUATIONS.

W9-AYB-533

Personal stories written by patients provide meaningful and illuminating accounts of their experience with illness.

Nursing Care Plans are now easy to read and clearly present the rationale for each action.

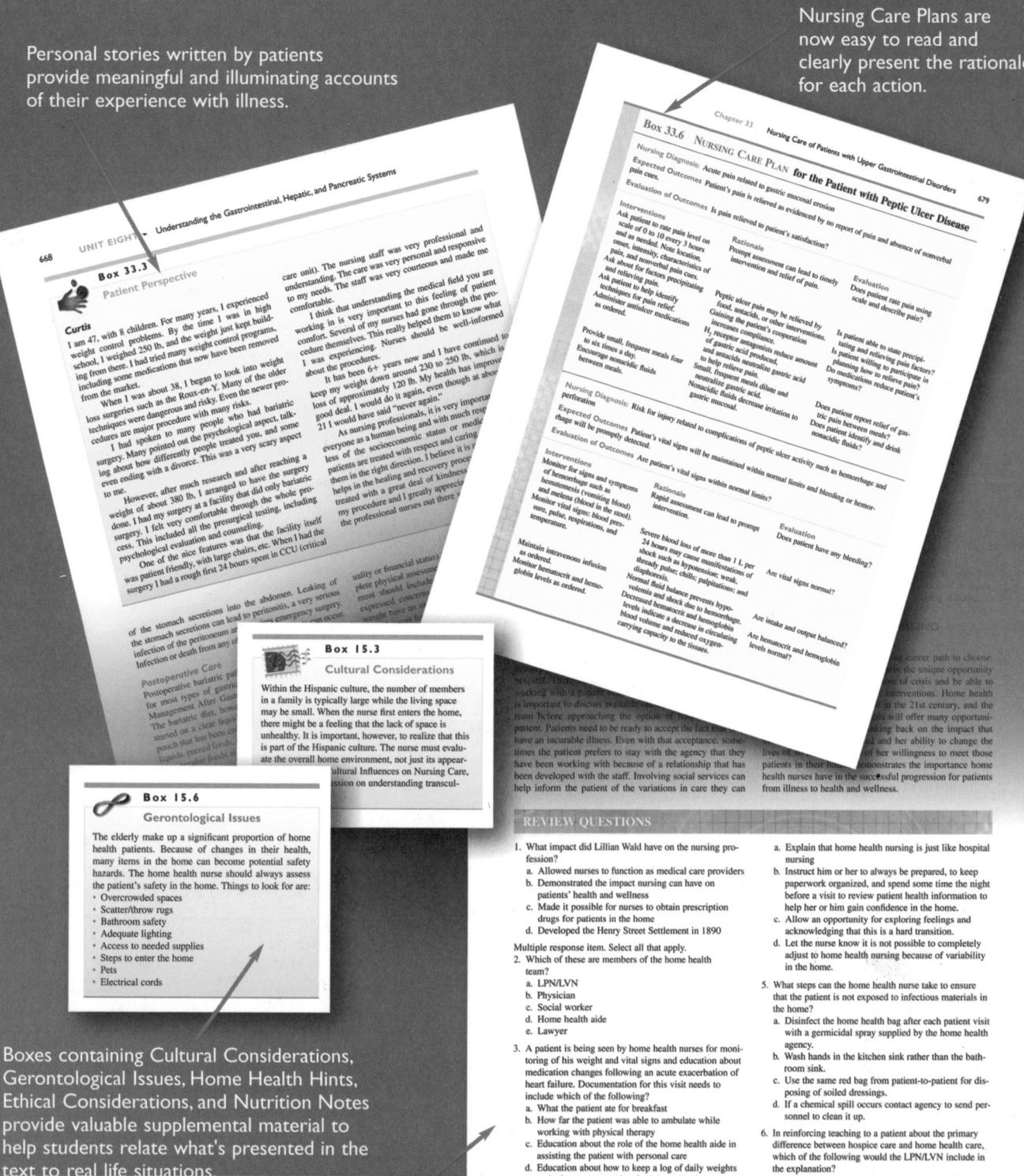

Boxes containing Cultural Considerations, Gerontological Issues, Home Health Hints, Ethical Considerations, and Nutrition Notes provide valuable supplemental material to help students relate what's presented in the text to real life situations.

Each chapter concludes with Review Questions that reflect the alternate format NCLEX-PN type questions.

NEW! STUDENT CD-ROM

- **UNIT ANALYSIS TUTORIAL**
  - An easy method for calculating drug dosages and IV rates

- **STUDENT TEST BANK**
  - 500 NCLEX-style questions with difficulty levels
  - 100 fill-in-the-blank unit analysis questions

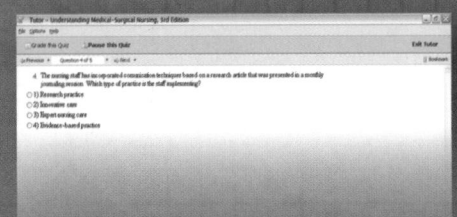

- **INTERACTIVE EXERCISES**
  - Over 170 interactive exercises that include: fill-in-the-blank, picture match, flash cards, and case studies

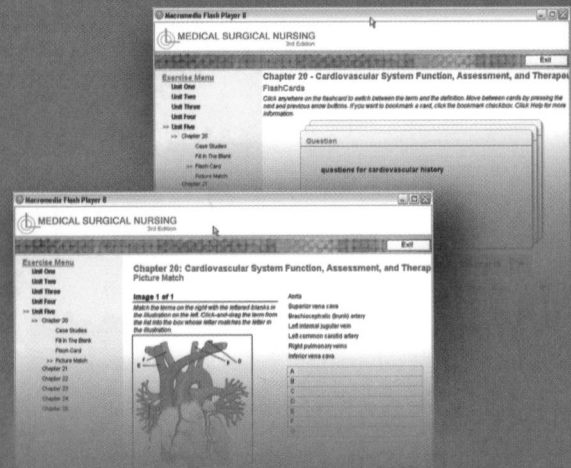

- **MEDIA BANK**
  - 39 stereophonic audio clips (heart, lung, bowel sounds, etc.)

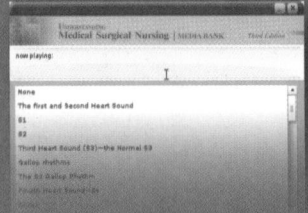

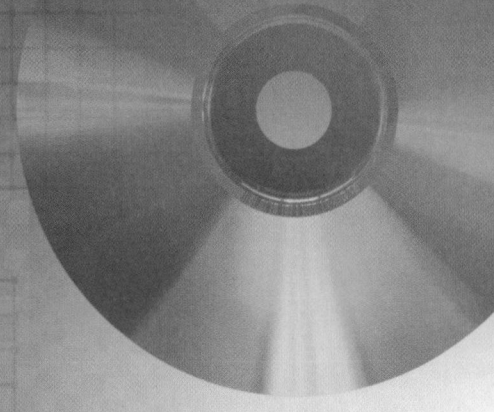

ADDITIONAL LEARNING TOOLS

THE THIRD EDITION NOW PACKS A POWERFUL VIRTUAL PUNCH WITH A STUDENT CD AND BONUS MATERIAL ON THE WEB.

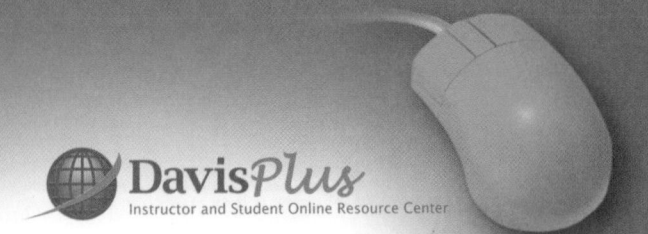

DavisPlus
Instructor and Student Online Resource Center

NEW! DAVISPLUS ONLINE RESOURCES

- **HTTP://DAVISPLUS.FADAVIS.COM**
- **20 NCLEX-TYPE QUESTIONS**
- **10 UNIT ANALYSIS QUESTIONS**
- **OVER 30 ANIMATIONS**

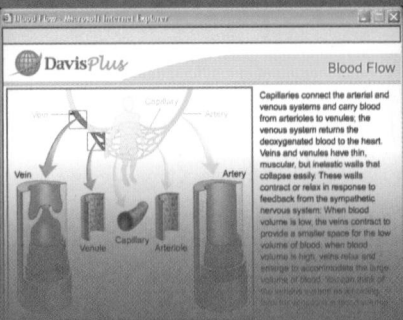

CONTENTS IN BRIEF

UNDERSTANDING
Medical Surgical
Nursing

THIRD EDITION

LINDA S. WILLIAMS, MSN, RNBC
Professor of Nursing
Jackson Community College
Jackson, Michigan

PAULA D. HOPPER, MSN, RN
Professor of Nursing
Jackson Community College
Jackson, Michigan

F. A. DAVIS COMPANY • Philadelphia

F. A. Davis Company
1915 Arch Street
Philadelphia, PA 19103
www.fadavis.com

Copyright © 2007 by F. A. Davis Company

Printed in the United States of America

Last digit indicates print number: 10 9 8 7 6 5 4 3

Acquisitions Editors: Lisa B. Deitch/Jonathan Joyce
Director of Content Development: Darlene D. Pedersen
Special Projects Editor: Shirley A. Kuhn
Senior Project Editor: Ilysa H. Richman
Art and Design Manager: Carolyn O'Brien

As new scientific information becomes available through basic and clinical research, recommended treatments
and drug therapies undergo changes. The author(s) and publisher have done everything possible to make
this book accurate, up to date, and in accord with accepted standards at the time of publication. The author(s),
editors, and publisher are not responsible for errors or omissions or for consequences from application of the
book, and make no warranty, expressed or implied, in regard to the contents of the book. Any practice
described in this book should be applied by the reader in accordance with professional standards of care used
in regard to the unique circumstances that may apply in each situation. The reader is advised always to check
product information (package inserts) for changes and new information regarding dose and contraindications
before administering any drug. Caution is especially urged when using new or infrequently ordered drugs.

ISBN 13: 978-0-8036-1491-8
ISBN 10: 0-8036-1491-8

Library of Congress Cataloging-in-Publication Data

Understanding medical-surgical nursing / [edited by] Linda S. Williams, Paula D.
Hopper. — 3rd ed.
    p. ; cm.
  Includes bibliographical references and index.
  ISBN 0-8036-1491-8
 I. Nursing. 2. Surgical nursing. I. Williams, Linda S. (Linda Sue), 1954-
II. Hopper, Paula D.
 [DNLM: 1. Nursing Care. 2. Nursing. WY 100 U548 2007]
 RT41.W576 2007
 617'.0231—dc22
                                                                    2006035577

Preface

Welcome to the third edition of *Understanding Medical Surgical Nursing!* We have fully updated all the material, and have added exciting new information on home health care, end-of-life care, disaster response and bioterrorism, stroke, and more.

We continue to work hard to provide a text written at an understandable level, with features that help students understand, apply, and practice the challenging content required to function as practical/vocational nurses. We are thankful to the many students who tell us they find the book very readable, and actually enjoyable. We are overjoyed to hear from several nursing programs that their NCLEX scores soared after adopting this textbook.

We continue to emphasize understanding, critical thinking, and application throughout the book. We believe that a student who learns to think critically will be better able to apply information to new situations. We hope both students and instructors find this third edition a practical tool for learning and understanding medical-surgical nursing.

FEATURES OF THE BOOK

We have kept our most popular features from the first two editions, and added new ones based on reader input.

- *Questions to Guide Your Reading* begin each chapter. In our experience, the standard objectives found in many textbooks have little meaning and provide little assistance to students. Literature suggests that comprehension increases when students read guiding questions before reading the text. So we have provided a series of questions that students should keep in mind as they read. These questions can be translated easily back into objectives by instructors who prefer this format.
- Special features written by actual patients, called *Patient Perspectives,* were added in the second edition. Many more have been added to this edition. These stories help to make patients' experiences with illness more meaningful and personal for students.
- Web links are included in the text to help students do further research on topics of interest. Every effort was made to use only major established web sites that are unlikely to change in the near future.
- One of our most popular features, Critical Thinking Exercises, has been expanded to help students practice and think about what they are learning. We have added more math calculations and documentation practice to Critical Thinking Exercises where applicable.
- Review questions at the end of each chapter have been updated and include alternate format items to reflect NCLEX-PN.
- Suggested Answers for the Critical Thinking Exercises and Review Questions are included. Research supports the importance of immediate feedback to reinforce learning, so we feel strongly that students should have access to correct answers while they are studying, without having to wait for their next instructor contact. Since there can be many answers to some of the critical thinking questions, we have provided sample answers to help stimulate students' thinking.
- The effects of aging on body systems have been converted from text format to a mindmap format. We believe this visual representation is easier to understand and apply than the traditional text.
- We have changed our Nursing Process format from text to bullet lists. It is very easy to read, clearly stands out, and makes interventions with rationale very clear to students.
- More Learning Tips, a very popular feature in past editions, have been added. New to the third edition are Nursing Care Tips and Safety Tips.
- JCAHO National Patient Safety Goals are reflected in many of the safety tips to give students an introduction to these safety goals.
- Nursing assessment, laboratory tests, and medications have been placed in consistent tables that are easy to read and understand.

- Summary boxes including nursing diagnoses have been expanded and included for most major disorders.
- A pronunciation key for new words is found at the beginning of each chapter.
- A review of anatomy and physiology is presented at the beginning of each unit.
- Word-building footnotes are found throughout the chapters to make complex medical terminology easier to understand.
- Nursing care plans with geriatric considerations have been updated.
- Boxed presentations of Cultural Considerations, Gerontological Issues, Home Health Hints, Ethical Considerations, and Nutrition Notes provide valuable supplemental information and help students relate text material to real life situations.
- Many new photographs and drawings have been added to illustrate important concepts.
- A comprehensive, updated glossary of new words is included in the appendix.

TO STUDENTS: HOW TO USE THIS BOOK

As you begin each chapter, carefully read the section labeled *Questions to Guide your Reading.* Then, when you are finished reading each chapter, go back and make sure you can answer each question.

You will find a list of new words and their pronunciations at the beginning of each chapter. These words appear in bold at their first use in a chapter, and they also appear in the glossary at the end of the book. By learning the meanings of these words as you encounter them, you will increase your understanding of the material.

You also will encounter other learning tips to increase your understanding and retention of the material. You may want to develop your own memory techniques in addition to those provided. (If you think of a good one, send it to us and you may find it in the next edition!) Many of the learning tips have been developed and used in our own classrooms. We find them helpful in fostering understanding of complex concepts or as memory aids. However, we want to stress that memorization is not the primary focus of the text but rather a foundation for understanding and thinking about more complex information. Understanding and application will serve you far better than memorization when dealing with new situations.

Each chapter includes critical thinking case studies designed to help you apply material that has been presented. A series of questions related to the case study will help you integrate the material with what you already know. These questions emphasize critical thinking, which is based on a foundation of recall and understanding of material. To enhance your learning, try to answer the questions before looking up the answers at the end of the chapter.

Review questions appear at the end of each chapter to help you prepare for chapter tests, and also for the NCLEX-PN. Again, to assess your learning, try to answer the questions before looking up the answers at the back of the book.

A bibliography at the end of each unit provides sources for additional reading material. Web sites have been included in many chapters. We believe it is important for you to interact with current technology to expand your information resources.

The following appendices are included for easy reference:

- NANDA nursing diagnoses
- Lab values
- Common medical abbreviations (Although it is still important to know the abbreviations, many can increase risk of errors. Check www.JCAHO.org for a list of abbreviations to avoid.)
- Common prefixes and suffixes to help learn word building techniques

SUPPLEMENTAL MATERIALS

- A new *Electronic Student Guide* is included with the book. This provides practice in the form of objective (fill-in, labeling, and flashcard) exercises, and case studies. There are also review questions and a practice NCLEX test. We have also included a brief math tutorial using Unit Analysis, and practice calculation problems. Answers are provided to all exercises for immediate feedback.
- A paperback *Student Workbook* is available to provide the student additional contact and practice with the material. Each chapter includes vocabulary practice, objective exercises, a case study or other critical thinking practice and review questions written in NCLEX-PN format. Answers provide immediate feedback. Rationales are provided for non-anatomy review question answers.
- An *Instructor's Resource Disk* includes an *Electronic Instructor's Guide* that provides materials for use in the classroom. Each chapter has a chapter outline with suggested classroom activities. Also included are student activities for printing and using for individual practice or for collaborative learning activities. These activities help the student to interact with the material, understand it, and apply it. Many of the activities are based on real patient cases and have been used with our own practical nursing students. Feedback from students has helped to refine the exercises. We believe the use of collaborative learning has greatly enhanced our students' success in achieving their educational and licensure goals. Another benefit is the sense of community the students develop as a result of working in groups. A brief introduction and guidelines for using collaborative learning techniques is

included. Also included is an expanded *Electronic Test Bank*, available to instructors who adopt the textbook, which provides test questions that assist students to prepare for NCLEX-PN. These questions have been prepared according to test item writing protocols. The questions are in multiple choice and alternate format, and test recall, application, and analysis of material. Many of the test questions have been developed, used and refined by the authors in their own medical-surgical courses

for practical nursing students. The program allows instructors to choose and modify the questions that best suit their classroom needs. Finally, for the instructor's convenience, there is a comprehensive *Power Point* program for classroom presentations. Images from the text have been added for the third edition. Each presentation can be modified, reduced, or expanded by individual instructors to suit their needs.

Acknowledgements

Many people helped us make this book a reality. First and foremost are our students, who provided us with the inspiration to undertake this project. We hope that they continue to find this text worth reading.

The F.A. Davis Company has been an exceptional publishing partner. We feel fortunate to have had their continued enthusiasm and confidence in our book. The staff at F.A. Davis has guided us through this project for three editions to help us create a student-friendly book that truly promotes understanding of medical-surgical nursing.

Lisa Deitch, Shirley Kuhn, Ilysa Richman, Darlene Pedersen, Doris Wray, and many others have been extremely patient and kind as we worked hard to provide a quality text and meet deadlines.

We thank the staff of W.A. Foote Memorial Hospital in Jackson, Michigan for allowing us access to their facility and patients for a great photo shoot. Our photographer, Robert Conway, did a terrific job of obtaining some challenging shots.

Contributors from across the United States and Canada, including many well-known experts in their fields, brought expertise and diversity to the content. Their hard work is much appreciated. Reviewers from throughout the United States provided insights that enhanced the quality of the text. Elizabeth Hopper provided invaluable organizational assistance.

Many of our co-workers have contributed to this book and given us ongoing encouragement and validation of the worthiness of this project. Elizabeth Ackley, Marina-Martinez Kratz, Sharon Nowak, Debra Perry-Philo, Carroll Lutz, Suzanne Fox, Linda Nabozny, and Anna Ricks were especially helpful in providing material, advice, and encouragement.

We wish to thank everyone who played a role, however large or small, in helping us to provide a tool to help students realize their dreams of becoming an LPN or LVN. We hope this book will help train nurses who can provide safe and expert care because we have helped them to learn to think critically.

Contributors

Nancy Ahern, RN, MSN
Instructor and Program Coordinator
University of Central Florida
Cocoa, Florida

Brenda Anderson
St. Bernards Medical Center
Patient Care Manager-Education
Jonesboro, Arizona

Debra Aucoin-Ratcliff, RN, BSN, MN, DNPc
Nursing Faculty
American River College
Sacramento, California

Cynthia Francis Bechtel, MS, RN, CNE, CEN, EMT-I
Associate Professor
Anna Maria College
Paxton, Massachusetts

Virginia Birnie, RN, BScN, MSN
Nursing Instructor
Camosun College
Victoria, British Columbia
Canada

Janice L. Bradford, MS
Assistant Professor
Jackson Community College
Jackson, Michigan

Lucy L. Colo, RN, MSN
Faculty
Huron School of Nursing
East Cleveland, Ohio

Linda Hopper Cook RN, MN, PhD Candidate
Instructor
Grant MacEwan College School of Nursing
Edmonton, Alberta
Canada

Mary Dillinger, MS, RN, ACRN
Clinical Nurse Specialist
Munson Medical Center
Traverse City, Michigan

Susan Garbutt, RN, MSN, CIC
Faculty
St. Petersburg College
St. Petersburg, Florida

Karen P. Hall, RN, MSHSA, CNA-BC
Director of Patient Care Services
Doctors Medical Center
Modesto, California

Wendy Hockley, LPN, BS, MA
Manager
WA Foote Memorial Hospital
Jackson, Michigan

Lenetra Jefferson, MSN, RN, LMT, PhD Candidate
Educational Coordinator
Delgado Community college
New Orleans, Louisana

Jean Jeffries, BSN, RN
Registered Nurse
Huntsville Hospital
Huntsville, Alabama

Rodney B. Kebicz, RN, BN, MN
Instructor
Assiniboine Community College
Winnipeg, Manitoba
Canada

Lynn Keegan, RN, PhD, AHN-BC, FAAN
Director
Holistic Nursing Consultants
Port Angeles, Washington

Marty Kohn, RN, BSN, MS, FNP-CWOCN
Nurse Practitioner Wound Care Center
Foote Hospital
Jackson, Michigan

Linda Marie Lowe, RN, BSN
Assistant Professor
University of Northern British Columbia
Prince George, British Columbia
Canada

Carroll Lutz, BSN, MA, RN
Associate Professor Emerita
Jackson Community College
Jackson, Mississippi

Marina Martinez-Kratz, RN, BSN, MS
Professor
Jackson Community College
Jackson, Michigan

Maureen McDonald, MS, RN
Professor
Massasoit Community College
Brockton, Massachusetts

Kelly McManigle, BSN, MSN
Nursing Faculty
Manatee Technical Institute
Bradenton, Florida

Betsy Murphy, FNP, CHPN
Business Relations
Capital Hospice
Fairfax, Virginia

Sharon M. Nowak, RN, MSN
Associate Professor
Jackson Community College
Jackson, Michigan

Lazette V. Nowicki, RN, MSN
Adjunct Nursing Faculty
American River College
Sacramento, California

Debra Perry-Philo, BSN, MSN
Nursing Faculty
Jackson Community College
Jackson, Michigan

Lynn Dianne Phillips, RN, MSN, CRNI
Nursing Instructor
Butte College
Oroville, California

MaryAnne Pietraniec-Shannon, PhD, APRN, BC
Professor
Lake Superior State University
Sault Sainte Marie, Michigan

Ruth Remington, PhD, APRN, BC
Assistant Professor
University of Massachusetts, Lowell
Lowell, Massachusetts

Patrick M. Shannon, JD, EdD, MPH
Attorney
Bay Mills Community College
Brimley, Michigan

Susan Smith, BS, MS, RNC, CAN
President/Educator
SK Smith Consulting
Warriors Mark, Pennsylvania

Rita Bolek Trofino, MNEd, RN
Director of Healthcare Programming and Initiatives
Pennsylvania Highlands Community College
Johnstown, Pennsylvania

Deborah L. Weaver, RN, PhD
Associate Professor
Valdosta State University
Valdosta, Georgia

Jennifer Whitley, RN, MSN, CNOR
Educator
Huntsville Hospital
Huntsville, Alabama

Bruce K. Wilson, PhD, RN, CNS
Professor
University of Texas-Pan American
Edinburg, Texas

Contributors to Previous Editions

We would like to acknowledge and thank the following individuals for their contributions to the first two editions. All contributions have helped to make *Understanding Medical Surgical Nursing* what it has evolved into today.

Jeanette Acker, RN, BSN
Manager, Stepdown Unit
W.A. Foote Memorial Hospital
Jackson, Michigan

Betty J. Ackley, RN, MSN, EdS
Professor of Nursing
Jackson Community College
Jackson, Michigan

Joseph Catalano, RN, PhD
Professor of Nursing
East Central University
Ada, Oklahoma

Elizabeth Chapman, RN, MS, CCRN
Nursing Faculty
Mississippi Gulf Coast Community College
Gulfport, Mississippi
ICU Staff Nurse
Hancock Medical Center
Bay St. Louis, Mississippi

Kathleen R. Culliton, APRN, MS, GNP
Assistant Professor
Weber State University
Ogden, Utah

Constance Monlezun Darbonne, RN, MPH, CFNP
Family Nurse Practitioner
Clinical Instructor, Community Health
McNeese State University
Lake Charles, Louisiana

Sharon Gordon Dawson, RN, MSN, CNOR
Educator, Surgical Services
Swedish Medical Center
Englewood, Colorado

Vera Dutro, RN, BSN, OCN
Infusion Nurse
Zanesville Infusion Therapy
Zanesville, Ohio

Rowena Elliott, MS, RN, CNN, C, CLNC
Assistant Professor
University of Mississippi
Jackson, Mississippi

Mary Friel Fanning, RN, MSN, CCRN
Director, Adult Cardiac Nursing Units
West Virginia University Hospitals
Morgantown, West Virginia

Donna D. Ignatavicius, MS, RN, CM
Clinical Nurse Specialist in
    Medical/Surgical/Gerontological Nursing
Calvert Memorial Hospital
Owner/Consultant, DI Associates
Prince Frederick, Maryland

Cheryl L. Ivey, RN, MSN
Department Director
Emory University Hospital
Atlanta, Georgia

Josephine Whitney Johns, RN, OCN, CRNI
South Mississippi Home Health
Oncology Specialty Nurse
Board of Director, Mississippi Cancer Pain Initiative
Co-founder, Mississippi Gulf Coast Chapter
Oncology Nurse Association
Gulfport, Mississippi

Elaine Kennedy, EdD, RN
Professor of Nursing
Wor-Wic Community College
Salisbury, Maryland

Gail Ladwig, RN, MSN, CHTP
Associate Professor of Nursing
Coordinator JCC/UM BSN Transfer Program
Jackson Community College
Jackson, Michigan

Diane Lewis, RN, MS
Hospice of Grant/Riverside Methodist Hospitals
Westerville, Ohio

Gary S. Lott, RN, MS
Instructor of Nursing
Mississippi Gulf Coast Community College
Gulfport, Mississippi

Sharon D. Martin, MSN, BSN, APRN, BC
Associate Professor of Nursing
Saint Joseph's College
Standish, Maine

Deborah J. Mauffray, RN, MSN, CNS, CDE, CWOCN
Clinical Nurse Specialist in Wound, Ostomy, and
    Incontinence
Memorial Hospital at Gulfport
Gulfport, Mississippi

Cindy Meredith, MSN, RN
Director and Instructor of Nursing
Spring Arbor University
Spring Arbor, Michigan

Marsha A. Miles, RN, MSN, CCRN
Instructor
Valdosta State University
College of Nursing
Valdosta, Georgia

Debbie Millar, MEd, BScN, RN, MBA Candidate
Clinical Educator
Humber River Regional Hospital
Toronto, Ontario
Canada

Kathy Neeb, ADN, BA
RN Consultant
North Memorial Occupational Health Clinic
Robbinsdale, Minnesota

Winifred J. Ellenchild Pinch, EdD, MEd, MS, RN, BS
Professor
Creighton University
Omaha, Nebraska

Larry Purnell, PhD, MSN, BSN, FAAN
Professor
University of Delaware
Sudlersville, Maryland

Deborah L. Roush, RN, MSN
Assistant Professor
Valdosta State University
College of Nursing
Valdosta, Georgia

Valerie C. Scanlon, PhD
Professor
College of Mount St. Vincent
Bronx, New York

Kate Schmitz, RN, MS
Clinical Nurse, Emergency Department
St. Joseph Hospital
Creighton University Medical Center
Omaha, Nebraska

Sally Schnell, RN, MSN, CNRN
Professional Education Coordinator
Regional Organ Bank of Illinois
Chicago, Illinois

Jill Secord, RN, BSN, CRNI
University of Michigan Health System—-M-CARE
Jackson, Michigan

George B. Smith, MSN, BSN, ADN
Nursing Faculty
Hillsborough Community College
Tampa, Florida

Martha Spray, RN, BSN, MS
Adult PN Instructor
Mid East Ohio Vocational School
Zanesville, Ohio

Rose Utley, PhD, RN
Associate Professor
Southwest Missouri State University
Rogersville, Missouri

Kathleen Kelley Walsh, RN, MS
Professor of Nursing
Jackson Community College
Jackson, Mississippi

JoAnn Widner, RN, MS
Health Educator
Central North Alabama Health Services, Inc.
Huntsville, Alabama

Reviewers

Deborah L. Benns, MSN, BSN, BA, RN
Nursing Professor
Rend Lake College
Ina, Illinois

William Beiswenger, RN, MA, CDE
Certified Diabetes Educator
W.A. Foote Memorial Hospital Diabetes Center
Jackson, Michigan

Nicholle Bieberdorf, RN, BAN
Practical Nursing Instructor
Northwest Technical College
Bemidji, Minnesota

L. Adrienne Bowlus, MSN, RN
Instructor
Apollo School of Practical Nursing
Lima, Ohio

Rosemary Brown, RN, MSN, FNP-C
Program Coordinator
Idaho State University
Pocatella, Idaho

Monica Cauley, RN, MSN, GNP/GCNS
Chair, Health Science
Larleen B. Wallace Community College, MacAuthor
   Campus
Opp, Alaska

Jessie Chatman Williams, RN, MA
Nursing Instructor
Mineral Area College
Park Hills, Missouri

Michelle Colleran Cook, MS, RN
Nursing Professor
MassBay Community College
Framingham, Massachusetts

Robin S. Culbertson, RN, MSN, EDS
Nursing Instructor
Okaloosa Applied Technology Center
Fort Walton Beach, Florida

Kim DeEll, RN, BSN
Nursing Instructor
Malaspina University College
Duncan, British Columbia, Canada

Carol Duell, MSN, CRNP
Nursing Instructor
Eastern Center for Arts and Technology
Willow Grove, Pennsylvania

Theresa Ellis, MSN, CS
Clinical Quality Specialist
Foote Hospital
Addison, Michigan

Andi Foley, RN, BSN, CEN
Charge RN
Lakeland Regional Medical Center
Lakeland, Florida

Madeline Gervase, MSN, CCRN, FNP, RN
Assistant Professor
Union County College
Plainfield, New Jersey

Tracey A. Hartke, MSN, RN
Front Range Community College
Westminster, Colorado

Dorothy A. Hogan, RN, MN
Nursing Faculty
Wayne Community College
Goldsboro, North Carolina

Phyllis Sue Howard, RN, BSN
Administrator, PN Program
Ashland Community & Technical college
Ashland, Kentucky

Connie Hunt, RN, BSN
Instuctor, Practical Nursing
Indian Capital Technology Center
Stilwell, Oklahoma

Theresa Isom, AD, BS, MS
Nursing Coordinator
Tennessee Technology Center at Memphis
Memphis, Tennessee

Jaclynn A. Johnson, RNC, MSN
Lead Instructor, 1st Level Nursing
La Junta, Colorado

Ethel M. Jones, RN, MSN, Ed. S., DSNc
Coordinator, Practical Nursing
H. Councill Trenholm State Technical College
Montgomery, Alabama

Linda Kimble, MSN, RN, CNP
Director
The Robert T. White School of Practical Nursing
Alliance, Ohio

Ellen Anne Kliethermes, RN
Instructor
Nichols Career Center
Loose Creek, Missouri

Cynthia L. Lapp, RN, BS
LPN Instructor – Level 2
Charles H. Bohlen Jr. Technical Center
Watertown, New York

Cathy A. Learn, RN, MSN, MA
Director, Nursing
Mid East Career and Technology Schools
Zanesville, Ohio

Patricia B. Lisk, RN, BSN
Instructor
Augusta Technical College
Augusta, GA 30906

Linda K. Maranville, RN, BSN, PHN
Instructor
American Career College
Los Angeles, California

Patricia Marrow, RN, BSN, MA
Nursing Educator, LPN Program
Daytona Beach Community College
Daytona Beach, Florida

Mary Patricia Norrell, RNC, BSN, MS
Chair, Practical Nursing Program
Ivy Tech State College
Columbus, Indiana

Darlene D. Pedersen, MSN, APRN, BC
Director and Psychotherapist
PsychOptions
Philadelphia, Pennsylvania

Candace J. Pritchard, BSN, RN
Instructor, Practical Nursing
Pickens Technical College
Aurora, Colorado

LuAnn J. Reicks, RNBC, BS, MSN
Professor; PN Coordinator
Iowa Central Community College
Fort Dodge, Iowa

Carleen J. Ronchetti, RN, MS
Nursing Instructor
Lake Superior College
Duluth, Minnesota

Denise Root, RN, ADN, BSN, MSN
Director, Nursing Department
Otero Junior College
LaJunta, Colorado

Glynda Renee Sherrill, RN, BSN,
PN Instructor
Indian Capital Technology Center
Tahlequah, Oklahoma

Penny Snyder, RN, BSN
Assistant Professor
North Central State College
Mansfield, Ohio

Frances Swasey, RN, MN
Chair, Nursing Department
College of Eastern Utah
Price, Utah

Beverley D. Turner, RN, MA
Campus Director
Desert Career College
Palm Springs, California

Rita Van Horn, RN, PHD
Director of Nursing
Bellingham Technical College
Bellingham, Washington

Catherine Wardlow, RN, BS, Med, MS
Practical Nursing Instructor
Francis Tuttle Technology Center
Oklahoma City, Oklahoma

Deborah L. Weaver, RN, PHD
Associate Professor, Nursing
Valdosta State University
Valdosta, Georgia

Martha Williams, BA, RN
Professor
Central Texas College
Brady, Texas

Christina Wilson, RN, BAN, PHN
Faculty, Practical Nursing Department
Anoka Technical College
Anoka, Minnesota

Contents

unit ONE

UNDERSTANDING HEALTH CARE ISSUES

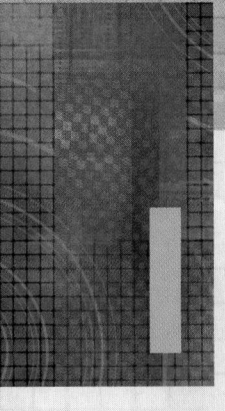

Critical Thinking and the Nursing Process

PAULA D. HOPPER
AND LINDA S. WILLIAMS

QUESTIONS TO GUIDE YOUR READING

1. How is critical thinking of value in the nursing process?

2. What are objective and subjective data?

3. How can the documentation of data be improved?

4. How would you prioritize patient care based on Maslow's hierarchy of human needs?

5. What is your role as a licensed practical nurse/licensed vocational nurse in using the nursing process?

6. What is a nursing diagnosis?

7. What is the evaluation phase of the nursing process?

Excellence in the delivery of nursing care requires good thinking. Each day nurses make many decisions that will affect the care of their patients. For those decisions to be effective, the thought processes behind them must be sound.

CRITICAL THINKING AND SAFE CARE

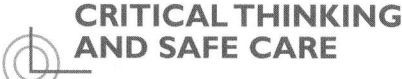

Nurses must learn to think critically. This means they must use their knowledge and skills to make the best decisions possible in patient care situations. Halpern[1] says that "**critical thinking** is the use of those cognitive [knowledge] skills or strategies that increase the probability of a desirable outcome." Critical thinking is sometimes called directed thinking because it focuses on a goal. Other terms used when talking about critical thinking include *reasoning, common sense, analysis,* and *inquiry.* Good thinking requires critical thinking attitudes and skills, which are described below. It also requires a good knowledge base, so your thinking is based upon correct factual material. These are the topics of the rest of this book.

Critical Thinking Attitudes

Researchers have identified attitudes that are associated with good critical thinking. Green identifies seven attitudes, summarized below.[2]

Intellectual Humility

Have you ever known people who think they "know it all"? They do not have intellectual humility. People with intellectual humility have the ability to say, "I am not sure about that…. I need more information." Certainly, we want our patients to think we are smart and know what we are doing, but patients also respect nurses who can say, "I do not know; let me find out." It is unsafe to care for patients when you are not sure of what you need to do.

Intellectual Courage

Intellectual courage allows you to look at other points of view even when you do not agree with them at first. Maybe you really believe that 8-hour shifts are best for nurses, and have a lot of good reasons for your belief. But if you have intellectual courage, you will be willing to really listen to the arguments for changing to 12-hour shifts. Maybe you will even be convinced. Sometimes you have to have the courage to say, "Okay, I see you were right after all."

Intellectual Empathy

Consider the patient who snaps as you enter her room, "I've been waiting all morning for my bath. If you do not help me with it right now I am going to call your supervisor." The first response that comes into your head is, "I have five other patients; you are lucky I am here now!" But, if you have intellectual empathy, you will be able to think, "If I were this patient, who is in chronic pain and is tired of being in the hospital, how would I feel?" It might change how you respond.

Intellectual Integrity

Your patient seems to ask a hundred questions when you bring her a medication that has been newly prescribed for her high blood pressure. But later you notice she is taking an herbal remedy from her purse. It is good that she is asking a lot of questions about her drug, which has been tested extensively by the Food and Drug Administration (FDA). Herbal remedies are not held to the same standards as medications in the United States. Someone with intellectual integrity would want the same kind of proof that both types of medications are safe and effective before using them.

Intellectual Perseverance

Do not give up. Consider this scenario. You have concerns about some side effects you have noticed when you administer a new drug to your patients. You mentioned it to the physician and he said not to worry about it, but you are still concerned. If you have intellectual perseverance, you might do some research on the web, then go to your supervisor or the pharmacist to discuss your concerns.

Faith in Reason

If you have faith in reason, you believe in your heart that good thinking, and reason, will indeed result in the best outcomes for your patients. And if you really believe, you will be more likely to attend a seminar or read an article on critical thinking skills.

Intellectual Sense of Justice

One of your co-workers wants to change the medication administration schedule on your unit. She says it is because it will be better for the patients, but you think it might be because it fits her break schedule better. If you have an intellectual sense of justice, you will be sure that your thinking is not biased by something that you just want for yourself, like your co-worker seems to be doing. You should examine your own motives as well as those of others when you are making decisions.

So, what does this all mean to you as a nursing student? The term "metacognition" means to "think about thinking." It is important for you to try to develop the attitudes of a critical thinker, and to learn to think clearly and critically about your patient care. In order to do that, you need to constantly think about your thinking. Are you practicing intellectual humility? Are you trying to be courageous and empathetic? These attitudes create an excellent base on which to build a nursing knowledge base, and on which to develop further thinking skills.

Knowledge Base

Nurses must have a good knowledge base in order to safely care for their patients. You could not drive a car without first learning the basics of how a car works and how to follow the rules of the road. In the same way, you must understand the human body in health and illness before you can understand how to take care of an ill patient. This is the reason you are going to school and studying this book.

Information is found in many places; some information is good, and some is not as good. For example, health information found on a website may have been put there by a major university medical school, or it may have been put there by a patient who has a particular disorder. You may learn about a patient's experience by reading his or her website, but you certainly would not base care of your patients on this one person's personal experience.

The best knowledge upon which to base your practice comes from research. Nurse researchers try new methods for taking care of patients and compare them with traditional methods to determine what works best. For example, for many years nurses were taught to massage patients' reddened bony prominences to prevent pressure ulcers. Through research, we now know that this practice should be avoided because it can further harm tissue that is already damaged.

When nursing care is based on good, well-designed research studies, it is called **evidence based practice**. As nurses, we need to use as many interventions as we can that have been researched. Other interventions, until they are validated by research, have to be based on our best critical thinking skills. Some expert organizations are beginning to "bundle" best practice strategies together to increase their use. Bundles are groups of interventions that, when used together, have been shown to improve patient outcomes. To find more information on bundles, go to http://www.ihi.org/ihi and type "bundles" in the search window. It is nice to be able to tell a patient or family member that "Your loved one is being cared for based on the latest research recommendations."

Concern for Patient Safety

Safety is on everyone's mind. Many people know of someone who has been affected by a medical error or who has been unhappy with their care. Health-care providers are being held accountable for safe care by society. As a result, guidelines to reduce errors in health care and improve patient outcomes have been developed. The Joint Commission on Accreditation of Hospitals and Organizations (JCAHO) is an organization that accredits health-care agencies. JCAHO's 2006 patient safety goals can be found at http://www.jcipatientsafety.org. As you will see, care in various health-care settings is addressed in these goals. Following is an example of one of the goals which you will find throughout the book as safety tips.

These goals are throughout the book to increase your awareness and understanding of them. They address important areas of concern such as using medications safely, correctly identifying patients, identifying operative sites correctly, improving communication, reducing fall injuries, and reducing risk for infections in institutionalized elderly persons to name a few. So become familiar with them and look for annual updates on the web. Of course, it takes critical thinking to use them at the right times and in the right circumstances. Using them appropriately helps you provide safer care with fewer errors, which your patients appreciate.

SAFETY TIP

Use at least two patient identifiers (neither to be the patient's room number) when taking blood samples and other specimens for clinical testing, or providing any other treatments or procedures (JCAHO, 2006). 2006 National Patient Safety Goals from www.jcaho.org

Critical Thinking Skills
Problem Solving

Problem solving is one type of critical thinking skill. Nurses solve problems on a daily basis. However, a problem can be handled in a way that may or may not help the patient. For instance, consider Mr. Frank, who is in pain and requests pain medication. You check the medication record and find that his analgesic medication is not due for another 40 minutes. You can choose to manage this problem in a variety of ways. One obvious approach is to return to Mr. Frank and tell him that it is not time for the pain medication and that he will have to wait. This may solve your problem (you can move on to the next patient), but it does not solve the problem in an acceptable way for Mr. Frank. An alternative approach is to use a standard problem-solving method:

1. Gather **data.** When Mr. Frank requests pain medication, the first thing you do is obtain more data. As a good critical thinker, you can use intellectual empathy as well as your knowledge base about pain to decide what additional data you need. You decide to use a pain-rating scale on which the patient rates pain on a scale of 0 (no pain) to 10 (the greatest pain possible). Mr. Frank states that his pain is in his back and rates it as an 8 on the 10-point scale. You check his history and find he has compression fractures of his spine. Your empathetic attitude tells you that waiting for 40 minutes to relieve his pain is not acceptable. You next go to the medication record and find that he has no alternative pain medications ordered.

2. Identify the problem. Here you use your knowledge base to draw the conclusion that Mr. Frank is in acute pain, and the current medication orders are not sufficient to provide pain relief.

3. Decide what outcome (sometimes called a goal) is desirable. The outcome should be determined by you (the nurse) and the patient working together. The patient is intimately involved in this situation and deserves to be consulted. In this case you talk to Mr. Frank and determine that he needs pain relief now; he cannot wait until the next scheduled dose of medication. He states that he is able to tolerate a pain rating of 3 or less on a 10-point scale.

4. Plan what to do. Formulate and evaluate some alternative solutions. For example, you can decide to tell Mr. Frank that he has to wait 40 minutes;

however, this will not help him reach his desired outcome of pain control. Giving the medication early might relieve his pain, but this would not be following the physician's orders and may have harmful effects for Mr. Frank. You could decide to try some non–drug pain-control methods, such as relaxation, distraction, or imagery. These might be helpful, but you recall from pharmacology class that complementary methods should be used in conjunction with, not in place of, medications. Another alternative is to report to the physician that Mr. Frank's pain is not controlled with the current pain-control regimen. Once you have several alternative courses of action, decide which will best help the patient. Then you can discuss those options with the registered nurse (RN) and together decide the best thing to do; in this case, you might decide to have the RN contact the physician while you work with the patient on relaxation exercises. You might decide to ask Mr. Frank if he would like to listen to some of the music his wife brought in for him. You can also tell Mr. Frank that the physician is being contacted. This would assure him that his pain-relief needs are being taken seriously.

5. Implement the plan of care. The RN enters the room and informs you and the patient that the physician has changed the analgesic orders. You obtain and administer the first dose of the new analgesic, being sure to explain its effects and side effects to Mr. Frank. The RN also informs Mr. Frank that the physician has ordered a consultation with the pain clinic.

6. Evaluate the plan of care. Did the plan work? As you reassess Mr. Frank 30 minutes later, he rates his pain level at 2. You think back to the desired outcome, compare it with the current data collected, and determine that your **interventions** were successful.

Can you see how using good thinking attitudes, a good knowledge base, and the problem-solving process led to a better outcome than simply choosing the first obvious option? You were able to effect a positive change: assisting a patient in achieving pain relief. And you have undoubtedly earned Mr. Frank's trust in the process. Problem solving is how nurses make decisions on a daily basis. This is known as the *nursing process.*

Other Critical Thinking Skills

Problem solving is just one critical thinking skill. There are many others that are beyond the scope of this book. Following are a few questions to ask yourself as you continue to develop your critical thinking. There are many more questions you might ask. These are not in any order, nor would they all be asked for a given situation. They are just some ideas to get you started.

- Have I thought this through?
- What information do I need?
- How do I know?

- Is someone influencing my thinking in ways I am not aware of?
- What conclusions can I draw from the information I have?
- Am I basing this decision on assumptions that may or may not be true?
- Am I thinking creatively about this, or am I in a rut?
- Is there an expert I can consult that can help me think through this?
- Is there any research or evidence that this is true?
- Am I too stressed or tired to think carefully about this right now?

NURSING PROCESS

Previously you used the **nursing process** to solve a real problem. The nursing process is an organizing framework that links the process of thinking with actions in nursing practice. The nursing process can be used to assess patient needs, formulate nursing diagnoses, and plan, implement, and evaluate care. As a nursing student, you consciously use the nursing process with each patient problem. With experience, you will internalize the nursing process and use it without as much conscious effort.

Role of the Licensed Practical Nurse and Licensed Vocational Nurse

The licensed practical nurse (LPN) or licensed vocational nurse (LVN) carries out a specific role in the nursing process, as described in Table 1.1. The LPN/LVN collects data, assists in formulating nursing diagnoses, assists in determining outcomes and planning care to meet patient needs, implements patient care interventions, and assists in evaluating the effectiveness of nursing interventions in achieving the patient's outcomes. It is the role of the LPN/LVN to provide direct patient care. This gives the LPN/LVN an opportunity to develop a relationship with the patient that aids in assisting in the other parts of the nursing process. The LPN/LVN and the RN work as a team to analyze data and develop, implement, and evaluate the plan of care (Fig. 1.1).

TABLE 1.1 ROLE OF THE LPN/LVN IN THE NURSING PROCESS

Steps of the Process	Role of the LPN/LVN
Assessment	Assists in collecting data
Nursing Diagnosis	Assists in choosing appropriate nursing diagnoses
Planning Care	Assists in developing outcomes and planning care to meet outcomes
Implementation	Carries out those portions of the plan of care that are within the LPN/LVN's scope of practice
Evaluation	Assists in evaluation and revision of the plan of care

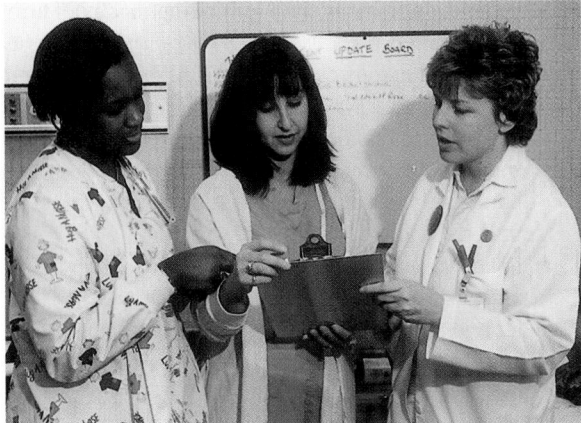

FIGURE 1.1 The nursing care team collaborating on a nursing care plan.

Data Collection

The first step in the nursing process is data collection. The LPN/LVN assists the RN in collecting data from a variety of sources. Data are divided into two types: **subjective data** and **objective data.**

Subjective Data

Information that is provided verbally by the patient is called subjective data. Symptoms are subjective data. Subjective data are often placed in quotes, such as "I have a headache" or "I feel out of breath." You must listen carefully to the patient and understand that only the patient truly knows how he or she feels.

When collecting subjective data, begin with the patient's main concern. Focus on the reason the patient is seeking health care. The question, "What happened that made you decide to come to the hospital (clinic, office)?" can be helpful.

Once the patient has identified the main concern, further questioning can elicit more pertinent information. Use the letters of the "WHAT'S UP?" questioning format to remember questions to ask the patient (Box 1.1 What's Up? Guide to Symptom Assessment). Asking the right questions can help you obtain better data with which to make the best decisions.

Next, obtain a patient history. This is done by asking the patient and family questions about the patient's past and present health problems, including specific questions about each body system, family health problems, and risk factors for health problems. The patient's medical record may also be consulted for background history information.

In addition to assessment related to physiological functioning, ask the patient about personal habits that relate to

LEARNING TIP

Practice assessing a symptom on a classmate. Ask the "WHAT'S UP?" questions.

Box 1.1

WHAT'S UP? Guide to Symptom Assessment

W—Where is it?

H—How does it feel? Describe the quality.

A—Aggravating and alleviating factors. What makes it worse? What makes it better?

T—Timing. When did it start? How long does it last?

S—Severity. How bad is it? This can often be rated on a scale of 0 to 10.

U—Useful other data. What other symptoms are present that might be related?

P—Patient's perception of the problem. The patient often has an idea about what the problem is, or the cause, but may not believe that his or her thoughts are worth sharing unless specifically asked.

---

health, such as exercise, diet, and the presence of stressors, per institutional assessment guidelines. Finally, assess the patient's family role, support systems, and cultural and spiritual beliefs.

Objective Data

Objective data are pieces of factual information obtained through physical assessment and diagnostic tests and are observable or knowable through the five senses. Objective data are sometimes called *signs*. Examples of objective data include the following:

- 3-cm red lesion
- Respiratory rate 36
- Blood glucose 326 mg/dL
- Patient is moaning

Note that these are all observable or measurable by a nurse and do not require explanation by the patient.

Objective data are gathered through physical assessment. Inspection, palpation, percussion, and auscultation techniques are used to collect objective data (Fig. 1.2). Give special attention to areas that the patient has identified as potential problems.

Documentation of Data

Collected data are documented in the patient's medical record. Identification of any significant problem or variation from normal is reported immediately to an RN or physician and then documented. The recorded data should be accurate and concise. You should document exactly what you observed or heard stated by the patient, significant other, or health team members. Avoid interpreting the data and using words that have vague meanings in your documentation. For example, "nailbed color is pink" gives clearer information than "nailbed color is normal." "Capillary refill is 2 seconds" provides more precise data than "capillary refill is good." The statement "the wound looks better" is not meaningful unless the wound has been previously observed by the

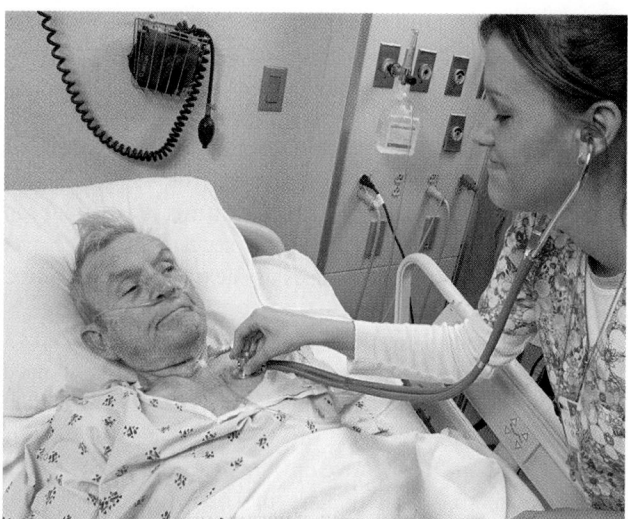

FIGURE 1.2 Nurse auscultating patient's chest.

reader. Stating that "the wound is 1 by 2 inches, red, with no drainage or odor" provides data with which to compare the future status of the wound and determine whether it is responding to treatment. When documenting subjective data, use direct quotations from the patient whenever possible. Quotes accurately represent the patient's view and are least open to interpretation. Meaningful documentation promotes continuity of patient care.

LEARNING TIP

Documenting exactly what is observed is more appropriate, easier, and less time consuming than seeking other words or ways to state observations. Beginners may be tempted to search for elaborate phrases or words when simple, direct words are best. Stating exactly what is seen or heard usually provides the most clear and accurate information.

Nursing Diagnosis

Once data have been collected, the LPN/LVN assists the RN to compare the findings with what is considered "normal." Data are then grouped, or clustered, into sets of related information that identify problems.

According to the North American Nursing Diagnosis Association (NANDA), a **nursing diagnosis** is a clinical judgment about individual, family, or community response to actual or potential health problems or life processes. Nursing diagnoses are standardized labels that make an identified problem understandable to all nurses. Nursing diagnoses are the foundation used to select interventions to achieve a desired outcome. A list of NANDA-approved nursing diagnoses can be found in Appendix A of this book.

Nursing actions are either independent or collaborative. Independent nursing actions can be initiated by the nurse.

Examples of independent nursing actions include teaching the patient deep breathing exercises, turning a patient every 2 hours, teaching about medications, and giving a back rub for comfort. Collaborative actions require a physician's order to perform them in response to both nursing and medical diagnoses. Examples of this are giving prescribed medications, applying antiembolism stockings, requesting a referral to physical therapy, and inserting a urinary catheter.

A diagnosis is considered "nursing" instead of "medical" if the interventions necessary to treat the problem are primarily independent nursing functions. Even with independent nursing functions, nurses often consult with physicians about plans of care. When the physician directs most of the care related to a particular health problem, it is a medical diagnosis rather than a nursing diagnosis. For example, a patient with pneumonia (a medical diagnosis) has many needs that depend on physician orders, such as respiratory treatments and antibiotics. The nurse, however, can provide important assessment findings related to the health problem and provide nursing measures such as encouraging fluid intake, coughing, and deep breathing. When the physician and nurse work closely together on a patient problem, it is referred to as a collaborative problem.

One of the NANDA nursing diagnoses is acute pain. In Mr. Frank's example, the pain was assessed as a health problem, and a plan of care was developed to manage the pain. The physician was contacted for analgesic orders, and independent nursing actions were used, including relaxation and distraction. These independent nursing actions did not require a physician's order.

A well-written nursing diagnosis helps guide development of a plan of care. The three parts to a diagnosis follow:
- Problem—the nursing diagnosis label from the NANDA list
- Etiology—the cause or related factor (usually preceded by the words "related to")
- Signs and symptoms—the subjective or objective data that are evidence that this is a valid diagnosis (often preceded by the words "as evidenced by")

CRITICAL THINKING

Nursing Diagnosis

■ Which of the following are NANDA nursing diagnoses? Which are medical diagnoses?
1. Impaired mobility   N
2. Ineffective coping   N
3. Herniated disk   med
4. Fractured femur   med
5. Diabetes   med
6. Impaired gas exchange   N
7. Appendicitis   med
8. Health-seeking behaviors   N

Suggested answers at end of chapter.

The statement of problem, etiology, and signs and symptoms is called the PES format. Look again at the case study of Mr. Frank. A diagnosis using this format might read as follows: "Acute pain related to muscle spasms and nerve compression as evidenced by patient's pain rating of 8." Note how the complete diagnosis gives you more helpful information than simply the label "pain." This additional information helps determine an appropriate outcome and guides intervention selection.

Plan of Care

Once nursing diagnoses are identified, an individualized plan of care to help the patient meet his or her care needs is designed. It is important to include the patient in the development of the plan of care. The patient must be in agreement with the plan for it to be successful in meeting the desired outcomes. The first step in planning care after diagnoses are selected is to prioritize the diagnoses and develop outcomes, or goals, for each. Actions that will help the patient meet the desired outcomes can then be determined.

Prioritizing Care

Once you know what problems need to be addressed, you must decide which problem or intervention needs to be taken care of first. You and the patient decide together which problems take priority. Maslow's hierarchy of human needs is one commonly used psychological theory that can be used as a basis for determining priorities (Fig. 1.3). According to

Maslow, humans must meet their most basic needs (those at the bottom of the triangle) first. They can then move up the hierarchy to meet higher level needs.

Physiological needs are the most basic. For example, a person who is short of breath cannot attend to higher level needs because the physiological need for oxygen is not being met. Once physiological needs are met, the patient can concentrate on meeting safety and security needs. Love, belonging, and self-esteem needs are next; self-actualization needs are the last to be met.

Throughout life, individuals move up and down Maslow's hierarchy in response to life events. If a need occurs on a level below the patient's current level, the patient will move down to the level of that need. Once the need is fulfilled, the person can move upward on the hierarchy again.

In a nursing plan of care the patient's most urgent problem is listed first. According to Maslow's hierarchy of human needs, this usually involves a physiological need such as oxygen or water because these are life-sustaining needs. If several physiological needs are present, life-threatening needs are ranked first, health-threatening needs are second, and health-promoting needs, although important, are last.

Once physiological needs are met, needs related to the next level of the hierarchy, safety and security, can be addressed. Remaining diagnoses are listed in order of urgency as they relate to the hierarchy. Needs can occur simultaneously on different levels and must be addressed in a holistic manner, with prioritization guiding the care provided.

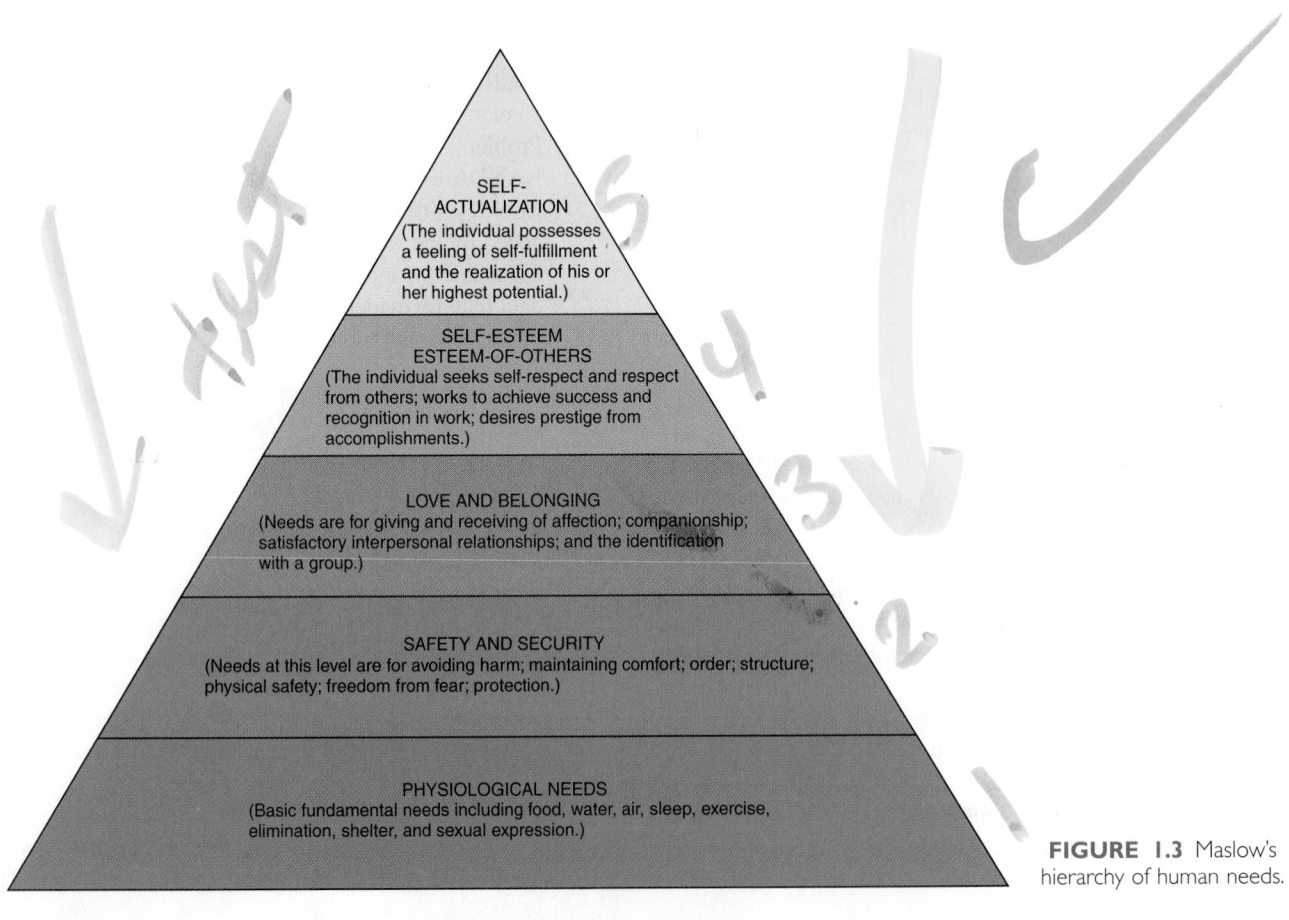

FIGURE 1.3 Maslow's hierarchy of human needs.

LEARNING TIP

If you are developing a plan of care for a patient with complex needs and are not sure where to start, go back to the assessment phase. Often additional information can help you better understand the patient's needs and develop a plan of care that is individualized to the patient's specific problem areas.

Establishing Outcomes

An outcome is a statement that describes the patient's desired goal for a problem area. It should be measurable, be realistic for the patient, and have an appropriate time frame for achievement. *Measurable* means that the outcome can be observed, or is objective. It should not be vague or open to interpretation, with the use of subjective words such as *normal, large, small,* or *moderate.* Consider, for example, two outcomes:

- The patient's shortness of breath will improve.
- The patient will be less short of breath within 15 minutes as evidenced by the patient rating the shortness of breath at less than 3 on a scale of 0 to 10, respiratory rate between 16 and 20, and relaxed appearance.

Although the first outcome seems appropriate, in reality it is difficult to know when it has been met. There is nothing to objectively indicate when the problem has been resolved. The second outcome is objective. You can see that when the patient rates his or her shortness of breath less than 3, is breathing at a rate of 16 to 20, and appears relaxed, the desired outcome will have been met. The outcome is realistic, and the 15-minute time frame ensures that the patient's distress is minimized. If the plan of care does not achieve the desired outcome in the given time frame, it should be evaluated and revised as needed.

When determining criteria for a measurable outcome, look at the signs and symptoms portion of the nursing diagnosis. The resolution or continuation of the signs and symptoms identified in the NANDA nursing diagnoses are evidence that nursing interventions were effective. If the desired outcome is not achieved, reevaluation of the problem and interventions is needed. Look at another outcome example to see how criteria are used for measurement:

> Nursing diagnosis—Ineffective airway clearance related to excess secretions as evidenced by coarse crackles and nonproductive cough.
> Outcome—Demonstrates clear lung sounds and productive cough within 8 hours.

Identifying Interventions

Interventions are the actions you take to help the patient meet the desired outcome. Therefore, interventions are considered goal directed. Any intervention that does not contribute to meeting the outcome should not be part of the plan of care.

One way to create a plan is to include interventions that can be categorized as "take, treat, and teach." In the first intervention category, "take," or identify data that should be routinely collected related to the problem. Next, "treat" the problem by identifying deliberate actions to help reach the outcome. Last, identify what to "teach" the patient and family for the patient to learn to care for himself or herself.

Look again at the nursing diagnosis of impaired airway clearance. A plan of care for this problem using the take, treat, and teach method might look like the following:

Take: Auscultate lung sounds every 4 hours and prn.
Assess respiratory rate every 4 hours and prn.
Treat: Provide 2 L of fluids every 24 hours.
Offer expectorant as ordered.
Provide cool mist vaporizer in room.
Teach: Teach the patient the importance of fluid intake.
Teach the patient to cough and deep breathe every 1 to 2 hours.

In addition to identifying interventions, it is important to understand how and why they will work. This is called identifying rationales. For example, assess lung sounds and respiratory rate every 4 hours because increased crackles and respiratory rate indicate retained secretions. Fluids are provided to help liquefy secretions and ease their removal. Sound rationale that is evidence (research) based should guide the selection of each nursing intervention.

Implementation

Once the plan of care has been identified, it must be communicated to the patient, family, and health team members and then implemented. One way a plan of care is communicated is by writing it as a nursing care plan. The nursing care plan is documented on the patient's medical record and allows other nurses to know the patient's priority problems, the desired outcomes, and the plan for meeting the outcomes. In this way, all nurses can provide consistent care for the patient.

When implementing the plan of care, the actions listed as interventions are performed. The patient's response to

Be able to do ✓ *Test*

CRITICAL THINKING

Prioritizing Care

■ Based on Maslow's hierarchy of needs, list the following nursing diagnoses in order from highest (1) to lowest (5) priority. Give rationales for your decisions.

4 Deficient knowledge
2 Constipation
5 Disabled family coping
3 Anxiety
1 Ineffective airway clearance

Suggested answers at end of chapter.

each intervention is noted and documented. This documentation provides the basis for **evaluation** and revision of the plan of care.

Evaluation

The last step of the process is evaluation. Evaluation examines both outcomes and interventions. The nurse continuously evaluates the patient's progress toward the desired outcomes and the effectiveness of each intervention. If the outcomes are not reached within the given time frame, or if the interventions are ineffective, the plan of care is revised. Any part of the plan of care can be revised, from the diagnosis or desired outcome to the interventions. Acute care institutions require review and updating of the plan of care every 24 hours.

SUGGESTED ANSWERS TO

CRITICAL THINKING

■ *Nursing Diagnosis*
1. Impaired mobility = nursing
2. Ineffective coping 5 nursing
3. Herniated disk = medical
4. Fractured femur = medical
5. Diabetes = medical
6. Impaired gas exchange = nursing
7. Appendicitis = medical
8. Health-seeking behaviors = nursing

■ *Prioritizing Care*
1 Ineffective airway clearance—physiological need that can be life threatening
2 Constipation—physiological need that can be health-threatening
3 Anxiety—safety and security need
4 Deficient knowledge—safety and security need
5 Disabled family coping—love and belonging need

REVIEW QUESTIONS

1. In which of the following ways is critical thinking useful to the nursing process?
   a. It highlights the obvious solution to a problem.
   b. It can lead to a better outcome for the patient.
   c. It simplifies the process.
   d. It helps the nurse arrive at a solution more quickly.

2. Which nurse is exhibiting intellectual humility?
   a. The nurse who is an expert at wound care.
   b. The nurse who reports an error to the supervisor.
   c. The nurse who tries to empathize with the patient.
   d. The nurse who asks a co-worker about a new procedure.

3. Which of the following pieces of information is considered objective data?
   a. The patient's respiratory rate is 28.
   b. The patient states, "I feel short of breath."
   c. The patient is short of breath.
   d. The patient is feeling panicky.

4. An LPN/LVN is collecting data on a newly admitted patient who has an ulcerated area on his left hip. It is 2 inches in diameter and 1 inch deep, with yellow exudate. Which of the following statements best documents the findings in the patient's database?

   a. Wound on left hip, 2 inches diameter, 1 inch deep, infected
   b. Left hip wound is large, deep, and has yellow drainage
   c. Pressure ulcer on left hip, yellow drainage
   d. Wound on left hip 2 inches in diameter, 1 inch deep, yellow exudate

5. A 34-year-old mother of three children is admitted to a respiratory unit with pneumonia. Based on Maslow's hierarchy of needs, which of the following patient problems should the nurse address first?
   a. Frontal headache from stress of hospital admission
   b. Anxiety related to concern about leaving children
   c. Shortness of breath from newly diagnosed pneumonia
   d. Deficient knowledge about treatment plan

6. Place the steps of the nursing process in correct chronological order of use. Use all options.
   2 a. Nursing Diagnosis
   5 b. Evaluation
   1 c. Assessment
   3 d. Planning Care
   4 e. Implementation

7. Which of the following parts of the nursing process can be carried out by an LPN/LVN?
   a. Implementation of interventions
   b. Nursing diagnosis ✓
   c. Analysis of data
   d. Evaluation of outcomes

8. Which of the following is a nursing diagnosis?
   a. Stroke
   b. Renal failure
   c. Fracture
   d. Acute pain

9. A nurse teaches a patient the importance of stopping smoking. Which of the following patient responses would best indicate to the nurse the effectiveness of the instruction?
   a. "I have a brother who died of lung cancer. I know smoking is bad."
   b. "I tried to quit 5 years ago, and I really would like to, but it is very hard."
   c. "Thank you for the information. I will call the Smoke Stoppers organization today."
   d. "I know you are right; I should stop smoking."

References

1. Halpern, D: Thought and knowledge: an introduction to critical thinking, ed 3. Lawrence Erlbaum Associates, Mahwah, NJ, 1996, p 5.
2. Green, Carol J. Critical Thinking in Nursing. Prentice Hall Health, Upper Saddle River, NJ, 2000.
3. North American Nursing Diagnosis Association (NANDA): Nursing Diagnosis: Definitions and Classification, 2005–2006. Philadelphia, 2005.

Bibliography

1. Ackley, BJ, and Ladwig, GB: Nursing Diagnosis Handbook, ed. 7. Mosby, St. Louis, 2006.
2. Paul, Richard: The state of critical thinking today. New Directions for Community Colleges, no. 130, Summer 2005.

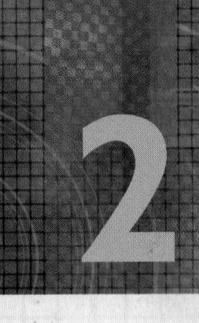

2

Issues in Nursing Practice

LENETRA JEFFERSON, LINDA MARIE LOWE, AND PATRICK M. SHANNON

KEY TERMS

administrative laws (ad-MIN-i-STRAY-tive LAWZ)
autocratic leadership (AW-tuh-KRAT-ik LEE-der-ship)
autonomy (AW-taan-o-MEE)
beneficence (buh-NEF-i-sens)
civil law (SIV-il LAW)
code of ethics (KOHD OF ETH-icks)
confidentiality (KON-fi-den-she-AL-i-tee)
criminal law (KRIM-i-nuhl LAW)
delegation (DELL-a-GAY-shun)
democratic leadership (DEM-ah-KRAT-ik LEE-der-ship)
deontology (DEE-on-TOL-o-gee)
diagnosis-related groups (DYE-ag-NOH-sis ree-LAY-TED GROOPS)
distributive justice (dis-TRIB-yoo-tiv JUS-tiss)
empathy (EM-puh-thee)
ethical (ETH-i-kuhl)
feminist (FEM-uh-nist)
fidelity (fi-DEL-i-tee)
health (HELLTH)
illness (ILL-ness)
justice (JUS-tiss)
laissez-faire leadership (LAYS-ay-FAIR LEE-der-ship)
leadership (LEE-der-ship)
liability (LYE-uh-BIL-i-tee)
limitation of liability (LIM-i-TAY-shun OF LYE-uh-BIL-i-tee)
malpractice (mal-PRAK-tiss)
morality (muh-RAL-i-tee)
negligence (NEG-li-jens)
nonmaleficence (NON-muh-LEF-i-sens)
paternalism (puh-TER-nuhl-izm)
principles (prin-SI-plz)
respondeat superior (res-POND-ee-et sue-PEER-ee-or)
standard of best interest (STAND-erd OF BEST IN-ter-est)
summons (SUM-muns)
theorists (THEE-or-RISTS)
torts (TORTS)
utilitarian (yoo-TILL-i-TAR-i-en)
values (VAL-yooz)
veracity (vuh-RAS-i-tee)
welfare rights (WELL-fare RIGHTS)

QUESTIONS TO GUIDE YOUR READING

1. What are factors influencing changes in the health-care delivery system?

2. What is the LPN/LVN's role in the health-care delivery system?

3. What are three leadership styles?

4. What is the LPN/LVN's role in leadership?

5. Why are ethics important in health care?

6. What is an example of a character trait and how does it relate to nursing?

7. What are the definitions of the four major principles in ethics and how would you apply one to an ethical dilemma?

8. What are the steps of the ethical decision-making model?

9. Where is the regulation of nursing practice defined?

10. How can you provide quality care and limit your liability?

11. How would you define HIPAA (Health Insurance Portability and Accountability Act of 1996)?

HEALTH-CARE DELIVERY

The **health**-care delivery system continues to experience rapid and dramatic changes from acute care to outpatient and community settings. As nursing adapts to these changes, it is important to understand wellness and **illness** treatments, factors that influence health care, and application of principles of cultural diversity during care.

Health-Illness Continuum

The World Health Organization in the preamble of its constitution defines health as a "state of complete physical, mental and social well-being and not merely the absence of disease and infirmity." This definition provides a narrow view of health that does not provide for chronic illness effects or fluctuating levels of wellness. The health-illness continuum, in contrast, addresses various levels of health that are continually shifting for an individual. One end of the continuum represents high-level health and the other end poor health with impending death. Individuals move along the continuum throughout their lives.

Health-Care Delivery Systems

A focus on prevention and providing services from birth to death under one integrated system is an approach being used in some health-care systems. Hospital consolidations have resulted in development of health-care systems that may cover large geographic areas. The hospital then provides the integrated care delivery network for the system (Fig. 2.1).

Factors Influencing Health-Care Change

Changing characteristics of the American population influence the health-care delivery system. These changing characteristics include increasing size of the national population, the increasing number of elderly people, the birth rate decline, the increase in the number of uninsured or underinsured, and increased cultural diversity. The size of the American population is projected to increase to over 350 million people by the year 2020.[1] The health-care needs of the elderly can be complex and chronic, which places increased demands on the health-care system. The declining birth rate means there will be fewer school-age children and fewer people in the future to care for the elderly. The increase in the uninsured places additional strains on the system, and the increase in cultural diversity impacts how health care is delivered.

The change in how diseases are being treated today greatly influences health-care delivery. Chronic diseases are the most frequently treated conditions. Increasing numbers of infectious diseases, such as AIDS, tuberculosis, and resistant infectious organisms are also challenging the health-care system.

Additionally, the development of new technology for communicating information and designing medical equipment for testing and treatment is changing the health-care industry. New expensive technology is continually being introduced that quickly outdates equipment in use. This makes change and relearning a constant in today's health-care environment.

ECONOMIC ISSUES

The health-care system is mainly funded by the government and private insurers. Costs have risen dramatically in recent years. Access to care is not available to everyone and is often linked to availability of resources. Preventive care is not an option for many people. Treatment is often sought in the costly emergency room after a medical problem has become complex.

Medicare and Diagnosis-Related Groups (DRGs)

Medicare was created in 1966 to provide health insurance as part of the Social Security Act. It is run by the United States government and currently covers all individuals age 65 and over and disabled people under 65 years of age who are eligible for Social Security. It is funded by a deduction from every person's paycheck that is matched by the government. There are two parts of coverage in the original Medicare plan. Part A covers inpatient hospital care, skilled nursing facilities, hospice services, and some home care. There is no premium or deductible for Part A. Part B is medical insurance that covers physician costs, outpatient services, some home care, supplies, and other things not covered by Part A. Some preventive services may also be covered. A monthly premium and yearly deductible are paid for Part B coverage. For more information, visit www.medicare.gov.

New prescription drug coverage for everyone with Medicare coverage became available January 1, 2006. For more information on this coverage visit www.medicare.gov.

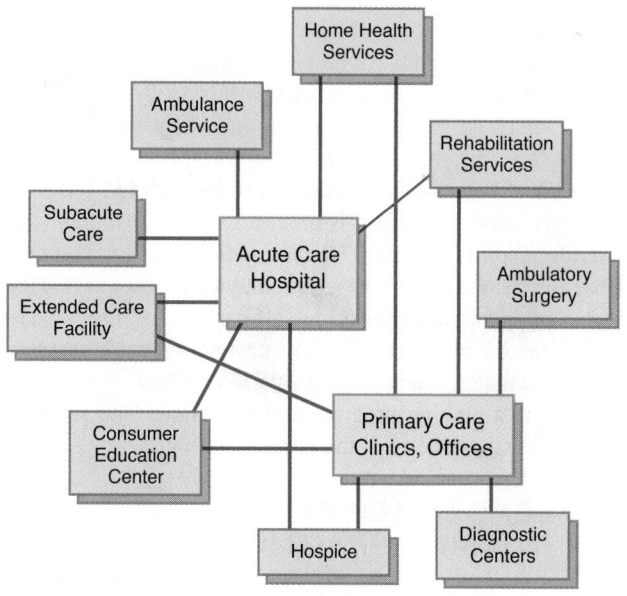

FIGURE 2.1 An integrated health-care system.

Congress created the DRG payment system in 1983 for 470 diagnostic categories to help control costs in the Medicare program, which previously had no reimbursement limits. All hospitals are paid the same fee for patients in the same diagnostic category regardless of length of stay and supply costs. Hospitals lose money if the patient's costs exceed the DRG payment but make money if the costs are less than the payment. The incentive to deliver more cost-effective care within the DRG payment system lies with the hospital. Effective discharge planning and nursing involvement in maintaining quality but cost-effective care are essential in this payment system.

Medicaid

The Medicaid payment system was also created in 1966 to provide health insurance as part of the Social Security Act for low-income or disabled persons under 65 years of age and their dependent children. Some low-income people over 65 years of age may also qualify. Medicaid funding comes from federal, state, and local taxes. Medicaid benefits vary from state to state.

Managed Health Care

There are a variety of organizations that consist of groups of health-care providers who provide all or most of the health care required for a group of people in an effort to contain costs. Health maintenance organizations (HMOs) were first begun in the 1930s, but did not flourish until the 1970s. Their emphasis is on wellness, health promotion, and illness prevention. Preferred provider organizations (PPOs) are much newer. A PPO is a network of providers who provide care to plan members at set discounted rates. The early movement to contain health-care costs led to the formation of HMOs and then PPOs. HMOs deliver multiple forms of health-care services to individuals who enroll in this prepaid group practice health program. The purpose of the HMO is to reduce overlapping services and provide quality and cost-effective care. Healthy patients require fewer services so preventive care is promoted. PPOs are a method of reducing costs to businesses that insure employees. Hospitals and physicians develop a contract with employers to provide services at a negotiated fee.

LEARNING TIP

To understand what the term *managed care* means, reverse the words: *Care management.*

As managed care is implemented, trends are emerging. The need for hospital beds is decreasing. Shorter lengths of stay for more acutely ill patients are being seen. Discharged patients are requiring more home care for more complex needs. Home care is rapidly expanding to meet this need. Case management is a strategy for providing patient care to ensure that the best patient outcome is achieved while controlling costs. The health-care industry is being challenged to provide cost-effective care while maintaining quality health care that meets the needs of the patient.

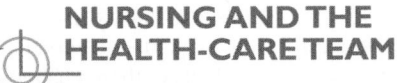

NURSING AND THE HEALTH-CARE TEAM

Nursing is an integral part of the health-care network. Nurses work as Licensed Practical Nurses (LPNs) or Licensed Vocational Nurses (LVNs); Registered Nurses (RNs); or Registered Nurses with advanced practice skills that include Nurse Practitioners (NPs), Clinical Nurse Specialists (CNSs), Certified Nurse Midwives (CNMs), and Certified Registered Nurse Anesthetists (CRNAs). The LPN/LVN provides direct patient care under the direct supervision of a registered nurse or physician. Certified nursing assistants are trained to assist nurses in providing health care to patients.

Nurses work in collaboration with other members of the health-care team to meet patient health-care needs. Educational requirements, titles, and duties are described for some health-care team members. Licensed *physicians* provide medical care to patients after graduating from a college of medicine or osteopathic medicine. *Physician assistants* after graduating from a physician's assistant program work under the supervision of a physician and perform certain physician duties such as history taking, injections, and suturing of wounds. Licensed *pharmacists* complete 5 or 6 years of college and dispense medications from prescriptions, consult with physicians, and provide medication information to patients. *Social workers* usually have a master's degree in social work and treat psychosocial problems of patients and their families. *Dietitians* provide nutrition information, analyze nutritional needs, and calculate special dietary needs. Licensed *physical therapists* complete a college physical therapy program and assist patients in reducing physical disability, bodily malfunction, movement dysfunction, and pain through evaluation, education, and treatment. *Physical therapy assistants*, whose educational requirements vary, may complete 2 years of education and be licensed and then work under the supervision of a physical therapist. *Respiratory therapists* have a 2-year college degree, may be registered (RRT), and work with patients who have respiratory problems. *Respiratory therapy technicians* have 1 year of education, may be certified (CRTT), and work under the supervision of a respiratory therapist to provide respiratory care. *Occupational therapists* complete a bachelor's or master's program, may be registered (OTR), and assist patients in restoring self-care, work, and leisure skills from developmental deficits or injury. *Health unit secretaries* manage the clerical work. *Student nurses* are enrolled in a nursing program and work under the supervision of nursing faculty in the clinical setting.

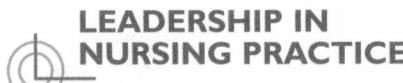

LEADERSHIP IN NURSING PRACTICE

Leadership skills are necessary for the LPN/LVN to effectively guide patient care and achieve goals. Leadership involves decision making, communicating, motivating, and guiding others. The leadership process seeks to change behaviors in others in order to accomplish goals.

Anyone who influences others to achieve goals is a leader. Effective leaders must be knowledgeable in the management process and able to make decisions. They should be role models and an inspiration to others. Positive thinking and the use of humor are valuable assets of good leaders. Ultimately leaders must earn the respect of their co-workers to be successful. In order to prepare for a leadership role, you should understand and apply the following principles of leadership.

Leadership Styles

There are three leadership styles: **autocratic, democratic,** and **laissez-faire.**

Autocratic Leadership Style

An autocratic leader has a high degree of control. Almost no control is given to others. In autocratic leadership, the leader determines the goals and plans for achieving the goals. Others are instructed what to do but are not asked to provide input. The group usually achieves high-quality outcomes under this style of leadership. This is an efficient leadership style for situations when decisions must be made quickly as in an emergency such as evacuation of a building or a code for cardiac arrest.

Democratic Leadership Style

A democratic leader has a moderate degree of control. Others are given some control and freedom. In democratic leadership, participation is encouraged in determining goals and plans for achieving the goals (Fig. 2.2). Decisions are made within the group. The leader assists the group by steering and teaching rather than dominating. The leader shares responsibility with the group. The group usually achieves high-quality outcomes and is more creative under this style of leadership. This is an efficient leadership style for most situations. Group members are more satisfied and motivated to achieve goals because they are active participants.

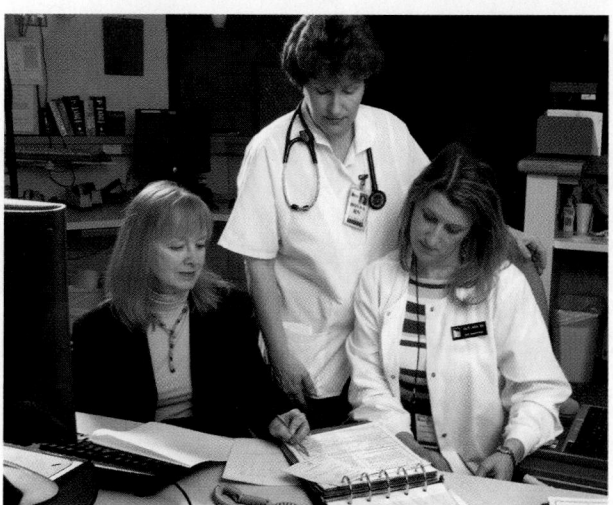

FIGURE 2.2 Group participation in decision making.

Laissez-Faire Leadership Style

A laissez-faire leader exerts no control over the group. Others are given complete freedom under this leadership style. With laissez-faire leadership, no one is responsible for determining goals and plans for achieving the goals. This produces a feeling of chaos. If decisions are made, the group makes them. Very little is accomplished under this leadership and the quality of outcomes is poor.

Management Functions

There are five major components in the management process. They include planning, organizing, directing, coordinating, and controlling.

Planning

The first step of the management process is planning. A plan must be developed to ensure that desired patient care outcomes are achieved. To formulate the plan, desired outcomes or problems are identified and data are collected about them. Alternatives or solutions are considered using the collected data and input from others. A decision is then made about the best option or course of action. The leader should ensure that the choice is realistic and can be implemented. Involving others in the planning and decision-making process from beginning to end can assist in greater acceptance at the time of implementation.

Organizing

The purpose of organizing, the second step in the management process, is to provide an orderly environment that promotes cooperation and goal achievement. Providing a framework for goals and the activities that accomplish them is the initial step in organization. Policies and procedures provide this framework as well as guidance for those carrying out tasks designed to accomplish the organization's goals.

Directing

Making assignments is the primary function of directing. Nurses make assignments for patient care. One person, usually the nurse in charge or the team leader, makes the assignments. State Nursing Practice Acts define who can make assignments and delegate care. Communication is important in directing. Assignments must be clearly and specifically stated. The individual making assignments must be sure that they are correctly understood and should seek out the receiving person for clarification. Effective directing can be accomplished by providing verbal and written assignment information, making requests rather than giving orders, and giving instructions as needed.

Coordinating

Coordination is the process of looking at a situation to ensure that it is being handled in the most effective way for the organization or coordinating services for a patient. The nurse may assess a particular activity or issues related to patient care assignments. In a long-term care facility, for example, the nurse may want to review skin assessment and care throughout the facility to see if it is being done consis-

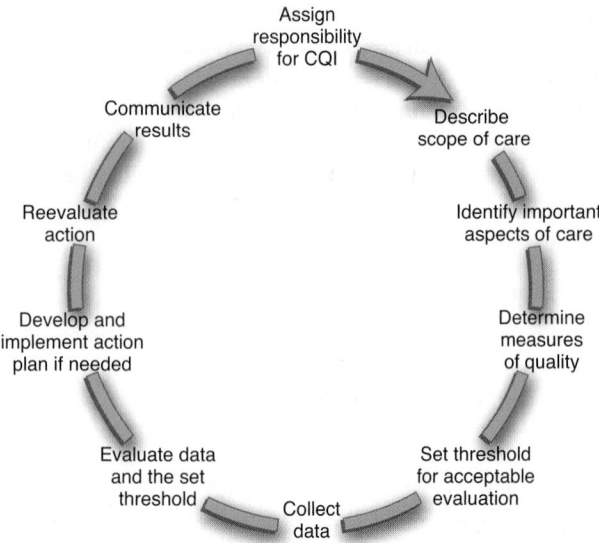

FIGURE 2.3 A continuous quality management model.

tently and uniformly. If a concern is found, problem-solving techniques are used.

Controlling

The final phase of the management process is controlling to evaluate the accomplishment of the organization's goals. Continuous quality improvement is linked with controlling. If the organization's efficiency or ability to reach its goals is impaired, the use of the continuous quality improvement model can facilitate correction of the concern (Fig. 2.3).

Leadership and Delegation for the LPN/LVN

LPN/LVNs are leaders and managers for the care of the patients to whom they are assigned under the supervision of a registered nurse, physician, or dentist. Beyond this application of a leader and manger role for the LPN/LVN, state nurse practice acts specify if the LPN/LVN can assume other leader or manager roles. Within this dependent role, some application of **delegation** may be allowed.

LEARNING TIP

Review your state nurse practice act. Does your state allow LPN/LVNs to delegate? If so, to whom and what can be delegated?

Delegation is the act of empowering another person to act. Delegation occurs in a downward manner, meaning RNs delegate to LPN/LVNs and unlicensed assistive personnel (UAP) and LPN/LVNs, in certain circumstances, delegate to LPN/LVNs and UAPs (see below). When delegation occurs, responsibility for the care is transferred to the delegate but accountability for the care remains with the delegator.

The LPN/LVN might function as a team leader or charge nurse primarily in the long-term care setting, requir-

ing some use of delegation to UAPs. When the LPN/LVN acts as a team leader or charge nurse, a registered nurse delegates the authority to provide supervision and delegation of tasks. Team leaders are responsible for the coordination and delivery of patient care to each of the patients assigned to the team. They assess the patients assigned to the team to plan appropriate care and contribute to the nursing care plan. Team leaders receive information from team members and communicate patients' needs to appropriate individuals. Since team leaders guide patient care provided by the team, they must be knowledgeable about safety policies, patients' rights, and the accountability of being a team leader. All patients are entitled to quality care and treatment with dignity and respect. The team leader is accountable for all care provided by the team. Supervision involves initial direction for the task and then monitoring of the task and outcome at intervals. At the end of the team's work shift, team leaders are responsible for transferring patient care to the oncoming team. This transfer of care is accomplished by reporting the patient's condition, status, and needs to the oncoming team leader (Fig. 2.4). Institutional policy specifies whether the RN or LPN/LVN communicates the report.

Within the leadership role, the LPN/LVN must decide when delegation would most benefit the situation and the patient. The nurse must follow the state practice act and the scope of practice when making any decisions regarding delegation. Consult the charge nurse, team leader, and nurse practice act for your state when deciding if delegation is appropriate. Ultimately, the nurse must ask several important questions to determine when delegation would best benefit the situation. These questions include:

- Does the state practice act allow for delegation in this situation?
- Is the person whom I am delegating to have the knowledge and education to perform this skill and is it documented for me to have access to make the decisions regarding delegation?

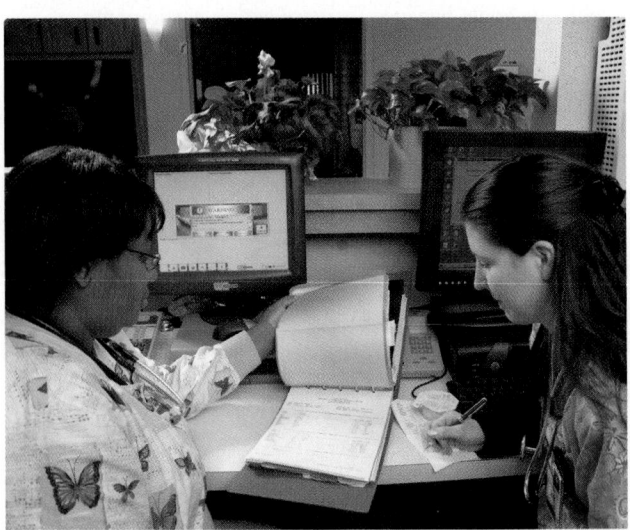

FIGURE 2.4 Communication of the patient's status when transferring the patient's care to another team leader.

- Would it benefit the patient if I delegated this skill to the support person?

Delegation Process

Delegation is a complex process. When delegation is considered, the following steps should be considered that encompass the decision to delegate, what to delegate, and to whom delegation can be made:

1. Know your state practice act rules for delegation. The LPN/LVN scope of practice usually does not provide for the legal authority for the LPN/LVN to delegate. However, some state board rules allow LPN/LVNs to delegate tasks that are within the LPN/LVN's scope of practice as long as the RN has given the LPN/LVN the authority to delegate the tasks.
2. Identify the skills of the person to whom you may delegate to determine if he or she has the knowledge and ability to carry out the task. When selecting a delegatee for a particular task, consider if there is potential for harm to the patient during the task, whether it is a complex task that will require problem solving, how predictable the outcome is, and how much interaction with the patient is needed. Match the skills and talents of the delegatee to the task being delegated. Remember, nursing judgment can never be delegated.
3. Use The National Council of State Boards of Nursing's five rights of delegation for the decision-making process for delegation.[2] Following these guidelines will give you a framework for your decision-making process and comfort in knowing you utilized them to make good choices.
   - Right task—is it appropriate to delegate?
   - Right circumstances—is this situation safe and appropriate for delegating?
   - Right person—is this delegatee the appropriate person for the task and this patient's needs?
   - Right communication—is there clear understanding between you and the delegatee for terms used, communication, and reporting needs?
   - Right supervision—is it defined how and when direct supervision will occur?

Delegation requires trust. You should be comfortable with your delegatee and know that you understand each other's methods of communicating so that miscommunications do not occur.

When you first begin your career, the process of delegating may seem difficult. As with any skill, it takes practice to feel confident in carrying out the process.

CAREER OPPORTUNITIES FOR LPN/LVNS

Today, LPNs can choose to work in a variety of settings in acute care or long-term care or expand their roles through additional education. Many schools provide for an acceler-ated educational tract for LPN/LVNs seeking to become registered nurses with either an associate degree or a bachelor's degree. Advanced educational opportunities include a masters degree in nursing or a doctor of philosophy degree. Check with colleges/universities to see which program would best meet your needs for continuing your education. Other career opportunities include massage therapist or roles previously mentioned in the chapter. Travel nursing is one of the fastest growing areas within the health-care delivery system. It is an exciting way to see the world while working. Since licensure in other states is required, you should check these requirements with travel nursing agencies if you are interested in travel nursing.

The LPN/LVN of today must be equipped with knowledge and skills to be able to sufficiently function within a health-care delivery system. An understanding of leadership, delegation, and career opportunities will provide a basis to begin your journey in practicing as a LPN/LVN. We wish you well on your journey!

ETHICS AND VALUES

Preamble

> … *just because we are able to do something does not mean that it is right to do it. Moreover, what is possible and even legal might not be ethical. Therefore, we must ask, especially regarding the new science: Is it right? Is it ethical?*

> MARGARET SOMERVILLE, THE ETHICAL CANARY, XIII[3]

The term "ethics" itself is a branch of philosophy that seeks to understand the nature, purposes, justification, and founding **principles** of moral rules and the systems they comprise.[4] We know that every society has a fairly regulated set of moral rules or guidelines that secure the boundaries of what is considered acceptable behavior. Often these rules are about *behavior*. Such examples of behaviors are:

- Harming other people (e.g., homicide, rape, theft)
- Concerning oneself with the well-being of others (e.g., helping others, responding to people in distress)
- Actions that touch on issues of respect for other persons (e.g., segregation, using other people for one's own ends without concern for their welfare)

Often the rules about such behavior are expressed in statements about what you *ought* to do or *should* do. These rules fit together, fairly consistently, to form the moral code by which a society lives.

One of the most exciting and challenging areas of nursing practice today is bioethics. Bioethics is a branch of ethics that studies moral **values** in the biomedical sciences. In the current practice of nursing, the term *bioethics* has come to be most closely associated with ethics in health-care: life and life choices as affected by health, sickness, disease, or trauma. Ethics is the study of systems of traditions, values, and beliefs as they relate to persons and their relationships with one another. To use words such as "good" and "bad" does not give the whole picture. Maybe there has to be a decision made about a patient and possibly the choice that we have to make may be the least harmful. What *should* we do? and What *ought* we to do? are part of ethics and we are responsible for knowing *why* we might take the intended action or decision.

Morals or **morality** are also related to ethics. Some individuals use the terms *ethics* and *morals* interchangeably; however, *morals* more specifically refers to our personal values, the standards set by our own conscience, and our personal choices of what *we* consider *good* and *bad*, *right* and *wrong*.

Values are standards, ideals, or concepts that give meaning to an individual's life. Values are most commonly derived from societal norms, religion, and family traditions. They serve as a guide for making decisions and taking certain actions in everyday life. Individuals can change their value systems when they experience life-changing events. Values are not usually written down, but it can be helpful to make a list of your values and attempt to rank them by priority. Value conflicts often occur in everyday life and can force an individual to select a higher priority value over a lower priority value. For example, a nurse who values both her career and her family may be forced to decide between going to work or staying home with a sick child.

Values exist on many different levels. Individuals have personal values that govern their lives and actions. Many groups and organizations have values that may or may not be identical to personal values. When a person becomes a member of a group or organization, he or she agrees to accept the values of the group. Examples of groups include clubs, churches and religious organizations, political parties, and professions. The values of a profession are usually outlined in a **code of ethics.** Failure to adhere to a code of ethics of a profession may be an indication that the individual really does not want to belong, or possibly *cannot* belong, to that group. Society as a whole has values. As a member of a society or country, an individual accepts the values of that culture. Finally, societal values may change with the adoption of new laws.

Ethical issues surround us throughout our entire lifetime. Bioethical issues are particularly prevalent in our professional lives for several reasons. Health care has the potential to affect us and our patients at every milestone of human development. Life and death issues and decisions can be especially difficult for health-care professionals, who may be faced with these issues every day. Today's sophisticated technology and complex treatments, which are advancing exponentially, present other challenges. When sophisticated interventions are available, one obvious ethical question is, should we use them? Ethical issues are raised when the organization of health-care delivery systems becomes more complex as mergers and alliances come and go. Despite the large percentage of our country's wealth dedicated to health care, financial resources are not unlimited. How those resources are allocated can be troublesome,

with the needs and desires of many different groups and organizations competing for a slice of the pie.

Although bioethical issues abound, not all issues are problems and not all ethical problems make headline news. Nurses are involved in ethical decision-making every day that may not become problems. A promise might be extended to return to the patient and assess whether or not the pain medication was effective. Patients might share information that they want to remain confidential. A family agrees to a "do not resuscitate" (DNR) order for their loved one when they believe there is no hope for recovery. A young man in the prime of life is given cardiopulmonary resuscitation (CPR) when he suddenly goes into respiratory failure on the day of his proposed discharge. These examples usually are not problems but, depending on the situation, can develop into ethical dilemmas.

An ethical dilemma is created when:
- The required moral action is not clear
- Individuals in the situation do not agree on the proposed solution
- Neither of the available choices seems to offer a "best" option

It should be borne in mind that although while clinical decision making has been seen traditionally as the responsibility of the doctor, the consequences of those decisions fall largely on the nurses who are caring for such patients.

Potential solutions may appear to be equally good or, worse, equally risky: A promise cannot be kept; information cannot remain confidential; DNR orders may not be acceptable for some individuals. Not every patient should be the recipient of CPR endeavors, even those who are very young. When patients are conscious, their choices are usually respected, but on occasion even that premise can be difficult to apply. Often groups of individuals must work together to resolve a conflict that occurs if there is disagreement between physicians and families, nurses and physicians, or among family members.

A basic mastery of several elements enhances your ability to perform competently when bioethical issues present themselves and decision making is the focus. Understanding the ethical component of your nursing role is a first step. Discovering how your personal *value set* influences your nursing practice. Acquiring knowledge about relevant ethical material is also essential. An ethical decision-making process is a useful tool for examining ethical dilemmas. Together these elements provide a foundation from which you can begin to explore the meaning of bioethics in nursing practice today. For more information about bioethics, visit the *America Journal of Bioethics Online* at http://www.ajobonline.com or try The Center for Bioethics and Human Dignity at http://www.cbhd.org

Ethical Obligations and Nursing

As a nurse, you are an invaluable member of the health-care team. Members of the team contribute to patient care according to their educational preparation and assigned responsibilities. A common goal among all health team members is to provide holistic care to the patient because not only is the individual's mind, body, and spirit affected by disease or trauma, the disease process impacts upon the patient's family and community. A central component of that holistic care encompasses your responsibility to practice ethically.

In addition to practicing within the law, nurses have ethical obligations related to the law. First, if the law is considered unethical or has serious limitations, a basic moral obligation of the nurse, if not the health-care profession as a whole, is to make an effort to change that law. As a by-product, laws can sometimes unfairly affect health care in relation to accessing, services, subsidizing health care, or allocating health care dollars. Laws sometimes can be unethical because they are enacted based on power, authority, and political influences rather than high moral standards. Laws are created to reflect current common ethical beliefs (e.g., do not kill, do not steal) and values. However, in a democratic society with a diverse population such as in the United States, there are serious questions about the degree to which society should enforce moral behavior through the law and vice versa.

Nursing Code of Ethics

Some of the major ethical obligations of nursing practice are addressed within the nursing code of ethics. As a professional guide for ethical practice, the National Association for Practical Nurse Education and Service (NAPNES) developed a code of ethics for the licensed practical nurse/licensed vocational nurse (LPN/LVN). Like all codes of ethics, this code is an important document because it is a public statement of the basic ethical principles and standards for LPN/LVNs. An organization's code of ethics should be supported by the majority of its members. The code should provide guidance for appropriate decision-making based upon the laws and expectations of that time. A code of ethics also provides a base for professional self-evaluation and reflection regarding ethical practice.[5] Finally, the code of ethics is the tool by which the public can hold the professional accountable.

A code does not dictate a particular action, nor is it a legal document, although the code should not be in conflict with the law. The code is not enforced by any organization, and no punishment exists if a nurse fails to adhere to it. A code must be interpreted because it usually contains broad statements, but it does serve as a general guideline for professional ethical issues. Over time, the opinion of society changes and, as such, the codes are revised and updated. Although the Hippocratic oath (400 BC), the earliest Western code of ethics for physicians, contains fundamental moral advice, the passage of time and the occurrence of notable events make it incomplete for medical practice today. Changes in society prompt us to examine the profession's ethical standards and update them appropriately. There are several websites that offer information and guidance. The most important website for nurses is the American Nurses Association website (http://www.nursingworld.org/). This

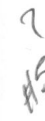

website has a section that is entitled "The Centre for Ethics and Human Rights" dedicated to current statements on ethical dilemmas that contains the code of ethics for nurses. This can be found at http://www.nursingworld.org/ethics/code/protected_nwcoe303.htm

Virtues

Particular ethical obligations can be summarized in the form of virtues. Each individual is endowed with specific character traits. As we grow, develop, and experience life, we acquire certain other character traits. Virtues are character traits most often associated with one's values and morality or conscience and are different from the skills that we acquire as nurses. Skills are used to implement various actions, something we do, whereas virtues define who we are. The Nightingale Pledge is implicit in its expectation of certain virtues possessed by graduating nurses. Such virtues include faith, loyalty, trustworthiness, and temperance.[6] These are all ideal traits, and although we may strive to act as virtuous persons, we are human and may not always succeed. The code of ethics specifically invokes faithfulness and respect for patient choice and acts as a constant reminder to that high standard to which we should always strive to maintain.

In addition, it should be remembered that virtues are related to roles and responsibilities and are therefore time dependent. For example, in the early decades of organized nursing in the United States, nurses occupied a handmaiden role relative to the physician. Obedience to the physician was considered a virtue, but such obedience is no longer held as a virtue by nurses.

FIDELITY (ALSO A PRINCIPLE). Fidelity is the obligation to be faithful to commitments made to self and others. In health care, fidelity includes faithfulness or loyalty to agreements and responsibilities accepted as part of the practice of nursing. It also means *not* promising a patient something that one cannot deliver or what they do not control (for example, a patient asks not to be resuscitated if they have a cardiac arrest, but the physician has not been consulted). Fidelity is the main support for the concept of accountability, although conflicts in fidelity might arise because of obligations owed to different individuals or groups. For example, nurses have an obligation of fidelity to the patients they care for to provide the highest quality care possible, as well as an obligation of fidelity to their employing institution to follow its rules and policies. Nurses can have an ethical dilemma when a hospital's policy on staffing creates a situation that does not allow the nurses to provide the quality of care they feel is necessary.

Maintaining a patient's privacy and **confidentiality** is related to fidelity (Fig. 2.5). Privacy and confidentiality may or may not be explicit promises. Nurses are obligated to only discuss the patient under circumstances in which it is necessary to deliver high-quality *holistic* health care such as:

- When given specific instructions to do so by the patient

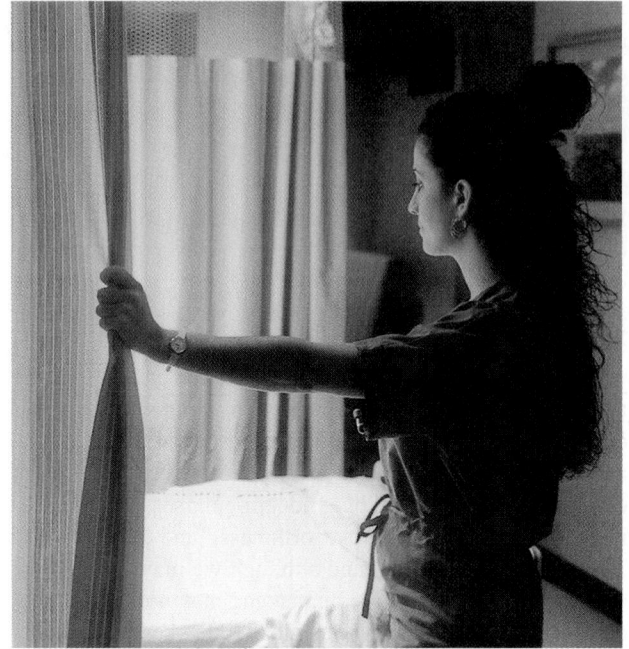

FIGURE 2.5 Maintaining privacy is a patient right and conveys caring to the patient.

- When there is the grave possibility of harm coming to either the patient or others
- When legally mandated to do so

Confidentiality also includes the necessary communication of information through the posting of unit census and various schedules for tests, procedures, or special examinations (operating room, physical therapy, radiology), storage and access of patient information through computers, and the transmission of patient information via fax machines. Many individuals have legitimate access to the patient's chart in addition to direct caregivers: faculty members in the course of making student assignments, accrediting agencies, risk managers, quality assurance personnel, insurance companies, and researchers. Each is obligated to maintain patient confidentiality to the extent that concealing information:

- Does not compromise mandated reports (communicable diseases or gunshot wounds)
- Considers various releases already granted by the patient (such as when insurance coverage was obtained)
- Ensures gathering data in the aggregate without identification of specific patients (research or institutional statistics)

Other forms of necessary communication include regular shift changes and case conferences. Care should be taken to hold these information-sharing events in settings where the discussion remains private.

VERACITY. **Veracity** is the virtue of truthfulness. Within health care, it requires health-care providers, whenever possible, to tell the truth and not intentionally deceive or mislead patients. As with other rights and obligations, there are limitations to this virtue. The primary limitation occurs when telling patients the truth would seriously harm their ability to recover, or when the truth may produce greater illness (this can be considered under the principle of **nonmaleficence** or doing no harm, which finds its origins in the Hippocratic Oath). Another difficult situation may be created in relation to diagnostic information. Although giving diagnostic information is the responsibility of the physician or registered nurse (RN), LPN/LVNs sometimes find themselves caught in situations in which they must deal with patients' questions. If LPN/LVNs feel uncomfortable about reinforcing physician or RN explanations about unpleasant information, they may avoid answering patients' questions directly. However, patients do have a right to know this information.

INTEGRITY. Integrity is a holistic, unwavering moral sense of self. Each individual has a cluster of values, beliefs, and traditions that form the basis for moral decision making; in a sense, the conscience. This sense of self can be compromised when the nurse is requested to act in a manner that requires setting aside or acting against values, beliefs, or traditions. The nurse who believes in the sanctity of life and that human life begins at conception, may not be able to maintain integrity if required to participate in abortion procedures. However, this nurse also has the responsibility not to accept a professional position where abortion is an issue, as a nurse cannot abandon a patient in need of nursing services. The nurse with integrity is faithful to professional responsibilities and obligations.

COMPASSION. Compassion or caring is a central virtue in nursing. Some label this **empathy** and connect it to the ability of a nurse to identify with a patient's suffering, pain, or disability. The difference between the two virtues is that in compassion, the nurse wishes to alleviate discomfort.[7] Patients are comforted by the compassionate nurse, and such nurturing can assist in the healing process. A nurse without any emotion robs patients of the full potential for healing that is only possible when all parties are actively engaged in all aspects of the relationship. Compassion should not be so dominant that it clouds judgment and prevents effective and efficient provision of nursing services. Compassion, in order to be effective, needs to be tempered with rationality.

DISCERNMENT. Discernment has been described as practical wisdom or common sense. This is the ability to understand, to have insight into the hidden, as well as the obvious elements of a situation. A nurse who has a discerning approach is one who is sensitive to the patient's actions and responses and does not necessarily accept what is seen at face value. Verbal, nonverbal, and subconscious communication, as well as concrete signs and symptoms, all contribute to the overall evaluation of the patient by the discerning nurse. This is sometimes translated as practical wisdom because this type of nurse has a depth of understanding of patients that leads to the selection of the appropriate action, which in turn is implemented in a caring manner. It can be argued that possessing a discerning nature is a product of experience and knowledge, for in nursing it is not enough to act upon *gut* instinct but to base opinion and action upon accepted approaches.

TRUSTWORTHINESS. It is vital that as health-care workers we inspire confidence in the patients we care for. We need to be considered trustworthy in order to have a true partnership with our patients. Sometimes, certain nurses may be preferred by patients because they convey a sense of confidence with the care they provide, and when one thinks that in many situations, patients' lives are truly in the nurse's hands, this preference is well grounded. When a patient feels that a nurse is worthy of their trust, an ease develops within the relationship that decreases stress and anxiety that diagnoses and treatment plans often bring. As a result, the patient develops more effective coping mechanisms. Indeed, studies have shown that it is the erosion of trust that is cited as a major factor in the escalating lawsuits that have been initiated against health professionals.

RESPECTFULNESS. Respectfulness is an attitude of a nurse toward the patient that indicates valuing that patient and their feelings as a unique individual. All patients should be treated with dignity and their autonomy acknowledged. Nurses are obligated to make an effort to identify their own biases and prejudices and work to avoid stereotyping and "isms" in patient relationships (e.g., classism, sexism, racism, ageism, and ethnocentrism), as well as eliminate discrimination based on religion, sexual orientation, or disability. Attentiveness to bias and discrimination is not limited to private interactions, but nurses are also responsible for drawing attention to unacceptable statements or negative actions that reflect disrespect for race, religion, gender, class, age, culture, sexual orientation, or disability in any health-care situation.

Rights

Rights represent at least two ways to think about what we are owed or what we deserve. Harris (2001) puts forward the position that if all people are considered valuable and equal, then it follows that there are rights possessed by people by virtue of their humanity.[4] These basic rights could be translated into goods and services (such as the right to clean water, the right to food). These are positive rights, and because something needs to be provided, there is a responsibility for someone to furnish these items. Second, other rights can be determined to protect us (e.g., right to privacy, right to self-determination). These are negative rights preventing some action that would intrude on our lives or prevent us from acting as we choose.

Laws guarantee some rights. Others are moral rights based on values and ethical principles but are not enforceable by law. "Basic human rights" is a common phrase that we hear when discussing the condition of various people around the world, especially when those rights are compromised. The United Nations has a document, "The Universal Declaration of Human Rights," that serves to represent what all people should be provided with or protected from.

In health care, there are increasingly heated discussions about rights of patients. It is true that in the past, patients were seen simply as passive recipients of whatever treatments or actions professionals determined necessary for their conditions. Now, professionals recognize patient autonomy and patients' active participation in health care.[8] The American Hospital Association (AHA) first devised a patients' bill of rights in 1973, which formally began recognition of what patients are entitled to but may not always receive. The revised bill includes statements on confidentiality, informed consent, and the right to refuse treatment. The 2005 version can be found at http://www.aha.org/aha/ptcommunication/partnership/index.html. It is an easy to understand brochure entitled "The Patient Care Partnership: Understanding Expectations, Rights and Responsibilities." The brochure is available in multiple languages. Many health-care organizations followed the patient bill of rights with other more specific bills of rights, such as those developed by nursing homes and veterans' hospitals.

In bioethics many issues can be framed within a rights context. An important rights issue is whether people have a "right" to health care. Such a right is discussed at every level of society, from local governments that determine services they will provide in city clinics and public schools to the federal government, which periodically grapples with the debate on national health insurance. Another prominent dispute is the "right to die" with dignity, which is arousing more interest as the largest cohort (the "baby boomers") edge toward the later decades of life. Combined threats of the loss of autonomy and the possibility of being subjected to endless, painful technological interventions while dying rightfully substantiates such concerns. By contrast, the "right to life" is another central concept in our society as groups organize politically to prevent abortions and overturn the *Roe v. Wade* decision of the Supreme Court.[9] This right also extends to discussions of reproductive rights and the health care of pregnant women. These are but a few examples of rights issues and potential conflicts. Others can be identified as various areas in medical surgical nursing are explored.

Building Blocks of Ethics

The discipline of ethics, especially health-care ethics, provides us with useful tools and knowledge that can assist us when we encounter difficult situations. The professional's understanding of basic concepts, presented here in the form of ethical principles and ethical theories, helps specifically target the ethical components of the problem. Principles and theories offer frameworks for ethical problem solving. However, knowledge about "ethics" cannot in itself provide all the answers to a problem or dilemma. What such knowledge *does* do is assist us in focusing upon the ethical aspects of each case. When we apply appropriate ethical rationale in our problem solving, we become grounded within this analytical framework. Such frameworks have the ability to make us look at many facets of an ethical problem, and presenting a particular position relative to a situation or describing values, beliefs, and traditions using these common ethical terms helps clarify discussions and possibly prevents escalating arguments. When one becomes familiar with health-care ethics, problems with communication, management of the unit, and legislation or the law can more easily be separated from the ethical dimension and resolved in their own problem-solving session.

Ethical Principles

Ethical principles derive from moral theory and have two purposes. The first is to provide some framework for society's moral conduct. Second, they enable us in taking consistent positions and approaches to moral dilemmas. Ethical principles can be found in many professional codes of conduct. The ethical principles that are widely used when examining bioethical and health-care dilemmas include autonomy, beneficence, nonmaleficence, and justice. Given these ethical principles' prominence in the bioethical literature, a basic understanding of them is necessary.

AUTONOMY. According to ethicists (and. e.g., behaviorists, social scientists, psychologists), what makes human beings different from nonhumans is that people have dignity based on their ability to choose freely what they will do with their lives. **Autonomy** is the right of self-determination, independence, and freedom founded on the notion that humans have value, worth, and moral dignity. Autonomy in health care refers to those individuals who are considered capable and competent making health-care decisions for themselves. Health-care providers do not have to agree with such decisions, but we must respect the autonomy of the person making that choice. Preventing patients from making autonomous decisions or deciding for patients without regard for their preferences is **paternalism.** Autonomy also encompasses the professional's self-determination and freedom.

Autonomy, as with most rights, is not an absolute right, and under certain conditions, limitations can be imposed on autonomy. Generally, these limitations occur when an individual's autonomy interferes with the rights, health, or well-being of others. For example, patients generally have an autonomous right to refuse any or all treatments. This autonomous right is guaranteed by federal legislation known as the Patient's Self-Determination Act. However, in the case of contagious diseases that affect society, such as tuberculosis (TB), an individual can be forced by the health-care and legal systems to take medications to cure the disease. Individuals can also be quarantined to prevent the spread of disease.[10]

BENEFICENCE. This principle proposes that one must take a positive action that does good for another and act in a way that will prevent harm to others. Within health care, **beneficence** is the principle of considering and offering treatments that are likely to provide relief.[11] At this point, it should be mentioned that the provision of *good* care means not just the provision of a technologically competent care of patients, but care that includes a respect for the patient's

beliefs, feeling, and wishes, as well those of their family and significant others. A common problem encountered when applying the principle of beneficence, is just *what* is good for another and who is the best person to make this decision.

NONMALEFICENCE. Nonmaleficence, one of the oldest obligations in health care, dating back to the Hippocratic Oath (400 BC), is related to beneficence and in a sense it is the opposite side of the coin as it is difficult to speak of one concept without mentioning the other. According to Burkhardt and Nathaniel,[12] nonmalificence

> ... requires us to act in such a manner as to avoid causing harm to patients. Included in this principle are deliberate harm, risk of harm, and harm that occurs during the performance of beneficial acts.

It is the requirement that health-care providers do no harm to their patients either *intentionally* or *unintentionally* (which can be quite difficult!). In current health-care practice, the principle of nonmaleficence may be intentionally violated in order to produce a greater good in the long-term treatment of the patient. For example, a patient may undergo a painful and debilitating or mutilating surgery to remove a cancerous growth, thereby avoiding death and prolonging life.

By extension, the principle of nonmaleficence also requires a nurse to protect from harm those who cannot protect themselves. This protection from harm includes groups such as children, the mentally incompetent, the unconscious, and those who are too weak or debilitated to protect themselves.

JUSTICE. Justice is based upon the principle of fairness and equality. Concerns for justice may focus upon how we treat individuals and groups in society (psychologically, socially, legally, politically). How we distribute material resources such as health care (**distributive justice**) and burdens (taxes) equitably, and the appropriate compensation to those who have been harmed. When the patient makes an appointment for 9 a.m. at the outpatient clinic and his or her neighbor makes a 10 a.m. appointment, each expects to be seen by the primary care provider at the designated time unless some emergency prevails. Unequal treatment would result if a walk-in who has no pressing problem is seen by the provider in place of the 9 a.m. appointment, forcing each subsequent appointment to be delayed beyond the prearranged time. Distribution of material resources can be complex because it involves not only benefits (what we receive) but also burdens (what we may be taxed for but then do not receive). Burdens are not just monetary, but also include such factors as the unequal participation of individuals in medical research and the sacrifices family members make when caring for disabled individuals in the home.

One of the most serious limitations of these principles is the lack of any built-in priority when applying them to an

---

autonomy: auto—self + nimos—rule
beneficence: bene—good + facere—to do

nonmaleficence: non—not + maleficentia—evil doing

ethical dilemma. Autonomy is not automatically prioritized over justice or beneficence over nonmaleficence. However, these principles are helpful in categorizing various preferences and positions when examining a dilemma, and their categorization can lead to a clarification of various disagreements among participants in the ethical discussion. Working with principles moves the discussion to a focus on ethics rather than a particular personal viewpoint or feeling. Such a strategy can also avoid a power struggle between participants who simply want to win the argument. An example of an ethical dilemma is the following scenario. A nurse attempts to support a patient's refusal of surgery, while the physician claims that the patient must have surgery or she will lose her leg. Realizing that the nurse is arguing the case from the perspective of the patient's autonomy (self-determination), whereas the physician's desire to perform surgery is attributable to beneficence (obligation to come to the assistance of those in need[13]), moves the discussion to one based on conflicting principles rather than conflict between individuals. From this point of clarification, the discussion can focus on autonomy and beneficence and the rationale for the possible prioritizing of one principle over the other. This strategy does not resolve the dilemma, but it makes it less personal and forces participants to develop sound, ethical rationales for their solutions.

Ethical Theories

Ethical theories are concepts that are more complete than principles for analyzing ethical dilemmas. Such theories are used to explain variables, guide inquiry, and provide a foundation from which considered and thought-provoking questions emanate. However, only a brief description is included here; a more in-depth understanding can be obtained from other resources, such as the Web links, journals, and many books on the topic.

Two of the major theories used in bioethics are defined first, and then a subcategory of theories collectively known as feminist theories are introduced; finally, recognition of the relationship of theology or religion to bioethics completes this section.

UTILITARIANISM. Utilitarian theory is grounded in the premise that actions are judged right or wrong based purely upon their consequences and therefore outcomes are the most important elements to consider in decision making.[14] Right actions are morally preferred if they produce more happiness or greater benefits than unhappiness or burdens, and in utilitarianism, each person's happiness is equally important. This approach may be used by institutions and organizations under the guise of cost-benefit ratios. A hospital that has the responsibility to care for hundreds of patients is not as concerned with the individual patient who unfortunately is caught in the bureaucracy of its functioning. This is not to say that all institutions operate on this theory at all times, but in general, rules, policies, and procedures are developed with the majority in mind. There are several major criticisms of this theory. One is that an individual is often sacrificed for the good of the majority (often seen in

wartime). The second is that it can be difficult to predict outcomes, especially when human nature is involved.

DEONTOLOGY. Deontology is a philosophical theory requiring human actions and attitudes to be based on *duty* and the moral worth of an action (the result) should not be judged only in terms of its consequences. For example, health professionals might operate by a rule that indicates that a moral person never lies. No matter how much the truth might hurt, the truth is revealed. Another rule might be to never use people as a means to an end. Translated this means that regardless of the benefits, individuals cannot be forced to participate in medical research studies to benefit others. An individual's right to voluntarily participate in research must be respected. Research does not have to benefit the individual participant as long as this is understood by the individual. However, the individual cannot be used simply to meet the investigator's needs. Acting morally only because one has a duty to do so, without any consideration of the outcome, is a serious limitation of this theory.

FEMINIST THEORIES. Feminist approaches challenge traditional theories in that they focus upon gender bias, discrimination, and prejudice in addition to the more serious actions of oppression and violence against women. The rise of such theories can find their origins in Carol Gilligan's original hypothesis that the moral orientation of a person is associated with their gender. In other words, the judgments of women are predominantly oriented toward the value of care and the judgments of men predominantly toward the value of justice.[15]

This view is important because of existing power differentials among the providers and recipients of health care, as well as the previous treatment of normal development, injury, illness, disease, and dying in women. Current, or *third wave* feminist theories are really a group of various approaches to ethical problems and decision-making rather than one uniform approach.[16] Feminists may use utilitarian and deontological theories, as well as various other approaches, to develop a systematic organization of ethical rules and principles. Some feminist theories focus on feminine attributes (emotional attachment, caring, prominence of relationships, and connection with people), emphasizing their importance in ethical decision-making. In general, those who support this approach observe the devaluing of these attributes in society. Caring, as an example of one attribute, is important personally, but supporters recognize that caring is not systematically rewarded in our society. Other theories are more politically oriented and concentrate their energies on developing approaches to ethical decision making that minimize the subordination and marginalization of women, whatever other principles they support. For example, in a liberal approach to ethical decision making, human beings have a political responsibility to organize and maintain a particular society based on freedom and the various perceived rights that one has. Rules are supposed to protect privacy. From a feminist perspective, the liberal approach focuses on making sure that women are included in the political processes when such rules are made, helping to develop a balanced legislation, this serves to shape the communities in which we live. In health care a liberal feminist approach focuses on providing women with educational and promotional opportunities for leadership positions in health-care systems. In leadership positions, it is hoped that women will use their power and authority in order to make the health-care system more accommodating for other women.

THEOLOGICAL PERSPECTIVES. Theological perspectives include the many religious traditions represented in our culture. Religious teachings are key concepts for ethical decision making for some individuals. In fact, many individuals consider these teachings as a divine source of values and morals. Jehovah's Witness believers' rejection of blood transfusions is a common example of how religious beliefs affect health-care decision making. This religious group has collected a large amount of information about blood substitutes and alternative therapies. Leaders of Jehovah's Witnesses are prepared to provide education for health professionals about their beliefs and acceptable interventions. In another area, a number of religious traditions oppose abortion, which affects both health professionals and patients. Euthanasia is an issue addressed by numerous organized religious groups, which in turn can affect how patients make decisions regarding end-of-life issues. One of the difficulties with religious traditions is that it is not simply the official church teaching that is involved, but the individual member's interpretation of that teaching. Assessment of the importance of this dimension of the patient's life is important in the ethical analysis.

Ethical Decision Making

A variety of models and frameworks for ethical decision making are available. The steps listed in this section are a combination of several ideas that have been suggested. In its simplest form, ethical decision making is an informed problem-solving process. Similar to the nursing process, as discussed in the first chapter, the steps described in this section take the user through a set of strategies that assist in approaching a problem in an organized and systematic manner. Nurses applying these steps use critical thinking skills in order to be as logical and objective as possible. This is not to say that feelings and emotions are to be put aside. Indeed such feelings and associations as bonding, love, commitment, and other sentiments define our humanity. However, a balanced perspective is the goal, which includes respecting these feelings without allowing them to overshadow the process and the outcome. Although making the final decision may not be easy, the user knows that once these steps have been completed, the situation has been thoroughly examined and all viable and reasonable aspects explored before the decision was made.

Step 1: Gather and Verify the Information
Many kinds of information can contribute to an in-depth understanding of the situation, which provokes an ethical dilemma. Basically one needs to know who is involved, what is involved, and the context of the problem. Foremost is information about the patient—what the patient says when conscious and competent. Determining competency itself can be an involved and frustrating process, especially when there are competing parties involved (e.g., a disagreement in a family about the competency of a parent). The chart is an obvious resource for clinical data, but so are the health professionals who are assigned to the patient because not every individual records all that is known about the patient. When appropriate, health-care records from previous hospitalizations may be helpful, as well as charts from other institutions and agencies. External factors also need to be included, such as legal aspects, governing policies and procedures of the institution, and available resources. The amount of information gathered depends on the time frame and urgency of the decision.

Step 2: Clarify the Values of All the Participants
The values, beliefs, and traditions of all participants are important, especially those of the patient, but more so when the patient is unconscious or incompetent (often called *non compos mentis* from the Latin *non* meaning not, *compos* in control, and *mentis* mind) and a group is attempting to reach a consensus based on some understanding of the patient. Advance directives or a living will prepared by the patient are often helpful as guides when the patient can no longer express personally held ethical beliefs (see Chapter 16). In addition, it is important to realize that sometimes the advance directive of a patient may be the polar opposite of the wishes of family. For example, a patient with a preexisting condition such as Parkinson's disease may not wish aggressive action to be taken and wants to be allowed to die should he or she have a massive heart attack. The family, not wishing to let go of their loved one, may fight to keep the patient alive. Determining the ethical orientation of all participants clarifies their perspectives and moves decision making to a more objective level. Decision makers must be especially aware of assumptions, stereotyping, biases, and prejudices related to socioeconomic status, ethnic identification, gender, sexual and religious preferences, and other common characteristics of the participants.

Step 3: Identify the Ethical Dilemma and the Conflicts in Values
Separating the ethical aspects from the nonethical facets facilitates the decision-making process. For example, a conflict can arise as a result of gaps in communication rather than a conflict of ethical principles. When the communication channels are open and the decision-making process is transparent, it no longer is an issue. Sometimes both nonethical and ethical aspects need to be addressed in a parallel fashion to reach a resolution of the situation. The importance of various ethical values for each participant should be explored.

Step 4: Examine Possible Actions and the Consequences of Each Action
There is no magic number of "possible actions," but it is easy to pose solutions at the extremes of possible actions.

Consider informing the patient as an example. The two obvious solutions are to tell and not to tell. But in clinical practice it is not that simple, and it is more useful also to pose solutions that are between the extremes. Suppose the issue is a critically injured patient who wants to know the condition of her spouse and child, who were also in the automobile accident. Her spouse was killed and her child is in critical condition. At the moment, her own status is unstable and telling her might have a deleterious effect on her own health. Telling her is certainly an option, just one with certain limitations at that time. Not saying anything in response to her question is a possibility but seems to show a lack of respect for her dignity as a person and her right to information. What might be some possible actions in between those extremes? Is there some response that tells part of the information while avoiding the worst part, her spouse's death? Even if the partial truths seem unacceptable at first glance, they ought to be added to the list of possible actions. Examination of a range of possible actions aids in identifying where the line is drawn for determining morally acceptable choices versus those not morally acceptable or for creating a list of each choice's risks and benefits.

Step 5: Determine the Ethical Foundation for Each Action

Each action should be based on selected ethical values, principles, or theories. Perhaps the code of ethics lends some support as ethical rationale. One strategy that is proposed on occasion, especially for an incompetent or unconscious patient, is an application of the **standard of best interest**. The best interest standard involves the determination of what action is in the best interest of the patient given the information that is known about the patient and the situation. Family members together with health-care providers usually make the best interest determination. Ideally, this decision is made in an objective manner, setting aside any special interests of the family or health professionals. For example, it may be in the best interest of the patient to be discharged and go home so that recovery can be optimized in that setting. Family members themselves may have other goals that make placement in a long-term care facility better for them. Health professionals may be pressured by administrative personnel to simply arrange a discharge, regardless of where the patient might be discharged to or what might be best for the patient, because of utilization review and financial reimbursement considerations. Under the best interest standard, the optimal placement is in the home because it is considered to have the best outcome for the patient.

Step 6: Determine the Best Action with the Strongest Ethical Support

Each action is judged based on its risks, benefits, and supporting rationale. The actions are then ranked in order of their priority. Strong ethical support for the first priority is required, as well as a reasonable potential for the action to be implemented. For example, if placement in a nursing home after discharge from the acute care facility is considered to be the best solution for a patient, but there is no room avail-

able in the potential facilities, that action must be set aside. If the preferred action fails, it is possible to move to choice number two. The designation of these priorities does not necessarily mean that their supporting ethical rationale always results in the same ranking, nor does it mean that principles or theories are always in opposition to one another.

Utilitarians and deontologists may disagree about the important principles in decision making. However, it should not be assumed that different **theorists** cannot reach a mutually agreeable decision. Although their rationale for the decision may differ, the final solution each proposes may be identical. A case in point involves the relief of pain and suffering. The deontologist might argue that there is a duty among health professionals to provide pain medications and make patients comfortable. This action shows respect for the value and dignity of the individual. A utilitarian might argue that pain and suffering should be relieved because doing so creates a positive outcome: the patient is more comfortable without pain and the family is helped too in that they do not have to watch a loved one suffer. In an even broader context, the more pain and suffering that is relieved, the greater the number of patients who benefit. So both theorists support the same action, but for different reasons.

Even theorists, such as utilitarians, can disagree among themselves. A classic case involving confidentiality was solved based on utilitarian concepts, yet both the ruling vote and the dissenting vote were based on utilitarian principles.[17] The majority opinion of the court indicated that more good would be created by disregarding confidentiality obligations because overriding the patient's confidentiality would have saved the life of a third person who the patient threatened to murder. The minority opinion of the court stated that confidentiality should not be breached because it gave society the message that psychiatrists would not keep patient confessions secret and therefore would inhibit most individuals who have psychiatric problems from seeking professional help.

Step 7: Implement the Action

Needless to say, the selected action needs to be carried out. Responsibilities for the professionals and others in the situation can be assigned. Assigning a coordinator for the implementation of the action, especially if several individuals have responsibilities for portions of the action, enhances the potential for success, ensuring that someone will check on the process of implementation and that the action is evaluated.

Step 8: Evaluate the Outcome

We can learn from success and failure. Successful resolution of an ethical dilemma provides us with knowledge for the next ethical dilemma. Although no two dilemmas are exactly alike, selected features of a particular dilemma may parallel a subsequent situation and assist in solving the new dilemma. Failures also teach us a lesson. Retracing all the steps of the ethical decision-making process may provide insight and greater understanding of what steps of the process could have been better implemented. Evaluation is also important because the next time we confront a similar dilemma we may not have the luxury of examining the new dilemma in as much detail. Prior experience enables us to face new dilemmas more confidently and to determine the better action more quickly. It is also important when making important decisions such as these that involve the life and care of vulnerable populations that absolute transparency is evident. Patients and family members have the right to know how and why decisions are made, especially if it is a resource allocation decision. One caution, however: It is very important to evaluate the outcome when decisions are made and the action taken within a limited time frame.

 LEGAL CONCEPTS

To promote harmony, safety, and productivity as members of a society, we create rules. The rules of society can be informal or formal. An informal social rule, for example, is opening a door for someone. A criminal statute (law) is an example of a formal rule of society. Social rules or codes promote our social well-being. It would be unsafe to live in a community that existed without rules. All societies must require minimum standards of conduct for their members. Laws are the governmental mandates of a society that define individuals' duties to themselves, their neighbors, and the government. The failure to adhere to laws can result in punishment that may include imprisonment or monetary fines.

CRITICAL THINKING

Ethical Decisions

1. Identify a health-care–related ethical dilemma you have encountered as a student. How did you solve the dilemma? What expert resources did you use?
2. Apply the ethical decision-making model to the ethical dilemma. How are your decision-making process and proposed actions different when using the model?

Regulation of Nursing Practice

Nursing is a licensed health-care profession. Nurses must be licensed by their state to practice nursing. The rationale for state licensure is to improve the quality of health-care services and to protect the public. As such, state governments have created licensing boards to establish the entry-level requirements for nurses. These licensing boards also establish regulations that define the scope of appropriate nursing practice for licensed nurses. These licensing regulations are found in state nursing practice laws and within regulations that are made by the licensing agency.

The state nursing practice laws and the attendant nursing regulations establish the parameters within which nurses must practice to obtain and maintain state license. These regulations are referred to as **administrative laws.** These

considerations and mandates can be the basis for disciplinary actions by the licensing body. The failure to adhere to the regulatory mandates of the nursing licensing body can result in the loss of the privilege to practice nursing. Unprofessional conduct and conviction of a crime are examples of possible violations of nursing regulations.

Health Insurance Portability and Accountability Act of 1996 (HIPAA)

Since 1996, the federal government has regulated the distribution of personal health information. Licensed nurses along with other health workers are required to follow the requirements established by the Health Insurance Portability and Accountability Act of 1996 (HIPAA). This Act creates civil and criminal liability for health-care workers who wrongfully disclose an individual's health information. HIPAA has created a national standard for the protection of individual health information. The Department of Health and Human Services has developed a privacy rule that has, for the first time, established a basis for the federal protection of private health information. Licensed nurses must be sensitive to these legal limitations for the distribution of personal health information. Depending upon the seriousness of the violation of the HIPAA standards, one may be sentenced to up to 10 years in prison. HIPAA establishes very stringent guidelines. Licensed nurses should review their employer's HIPAA compliance policies and adhere to them. For more information on HIPAA and how it impacts health-care information and workers, please see the United States Department of Human Services website at www.hhs.gov/ocr/hipaa.

Nursing Liability and the Law   #10?

Liability refers to the level of responsibility that society places on individuals for their actions. In recent years, this responsibility has been interpreted to mean the financial responsibility owed to those who are injured by wrongful actions. Laws establish liability or responsibility for these wrongful actions. Following the law is a major part of the practice of nursing.

Administrative laws establish the licensing authority of the state to create, license, and regulate the practice of nursing. **Criminal law** regulates behaviors for citizens within this coountry. **Civil law** provides the rules by which individuals seek to protect their personal and property rights.

Criminal and Civil Law

All individuals, regardless of their occupations, are required to obey the criminal laws of the government. Criminal laws establish the rules of social behavior and define the punishment for the breaking of those rules, which can result in imprisonment or monetary fines.

Criminal law is different from civil law in the nature of remedies that are used for punishment. A crime is viewed as an action taken by an individual against society that the government will prosecute and punish. The breaking of a criminal law may result in criminal punishment and civil liability. For instance, an intoxicated driver may go to jail for a crime and also be held civilly liable for any personal injury that resulted. Examples of criminal acts are assault, battery, rape, murder, and larceny.

Civil laws dictate how disputes are settled among individuals and how liability is assigned for wrongful actions. For health-care workers, civil liability is a constant concern. The potential for civil liability is demonstrated by an increased use of health-care procedures such as diagnostic testing, which results in higher health-care costs. Civil liability is a method by which a patient can seek financial recovery for injuries and losses caused by the wrongful action or lack of action by a health-care worker.

A civil liability suit begins with the filing of a complaint with a court. A copy of the complaint must be given or served by the plaintiff to the defendant. A **summons,** which is a notice to defendants that they are being sued, is attached to the complaint. The complaint describes the claim being made by the plaintiff, and the summons instructs the defendant that the complaint must be answered within a specified period, usually 20 to 30 days. Nurses served with a summons relating to work should notify their employers and take these documents seriously. The nurse must ensure that the summons is answered. If the employer does not answer the summons, the nurse must seek legal counsel to answer the summons within the specified time. If the nurse fails to answer the summons and complaint, it may result in a default judgment, which is acknowledgment of liability.

Civil wrongs caused by the act or omission of a health-care worker can be physical, emotional, and financial in nature. The person claiming a civil cause of action and injury is the plaintiff, and the person alleged to have caused the injury is the defendant. Lawsuits involving civil wrongs are called **torts.** The institution that employs the worker may also become liable for the acts or omissions of its employees. This theory of law is called **respondeat superior.** It is important for employees to understand that their work may result in civil liability for their employers.

Civil or tort liability for health-care workers can be based on intentional actions, unintentional actions, and even the omission of action. **Malpractice** may be defined as a breach of the duty that arises out of the relationship that exists between the patient and the health-care worker. This term includes liability that may arise from intentional torts and unintentional torts. Intentional torts are lawsuits wherein the defendant is accused of intentionally causing injury to the plaintiff. Examples of intentional torts are assault, battery, defamation, false imprisonment, outrage, invasion of privacy, and wrongful disclosure of confidential information (Box 2.1 Intentional Torts).

Negligence

An unintentional tort is known as **negligence.** Negligence occurs when injury results from the failure of the wrongdoer to exercise care. This failure to follow due care in the protection of the person injured is referred to as a breach of duty. Professionals owe a higher duty of care to their patients. The failure of a health-care professional to follow

---

Box 2.1

Intentional Torts

Assault	Unlawful conduct that places another in immediate fear of an unlawful touching or battery; real threat of bodily harm
Battery	Unlawful touching of another
Defamation	Wrongful injury to another's reputation or standing in a community; may be written (libel) or spoken (slander)
False Imprisonment	Unlawful restriction of a person's freedom
Outrage	Extreme and outrageous conduct by a defendant in the care of the patient or the body of a deceased individual
Invasion of Privacy and Wrongful Disclosure of Confidential Information	Liability when a patient's privacy is invaded physically or when records are released without authority

---

a prescribed duty of care is called malpractice. Professional negligence, therefore, is referred to as malpractice (Box 2.2, Components Necessary for a Finding of Negligence). All professionals, including LPN/LVNs, are responsible for their own actions whether they are intentional or negligent in nature. Although the employing agency is also responsible for the actions of its employees, employees always remain responsible for their own actions as well.

Limitation of Liability

All professions are concerned with the **limitation of liability.** Some examples of liability limitations are ensuring patient rights, accurately documenting procedures, following institutional policies, acquiring individual malpractice or liability insurance, pursuing continuing education, and practicing in accordance with the current standards of the nursing profession. Some states have enacted tort reform legislation. Much of this legislation is directed at limiting liability for health-care professionals and institutions. Examples of this reform legislation are limitations on the

---

Box 2.2

Components Necessary for a Finding of Negligence

- A duty of care owed to patients
- A breach of duty to exercise care
- Injury and damages occurring from this breach of duty

dollar amount allowable for a patient's damages, shortening the time in which a patient can file a lawsuit, and requiring stringent expert medical evaluation of a claim before a lawsuit can be filed.

All patients are entitled to quality care and treatment with dignity and respect. To provide quality care and limit liability, understand and provide the rights your patient is entitled to and question directions that are controversial, given verbally, concern situations of high liability, or involve a discrepancy between the direction and standard policy. Rights are defined as something due an individual according to just claims, legal guarantees, or moral and ethical principles. **Welfare rights,** also called legal rights, are rights that are based on a legal entitlement to some good or benefit. These rights are guaranteed by laws such as the Bill of Rights and if violated can come under the powers of the legal system. For example, citizens of the United States have a right to equal access to employment regardless of race, sex, or religion. The type of treatment and care a patient has the right to expect is outlined in the patient bill of rights. Stay informed on the status of patient rights' legislation as

you will be expected to follow it. Knocking before entering a patient's room and introducing oneself to the patient are examples of a patient's rights.

Documentation is a legal record of your actions. Document nursing actions based on orders given, as well as the name and title of the person who gave the verbal direction. Documentation must be clear, honest, and accurate. Always practice at a level that is generally accepted by the nursing profession. Failure to adhere to acceptable practice standards is cause for concern and can create potential liability for both you and the health-care institution.

It is important to understand that some employers do not provide malpractice insurance for their nursing employees. Always ask an employer exactly who is covered under the employer's liability insurance. If nursing employees are covered, the employer's insurance provides coverage from liability only as long as the employee follows the employer's work policies. For this reason, employer-provided liability insurance is not personal liability insurance. As a result, LPN/LVNs often carry personal liability insurance.

REVIEW QUESTIONS

1. Factors influencing health care changes include which of the following?
   a. Increasing birth rate
   b. Increasing cultural diversity
   c. Decreasing elderly population
   d. Decreasing population size in America

2. Which of these actions would the nurse correctly interpret as falling within the scope of practice of the LPN/LVN?
   a. Performing an admission physical assessment on a critical care patient
   b. Administering IV push morphine
   c. Ambulating a 1-day postoperative patient
   d. Developing the plan of care for a newly admitted surgical patient

3. Which of the following describes how an autocratic leader makes decisions?
   a. Seeks information from all staff members
   b. Uses own knowledge to decide
   c. Forms focus groups to gather information
   d. Forms a staff committee to provide input

4. Which of these situations would be an appropriate example of a leadership role for the LPN/LVN?
   a. Consulting with an RN to modify care for assigned patient
   b. Performing an annual employee evaluation on a nursing assistant
   c. Supervising the RN and LPN/LVN staff on a surgical unit
   d. Interviewing new graduate RN for a staff position

5. As a nurse provides care to patients, it is important to have an understanding of ethics for which of the following reasons?
   a. Resources are unlimited and available to everyone.
   b. Technological interventions are always desirable.
   c. Health-care systems are being simplified.
   d. A health crisis can occur at any stage of human development.

6. The nurse is planning quality care for a patient without regard to race, ethnicity, and gender. Which of the following ethical obligations does this exhibit?
   a. Fidelity
   b. Integrity
   c. Respectfulness
   d. Compassion

7. A patient's family requests that a feeding tube be inserted. The patient has an advance directive indicating that a feeding tube is not to be inserted. As the nurse and physician consider what is best for the patient in this ethical dilemma, which of the following principles is represented?
   a. Autonomy
   b. Beneficence
   c. Nonmaleficence
   d. Justice

8. The nurse reviews the advance directive for a patient who is comatose. Which of the steps in the ethical decision making process is the nurse performing?
   a. Clarifying the values of all participants.

b. Examining possible actions and the consequences of each.

c. Determining best action with strongest ethical support.

d. Implementing the outcome.

9. The nurse has a question about how a nursing license is regulated. In which of the following documents will the nurse find this information?

a. An institutional policy

b. Nursing ethics code

c. State nursing practice laws

d. National nursing standards

Multiple response item. Select all that apply.

10. In providing professional nursing care, the nurse understands that the law of negligence requires which of the following to create liability?

a. A duty of care owed

b. Assault

c. Ethical violations

d. A breach of duty

e. Injury and damages

f. A crime

11. The Health Insurance Portability and Accountability Act of 1996 requires licensed professional nurses to do which of the following?

a. Maintain continuing nursing education credit hours.

b. Protect the privacy of an individual's personal health information.

c. Limit nursing work hours to no more than 35 hours per week.

d. Forgo membership in any union or collective bargaining agreement unit.

References

1. United States Department of Health and Human Services. Public Health Service. Healthy People 2010: National Health Promotion and Disease Prevention Objectives. U.S. Government Printing Office, Washington, DC, 2000.

2. National Council of State Boards of Nursing. Delegation: Concepts and decision-making process. Issues, 16(4):1, 1995.

3. Somerville, M: The Ethical Canary. Penguin Books, Toronto, 2000, p. xiii.

4. Harris, J: The Value of Life: An Introduction to Medical Ethics. Routledge, London, 2001.

5. Canadian Nurses Association Code of Ethics for Registered Nurses 2005.

6. Burkhardt M, and Nathaniel K: Ethics and Issues in Contemporary Nursing. Delmar, NY, 2002, p. 50.

7. www.dictionary.com Keyword = compassion

8. Jones, R et al: Changing face of medical curricula. Lancet 357:699, 2001.

9. http://www.tourolaw.edu/patch/Roe/#rop

10. Guido, GW: Legal and Ethical Issues in Nursing. Prentice Hall Health, Upper Saddle River, New Jersey, 2001.

11. Looney, E: Ethical Issues in Palliative Care: Understanding the Basics—Part I: Topics Clin Nutr 15:(2), 2000.

12. Burkhardt, M, and Nathaniel, K: Ethics and Issues in Contemporary Nursing. Delmar, NY, 2002.

13. Keatings, M, Smith, O: Ethical and Legal Issues in Canadian Nursing. Saunders, Toronto, 2000.

14. Russo, M, Szymanski, S, and Sunal, D: Teaching Bioethics. Science Activities 41:5–12, 2004.

15. Schwickert, E: Translated by Sarah Clark Miller: Gender, Morality, and Ethics of Responsibility: Complementing Teleological and Deontological Ethics. Hypatia 20:164–187, 2005.

16. Kinser, A: Negotiating Spaces For/Through Third-Wave Feminism. NWSA J 16:124, 2004.

17. Tarasoff v. Regents of the University of California. 17 Cal. 3d 425, 1976.

Resources

1. www.nflpn.org

2. http://ethics.acusd.edu/video/Catalogue/all.asp Watch expert presenters discussing aspects of ethics, both in the health-care field, and general philosophy.

3. Nursing Ethics Network provides a host of links for information on ethical decision making for health-care professionals. Go to http://jmrileyrn.tripod.com/nen/nen.html

4. When making difficult ethical decisions, David Seedhouse and Lisetta Lovett's "Ethical Grid," which can be found in Practical Medical Ethics, Seedhouse D, and Lovett, L (eds.). John Wiley & Sons, Chichester, UK, 1993, is a great resource.

5. For an interesting perspective on approaches to bioethics, including feminist and womanist theory, see Karen Lebacqz's Bioethics—Eleven Approaches in Dialog: A Journal of Theology 43:100–106, 2004.

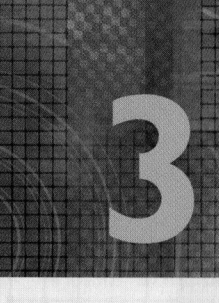

3

Cultural Influences on Nursing Care

NANCY AHERN

KEY TERMS

acculturation (uh-KUL-chur-AY-shun)
beliefs (bee-LEEFS)
cultural (KUL-chur-uhl)
cultural assimilation (KUL-chur-uhl uh-SIM-uh-LAY-shun)
cultural awareness (KUL-chur-uhl a-WARE-ness)
cultural competence (KUL-chur-uhl KOM-pe-tens)
cultural conflict (KUL-chur-uhl KON-flikt)
cultural diversity (KUL-chur-uhl di-VER-si-tee)
cultural sensitivity (KUL-chur-uhl SEN-si-TIV-i-tee)
cultural shock (KUL-chur-uhl)
culture (KUL-chur)
customs (KUS-tums)
ethnic (ETH-nick)
ethnocentrism (ETH-noh-SEN-trizm)
generalizations (JEN-er-al-i-ZAY-shuns)
stereotype (STER-ee-oh-TIGHP)
traditions (tra-DISH-uns)
values (VAL-yooz)
worldview (WERLD-vyoo)

QUESTIONS TO GUIDE YOUR READING

1. What are the meanings of the concepts common to culture and ethnicity?

2. What are examples of cultural characteristics, values, beliefs, and practices?

3. What are attributes of culturally diverse patients and their families and how do they affect nursing care?

4. What data should you collect from culturally diverse patients and their families?

5. How can you provide a holistic approach to patient care according to cultural characteristics and attributes?

CASE STUDY

Your clinical instructor has assigned you to provide care to Mary Williams, a 72-year-old African American woman. Ms. Williams has diabetes and hypertension (high blood pressure). She was admitted to the hospital for gangrene of her left foot. When you enter her room, you find Ms. Williams anxious and crying. She tells you that she is scheduled for surgery later in the day. When asked about her foot, she tells you that she has been applying a poultice to draw out the germs but it has not worked yet. She adds that she has been praying for the cure that she knows will come. As you are collecting history information about her diabetes, Ms. Williams admits that her doctor told her to attend diabetes classes years ago but she stopped going because she didn't like what she heard. She quickly changes the subject, wanting to talk about nothing but her grandchildren. Your attempts to complete preoperative teaching are unsuccessful.

    Cultural diversity in the United States is increasing. The United States has become a multicultural society. Immigration from Spanish-speaking and Asian countries has resulted in dramatic shifts in census numbers. Table 3.1 illustrates the changes and projections in racial and ethnic makeup in the United States by the year 2010. As a result, **cultural** and **ethnic** differences between nurses and their patients are becoming more evident and must be recognized. Thus there is a need for you to become knowledgeable about **cultures** other than your own. This chapter provides you with the basics of culture and its impact on health promotion and wellness.

CONCEPTS RELATED TO CULTURE

Culture refers to the socially transmitted behavior patterns, **beliefs, values, customs,** arts, and all other characteristics of people that guide their view of the world **(worldview).** Cultural beliefs, values, customs, and **traditions** are primarily learned within the family on an unconscious level. They can also be learned from the community in which one lives, in religious organizations, and in schools. As you try to understand more about culture, keep in mind that it contains a number of characteristics (Box 3.1, Characteristics of Culture). All individuals and groups have the right to maintain their cultural practices as they feel are appropriate.

Box 3.1

Characteristics of Culture

- *Culture is learned.* Learning occurs through life experiences shared with other members of the culture.
- *Culture is taught.* Cultural values, beliefs, and traditions are passed down from generation to generation either formally (e.g., in schools) or informally (e.g., in families)
- *Culture is shared by its members.* Cultural norms are shared through teachings and social interactions.
- *Culture is dynamic and adaptive.* Cultural customs, beliefs, and practices are not static, but change over time and at different rates. Cultural change occurs with adaptation in response to the environment.
- *Culture is complex.* Cultural assumptions and habits are unconscious, which may make it difficult for members of the culture to explain to others.
- *Culture is diverse.* Culture demonstrates the variety that exists between groups and among members of a particular group.
- *Culture exists at many levels.* Culture exists in material (e.g., art, dress, or artifacts) and nonmaterial (as language, traditions, customs, beliefs, and practices) levels.
- *Culture has common beliefs and practices.* Members of the culture share the same beliefs, traditions, customs, and practices as long as they continue to be adaptive and satisfy their needs. Some members do not always follow all of these, but many do.
- *Culture is all encompassing.* Culture can affect everything its members think and do.
- *Culture provides identity.* Cultural beliefs provide identity for its members as long as there is no conflict with the dominant culture or lack of gratification by its members.

Culture has strong influences on a patient's understanding of health and responses to nursing care. You must understand the impact diversity can have on health behaviors in order to better meet the needs of your patients (Fig. 3.1). As you learn more about ethnic and cultural groups, you will be challenged to look at the differences and similarities across cultures.

TABLE 3.1 UNITED STATES DEMOGRAPHIC PERCENTAGES 1995–2010[3]

Race/National Origin	1995	2000	2005 Projections	2010 Projections
White, non-Hispanic	73.6	71.3	69.3	67.3
Spanish/Hispanics/Latinos	10.3	11.9	13.3	14.6
Black, non-Hispanic	12.0	12.2	12.3	12.5
American Indian or Alaska Native, non-Hispanic	0.7	0.7	0.8	0.8
Asian and Pacific Islander, non-Hispanic	3.4	3.8	4.3	4.8

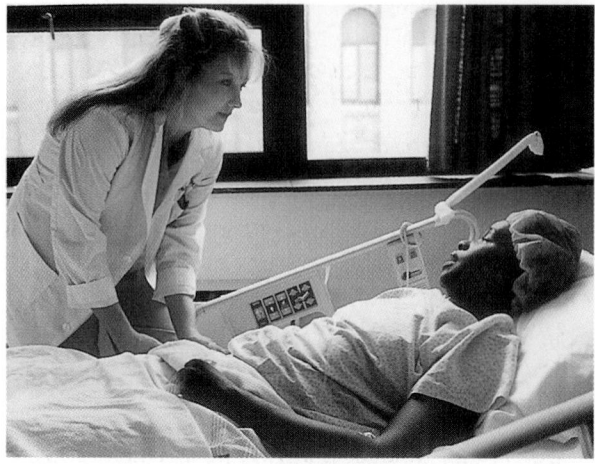

FIGURE 3.1 The nurse must assess patients' special needs related to their cultural backgrounds.

Look for a minute at our patient, Ms. Williams. Did she behave as you would have in a similar situation? How do you think the characteristics of her culture affected her behavior?

While the terms **cultural sensitivity, cultural awareness,** and **cultural competence** are similar, they have different meanings. *Cultural sensitivity* is knowing politically correct language and not making statements that may offend another person's cultural beliefs. *Cultural awareness* focuses on history and ancestry and emphasizes an appreciation for and attention to arts, music, crafts, celebrations, foods, and traditional clothing. *Cultural competence* includes the skills and knowledge required to provide effective nursing care. In order for you to be culturally competent, you need to:

- Have an awareness of your own culture and not let it have an undue influence on your patient.
- Have specific knowledge about your patient's culture.
- Accept and respect cultural differences.
- Adapt your nursing care (when appropriate) to your patient's culture.

We will discuss more about cultural competence later in the chapter.

Even though you may have knowledge about another culture, there are barriers that can cause you not to appreciate cultural differences, especially ethnocentrism and stereotyping. **Ethnocentrism** is the tendency for human beings to think that their ways of thinking, acting, and believing are the only right, proper, and natural ways. Ethnocentrism perpetrates an attitude that beliefs that differ greatly from your own are strange or bizarre and therefore wrong. Additionally, you must be careful not to **stereotype** your patient. A stereotype is an opinion or belief about a group of people that is ascribed to an individual. For example, the statement "All Chinese people prefer traditional Chinese medicine" is a stereotype. This stereotype is not true. Although many Chinese people may prefer traditional Chinese medicine for some health conditions, not all Chinese people prefer

traditional Chinese medicine. Some Chinese people prefer the Western medicine that is practiced in the United States.

However, you can still make **generalizations** about an ethnic individual without stereotyping. Whereas a generalization, or assumption, may be true for the group, it does not necessarily fit the individual. Therefore, you must seek additional information to determine whether the generalization fits the individual. The challenge is for you to understand the patient's cultural perspective. If you have specific cultural knowledge, you can improve therapeutic interventions by becoming a co-participant with patients and their families. To do this, it is very important that you develop a personal, open style of communication and be receptive to learning from patients from cultures other than your own (Fig. 3.2).

A few additional terms are important for your understanding of culture relate to the socialization process of those who are learning to become a member of a society or group. As people immigrate to a new country they gradually accept the new culture through a learning process. They learn to accept their own beliefs and those of their new country. This is known as **acculturation**. This occurs because the new member must learn enough of the new culture to survive. A step further is when **cultural assimilation** occurs. This happens when the new member takes on the dominant culture's values, beliefs, and practices. This process could potentially be viewed as negative as the person may lose some of his rich heritage to become more like the dominant culture. Imagine for a moment that you have moved to China. At first you eat the food and attempt to understand the language of your new country. Over time, you may learn to cook the food, speak the language, and perhaps blend some of the Chinese beliefs, tradition, and practices with your own. As this practice continues to occur, acculturation is evident. This process may not always be smooth. When one's culture conflicts with the new culture **cultural conflict**

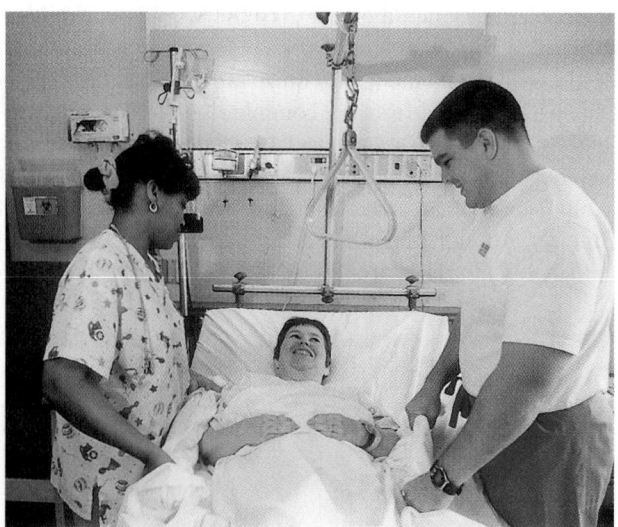

FIGURE 3.2 Health-care workers may come from a variety of cultural backgrounds.

occurs. Worse than that, **cultural shock** happens when values, beliefs, and practices sanctioned by the new culture are very different from the ones of the native culture. Let's look at another example. Chi Ling is a four-year-old boy who is a recent immigrant enrolled in a new school. He is alone and afraid although he is surrounded by other boys and girls his age. It is lunchtime and although his teacher is trying to help him with his food, he starts crying. The fork and spoon are foreign to him. At home he is used to eating his lunch with chopsticks. In addition he does not understand the words spoken to him. Little Chi is experiencing cultural shock.

HEALTH-CARE VALUES, BELIEFS, AND PRACTICES

Cultural values, beliefs, and practices are important in health care. Values can help shape one's beliefs and practices. Do you know what your values are regarding health and illness? A *value* can be defined as a principle or standard that has meaning or worth to an individual.[1] "Cleanliness" is an example of a value. A *belief* is something that an individual accepts as true (e.g., "I believe that germs cause illness and disease"). A *practice* is a set of behaviors that one follows; for example, washing hands before eating. It is important for you to understand the differences between these terms as we will be discussing them as they relate to cultural groups.

In order for you to be able to provide culturally competent care, you need to know how the people you encounter define health and illness. It is generally known that people follow one of the three major health belief systems: scientific (Western medicine or biomedical), spiritual, or holistic. You are already familiar with the scientific health system which dominates health care in Western societies. Belief in supernatural forces dominates the spiritual system, which is considered by many to be an alternative health-care system. (Some experts call this magicoreligious, but this is an offensive term to some religious individuals.) The holistic belief system focuses on the beliefs for the need of balance and harmony of the body and spirit with nature.

Health care typically focuses on the prevention of illness, health promotion, and acute care practices while considering traditional, religious, and biomedical (scientific) beliefs. Additionally, individual responsibility for health, self-medicating practices, views toward mental illness, and the patient's response to pain and the sick role are shaped by one's culture. Most societies combine biomedical health care with traditional, folk, and religious practices, such as praying for good health and wearing charms or amulets to ward off diseases and illnesses. There are many examples of individual and family folklore practices for curing or treating specific illnesses. Think for a minute about such practices that you may perform. What do you do for a fever or a sore throat? Does chicken noodle soup come to mind? Many times folk therapies are handed down from family members and may have their roots in religious beliefs. Examples of folk medicines include covering a boil with axle grease, wearing copper bracelets for arthritic pain, and drinking herbal teas. As an addition to biomedical treatments, many people use complementary therapies, such as acupressure, reflexology, and other traditional therapies specific to the cultural group.

Often folk practices are not harmful and can be added into the patient's plan of care. However, some may conflict with prescription medications, intensify the treatment effect, or cause an overdose. It is essential to inquire about the full range of therapies being used by your patients, such as food items, teas, herbal remedies, nonfood substances, over-the-counter (OTC) medications, medications prescribed by others, and medications borrowed from others. If patients feel that you do not accept their beliefs and practices, they may be less open to sharing information and less compliant with prescribed treatment. You should try to encourage your patients' practices that could be helpful and discourage those that may be harmful. Before encouraging or discouraging such practices, you will need to discuss them with the appropriate health-care team member. Think about Ms. Williams. Does she use any folk practices? How would you address this specific situation?

Before moving on, we need to discuss the subjects of mental illness and cultural responses to pain and the sick role. Mental illness may be seen by many as being unimportant compared with physical illness. Mental illness is culture bound. What may be perceived as a mental illness in one society may not be considered a mental illness in another society. Among some cultures, having a mental illness or an emotional difficulty is considered a disgrace and is taboo. As a result, the family is likely to keep the mentally ill or handicapped person at home as long as they possibly can.

Cultural responses to pain and the sick role can vary among cultures. For example, some individuals are expected to openly express their pain. Others are expected to suffer their pain in silence. For some, the sick role is readily accepted, and any excuse is accepted for not fulfilling daily obligations. Others minimize their illness and make extended efforts to fulfill their obligations.

Nursing Assessment and Strategies

To begin your assessment of your patient's health beliefs, ask the following questions:

- What do you usually do to maintain your health?
- What do you usually do when you are sick?
- What kind of home treatments do you use when you are sick?
- Who is the first person you see when you are sick?
- What do you do when you have pain?
- Do you wear charms or bracelets to ward off illness?
- Do you take herbs or drink special teas when you are sick? What are they?
- Do you practice special rituals or prayers to maintain your health?

Cultural Self-Enrichment Exercise:
HOW YOUR CULTURAL BELIEFS AFFECT YOUR HEALTH BEHAVIORS
- How do you define health for yourself?
- How do you define illness for yourself?
- Identify preventive health-care practices that you use.
- When you see a health-care provider for a minor illness, what do you expect the health-care provider to do for you?
- Identify your self-medicating behaviors.
- What home remedies do you use when you are ill?
- What meaning does pain have to you? What measures do you use when you are in pain?
- What are your personal views toward autopsy, organ donation, organ transplantation, and receiving blood or blood products?

Cultural Self-Assessment Exercise:
WHAT IS YOUR CULTURAL BACKGROUND?
- How do you identify yourself in terms of racial, cultural, or ethnic background? From what country did your ancestors originate? Were your parents from the same or similar ethnic backgrounds?
- What stories do you remember that your parents, grandparents, or other relatives told about relocating in the United States? Do you know why they originally came to America?
- How do these stories compare with those of others from similar backgrounds?
- How do these stories compare with those of others from different backgrounds?

Remember, one's values and beliefs are not better than another's—they are just different.

CHARACTERISTICS OF CULTURAL DIVERSITY

Primary and secondary characteristics of diversity affect how people view their culture. The primary characteristics of diversity include nationality, race, skin color, gender, age, and religious affiliation. Secondary characteristics include socioeconomic status, education, occupation, military experience, political beliefs, length of time away from the country of origin, urban versus rural residence, marital status, parental status, physical characteristics, sexual orientation, and gender issues.

Culturally diverse care needs to take into account seven cultural phenomena that may vary with use but can be seen in all cultural groups: (1) communication, (2) space, (3) time orientation, (4) social organization, (5) environmental control/health beliefs, (6) biological variations, and (7) death and dying issues.

Communication Styles

Communication styles include verbal and nonverbal variations. Verbal communication includes spoken language, dialects, and voice volume. Dialects are variations in grammar, word meanings, and pronunciation of spoken language. Nonverbal communication includes the use and degree of eye contact, the perception of time, and physical closeness when talking with peers and perceived superiors. In some societies, people are expected to maintain eye contact without staring, which denotes that they are listening and can be trusted. However, in other societies, as a sign of respect, people should not maintain eye contact with superiors such as teachers and those in positions of higher status.

Nursing Assessment and Strategies
Ask the following questions:
- By what name do you prefer to be called?
- What language do you speak at home?

Cultural Self-Enrichment Exercise:
COMMUNICATION
- How many languages do you speak? Do you speak a dialect of your dominant language? Does it interfere with communication with your patients?
- Do you speak in a soft, medium, or loud tone of voice? Does this tone change in different situations? How close do you stand when you speak with close friends? Does this distance change when you converse with your teacher, your religious leader, or a politician?
- Identify characteristics from your worldview in terms of being present, past, and future oriented.
- By what name do you prefer to be called? Why? Does this change in different situations?

Be sure to do the following:
- Take cues from the patient for voice volume.
- Be an active listener, and become comfortable with silence.
- Avoid appearing rushed.
- Be formal with greetings until told to do otherwise.
- Take greeting cues from the patient.
- Speak slowly and clearly. Do not speak loudly or with exaggerated mouthing.
- Explain why you are asking specific questions.
- Give reasons for treatments.
- Repeat questions if necessary.
- Provide written instructions in the patient's preferred language.
- Obtain an interpreter if necessary.

Space

Space refers to one's "personal space." Are you aware of your comfort zone? In other words, how close can someone get to you before you feel less safe and secure? Like you, most people have such a comfort space. Personal space tends to be different when speaking with close friends versus strangers. For example, people from the Middle East tend to stand close together when talking, while others from European countries such as Germany require a much larger space. The need for space is important for the patient's privacy, autonomy, security, and self-identity. Understanding your patients' meaning of space can be important when you are trying to assess, treat, and teach them.

Cultural Self-Enrichment Exercise: SPACE

- Are you aware of your comfort zone? Is it different for close friends/family and strangers?
- How does it make you feel when someone violates your comfort zone?
- Do you respect other individuals' space when you communicate with them?
- How do you determine that you are protecting another's personal space?
- How do you feel when someone touches you?
- Do you have a firm handshake?

Nursing Assessment and Strategies

Ask the following questions:

- Are you comfortable?
- Do you have any concerns that you would like to discuss?

Be sure to do the following:

- Make sure you patients are comfortable before you interview them.
- Maintain appropriate physical distance (observe for cues).
- Be aware of cultural differences.
- Be aware of physical objects that may be a barrier to comfort.
- Make sure that the patient's physical environment is arranged to assure safety, security, and familiarity.

Time Orientation

Time orientation (past, present, future) can vary among people from different cultures. The perception of time has two dimensions. The first dimension is related to clock versus social time. For example, some cultures have a flexible orientation to time and events, and appointments take place when the person arrives. An event scheduled for 2 p.m. may not begin until 2:30 or when a majority of the people arrive. For others, time is less flexible, and appointments and social events are expected to start at the agreed-on time. For many, social events may be flexible, whereas medical appointments and business engagements start on time.

The second dimension of time relates to whether the culture is predominantly concerned with the past, present, or future. Past-oriented individuals maintain traditions that were meaningful in the past and may worship ancestors. Present-oriented people accept the day as it comes, with little regard for the past; the future is unpredictable. Future-oriented people anticipate a bigger and better future and place a high value on change. However, some individuals balance all three views—they respect the past, enjoy living in the present, and plan for the future.

Hospitals, clinics, and physicians' offices maintain a tight time schedule. It is therefore important that you understand the patient's time orientation so that you can prepare them for the timing of appointments, tests, and treatments. In addition, it is important that you know their usual routines so that you can incorporate these as much as possible in their daily care.

Cultural Self-Enrichment Exercise: TIME ORIENTATION

- Are you aware of your time orientation (past, present, future)?
- Are you usually on time for appointments?
- Are your biological capacities (e.g., sleep and rest, eating) affected by your body rhythms?
- Do you have routines that you need to follow at certain times of the day?

Nursing Assessment and Strategies

Ask the following question to understand your patients' time orientation:

- Are you normally on time for appointments?
- Are there any routines that you need to follow?
- What time do you usually eat your meals? Take your bath?

Be sure to do the following:

- Have a clock in the patient's room.
- Assess for orientation and reorient to time as needed.
- Prepare patients ahead of time before a procedure or test.
- Give time options when appropriate.

Social Organization

Family organization includes the perceived head of the household, gender roles, and roles of the elderly and extended family members. The head of the household may be patriarchal (male dominated), matriarchal (female dominated), or egalitarian (shared equally between men and women). An awareness of the family dominance pattern is important for determining which family member to speak to when health-care decisions have to be made. Confidentiality issues can complicate this issue. Be sure to follow your institution's policies when communicating with family members. You may need to obtain the patient's permission before planning care with family members.

In some cultures, specific roles are outlined for men and women. Men are expected to protect and provide for the family, manage finances, and deal with the outside world. Women are expected to maintain the home environment, including child care and household tasks. You must accept that not all societies share or even desire an egalitarian family structure.[1]

Roles for the elderly and extended family vary among culturally diverse groups. In some cultures, the elderly are seen as being wise, are deferred to for decision making, and are held in high esteem. Their children are expected to provide for them when they are no longer able to care for themselves. In other cultures, although the elderly may be loved by family members, they may not be given such high regard and may be cared for outside the home when self-care becomes a concern.

The extended family is very important in some groups, and a single household may include several generations living together out of desire rather than out of necessity. The extended family may include both blood-related and non–blood-related individuals who are provided with family status. For others, each generation lives separately and has its own living space.

You can assist your patients with their treatment plans when you have a better understanding of the family dynamics. It is important to know who to include for planning of care, discharge planning, and patient teaching. This will also help the appropriate hospital personnel to assist the patient and family to plan for home care.

Nursing Assessment and Strategies

Ask the following questions:
- Who makes the decisions in your household?
- Who takes care of money matters, does the cooking, or is responsible for child care?
- Who decides when it is time to see a health-care provider?
- Who lives in your household? Are they all blood related?

Be sure to do the following:
- Observe the use of touch between family members.
- Allow family members to decide where they want to stand or sit for comfort.

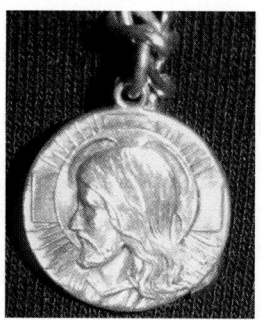

FIGURE 3.3 Religious artifacts are central to many people's health and illness practices.

Environmental Control

Environmental control refers to one's perception of his or her ability to plan for activities that control nature or direct environmental factors. This concept is broader than where an individual lives, but it implies the systems and processes that affect individuals. While systems can include such things as cultural health beliefs and practices, processes can consist of interactions between individuals, families, and groups. Consideration is given to cultural values and beliefs, especially as they are different from those of the dominant health-care view (scientific, biomedical). Distinctions are made between health and illness and what individuals do to promote or maintain health and to prevent and treat illnesses. Not all of your patients will turn to the scientific health-care system or provider. In fact, many individuals try some form of alternative therapy before seeking treatment If you use, for example, herbs or over-the-counter medications, you are doing just that. People also use alternative therapies and religious systems such as prayer in combination with the scientific medical system. Religious beliefs and practices may be very important to patients (Fig. 3.3).

Nursing Assessment and Strategies

Ask the following questions:
- How do you define health? Illness?
- Do you have any special beliefs about health and illness?

Cultural Self-Enrichment Exercise: SOCIAL ORGANIZATION
- Who is considered the head of the household in your family?
- Are there specified gender roles for family members?
- What are the roles of the elderly in your family?
- Do you identify with an extended family? Are they all blood relatives? What roles do they play?
- What kind of decisions do men make and what kind of decisions do women make?

Cultural Self-Enrichment Exercise: ENVIRONMENTAL CONTROL
- How do you define health and illness?
- What are your health and illness values, beliefs, and practices?
- What do you do when you are sick?
- Do you use alternative or religious practices for healing?
- How do you tolerate pain? What do you do for pain?
- How do you handle grief?
- How are your health and illness values, beliefs, and practices different from others in your dominant culture?

- What do you do to keep well?
- When you feel ill, what is the first thing you do to get better?
- How do you deal with pain?
- How do you and your family express grief?
- Are there any cultural beliefs or practices that I need to know about in order to plan your care?

Be sure to do the following:

- Be aware of possible cultural beliefs and practices.
- Never stereotype what you know about different cultures; always ask for specifics.
- Perform a cultural assessment on all of your patients.
- Determine how your patients view health and illness.
- Ask if they have received any treatments for their illness of any kind.
- Ask about religions beliefs and practices.
- Encourage helpful practices and discourage those that are harmful.

Health-Care Practitioners

Health-care practitioner choices are made based on the patient's perceived status and previous use of traditional, religious, and biomedical health-care providers. In Western societies, educated health-care providers are treated with great respect. However, some people prefer traditional healers because they are known to the individual, family, and community.

It is important to respect differences in gender relationships when providing care. Some people may be especially modest because of their religion, seeking out same-gender nurses and physicians for intimate care. Respect these patients' modesty by providing privacy and assigning a same-gender care provider when possible.

Cultural Self-Enrichment Exercise
HEALTH-CARE PRACTITIONERS
- What complementary health-care practitioners have you used? Were they successful?
- Identify complementary health-care practitioners used by your friends. Were they successful?
- When you are ill and need to see a health-care provider, do you prefer a same-gender provider? Why or why not?

Nursing Assessment and Strategies
Ask the following questions of your patients:
- What health-care providers besides physicians and nurses do you see when you are ill?
- Do you object to male or female health-care providers giving physical care to you?

Be sure to do the following:
- Observe for alternative care providers who may visit the patient in the health-care facility.

Biological Variations

Biological variations refer to ways in which people are different from one another physiologically and genetically. These differences can make them more susceptible to certain illnesses and diseases, and may also influence the effectiveness of different medications. Differences in biological variations can include (1) body build and structure, (2) skin color, (3) vital signs, (4) laboratory values, (5) susceptibility to disease, and (6) nutritional variations. Darker skin color can challenge you to be more observant when you are assessing the skin color of your patient. Laboratory test results can also be different in a number of cultures. For example, American Indians and Hispanic Americans may have higher blood glucose levels than whites.

Also included with biological variations are differences in nutritional practices. Nutritional practices are currently being scrutinized in our society. These practices include the meaning of food to individuals, food choices and rituals, food taboos, and how food and food substances are used for health promotion and wellness. Cultural beliefs influence what people eat or avoid. In addition to being important for survival, food offers security and acceptance, plays a significant role in socialization, and can serve as an expression of love.

Culturally congruent dietary counseling, such as changing amounts and preparation practices and including ethnic food choices, can reduce health risks. Whenever possible, you should determine a patient's dietary practices. Culturally diverse patients may refuse to eat on a schedule of American mealtimes or eat American foods. Counseling about food group requirements or dietary restrictions must respect an individual's cultural background. Most cultures have their own nutritional practices for health promotion and disease

Cultural Self-Enrichment Exercise:
BIOLOGICAL VARIATIONS
- Do you know of any diseases or illnesses you are prone to because of your cultural background?
- Are you at ideal body weight for your height?
- What are your activity habits? Do they need to be improved?
- What is the meaning of food in your culture?
- Are there any dietary deficiencies or food limitations for you?
- What cultural or ethnic foods do you prepare at home?
- When you eat out for lunch or dinner, what are your favorite ethnic foods? Which ethnic foods do you not like? Why?
- What dietary practices do you engage in when you are ill?
- What kinds of foods do you eat to stay healthy?
- In your culture or personal belief system, are there any foods that are restricted or taboo?

prevention. For many, a balance of different types of foods is important for maintaining health and preventing illness. Common folk practices recommend specific foods during illness and for prevention of illness or disease. Therefore, a thorough history and assessment of dietary practices can be an important diagnostic tool to guide health promotion.

Nursing Assessment and Strategies

Ask the following questions of your patients:
- Are you at risk for any diseases or genetic disorders related to your cultural background?
- Are you satisfied with your weight?
- Are you active? What is you normal exercise pattern?
- Do you protect your eyes and skin from the sun? From possible injuries?
- Do you have any drug or food allergies?
- Has anyone in your family had any major illnesses?
- What do you eat to stay healthy?
- What do you eat when you are ill?
- Are there certain foods that you do not eat? Why?
- Do certain foods cause you to become ill? What are they?
- Who prepares the food in your household?
- Who purchases the food in your household?

Be sure to do the following:
- Teach about any biological variations that may pertain to your patient.
- Determine usual eating patterns and teach good nutrition habits, taking into account patient preferences. Refer to the dietician if appropriate.

Death and Dying and End of Life Issues

Death rituals of cultural groups are the least likely to change over time. To avoid cultural taboos, you must become knowledgeable about rituals surrounding death and bereavement. For some, the body should be buried whole. Therefore, an amputated limb may be buried in a future grave site, and organ donation would probably not be acceptable. Cremation may be preferred for some, whereas for others it is taboo and burial is the preferred practice. Views on autopsy vary accordingly. Some cultural groups have elaborate ceremonies that last for days in commemoration of the dead. To some individuals these rituals appear to be a celebration, and in a sense they are a celebration of the person's life rather than a mourning of the person's death. If you are uncertain, find out from the family if there is anything that the health-care team can do to facilitate cultural practices.

The expression of grief in response to death varies within and among cultural and ethnic groups. For example, in some cultures, loved ones are expected to suffer the grief of death in silence, with little display of emotion. In other cultures, loved ones are expected to demonstrate an elaborate display of emotions to show that they cared for the individual. These variations in the grieving process may cause confusion if you perceive some individuals as overreacting and others as not caring. You must accept that there are culturally diverse behaviors associated with the grieving process. Bereavement support strategies include being physically present, encouraging reality orientation, openly acknowledging the family's right to grieve as they need to, assisting the family to express their feelings, encouraging interpersonal relationships, promoting interest in a new life, and making referrals to other staff and spiritual leaders as appropriate.

At times you may also be somewhat involved with other end-of-life decisions. Some of these may include advanced directives, resuscitation status, and organ transplantation.

Cultural Self-Enrichment Exercise:
DEATH AND DYING
- What are the usual burial practices in your family?
- What is expected of family members and friends after a loved one dies?
- How is grief expressed in your family? Are there different expectations for men and women?
- Are any specific rituals associated with death?
- Do you believe in organ transplantations?
- Do you have advance directives?

Nursing Assessment and Strategies

Ask the following questions of your patients:
- What are the usual burial practices in your family?
- Do you believe in autopsy?

Be sure to do the following:
- Observe expressions of grief. Support the family in their expression of grief.
- Observe for differences in the expression of grief among family members.
- Offer to obtain a religious counselor/spiritual leader if the family wishes.

ETHNIC AND CULTURAL GROUPS

Cultural Groups in the United States

This chapter describes selected attributes of some of the cultural groups in the United States. These groups include European Americans (white), Spanish/Hispanics/Latinos, African Americans (black), American Indians/Alaskan Native, Arab Americans, and Asian/Pacific Islander Americans. The groups described here by no means represent all the cultural groups in North America; they do, however, represent the largest population percentages in the United States. As of the 2000 census, the federal government initiated new terminology for classifying people of diverse racial and ethnicity and it is used in this chapter.

Attributes presented for each group include communication styles, space, time orientation, social organization, environmental control, biological variation, health-care beliefs, traditional health-care practitioners, and death and dying issues. Traditional health-care practitioners are those practitioners from the patient's native culture, such as shamans, herbalists, and other traditional healers. Racial and ethnic biological variations, susceptibility to disease, and genetic diseases are covered to a greater extent elsewhere in this textbook. (See Box 3.2 Ethical Consideration—Cultural Stereotyping and Box 3.3 Gerontological Issues.)

Cultural Self-Assessment Exercise
- Identify your primary and secondary cultural characteristics. How do they affect your world-view?
- Share these views with others in your class.

European Americans
European American is the term used to describe people living in the United States whose heritage is from the countries of England, Scotland, Wales, Ireland, Norway, Switzerland, France, Sweden, the Netherlands, Belgium, and other northern European countries. European American groups include the white ethnic groups. Many of the descendants of these original European immigrants practice the unique attributes of the subcultures from which they originate. There is much diversity in the primary and secondary characteristics of diversity within this cultural group.

Many European Americans maintain the value of individualism over group norms and are activity oriented. Most European Americans practice Western medicine that uses high technology and emphasizes scientific discovery.[1] (See Box 3.4 Cultural Consideration.)

Spanish/Hispanics/Latinos
The term *Spanish/Hispanics/Latinos* is used to describe people whose cultural heritage has a strong Spanish influence. However, many people in this group prefer to identify themselves as Chicano or with terms that provide a country of origin, such as *Mexican, Peruvian, Puerto Rican,* and *Cuban.*[1] The population breakdown of Spanish/Hispanics/Latinos populations in the United States are Mexican Americans (67%), Puerto Ricans (9%), Central and South Americans (14%), Cubans (4%), and other groups, including Caribbean (7%).[2] Hispanics immigrate from any number of Central and South American countries, the Caribbean,

---

Box 3.2

Ethical Consideration—Cultural Stereotyping

Sharon, an experienced Licensed Practical Nurse, was on duty on the labor and delivery unit when Ruth and her husband Aaron arrived. Ruth was flushed and distressed and obviously in labor. Aaron was bending over his wife, attempting to coach her breathing, and trying to keep calm. The child was very early, only 30 weeks' gestation. Aaron was wearing a yarmulke, so Sharon assumed they were Jewish.

The usual expectation in labor and delivery is the arrival of a beautiful healthy child. Ruth and Aaron were no exception. Unfortunately, their infant son was stillborn due to gross prematurity and a "true knot" in the cord that had denied oxygen to the baby during the latter stages of the labor and delivery. After the delivery, Ruth was transferred to the medical-surgical unit for postpartum care, a practice commonly followed when stillbirths occur.

Sharon decided that she could make the situation a little easier for the couple by arranging care of the stillborn child. She expected that the parents would want help with contacting a funeral home and other details. She had done this many times before and it seemed to help the grieving parents when she took some of the burden from them by initiating the process.

Sharon told Ruth she had made some preliminary phone calls that would start the process of a funeral and accompanying activities. Ruth looked distressed, and Sharon misinterpreted this expression as her unfamiliarity with the funeral home that would be handling the arrangements.

Sharon tried to reassure Ruth, stating that she had been present at many funerals of children who had died either before, during, or after birth and the funeral home she had called was reputable and respectful. Sharon recounted her personal experience of these events and stated that sometimes the ritual of the wake, the burial, and the gathering afterward were therapeutic, bringing some closure. Aaron, who was visiting at the time, called Sharon out of the room and indicated his very strong displeasure that Sharon had begun arrangements. He explained rather tersely that he had contacted his rabbi, who as *mara d'atra* [halakhic authority] held the position of authority in Aaron and Ruth's community. The rabbi had made a *p'sak* [ruling/decision]. This *p'sak* meant that although the child was both premature and dead at birth, it was to be treated as a fetus. As such, it would be the family that would conduct the funeral, and there would be no ceremony attached. Aaron turned his back on Sharon and went back into the room.

Sharon completed her shift without additional communication with the couple, and Ruth was discharged before Sharon returned the next day. Sharon was plagued with a feeling that she had made a major error in caring for this woman and had failed to meet her emotional needs.

It is evident from this case that several major ethical principles were either ignored or transgressed. What do you think they were and why? (Suggested answers at end of chapter.)

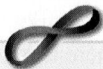

Box 3.3

Gerontological Issues

Aging, Ethnicity, Health, and Illness

Compared with white or European American older adults, ethnic minorities are more likely to:
- Live in poverty
- Have a shorter life expectancy
- Experience debilitating disease processes or functional disability at a higher rate and at an earlier age
- Have difficulty accessing health-care services

　　Remember that older adults need to be assessed within their personal cultural context. Avoid generalizing cultural practices to individuals or families without first assessing whether this practice or belief is true for them. For example, it would be wrong to assume that an older Mexican American woman who lives with her extended family will get the family's support for assistance with bathing and other activities of daily living. If an older Chinese woman uses herbs and folk treatments for common complaints, it does not mean that she will not use the services, treatments, or medications of Western medicine. Always assess individual preferences.

and other Spanish-speaking countries. Thus, there is much diversity in the Spanish/Hispanics/Latino population in the United States.

　　Some Spanish/Hispanics/Latinos speak only Spanish, only English, or both Spanish and English, while others speak neither Spanish nor English but rather an Indian dialect. The spoken language depends on individual circumstances and the length of time spent in the United States. Spanish is the second most common spoken language in the United States.

　　Spanish/Hispanics/Latinos compose approximately 13% of the U.S. population; they recently became the majority minority population. They live in all 50 states with more than 90% living in and around cities. Four of every five Spanish/Hispanics/Latinos are born and raised in the United States. Many of these individuals have come from poverty; for them money has little value. They sacrifice for their basic needs (Figs. 3.4 and 3.5).

　　The majority of Spanish/Hispanics/Latinos practice adaptations from the Roman Catholic religion. Their close relationship with God makes it acceptable for people to experience visions and dreams in which God or the saints speak directly to them. Thus, health-care providers must be careful not to attribute these culture-bound visions to hallucinations that indicate a need for psychiatric services.[1] (See Box 3.4, Cultural Consideration.)

African Americans/Blacks

African Americans/blacks are the second largest ethnic group in the United States and represent more than 100 racial strains.[1] They make up 12.3% of the population.[3]

(Text continued on page 45)

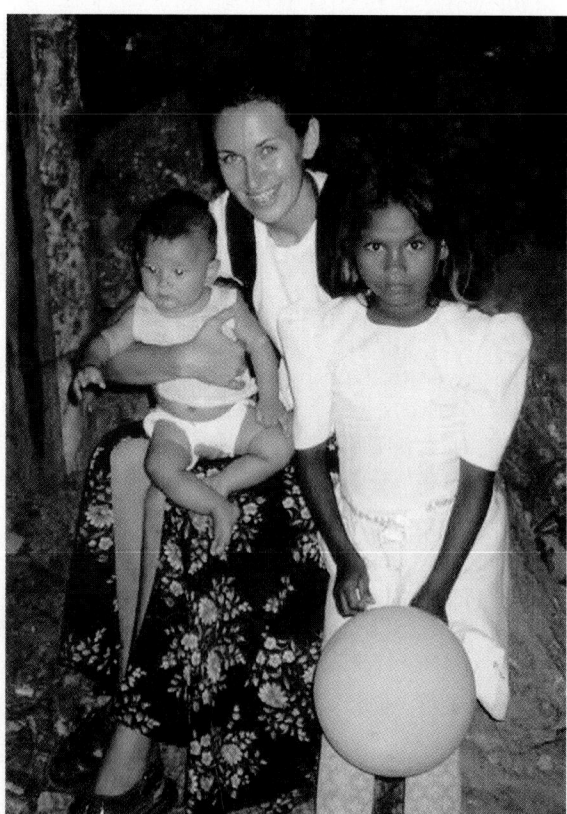

FIGURE 3.4 Honduras couple waits to get married until they can afford a celebration (at 100 years young).

FIGURE 3.5 Many mission workers have helped with health-care needs in Central and South American countries.

Box 3.4

Cultural Consideration*[1,5,6]

	European Americans (White)	Spanish/Hispanics/Latinos	African Americans (Black)	American Indian/Alaskan Natives	Arab Americans	Asian/Pacific Islanders
Communication	Primary language is usually English; often speak own national language. Eye contact should be maintained, without staring. Loud voice volume is the norm.	Primary language either English, Spanish, or Portuguese (many dialects). Dramatic body language. Some believe direct eye contact can cause illness ("evil eye").	Primary language is usually English. May speak "black English" occasionally depending on the situation. Usually loud voice volume. Nonverbal communication important; direct eye contact may be interpreted as aggression.	English, tribal languages. Silence. Talking loudly may be considered rude. Use body language. Avoid eye contact.	Primary language is Arabic. Most speak some English. May use spirited, loud voice. May be reluctant to disclose personal information. Maintain intense eye contact.	English (may prefer national language and specific to each country); many dialects. Loud talking is considered rude. Silence is acceptable. Avoid eye contact. Avoid use of "no."
Space	Depends on area; tend to avoid physical closeness. Handshake proper.	Value physical closeness and touching.	Close personal space. Touch frequently with friends, less so with strangers. Touching another's hair considered improper.	Space very important; has no boundaries. Touch is not acceptable from strangers. Pointing and direct eye contact may be considered rude.	Stand very close when talking. Touch only between same gender.	Avoid physical closeness and touching.
Time Orientation	Future over present	Present	Present over future	Usually present	Present or future	Present
Social Organization	Nuclear family basic, extended family important. Man dominant figure. Judeo-Christian religions.	Nuclear family basic, extended family highly valued. Man is decision maker; woman is homemaker.	Many female single-parent families. Large, extended families important.	Extended family basic unit. Very family oriented. Elders honored.	Patriarchal household, with well-defined gender roles. Elders respected and cared for by family.	High value on immediate and extended family. Hierarchical family structure.

(Continued on following page)

Box 3.4 (Continued)

Cultural Consideration*[1,5,6]

	European Americans (White)	Spanish/ Hispanics/ Latinos	African Americans (Black)	American Indian/ Alaskan Natives	Arab Americans	Asian/Pacific Islanders
	Community social organizations important. Many concerned with status.	Catholicism.	Strong social and church affiliations Protestant (often Baptist).	Strong community affiliations. Sacred myths and legends.	Extended family important; may live in close proximity. May be Christian, Jewish, or Muslim.	Family honor and loyalty honored. Tradition important. Male has power; woman is obedient. High value placed on children and education. Christianity, Buddhism, Taoism, and Islamic religions
Environmental Control/Health Beliefs	Rely primarily on modern health-care system. Value individual responsibility for health. Believe human can control nature. Have strong belief and value in technology. Most use folk remedies or OTCs before seeing a health-care provider. Use of prayers and religious symbols for good health. Have controlled expression of pain but need little encouragement for pain relief.	Traditional health and illness beliefs. Folk medicine traditions. Health beliefs are strongly affected by religion, believing in God's will. May have shrines or statues in the home to pray for good health. Theory of hot and cold foods used for health maintenance and treatment of disease. Expressive with pain.	Traditional health and illness beliefs. Folk medicine tradition. May believe that serious illness sent from God. Use prayers for prevention and health recovery. Pain is seen as a sign of illness. Sick role not seen as a burden. Folk healers. A respected elderly female community member commonly	Traditional health and illness beliefs. Folk medicine traditions. Promote harmony with nature. Inanimate objects ward off evil spirits. Elderly may request same-gender direct-care provider. Pain is something to be endured. Sick role not usually supported. Traditional healers: shamans, medicine man, diviners, crystal gazers.	Focus on acute care over prevention. Illness may be considered punishment for sins. May pray five times a day for health. Acceptable to purchase organs for transplantation. Sick role supported.	Traditional health and illness beliefs. Traditional medicine traditions. Good health is a gift from ancestors. Imbalances in the yin and yang cause illness. Believe blood is the source of life and is not replenished. Amulets worn to ward off disease. Traditional healers: doctors, herbalists, acupuncturists who use such therapies as acupuncture, acumassage, coining, and cupping.

	European Americans (White)	Spanish/Hispanics/Latinos	African Americans (Black)	American Indian/Alaskan Natives	Arab Americans	Asian/Pacific Islanders
	Sick role not well accepted except with a major illness. Traditional healers: Western-educated health-care providers; recent trend to use complementary therapists.	Easily enter the sick role. Traditional healers: curandero, espiritisa, patera, senora.	sought for initial health care. Use spiritualists, voodoo priest or priestess, or root doctor.			
Biological Variations	Nutritional preferences include meats (especially red) and carbohydrates. Diets tend to be high in fat and sodium; Eating and drinking may be social rituals. Culture stresses thinness to be attractive. Susceptibility: heart disease, breast cancer, diabetes mellitus, thalassemia, Tay-Sachs disease (Eastern European Jewish).	Nutritional preferences include spicy and fried foods, beans, and rice. Important for food to be served warm. Many subscribe to the hot and cold theory (e.g., illness caused when body is exposed to imbalance of hot/cold substances). Food choices vary by specific country.	Nutritional preferences include fried foods, barbecued foods, greens, legumes. Diet commonly high in fat and sodium. Food selections may vary according to socioeconomic status and rural versus urban residence. Being overweight is seen as positive. Food is seen as a symbol of health and wealth.	Nutritional preferences vary greatly depending on location and tribe. Nontraditional diets tend to be high in fat and commonly lack fruits and vegetables. Herbs used to cleanse the body of evil spirits and poison. Susceptibility: heart disease, alcoholism, liver disease, diabetes mellitus, tuberculosis, arthritis, glaucoma.	Nutritional preferences include fresh meats and vegetables; may avoid pork and alcohol (Islam). High risk for diabetes, hypertension, hypercholesterolemia. Less likely than general population to smoke, drink alcohol, or use illicit drugs.	Nutritional preferences include raw fish and rice. Foods are balanced between the yin and yang. Diet is high in salt. Food is fundamental form of socialization Susceptibility: lactose intolerance, thalassemia, liver and stomach cancer, hypertension, coccidioidomycosis.

(Continued on following page)

Box 3.4 (Continued)

Cultural Consideration*[1,5,6]

	European Americans (White)	Spanish/ Hispanics/ Latinos	African Americans (Black)	American Indian/ Alaskan Natives	Arab Americans	Asian/Pacific Islanders
			Susceptibility: keloid formation, lactose intolerance, sickle cell anemia, glucose-6-phosphate dehydrogenase deficiency, thalassemia, sarcoidosis, hypertension, coccidioidomycosis, esophageal and stomach cancers.			
		Susceptibility: lactose intolerance, diabetes mellitus, parasites, coccidiodomycosis, gout.				
Death and Dying Issues	Autopsy and burial or cremation usually connected with religious practices or individual decisions. Have varied expressions of grief. Men are expected to be in more control of grief than women.	Burial is the usual practice, rarely cremation; many resist autopsy, the body should be buried whole. May have elaborate ceremonial burial. Women very expressive with grief; men are expected to maintain control.	Death does not end connection between people; body is kept intact after death; prefer no autopsy. Relatives may communicate with the dead person. Offer eulogy at burial with religious songs. Usually prefer burial. Express grief openly.	Believe body should go into the after-life whole. Some engage in a cleansing ceremony after touching a dead body. Tribal laws may dictate cremation versus burial. Openly express grief.	Believe death is God's will. At time of death, bed should face the holy city of Mecca (for Muslims). May perform ritual washing of the body after death. Cremation or autopsy not acceptable. May weep with grief, but limited.	Autopsy not understood by many. Cremation acceptable, but burial also common. Extended grieving time (7 to 30 days) for the more traditional. Expression of grief is highly varied between men and women and among specific countries.

*While many other cultural groups are represented in the United States, the most common are presented here.

Although African Americans/blacks live in all 50 states, more than half live in the South. It is important to understand that not all people with black skin identify themselves as African American. Many black-skinned people from the Caribbean prefer terms more specific to their identity, such as *Haitian, Jamaican,* or *West Indian.*

African Americans/blacks have been called by many names. Their ancient African name is Nehesu or Nubian. During slavery days in America, they were called *Negro,* a Spanish-Portuguese word meaning "black." After emancipation in 1863, they were called *colored,* a term adopted by the First Colored Men's Convention in the United States in 1831. The United States Bureau of the Census adopted the word *Negro* in 1880. During the civil rights movements in the 1960s, the term *black* was used to signify a philosophy of life instead of color. In the 1970s, these ethnic peoples referred to themselves as African Americans because they were proud of both their African and American heritages. In 1988, the term *African American* was widely adopted in the United States by individuals whose ancestry originated from Africa. These terms continue to cause confusion when people attempt to use the "politically correct" term for this group in the United States. Additionally, titles such as the National Black Nurses Association and the National Association for the Advancement of Colored People (NAACP) still exist.[1]

African Americans/blacks are underrepresented in colleges and universities, managerial and administrative positions, and the health-care professions. They are overrepresented in high-risk, hazardous occupations such as the steel and tire industries, construction industries, and high-pollution factories (See Box 3.4 Cultural Consideration.)

CRITICAL THINKING

■ Now that you have learned more about the black culture, let's look at Ms. Williams again. Review Box 3.4 Cultural Consideration and answer the following questions:
1. What does your interaction with Ms. Williams tell you about her time orientation?
2. What is evident about her social organization?
3. What biological variations may Ms. Williams demonstrate that are likely due to her culture?

American Indians/Alaskan Natives

There are more than 400 American Indian/Alaskan Native tribes in the United States, totaling 0.8% of the population.[3] Although there are similarities among Native Americans, each tribe has its own unique perspective on health and illness. Many traditional American Indians/Alaskan Natives live on reservations; others live in urban areas and practice few of their traditions. Many American Indians/Alaskan Natives have a strong belief that illness is caused by an imbalance with nature and the universe. Tribal identity is maintained through powwows, ceremonial events, and arts and crafts that are taught to children at a young age. Communicating with nature is important for maintaining life forces.[1] American Indians/Alaskan Natives are the original inhabitants of North America.

American Indians/Alaskan Natives are underrepresented in all the health professions. They are consistently identified as the most underrepresented minority group in institutions of higher learning.[4] (See Box 3.4 Cultural Consideration.)

Arab Americans

Arab Americans are a large and diverse population, with over 3,000,000 in the United States. Some common bonds include the Arabic language and the Islamic religion. Arab Americans include people from Morocco, Algeria, Tunisia, Libya, Sudan, and Egypt and the western Asian countries of Lebanon, occupied Palestine, Syria, Jordan, Iraq, Iran, Kuwait, Bahrain, Qatar, United Arab Emirates, Saudi Arabia, Oman, and Yemen. Many early Arab immigrants were Christians from Lebanon and Syria.

Although many Arab Americans favor professional occupations, many are underemployed, have their own businesses, and work in a variety of other occupations. Arab Americans, whether born in the United States or in Arab countries, are more educated than the average American. They are more likely to be in managerial and professional specialty occupations than any other ethnic group in America. However, a significant number of primarily foreign-born Arab Americans are unemployed and live in poverty.

Asian Americans/Pacific Islanders

This large group is far from homogeneous. The term *Asian,* as used in most references, includes 32 different groups. These groups include Asians, Pacific Islanders, Indochinese, and other Asian groups. Asians include people from Korea, Japan, and 54 ethnic groups from China. Pacific Islanders include Hawaiians, Polynesians, Filipinos, Malaysians, and Guamanians. Indochinese populations include Cambodian, Vietnamese, Hmong, and Laotian. Other Asian groups include Asian Indian, Pakistani, and Thai.

Although it is difficult to determine exact numbers of Asians from specific countries because of the method of keeping population statistics, they are a significant and fast-growing population in the United States. It is important for many Asian patients to "save face." Individual shame is shared with the family and community. Most Asians see the nurse as an authority figure. Although known by different names, most Asian cultures practice the *yin* and *yang* balance of forces for illness prevention and maintaining health. Yin is considered female and represents cold and weakness. Yang is considered male and represents strength and warmth. Foods and all forces are classified as yin or yang and must be balanced or illness occurs. Yin and yang forces are major components of traditional Chinese medicine, which includes acupressure, acumassage, and cupping. (See Box 3.4 Cultural Consideration.)

CULTURALLY COMPETENT CARE

The American Nurses' Association supports the need for nurses to understand cultural diversity and to become culturally competent. However, there is no real agreement as to how your knowledge, skills, and attitudes will best help these diverse populations. You certainly cannot achieve cultural competence overnight; it is a developmental process. Each time you care for a patient from a different culture, you learn more, become more aware and sensitive to individual needs, and move toward becoming culturally competent.

There are a number of models and theories that describe cultural competence. In addition, you will find that there a number of good resource books and websites that will assist you on this journey.

The following strategies for culturally competent care may be helpful:

- Consider each of your clients as unique, influenced but not defined by their culture.
- Know your own cultural values, beliefs, and practices and appreciate how they may be different from those of others.
- Never let your own biases about people and groups stand in the way of good care.
- Learn as much as you can about cultural groups in your community.
- Make an effort to include beliefs and practices from other cultures into your care when appropriate.
- Try to encourage helpful cultural practices and discourage harmful ones.
- Be aware of how you communicate with others; be aware of verbal and nonverbal patterns.
- Respect your patients regardless of their cultural background.
- Learn from your mistakes.

The list does not include everything you can do. Can you think of other strategies?

CRITICAL THINKING

The Lopez Family

■ Jose, age 23, and his wife, Louisa, age 19, immigrated to the United States 3 years ago from Mexico. They have two children, Maria, 3 years old, and Jesus, 6 months old. The young couple brings the children to the emergency room for the treatment of ear infections. Jose informs you that Maria is complaining of a sore throat and ear pain and Jesus is "fussy" and not eating. He states that he has been to his *curandero*,

but neither child has improved. You also notice that the children are dressed in heavy clothing, although it is quite warm outside. When you question the parents, Louisa responds that they are "cold."

Jesus is admitted to the hospital for dehydration. As you are admitting the infant to your unit, you are aware that Jose is answering all of your questions and making decisions for Jesus' care. He states that they will all need to spend the night with Jesus. Jose further adds that Jesus needs more clothes on and that the temperature in the room needs to be increased. The parents refuse the warmed bottle of formula for Jesus but ask for it to be chilled. Louisa sits in the corner of the room chanting, crying, and rubbing some beads.

1. What nonverbal communication characteristics do these parents display that are common among people of Spanish descent?
2. Why do you think the children are dressed inappropriately for the weather?
3. Do Jose's demands mean that he is uncooperative and trying to control the care of his son?
4. Why do you think Jose refused his son's warm bottle?
5. What is the significance of Louisa's behavior?
6. What might you do to improve Jesus' care?
7. How will you handle the father's request for the entire family to stay in your patient's room?
8. How can you become more culturally competent in this situation?

Suggested answers at end of chapter.

Home Health Hints

- The effect of the patient's cultural beliefs and practices related to health care are more evident when care is provided in the home. The nurse must adapt care to the patient's environment rather than the patient adapting to the nurse's hospital environment. The nurse is a guest in the patient's house.
- When scheduling a home visit, it is important to find out the primary language spoken in the home. It is also helpful to carry a translation book when the language is known. If necessary, arrange to have an interpreter, either a family member or co-worker, available to ensure understanding of what is discussed.
- Be aware of the cultural significance of family hierarchy. If possible, avoid having children translate for parents.

REFLECTIONS ON CASE STUDY

After learning more about culture, how do you think the characteristics of Ms. Williams's culture affected her behavior? At her age, it is evident that she has learned many of her beliefs and practices about health and illness from others. While many of her behaviors can be explained by fear and denial, it is probable that other things are going on in this situation. Ms. Williams may feel more comfortable with people of her own culture, at least when it comes to asking for health information. Like a number of other cultures, your patient may not trust biomedical or Western medicine treatments. She may be more comfortable with the practices and healers that she knows better. Can you think of other explanations?

Rarely do practicing nurses have the luxury to assess each patient comprehensively on a first encounter. The essentials for culturally competent care are obtained as needed. As you meet patients from other cultures, continue to learn about theses new cultures. Astute observations, an openness to diversity, and a willingness to learn from patients are what you need for effective cross-cultural competence in clinical practice. Through these avenues, you can provide culturally competent nursing care. Cultural competence is not a luxury; it is a necessity.

Remember that it is important that you acknowledge that there are similarities within a group. This does not mean that ALL of the people in the group have all of those characteristics. You must see each of your patients as being unique. In summary, let's take a trip to BALI:

Be aware of your own cultural heritage.

Appreciate that your patient is unique; influenced, but not defined by his culture.

Learn about your patient's cultural group.

Incorporate your patient's cultural values, beliefs, and practices into their plan of care.

REVIEW QUESTIONS

1. A nurse who assumes all patients have the same beliefs as his or her own culture is exhibiting
   a. Cultural stereotyping.
   b. Ethnocentrism.
   c. Cultural sensitivity.
   d. Cultural dominance.

2. A 12-year-old Mexican child needs an appendectomy. His parents bring in the priest from their church to pray over the child. The prayers are continuing when it is time to take the child to surgery. How should the nurse respond?
   a. Gently tell the parents that they must stop praying so the child can be taken to surgery.
   b. Give the parents and priest as much time as they need for prayers prior to surgery.
   c. Tell the parents that the child could die from a ruptured appendix if surgery is delayed.
   d. Permit the parents and priest to stay and pray as the child goes into surgery.

3. An Osage American Indian woman is slow at giving responses and does not maintain eye contact with you when you are doing her intake interview. Which of the following interpretations of her behavior is most likely accurate?
   a. Direct eye contact may be interpreted as rude in her culture.
   b. She does not want to answer personal questions.
   c. She does not understand you.
   d. She does not want to talk with a nurse and prefers a physician.

4. An Arab American man is refusing his dinner tray, which consists of potatoes with cheese, a slice of ham, and green beans. What knowledge should guide the nurse's data collection related to this incident?
   a. Arabs do not like foods from different sources on the same plate.
   b. Some Arabs do not eat dairy products.
   c. Islamic Arabs may not eat pork.
   d. Arabs generally do not eat vegetables.

5. A Puerto Rican man has been admitted for reconstructive orthopedic surgery on his knee. His wife brings jars of special blends of spices that he wants to put on his food because the hospital food is too bland. He is on a general diet. What action should you take?
   a. Allow him to use them.
   b. Carefully explain that family cannot bring food items to the hospital.
   c. Have the dietitian speak with the family.
   d. Report the situation to the physician.

References

1. Purnell, L, and Paulanka, B (eds.): Transcultural health care: A culturally competent approach. F.A. Davis, Philadelphia, 2003.
2. United States Bureau of Census (2003): The Hispanic Population in the United States: March 2002. Available at http://www.census.gov/prod/2003pubs/p20-545.pdf.
3. United States Bureau of Census (2003): U.S. census data. Available at http://www.census.gov.
4. Preito, D: American Indians in medicine: The need for Indian healers. Academic Med 64:388, 1989.
5. Giger, J. N., ad Davidhizar, R: Transcultural Nursing: Assessment and Intervention, ed. 3. Mosby, St. Louis, 1999.
6. Spector, RE: Cultural Diversity in Health and Illness, ed. 6. Upper Saddle River, NJ, Prentice Hall, 2004.

ETHICAL CONSIDERATION DISCUSSION

It is evident from this story that the traditional American or Christian conception of the rituals associated with the death of a child may not be held by other cultures, including this Jewish patient and her husband. Upon reflection, Sharon realized that she had not respected this couple's **autonomy,** or even provided an environment that would foster the **creation of autonomy**. She had failed to **minimize harm,** failed to produce the most **beneficial outcome** for Aaron and Ruth, and had not familiarized herself with the wishes of the couple.

Sharon did not serve her clients' needs first. She should have determined what Ruth and Aaron needed at that sensitive time. Instead, she assumed she knew what was required and subsequently made poor choices for her clients. Were her clients harmed? If Sharon had known that there were significant religious protocols to be observed in this situation, would she have gone ahead and made phone calls, in essence, to interfere with the designated roles of the parents? Sharon did cause some anxiety in this case. Sharon could have been most helpful by asking respectful questions about what she could do to assist the couple during this sad time. Aaron and Ruth may indeed have asked Sharon to be involved in the preparations and funeral.

Instead of holding assumptions and applying our own vision of what a client may need, nurses need to assess a family's values, gather appropriate information about their culture, and find what the role expectations are in each situation. There should be an atmosphere of mutual respect and open communication. Patients' values and preferences cannot be assumed, even when nurses can correctly identify the culture of the family. Cultural stereotyping is a mistake that is easy to make. However, if we approach our clients with an open and nonjudgmental attitude, we will be able to gather the data that is essential to providing culturally competent nursing care.

SUGGESTED ANSWERS TO

CRITICAL THINKING

■ Ms. Williams

1. Ms. Williams's time orientation is the present. She is not only concerned with the future effects of her uncontrolled diabetes.
2. Family is very important. She prays for healing.
3. We do not know Ms. William's weight, but overweight is seen as positive, and excess weight is a risk factor for diabetes and hypertension.

■ The Lopez Family

1. Jose's behavior indicates that he is the primary decision maker and in charge of this situation. Louisa's crying is normal. She is most likely praying.
2. This may relate to the couple's beliefs in the hot and cold theory.
3. His role as father may dictate that he should maintain control. He probably does not mean to be uncooperative.
4. Again, this may be related to hot and cold beliefs about treatment of diseases.
5. Culture-bound role does not dictate that she assume control of the situation. She is upset and praying.
6. Attempt to incorporate the family's cultural beliefs and practices when possible.
7. Explain that it would not be good for Maria to remain in the hospital, because she will be at greater risk for exposure to infection. Ask if there are other relatives who can care for Maria. Find out if the parents can divide their time with their son.
8. Be aware of your own cultural beliefs, appreciate you patient's culture, learn more about the Lopez family's culture (ask questions), and include their beliefs and practices when possible. Explain when other practices cannot be followed. Ask for alternatives.

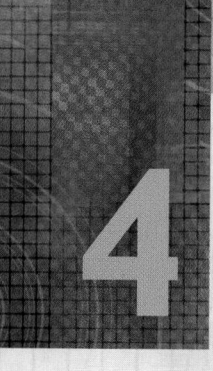

4

Alternative and Complementary Therapies

LYNN KEEGAN

KEY TERMS

acupuncture (ak-yoo-PUNGK-chur)
allopathic (AL-oh-PATH-ik)
Ayurvedic (AY-YUR-VAY-dik)
chiropractic (ky-roh-PRAK-tik)
homeopathy (HO-mee-AH-pa-thee)
naturopathy (NAY-chur-AH-pa-thee)
osteopathic (AHS-tee-ah-PATH-ik)

QUESTIONS TO GUIDE YOUR READING

1. What is the difference between an alternative and complementary therapy?

2. What are some systems of health care that have contributed to the development of new therapies?

3. How can the different types of therapies be classified?

4. What are some safety issues in alternative and complementary therapies?

5. What is the role of the licensed practical nurse/licensed vocational nurse (LPN/LVN) in assisting a patient with alternative and complementary therapies?

Health care in the 21st century requires that nurses recognize the shift of thinking toward the incorporation of alternative and complementary approaches to care. Nurses at all levels and in every area of practice are answering the call to use new methods to care for the ill and to enhance the health of those who are well.

Holistic nursing was a precursor to many of the now popular alternative and complementary therapies. It was introduced in the 1970s and has been growing ever since. Holistic nursing is simply defined as caring for the whole person—body, mind, and spirit—in a constantly changing environment.

ALTERNATIVE OR COMPLEMENTARY: WHAT'S THE DIFFERENCE?

The words *alternative* and *complementary* are sometimes used interchangeably, but they are not the same. *Alternative* therapy, sometimes called "unconventional" therapy, refers to a therapy used instead of conventional or mainstream therapy. An example is using **acupuncture** instead of analgesics. *Complementary therapy* refers to a therapy used in addition to a conventional therapy. For example, a nurse might suggest guided imagery, music, and relaxation techniques for pain control in addition to prescribed drug therapy.

A good all-around website for alternative and complementary medicine is http://www.healthy.net. To learn about holistic nursing and complementary therapies, visit the American Holistic Nurses Association at http://www.ahna.org.

INTRODUCTION OF NEW SYSTEMS INTO TRADITIONAL AMERICAN HEALTH CARE

There are many new and different philosophies within the scope of expanded medical and nursing practice. These systems reflect cultures and attitudes in healing that range from East to West and from ancient to modern.

In the United States, the primary system of medicine is just called *medicine,* although some people refer to it as **allopathic** medicine. A number of other schools of thought and philosophies are also being increasingly used. The most frequently seen new systems include **Ayurvedic,** Chinese, **chiropractic,** naturopathic, American Indian, and **osteopathic** medicine. Each philosophical system can stand alone or, as in most instances in the United States, be used in combination with other systems. Most of these recently introduced systems use alternative and complementary therapies.

Allopathic/Western Medicine

we do this

The most common name for allopathic medicine is *Western medicine.* Other commonly used terms for Western medicine are *conventional medicine* and *mainstream medicine.* Many people have not heard the term *allopathic* because most doctors and nurses do not refer to themselves or their practice by this name. Practitioners of other systems of medicine more often use the term when referring to what most of us consider mainstream medicine. Allopathy is a method of treating disease with remedies that produce effects different from those caused by the disease itself. For example, when a patient has a bacterial infection, a Western medical practitioner prescribes an antibiotic to eliminate the invading pathogen.

Practitioners of Western medicine are medical doctors, nurses, and allied health personnel. This system of medicine uses scientific data to determine the validity of a diagnosis and the effectiveness of treatment. It is evidence-based medicine. This means that peer-reviewed medical literature is very important. In scientific investigations, results can be verified and reproduced through various types of studies and statistical analyses. Practitioners use a variety of therapies, including drugs, surgery, and radiation therapy. Western medicine practitioners have made most of the significant advances and developments in modern medicine.

For further information see the American Medical Association site at http://www.ama-assn.org.

Ayurvedic Medicine

Ayurveda is the ancient Hindu system of medicine, which originated in India. Its main goals are to maintain the health of healthy people and cure the illnesses of sick people. Ayurveda maintains that illness is the result of falling out of balance with nature. Diagnosis is based on three metabolic body types call *doshas.* An Ayurvedic doctor determines which dosha type is most appropriate for the patient: vata, pitta, or kapha. Treatment usually involves prescribing a diet, herbal remedies, breath work, physical exercise, yoga, meditation, massage, and a rejuvenation or detoxification program.

Ayurveda is rapidly becoming more popular in America. The books and videos of Deepak Chopra are examples of this increasingly popular system of therapy. An introduction to Ayurveda can be found at http://www.ayurveda.org.

Traditional Chinese Medicine

Traditional Chinese medicine is thousands of years old and involves such techniques and practices as acupuncture, acupressure, herbs, massage, and qi gong. The diagnosis and treatment of disturbances of qi (pronounced "chee")—or vital energy—is a distinctive characteristic of Chinese medicine.

Acupuncturists, one segment of traditional Chinese medicine practitioners, claim to be able to tell much about a

---

acupuncture: acus—needle + punctura—puncture
allopathic: allos—other + pathic—disease or suffering
Ayurvedic: ayu—life + veda—knowledge or science
chiropractic: cheir—hand + pracktos—to do
osteopathic: osteo—bone + pathy—disease

patient's state of health by checking pulses, looking at the color of the tongue, checking facial color, assessing voice and smell, and asking a variety of questions. To treat patients, acupuncturists insert one or more needles along the meridians (pathways) where qi flows (Fig. 4.1). Many acupuncturists also prescribe herbal remedies as well.

Chiropractic Medicine

Daniel David Palmer founded chiropractic therapy in 1895. Chiropractic medicine holds that illness is a result of nerve dysfunction. The main treatment modality of chiropractors is manual adjustment and manipulation of the vertebral column and the extremities. They use direct hand contact and mechanical and electrical treatment methods to manipulate joints. The goal is to remove the interference with nerve function so the body can heal itself. Chiropractors do not perform surgery, nor do they prescribe drugs. See the American Chiropractic Association site at http://www.amerchiro.org.

Homeopathic Medicine

Homeopathy was developed by Samuel Hahnemann in Germany in the early 19th century. Homeopathy is based on Hahnemann's principle that "like cures like," meaning that tiny doses of a substance that create the symptoms of disease in a healthy person will relieve those symptoms in a sick person.

Although there are schools and courses to train homeopaths, no diploma or certificate from any school or program is a license to practice homeopathy in the United States. Medical doctors and doctors of osteopathy are granted certificates of competency to practice homeopathy. Other health-care practitioners may be allowed to use homeopathy within the scope of their state licenses.

See The National Center for Homeopathy website at http://www.homeopathic.org. This site has a research section with annotated listings from the medical literature discussing the value of homeopathy. In addition, there is a good review of licensing laws regarding homeopathy.

Naturopathic Medicine

Naturopathy primarily uses natural therapies such as nutrition, botanical medicine (herbs), hydrotherapy (water-based therapy), counseling, physical medicine, and homeopathy to treat disease, promote healing, and prevent illness.

homeopathy: homeo—like + pathos—disease

naturopathy: naturo—nature + pathy—disease

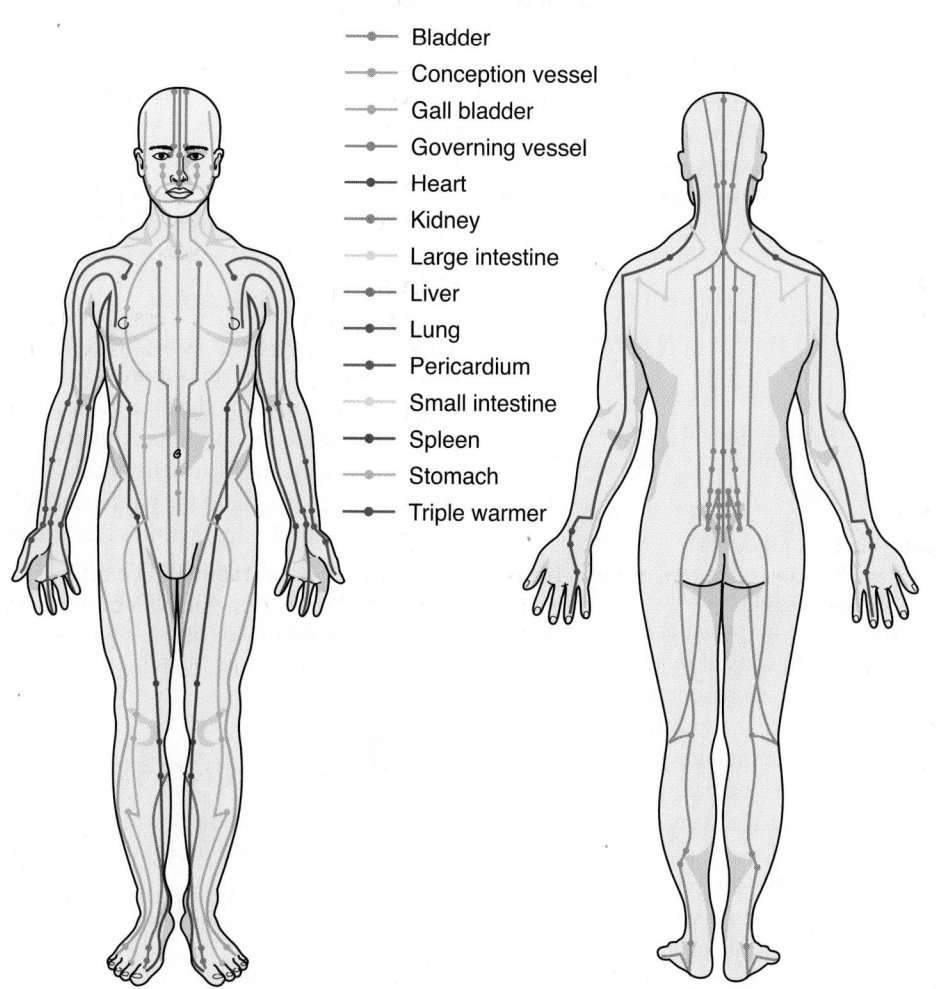

Bladder
Conception vessel
Gall bladder
Governing vessel
Heart
Kidney
Large intestine
Liver
Lung
Pericardium
Small intestine
Spleen
Stomach
Triple warmer

FIGURE 4.1 Qi meridians are used in the Chinese medicine techniques of acupressure and acupuncture.

Naturopathic physicians have a doctor of naturopathy (ND) degree and can be licensed in 11 states. There are three schools of naturopathic medicine in the United States. For more information about naturopathy, visit http://www.natur-opathic.org.

American Indian Medicine

American Indian medical practices vary from tribe to tribe. In general, American Indian medicine is a community-based system with rituals and practices such as the sweat lodge, herbal remedies, the medicine wheel, the sacred hoop, the "sing," and shamanistic healing. For example, an ill person may be placed in a small, enclosed sweat lodge while singing or chanting is done outside the lodge. It is believed that toxic substances are drawn out in the sweat of the person inside the lodge. After the ceremony, the ill person may be placed on a cot outside and be prayed over. You can learn more about American Indian Medicine at the Association of American Indian Physicians' website at http://www.aaip.com.

Osteopathic Medicine

Osteopathic medicine was founded in the United States in 1874 by Andrew Taylor Still, a frontier physician who was dissatisfied with the state of medicine at that time. This practice of medicine emphasizes the interrelationship of the body's nerves, muscles, bones, and organs. The osteo-pathic philosophy involves treating the whole person, recog-nizes the body's ability to heal itself, and stresses the importance of diet, exercise, and fitness with a focus on pre-vention. For more information about osteopathy, visit the American Osteopathic Association website at http://www.aoa-net.org.

ALTERNATIVE AND COMPLEMENTARY THERAPIES

Discussion of all alternative and complementary therapies is beyond the scope of this text. Table 4.1 is a summary of the most commonly used therapies.

Herbal Therapy

Many people use herbs for healing. However, when doing so, the patient should only take herbs under the supervision of a health-care provider. Herbs can aid in healing, but they also can harm. Some of the more common herbs are described in Table 4.2. Figure 4.2 shows echinacea, an herb commonly prepared for use as an immune system booster.

It is important to note that herbal remedies are not foods. They have potent medicinal effects and can interact with prescribed medications and even surgery. This can be problematic, both because herbs are readily available in health food stores and drugstores and because many patients do not tell their doctors or nurses about their herb use. Be sure to assess patients' use of herbs and supplements, and educate them about the need to inform primary care providers when using herbs.

TABLE 4.1 CATEGORIES AND TYPES OF ALTERNATIVE AND COMPLEMENTARY THERAPIES

Category of Therapy	Types of Individual Therapies
Herbal medicine and nutritional supplements	Herbal medicine
	Nutrition and special diet thera-pies
	Nutritional supplements
Mind-body therapies	Art therapy
	Music/sound therapies
	Guided imagery
	Hypnosis and hypnotherapy
	Meditation and relaxation
Posture and mobility therapies	Movement therapies
	Tai chi and qi gong
	Yoga
Touch therapies and bodywork	Massage and related massage therapies
	Acupressure
Energetic therapies	Biofeedback
	Healing touch
	Magnet therapy
	Polarity therapy
	Reiki
	Spiritual healing
	Therapeutic touch
Miscellaneous therapies	Aquatherapy/hydrotherapy
	Aromatherapy
	Chanting
	Chelation therapy
	Colon therapy
	Kinesiology
	Light therapy
	Pet therapy

Relaxation Therapies

Progressive Muscle Relaxation

Progressive muscle relaxation is a simple technique that anyone can learn. It is the process of alternately tensing and relaxing muscle groups. Often this process is performed in a systematic manner, such as from head to toe. The purpose of the technique is to help the participant identify subtle levels of mental and physical tension that accompany mental and emotional stress. When our conscious awareness of the ten-sions increases, we can learn to relax and thus reduce the effects of stress and tension. The idea is to become aware of the ability to fine tune the relaxation response.

LEARNING TIP

Try using progressive muscle relaxation the next time you are anxious during a nursing examination.

Guided Imagery

Guided imagery is another example of a complementary therapy that many nurses use. Guided imagery involves

TABLE 4.2 COMMON HERBS AND THEIR INTENDED PROPERTIES AND USES

Herb	Purported properties/uses
Aloe vera	Soothing agent, used for skin lesions; toxin absorber
Bee pollen	Increases energy, stamina, and strength
Capsaicin	For tenderness and pain of osteoarthritis, fibromyalgia, diabetic neuropathy, and shingles
Chamomile	For anxiety, stomach distress, and infant colic
Echinacea	Antiviral; used for colds, flu, and other infections
Feverfew	Anti-inflammatory; used for migraine headaches and as an appetite stimulant; promotes menstruation, eliminates worms, suppresses fever
Ginger	For nausea and vomiting, hypertension, and high cholesterol
Ginkgo	May improve memory and help cognitive function in Alzheimer's disease
Kava	For anxiety, insomnia, low energy, muscle tension
St. John's wort	For mild to moderate depression; viral infections, including human immunodeficiency virus (HIV); and herpes

using mental images to promote physical healing or changes in attitudes or behavior (Box 4.1 Guided Imagery). Practitioners may lead patients through visualization exercises or offer instruction in using imagery as a self-help tool. Guided imagery is often used to alleviate stress and to treat stress-related conditions such as insomnia and high blood pressure. People with cancer, acquired immunodeficiency syndrome (AIDS), chronic fatigue syndrome, and other disorders can use specific images to boost the immune system. Guided imagery is often an added layer of therapy for someone who has learned the progressive relaxation skill discussed previously.

A common guided imagery technique begins with a general relaxation process. For those new to the process, it is good to begin with the progressive muscle relaxation as explained above. Guided imagery works best when all the senses are used. This exercise is very basic but gives an idea of how the technique works. When used for healing, many more steps are involved. For additional information read journal articles, books, and Internet sites. It is important to note that with this and any of the alternative and complementary therapies, you must have some training and skill before using the technique with patients. Find more on guided imagery at http://www.healthy.net; type "guided imagery" into the search window.

LEARNING TIP

When you are stumped on a test question, close your eyes and imagine yourself asking the question of your favorite instructor. Imagine what his or her answer would be.

Box 4.1

Guided Imagery

Assist your patient to progress through the following steps:

- Assume a comfortable position in a quiet environment.
- Close your eyes and keep them closed until the exercise is completed.
- Breathe in and out deeply to the count of four, repeating this step four times.
- When relaxed, think of a favorite peaceful place and prepare to take an imaginary journey there.
- Picture what this place looks like and how comfortable you feel being there.
- Listen to all the sounds; feel the gentle, clean air; and smell the pleasant aromas.
- Continue to breathe deeply, and appreciate the feeling of being in this special place.
- Feel the sense of deep relaxation and peace of this place.
- As you continue to breathe deeply, slowly and gently bring your consciousness back to the setting in this room.
- Slowly and gently open your eyes, stretch, and think about how relaxed you feel.

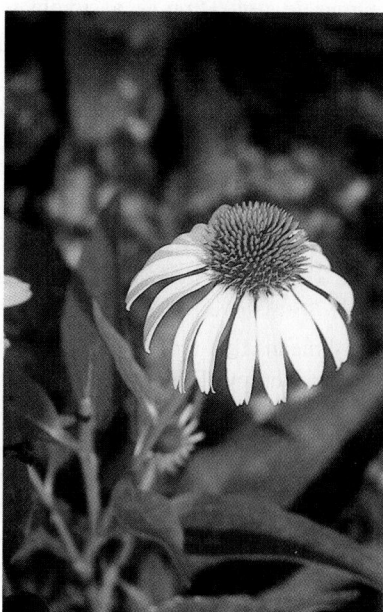

FIGURE 4.2 Echinacea is a commonly used herb for colds and flu.

Biofeedback

Biofeedback might be considered the third tier of learning of progressive relaxation. It is a technique used especially for stress-related conditions such as asthma, migraines, insomnia, and high blood pressure. Biofeedback is a way of monitoring and controlling tiny metabolic changes in one's body with the aid of sensitive machines that provide feedback. (See Box 4.2 Patient Perspective.)

Massage Therapy

Massage is the use of touch to achieve therapeutic results, and may include pressure, friction, and kneading of the body. Massage may be used to relax muscles, reduce anxiety, increase circulation, and reduce pain.

Massage also provides a caring form of touch. In the past, a back massage was a nightly routine for hospitalized patients, helping them relax for sleep. Sadly, today, patients are often not touched except for technical procedures.

You can learn basic massage techniques in nursing school. Or you may also choose to obtain formal massage therapy education in order to practice more advanced techniques.

SAFETY TIP

Do not use firm massage on a patient taking anticoagulant agents or a patient with a low platelet level. Tissue injury could cause bleeding.

Aquatherapy

If you have ever sat in a warm tub, you already know how good it can feel when your muscles are tired or aching, and how mentally relaxing it can be. People who suffer from arthritis or other chronic pain understand how warm water can ease their discomfort. Relaxing in water feels good for three reasons: warmth, water movement causing massage, and buoyancy.

Long before there were analgesics, the human body relied on its own naturally occurring, internally generated, painkilling chemicals called endorphins. Through research we now know that warm water stimulates the release of endorphins. They are released in response to both acute and chronic pain. The most recognized methods to release endogenous (naturally occurring) endorphins are physical exercise, acupuncture, and electrical nerve stimulation. Any type of skin stimulation, even the mechanical impact of water, can cause the release of endorphins. However, pain reduction is only part of the healing process. Ultimately, blood flow is what brings nutrients to damaged cells and facilitates healing. When the body is immersed in warm water, the blood vessels nearest the skin relax, allowing more blood to flow. The results are fatigue relief, faster tissue repair, and relief of pain.

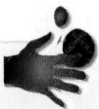

Box 4.2

Patient Perspective

Polly

I am scared to death of flying. The minute I get on an airplane, I feel jittery, my heart races, and I can't calm down until we are safely back on the ground. Several years ago, I decided to try biofeedback therapy to overcome this fear.

My therapist was wonderful. She immediately put me at ease, and assured me I wasn't a crazy person to be afraid to fly. She then put a temperature sensor on my finger (my hands were usually pretty cold). In her calm, soft voice, she guided me through a relaxation exercise, using imagery and progressive muscle relaxation. By the time we were finished, my hands would be several degrees warmer than when we had started! This showed my vessels were dilating, a sign that my sympathetic nervous system was slowing down its activity. So, I felt calmer. The sensor gave me feedback that told me when my relaxation was working well. We did this every week for a couple of months, until I got really good at warming my hands and relaxing.

Now when I fly, I close my eyes, imagine a peaceful scene and use my relaxation techniques. I still don't like it much, but at least I feel a bit calmer!

Heat and Cold Application

Local application of heat or cold provides additional methods of skin stimulation. A warm compress can soothe sore muscles and dilate vessels in a defined area, bringing healing circulation as well as endorphin release. Ice or a cold gel pack can help numb an area. It also causes overdilated vessels to constrict, yielding relief from pain and throbbing of overstimulated nerve endings. Ice can be helpful on an acute injury and for some types of headaches. Check institution policy before applying heat or cold—a physician's order may be required.

SAFETY AND EFFECTIVENESS OF ALTERNATIVE THERAPIES

Safety generally means that the benefits outweigh the risks of a treatment or therapy. If your patient is interested in using an alternative or complementary therapy, first counsel the patient to talk with the primary care provider. The patient also should ask the practitioner of the therapy about its safety and effectiveness. Patients should tell their primary care providers and alternative practitioners about all therapies they are receiving because this information may be used to consider the safety of their entire treatment plan.

The patient should be as informed as possible and continue gathering information even after a practitioner has

Box 4.3

Questions Patients Should Ask Before Starting an Alternative or Complementary Therapy

1. What will this therapy do for me?
2. What are the advantages of this therapy?
3. What are the disadvantages?
4. What are the side effects?
5. What risks are associated with this therapy?
6. How much will it cost? Will my insurance cover the cost?
7. How long will it take? How many treatments will be necessary?
8. How will it interact with my other therapies and medications?
9. What research has been done on this therapy?

been selected. You can find information about specific therapy or therapies in journal articles and books. (See Box 4.3 Questions Patients Should Ask Before Starting an Alternative or Complementary Therapy.)

 ROLE OF THE LPN/LVN

Patients may ask you about the use of an alternative or a complementary therapy. Because the safety and effectiveness of many therapies is still unknown, advising patients presents a challenge. The following steps are suggestions for helping to advise patients regarding the use of these kinds of therapies:

1. Take a close look at the background, qualifications, and competence of the proposed practitioner. Check credentials with a state or local regulatory agency with authority over the area of practice they seek. Are they licensed or certified? By whom?
2. Visit the practitioner's office, clinic, or hospital. Evaluate the conditions of the setting.
3. Talk with others who have used this practitioner.
4. Consider the costs. Are the treatments covered by insurance, or is it direct pay?
5. Discuss use of an alternative or complementary therapy with their primary care provider.

 NURSING APPLICATIONS

There are ways to gain confidence with alternative and complementary therapies:

1. Begin by trying one or two of these therapies yourself. Start by choosing a basic therapy such as massage, music, or guided imagery. Follow the guidelines listed in Box 4.3 (Questions Patients Should Ask Before Starting an Alterna-

tive or Complementary Therapy) to make sure it is a safe strategy. Not only will you encounter the benefits firsthand, but you will also come away with a better understanding of what patients experience.
2. Ask your patients if they use any alternative or complementary therapies and what their responses to them have been. Try to eliminate any preconceived notions you might have. Your patients will feel more comfortable mentioning them to you if they feel you understand the treatment and why they decided to use it.
3. If you decide to become involved, get adequate instruction in the therapies before you administer them. Many universities and agencies offer continuing education courses on these therapies, and some nursing schools incorporate alternative and complementary therapies in their skills courses.

If you wish to incorporate alternative and complementary therapies into your practice, be sure to check your state's nurse practice act for any regulations. Discuss them with the patient and his or her primary care provider before using them. If you work for a hospital or other health care institution, also check institutional policy.

As the public understands more about alternative and complementary therapies, you can expect to see even greater demand for these treatments. Nurses have been in the forefront of developing the holistic philosophy that has now become an accepted standard of care.

CRITICAL THINKING

Mr. Jones

■ Mr. Jones asks you whether he should stop his chemotherapy and try magnet therapy for his prostate cancer. How do you respond?

Suggested answers at end of chapter.

 ### Home Health Hints

- When taking a health history, ask the patient or caregiver about the use of complementary or alternative therapies because these may influence the effects or side effects of some prescription medications.
- Be mindful of the importance of complementary and alternative therapies to the patient's health-care belief system.
- Consider the alternative practitioner as part of the patient's health care team.
- Discuss concerns regarding potential interactions with the registered nurse or physician.

SUGGESTED ANSWERS TO

CRITICAL THINKING

■ *Mr. Jones*

As with all medical treatments, it is important to support the established therapy the physician has prescribed. Therefore a good response might be the following:

"Mr. Jones, chemotherapy is an established medical treatment for your condition. There is a lot of evidence for its effectiveness in the medical literature. If you want to supplement your therapy, there may be some other treatments you can add. I suggest that you discuss your feelings about seeking some additional treatments with your doctor."

REVIEW QUESTIONS

1. Which of the following statements best defines a complementary therapy?
   a. An alternative treatment that is used in place of a conventional treatment
   b. A treatment that is often dangerous and should be avoided
   c. A treatment that can be used in addition to a conventional treatment
   d. A treatment that is used after conventional treatments have failed

2. Which of the following therapies is most likely to use research-based interventions?
   a. Naturopathy
   b. Osteopathy
   c. Allopathy
   d. Homeopathy

3. A patient with high blood pressure tells his nurse he has been taking a ginger supplement in addition to his prescribed medications at home. What is the best response by the nurse?
   a. "Nonprescription supplements can interact with prescription medications. You should not take it any longer."
   b. "Ginger can be effective for hypertension. Be sure to monitor your blood pressure while you are taking it."
   c. "Ginger is a safe supplement because it is a food. It should not interact with your medications."
   d. "You should check with your physician to make sure the ginger doesn't interact with your other medications before you continue to take it."

4. Which of the following complementary therapies are considered relaxation therapies? Select all that apply.
   a. Progressive muscle relaxation
   b. Tai chi
   c. Biofeedback
   d. Homeopathic therapies
   e. Guided imagery

5. Which of the following statements best describes the most important role of the LPN in alternative and complementary therapies?
   a. The LPN should become familiar with and practice at least one alternative or complementary therapy.
   b. The LPN should become adept at collecting and reporting data related to patients' use of alternative and complementary therapies.
   c. The LPN should discourage use of alternative and complementary therapies because they can interact negatively with conventional therapies.
   d. The LPN does not need to become involved in alternative and complementary therapies.

Unit I Bibliography

1. Colbath, JD, and Prawlucki, PM (eds): Holistic nursing care (collection of 12 articles). Nurs Clin North Am. 36;, 2001.
2. Dossey, B, Keegan, L, and Guzzetta, C. Holistic Nursing: A Handbook for Practice, ed 4, Jones and Bartlett, Sudbury, MA, 2005.
3. Keegan, L: Healing with Alternative and Complementary Therapies. Delmar, Albany, NY, 2001.
4. Keegan, L, and Keegan, G. T. Healing Waters. New York, Berkley, 1998.
5. Pettigrew, A, King, M, McGee, K, Rudolph, C: Complementary therapy use by women's health clinic clients. Alternative Ther 10: 2004.
6. Tedesco, P, and Cicchetti, J: Like cures like: Homeopathy. Am J Nurs,101: 2001.
7. Waddell, DL, Hummel, ME, and Sumners, AD: Three herbs you should get to know. Am J Nurs 101: 2001.
8. Walker, MJ, and Walker, JD: Healing Massage: A simple approach. Albany, NY, Thomson Delmar Learning, 2003.
9. Wenk-Sormaz, H: Meditation can reduce habitual responding. Alternative Ther. 11: 2005.

unit TWO

UNDERSTANDING HEALTH AND ILLNESS

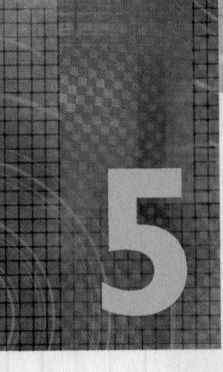

5

Nursing Care of Patients with Fluid, Electrolyte, and Acid-Base Imbalances

BRUCE K. WILSON

KEY WORDS

acidosis (ass-i-DOH-sis)
alkalosis (al-ka-LOH-sis)
anion (AN-eye-on)
antidiuretic (AN-ti-DYE-yoo-RET-ik)
cation (KAT-eye-on)
dehydration (DEE-high-DRAY-shun)
diffusion (di-FEW-zhun)
dysrhythmia (dis-RITH-mee-yah)
edema (e-DEE-ma)
electrolytes (ee-LEK-troh-lites)
extracellular (EX-trah-SELL-yoo-lar)
filtration (fill-TRAY-shun)
hydrostatic (HIGH-droh-STAT-ik)
hypercalcemia (HIGH-per-kal-SEE-mee-ah)
hyperkalemia (HIGH-per-kal-EE-mee-ah)
hypermagnesemia (HIGH-per-MAG-nuh-ZEE-mee-ah)
hypernatremia (HIGH-per-nuh-TREE-mee-ah)
hypertonic (HIGH-per-TAHN-ik)
hyperventilation (HIGH-per-VEN-ti-LAY-shun)
hypervolemia (HIGH-per-voh-LEE-mee-ah)
hypocalcemia (HIGH-poh-kal-SEE-mee-ah)
hypokalemia (HIGH-poh-kuh-LEE-mee-ah)
hypomagnesemia (HIGH-poh-MAG-nuh-ZEE-mee-ah)
hyponatremia (HIGH-poh-nuh-TREE-mee-ah)
hypotonic (HIGH-poh-TAHN-ik)
hypovolemia (HIGH-poh-voh-LEE-mee-ah)
interstitial (IN-ter-STISH-uhl)
intracellular (IN-trah-SELL-yoo-ler)
intracranial (IN-trah-KRAY-nee-uhl)
intravascular (IN-trah-VAS-kyoo-lar)
isotonic (EYE-so-TAHN-ik)
osmosis (ahs-MOH-sis)
osteoporosis (AHS-tee-oh-por-OH-sis)
semipermeable (SEM-ee-PER-mee-uh-bull)
transcellular (trans-SELL-yoo-lar)

QUESTIONS TO GUIDE YOUR READING

1. What are the purposes of fluids and electrolytes in the body?

2. What are the signs and symptoms of common fluid imbalances?

3. Which patients are at the highest risk for dehydration and fluid excess?

4. What data should you collect in patients with fluid and electrolyte imbalances?

5. What are therapeutic interventions for patients with fluid and electrolyte disturbances?

6. What are education needs of patients with fluid imbalances?

7. What are common causes, signs and symptoms, and treatments for sodium, potassium, calcium, and magnesium imbalances?

8. Which foods have high sodium, potassium, and calcium content?

9. What are common causes of acidosis and alkalosis?

10. How do arterial blood gases change for each type of acid-base imbalance?

The body undergoes continuous dynamic change. The proper amount of fluid is needed to support these changes and to transport building and waste materials. Approximately 60% of a young adult's body weight is water. Elderly people are less than 50% water, and infants are between 70% and 80% water. Women have less body water because they have more fat than men. Fat cells do not contain water.

In addition to water, body fluids also contain solid substances that dissolve, called solutes. Some solutes are **electrolytes** and some are nonelectrolytes. Electrolytes are chemicals that can conduct electricity when dissolved in water. Examples of electrolytes are sodium, potassium, calcium, magnesium, acids, and bases; these are discussed later in this chapter. Nonelectrolytes do not conduct electricity; for example, glucose and urea.

FLUID BALANCE

Fluids are located both inside the cells (**intracellular** fluid [ICF]) and outside the cells (**extracellular** fluid [ECF]). ECF can be further divided into three types: **interstitial** fluid, **intravascular** fluid, and **transcellular** fluid (Fig 5.1).

Interstitial fluid is the water that surrounds the body's cells and includes lymph. Fluids and electrolytes move between the interstitial fluid and the intravascular fluid, which is the plasma of the blood. Transcellular fluids are those in specific compartments of the body, such as cerebrospinal fluid, digestive juices, and synovial fluid in joints.

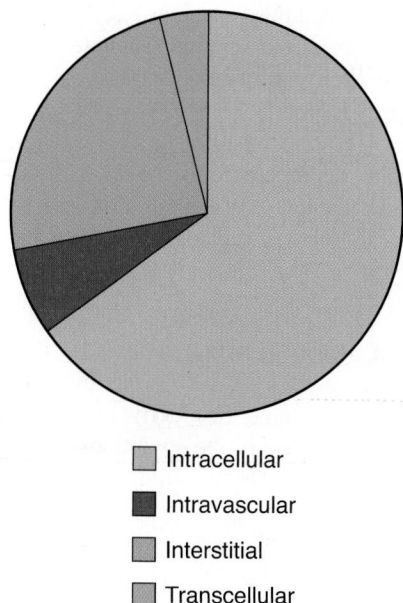

☐ Intracellular
■ Intravascular
☐ Interstitial
☐ Transcellular

FIGURE 5.1 Normal distribution of total body water.

intracellular: intra—within + cellular—cell
extracellular: extra—outside of + cellular—cell
interstitial: inter—between + stitial—tissue
intravascular: intra—within + vascular—blood vessel
transcellular: trans—across + cellular—cell
electrolyte: electro—electricity + lyte—dissolve

Control of Fluid Balance

The primary control of water in the body is through pressure sensors in the vascular system, which stimulate or inhibit the release of **antidiuretic** hormone (ADH) from the pituitary gland. A diuretic is a substance that causes the kidneys to excrete more fluid. ADH works in just the opposite way. ADH causes the kidneys to retain fluid. If fluid pressures within the vascular system decrease, more ADH is released and water is retained. If fluid pressures increase, less ADH is released and the kidneys eliminate more water.

Movement of Fluids and Electrolytes in the Body

Fluids and electrolytes move in the body by active and passive transport systems. Active transport depends on the presence of adequate cellular adenosine triphosphate for energy. The most common examples of active transport are the sodium-potassium pumps. These pumps, located in the cell membranes, cause sodium to move out of the cells and potassium to move into the cells when needed.

In passive transport, no energy is expended specifically to move the substances. General body movements aid passive transport. The three passive transport systems are **diffusion, filtration,** and **osmosis.**

Diffusion is a process in which the substance moves from an area of higher concentration to an area of lower concentration. If you pour cream into a cup of coffee, the movement of the molecules causes the cream to eventually be dispersed throughout the beverage. If you stir the coffee, this process occurs at a faster rate. Body movement assists passive transport, like stirring the coffee. It causes the diffusion to occur at a faster rate.

Filtration is the movement of both water and smaller molecules through a **semipermeable** membrane. The semipermeable membrane works like a screen that keeps the larger substances on one side and permits only the smaller molecules to filter to the other side of the membrane. Filtration is promoted by **hydrostatic** pressure differences between areas.

Hydrostatic pressure is the force that water exerts; sometimes called water pushing pressure. In the body, filtration is important for the movement of water, nutrients, and waste products in the capillaries. The capillaries serve as semipermeable membranes allowing water and smaller substances to move from the vascular system to the interstitial fluid, but larger molecules and red blood cells remain inside the capillary walls.

Osmosis is the movement of water from an area of lower substance concentration to an area of higher concen-

antidiuretic: anti—against + diuretic—urination
diffusion: diffuse—spread, scattered
filtration: filter—strain through
osmosis: osmo—impulse + osis—condition
semipermeable: semi—half or part of + permeable—passing through
hydrostatic: hydro—water + static—standing

tration. The substances exert an osmotic pressure sometimes called water pulling pressure. The term *osmolarity* refers to the concentration of the substances in body fluids. The normal osmolarity of the blood is between 270 and 300 milliosmoles per liter (mOsm/L).

Another term for osmolarity is *tonicity.* Fluids or solutions can be classified as **isotonic**, **hypotonic,** or **hypertonic.** A fluid that has the same osmolarity as the blood is called isotonic. For example, a 0.9% saline solution (normal saline) is isotonic to the blood and is often used as a solution for intravenous (IV) therapy. A solution that has a lower osmolarity than blood is called hypotonic. When a hypotonic solution is given to a patient, the water leaves the blood and other ECF areas and enters the cells. Hypertonic solutions exert greater osmotic pressure than blood. When a hypertonic solution is given to a patient, water leaves the cells and enters the bloodstream and other ECF spaces.

Fluid Gains and Fluid Losses

Water is very important to the body for cellular metabolism, blood volume, body temperature regulation, and solute transport. Although people can survive without food for several weeks, they can survive only a few days without water.

Water is gained and lost from the body every day. In addition to liquid intake, some fluid is obtained from solid foods. When too much fluid is lost, the brain's thirst mechanism tells the individual that more fluid intake is needed. Older adults are more prone to fluid deficits because they have a diminished thirst reflex and their kidneys do not function as effectively. An adult loses as much as 2500 mL of sensible and insensible fluid each day. Sensible losses are those of which the person is aware, such as urination. Insensible losses may occur without the person recognizing the loss. Perspiration and water lost through respiration and feces are examples of insensible losses.

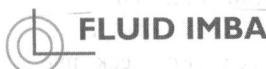 FLUID IMBALANCES

Fluid imbalances are common in all clinical settings. Elderly people are at the highest risk for life-threatening complications that can result from either fluid deficit, more commonly called **dehydration,** or fluid excess. Infants are at risk for fluid deficit because they take in and excrete a large proportion of their total body water each day.

Dehydration

Although there are several types of dehydration, only the most common type is discussed in this chapter. Dehydration occurs when there is not enough fluid in the body, especially in the blood (intravascular area).

Pathophysiology and Etiology

The most common form of dehydration results from loss of fluid from the body, resulting in decreased blood volume.

---

isotonic: iso—equal + tonic—strength

hypotonic: hypo—less than + tonic—strength

hypertonic: hyper—more than + tonic—strength

dehydration: de—down + hydration—water

Box 5.1

Common Causes of Dehydration

Long-term nothing by mouth (NPO) status
Hemorrhage
Profuse diaphoresis (sweating)
Diuretic therapy
Diarrhea
Vomiting
Gastrointestinal suction
Draining fistulas
Draining abscesses
Severely draining wounds
Systemic infection
Fever
Frequent enemas
Ileostomy
Cecostomy
Diabetes insipidus

This decrease is referred to as **hypovolemia.** Hypovolemia occurs when the patient is hemorrhaging or when fluids from other parts of the body are lost. For example, severe vomiting and diarrhea, severely draining wounds, and profuse diaphoresis (sweating) can cause dehydration.

Hypovolemia may also occur when fluid from the intravascular space moves into the interstitial fluid space. This process is called third spacing. Examples of conditions in which third spacing is common include burns, liver cirrhosis, and extensive trauma. See Box 5.1 for Common Causes of Dehydration.

As described previously in this chapter, the body initially attempts to compensate for fluid loss by a number of mechanisms. If the cause of dehydration is not resolved or the patient is not able to replace the fluid, a state of dehydration occurs.

Prevention

You can help prevent dehydration by identifying patients who have the highest risk for developing this condition. High-risk patients include the elderly, infants, children, and any patient who has one of the conditions listed in Box 5.1 (Common Causes of Dehydration). Also see Box 5.2, Gerontological Issues.

Adequate hydration is another important intervention to help prevent dehydration. You should encourage patients to drink adequate fluids. Adults need 30 mL/kg /day of fluids. If a patient is unable to take enough fluid by mouth, alternate routes may be necessary.

Signs and Symptoms

Thirst is the initial symptom experienced by otherwise healthy adults in response to hypovolemia. As the percentage of water in the blood goes down, the percentage of other substances goes up, resulting in the thirst response. As the

---

hypovolemia: hypo—less than + vol—volume + emia—blood

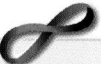

Box 5.2

Gerontolical Issues

As a person ages, total body water decreases from 60% to 50% of total body weight. The age-related decrease in total body water is secondary to an increase in body fat and a decrease in thirst sensation. These factors increase the risk of developing dehydration.

Manifestations of dehydration in an older adult are different from typical manifestations in a younger person, and may include altered mental status, lightheadedness, and syncope. These occur because a patient with hypovolemia has an inadequate circulatory volume and, therefore, oxygen supply to the brain.

blood volume decreases, the heart pumps the remaining blood faster but not as powerfully, resulting in a rapid, weak pulse and a low blood pressure. The body pulls water into the vascular system from other areas, resulting in decreased tear formation, dry skin, and dry mucous membranes.

The individual with dehydration has poor skin turgor. Turgor is poor if the skin is pinched and a small "tent" remains (called *tenting*). Temperature increases because the body is less able to cool itself through perspiration. Temperature may not appear elevated in an elderly person because an elder's normal body temperature is often lower than a younger person's. Urine output decreases and the urine becomes more concentrated as water is conserved. Dehydration should be considered in any adult with a urine output of less than 30 mL per hour. The urine may appear darker because it is less diluted. The patient becomes constipated as the intestines absorb more water from the feces. A major method of evaluating dehydration is weight loss. A pint of water weighs approximately 1 pound. Symptoms of dehydration in the elderly may be atypical (see Box 5.2, Gerontological Issues).

Complications

If dehydration is not treated, lack of sufficient blood volume causes organ function to decrease and eventually fail. The brain, kidneys, and heart must be adequately supplied with blood (perfused) to function properly. The body protects these organs by decreasing blood flow to other areas. When these organs no longer receive their minimum requirements, death results.

LEARNING TIP

The magic fluid number is 30: Healthy adults should drink approximately 30 mL of fluid per kilogram of body weight per day, and they should urinate at least 30 mL per hour. Of course, this is just a basic rule of thumb and may vary based on the person's individual circumstances.

Diagnostic Tests

The patient with dehydration usually has an elevated blood urea nitrogen (BUN) level and elevated hematocrit. Both values are increased because there is less water in proportion to the solid substances being measured. The specific gravity of the urine also increases as the kidneys attempt to conserve water, resulting in a more concentrated urine.

Therapeutic Interventions

The goals of therapeutic interventions are to replace fluids and resolve the cause of dehydration. In a patient with moderate or severe dehydration, IV therapy is used. Isotonic fluids that have the same osmolarity as blood are typically administered.

PATIENT SAFETY TIP

Use at least two patient identifiers (neither to be the patient's room number) whenever administering medications or blood products; taking blood samples and other specimens for clinical testing, or providing any other treatments or procedures. 2006 National Patient Safety Goals from www.jcaho.org

Nursing Process

Nurses can play a major role in identifying and caring for patients who are dehydrated.

ASSESSMENT/DATA COLLECTION. Assess the patient for signs and symptoms of dehydration. All the classic signs and symptoms may not be present.

When assessing an elderly patient for skin turgor (tenting), assess the skin over the forehead or sternum. The skin over these areas usually retains elasticity and is therefore a more reliable indicator of skin turgor. Also check mucous membranes, which should be moist.

Weight is the most reliable indicator of fluid loss or gain. A loss of 1 to 2 pounds or more per day suggests water loss rather than fat loss. The patient in the hospital setting should be weighed every day. The patient in the nursing home or home setting should be weighed at least three times a week if the patient is at risk for fluid imbalance. Weigh the patient before breakfast using the same scale each time. Intake and output are also typically measured (Box 5.3 Cultural Consideration).

NURSING DIAGNOSES, PLANNING, AND IMPLEMENTATION. Actual or risk for deficient fluid volume related to fluid loss or inadequate fluid intake. The primary nursing diagnosis and interventions for the patient with dehydration include:

EXPECTED OUTCOME: The patient will be adequately hydrated as evidenced by stable weight, moist mucous membranes, and elastic skin turgor.

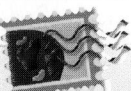

Box 5.3

Cultural Considerations

Muslims who celebrate Ramadan fast for 1 month from sunup to sundown. Although the ill are not required to fast, the pious may still wish to do so. Fasting may include not taking fluids and medications during daylight hours. Therefore, the nurse may need to alter times for medication administration, including intramuscular medication. Special precautions may need to be taken to prevent dehydration in Muslim patients.

Monitor daily weights and input and output (I&O) *so problems can be detected and corrected early.*

Plan with the patient and other members of the health-care team the type and timing of fluid intake. *Planning with the patient increases the likelihood the plan is followed.*

Offer fluids often to the confused patient *since he or she may not drink independently.*

Correct the underlying cause of the fluid deficit, *so it does not recur.*

Be careful not to overhydrate the patient, *so fluid excess does not occur.*

See Box 5.4, Best Practice Recommendations for Maintaining Oral Hydration in Older People.

EVALUATION. The patient who is adequately hydrated will have elastic skin turgor, moist mucous membranes, and stable weight.

Patient Education

The patient, family, and significant others need to be taught the importance of reporting early signs and symptoms of dehydration to a physician or other health care provider. At home or in the nursing home, infections often cause fever

CRITICAL THINKING

Mrs. Levitt

■ Mrs. Levitt is a 92-year-old widow who has been in a nursing home for 4 years. Today she complains that her urine smells bad and that her heart feels like it is beating faster than usual. You suspect that she is becoming dehydrated. You check her urine and find that it is a dark amber color and has a strong odor. Her heart rate is 98, blood pressure 126/74, respiratory rate 20, and temperature 99.2.

1. What other data should you collect, and what results do you expect?
2. Which interventions should you provide at this time?
3. How should you document your findings?

Suggested answers at end of chapter.

Box 5.4

Best Practice Recommendations for Maintaining Oral Hydration in Older People

- A fluid intake sheet is the best method of monitoring daily fluid intake.
- Urine specific gravity may be the simplest, most accurate method to determine patient hydration status.
- Evidence of a dry furrowed tongue and mucous membranes, sunken eyes, confusion, and upper body muscle weakness may indicate dehydration.
- Regular presentation of fluids to bedridden older people can maintain adequate hydration status.
- Owing to the observation that medication time can be an important source of fluids, fluids should be encouraged at this time.

Source: Adapted from Joanna Briggs Best Practice Recommendations: Maintaining Oral Hydration in Older People, 5:6, 2001.

and sepsis, a serious condition in which the infection invades the bloodstream. The body attempts to decrease the temperature through perspiration. The patient becomes dehydrated as a result and can become increasingly ill.

Fluid Excess

Fluid excess, sometimes called overhydration, is a condition in which a patient has too much fluid in the body. Most of the problems related to fluid excess result from too much fluid in the bloodstream or from dilution of electrolytes and red blood cells.

Pathophysiology and Etiology

The most common result of fluid excess is **hypervolemia** in which there is excess fluid in the intravascular space. Healthy adult kidneys can compensate for mild to moderate hypervolemia. The kidneys increase urinary output to rid the body of the extra fluid.

The causes of fluid excess are related to excessive intake of fluids or inadequate excretion of fluids. Conditions that can cause excessive fluid intake are poorly controlled IV therapy, excessive irrigation of wounds or body cavities, and excessive ingestion of water. Conditions that can result in inadequate excretion of fluid include renal failure, heart failure, and the syndrome of inappropriate antidiuretic hormone. These conditions are discussed elsewhere in this book.

Prevention

One of the best ways to prevent fluid excess is to avoid excessive fluid intake. For example, you should monitor the

hypervolemia: hyper—more than + vol—volume + emia—blood

patient receiving IV therapy for signs and symptoms of fluid excess. In at-risk patients, an electronic infusion pump or a quantity-limiting device, such as a burette, should be used to control the rate of infusion.

Also monitor the amount of fluid used for irrigations. For example, when a patient's stomach is being irrigated (gastric lavage), be sure an excessive amount of fluid is not absorbed.

Signs and Symptoms

The vital sign changes seen in the patient with fluid excess are the opposite of those found in patients with dehydration. The blood pressure is elevated, pulse is bounding, and respirations are increased and shallow. The neck veins may become distended, and pitting edema in the feet and legs may be present. The skin is pale and cool. The kidneys increase urine output, and the urine appears diluted, almost like water. The patient rapidly gains weight. In severe fluid excess, the patient develops moist crackles in the lungs, dyspnea, and ascites (excess peritoneal fluid).

Complications

Acute fluid excess typically results in congestive heart failure. As the fluid builds up in the heart, the heart is not able to properly function as a pump. The fluid then backs up into the lungs, causing a condition known as pulmonary edema. Other major organs of the body cannot receive adequate oxygen, and organ failure can lead to death.

Diagnostic Tests

In the patient experiencing fluid excess, the BUN and hematocrit levels tend to decrease from hemodilution. The plasma content of the blood is proportionately increased when compared with the solid substances. The specific gravity of the urine also diminishes as the urinary output increases.

Therapeutic Interventions

Once the patient's breathing has been supported, the goal of treatment is to rid the body of excessive fluid and resolve the underlying cause of the excess. Drug therapy and diet therapy are commonly used to decrease fluid retention.

POSITIONING. To facilitate ease in breathing, the head of the patient's bed should be in semi-Fowler's or high Fowler's position. These positions allow greater lung expansion and thus aid respiratory effort. Once the patient has been properly positioned, oxygen therapy may be necessary (Fig. 5.2).

OXYGEN THERAPY. Oxygen therapy is typically used to ensure adequate perfusion of major organs and to minimize dyspnea. If the patient has a history of chronic obstructive pulmonary disease, such as emphysema or chronic bronchitis, do not administer more than 2 L per minute of oxygen. At higher oxygen doses, the patient may lose the stimulus to breathe and may suffer respiratory arrest.

DRUG THERAPY. Diuretics are frequently administered to rapidly rid the body of excess water. A diuretic is a drug that

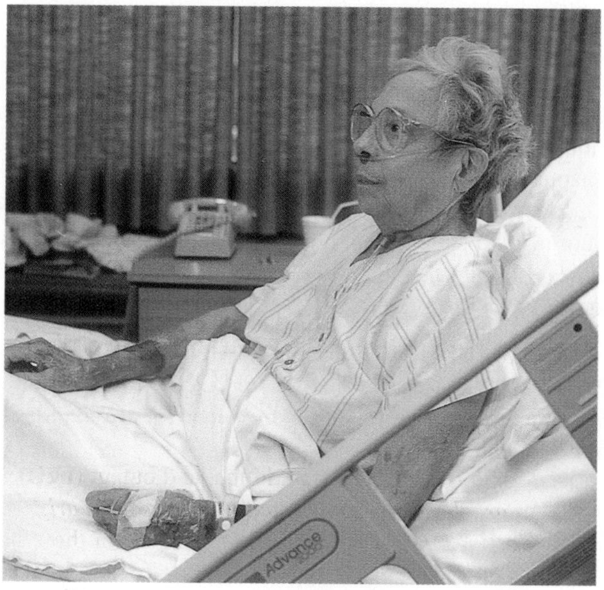

FIGURE 5.2 Patient in high Fowler's position with oxygen.

increases elimination by the kidneys. The drug of choice for fluid excess when the patient has adequately functioning kidneys is usually furosemide (Lasix). Furosemide is a loop (high-ceiling) diuretic that causes the kidneys to excrete sodium and water. Sodium (Na^+) and water tend to move together in the body. Potassium (K^+), another electrolyte, is also lost, which can lead to a potassium deficit, which is discussed later in this chapter.

Furosemide may be given by the oral, intramuscular, or IV route. The oral route is used most commonly for mild fluid excess. IV furosemide is administered by a registered nurse (RN) or physician for severe excess. The patient should begin diuresis within 30 minutes after receiving IV furosemide. If not, another dose is given. Strict intake and output should be monitored when a patient is receiving IV furosemide.

DIET THERAPY. Mild to moderate fluid restriction may be necessary, as well as a sodium-restricted diet. In collaboration with the dietitian, a physician prescribes the specific restriction necessary, usually a 1- to 2-g Na^+ restriction for severe excess. Different diuretics result in differing electrolyte elimination. Specific diet therapy depends on the medications the patient is receiving and the patient's underlying medical problems.

Nursing Process

The nurse plays a pivotal role in the care of a patient with fluid excess. Prompt action is needed to prevent life-threatening complications.

ASSESSMENT/DATA COLLECTION. Observe a patient who is at high risk for fluid excess and monitor fluid I&O carefully. If the patient is drinking adequate amounts of fluid (1500 mL per day or more) but is voiding in small amounts, the fluid is being retained by the body.

Assess for edema, which is fluid that accumulates in the interstitial tissues. If the edema is pitting, a finger pressed

---

edema: swelling

against the skin over a bony area such as the tibia leaves a temporary indentation. For patients in bed, check the sacrum for edema. For patients in the sitting position, check the feet and legs. Also assess lung sounds since excess fluid accumulation in the lungs can cause crackles (see Chapter 29).

As mentioned earlier, weight is the most reliable indicator of fluid gain. A gain of 1 to 2 pounds or more per day indicates fluid retention even though other signs and symptoms may not be present.

NURSING DIAGNOSES, PLANNING, AND IMPLEMENTATION. Actual or risk for excess fluid volume related to excessive fluid intake or inadequate excretion of body fluid

EXPECTED OUTCOME: Patient will return to a normal hydration status as evidenced by return to weight that is normal for patient, absence of edema, and clear lung sounds.

- Weigh the patient daily and report any increase to the physician. *Increased weight indicates fluid retention.*
- Implement fluid restriction as ordered *to reduce excess.* Work with the patient and RN to determine how it should be implemented. For example, if a patient is on a 1000 mL per day fluid restriction, you might plan for 150 mL with each meal, 450 mL to be given to the patient to use as he or she likes during the day, and 100 mL to be used during the night. Be sure to include the patient in your planning, and remember to reserve enough fluid for swallowing medications. Post a sign in the patient's room so other caregivers know how much fluid the patient can have.
- Administer diuretics as ordered, and monitor patient response. Be sure to monitor potassium in patients receiving potassium-losing loop or thiazide diuretics. *Diuretics promote diuresis.*
- Report urinary output below 30 mL per hour to the physician or RN *because it may signify increasing renal complications.*

EVALUATION. If interventions have been effective, the patient will return to his or her normal weight with clear lung sounds and no edema. Many patients must remain on drug and diet therapy after hospital discharge to prevent the problem from recurring.

Patient Education

In collaboration with the dietitian, the patient, family, or other caregiver should be instructed about the fluid and sodium restrictions to prevent further problems (Box 5.5 Nutrition Notes). High-sodium foods to avoid are listed in Box 5.6 Common Food Sources of Sodium.

Teaching caregivers about diuretic therapy is essential to prevent electrolyte imbalances. If a potassium-losing diuretic is prescribed, teach which foods are high in potassium, such as oranges and other citrus fruits, melons, bananas, and potatoes (Box 5.7 Food Sources of Potassium).

The patient's serum potassium level must be periodically monitored by a physician or home-care nurse. If it becomes too low, an oral potassium supplement is needed.

The family or other caregiver also needs to be taught common signs and symptoms of fluid excess that should be reported to a physician or other health-care provider. Of special importance is weight gain. The patient should be weighed at least three times a week in the home or nursing home if he or she is at high risk for fluid excess, and weight gain should be reported.

CRITICAL THINKING

Mr. Peters

■ Mr. Peters is a 32-year-old man with a congenital heart problem. He has been recovering from congestive heart failure and fluid excess. Today, his blood pressure is higher than usual and his pulse is bounding. He is having trouble breathing and presses the call light for your assistance.

1. What should you do first when you assess Mr. Peters's condition?
2. What questions should you ask him?
3. What other assessments should you perform?

Suggested answers at end of chapter.

 ELECTROLYTE BALANCE

Natural minerals in food become electrolytes or ions in the body through digestion and metabolism. Electrolytes are usually measured in milliequivalents per liter (mEq/L) or in milligrams per deciliter (mg/dL).

Electrolytes are one of two types: **cations,** which carry a positive electrical charge, and **anions,** which carry a negative electrical charge. Although there are many electrolytes in the body, this chapter discusses the most important ones, including sodium (Na^+), potassium (K^+), calcium (Ca^{2+}), and magnesium (Mg^{2+}). These electrolytes are maintained in different concentrations inside the cell and outside the cell because of pumps in the cell wall (Fig. 5.3).

 ELECTROLYTE IMBALANCES

The two types of electrolyte imbalances are deficit and excess. In general, if a patient experiences a deficit of an electrolyte, the electrolyte is replaced either orally or intravenously. If the patient experiences an excess of the electrolyte, treatment focuses on getting rid of the excess, often by the kidneys. The underlying cause of the imbalance must also be treated.

The most important aspect of nursing care is prevent-

---

cation: cat—descending + ion—carrying
anion: an—without + ion—carrying

Box 5.5

Nutrition Notes

Reducing Sodium Intake

Many foods, such as dairy products, grain products, and some vegetables, are naturally high in sodium, but the major sources of sodium in the diet are salted and processed foods, including baked goods and condiments. For example, American cheese has more sodium than Cheddar, and cured ham has more than fresh pork. Drinking water may contain significant amounts of sodium, particularly if it is a softened or mineral water. Because of the numerous "hidden" sources of sodium, patients on low-sodium diets benefit from education by a dietician.

The Adequate Intake (AI) of sodium is 1.5 g per day for adults through age 49, 1.3 g for those 50 to 70 years of age, and 1.2 g for those 71 years of age and older. The upper tolerable intake level (UL) for sodium is 2.3 g per day, obtainable in slightly more than teaspoon of salt. None of these amounts applies to individuals losing large amounts of sweat daily or to unacclimatized persons exercising in a hot environment.

Specific definitions for reduced sodium food products have been adopted. Note that serving size is an important variable.

- Salt or sodium free: <5 mg sodium per serving
- Very low sodium: <35 mg sodium per serving (per 100 g if main dish)
- Low sodium: <140 mg sodium per serving (per 100 g if main dish)

Box 5.6

Common Food Sources of Sodium*

Food Group	Serving Size	Range (mg)
Breads, all types	1 oz	95–210
Frozen pizza, plain, cheese	4 oz	450–1200
Frozen vegetables, all types	1/2 cup	2–160
Salad dressing, regular fat, all types	2 tbsp	110–505
Salsa	2 tbsp	150–240
Soup (tomato), reconstituted	8 oz	700–1260
Tomato juice	8 oz (~1 cup)	340–1040
Potato chips[†]	1 oz (28.4 g)	120–180
Tortilla chips[†]	1 oz (28.4 g)	105–160
Pretzels[†]	1 oz (28.4 g)	290–560

*The ranges of sodium content for selected foods available in the retail market. This table is provided to exemplify the importance of reading the food label to determine the sodium content of food, which can vary by several hundreds of milligrams in similar foods.

[†]All snack foods are regular flavor, salted.

Source: Agricultural Research Service Nutrient Database for Standard Reference, Release 17 and recent manufacturers label data from retail market surveys. Serving sizes were standardized to be comparable among brands within a food. Pizza and bread slices vary in size and weight across brands.

Note: None of the examples provided was labeled low-sodium.

---

ing and assessing electrolyte imbalances. High-risk patients should be identified and monitored carefully. Serum electrolytes are measured on a regular basis. As a general rule, patients should be checked for electrolyte imbalance when there is a change in their mental state (either increased irritability or decreased responsiveness) or when muscle function changes. Patient education is another important nursing role for patients with electrolyte imbalances.

Sodium Imbalances

The normal level of serum sodium is 135 to 145 mEq/L. Because sodium is the major cation in the blood, it helps maintain serum osmolarity. Therefore, sodium imbalances are often associated with fluid imbalances, described earlier in this chapter. Sodium is also important for cell function, especially in the central nervous system. The two sodium imbalances are **hyponatremia** (sodium deficit) and **hypernatremia** (sodium excess).

---

hyponatremia: hypo—less than + natr—sodium + emia—blood

hypernatremia: hyper—more than + natr—sodium + emia—blood

Hyponatremia

Hyponatremia occurs when the serum sodium level is less than 135 mEq/L.

PATHOPHYSIOLOGY AND ETIOLOGY. Many conditions can lead to either an actual or a relative decrease in sodium. In an actual decrease, the patient has inadequate intake of sodium or excessive sodium loss from the body. As the percentage of sodium in the ECF decreases, water is pulled by osmotic pressure into the cells. In a relative decrease, the sodium is not lost from the body but leaves the intravascular space and moves into the interstitial tissues (third spacing). Another cause of a relative decrease occurs when the plasma volume increases (fluid excess), causing a dilutional effect. The percentage of sodium compared with the fluid is diminished.

PREVENTION. Additional sodium is commonly administered to patients at high risk for hyponatremia (Box 5.8 Conditions that Place Patients at Risk for Hyponatremia), usually by the IV route. Individuals who have high fevers or who engage in strenuous exercise or physical labor, especially in the heat, need to replace both sodium and water. Hyponatremia is especially dangerous for the elderly patient.

Box 5.7

Food Sources of Potassium*

Food, Standard Amount	Potassium (mg)	Calories
Sweet potato, baked, 1 potato (146 g)	694	131
Beet greens, cooked, 1/2 cup	655	19
Potato, baked, flesh, 1 potato (156 g)	610	145
Yogurt, plain, nonfat, 8-oz container	579	127
Prune juice, 3/4 cup	530	136
Soybeans, green, cooked, 1/2 cup	485	127
Bananas, 1 medium	422	105
Spinach, cooked, 1/2 cup	419	21
Tomato juice, 3/4 cup	417	31
Tomato sauce, 1/2 cup	405	39
Milk, non-fat, 1 cup	382	83
Pork chop, center loin, cooked, 3 oz	382	197
Apricots, dried, uncooked, 1/4 cup	378	78
Cantaloupe, 1/4 medium	368	47
1%-2% milk, 1 cup	366	102-122
Kidney beans, cooked, 1/2 cup	358	112
Orange juice, 3/4 cup	355	85
Split peas, cooked, 1/2 cup	355	116

*Food sources of potassium ranked by milligrams of potassium per standard amount, also showing calories in the standard amount. (The adequate intake [AI] for adults is 4,700 mg/day potassium.)

Source: Nutrient values from Agricultural Research Service (ARS) Nutrient Database for Standard Reference, Release 17. Foods are from ARS single nutrient reports, sorted in descending order by nutrient content in terms of common household measures. Food items and weights in the single nutrient reports are adapted from those in 2002 revision of USDA Home and Garden Bulletin No. 72, Nutritive Value of Foods. Mixed dishes and multiple preparations of the same food item have been omitted from this table.

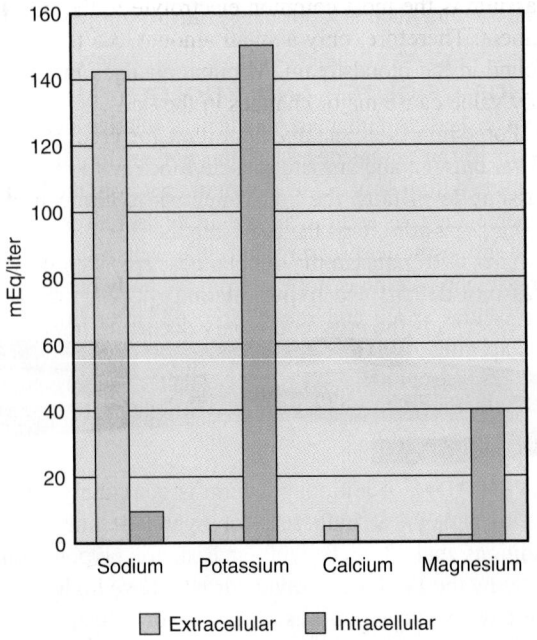

FIGURE 5.3 Extracellular and intracellular electrolytes.

SIGNS AND SYMPTOMS. Unfortunately, the signs and symptoms of hyponatremia are vague and depend somewhat on whether a fluid imbalance accompanies the hyponatremia. The patient with sodium and fluid deficits has signs and symptoms of dehydration (discussed previously). The patient with a sodium deficit and fluid excess has signs and symptoms associated with fluid excess.

In addition, the patient experiences mental status changes, including disorientation, confusion, and personality changes caused by cerebral edema (fluid around the brain). Weakness, nausea, vomiting, and diarrhea may also occur.

COMPLICATIONS. In severe hyponatremia, respiratory arrest or coma can lead to death. The patient who also has fluid excess may develop pulmonary edema, another life-threatening complication.

DIAGNOSTIC TESTS. The primary diagnostic test is to obtain the serum sodium level, which is lower than the normal value when hyponatremia is present. The serum osmolarity also decreases in patients with hyponatremia. Other laboratory tests may be affected if the patient

Box 5.8

Conditions that Place Patients at High Risk for Hyponatremia

Nothing by mouth (NPO)
Excessive diaphoresis (sweating)
Diuretics
Gastrointestinal suction
Syndrome of inappropriate antidiuretic hormone
Excessive ingestion of hypotonic fluids
Freshwater near-drowning
Decreased aldosterone

experiences an accompanying fluid imbalance. Serum chloride (Cl^-), an anion, is often depleted when sodium decreases because these two electrolytes commonly combine as NaCl (salt in solution, or saline).

THERAPEUTIC INTERVENTIONS. Therapeutic interventions focus on resolving the underlying cause of hyponatremia and replacing the lost sodium. The physician orders IV saline for patients who have hyponatremia without fluid excess.

For patients who have a fluid excess, a fluid restriction is often ordered. Diuretics that rid the body of fluid but do not cause sodium loss may also be used. For patients with cerebral edema, steroids may be prescribed to reduce **intracranial** swelling. I&O are strictly monitored, and the patient is weighed daily.

Hypernatremia

Hypernatremia occurs when the serum sodium level is above 145 mEq/L.

PATHOPHYSIOLOGY AND ETIOLOGY. Serum sodium increase may be an actual increase or a relative increase. In an actual increase, the patient receives too much sodium or is unable to excrete sodium, as seen in renal failure. In a relative increase, the amount of sodium does not change but the amount of fluid in the intravascular space decreases. The percentage of sodium (solid) is increased in relationship to the amount of plasma (water).

In mild hypernatremia, most excitable tissues, such as muscle and neurons of the brain, become more stimulated. The patient becomes irritable and has tremors. In severe cases, these tissues fail to respond.

PREVENTION. Prevention of hypernatremia is not as simple as prevention of hyponatremia. Most patients have a sodium excess as a result of an acute or chronic illness. Patients with a potential for electrolyte imbalance must always have their IV fluids carefully regulated.

SIGNS AND SYMPTOMS. Thirst is usually one of the first symptoms to appear. If you eat salty foods, such as potato

chips, the amount of sodium in the body increases and you become thirsty. Other signs and symptoms of hypernatremia are vague and nonspecific until severe excess is present. Like the patient with a sodium deficit, the patient experiencing sodium excess has mental status changes, such as agitation, confusion, and personality changes. Seizures may also occur.

At first, muscle twitches and unusual contractions may be present. Later, skeletal muscle weakness occurs that can lead to respiratory failure. If fluid deficit or fluid excess accompanies the hypernatremic state, the patient also has signs and symptoms associated with these imbalances.

COMPLICATIONS. The patient experiencing severe hypernatremia may become comatose or have respiratory arrest as skeletal muscles weaken.

DIAGNOSTIC TESTS. The most reliable diagnostic test is the serum sodium level, which indicates an increase above the normal level. Serum osmolarity may also increase. If the patient has a fluid imbalance, other laboratory values, such as BUN, hematocrit, and urine specific gravity, are affected (see earlier discussion).

THERAPEUTIC INTERVENTIONS. If a fluid imbalance accompanies hypernatremia, it is treated first. For example, fluid replacement without sodium in a patient with dehydration should correct a relative sodium excess. If the kidneys are not excreting adequate amounts of sodium, diuretics may help if the kidneys are functional. If the kidneys are not functioning properly, dialysis may be ordered. I&O and daily weights are strictly monitored.

The cause of hypernatremia is also treated in an attempt to prevent further episodes of this imbalance. For some patients, a sodium-restricted diet is prescribed.

Potassium Imbalances *Important for heart* 3.5.

Potassium is the most common electrolyte in the ICF compartment. Therefore, only a small amount, 3.5 to 5 mEq/L, is found in the bloodstream. Minimal changes in this laboratory value cause major changes in the body.

Potassium is especially important for cardiac muscle, skeletal muscle, and smooth muscle function. As the serum potassium level falls, the body attempts to compensate by moving potassium from the cells into the bloodstream.

The two potassium imbalances are **hypokalemia** (potassium deficit) and **hyperkalemia** (potassium excess). Hypokalemia is the most commonly occurring imbalance.

Hypokalemia

Hypokalemia occurs when the serum potassium level falls below 3.5 mEq/L.

PATHOPHYSIOLOGY AND ETIOLOGY. Most cases of hypokalemia result from inadequate intake of potassium or

intracranial: intra—within + cranial—cranium (skull)

hypokalemia: hypo—less than + kal—potassium + emia—blood

hyperkalemia: hyper—more than + kal—potassium + emia—blood

excessive loss of potassium through the kidneys. Hypokalemia most often occurs as a result of medications. Potassium-losing diuretics (e.g., furosemide [Lasix]), digitalis preparations (e.g., digoxin [Lanoxin]), and corticosteroids (e.g., prednisone [Deltasone]) are examples of drugs that cause increased excretion of potassium from the body. Potassium may also be lost through the gastrointestinal (GI) tract, which is rich in potassium and other electrolytes. Severe vomiting, diarrhea, and prolonged GI suction cause hypokalemia (Box 5.9. Patient Perspective). Major surgery and hemorrhage can also lead to potassium deficit.

PREVENTION. Most patients having major surgery receive potassium supplements in their IV fluids to prevent hypokalemia. For patients receiving drugs known to cause hypokalemia, foods high in potassium may prevent a deficit (see Box 5.7, Food Sources of Potassium). Patients receiving digitalis must be closely monitored because hypokalemia can enhance the action of digitalis and cause digitalis toxicity.

SIGNS AND SYMPTOMS. Many body systems are affected by a potassium imbalance. Muscle cramping occurs with either a deficit or an excess of potassium. Vital signs change because the respiratory and cardiovascular systems need potassium to function properly. Skeletal muscle activity diminishes, resulting in shallow, ineffective

respirations. The pulse is typically weak, irregular, and thready because the heart muscle is depleted of potassium. A major danger is an irregular heartbeat (**dysrhythmia**), which can lead to a cardiac arrest. Orthostatic (postural) hypotension may also be present.

The nervous system is usually affected as well. The patient experiences changes in mental status followed by lethargy. The motility of the GI system is slowed, causing nausea, vomiting, abdominal distention, and constipation. Vomiting may further increase potassium loss.

COMPLICATIONS. If not corrected, hypokalemia can result in death from dysrhythmia, respiratory failure and arrest, or coma. The patient must be treated promptly before these complications occur.

DIAGNOSTIC TESTS. The primary laboratory test is to obtain a serum potassium level. The patient's electrocardiogram (ECG) may show cardiac dysrhythmias associated with potassium deficit. In addition to a decrease in the serum potassium level, the patient may have an acid-base imbalance known as metabolic **alkalosis,** which commonly accompanies hypokalemia. In metabolic alkalosis, the serum pH of the blood increases (above 7.45) so that the blood is more alkaline than usual. Acid-base imbalances are discussed later in this chapter.

THERAPEUTIC INTERVENTIONS. The goal of treatment is to replace potassium in the body and resolve the underlying cause of the imbalance. For mild to moderate hypokalemia, oral potassium supplements are given.

For severe hypokalemia, IV potassium supplements are given. Because the kidneys eliminate excess potassium, potassium should be added to IV fluids only after the patient has voided. Potassium is a potentially dangerous drug, especially when administered intravenously. In too high a concentration, it causes cardiac arrest. Only IV solutions which are premixed and carefully labeled should be used. Potassium is *never* given by IV push. The patient's laboratory values must be monitored carefully to prevent giving too much potassium. Administration of IV potassium is done by a registered nurse.

Teach the patient about the side effects of oral potassium and precautions associated with potassium administration. Box 5.10 (Tips for Receiving Oral Potassium Supplements) summarizes the precautions you need to be aware of when giving oral potassium supplements.

Hyperkalemia   give diarctics

Hyperkalemia is a condition in which the serum potassium level exceeds 5 mEq/L. It is rare in a person with healthy kidneys.

PATHOPHYSIOLOGY AND ETIOLOGY. Hyperkalemia may result from an actual increase in the amount of total body potassium or from the movement of intracellular

---

Box 5.9

Patient Perspective

Patricia

I take hydrochlorothiazide for my high blood pressure. Since it can make me lose potassium, I also take a potassium supplement. So I thought I was all set. But recently I ate something that did not agree with me, and had diarrhea for a couple of days. One morning as I was driving to work, I felt so weak it made me frightened. I drove back home and asked my husband to drive me to work. I arrived safely, but as I walked down the hallway, I again felt so weak I had to sit down. I felt like I could not put one foot in front of the other. I kept thinking "this is all in my head." I decided maybe I was dehydrated from the diarrhea, so I drank a bottle of Gatorade and a glass of orange juice. Slowly I began to feel a bit better, and made it through the day. After work I had to take my daughter to the doctor, so I asked about my symptoms. I was sent to the lab where I had my potassium level checked and it was 3.1! Normal is 3.5 to 5 mEq/L. Mine must have been even lower before I drank the juice and Gatorade. I learned that I probably lost a lot of potassium because of the diarrhea. I also learned that low potassium made my muscles weak and could have affected my heart function. Next time I have diarrhea, I plan to call my doctor.

---

dysrhythmia: dys—bad or disordered + rhythmia—measured motion

alkalosis: alkal—alkaline + osis—condition

Box 5.10

Tips for Patients Receiving Oral Potassium Supplements

- Do not substitute one potassium supplement for another.
- Dilute powders and liquids in juice or other desired liquid to improve taste and to prevent gastrointestinal irritation. Follow manufacturer's recommendations for the amount of fluid to use for dilution, most commonly 4 oz per 20 mEq of potassium.
- Do not drink diluted solutions until mixed thoroughly.
- Do not crush potassium tablets, such as Slow-K or K-tab tablets. Read manufacturer's directions regarding which tablets can be crushed.
- Administer slow-release tablets with 8 oz of water to help them dissolve.
- Do not take potassium supplements if taking potassium-sparing diuretics such as spironolactone or triamterene.
- Do not use salt substitutes containing potassium unless prescribed by the physician.
- Take potassium supplements with meals.
- Report adverse effects, such as nausea, vomiting, diarrhea, and abdominal cramping, to the physician.
- Have frequent laboratory testing for potassium levels as recommended by the physician.

Source: Adapted from Lee, CA, Barrett, CA, and Ignatavicius, DD: Fluids and Electrolytes: A Practical Approach, ed 4. F.A. Davis, Philadelphia, 1996.

potassium into the blood. Overuse of potassium-based salt substitutes or excessive intake of oral or IV potassium supplements can cause hyperkalemia. Use of potassium-sparing diuretics (e.g., spironolactone [Aldactone]) may also contribute to hyperkalemia. Patients with renal failure are at risk for hyperkalemia because the kidneys cannot excrete potassium.

Movement of potassium from the cells into the blood and other ECF is common in massive tissue trauma and metabolic **acidosis.** Metabolic acidosis is an acid-base imbalance commonly seen in patients with uncontrolled diabetes mellitus. Acid-base imbalances are discussed later in this chapter.

PREVENTION. For patients receiving potassium supplements, hyperkalemia can be prevented by monitoring serum electrolyte values and the patient's signs and symptoms.

SIGNS AND SYMPTOMS. Most cases of hyperkalemia occur in patients who are hospitalized or those undergoing therapeutic interventions for a chronic condition. The classic

manifestations are muscle twitches and cramps, later followed by profound muscular weakness; increased GI motility (diarrhea); slow, irregular heart rate; and decreased blood pressure.

COMPLICATIONS. Cardiac dysrhythmias and respiratory failure can occur in severe hyperkalemia, causing death.

DIAGNOSTIC TESTS. In addition to an elevated serum potassium level, an irregular ECG is associated with hyperkalemia. If the patient also has metabolic acidosis, the serum pH falls below 7.35.

THERAPEUTIC INTERVENTIONS. For mild, chronic hyperkalemia, dietary limitation of potassium-rich foods may be helpful. Potassium supplements are discontinued, and potassium-losing diuretics are given to patients with healthy kidneys. For patients with renal problems, a cation exchange resin, such as sodium polystyrene sulfonate (Kayexalate), is administered either orally or rectally. This drug releases sodium and absorbs potassium for excretion through the feces and out of the body.

In cases in which cellular potassium has moved into the bloodstream, administration of glucose and insulin can facilitate the movement of potassium back into the cells. During treatment of moderate to severe hyperkalemia, the patient should be in the hospital on a cardiac monitor.

Calcium Imbalances

Calcium is a mineral that is primarily stored in bones and teeth. A small amount is found in ECF. The normal value for serum calcium is 9 to 11 mg/dL, or 4.5 to 5.5 mEq/L. Minimal changes in serum calcium levels can have major negative effects in the body.

Calcium is needed for the proper function of excitable tissues, especially cardiac muscle. It is also needed for adequate blood clotting. The two calcium imbalances are **hypocalcemia** and **hypercalcemia.**

Hypocalcemia

Hypocalcemia occurs when the serum calcium falls below 9 mg/dL, or 4.5 mEq/L.

PATHOPHYSIOLOGY AND ETIOLOGY. Although calcium deficit can be acute or chronic, most patients develop hypocalcemia slowly as a result of chronic disease or poor intake. The woman who is postmenopausal is most at risk for hypocalcemia. As a woman ages, calcium intake typically declines. The parathyroid glands recognize this decrease and stimulate bone to release some of its stored calcium into the blood for replacement. The result is a condition known as **osteoporosis**, in which bones become porous and brittle and fracture easily. The woman who is

---

hypocalcemia: hypo—less than + calc—calcium + emia—blood

hypercalcemia: hyper—more than + calc calcium + emia—blood

osteoporosis: osteo—bone + porosis—porous

acidosis: acid—acidic + osis—condition

postmenopausal has a decreased level of estrogens, hormones that help prevent bone loss in the younger woman. Immobility or decreased mobility also contributes to bone loss in many patients. The patients at highest risk for osteoporosis are thin, petite, Caucasian women.

Hypocalcemia can also result from inadequate absorption of calcium from the intestines, as seen in patients with Crohn's disease, a chronic inflammatory bowel disease. An insufficient intake of vitamin D prevents calcium absorption as well. Conditions that interfere with the production of parathyroid hormone, such as partial or complete surgical removal of the thyroid or parathyroids, can also cause hypocalcemia.

Finally, patients with hyperphosphatemia (usually those with renal failure) often experience hypocalcemia. Calcium and phosphate have an inverse relationship. When one of these electrolytes increases, the other tends to decrease and vice versa.

PREVENTION. In the United States, the typical daily calcium intake is less than 550 mg. The adequate intake (AI) of calcium for adults ages 19 to 50 is 1000 mg; the AI for adults over age 50 is 1200 mg.

Hypocalcemia can be prevented in premenopausal and postmenopausal women by consuming calcium-rich foods and by taking calcium supplements. These supplements can be purchased over-the-counter in any pharmacy or large food store. An inexpensive source of calcium for patients who do not require vitamin D supplementation is calcium carbonate (Tums), which provides 240 mg of elemental calcium in each tablet.

Vitamin D supplementation may be required in addition to calcium for homebound or institutionalized patients who have no exposure to the sun. The ultraviolet light causes the skin to manufacture vitamin D.

SIGNS AND SYMPTOMS. Chronic hypocalcemia is usually not diagnosed until the patient breaks a bone, usually a hip. Acute hypocalcemia, which can occur after surgery or in patients with acute pancreatitis, has several signs and symptoms. These include increased and irregular heart rate, mental status changes, hyperactive deep tendon reflexes, and increased GI motility, including diarrhea and abdominal cramping. Two classic signs that can be used to assess for hypocalcemia are Trousseau's sign and Chvostek's sign.

To test for Trousseau's sign, inflate a blood pressure cuff around the patient's upper arm for 1 to 4 minutes. In a patient with hypocalcemia, the hand and fingers become spastic and go into palmar flexion (Fig. 5.4). A positive Chvostek's sign test also indicates calcium deficit. To test for this sign, tap the face just below and in front of the ear. Facial twitching on that side of the face indicates a positive test (Fig. 5.5).

> **LEARNING TIP**
>
> You can remember which sign is **CH**vostek's sign because it causes spasm near the **CH**eek.

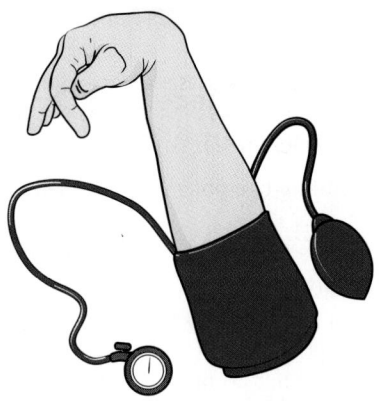

FIGURE 5.4 Trousseau's sign.

COMPLICATIONS. In severe hypocalcemia, seizures, respiratory failure, or cardiac failure can occur and lead to death if not aggressively treated. The patient may have a sudden laryngospasm that will stop air from entering the patient's lungs.

DIAGNOSTIC TESTS. The patient with hypocalcemia has a lowered serum calcium and an abnormal ECG. The parathyroid hormone level may be increased because it stimulates bone to release more calcium into the blood.

THERAPEUTIC INTERVENTIONS. In addition to treating the cause of hypocalcemia, calcium is replaced. For mild or chronic hypocalcemia, oral calcium supplements with or without vitamin D are given. Calcium supplements should be administered 1 to 2 hours after meals to increase intestinal absorption.

For patients with acute or severe hypocalcemia, IV calcium gluconate or calcium chloride is given. When a patient has had thyroid or parathyroid surgery, this medication must be readily available for emergency use.

For patients with hyperphosphatemia, usually those with renal failure, aluminum hydroxide is used to bind the excess phosphate for elimination via the GI tract. As the phosphate decreases, the serum calcium begins to increase closer to normal levels.

Diet therapy is an important part of treatment. Teach the patient, family, or other caregiver which foods are high in calcium (Table 5.1). Many foods today are fortified with

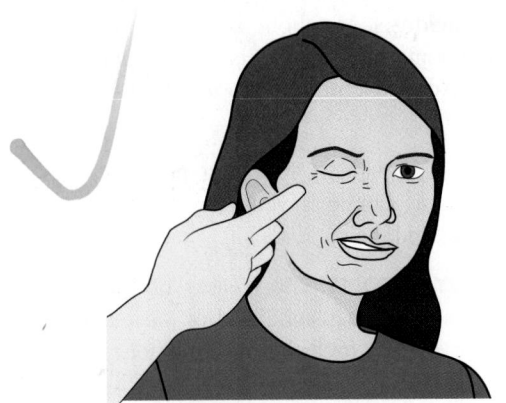

FIGURE 5.5 Chvostek's sign.

calcium. Vitamin D foods are also encouraged, especially milk and other dairy products. For patients experiencing difficulty digesting dairy products and those who choose not to use dairy products, special attention must be paid to including other dietary calcium sources.

CRITICAL THINKING

Mrs. Wright

■ Mrs. Wright is a 77-year-old petite Caucasian woman who lives alone at home. She is on a fixed income and rarely eats calcium-rich foods. She recently fell and broke her hip. After surgery she returned home under the care of a home health agency.

1. What made the patient at high risk for a fracture?
2. What would you expect her serum calcium level to have been before the fall?
3. What patient teaching related to diet and calcium supplements should the home health-care nurse include during his or her home visits?

Suggested answers at end of chapter.

Hypercalcemia   give Lastix

Hypercalcemia occurs when the serum calcium is above 11 mg/dL, or 5.5 mEq/L.

PATHOPHYSIOLOGY AND ETOLOGY. Chronic hypercalcemia can result from excessive intake of calcium or vitamin D, renal failure, hyperparathyroidism, cancers, and overuse or prolonged use of thiazide diuretics, such as hydrochlorothiazide (HydroDiuril). Acute hypercalcemia can occur as an emergency in patients with invasive or metastatic cancers.

PREVENTION. Although many causes of increased calcium cannot be prevented, a person receiving calcium supplements should be monitored carefully. Some women believe that if 2 or 3 tablets a day are helpful, consuming twice that much will help even more. The result can be serum calcium excess. Educating the public about the proper amount of calcium needed each day and the danger of too much calcium is very important.

SIGNS AND SYMPTOMS. Patients who have mild hypercalcemia or a slowly progressing calcium increase may have no obvious signs and symptoms. However, acute hypercalcemia is associated with increased heart rate and blood pressure, skeletal muscle weakness, and decreased GI motility.

COMPLICATIONS. In some cases, the patient may experience renal or urinary calculi (stones) resulting from the build-up of calcium. In more severe cases of acute hypercalcemia, the patient may experience respiratory failure caused by profound muscle weakness or heart failure caused by dysrhythmias.

THERAPEUTIC INTERVENTIONS. Patients with severe hypercalcemia should be hospitalized and placed on a cardiac monitor. Unless contraindicated by other conditions, the primary treatment is to give large amounts of fluids and

---

TABLE 5.1 FOOD SOURCES OF CALCIUM*

Food, Standard Amount	Calcium (mg)	Calories
Fortified ready-to-eat cereals (various), 1 oz	236–1043	88–106
Plain yogurt, nonfat (13 g protein/8 oz), 8-oz container	452	127
Romano cheese, 1.5 oz	452	165
Pasteurized processed Swiss cheese, 2 oz	438	190
Swiss cheese, 1.5 oz	336	162
Sardines, Atlantic, in oil, drained, 3 oz	325	177
Pasteurized process American cheese food, 2 oz	323	188
Mozzarella cheese, part-skim, 1.5 oz	311	129
Cheddar cheese, 1.5 oz	307	171
Fat-free (skim) milk, 1 cup	306	83
1% low-fat milk, 1 cup	290	102
Low-fat chocolate milk (1%), 1 cup	288	158
2% reduced fat milk, 1 cup	285	122
Whole milk, 1 cup	276	146
Molasses, blackstrap, 1 tbsp	172	47
Spinach, cooked from frozen, 1/2 cup	146	30
Ocean perch, Atlantic, cooked, 3 oz	116	103
Oatmeal, plain and flavored, instant, fortified, 1 packet prepared	99–110	97–157
Okra, cooked from frozen, 1/2 cup	88	26
Soybeans, mature, cooked, 1/2 cup	88	149

*Food sources of calcium ranked by milligrams of calcium per standard amount; also calories in the standard amount. The bioavailability may vary. (The adequate intake [AI] for adults is 1000 mg/day.)

Source: Adapted from Nutrient Values from Agricultural Research Service (ARS) Nutrient Database for Standard Reference, Release 17. Foods are from ARS single-nutrient reports, sorted in descending order by nutrient content in terms of common household measures. Food items and weights in the single nutrient reports are adapted from those in 2002 revision of USDA Home and Garden Bulletin No. 72, Nutritive Value of Foods. Mixed dishes and multiple preparations of the same food item have been omitted from this table.

promote diuresis. Saline infusions are the most useful solutions to promote renal excretion of calcium.

The physician also discontinues thiazide diuretics if the patient was receiving them and prescribes diuretics that promote calcium excretion, such as furosemide (Lasix). Other drugs that bind with calcium to lower calcium levels may also be used, such as plicamycin (Mithramycin, Mithracin) and D-penicillamine (Cuprimine).

If hypercalcemia is so severe that cardiac problems are present, hemodialysis, peritoneal dialysis, or ultrafiltration may be necessary to cleanse the blood of excess calcium. (See Chapter 37 for discussion of these procedures.)

Magnesium Imbalances

Magnesium and calcium work together for the proper functioning of excitable cells, such as cardiac muscle and nerve cells. Therefore, an imbalance of magnesium is usually accompanied by an imbalance of calcium.

The normal value for serum magnesium is 1.5 to 2.5 mEq/L. The magnesium imbalances are called **hypomagnesemia** and **hypermagnesemia.**

Hypomagnesemia

Hypomagnesemia occurs when the serum magnesium level falls below 1.5 mEq/L. It results from either a decreased intake or an excessive loss of magnesium. Causes of inadequate intake include malnutrition and starvation diets. Patients with severe diarrhea and Crohn's disease are unable to absorb magnesium in the intestines.

One of the major causes of hypomagnesemia is alcoholism, which causes both a decreased intake and an increased renal excretion of magnesium. Certain drugs, such as loop (high-ceiling) and osmotic diuretics, aminoglycosides (e.g., gentamicin), and some anticancer agents (e.g., cisplatin), can increase renal excretion of magnesium.

The signs and symptoms of hypomagnesemia are similar to those for hypocalcemia, including positive Trousseau's and Chvostek's signs, described earlier in this chapter.

The goal of management is to treat the underlying cause and replace magnesium in the body. Magnesium sulfate is administered intravenously. If the serum calcium is also low, calcium replacement is prescribed. The patient is placed on a cardiac monitor because of magnesium's effect on the heart. Life-threatening dysrhythmias can lead to cardiac failure and arrest.

Hypermagnesemia

Hypermagnesemia results when the serum magnesium level increases above 2.5 mEq/L. The most common cause of hypermagnesemia is increased intake coupled with decreased renal excretion caused by renal failure.

Signs and symptoms are usually not apparent until the serum level is greater than 4 mEq/L. Then the signs

and symptoms include bradycardia and other dysrhythmias, hypotension, lethargy or drowsiness, and skeletal muscle weakness. If not treated, the patient experiences coma, respiratory failure, or cardiac failure.

When kidneys are functioning properly, loop diuretics such as furosemide (Lasix) and IV fluids can help increase magnesium excretion. For patients with renal failure, dialysis may be the only option.

ACID-BASE BALANCE

The cells of the body function best when the body fluids and electrolytes are within a very narrow range. Hydrogen (H^+) is another ion that must stay within its normal limits. The amount of hydrogen determines whether a fluid is an acid or base.

An acid is a substance that releases a hydrogen ion. The stronger the acid, the more hydrogen ions are released. A common acid in the body is hydrochloric acid (HCl), which is found in the stomach. A base is a substance that binds hydrogen. A common base in the body is bicarbonate (HCO_3^-). *Alkali* is another word for base.

Sources of Acids and Bases

Acids and bases are formed in the body as part of normal metabolic processes. Acids are formed as end products of glucose, fat, and protein metabolism. These are called fixed acids because they do not change once they are formed. A weak acid, carbonic acid, can be formed when the carbon dioxide resulting from cellular metabolism combines with water. This acid can again change to bicarbonate (a base) and hydrogen and therefore is not a fixed acid.

The ECF maintains a delicate balance between acids and bases. The strength of the acids and bases can be measured by pH. The pH of a solution can vary from 0 to 14, with 7 being neutral, 0 to 6.99 being acid, and 7.01 to 14 being base, also called alkaline. The normal serum pH is 7.35 to 7.45, or slightly alkaline. It must remain in an extremely narrow range to sustain life. A pH lower than 6.9 or higher than 7.8 is usually fatal.

Control of Acid-Base Balance

As discussed in the sections on fluid and electrolyte balance, the body has several ways in which it tries to compensate for changes in the serum pH. Three major mechanisms are used: cellular buffers, the lungs, and the kidneys.

Cellular buffers are the first to attempt a return of the pH to its normal range. Examples of cellular buffers are proteins, hemoglobin, bicarbonate, and phosphates. These buffers act as a type of sponge to "soak up" extra hydrogen ions if there are too many (too acidic) or release hydrogen ions if there are not enough (too alkaline).

The lungs are the second line of defense to restore normal pH. When the blood is too acidic (pH is decreased), the lungs "blow off" additional carbon dioxide through rapid, deep breathing. This reduces the amount of carbon dioxide available to make carbonic acid in the body. If the blood is

---

hypomagnesemia: hypo—less than + magnes—magnesium + emia—blood

hypermagnesemia: hyper—more than + magnes—magnesium + emia—blood

too alkaline (pH is increased), the lungs try to conserve carbon dioxide through shallow respirations.

The kidneys are the slowest to respond to changes in serum pH, taking as long as 24 to 48 hours to assist with compensation. The kidneys help in a number of ways, including regulating the amount of bicarbonate (base) that is kept in the body. If the serum pH lowers and becomes too acidic, the kidneys reabsorb additional bicarbonate rather than excreting it so that it can help neutralize the acid. If the serum pH increases and becomes too alkaline, the kidneys excrete additional bicarbonate to get rid of the extra base. The kidneys also buffer pH by forming acids and ammonium (a base).

Acidosis or alkalosis that is corrected for by the body is referred to as compensated. The pH is returned to normal or near normal, but the P_{CO_2} and H_{CO_3} are abnormal.

ACID-BASE IMBALANCES

Most acid-base imbalances are caused by a number of acute and chronic illnesses or conditions. The primary treatment for each of the imbalances is to manage the underlying cause, which corrects the imbalance. The role of the nurse is to identify patients at risk and monitor laboratory test values for significant changes.

The laboratory tests that are used to evaluate acid-base balance are called arterial blood gases (ABGs). As the name implies, the blood sample that is analyzed must be from an artery rather than a vein. The femoral, brachial, and radial arteries are most often used to obtain the sample. Table 5.2 lists ABG values and what they indicate.

The two broad types of acid-base imbalance are acidosis and alkalosis. Each of these types can occur suddenly, which is called an acute imbalance, or develop over a long period, referred to as a chronic imbalance.

When the serum pH falls below 7.35, the patient has acidosis because the blood becomes more acidic than normal. Too much acid in the body or too little base causes acidosis. Acidosis can be divided into two types: respiratory and metabolic. Respiratory acidosis is caused by problems occurring in the respiratory system. Metabolic acidosis is the result of problems in the rest of the body.

When the serum pH increases above 7.45, the patient has alkalosis because the blood becomes more alkaline or basic. Alkalosis is caused by too little acid in the body or too much base. It can also be divided into two types: respiratory alkalosis and metabolic alkalosis.

Respiratory Acidosis

As the name indicates, the primary cause of this type of acidosis is respiratory problems. Carbon dioxide is not adequately "blown off" during expiration, causing a build-up of carbon dioxide in the blood. As mentioned earlier, carbon dioxide mixes with water to create a weak acid in the body, thus increasing the acidity of the blood.

Acute respiratory acidosis is caused by hypoventilation, usually as a result of an acute flare up of chronic respiratory disease, drugs, or neurological problems that depress breathing. Patients with chronic respiratory disease may have chronic respiratory acidosis.

The signs and symptoms of respiratory acidosis involve the central nervous system and the musculoskeletal system. As carbon dioxide increases, mental status is altered, progressing from confusion and lethargy to stupor and coma if not treated. The lungs are not able to get rid of excess carbon dioxide. Instead respirations become more depressed and shallow as muscle weakness worsens.

The treatment of respiratory acidosis is aggressive management of the underlying respiratory problem, discussed in the respiratory unit (Unit Seven) of this text.

Metabolic Acidosis

Metabolic acidosis can result from too much acid in the body (usually fixed acids) or too little bicarbonate in the body. Uncontrolled diabetes mellitus and end-stage renal failure are the two most common causes of metabolic acidosis resulting from increased fixed acids.

The GI tract is rich in bicarbonate. Patients experiencing severe diarrhea or prolonged nasointestinal suction are at high risk for metabolic acidosis as a result of bicarbonate (base) loss. The serum pH decreases as the bicarbonate level decreases (see Table 5.2). As mentioned earlier in the discussion on hyperkalemia, serum potassium tends to increase in the presence of metabolic acidosis. Excess hydrogen in the ECF moves into the cells in exchange for potassium, which leaves the cells and enters the blood. In a sense, this is a way of compensating for the acidotic state.

TABLE 5.2 ARTERIAL BLOOD GAS VALUES AND CHANGES IN ACID-BASE IMBALANCES

	pH	P_{CO_2}	H_{CO_3}
Normal values	7.35–7.45	32–45 mm Hg	20–26 mEq/L
Respiratory acidosis	↓	↑	Normal
Respiratory acidosis with compensation	Nearly normal	↑	↑
Respiratory alkalosis	↑	↓	Normal
Respiratory alkalosis with compensation	Nearly normal	↓	↓
Metabolic acidosis	↓	Normal	↓
Metabolic acidosis with compensation	Nearly normal	↓	↓
Metabolic alkalosis	↑	Normal	↑
Metabolic alkalosis with compensation	Nearly normal	↑	↑

The signs and symptoms are similar to those associated with respiratory acidosis, with the exception of the respiratory pattern. To help compensate for the acidotic state, the lungs get rid of extra carbon dioxide through Kussmaul's respirations. Kussmaul's respirations are deep and rapid and can occur only in patients with healthy lungs.

The treatment for the patient with metabolic acidosis is management of the underlying disease or condition. Information about disease management, such as diabetes, is found elsewhere in this book.

Respiratory Alkalosis

Respiratory alkalosis occurs when there is excessive loss of carbon dioxide through **hyperventilation.** Patients may hyperventilate when they are severely anxious or fearful. Patients who hyperventilate have rapid shallow respirations, are light-headed, and may become confused. The heart rate increases and the pulse becomes weak and thready. The serum pH is increased and the $Paco_2$ is very low. Mechanical ventilation can also cause respiratory alkalosis, and it can occur as a result of being at high altitudes. You may have experienced this while deep breathing during a pulmonary examination.

Respiratory alkalosis is treated by having patients hold their breath or rebreathe their own carbon dioxide with the use of either a rebreathing mask or a plain paper bag. The underlying cause must also be treated.

---

hyperventilation: hyper—more than ventilation—air

Metabolic Alkalosis

Metabolic alkalosis results from excessive ingestion of bicarbonate or other bases into the body or loss of acids from the body. Overuse or abuse of antacids or baking soda (sodium bicarbonate) can lead to metabolic alkalosis. Because the stomach contains hydrochloric acid, prolonged vomiting or nasogastric suction can cause loss of acid and also lead to metabolic alkalosis.

The serum pH is increased, as is bicarbonate. As discussed under potassium imbalances, the serum potassium decreases. Hydrogen from the ICF moves into the blood in exchange for potassium, which moves from the blood into the cells. This is one way that the body works to keep an acid-base balance. Hypocalcemia may also accompany hypokalemia.

The signs and symptoms of metabolic alkalosis are related to hypokalemia and hypocalcemia rather than the alkalotic state itself. Treatment involves identifying the underlying cause and managing it as quickly as possible.

Compensation

If the respiratory system is compensating for metabolic acidosis the Pco_2 will be decreased to return the pH to normal or near normal. In a similar fashion, if there is metabolic alkalosis, the breathing pattern will change to conserve CO_2 and restore the pH level. In chronic respiratory conditions, the kidneys conserve HCO_3 to buffer in the case of respiratory acidosis and excrete HCO_3 in cases of chronic respiratory alkalosis.

REVIEW QUESTIONS

1. Which of the following are functions of sodium in the body? Choose all responses that are correct.
   a. Maintenance of serum osmolarity
   b. Formation of bones and teeth
   c. Control of bronchodilation
   d. Control of serum glucose
   e. Maintenance of cellular function

2. A 93-year-old patient with diarrhea and dehydration is admitted to the hospital from an extended care facility. For which of the following symptoms of dehydration should the nurse assess?
   a. Pale-colored urine, bradycardia
   b. Disorientation, poor skin turgor
   c. Decreased hematocrit, hypothermia
   d. Lung congestion, abdominal discomfort

3. Which patient is most at risk for fluid excess?
   a. An infant with pneumonia
   b. A teen with multiple injuries following an automobile accident
   c. A middle-aged man who has just had surgery
   d. An elderly patient receiving IV therapy

4. Which of the following is the most reliable way to monitor a patient's fluid status?
   a. I&O
   b. Skin turgor
   c. Daily weights
   d. Lung sounds

5. When caring for a patient with fluid excess, which of the following interventions will help relieve respiratory distress?
   a. Elevate the head of the bed.
   b. Encourage the patient to cough and deep breathe.
   c. Increase fluids to promote urine output.
   d. Perform percussion and postural drainage.

6. A patient is being discharge following hospitalization for fluid imbalance. Which instruction by the nurse should take priority?
   a. "Weigh yourself every day and report changes."
   b. "Call your doctor immediately if you feel weak or fatigued."
   c. "Drink eight glasses of water a day."
   d. "Measure everything you drink, and measure how much you urinate each day."

7. A patient is being treated for hypokalemia. When evaluating his response to potassium replacement therapy, which of the following changes in his assessment should you observe for?
   a. Improving visual acuity
   b. Worsening constipation
   c. Decreasing serum glucose
   d. Increasing muscle strength

8. A patient is being placed on a potassium-losing diuretic. Which foods are high in potassium and should be recommended to the patient by the nurse? Choose all responses that are correct.
   a. Bread
   b. Potato

   c. Tomato juice
   d. Banana
   e. Gelatin

9. Which patient is at risk for respiratory acidosis?
   a. The patient with uncontrolled diabetes mellitus.
   b. The patient with chronic pulmonary disease.
   c. The patient who is very anxious.
   d. The patient who overuses antacids.

10. Which pH value represents acidosis?
    a. 7.26
    b. 7.35
    c. 7.4
    d. 7.49

Bibliography

1. Beers, MH, and Berkow, R (eds): The Merck Manual of Diagnosis and Therapy, 17th Centennial Edition. Retrieved 6/30/05 from http://www.merck.com/mrkshared/mmanual/home.jsp.
2. Carpenito-Moyet, LJ (ed): Nursing Diagnosis: Application to Clinical Practice, ed. 10. Lippincott Williams & Wilkins, Philadelphia, 2004.
3. Dietary Guidelines for Americans 2005. US Department of Health and Human Services, US Department of Agriculture. Retrieved 6/30/05 from www.healthierus.gov/dietaryguidlines.
4. Hamilton, S: Detecting dehydration and malnutrition in the elderly. Nursing 31:56–57, 2001.
5. Kee, JL, Paulanka, BJ, and Purnell, LD: Handbook of Fluids, Electrolytes and Acid-Base Imbalances, ed. 2. Thompson, Clifton Park, NY, 2004.
6. Munden, J (ed): Professional Guide to Diagnostic Tests. Lippincott Williams and Wilkins, Philadelphia, 2004.
7. Purnell, LD, and Paulanka, BJ: Guide to Culturally Competent Health Care. F.A. Davis, Philadelphia, 2005.
8. Schnell, ZB, Van Leeuwen, AM, and Kranpitz, TR: Davis's Comprehensive Laboratory and Diagnostic Handbook With Nursing Implications. F.A. Davis, Philadelphia, 2003.

SUGGESTED ANSWERS TO

CRITICAL THINKING

■ Mrs. Levitt

1. Check her weight and compare it with her previous weights. Dehydration is associated with weight loss. Monitor mental status for disorientation. Check skin turgor for tenting. Continue to monitor vital signs.
2. Encourage increased fluid intake; notify the RN or physician if Mrs. Levitt is unable to take in additional fluids or if the fluids do not normalize assessment findings.
3. S: "My urine smells bad, and my heart is beating fast."

   O: Pt's urine is dark amber and strong smelling. VS P 98, BP 126/74, RR 20, T 99.2. Fluids encouraged. RN notified.

■ Mr. Peters

1. Raise the head of the bed to assist breathing.
2. Questions to ask might include the following: When

did your symptoms begin? Have you had these symptoms before? (If the patient is too dyspneic to answer, do not ask many questions.)
3. Check breath sounds for crackles, observe for dependent edema and ascites, observe for distended neck veins, assess skin for color and temperature, check weight and compare with previous weight, and monitor I&O.

■ Mrs. Wright

1. The patient is at high risk for osteoporosis, and thus fracture, because she is an elderly, petite, Caucasian woman.
2. Her serum calcium levels would be low or low normal, since the body will mobilize calcium in the bones in an attempt to maintain serum calcium levels.
3. Teach her about consuming foods high in calcium, the need to be compliant with taking her calcium supplements, and to take them 1 to 2 hours after meals for best absorption by the body.

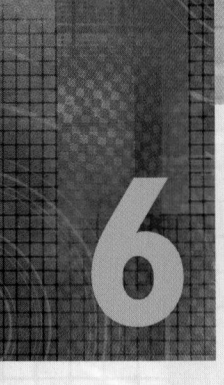

6

Nursing Care of Patients Receiving Intravenous Therapy

LYNN DIANNE PHILLIPS

KEY TERMS

bolus (BOH-lus)
cannula (KAN-yoo-lah)
extravasation (eks-TRA-vah-ZAY-shun)
intravenous (IN-trah-VEE-nus)
phlebitis (fla-BYE-tis)

QUESTIONS TO GUIDE YOUR READING

1. How is the practice of intravenous therapy regulated?

2. What are the indications for intravenous therapy?

3. What factors influence the condition, size, and long-term use of veins?

4. What steps are used for insertion of an intravenous catheter?

5. What techniques can be used for visualization of difficult veins?

6. How will you know if your nursing interventions to prevent complications of intravenous therapy are effective?

7. How will you calculate a drip rate for a patient receiving a parenteral solution?

8. What is the difference between isotonic, hypertonic, and hypotonic solutions?

9. How would you explain the basic differences between central venous access devices: percutaneous catheters, peripherally inserted central catheters, tunneled catheters, and implanted ports?

CASE STUDY

Mrs. Brown, 85 years old, is admitted to the hospital with weight loss of 6% of her total body weight due to gastroenteritis. Her blood pressure is 102/80, pulse is 96 beats per minute, and respirations are 14 per minute. Her physical assessment shows decreased turgor over the sternum, dry, cracked lips, and a weak, thready pulse. The physician has ordered an IV to be started of 5% dextrose and 0.45% sodium chloride at 100 mL per hour. As you read this chapter, reflect on the challenges of fluid volume deficit in the elderly and initiation of infusion therapy.

Intravenous (IV) therapy is the administration of fluids or medication via a needle or catheter (sometimes called a **cannula**) directly into the bloodstream. The practice of IV therapy is governed by state nurse practice acts as statutory laws. Some states now include IV therapy within the licensed practical nurse (LPN) and licensed vocational nurse (LVN) roles. The practice acts define the parameters within which individuals are qualified and licensed to practice nursing in a particular state and serve to codify the nursing obligation to act in the best interest of society.

Various specialty organizations, such as the Infusion Nurses Society (INS, http://www.ins1.org), set forth guidelines for standards of practice for infusion therapy. The Centers for Disease Control and Prevention (CDC, http://www.cdc.gov/niosh/2000-108.html) provides information on needlestick injuries, which can occur during initiation of IV therapy. The Occupational Safety and Health Administration (OSHA, http://www.osha.gov) oversees workplace safety including safety issues related to IV therapy, and the American Society for Parenteral and Enteral Nutrition (ASPEN, http://www.clinnutr.org) provides resources related to IV nutrition.

INDICATIONS FOR INTRAVENOUS THERAPY

Patients receive a variety of substances via IV therapy, including fluids, electrolytes, nutrients, blood products, and medications. Patients can receive life-sustaining fluids, electrolytes, and nutrition when they are unable to eat or drink adequate amounts. The IV route also allows rapid delivery of medication in an emergency. Many medications are faster acting and more effective when given via the IV route. Other medications can be administered continuously via IV to maintain a therapeutic blood level. Patients with anemia or blood loss can receive lifesaving IV transfusions. Patients who are unable to eat for an extended period can have their nutritional needs met with total parenteral nutrition (TPN).

When a patient needs intermittent rather than continuous IV therapy, access to the venous system can be provided by a locking device whereby an IV catheter is inserted and capped with a port or cap that seals after each use. (See the Intermittent Infusion section later in this chapter.) This is to provide access to the bloodstream for intermittent or emergency medications, without the need for continuous fluid infusion.

TYPES OF INFUSIONS

Continuous Infusion

In a continuous infusion, the physician orders the infusion in milliliters (mL) to be delivered over a specific amount of time; for example, 100 mL per hour. The infusion is kept running constantly until discontinued by the physician. An IV controller or roller clamp allows the solution to infuse at a constant rate.

Intermittent Infusion

Intermittent IV lines are "capped off" with an injection port and used only periodically. Thus intermittent IV therapy is administered at prescribed intervals. You must ensure that an intermittent catheter is patent (not occluded with a clot) before injecting a drug or solution. Draw back with a syringe to check for backflow of blood before injection.

Sites that are capped with an injection cap are called saline or heparin locks. A diluted solution of heparin, an anticoagulant, may be used to "flush" the catheter after each use and every 8 hours or according to institution policy. However, many institutions are changing this practice and specifying saline solution for flushes, which is believed to be safer and less costly. In 2000 Standards of Practice,[1] the INS recommends the use of saline (0.9% sodium chloride) solution for maintaining peripheral locking devices, whereas heparin is recommended for central venous access devices. Check your institution's policy for specific guidelines.

Regular flushing ensures catheter patency. Flushing also prevents the mixing of incompatible medications and solutions. Positive pressure must be maintained in the lumen of the catheter during the administration of the flush solution to prevent a backflow of blood into the catheter lumen. This is accomplished by continuing to slowly inject the saline or heparin solution even as the catheter is withdrawn from the cap. Intermittent catheters should be flushed after administration of IV medication, blood sampling, and conversion from continuous to intermittent IV therapy.

If resistance is met while a catheter is being flushed, a clot may be occluding the catheter. Do not exert pressure on the syringe plunger in an attempt to restore patency because doing so may dislodge the clot into the vascular system or rupture the catheter.

Some medications that are given intermittently are not compatible with heparin and therefore are given by the SASH method as follows:

1. Flush with Saline solution.
2. Administer the medication.
3. Flush with Saline solution.
4. Flush with Heparin solution.

---

intravenous: intra—within + venous—vein
cannula: tube or sheath

NURSING CARE TIP

Always check for catheter patency before injecting any substance into the circulatory system.

Bolus

A **bolus** drug (sometimes called an IV push or IVP drug) is
injected slowly via a syringe into the IV site or tubing port.
It provides a rapid effect because it is delivered directly into
the patient's bloodstream. Bolus drugs can be dangerous if
they are given incorrectly, and a drug reference should
always be checked to determine the safe amount of time over
which the drug can be injected. IV push drugs are usually
administered by registered nurses (RNs) and are not within
the scope of practice of the LPN/LVN in many states.
However, you should be aware of the drugs being given so
you can assist in observing the patient for desired or adverse
effects.

Piggy Back/Secondary Infusion

Some IV medications, such as antibiotics, need to be infused
over a short period of time. For example, an antibiotic may
be mixed with 50 mL of dextrose solution and infused over
30 minutes. This may be done as an intermittent infusion, as
described above. If the patient already has a primary continuous IV infusing, the antibiotic (secondary) infusion can be
"piggybacked" into the primary IV line. In order for the piggyback medication to infuse, it must hang higher than the
primary infusion (Fig. 6.1). Piggyback medications can be
infused using either gravity or a controller. The medication
in the piggyback must be compatible with any other solution
that is in the primary IV tubing.

METHODS OF INFUSION

Gravity Drip

Gravity can be used to drip a solution into a vein (see Fig.
6.1). The solution is positioned about 3 feet above the infusion site. If it is positioned too high above the patient, the
infusion may run too fast. Positioned too low, it may run too
slowly. Flow is controlled with a roller, screw, or slide
clamp. A mechanical flow device can be added to achieve
accurate delivery of fluid with minimal deviation.

Calculating Drip Rates

When using a gravity set, the nurse must calculate the drops
(gtt, L. *guttae*) required per minute to deliver fluid at the
ordered rate. Commercial parenteral administration sets vary
in the number of drops delivering 1 mL. Sets typically
deliver 10, 15, 20, or 60 drops per milliliter of fluid. For
example, to deliver 100 mL per hour using a set with 10-drop
factor tubing, a flow rate of 17 drops per minute is necessary.

bolus: mass or lump

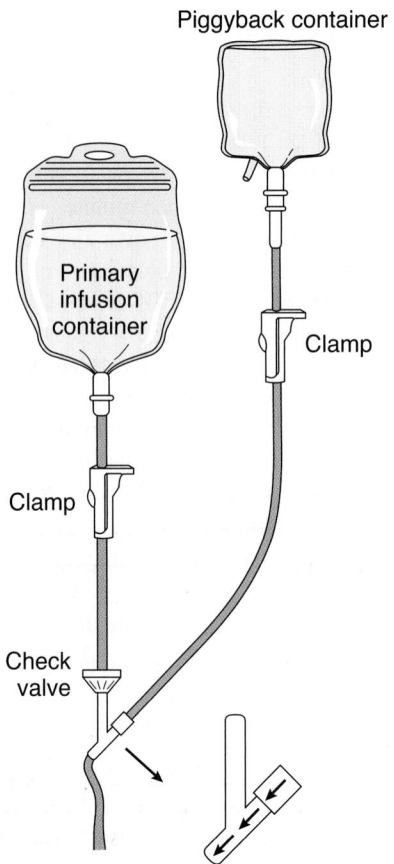

FIGURE 6.1 Gravity drip setup with piggyback infusion.

To administer the same amount using a set with 15-drop factor tubing, a flow rate of 25 drops per minute is necessary.
Check the label on the administration set to determine how
many drops per milliliter (drop factor) are delivered by the
set. Sets delivering 10, 15, or 20 drops per minute are called
macrodrip sets, and are used for fluids that need to be infused
more quickly. Sets delivering 60 drops per milliliter are
called minidrip or microdrip sets and are used for solutions
that need to be infused more slowly.

　　To determine drops per minute of an IV solution, the
nurse needs to know the amount of fluid to be given in a
specified time interval and the drop factor of the administration set to be used. The formula for determining drops per
minute is as follows:

mL	1 hr	gtt	= gtt per minute
hr or hrs	60 min	1 mL	

If a controller or pump is being used, the calculation is even
easier:

$$\frac{\text{Total mL}}{\text{Total number of hours}} = \text{mL per hour}$$

Sample problems:
Order:　　　Zinacef 1 g in D5W 100 mL over 1 hour
Drop factor:　　10 gtt/mL

$$\frac{100\ mL}{1\ hr} \cdot \frac{1\ hr}{60\ min} \cdot \frac{10\ gtt}{1\ mL} = 16.66\ or\ 17\ gtt\ per\ minute$$

Order: Normal saline 1000 mL over 8 hours

$$\frac{1000\ mL}{8\ hours} = 125\ mL\ per\ hour$$

Factors Affecting Flow Rates

CHANGE IN CATHETER POSITION. A change in the catheter's position may push the bevel either against the wall of the vein, which will decrease the flow rate, or away from the wall of the vein, which may increase the flow rate. Careful taping and avoidance of joint flexion above the site minimizes this problem. Patients may need to be reminded to keep flexion to a minimum when an IV is placed near a joint.

HEIGHT OF THE SOLUTION. Because infusions flow by gravity, a change in the height of the infusion bag or bottle or a change in the level of the bed can increase or decrease the flow rate. The flow rate increases as the distance between the solution and the patient increases. A patient may alter the flow rate greatly simply by standing up. The ideal height for a solution is 3 feet above the level of the heart.

PATENCY OF THE CATHETER. A small clot or fibrin sheath may occlude the catheter lumen and decrease or stop the flow rate. Clot formation can result from irritation, increased venous pressure, or backup of blood into the line. Avoid use of a blood pressure cuff on the affected extremity because of the resulting transient increase in venous pressure. A regular flush schedule helps maintain patency. NEVER exert pressure with a saline or heparin flush in an attempt to restore patency; doing so may dislodge a clot into the vascular system or rupture the catheter.

Electronic Control Devices

Electronic pumps and controllers regulate the rate of infusion (Fig. 6.2). Controllers measure the amount of solution delivered and depend on gravity to deliver the infusion. Pumps use positive pressure to deliver the solution. Pumps are often used for central lines to help overcome the high pressure of the central circulation.

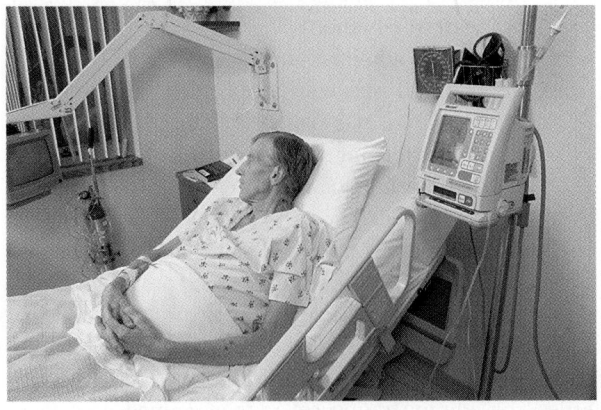

FIGURE 6.2 Infusion pump.

Pumps and controllers are used for the infusion of precise volumes of solution. Institution policy often dictates use of controllers for infusion of potent medications, such as heparin, concentrated morphine, and chemotherapy solutions, and for very fast or slow rates. Some electronic infusion devices are portable and are designed to be worn on the body. These are called ambulatory infusion devices. It is important to know the type of pump being used and its manufacturer's guidelines.

Filters

It is recommended by the Infusion Nursing Standards of Practice that filters be used routinely for the delivery of IV therapy. Filters fit onto the IV tubing between the solution and the insertion site and remove contaminants from the IV fluid. A 0.22-μm filter removes bacteria and fungi from IV fluids. Check institution policy and manufacturers' guidelines for use of filters.

TYPES OF FLUIDS

Fluids and electrolytes administered intravenously pass directly into the plasma space of the extracellular fluid compartment. They are then absorbed based on the characteristics of the fluid and the hydration status of the patient. The most commonly infused fluids are dextrose and sodium solutions. These are called crystalloid solutions.

Dextrose Solutions

Dextrose in water is available in many concentrations and provides carbohydrates in a readily usable form. Solutions of 2.5%, 5%, and 10% dextrose in water are used for continuous peripheral infusions. Concentrations of 20% and above must be given into a large vein and are infused via a central line. These high concentrations can be used for treating hypoglycemia or in combination with TPN because they supply a large number of calories.

Sodium Chloride Solutions

Sodium chloride solutions are available in concentrations of 0.25%, 0.33%, 0.45%, 0.9% (normal saline), 3%, and 5%. Combination dextrose and sodium chloride solutions, such as 5% dextrose with 0.45% sodium chloride (often referred to as "D5 and a half"), are commonly used.

Electrolyte Solutions

Electrolyte solutions are used to replace lost fluids and electrolytes. Lactated Ringer's solution is an example of a premixed electrolyte solution. Potassium is an electrolyte that is commonly added to a solution to replace deficits. Potassium is limited to 10 to 20 mEq per hour and is never administered as an IV bolus because of the risk of cardiac complications and death with rapid infusion.

Tonicity of IV Solutions

Intravenous fluids may be classified as isotonic, hypotonic, or hypertonic. (See Chapter 5 to review these concepts.)

Isotonic fluids have the same concentration of solutes to water as body fluids. Hypertonic solutions have more solutes (i.e., are more concentrated) than body fluids. Hypotonic solutions have fewer solutes (i.e., are less concentrated) than body fluids. Water moves from areas of lesser concentration to areas of greater concentration. Therefore, hypotonic solutions send water into areas of greater concentration (cells), and hypertonic solutions pull water from the more highly concentrated cells.

Isotonic Solutions

Normal saline (0.9% sodium chloride) solution is an isotonic solution that has the same tonicity as body fluid. When administered to a patient requiring water, it neither enters cells nor pulls water from cells; it therefore expands the extracellular fluid volume. A solution of 5% dextrose in water (D5W) is also isotonic when infused, but the dextrose is quickly metabolized, making the solution hypotonic.

Hypotonic Solutions — *draws out into cells*

Hypotonic fluids are used when fluid is needed to enter the cells, as in the patient with cellular dehydration. They are also used as fluid maintenance therapy. An example of a hypotonic solution is 0.45% sodium chloride solution.

Hypertonic Solutions — *pulling back into blood stream*

Examples of hypertonic solutions include 5% dextrose in 0.9% sodium chloride and 5% dextrose in lactated Ringer's solution. Hypertonic solutions are used to expand the plasma volume, as in the hypovolemic patient. They are also used to replace electrolytes.

INTRAVENOUS ACCESS

Intravenous therapy can be administered into the systemic circulation via the peripheral or central veins. Peripheral veins lie beneath the epidermis, dermis, and subcutaneous tissue of the skin. They usually provide easy access to the venous system. Central veins are located close to the heart. Special catheters that end in a large vessel near the heart are called central lines. This chapter primarily discusses peripheral catheters. The definitions of the various central venous access devices are discussed briefly at the end of the chapter.

ADMINISTERING PERIPHERAL INTRAVENOUS THERAPY

Starting a Peripheral Line

The Phillips 15-step approach to starting a peripheral line offers an organized and thorough method, as described in Table 6.1. Remember to always check your institution's policy before performing any procedure.

Check Physician's Order

A physician's order is necessary to initiate IV therapy. According to the INS, a prescriber's verbal order written by a nurse in the medical record in a hospital setting should be

TABLE 6.1 PHILLIPS 15-STEP METHOD FOR STARTING A PERIPHERAL LINE

Phase	Step
Precatheterization (preparation)	1. Check physician's order.
	2. Wash your hands for 15 to 20 seconds.
	3. Prepare the equipment.
	4. Assess the patient.
Catheterization (venipuncture)	5. Select the site and dilate the vein.
	6. Select the needle (catheter).
	7. Put on gloves.
	8. Prepare the site.
	9. Enter the vein using the direct or indirect method.
	10. Stabilize the catheter with tape, and apply a dressing.
Postcatheterization (cleanup)	11. Label the site, tubing, and bag.
	12. Properly dispose of used equipment.
	13. Educate the patient.
	14. Calculate the drip rate, if applicable.
	15. Document the procedure.

Source: Phillips, L: Manual of IV Therapeutics, ed. 4. F.A. Davis, Philadelphia, 2005.

signed by the prescriber within an appropriate time (according to institution policy). The order should include solution, volume, rate, and route. If medication is ordered, the order should also include the medication, dosage, and frequency.

Wash Hands

Before beginning the procedure, wash your hands for 15 to 20 seconds. Wear gloves when inserting the catheter and any time you have a risk of exposure to body fluid.

Gather Equipment

Obtain the following equipment and inspect it for integrity:
- Clean gloves
- Prepping solution (70% isopropyl alcohol, povidone-iodine [Betadine], or chlorhexidine)
- Sterile 2-inch by 2-inch gauze pads
- $1/_2$-inch or 1-inch tape
- Disposable latex (or nonlatex, in the case of allergy) tourniquet
- Catheters (over-the-needle sizes 18, 20, 22, and 24 are the most common)
- Appropriate administration set
- IV solution (inspected for puncture holes, visible contamination, and expiration date)
- prn device (locking device) if the catheter is maintained as a saline lock
- IV pole if needed

Some institutions have IV start kits that contain a tourniquet, gloves, alcohol, bandages, and prepping solution.

Once the solution is verified and inspected for integrity, the administration set is spiked to puncture the solution bag or bottle, taking care to keep the spike and the bag opening sterile. The administration set is then primed with the IV solution ordered by the physician.

PATIENT SAFETY TIP

Comply with current Centers for Disease Control and Prevention (CDC) hand hygiene guidelines (2006 National Patient Safety Goals from www.jcaho.org).

The CDC recommends the following for hand hygiene[2]: Decontaminate hands after removing gloves

- Before eating and after using a restroom, wash hands with a nonantimicrobial soap and water or with antimicrobial soap and water.
- Antimicrobial-impregnated wipes may be considered as an alternative to washing hands with nonantimicrobial soap and water.
- When using an alcohol-based hand gel, apply product to palm of one hand and rub hands together, covering all surfaces of hands and fingers until hands are dry.

Assess and Prepare Patient

Several factors should be considered before venipuncture. The type of solution, condition of vein, duration of therapy, catheter size needed, patient age, patient activity, presence of disease or previous surgery, presence of a dialysis shunt or graft, medications being taken by the patient (such as anticoagulants), and allergies must be assessed before a venipuncture. Provide privacy for the procedure, explain the procedure to the patient, and evaluate the patient's knowledge of the procedure by talking with the patient before assessing the upper arms for suitable venipuncture sites.

Select Site and Dilate Vein

Proper vein selection is important to accommodate the prescribed therapy and to minimize potential complications (Box 6.1 Considerations for Vein Selection). Avoid use of an arm on the side where the patient has had a mastectomy, has a dialysis access site, or is scheduled for a surgical procedure. The patient's condition and diagnosis, age, vein condition, size, location, and type and duration of therapy should

Box 6.1

Considerations for Vein Selection

- Age of patient
- Availability of sites
- Size of catheter to be used
- Purpose of infusion therapy
- Osmolarity of solution to be infused
- Volume, rate, and length of infusion
- Degree of mobility desired

Box 6.2

General Considerations When Initiating Intravenous Therapy

1. Use veins in the upper part of the body.
2. When multiple sticks are anticipated, make the first venipuncture distally and work proximal with subsequent punctures.
3. If therapy will be prescribed for longer than 3 weeks, a long-term access device should be considered.
4. Avoid using venipunctures in affected arms of patients with radical mastectomies or a dialysis access site.
5. If possible, avoid taking a blood pressure on the arm receiving an infusion because the cuff interferes with blood flow and forces blood back into the catheter. This may cause a clot or cause the vein or catheter to rupture.
6. No more than two attempts should be made at venipuncture before getting help.
7. Immobilizers should not be placed on or above an infusion site.

be considered before initiation of intravenous therapy (Box 6.2 General Considerations When Initiating Intravenous Therapy). The vein should be able to accommodate the gauge and length of catheter used.

Hand veins are used first if long-term intravenous therapy is expected (Box 6.3 Cultural Considerations). This allows each successive venipuncture to be made proximal to the site of the previous one, which eliminates the passage of irritating fluids through a previously injured vein and discourages leakage through old puncture sites. Hand veins can be used successfully for most hydrating solutions, but they are best avoided when irritating solutions of potassium or antibiotics are anticipated.

Vein size must also be considered. Small veins do not tolerate large volumes of fluid, high infusion rates, or irritating solutions. Large veins should be used for these purposes. Figure 6.3 shows peripheral veins that may be used for IV therapy.

If veins are constricted, venipuncture is more difficult. Fever, anxiety, and cold temperatures can cause veins to

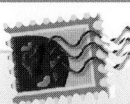

Box 6.3

Cultural Considerations

Among the Vietnamese, the head is considered sacred. Thus, the practice of starting IV lines in the scalp may cause a Vietnamese patient significant anxiety. Consider other sites first. If the patient must have an IV line in the scalp, carefully explain why it is necessary.

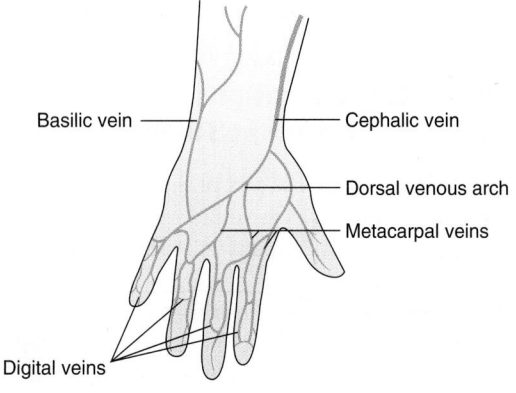

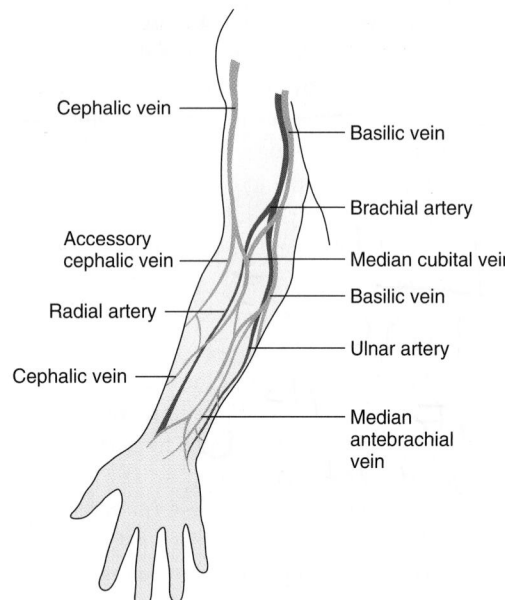

FIGURE 6.3 Peripheral veins used for IV therapy. (Modified from Phillips, L: Manual of IV therapeutics [4th ed.]. FA Davis, Philadelphia, 2005.)

constrict. Smoking before the insertion of an IV line also causes veins to constrict.

DILATE VEIN. A tourniquet helps to dilate and stabilize the vein, easing venipuncture and threading of the catheter. Place the tourniquet 6 to 8 inches above the insertion site. If the tourniquet is too close to the insertion site, it will create

NURSING CARE TIP

Many patients know from experience that their veins are difficult to access. Asking the patient for his or her "best vein" may decrease the number of attempts prior to successful IV catheterization. In addition, when selecting a hand vein, consider avoiding the patient's dominant hand to avoid possible accidental patient removal of the IV.

too much pressure and cause the vein to burst. The tourniquet should be tight enough to impede venous flow while maintaining arterial flow. A tourniquet should be at least 1 inch wide and should not be left on for more than 3 minutes to prevent impaired blood flow to the extremity.

Occasionally, additional techniques are necessary to distend the vein. Placing the arm in a dependent position or placing a warm towel over the site for several minutes before applying the tourniquet help to dilate a vein. The whole extremity must be warmed to improve blood flow to the area. Opening and closing the fist pumps blood to the extremity and increases blood flow to help dilate the vein. A blood pressure cuff inflated to 30 mm Hg is an appropriate method for vein dilation, especially with fragile veins in the elderly. Box 6.4 (Techniques for Patients with Difficult Venous Access) lists additional tips for difficult to find veins.

NURSING CARE TIP

Use a tourniquet only once. Using the same tourniquet on more than one patient can result in cross contamination. Tourniquets may be sources of latex exposure; use a nonlatex tourniquet or blood pressure cuff technique for patients with latex allergy.

Choose the Catheter
Needles have been largely replaced with flexible plastic catheters that are inserted over a needle (Fig. 6.4B). The needle (or stylet) is removed after the catheter is in place. These are available in a variety of sizes (gauges) and lengths. For patient comfort, choose the smallest gauge catheter that will work for the intended purpose. Use smaller gauge catheters (20 to 24 gauge) for fluids and slow infusion rates. Use larger catheters (18 gauge) for rapid fluid administration and viscous solutions such as blood. Also consider vein size when choosing a catheter gauge. Refer to institution policy and equipment stock for specific recommendations. Keep in mind that the INS recommends that short peripheral catheters be removed every 72 hours and immediately upon suspected contamination.

Gloves
The CDC recommends following standard precautions whenever exposure to blood or body fluids is likely. Wearing latex or vinyl gloves provides basic protection from blood and body fluids.

Prepare the Site
Clean the peripheral insertion site with an antimicrobial solution before catheter placement. If the patient's skin is dirty, wash it with soap and water before applying the antimicrobial solution. If the patient has excess hair, it can be clipped with scissors. Be sure to follow institution policy when choosing a solution. Most institutions use an alcohol-

Box 6.4

Techniques for Patients with Difficult Venous Access

Altered Skin Integrity (Lesions, Burns, or Disease Process)
- Use indirect light (tangential lighting)
- Do not flatten veins or cause damage to skin
- Use light directed toward the side of patient's extremity to illuminate the blue veins (*Note*: also can be used on dark-skinned individuals.)

Hard sclerosed vessels (related to disease process, personal misuse, frequent drug therapy)
- Assess for collateral circulation.
- Use multiple tourniquet technique to increase oncotic pressure inside the tissue, forcing small vessels of periphery to be visualized.
  - Place one tourniquet high on arm for 2 minutes and leave in place; stroke downward toward hand.
  - After 2 minutes, place a second tourniquet at mid arm just below the antecutital fossa; leave along with first tourniquet for 2 minutes
  - This should bring peripheral veins into view; if necessary, place a third tourniquet at wrist.
  - Do not leave on more than 6 minutes total.

Obesity or Edema
- Use 2-inch catheter
- Use multiple tourniquet technique
- Displace edema to side to visualize veins

Source: Phillips, LD: Manual of IV Therapeutics, ed. 4. F.A. Davis, Philadelphia, 2005.

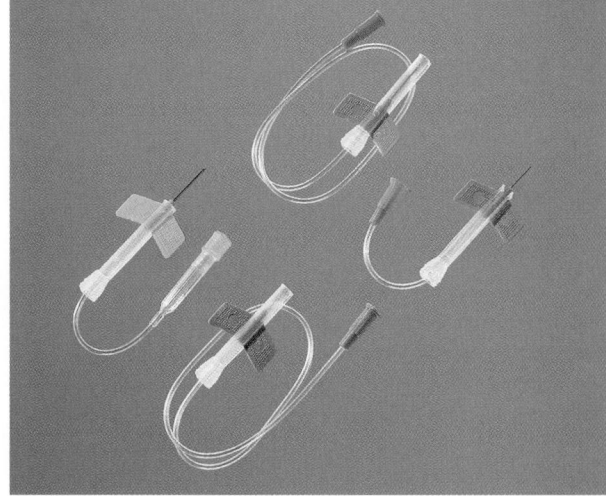

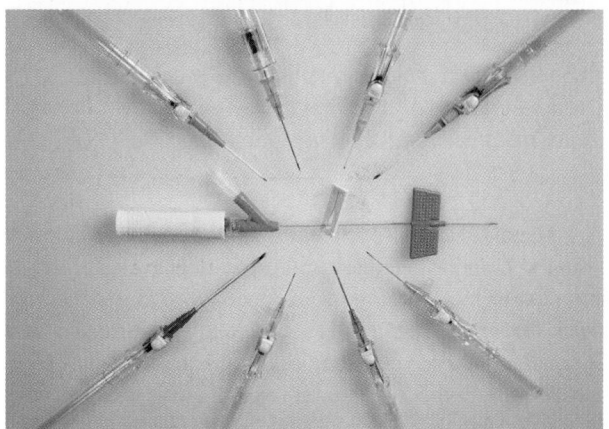

FIGURE 6.4 (A) SAF-T EZ set IV needles. (B) BD IV Safety Catheters. *(Courtesy Becton Dickinson, Franklin Lakes, N.J.)*

or iodine-based product. A newer preparation called ChloraPrep (Medi-Flex Hospital Products, Inc., Leawood, KS) is a chlorhexidine preparation solution that does not stain the skin or cause the irritation to the skin that Betadine products can. Avoid using alcohol after an antimicrobial preparation because alcohol negates the anti-infective action of the prep agent.

Apply the solution in a circular motion, starting at the intended site and working outward to clean an area 2 to 3 inches in diameter. If alcohol is used, it should be applied with friction for at least 30 seconds or until the final applicator is visually clean. Blotting of excess solution at the insertion site is not recommended. Allow the solution to air dry completely.

Insert the Catheter

Venipuncture can be performed using a direct (one-step) or indirect (two-step) method. The direct method is appropriate for small-gauge catheters, fragile hand veins, or rolling veins. The indirect method can be used for all venipunctures.

Hold the catheter with the bevel (slanted opening) of the needle facing up. With the tourniquet in place, enter the vein using either the direct or indirect approach. When using

the direct entry approach, hold the needle at a 30- to 45-degree angle directly above the vein and then penetrate the skin and vein in one motion (Fig. 6.5). When using some newer catheters, the angle of insertion is minimal.

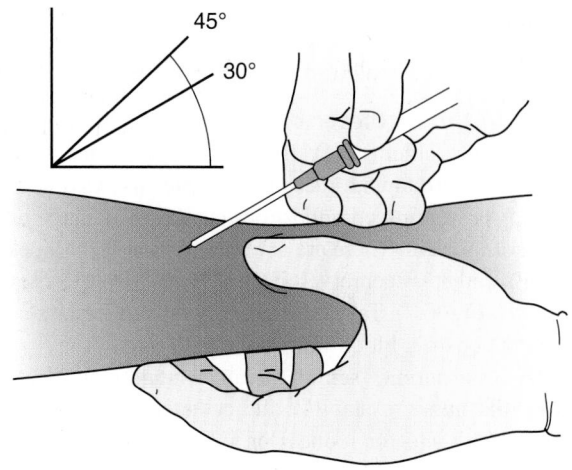

FIGURE 6.5 Insert the needle of choice bevel up at a 30- to 45-degree angle, depending on the vein location and catheter.

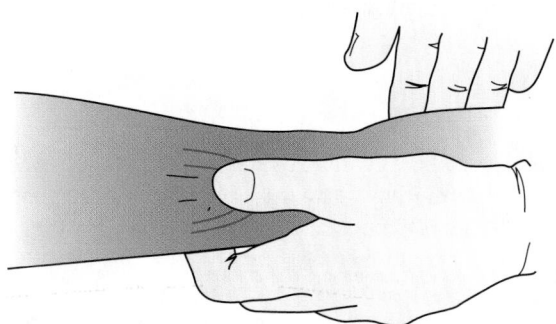

FIGURE 6.6 Pull skin below the intended puncture site using a downward motion to stabilize the skin and prevent the vein from rolling.

 NURSING CARE TIP

Use traction (a downward pulling motion to make the skin taut below the puncture site) before venipuncture to stabilize the skin and prevent the vein from rolling during venipuncture (Fig. 6.6).

The indirect approach may help decrease vein collapse. To use it, hold the needle at a 30- to 45-degree angle over the skin next to (not over) the vein. Once the skin is punctured, lower the needle angle and locate and puncture the vein. Depending on the type of device used, a small flash of blood may be seen in the tubing or at the hub of the catheter when the needle is in the vein. The angle of the needle is then lowered so that it is parallel with the skin as it is threaded into the lumen of the vein. If a catheter-over-needle device is used, the needle is advanced $^1/_4$ inch and then the catheter is advanced for its remaining length as the metal needle (stylet) is withdrawn.

The tourniquet is then released, and the IV solution or injection cap is connected to the hub of the catheter. Blood may ooze from the hub at this time. If an injection cap is being used, the catheter is flushed with 0.9% sodium chloride solution to check for patency. A smooth, easy flush and no signs of infiltration indicate that the catheter is patent and that the prescribed solution can be administered.

Stabilize the Catheter and Dress the Site

A common problem in IV therapy is dislodgement of the catheter. Secure taping keeps the catheter in place and stable, thus preventing complications caused by damage to the intima of the vein. There are several different techniques for taping a catheter securely, including the U, H, and chevron methods (Fig. 6.7). Take care to apply tape in a manner that does not constrict blood flow to the extremity.

A transparent, semipermeable membrane dressing allows the nurse to stabilize the catheter and monitor the venipuncture site for redness or swelling and provides an occlusive dressing for the site. Another acceptable method of dressing management is the use of sterile 2-inch by

U Method	H Method	Chevron Method
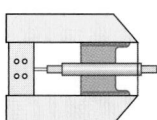		
Use for Winged Set	**Use for Winged Set**	**Use for Winged Set**
1. Cut three strips of 1/2-in tape. With sticky side up, place one strip under tubing.	1. Cut three strips of 1-in tape.	1. Cover the venipuncture with transparent dressing or 2 x 2 gauze dressing.
2. Bring each side of the tape up, folding it over the wings of the needle. Press it down, parallel with the tubing.	2. Place one strip of tape over each wing, keeping the tape parallel with the needle.	2. Cut a long 5- to 6-in strip of 1/2-in tape. Place one strip of tape, sticky side under hub, parallel with the dressing.
3. Loop the tubing and secure it with a piece of 1-in tape.	3. Place another strip of tape perpendicular to the first two. Place over the wings to stabilize wings and hub.	3. Cross the end of the tape over the opposite side of the needle so that the tape sticks to the patient's skin.
		4. Apply a piece of 1-in tape across the wings of the chevron. Loop the tubing and secure it with another piece of 1-in tape.

* For all methods, include on the last piece of tape the date, time and insertion, size of gauge, length of needle or catheter, and your initials.

FIGURE 6.7 Taping techniques for IV access devices. *(Modified from Phillips, L: Manual of IV therapeutics [4th ed.]. FA Davis, Philadelphia, 2005.)*

2-inch gauze over the venipuncture site and a piece of 1-inch tape over the gauze. Band-Aids are not acceptable dressings over catheters.

Arm boards are not used routinely. However, if a confused patient places the IV site in danger, the extremity can be immobilized as a last resort; this requires a physician's order.

Label the Site

The IV setup should be labeled in three areas: the insertion site, the tubing, and the solution container. Once the venipuncture procedure is completed, label the setup with the date, time, catheter type and size, and your initials.

Dispose of Equipment

All needles, catheters, and blood-contaminated equipment should be disposed of according to institution policy in a tamper-proof, nonpermeable container.

Educate the Patient

Patients have the right to receive information on all aspects of their care in a manner they can understand. They also have the right to accept or refuse treatment. Explain the rationale for the IV therapy that has been ordered. Explain your actions as you start the IV, and be sure the patient understands how to protect the site and problems to report.

Calculate Drip Rate

All IV infusions should be monitored frequently for accurate flow rates and complications associated with infusion therapy. (See the section on calculating drip rates earlier in this chapter.)

Document

Document your actions and the patient's response in the medical record according to institution policy. All IV solutions are also documented on the medication administration record. Include the following:

- Date and time of insertion
- Manufacturer's brand name and style of device
- Gauge and length of the device
- Location of the accessed vein
- Solution infusing and rate of flow
- Method of infusion (gravity or pump)
- Number of attempts needed for a successful IV start
- Patient's response and specific comments related to the procedure
- Signature

CRITICAL THINKING

Mrs. Green

■ Mrs. Green is admitted with a diagnosis of symptomatic anemia and has an atrioventricular (AV) dialysis shunt in her left arm. An IV line is ordered for administration of 2 units of packed red blood cells. What must be taken into consideration when assessing Mrs. Green for an appropriate venipuncture site?

Suggested answers at end of chapter.

NURSING PROCESS FOR THE PATIENT RECEIVING IV THERAPY

Assessment/Data Collection

A patient receiving IV therapy is assessed routinely. IV therapy is a medical intervention, and the nurse is responsible primarily for appropriate monitoring, documenting, and reporting related to the therapeutic goals. Some institution policies require assessment as often as every hour. Assessment should be systematic and thorough. It begins with observation and evaluation of the patient for signs of fluid imbalance. This is especially important when caring for an older patient (Box 6.5 Gerontological Issues). Daily weights and measurement of intake and output help determine whether the patient is retaining too much fluid. Skin turgor, mucous membrane moisture, vital signs, and level of consciousness also indicate hydration status. New onset of fine crackles in the lungs can indicate fluid retention. Table 6.2 lists other symptoms of complications, along with prevention and treatment strategies.

Inspect the site for redness or swelling, evaluate the integrity of the dressing, and document your findings. Inspect the tubing to ensure tight connections and the absence of kinks or defects. Inspect the solution container and compare it with the physician's order for type, amount, and rate. Report complications to the RN or physician.

Nursing Diagnosis, Planning, and Implementation

Priority nursing diagnoses for IV-related issues include:
Fear related to insertion of catheter

EXPECTED OUTCOME: *The patient will be able to cooperate with the procedure; patient will verbalize minimal fear.*

- Explain the IV therapy to the patient. *Lack of knowledge is associated with fear.*

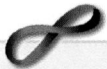

Box 6.5

Gerontological Issues

Care of the Older Adult Receiving Intravenous Therapy

When an older patient is receiving IV fluids, the nurse must regularly assess the patient for potential fluid volume excess. Symptoms of fluid volume excess include:

- elevated blood pressure.
- increasing weight.
- full bounding pulse.
- shallow but rapid respirations.
- jugular-venous distention.
- increased urine output.
- development of moist crackles in the lungs.

If these signs are present:
- Immediately notify the RN or turn down the IV to a minimum drip rate (1 mL per minute); do not discontinue the IV because the physician may want to administer IV diuretics.
- Position the patient to maximize lung expansion.
- Check peripheral oxygen saturation with an oximeter.
- Apply oxygen by mask or nasal cannula if indicated and per institution guidelines.
- Closely monitor patient's vital signs, level of consciousness, and oxygen saturation along with fluid output.
- Assist the physician or RN with IV push administration of diuretic medication such as furosemide if ordered.

TABLE 6.2 COMPLICATIONS OF PERIPHERAL IV THERAPY

Local Complications of IV Therapy

Complication	Signs and Symptoms	Treatment	Prevention
Hematoma	Ecchymoses Swelling Inability to advance catheter Resistance during flushing	Remove catheter Apply pressure with 2×2 Elevate extremity	Use indirect method of venipuncture Apply tourniquet just before venipuncture
Thrombosis	Slowed or stopped infusion Fever/malaise Inability to flush catheter	Discontinue catheter Apply cold compress to site Assess for circulatory impairment	Use pumps Choose microdrip sets with gravity flow if rate is below 50 mL/hr Avoid flexion areas
Phlebitis	Redness at site Site warm to touch Local swelling Pain Palpable cord Sluggish infusion rate	Discontinue catheter Apply cold compress initially; then warm Consult physician if severe	Use larger veins for hypertonic solutions Choose smallest catheter appropriate Use good hand hygiene Add buffer to irritating solutions Change solutions and containers every 24 hr Rotate infusion sites every 72–96 hours
Infiltration (Extravasation)	Coolness of skin at site Taut skin Dependent edema Backflow of blood absent Infusion rate slowing	Discontinue catheter Apply cool compress Elevate extremity slightly Follow extravasation guidelines Have antidote available	Stabilize catheter Place catheter in appropriate site Avoid antecubital fossa
Local Infection	Redness and swelling at site Possible exudate Increase WBC count Elevated T lymphocytes	Discontinue catheter and culture site and catheter Apply sterile dressing over site Administer antibiotics if ordered	Inspect all solutions Use sterile technique during venipuncture and site maintenance
Venous Spasm	Sharp pain at site Slowing of infusion	Apply warm compress to site Restart infusion in new site if spasm continues	Take thorough history Verify allergies Use proper patient identification Warm solutions with appropriate warming device if appropriate.

Systemic Complication of Peripheral IV Therapy

Complication	Signs and Symptoms	Treatment	Prevention
Septicemia	Fluctuating temperature Profuse sweating Nausea/vomiting Diarrhea Abdominal pain Tachycardia Hypotension Altered mental status	Restart new IV system Obtain cultures Notify physician Initiate antimicrobial therapy as ordered Monitor patient closely	Use good hand hygiene Carefully inspect fluids Use Luer-Loks Cover infusion sites with appropriate dressings Follow standards of practice related to rotation of sites/hang time of infusions Use appropriate preparation solutions
Fluid Overload	Weight gain Puffy eyelids Edema Hypertension Changes in input and output (I&O) Rise in central venous pressure (CVP) Shortness of breath Crackles in lungs Distended neck veins	Decrease IV flow rate Place patient in high Fowler's position Keep patient warm Monitor vital signs Administer oxygen Use microdrip set or controller	Monitor infusion Maintain flow at prescribed rate Monitor I&O Know patient's cardiovascular history Do not "catch up" infusion if behind schedule
Air Embolism	Lightheadedness Dyspnea, cyanosis, tachypnea, expiratory wheezes, cough Mill wheel murmur, chest pain, hypotension Changes in mental status Coma	Call for help! Place patient in Trendelenburg's position Administer oxygen Monitor vital signs Notify physician	Remove all air from administration sets Use Luer-Loks Attach piggyback to appropriate port

Complications	Signs and Symptoms	Treatment	Prevention
Speed Shock	Dizziness Facial flushing Headache Tightness in chest Hypotension Irregular pulse Progression of shock	Call for help! Give antidote or resuscitation medications	Reduce the size of drops by using microdrip set Use electronic infusion device (EID) Monitor infusion sites Dilute IV push mediations if possible, give slowly
Catheter Embolism	Sharp sudden pain at IV site Rough, uneven catheter noted on removal Chest pain Tachycardia	Apply tourniquet above elbow Contact physician Start new IV Measure remainder of catheter	Use radiopaque catheters! Do not apply pressure over site. Avoid joint flexions. Never reinsert stylet that has been removed from sheath

Source: Adapted from Phillips, LD: IV Notes. Philadelphia F.A. Davis, 2005, Table 9–9, pp. 396–398.

- Insertion procedure
- Rationale for IV therapy
- Care of the IV
- Importance of reporting pain or swelling, or pump alarm
- Use techniques to minimize discomfort. *Pain may increase fear.*

Impaired physical mobility related to placement and maintenance of IV catheter

EXPECTED OUTCOME: The patient will experience minimal inability to move; the patient will not experience complications related to immobility.

- Use insertion site away from joints if at all possible. *Joint areas are mobile and it will be difficult to maintain an intact site.*
- If you must use a mobile site, such as the antecubital fossa or wrist area, immobilize with arm board or gauze wrapping *to reduce catheter movement.*
- If site must be wrapped, be sure to leave insertion site visible or remove dressing to view site according to agency policy. *The site must still be visualized for complications even if it is covered.*
- Assist patient with activities of daily living (ADLs). *The patient may have difficulty with ADLs if movement is limited.*

Risk of infection related to broken skin or traumatized tissue

EXPECTED OUTCOME: The patient will be free from infection as evidence by no redness, swelling, or purulence at IV insertion site, no fever, and normal white cell count.

- Monitor for signs of infection so the IV can be changed and infection treated quickly if it occurs
- Use good handwashing and strict aseptic techniques during catheter insertion to prevent introduction of pathogens.
- Change catheter, tubing, and solutions regularly according to agency policy *to prevent growth of microorganisms.*

Evaluation

The RN is responsible for evaluation and thus monitors the patient for evidence that the goals of therapy are being met

and that complications are avoided. The LPN/LVN collects data that contribute to the evaluation. For example, if antibiotic therapy is administered, monitor the patient's temperature and other signs that the infection is resolving. If IV therapy is ordered to correct dehydration, monitor skin turgor, vital signs, and other appropriate signs of improved fluid balance. Document all findings and report them to the RN.

CRITICAL THINKING

Mr. Rick

■ Mr. Rick's IV has blood backed up in the tubing. When you open the clamp to increase the flow, nothing happens. What should you do?

Suggested answer at end of chapter.

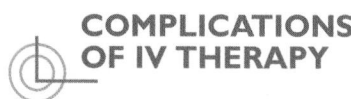

COMPLICATIONS OF IV THERAPY

See Table 6.2 for complications, their prevention, and treatment. Any complication or unusual incident should be reported to the physician, and an incident report should be prepared according to institution policy. This applies to the hospital and the home situation.

CRITICAL THINKING

Mrs. Gonzalez

■ Mrs. Gonzalez is receiving 5% dextrose in water at 83 mL per hour. One hour after the infusion starts, she complains of pain at the site. The site is cool to the touch and swollen, and the infusion rate is sluggish.

1. What might be happening?
2. How do you further assess the patient?
3. What action do you take?
4. How should you document your findings?

Suggested answers at end of chapter.

⊕ ALTERNATIVE ACCESS ROUTES

The role of the LPN/LVN in central venous access in most states is limited to assisting the RN with assessments. It is important for you to be able to recognize the different central venous access devices.

Central Venous Catheters

Central venous catheters terminate in the superior vena cava near the heart (Fig. 6.8). They are used when peripheral sites are inadequate or when large amounts of fluid or irritating medication must be given. Central catheter devices include a percutaneous catheter, peripherally inserted central catheter (PICC), tunneled catheter, and implanted port. These devices can have one, two, or three lumens in the catheter or one or more port chambers. Each lumen exits the site in a separate line, called a tail. Multilumen catheters allow for the administration of incompatible solutions at the same time.

Be careful not to confuse a central catheter with a dialysis catheter. Dialysis catheters should be used only for dialysis and not for IV therapy, and should be accessed only by physicians or specially trained dialysis nurses.

Percutaneous Central Catheter

A percutaneous central catheter is inserted by a physician into the jugular or subclavian vein. After insertion, correct placement is determined by x-ray before the catheter is used. These short-term central venous catheters may remain in place up to several weeks, but usual placement time is 7

days. These catheters are inserted at the bedside and are cost effective for short-term central venous access in the acute care setting.

hands, Brachial

Peripherally Inserted Central Catheter (PICC)

A PICC line is a long catheter that is inserted in the arm and terminates in the central circulation. This device is used when therapy will last more than 2 weeks or the medication is too caustic for peripheral administration. Specially trained RNs insert PICC lines. They can be left in place for long periods, minimizing the trauma of frequent IV insertions. Consult with a physician if long-term therapy is anticipated.

It is important to follow the manufacturer's recommended guidelines for flushing the catheter and to be aware of your institution's policy. An RN removes the PICC or midline catheter when therapy is terminated. An LPN/LVN may assist the RN with this procedure if the state nursing practice act permits.

Tunneled Catheters

Central venous tunneled catheters (CVTCs) are intended for use for months to years to provide long-term venous access. CVTCs are composed of polymeric silicone with a Dacron polyester cuff that anchors the catheter in place subcutaneously. The catheter tip is placed in the superior vena cava.

Advantages of a CVTC are that a break or tear in a catheter is easy to repair, and they can be used for many purposes. Disadvantages include weekly site care, cost of maintenance supplies, and they can affect the patient's body image (see Fig. 6.8).

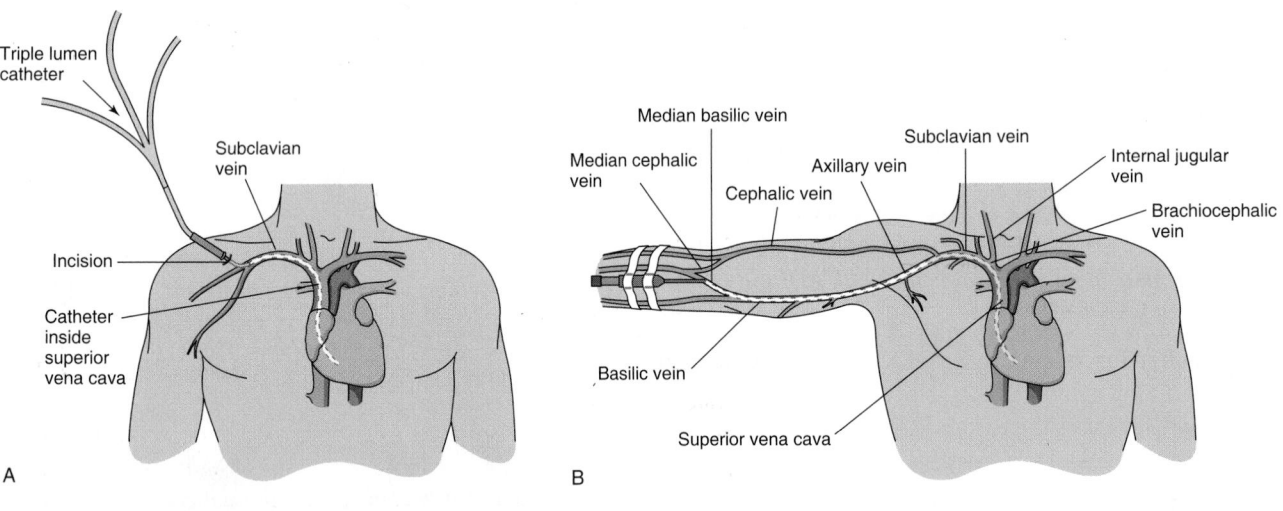

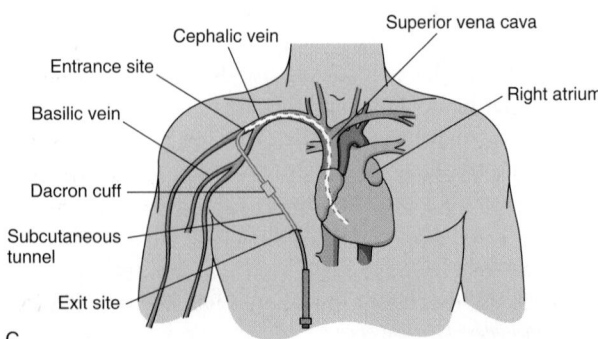

FIGURE 6.8 Central lines. (A) Triple-lumen subclavian catheter. (B) PICC line. (C) Tunneled catheter. *(B and C modified from Phillips, L: Manual of IV therapeutics [4th ed.]. FA Davis, Philadelphia, 2005.)*

Ports

A port is a reservoir that is surgically implanted into a pocket created under the skin, usually in the upper chest. An attached catheter is tunneled under the skin into a central vein. An advantage of a port is that, when not in use, it can be flushed and left unused for long periods. Because the port is under the skin, the patient can swim and shower without risk of contaminating the site.

Ports come in a variety of sizes and styles and are now being used in many areas of the body. Ports can be used to administer chemotherapeutic agents and antibiotics that are toxic to tissues and are suitable for long-term therapy. Ports should be accessed only by specially trained RNs. Most ports require the use of special noncoring needles that are specifically designed for this purpose. Regular needles can cut a "core" in the septum (self-sealing covering), which can travel through the catheter and cause an embolism.

Nursing Management of Central Access Devices

Central lines have sterile, occlusive dressings to protect the site. Sterile gloves and mask should be worn during the dressing change. Whenever tubing is disconnected for changing, the patient is instructed to perform Valsalva's maneuver if able. This maneuver increases thoracic pressure and prevents air from entering the central line. Institution policy directs specific dressing and tubing change procedures.

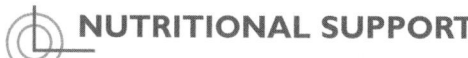

NUTRITIONAL SUPPORT

Total parenteral nutrition (TPN) is complete IV nutrition that is administered to patients who are unable to take adequate nutrients via the enteral route (mouth or tube feeding). TPN may be used to promote wound healing or to help a patient achieve optimal weight before surgery, or it may be used to avoid malnutrition from chronic disease or after surgery. Patients with ulcerative colitis, trauma, or cancer cachexia are candidates for TPN. Every effort should be made to return a patient on TPN to oral or tube feedings as soon as possible (Box 6.6, Nutrition Notes).

TPN provides and maintains the essential nutrients required by the body. Solutions contain carbohydrates, amino acids, lipid emulsions, electrolytes, trace elements, and vitamins in varied amounts according to the patient's needs. Parenteral nutrition requires filtration and an electronic infusion device for administration. In the home setting an ambulatory infusion device is used to allow the patient more mobility.

Initial assessment includes the patient's height, daily weight, nutritional status, and current laboratory values. Because of the high glucose concentration of TPN, the patient is at risk for infection and blood glucose disturbances. Insulin therapy may be necessary during TPN administration. Ongoing assessments include blood glucose levels according to institution policy and monitoring for signs and symptoms of infection, hyperglycemia, and hypo-

---

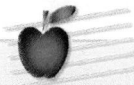

Box 6.6

Nutrition Notes

Total Parenteral Nutrition

Serious metabolic complications of total parenteral nutrition can occur quickly. Rapid shifts in potassium, magnesium, phosphorus, and glucose among the body's fluid compartments can become life-threatening. Glucose in excess of the body's needs can produce carbon dioxide retention, hyperlipoproteinemia, and fatty deposits in the liver. Therefore, administration of TPN requires careful monitoring. The goal is to provide sufficient nutrients but not excessive amounts that create physiological stress.

To avoid complications, TPN infusions are started slowly at low concentrations. Adjustments are made cautiously, changing one component (amount, concentration, or rate) at a time and observing the patient's reaction. In particular, nurses and pharmacists involved in home parenteral nutrition need to carefully follow agency guidelines for mixing and storing TPN since problems can occur with degradation of components. Serious complications including death can occur when guidelines are not carefully observed. In addition, administration of drugs in TPN (or mixing in the same tubing) should be avoided if at all possible.

In a patient whose only nutrition is obtained from TPN, the gastrointestinal cells will atrophy. Therefore, the patient must be weaned from parenteral feeding while oral or tube feedings are slowly restarted. As gastrointestinal intake increases, TPN is decreased. Sometimes, when circumstances permit, gastrointestinal function can be maintained throughout TPN administration by giving the patient a liquid or light diet along with TPN.

---

glycemia. When TPN therapy is begun, the rate is increased gradually to the prescribed rate to help prevent hyperglycemia. When it ends, the rate is gradually decreased to prevent hypoglycemia.

When nutritional solutions contain final concentrations exceeding 10% dextrose or 5% protein, they must be administered via a central catheter. When final concentrations are less than 10% dextrose or 5% protein, they may be administered through a peripheral vein. Peripheral therapy is a short-term intervention because it does not provide adequate nutrition over an extended period.

It is essential that the entire health-care team be involved in TPN therapy because TPN is total replacement for food. The pharmacist, dietitian, physician, and nurse communicate in a team conference to discuss the assessment, plan, and outcome criteria. Many institutions have nutrition teams that assess the appropriateness of TPN for individual patients.

HOME INTRAVENOUS THERAPY

As health-care costs continue to escalate, patients are using more alternatives to hospitalization. Subacute care, skilled nursing care in nursing homes, and home health care are growing. Home IV therapy allows many patients the benefit of early discharge and the ability to accomplish health care in the privacy and comfort of their own homes. Some home health agencies employ nurses to instruct patients and their families in the administration of home IV therapy (see Home Health Hints).

Home IV antibiotic therapy is becoming the method of choice in the long-term treatment of a number of infections, including bacterial endocarditis, osteomyelitis, and septic arthritis. Other patients with chronic diseases choose to receive TPN at home. The health team can assess patients and their families for their ability to manage home IV therapy.

REFLECTIONS ON CASE STUDY

Think again about Mrs. Brown from the beginning of the chapter. She will need monitoring of intake and output, daily weights, and close monitoring of her IV infusion. You should anticipate that serum electrolytes, BUN, and creatinine laboratory studies will be ordered. When initiating the infusion, use care in application of a tourniquet because elderly skin is thin and bruising can occur. Choose a number 20- or 22-gauge catheter to start the infusion. Once it is started, continue to monitor weights and lung sounds because elderly patients can quickly go from fluid depletion to fluid overload (see Box 6.5 Gerontological Issues).

Home Health Hints

- If IV therapy is to be continued after hospital discharge, assist the RN in teaching the patient and caregiver the skills to oversee the IV therapy. Obtain a referral for a home-care nurse to continue monitoring and teaching after discharge.
- In addition to basic IV care, teach the caregiver the effects and side effects of the medications and signs and symptoms that should be reported to the nurse or doctor.
- Instruct the home-care patient to refrain from smoking for at least 30 minutes before IV insertion to prevent vasoconstriction and ensure successful venipuncture.
- Instruct the patient to cover the IV site with a stretch bandage such as Spandage to prevent tugging at the catheter site.
- Help the patient and caregiver identify a safe place to keep supplies. Make sure they understand the recommendations for storage of IV medications since some medications require refrigeration.
- Supplies should include a biohazard container. Home health agencies will supply these containers. The nurse is responsible for returning filled boxes to his or her agency for disposal.

REVIEW QUESTIONS

1. Which of the following is the best resource for the nurse who has a question about implementation of IV therapy at a specific institution?
   a. An experienced nurse
   b. Institution policy
   c. The physician
   d. INS standards

2. Which patients have a need for IV therapy? Choose all that apply.
   a. An 88-year-old man admitted to the hospital with dehydration
   b. A 21-year-old woman with an eating disorder and severe weight loss
   c. A 58-year-old woman with pneumonia that has been unresponsive to oral antibiotics
   d. A 37-year-old man recovering from a fall and broken arm
   e. A 4-year-old brought to the emergency room because of prolonged vomiting

   f. A patient with fluid overload who requires fast acting diuretic therapy

3. A patient requests that an IV not be initiated in his hand. Which site is the next best choice?
   a. Forearm
   b. Antecubital fossa
   c. Upper arm
   d. Lower extremity

4. Place the steps for insertion of a peripheral IV catheter in chronological order. Use all the options.
   a. Put on gloves
   b. Check physician's order.
   c. Prepare insertion site.
   d. Label the dressing.
   e. Wash hands.
   f. Dilate the vein.
   g. Document the procedure.

h. Insert the catheter.

i. Stabilize the site with tape.

5. The nurse must initiate an infusion on a 21-year-old man who has a history of drug abuse, a diagnosis of septicemia, and multiple tattoos over his arms. What would be the best approach to be able to visualize and initiate a peripheral IV?
   a. Place the arm in a dependent position.
   b. Use a blood pressure cuff.
   c. Use the multiple tourniquet technique.
   d. Have another nurse hold the patient's arm.

6. A patient receiving IV therapy via a central line develops hypotension, cyanosis, and tachycardia. The nurse notes a crack in the IV tubing. Which of the following actions should the nurse take first?
   a. Have the RN call the physician.
   b. Clamp the tubing and administer oxygen.
   c. Raise the head of the bed.
   d. Slow the infusion and lay the patient flat.

7. Which of the following solutions is isotonic?
   a. 0.45% NS
   b. D5/0.2% NS
   c. D5/0.45% NS
   d. 0.9% NS

8. The nurse is assessing a patient and notes a silicone catheter taped to his chest, and can feel the catheter under the skin. This type of catheter would be a:
   a. Peripherally inserted central catheter
   b. Implanted port
   c. Central venous tunneled catheter
   d. Percutaneous catheter

9. The physician orders 5% dextrose in water at 100 mL per hour. What is the drip rate using tubing with a drop factor of 20? 32 gtt per minute

10. A patient is to receive 1000 mL normal saline over 12 hours. How many mililiters per hour should be set on the controller? ___ mL/hour

References

1. Intravenous Nursing Sttandards of Practice. Infusion Nurses Society, Norwood, MA, 2000.
2. U.S. Centers for Disease Control and Prevention. Guideline for Hand Hygiene in Health-Care Settings. Atlanta: U.S. Department of Health and Human Services 51(RR16), 2002, pp 1–44.

Bibliography

1. American Society for Parenteral and Enteral Nutrition http://www.clinnutr.org
2. Centers for Disease Control and Prevention, Division of HIV/AIDS Prevention, National Center for HIV, STD and TB Prevention: Surveillance Report, 9(1), 1997.
3. Phillips, LD: Manual of IV Therapeutics, ed. 4. F.A. Davis, Philadelphia, 2005.
4. Phillips, LD: IV Notes. F.A. Davis, Philadelphia, 2005.

SUGGESTED ANSWERS TO

CRITICAL THINKING

■ Mrs. Green

Consider the following when assessing the patient for an appropriate venipuncture site:
1. An 18-gauge catheter should be used for blood administration whenever possible.
2. The catheter should not be inserted in the arm that has the shunt.
3. The catheter should be placed in the forearm. Hand veins are too small to accommodate the delivery of blood.

■ Mr. Rick

Your patient's IV line is likely clotted. If it has been so for a long time, it will not be salvageable. Do not flush it because doing so can dislodge the clot into the circulation. Discontinue the IV and insert a new catheter.

■ Mrs. Gonzalez

1. The IV fluid may be leaking at the insertion site and flowing into the subcutaneous tissue, a problem known as **extravasation.**
2. Consider whether the pain could be caused by the build-up of fluid under the skin.
3. Compare the insertion site with the opposite limb. If the IV solution has infiltrated, stop the infusion, discontinue the catheter, and restart the catheter in a new site.
4. "Patient complains of pain at IV site in right arm; area is cool to touch and edematous in 4.5-cm area around site. Flow rate sluggish. Infusion discontinued; IV restarted in left arm with 22-gauge catheter. Infusing well with no signs of infiltration."

extravasation: extra—outside + vas—vessel + tion—condition

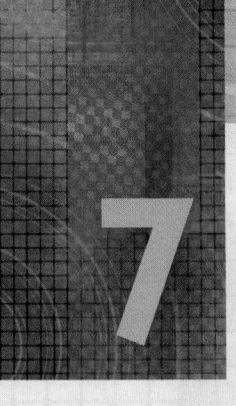

7

Nursing Care of Patients with Infections

SUSAN GARBUTT

KEY TERMS

aerobic (air-O-bick)
anaerobic (ann-air-OH-bick)
antibodies (AN-ti-baw-dees)
antigen (AN-tih-jen)
asepsis (ah-SEP-sis)
bacteria (back-TEER-e-ah)
colonization (collin-i-ZAY-shun)
dormant (DOOR-mant)
flora (FLOOR-ah)
fungi (FUNG-guy)
hand hygiene (hand HY-jeen)
host (HOE-st)
morbidity (more-BID-it-ee)
mortality (more-TAL-it-ee)
nosocomial infection (no-zoh-KOH-mee-uhl
    in-FECK-shun)
pathogen (PATH-o-jen)
personal protective equipment (PUR-
    sun-al pro-TEK-tiv i-KWIP-ment)
phagocytosis (fay-go-sigh-TOH-sis)
protozoa (pro-tow-ZOH-ah)
reservoir (REZ-er-vwar)
rickettsia (ra-KET-see-ah)
sepsis (SEP-sis)
standard precautions (STAN-derd pre-
    KAW-shuns)
Staphylococcus (staff-il-oh-KOCK-us)
vector (VECK-tur)
virulence (VEER-you-lence)
virus (VIGH-rus)

QUESTIONS TO GUIDE YOUR READING

1. What are the links in the chain of infection?

2. How can you interrupt the routes of transmission of infectious disease?

3. How can you assist the body's defense mechanisms to fight infectious disease?

4. What are the signs and symptoms of a localized versus a generalized infection?

5. What are principles of anti-infective medication administration?

6. What nursing care will you provide for a patient with an infectious disease?

7. How will you know if your nursing care has been effective?

THE INFECTIOUS PROCESS

Events leading to an infection are shown in Figure 7.1. To prevent an infection, links in the chain of events must be broken. If an infection occurs, treatment focuses on breaking the chain of infection to prevent the spread of infection to others (Box 7.1, Cultural Considerations).

A **pathogen** causes disease. When pathogenic microbes are present in the body without causing symptomatic infection, it is referred to as **colonization.** When an infection occurs without producing symptoms, it is known as a subclinical infection. Identification of a subclinical infection is made from a **host's** increased antibody level for the microbe. An infection causes signs, symptoms, and injury to the host.

Reservoir

A **reservoir** is the place in the environment where infectious agents live, multiply, and reproduce so they can be transmitted to a susceptible host. A reservoir can be animate, such as people, insects, animals, and plants, or inanimate, such as water, soil, or medical devices.

Causative Agents

Microorganisms that cause infection include **bacteria, viruses, fungi, protozoa,** helminths, and prions (Table 7.1). Microbes that occur naturally in or on a particular body part are known as normal **flora.** They are usually harmless, or nonpathogenic, because they do not normally produce disease in a healthy person. Normal flora are helpful to the human host. For example, intestinal flora (bacteria) assist in

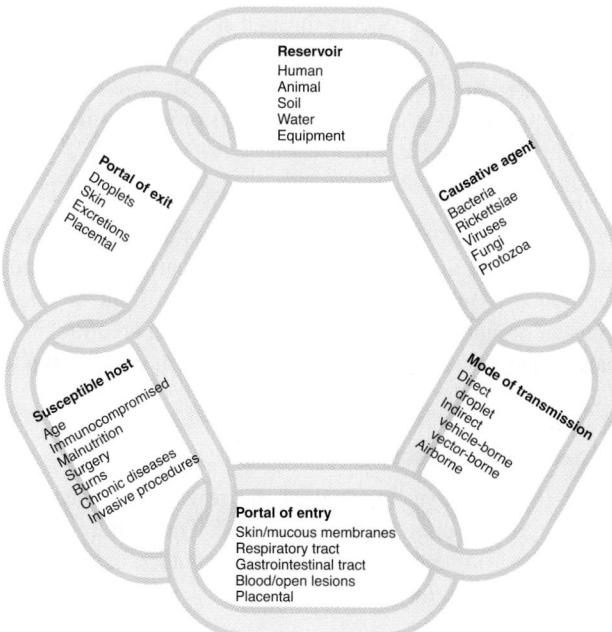

FIGURE 7.1 Chain of events in the infectious process.

protozoa: proto—first + zoon—animal

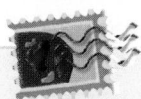
vitamin K production, a necessary nutrient for normal blood clotting. However, if these bacteria get into another area of the body, such as the blood, they may produce disease and are then referred to as pathogens.

Bacteria

Bacteria are single-celled organisms that usually reproduce by simple cellular division. Bacteria may depend on a host or may live and reproduce outside a host. Most bacteria produce cell walls that are susceptible to antibiotics. However, bacteria can mutate in order to survive.

Bacteria are named according to their shape (spherical [coccus], rod [bacillus], and spiral [spirillum]) and classified according to their staining properties (Gram's method, acid-fast staining). Bacteria respond to stains in one of three ways: gram-positive bacteria stain purple; gram-negative bacteria lose purple stain when exposed to alcohol but stain red with a second dye; and acid-fast bacteria keep purple stain when an acid is applied.

Bacterial growth depends on oxygen, nutrition, light, temperature, and humidity. **Aerobic** bacteria, such as those found on the skin, need oxygen to live. **Anaerobic** bacteria, such as bacteria in the gastrointestinal tract, live without oxygen. Most bacteria that inhabit humans grow best at body temperature, 98.6°F (37°C).

Rod-shaped bacteria form spores that are thick walled and hard to kill. Spores remain in a resting state until favor-

TABLE 7.1 COMMON INFECTIONS

Microorganism	Type or Site of Infection
Gram-Positive Bacteria	
Staphylococcus aureus	Pneumonia, cellulitis, peritonitis, toxic shock
Staphylococcus epidermidis	Postoperative bone/joints, IV line–related phlebitis
Staphylococcus pneumoniae	Pneumonia, meningitis, otitis media, sinusitis, septicemia
Gram-Negative Bacteria	
Escherichia coli	Urinary tract, pyelonephritis, septicemia, gastroenteritis
Klebsiella pneumoniae	Pneumonia and wounds
Legionella pneumophila	Pneumonia
Neisseria gonorrhoeae	Gonorrhea
Pseudomonas aeruginosa	Wounds, urinary tract, pneumonia, IV lines
Salmonella enteritidis	Gastroenteritis, food poisoning
Viruses	
Herpes virus group	Cold sores/fever blisters, genital herpes
Epstein-Barr	Infectious mononucleosis
Varicella zoster	Skin (chickenpox and shingles)
Hepatitis (A, B, C, D, E)	Liver
Human immunodeficiency virus	Acquired immunodeficiency syndrome
Influenza (A, B, C)	Bronchiolitis, pneumonia
Rubella	German measles
Rubeola	Measles
Protozoa	
Giardia lamblia	Gastroenteritis
Trichomonas vaginalis	Trichomoniasis
Dientamoeba fragilis	Diarrhea, fever
Entamoeba histolytica	Amebic dysentery
Toxoplasma gondii	Toxoplasmosis
Plasmodium falciparum	Malaria
Fungi	
Candida albicans	Nailbed, thrush, vaginitis
Histoplasma capsulatum	Pneumonia

able conditions exist that allow the organism to resume normal function. Prolonged exposure to high temperature destroys spores on surgical equipment. Bleach is used in patient rooms to kill spores from *Clostridium difficile* (*C. diff*).

RICKETTSIAE. Rickettsiae are a type of bacteria that must be inside living cells to reproduce. Rickettsiae **vectors** (living organisms that transmit disease) are infected fleas, ticks, mites, and lice that bite humans. Several diseases are caused by **rickettsiae.** Rocky Mountain spotted fever, caused by *Rickettsia rickettsii,* whose reservoirs (the places in nature where the organism usually lives and multiplies without causing disease) are rodents and dogs, is transmitted to humans by a tick bite.

Viruses

Viruses are organisms smaller than bacteria that depend on host cells to live and reproduce (see Table 7.1). Invaded host cells make more virus material. The new viral particles are then released either by destroying the host cell or by forming small buds that break away to infect other cells.

When a virus enters a cell, it may immediately trigger disease or remain **dormant** (inactive) for years without causing illness. An example of this is *human herpesvirus 3* (varicella zoster virus), which can cause disease quickly (chickenpox) or remain dormant for years, eventually erupting in the disease called shingles. Antibiotics are not effective against viruses. Newer antiviral drugs are used to decrease symptoms caused by viruses and to decrease the viral load (the number of viral cells in the patient's blood).

Fungi

Fungi are a group of organisms that includes yeasts, molds, and mushrooms and can produce highly resistant spores (see Table 7.1). Because fungi do not contain chlorophyll, they must obtain food from living organisms or dead organic matter. Normal flora of the mouth, skin, vagina, and intestinal tract include many fungi. Most fungi are not pathogenic, and serious fungal infections are rare. Antifungal medications treat fungal infections.

Protozoa

Protozoa are single-celled parasitic organisms with flexible membranes that live in the soil and obtain nourishment from dead or decaying organic material (see Table 7.1). Protozoa infect humans through fecal-oral contamination or through ingestion of food or water contaminated with cysts or spores, through host-to-host contact, or by the bite of a mosquito or other insect that has previously bitten an infected person.

Helminths

Helminths are wormlike parasitic animals: roundworms, flatworms, tapeworms, pinworms, hookworms, and flukes. Disease transmission occurs through skin penetration of larvae or ingestion of helminth eggs. Trichinellosis (caused by the roundworm *Trichinella spiralis*) is a disease caused by eating raw or undercooked meat of pigs or wild animals that contain *Trichinella* larvae.

Prions

Prions are recently identified organisms or agents thought to be unique proteins with long incubation periods. How they reproduce is unknown. Research will shed light on these unusual organisms or protein particles, which are thought to cause mad cow disease and the human dementia known as Jakob-Creutzfeldt syndrome.

Mode of Transmission

Once the causative agent exits the reservoir, a means of transfer to a susceptible host is needed. Transmission methods for microorganisms include direct contact, indirect contact, and through the air.

Direct Contact

Direct transmission occurs through touching, biting, kissing, sexual contact, or droplet spray into the eyes or on mucous membranes while sneezing, coughing, spitting, singing, or talking. Droplet spread is usually limited to 3 feet or less. Illnesses spread by direct transmission may include influenza, impetigo, scabies, conjunctivitis, pediculosis, herpes, *C. difficile,* and all sexually transmitted diseases, including human immunodeficiency virus (HIV). Protect yourself and your patients from direct transmission with hand washing, aseptic technique, and use of **personal protective equipment** (PPE) (gloves, surgical masks, goggles, gowns, and booties). PPE is selected and used based on the task to be performed and the isolation precautions (standard precautions and/or transmission-based precautions)

Indirect Contact

Indirect transmission is either vehicleborne or vectorborne. Vehicleborne transmission is the spread of an infectious organism by contact with a contaminated object, such as a toy, soiled bedding, dressings from a wound, surgical instruments, water, food, and biological products such as blood, serum, plasma, tissues, and organs. Vehicleborne illnesses include conjunctivitis, trichinellosis, HIV, and hepatitis A, B, C, D, and E. Vehicle transmission can be avoided through proper hand washing, thorough cleaning of the patient environment, and provision of clean water and food supplies. Vectorborne transmission is the spread of infectious organisms through a living source other than humans, such as an insect, flea, mouse, or rat. Diseases spread through vectors include malaria, plague, and Lyme disease. Vector transmission can be reduced with insect repellants, avoidance of infested areas, and rodent control.

Airborne

Airborne transmission is different from droplet transmission (see Direct Contact discussed earlier) because the particles floating in the air are much smaller, remain suspended in the air for a long time, and may travel large distances. Airborne organisms can be inhaled or deposited on the mucous membrane of a susceptible host. Measles, chickenpox, and tuberculosis are transmitted by airborne transmission. Airborne transmission is prevented with the use of high-efficiency particulate air (HEPA) respirators (also known as a tuberculosis [TB] mask). HEPA respirators filter the tiniest particles from the air, unlike surgical masks, which can allow such particles to pass into the respiratory system of a host. Institutions provide individual fit testing and training for HEPA respirator use for each health care worker.

NURSING CARE TIP

If you provide care for patients with suspected or confirmed diseases that are spread through airborne transmission, such as TB, be sure you have your own fit-tested HEPA mask to wear. Do not use other masks because they do not provide adequate protection. If you cannot obtain your own fit-tested mask, you should not enter the patient's room.

Multiple Modes of Transmission

Many diseases have multiple modes of transmission requiring a variety of protective techniques. For example, chickenpox is transmitted by direct contact, indirect contact, and airborne transmission. It is no wonder 80% to 90% of susceptible persons exposed develop the disease. Understanding the modes of transmission of a particular disease allows you to use the appropriate means of protection without using unnecessary supplies that increase costs.

Portal of Entry

To produce disease, organisms must gain entry into a susceptible host. Routes of entry into a susceptible host include the respiratory tract, skin (usually nonintact), mucous membranes, gastrointestinal tract, genitourinary tract, and placenta. Once the organism enters the host, it may lead to disease, depending on the condition of the host and many other factors, such as the **virulence** of the organism.

Susceptible Host

The body has many defense mechanisms to prevent infection, such as intact skin and mucous membranes and a functioning immune system. A breakdown in these defenses increases the possibility of infection. Factors that increase susceptibility to infection are very young age, old age, malnourishment, immunocompromise, chronic disease, stress, and invasive procedures (Box 7.2, Gerontological Issues).

Portal of Exit

The portal of exit is the route by which the infectious agent leaves the host, who has become a reservoir for infection: respiratory tract, skin, mucous membranes, gastrointestinal tract, genitourinary tract, blood, open lesions, or placenta.

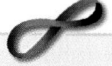

Box 7.2

Gerontological Issues

Infection and Older Adults

Often an older patient may not have typical symptoms of an infection. For example, a serious bacterial infection may cause no elevation in temperature. In fact, a fever is not a common complaint or sign of infection for an older adult.

This difference among older adult patients may cause significant delay in providing appropriate treatment and care. Be alert for the following in the older adult patient, which may indicate an infection:

- Behavioral change, such as pacing or irritability.
- Masking of the symptoms of infection by a chronic disease. For example, the inflammation and pain of degenerative joint disease may make it difficult for a patient to recognize an infection in an affected joint.

THE HUMAN BODY'S DEFENSE MECHANISMS

Skin and Mucous Membranes

Intact skin and mucous membranes are the body's first line of defense against infection. Oral mucous membranes have many layers, making it difficult for organisms to enter the body. The skin has acidic (pH <7) properties that render some organisms unable to produce disease. For example, many bacteria prefer an alkaline (pH >7) environment for reproduction. There is also an abundance of normal flora that impairs the growth of pathogens both on the skin and in the gastrointestinal (GI) tract.

Cilia

Cilia are hairlike structures lining upper respiratory tract mucous membranes that protect the lungs. Cilia trap mucus, pus, dust, and foreign particles to prevent them from entering the lungs. Then the cilia push the trapped particles up to the pharynx with wavelike movements for expectoration.

Gastric Juices

Gastric juices inside the stomach are very acidic (pH 1 to 5). This acidic environment destroys most organisms that enter the stomach.

Immunoglobulins

Immunoglobulins are proteins found in serum and body fluids that may act as **antibodies** to destroy invading organisms and prevent the development of infectious disease. Antibodies are proteins that are produced by B lymphocytes when foreign **antigens** of invading cells are detected. Antigens are markers on the surface of cells that identify cells as being the body's own cells (autoantigens) or as being foreign cells (foreign antigens). Antibodies combine with specific foreign antigens on the surface of the invading organisms, such as bacteria or viruses, to control or destroy them. Antigens are neutralized or destroyed by antibodies in several ways. Antibodies can initiate destruction of the antigen, neutralize toxins released by bacteria, promote antigen clumping with the antibody, or prevent the antigen from adhering to host cells.

Leukocytes and Macrophages

Leukocytes (white blood cells) are the primary cells that protect against infection and tissue damage. There are five types of leukocytes:

- Neutrophils are phagocytic cells focusing on bacteria and small particles.
- Monocytes become macrophages and are mainly phagocytic on tissue debris and large particles.
- Lymphocytes' functions include antigen recognition and antibody production.
- Basophils respond to inflammation from injury.
- Eosinophils destroy parasites and respond in allergic reactions.

After recognizing a foreign antigen, neutrophils and macrophages engulf and digest it, a process known as **phagocytosis.** The macrophages move the antigen fragments to their surface to be recognized by T lymphocytes to further stimulate action of the immune system. Phagocytes ingest and destroy bacteria, damaged or dead cells, cellular debris, and foreign substances.

Lysozymes

Lysozymes are bactericidal enzymes present in white blood cells and most body fluids, such as tears, saliva, and sweat. These enzymes dissolve the walls of bacteria, destroying them.

Interferon

If an invading organism is a virus, white blood cells and fibroblasts release interferon (a group of antiviral proteins). Interferon aids in the destruction of infected cells and inhibits production of the virus within infected cells. Tumor cell growth may also be inhibited by interferon.

Inflammatory Response

The inflammatory response occurs as a result of any bodily injury. This response can be caused by pathogens, trauma, or other events causing injury to tissues. Infection may or may not be present.

Vascular Response

The first step of the inflammatory process is local vasodilation, which increases blood flow to the injured area. Pathogenic organisms can trigger the first step of the inflammatory process. Increased blood flow creates redness and heat at the injury. The increase in blood flow brings more plasma to the area to nourish tissue and carry waste and debris away.

Inflammatory Exudate

The second step of the inflammatory process is increased permeability of the blood vessels, which allows plasma to move out of the capillaries and into the tissues. Swelling occurs, resulting in pain from pressure on nearby nerve endings.

Phagocytosis and Purulent Exudate

The final step of the inflammatory process is the destruction of pathogenic organisms and their toxins by leukocytes. During this process, a purulent exudate (pus) may form that contains protein, cellular debris, and dead leukocytes.

Immune System

The immune system is the body's final line of defense against infection. Immune cells and lymphoid tissue work with the body's other defense mechanisms. Immune cells include lymphocytes (T cells, B cells, and natural killer cells), which have protective functions related to specific antigens. Macrophages assist T and B lymphocytes.

---

phagocytosis: phagein—to eat + cytos—cell + osis—condition

The lymphoid organs are the thymus, which is vital to the development of the immune system, and the bone marrow, which produces leukocytes. Other lymphoid structures include the spleen, tonsils, intestinal lymphoid tissue, and lymph nodes, where immune cells grow and whose filtering of foreign materials prevents them from entering the bloodstream. The spleen destroys old or damaged red blood cells and contains large amounts of lymphocytes.

The immune system is a finely tuned network that functions together to protect the body from invasion by pathogenic organisms. When this network breaks down, infectious disease can result.

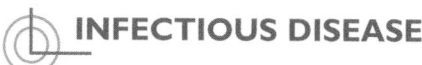

INFECTIOUS DISEASE

General Clinical Manifestations of Infections

Localized Infection

Localized infection is caused by an increase of microbes in one area that triggers the inflammatory response. Manifestations of a local infection include pain, redness, swelling, and warmth at the site. Pain is most severe when the infection occurs in closed cavities. Redness and swelling are seen when surface structures are involved. Warmth may be felt at the site. Body temperature may rise, producing an antimicrobial effect.

Generalized Infection

Generalized infections occur when there is systemic or whole body involvement. Symptoms of generalized infection may include headache, malaise, muscle aches, fever, and anorexia. As the infection progresses, there can be an increase in fever, elevated white blood cell count, decreased blood pressure, mental confusion, tachycardia, and shock. **Sepsis** is the term used for an infection that has spread to the bloodstream.

Laboratory Assessment

Several methods are used to identify pathogens. One method is performing a microscopic examination, such as Gram's method of staining. Another method is culture and sensitivity (C&S). Organisms found in the culture specimen are grown on a laboratory plate and identified within 24 to 48 hours. A sensitivity examination is then done, which exposes any organism to many antibiotics to determine which antibiotic will be most effective for treatment.

A serum antibody test measures reaction to a certain antigen. A positive result on this test does not always mean an active infection is present. It can simply mean there has been an exposure to the antigen, so it is not as accurate as a culture.

A complete blood cell count with differential (CBC with diff) is usually obtained when an infectious disease is suspected. The five different types of leukocytes and their levels are identified. Elevations in specific leukocytes occur based on the type and severity of the pathogen.

Erythrocyte sedimentation rate (ESR, sed rate) is an early screening test for inflammation but not a definitive test for infection. During the inflammatory process, red blood cells become heavier and during the test settle to the bottom of a tube. The ESR measures in millimeters per hour the speed at which the red blood cells settle in the tube. The faster the settling, the greater the inflammation.

Other tests such as x-rays, computed tomography (CT), and magnetic resonance imaging (MRI) are helpful in identifying, abscesses (walled-off infections). Skin tests diagnose infections, such as the purified protein derivative (PPD) skin test, which screens for tuberculosis. (See Chapter 31.)

Immunity

Immunity is the ability of the body to protect itself from disease. (See Chapter 17.) There are several types of immunity:
- Natural immunity occurs in species and prevents one species from contracting illnesses found in another species.
- Innate immunity is genetic, hereditary immunity is that which a person is born with.
- Acquired immunity is obtained either actively or passively through exposure to an organism, from a vaccine, or from an injection of immunoglobulins (antibodies) or is passed from mother to baby.

Types of Diseases

There are many types of infectious diseases. Those discussed are found in the chapters related to the body system they affect. For respiratory diseases such as tuberculosis, see Chapter 31; for bloodborne diseases such as HIV, see Chapter 19; for hepatitis, see Chapter 35. Mononucleosis is discussed below.

Mononucleosis

Infectious mononucleosis (referred to as mono or the kissing disease) is an infection that is usually caused by the Epstein-Barr virus (a herpesvirus). Mononucleosis is a contagious disease that anyone may develop. However, it is mainly diagnosed in young adults. Most adults have been exposed to the virus and have antibodies to it but never develop the disease. The virus remains in the body for a lifetime but rarely causes another infection.

Mononucleosis is primarily spread through person-to-person contact, mainly through saliva. Sharing utensils, food, or beverages can transmit the disease. Coughing or sneezing of small droplets of infected saliva or mucus into the air allows the virus to be inhaled by others.

The incubation period for mononucleosis is 4 to 8 weeks after exposure. Symptoms during the first 3 days include extreme fatigue, loss of appetite, and chills. Then a severe sore throat, headache, high fever, reddened throat and tonsils with a white coating, generalized lymphadenopathy (enlarged lymph nodes in two different sites other than inguinal nodes), or diarrhea occur. The spleen enlarges 50% of the time. Occasionally, a rash develops similar to the measles.

Signs and symptoms, as well as diagnostic tests, confirm mononucleosis. Lymphocyte levels are elevated. The monospot and heterophile antibody tests confirm mononucleosis.

Usually no specific treatment is needed. The illness runs its course as other viral illnesses do. Antiviral drugs are not effective. Symptoms are treated as needed with supportive care. Fatigue may last for months. Rest is important. If the spleen is enlarged, contact sports, lifting, and straining are avoided to prevent trauma and rupture. Mild inflammation of the liver or hepatitis may occur, but no treatment is usually required. Other complications are rare.

INFECTION CONTROL IN THE COMMUNITY

Many levels of organizations work closely together to control communicable diseases. The World Health Organization (WHO) and the Centers for Disease Control and Prevention (CDC) teach standards to prevent and control diseases and monitor disease outbreaks. Local health departments teach how to prevent and control the spread of disease. Community immunization programs have helped reduce infectious diseases.

Although requirements vary from state to state, most elementary schools require some proof of childhood immunization. Many colleges also require or recommend immunization to help control the outbreak of diseases such as measles and meningitis. In addition, educating the public about the importance of hand hygiene, immunization, clean water, safe food handling techniques, and safer sex precautions in preventing the spread of disease is essential.

Both the hospital and home health-care nurse have a responsibility to provide infection control teaching for the patient with an infection and his or her family. Such techniques may include use of disposable dishes and utensils and disposable gloves and proper disposal of contaminated items. Techniques used should be specific to the interruption of the transmission of the particular disease.

INFECTION CONTROL IN HEALTH–CARE AGENCIES

If on admission to a hospital or health-care agency a patient already has an infection, it is referred to as a community-acquired infection. An infection that develops as a result of the stay in the hospital or health-care agency is called a **nosocomial infection.** The host's condition plays a major role in whether or not an infection is acquired. Patients in the hospital are commonly debilitated, malnourished, or immunocompromised. Multiple antibiotic therapy also increases susceptibility to other types of infection and promotes the resistance of pathogens to antibiotics. Therefore, the risk of developing a nosocomial infection is very high. Some areas within an institution tend to have an increased number of nosocomial infections, such as intensive care, neonatal, dialysis, oncology, and burn units. Patients in these areas tend to undergo more invasive procedures and are debilitated, increasing susceptibility to infection.

Several pathogens are commonly responsible for causing nosocomial infections:

- *Escherichia coli* (*E. coli*) is the most common pathogen causing nosocomial urinary tract infections. *E. coli* normally lives in the healthy intestinal tract of humans. *E. coli* can be spread by the patient, by the unwashed hands of a health-care worker, or through contaminated food and water.
- ***Staphylococcus*** *aureus* (commonly known as staph) is the most common pathogen causing nosocomial surgical wound infections and nosocomial septicemia. Staph usually lives in the nose and on the skin of healthy people. (Some highly pathogenic strains of staph are also emerging in the world.)
- *Pseudomonas aeruginosa* is the most common pathogen in nosocomial pneumonia. It is found in soil, around water, and in the health-care setting around sinks, water, irrigating solutions, and nebulizers on respiratory equipment.

The single most effective way to prevent and control the spread of infection is by effective hand hygiene. Most organisms in the institutional setting are transmitted via the hands of health-care workers. Hands *must* be washed before and after every patient contact to prevent the direct transmission of organisms (Fig. 7.2). Patients may also transmit organisms with inadequate hand washing. Teach patients the importance of hand washing after handling their own secretions. The use of gloves decreases the transmission of organisms, but CDC guidelines also require hand washing before and after glove use.

SAFETY TIP

Proper hand washing requires wetting the hands, soaping, and lathering, with at least 15 seconds of rubbing your hands together, covering all surfaces. Interlace your fingers to cleanse between them, rub your nails against your palms to clean under the nails, and then rinse your hands with fingertips pointed downward under running water. Dry your hands with clean disposable paper towels. Use the paper towel to turn off the faucet. Apply lotion to your hands to prevent drying and cracking in which infection could develop. Avoid hot water as it causes drying (CDC, 2002).

Asepsis

The concept of **asepsis** (freedom from organisms) is important for all health-care workers who have direct or indirect patient contact. For hospitalized patients, the most common sites for infectious diseases are the genitourinary tract, respiratory tract, bloodstream, and surgical wounds. Be aware of patients at risk of developing these infections and protect them with aseptic techniques.

Medical Asepsis

Medical asepsis is commonly referred to as clean technique. The goal is to reduce the number of pathogens or prevent the transmission of pathogens from one person to another. Frequent, proper hand hygiene is one of the best ways to achieve this goal. Gowns, gloves, masks, and protective eyewear or rooms with special ventilation may also be helpful (Fig. 7.3). Disinfectants and precautions as defined by the CDC are also crucial tools. Techniques used should be appropriate to interrupt the spread of the known pathogen. As part of medical asepsis you should keep your own body and clothing clean to prevent spread of infection to patients, yourself, and your family (Box 7.3 Guidelines to Prevent Spread of Infection to the Patient, Self, and Family).

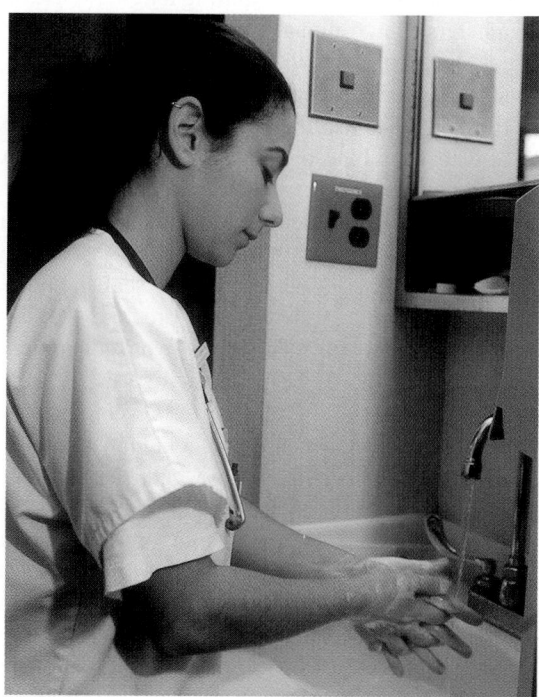

FIGURE 7.2 Frequent hand washing by health care workers helps reduce the spread of microorganisms.

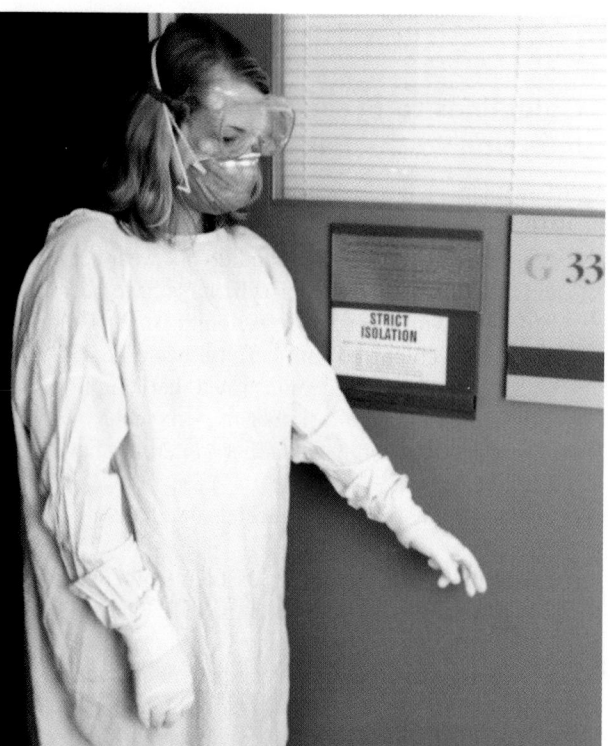

FIGURE 7.3 Gloves, gowns, masks, goggles, and face shields help prevent the spread of infection to health care workers and patients.

Surgical Asepsis

Surgical asepsis (sterile technique) refers to an item or area that is free of all microorganisms and spores. Surgical asepsis is used in surgery and to sterilize equipment. Articles can be subjected to intense heat or chemical disinfectants to destroy all organisms. The use of pressurized steam sterilizers, called autoclaves, kills even the most powerful organisms. Some equipment cannot be exposed to moist heat, so gas sterilizers are used instead. Once these articles are sterilized, they are dated, packaged, and sealed. Once a package is opened or outdated, it is no longer considered sterile. Sterile technique is rarely required in the home-care setting.

Infection Prevention Guidelines

The CDC guidelines for infection control and isolation precautions are used in hospital and health-care agency policies. CDC and agency guidelines are continuously updated and should be followed for your protection, as well as your patients'. Current CDC guidelines for isolation precautions in hospitals include two tiers of precautions: standard precautions and transmission-based precautions (Table 7.2). Visit http://www.cdc.gov/ncidod/hip/Guide/guide.htm for more details.

Standard Precautions

Standard precautions are used in the care of *all patients*. These precautions require you to assume that all patients are infectious regardless of their diagnosis. Standard precautions apply to blood, secretions, excretions, open skin, mucous

Box 7.3

Guidelines to Prevent Spread of Infection to the Patient, Self, and Family

- Bathe daily and wear a clean uniform/clothing every day.
- Keep your fingernails short and do not wear acrylic nails. Both long nails and acrylic nails have been associated with spread of infection to patients and they can be colonized with harmful bacteria. Multiple studies have demonstrated that long fingernails and artificial nails harbor bacteria and have caused infections in patients that sometimes have resulted in death.
- Avoid wearing rings and bracelets that harbor organisms.
- Cleanse your stethoscope at least daily and in between patient use with alcohol. VRE bacteria have been cultured from stethoscopes in a hospital setting.
- Wash your hands between each patient contact. Hand washing is recognized as the single most important action to take to prevent spread of infection. If you are unable to use soap and water, use a nondrying alcohol hand gel, which has been shown to be effective in cleansing hands and preventing drying of the skin.
- Follow prescribed isolation precautions for your protection, as well as that of the patient.
- Remove your uniform and bathe/shower when you come home from work. This will decrease the spread of antibiotic-resistant bacteria to your home and your family. Keep your nursing shoes clean and put away from the rest of the family.

membranes, and all body fluids, excluding sweat. All patients with draining wounds or secretions of body fluids are considered infectious until an infection is confirmed or ruled out. Using gloves, gowns, masks, goggles, face shields, and, most important, hand washing helps prevent the spread of infection to health-care workers and other patients.

CRITICAL THINKING

■ Which of the following patients is at greatest risk for infection and why?
1. Mr. Ashland, age 55, is hospitalized for a hernia repair. He is overweight and has adult-onset diabetes.
2. Mrs. Burrows, age 72, is hospitalized for a broken hip. She is thin, frail, has dementia, and has undergone placement of a urinary catheter.
3. Jackson Dunn, age 2, is hospitalized for minor surgery. Jackson is thin and small for his age.

Suggested answers at end of chapter.

Transmission-Based Precautions

Transmission-based precautions are used for patients with specific communicable diseases that can be transmitted to others. Transmission-based precautions are an additional layer of protection used in addition to standard precautions.

Prevention of Respiratory Tract Infections

Nosocomial pneumonia has been linked with the highest infection mortality rate in hospitalized patients. Patients who are at highest risk for pneumonia are those with endotracheal, nasotracheal, or tracheostomy tubes because these invasive tubes bypass the normal defenses of the upper respiratory tract. Strategies to prevent infections such as ventilator-associated pneumonia (VAP) are being "bundled" together to get health-care workers to remember to use these strategies. For more information on VAP bundles, visit http://www.ihi.org/IHI and put "VAP bundle" in search or visit http://www.ihi.org/NR/rdonlyres/35B687FE-D4D0-44E5-A671-E76D74BB8D9F/0/VAP.pdf#search='canadian%20vap%20bundle'

Prevention of Genitourinary Tract Infections

The most common hospital-acquired infection is a urinary tract infection. Patients with urinary catheters are at the greatest risk. The urinary tract is normally a sterile tract, but insertion of a catheter into the bladder may allow organisms to enter. Institutional policy on appropriate use of urinary catheters differs, and you should follow the policy of your particular institution. Appropriate uses of catheters include use in patients with urinary obstructions, neurogenic bladder conditions, and in those in shock.

Indwelling urinary catheters should be removed as soon as possible. For patients requiring long-term use of urinary catheters, intermittent catheterization is preferred because it has been shown to significantly reduce the risk of infection. Using strict aseptic technique while inserting and caring for the catheter in the health-care agency is imperative. The catheter tubing must be securely anchored to the patient's leg, according to agency protocol, so it does not move in and out of the urethra. Movement can encourage organisms to enter the urinary tract.

The closed urinary drainage system seal should never be opened. If intermittent irrigation is ordered, sterile technique must be used to protect both ends from contamination. The drainage bag should be positioned so that it is never higher than the level of the bladder to prevent backflow of urine into the bladder, which could contaminate the sterile urinary tract. If an indwelling urinary catheter and drainage system is used long term, the catheter and the entire system should be changed regularly using sterile technique. Standards in home care differ from institutional care because patients are generally at lower risk of infection within their own environment.

All long-term indwelling urinary catheters are considered colonized, but only a few will cause infection in the patient. Remember that the most crucial point at which

TABLE 7.2 STANDARD PRECAUTIONS AND TRANSMISSION-BASED PRECAUTIONS

Standard Precautions

Use standard precautions for all patient care. Combine standard precautions with transmission-based precautions as needed based on the patient's illness.

Hand washing	Wash hands with nonmicrobial soap unless specially contraindicated before and after using gloves, between patients, and between procedures on same patient.
Gloves	Wear gloves before contact with any body fluids or substances.
Mask, Eye Protection, Face Shield	Use protective equipment for patient care if splashes or sprays of blood or body fluids are likely.
Gown	Wear gown to protect skin/prevent soiling of clothing for patient care if splashes or sprays of blood or body fluids are likely.
Occupational Health and Bloodborne Pathogens	Dispose of sharps properly; do not recap needles.
Patient Care Equipment	Clean reusable equipment before reuse. Discard single-use items properly.
Linen	Handle linen to avoid clothing contamination.
Patient Placement	Use private room for infectious patients.

Transmission-Based Precautions

Airborne Precautions

Examples: measles, tuberculosis, varicella (chickenpox, shingles)

Patient placement	Provide private room with regulated air flow. Keep door closed.
Respiratory protection	Do not enter room if susceptible to measles or chickenpox unless no immune caregivers available. If susceptible, wear fit-tested N95 or HEPA respirator.
Patient transport	Limit patient transport to essential purposes. Place surgical mask on patient.

Droplet Precautions

Examples: diphtheria (pharyngeal), *Haemophilus influenzae* (epiglottitis, meningitis, pneumonia, sepsis), influenza, mumps, mycoplasma pneumonia, *Neisseria meningitidis* (meningitis, pneumonia, sepsis), pertussis, pneumonic plague, rubella, streptococcal pneumonia

Patient placement	Provide private room or separation of at least 3 feet between the infected patient and other patients.
Mask	Wear mask for patient care if within 3 feet of patient.
Patient transport	Limit patient transport to essential purposes. Place surgical mask on patient.

Contact Precautions

Examples: cellulitis, *Clostridium difficile*, skin infections (diphtheria, herpes simplex virus, impetigo, pediculosis, scabies. conjunctivitis, viral hemorrhagic infections (Ebola, Lassa, or Marburg), herpes zoster

Patient placement	Provide private room or place with patient with same infection and no other infection.
Hand washing, gloves, gown	Protect self and others from contaminated items.
Patient transport	Limit patient transport.
Patient care equipment	Dedicate the use of noncritical patient care equipment to a single patient.

Data from Public Health Service, US Department of Health and Human Services, Centers for Disease Control and Prevention, Atlanta, and Garner JS, Hospital Infection Control Practices Advisory Committee: Guideline for isolation precautions in hospitals. Infect Control Hosp Epidemiol 17:53, 1996; and Am J Infect Control 24:24, 1996 Accessed on August 15, 2005 at http://www.cdc.gov/ncidod/hip/ISOLAT/std_prec_excerpt.htm

bacteria may enter the patient is during the insertion of the catheter, so excellent technique is required. Another point to remember is that the urinary tract is highly vascular (many blood vessels close to the surface), so that an infection in this tract can easily result in bacteremia (bacteria in the

SAFETY TIP

Catheters should be used only when necessary because of the **morbidity** and **mortality** associated with infections that develop from them.

CRITICAL THINKING

Mr. Carson

■ While working in an extended-care facility you see Mrs. Brandt, nursing assistant, wheeling Mr. Carson to activities. He has a long-term urinary catheter. The urine bag is hung on the arm of the wheelchair with a cloth partially covering it. What is your responsibility in this situation?

Suggested answers at end of chapter.

blood), which can then progress to septicemia (infection in the blood), a potentially life-threatening condition.

Prevention of Surgical Wound Infections

The initial dressing for surgical wounds is applied in the operating room using sterile aseptic technique. Postoperative orders indicate when to change the dressing. Sterile technique should be used. The wound is monitored with every dressing change for signs of infection.

Protection from Septicemia (Sepsis)

Septicemia (commonly called blood poisoning) is a blood infection with a variety of causes, including infection in another body site and contamination of invasive catheters and solutions (central lines, arterial lines, pulmonary artery catheters, urinary catheters). Insertion and care of these catheters require sterile technique and careful observation for infection signs. All solutions should be examined for expiration date, signs of contamination, cloudiness, particles, or discoloration before use. Indications of sepsis such as fever, tachypnea, tachycardia, hypotension, and elevated white blood cell count should be reported promptly to the physician for immediate treatment. Blood cultures may be ordered. Antibiotics are used to treat sepsis. An intravenous (IV) drug, drotrecogin alfa (activated) (Xigris), is available to treat severe sepsis when death is likely. Drotrecogin alfa (activated) is given for 96 hours. It is associated with a risk of bleeding. Drotrecogin alfa (activated) has reduced mortality in patients, which may be due to its anti-inflammatory effects.

ANTIBIOTIC-RESISTANT INFECTIONS

Antibiotic-resistant infections are on the rise. These types of infections result in increased health-care costs, morbidity (death), and mortality (illness). Methods to prevent these infections include not using antibiotics in animal feed, teaching patients to take all prescribed medications exactly as ordered, and avoiding the use of antibiotics for viral infections (common cold or flu). American College of Physicians/American Society of Internal Medicine guidelines suggest that most upper respiratory infections do not require antibiotic treatment. For healthy adults with the symptoms of bronchitis, sinusitis, pharyngitis, and other upper respiratory infections, over-the-counter cold symptom remedies and saltwater gargles should be used for symptom relief.

Two infections that are on the rise include methicillin-resistant *Staphylococcus aureus* (MRSA) and vancomycin-resistant enterococci (VRE). For more information on antibiotic resistance, visit the World Health Organization at http://www.who.int/csr/en/.

Methicillin-Resistant *Staphylococcus Aureus*

A serious antibiotic-resistant infection is caused by methicillin-resistant *S. aureus* (MRSA). MRSA is difficult to treat

NURSING CARE TIP

Antibiotics are not effective against viral infections such as colds or the flu. People need to be educated that antibiotics do not work on viral infections. The misuse of antibiotics is creating antibiotic-resistant "superbugs." People should not ask health-care providers for antibiotics to treat viral infections. Use of antibacterial products such as antibacterial soaps may also contribute to the superbug problem. Nurses play a vital role in educating people of this growing problem.

and has a high mortality rate. MRSA affects mainly the elderly and the chronically ill. Vancomycin hydrochloride, a potent and expensive antibiotic, can be used intravenously to treat MRSA. Fear exists that the bacteria will further mutate to become resistant to all currently available antibiotics. A few isolated cases of this have been documented worldwide. The risk that these resistant organisms will spread is real, which will return us to the preantibiotic days when *S. aureus* was a killer.

Vancomycin-Resistant Enterococci

Vancomycin-resistant enterococci (VRE) infections are common. Although enterococci are normal flora in the GI and female genital tracts, VRE are a new pathogenic strain. VRE are transmitted via direct or indirect contact. Patients at risk for VRE infections include those with indwelling urinary or central venous catheters, the immunocompromised or critically ill, those receiving multiple antibiotics or vancomycin therapy, surgical patients, and those with extended hospital stays. Preventive VRE measures focus on proper hand hygiene, education of health-care workers, aggressive infection-control methods, and restricting use of vancomycin. Patients with VRE should be isolated, and current CDC and institutional isolation policies should be strictly followed (Fig. 7.4). Treatment is difficult, involving combination antibiotic therapy, although VRE may also be resistant to other antibiotics.

Quinupristin/dalfopristin (Synercid) is an intravenous drug for VRE treatment. Linezolid (Zyvox) can treat both

---

Antibiotic-Resistant Organism Precautions

Visitors: Report to the Nurses' Station before entering the room.

1. **Private** room required.
2. **Gloves** <u>must</u> be worn by <u>all hospital personnel</u> entering room.
3. **Wash Hands** on entering and leaving room.
4. **Gowns:** required **IF** contamination of clothing is likely.
5. **Decontaminate All Equipment** used in the room before removal from the room.

FIGURE 7.4 Antibiotic-resistant organism precautions for vancomycin-resistant enterococci (VRE).

VRE and MRSA and should ideally be used only for these serious infections so that resistance does not develop. Research is ongoing to develop more antibiotics for resistant organisms, but antibiotic-resistant bacteria remain a very serious threat to the health of the world population.

THERAPEUTIC INTERVENTIONS FOR INFECTIOUS DISEASES

Treatment is begun once an infectious organism and the affected body system are identified. The type of organism and site of infection are important in selecting an appropriate medication. The drug of choice must be able to destroy (or control) the pathogen:

- Antibiotics treat bacterial infections, not viruses, fungi, helminthes, or prions.

- Antiviral medications treat viral infections, but their use is aimed at symptom control rather than cure.
- Antifungal drugs are available for fungal infections, but cure may require extended use.

Cost effectiveness is another concern when selecting a medication. Newer anti-infectives can be very expensive.

Antibiotics can be classified as either bactericidal or bacteriostatic (Table 7.3). Bactericidal agents kill bacteria, whereas bacteriostatic agents inhibit or retard bacterial growth, leaving the final destruction of the bacteria up to the infected host's immune system. Bacteriostatic agents may be less helpful for the patient who is immunocompromised.

When preparing to give an antibiotic, first ask about allergies a patient may have. Patients may have allergies to one antibiotic group that prevents the use of chemically similar drugs. Therefore, all allergies should be reported to the health-care provider.

TABLE 7.3 MEDICATIONS FOR TREATING INFECTIOUS DISEASE

Type and Examples/Uses	Nursing Implications	Patient Teaching
	Bactericidal Antibiotics	
Penicillins amoxicillin (Amoxil), ticarcillin (Ticar), penicillin G, ampicillin (Omnipen) • Most effective against gram-positive organisms.	• Most widely used antibiotic. • Monitor patient for allergic reaction (rash, hives, itching) or anaphylactic shock (fever, chills, trouble breathing, lower blood pressure, tight throat). Keep epinephrine available. • If signs of allergic reaction occur, stop parenteral drug and notify primary care provider immediately. • Watch for superinfection.	• Review signs of allergic reactions. • Tell patient and family to stop drug and call primary care provider if allergy signs occur. • Tell patient to notify primary care provider if white patches appear in mouth or vagina becomes irritated.
Cephalosporins *cephalothin (Keflin), cefazolin (Ancef), cefaclor (Ceclor), ceftriaxone (Rocephin)* • First-generation drugs are most effective against gram-positive organisms. • Second- and third-generation drugs are more effective against gram-negative organisms.	• Patient with penicillin allergy may have cross allergy to cephalosporins. • Common side effects include GI disturbance, phlebitis, pain at injection site, rash, and hives. • Less common but serious side effects include kidney and liver damage and superinfection. • Monitor blood urea nitrogen, creatinine, lactic dehydrogenase, aspartate aminotransferase, and alanine aminotransferase to detect kidney or liver damage.	• Tell patient to take drug on an empty stomach, 1 hour before or 2 hours after meals, to increase absorption. • Tell patient to take drug at specified intervals over 24-hour period.
Aminoglycosides amikacin (Amikin), gentamicin (Garamycin), tobramycin (Nebcin) • Used to treat gram-negative organisms.	• Usually given parenterally because they are not absorbed well in GI tract. • Monitor peak and trough levels to keep drug in therapeutic range. • Assess patient's kidney function. • Check for ototoxicity (ringing in ears, deafness). • Don't mix or infuse with any other drug.	• Tell patient to report signs of allergy, tinnitus, vertigo, or hearing loss. • Tell patient to obtain daily weights because weight gain may indicate kidney problems.

(Continued on following page)

TABLE 7.3 **MEDICATIONS FOR TREATING INFECTIOUS DISEASE** *(Continued)*

Type and Examples/Uses	Nursing Implications	Patient Teaching
Fluoroquinolones ciprofloxacin (Cipro), levofloxacin (Levaquin), norfloxacin (Noroxin), ofloxacin (Floxin), trovafloxacin (Trovan) • Used to treat a variety of infections, such as bronchitis, bone and joint infection, pneumonia, tuberculosis, sexually transmitted disease, and urinary tract infection.	• Give drug on an empty stomach. • Monitor liver function and report signs of dysfunction (fatal hepatitis may occur). • Do not give with antacids that contain aluminum, calcium, or magnesium.	• Tell patient to take with a full glass of water; encourage fluids. • Tell patient to report side effects: swelling of face/throat, trouble swallowing, shortness of breath, itching, hives, pain in shoulder, hands, or heel tendons. • Explain that drug may cause drowsiness and increase sensitivity to light. Advise sun protection.
	Bacteriostatic Antibiotics	
Tetracyclines tetracycline HCl, doxycycline (Vibramycin), minocycline HCl (Minocin) • Treat most gram-positive and gram-negative organisms.	• Tetracycline HCl comes only in oral form. The others are usually given IV because intramuscular route leads to poor absorption. • Give 1 hour before or 2 hours after meals. • Do not give with milk, milk products, or antacids because they impair absorption. • GI disturbances are the most common side effect. • Tetracyclines increase anticoagulant activity. Monitor prothrombin time, international normalized ratio, partial prothrombin time as ordered.	• Suggest eating crackers and juice (but not a full meal) to reduce GI upset. • Tell patient to avoid prolonged sun exposure during therapy.
Erythromycin E-mycin, EES, erythromycin • A broad-spectrum antibiotic effective against many gram-negative and gram-positive organisms.	• Give on an empty stomach 1 hour before or 2 hours after meals. • Give with a full glass of water (not with acidic fruit juices, such as orange juice or grapefruit juice). • When giving drug IV, administer slowly to decrease vein irritation.	• Urge patient to take drug around the clock and complete entire course of treatment. • Explain that gastric distress is common but not a reason to stop the drug. • Suggest that patient contact primary care provider if side effects are intolerable.
Sulfonamides sulfamethoxazole (Gantanol), sulfasalazine (Azulfidine), sulfisoxazole (Gantrisin), trimethoprim sulfamethoxazole (Bactrim, Septra) • Effective against most gram-positive and many gram-negative organisms.	• Commonly used with urinary tract infections, *Pneumocystis carinii* pneumonia, and otitis media. • Common side effects include rash, pruritus, nausea, vomiting, phlebitis, signs of bleeding. • IV drug should be given over 1 hour. • Monitor intake and output • Fluid intake should be at least 1500 mL daily. • Bleeding time may increase, so use caution with anticoagulants. • Phenytoin (Dilantin) toxicity may be increased. • The risk of hypoglycemia may be increased.	• Instruct patient to take drug on an empty stomach 1 hour before or 2 hours after meals. • Tell patient to take with a full glass of water; encourage fluids. • Advise against prolonged exposure to the sun. • Tell patient to stop drug and call primary care provider if signs of allergic reaction or bleeding occur.
	Antifungal Agents	
Amphotericin B • Interferes with the cell wall structure of the fungus, causing it to die.	• Given parenterally and reserved for life-threatening fungal infections. Monitor patient during first hour of infusion for febrile reaction. • Monitor injection site often because drug is very irritating to tissues.	• Explain the purpose of treatment and need for long-term IV therapy. • Instruct patient and family on side effects and possible discomfort at IV site.

Type and Examples/Uses	Nursing Implications	Patient Teaching
	• Report side effects: nausea, vomiting, diarrhea. • Monitor intake and output, blood urea nitrogen (BUN), and creatinine levels for signs of kidney damage. • Obtain daily weight because fluid retention follows kidney damage. • Encourage 2000–3000 mL of fluid daily to help flush drug through kidneys.	
Fluconazole (Diflucan)	• Can be given either parenterally or orally.	• Tell patient to take drug at same time each day and not to double a dose if one is missed.
• Used to treat candidal and urinary tract infections, as well as cryptococcal meningitis.	• Cultures are obtained before giving drug.	• Teach patient and family to notify the primary provider at the first sign of yellow skin, dark urine, or pale stools (signs of liver damage).
	• Monitor BUN and creatinine. Use cautiously if patient has renal impairment. • Monitor liver function. • Monitor side effects: hepatotoxicity, nausea, vomiting, diarrhea, abdominal discomfort.	

Many antibiotics are metabolized by the liver and excreted by the kidneys. Disorders of these organs may require lower doses. Antibiotic levels fluctuate greatly depending on organ function, age, sex, health, and other factors. Antibiotic peak (highest blood level) and trough levels (lowest blood level) need to be monitored to prevent toxicity and damage to major organs.

General Principles

Nurses are responsible for administering medications correctly, including giving the correct dose and for teaching the patient the importance of taking these medications properly. Certain nursing and patient teaching responsibilities relate to *all* anti-infective medications. Consult drug references for further information before giving anti-infectives.

Nursing Responsibilities
- All patient allergies are noted, especially any documented allergy to the specific drug ordered or cross allergies to the drug ordered, and the primary care provider is notified of allergy before treatment is started.
- Monitor and report any side effects or signs of allergic response, especially anaphylactic reactions.
- Observe and report any signs of superinfection (one that occurs as a result of antibiotic use). For example, thrush may develop as antibiotics disrupt the normal flora of the GI tract.

Patient Education
- Stress to the patient and family the need to take *all* the medication exactly as prescribed. Explain that stopping treatment when the patient feels better results in potential relapse with more resistant organisms.

- Explain what signs and symptoms to watch for (allergic and nonallergic side effects) and what to do about them, especially when to call the primary care provider.

SAFETY TIP

Always review and know the normal dose of a medication before giving the medication. You are responsible for any medication you give, even if the dose was ordered incorrectly and you were following the order. If the dose is outside the normal range, do not give it. Consult with the RN, pharmacist, or supervisor who should contact the ordering physician for clarification. Always reviewing medication doses prior to giving them keeps your patient and your nursing license safe.

 NURSING PROCESS

General Infections

Assessment/Data Collection
It is important to recognize the earliest signs and symptoms of infection. Early detection can help provide early treatment to prevent major complications and reduce costs. Providing emotional support to the patient is also important (Box 7.4, Patient Perspective). Patients who are prone to infection because of immunosuppression should take special precautions to prevent infection (Box 7.5, Teaching Points to Prevent Infection in the Older Adult, Debilitated, or Immunocompromised Patient).

CRITICAL THINKING

Mr. Cheevers

■ Mr. Cheevers is admitted to the hospital for IV antibiotic therapy. He states that he has no allergies. One hour after the infusion begins, you happen to meet the nursing assistant coming down the hall with a blanket. He casually says, "Mr. Cheevers is very cold. I'm bringing him a blanket. He is also restless and a bit short of breath." What is your responsibility in this situation?

Suggested answers at end of chapter.

Nursing Diagnosis, Planning, and Implementation
Risk for infection related to external factors

EXPECTED OUTCOME: The patient remains free from symptoms of infection.

- Follow current hand hygiene guidelines *to reduce spread of infection.*
- Use standard precautions and transmission-based precautions *to prevent the transmission of organisms.*
- Observe and report signs of infection such as redness, warmth, and fever, especially for neutropenic

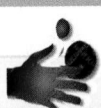

Box 7.4

Patient Perspective

Emotions of Chronic Infection
Edie

It was back! I wasn't sure I could deal with it one more time. I've been hospitalized four times with this same infection (cellulitis) in my leg. It feels like I've lost my life. I can't count on being able to do anything and go anywhere because the infection just keeps coming back.

My left leg is now all swollen, reddened, discolored, and very painful. I can tell when I'm infected by more than the pain in the leg. I feel weak, kind of spacey, and once I passed out. I'm so sick of going into the emergency room—waiting forever to get admitted, all the IV starts and blood draws. With these infections, I've had a PICC (peripherally inserted central catheter) line twice. I've been sent home on IV antibiotics, sometimes for weeks at a time. I've learned how to hang my own IV antibiotics; in fact, I've learned much more than I ever wanted to.

My cellulitis is associated with chronic lymphedema, causing swelling in my legs. I'm working hard to keep the swelling down, so that the infection doesn't reoccur. Wish me luck and keep giving me psychosocial support during your nursing care. I'm not sure how I will be able to deal with this much longer.

Box 7.5

Teaching Points to Prevent Infection in the Older Adult, Debilitated, or Immunocompromised Patient

- Wash your hands frequently, using proper technique.
- Avoid crowds or anyone with an infection.
- Stay well nourished because food helps keep the immune system healthy.
- Have a flu shot yearly and a pneumonia shot as recommended by your primary care provider.
- Wash raw fruits and vegetables thoroughly, cook food thoroughly, and store food safely to prevent food poisoning. (NOTE: with severe immunocompromization, raw foods, soft cheeses, and yogurt may be contraindicated.)
- If your immune system is depressed, notify your primary care provider about any elevated temperature, even in the absence of other symptoms. People with depressed immune function cannot mount the usual immune response to infection, and a low-grade fever may be the only sign of infection.

patients *as they do not have normal inflammatory response and low-grade fever is often the only sign.*
- Use oral thermometers for critically ill adults. *Oral thermometers are best practice if pulmonary artery catheters are not available for core body temperature.*
- Monitor laboratory values of white blood cell counts and cultures *as they correlate to patient's immune function for planning care.*

Evaluation
If interventions have been successful, the patient remains free from symptoms of infection.

Imbalanced nutrition: less than body requirements related to problems eating or digesting food

EXPECTED OUTCOME: The patient maintains ideal body weight for height and weight and eats a balanced diet.
- Identify and provide foods patient enjoys with pleasant presentation *as patient will be more likely to try to eat enjoyed foods in a clean, odor-free environment.*
- Explain and ensure that a balanced diet with protein, fatty acids, and vitamins is available and should be eaten. *These nutrients are needed for healthy immune system function.*
- Monitor and document patient intake *to provide accurate nutritional assessment.*
- Provide antiemetics as ordered *to control nausea and vomiting and improve nutritional intake.*

Evaluation

If interventions have been effective, patient's body weight will be maintained within ideal body weight range and patient will eat a balanced diet. Patient will be free of signs and symptoms of infection.

Deficient knowledge related to disease process and treatment

EXPECTED OUTCOME: The patient describes therapy and carries out treatment.

- Explain infection and prevention of infectious diseases. *Patients' understanding of how infections occur helps them in controlling their risk for developing an infection.*
- Recommend responsible use of antibiotics *to prevent resistant organisms.*
- Explain medications, side effects, and symptoms to report *to promote compliance with treatment and safe medication use.*
- Teach patients how to participate in their own care and have them assist in the development of their plan of care *to promote compliance with treatment.*

Evaluation

If interventions have been effective, the patient will state understanding of therapy and plan and carry out treatment plan.

Respiratory Tract Infections

Assessment/Data Collection

Patients with respiratory tract infections may have a cough, a congested or runny nose, a sore throat, chest congestion, or chest pain. The throat may be reddened, or there may be white patches in the back of the throat. Lung sounds can include crackles, rhonchi, or wheezing. Ask patients if they have a productive cough and the amount, frequency, and color of the sputum. A sputum culture is obtained to identify the presence of pathogenic organisms for appropriate treatment.

Nursing Diagnosis, Planning, and Implementation
Risk for infection related to external factors

EXPECTED OUTCOME: The patient remains free from symptoms of infection.

- Encourage coughing and deep breathing *to keep airways clear and prevent atelectasis.*
- Provide oral care with toothbrush or suction-type toothbrush regularly to remove plaque *since Toothettes do not remove plaque, which has been found to contribute to pneumonia development.*
- Encourage fluids if not contraindicated. *Dehydration is associated with dry, sticky secretions that are difficult to cough up.*
- Provide pain relief *so patient will take deep breaths.*
- Elevate head of bed 30 degrees or more when a tube feeding is infusing *to prevent aspiration pneumonia.*
- Use sterile water rather than tap water from faucet

for oral care for immunocompromised patients *to prevent nosocomial pneumonia infection.*

Evaluation

If interventions have been effective, oxygen saturation will be above 90%, with report of decreased dyspnea. Respirations will be even and unlabored and patient will be free of signs and symptoms of infection.

Gastrointestinal Tract Infections

Assessment/Data Collection

The symptoms of GI tract infections may include nausea, vomiting, diarrhea, cramping, and anorexia. Patients may have frequent episodes of emesis and diarrhea and need to be monitored for signs of dehydration resulting from the loss of fluid. Stool cultures may be ordered.

Nursing Diagnosis, Planning, and Implementation
Risk for infection related to external factors

EXPECTED OUTCOME: The patient remains free from symptoms of infection.

- Encourage fluid intake *to replace fluid lost during fever, vomiting, and diarrhea.*
- Follow standard precautions to prevent the spread of C. diff, especially for older and immunocompromised patients. *C. diff does not usually cause infection in healthy adults.*

Evaluation

Patient will be free of infection and nausea, vomiting, diarrhea, cramping, anorexia, and dehydration if interventions have been successful.

Genitourinary Tract Infection

Assessment/Data Collection

Symptoms of a urinary tract infection (UTI) can include voiding urgency, frequency, burning, flank pain, change in color of urine, foul odor of urine, and confusion or change in mental status for the older adult. Monitor frequency, amount, color, and odor of the urine. Urinalysis and urine cultures may be ordered.

Nursing Diagnosis, Planning, and Implementation
Risk for infection related to external factors

EXPECTED OUTCOME: The patient remains free from symptoms of infection.

- Do not request and avoid use of urinary catheters unless no other options *as patients are more likely to develop bacteremia.*
- Use sterile technique for inserting urinary catheters *to prevent nosocomial infections.*
- Avoid contamination when emptying urinary catheter bags *to prevent nosocomial infections.*
- Use evidence-based facility policy for identifying and managing symptoms related to the urinary tract. *Evidence-based practice improves quality of care and reduces variability in management.*

- Standard diagnostic criteria should be used to identify, document, and communicate to physicians detailed symptoms such as fever or hematuria and not urine odor, urine color, clarity, or culture results alone *as they cannot distinguish symptomatic from asymptomatic infections and the need for medication.*
- Education of patients, residents, families, and staff should be given on evidence-based practice for UTI identification and management *to promote appropriate practices.*

Evaluation

If interventions have been effective, patient will have normal urine output without symptoms of infection such as urgency, frequency, burning, flank pain, change in color of urine, foul odor of urine, or confusion or change in mental status.

REVIEW QUESTIONS

1. Place the links in the chain of infection in their proper order of occurrence in causing an infection.
   a. Portal of Entry
   b. Causative Agents
   c. Mode of Transmission
   d. Portal of Exit
   e. Reservoir
   f. Susceptible Host

2. Which of the following is the most important technique for the nurse to use during patient care to prevent infection transmission?
   a. Wear gloves
   b. Wear gown
   c. Wash hands
   d. Wear mask

3. Which of the following nursing actions should the nurse include in the plan of care to help maintain the body's first line of defense against infection?
   a. Help the patient cough and deep breathe.
   b. Apply lotion to clean skin.
   c. Give an antibiotic as ordered
   d. Help the patient void.

4. Which of the following patient temperature readings would be the priority for the LPN/LVN to report to the registered nurse?
   a. Temperature 97°F (36.1°C) for older patient with hypertension
   b. Temperature 98.9°F (37°C) for first day postoperative patient
   c. Temperature 99.6°F (37.5°C) for patient with neutropenia
   d. Temperature 100°F (37.7°C) for patient with appendcitis

5. The nurse is to give a newly ordered antibiotic to a patient with a wound infection. Which of the following should the nurse do first?
   a. Check all patient allergies.
   b. Check the patient's temperature.
   c. Change dressing and note wound appearance.
   d. Give antibiotic before meal time.

6. Which of the following is the most important action for the nurse to use to prevent a hospital-acquired urinary tract infection in a patient with an indwelling urinary catheter?
   a. Ensure an adequate intake of IV and oral fluids.
   b. Use clean technique for catheter insertion.
   c. Position drainage bag higher than bladder level.
   d. Maintain a closed urinary drainage system.

7. Which of the following statements indicates to the nurse that the patient understands the general principles of appropriate antibiotic use?
   a. "I'll take this until I start feeling better."
   b. "I have pills left over from the last time I had this infection."
   c. "I'll take all of this as it says to on the medication label."
   d. "I take only half of a pill to reduce the cost of the pills."

Bibliography

1. Arnold SR, Straus S, Arnold S: Interventions to improve antibiotic prescribing practices in ambulatory care. Cochrane Database Syst Rev (4):CD003539, 2005.
2. Arroll, B, and Kenealy, T: Antibiotics for the common cold (Cochrane Review). In: *The Cochrane Library,* 1, Update Software, Oxford, UK, 2002.
3. Belliveau P, DeBellis, R: Management of nosocomial urinary tract infections in adult patients. J Clin Outcomes Manage 12:306, 2005.
4. Bjerke, NB: The evolution: Handwashing to hand hygiene guidance. Crit Care Nurs Q 27:295–307, 2004.
5. Brown, M, and Willms, D: Colonization of Yankauer suction catheters with pathogenic organisms. Am J Infect Control 33:483–485, 2005.
6. Ford-Thomas, C: Review: multivitamins and mineral supplements do not reduce infections in elderly people. Evid Based Nurs 9:24, 2006. doi:10.1136/ebn.9.1.24
7. Gagan, MJ: Review: probiotics are effective in preventing antibiotic associated diarrhoea. Evid Based Nurs 6:16, 2003.
8. Girou, E, Chai SH, Oppein F, et al: Misuse of gloves: the

foundation for poor compliance with hand hygiene and potential for microbial transmission? J Hosp Infect 57:162–169, 2004.

9. Goldrick BA: MRSA, VRE, and VRSA: How do we control them in nursing homes? Am J Nurs 104:50–51, 2004.

10. Gupta, A, Della-Latta, P, Todd, B, et al: Outbreak of extended-spectrum beta-lactamase-producing *Klebsiella pneumoniae* in a neonatal intensive care unit linked to artificial nails. Infect Control Hosp Epidemiol 25:210–215, 2004.

11. Jumaa, PA: Hand hygiene: simple and complex. Int J Infect Dis 9:3–14, 2005.

12. Klevens, RM, Edwards, JR, Tenorea, FC, et al: Changes in the epidemiology of methicillin-resistant *Staphylococcus aureus* in intensive care units in US hospitals, 1992–2003. Clin Infect Dis 42(3):389–391, 2006.

13. Mody L, McNeil SA, Sun R, et al: Introduction of a waterless alcohol-based hand rub in a long-term-care facility. Infect Control Hosp Epidemiol 24:165–171, 2003.

14. Stirling, B, Littlejohn, P, and Willbond, ML: Nurses and the control of infectious disease. Understanding epidemiology and disease transmission is vital to nursing care. Can Nurse 100:16–20, 2004.

Reference

1. Guideline for Hand Hygiene in Health-Care Settings MMWR October 25, 2002/51(RR16):1. CDC, 2002 accessed on 8/9/05 at http://www.cdc.gov/mmwr/preview/mmwrhtml/rr5116a1.htm

SUGGESTED ANSWERS TO

CRITICAL THINKING

■ *Mrs. Sampson*

1. Hand washing reduces the microorganisms on the nurse's hands to help reduce their transmission from patient to patient. This helps prevent exposure to pathogens and infection.

2. Risk for infection.

3. Reverse isolation, the goal of which is to protect the patient from exposure to organisms rather than to protect others from exposure to the patient.

■ *Who Is at Greatest Risk of Infection?*

1. Mr. Ashland has two risk factors: chronic disease and probably stress.

2. Mrs. Burrows has many risk factors, including old age, debilitated condition, probable malnourishment, probable stress, and an invasive procedure. This patient is at greatest risk.

3. Jackson has four risk factors: his young age, probable stress, possible malnourishment, and an invasive procedure.

■ *Mr. Carson*

1. Ask the nursing assistant about the urinary bag placed above the patient's bladder. Explain that the bag should always stay below the level of the bladder both for proper drainage and for infection control.

2. Assist the nursing assistant in repositioning the bag properly.

3. Let Mr. Carson's primary nurse know about the potential backflow of urine so that he can be assessed in the next few days for signs of a bladder infection.

■ *Mr. Cheevers*

Mr. Cheevers may be experiencing signs of allergic reaction to the medication. The fact that he has no history of allergy is no guarantee that he is not experiencing one now. He needs to be evaluated immediately, and if allergy is suspected, the IV should be stopped and the primary care provider notified. Epinephrine should be on hand to treat the patient for anaphylaxis. The primary nurse needs to be alerted to the situation in the event that it worsens. Later the nursing assistant can be instructed about the signs of allergic response.

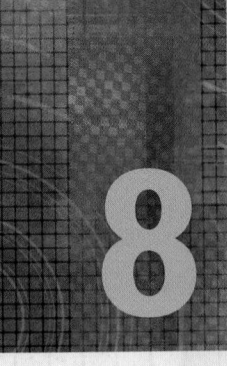

8

Nursing Care of Patients in Shock

CYNTHIA FRANCIS BECHTEL

KEY TERMS

acidosis (ass-i-DOH-sis)
acute pulmonary hypertension (ah-KEWT PULL-muh-NAIR-ee HIGH-per-TEN-shun)
anaerobic (AN-air-ROH-bick)
anaphylaxis (AN-uh-fi-LAK-sis)
bronchospasm (BRONG-koh-spazm)
cardiac output (KAR-dee-ack OWT-put)
cardiogenic (KAR-dee-oh-JEN-ick)
cyanosis (SIGH-uh-NOH-sis)
distributive (dis-TRIB-yoo-tiv)
dysrhythmia (dis-RITH-mee-yah)
epinephrine (EP-i-NEFF-rin)
extracardiac (EX-trah-KAR-dee-ack)
hypotension (HIGH-poh-TEN-shun)
hypovolemic (HIGH-poh-voh-LEEM-ick)
ischemia (iss-KEY-mee-ah)
lactic acid (LAK-tik ASS-id)
laryngeal edema (lah-RIN-jee-uhl uh-DEE-muh)
myocardium (MY-oh-KAR-dee-um)
myocarditis (MY-oh-kar-DYE-tis)
neurogenic (NEW-roh-JEN-ick)
norepinephrine (NOR-ep-i-NEFF-rin)
oliguria (AWH-li-GYOO-ree-ah)
perfusion (per-FEW-shun)
pericardial tamponade (PER-ih-KAR-dee-uhl TAM-pon-AID)
sepsis (SEP-sis)
tachycardia (TAK-ih-KAR-dee-yah)
tachypnea (TAK-ip-NEE-ah)
tension pneumothorax (TEN-shun NEW-moh-THOR-raks)
thrombi (THROM-bye)
toxemia (tock-SEE-me-ah)
trauma (TRAW-mah)
Trendelenburg (tren-DELL-en-berg)
urticaria (UR-ti-CARE-ee-ah)

QUESTIONS TO GUIDE YOUR READING

1. How would you explain the pathophysiology of shock and compensatory mechanisms?

2. What are the etiologies, signs, and symptoms of the four categories of shock?

3. What data should you collect when caring for patients with shock?

4. What are current therapeutic interventions for shock?

5. What nursing care should you provide for patients with shock?

6. How would the nurse prioritize care for a client in shock?

7. What findings would demonstrate a positive response to therapeutic interventions for shock?

Shock is a life-threatening condition. A patient in shock is in a state of circulatory collapse that results in organ damage and death without immediate treatment. Massive bleeding, overwhelming infection, severe allergic reactions, and cardiac failure are examples of conditions that may lead to shock. No matter what its source, shock is a medical emergency that requires rapid, comprehensive intervention in collaboration with the health care team.

Shock is defined as "inadequate tissue **perfusion**," in which there is insufficient delivery of oxygen and nutrients to the body's tissues and inadequate removal of waste products from these tissues. All body systems are affected by reduced oxygen supplies. The resulting injury to the body can be treated in the early stages of shock, but if shock is prolonged, it leads to irreversible cell damage and death. By the time blood pressure drops, cellular and tissue damage have already occurred. Therefore, it is important to identify patients at risk for shock and carefully assess them to detect early symptoms.

 ## PATHOPHYSIOLOGY OF SHOCK

Tissue perfusion and blood pressure are maintained in the body by three mechanisms: (1) adequate blood volume, (2) an effective cardiac pump, and (3) effective blood vessels. The body is able to compensate for failure of one of these mechanisms by making a change in one or both of the other two. Shock occurs when compensatory mechanisms fail, resulting in inadequate tissue perfusion. Common causes of shock include inadequate **cardiac output** caused by heart failure, a sudden loss of blood volume resulting from hemorrhage, or a sudden decrease in peripheral vascular resistance caused by **anaphylaxis, sepsis,** and neurological alterations.

Metabolic and Hemodynamic Changes in Shock

When blood pressure falls, the body responds by activating the sympathetic nervous system. **Epinephrine** and **norepinephrine** are released from the adrenal medulla and increase cardiac output by causing the heart to beat faster and stronger. Blood is shunted away from the skin, kidneys, and intestines to preserve blood flow to the brain, liver, and heart. Epinephrine, cortisol, and glucagon raise blood glucose levels to supply cells with fuel. Stimulation of the renin-angiotensin-aldosterone system from decreased cardiac output causes vasoconstriction and retention of sodium and water to decrease further fluid loss. Respiratory rate increases to deliver more oxygen to the tissues. Together these compensatory responses produce the classic signs and symptoms of the initial stage of shock: **tachycardia, tachypnea,** restlessness, anxiety, and cool, clammy skin with

pallor. If oxygen delivery remains inadequate, signs and symptoms of progressive and irreversible shock stages are seen (Table 8.1).

> ## CRITICAL THINKING
>
> ### Classic Signs of Shock
>
> ■ What is the cause and compensatory purpose of each of the classic signs of shock: tachycardia, tachypnea, **oliguria,** pallor, and cool, clammy skin?
> *Suggested answer at end of chapter.*

> ## ↘ LEARNING TIP
>
> Tachycardia is a compensatory mechanism that is usually the first sign of shock. When a patient develops sustained tachycardia, it is a signal that the patient's condition is changing. Be aware that elderly patients cannot tolerate tachycardia very long because their ability to adapt to stress is reduced.
>
> Consider the cause of the tachycardia. For example, a surgical patient who develops tachycardia may be hemorrhaging and should be assessed for bleeding. Be aware that with internal hemorrhaging there may not be any visible signs of bleeding. Changes in vital signs may be the only evidence.
>
> Provide prompt intervention, such as applying direct pressure to an area of hemorrhage, and implement the physician's orders immediately.

Inadequate tissue blood flow causes an important change in cellular metabolism. When cells are deprived of oxygen, they shift to **anaerobic** metabolism to continue to receive nutrition and energy. As you may recall, anaerobic metabolism is an inefficient form of metabolism that can supply the energy needs of the cell for a few minutes only. After that, the body's metabolic rate and temperature begin to fall as a result of reduced energy production. Anaerobic metabolism results in the production of **lactic acid** as an unwanted by-product. Unless the lactic acid can be circulated to the liver and thus removed from the bloodstream, the blood becomes increasingly acidic. **Acidosis,** which is a fall in blood pH below 7.35, is one of the classic signs of shock.

Effect on Organs and Organ Systems

Prolonged shock causes extensive damage to the organs and organ systems (Table 8.2). Inadequate blood flow results in

---

anaphylaxis: an—without + phylaxis—protection
tachycardia: tachy—fast + cardia—heart
tachypnea: tachy—fast + pnea—breathing

oliguria: olig—few + uria—urine
anaerobic: an—without + aerobic—presence of oxygen
acidosis: acid—sour + osis—condition

TABLE 8.1 SIGNS AND SYMPTOMS OF SHOCK STAGES

Signs and Symptoms	Stages		
	Mild/Compensated *Able to maintain BP and tissue perfusion*	*Moderate/Progressive* *Compensatory mechanisms start to fail*	*Severe Irreversible/Decompensated* *Do not respond to treatment* *Death is imminent*
Heart Rate	Tachycardia	Tachycardia >150 bpm	Slowing
Pulses	Bounding	Weaker, thready	Absent
Blood Pressure			
Systolic	Normal	Below 90 mm Hg In hypertensive 25% below baseline	Below 60 mm Hg
Diastolic	Normal	Decreased	Decreasing to 0
Respirations	Elevated	Tachypnea, crackles	Slowing
Depth	Deep	Shallow	Irregular, shallow
Temperature	Varies	Decreased May elevate in septic shock	Decreasing
Level of consciousness	Anxious, restless, irritable, alert, oriented, impending sense of doom	Confused, lethargy	Unconscious, comatose
Skin and Mucous Membranes	Cool, clammy, pale	Cold, moist, clammy, pale	Cyanosis, mottled, cold, clammy
Urine Output	Normal	Decreasing to less than 20 mL/hr	15 mL/hr decreasing to anuria
Bowel Sounds	Normal	Decreasing	Absent

CRITICAL THINKING

Anaerobic Metabolism

■ Why is anaerobic metabolism necessary and helpful if it produces the complication of metabolic acidosis?
Suggested answer at end of chapter.

tissue **ischemia** and injury. Because blood is shunted away from the kidneys early in shock to save fluid and provide oxygen to vital organs, the kidneys commonly are injured first. The kidneys can tolerate reduced blood flow for about 1 hour before sustaining permanent damage. Cells in the kidneys die when there is a lack of oxygen and nutrients. If there is widespread damage to the kidneys, complete renal failure is likely. Renal failure resulting from inadequate blood flow to the kidneys can be prevented and treated by replacing lost fluids.

Several organs of the gastrointestinal system may be injured early in shock. Inadequate circulation to the intestines may result in injury of the mucosa and may even cause paralytic ileus. **Toxemia** may result when the body absorbs into the circulation normally occurring bacteria and endotoxins from inside the bowel. The liver may be injured both by ischemia and by toxins created by the shock state as blood is circulated through it for cleansing. Signs and symptoms of liver injury include decreased production of plasma proteins, abnormal clotting (because clotting factor production by the liver is impaired), and elevated serum levels of ammonia, bilirubin, and liver enzymes.

The immune system is also affected by shock. Many of the body's defenses become depleted from shock, leaving the body vulnerable to infection. Also, if the liver has been damaged, it is unable to assist the immune system in providing defense.

The body attempts to preserve blood supply to the heart and brain because these are vital organs that require a continuous supply of oxygen. Shock places extra demands on the heart itself, creating a situation in which the heart is in extra need of oxygen at a time when oxygen supplies are already low. When the **myocardium** receives inadequate oxygenation, cardiac output decreases and shock worsens.

TABLE 8.2 EFFECT OF SHOCK ON ORGANS AND ORGAN SYSTEMS

Lungs	Acute respiratory failure Acute respiratory distress syndrome
Renal	Renal failure
Heart	Dysrhythmias, myocardial ischemia, and myocardial depression
Liver	Abnormal clotting; decreased production of plasma proteins; elevated serum levels of ammonia, bilirubin, and liver enzymes
Immune System	Depletion of defense components
Gastrointestinal System	Mucosal injury, paralytic ileus, pancreatitis, absorption of endotoxins and bacteria
Central Nervous System	Ischemic damage, necrosis, brain death

The pumping ability of the heart can be further depressed by acidosis, toxins released into the blood from ischemic tissues, or ischemia-induced **dysrhythmias.** If the brain is deprived of circulation for more than 4 minutes, brain cells die from a lack of oxygen and glucose. Lengthy shock may result in brain death.

COMPLICATIONS FROM SHOCK

Acute respiratory distress syndrome (ARDS), disseminated intravascular coagulation (DIC), and multiple organ dysfunction syndrome (MODS) are three especially grave conditions that may follow a prolonged episode of shock. Patients with ARDS usually develop respiratory failure despite high levels of supplemental oxygen and mechanical ventilation. DIC results from ischemic damage to the endothelial lining of blood vessels. The formation of multiple tiny **thrombi,** microscopic debris, and depletion of tissue clotting factors cause abnormal bleeding and additional tissue damage. DIC itself may cause shock and death. MODS is a major cause of death following shock. When an organ has inadequate perfusion it fails, which may increase the rate of failure of other organs. It usually begins with respiratory failure, followed by failure of the kidneys, heart, liver, and finally cerebral and gastrointestinal function.

 LEARNING TIP

To understand what *disseminated intravascular coagulation* means, define each of the words and then put the definitions together.

Disseminated = scattered or widespread

Intravascular: intra = inside + vascular = vessels

Coagulation = clotting

These definitions put together tell you that DIC is scattered, widespread clotting inside the vessels.

At first, hemorrhage does not seem reasonable in light of a clotting problem, but if you think about what is occurring, it does make sense. When many clots form throughout the body in response to stressors, few clotting factors remain available to form the clots needed to prevent hemorrhage. As a result, hemorrhage is a risk in DIC.

CLASSIFICATION OF SHOCK

The different forms of shock are classified by their cardiovascular characteristics (Table 8.3). The four shock categories are:

- **Hypovolemic** shock caused by a decrease in the circulating blood volume

- **Cardiogenic** shock caused by cardiac failure
- **Extracardiac** obstructive shock caused by a blockage of blood flow in the cardiovascular circuit outside the heart
- **Distributive** shock caused by excessive dilation of the venules and arterioles

Most cases of clinical shock show only some components of each of these categories. However, this classification system is helpful in understanding shock. The hallmark characteristic, exhibited in all forms of shock, is a decrease in blood pressure usually below the level required to provide an adequate supply of blood to the tissues.

Hypovolemic Shock

Any severe loss of body fluid may lead to hypovolemic shock. Hypovolemic shock can be caused by dehydration; internal or external hemorrhage; fluid loss from burns, vomiting, or diarrhea; or loss of intravascular fluid into the interstitium as a result of sepsis or **trauma.** Clinical signs and symptoms include pale, cool, clammy skin; tachycardia; tachypnea; flat, nondistended peripheral veins; decreased jugular vein circumference; decreased urine output; and altered mental status. The body is usually able to compensate for blood loss of less than 15% or 750 mL. The initial symptom may only be tachycardia. At 20% to 25% blood loss, tachycardia and mild to moderate **hypotension** are present. With a loss of 40% or greater (2000 mL), all clinical signs and symptoms of shock are present. Volume loss may not be the only contributing factor to hypovolemic shock, but also the patient's age, health status, and the time frame for fluid loss can be factors.

Cardiogenic Shock

Cardiogenic shock results when the heart fails as a pump. It occurs in 5% to 10% of patients with acute myocardial infarction (AMI). In most cases, approximately 40% of the myocardium must be lost to produce cardiogenic shock. Patients with cardiogenic shock have signs and symptoms similar to hypovolemic shock, except that they may display distended jugular and peripheral veins, as well as other symptoms of heart failure, such as pulmonary edema. The presence of pulmonary edema is what differentiates cardiogenic shock from other forms of shock. Other causes of cardiogenic shock include rupture of heart valves, acute **myocarditis,** end-stage heart disease, severe dysrhythmias, or traumatic injury to the heart.

Obstructive Shock

Extracardiac obstructive shock occurs when there is a blockage of blood flow in the cardiovascular circuit outside the heart. Several conditions may cause obstructive shock. **Pericardial tamponade,** which is the filling of the pericardial sac with blood, compresses the heart and limits its filling capacity. **Tension pneumothorax** compresses the heart from an abnormal collection of air in the pleural space and interferes with normal cardiac functioning. **Acute pulmonary hypertension,** a sudden abnormally elevated pressure in the pulmonary artery, increases resistance for blood

TABLE 8.3 CATEGORIES OF SHOCK

Category	Causes	Signs and Symptoms
Hypovolemic Shock	Any severe loss of body fluid; dehydration, internal or external hemorrhage, fluid loss from burns or from vomiting or diarrhea, or loss of intravascular fluid into the interstitium.	Tachycardia, tachypnea, hypotension, cyanosis, oliguria, flat nondistended peripheral veins, decreased jugular veins, and altered mental status.
Cardiogenic Shock	Myocardial infarction, myocarditis, end-stage cardiomyopathy, severe dysrhythmias, valvular disease, severe electrolyte imbalance, and drug overdoses.	Dysrhythmias, labored respirations, hypotension, cyanosis, oliguria, altered mental status, possibly distended jugular and peripheral veins, and symptoms of congestive heart failure.
Obstructive Shock	Any block to the cardiovascular flow. Pericardial tamponade, tension pneumothorax, intrathoracic tumors, massive pulmonary emboli, and large systemic emboli.	Tachycardia, tachypnea, hypotension, cyanosis, oliguria, and altered mental status; jugular veins may be distended.
Distributive Shock	Any condition causing massive vasodilation of the peripheral circulation. Subcategories include anaphylactic, septic, and neurogenic shock.	See subcategories below.
Anaphylactic shock	Insect stings, antibiotics, anesthetics, contrast dye and blood products are typical allergens.	Tachycardia, tachypnea, hypotension, cyanosis, oliguria, and altered mental status. May also have urticaria, pruritus, angioedema, laryngeal edema, and severe bronchospasm. If conscious, may be extremely apprehensive and complain of a metallic taste.
Septic shock	Massive release of chemical mediators and endotoxins causes loss of vascular autoregulatory control and loss of fluid into the interstitium. Bacteria, especially gram-negative strains, protozoans, and viruses.	Early or warm phase: blood pressure, urine output, and neck veins may be normal. Skin warm and flushed with full veins. Fever usually present, although temperature may be subnormal. Late phase: tachycardia, tachypnea, hypotension, oliguria, flat jugular and peripheral veins, and cool clammy skin. Normal or subnormal temperature.
Neurogenic shock	Dysfunction or injury to the nervous system. Spinal cord injury, general anesthesia, fever, metabolic disturbances, and brain injuries.	Early phase: hypotension and altered mental status, bradycardia, and skin that is warm and dry. Late phase: tachycardia, tachypnea, and cool clammy skin.

flowing out the right side of the heart. All these conditions decrease cardiac output, which can lead to shock. Tumors or large emboli may also cause shock. Signs and symptoms of obstructive shock are similar to those of hypovolemic shock, except that jugular veins are usually distended.

Distributive Shock

Distributive shock occurs when peripheral vascular resistance is lost because of massive vasodilation of the peripheral circulation. Distributive shock includes anaphylactic, septic, and **neurogenic** shock.

Anaphylactic Shock

Anaphylactic shock, the most severe type of distributive shock, occurs when the body has an extreme hypersensitivity reaction to an antigen. Death from anaphylactic shock may occur in minutes. It occurs most commonly from insect stings, antibiotics (especially penicillins), shellfish, peanuts, anesthetics, contrast dye, and blood products. The signs and symptoms are similar to those seen in hypovolemic shock. Additionally, patients may have symptoms specific to allergic reactions, including **urticaria,** pruritus, wheezing, **laryngeal edema, angioedema,** and severe **bronchospasm.** If conscious, patients may be extremely apprehensive and short of breath, and they may complain of a metallic taste.

Septic Shock

Septic shock, the most common type of distributive shock, is caused by systemic infection and inflammation. Extensive release of chemical mediators and endotoxins causes dilation of blood vessels and loss of fluid into the interstitial space. Most cases of sepsis are caused by gram-negative bacteria, although other bacteria and viruses may be the cause. In recent years, the number of cases of gram-negative shock has been decreasing, whereas there has been an alarming increase in the number of cases of septic shock from multidrug-resistant bacteria and fungi. Septic shock is the leading cause of death among critical care patients. Predisposing conditions include trauma, diabetes mellitus, corticosteroid therapy, immunocompromise (e.g., as seen in patients with human immunodeficiency virus [HIV] and in those undergoing chemotherapy treatment for cancer), burns, malnutrition, and invasive catheters.

During the early, or warm, phase of septic shock (which may be referred to as "pink" shock), blood pressure, urine output, and neck vein size may be normal, but the skin is warm and flushed owing to vasodilation. Fever is present in the majority of patients, although some may have a subnormal temperature. Left untreated, septic shock progresses to a second phase with signs and symptoms similar to hypovolemic shock: hypotension, oliguria, tachycardia, tachypnea, flat jugular and peripheral veins, and cold, clammy skin. Body temperature may be normal or subnormal.

Neurogenic Shock

Neurogenic shock occurs when dysfunction or injury to the nervous system causes extensive dilation of peripheral blood vessels. It is a rarer form of shock, occurring most commonly as a result of injury to the spinal cord (referred to as spinal shock). It occurs due to factors that either stimulate the parasympathetic nervous system or block the sympathetic nervous system. Other causes include general anesthesia, fever, metabolic disturbances, and brain contusions and concussions. Signs and symptoms include hypotension and altered mental status and, during the early phases, bradycardia and warm, dry skin. As shock progresses, however, tachycardia and cool, clammy skin develop.

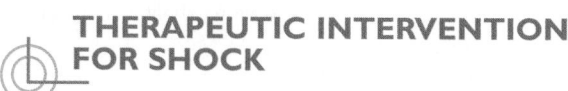

THERAPEUTIC INTERVENTIONS FOR SHOCK

Because of the emergency nature of shock, the exact nature of the shock must be determined while interventions such as ventilatory and circulatory support are being implemented (Table 8.4). Life-threatening symptoms must be treated immediately (Table 8.5). Medications that are used in shock are listed in Table 8.6. The order of interventions and testing is guided by the stability of the patient. Intervention priorities are as follows:

1. Airway
2. Breathing and respiratory support
3. Cardiovascular support
4. Maintenance of circulatory volume
5. Control of bleeding if present
6. Assessment of neurological status
7. Treatment of life-threatening injuries
8. Determination and treatment of the cause of shock

Modified Trendelenburg Position

Research studies have not demonstrated that the Trendelenburg position or the modified Trendelenburg position is

TABLE 8.4 ASSESSMENT OF THE PATIENT IN SHOCK

Signs and Symptoms	Tachycardia, tachypnea, hypotension, oliguria, cyanosis, altered mental status
Diagnostic Tests	
Laboratory Tests	Complete blood count, serum osmolarity, blood chemistries, prothrombin time, partial thromboplastin time, blood typing and crossmatch, serum lactate, arterial blood gases, cardiac isoenzymes, urinalysis
Imaging	Chest x-ray, spinal films, computed tomography, echocardiogram
Monitoring	Electrocardiogram, arterial pressure monitor, central venous pressure, pulmonary artery catheter, gastric pH

TABLE 8.5 THERAPEUTIC INTERVENTIONS FOR SHOCK

Respiratory support	Oxygen (nasal cannula, face mask, non-rebreather mask, assisted ventilations with bag-valve-mask, ventilator) SpO_2 >90%
Cardiovascular support	Venous lactic acid <2.2 mmol/L Vasopressor medication (dopamine) if fluid resuscitation not effective Revascularization of heart in cardiogenic shock via angioplasty with or without stent or fibrinolytic therapy (alteplase) Antidysrhythmics Positive inotropes
Adequate circulatory volume	1–3 L IV fluids Crystalloid fluids: normal saline (0.9% sodium chloride) or lactated Ringer's solution. 3 mL crystalloid solution for every 1 mL fluid lost Blood or blood products Urine output >30 mL/hour Hemoglobin >10 g/dL
Control of bleeding	Pressure dressings Surgical intervention
Treatment of life-threatening injuries	Surgical interventions Medications
Determination and treatment of causes of shock	Septic shock: antibiotics Cardiogenic shock: morphine, diuretics, nitrates Anaphylactic shock: epinephrine, diphenhydramine (Benadryl), methylprednisolone (Solu-Medrol), aminophylline

beneficial in improving cardiac output in shock. In fact, these positions actually can have negative effects such as compromising respirations among other effects. Although you may still see these positions used, it is important to follow valid research results for the best patient outcomes. In cardiogenic shock, any position that increases blood flow to the compromised heart increases the heart's workload. This could overwhelm or flood the heart so that it is unable to keep up with the blood volume returning to it. The result could be death.

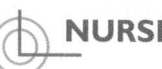

NURSING PROCESS

Assessment/Data Collection

Assessment of the patient in shock must be carried out quickly and should always start with the ABCDs: airway, breathing, circulation, and disability.

Airway is assessed for patency and opened as necessary. A compromised airway must be treated immediately with the head-tilt/chin-lift method, an oral or nasal airway, or endotracheal intubation.

Breathing is assessed for rate, depth, and symmetry of chest movement. The patient is observed for use of accessory muscles. Lung sounds are auscultated. Crackles may be

TABLE 8.6 MEDICATIONS USED FOR SHOCK

Medication Class/Action	Examples	Route	Side Effects	Nursing Implications
Autonomic nervous system agents				
Alpha and beta adrenergic agents				
Strengthens myocardial contraction and increases systolic BP and increases cardiac output	Epinephrine Dopamine Norepinephrine	IV IV IV	Nervousness Palpitations Tachycardia Tremors	Correct hypovolemia before giving medications in shock Monitor VS frequently Monitor intake and output
Used for bronchodilation	Epinephrine	SC/IM		First drug given in anaphylactic shock Give with TB syringe
Beta adrenergic agent Increases cardiac output in cardiogenic shock Constricts bronchial arterioles Inhibits histamine release Relieves bronchospasm in Rx of anaphylactic shock	Dobutamine	IV	Increased heart rate Anginal pain	Monitor VS frequently Monitor intake and output
Antihistamine	Benadryl	IV/PO	Drowsiness Tachycardia Dry mouth	Monitor VS Caution about activity with drowsiness
Anti-inflammatory Control of severe allergic reactions	Methyprednisilone (Solu-medrol)	IV	Side effects usually occur with long-term use	
Cogin A new class of agents that inhibits coagulation, decreases the inflammatory response, and promotes fibrinolysis in sepsis Increases survival in patients with severe sepsis	Xigris/Drotrecogin alfa	IV infusion for 96 hr	Bleeding	Contraindicated in patients with active bleeding or high risk of bleeding

IV = intravenous; PO = oral; Rx = treatment; SC = subcutaneous; VS = vital signs.

found in the patient with cardiogenic shock or in the patient who has received too much intravenous (IV) fluid. Wheezing may be present in the patient with anaphylactic shock.

Circulation is assessed with blood pressure. A narrowing pulse pressure may be present before a drop in systolic pressure and indicates a decrease in cardiac stroke volume and peripheral vasoconstriction. Peripheral pulses are palpated. Tachycardia is the first sign of shock. However, patients on medications that block the sympathetic nervous system response will not exhibit tachycardia. The pulse is assessed for quality; commonly it is weak and thready in a patient with shock. As shock progresses, the peripheral pulses become bradycardic or absent. A capillary refill greater than 3 seconds indicates inadequate circulation. Capillary refill has been found to be an unreliable indicator of shock in adults, especially elderly people. Other observations regarding circulation include distended neck veins, which may be collapsed or full; skin that may be cool, pale, and diaphoretic; presence of **cyanosis;** mucous membranes that may be pale and dry; and thirst. Rapidly scan the entire body for evidence of bleeding or other injuries. Palpate the abdomen for signs of internal bleeding, such as a tender, distended, boardlike abdomen.

CRITICAL THINKING

Beta Blockers

■ A patient who takes a beta blocker is being monitored for septic shock. What sign of shock do you understand will not be present in a patient taking a beta blocker?

Suggested answer at end of chapter.

Disability is assessed by determining the patient's level of consciousness (LOC). A decrease in LOC indicates disability. This disability can range from lethargy to coma.

All four limbs are assessed for circulation, sensation, and mobility (CSM). Bilateral responses are compared for

NURSING CARE TIP

There is usually a loss of peripheral pulses in the patient whose systolic blood pressure has dropped below 80. If you are able to palpate radial pulses on your patient, you know that the systolic blood pressure is at least 80.

NURSING CARE TIP

To assess level of consciousness, determine if the patient is alert by asking his or her name, the date, and the location. If the patient can answer all three questions, he or she is "alert and oriented × 3 (person, place, time)."

equality. Circulation is assessed by palpating pulses for presence and quality. Sensation is determined by touching the patient's hands and feet and asking what the patient feels and if there is any numbness or tingling. Mobility (motor ability) is assessed by having the patient move all four limbs and wiggle the fingers and toes. Have the patient push with his or her feet against your hands and squeeze two of your fingers to assess strength.

A "head-to-toe" approach can follow the primary ABCD assessment. The presence, severity, and location of pain or nausea and vomiting are assessed. Bowel sounds are auscultated to determine whether they are normal, absent, hyperactive, or hypoactive. When an indwelling urinary catheter has been placed, the color of the urine and the rate of urine output are noted. Body temperature should be noted.

Nursing Diagnosis, Planning, Implementation, and Evaluation

See Table 8.7 for a summary of shock.

See Box 8.1 Nursing Care Plan for the Patient in Shock.

LEARNING TIP

Here is a saying to help you remember blood pressure effects in shock:

If they're 90/60, they're getting kinda sickly. Say it again. If they're 90/60, they're getting kinda sickly.

CRITICAL THINKING

Mr. Hall

■ Mr. Hall, who is 55 years old, has suffered an acute myocardial infarction. He is complaining of chest pain (rated 10 out of 10 on the pain rating scale) and difficulty breathing. His SpO_2 is 89%. Crackles are heard on auscultation of breath sounds. The electrocardiogram shows an irregular and rapid heartbeat. He is restless and apprehensive.

1. Name three nursing priorities for Mr. Hall's care.
2. What type of IV fluid and rate is appropriate for Mr. Hall?
3. What signs and symptoms indicate Mr. Hall is in cardiogenic shock?

Suggested answers at end of chapter.

TABLE 8.7 SHOCK SUMMARY

Signs and symptoms	Tachycardia Tachypnea Hypotension Oliguria Cyanosis Altered mental state
Diagnostic tests	Decreased hemoglobin Increased lactic acid Decreased hematocrit in hemorrhage Increased WBC in sepsis Decreased pH in metabolic acidosis
Therapeutic interventions	Oxygen IV fluids Vasopressor medications Treat underlying cause
Complications	Acute respiratory distress syndrome (ARDS) Disseminated intravascular coagulation (DIC) Multiple organ dysfunction syndrome (MODS)
Possible nursing diagnoses	Ineffective tissue perfusion (renal, cerebral, cardiopulmonary, gastrointestinal, peripheral) Fear

CRITICAL THINKING

Mrs. Neal

■ Mrs. Neal, who is 45 years old, came to the emergency room in severe hypovolemic shock after sustaining several bleeding wounds in an automobile accident. Her shock is resolving after receiving several transfusions and surgical repair of her injuries. She has just been admitted to the surgical unit for postoperative care.

1. What postoperative nursing assessments should be performed first?
2. Mrs. Neal's family is very alarmed by her condition. What interventions can you provide to decrease their anxiety?
3. What postoperative complications may develop in Mrs. Neal?
4. What documentation is appropriate for Mrs. Neal?

Suggested answers at end of chapter.

BOX 8.1 NURSING CARE PLAN for the Patient Experiencing Shock

Ineffective Tissue Perfusion (Renal, Cerebral, Cardiopulmonary, Gastrointestinal, Peripheral) related to hypovolemia or inadequate cardiac output or inadequate vascular tone

Expected Outcomes Patient demonstrates adequate tissue perfusion

Evaluation of Outcome Is patient's skin warm/dry, peripheral pulses present/strong? Are vital signs within patient's normal range? Are lung sounds normal, intake/output balanced, edema absent, pain/discomfort absent? Is patient alert and oriented?

Interventions	Rationale	Evaluation
Maintain airway and provide oxygenation.	Ensures adequate oxygenation and tissue perfusion.	Is SpO_2 >90%? Is skin pink? Are respirations between 12 and 20? Are lung sounds clear?
Monitor vital signs.	Changes in vital signs, which indicate change in condition, can be detected early and treated promptly.	Is heart rate between 60 and 100 beats per minute? Is heart rhythm regular? Are peripheral pulses strong? Is systolic blood pressure (BP) >100 mm Hg? Is patient alert and oriented $\times$ 3?
Monitor intake and output.	Provides adequate cardiac output to perfuse tissues. Assesses renal function. Urine output is an indicator of renal function.	Is urinary output >30 mL/hr?
Provide adequate fluid intake.	Maintains volume.	Are mucous membranes moist? Is skin turgor < 3 seconds?
Position patient appropriately (head elevated for patients with shortness of breath, increased intracranial pressure).	Proper positioning promotes circulation and helps prevent skin breakdown.	Is edema noted? Is skin breakdown noted?
Provide quiet, restful environment.	Conserves energy and lowers tissue oxygen demands.	Is patient resting comfortably without anxiety?
Maintain body temperature with warmed IV fluids, room temperature, blankets.	Recovery is aided by normal body temperature.	Is body temperature within normal limits?
Assess for pain and provide pain relief measures.	Pain increases tissue demands for blood and oxygen.	Is patient pain free?
Geriatric		
Change positions slowly.	Age-related losses of cardiovascular reflexes can result in hypotension.	Is systolic BP >100 mm Hg?

Decreased Cardiac Output related to reduced circulating blood volume

Expected Outcomes: Patient has adequate cardiac output as evidenced by vital signs and cardiac rhythm within normal limits (WNL).

Evaluation of Outcome Are blood pressure, heart rate, and cardiac rhythm within normal limits?
Are nailbeds and/or skin pink?
Is skin warm and dry?

Interventions	Rationale	Evaluation
Monitor heart rate and cardiac rhythm with ECG and report abnormalities.	Changes in heart rate and cardiac rhythm can be detected immediately and treated appropriately.	Is heart rate and rhythm normal?
Assess skin/nailbed color, capillary refill and peripheral pulses and report abnormalities.	Inadequate perfusion is first evident in skin/nailbeds and peripheral pulses.	What color and temperature is the skin/nailbeds? Is capillary refill normal? Are peripheral pulses present? Is heart rate and rhythm normal?
Give cardiovascular medications and oxygen as ordered.	Cardiac function can be supported with medications. Supplemental oxygen increases oxygenation of heart and tissues.	
Reduce myocardial oxygen demand by utilizing comfort measures to alleviate pain and anxiety, and by keeping the body at an appropriate temperature.	Pain, anxiety, and cold all increase tissue demands for blood and oxygen, which places increased workload on the heart to supply it.	Is body temperature within normal limits? Is the patient free of pain and anxiety?

Fear related to severity of condition and unknown outcome

Expected Outcomes Patient states fear is reduced.

Evaluation of Outcomes Does patient state fear is decreased?

Interventions	Rationale	Evaluation
Provide explanations for procedures, the condition and its treatment.	Knowledge allows a feeling of control and reduces fear.	Does patient state fear is reduced?

Deficient Knowledge related to unfamiliar condition of shock

Expected Outcomes Patient explains shock and its treatment.

Evaluation of Outcomes Can patient explain shock and how it is treated?

Interventions	Rationale	Evaluation
Assess patient's ability to learn and identify barriers to learning.	For learning, the patient must be ready to learn. Barriers such as life style changes or the shock of the diagnosis may decrease learning.	Is patient alert and stable? Does patient indicate willingness to learn? Does patient express concerns about condition?
Provide information that is most relevant to patient first.	Giving necessary information first meets patient's immediate needs.	Does patient state understanding of important information?
Allow time for questions and clarification.	Clarification ensures accurate information is learned.	Does the patient state accurate information?

REVIEW QUESTIONS

1. Which of the following mechanisms does the body use to compensate for shock?
   a. Peripheral nervous system depression
   b. Central nervous system depression
   c. Sympathetic nervous system stimulation
   d. Parasympathetic nervous system stimulation

2. Which of the following findings would the nurse recognize as specifically occurring with anaphylactic shock?
   a. Wheezing
   b. Hypotension
   c. Tachycardia
   d. Oliguria

3. Which of the following conditions causes the decreased level of consciousness commonly found in patients experiencing shock?
   a. Severe pain
   b. Endotoxins
   c. Cerebral edema
   d. Cerebral hypoxia

4. Which of the following nursing diagnoses is most appropriate to include in the plan of care for a patient experiencing shock?
   a. Fatigue
   b. Ineffective tissue perfusion
   c. Ineffective health maintenance
   d. Hopelessness

5. A patient who is found lying in a pool of blood from a leg incision that has opened is restless and confused. The nurse calls for help and takes vital signs. Which of the following treatments for shock would the nurse anticipate would be ordered first?
   a. IV fluids
   b. Oxygen
   c. Vasopressor medications
   d. Antibiotics

6. Which patient would be a priority for the nurse to see?
   a. A patient who was in a motor vehicle accident, blood pressure 140/80, pulse 98, respirations 22
   b. A patient who had chest pain with blood pressure 108/68, pulse 84, respirations 16
   c. A patient who slipped and fell with blood pressure 112/74, pulse 68, respirations 14
   d. A patient who is one day post op, blood pressure 90/58, pulse 118, respirations 24

7. Which of the following findings would indicate to the nurse that therapeutic interventions are effective in shock?
   a. Heart rate 110
   b. SpO_2 89%
   c. Systolic blood pressure 108
   d. Respiratory rate 22

8. Place in correct order of occurrence systolic blood pressure progression through the three stages of shock beginning with mild, moderate, and severe. Use all options.
   a. Below 60 mm Hg
   b. Normal
   c. Below 90 mm Hg

SUGGESTED ANSWERS TO

CRITICAL THINKING

■ *Classic Signs of Shock*

Tachycardia is caused by decreased cardiac output and reduced tissue oxygenation. Its purpose is to increase cardiac output and oxygen delivery by causing more heart beats to pump out blood from the heart.

Tachypnea is caused by decreased tissue oxygenation. Its purpose is to increase respirations so more oxygen is available for delivery to tissues.

Oliguria is caused by a reduced blood flow to the kidneys. Its purpose as a compensatory mechanism is to conserve as much fluid as possible to help maintain a normal blood pressure.

Pallor is caused by reduced blood volume or flow. When pallor results from compensation, it is due to peripheral vasoconstriction that occurs to shunt blood volume to the vital organs.

Cool, clammy skin is the result of decreased blood flow to the skin and the release of moisture (sweat) from the skin. The sympathetic nervous system causes these compensatory mechanisms; peripheral vasoconstriction shunts blood to the vital organs, and sweating cools the body in anticipation of the fight or flight response, which generates body heat when it occurs.

■ *Anaerobic Metabolism*

Anaerobic metabolism is the source of nutrition and energy for the cell that prevents cellular death when oxygen is not available. It is a short-term compensatory mechanism to save the cell until oxygen becomes available again.

■ *Beta Blockers*

Tachycardia will not be present. Beta blockers block the response of the sympathetic nervous system, which is activated in shock.

■ *Mr. Hall*

1. Nursing priorities for Mr. Hall include relief of chest pain and anxiety, stabilization of cardiac rhythm and vital signs, and adequate tissue oxygenation.

2. Because Mr. Hall's lung sounds reveal crackles, indicating fluid in the lungs, he should not be given IV fluids. He should have an IV access to give IV medications as needed. He already has too much fluid for his heart to handle, and giving him IV fluids could be life threatening.

3. Signs of cardiogenic shock include decreased blood pressure; increased heart and respiratory rates; cyanosis; decreased urine output; cool, pale skin; and decreased mental status.

■ *Mrs. Neal*

1. Assessment of respiratory status and cardiovascular status, inspection of surgical wounds for bleeding, assessment of mental status, and need for pain relief should be performed first.

2. Explain the cause of shock and all interventions, rationales, and desired outcomes. Keep the environment calm, provide for privacy, and answer all questions in a matter-of-fact and reassuring manner. Allow Mrs. Neal's family to visit.

3. Unrelieved pain, bleeding, infection, and respiratory complications are possible.

4. Airway: rate, depth, regularity of respirations; breath sounds, SpO_2. Vital signs: cardiac rhythm, quality of pulses, skin color, blood pressure, body temperature. Urine output: oral and IV intake, fluid balance. Pain: measures to relieve pain and evaluation of those measures. Dressings: any bleeding. Bowel sounds.

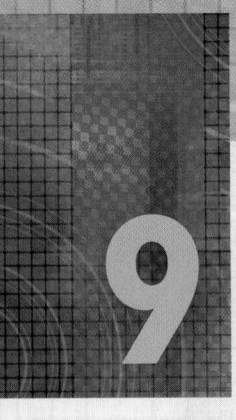

9

Nursing Care of Patients in Pain

KAREN P. HALL

KEY TERMS

addiction (uh-DIK-shun)
adjuvant (ad-JOO-vant)
agonist (AG-un-ist)
analgesic (AN-uhl-JEE-zik)
antagonist (an-TAG-on-ist)
breakthrough (BRAYK-THROO)
ceiling effect (SEE-ling e-FEKT)
endorphins (en-DOR-fins)
enkephalins (en-KEF-e-lins)
equianalgesic (EE-kwee-AN-uhl-JEE-zik)
malingerer (muh-LING-ger-er)
neuropathic (NEW-roh-PATH-ik)
nociceptive (NOH-see-SEP-tiv)
opioid (OH-pee-OYD)
pain (PAYN)
patient-controlled analgesia (PAY-shunt kon-
    TROHLD AN-uhl-JEE-zee-ah)
physical dependence (FIZ-ik-uhl dee-PEN-dens)
prostaglandins (PRAHS-tah-GLAND-ins)
pseudoaddiction (sue-doh-ah-DIK-shun)
psychological dependence (SY-ko-LAW-jick-al dee-
    PEN-dens)
suffering (SUFF-er-ing)
tolerance (TAWL-er-ens)
transdermal (trans-DER-mal)

QUESTIONS TO GUIDE YOUR READING

1. How is pain defined?

2. What are the common myths and barriers to the effective management of pain?

3. What are the differences between addiction, physical dependence, and tolerance?

4. What is current knowledge of the basic physiology of the pain response?

5. What are characteristics that help to define acute, chronic nonmalignant, and cancer pain?

6. What should be included in a basic pain assessment?

7. How is the World Health Organization analgesic ladder used for the treatment of pain?

8. What are the three classes of analgesics and their uses?

9. What are commonly used pain medication treatment modalities and their appropriate use?

10. How and when are nondrug pain management techniques utilized?

11. How does ethical decision making play a role in the care of the patient in pain?

THE PAIN PUZZLE

Pain is the most common reason patients seek medical advice. However, despite the widespread nature of the problem, pain is often untreated or undertreated. The care of patients with pain is challenging and requires a systematic approach to assessment and treatment.

Decisions about pain management require careful assessment of the patient's condition and attention to the ethical principles that influence patient care. Providing information and giving the patient choices helps maintain the patients autonomy. Just as risks, benefits, and alternatives to surgery and anesthesia are discussed with the patient, so should pain management options be discussed in the process of obtaining informed consent. Nurses often worry about overmedicating patients, thinking that they are "doing good" (beneficence) or "doing no harm" (nonmaleficence) by withholding medication from a patient they do not believe is in pain (Box 9.1 Ethical Consideration). It is important to learn as much as you can about pain and pain management so you can effectively advocate for your patients, assist with patient education, and provide appropriate resources.

The Joint Commission for Accreditation of Healthcare Organizations (JCAHO) published pain management standards in 2000 and began assessing the management of pain in hospitals and other health-care organizations based on these standards in January 2001. These standards support the importance of the appropriate and effective management of pain. They address assessment and the safe pharmacological management of pain, as well as patient and family teaching, postoperative pain, management of opioid-induced side effects, discharge planning, and process improvement. These guidelines are available through the JCAHO.org website.

For more information on pain management, visit the following Web sites. For some sites, it may be necessary to type "pain" in the search window.

> http://www.ahrq.gov
>
> http://www.ampainsoc.org
>
> http://www.cancer.org
>
> http://www.iasp-pain.org
>
> http://www.jcaho.org
>
> http://www.who.org

Cultural differences must be considered when planning care for the patient in pain. People from various cultures have different ways of expressing pain (Box 9.2 Cultural Considerations). Some may be dramatic and emotional; others tend to be stoic and quiet. Knowledge of widely accepted information about different ethnic and cultural groups can be useful in understanding a patient's experience and what care might be considered acceptable. It is important, however, to assess a patient's pain care needs individually and not make assumptions based on culture or ethnicity alone.

Because of the importance of controlling health-care costs, the entire health team must provide care in the most cost-effective manner possible while continuing to provide the best quality of care. Effective pain management can help reach those goals by enhancing comfort, minimizing side effects of **opioids** and complications related to inadequate pain control, and reducing the lengths of hospital stays.

(Text continued on page 125)

Box 9.1

Ethical Consideration—Controlling Pain

A patient was admitted from home to the medical unit 2 days after his 83rd birthday with a diagnosis of metastatic cancer of the pancreas. He had several full-course treatments of chemotherapy and radiation during the previous year with only temporary remissions of the disease. His condition deteriorated rapidly during the previous month, and his family was no longer able to care for him. The patient's physician expected him to die within a few weeks and admitted him to the hospital, primarily for pain control. On admission, the physician ordered morphine sulfate (MS) 5 mg IV to be given every 2 hours around the clock.

Although this seemed like a relatively large dose of a strong opioid medication to be given this frequently, the patient tolerated the treatment for the first 36 hours, and reported a significant reduction in his pain. On the third morning after his admission, he was difficult to arouse for his morning vital signs and breakfast. When his nurse, Kathy, finally did manage to awaken him, he was disoriented, his blood pressure was 82/50, and his respirations were shallow and 10/min. He still complained of generalized pain and asked for more medication.

Kathy did not give the patient his scheduled 0800 dose of MS. She phoned the physician and reported her assessment of the patient, expressing her belief that continuing the medication at the previously prescribed dose and frequency would be fatal to this patient. The physician, who had been up most of the night with an emergency patient, told her that the patient was dying and that she should administer the medication immediately. In this situation:

- What are Kathy's ethical obligations in this case (to self, patient, and community)?
- How should she weigh the risks and benefits of providing adequate pain medication given the possible side effect of hastening the patient's death?
- If Kathy has a moral objection to carrying out a physician's order, what are her options?
- How can Kathy find a way to start meaningful dialogue about such issues with the physician?

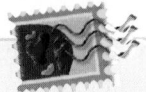

Cultural Considerations

The pain experience may differ between and among individuals of differing cultural, ethnic, or religious groups. Remember that individuals within groups can vary, and not all fit the general descriptions provided below. (See Chapter 3.)

Culture	Expression and Meaning of Pain	Patient Preferences	Assessment	Interventions
Native American	Frequently do not request pain medicine and are undertreated. May not realize that they can ask for pain medicine. Many believe pain is something that must be endured. May describe pain in general terms such as "not feeling good." The word for pain varies according to the tribal language.	Many prefer traditional herbal medicines. May complain to family member or visitor, who relays message to caregiver.	Frequently ask patient and family members or visitors if patient has pain. Observe for nonverbal clues of pain.	Explain that the control of pain can promote healing. Offer pain medicine as needed. Allow adequate time for response; silence is valued. Maintain a calm, relaxing environment. Incorporate traditional practices for pain relief if not harmful.
European American	Strong sense of stoicism, especially in men. Fear of being dependent may decrease use of pain medicine. Many have fear of addiction. May continue to work and carry out daily activities and minimize pain.	May prefer relaxation and distractions as means of pain control.	Observe for nonverbal signs of pain. Use visual analog or numerical pain scales to assess severity of pain.	Encourage use of pain medicine as needed. Incorporate distraction and relaxation techniques.
African American	Usually openly and publicly display pain, but this is highly variable. Many, especially the elderly, fear that medication may be addictive. Many believe that suffering and pain are inevitable and should be endured.	May focus on spirituality and religious beliefs to endure pain. Prayers and the laying on of hands are thought to relieve pain if the client has enough faith.	Observe for verbal and nonverbal expressions of pain. Use of pain scales is helpful.	Offer pain medication as needed. Allow meditation and prayer along with pain medication. Support patient's spiritual practices.
Hispanic American	Puerto Ricans tend to be expressive of pain and discomfort. Moaning, groaning, and crying are culturally accepted ways of dealing with and reducing pain. Mexicans may bear pain stoically because it is "God's will." Many feel that pain and suffering are a consequence of immoral behavior. For men, expressing pain shows weakness. The Spanish word for pain is *dolar*.	Prefer oral or intravenous medication for pain. Heat, herbal teas, and prayer are used to manage pain.	Visual analog and numerical scales may be helpful. Observe and compare verbal and nonverbal behaviors indicating pain.	Do not censor verbal expression of pain. Incorporate traditional practices as permitted. For individuals who are stoical with pain, encourage pain medicine frequently. Explain that pain control can hasten healing.

Culture	Expression and Meaning of Pain	Patient Preferences	Assessment	Interventions
Asian American	Chinese and Koreans tend to be stoical, and describe pain in terms of diverse body symptoms instead of locally. Filipinos may view pain as a part of living an honorable life. Some view this as an opportunity to reach a fuller life and to atone for past transgressions. Frequently stoic and tolerate pain to a high degree. Some moan as an expression of pain. For asians, bearing pain is a virtue and a matter of family honor. Some, especially older individuals, may fear addiction.	Prefer oral or intravenous pain medications. May like warm compresses. For Koreans, intramuscular injections may be seen as an invasion of privacy. Vietnamese maintain self-control as a means of pain relief.	Observe for nonverbal signs of pain. Vietnamese may not understand numerical scale of rating pain. Observing facial expression may provide a good indicator of pain.	Incorporate traditional healing methods as much as possible. Offer and encourage pain medicines to promote healing.
Arab American	See pain as something to be controlled. May express pain openly to family with elaborate verbal expressions, less so with caregivers. May use terms such as fire, hot, and cold.	Intramuscular or intravenous usually preferred over oral medications.	Compare verbal and nonverbal characteristics of pain to determine degree of pain.	Engage family to help with distraction and relaxation techniques. Administer medication promptly.

It is not possible to record a patient's pain on a machine or measure it as with a blood or urine sample. It is difficult to objectively gauge the effect of a nursing intervention on pain, whether the intervention is medication or nondrug therapy. Pain and its treatment can be likened to a difficult puzzle that requires many pieces to solve.

In this chapter, the many challenges of pain assessment and treatment are discussed. Some of the tools needed to effectively deal with these challenges are presented. Common myths and barriers that continue to affect nursing practice are clarified.

DEFINITIONS OF PAIN

According to Margo McCaffery, a well-known consultant in the care of patients with pain, "Pain is whatever the experiencing person says it is, existing whenever the experiencing person says it does."[1] This is a reminder to nurses to accept the patient's report of pain.

In 1979, pain was defined by the International Association for the Study of Pain (IASP) as "an unpleasant sensory and emotional experience associated with actual or potential tissue damage or described in terms of such damage."[2] This definition indicates that pain is complex, and is not only physical but has emotional and other components as well.

Why does it exist? Pain is a protective mechanism or a warning. Pain in the presence of injury may help to prevent further injury. Consider the patient who experiences a fracture and holds it still to prevent further damage or a child who touches a hot stove and pulls his or her hand away before a serious burn occurs.

Why is untreated or undertreated pain a bad thing? Complications can occur when pain is experienced. The body produces a stress response in the presence of pain during which harmful substances are released from injured tissue. Reactions include breakdown of tissue, increased metabolic rate, impaired immune function, and negative emotions. In addition, pain prevents the patient from participating in self-care activities such as walking, deep breathing, and coughing. Consider the patient who has had chest surgery and then has to cough and deep breathe. It hurts! Because he or she hurts nursing pain, the patient tries not to cough, turn, or even move. Retained pulmonary secretions and pneumonia can develop. If the patient does not move around, return of bowel function is delayed and an ileus can result. When pain is well controlled, complications can be avoided and patients are able to do what they need to do to get well and go home from the hospital or continue with recovery activities. The concept of "balanced analgesia" (see Options for Treatment below) emphasizes pain relief and control of adverse effects by combining analgesics from different classes of medications rather than using opioids alone.

Suffering often accompanies pain, but not all pain has the element of suffering. Suffering can exist without pain and pain without suffering. Suffering represents a threat to one's self-image or life. According to the latest cancer pain guidelines from the Agency for Health Care Research and Quality (AHCRQ), suffering is defined as the state of severe distress associated with events that threaten the intactness of the person.[3] Pain can be a constant reminder for patients with cancer that they have a life-threatening illness. Suffering can often be relieved if patients believe that their pain can be relieved.

MYTHS AND BARRIERS TO EFFECTIVE PAIN MANAGEMENT

Treatment of patients in pain is influenced by a number of factors, including the nurse's personal experiences with pain. Why are some patients not believed when they report pain? Why do some nurses and other health-care team members insist that patients behave a certain way before they are believed? Common myths about pain may impair the nurse's ability to be objective about pain and create barriers to effective treatment. Because there is no objective measure for pain, nurses may rely on what is comfortable rather than what has been proven to be effective.

Myth: A person who is laughing and talking is not in pain.

Fact: A person in pain is likely to use laughing and talking as a form of distraction. This can be very effective in the management of pain, especially when used in conjunction with appropriate drug therapies. Patients may be more easily distracted when they have visitors and may ask for pain medication as soon as their family or significant other goes home.

Myth: If morphine is given too early to the patient with cancer pain, it will not work when the patient really needs it, toward the end, when the pain is worse.

Fact: Morphine is an opioid **agonist.** Opioid doses can be escalated (titrated upward) indefinitely as needed as the patient's pain increases. There is no **ceiling effect,** or maximum effective dose. Side effects such as sedation or clinically significant respiratory depression may temporarily limit the dose or the rate at which the dose can be increased.

Myth: Respiratory depression is common in patients receiving opioid pain medications.

Fact: Respiratory depression is uncommon in patients receiving opioid pain medications. If patients are monitored carefully when they are at risk, such as with the first dose of an opioid or when a dose is increased, respiratory depression is preventable. A patient's respiratory status and level of sedation (LOS) should be routinely monitored using an LOS scale.

Myth: Pain medication is more effective when given by injection.

Fact: Intramuscular (IM) injections are not recommended because they are painful, have unreliable absorption from the muscle, and have a lag time to peak effect and rapid falloff compared with oral administration. Oral administration is the first choice if possible; the intravenous (IV) route has the most rapid onset of action and is the preferred route for postoperative administration.

Myth: Teenagers are more likely to become addicted than older patients.

Fact: Addiction to opioids is very uncommon in all age groups when taken for pain by patients without a prior drug abuse history.

MORE PAIN-RELATED DEFINITIONS

Nurses often express concern about patients who require large amounts of pain medication or know exactly when their next dose of pain medication is due. Nurses may say that such patients are addicted or that they are "clock watchers," but do we really know what that means? Patients are expected to be informed about their medications and involved in their care, but when they know when their medications are due, we may become suspicious. In truth, if a patient is watching the clock, the most likely reason is because he or she is in pain. The most common reason that patients ask for more pain medicine is because they have increased pain. It is important to understand the differences between **addiction,** **physical dependence,** and **tolerance.** When talking with patients and teaching them about their medications, it is important to help them understand these differences as well. Addiction is something many patients fear.

CRITICAL THINKING

Mrs. Smithers and Mr. Barnett

■ Mrs. Smithers had an abdominal hysterectomy and is sitting up in bed the morning after surgery, putting on her makeup. On morning rounds she is smiling but reports that her pain is at 6 on a scale of 0 to 10. Mr. Barnett has just been transferred from the surgical intensive care unit the day after surgery for multiple injuries. He is moaning and reports his pain at 6 on a scale of 0 to 10. Which of these patients is really having as much pain as they say they are? How can you make that judgment?

Suggested answers at end of chapter.

Tolerance simply means that it takes a larger dose to provide the same level of pain relief. Physical dependence is a physiological phenomenon that most people experience after a few weeks of continuous opioid use. If an opioid is abruptly discontinued after a few weeks of use, the patient may experience a withdrawal syndrome, exhibiting symptoms such as sweating, tearing, runny nose, restlessness, irritability, tremors, dilated pupils, sleeplessness, nausea, vomiting, and diarrhea. These symptoms can be prevented by slowly weaning a patient from an opioid rather than stopping it suddenly.

Psychological dependence is a better term for addiction and is defined as a pattern of compulsive drug use characterized by a continued craving for an opioid and the need to use the opioid for effects other than pain relief. The patient who is psychologically dependent continues to use the drug despite harmful effects.

Pseudoaddiction has been described in patients who are receiving opioid doses that are too low or spaced too far apart to relieve their pain, and certain behavioral characteristics resembling psychological dependence, such as drug-seeking behaviors, have developed. The difference is, in the patient with this phenomenon, the drug seeking behaviors cease when the pain is relieved.

MECHANISMS OF PAIN TRANSMISSION

Many theories of how pain is transmitted are described in the literature. The specificity theory, developed by Descartes in 1644, proposed that body trauma sends a message directly to the brain, causing a sort of "bell" to ring, prompting a response from the brain. In 1965, Melzack and Wall proposed the gate control theory, which describes the dorsal horn of the spinal cord as a gate, allowing impulses to go through when there is a pain stimulus and closing the gate when those impulses are inhibited. The gate control theory stimulated massive research on the physiology of pain and is still considered in research.

Much more is known about the transmission of pain today. **Endorphins** are endogenous (naturally occurring) chemicals that act like opioids to inhibit pain impulses in the spinal cord and brain. Unfortunately, they degrade too quickly to be considered effective **analgesics.** Endorphins are the chemicals that stimulate the long-distance runner's "high." **Enkephalins** are one type of endorphin.

Pain is transmitted through the dorsal horn of the spinal cord and other points in the central nervous system to higher centers of the brain with the influence of chemicals known as neurotransmitters, which are released from damaged tissue. These chemicals include **prostaglandins,** substance P, and others. Many treatments and analgesics are designed, based on known principles, to inhibit the release of these chemicals at different points along the pain pathway. It is also now understood that men and women respond differently to painful stimuli and to pain management interventions.

Mechanisms of pain transmission are **nociceptive** and **neuropathic.** *Nociception* refers to the body's normal or physiological reaction to noxious stimuli, such as tissue damage, with the release of pain-producing substances. Nociceptive pain in the visceral organs may be referred to other parts of the body (Fig. 9.1). Neuropathic pain is pain associated with injury to either the peripheral or central nervous system. Unlike nociceptive pain, neuropathic, or nonphysiologic, pain is not usually localized, and it may spread to involve other areas along the nerve pathway.

TYPES OF PAIN

Pain is often categorized according to whether it is acute, cancer related, or chronic nonmalignant. Acute pain is des-

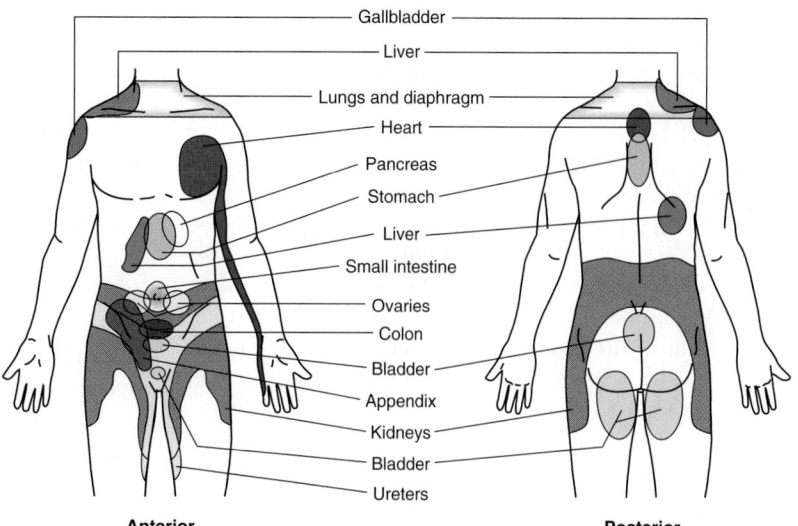

FIGURE 9.1 Sites of referred pain.

Anterior

Posterior

---

pseudoaddiction: pseudo—false + addiction—psychological dependence

nociceptive: noci—pain + ceptive—reception
neuropathic: neuro—nerves + pathy—disease, suffering

cribed as pain that follows injury to the body, prompting an inflammatory response, and subsides as healing takes place. It may be associated with short-term, objective, physical signs such as increased heart rate and elevated blood pressure. Examples of acute pain include pain related to fractures, burns, or other trauma.

Cancer pain may be acute, chronic, or intermittent and often has a definable cause such as tumor invasion or neuropathy caused by the cancer treatment.

Chronic nonmalignant pain persists beyond the time when healing usually takes place, such as low back pain, the pain accompanying arthritis, and phantom limb pain. Chronic nonmalignant pain may have nociceptive as well as neuropathic components and may require a variety of medications and nondrug treatments. Because of the body's ability to adapt, patients with chronic nonmalignant pain or chronic cancer pain may not appear to be in pain. The physiological responses that accompany acute pain, such as elevated heart rate and blood pressure, cannot be sustained without harm to the body, so the body adapts and the vital signs return to normal. The nurse must guard against labeling these patients as **malingerers** (pretending to be in pain) or drug seeking.

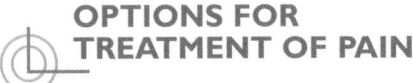

OPTIONS FOR TREATMENT OF PAIN

Analgesics

Medications that relieve pain are called analgesics. Analgesics are the largest pieces of the pain management puzzle. There are three main classes of analgesics: opioids, nonopioids, and **adjuvants.** Opioids are classified by their ability to bind to opioid receptors in the brain and spinal cord, as well as other areas of the body, inhibiting the perception of pain. Nonopioids include nonsteroidal anti-inflammatory drugs (NSAIDs) and acetaminophen (Tylenol). Adjuvants include categories of drugs that were originally developed for a different purpose but have been found to have pain-relieving properties in certain painful conditions.

Nonopioids

Nonopioids are generally the first class of drugs used for treatment of pain. They can be useful for acute and chronic pain from a variety of causes, such as surgery, trauma, arthritis, and cancer. These medications are limited in their use because they have a ceiling effect to analgesia. A ceiling effect indicates that there is a dose beyond which there is no improvement in the **analgesic** effect and there may be an increase in adverse effects. When used in combination with opioids, care must be taken to ensure that the dose of the nonopioid drug does not exceed the maximum safe dose for a 24-hour period. For example, if a patient receiving two acetaminophen with hydrocodone (Vicodin) tablets every 4 hours continues to experience pain, the dose cannot be increased because of the potential toxic effects of the aceta-

TABLE 9.1 ADVERSE EFFECTS OF NONOPIOIDS

Drug	Adverse Effects
NSAIDs (including aspirin)	Gastrointestinal (GI) irritation and bleeding Inhibition of platelet aggregation, increasing risk of GI bleeding Renal insufficiency in some patients, especially the elderly Patients with asthma at risk for hypersensitive reactions
Acetaminophen	Necrosis of the liver with overdose

minophen (Table 9.1). Nonopioids do not produce tolerance or physical dependence. Most do have antipyretic (fever-reducing) effects. This class of drugs works primarily at the site of injury, or peripherally, rather than in the central nervous system as opioids do. NSAIDs block the synthesis of prostaglandin, one of many chemicals necessary for pain transmission. In general, it is helpful to include a nonopioid in any analgesic regimen, even if the pain is severe enough to require the addition of an opioid. See Table 9.2 for examples of nonopioid analgesics.

Opioids

Opioids are drugs that have actions similar to morphine. They are added to nonopioids for pain that cannot be managed effectively by nonopioids alone. Opioids are classified as full agonists, partial agonists, or mixed agonists and **antagonists.** Full agonists have a complete response at the opioid receptor site; the partial agonist has a lesser response. The mixed agonist and antagonist activates one type of opioid receptor while blocking another.

Opioids alone have no ceiling effect to analgesia. Doses can safely be increased to treat increasing pain if the patient's respiratory status and level of sedation are stable. See Box 9.3 (Common Adverse Effects of Opioids) for adverse effects of opioids. Controlled-release opioids such as oxycodone (Oxycontin) and morphine (MS Contin) are effective for prolonged, continuous pain.

Controlled- or time-release medication should never be crushed, but always taken whole. Whenever a controlled-release preparation is used, it is important to have an immediate-release medication available for **breakthrough** pain, such as oral morphine solution (OMS) or oxycodone (Oxy-IR).

Morphine is the drug of choice for the treatment of moderate to severe pain. It is the drug used as a standard against which all other analgesics are compared. (See Table 9.3 for **equianalgesic** doses of medications.) Morphine is long acting (4 to 5 hours) and available in many forms, making it convenient, as well as affordable, for the patient. It has a slower onset than many other opioid agonists.

equianalgesic: equi—equal + analgesic—relieving pain

TABLE 9.2 ANALGESIC AGENTS

Medication Class/ Action	Drug Examples	Route	Common Side Effects	Nursing Implications
Salicylates Peripherally acting analgesics; reduce pain, fever, inflammation	Aspirin	PO, PR	Tinnitus, GI upset and bleeding, renal impairment	Give with food. Decreases platelet aggregation, so watch for bleeding.
NSAIDS Peripherally acting analgesics; reduce pain, fever, inflammation	Ibuprofen (Motrin) Ketorolac (Toradol) Naproxen (Naprosyn)	PO PO, IM, IV PO	GI upset and bleeding, renal impairment	Give with food. Decrease platelet aggregation, so watch for bleeding.
Second-Generation NSAIDS COX-2 inhibitors; reduce pain and inflammation, no effect on platelet aggregation	Celecoxib (Celebrex)	PO	Abdominal pain, renal impairment, GI upset and bleeding, but less risk for bleeding than 1st generation NSAIDS.	Rofecoxib (Vioxx) and Valdecoxib (Bextra) have been removed from the market owing to increased risk for MI and stroke. Research is ongoing to determine if all COX-2 inhibitors have this effect.
Acetaminophen Relieves pain and fever; no anti-inflammatory or antiplatelet effect	Acetaminophen (Tylenol)	PO, PR	Liver toxicity and failure	Maximum safe dose is 4 g per day.
Opioids Bind to opiod receptors in the CNS to alter perception of pain.	Codeine (Tylenol #3 is acetaminophen with codeine) Fentanyl (Sublimaze, Duragesic) Hydromorphone (Dilaudid) Meperidine (Demerol) Methadone (Dolophine) Morphine Oxycodone (Vicodin is aceta-minophen with hydro-codone)	PO, PR, IM, SQ, IV, Epidural PO, IV, IM, Patch PO, PR, IV, IM PO, IV, IM, SQ PO, IM, SQ PO, IM, SQ, IV PO	Respiratory depression, sedation, hypoten-sion, constipation	Monitor vital signs, level of sedation, and respiratory status. Encourage fluids and fiber to prevent con-stipation. Avoid use of meperidine in elderly.

TABLE 9.3 EQUIANALGESIC CHART*

Drug	Parenteral (IM/IV/SQ)	Oral Dose	Conversion Factor (Parenteral to PO)
Morphine	10 mg	30 mg	3
Codeine	130 mg	200 mg NR	1.5
Hydromorphone (Dilaudid)	1.5 mg	7.5 mg	5
Methadone (Dolophine)	10 mg	20 mg	2
Meperidine (Demerol)	75 mg	300 mg NR	4

NR = Not recommended at that dose.

*Approximate doses of medications in milligrams to equal same amount of pain relief.

Source: Adapted from McCaffery, M: Pain: Assessment and Use of Analgesics (conference). Fall 1996.

Hydromorphone (Dilaudid) is commonly used for moderate to severe pain as well. It is shorter acting than morphine and has a somewhat faster onset. It is a good option for pain management in most patients

Meperidine (Demerol), also an opioid agonist, should be reserved for healthy patients requiring opioids for a short period or for those who have unusual reactions or allergic responses to other opioids. When broken down in the body, it produces a toxic metabolite called normeperidine. Normeperidine is a cerebral irritant that can cause adverse effects ranging from dysphoria and irritable mood to seizures. Normeperidine has a long half-life even in healthy patients, so those with impaired renal function are at increased risk. Meperidine use should be avoided in patients over the age of 65, in those with impaired renal function, and in those receiving monoamine oxidase inhibitor (MAOI) antidepressants. Additionally, the effective dose of

SAFETY TIP

It is important to monitor a patient's level of sedation and respiratory status whenever administering opioids. Increased sedation, decreased respiratory effort, and constricted pupils can be signs of opioid overdose. Careful monitoring and dosage adjustments of opioids can prevent opioid-induced respiratory depression.

oral meperidine is three to four times the parenteral dose, and is not recommended.

Fentanyl (Sublimaze, Duragesic) can be administered parenterally, intraspinally, or by **transdermal** patch (Duragesic patch). Fentanyl is commonly used intravenously with anesthesia for surgery and also for relief of postoperative pain via the intravenous route. **Patient-controlled analgesia** (PCA) or epidural route (discussed later in this chapter) IV fentanyl is very short acting and must be administered more frequently than other opioids to maintain an effective level of analgesia. The fentanyl patch is useful for the patient with stable cancer pain and requires dosing only every 3 days.

Methadone (Dolophine) is a potent analgesic that has a longer duration of action than morphine. It has a very long half-life and accumulates in the body with continued dosing. Dosing intervals may be lengthened after pain relief has been achieved. Methadone is well absorbed from the gastrointestinal tract and is very effective when given orally at

CRITICAL THINKING

Mrs. Shepard

■ Mrs. Shepard is 92 years old and has undergone an open cholecystectomy. Her continuous epidural infusion of analgesic has been discontinued. The physician has ordered oral acetaminophen with hydrocodone every 3 to 4 hours as required for pain. This is her second postoperative day, and she refuses to get out of bed because her pain is 7 on a scale of 0 to 10.

The medication record shows that Mrs. Shepard has not received any pain medication since the continuous epidural infusion was stopped 3 hours ago.

1. Why is Mrs. Shepard in so much pain?
2. What complications can occur as a result of her pain?
3. Each analgesic tablet contains 500 mg of acetaminophen and 5 mg hydrocodone. The maximum daily dose of acetaminophen is 4 g. If she takes one tablet every 3 hours, is her dose safe?
4. What can be done to relieve her pain and better prevent it in the future?

Suggested answers at end of chapter.

doses similar to the parenteral dose. Methadone is also used in drug treatment programs during detoxification from heroin and other opioids. Patients on methadone maintenance can present a unique challenge when admitted to the hospital. It is important to continue the maintenance dose even if additional pain medications are required after surgery or trauma. See Table 9.2 for examples of opioids.

Opioid Antagonists

Naloxone (Narcan) is a pure opioid antagonist that counteracts, or antagonizes, the effect of opioids. It is often used in the emergency department setting for treatment of opioid overdose. Caution must be used when naloxone is given to a patient receiving opioids for the treatment of pain. If too much naloxone is given too fast, it can reverse not only the respiratory depression and sedation but the analgesia as well.

Some antagonists are shorter acting than the opioid that is being used. If the antagonist is given because of respiratory depression, the dose may need to be repeated because its effect may wear off before that of the opioid.

Some analgesics are classified as combined agonist and antagonist. These drugs bind with some opioid receptors and block others. The most commonly used agonist-antagonist drugs are butorphanol (Stadol) and nalbuphine (Nubain).

How does this information translate into nursing practice? Consider, for example, a patient who is taking sustained-release morphine every 12 hours to control metastatic bone pain and is experiencing breakthrough pain between doses. You observe that butorphanol has been ordered for pain by another doctor and administer it. The butorphanol will antagonize, or counteract, the effects of the morphine, and the patient may develop acute pain. It is important to be informed about the actions of all drugs that are administered and to be aware of possible drug interactions that may interfere with patient care.

Agonist-antagonist drugs are also used sometimes to counteract opioid adverse effects. Nalbuphine (Nubain) can be used to treat itching and nausea that may accompany the administration of opioids. A smaller dose can be given so that the analgesia is not reversed completely along with the reversal of the adverse effect.

Analgesic Adjuvants

Adjuvants are classes of medications that may potentiate the effects of opioids or nonopioids, have analgesic activity themselves, or counteract unwanted effects of other analgesics. Adjuvants are especially important when treating pain that does not respond well to traditional analgesics alone. Examples of adjuvants are steroids, benzodiazepines, antidepressants, and anticonvulsants.

Steroids can be used to treat a variety of pain conditions, including acute and chronic cancer-related pain. They may be used as part of actual cancer treatment because of their toxicity to some cancer cells, or they may reduce pain by decreasing inflammation and the resultant compression of healthy tissues. Their use is standard emergency practice in the treatment of suspected spinal cord compression. Patients with pain caused by malignant lesions pressing on nerves such as the brachial or lumbosacral plexus may receive large doses of steroids.

Benzodiazepines such as midazolam (Versed) or diazepam (Valium) are effective for the treatment of anxiety or muscle spasms associated with pain. These drugs do not provide pain relief except in the treatment of muscle spasms. Benzodiazepines may cause sedation, which limits the amount of opioid that may be safely given.

Tricyclic antidepressants such as amitriptyline, imipramine, desipramine, and doxepin have been shown to relieve pain related to neuropathy and other painful nerve-related conditions. These medications must be taken for days to weeks before they are fully effective, and patients must be instructed to continue the medications even if they seem ineffective at first. Additional benefits of this class of medications may include mood elevation and improved ability to sleep.

Anticonvulsants such as carbamazepine (Tegretol) and gabapentin (Neurontin) are often used to relieve the sharp or cutting pain caused by peripheral nerve syndromes. Again, these medications must be taken regularly before full benefit is realized.

Stimulants such as methylphenidate hydrochloride (Ritalin) or caffeine-containing medications may be used to counteract the sedating effects of opioids in some patients.

A "balanced analgesia" approach should be used, combining analgesics and adjuvants from different classes to minimize opioid adverse effects, such as nausea and vomiting or sedation (Box 9.3, Common Adverse Effects of Opioids) while maximizing pain relief. For example, an opioid and a nonopioid given together can provide pain relief with an overall lower dose of each medication than if they were given alone. Because these drugs have different mechanisms of action and different adverse effects, it is possible to give lower doses of opioids providing an "opioid sparing" effect. If doses can be reduced in this manner additional, sedating medications such as antiemetics and antihistamines may be avoided.

World Health Organization Analgesic Ladder

In 1990, the World Health Organization (WHO) developed the WHO analgesic ladder, which involves choosing among three levels of treatments based on intensity of pain (Fig.

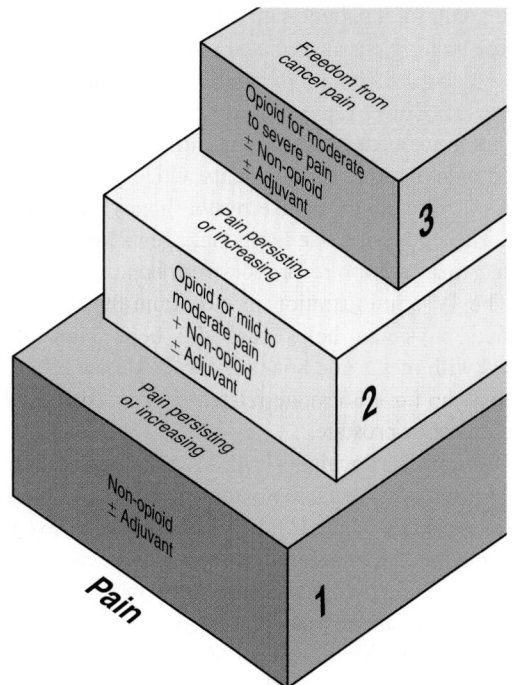

FIGURE 9.2 World Health Organzation three-step analgesic ladder.

9.2). The ladder, which helps direct the interventions required when using medications to treat pain, was developed for the treatment of cancer pain but can be used when treating other types of pain as well.

When experiencing mild pain (level I on the WHO ladder), the patient can usually sleep, perform activities of daily living, and even work. The first level of the ladder addresses the use of nonopioid analgesics. When pain is unrelieved by maximum around the clock (ATC) dosing, the treatment moves up the ladder to level II (mild to moderate pain) and adds an opioid analgesic. The patient with mild to moderate pain may not be able to sleep or may have trouble working and staying focused. If pain increases beyond that which is controlled by the level II analgesics, it is time to move on to level III. At this level, the pain is moderate to severe and is affecting the quality of the patient's life, and he or she may not be able to perform activities of daily living. At any level, an adjuvant analgesic may be appropriate.

Analgesics should be given on an ATC basis to prevent breakthrough pain, especially for cancer and chronic nonmalignant pain. For patients experiencing surgical or traumatic pain, analgesics should be given ATC until the pain decreases to a level that allows medications to be given as required (e.g., prn, such as prior to physical therapy). When using the WHO ladder, it is important to keep in mind that it is not necessary to start at level I if the patient is having severe pain. Analgesics from level III on the WHO ladder may be the starting point for some patients.

Other Interventions

Other pain treatments include the use of radiation therapy or antineoplastic chemotherapy to help shrink tumors that are

---

Box 9.3

Common Adverse Effects of Opioids

Sedation
Respiratory depression*
Constipation
Nausea, vomiting
Itching
Constricted pupils*

---

*These effects are not common, but they alert the nurse to possible overdose.

causing pain for a patient with cancer. Chemotherapy is also used for treating pain associated with connective tissue disorders such as rheumatoid arthritis or systemic lupus erythematosus. Bowel regimens, laxatives, enemas, or antigas medication to decrease abdominal fullness may also be considered pain treatments. In patients with osteoporosis, drugs that result in calcium uptake by the bones can aid in pain relief. These may include hormonal agents and medications that decrease calcium resorption from bone.

The IV administration of strontium-89 chloride by a qualified physician helps ease the bone pain of some patients with metastatic bone cancer. It is most effective for patients who have hormone-related cancers, such as cancer of the breast or prostate.

Lidocaine/prilocaine (EMLA, a eutectic mixture of local anesthetics) cream is a topical local anesthetic that decreases pain associated with procedures such as venipunctures and lumbar punctures. It is most effective if left in place for 1 hour before the procedure and covered with a semipermeable membrane dressing such as Tegaderm or Opsite before the needle stick. EMLA and tetracaine gel are effective topical local anesthetics and safe for use in children. A lidocaine patch is available for patients with postherpetic nerve pain.

Placebos

Use of placebos involves the administration of an inactive substitute such as normal saline in place of an active medication. In the past, placebos were sometimes given in an attempt to determine whether a patient's pain was "real." This is unethical and inappropriate unless the patient has given written consent. The use of placebos is a denial of the patient's report of pain. If a placebo is ordered for a patient, discuss concerns with the physician and nurse supervisor. Placebos are used in drug studies (clinical trials) to compare a new drug with an inactive substance. In studies, patients are informed that they may be receiving a placebo.

Routes for Medication Administration

Analgesics can be administered by almost any route. The oral route is desired in most instances because it is easy and painless for the patient and can be used at home. See Table 9.4 for a comparison of the various routes.

Nondrug Therapies

Nondrug treatments are usually classified as cognitive-behavioral interventions or physical agents. The goals of these two groups of treatments are different. Cognitive-behavioral interventions can help patients understand and cope with pain and take an active part in its assessment and control. The goals of physical agents may include providing comfort, correcting physical dysfunction, altering physiological response, and reducing fear that might be associated with immobility. Nondrug therapies should be used in conjunction with drug therapies and are not expected to relieve pain alone.

Cognitive-Behavioral Interventions

Included in this group are interventions such as educational information, relaxation exercises, guided imagery, distraction (e.g., music, television), and biofeedback. These treatments require extra time for detailed instruction and demonstration. The use of these modalities must be acceptable to the patient to be useful.

Providing patients with educational information about what to expect and how patients can participate in their own care has been shown to decrease patients' reports of postoperative pain and analgesic use. Relaxation can be accomplished through a variety of methods. The patient may prefer a relaxation exercise with a script that can be practiced and used the same way each time or simply the use of a favorite piece of music that allows a state of muscle relaxation and freedom from anxiety. Guided imagery uses the patient's imagination to take the patient away from the pain to a favorite place, such as a beach in Tahiti. The success of guided imagery does not mean that the pain is in any way imaginary. The use of distraction is commonly used by patients to focus their attention on something other than the pain. Patients watch a favorite television program or laugh with visitors when they are in pain. When the program is over or the visitors leave, the patient may notice the pain again and ask for a dose of pain medication.

Biofeedback is sometimes used in chronic pain programs to show patients how to teach their bodies to respond to different signals. Biofeedback has been very useful in patients with migraine headaches. When patients experience the aura that many migraine sufferers get before the headache, they begin the exercise that relaxes them and prevents the migraine.

Physical Agents

Physical agents can contribute directly to the patient's comfort. Examples of physical agents include applications of heat or cold, massage, exercise, immobilization, and transcutaneous electrical nerve stimulation (TENS).

The application of heat to sore muscles and joints is effective for pain relief. Heat works to increase circulation, induce muscle relaxation, and decrease inflammation when applied to a painful area. Heat can be applied using dry or moist packs or wraps or in a bath or whirlpool. Heat is contraindicated in conditions that would be worsened by its use, such as in an area of trauma, because of the possibility of increased swelling caused by vasodilation. To prevent burns, heat should not be applied over areas of decreased sensation.

Cold can reduce swelling, bleeding, and pain when used to treat a new injury. Cold can be applied by a variety of methods, such as cold wraps and cold packs, as well as localized ice massage. Patients often choose heat over cold if they have the choice. Cold is better tolerated over a small area. Alternating heat and cold therapies is most effective if not contraindicated.

Massage and exercise are used to stretch and regain muscle and tendon length, and to relax muscles. Massage pressure can be superficial or deep. It is important that

TABLE 9.4 ROUTES FOR ANALGESIC ADMINISTRATION

Route	Uses	Advantages	Disadvantages	Nursing Considerations
Oral	Preferred route in most cases	Convenient, inexpensive	Slower onset than IV	Can provide consistent blood levels when given ATC
Rectal	May be used to provide local or systemic pain relief	Can be used when patient is unable to take oral medication	May be difficult for patient or family to self-administer	Some oral preparations can be given rectally
Transdermal patch	Chronic pain	Easy to apply; delivers pain relief for three days without patch change.	12-hour delay before effective drug level reached, and delay in excreting once removed. Patient must be closely monitored and alternative routes may be needed when starting and stopping therapy.	May be less effective in smokers owing to circulatory alterations. Absorption may be erratic. Absorption may be increased with fever. Use caution not to touch medication when applying. Follow drug manufacturer's instructions for administration.
Intramuscular	Acute pain	Rapid pain relief	Painful	Use only if other routes cannot be used.
Intravenous	Preferred route for postoperative and chronic cancer pain for patients who cannot tolerate oral route.	Provides rapid relief; continuous infusion provides steady drug level	Difficult to use in home care setting; requires training.	Follow drug manufacturer instructions for administration.
Patient controlled Intravenous	Used to allow patient control over administration schedule	Patient can simply push a button to administer a dose of opioid	Requires special training. Pump must be programmed correctly.	An hourly limit and lockout interval are programmed into the pump to prevent the patient from accidentally overdosing. Teach patient and family that only the patient should push the button.
Subcutaneous	May be used if IV route is problematic	Can deliver effective pain relief	Injection may be painful	May be effective for treatment of chronic cancer pain
Intraspinal (epidural or subarachnoid)	Catheter into epidural or subarachnoid space may be used for traumatic injuries or chronic pain unrelieved by other methods; may also be used for orthopedic procedures.	May be able to control pain with lower doses of opioid because relief is delivered closer to site of pain. Fewer systemic side effects.	Requires single or continuous injection in back; may be associated with intense itching.	Steroids may be administered with opioid to reduce pain by treating inflammation.

massage is acceptable and not offensive to the patient. Immobilization is used following a variety of orthopedic procedures, as well as fractures and other injuries worsened by movement.

Physical agents are readily available, inexpensive, and require little preparation or instruction. But always remember, it is important to use nondrug treatments to enhance appropriate drug treatments, not as a substitute.

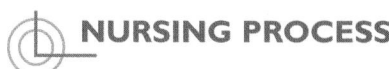

NURSING PROCESS

Assessment/Data Collection

Accurate assessment of pain is essential to effective treatment. Without appropriate assessment, it is not possible to intervene in a way that meets the patient's needs. The American Pain Society recommends that nurses consider pain the "fifth vital sign."[4] That way it will be routinely assessed whenever other vital signs are assessed. The WHAT'S UP? format found in Chapter 1 can assist you in performing a complete and effective assessment (Table 9.5). Following are some additional key points for assessing pain and putting together more pieces of the pain puzzle.

Accept the Patient's Report of Pain

Pain is what the patient says it is, not what the nurse or physician thinks it should be. When a member of the healthcare team distrusts the patient's report of pain, the patient can usually sense that he or she is not believed. The patient may compensate by either underreporting pain or, less com-

TABLE 9.5 WHAT'S UP? FORMAT FOR ASSESSMENT OF PAIN

W—Where is the pain? Be specific. Use drawing of body if necessary.

H—How does the pain feel? Is it shooting, burning, dull, sharp?

A—Aggravating and alleviating factors. What makes the pain better? Worse?

T—Timing. When did the pain start? Is it intermittent? Continuous?

S—Severity. How bad is the pain on a 0 to 10 (0 to 5; faces) scale

U—Useful other data. Are you experiencing any other symptoms associated with the pain or pain treatment? Itching, nausea, sedation, constipation?

P—Perception. What is the patient's perception of what caused the pain?

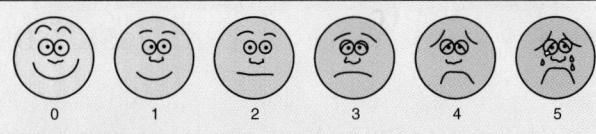

1) Explain to the child that each face is for a person who feels happy because he or she has no pain (hurt, or whatever word the child uses) or feels sad because he or she has some or a lot of pain.
2) Point to the appropriate face and state, "This face is . . .":
0—"very happy because he doesn't hurt at all."
1—"hurts just a little bit."
2—"hurts a little more."
3—"hurts even more."
4—"hurts a whole lot."
5—"hurts as much as you can imagine, although you don't have to be crying to feel this bad."
3) Ask the child to choose the face that best describes how he or she feels. Be specific about which pain (e.g., "shot" or incision) and what time (e.g., now? earlier before lunch?).

FIGURE 9.4 Wong-Baker faces. *(From Wong, DL: Whaley & Wong's Essentials of Pediatric Nursing, ed. 5. Mosby, St. Louis, 1997.)*

monly, anxiously overreporting. Patients may try to hide their pain for fear of being thought of as a complainer or drug seeker.

Obtain a Pain History

Information is obtained from the patient about the pain he or she is experiencing. Allowing the patient to describe the pain in his or her own words helps establish a trust relationship between you and the patient. This is also the time to discover the effects the pain is having on the patient's quality of life. Does the pain prevent the patient from eating, sleeping, or participating in work or family activities? Are there adverse effects such as nausea and vomiting or constipation that need to be addressed? Emotional and spiritual distress and coping abilities should be assessed. Ask the patient about how he or she has coped with pain previously and what treatment measures have been effective in the past as well as those that have not been effective. A thorough history is essential so you can individualize pain interventions to fit the patient's needs.

A variety of tools are available to assist in accurate and complete pain assessment. You should become familiar with the tool used in your setting and use it consistently. It is of utmost importance that all health-care personnel caring for the patient use the same pain rating scale, whether it is a numerical scale (e.g., 0 to 5 or 0 to 10), a visual analog scale (Fig. 9.3), or the Wong-Baker faces scale (Fig. 9.4). Whatever scale is used, it must be one that has been validated with research. The faces scale was developed for use in children, but has also been shown to be a valid instrument

for use in the elderly. Some scales are cute and interesting but may not be valid or even useful. The best tools are simple and easy to use. Longer questionnaires, although valid, require more time and may cause distress for the patient in acute pain but may be helpful when doing a complete pain history (Fig. 9.5). A scale should also be used to monitor the patient's level of sedation following opioid administration (Fig. 9.6). Any unexpected decrease in the patient's level of consciousness should be reported promptly to the registered nurse (RN) or physician.

It is important to use the patient's own descriptions and words when taking the pain history, such as *aching, knifelike,* or *throbbing.* This is also true when the patient is experiencing neuropathic (non-physiological) pain, which can be difficult to define. Terms commonly used to describe neuropathic pain include *burning, shocklike,* and *tingling.*

Do a Complete Physical Assessment

A good physical assessment is necessary to determine the effect of the pain and pain treatments on the body. It helps identify all the pain sites and helps you to prioritize the seemingly overwhelming task of helping the patient achieve acceptable pain relief and good qualify of life. As discussed previously, the patient with acute pain may exhibit signs such as grimacing and moaning or elevated pulse and blood pressure, but these signs cannot be relied on to "prove" that the patient is in pain. The only reliable source of pain assessment is the patient's self-report (Box 9.4, Gerontological Issues).

Nursing Diagnosis, Planning, and Implementation

See Box 9.5, Nursing Care Plan for the Patient in Pain. Some additional principles to consider during planning and implementation follow.

Set Goals with the Patient

Establish a pain control goal during the planning phase. The patient must be asked to determine an acceptable level of

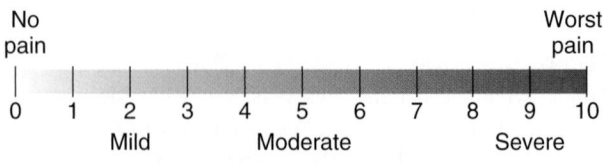

No pain   Worst pain

0   1   2   3   4   5   6   7   8   9   10
          Mild   Moderate   Severe

FIGURE 9.3 Pain scale.

Pain Assessment Chart (For Admission and/or Follow-up)

1. Patient _____ 2. DX _____

Assessment on Admission

Date _____/_____/_____   Pain ☐   No Pain ☐   Date of Pain Onset _____/_____/_____

1. Location of Pain (indicate on drawing)

2. Description of Predominant Pain (in patient's words) _____

_____

_____

3. Intensity [Scale 0 (no pain) — 10 (most intense)] _____

_____

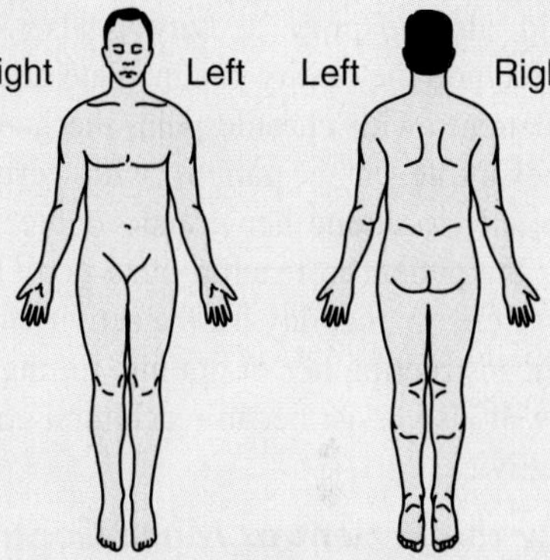

4. Duration and when occurs _____

5. Precipitating Factors _____

_____

6. Alleviating Factors _____

_____

7. Accompanying Symptoms

GI: Nausea ☐   Emesis ☐   Constipation ☐   Anorexia ☐

CNS: Drowsiness ☐   Confusion ☐   Hallucinations ☐

Psychosocial: Mood _____   Anger _____

Anxiety _____   Depression _____

Relationships _____

_____

8. Other Symptoms

Sleep _____   Fatigue _____

Activity _____   Other _____

9. Present Medications _____

_____

_____

Doses and times medicated last 48 hours _____

_____

10. Breakthrough Pain _____

_____

Signature: _____

FIGURE 9.5 Pain assessment chart. *(Modified from The Purdue Frederik Company, Norwalk, CN.)*

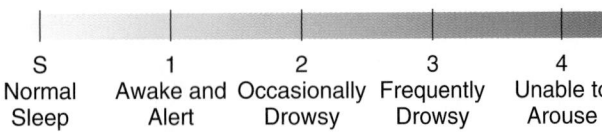

S	1	2	3	4
Normal Sleep	Awake and Alert	Occasionally Drowsy	Frequently Drowsy	Unable to Arouse

FIGURE 9.6 Level of sedation scale.

pain if complete freedom from pain is not possible. Education is important when helping the patient set a realistic pain control goal. Although a goal of zero pain is desirable, it may not be possible or safe. On the other hand, a patient may choose a pain goal of 6 but be unable to get out of bed and do other recovery activities. Patients should also identify activity goals. After surgery, goals may include the ability to ambulate and sleep without pain. For patients with chronic pain, the goals may be different. For example, if a patient with terminal cancer wants to be able to attend her granddaughter's wedding, you can assist the patient in reaching that goal. She can be taught to reserve energy that day for the activity that is most important to her. Instructing her in optimal timing of her pain medication will also assist her in reaching a good comfort level for the activity.

Allow the Patient as Much Control as Possible

Pain can bring forth feelings of helplessness and hopelessness. Giving patients pain management options allows them to maintain some control. It is also the nurse's responsibility to teach patients about the goals of pain management and why it is an important part of care. If patients understand

Box 9.4

Gerontological Issues

The older patient may have different manifestations of pain than a younger patient. Older patients who are confused may be unable to tell you that they are feeling pain. Consider incidents of restlessness and confusion as possible signs of pain. Pulling at dressings, tugging at IV sites, and trying to climb over the side rails to get out of bed can also be symptoms of discomfort. Any change in the patient's behavior may be indicative of discomfort. Remember to take more time when assessing pain in the older patient as they may need more time to process what you are asking.

You can anticipate pain and provide relief measures to prevent severe pain. A trial dose of pain medication may help to determine if the patient's behavior is because of pain. Pain medications and basic comfort care can be administered routinely if pain is likely. Nagging achiness in hands and feet is often noted as a reason for decreased activity, inability to sleep, and altered functional ability. A hand or foot massage using lotion and gentle massage strokes is often a very relaxing comfort measure.

Opioid analgesic doses may need to be decreased initially as they tend to work longer and stronger in the older patient.

BOX 9.5   NURSING CARE PLAN **for the Patient in Pain**

Nursing Diagnosis: Pain

Expected Outcomes: Pain is at a level that is acceptable to the patient. Patient is able to participate in activities that are important to him or her.

Evaluation of Outcomes: Is pain at a level that is acceptable to the patient? Is the patient able to participate in activities that he or she has identified as important?

Intervention	Rationale	Evaluation
Assess pain based on patient report. Use the WHAT'S UP format.	Patient's pain is defined as what the patient says it is, when the patient says it is occurring.	Does the patient verbalize his or her pain?
		Does the patient use verbal or nonverbal messages that imply trust in nurse's belief of pain report?
Teach the patient to use a pain rating scale. Use the same scale consistently.	A rating scale is the most reliable method for assessing pain severity.	Does the patient understand the use of the scale and use it to report pain?
Determine with patient what is an acceptable pain level.	Only the patient can decide what pain level is acceptable.	Is the patient's pain at an acceptable level?

Intervention	Rationale	Evaluation
Assess whether pain is acute, chronic, or both.	Acute and chronic pain may present differently and may require different interventions.	Has acute versus chronic pain been identified? Are treatments appropriate?
Assess need for and offer emotional and spiritual support for the experience of pain and suffering.	Pain, as well as disease processes, can be accompanied by feelings of powerlessness and distress.	Does the patient appear emotional, angry, or withdrawn? Does the patient have difficulty making decisions? Is the patient-nurse relationship therapeutic?
Give analgesics before pain becomes severe. For moderate to severe pain, give analgesics ATC.	Severe pain is more difficult to relieve.	Is analgesic schedule effective?
Combine opioid and nonopioid analgesics as ordered.	Balanced analgesia provides optimum pain relief with fewer side effects.	Is the analgesic combination effective?
Assess for pain relief approximately 1 hour after administration of oral analgesics, or 30 minutes after IV analgesics.	If pain is not relieved, additional measures will be needed.	Does patient report acceptable level of relief?
Observe for anticipated adverse effects of pain medication.	Many pain medications cause nausea and constipation. The nausea usually subsides after several days, but the constipation does not.	Are adverse effects occurring? Can they be managed? Does medication regimen need to be adjusted?
If opioids are being used, assess for respiratory depression and level of sedation at regular intervals.	High doses or sudden increases in does of an opioid can result in respiratory depression and increased sedation.	Is the patient's respiratory rate greater than 8 per minute or above the parameter ordered by the physician? Is the patient alert and oriented?
Institute measures to prevent constipation: 8 to 10 glasses of fluid daily (unless contraindicated), fiber in meals, fiber or bulk laxatives, and exercise as tolerated.	A common side effect of opioids is constipation.	Are the patient's bowels moving according to his or her usual pattern?
Teach patient alternative (nondrug) pain relief interventions, such as relaxation and distraction, to be used with medication.	Alternative interventions can help the patient feel in control and may help reduce the perception of pain.	Does the patient use alternative interventions effectively?
Assess whether patient is taking pain medications appropriately, and if not, assess reasons. Instruct in how to manage pain interventions.	Pain medications must be taken appropriately to be effective.	Is the patient able to manage the pain control regimen? Are adjustments necessary?

that the health care provider's goals and theirs are the same, they are likely to cooperate with and contribute to the pain management plan.

Understand that Pain Affects the Whole Family

It is important to include the whole family in the plan. Understanding family dynamics helps the nurse in implementing an effective pain management plan. Cultural influences are also important to consider (see Chapter 3). It is difficult for family members to see loved ones in pain.

Including them in the planning helps them feel that they can help make the patient more comfortable. (See Home Health Hints.)

Pain is Exhausting

Pain may keep the patient from sleeping. This cycle of sleeplessness and pain must be interrupted to help the patient. The need for adequate rest must not be ignored. This is often an ongoing problem for the patient with chronic nonmalignant pain or chronic cancer pain, and it is perhaps more difficult to manage. The patient must get at least 4 to 6 hours of uninterrupted sleep to be relaxed enough to break the cycle. Controlled-release opioids may help maintain pain relief, allowing the patient to sleep. If controlled-release medications are not used, it may be necessary to wake a patient to administer pain medication so that the pain does not get out of control. The addition of a sedative may be necessary to allow the patient to sleep.

A Team Approach to Pain Management

A plan must be developed using an interdisciplinary approach, including the patient and family, the nurse, and the physician. Other team members, such as the occupational and physical therapist, chaplain, social worker, and pharmacist, should be included as appropriate. Communication is the important link allowing the team to be effective in creating a plan that works for the patient. Plans must be individualized to meet the special needs of each patient and vary greatly depending on the characteristics of pain the patient is experiencing and the effect on the patient.

Patient Education

Patients must be informed about the medications they are taking for pain management so they can take an active role in their care. Patients informed about the goals of pain management are more likely to report unrelieved pain so that they can receive prompt and effective treatment. Goals include a satisfactory comfort level with minimal side effects and complications of pain and its treatment, as well as a reduced period of recovery.

CRITICAL THINKING

Mr. Sebastian

■ Mr. Sebastian is a 75-year-old man who has been diagnosed with lung cancer and is anxious about leaving the hospital to return home following a thoracotomy. The nursing assessment reveals the need for home health care for dressing changes and teaching about the medications he will need at home. While in the hospital, Mr. Sebastian has required 5 mg of morphine IV every 4 hours around the clock.

1. The morphine is available in syringes prefilled with morphine grains 1/6 per mL. How many mililiters should the nurse administer?
2. What discharge instructions must be given to Mr. Sebastian and his wife before sending him home?
3. How might his pain be managed at home to prevent unnecessary readmissions to the hospital?

Suggested answers at end of chapter.

CRITICAL THINKING

Mrs. Zales

■ Mrs. Zales, a 32-year-old woman, was admitted for a hysterectomy after being treated for painful endometriosis for 12 months. After her surgery she had a PCA pump with hydromorphone, which was effective in relieving her pain. Forty-eight hours after surgery the surgeon discontinued the PCA pump and ordered oral hydrocodone with acetaminophen. It was ineffective, so an order for hydromorphone, 2 to 4 mg orally every 3 to 4 hours as needed, was added. The nurses gave only one dose of the hydromorphone, then, thinking that her pain should be lessening, switched Mrs. Zales back to the hydrocodone with acetaminophen. By the next morning she was in severe pain, and the on-call physician ordered IM meperidine and promethazine (Phenergan). Mrs. Zales's discharge was delayed until her pain could be controlled.

What do you think happened? How could the delayed discharge have been avoided?

Suggested answers at end of chapter.

CRITICAL THINKING

Ms. Jackson

■ Ms. Jackson had abdominal surgery 2 days ago. She has been receiving morphine via IV PCA at an average of 2.5 mg per hour for the last 6 hours. She rates her pain at 3 on a scale of 0 to 10. She is to be discharged today. Her physician has ordered codeine 30 mg with acetaminophen (Tylenol with codeine No. 3), 1 or 2 tablets every 4 hours as needed for pain at home.

Will Ms. Jackson be comfortable at home? Why or why not?

Suggested answers at end of chapter.

NURSING CARE TIP

Many medication interventions are available for the treatment of pain. Whenever possible, administer analgesics by the mouth, by the WHO ladder, and by the clock.

ETHICAL CONSIDERATION DISCUSSION

This is a complex case. Not only are we looking at professional ethical obligations as dictated by her regulatory body; we have to consider Kathy's personal values. There may be a conflict. Kathy may believe that life is valuable and worth preserving at any cost, and that the administration of a medication that will shorten life or even precipitate a death cannot be an activity that she can become involved in. Her beliefs may prohibit her from taking many jobs where end of life issues are part of daily routine (such as abortion clinics, palliative care units, long-term care units, and emergency rooms).

If Kathy has moral objections to administering what she considers to be a lethal dose of medication, she should seek out her supervisor in order to explain her difficulty with the order. She may be able to withdraw from assisting with or performing procedures that are against her personal moral values. This task can be undertaken by a nurse who has no moral objections, provided that there is a nurse available. The supervisor may choose to administer the medication himself or herself, or to pursue alternate outcomes, such as contacting the palliative care team or an alternate physician if possible. Kathy might consider talking with the physician or forming a group on the unit to discuss the issues and develop some unit guidelines for such cases.

Situations like this are an everyday occurrence. A nurse should assess the work environment before committing to work on a unit. Kathy may be able to inform her supervisor and colleagues that under certain circumstances, she will not participate in a treatment regimen and will need to rely upon the team to support that decision and assist with finding alternate methods of delivering care. She should recognize, however, that sometimes there is no one else available to administer medications or perform procedures. At that point, she would have to think carefully about her professional obligations; that is, to whom does she owe the primary obligation . . . to the patient or to her own moral code? And what is that obligation? In the end, if Kathy is unable to function effectively on this unit, she may need to seek employment elsewhere.

It is important to provide the patient with information about a drug's common adverse effects, the frequency of the dose and its duration of action, and potential drug-drug and food-drug interactions if indicated. There are many special considerations for medications such as control release oral agents and transdermal patches; care must be taken to include these in the education plan for the patient using these medications at home. Drug-specific instructions are found in drug handbooks. Education must be presented at a level that the patient can understand. Informed patients use their medications more effectively and safely.

Evaluation

The final phase of the nursing process is evaluation. Once the plan of care has been implemented, evaluate whether the patient's goals have been met. Has the patient's identified goal for an acceptable level of pain been met? How were the pain treatments tolerated? Was the patient able to participate in activities that he or she identified as important? The plan should be continuously updated based on the evaluation.

Home Health Hints

- Emotional or spiritual distress and fear related to dependence on family caregivers may alter the patient's perception or report of pain. Some patients may feel pain more intensely because of the influence of fear, and others may underreport if they are trying to protect family members.
- Several alternative measures are easily taught to patients and caregivers in the home. For example, ice can be made in paper cups and used for a cold massage of a painful area.
- Medical massage therapy is growing in popularity for the treatment of chronic pain. Remember a physician's order might be necessary for this type of treatment. Discuss this option with the registered nurse, patient, and caregiver to help identify if this intervention is appropriate for your patient.

REVIEW QUESTIONS

1. A patient is walking up and down the hall and visiting with other patients. He is laughing and joking. He approaches the nurse's station, asks for his pain shot, and reports that his pain is 6 on a scale of 0 to 10. Based on McCaffery's definition of pain, which of the following assumptions by the nurse is most likely correct?
   a. The patient is not really in pain but just wants his medication.
   b. The patient is having pain at a level of 6 on a scale of 0 to 10.
   c. The patient is in minimal pain and should receive a pill instead of a shot.
   d. The patient is in pain but does not need his pain medication yet.

2. A patient with terminal cancer has been requiring 5 mg of IV morphine every 1 to 2 hours to control pain, yet is engrossed in a movie on television and appears to be in no pain. Which of the following explanations of this behavior is most likely correct?
   a. Denial of pain is common in patients with cancer.
   b. The cancer treatment is working and the pain is improving.
   c. The patient is hiding the pain in order to finish watching the movie undisturbed.
   d. Distraction can be an effective treatment for pain when used with appropriate drug treatments.

3. Which patient is exhibiting tolerance to opioid analgesics?
   a. The patient who requests opioid analgesics frequently because of severe acute pain.
   b. The patient who refuses opioid analgesics because of fear of addiction.
   c. The patient who needs increasing doses of opioids to achieve the same level of pain relief.
   d. The patient who requests opioid analgesics even when not in pain in order to feel euphoric.

4. A patient has incisional pain following total hip replacement surgery. Which of the following types of pain is the patient experiencing?
   a. Nociceptive/physiological
   b. Neuropathic/ nonphysiological
   c. Chronic nonmalignant

5. With which type of pain is the patient least likely to present with outward signs such as moaning or changes in vital signs?
   a. Acute pain
   b. Chronic nonmalignant pain
   c. Cancer pain

6. Which of the following methods is the most reliable way to assess a patient's pain?
   a. Ask the patient to describe the pain.
   b. Observe the patient for physical signs of pain such as moaning or grimacing.
   c. Ask the patient to rate his or her pain using a valid assessment scale.
   d. Ask a family member to rate the patient's pain.

7. According to the World Health Organization analgesic ladder, at what point in a patient's pain experience is it appropriate to use adjuvant treatments? Choose all answers that are correct.
   a. In addition to analgesics for early, mild pain
   b. As an alternative to analgesics for moderate to severe pain
   c. In addition to analgesics for pain that is persistent despite treatment
   d. In addition to analgesics for pain that is growing increasingly more severe

8. A patient is hospitalized following a motor vehicle accident. He has multiple orthopedic injuries and is in acute pain. He has an order for morphine 6 mg IV every 4 hours as needed. He can also have a nonopioid oral analgesic every 4 hours as needed. In order to reduce the risk of adverse effects and maintain an acceptable level of sedation and pain control, which of the following analgesic schedules will be most effective?
   a. Offer the opioid every 4 hours.
   b. Tell him to put on his light when he feels pain, and give the drugs immediately when he requests them.
   c. Give both the IV opioid and the PO nonopioid every 4 hours ATC.
   d. Alternate the IV analgesic with the nonopioid oral analgesic.

9. Mr. Lawrence is an 88-year-old man admitted with a broken hip after a fall. He has an order for meperidine 50 to 75 mg IM q4–6hr prn pain. As his nurse, which of the following actions should you take?
   a. Give the meperidine every 4 hours ATC.
   b. Offer the meperidine every 6 hours because you know that his liver and kidney function may be diminished.
   c. Administer an NSAID with the meperidine for added pain relief.
   d. Talk to the RN or physician about getting an order for a different analgesic.

10. A patient is started on gabapentin (Neurontin) 300 mg by mouth three times daily for chronic nerve pain related to diabetic neuropathy. Which instruction should the nurse provide?
    a. "Take the medication at the first sign of any pain, up to three times daily."

b. "Take one capsule every eight hours continuously to keep the pain under control."

c. "Take the medication only when you need it, to prevent becoming addicted."

d. "Take one capsule three times a day, then discontinue it when the pain is under control."

11. A nurse receives an order to administer 1 mL of sterile normal saline IM to a patient suspected of opioid abuse. Which response by the nurse is appropriate first?

a. Administer the saline and carefully document the patient's response in the medical record.

b. Administer the saline but inform the patient exactly what it is and why it was ordered.

c. Refuse to administer the medication and inform the physician that the order is inappropriate.

d. Share concerns about the order with the supervisor and explain why the nurse cannot in good conscience administer the saline.

12. A nurse needs to administer morphine 10 mg IM. It is supplied as grains 1/4 per mL. How many milliliters should the nurse prepare for injection?
_____ mL

References

1. McCaffery, M, and Pasero, C: Pain: Clinical Manual, ed 2. Mosby, St Louis, 1999.
2. International Association for the Study of Pain: http://www.iasp-pain.org, January 2006.
3. Agency for Health Care Policy and Research: AHCPR Clinical Practice Guideline: Management of Cancer Pain. US Depart-ment of Health and Human Services, Rockville, MD, 1994.
4. American Pain Society: Pain: The Fifth Vital Sign. http://www.ampainsoc.org/advocacy/fifth.htm, January 2006.

SUGGESTED ANSWERS TO

CRITICAL THINKING

■ Smithers and Barnett

It is important to accept both patients' pain reports. Assessment should be based on what the patient says rather than what is observed. Each patient copes with his or her pain in a unique way, and the nurse cannot judge whether one is in more pain than the other.

■ Mrs. Shepard

1. Pain medication is most effective when given on a routine schedule around the clock to avoid breakthrough pain. Mrs. Shepard's epidural infusion should continue to relieve her pain for a time, up to several hours after it is discontinued, depending on the medication used. The oral medication is most effective when given at the time the epidural is stopped so that it is taking effect as the epidural effects wear off. See Box 9.4 (Gerontological Issues) for special considerations for the older patient.

2. Pain prevents patients from moving freely. Postoperative complications such as retained pulmonary secretions and ileus can occur when patients are immobile. Effective pain management can help prevent these complications.

3. If she takes a dose every 3 hours, then she will receive eight doses in 24 hours: 500 mg × 8 = 4000 mg or 4 g, which is the maximum safe dose. Recall that elderly patients metabolize and excrete medications more slowly than younger patients. If she will need the hydrocodone/acetaminophen more than a few days, it would be wise to consult with the physi-

cian about giving the opioid and acetaminophen separately.

4. Mrs. Shepard should be instructed what her role will be when her pain management regimen is altered. Does she have to ask for the pain medication or will it just be brought to her? Patient and family education is vital to success in management of a patient's pain.

■ Mr. Sebastian

1.
$$\frac{5 \text{ mg}}{} \left| \frac{1 \text{ grain}}{60 \text{ mg}} \right| \frac{1 \text{ mL}}{\text{grains } 1/6} = 0.5 \text{ mL}$$

2. Home instruction regarding ATC administration of pain medication is indicated, as well as effects and side effects to report. He will also need to implement measures to prevent constipation.

3. MS Contin, a long-acting form of morphine, may be an option for Mr. Sebastian, along with an immediate-release preparation for breakthrough pain. Also, information about what to do and who to contact if pain becomes unmanageable is necessary to help prevent readmissions to the hospital.

■ Mrs. Zales

Mrs. Zales was probably tolerant to opioids because of her need for medication for chronic pain over the last year. For this reason, she needed more medication than a nontolerant patient who does not usually use opioids. Also, the belief that promethazine and other phenothiazines potentiate opioids is a myth. They do cause increased levels of sedation and may limit the amount

(Continued on following page)

of opioid that can be given safely. IM injections are not recommended because they are painful, absorption is not predictable, and there is a delay between injection and relief. Nurses often base the treatment of a patient's pain on what they usually do or what they think should be effective rather than on sound pain management practices and principles. A more rational approach to Mrs. Zales would have been regular pain assessment with ATC treatment until pain began to subside. If her pain level had been better controlled, she might have been discharged on oral analgesics without the delay.

■ *Ms. Jackson*

Using an equianalgesic conversion, we can determine whether Ms. Jackson is likely to have good pain relief based on her requirement with the PCA. Her current pain level of 3 shows that the morphine has been effective. Remember that the pump keeps a history of what the patient uses, which is the best indicator of what the patient needs. Ms. Jackson has used 15 mg of morphine during the past 6 hours. An equianalgesic dose of Tylenol with codeine No. 3 would be almost 200 mg of codeine, but only 30 to 60 mg has been ordered. In addition, if Ms. Jackson takes enough Tylenol with codeine No. 3 to get 200 mg of codeine, she will receive a dangerous dose of both the codeine and the acetaminophen. The physician needs to be contacted for different analgesic orders.

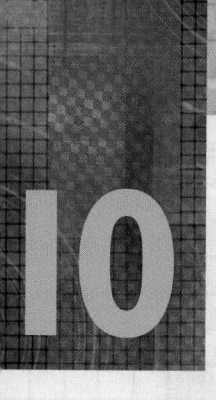

10

Nursing Care of Patients with Cancer

LUCY L. COLO AND JANICE L. BRADFORD

KEY TERMS

alopecia (AL-oh-PEE-she-ah)
anemia (uh-NEE-mee-yah)
anorexia (AN-oh-REK-see-ah)
benign (bee-NINE)
biopsy (BY-ahp-see)
cancer (KAN-sir)
carcinogen (kar-SIN-oh-jen)
chemotherapy (KEE-moh-THER-uh-pee)
contact inhibition (kon-takt in-huh-BIH-shun)
cytotoxic (SIGH-toh-TOCK-sik)
desquamation (dee-skwa-MAY-shun)
in situ (in-SIT-yoo)
leukopenia (LOO-koh-PEE-nee-ah)
malignant (muh-LIG-nunt)
metastasis (muh-TASS-tuh-sis)
mucositis (MYOO-koh-SIGH-tis)
nadir (NAY-dir)
neoplasm (NEE-oh-PLAZ-uhm)
neutropenia (noo-troh-PEE-nee-ah)
oncology (on-CAW-luh-gee)
oncovirus (ON-koh-VIGH-russ)
palliation (pal-ee-AY-shun)
radiation therapy (RAY-dee-AY-shun THER-uh-pee)
stomatitis (STOH-mah-TIGH-tis)
thrombocytopenia (THROM-boh-SIGH-toh-PEE-nee-ah)
tumor (TOO-mur)
vesicant (VESS-i-kant)
xerostomia (ZEE-roh-STOH-mee-ah)

QUESTIONS TO GUIDE YOUR READING

1. What are the normal structures and functions of the cell?

2. What changes occur in the cell when it becomes malignant?

3. Which medications are commonly used as chemotherapeutic agents?

4. What are the special nursing needs of the patient receiving chemotherapy or radiation therapy?

5. Which data should you collect when caring for a patient with cancer?

6. What are nursing interventions for common oncological emergencies?

7. How will you know if your nursing interventions have been effective?

8. What is the role of hospice in providing care for patients with advanced cancer?

REVIEW OF NORMAL ANATOMY AND PHYSIOLOGY OF CELLS

Cells are the smallest living structural and functional subunits of the body. Although human cells vary in size, shape, and certain metabolic activities, they have many characteristics in common.

Cell Structure

Human cells have a cell membrane, cytosol, cell organelles, and, with the exception of mature red blood cells, a nucleus. In the mature red blood cell, the nucleus has been lost. Each cell structure has a specific and vital function. The cell membrane forms the outer boundary of the cell and is made up of phospholipids, proteins, and cholesterol. Proteins serve four different purposes: (1) Some are channels or transporters to permit movement of materials, (2) some are enzymes catalyzing reactions, (3) some are receptor sites for hormones to trigger a cell's activity, and (4) some are antigens to identify the cell as belonging in the body.

A cell membrane is selectively permeable, meaning that not all substances pass through equally. The lipids in the membrane permit the diffusion of lipid-soluble materials into or out of the cell. Materials may enter or leave a cell in a variety of ways, such as diffusion, osmosis, active transport, pinocytosis, and phagocytosis.

Cytosol and Cell Organelles

Cytosol is a watery solution of minerals, gases, and organic molecules that is found between the cell membrane and the nucleus. Chemical reactions (such as the synthesis of adenosine triphosphate [ATP] in glycolysis) take place in the cytosol. Cell organelles are subcellular structures with specific functions, which are shown in Figure 10.1. Many cell organelles are found in the cytosol.

Nucleus

The nucleus of a cell is surrounded by a double-layered nuclear membrane with many pores. Inside the nucleus are one or more nucleoli and the chromosomes of the cell.

A nucleolus is a small sphere made of deoxyribonucleic acid (DNA), ribonucleic acid (RNA), and protein. The nucleoli form a type of RNA called ribosomal RNA, which is part of the cell organelle called the ribosome and is involved in protein synthesis.

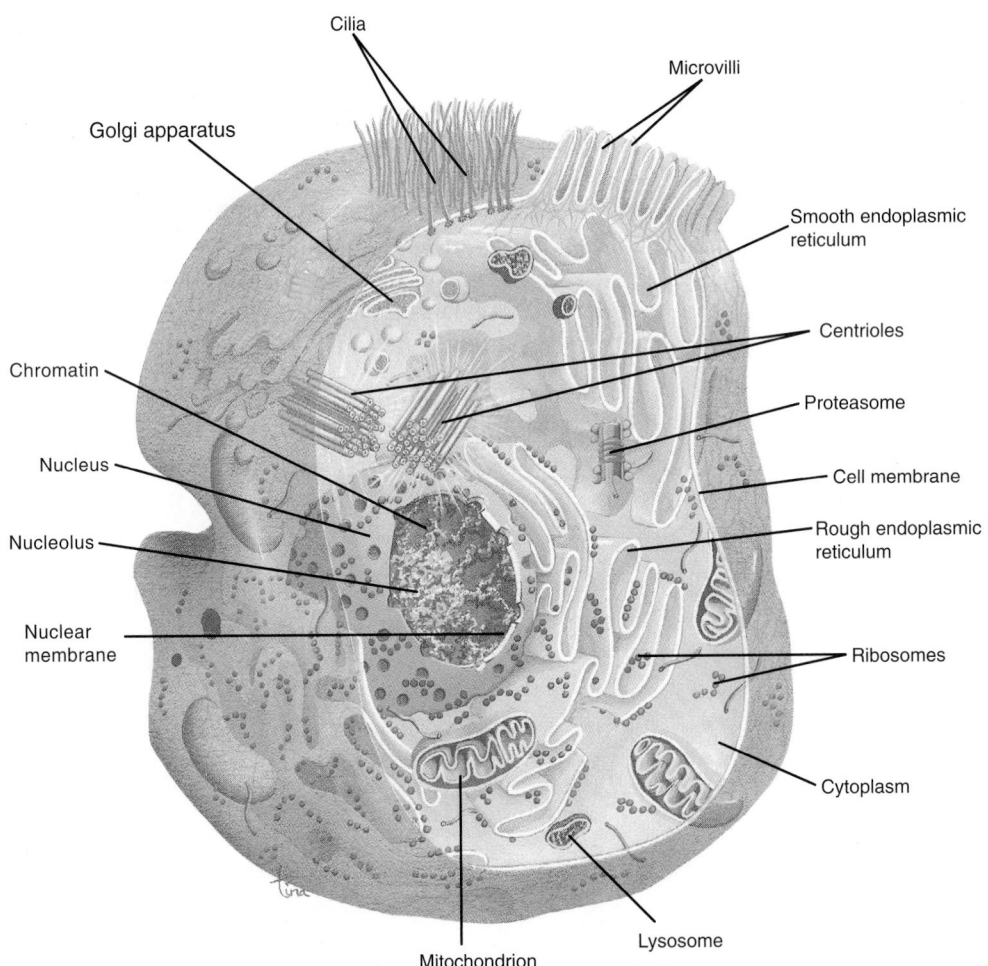

FIGURE 10.1 Schematic diagram of a typical human cell. *(From Scanlon, V, and Sanders, T: Essentials of Anatomy and Physiology, ed. 4. F.A. Davis, Philadelphia, 2003.)*

The nucleus is the control center of the cell because it contains the chromosomes. The 46 chromosomes of a human cell are made of DNA and protein. DNA is the genetic code for the characteristics and activities of the cell. Specific regions of DNA are called genes; a gene is the code for one protein. Not all the genes in any cell are active—only those relative few needed for the proteins to carry out their specific functions. These proteins may be structural, such as the collagen of connective tissue, or functional, such as the hemoglobin of red blood cells. Important functional proteins are the enzymes that catalyze the specific reactions characteristic of each type of cell.

Genetic Code and Protein Synthesis

The genetic code of DNA is the code for the amino acid sequences needed to synthesize a cell's proteins (Fig. 10.2). A complementary copy of the DNA's gene is made by a molecule called messenger RNA (mRNA). The mRNA then moves to the cytoplasm of the cell and attaches to the ribosomes. Transfer RNA (tRNA) molecules bring the necessary amino acids to the proper places on the mRNA molecule, and enzymes of the ribosomes catalyze the formation of peptide bonds to link the amino acids into the primary structure of a protein.

As with any complex process, mistakes are possible. Should there be a mistake in the DNA code, the process of protein synthesis may go on anyway, but the resulting protein will not function normally; this is the basis for genetic diseases. DNA mistakes acquired during life are called mutations. A mutation is any change in the DNA code. Ultraviolet rays or exposure to certain chemicals may cause structural changes in the DNA code. These changes may kill the affected cells or may irreversibly alter their function. Such altered cells may become **malignant,** being unable to function normally but very active; this is the basis of some forms of **cancer.**

Mitosis

Mitosis is the process by which a cell reproduces itself. One cell, after its 46 chromosomes have duplicated themselves, divides into two cells, each with a membrane, cytoplasm, and organelles from the original cell and a complete set of chromosomes. Mitosis is necessary for the growth of the body and the replacement of dead or damaged cells. Some cells are capable of mitosis and others are not. Cells of the epidermis of the skin undergo mitosis continuously to replace the superficial cells that are constantly worn off the skin surface. The same is true of cells that line the stomach

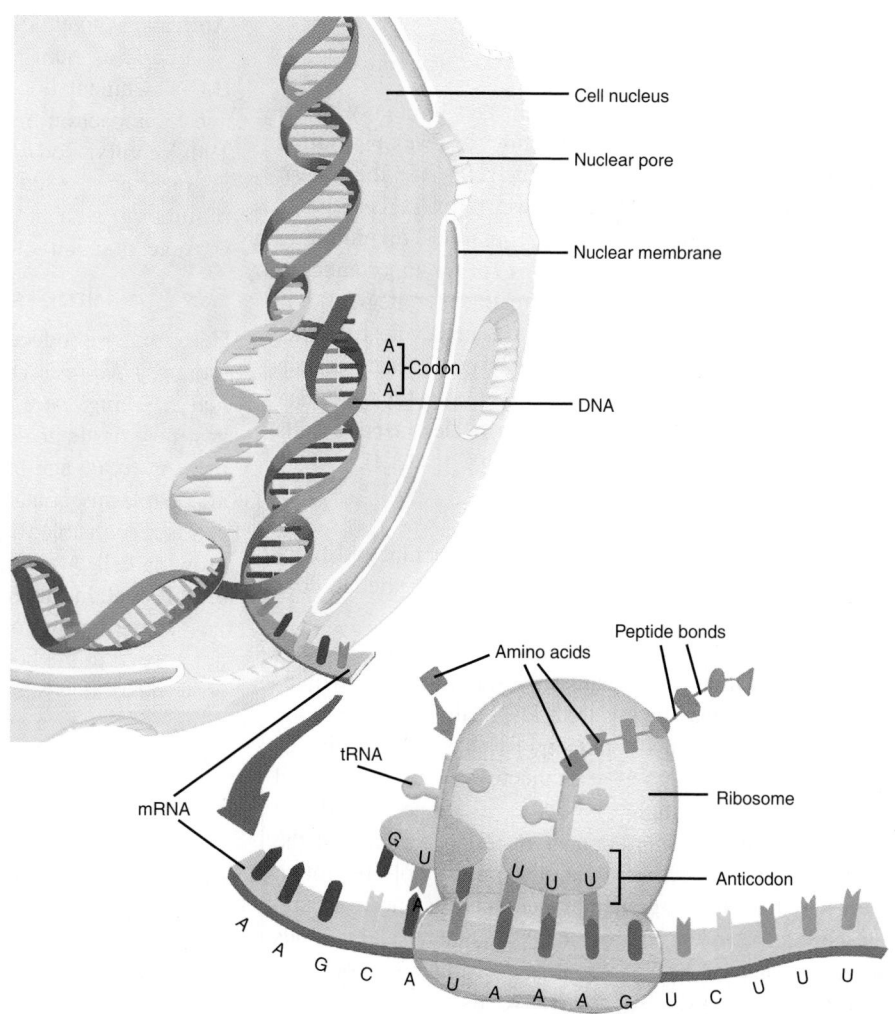

FIGURE 10.2 Schematic diagram of the process of protein synthesis. *(From Scanlon, V, and Sanders, T: Essentials of Anatomy and Physiology, ed. 4. F.A. Davis, Philadelphia, 2003.)*

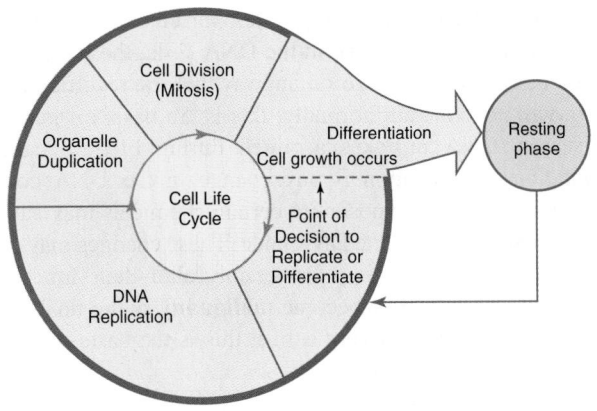

FIGURE 10.3 Cell cycle.

and intestines. Cells in the red bone marrow also divide frequently; red blood cells have a fixed life span (about 120 days) and must be replaced. Some cells seem to be capable of only a limited number of divisions, and when that limit has been reached, the cells die and are not replaced.

Other cells do not undergo mitosis to any great extent after birth. Nerve cells (neurons) are unable to divide (except for in the hippocampus), and muscle cells have very limited mitotic capability. When such cells are lost through injury or disease, the loss of their function in the individual is usually permanent.

Cell Cycle

The cell cycle involves a series of changes through which a cell progresses, starting from the time it develops until it reproduces itself. The duration of the cell's life, the time it takes for mitosis to occur, the growth ratio (percentage of cycling cells), the frequency of cell loss, and the doubling time (time for a **tumor** to double its size) are important concepts related to tumor growth and treatment strategies.

Cells can occupy three places in the cell cycle: cells that are actively dividing, cells that leave the cycle after a certain point and die, and cells that temporarily leave the cycle and remain inactive until reentry into the cycle. Inactive cells continue to synthesize RNA and protein (Fig. 10.3).

Cells and Tissues

A tissue is a group of cells with similar structure and functions. The four groups of human tissues are epithelial, connective, muscle, and nervous tissue

Epithelial tissues form coverings and linings throughout the body. Often the cells are capable of mitosis, and damage to the tissue may be repaired. The healing of a cut to the skin is a typical example. Epithelial tissue also forms glands.

There are many types of connective tissues with varied functions. For example, blood is a connective tissue involved in the transportation of materials throughout the body. Fibrous connective tissue, made mostly of the protein collagen, forms strong membranes such as those around muscles, attaching structures such as ligaments and tendons and the dermis of the skin. Bone and cartilage support connective tissues. Adipose connective tissue stores fat as

potential energy. Many kinds of connective tissue cells are capable of mitosis.

There are three kinds of muscle tissue: skeletal muscle, smooth muscle, and cardiac muscle. Skeletal muscle tissue makes up the voluntary muscles attached to the skeleton. Smooth muscle is found in viscera such as the stomach and intestines, the walls of arteries and veins, the walls of the bronchial tubes, and the uterus. Cardiac muscle forms the walls of the heart. As mentioned, the cells of muscle tissue have little ability to reproduce themselves.

Nervous tissue is made of neurons and supporting neuroglial cells. Although mature neurons are not capable of mitosis, many neuroglia are capable. It is the neuroglia, not neurons, that usually form the tumors that develop in the central nervous system.

INTRODUCTION TO CANCER CONCEPTS

Oncology is the branch of medicine dealing with tumors. Oncology nursing is also called cancer nursing; it is an important component of medical-surgical nursing care. See Box 10.1 Cancer Resources. Cancer is second only to heart disease in mortality rates in the United States. The American Cancer Society reports that an estimated 10 million Americans alive today have a history of cancer.

Early accounts of cancer date back to the 17th century B.C. Documentation of the benefits of early cancer detection and its impact on treatment exist from the beginning of the 19th century. Today, microscopic technology and genetic engineering provide physicians with a better understanding of tumor growth and cell activity and a means for early cancer detection and intervention.

Benign Tumors

Cells that reproduce abnormally result in **neoplasms,** or tumors. *Neoplasm* is a term that combines the Greek word *neo,* meaning "new," and *plasia,* meaning "growth," to suggest new tissue growth. The new growth results in enlargement of tissue and the formation of an abnormal mass. Not all neoplasms contain cancer cells; however, a neoplastic cell is responsible for producing a tumor and shows a lively growing cell. A neoplastic growth is very difficult to detect until it contains about 500 cells and is approximately 1 cm.

A **benign** tumor is defined as a cluster of cells that is not normal to the body but is noncancerous. Benign tumors grow more slowly and have cells that are the same as the original tissue. An organ containing a benign tumor usually continues to function normally.

Cancer

Cancer is a group of cells that grows out of control, taking over the function of the affected organ. Cancer cells are described as poorly constructed, loosely formed, and with-

---

oncology: onco—mass + logy—word, reason
neoplasm: neo—new + plasm—form

out organization. An organ with a cancerous tumor eventually ceases to function. A simplistic definition is "confused cell." *Malignant,* a term often used as a synonym for cancer, is defined as a growth that resists treatment and tends to worsen and threaten death. A comparison of benign and malignant tumors is found in Table 10.1.

LEARNING TIP

Cancer is not contagious.

Pathophysiology

Cancer is not one disease, but many diseases with different causes, manifestations, treatments, and prognoses. There are more than 100 different types of cancer caused by mutation of cellular genes. Cancer takes on the characteristics of the cell it mutates and then takes on characteristics of the mutation. Growth-regulating signals in the cell's surrounding environment are ignored as the abnormal cell growth increases. Normal cells are limited to about 50 to 60 divisions before they die. Cancer cells do not have a division limit and are considered immortal.

The progression from a normal cell to a malignant cell follows a pattern of mutation, defective division and abnormal growth cycles, and defective cell communication. Cell mutation occurs when a sudden change affects the chromosomes, causing the new cell to differ from the parent. The malignant cell's enzymes destroy the gluelike substance found between normal cells, which disrupts the transfer of information used for normal cell structure.

Cancer cells also lack **contact inhibition**. This is a property of normal cells in which contact by the cell with another cell or tissue signals cells to stop dividing. Since cancer cells do not possess contact inhibition, they continue to divide and invade surrounding tissues.

Etiology

Cancer cell growth and reproduction involves a two-step process. The first step in cancer growth is called initiation. Initiation causes an alteration in the genetic structure of the cell (DNA). Cell alteration is associated with exposure to a **carcinogen**. The cellular change primes the cell to become cancerous.

Promotion is the second type of cancer cell growth. It occurs after repeated exposure to carcinogens causes the initiated cells to mutate. During the promotion step, a tumor forms from mutated cell reproduction.

A healthy immune system can often destroy cancer cells before they replicate and become a tumor. It is important to remember that any substance that weakens or alters the immune system puts the individual at risk for cell mutation. Medical researchers support the theory that cancer is a symptom of a weakened immune system.

Risk Factors

Increased risk of cancer is linked to many environmental factors. An evaluation of cancer begins with assessment of well-known risk factors such as specific viruses; exposure to radiation, chemicals, and irritants; genetics; diet; and general immunity. Certain racial and ethnic groups also are at higher risk for some types of cancer (Box 10.2 Cultural Considerations).

---

carcinogen: karkinos—cancer, crab + genesis—birth

TABLE 10.1   BENIGN AND MALIGNANT TUMORS

	Benign	Malignant
Growth Rate	Typically slow expansion	Often rapid with cell numbers doubling normal cell growth; malignant cells infiltrate surrounding tissue
Cell Features	Typical of the tissue of origin	Atypical in varying degrees of the tissue or origin; altered cell membrane; contains tumor-specific antigens
Tissue Damage	Minor	Often causes necrosis and ulceration of tissue
Metastasis	Not seen; remains localized at site of origin	Often spreads to form tumors in other parts of the body
Recurrence after Treatment	Seldom recurs after surgical removal	Recurrence can be seen after surgical removal and following radiation and chemotherapy
Related Terminology	Hyperplasia, polyp, and benign neoplasia	Cancer, malignancy, and malignant neoplasia
Prognosis	Not injurious unless location causes pressure or obstruction to vital organs	Death if uncontrolled

VIRUSES. Certain viruses, such as the **oncoviruses** (RNA-type viruses), are linked to cancer in humans. Retrovirus is an enzyme produced by RNA tumor viruses and is found in human leukemia cells.

The Epstein-Barr virus (EBV), which causes infectious mononucleosis, is also associated with Burkitt's lymphoma. Herpes simplex virus 2 has been associated with cervical and penile cancers. Papillomavirus, associated with genital warts, is considered one cause of cervical cancer in women. Chronic hepatitis B is linked with liver cancer.

RADIATION. There is an increased incidence of cancer in persons exposed to prolonged or large amounts of radiation.

---

oncovirus: onco—mass + virus

Ionizing radiation involving ultraviolet rays such as sunlight, x-rays, and alpha, beta, and gamma rays plays a major role in promoting leukemia and skin cancers, primarily melanomas.

Persons exposed to radioactive materials in large doses, such as a radiation leak or an atomic bomb, are at risk for leukemia and breast, bone, lung, and thyroid cancer. Controlled **radiation therapy** is used to treat cancer patients by destroying rapidly dividing cancer cells. Radiation can also damage normal cells. The decision to use radiation is made after careful evaluation of the tumor's location and vulnerability to other treatments.

CHEMICALS. Chemicals are present in air, water, soil, food, drugs, and tobacco smoke. Chemical carcinogens are

---

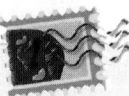

Box 10.2

Cultural Considerations

Many racial and ethnic groups in the United States have high rates of cancer. Although risk factors for the development of specific cancers are similar, barriers to prevention and nursing strategies to reduce risk factors vary among ethnicities.

Europeans

Foreign-born and first-generation white men from Norway, Sweden, and Germany have an increased risk of stomach cancer. This suggests an interrelation among ethnic, geographical, and dietary risk factors as the cause of this high incidence of stomach cancer. Assessing for these data among these populations may assist in the diagnostic process.

Recent Eastern European immigrants may be a risk for thyroid cancer and leukemia because of the current industrial pollution and radiation exposure from the Chernobyl nuclear disaster in the former USSR in 1986. Some contamination occurred in Estonia, Latvia, Lithuania, and Poland. This may constitute a health hazard and may affect both recent immigrants and visitors to these countries. It is essential that healthcare providers carefully screen individuals for these cancers.

African Americans

Cancer sites among African Americans include the prostate, breast, lung, colon, rectum, cervix, pancreas, and esophagus. Because African Americans are overrepresented in the working class, they experience increased exposure to hazardous occupations. For example, African American men are at a higher risk for developing cancer related to their high representation in the steel and tire industries and in factories manufacturing chemicals and pesticides. They have the highest overall cancer rate, the highest overall mortality rate, and their 5-year survival rate is 30% lower than that of European

Americans. In general, African Americans report later for treatment than European Americans. Colon tumors are deeper within African Americans, making detection on digital examination more difficult. Poverty, a diet high in fat and low in fiber, and lower levels of thiamine, riboflavin, vitamins A and C, and iron may increase cancer risk among African Americans. Additionally, cigarette smoking, inner city living with pollution, obesity, and alcohol consumption increase African Americans' risk for developing cancer.

Lack of medical care access acts as a barrier to prevention among African Americans. Survival, not prevention, is the priority for some. Additional barriers include a lack of cancer risk teaching and detection in some African American communities, lack of health insurance, and little stigma attached to alcohol consumption and smoking. Strong family ties encourage seeking health care from family members before professionals.

Primary strategies for cancer prevention and increasing survival among African Americans include using African American professionals as speakers in community activities, using church-based information dissemination, providing forums in African American communities, and addressing smoking advertisements in African American communities. Additional strategies include involving granny healers and ministers, changing food preparation practices and amounts rather than changing cultural food habits, involving extended family members in educational campaigns, and using high-profile African Americans such as sports leaders and actors in media campaigns.

Hispanics

Hispanic populations in the United States have an increased incidence for some types of cancer. Cervical cancer is increased among Central and South American women. Pancreatic, liver, and gall-bladder cancer is increased among Mexican Americans. Many Mexican Americans are less aware of the early warning signs of cancer; many are more fearful of getting cancer than the general public; and many work in mining, factories using chemicals, and farming using pesticides.

Barriers to preventive health care among many Hispanics include high poverty rates, low educational rates, a preference for health-care providers who understand Spanish, a preference for health-care information presented in Spanish, a delay in seeking treatments for symptoms, and using lay healers as a first choice in health care. Additionally, many have a fear of surgical intervention with a body cavity left open to air and have decreased access to health care. For some, an undocumented immigration status creates a fear of reprisal.

Nursing approaches effective among Hispanics include educating lay healers regarding cancer prevention and early warning signs of cancer, using bilingual health-care providers, using Hispanic health-care providers whenever available, using respected Hispanic community leaders in educational programs, presenting videos in Spanish using Hispanic actors, educating the entire family because of close family networks, and connecting with Hispanic community churches, restaurants, and stores. Additionally, the nurse can use the 1-800-4-CANCER telephone number for Spanish translation and counseling, become involved with Hispanic community movements, and provide information in community and regional Hispanic newspapers and community publications.

Asians and Pacific Islanders

Cervical, liver, lung, stomach, multiple myeloma, esophageal, pancreatic, and nasopharyngeal cancer are higher among Chinese Americans. Chinese American women have a 20% higher rate of pancreatic cancer. High rates of stomach and liver cancer in Korea predispose recent immigrants to these conditions. Thus, the nurse needs to assess and teach newer immigrants regarding these types of cancer.

High rates of stomach, breast, colon, and rectal cancer common among Japanese people may be related to the high sodium content of the Japanese diet, a genetic predisposition, consumption of salted fish and contaminated grain, hepatitis B, smoking, vitamin A deficiency, low vitamin C intake, chronic esophagitis, and pulmonary sequelae of cigarette smoking. Barriers to prevention include the following: prevention models are not native to their culture; there may be a lack of trust in Western medicine; they have decreased access to health care; some are unable to speak the English language; and for some, an undocumented immigration status creates a fear of reprisal.

Nursing approaches to improve cancer risk prevention among Asians and Pacific Islanders include education about prevention versus acute care practice, educating native healers, involvement in community with respected native leaders, videos and literature in native language, and incorporating native healing practices such as traditional Chinese medicine.

Native Americans

Native American populations have an increased risk for skin, pancreatic, gallbladder, liver, and prostate cancer. Risk factors for the development of cancer include obesity, a diet high in fat, high rates of alcohol consumption, and high rates of smoking. Barriers to prevention include a lack of Native American health-care providers, health care providers' unfamiliarity with Native American cultures, lack of financial resources, and a lack of integration of Native American healing practices into prevention practices. Nursing approaches to decrease cancer risk prevention among Native American populations include the following: incorporate prevention into Native American healing practices; educate Native American lay healers regarding cancer prevention practices; work with tribal community leaders; respect modesty, gender roles, and tribal customs; work with the Indian Health Service and Bureau of Indian Affairs; encourage traditional customs of physical fitness and exercise; and encourage dietary portion control and healthy food preparation practices instead of changing cultural food habits.

---

implicated as triggering mechanisms in malignant tumor development. Length of exposure time and degree of exposure intensity to chemical carcinogens are associated with risk for cancer development.

Smoking accounts for 87% of lung cancer worldwide.[1] Chemical agents, such as those in tobacco, are more toxic when used with alcohol. Alcohol and tobacco are the most frequent causes of cancers of the mouth and throat. Chemicals used in manufacturing, such as vinyl chloride, are associated with liver cancer.

IRRITANTS. Chronic irritation or inflammation caused by irritants such as snuff or pipe smoke often cause cancer in local areas. Nevi (moles) that are chronically irritated by clothing, especially clothing contaminated by chemical residue, may become malignant. Asbestos found in temperature and sound insulation has been proven to cause a particularly destructive type of lung cancer.

GENETICS. Genetics plays a large part in cancer formation. Certain breast cancers are linked to a specific gene mutation.

Skin and colon cancers have a genetic tendency. People with Down's syndrome (a chromosomal abnormality) have a higher risk of developing acute leukemia.

DIET. Diet is a large factor in both cause and prevention of malignancies. People who eat high-fat, low-fiber diets are more prone to develop colon cancers. Diets high in fiber reduce the risk of colon cancer. High-fat diets are linked to breast cancer in women and prostate cancer in men. Consumption of large amounts of pickled, smoked, and charbroiled foods has been linked with esophageal and stomach cancers. A diet low in vitamins A, C, and E is associated with cancers of the lungs, esophagus, mouth, larynx, cervix, and breast.

HORMONES. Hormonal agents that disturb the balance of the body may also promote cancer. Long-term use of the female hormone estrogen is associated with cancer of the breast, uterus, ovaries, cervix, and vagina. It has been found that children born of mothers who took diethylstilbestrol (DES) during pregnancy have an increased incidence of reproductive cancers. DES is a synthetic hormone with estrogenlike properties used in the past to prevent miscarriage.

Tumors of the breast and uterus are tested for estrogen or progesterone influence. If a breast tumor is malignant, the tumor is tested and treatment varies depending on whether it is positive for estrogen or progesterone dependence.

IMMUNE FACTORS. A healthy immune system destroys mutant cells quickly on formation. An individual with altered immunity is more susceptible to cancer formation when exposed to small amounts of carcinogens compared with someone with a healthy immune system. Immune system suppression allows malignant cells to develop in large numbers.

Altered immunity is noted in persons with chronic illness and stress. An increased risk of cancer follows a traumatic, stressful period in life, such as the loss of a mate or a job. Failure to decrease stress productively contributes to a higher incidence of chronic illnesses. Thus, a cycle of stress, illness, and increased cancer risk develops. Individuals with acquired immunodeficiency syndrome (AIDS) have a compromised immune system and an increased risk for certain cancers. A decline in the immune system is also noted as the body ages. A weaker immune system contributes to chronic illnesses and cancers associated with the elderly population.

Cancer Classification

Cancers are identified by the tissue affected, speed of cell growth, cell appearance, and location. Neoplasms occurring in the epithelial cells are called carcinomas. Carcinoma is

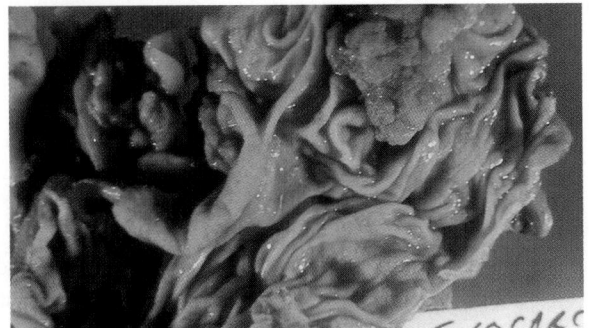

FIGURE 10.4 Adenocarcinoma of the caecum. *(Photo courtesy Dinesh Patel, MD. Medical Oncology, Internal Medicine, Zanesville, OH.)*

the most common type of cancer and includes cells of the skin, gastrointestinal system, and lungs (Figs. 10.4 and 10.5). Cancer cells affecting connective tissue, including fat, the sheath that contains nerves, cartilage, muscle, and bone, are called sarcomas. *Leukemia* is the term used to describe the abnormal growth of white blood cells. Cancers involving cells of the lymphatic system, lymph nodes, and spleen are called lymphomas. See Table 10.2 for cancer types based on origin.

Spread of Cancer

Neoplastic cells that remain in one area are considered localized, or **in situ,** cancers. These tumors may be difficult to visualize on clinical examination and are detected through microscopic cell examination. In situ tumors are often removed surgically and require no further treatment. **Metastasis** is the term used to describe the spread of the tumor from the primary site into separate and distant areas.

Metastasis is the stage at which cancer cells acquire invasive behavior characteristics and cause the surrounding tissue to change (Fig. 10.6). Metastasis occurs primarily because cancer cells break away more easily than normal cells and can survive for a time independently from other cells. There are three steps in the formation of a metastasis.

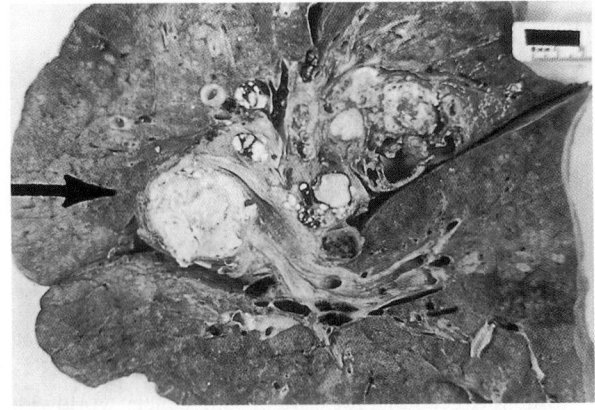

FIGURE 10.5 Lung cancer. *(Photo courtesy Dinesh Patel, MD. Medical Oncology, Internal Medicine, Zanesville, OH.)*

in situ: in—in + situ—position
metastasis: meta—beyond + stasis—stand

LEARNING TIP

An individual's cancer risk is viewed as the balance between exposure and susceptibility to carcinogens.

TABLE 10.2 TUMOR DESCRIPTION

Tumor Type	Character	Origin
Fibroma	Benign	Connective tissue
Lipoma	Benign	Fat tissue
Carcinoma	Cancerous	Tissue of the skin, glands, and digestive, urinary, and respiratory tract linings
Sarcoma	Cancerous	Connective tissue, including bone and muscle
Leukemia	Cancerous	Blood, plasma cells, and bone marrow
Lymphoma	Cancerous	Lymph tissue
Melanoma	Cancerous	Skin cells

Cancer cells are able to (1) invade blood or lymph vessels, (2) move by mechanical means, and (3) lodge and grow in a new location.

Metastatic tumors carry with them the cell characteristics of the original or primary tumor site. As a result, surgeons are able to determine the original tumor site based on metastatic cell characteristics. For example, lung tissue found in the brain suggests a primary lung tumor with metastasis to brain tissue. Common sites of metastasis are the lungs, liver, bones, and brain.

Incidence of Cancer

Cancer affects all age groups, although the incidence is higher in people ages 60 to 69. The second highest age group is ages 70 to 79. Men have a higher incidence of cancer than women. Cancer in people over age 60 is thought to occur from a combination of exposure to carcinogens and weakening of the body's immune system.

Some cancers, such as Wilms's tumor of the kidney and acute lymphocytic leukemia, occur more commonly in young people. The cause of tumors in young people is not well understood, but genetic predisposition tends to be a major factor.

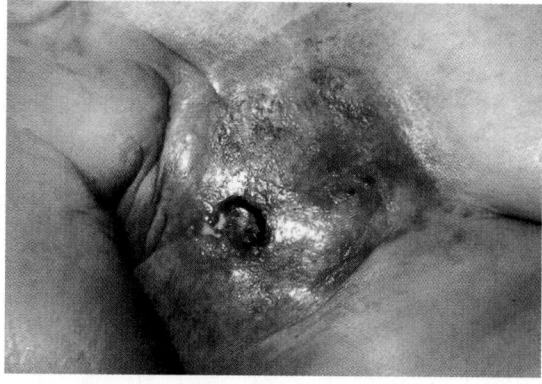

FIGURE 10.6 Invasive metastasis to skin area following mastectomy for breast cancer. *(Photo courtesy Dinesh Patel, MD. Medical Oncology, Internal Medicine, Zanesville, OH.)*

The most common type of cancer in adults is skin cancer; it is also considered to be the most preventable. Exposure to ultraviolet radiation (sunlight) increases the risk of skin cancer. Wearing protective clothing and sunscreen can greatly reduce the risk of skin cancer.

Lung cancer is responsible for the highest mortality rate in both men and women and also is commonly preventable. Cigarette smoking is the main cause, along with air pollution and exposure to chemical agents.

Men have a high incidence of prostate cancer between ages 60 and 79. Cancer of the colon and rectum has been linked to the consumption of high-fat, low-fiber diets and ranks as the third highest cancer in men.

The highest incidence of cancer in women is in the lungs, and the second highest is in the breast. Women with a family history of breast cancer have a greater risk than those with no family history. Commercial testing for the oncogene linked with breast cancer is available and marketed for high-risk women, especially those in the Ashkenazi Jewish population. Genetic testing is done through genetic counseling programs, and the cost ranges from $700 to $2400, depending on the geographical region. See Figure 10.7 for estimated new cancer cases and deaths for 2005.

Mortality Rates

Cancer survival rates have improved over the past 30 years, and since the 1990s the number of cancer deaths has decreased for both men and women. A 5-year period is used to monitor cancer patients' progress following diagnosis and treatment. Survival statistics are based on persons living 5 years in remission. Remission is considered to have occurred when all signs and symptoms of cancer have disappeared, even though there still may be cancer in the body.

For more information about cancer incidence and mortality data, visit the National Cancer Institute website at http://www.nci.nih.gov or the National Coalition for Cancer Survivorship website at http://www.cansearch.org.

Detection and Prevention

Nurses play an important role in preventing and detecting cancer. You can help educate patients about risk factors, self-examination, and cancer screening programs. Early diagnosis and treatment provide time to stop the progression of cancer.

EARLY DETECTION. An annual physical examination helps medical personnel detect the seven warning signals of cancer promoted by the American Cancer Society. The warning signals can be remembered with the mnemonic CAUTION:

- **C**hange in bowel or bladder habits
- **A** sore that fails to heal
- **U**nusual bleeding or discharge
- **T**hickening or lump in breast or other tissue
- **I**ndigestion or swallowing difficulties
- **O**bvious change in wart or mole
- **N**agging cough or hoarseness

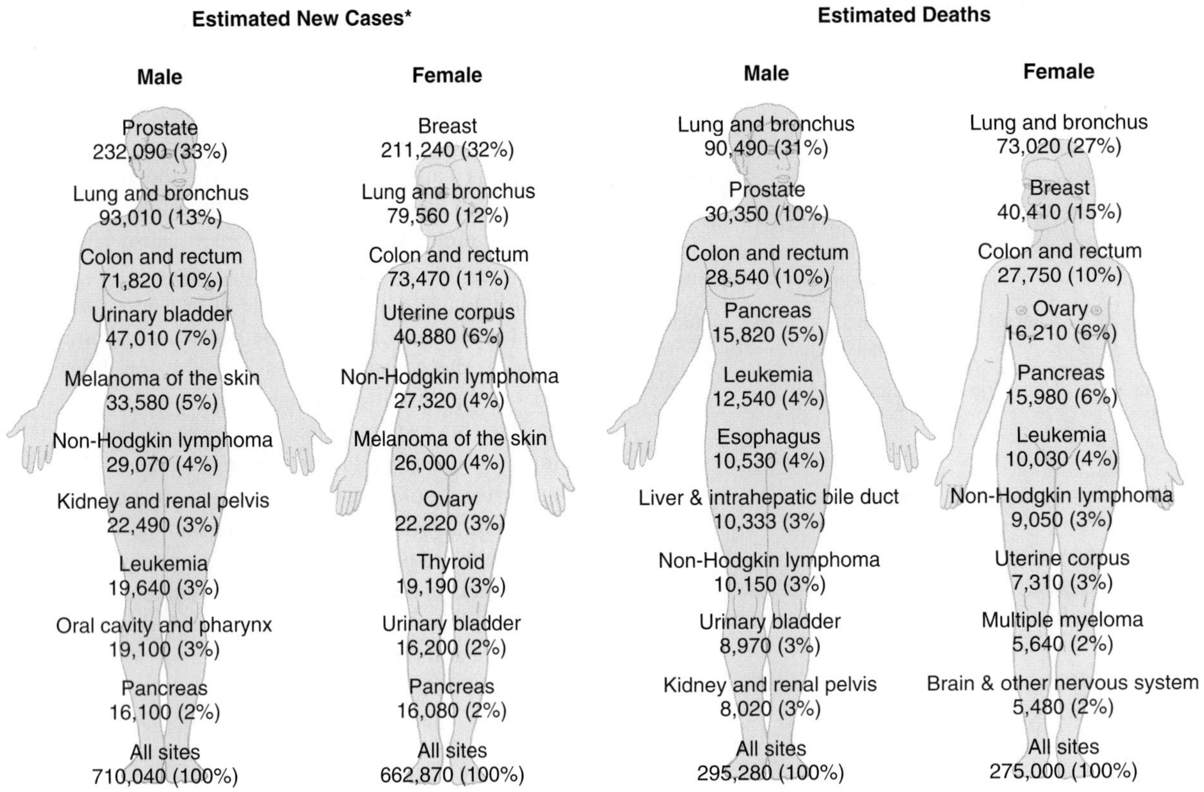

Estimated New Cases*

Male	Female
Prostate 232,090 (33%)	Breast 211,240 (32%)
Lung and bronchus 93,010 (13%)	Lung and bronchus 79,560 (12%)
Colon and rectum 71,820 (10%)	Colon and rectum 73,470 (11%)
Urinary bladder 47,010 (7%)	Uterine corpus 40,880 (6%)
Melanoma of the skin 33,580 (5%)	Non-Hodgkin lymphoma 27,320 (4%)
Non-Hodgkin lymphoma 29,070 (4%)	Melanoma of the skin 26,000 (4%)
Kidney and renal pelvis 22,490 (3%)	Ovary 22,220 (3%)
Leukemia 19,640 (3%)	Thyroid 19,190 (3%)
Oral cavity and pharynx 19,100 (3%)	Urinary bladder 16,200 (2%)
Pancreas 16,100 (2%)	Pancreas 16,080 (2%)
All sites 710,040 (100%)	All sites 662,870 (100%)

Estimated Deaths

Male	Female
Lung and bronchus 90,490 (31%)	Lung and bronchus 73,020 (27%)
Prostate 30,350 (10%)	Breast 40,410 (15%)
Colon and rectum 28,540 (10%)	Colon and rectum 27,750 (10%)
Pancreas 15,820 (5%)	Ovary 16,210 (6%)
Leukemia 12,540 (4%)	Pancreas 15,980 (6%)
Esophagus 10,530 (4%)	Leukemia 10,030 (4%)
Liver & intrahepatic bile duct 10,333 (3%)	Non-Hodgkin lymphoma 9,050 (3%)
Non-Hodgkin lymphoma 10,150 (3%)	Uterine corpus 7,310 (3%)
Urinary bladder 8,970 (3%)	Multiple myeloma 5,640 (2%)
Kidney and renal pelvis 8,020 (3%)	Brain & other nervous system 5,480 (2%)
All sites 295,280 (100%)	All sites 275,000 (100%)

*Excludes basal and squamous cell skin cancers and in situ carcinoma except urinary bladder.
Note: Percentages may not total 100% due to rounding.

FIGURE 10.7 Estimated new cancer cases and deaths by sex, United States, 2005. *(Cancer Facts and Figures, American Cancer Society, 2005.)* http://www.cancer.org/downloads/STT/CAFF2005f4PWSecured.pdf, page 10.

The American Cancer Society[2] recommends monthly breast self-examination after puberty for both men and women, and monthly self-testicular examination for men (see Chapter 41 for information on how to do self-examinations).

Mammography (a specific x-ray of breast tissue used to detect a mass too small for palpation) is recommended annually in women after age 40. However, if a woman is at risk for breast cancer because of family history, the frequency of screening should be discussed with her doctor. Routine pelvic examinations no longer have a recommended frequency. This is a matter to be discussed between a woman and her doctor. Initial Papanicolaou testing (Pap smear) is currently recommended to begin no later than age 21. If a woman has three normal results in a row, screening can be done every 2 to 3 years unless there are risk factors present. Once a woman is past the age of 70 and has had three normal Pap tests in a row within the past 10 years, she can choose to stop screening. Cytological examination of cervical cells increases the chance of diagnosing cervical cancer in situ.

The American Cancer Society recommends one of the following five options to screen for colorectal cancer, beginning at age 50:

1. An annual stool test for blood
2. A flexible sigmoidoscopy every 5 years
3. A yearly stool test for blood and flexible sigmoidoscopy every 5 years
4. A double-contrast barium enema every 5 years
5. A colonoscopy every 10 years

Option 3 is preferred. Screening should begin earlier and take place more frequently in high-risk people.

Screening for prostate cancer is important for men beginning around age 50. Digital rectal examination and prostate-specific antigen (PSA) blood testing is recommended annually for men older than 50 who have a life expectancy of at least 10 years and for younger men who are at higher risk. See Box 10.3 Gerontological Issues for specific screening recommendations for older adults.

GENETIC TESTING. Currently, much attention is directed toward genetic testing and identification of persons at risk for cancer. Genetic testing technology poses both legal and ethical questions concerning confidentiality and insurance cost issues. The cooperation of family members is important because genetic testing is done after a family member has been diagnosed with cancer. Family members may experience a variety of emotions surrounding the increased risk for themselves and their guilt over the role they may have played in increasing the risk for their children.

HEALTHY LIFESTYLE. Promotion of healthy lifestyles, including proper diet and exercise, helps strengthen the

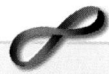

Box 10.3

Gerontological Issues

Screening Guidelines

Use the following American Cancer Society guidelines for older adults

Colorectal cancer:
- Sigmoidoscopy, every 5 years, and/or
- Fecal occult blood test yearly, or
- Double contrast barium enema every 5 years, or
- Colonoscopy every 10 years

Breast cancer:
- Breast self-examination monthly
- Breast clinical examination yearly
- Mammogram yearly

Prostate cancer:
- Prostate exam (digital rectal exam) yearly
- Prostatic surface antigen yearly

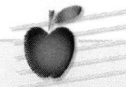

Box 10.4

Nutrition Notes

Reducing Cancer Risk

Encourage patients to consume these foods:
- Fruits and vegetables, especially those rich in vitamin C or carotene
- Cruciferous vegetables (cabbage, broccoli, Brussels sprouts)
- Whole grains
- Grilled meats that have been
  - Precooked in a microwave oven.
  - Marinated but basted only with fresh marinade, not that used to steep raw meat

Encourage patients to limit these foods:
- Excessive meat, especially when smoked, salted, charbroiled, or cooked at high temperatures
- Excessive fat (more than 30% of daily calories)
- Excessive calories
- Alcohol

immune system and reduce cancer risk. The American Cancer Society promotes smoking cessation campaigns and supports the effort by stating that smoking is the most preventable cause of death from lung cancer. Second-hand smoke contributes to an increased risk of lung cancer in nonsmokers as well.

PROTECTANT FOODS. There has been a lot of attention in the news in areas of diet and cancer risk. This is an area where much research is being done. The American Cancer Society does provide information about diet and cancer. This includes discussion about folic acid, omega-3 fatty acids, and antioxidants, to name a few. A diet poor in folic acid can lead to development of cancers of the colon and breast. It is recommended that folic acid is best obtained by eating fruits, vegetables, and enriched grain products.

People who ingest a high saturated fat diet are at a greater risk of obesity, which can be a risk factor for some types of cancer. However, ingestion of omega-3 fatty acids in animals has been studied and shown to suppress the incidence of certain cancers. These findings are being researched for application in humans. Foods rich in omega-3 fatty acids include fish.

Eating antioxidant-rich foods like vegetables and fruits has been shown to have some effect on lowering the risk of cancer. Antioxidants include vitamins C and E, selenium, and carotenoids. However, no study has yet confirmed that this same effect could come from ingesting supplements containing antioxidants.

Most research points to the benefit of eating a balanced diet rather than using supplements to prevent cancer (Box 10.4 Nutrition Notes).

VACCINES. Preventive cancer vaccines are being developed for cancers associated with specific viruses. At present, most cancer vaccines are therapeutic rather than prophylactic and are used to stimulate the patient's immune system to destroy cancer cells. Vaccine therapy for malignant melanoma and lymphoma is being tested.

Diagnosis of Cancer

A diagnosis of cancer can be a very frightening experience (Box 10.5 Patient Perspective). Often people try to mask symptoms because they are so frightened of the disease. A careful and thorough assessment of the patient's present and past medical and surgical histories and pertinent family history should be obtained. A complete physical examination provides both objective and subjective data. The most conclusive information about the health of tissue is acquired by examining cell activity through biopsy.

BIOPSY. Accurate identification of a cancer can be done only by **biopsy** (surgical removal of tissue cells). Microscopic examination of a piece of suspected tissue or aspirated body fluid can confirm the presence of mutant cells. A biopsy is commonly done in a physician's office or outpatient surgery department.

Incisional biopsy is an invasive procedure that involves the surgical removal of a small amount of tissue for inspection. Tissue can also be removed during endoscopic procedures (insertion of a tube to observe the inside of a hollow organ or cavity), such as a lung biopsy done during bronchoscopy. Excisional biopsy is used to remove an entire tissue mass. Needle aspiration biopsy involves insertion of a needle into tissue for fluid or tissue aspiration (Fig. 10.8). This procedure is less invasive than incisional or excisional biopsy. Transcutaneous aspiration involves the insertion of a fine needle into tissue such as breast, prostate, or salivary gland and is used for diagnosing metastatic cancers. Frozen section biopsy provides immediate evaluation of the tissue sample during a surgical procedure. By freezing the

Box 10.5

Robyn

I am a 43-year-old woman with three children and in the prime of my life, at least I thought. That was before I was diagnosed with cancer in my left breast. I was breast-feeding at the time I felt the lump and, although I went for a biopsy, I felt sure the lump resulted from a blocked milk duct or fibroid cyst. But, unbelievably, the biopsy came back positive for cancer. My whole life flipped upside down. I was devastated.

I was scheduled for surgery within a week, and my emotions were in complete turmoil. I felt nauseated all the time, vomited almost every morning, and had diarrhea daily. My stomach felt like it had a pot of bees inside. I never cried so much in my life. Thinking about all the tests, the surgery, and the untold ways my life could be affected made me a nervous wreck. Finally, I got down on my knees and turned this whole crisis over to God. I couldn't handle it anymore, so I asked God to give me peace, and I placed all my trust and faith in Him. It worked, and I was finally able to get control and face this thing head on.

As I went for further testing, the nurses and technicians I met were all very helpful and informative. Some actually broke down with me because they had endured this same disease. We would hold each other and then exchange phone numbers just to "talk" if I needed it. It was very encouraging to know these women had made it through, and I could too.

The surgery went smoothly, and I was released the next day. There wasn't much discomfort, and I felt good physically. The nerve was removed and a scar runs from the center of my chest down under my armpit. I was able to return to work in 3 weeks. The doctor gave me a prescription for a prosthesis as soon as the drains were removed and I began healing. We went to a specialty place to be fitted, and, although the prosthesis was nothing like the real thing, I looked normal and it helped to build my confidence.

The impact on my family was one of complete bewilderment because I had no family history of this type of cancer. Everyone tried to help with positive sentiments like we caught it early, breast cancer has a high cure rate, periodic follow-up can keep you cancer free, and so on. My husband and children supported and comforted me. I tried to focus on them because I want to be there for them when they graduate, get married, etc. My mother and sister helped get me to all my appointments and filled my prescriptions.

Chemo was advised as a follow-up treatment, and I was scheduled for four rounds, one every 3 weeks. This was undoubtedly the worst thing I have ever endured. Not even giving birth can compare to the way chemo makes you feel. I had a very bad experience the first round and was extremely sick and unable to eat for 5 days. I wondered why I didn't just die from the cancer because I felt that this was killing me. Before the second round, I told the doctor how violently ill I'd been and she adjusted the dosages of some of the drugs. I was very groggy; although I didn't vomit, I still wasn't feeling myself. For the third round, they changed a medication and I withstood the side effects a lot better—although I was still nauseated, light-headed, fatigued, and unable to focus, eat, or taste anything. At times, it was hard just to put one foot in front of the other. They prepared me for the loss of my hair, but you really don't know how hard that is until it starts coming out in globs. Not just the loss, but then you have such a long time to wait for it to grow back. When the chemo is over, it's hard to look back and feel the way you did then, but when you look in the mirror and your hair is still gone, it's a hard reminder.

All through being diagnosed and dealing with breast cancer I have felt a tremendous outpouring of love and caring, not only from my immediate family but also from my church family. I was never so well taken care of. All the hugs, cards, calls, food, and flowers brought to the house encouraged me tremendously. It makes it a little easier to cope when you know you have so many people who care and are concerned enough to take time out of their daily lives to give you support.

I'm lucky because my sister is an RN and prepared me for many of the side effects and difficulties. She also was there to help ask questions and get information from other survivors that kept me in a positive frame of mind. I know that without her help and God's grace and peace my recovery would not have been so easy. Looking back I can't really feel all those terrible emotions and symptoms, but I still am afraid of the unknown. It is not easy when it is you and not someone else this happens to.

Now that I'm through the worst part of this, I take positive steps every day to enjoy the little things in life. I feel that the more you keep involved in everyday activities and become educated about the disease and its treatments, the easier it is to deal with. I am taking a drug called tamoxifen now and will be for 5 years. Two of the side effects are hot flashes and sweats. If this is all I have to deal with, however, praise God. My prognosis is very good, and I am expecting a complete cure because I am a survivor.

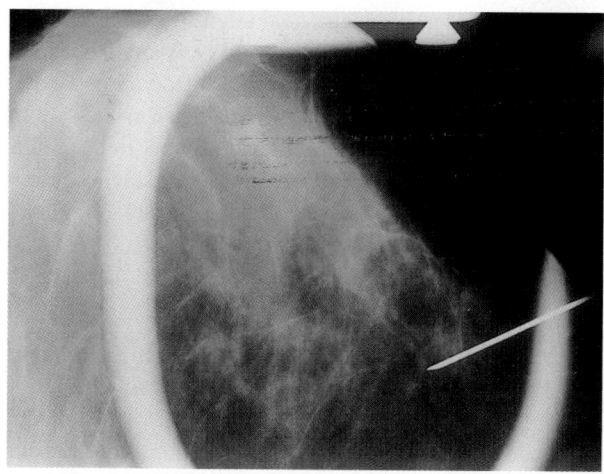

FIGURE 10.8 Fine-needle breast biopsy. (Photo courtesy Dinesh Patel, MD. Medical Oncology, Internal Medicine, Zanesville, OH.)

tissue sample for microscopic examination, a quick analysis is possible, which helps direct the remainder of the surgical procedure. Frozen section biopsy is especially useful in the diagnosis and surgical intervention of breast cancer.

Stereotactic biopsy is a safe and efficient procedure for evaluating lesions in the brain and breast. The procedure is done by a specially trained radiologist. The biopsy site must be firmly immobilized. The lesion is scanned for location, and a small incision is made for easy insertion of a small fiberoptic instrument (Fig. 10.9). Stereotactic biopsy of the brain involves a local anesthetic because a small hole in the skull is made. Breast stereotactic biopsy uses pressure exerted by a mammogram machine to secure the breast; anesthesia may not be necessary.

LABORATORY TESTS. Blood, serum, and urine tests are important in establishing baseline values and general health status. Laboratory values are used with other assessment findings. An elevated white blood cell (WBC) count is

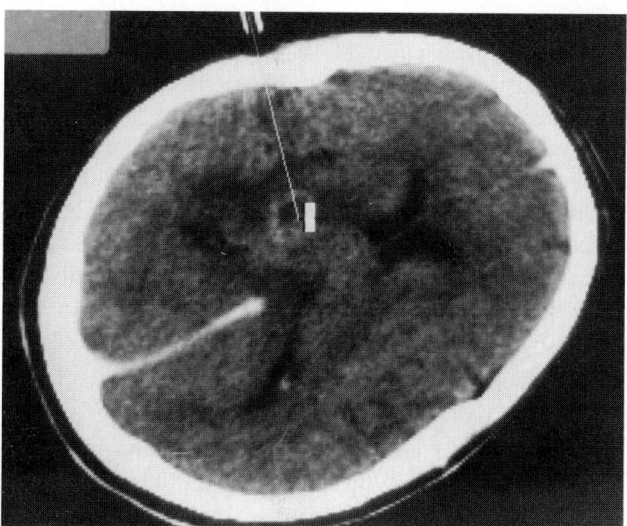

FIGURE 10.9 Stereotactic biopsy of a brain lesion. (Photo courtesy Dinesh Patel, MD. Medical Oncology, Internal Medicine, Zanesville, OH.)

expected if the patient has evidence of infection; however, an increase in WBCs without infection raises suspicion of leukemia. Fifty percent of patients with liver cancer have increased levels of bilirubin, alkaline phosphatase, and glutamic-oxaloacetic transaminase.

Bone marrow aspiration is done to learn the number, size, and shape of red and white blood cells and platelets. Bone marrow aspiration is a major tool for diagnosis of leukemia. (See Chapter 27 for a description of this test and related nursing care.)

Tumor markers, also called biochemical markers, are proteins, antigens, genes, hormones, and enzymes produced and secreted by tumor cells. Tumor markers help confirm a diagnosis of cancer, detect cancer origin, monitor the effect of cancer therapy, and determine cancer remission. Some examples of tumor markers include the following:

- Prostatic acid phosphatase (PAP)—high levels noted in prostate cancer
- PSA—elevated levels associated with prostate cancer
- Cancer antigen (CA) 15-3—elevated levels noted in breast cancer; useful in monitoring patient response to therapy for metastatic breast cancer
- CA 125—increased levels in ovarian, cervical, liver, and pancreatic cancers
- CA 19-9—used to diagnose and evaluate colorectal, pancreatic, and hepatobiliary cancers
- Alpha-fetoprotein (AFP)—elevated in hepatocellular cancer
- Carcinoembryonic antigen (CEA)—increased levels suggest tumor activity

CYTOLOGICAL STUDY. Cytology is the study of the formation, structure, and function of cells. Cytological diagnosis of cancer is obtained primarily through Pap smears of cells shed from a mucous membrane (e.g., cervical or oral smear). Test results are based on the degree of cell abnormality. Normal results reflect no cellular changes. Slight cellular changes are considered normal, with a possible link to abnormal cells seen in infection. Significant cellular changes reflect a higher probability of precancerous or cancerous activity. Infection causes cellular changes and contributes to an increase in abnormal cells detected.

RADIOLOGICAL PROCEDURES. X-ray examination is a valuable diagnostic tool in detecting cancer of the bones and hollow organs. Routine chest x-ray examination is one diagnostic test used in detecting lung cancer. Mammography is a reliable and noninvasive low-radiation x-ray procedure for detecting breast masses (Fig. 10.10). Breast tissue is compressed to allow better visualization of the soft tissue. You must alert patients that soft tissue compression causes a degree of discomfort, but the compression is necessary to obtain an accurate picture. Assure the patient that the discomfort is brief. See Chapter 41 for more information on mammography.

Contrast media x-ray studies are used to detect abnormalities of bone and the gastrointestinal and urinary sys-

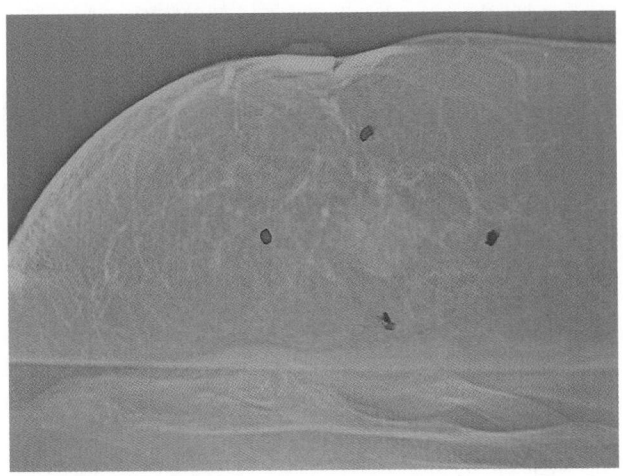

FIGURE 10.10 Mammogram. *(Photo courtesy Dinesh Patel, MD. Medical Oncology, Internal Medicine, Zanesville, OH.)*

tems. Contrast media can be given by various methods. Barium is given orally for visualization of the esophagus and stomach or rectally for visualization of the colon (e.g., a barium enema). Intravenous injection of contrast media is used for lung and brain scans.

Computed tomography (CT) provides a three-dimensional, cross-sectional, computerized picture of the body. CT scans are important in the diagnosis and staging of malignancies and can detect minor variations in tissue thickness. The use of a contrast medium enhances the accuracy of an abdominal CT scan. CT scans are also used to improve the accuracy of inserting a fine needle for biopsy.

NUCLEAR IMAGING PROCEDURES. Nuclear medicine imaging involves camera imaging of organs or tissues containing radioactive media. Radioactive compounds are given intravenously or by ingestion. These studies are highly sensitive and can detect sites of abnormal cell growth months before changes are seen on an x-ray.

Positron emission tomography (PET) scanning provides information about cellular biochemical and metabolic activity. Patients are given biochemical compounds, and images are made of the tissue through gamma-camera tomography. PET scans have been useful in brain imaging as well as the detection of the spread of cancers of the lung, ovaries, colon, rectum, and breast.

ULTRASOND PROCEDURES. Ultrasonography uses high-frequency sound waves to provide images of deep soft-tissue structures in the body. The procedure is noninvasive and does not use x-rays. Echoes from high-frequency sound waves outline tissue density and masses. This technology helps detect tumors of the pelvis and breast. Ultrasound may also be used to distinguish between benign and malignant breast tumors.

MAGNETIC RESONANCE IMAGING. Magnetic resonance imaging (MRI) creates sectional images of the body. MRI can be done with or without contrast dye and does not use radiation. The patient is placed in a cylinder-shaped magnetic field. The magnetic field aligns the nuclei of body cells in one direction. The magnetized cells are then excited by radiofrequency pulses. Images are made as cell nuclei change their alignment. MRI is valuable in the detection, localization, and staging of malignant tumors in the central nervous system, spine, head, and musculoskeletal system. MRI cannot be used in patients with pacemakers, implanted pumps, surgical clips, metal knees or hips, or in some cases tattooed eyeliner because metals are attracted by the magnet.

ENDOSCOPIC PROCEDURES. An endoscopic examination allows the direct visualization of a body cavity or opening. The procedure involves the insertion of a flexible endoscope containing fiberoptic glass bundles that transmit light and can produce an image. Endoscopy enables the surgeon to biopsy abnormal tissue and is used to detect lesions of the throat, esophagus, stomach, colon, and lungs.

Oral endoscopic procedures require patient preparation to reduce the risk of aspirating stomach secretions. The patient is given nothing to eat or drink before and immediately after the examination. A local anesthetic is used during the examination to anesthetize the throat. Following the procedure, oral food and fluids are withheld until the gag reflex returns to prevent aspiration. The gag reflex is assessed by touching a cotton-tipped swab to the back of the throat to stimulate the reflex after the procedure.

Staging and Grading

Tumor staging is used to determine the stage of solid-tumor masses, providing valuable information to guide treatment plans. Tumor staging is important in the development of an international system that can compare statistics among cancer centers. The most common system used for staging tumors is the tumor, node, metastasis (TNM) system.

This staging system classifies solid tumors by size and tissue involvement. TNM stages are T0 (no tumor), Tis (tumor in situ), and T1 through T4 (progressive increase in tumor size or involvement). Extent of lymph node involvement ranges from N0, no nodes, to N4, a large amount of lymph node involvement. Metastasis is described as M0, no metastasis, to M1, metastasis to some area (Table 10.3).

There is also a rating or grading system to define the cell types of tumors. Tumors are classified according to the percentage of cells that are differentiated (mature). If the tissue of a neoplastic tumor closely resembles normal tissue, it is called well differentiated. A poorly differentiated tumor is a malignant neoplasm that contains some normal cells, but most of the cells are abnormal. The better defined or differentiated the tumor, the easier it is to treat.

Treatment for Cancer

There are three main types of treatment for cancer: surgery, radiation therapy, and **chemotherapy.** To find out more about cancer treatment options, visit the American Cancer Society website at http://www.cancer.org.

---

chemotherapy: chemo—chemistry + therapy—treatment

TABLE 10.3 TUMOR, NODE, METASTASIS CLASSIFICATION, STAGING, AND TISSUE INVOLVEMENT

Classification	Staging	Tissue Involvement
Primary tumor (T)		
T_{is}	Stage I	Tumor in situ; indicates no invasion of other tissues
T_1, T_2, T_3, T_4	Stage II	Ranges indicate progressive increase in tumor size with local metastasis
Regional lymph node involvement (N)		
N_0	No nodes	
$N_1, N_2, N_3,$	Stage III	Metastasis to regional lymph nodes
Metastasis (M)		
M_0	No metastasis	
M_1	Stage IV	Distant metastasis

SURGERY. Surgery can be curative when it is possible to remove the entire tumor. Skin cancers and well-defined tumors without metastasis can be removed without any additional intervention. Other tumors may be removed as much as possible, with follow-up chemotherapy or radiation to treat the remaining tumor cells.

Prophylactic surgery is used to remove moles or lesions that have the potential to become malignant. Colon polyps are often removed to prevent malignancies from developing, especially if the polyps are considered premalignant. An extreme example of prophylactic surgery is a woman who elects to have a mastectomy (surgical removal of the breast) because of a high incidence of breast cancer in her family.

Surgery may also be done for **palliation** (symptom control). Surgical removal of tissue to reduce the size of the tumor mass is helpful, especially if the tumor is compressing nerves or blocking the passage of body fluids. The goals of palliative surgery are to increase comfort and quality of life.

Reconstructive surgery can be done for cosmetic enhancement or for return of function of a body part. Facial reconstruction is important for a patient's self-image after removal of head or neck tumors. Women can elect to have breast reconstruction after mastectomy.

Surgical intervention for cancer treatment is typically not an emergency intervention, which allows patients and medical personnel time for planning. Autologous blood donation (blood donated by the patient before surgery) has become popular and reduces the risk of exposure to bloodborne infections. The American Red Cross and many hospitals have programs specifically designed for autologous blood donation and accept donations from 30 days to 72 hours before surgery.

You can play a major role in reducing the patient's fears about postoperative pain. Patient-controlled analgesia (PCA) provides patients with some control over their pain.

Therapies such as deep relaxation, imagery, and hypnosis can be used with traditional pain control measures.

It is important to encourage patients to express and discuss their fears. Patients with a limited understanding of cancer may fear that tissues will not heal postoperatively. Provide information about wound care, including dressing changes and drainage tubes, to increase the patient's knowledge base and sense of control. Visual aids concerning tumor site and surgical procedures are valuable teaching tools.

Patients who are undernourished are poor surgical candidates and require intervention such as enteral or parenteral nutrition before and after surgery. Patients with cancer are also at increased risk for postoperative deep vein thrombosis (DVT). Preoperative teaching includes the importance of leg movement, early ambulation, wearing antiembolism stockings, and recognizing symptoms of DVT, such as calf pain or a cramping sensation in the calf muscle when the foot is dorsiflexed.

RADIATION. Radiation is used commonly in the treatment of cancer for control or palliation, or it can be curative if the disease is localized. The decision to use radiation is commonly based on cancer site and size. Radiation destroys cancer cells by affecting cell structure and the cell environment. It is used in fractionated (divided) doses to prevent destructive side effects; however, side effects can occur in the area being treated because of damage to normal cells.

The size of a large tumor can be decreased with radiation before surgery, making surgical intervention more effective and less dangerous. Palliative radiation is used to reduce the size of a large cancerous lesion and consequently reduce pressure and pain. Radioisotopes inserted into cancerous tissue during surgery help destroy the cancerous cells without removing the organ.

Nursing Care of the Patient Receiving Radiation Treatment. Symptoms of tissue reaction to radiation treatment can be expected about 10 to 14 days after the start of the treatment program and continue up to 2 weeks after treatment is completed. Typical reactions and appropriate nursing interventions include the following:

- Fatigue. Encourage the patient to nap frequently and prioritize activities. Reassure the patient that the feeling will go away when the treatments are completed.
- Nausea, vomiting, and **anorexia.** Encourage the patient to take prescribed medication for nausea and vomiting. Anorexia can be eased by giving small amounts of high-carbohydrate, high-protein foods and avoiding foods high in fiber.
- **Mucositis** (inflammation of the mucous membranes, especially of the mouth and throat). Encourage the patient to avoid irritants such as smoking, alcohol, acidic food or drinks, extremely

---

anorexia: an—not + orexis—appetite
mucositis: muco—mucous (membrane) + itis—inflammation

hot or cold foods and drinks, and commercial mouthwash. Advise the patient to perform mouth care before meals and every 3 to 4 hours. A neutral mouthwash is appropriate and can be made by using 1 ounce of diphenhydramine hydrochloride (Benadryl) elixir diluted in 1 quart of water or normal saline solution. Agents that coat the mouth, such as Maalox, are sometimes used. Lidocaine hydrochloride 2% viscous has an anesthetic effect on the mouth and throat.

- **Xerostomia** (dry mouth). Encourage frequent mouth care. Saliva substitute is available over-the-counter and is helpful, especially at night when patients complain of a choking sensation from extreme dryness.
- Skin reactions. These can vary from mild redness to moist **desquamation** similar to a second-degree burn. Skin surfaces that are especially warm and moist, such as the groin, perineum, and axillae, have poor tolerance to radiation. Prophylactic skin care includes keeping skin dry; keeping it free from irritants, such as powder, lotions, deodorants, and restrictive clothing; and protecting it against exposure to direct sunlight. Irradiated skin can be fragile during treatment. It is important to wash these areas gently with mild soap and water, rinse well, and pat dry. The skin may have markings and tattoos to delineate the treatment field. Take care not to wash off the markings.
- Bone marrow depression. This reaction occurs with both radiation and chemotherapy. Weekly blood cell counts are done to detect low levels of WBCs, red blood cells, and platelets. Transfusions of whole blood, platelets, or other blood components may be necessary.

---

xerostomia: xero—dry + stoma—mouth

Safety Considerations. Radiation may be administered externally or internally. External radiation is given by a trained medical specialist in a designated area in the hospital or clinic. Internal radiation is administered to patients admitted to a health-care facility.

Safety guidelines must be followed when caring for a patient with radioactive materials implanted into tissue or body cavities or administered orally or intravenously because the patient will be radioactive. Nursing responsibilities include knowledge about the following:

- Radiation source being used
- Method of administration
- Start of treatment
- Length of treatment
- Prescribed nursing precautions

Personnel involved with radiation therapy must recognize the three primary factors in radiation protection: time, distance, and shielding. These three factors depend on the type of radiation used. *Time* involves the time spent administering care, *distance* involves the amount of space between the radioisotope and the nurse, and *shielding* involves the use of a barrier such as a lead apron.

You must work efficiently when caring for patients who are receiving radioisotopes that are releasing gamma rays. Your exposure to radiation is proportionate to the time spent and the distance from the radiation source. For example, you will receive less exposure standing at the foot of the bed of a patient with radioisotopes inserted into the head than if you stand at the head of the bed (Fig. 10.11). Time and distance are used to protect the nurse, visitors, and other personnel.

It is important to teach the patient and family members the reason nursing care focuses on providing only essential care. Speedy nursing encounters and visitor restrictions are better accepted and less likely to promote feelings of isolation when patients understand the reasons behind them.

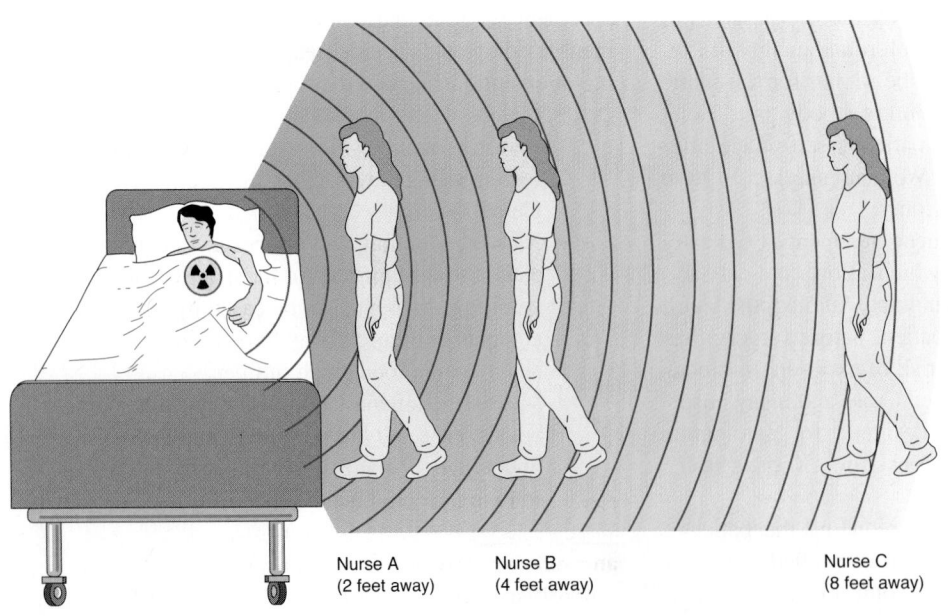

Nurse A
(2 feet away)

Nurse B
(4 feet away)

Nurse C
(8 feet away)

FIGURE 10.11 Radiation distancing. Nurse B receives less radiation than Nurse A, and Nurse C receives less radiation than Nurse B.

Drainage from the site of a radioactive colloid injection is considered radioactive, and the physician must be informed immediately. Dressings contaminated with radioactive seepage must be removed with long-handled forceps. Radioactive materials must never be touched with unprotected hands; shielding is required to prevent exposure to radiation. Contamination from radioisotope applicators or interstitial implants cannot occur when the capsule is intact; contamination occurs when the capsule is broken.

SAFETY TIP

Remember to use the principles of time, distance, and shielding to protect yourself from radiation exposure.

CHEMOTHERAPY. Chemotherapy is chemical therapy that uses **cytotoxic** drugs to treat cancer. Cytotoxic drugs can be used for cure, control, or palliation of cancerous tumors and are described according to how they affect cell activity. For example, alkylating agents bind with DNA to stop the production of RNA; antimetabolites substitute for nutrients or enzymes in the cell life cycle; mitotic inhibitors interfere with cell division; antibiotics inhibit DNA and RNA synthesis; and hormonal agents alter the hormonal structure of the body. Chemotherapy is usually more effective when multiple drugs are given in multiple doses. Examples of specific drugs and their adverse effects are provided in Table 10.4.

The effects of chemotherapy are systemic unless used topically for skin lesions. Chemotherapy is used preoperatively to shrink tumors and postoperatively to treat residual tumors. Factors influencing the effectiveness of chemotherapy are tumor type, available chemotherapeutic drugs, and genetics.

Combination Chemotherapy. Combination chemotherapy means that two or more antineoplastic agents are used together to treat a particular type of cancer. This can expose a larger number of cells at different points in the cell cycle to more than one kind of chemotherapy. Combining drugs also decreases the side effects of therapy and decreases the possibility of the tumor becoming resistant to the therapy.

In order for drugs to be combined this way, there are several criteria that need to be met. These include being effective when used alone to treat certain cancers and having different toxicities that would limit their use. For example, if three drugs that are all cardiotoxic are given, the patient is more likely to develop cardiotoxicity. Patients are still monitored for toxic effects from the treatment as well as improvement in their status.

Routes of Administration. Chemotherapy may be given via oral, intramuscular, intravenous, or topical routes. The

dosage of medication is regulated by the size of the individual and the toxicities of the drug. The administration of intravenous chemotherapeutic agents requires specialized training and knowledge of antineoplastic drugs.

Vesicant drugs are given only by the intravenous route. These drugs cause blistering of tissue that eventually leads to necrosis if they infiltrate, or leak out of the blood vessel, into soft tissue (Fig. 10.12). Skin grafts may be necessary if tissue damage is extensive.

Central Lines. Central lines are intravenous catheters that terminate in the superior vena cava near the right atrium of the heart. This is a large vessel that allows for dilution of vesicant drugs and reduces the risk of infiltration. Central lines may be external, with the distal end of the catheter exiting the skin, or internal, with the distal catheter ending in an implanted port. See Chapter 6 for additional information on central lines.

Side Effects. Toxicities in patients receiving chemotherapy vary according to the medications given; however, some general side effects are commonly associated with chemotherapeutic drugs. Fast-growing epithelial cells, such as those of the hair, blood, skin, and gastrointestinal tract, are generally affected by both chemotherapy and radiation.

Hematologic System. Chemotherapy is toxic to the bone marrow, which is where the blood cells are produced. Numbers of blood cells (especially white cells) drop after approximately 7 to 14 days, depending on the drug. This time period when the cell counts are lowest is called the **nadir.** This is then the time when patients are most at risk for developing complications. Patients may develop low white blood cell counts **(leukopenia),** increasing their susceptibility to infection and sepsis. A reduction in platelets **(thrombocytopenia)** increases the risk of bruising and bleeding and can require platelet transfusions. Increased risk

(Continued on page 162)

LEARNING TIP

When assessing patients with possible side effects of chemotherapy and radiation, use the mnemonic BITES:

B—Bleeding suggests low platelet count.
I—Infection suggests low WBC count and a risk for infection.
T—Tiredness suggests anemia.
E—Emesis places the patient at risk for altered nutrition and fluid and electrolyte imbalance.
S—Skin changes may be evidence of radiation reaction or skin breakdown.

---

cytotoxic: cyto—cell + toxic—poison

vesicant: vesicate—to blister
leukopenia: leuko—white cells + penia—lack
thrombocytopenia: thrombo—clot + cyte—cell + penia—lack

TABLE 10.4 CHEMOTHERAPY MEDICATIONS

Medication Class/Action	Examples	Route	Side Effects	Nursing Implications
Antitumor Antibiotics Damage cells' DNA and the ability to make DNA and RNA	Bleomycin (Blenoxane)	IM or IV	Fever, chills, cough, shortness of breath; in severe cases, pulmonary fibrosis, pain at the tumor site, anaphylaxis	Observe for changes in respiratory status related to pulmonary toxicity. Observe for anaphylaxis.
	Doxorubicin (Adriamycin)	IV	Red urine, nausea and vomiting, alopecia, cardiac damage	This drug is a vesicant and should be given through a running IV or a central line if it is a continuous infusion. Monitor cardiac status. Lifetime dose is 550 mg/m^2.
	Mitoxantrone (Novantrone)	IV	Headache, dyspnea, diarrhea, nausea, vomiting, stomatitis, alopecia, fever, bone marrow suppression, allergic reactions from itching to angioedema	Urine may be a blue-green color for 24 hours after the dose is given. Monitor WBC and platelet count prior to each dose. Observe for signs of allergic reaction. Teach patient signs of bleeding.
Antimetabolites Resemble normal metabolites needed for cell function. Once they can trick the cell into gaining entry, cell division becomes impaired.	Capecitabine (Xeloda)	PO	Bone marrow depression, nausea, vomiting, stomatitis, hand and foot syndrome	Monitor WBC and platelet count throughout therapy. Teach the patient signs of infection and bleeding. Teach the patient about mouth care. Drug should be taken after a meal with plenty of water. Teach the patient about hand and foot syndrome and to notify MD if it should occur.
	Cytabine (Cytosar)	IV	Fever, chills, unusual bleeding or bruising, sore throat, tiredness, nausea and vomiting	Monitor CBC prior to each dose. Instruct the patient of signs of infection or bleeding. Instruct patient to call MD for any temperature increases greater than 37.8°C (100.0°F).
	Fluorouracil (5-FU)	IV	Diarrhea, loss of appetite, alopecia, nausea and vomiting, skin sensitivity, stomatitis	Monitor CBC prior to dose. Nadir occurs in 10–14 days. Instruct about mouth care.
	Gemcitabine (Gemzar)	IV	Dyspnea, edema, nausea, vomiting, diarrhea, stomatitis, hamaturia, alopecia, bone marrow suppression	Monitor CBC prior to each dose. Premedicate with antiemetics. Instruct patient to report any flu like symptoms to MD.
Alkylating Agents Cause the DNA strands to bind together and prevent the cell from dividing.	Carmustine (BCNU)	IV	Fever and chills, nausea and vomiting, pulmonary toxicity, vision changes	This drug is an irritant. The patient may have pain at the injection site from the drug. Nadir occurs in 3–5 weeks. Monitor labs prior to each dose. Monitor respiratory status.
	Cisplatin (Platinol)	IV	Ototoxicity, fever and chills, tinnitus, nausea and vomiting	Monitor neurological status, renal function studies. Premedicate with antiemetics. Monitor for signs of anaphylaxis. Nadir occurs in 2–3 weeks; monitor CBC prior to each dose.
	Cyclophosphamide (Cytoxan)	IV, PO	Nausea and vomiting, hematuria, alopecia, bone marrow depression	Monitor CBC prior to each dose. Monitor BUN and creatinine. Teach the patient to drink at least 3 L of fluid a day and to void every 2 hours. This drug requires hydration prior to and after drug is given. Oral form should be taken early in the morning so that the drug does not build up in the bladder during the night.
	Ifosfamide (Ifex)	IV	CNS toxicity, nausea, vomiting, hemorrhagic cystitis, alopecia	Monitor urine for blood. This drug requires hydration before and after each dose. Premedicate with antiemetics. Monitor CBC.

Medication Class/Action	Examples	Route	Side Effects	Nursing Implications
Antimitotic Agents Come from plant sources. Prevent mitosis from occurring in the cell and then cells cannot divide.	Docetaxel (Taxotere)	IV	Fatigue, edema, nausea and vomiting, stomatitis, anemia, thrombocytopenia, myalgia, alopecia, hypersensitivity, anaphylaxis, bone marrow depression, neuropathy	Patient must take dexamethasone starting 1 day prior to the scheduled chemotherapy to prevent hypersensitivity. Monitor CBC. Nadir occurs on day 7. Monitor weight. Monitor skin for changes. Monitor for changes in neurological status from baseline.
	Paclitaxel (Taxol)	IV	Nausea, vomiting, myalgia, cardiac toxicities, hypersensitivity or anaphylaxis, neuropathy, alopecia, stomatitis, hypotension	Premedicate with antiememtic and dexamethasone. Monitor for signs of hypersensitivity. Monitor CBC and platelet counts. Monitor neurological status for changes from baseline. Teach the patient about mouth care. Monitor vital signs for changes.
	Vincristine (Oncovin)	IV	Constipation, difficulty walking, tingling in fingers and toes	This drug is a vesicant and should be given through a running IV. Assess for neuropathies or changes in neurological status from baseline. Monitor CBC, platelets.
	Vinorelbine (Navelbine)	IV	Fatigue, constipation, nausea, alopecia, bone marrow suppression, neuropathy, nausea, vomiting, stomatitis	This drug is a vesicant. When giving through a running IV, use the port closest to the IV bag rather than the patient. Monitor CBC prior to each dose. Nadir occurs in 7–10 days. Teach patient signs of infection and bleeding. Monitor neurological status and changes from baseline. Teach the patient about mouth care.
Topoisomerase Inhibitors Inhibit topoisomerase (the enzyme needed for DNA to copy) and cause cell death.	Etoposide (VP-16)	IV	Nausea and vomiting, alopecia, numbness and tingling in fingers and toes, bone marrow depression	Premedicate for nausea. Nadir occurs in 10–14 days; monitor CBC prior to each cycle. Monitor neurological status and changes from baseline.
	Irinotecan (Camptosar)	IV	Dizziness, headache, insomnia, dyspnea, edema, nausea, vomiting, diarrhea, stomatitis, alopecia, bone marrow suppression, weight loss	Teach measures to control diarrhea and to notify MD if it occurs. Monitor CBC prior to each dose.
	Topotecan (Hycamtin)	IV	Headache, dyspnea, nausea, vomiting, diarrhea, hair loss, bone marrow suppression	Monitor CBC. Premedicate for nausea.
Hormones	Tamoxifen (Nolvadex)	PO	Hot flashes, weight gain, nausea, bone pain	Anticoagulants increase the PT. Instruct the patient not to take antacids within 2 hours of taking tamoxifen. May cause bony pain but the discomfort is temporary.
Miscellaneous Agents Work by interfering with enzyme systems or metabolic pathways in the cells	Hydroxyurea (Hydrea)	PO	Fever and chills, sore throat, drowsiness, diarrhea, nausea and vomiting	Monitor WBC. Monitor metabolic panel for signs of tumor lysis syndrome. Monitor neurological status and changes from baseline.
	Procarbazine (Matulane)	PO	Bone marrow depression, MAO inhibitor, drowsiness, nausea and vomiting, peripheral neuropathy	Monitor CBC prior to each cycle. Premedicate as needed for nausea. Monitor neurological status and changes from baseline.
	Thalidomide (Thalomid)	PO	Birth defects, peripheral neuropathy, drowsiness, rash, constipation, **neutropenia**	Pregnancy test done before beginning therapy. CONTRAINDICATED IN PREGNANCY. Monitor neurological status and changes from baseline. Teach patient to report any rash to MD. Instruct about measures to prevent constipation. Monitor CBC throughout therapy.

CBC = complete blood count; CNS = Central nervous system; GI = gastrointestinal; IM = intramuscular;
IV = intravenous; MAO = monoamine oxidase inhibitor; PT = prothrombin time.

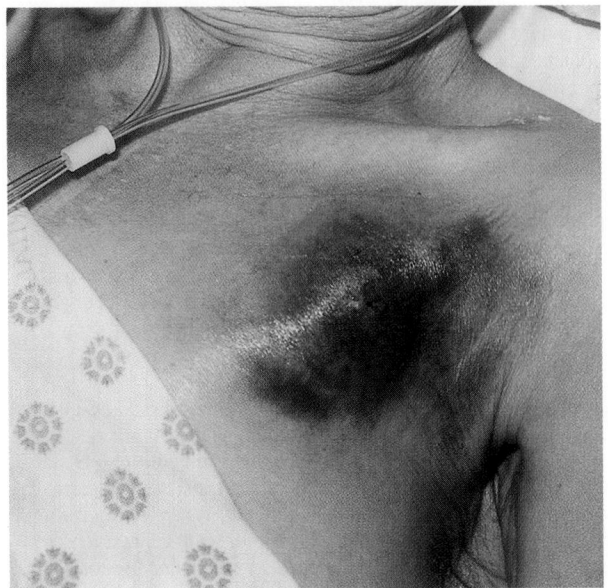

FIGURE 10.12 Necrosis of skin tissue resulting from administration of a vesicant chemotherapy drug. *(Photo courtesy Dinesh Patel, MD. Medical Oncology, Internal Medicine, Zanesville, OH.)*

of **anemia** occurs with the reduction of red blood cells and may require blood transfusions. See Table 10.5 for medications that can be used to stimulate production of these cells.

Gastrointestinal System. The gastrointestinal tract is susceptible to the toxicity of chemotherapy drugs. Patients often become nauseated and vomit or experience diarrhea. **Stomatitis** is a common complaint and is discussed under side effects of radiation. These side effects can be controlled with medication.

Hair. **Alopecia**, or hair loss, is common with many (but not all) chemotherapeutic drugs. This is a temporary condition, and growth of the new hair usually starts when the chemotherapeutic medication is stopped. Alopecia involves the entire body and includes eyebrows, eyelashes, and axillary and pubic hair. Hair regrowth may be of different color or texture than the original hair. It is not uncommon for individuals who originally had straight hair to regrow curly hair.

Reproductive System. The effects of chemotherapy or radiation can cause temporary or permanent alterations of the reproductive system. Occasionally, patients are rendered sterile because of the treatment. Issues concerning fertility should be discussed with the patient before treatment. Measures such as freezing ova and the use of sperm banks provide options for the patient and his or her partner.

Neurological System. Drugs may affect the neurological system. An adverse reaction to vincristine is neurotoxicity, which may result in tingling or numbness in the extremities and in severe cases may cause footdrop from muscle weakness.

---

anemia: an—not + emia—blood
stomatitis: stoma—mouth + itis—inflammation

Less common complications include renal toxicities, such as pain and burning on urination, and hematuria. Doxorubicin (Adriamycin) has been associated with permanent heart damage, and bleomycin can cause pulmonary fibrosis.

Severe toxic side effects can be controlled by carefully limiting the amount of medication given and constantly monitoring the patient for complications.

New Treatments Being Researched

New therapies for cancer are constantly being researched. Hyperthermia has been used with radiation and chemotherapy. It has been beneficial in some types of cancer but is seldom used except in investigational studies.

Biological response modifiers (such as interferons) are drugs used to stimulate the immune system. These drugs are used commonly for specific types of cancer and have produced some beneficial results. They are also being used in many investigational studies. Go to www.cancer.gov for information on current clinical trials.

NURSING PROCESS FOR THE PATIENT WITH CANCER

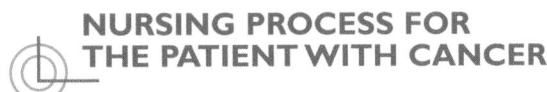

Assessment/Data Collection

Patients with cancer are assessed for many different problems associated with cancer and its treatment. Thorough assessment will assist the health team to build a plan of care relevant to the patient's needs.

Monitor laboratory studies. The normal platelet level is 150,000 to 300,000/mm³. Potential for bleeding exists when the platelet count is 50,000; risk for spontaneous bleeding occurs when the count is less than 20,000. Monitor the white blood cell count for risk for infection and the red cell count for anemia.

Monitor the patient's weight and note complaints of nausea, changes in taste, vomiting, and diarrhea related to either the disease or treatment. Monitor oral mucosa for lesions or inflammation. Also monitor for signs of dehydration. Box 10.6 (Nutrition Notes) presents criteria for determining whether a patient needs nutritional support.

Psychosocial issues related to cancer are as varied as the persons afflicted with the disease. You can help the patient explore perceptions about quality of life. Culture and age affect cancer perceptions (e.g., in a culture in which life expectancy is short, possible death from cancer in the later years is not a significant threat). Assess the patient's ability to cope and what coping strategies have been effective in the past. Determine what information the patient has received and understands about his or her disease and prognosis.

Assess the roles of the patient and caregiver in the family. Be aware of whether the caregiver is able to be at home or whether he or she must work outside the home and care for the patient. Isolation can be either self-imposed or imposed by friends and family, as terminal illness issues are confronted. It can be very frustrating to see a loved one decline with cancer; often people say they are "afraid of say-

TABLE 10.5 COLONY-STIMULATING FACTORS

Medication Class/Action	Examples	Route	Side Effects	Nursing Implications
Granulocyte Colony-Stimulating Factor (G-CSF) Stimulates proliferation of stem cells into granulocytes (neutrophils).	Filgrastim (Neupogen) Pegfilgrastim (Neulasta)	IV, SC	Bone pain	Monitor CBC. Teach self- administration of SC medication if to be given at home.
Granulocyte-Macrophage Colony-Stimulating Factor (GM-CSF) Stimulates proliferation of stem cells into neutrophils, monocytes, macrophages, and eosinophils.	Sargramostim (Leukine)	IV, SC	Headache, itching, rash, bone or joint pain, muscle ache, dyspnea	Monitor vital signs and respiratory status during IV infusion. Monitor CBC. Teach self- administration of SC medication if to be given at home.
Erythropoietin Stimulates proliferation of stem cells into red blood cells.	Epoetin alfa (Epogen, Procrit)	IV, SC	Hypertension, seizure	Monitor blood pressure and hematocrit. Teach self-administration of SC medication if to be given at home.
Interleukin-11 Stimulates production of platelets.	Oprelvekin (Neumega)	SC	Dizziness, weakness, conjunctival hemorrhage, dyspnea, cough, pleural effusion, dysrhythmia, edema, syncope, anorexia, constipation, diarrhea, vomiting, alopecia, rash, bone and muscle pain, chills, fever, infection, pain	Monitor for fluid retention. Monitor CBC, platelet count. Teach self- administration of SC medication if to be given at home.

ing or doing the wrong thing" so they "just stay away." Listen for cues from patients expressing self-blame, anger, or depression. It is important to recognize signs of depression and suicidal tendencies.

Assess for fatigue and anxiety in the patient being treated for cancer. A decline in sexual desire is not uncommon during cancer treatment. Assess for anxiety about sexual intercourse, including fears concerning contracting cancer from the patient and fears that sexual intercourse will make the cancer worse.

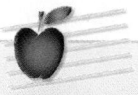

Box 10.6

Nutrition Notes

Assessing the Need for Nutritional Support

Intensive nutritional support may not benefit all cancer patients because the tumor interferes with the patient's utilization of nutrients. Clinical judgment is required to analyze the patient's needs and expected response. In general, if any of the following findings are present, you should talk with the dietitian or physician about the need for nutritional support.
- Weight 5 kg (11 lb) below a healthy body weight
- Serum albumin less than 3 g/dL
- Location of cancer (head and neck, gastrointestinal system)

Assess the patient's feelings about any actual or perceived change in appearance due to surgery, radiation, or chemotherapy.

Nursing Diagnosis, Planning, and Implementation

See Box 10.7 Nursing Care Plan for the Patient with Cancer for top nursing care priorities. Additional nursing diagnoses are presented below. Also see Box 10.8 Cancer Survivor's Bill of Rights.

Ineffective protection related to thrombocytopenia associated with chemotherapy and radiation

EXPECTED OUTCOME: The patient will be free of bleeding.
- Monitor platelet counts. *Platelet count of <50,000 indicates potential for bleeding*
- Teach self-administration of oprelvekin (Neumega) as ordered. *Oprelvekin stimulates production of platelets.*
- Test all urine and stool for occult blood *to detect the presence of blood.*
- Avoid giving intramuscular, subcutaneous, or rectal medications. *Medications given via invasive routes can cause bleeding.*
- Apply pressure for at least 5 minutes to venipuncture or injection sites. *Pressure for a longer time*

(Text continued on page 166)

Box 10.7 NURSING CARE PLAN for the Patient with Cancer

Nursing Diagnosis: Risk For Ineffective Coping Related to the Diagnosis and Treatment of Cancer as Evidenced by Behaviors Such as Denial, Isolation, Anxiety, and Depression

Expected Outcomes Patient will cope effectively as evidenced by identifying stressors related to illness and treatment; communicating needs, concerns, and fears; and use of appropriate resources to support coping.

Evaluation of Outcomes Is patient able to identify stressors and communicate concerns? Does patient effectively draw upon past coping mechanism? Does patient have and appropriately use support systems?

Interventions	Rationale	Evaluation
Assess effective coping mechanisms used in the past and currently available to the patient.	Coping mechanisms that worked in the past may be helpful again, and the nurse can support appropriate choices.	Is the patient able to identify and draw on past coping mechanisms?
Use active listening skills to encourage the patient to express feelings and fears.	The patient must identify fears to be able to cope effectively with them.	Does the patient identify fears and concerns?
Assess the meaning of quality of life to the patient.	Once identified, the nurse can assist the patient to achieve quality-of-life goals.	Is the patient able to identify the meaning of quality of life? Are there ways the nurse can assist the patient to reach quality-of-life goals?
Assess for suicide risks.	A patient who feels hopeless may be at risk for suicide.	Is the patient at risk? Are suicide precautions necessary?
Explore outlets that promote feelings of personal achievement.	Personal achievement promotes self-esteem.	Does the patient have creative outlets that promote feelings of achievement? Can the nurse assist in implementing these activities?
Promote the use of humor.	Humor can be both distracting and therapeutic.	Does the patient use humor? Does it provide temporary distraction from concerns?

Nursing Diagnosis: Pain Related to Tissue Injury from Disease Process and Treatment

Expected Outcomes Patient will be pain free as evidenced by patient statement of comfort on pain scale.

Evaluation of Outcome Does patient state pain is controlled?

Interventions	Rationale	Evaluation
Assess the patient's pain including onset, location, duration, character, and aggravating and alleviating factors.	Assessment provides direction for the treatment plan.	Is assessment complete and used to guide treatment?
Ask patient to rate pain on a scale from 0 to 10 (0 = absence of pain; 10 = worst pain).	A pain rating should guide treatment and evaluate effectiveness of treatment.	Does patient use pain assessment scale effectively? Is patient in pain?
Monitor pain relief every 2 to 4 hours.	Alternative medications may be necessary for breakthrough pain.	Is PCA or epidural analgesic effective?
Administer analgesics as ordered, ATC.	Using an ATC schedule prevents pain from becoming severe.	Is patient's pain kept under control at all times?
Educate patient on use of PCA.	PCA allows the patient to be in control of own pain relief.	Does PCA keep patient pain free and able to participate in desired activities?

Interventions	Rationale	Evaluation
Monitor level of sedation and respiratory status if opioid dose is increased.	Patients who receive long-term opioid therapy develop a tolerance to the depressant effects of opioids.	Is patient alert with respiratory rate between 12 and 20?
Explain and encourage use of relaxation techniques and other complementary techniques.	Relaxation techniques can reduce pain intensity by reducing skeletal muscle tension.	Does patient use relaxation techniques effectively?
Use nonpharmacological interventions once the pain is controlled with medications.	Nonpharmacological interventions supplement but do not replace analgesics.	Does patient use non-pharmacological interventions? Do they help?

Nursing Diagnosis: Risk for infection related to diminished immunity and bone marrow suppression as a result of chemotherapy or radiation

Expected Outcomes The patient will be free and safe from infection as evidenced by being afebrile and stating self-care measures to protect from infection. Signs and symptoms of infection are identified and treated early.

Evaluation of Outcome Are signs and symptoms of infection absent? If present, are they reported quickly? Can the patient identify self—care measures for preventing infection?

Interventions	Rationale	Evaluation
Monitor body temperature every 4 hours.	Elevated body temperature is an early sign of infection.	What is the patient's temperature?
Monitor white blood cell count daily.	For the neutropenic patient, the WBC will not be elevated. Neutropenia is risk factor for infection.	Is the white cell count 5000 to 10,000/mm^3?
Assess for signs of inflammation or drainage at potential infection sites such as old aspirate sites, venipuncture sites, oral and rectal mucosae, perineal area, axillae, incisions, pierced earlobes, under breasts, and between toes.	Intact skin is the first line of defense against invading microorganisms.	Are there any sites that need special care to maintain skin integrity?
Monitor for signs of respiratory infection such as sore throat, cough, shortness of breath, and sputum production.	Nosocomial pneumonia has a high mortality and morbidity rate.	Are signs of respiratory infection present?
Monitor for signs of urinary tract infection including burning, pain, urgency, blood in urine.	GU tract is the most common site for nosocomial infection.	Are signs of urinary tract infection present?
Teach administration of G-CSF or GM-CSF as ordered.	These medications help the body produce more white blood cells. The patient may need to administer it subcutaneously at home.	Does patient demonstrate correct self-administration? Is white count improving?
Use good hand washing technique before interaction with the patient.	Appropriate hand hygiene can reduce the transmission of antimicrobial organisms.	Are you careful with your hand washing? Have you also instructed the patient, family, and nursing assistants about careful hand washing?
Limit visitors to only healthy adults.	Viral infection in an immunosuppressed patient has a high mortality rate.	Are the patient and family aware of visiting restrictions and rationale? Is there a sign on the door reminding visitors?
Keep fresh flowers and potted plants out of the patient's room.	Aspergillus is a fungus found in soil and water and can cause pneumonia.	Is the room free from potential sources of infection?

ATC = around the clock; G-CSF = granulocyte colony-stimulating factor; GM-CSF = granulocyte macrophage colony-stimulating factor; GU = genitourinary; PCA = patient-controlled analgesia.

Box 10.8

Cancer Survivor's Bill of Rights

The American Cancer Society promotes the following Survivor's Bill of Rights to promote cancer care.

1. Survivors have the right to assurance of lifelong medical care, as needed. the physicians and other professionals involved in their care should continue their constant efforts to be:
   * sensitive to the cancer survivor's lifestyle choices and need for self-esteem and dignity;
   * careful, no matter how long their patients have survived, to take symptoms seriously, and not dismiss aches and pains, for fear of recurrence is a normal part of survivorship;
   * informative and open, providing survivors with as much or as little candid medical information as they wish, and encouraging their informed participation in their own care;
   * knowledgeable about counseling resources, and willing to refer survivors and their families as appropriate for emotional support and therapy, which will improve the quality of individual lives.

2. Survivors will have the right to the pursuit of happiness. This means they have the right:
   * to talk with their families and friends about their cancer experience if they wish, but to refuse to discuss if that is their choice and not to be expected to be more upbeat or less blue than anyone else;

   * to be free of the stigma of cancer as a "dread disease" in all social relations;
   * to be free of blame for having gotten the disease and of guilt for having survived it.

3. In the workplace, survivors have the right to equal job opportunities. They have the right:
   * to apply for jobs worthy of their skills, and for which they are trained and experienced;
   * to be hired, promoted, and accepted on return to work, according to their individual abilities and qualifications, and not according to "cancer" or "disability" stereotypes;
   * to privacy about their medical histories.

4. Every effort should be made to assure all survivors adequate health insurance, whether public or private. This includes:
   * survivors have the right to be included in group coverage at the place of employment;
   * physicians, counselors, and other professionals must keep themselves and survivors informed and up to date on available group or individual health policy options;
   * social policy makers, both in government and in the private sector, must seek to broaden insurance programs like Medicare to include diagnostic procedures and treatment to help prevent recurrence and lessen survivor anxiety.

Source: From Cancer Survivor's Bill of Rights, American Cancer Society.

is needed at sites of invasive procedures to stop bleeding.
* Teach the patient about gentle mouth care including no flossing, a soft toothbrush, and wearing properly fitting dentures *to help prevent trauma and bleeding.*
* Avoid trauma to rectal tissue by avoiding rectal temperatures and enemas. Teach importance of avoiding anal intercourse. *Trauma to rectal tissue can cause bleeding to occur.*
* Instruct the patient not to take any salicylates or nonsteroidal anti-inflammatory medications *because they can interfere with platelet functions and cause bleeding in the GI tract.*
* Observe for bruising, petechiae, bleeding gums, tarry stools, and black emesis. *These are signs of bleeding.*
* Advise the patient to use an electric razor *to decrease trauma that could result in bleeding.*
* Teach the patient to avoid blowing his or her nose or inserting objects into the nose *to reduce trauma to nasal mucosa to prevent spontaneous bleeding.*

* Teach the patient to avoid intercourse for the duration of the thrombocytopenia *to decrease the probability of bleeding after intercourse.*

Nutrition, imbalanced: less than body requirements related to anorexia, nausea, or vomiting associated with disease, pain, and treatment

EXPECTED OUTCOME: The patient will have adequate caloric intake adequate to meet body requirements and balanced intake and output, as evidenced by stable weight and albumin ≥ 3g/dL.

* Monitor food and fluid intake and output every 8 hours. *This will provide objective data for the amount of nutrients and fluids taken in.*
* Weigh the patient daily. *Weight is an objective measurement to determine if intake is adequate enough to maintain weight.*
* Consult a dietitian for dietary supplements. *Dietitians can calculate the calories needed for adequate nutrition and make recommendations for supplements.*
* Consult with the physician for medications to con-

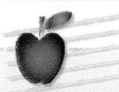

Box 10.9

Nutrition Notes

Treating Problems Related to Nutrition

Try these ideas if a cancer patient has problems with eating.

Early Satiety and Anorexia

- Select nutrient-dense foods. For example, fortify puddings and milkshakes with dry skim milk powder.
- Encourage appropriate exercise.
- Present food attractively.
- Remove covers from food containers away from the bedside if strong odors annoy the patient.
- Offer small, frequent meals.
- Encourage family to provide home-cooked food.
- If meals are rejected, offer 1 oz of a complete nutritional supplement every hour.

Bitter or Metallic Taste

- Cook in glass containers in a microwave oven.
- Serve food cold or at room temperature.
- See if the patient prefers eggs, fish, poultry, and dairy products to beef and pork.
- Experiment with sauces and seasonings. Sweet sauces and marinades may improve the palatability of meats.

Local Oral Effects

- Ulcerations—Offer soft, mild foods; cream sauces, gravies, and dressings for lubrication; cold foods for numbing; and straws for liquids. Avoid hot items, salty or spicy foods, and acidic juices. If an anesthetic mouthwash is prescribed, caution the patient to chew carefully to avoid biting the lips, tongue, or cheeks.
- Dry mouth—Offer frequent sips of water or artificial saliva. Lubricate with gravies, butter, margarine, milk, cream, or bouillon. Sugarless hard candy, chewing gum, or popsicles may stimulate saliva production.

- Dysphagia—Teach the patient to make swallowing a conscious act (inhale, swallow, exhale) and to experiment with head position. Offer foods with a smooth, even consistency. Thick liquids are easier to swallow than thin. Encourage dunking breads in a beverage to soften.

Nausea and Vomiting

- Administer antiemetics on a regular prophylactic schedule.
- Suggest dry crackers.
- Offer liquids between instead of with meals to reduce stomach volume and low-fat meals to facilitate stomach emptying.
- Instruct the patient to chew thoroughly, eat slowly, and rest afterward.
- Arrange meal schedule to take advantage of times when patient feels better.
- Avoid serving favorite foods when the patient is nauseous to avoid an association between those foods and vomiting.

Diarrhea

- Suggest a low-residue diet. (Citrotein and Enlive are clear liquid nearly complete nutritional supplements.)
- Try a lactose-free diet for temporary lactose intolerance.
- Propose pectin-containing foods (apples, strawberries, citrus fruits) to absorb water in the bowel.
- Recommend active cultures of yogurt to repopulate intestine.

Altered Immune Response

- Restrict fresh fruits and vegetables that cannot be peeled or adequately disinfected.
- Consider avoiding yogurt to prevent translocation of the bacteria to the bloodstream.

---

trol nausea, vomiting, and diarrhea. *If these symptoms are controlled, then the patient is better able to eat.*
- Keep the environment free of strong odors, such as disinfectants, perfumes, deodorizers, and body wastes. *Strong odors can induce nausea.*
- Provide room-temperature or cold foods and clear liquids. *These foods have fewer odors and may be more comfortable for the patient to eat.*
- Offer sour foods such as hard candy and lemon. *These may help control nausea.*

- Encourage listening to music or doing relaxation exercises. *These may provide distraction from pain and nausea.*
- Add nutmeg to foods. *Nutmeg may help slow down motility of the gastrointestinal tract and decrease the risk of nausea and vomiting.*
- Provide mouth care before meals. *Oral care allows for a better taste in the mouth, and saliva is necessary for digestion of food.*
- Provide small, high-calorie meals. *Smaller, more frequent meals prevent the patient from feeling full and wanting to vomit.*

- Administer pain medication before meals *to help reduce the impact of pain on the appetite.*
- Instruct the patient to avoid fluids with meals *to prevent premature feelings of fullness.*
- Teach the patient to avoid exercise before meals. *If the patient is fatigued, he or she will not have the energy to eat and digest food.*

See Box 10.9 (Nutrition Notes) for additional nutrition interventions.

Deficient self-care related to weakness and fatigue

EXPECTED OUTCOME: The patient will perform self-care activities to optimal potential.

- Assess what self-care activities the patient can do independently (bathing, grooming, feeding, toileting, ambulating). *By assessing what the patient can do independently, you can develop goals and interventions appropriate for this patient.*
- Teach self-administration of epoetin alfa as ordered. *Epoetin alfa stimulates production of red cells and can help fatigue related to anemia.*
- Identify and include the patient's strengths in self-care activities *to help increase the patient's independence.*
- Provide the tools necessary for the patient to assist with his or her own bathing, grooming, feeding, toileting, and ambulation. Physical and occupational therapy departments may be able to help identify assistive devices. *Adaptive and assistive devices can promote independence.*
- Teach the patient about options available for when he or she is no longer able to care for his or her own needs. *Support from other sources will help the patient conserve energy. Planning ahead can help reduce anxiety.*
- Instruct family members in how to assist in daily care. *Allowing family to assist in the daily care will promote their role as caregiver.*
- Consult home health-care or hospice nurses to assist with care needs upon discharge from the acute setting. *Support from these sources will assist the patient to maintain dignity when independence is no longer possible.*

Anticipatory grieving related to potential disease outcome

EXPECTED OUTCOME: The patient will be able to express feelings of guilt, anger, or sorrow and to share anticipated needs related to end-of-life care.

- Use therapeutic communication techniques to ask open-ended questions like, "What are your thoughts and fears?" *This can assist the patient to identify concerns, and also help the nurse to individualize nursing care.*
- Actively listen to the patient's grief. *Being present for the patient and just listening helps the patient communicate needs and fears.*
- Encourage family members to spend time with the patient to make end-of-life decisions. *More people would rather rely on family and friends than physicians to make end-of-life decisions.*
- Ask the patient about end-of-life decisions. Provide information as needed. *Knowing what a dying patient wants will help the nurse to develop the end-of-life care plan.*
- Contact the patient's minister or clergy if the patient agrees. *Religious beliefs can influence the patient's and/or family's grieving process.*
- Help the patient build memories by assisting to write letters, plan his or her funeral, or write an obituary. *These are ways to nurture the patient's relationship with family and to leave a memento behind.*

Caregiver role strain related to patient care and anticipated outcome

EXPECTED OUTCOME: The caregiver will identify resources available to assist in providing care for the patient.

- Observe the caregiver's ability to provide care for the patient. *The nurse needs to know if the caregiver will be able to handle the care needs.*
- Assist the caregiver to identify supports available to them. *Assistance to the caregiver can provide a break and decrease the risk of depression in the caregiver.*
- Instruct the caregiver in the resources available in the community. *Support groups can help the caregiver by providing an outlet for sharing their concerns and providing support.*
- Consult the multidisciplinary team to provide the services needed at time of discharge. *Preparing the caregiver for discharge needs/care with the proper resources will help the caregiver feel empowered to deliver the care.*

EXPECTED OUTCOME: Caregivers will maintain their physical and psychological health.

- Observe for signs of depression in the caregiver and intervene to help them cope. *The caregiver can develop a weakened immune system secondary to stress and depression.*
- Arrange for respite for the caregiver or encourage the caregiver to utilize this service. *Respite care can provide a break for the caregiver if they are willing to try it.*
- Encourage the caregiver to grieve over the patient. *Caregivers will grieve for the loved one's loss of function or role in the family.*

- Assist the caregiver with ways to decrease stress. *Encouraging caregivers to take the time to care for themselves will leave them with the energy they need to continue providing the care.*
- Actively listen to the caregiver's concerns. *Listening to the concerns of the caregiver can assist the nurse in assessing how well the caregiver is able to cope, and help in planning care.*

Social isolation related to changing relationships

EXPECTED OUTCOME: The patient will be able to identify feelings of isolation.

- Observe the patient for signs of barriers to social interaction such as incontinence, and lack of transportation, money, or support system. *Why a patient feels isolated can vary from one person to another but knowing the reason can help the nurse plan appropriate interventions.*
- Discuss causes of perceived or actual isolation. *How the patient is dealing with the illness will have an impact on how he or she manages the illness.*
- Listen to the patient describe reasons for isolation. *Listening and being present are ways to show caring.*

EXPECTED OUTCOME: The patient will be able to participate in chosen activities.

- Promote opportunities for the patient to interact socially such as mealtimes or therapy sessions. *The patient will feel less isolated if given an opportunity to participate in diversional activities.*
- Provide positive reinforcement to the patient when he or she initiates conversation with others. *Positive feedback by the nurse can impact the patient's sense of confidence.*
- Provide information about support groups and encourage the patient to contact these individuals. *Support groups can help the patient cope better with stressful events in their life.*

Ineffective sexuality pattern related to change in body functions

EXPECTED OUTCOME: The patient will have knowledge about limitations or changes in sexual activity during cancer treatment.

- Provide a private environment so that the patient feels comfortable discussing issues of sexuality. *Privacy is necessary so that there is a comfort level for the patient to express concerns.*
- Assess what the patient understands about sexuality during cancer treatment. *This discussion can clear up any misinformation the patient and partner may have regarding sexuality during therapy.*
- Encourage the patient to discuss concerns about

sexuality with his or her partner. *Communication is a key component of emotional intimacy.*
- Stress to the patient that cancer cannot be passed from person to person through sexual intimacy. *Cancer is not contagious.*
- Instruct the patient that sexual activity is usually safe during and after cancer treatment. *Sexual activity does not necessarily hurt the patient.*
- Advise the patient to abstain from sexual intercourse while his or her blood count is low to prevent the risk of secondary infections and bleeding. *A low WBC can put the patient at risk for infection. A low platelet count can put the patient at risk for bleeding.*
- Discuss with the patient that closeness and intimacy may still be desired even if sexual intercourse is not. *Closeness and touching are ways to be intimate without intercourse.*
- Instruct the patient and partner that pain during intercourse can be related to surgery or treatment and to take pain medication prior to sexual intercourse. *Pain medication prior to intercourse can make the patient more comfortable.*

Disturbed body image related to cancer and its treatment (e.g., surgical procedures such as an ostomy or loss of hair associated with chemotherapy)

EXPECTED OUTCOME: The patient will be able to accept the changes in body image resulting from cancer and its treatment.

- Allow the patient to discuss feelings of anger or depression and confirm that these feelings are normal when adjusting to body changes. *A patient may be better able to cope with body changes if he or she can talk about feelings and understand that the feelings are normal.*
- Encourage the patient to select a wig prior to hair loss. *Selecting a wig before the hair loss occurs allows the patient to find one resembling his or her own hair color and style.*
- Encourage the patient to provide own care to ostomy site or surgical wound when ready. *Encouragement and education about self-care will promote independence.*
- Provide resources such as Reach to Recovery (www.cancer.org, type in Reach to Recovery) and Look Good . . . Feel Better support groups (www.lookgoodfeelbetter.org/). *Support groups provide a forum for patients to share their experiences with others experiencing the same types of changes.*
- Provide information about community assistance/financial aid for programs or services. *Social workers can assist with community resources that can provide equipment or supplies for the patient.*

Evaluation

If the interventions have been effective, the patient does not experience any unusual bleeding or bruising. The patient and family are knowledgeable about risk factors associated with bleeding and about signs of bleeding to report promptly.

The patient is nourished and maintains weight within his or her normal limits. The patient maximizes his potential for self-care activities. The patient and caregiver have knowledge of available resources to assist with self-care activities in the home setting. Caregivers have the knowledge to be able to provide care for the patient. The patient is able to openly discuss feelings, and is able to spend time with family and loved ones to resolve any issues.

If interventions have been effective, the caregiver is able to utilize resources in the community to assist with the care of the patient, and maintain her or his own physical and psychological health while caring for the patient. The patient is able to discuss feelings of isolation and seek out activities to participate in. The patient maintains a healthy sexuality and is able to discuss feelings openly and honestly with her or his partner.

The patient is able to openly discuss concerns regarding body changes and is able to maintain control of his or her body. The patient has knowledge of community resources and support groups to assist with needs related to body image.

CRITICAL THINKING

Mrs. Jones

■ Mrs. Jones is admitted to your unit following a simple mastectomy for breast cancer. The tumor was staged as a T2, N0, M0. Estrogen and progesterone receptors were negative. A bone scan was negative for metastasis. She is scheduled for four chemotherapy treatments, 3 weeks apart. The medications prescribed are high doses of doxorubicin (Adriamycin) and cyclophosphamide (Cytoxan). A central line is inserted for chemotherapy.

1. What does the staging of Mrs. Jones's tumor mean?
2. What major side effects of her medications should you look for?
3. Why was a central line inserted?
4. What nursing diagnoses are appropriate for Mrs. Jones?

Suggested answers at end of chapter.

HOSPICE CARE OF THE PATIENT WITH CANCER

Patients who are considered terminal and have a life expectancy of 6 months or less are eligible for hospice care, which provides humanistic care for dying people and their families. The dying person is provided care in a home or homelike setting that promotes comfort and quality of life until death. Hospice care is offered as an inpatient or outpatient service (see Home Health Hints at the end of the chapter).

Inpatient services are used for symptom control and respite care for the family. Family and pets may be allowed to stay with the patient. Hospice care deals with the family in crisis and continues for up to 1 year after the patient dies, with follow-up counseling, listening, nurturing, and referrals.

Outpatient care is given in the home with family members providing the primary care. Support care is given by the hospice staff. Medications and supplies are furnished by the hospice service. At home, the patient can enjoy loved ones, pets, plants, music, and other personal possessions for as long as possible. See Chapter 16 Nursing Care of Patients at the End of Life for more information.

ONCOLOGICAL EMERGENCIES

Superior Vena Cava Syndrome

Superior vena cava syndrome (SVCS) occurs in patients with lung cancer when the tumor or enlarged lymph nodes block the circulation in the vena cava. This results in edema of the head and neck and may lead to seizures. Radiation therapy can be used to shrink the tumor and allow for circulation to resume naturally. Nursing interventions for the patient with SVCS include removing rings and restrictive clothing, avoiding taking blood pressure and venipunctures in the upper extremities, and elevating the head of the bed to decrease feeling of dyspnea.

Spinal Cord Compression

Spinal cord compression may develop in patients with bone metastasis when the bones collapse. This is a very painful problem and requires pain management while radiation is given to relieve the symptoms. Patients may develop some motor loss when this occurs. Often a myelogram or bone scan is used for diagnosis. Nursing care includes providing a safe environment, assistance with activity, and monitoring for changes in neurological status.

Hypercalcemia

Hypercalcemia occurs when the serum calcium level exceeds 11 mg/dL. Hypercalcemia is associated with the release of calcium into the blood from bone deterioration, or from ectopic secretion of parathyroid hormone by a tumor. It is common in patients with bone metastasis, especially metastasis from breast cancer. It can be treated with intravenous medication and hydration to lower the calcium levels. Nursing care includes monitoring intake and output, pain control, and changes in pulse rate and rhythm.

Pericardial Effusion/Cardiac Tamponade

Pericardial effusion, or cardiac tamponade, is a condition usually caused by direct invasion of the cancer, causing the pericardial sac to fill with fluid. Treatment involves draining the fluid from the heart sac by pericardiocentesis and using sclerosing agents to keep the pericardial sac from refilling with fluid. Nursing care for the patient with cardiac tamponade includes monitoring respiratory status, keeping the head of the bed elevated for maximum lung expansion, monitoring vital signs, monitoring intake and output, and assessing for edema.

Disseminated Intravascular Coagulation

Disseminated intravascular coagulation (DIC) involves an abnormal activation of the clot formation and fibrin mechanisms of the blood, resulting in the consumption of coagulation factors and platelets. Patients with DIC are at high risk for thrombus formation, infarctions, and bleeding. Treatment includes fresh frozen plasma and cryoprecipitates with heparin. Nursing interventions in the care of the patient with DIC include monitoring for bleeding, monitoring vital signs, assessing skin for signs of bleeding, accurate intake and output, and monitoring for changes in mental status.

Home Health Hints

- The home health or hospice nurse helps manage cancer pain in the home. Intramuscular dosing of pain medication should be avoided because of pain associated with injections and the burden this places on the caregiver. Oral or intravenous analgesics are preferred. For moderate to severe pain, medication dosing should be around-the-clock with prn doses for breakthrough pain.
- The nurse should anticipate constipation from opioid administration and treat prophylactically.
- Some patients are fearful about taking prescribed pain medications. Instruct them on the importance of taking the medications as ordered by the physician. It is important for the patient and caregiver to understand that it is easier to maintain pain relief then to try to gain control of and treat severe pain.
- Home health nurses are in key positions for making timely referrals for hospice care. Eligible clients are those who have a life expectancy of 6 months or less, have a desire for supportive care rather than continued treatments, and have a friend or relative who is willing to coordinate the care.

REVIEW QUESTIONS

1. Which of the following is the hereditary material of cells?
   a. Protein in the ribosomes
   b. DNA in the chromosomes
   c. RNA in the nucleus
   d. Ribosomes in the cytoplasm

2. A patient asks, "How do malignant tumors differ from benign tumors?" Which of the following statements by the nurse is most accurate? Select all that apply.
   a. Malignant tumors invade surrounding cells and tissues.
   b. Malignant tumors are generally encapsulated.
   c. Malignant tumors remain localized.
   d. Cells in malignant tumors stop dividing prematurely.
   e. Cells in malignant tumors lack contact inhibition.
   f. Malignant tumors have defective cell communication.

3. A patient has received vinorelbine (Navelbine) on day 1 of treatment. The nadir will occur in approximately 10 days. The patient is at greatest risk for which of the following complications at day 10?
   a. Infection
   b. Hair loss
   c. Diarrhea
   d. Myalgia

4. A female patient is starting on doxorubicin (Adriamycin). Which of the following nursing interventions will be most helpful as the patient plans for hair loss?
   a. Obtain a prescription for a hair growth product.
   b. Massage her scalp to increase circulation and delay hair loss.
   c. Teach her to apply ice to her scalp to prevent hair loss.
   d. Help her choose a wig before her hair loss begins.

5. Which of the following nursing actions is best before administering pain medication for cancer pain?
   a. Assess the patient's anxiety level.
   b. Assess the patient's understanding of the side effects of pain medication.
   c. Determine the patient's pain tolerance.
   d. Assess the success of past pain management measures.

6. The nurse notes that a patient undergoing treatment for bone cancer is having difficulty walking. For which oncologic emergency should the patient be assessed?
   a. Tumor lysis syndrome
   b. Hypercalcemia
   c. Spinal cord compression
   d. Superior vena cava syndrome

7. A patient receiving radiation therapy has reddened skin over the treated area. How will the nurse know if nursing interventions have been effective?
   a. The patient will be able to describe a proper skin care regimen.
   b. The nurse will keep the skin clean and dry.
   c. The patient's skin will remain intact without breakdown or infection.

d. The nurse will report the reddened area to the physician.

8. Which patient will benefit from hospice care?
   a. A patient who has liver cancer and is expected to live 4 to 6 weeks.
   b. A patient who is having multiple side effects from aggressive chemotherapy.
   c. A patient who is trying to make a decision about whether to have surgery that could cure his cancer but may risk serious loss of function.
   d. A patient who requires large doses of morphine to control pain related to his cancer and radiation treatment.

References

1. American Cancer Society: Cancer Prevention and Early Detection, Facts and Figures 2004. Accessed October 29, 2005 at www.cancer.org
2. American Cancer Society Cancer Detection Guidelines. Accessed July 9, 2005 at http//www.cancer.org/docroot/PED/content/PED_2_3X_ACS_Cancer_Detection_Guidelines_36.asp

Bibliography

1. American Cancer Society. www.cancer.org
2. It's Time to Focus on Lung Cancer. http://www.lungcancer.org/
3. Jemal, A, Murray, T, Ward E, et al: Cancer statistics, 2005. CA Cancer J Clin 55:19–23, 2005.
4. Lehne, R. Pharmacology for Nursing Care, ed. 5. Saunders, Philadelphia, 2004.
5. National Cancer Institute Cancer Information Service. http://cis.nci.nih.gov/

SUGGESTED ANSWERS TO

CRITICAL THINKING

■ *Mrs. Jones*

1. Mrs. Jones's tumor is beginning to invade surrounding tissue. There is no lymph node involvement and no metastasis.
2. Doxorubicin is commonly associated with red urine. Cyclophosphamide can cause blood in the urine. Both medications can cause nausea, vomiting, and alopecia. Both are vesicants.

3. Because the drugs are vesicants, it is important to inject them into a large vein.
4. Many diagnoses are appropriate, including acute pain related to surgical incision, disturbed body image related to alopecia and loss of a breast, imbalanced nutrition related to nausea and vomiting, risk for injury related to medication side effects, and deficient knowledge about cancer treatment and management of side effects.

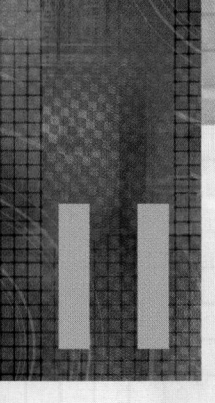

11

Nursing Care of Patients Having Surgery

LINDA S. WILLIAMS

KEY TERMS

adjunct (ADD-junkt)
anesthesia (AN-es-THEE-zee-uh)
anesthesiologist (an-es-THEE-zee-uhl-la-just)
aseptic (ah-SEP-tik)
atelectasis (AT-e-LEK-tah-sis)
debridement (da-breed-MAHNT)
dehiscence (dee-HISS-ents)
evisceration (E-VIS-sir-a-shun)
hematoma (HEE-muh-TOH-mah)
hypothermia (HIGH-poh-THER-mee-ah)
induction (in-DUCK-shun)
intraoperative (IN-trah-AHP-er-uh-tiv)
perioperative (PER-ee-AHP-er-uh-tiv)
postoperative (post-AHP-er-uh-tiv)
preoperative (pre-AHP-er-uh-tiv)
purulent (PURE-u-lent)
serosanguineous (SEER-oh-SANG-gwin-ee-us)
surgeon (SURGE-on)

QUESTIONS TO GUIDE YOUR READING

1. What are factors that influence surgical outcomes?

2. What is your role in each perioperative phase?

3. What is your role in obtaining informed patient consent?

4. How would you enhance learning for the elderly pre-operative patient?

5. What are some nursing interventions for common postoperative patient needs?

6. How will you know if your nursing interventions have been effective?

7. What are signs and symptoms of common postoperative complications?

8. What are the criteria for ambulatory discharge?

9. What is the role of the home health nurse in caring for postoperative patients?

The author acknowledges the contributions to this chapter by Linda Nabozny and Suzanne Fox.

Surgery is the use of instruments during an operation to treat injuries, diseases, and deformities.

Surgical procedures are named according to (1) the involved body organ, part, or location and (2) the suffix that describes what is done during the procedure (Table 11.1).

Physicians who perform surgery include **surgeons** or other physicians trained to do certain surgical procedures. Laser and scope technology continue to lead to new procedures that offer less risk, less invasion, faster recovery, and reduced hospitalization or ambulatory surgery. Robotic surgery is a newer area being explored. Today, surgery is a safe, effective treatment option because of medications such as antibiotics and anesthetics that allow a quicker recovery.

SAFETY TIP

A national partnership, the Surgical Care Improvement Project—A National Quality partnership (SCIP), began in 2005. The SCIP's goal is to improve the safety of surgical care by reducing postoperative complications by 25% by the year 2010. The partnership was developed by the Centers for Medicare & Medicaid Services (CMS) and the Centers for Disease Control and Prevention (CDC), and over 30 other national organizations are part of the partnership.

The four high-incidence and high-cost areas being examined by the SCIP are surgical site infections (SSIs), deep vein thrombosis (DVT), postoperative ventilator-related pneumonia, and adverse cardiac events. Methods for preventing SSIs include giving prophylactic antibiotics within 1 hour prior to surgery and controlling perioperative serum glucose during major cardiac procedures. DVT can be prevented by administering appropriate perioperative anticoagulants for those at risk. Examples of ways to prevent postoperative pneumonia are elevating the head of bed greater than or equal to 30 degrees for major postoperative surgical patients on a ventilator, if not contraindicated. Avoiding adverse cardiac events includes giving beta blockers during the perioperative period to eligible major noncardiac surgical patients and to surgical patients who have coronary artery disease. Look for updates on the committee's work at www.medqic.org/SCIP/

 SURGERY URGENCY LEVELS

Surgery is scheduled based on the urgency required for a successful outcome for the patient (Table 11.2). *Emergency,* or *immediate, surgery* is needed when life or limb is suddenly threatened and any delay in surgery would jeopardize

TABLE 11.1 SURGICAL PROCEDURE SUFFIXES

Suffix	Meaning	Word-Building Examples
-ectomy	Removal by cutting	crani (skull) + ectomy = craniectomy
		appen (appendix) + ectomy = appendectomy
-orrhaphy	Suture of or repair	colo (colon) + orrhaphy = colorrhaphy
		herni (hernia) + orrhaphy = herniorrhaphy
-oscopy	Looking into	colon (intestine) + oscopy = colonoscopy
		gastr (stomach) + oscopy = gastroscopy
-ostomy	Formation of a permanent artificial opening	ureter + ostomy = ureterostomy
		colo (colon) + ostomy = colostomy
-otomy	Incision or cutting into	oust (bone) + otomy = osteotomy
		thoro (thorax) + otomy = thoractomy
-plasty	Formation or repair	oto (ear) + plasty = otoplasty
		mamm (breast) + plasty = mammoplasty

the patient's life or limb. Examples of the need for emergency surgery are ruptured aortic aneurysm, ruptured appendix, traumatic limb amputation, or loss of pulse due to an extremity emboli. *Urgent surgery* is the need for an operation within 24 to 30 hours. Examples of this are fracture repair or an infected gallbladder. *Elective surgery* is that which can be planned and scheduled without any immediate time constraints. Examples of this are joint replacement, hernia repair, or skin lesion removal. *Optional surgery,* such as cosmetic surgery, is done at the request of the patient.

 PURPOSES OF SURGERY

Surgery is done for several reasons (see Table 11.2). *Preventive* surgery removes tissue before it causes a problem as in mole or polyp removal to prevent cancer development. *Diagnostic,* or *exploratory,* surgery takes tissue samples for study to make a diagnosis, uses scopes to look into areas of the body, or involves an incision to open an area of the body for examination. Examples of this surgery are a biopsy or exploratory laparotomy performed with a scope or incision. *Curative* surgery involves the removal of diseased or abnormal tissue as in an inflamed appendix, tumor, or a benign cyst or the repair of defects such as hernias or cleft palate. *Palliative* surgery is done when an underlying condition cannot be corrected but symptoms need to be alleviated. Examples of this are removal of part of a tumor that is causing pain or pressure, a rhizotomy which cuts a nerve root to relieve pain, insertion of a gastrostomy tube (feeding tube

TABLE 11.2 SURGERY URGENCY LEVEL AND PURPOSES

Urgency Level

Type	Definition	Examples
Emergent	Immediate surgery needed to save life or limb	Ruptured aortic aneurysm or appendix, traumatic limb amputation, loss of extremity pulse from emboli
Urgent	Surgery needed within 24–30 hours	Fracture repair, infected gallbladder,
Elective	Planned/scheduled, with no time requirements	Joint replacement, hernia repair, skin lesion removal

Handwritten: "Right away" under Emergent; "Broken hip" next to gallbladder; ", Lipo" next to skin lesion removal

Purposes of Surgery

Aesthetic	Requested by patient for improvement	Blepharoplasty, breast augmentation
Diagnostic	To obtain tissue samples, make an incision, or use a scope to make a diagnosis	Biopsy
Exploratory	Confirmation or measurement of extent of condition	Exploratory laparotomy
Preventive	Removal of tissue before it causes a problem	Mole or polyp removal
Curative	Removal of diseased or abnormal tissue	Inflamed appendix, tumor, benign cyst
Reconstructive	Correction of defects of body parts	Scar repair, total knee replacement
Palliative	Alleviation of symptoms without curing disease	Rhizotomy (cuts nerve root to relieve pain), partial tumor removal to relieve pain or pressure, gastrostomy tube for swallowing problem

inserted into the stomach through the abdominal wall) to provide tube feedings for a patient with swallowing problems, or formation of a colostomy (opening of the colon through the abdominal wall for fecal elimination) for an incurable bowel obstruction. *Cosmetic,* or *reconstructive,* surgery is done to improve appearance as in a face lift or mammoplasty, or to correct defects as in repair of scars.

 ## PERIOPERATIVE PHASES

There are three phases in the surgical process: **preoperative, intraoperative,** and **postoperative.** These phases together are referred to as **perioperative,** which is the time before, during, and after surgery. Each of the perioperative surgical phases has a defined time frame in which specific events related to surgery occur (Table 11.3).

TABLE 11.3 PERIOPERATIVE SURGICAL PHASES

Perioperative	All three phases surrounding and during surgery
Preoperative	Begins with decision for surgery and ends with transfer to the operating room
Intraoperative	Begins with transfer to operating room and ends with admission to postanesthesia care unit (PACU)
Postoperative	Begins with admission to PACU and continues until recovery is complete

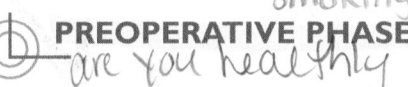

Handwritten: "Smoking effects surgery"

PREOPERATIVE PHASE
Handwritten: "are you healthy"

Your primary roles as a licensed practical nurse/licensed vocational nurse (LPN/LVN) in the preoperative phase are to:

- Assist in data collection for developing the patient's plan of care.
- Reinforce explanations and instructions given to the patient and family by the physician and registered nurse (RN).
- Provide emotional and psychological support for patients and their families.

Families of patients experience anxiety during surgery. You can help reduce the family's anxiety so that they are less anxious and able to assist the patient during recovery.

Other health team members assist in preparing the patient for surgery. The physician obtains a medical history, performs a physical examination, and orders diagnostic testing. Registered nurses perform a baseline preoperative assessment, provide explanations and instructions, offer patients and families emotional and psychological support to ease anxiety, develop a plan of care, and then verify the patient's name, surgical site (along with the patient), allergies, and related information when the patient arrives in the surgical area.

Factors Influencing Surgical Outcomes

When preparing a patient for surgery and assisting in the development of a nursing care plan, the goal is to identify and implement actions that reduce surgical risk factors. Preoperative care focuses on helping the patient achieve the best possible surgical outcome by being in the healthiest possible condition for surgery.

Emotional Responses

The word *surgery* causes a common emotional reaction in patients and their families. You need to be aware of these reactions to assist the patient in coping with them. If any of the patient's fears are extreme, such as a fear of dying or not waking up after surgery, the physician should be informed.

Surgical patients may experience various fears related to **anesthesia:** possible brain damage, feeling sensation during surgery, feeling loss of control, or a fear of not waking up. The patient should discuss these concerns with the

anesthesiologist. Listening to music or using guided imagery before surgery may reduce a patient's anxiety and help to calm the patient.

It is normal for patients to be concerned about pain. During surgery, the anesthesia provider gives medications to control pain. Nurses give prescribed analgesics for pain relief after surgery. Complementary techniques can also be used to help reduce pain, such as guided imagery or focused breathing.

Changes in body image may be a great fear for some patients. The thought of disfigurement, mutilation, bleeding, or having a scar causes great anxiety for some patients. Allow them to discuss these fears.

Age

Surgery can be a positive experience that promotes quality of life for many elderly patients. For healthy older patients, age alone does not mean that they are at greater surgical risk. Complications can occur, however, related to previous health status, immobilization occurring from surgery, normal aging changes reducing the effectiveness of deep breathing and coughing, and the effects of administered medications (Box 11.1 Gerontological Issues). Older patients may require a longer time to recover from anesthetic agents because of aging changes in drug metabolism and elimination.

Hydration and Nutrition

A normal fluid and electrolyte balance decreases complications. Patients should be well nourished to adequately heal and recover from surgery (Box 11.2 Nutrition Notes). Higher levels of protein (tissue repair and healing), vitamin C (collagen formation), and zinc (tissue growth, skin integrity, and cell-mediated immunity) are required. Obese or underweight patients may not heal as well and may have complications.

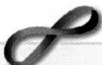

Box 11.1

Gerontological Issues

Surgical Considerations for the Older Adult

Older adults usually have limited physiological reserve, resulting in decreased ability to compensate for changes that occur during surgery. There is increased risk for hemorrhage, anemia, fluid/electrolyte imbalance, and infection. Increased risk for complications is secondary to age-related loss of blood vessel elasticity and decreased cardiac, respiratory, and renal reserves. Nursing interventions should be aimed at these age-related changes before, during, and after the surgical procedure to help reduce complications.

Preoperatively:
* Reassure the patient and family.
* Pad bony prominences to protect against pressure ulcers and muscle and bone discomfort.
* Teach what to expect before, during, and after surgery, diet changes, description and length of surgical procedure, activities in the recovery room, pain management, coughing and deep breathing exercises, procedures, and treatments (e.g., dressings, catheters).
* Ensure preoperative screening: blood work, radiographic studies, nutritional assessments, pulmonary function tests, electrocardiogram.

Intraoperatively:
* Assess patient for hypothermia (cool temperature in operating room, medications that slow metabolism).
* Assess patient for hypoxia (older adult may exhibit restlessness).
* Assess patient for hemorrhage.
* Assess patient's output (urine, drainage, bleeding, emesis).

Postoperatively:

Pain Control—Provide adequate pain relief so required postoperative activities, such as deep breathing, coughing, position changes, and exercise, can be performed more effectively.

Respiratory Function—Reduce respiratory complications by encouraging deep breathing and coughing:
* Do deep breathing and coughing after pain medication has begun to take effect because this will increase the older patient's ability to take deeper breaths. Assess the patient carefully when giving narcotic analgesics because they may cause respiratory depression.
* Use a pillow and instruct the patient to hold it firmly over abdominal or chest incisions to support the incision. Taking a deep breath increases chest expansion, as well as abdominal pressure, which may pull or stretch an incision.
* Older adults perform deep breathing and coughing exercises better if the nurse performs the exercises with them. For example, say the following:
  "Let's take a deep breath in through the nose, hold it and count to three, then slowly blow it out completely through the mouth. When you blow the air out, shape your lips like they are going to whistle. Great, let's do it again."

Mobility—Encourage mobility through the following nursing actions and observations:
* Use pillows to support the patient's body alignment; assist the patient to ambulate as soon as possible after surgery; and regularly help the patient with passive or active range of motion exercises, along with flexion and extension exercises, for legs and feet.
* Monitor for unilateral swelling of the leg and calf or groin pain, which may indicate deep vein thrombosis,

a risk related to venous pooling in the lower extremities. This risk is increased with postoperative inactivity.

• Assist the patient to change position at least every 2 hours. If patients lay in one position too long, pressure ulcers can develop. When tissues are compressed between bones and the bed surface, blood supply is reduced to the tissue and cells begin to die. This results in painful open wounds.

Bowel Function—Assess bowel sounds. It is common for patients to feel bloated after surgery. Increasing activity, such as walking—not just sitting in a chair—stimulates peristaltic action of the bowel. This helps expel flatus and reduce discomfort.

Urinary Function—Be aware of the following aspects of urinary function:

• It is common for individuals to have difficulty emptying their bladder after surgery. Patients who are sleeping but restless should be evaluated for bladder distention. It is often difficult to void on a bed pan or in a urinal in a supine position.

• Older men with an enlarged prostate may have even greater difficulty voiding if they have received medications that have urinary retention side effects.

• Assisting patients to sit or stand to use urinals, use a bedside commode, or ambulate to the bathroom promotes bladder emptying and helps avoid the use of urinary catheters.

• Measure urine output that is voided or from a catheter. Note the color and odor of the urine. Older adults are prone to dehydration, and this provides an indication of their hydration status for intervention.

Delirium—Perform the following nursing actions to minimize delirium:

• Monitor level of consciousness routinely. Provide a calm environment and orient patients to their environment. Restraints should not be used because they can worsen delirium.

• Recognize that urinary catheter presence can contribute to delirium, so methods to avoid the need for a catheter should be tried.

Obese patients have more respiratory problems and wound healing difficulties, such as delayed healing and wound **dehiscence** (opening of the incision). Emaciated individuals may have more infections and delayed wound healing because they lack the nutrients needed for tissue healing.

Smoking and Alcohol

Tobacco and alcohol use increases the surgical patient's risks. Smoking thickens and increases the amount of lung secretions and reduces the action of cilia that remove the secretions. Patients should be encouraged to avoid smoking for 24 hours before surgery or 3 to 4 weeks before surgery if they have a chronic lung disorder. Not smoking increases the action of the lungs' defense mechanisms and makes more hemoglobin available to carry oxygen during surgery. It also improves wound healing. Visit http://www.surgeon-general.gov/tobacco/hospital.htm for more information on smoking cessation.

Long-term alcohol use may cause nutritional deficiencies and liver damage, which can create bleeding problems,

---

Box 11.2

Nutrition Notes

Screening and Nourishing the Preoperative Patient

Mild to severe malnutrition affected 39% of patients undergoing gastrointestinal or orthopedic surgical procedures, but only about two-thirds of them received nutritional support and just 59% of the patients even had a weight recorded on their charts.[1] Patients with low serum albumin levels had more complications and slower recoveries from elective gastrointestinal surgery than patients with higher levels.[2]

Before elective surgery, the patient may have time to correct some nutritional deficiencies. Many patients are instructed to lose weight to reduce the risk of surgery. If they are anemic, an iron preparation can be administered. At least 2 to 3 weeks are required for objective evidence of the effectiveness of nutritional therapy. Before surgery on the gastrointestinal tract, a low-residue diet may be given for 2 to 3 days to minimize the feces in the bowel.

Preoperative fasting times have been reduced in recent years so that in many cases clear liquids may be consumed up to 2 hours before anesthesia, breast milk 4 hours, infant formula or a light meal 6 hours, and a regular meal 8 hours.[3] Clinical judgment is required regardless of the guidelines, which specifically exempt patients with gastromotility or metabolic disorders, those with potential airway problems, and women in labor.

Many botanical products sold in the United States over-the-counter as nutritional supplements profoundly affect body systems during surgery. So many people are taking botanical products that the American Society of Anesthesiologists[4] issued a warning to consumers of herbal medicine to stop taking the products 2 to 3 weeks before scheduled surgery. Possible interactions cited were an unintended deepening of anesthesia and problems with bleeding and blood pressure.

fluid volume imbalances, and drug metabolism alterations. In addition, alcohol interacts with medications and should be avoided before surgery.

Diseases

Chronic disorders may increase the patient's surgical risk unless they are well controlled. A preoperative assessment and clearance for surgery by the patient's physician may be needed. For diabetics, the stress of surgery can alter blood glucose levels. Patients with chronic lung disorders may have pulmonary complications from anesthesia. To help prepare patients with lung disorders for surgery, show them how to deep breathe and cough and use an incentive spirometer (Fig. 11.1).

Preadmission Surgical Patient Assessment

Nonemergent surgical patients have either a preadmission phone call or face-to-face interview with RNs in the preadmission testing (PAT) department. Patients have reduced anxiety and better understanding with prescreening.[5] The interview process includes a health history, identification of risk factors, patient and family teaching, discharge planning, and necessary referrals to social work, support groups, and educational programs. Laboratory tests, electrocardiograms (ECGs), chest x-rays, and other diagnostic testing are done based on the patient's needs. A urine or serum pregnancy test as appropriate for female patients may be done to prevent fetal exposure to anesthetics. Health information and diagnostic testing results are reviewed by anesthesia providers and interventions are ordered for abnormalities. Then a plan of care is developed.

Federal law says patients must be asked before surgery if they have a signed advance directive to place in the medical record. An advance directive (e.g., health-care durable power of attorney or living will) indicates a person's wishes for medical care if they become unable to speak for themselves. If there is no advance directive, written information on advance directives are provided. A health-care power of attorney allows patients to place someone of their own choosing, such as a relative or friend, in control of their medical decisions if they are unable to make them. A living will instructs the physician when to provide, withhold, or withdraw treatment that prolongs life and specifies types of treatment the patient wishes, such as comfort care only.

Preoperative Routines

Preoperative teaching provides information about common surgical preparation procedures and routines:

- Date and time of admission and surgery
- Admission procedures: arrive about 2 hours before surgery to allow preparation time
- Length of stay, items to bring and wear
- Recovery after surgery
- Family information: where to wait during surgery and who communicates patient's status to them
- Discharge criteria: if after outpatient surgery, a responsible adult must take the patient home

PREOPERATIVE INSTRUCTIONS. To reduce the risk of aspiration when anesthesia is started, as well as postoperative nausea and vomiting, the anesthesiologist orders fluid and food restrictions. The patient is told when to stop fluid and food intake (NPO), usually after midnight the night before surgery. If surgery is scheduled for the afternoon, clear liquids in the early morning may be allowed by the anesthesiologist. Patients may brush their teeth or rinse their mouth if no water is swallowed. Cancellation of surgery may result if the patient has not been NPO as ordered.

Any medications the patient is to take the morning of surgery, with an ounce of water, are explained. Special preparations, such as an enema, are also described. For abdominal or intestinal surgery, enemas are ordered to empty the bowel in order to reduce fecal contamination preoperatively and straining or distention postoperatively.

Instructions for postoperative care are given before surgery so the patient is alert when being taught and has time to learn. Patients should be told that active participation in postoperative care aids in their recovery. Teach patients how to report their pain level using a pain rating scale (such as a 0 [none] to 10 [severe] rating scale, a color-based rating scale, or a scale using pictures of faces showing varying degrees of frowning or smiling that indicate a certain pain level) so that prompt pain relief can be provided (see Chapter 9). Pain relief methods are described, such as analgesic injections, an epidural catheter, or patient-controlled analgesia (PCA). Anticipated dressings, tubes, casts, or special equipment, such as a continuous passive motion machine for total knee replacement, are also described. If needed, crutches are fitted to the patient, and their proper use is explained and demonstrated.

Postoperative exercises are taught to decrease complications. They include deep breathing and coughing, use of incentive spirometry, leg exercises, turning, and how to get

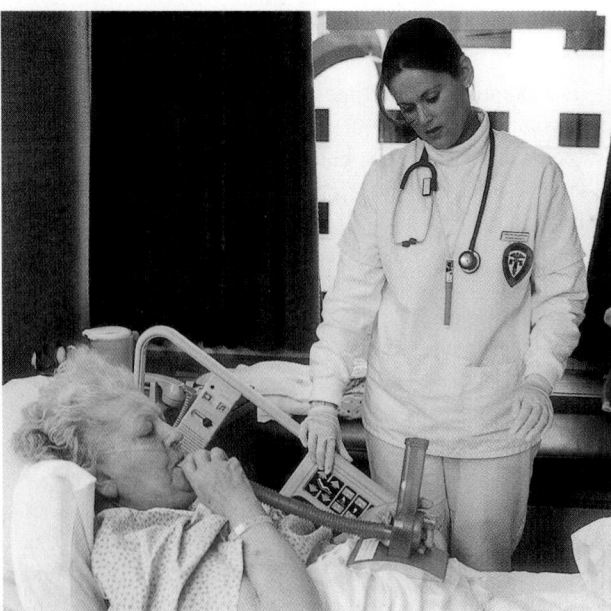

FIGURE 11.1 An incentive spirometer aids lung expansion.

out of bed. After an exercise is taught, the patient should perform a return demonstration so understanding and ability to perform the exercise correctly can be evaluated.

Deep breathing helps prevent the development of **atelectasis** (collapse of the lung caused by hypoventilation or mucous obstruction preventing some alveoli from opening and being fully ventilated) by expanding and ventilating the lungs. The patient is taught to sit up, exhale fully, take in a deep breath through the nose, hold the breath and count to three, and then exhale completely through the mouth. The patient is told to repeat this hourly while awake, in sets of five, for 24 to 48 hours postoperatively.

Incentive spirometry may also be ordered postoperatively to prevent atelectasis by increasing lung volume, alveoli expansion, and venous return. (see Fig. 11.1). Any patient can benefit from incentive spirometry, especially the elderly and those at increased risk for developing lung complications. The spirometer stays at the patient's bedside for hourly use while awake. Offer the spirometer to the patient each hour to ensure that it is used. Teach patients to do the following:

- Sit upright, at 45 degrees minimum, if possible.
- Take two normal breaths. Place mouthpiece of spirometer in mouth.
- Inhale until target, designated by spirometer light or rising ball, is reached, and hold breath for 3 to 5 seconds.
- Exhale completely.
- Perform 10 sets of breaths each hour.

Coughing moves secretions to prevent pneumonia. Teach patients how to cough effectively (Table 11.4). Give pain medication before coughing and offer reassurance that coughing should not harm the incision. Several sets of coughing are performed, if not contraindicated by the patient's condition (such as hernia repair or head injury), every 1 to 2 hours while the patient is awake.

Leg exercises, if not contraindicated, improve circulation and help prevent complications related to stasis of blood, such as emboli formation. Patients are told to lie down, raise the leg, bend it at the knee, flex the foot, extend the leg, and lower it to the bed. Each leg is exercised in sets of five. Foot circles are also done every hour while awake. Teach the patient to raise a leg slightly off the bed with toes pointed. Draw a circle in the air with the great toe, rotating to the right four times, then to the left. Repeat this five times and then do the same with the other foot.

Patients are taught that turning from side to side in bed is aided by bending the leg that is to be on top and placing a pillow between the legs to support the top leg. They are told, unless contraindicated, to use the bed rail to pull themselves over to the side. They are encouraged to deep breathe while turning instead of holding their breath to promote comfort.

To reduce the strain on the incision and to make it easier for patients to get out of bed, patients are instructed to turn to their side without pillows between their knees. Then

---

atelectasis: ateles—imperfect + ektasis—expansion

TABLE 11.4 TEACHING PATIENTS COUGHING TECHNIQUES

Procedure	Rationale
Have patient sit up and lean forward.	Promotes lung expansion and ability to generate forceful cough
Show patient how to splint incision with hands, pillow, or blanket.	Reduces incision pressure so it does not feel as if incision is opening
Have patient inhale and exhale deeply three times through mouth.	Helps expand lungs
Have patient take in deep breath and cough out the breath forcefully with three short coughs using diaphragmatic muscles. Take in quick deep breath through mouth, cough deeply, and deep breathe.	Generates forceful cough and expands lungs to help move secretions

they should place their hands flat against the bed and push up while swinging their legs out of bed and into a sitting position. Patients should be told to sit for a few minutes after changing position to avoid dizziness and falling. They should also deep breathe while sitting up to promote lung expansion.

DIAGNOSTIC TESTING. Patient preoperative diagnostic testing is based on the patient's age, medical history, assessment findings, and institutional protocols (Table 11.5). Abnormal findings are reported to the physician.

Preoperative Patient Admission

Upon admission for surgery, subjective and objective patient data are collected (Table 11.6). Ensure that patients have their contact lenses, glasses, or hearing aids for accurate communication. During the interview, note the patient's emotional reaction to surgery. If the patient is anxious, explore the cause of the anxiety and allow the patient to express concerns. Anxiety is a feeling of apprehension or uneasiness resulting from the uncertainties and risks associated with surgery, while fear, a feeling of dread from a source known to the patient, is an extreme reaction to surgery.

Nursing Process for Preoperative Patients
Nursing Assessment/Data Collection

SUBJECTIVE DATA. During data collection, it is important to ask the patient if there have been any personal or family problems with anesthesia. A rare hereditary muscle disease, malignant hyperthermia, can predispose the patient to a serious life-threatening reaction to certain anesthetic agents (discussed later). Prior surgeries are also recorded.

MEDICATIONS. All medications (herbs and over-the-counter, prescription, and recreational drugs) that the patient takes must be reviewed. Alterations in drug dosages and routes of administration may be required. You should ensure

TABLE 11.5 PREOPERATIVE DIAGNOSTIC TESTS

Diagnostic Test	Purpose
Chest x-ray	Detect pulmonary and cardiac abnormalities
Oxygen saturation	Obtain baseline level and detect abnormality
Serum Tests	
Arterial blood gases	Obtain baseline levels and detect pH and oxygenation abnormalities
Bleeding time	Detect prolonged bleeding problem
Blood urea nitrogen	Detect kidney problem
Creatinine	Detect kidney problem
Complete blood cell count	Detect anemia, infection, clotting problem
Electrolytes	Detect potassium, sodium, chloride imbalances
Fasting blood glucose	Detect abnormalities, monitor diabetes control
Pregnancy	Detect early, unknown pregnancy
Partial thromboplastin time	Detect clotting problem
INR, prothrombin time	Detect clotting problem, monitor warfarin therapy
Type and cross match	Identify blood type to match blood for possible transfusion
Urine Tests	
Pregnancy	Detect early, unknown pregnancy
Urinalysis	Detect infection, abnormalities

INR = International normalized ratio.

that the patient clearly understands all medication instructions. For example, patients taking an anticoagulant such as warfarin (Coumadin) may be told by their physician to decrease or stop it several days before surgery to avoid bleeding problems during surgery. Many herbs can interfere with medications used during surgery or increase bleeding times. Patients may be instructed to stop certain herbs several days or weeks before surgery.

Diabetic patients on insulin are usually given instructions by the physician to either hold their insulin or take half of their normal dose of insulin the day of surgery. On the day of surgery, blood glucose monitoring may be done every 4 hours or as ordered to ensure that blood glucose levels are maintained within a desired range.

Patients on chronic oral steroid therapy cannot abruptly stop their medication even though they are told to take nothing by mouth (NPO) before or after surgery. Serious complications, such as circulatory collapse, can develop if steroids are stopped abruptly. The physician should order a patient's steroid therapy to be given by a parenteral route if the patient is NPO, so that it is not interrupted. You should ensure that the steroid therapy is ordered and continued for the patient via an alternate route.

Patients should be asked about the use of drugs such as cocaine, marijuana, or opioids because these drugs can interact with anesthesia or other medications. To obtain honest, accurate information, patients should be told of this potential

TABLE 11.6 NURSING ASSESSMENT OF THE PREOPERATIVE PATIENT

Subjective Data: Health History Questions
Demographic information: Name, age, marital status, occupation, roles?
History of condition for which surgery is scheduled: Why are you having surgery?
Medical history: Any allergies, acute or chronic conditions, current medications, pain, or prior hospitalizations?
Surgical history: Any reactions or problems with anesthesia? Previous surgeries?
Tobacco use: How much do you smoke? Pack-year history (number of packs per day × number of years)?
Alcohol use: How often do you drink alcohol? How much?
Coping techniques: How do you usually cope with stressful situations? Support systems?
Family history: Hereditary conditions, diabetes, cardiovascular, anesthesia problems?
Female patients: Date of last menses and obstetrical information?

Objective Data: Body System Review
Vital signs, oxygen saturation
Height and weight
Emotional status: calm, anxious, tearful, affect
Neurological: ability to follow instructions
Skin: color, warmth, bruises, lesions, turgor, dryness, mucous membranes
Respiratory: infection: cough; breath sounds; chronic obstructive pulmonary disease; respiratory rate, pattern, and effort; barrel chest
Cardiovascular: angina, myocardial infarction, heart failure, hypertension, valvular heart disease, mitral valve prolapse, heart rate and rhythm, peripheral pulses, edema, jugular vein distention
Gastrointestinal: bowel sounds, date of last bowel movement, abdominal distention, firmness, ostomy
Musculoskeletal: deformities, weakness, decreased range of motion, crepitation, gait, artificial limbs, prostheses.

interaction. Information and questions should be stated in a nonjudgmental manner. For example, you should ask, "How much alcohol do you drink daily or weekly?" instead of "Do you drink alcohol?" The first statement assumes that people drink alcohol. This allows the patient who does not drink to indicate none and the patient who does to state an amount rather than having to say yes and then give an amount upon further questioning. More accurate responses are given because this approach is viewed more positively by the patient who consumes alcohol. Another example would be to ask the patient, "What roles do drugs or alcohol play in your life?"

OBJECTIVE DATA. A physical assessment of body systems is performed. This information can highlight risk factors for surgery, determine the type of anesthesia to be used, and assist in planning interventions to reduce risk factors. A cough, cold, or fever is reported to the physician because surgery may be delayed until the patient recovers from an acute infection. Dentures, bridges, capped teeth, and loose teeth are documented because they can become dislodged during intubation (insertion of endotracheal breathing tube) for general anesthesia, causing complications.

Nursing Diagnosis, Planning, and Interventions

Anxiety or fear related to potential change in body image, hospitalization, pain, loss of control, and uncertainties surrounding surgery.

EXPECTED OUTCOME: Patient will state reduced anxiety or fear.

- Inform patients about procedures and surgical routines, *which helps reduce anxiety.*
- Allow patients to express their concerns *to allow inaccurate information to be corrected.*
- If patients express extreme anxiety or fear, inform the physician *as complications or even death could result. When fear is excessive, the physician may reschedule the surgery until the patient is better able to cope.*

Deficient knowledge related to lack of prior experience with surgical routines and procedures

EXPECTED OUTCOME: Patient will demonstrate understanding of surgical information and routines.

- Patient anxiety levels should be considered when providing explanations *as learning can be affected by high anxiety levels.*
- Identify knowledge deficiencies with the patient *so that he or she is motivated to learn.*
- Reinforce information provided prior to admission and new information to patients *to promote informed choice and increase self-care abilities. Teaching is caring in action and empowers patients to be a participant in their care.*
- Include the patient's family or caregivers in teaching sessions *so they can assist the patient through the surgical experience.*
- Use a variety of teaching methods (discussion, written materials and instructions, models, and videos) *to allow for different learning styles and to reinforce learning.*
- Individualize explanations *so the patient is not overwhelmed.*
- Use teaching methods that adapt to aging changes that may affect learning. *Box 11.3 Gerontological Issues describes methods to provide a positive learning experience for the elderly patient.*
- Document teaching and patient understanding.

Evaluation

The goal of decreased anxiety is achieved if the patient states and demonstrates that anxiety is relieved. If the patient is able to learn during teaching sessions, anxiety is not a barrier to learning.

The goal for correcting deficient knowledge is reached if the patient states understanding of the information presented and accurately performs return demonstrations of presented information.

Preoperative Consent

Before performing surgery, it is the physician's responsibility to obtain voluntary, written, informed consent from the

---

Box 11.3
Gerontological Issues

Considerations for Elderly Patient Teaching Sessions

Environmental considerations:
- Comfortable: anxiety free, quiet, appropriate temperature
- Correctly lit: small, intense lighting with nonglare, soft white light (not fluorescent)
- Private: no distractions, no background noise, turn off pagers

Presentation considerations:
- Assess readiness to learn.
- Assess comfort and safety needs.
- Use past experience and relate to new learning.
- Base learning on assessment data and current knowledge base.
- Use simple, understandable words and avoid medical jargon.
- Use legible audiovisual materials: large print, black print on white nonglare paper.
- If using colors, remember that older adults see red, orange, and yellow best; blue, violet, and green are more difficult to see.
- Perform ongoing assessment of energy level of patient.
- Answer questions as they occur.

Presenter considerations:
- Have positive attitude and belief in self-care promotion for older adults.
- Earn trust by being viewed as credible, positive role model.
- Maintain professional appearance.
- Use knowledge of aging changes in presentation:
  - Speak slowly in low tone.
  - Sit near patient for best visibility.
  - Ensure that prostheses are in place: glasses, hearing aids.
  - Allow patient increased response time and use memory aids such as pictures or diagrams.
  - Use touch appropriately to convey caring.
- Teach most important information first.
- Present one idea at a time.
- Provide instruction using multiple senses (vision and hearing).
- Provide repetition.
- Ask for feedback to ensure comprehension.
- Provide feedback and positive reinforcement.

---

patient. The consent gives legal permission for the surgery and has two purposes. It protects the patient from unauthorized procedures, and it protects the physician, anesthesiologist, hospital, and hospital employees from claims of performing unauthorized procedures. A signed consent is needed for all invasive procedures, anesthesia, blood administration, and radiation or cobalt therapy.

Informed consent involves three elements:

1. The physician must tell the patient in understandable terms about the diagnosis, the proposed treatment and who will perform it, the likely outcome, possible risks and complications of treatment, alternative treatments, and the prognosis without treatment. If the patient has questions before signing the consent, the physician must be contacted to provide further explanation to the patient. It is not within the nurse's scope of practice to provide this information.

2. The consent must be signed before analgesics or sedatives are given because patients must demonstrate that they are informed and understand the surgery.

3. Consent must be given voluntarily. No persuasion or threats can be used to influence the patient. The patient can withdraw consent at any time, even after the consent form has been signed.

To ensure that patients are truly informed prior to signing a consent, in some institutions patients must take and pass a knowledge quiz, which can be given verbally. If they do not pass the quiz, then further explanation is required by the physician. Additionally, in the surgical holding area, patients verbally reconsent. They are asked, "Do you still remember what you were told about your surgery?"

It is often your role to obtain and witness the patient's or authorized person's signature on the consent form (Fig. 11.2). You should ensure that the person signing the consent form understands its meaning and that it is being signed voluntarily. If the patient is unable to read, the entire consent must be read to the patient before it is signed. Patients are unable to give consent if they are unconscious, are mentally incompetent, are minors, or have received analgesics or

drugs that alter central nervous system function within time frames specified by agency policy. Consent may be obtained in any of these cases from parents, next of kin, or legal guardians.

NURSING CARE TIP

Witnessing a Consent

As the patient's advocate you should ensure, before the consent is signed, that the patient is informed about the surgery and has no further questions for the physician.

If the patient does have questions, the consent should not be signed and the physician should be contacted to answer the patient's questions.

Your signature as a witness on a consent form indicates that you observed the informed patient or patient's authorized representative voluntarily sign the consent form. It does not mean that you informed the patient about the surgical procedure; that is the responsibility of the physician.

In a medical emergency, the patient may not be able to give consent. In this case, the next of kin or legal guardian may give telephone consent, or a court order can be obtained. If time does not permit this, the physician documents the need for treatment in the chart as necessary to save the patient's life or avoid serious harm, according to state law and institutional policy.

Preparation for Surgery

Preoperative Checklist

A preoperative checklist is usually completed and signed by the nurse (per agency policy) before the patient is transported from the unit to surgery (Fig. 11.3). The checklist provides guidance for preoperative preparation of the patient:

- An identification band is placed on the patient. A hospital gown is given to the patient to wear. Underwear is removed, depending on the type of surgery.
- Vital signs are taken and recorded as baseline information and to assess patient status.
- Makeup, nail polish, and artificial nails (if applicable) are removed to allow assessment of natural color and pulse oximetry for oxygenation status during surgery.
- Removal of hair pins, wigs, and jewelry prevents loss or injury. Rings such as wedding rings are taped in place if the patient does not want to take them off, except if the ring is on the operative side (arm or chest surgery), as edema may occur.
- Dentures, contact lenses, and prostheses are removed to prevent injury. Some patients are concerned about body image and do not want family

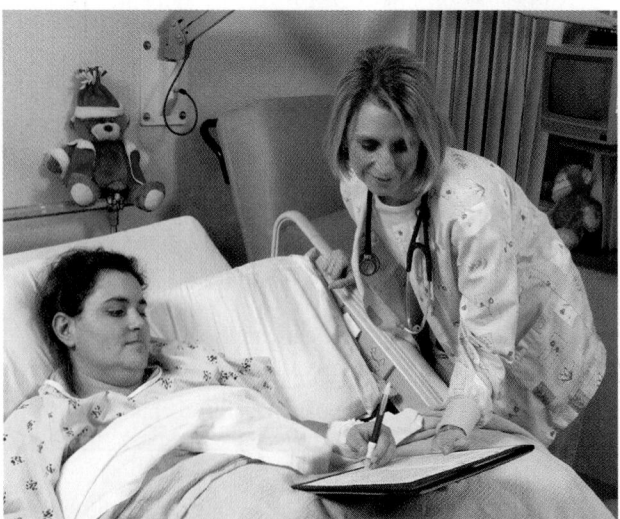

FIGURE 11.2 Nurse is witnessing signature of patient on surgical consent.

```
Pre-op Surgical Checklist                                    Client Name

_____  I.D. BAND ON                                 _____
_____  NPO AS ORDERED
_____  PRE-OP TEACHING COMPLETED
_____  INFORMED CONSENT SIGNED
_____  HISTORY AND PHYSICAL ON CHART
_____  ALLERGIES
_____  LAB RESULTS
_____      CBC: HGB _____ HCT _____ WBC _____ PLATELETS _____
_____      POTASSIUM _____
_____      URINALYSIS _____
_____      PREGNANCY TEST   SERUM _____ URINE _____
_____      PT _____ PTT _____ BLEEDING TIME _____
_____      TYPE AND SCREEN _____ CROSSMATCH _____-__ UNITS
_____  ECG ON CHART
_____  CHEST X-RAY REPORT ON CHART
_____  SHOWERED/BATHED
_____  HOSPITAL GOWN ON
_____  PREPS COMPLETED AS ORDERED
_____  ANTIEMBOLISM STOCKINGS
_____  JEWELRY TAPED/REMOVED: DISPOSITION _____
_____  VALUABLES: DISPOSITION _____
_____  DENTURES, PROSTHESIS REMOVED
_____  HAIR PINS, WIGS, MAKE UP, NAIL POLISH, ONE ACRYLIC NAIL REMOVED
_____  CONTACT LENSES REMOVED
_____  VOIDED
_____  VITAL SIGNS: T _____ P _____ R _____ BP _____
_____  PRE-OP MEDICATIONS GIVEN _____ SIDE RAILS UP _____
_____  IV STARTED _____
_____  EYE GLASSES AND HEARING AID(S) TO OR
_____  OLD CHART TO OR
_____  X-RAYS TO OR
_____  FAMILY LOCATION _____
_____  NEXT OF KIN _____
        CLIENT READY FOR SURGERY _____
            TIME _____        (NURSE SIGNATURE)
        COMMENTS:
```

FIGURE 11.3 Sample preoperative checklist form.

members to see them without dentures or makeup. Remove dentures after the family goes to the waiting room and insert them before the family sees the patient postoperatively.

- Glasses and hearing aids go with patients to surgery if they are unable to communicate without them. Label them with the patient's name and document where they go.
- All orders, diagnostic test results, consents, and history and physical (required on the chart) are reviewed for completion and documented on the checklist.
- Patient valuables are recorded and given to a family member or locked up per institutional policy by the nurse.
- Antiembolism devices are applied if ordered.
- Patients are asked to void before sedating preoperative medications are given, unless a urinary catheter is present, to prevent injury to the bladder during surgery.

Preoperative Medications

The final preparation before surgery is giving preoperative medications at the time ordered, usually 1 hour before, or on

TABLE 11.7 PREOPERATIVE MEDICATIONS

Category	Medication	Purpose
Narcotics	Morphine sulfate *Pain* Fentanyl (Sublimaze) Meperidine (Demerol) *pain*	Analgesia; enhancement of postoperative pain relief
Antianxiety and sedative hypnotics	Diazepam (Valium) Hydroxyzine hydrochloride (Vistaril) *increases anxiety* Lorazepam (Ativan) Midazolam (Versed) *pain/IV* Phenobarbital sodium (Luminal sodium)	Sedation; anxiety reduction
Anticholinergic	Atropine sulfate *— salvia/drys up/aspriate/dries secrection* Glycopyrrolate (Robinul) Scopolamine hydrobromide	Secretion reduction
Antiemetic	Droperidol (Inapsine) Ondansetron (Zofran) Metoclopramide (Reglan) Promethazine hydrochloride (Phenergan)	Control nausea and vomiting; may be effective into the postoperative period
Histamine (H₂) antagonist	Cimetidine (Tagamet) Famotidine (Pepcid) Ranitidine (Zantac)	Reduction of acidic gastric secretions in case aspiration occurs either silently or with vomiting.
Alkalinizing agent	Sodium citrate and citric acid (Bicitra)	Prevention of an asthmalike attack, pneumonitis, pulmonary edema, or severe hypoxia
Antibiotic	Cefazolin (Ancef) Cefoxitin (Cefotan) Ampicillin (Omnipen)	Prevention of postoperative infection

call to surgery (surgery calls to instruct that it is time to give the drugs) (Table 11.7). All medications administered are documented. The bed rails are raised for safety and the patient is instructed not to get up alone after medications are given.

Transfer to Surgery

When the surgery department is ready, the patient is taken to the surgical holding area on a stretcher (Fig. 11.4). The patient's chart, inhaler medications for those with asthma, and glasses or hearing aids also go to the surgical holding area. The patient can be accompanied by family members.

During surgery, the family waits in the surgical waiting area, which is a communication center where the family is kept informed regarding the patient's status. The physician

calls the family there when surgery is over. Families may be given beepers so that they can walk outside or to other areas of the hospital and still be reached.

After Transfer
After the patient goes to surgery, prepare the patient's room and necessary equipment so it is ready for the patient's return (Table 11.8).

INTRAOPERATIVE PHASE

When the patient is transferred to the operating table, the next phase of the perioperative period, the intraoperative phase, begins (Fig. 11.5). Surgery may take place in a hospital operating room (OR) or free-standing ambulatory or outpatient surgical centers (Fig. 11.6). Additionally, surgery is performed in physician's offices, cardiac catheterization laboratories, radiology centers, emergency rooms, and specialized units that perform endoscopy procedures.

The OR team members must perform a sterile surgical hand scrub to reduce the amount of microorganisms on their hands and arms. An antimicrobial soap scrub is used to reduce the chances of microorganism contamination. Jewelry (e.g., watches, rings, bracelets) is also removed. Fingernails are kept short and clean. Artificial nails and colored nail polish are not permitted. Gloves are worn by the OR team to keep the surgical field sterile.

The OR is designed to enhance **aseptic** technique. Clean and contaminated areas are separated. Special ventilation systems control dust and prevent air from flowing into

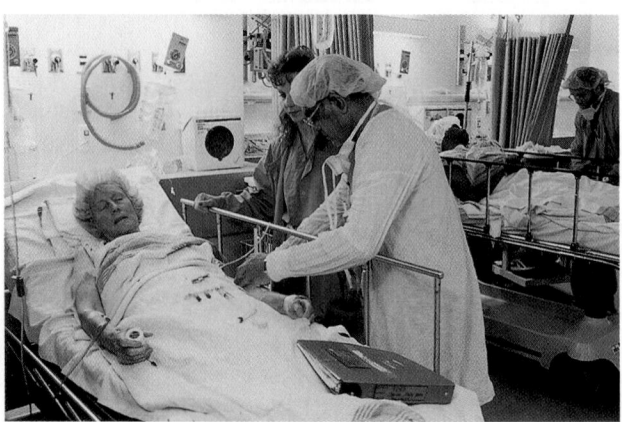
FIGURE 11.4 Surgical holding area.

TABLE 11.8 POSTOPERATIVE PATIENT HOSPITAL ROOM PREPARATION

After patient transfer to surgery, the nurse should prepare the patient's room for the patient's postoperative care needs to be ready for patient's return from the postanesthesia care unit.

Preparation	Rationale
	Bed
Bed linens should be clean and are changed if used before surgery by patient.	Reduces contamination of surgical wound
Place disposable, absorbent, waterproof pads on bottom sheet if drainage is expected.	Protects linen from wetness and soiling so a patient in pain does not have to be disturbed for linen change.
Apply lift sheet on bed of patient needing assistance with repositioning.	Makes lifting and turning easier for patient and nurse.
Have extra blankets available.	Patient may be cold or have a low temperature.
Fanfold top cover to end of bed or to side of bed away from patient transfer side.	Bed ready to receive patient on transfer from cart to bed. Allows covers to be easily pulled up over patient.
Obtain extra pillows as needed for positioning, elevating extremities, splinting during coughing.	Pillows help maintain position when patient is turned, elevate operative extremities for comfort and swelling reduction, or splint an incision during coughing.
	Equipment
Obtain IV pole.	Surgical patients have IV infusions postoperatively.
Have emesis basin at bedside.	Nausea or vomiting may occur, especially after movement during transfer.
Have tissues and washcloths in room.	Promotes comfort: washing face or a cool cloth on forehead.
Have urinal or bedpan available in room.	Patients may be unable to get out of bed for first voiding.
Prepare suction setup for tracheostomy, nasogastric tube, or drains as ordered.	Suction may be ordered related to surgical procedures: Sterile suction: tracheostomy
	Nasogastric tube: thoracic, abdominal, gastrointestinal surgery T-tube: cholecystectomy
Have oxygen set up as needed.	After tracheostomy, patients wear humidified oxygen mask.
Obtain special equipment as indicated by the surgical procedure.	Institutional policy and physician orders may require specialized equipment. Examples:
	Jaw surgery: suction, wire cutters, tracheostomy tray
	Tracheostomy: suction, extra tracheostomy set, tracheostomy care supplies
	Transurethral resection of prostate: irrigation supplies.
Have vital sign equipment available.	Promotes ability to promptly obtain vital signs.
	Documentation Forms
Obtain agency postoperative documentation forms and place in room	Promotes timely and accurate documentation of patient data.

IV = Intravenous.

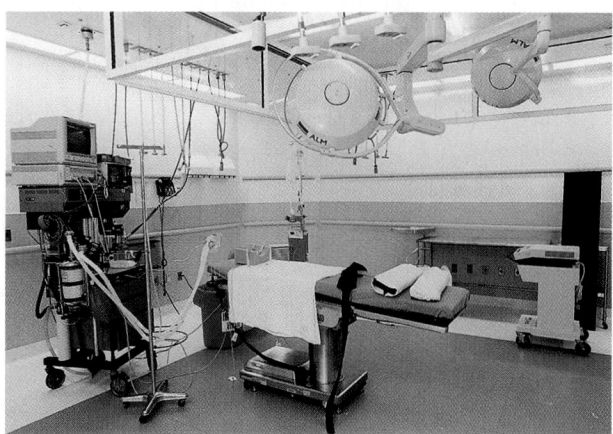

FIGURE 11.5 Operating room. Anesthesia equipment is on the left.

the OR from hallways. The temperature and humidity in the room are controlled to discourage bacterial growth. Everyone entering the OR wears surgical scrubs, shoe covers, caps, masks, and goggles to protect the patient from infection and themselves from bloodborne pathogens. Traffic in and out of the OR is limited. Strong disinfectants are used to clean the OR after each surgical case, and instruments are sterilized.

Before the patient arrives in surgery, a nursing plan of care is developed from preadmission assessment data. The OR is prepared based on the plan of care (Box 11.4 Nursing Care Plan). Attention is given to safety needs of the patient. Special needs are addressed, such as a tall patient's need for longer table length or an elderly patient's positioning needs resulting from osteoporosis. A surgical case cart containing sterile instruments required for the patient's case is prepared

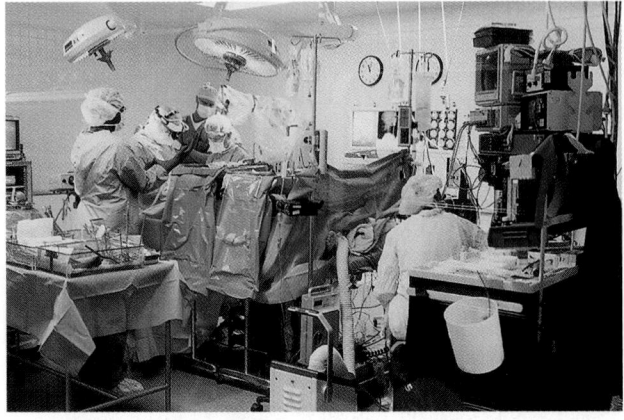

FIGURE 11.6 Operating room in use. Anesthesia is on the right.

ahead of time. Items such as needles and sponges are counted before surgery and again before closure of the incision to account for all of them and ensure that none has been left in the patient. To ensure safety, electrical equipment is checked for proper functioning.

Health-Care Team Member Roles

- Physician (medical doctor [MD], doctor of osteopathy [DO], oral surgeon, or podiatrist)
- Surgical (first) assistant: assists the physician and is either another physician, a specially trained registered nurse, or a physician's assistant

---

Box 11.4

Intraoperative Nursing Diagnoses and Expected Outcome

- Risk for perioperative-positioning injury related to positioning, chemicals, electrical equipment, and effect of being anesthetized
Free from injury

- Risk for impaired skin integrity related to chemicals, positioning, and immobility
Skin integrity is maintained

- Risk for deficient fluid volume related to NPO status and blood loss
Maintains blood pressure, pulse, and urine output within normal limits

- Risk for infection related to incision and invasive procedures
Is free of symptoms of infection

- Pain related to positioning, incision, and surgical procedure
Reports pain is relieved to satisfactory level

- Anesthesiologist: physician who specializes in anesthesia and supervises certified registered nurse anesthetists in the operating room
- Certified registered nurse anesthetist (CRNA): registered nurse trained and certified in the administration of anesthesia, usually at the master's degree level
- Registered nurse (RN): circulates in OR; roles include being patient's advocate, planning care, protecting patient safety, monitoring patient positioning, checking vital signs and making patient assessment, reducing patient's anxiety, monitoring sterility during surgery, preparing skin before incision, managing equipment such as by making sponge counts, documenting the procedure, and aiding health team communications
- Surgical (second assistant) technician: assists physician (may be an RN, LPN/LVN, or surgical technologist)

Patient Arrival in Surgery

The nurse greets the patient; verifies the patient's name, age, allergies, surgeon performing the surgery, informed consent, surgical procedure (right site, especially right or left when applicable), and medical history; answers questions; and alleviates anxiety. The patient is introduced to the anesthesiologist and CRNA, who also verify patient information and explain the type of anesthesia that is to be used. All surgical patients have intravenous (IV) fluids started. The patient may also receive prophylactic antibiotics. Taking a time out for everyone to stop and verify correct patient information can prevent adverse events.

SAFETY TIP

Eliminate wrong-site, wrong-patient, wrong-procedure surgery.

Create and use a preoperative verification process, such as a checklist, to confirm that appropriate documents (e.g., medical records, imaging studies) are available.

Implement a process to mark the surgical site and involve the patient in the marking process.

(2006 National Patient Safety Goals from www.jcaho.org)

As a patient enters the OR, he or she should be told what to expect:
- "The room may feel cool, but you can request extra blankets."
- "There is a lot of equipment in the room, including a table and large, bright overhead lights."

- "Several health-care team members will introduce themselves to you."
- "Your physician will greet you."

The patient is assisted onto the operating table, and a safety strap is carefully applied. Monitoring equipment is applied and readings recorded. Then the anesthesia provider begins anesthesia. When the anesthesia provider gives permission, the patient is carefully positioned to prevent pressure points that could cause tissue or nerve damage. Any necessary tubes that are not already in place, such as a nasogastric tube or urinary catheter, are inserted by the RN.

Patient allergies are rechecked. If the patient requires body hair removal, dry shaving with a safety razor should be avoided because of the potential for microabrasions and colonization by microorganisms. Hair should be removed with electric clippers or a depilatory, which is less harmful to the skin. Then a skin prepping solution that the patient is not allergic to, such as povidone-iodine, is used to cleanse the skin. (This may be done in preop holding or in surgery depending on the institution.) A large area surrounding the operative site is scrubbed to allow for extension of the incision. The scrub is completed in a circular motion from inside to outer edge. If an allergic reaction to the solution occurs, it can cause skin redness and blistering wherever the solution was used. After the skin is scrubbed, a sterile drape is applied with the incisional area left exposed.

SAFETY TIP

Improve the safety of using medications.

Label all medications, medication containers (e.g., syringes, medicine cups, basins), or other solutions on and off the sterile field in perioperative and other procedural settings.

(2006 National Patient Safety Goals from www.jcaho.org)

Anesthesia

Anesthesia is used for surgery to prevent pain and allow the procedure to be done safely. The type of anesthesia and the anesthetic agents are ordered by the anesthesia provider with input from the patient and physician (Box 11.5 Cultural Considerations).

There are two types of anesthesia: general and local (regional). General anesthesia (GA) causes the patient to lose sensation, consciousness, and reflexes. GA acts directly on the central nervous system. Local anesthesia blocks nerve impulses along the nerve where it is injected, resulting in the loss of sensation to a region of the body without the loss of consciousness.

General Anesthesia

General anesthesia is commonly given by an IV or inhalation route. GA is chosen when patients are anxious or do not

Box 11.5

Cultural Considerations

Care of the Patient Having Surgery

Chinese people show a greater increase in heart rate in response to atropine than Caucasian persons. Thus, the nurse needs to carefully monitor the pulse after atropine is given as a preoperative medication. Additionally, Chinese people are more sensitive to the sedative effects of diazepam (Valium) and require lower doses. Thus, the nurse needs to carefully monitor the Chinese patient for untoward effects of diazepam (Valium).

want local anesthesia, when the surgical procedure will take a long time and there is a need for muscle relaxation, or when the patient is unable to cooperate, as in head injury, muscle disorders, or impaired cognitive function.

INTRAVENOUS AGENTS. To begin most general anesthesia, the patient is induced (which means, anesthesia is caused) with a short-acting IV agent that provides a rapid, smooth **induction** (the period from when the anesthetic is first given until full anesthesia is reached). Because these agents last only a few minutes, they are used along with inhalation agents, which maintain anesthesia during surgery. After induction, the patient is intubated with an endotracheal (ET) tube to provide mechanical ventilation and anesthesia (Fig. 11.7).

INHALATION AGENTS. Maintenance of anesthesia is accomplished by using inhalation agents. These agents are delivered, controlled, and excreted through mechanical ventilation. Inhalation agents and the ET tube can be

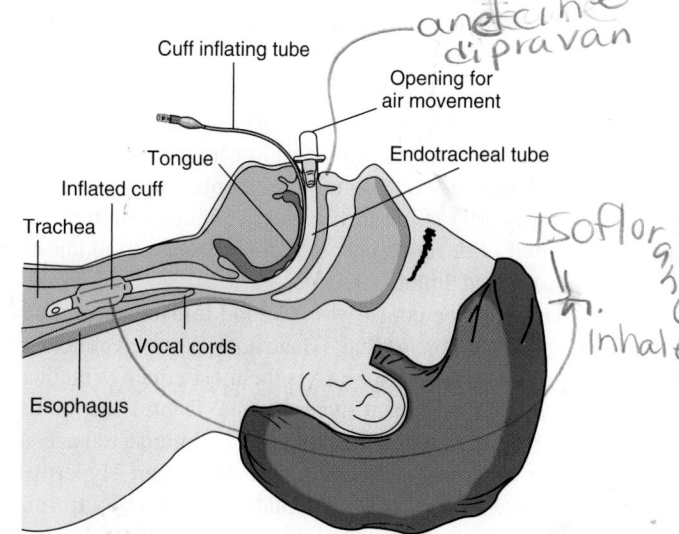

FIGURE 11.7 Endotracheal tube with cuff inflated.

---

induction: inductio—to lead in

irritating to the respiratory tract. Complications that can occur from their use include laryngospasm (sudden violent contraction of the vocal cords), laryngeal edema, irritated throat, or injury to the vocal cords. When the tube is removed, the nurse should closely monitor the patient and be prepared to provide respiratory support and assist with reintubation if complications arise.

in addition to

ADJUNCT AGENTS. An **adjunct** agent is a medication used along with the primary anesthetic agents. These medications can include narcotics to control pain, muscle relaxers to avoid movement of muscles during surgery, antiemetics to control nausea or vomiting, and sedatives to supplement anesthesia.

SAFETY TIP

Reduce the risk of surgical fires.

Educate staff, including operating licensed independent practitioners and anesthesia providers, about how to control heat sources and manage fuels, and establish guidelines to minimize oxygen concentration under drapes.

(2006 National Patient Safety Goals from www.jcaho.org)

Malignant Hyperthermia

Malignant hyperthermia (MH) is a rare hereditary muscular disease that can be triggered by some types of general anesthetic agents. Obtaining a history of anesthetic problems in the patient or family members can help detect the potential for development of this condition so that precautions can be taken. Those with a history of heat stroke are at increased risk for MH. A muscle biopsy can also diagnose this problem. Patients with this condition can undergo surgery safely with careful planning and choice of anesthetic agents by the anesthesia provider.

In MH, there is increased metabolism in muscles, which produces a very high fever and muscle rigidity, as well as tachycardia, tachypnea, hypertension, dysrhythmias, hyperkalemia, metabolic and respiratory acidosis, and cyanosis. MH is life threatening, so immediate treatment is required or death results. Surgery is stopped and anesthesia discontinued immediately. Oxygen at 100% is given. The patient must be cooled with ice and infusions of iced solutions. Dantrolene sodium (Dantrium), a muscle relaxant that relieves the muscle spasms, is the most effective medication for treating malignant hyperthermia. Dantrolene sodium is kept readily available in the OR and administered according to the treatment protocol of the Malignant Hyperthermia Association of the United States. For more information about malignant hyperthermia, visit www.mhaus.org.

Local (Regional) Anesthesia

Local anesthesia is selected when the patient is not anxious, can tolerate the local agent, and is not required by the sur-

gical procedure to be unconscious or relaxed. It is a good choice for some outpatient procedures or when the patient has not been NPO. The anesthesia provider, or sometimes the physician, administers local anesthesia.

Local anesthetic agents may include bupivacaine hydrochloride (Marcaine), lidocaine (Xylocaine), and dibucaine (Nupercainal). Topical administration places the agent directly on the surgical area. Local infiltration is achieved by injecting the medication into the tissue where the incision is to be made. A regional block is done by injecting the local agent along a nerve that carries impulses in the region where anesthesia is desired. There are several types of regional blocks. A nerve block is the injection of a nerve at a specific point. A Bier block is done by placing a tourniquet on an extremity to remove the blood and then injecting the local agent into the extremity. A field block is a series of injections surrounding the surgical area. A spinal or epidural block is injection of a local agent into an area around the spinal nerves.

SPINAL AND EPIDURAL BLOCKS. Injection of a local agent into the subarachnoid space produces spinal block (Fig. 11.8). Epidural block occurs when the local agent is injected into the epidural space. Spinal and epidural blocks are used mainly for lower extremity and lower abdominal surgery. Both motor and sensory function is blocked. The patient must be carefully monitored for complications. Hypotension results from sympathetic blockade causing vasodilation, which reduces venous return to the heart and therefore reduces cardiac output. Respiratory depression results if the block travels too far upward. As the block

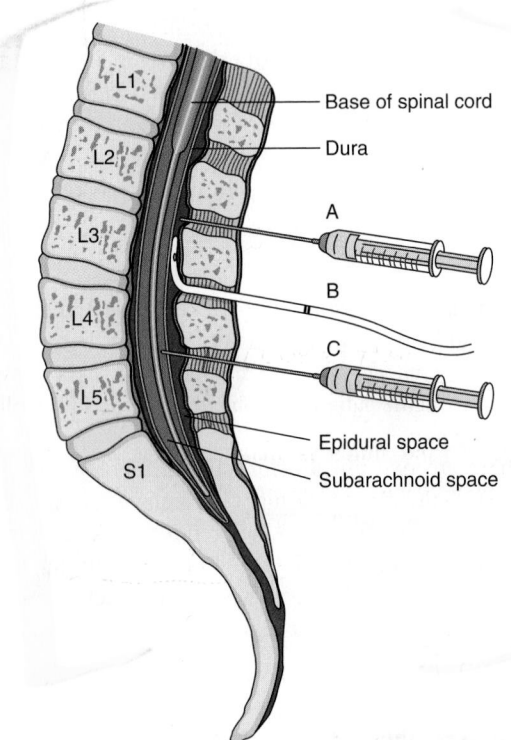

FIGURE 11.8 Injection of spinal anesthesia. *(A)* Epidural anesthesia. *(B)* Epidural catheter. *(C)* Spinal anesthesia.

[handwritten: 6–8hrs]

wears off, patients feel as if their legs are very heavy and numb. This is normal, and reassurance should be offered to the patient that this type of feeling does not last after the block wears off. *[handwritten: Lay flat will decrease headache]*

Complications. A postdural puncture headache may occur in 10% to 40% of patients caused by leakage of cerebrospinal fluid (CSF) from the needle hole in the dura that does not close when the needle is withdrawn. The use of a small-gauge spinal needle (less than 25 gauge) helps prevent headaches. Photophobia or double vision may also be present. Postanesthesia orders usually include methods to help reduce the pain of a headache, including positioning the patient flat and forcing fluids.

If a spinal headache develops, it may be severe and can last for weeks. Lying flat and prone (on abdomen) may help relieve the pain of the headache. Adequate fluid intake and analgesics may be ordered, and steroids may be helpful. If the headache continues, a blood patch treatment can be used to stop the CSF leakage. This treatment can be done by the anesthesiologist at the bedside or in the postanesthesia care unit (PACU). To create a blood patch, approximately 10 mL of the patient's own blood is injected into the epidural space at the previous puncture site. The injected blood forms a clot that "patches" the dural hole to prevent further CSF leakage. Pain relief should occur quickly if the patch is successful. Blood patch treatment can be repeated.

Conscious Sedation

[handwritten: Versed given IV]

Conscious sedation (sometimes called twilight sleep) is purposeful, minimal sedation that does not cause the complete loss of consciousness during selected medical, dental, or diagnostic procedures. Medications such as sedatives, hypnotics, and opioids are given to produce conscious sedation. Selection of patients who are eligible for conscious sedation is based on the procedure, the patient's general health, patient preference, and physician preference. Examples of short procedures for which conscious sedation is used are dental procedures, endoscopy (EGDs or colonoscopy), cardiac catheterization, cardioversion, and closed fracture reduction. During conscious sedation, patients are comfortable, respond purposefully, and maintain their own patent airway. Medications are ordered by the physician and usually administration by a specially trained registered nurse, as defined by agency and state scope of nursing practice.

A signed informed consent is obtained. Then an IV for medications and fluids is inserted before the procedure. Patient monitoring is done every 5 minutes to check vital signs, electrocardiogram, and oxygen saturation. Changes are reported to the physician. Oxygen may be given by nasal cannula or mask. Emergency equipment (e.g., airway suction, defibrillator, drugs) is on standby, according to advanced cardiac life support (ACLS) protocols.

After the procedure, the patient awakens easily and quickly. The patient is monitored every 15 to 30 minutes for response to the procedure and the drugs until the patient is fully awake and stable. The patient is ready for discharge when vital signs return to baseline and are stable, oral fluids

are retained, he or she has voided (if applicable), and written and oral discharge teaching is given to both the patient and the responsible adult to whom the patient is being discharged. The responsible adult and the patient must sign the instructions. Instructions include the following: an adult must drive the patient home and provide a safe environment; the patient must not and will not drive or operate heavy machinery or sign legal documents for 24 hours.

LEARNING TIP

In comparison with general anesthesia, conscious sedation:
- Is less invasive.
- Requires less medication.
- Causes less depression of the cardiovascular and respiratory systems.
- Allows the patient to more quickly return to a wakeful state.

Transfer from Surgery

When surgery is completed and anesthesia stopped, the patient is stabilized for transfer. After local anesthesia, the patient may return directly to a nursing unit. After general and spinal anesthesia, the patient goes to the PACU or, in some cases, the intensive care unit (ICU).

Patient safety, which is always a priority, is an important concern at this time. The patient is never left alone. Ensuring a patent airway and preventing falls and injury from uncontrolled movements are priorities. The anesthesia provider and OR nurses transfer the patient to the PACU and monitor the patient until the perianesthesia nurse is able to receive the report and assume care of the patient. This begins the final patient perioperative phase, the postoperative period.

SAFETY TIP

Improve the effectiveness of communication among caregivers.

Implement a standardized approach to "hand off" communications, including an opportunity to ask and respond to questions. (2006 National Patient Safety Goals from www.jcaho.org)

POSTOPERATIVE PHASE

The postoperative phase begins when the patient is admitted to the PACU or a nursing unit and ends with the patient's postoperative evaluation in the physician's office (Fig. 11.9). The family is updated on the patient's status by the physician as the patient is admitted to the PACU.

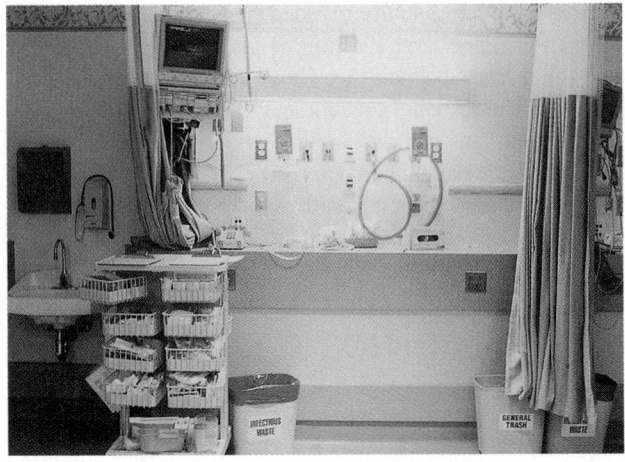

FIGURE 11.9 Postanesthesia care unit.

Admission to the Postanesthesia Care Unit

Stable, Need a Report

The perianesthesia nurse's goal is to promote safe recovery from anesthesia. The nurse's role in the PACU begins by receiving a patient report from the OR nurse and anesthesia provider. When the patient is admitted to the PACU, an admission assessment is done. The priority areas of patient assessment are the following:

- Respiratory status and patency of airway
- Vital signs including SaO_2
- Level of consciousness and responsiveness
- Surgical site incision/dressing/drainage tubes
- Pain level and pain management

Oxygen by nasal cannula or mask is given if the patient has had general anesthesia, or as ordered. Some patients who are still intubated may require mechanical ventilation. Continuous monitoring is done on all patients for ECG, pulse oximetry, and blood pressure measurements. The surgical site incision or dressing is assessed. Drainage and **hematoma** formation are documented and reported. Urinary catheter, drains, and nasogastric tubes are checked for function and patency as applicable.

The patient's body temperature is measured on admission to the PACU, and then blankets heated in blanket warmers are applied. If the patient's temperature is below normal, a warming blanket that can be set to a desired temperature is applied. Body temperature may be decreased as a result of a cool OR environment, anesthesia, cool IV solutions, and incisional openings, which allow heat loss. Patient recovery is aided by avoiding a decrease in body temperature during surgery. Using forced warm air before surgery to warm the patient, rather than warm blankets, has been shown to maintain body temperature best upon arrival in the PACU. Be aware that the elderly (and infants) are at increased risk of **hypothermia.** Temperature is measured again before PACU discharge because a normal body temperature is usually one of the discharge criteria.

Shivering may occur from anesthesia or as a result of being cold. It is important to control shivering because it increases oxygen consumption 400% to 500%. Meperidine (Demerol) is effective in relieving shivering when anesthesia is the cause. If the patient is cold, raising the body temperature is helpful to decrease shivering. It is important to provide supplemental O_2 during the episode of shivering and until the SaO_2 is normal.

See Box 11.6 Perianesthesia Nursing Responsibilities.

It is essential for nurses to wash their hands between patients in the PACU. Vital signs and assessment are done at least every 5 to 15 minutes, IV fluid infusion is maintained, and IV analgesics are given for pain as needed. Antiemetics are administered for nausea or vomiting. Deep breathing and coughing, if not contraindicated by the surgical procedure, are encouraged. Coughing increases pressure, which could cause harm to some surgical areas. Surgical procedures that prohibit coughing include hernia repair; eye, ear, intracranial, jaw, and plastic surgery. If the patient is no longer NPO, ice chips or sips of water may be offered when the patient is fully awake to promote comfort for a dry mouth. If ordered, postoperative therapies such as patient-controlled analgesia (PCA), which allows patients to administer their own pain medication (see Chapter 9), or continuous passive motion machines for joint replacement surgeries are begun in the PACU.

Nursing Process for Postoperative Patients in PACU

Various postoperative complications may occur in the PACU or later in the postoperative phase. The causes of these complications may be the surgical procedure, anesthesia, blood and fluid loss, immobility, unrelieved pain, or other diseases the patient may have. Nursing care focuses on preventing, detecting, and caring for these complications.

Respiratory Function

ASSESSMENT/DATA COLLECTION. Normal respiratory function can be altered in the immediate postoperative period by airway obstruction, hypoventilation, secretions, laryngospasm, or decreased swallowing and cough reflexes.

Box 11.6 *(all situations surrounding)*

Perianesthesia Nursing Responsibilities

- Airway maintenance
- Vital signs
- Respiratory assessment
- Neurological assessment
- Surgical site status
- General assessment
- Patient safety
- Monitoring anaesthetic effects
- Pain relief
- Assessing PACU discharge readiness

---

hematoma: heimatos—blood + oma—tumor

Respiratory function assessment includes respiratory rate, depth, ease, and pattern. Breath sounds, chest symmetry, accessory muscle use, and sputum are also observed.

NURSING DIAGNOSIS, PLANNING, AND IMPLEMENTATION. Ineffective breathing pattern related to anesthesia, pain, and analgesic/sedative medications

EXPECTED OUTCOME: Patients will maintain normal SaO_2 levels.

- Maintain oxygen therapy as ordered on all general anesthesia patients. *Hypoventilation can be an effect of anesthesia medications or analgesics, decreased level of consciousness, or an incision in the thorax causing painful respirations.*
- Encourage deep breathing *to expand the lungs.*
- Give analgesics carefully *to promote deep breathing but avoid respiratory depression.*
- Maintain CPAP/BiPap as needed *for those with sleep apnea. Patients with sleep apnea may bring their CPAP/BiPap machines with them for use.*
- Report respiratory depression to the anesthesiologist *for prompt treatment*

Ineffective airway clearance related to obstruction, anesthesia medications, and secretions

EXPECTED OUTCOME: Patients will have patent airway at all times.

- Ensure that patients maintain a patent airway *as airway obstruction is usually caused from relaxed muscles allowing tongue to block the pharynx in patients who have a decreased level of consciousness.*
- Use jaw-thrust method to manually open patient's airway *if patient has snoring respirations and has not completely emerged from anesthesia.*

Risk for aspiration related to depressed cough and gag reflexes and reduced level of consciousness

EXPECTED OUTCOME: Patients will have clear lung sounds.

- Position patients on their side, unless contraindicated, *to protect airway until they are awake.*
- Have suction equipment always available *to clear secretions or emesis.*

EVALUATION. The goal for ineffective airway clearance and aspiration is achieved if the patient's airway remains patent and lung sounds remain clear. The goal for ineffective breathing pattern is met if the patient's respiratory rate is within normal limits, no dyspnea is reported, and arterial blood gases are within normal limits.

Cardiovascular Function   *loosing Blood-hypovolemia*

ASSESSMENT/DATA COLLECTION. Alterations in cardiovascular function can include hypotension, dysrhythmias, and hypertension. Hypotension can be the result of blood and fluid volume loss or cardiac abnormalities. Shock can result from significant blood and fluid volume loss or from sepsis (see Chapter 8). Dysrhythmias may occur from hypoxia,

altered potassium or magnesium levels, hypothermia, pain, stress, or cardiac disease. New-onset hypertension can develop from pain, a full bladder, or respiratory distress. Cardiovascular function assessment includes heart rate, blood pressure, ECG, and skin temperature, color, and moistness. Vital signs are compared with baseline readings to determine if they are normal. Tachycardia, hypotension, pale skin color, cool, clammy skin, and decreased urine output indicate hypovolemic shock, which requires reporting and prompt treatment.

Nursing Diagnosis, Planning, and Implementation
Deficient fluid volume related to blood and fluid loss or NPO status

EXPECTED OUTCOME: Patients will maintain blood pressure, pulse, and urine output within normal limits.

- Check dressings and incisions for color and amount of drainage *to detect fluid loss.*
- Maintain IV fluids at ordered rate *to replace lost fluids but avoid fluid overload.*
- Monitor intake and output *to detect imbalances.*

EVALUATION. The goal for deficient fluid volume is met if vital signs and urine output are within normal limits.

NURSING CARE TIP

Tachycardia: An Early Warning Sign

Tachycardia is a compensatory mechanism designed to provide adequate delivery of oxygen in times of altered function. It is usually the earliest warning sign that an abnormality is occurring. It should be a red flag to assess the patient and ask yourself what this particular patient is likely to be experiencing that is compromising oxygenation, allowing you to begin prompt treatment.

PATIENT CONDITION	POSSIBLE CAUSES OF COMPROMISED OXYGENATION
Postoperative patient	Hemorrhage, respiratory depression, pain
Myocardial infarction patient	Cardiogenic shock, pain
Respiratory patient	Respiratory distress
Trauma patient	Hemorrhage, severe pain

Neurological Function
Until its effects wear off, anesthesia can alter neurological function. Patients may arrive in the PACU awake, arousable, or sleeping. If patients are sleeping, they should become more alert during their stay in the PACU. As emergence from anesthesia occurs, patients may become wild or agitated for a short period. This is referred to as emergence delirium. During this time it is important to provide safety measures

such as side rails and restraints with restraint protocols followed to protect IV lines and keep endotracheal tubes in place. Once resolved, the patient returns to a calm state and has no recollection of the episode. Movement, sensations, and perceptions may also be altered by anesthesia. Movement is the first function to return after spinal anesthesia.

For geriatric patients, it is important to review their history to understand if they have any cognitive or neurological deficits. Confused patients may be agitated or frightened when they awaken. It is helpful to know how caregivers normally communicate with the patient. You should understand that the patient may not be able to report pain or follow commands. If possible, it may be helpful to have a familiar relative or caregiver with the patient in the PACU to calm him and help him communicate. You should watch for nonverbal pain cues such as moaning, grimacing, rubbing an area, and restlessness. If patients have limited movements or sensations before surgery, you should know this to obtain an accurate assessment of anesthetic effects.

ASSESSMENT/DATA COLLECTION. A neurological assessment includes level of consciousness; orientation to person, place, time and event; pupil size and reaction to light; and motor and sensory function.

NURSING DIAGNOSIS, PLANNING, AND IMPLEMENTATION. Disturbed sensory perception related to decreased level of consciousness, amnesiac effects of anesthesia, or spinal anesthesia

EXPECTED OUTCOME: Patients will maintain safety and be free from injury.

- All patient data are verified until patients are awake and can communicate *to prevent errors.*
- Maintain patients' safety with side rails and extremities positioned in proper alignment and protected *until patients are fully awake or extremity movement and sensation return following spinal anesthesia.*
- Tubes, dressings, and IVs are secured and observed *to prevent dislodgement.*
- Provide orientation explanations as patients awaken and repeat until amnesiac anesthesia effects are no longer present. Examples of explanations include: "Mr. Smith, surgery is over; you are in the recovery room." "Your family is waiting for you and knows you are in the recovery room." "The doctor spoke with your family and told them how you are doing."

EVALUATION. The goal for disturbed sensory perception is met if the patient remains free from injury.

Pain *[handwritten: respiratory depression 12-20 Normal]*
ASSESSMENT/DATA COLLECTION. If patients are awake, they are asked to rate the presence of pain using a scale, such as 0 to 10, a pain scale using color, or pictures that rate pain. The location and character of the pain are documented. When patients are not fully awake, vital signs and nonverbal indications of pain should be monitored. Nonverbal indications of pain can include abnormal vital signs, restlessness, moaning, grimacing, rubbing, or pulling at specific areas or equipment.

NURSING DIAGNOSIS, PLANNING, AND IMPLEMENTATION. Pain related to tissue damage (mechanical [incision])

EXPECTED OUTCOME: The patient will report that pain is relieved at a satisfactory level.

- Monitor patient pain *as pain may result from surgical procedure, movement, deep breathing, anxiety, full bladder, positioning during surgery, nasogastric tubes, catheters, IVs, ET tubes, or prior medical conditions such as arthritis, cancer, or back pain.*
- Give IV narcotic analgesics promptly *for their rapid onset.*
- Begin PCA as ordered, *as it is started in PACU.*
- Reposition the patient, provide warmth, and empty full bladder *to help alleviate pain.*
- Play music in PACU, such as nature sounds or music by Mozart, dim lights, and reduce room noise *to help alleviate pain.*

EVALUATION. The goal for pain is met if patients report a decreased level of pain that is satisfactory to them. For example, the patient reports pain of 10 on a scale of 0 to 10. You medicate the patient, and 30 minutes later the patient rates pain as 2 on a scale of 0 to 10. The patient indicates that 2 is an acceptable pain level, so the goal is achieved.

Family Visitation

Family visitation in the PACU has been shown to be helpful to patients and their families. Allowing family visitation varies by hospital. Patients and families should be educated about the expectations for family visitation to keep it safe for the patient. During visitation, confidentiality of all patients must be ensured according to HIPAA (Health Insurance Portability and Accountability Act of 1996). Some patients do not want the surgical procedure revealed to their spouse or any family members.

Discharge from the Postanesthesia Care Unit

The length of stay in the PACU if the patient remains stable is normally about 1 hour. A postanesthesia recovery scale is used to score the patient's readiness to be discharged. The scale rates categories such as respiration, oxygen saturation, level of consciousness, activity, and circulation. The anesthesiologist discharges the patient for transfer to a nursing unit or home when discharge criteria are met (Table 11.9). The patient may be transferred to the ICU if patient status and/or frequent or invasive monitoring is needed.

Transfer to Nursing Unit

The perianesthesia nurse gives a report of the patient's condition to the unit nurse when the patient is transferred to the nursing unit. The patient is moved into bed on the nursing unit with assistance to prevent dislodging IVs, tubes, drains, or dressings. After patients are placed in bed, the following safety interventions are performed:

- The bed is placed in its lowest position, with the side rails raised.

TABLE 11.9 DISCHARGE CRITERIA FOR POSTANESTHESIA CARE UNIT OR AMBULATORY SURGERY

Vital signs stable
Patient awake or at baseline level of consciousness
Drainage or bleeding not excessive
Respiratory function not depressed
Oxygen saturation above 90%

Additional Criteria for Ambulatory Surgery
No nausea or vomiting
No IV narcotics within last 30 minutes
Voided if required by surgical procedure or ordered
Is ambulatory or has baseline mobility
Understands discharge instructions
Provides means of contact for follow-up telephone assessment
Released to responsible adult

- The nurse's call button is placed within easy patient reach and answered promptly.
- Patients are instructed that they should be assisted with ambulation when they get up.

When patients get up postoperatively, especially for the first time, they may be weak or dizzy. One or two health-care workers should assist the patient and allow the patient to dangle before standing (Fig. 11.10). These precautions can help prevent falls.

Nursing Process for Postoperative Patients

A complete patient assessment is performed after transfer to the nursing unit. Respiratory status, vital signs (including temperature), level of consciousness, surgical site, dressings, and pain assessment are noted. IV site, patency, and IV solution and infusion rate are assessed and monitored. Nasogastric tubes are hooked to suction or clamped as ordered. Drains and catheters are positioned to promote proper functioning.

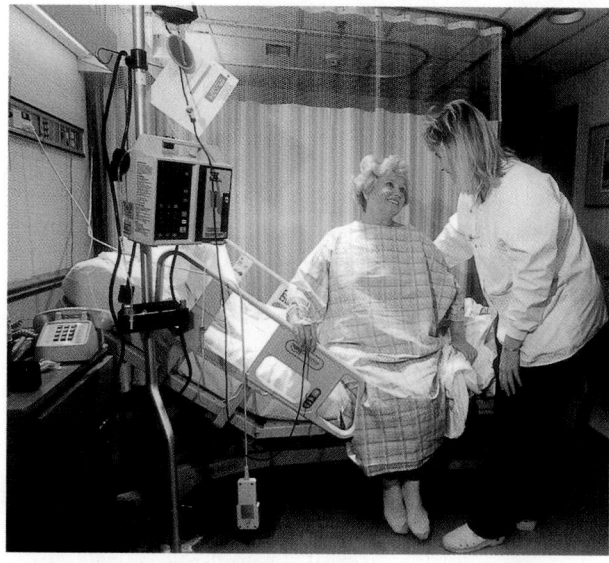

FIGURE 11.10 Postoperative patient dangling.

After discharge from the PACU, interventions to promote recovery include monitoring for complications (respiratory depression, hemorrhage, and shock), providing postoperative care, educating patients and their significant others, making necessary referrals, and providing home health care (Box 11.7 Nursing Care Plan for the Postoperative Patient).

Respiratory Function

ASSESSMENT/DATA COLLECTION. Regular monitoring of the patient's respiratory rate, depth, and effort and breath sounds as well as cough strength (if not contraindicated by the type of surgery, such as hernia repair or eye, ear, intracranial, jaw, or plastic surgery) should be done. Postoperative patients are at risk for developing atelectasis and pneumonia. They may have a weak cough as a result of being drowsy from anesthesia or analgesics. If fine crackles are heard in the lung bases, the patient should be encouraged to deep breathe or cough. Afterward you should listen again to see if the crackles have cleared. If the patient's airway is compromised, immediate action is taken to support the airway and the physician is notified.

NURSING DIAGNOSIS, PLANNING, AND IMPLEMENTATION. Ineffective breathing pattern related to pain and analgesic medications

EXPECTED OUTCOME: Patients will maintain normal Sao$_2$ levels and normal arterial blood gases.

- Maintain oxygen therapy as ordered on all general anesthesia patients. *Hypoventilation can be an effect of anesthesia medications or analgesics, or an incision in the thorax causing painful respirations.*
- Encourage deep breathing *to expand the lungs.*
- Give analgesics as needed *to promote deep breathing so the patient does not guard against deep respirations or coughing especially if incision is near the diaphragm.*

Ineffective airway clearance related to ineffective cough and secretion retention

EXPECTED OUTCOME: Patients will have patent airway and clear breath sounds at all times.

- Deep breathing and coughing is encouraged every hour while the patient is awake, especially through the first postoperative day. *Retained secretions can lead to mucous plugs that block bronchioles, causing alveoli to collapse and atelectasis. Infection can develop from the stasis of mucus, resulting in pneumonia.*
- Place incentive spirometer within patient's reach and encourage hourly use while awake *to prevent atelectasis.*
- Turn patient at least every 2 hours *to help expand the lungs and move secretions.*
- Ambulate patient as soon as possible *as immobility decreases movement of secretions.*

EVALUATION. If the patient's breath sounds are clear and arterial blood gases remain normal, the goals are met.

BOX 11.7   NURSING CARE PLAN for the Postoperative Patient

Nursing Diagnosis: Ineffective airway clearance related to ineffective cough and secretion retention

Expected Outcome Patient maintains a patent airway at all times. Breath sounds remain clear.

Evaluation Of Outcomes Is patient able to clear own secretions? Are breath sounds clear?

Interventions	Rationale	Evaluation
Monitor breath sound.	Abnormal breath sounds such as crackles or wheezes can indicate retained secretions.	Are breath sounds clear?
Encourage deep breathing and coughing and use of incentive spirometer hourly while awake.	Lung expansion helps prevent atelectasis and keeps lungs clear of secretions.	Does patient perform breathing and coughing and use incentive spirometer?
Ensure that patient's pain is relieved before activity.	Movement can cause or increase pain.	Does patient state pain is controlled before activity?
Encourage movement by turning every 2 hours and ambulating as able.	Movement promotes lung expansion and movement of secretions.	Is patient moving?

Nursing Diagnosis: Pain related to surgery, nausea, and vomiting

Expected Outcome Patient reports that pain management relieves pain satisfactorily and describes pain management plan.

Evaluation of Outcomes Does patient report satisfactory pain relief? Is patient able to describe pain management plan?

Intervention	Rationale	Evaluation
Assess pain using rating scale such as 0 to 10.	Self-report is the most reliable indicator of pain.	Does patient report pain using scale?
Provide analgesics prn.	Analgesics relieve pain.	Is patient's pain less after medication?
Provide antiemetics prn.	Antimetics relieve nausea and vomiting.	Is patient's nausea and vomiting less after medication?
Position patient comfortably.	Incisions, drains, tubing, equipment, and bed rest can cause discomfort, which positioning can relieve.	Does patient report positioning is comfortable?
Geriatric		
When assessing pain speak clearly and slowly so elderly patient can hear.	If elderly patient does not hear or misunderstands, pain may not be reported accurately to ensure appropriate intervention provided.	Does patient hear and report pain and relief accurately using pain scale?
Assess elderly patients' pain level regularly, observing nonverbal pain cues (restlessness, grimacing, moaning), especially for those cognitively impaired.	The pain of elderly patients is often underreported and undertreated, especially if cognitively impaired, and noting nonverbal cues can aid in pain treatment.	Are nonverbal cues present in elderly patients, especially those cognitively impaired?

Nursing Diagnosis: Risk for infection related to inadequate primary defenses from surgical wound

Expected Outcome Patient remains free from infection.

Evaluation of Outcomes Does patient remain free from infection?

Intervention	Rationale	Evaluation
Observe incision for signs and symptoms of infection.	Redness, warmth, fever, and swelling indicate infection.	Are signs and symptoms of infection present?
Monitor drainage and maintain drains.	Drains remove fluid from the surgical site to prevent infection development.	Are drainage amount and color normal for procedure?
Maintain sterile technique for dressing changes.	Sterile technique reduces infection development.	Is incision free of signs and symptoms of infection?

Circulatory Function

ASSESSMENT/DATA COLLECTION. Monitor the patient's circulatory status to detect and prevent hemorrhage, shock, and thrombophlebitis. Vital signs, Sao_2 and skin temperature, color, and moistness are observed and compared with baseline data and abnormal trends noted. Institutional policy is followed for frequency of patient vital sign monitoring. The incision or dressing is checked for drainage or hematoma formation. Drainage may leak down the patient's side and pool underneath the patient. While wearing gloves, feel underneath the patient or turn the patient to check for bleeding. Report any signs of hemorrhage or shock promptly.

The lower extremities of surgical patients are observed. Tenderness or pain in the calf may be the first indication of a deep vein thrombosis. Leg swelling, warmth, and redness, as well as fever, may also be present. Bilateral calf and thigh measurement is done daily if thrombophlebitis is suspected or diagnosed. Peripheral pulses and capillary refill are also checked.

NURSING DIAGNOSIS, PLANNING, AND IMPLEMENTATION. Deficient fluid volume related to blood and fluid loss or NPO status

EXPECTED OUTCOME: Maintain blood pressure and pulse within normal limits.

- Monitor dressings, incisions, drains, and tubes for color and amount of drainage and report bright red drainage or excessive drainage amounts immediately.
- Monitor intake and output *to detect imbalances.*
- IV fluids are maintained at the ordered rate *to maintain fluid volume.*

Ineffective tissue perfusion: peripheral or pulmonary related to interruption of blood flow during surgery, dehydration, and use of leg straps.

EXPECTED OUTCOME: Maintain normal tissue perfusion.

- Encourage leg exercises hourly while the patient is awake to prevent venous stasis and thrombosis.
- Assist with early postoperative ambulation as ordered to prevent thrombosis.
- Apply knee-length or thigh-length antiembolism

elastic stockings or intermittent pneumatic compression as ordered *to help prevent stasis of blood* (Fig. 11.11).
- Give low-dose heparin, low molecular weight heparin (enoxaparin [Lovenox]), warfarin, and plasma expanders such as dextran 40 and dextran 70 as ordered *to reduce clot formation.*
- Avoid pressure under the knee from pillows, rolled blankets, or prolonged bending of the knee and elevate legs *to help prevent venous stasis.*

EVALUATION. The goal for deficient fluid volume is met if vital signs and urine output are within normal limits. The goal for ineffective tissue perfusion is met if tissue blood flow remains normal.

Postoperative Pain

Pain is common after surgery, although each patient's pain experience varies. In addition to incisional pain, painful muscle spasms can occur. Nausea and vomiting, ambulation, coughing, deep breathing, and anxiety can cause discomfort and increase postoperative pain. Unrelieved pain has negative physiological effects. It also impairs deep breathing and coughing and hinders early ambulation, which may increase

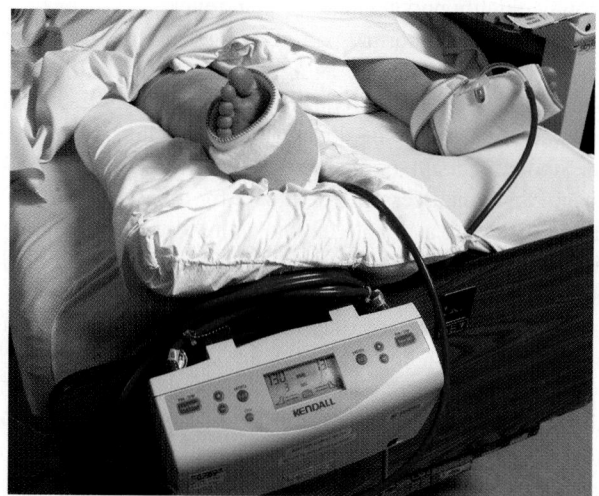

FIGURE 11.11 Postoperative patient wearing A-V Impulse System foot pump. The foot pump is used to prevent deep vein thrombosis, reduce pain and edema, and enhance arterial blood flow (*Kendall, Mansfield, MA*).

CRITICAL THINKING

Mrs. Owens

■ Mrs. Owens returned from a bowel resection 2 days ago. She is receiving 1000 mL of 0.9% normal saline over 10 hours.

1. As you monitor the patient you understand that the IV pump rate would be set at what rate?
2. How many milliliters should the nurse record as intake for 12 hours?

■ Intake and output for 12 hours:

Intake:
One 8-ounce (oz) cup of coffee
4 oz orange juice
6 oz of tomato soup
$^3/_4$ cup Jello
Two cups of water
1200 mL of 0.9% normal saline IV
Output:
1700 mL of urine

Suggested answers at end of chapter.

---

complications, length of hospital stay, and health-care costs. Nurses should understand that providing pain relief not only reduces suffering, it also has positive benefits for a quicker recovery. It is important for nurses to stay informed of advances in pain management and ensure that they make pain relief a priority in providing patient care. (See Chapter 9.)

ASSESSMENT/DATA COLLECTION. Nurses must be proactive and diligent in their provision of pain relief. Anticipating postoperative patients' pain by regularly monitoring their pain levels instead of waiting until it is the time for the next dose of pain medication is essential to provide quality nursing care for pain relief.

Pain is not a normal part of aging. Careful assessment of older patients' unique aging changes, chronic diseases, and pain relief needs is required to appropriately treat their postoperative pain. Cognitively impaired adults are at risk for undertreatment of their postoperative pain. You must ensure that you assess and treat pain for these patients. Pain rating scales are available for use with those who are cognitively impaired so that you can determine if they are experiencing pain.

If patients are not fully awake on transfer, vital signs and nonverbal indications of pain should be monitored. Nonverbal indicators of pain may include abnormal vital signs (usually elevated blood pressure, although hypotension can occur in some patients), restlessness, moaning, grimacing, and rubbing or pulling at specific body areas or equipment. Patients who are awake are asked the location of the pain, to rate the presence of pain, and to describe the pain quality, such as sharp, aching, throbbing, or burning, which is then documented.

NURSING DIAGNOSIS, PLANNING, AND IMPLEMENTATION. Pain related to tissue damage from surgery, muscle spasms, nausea, or vomiting

EXPECTED OUTCOME: The patient reports pain relief at a satisfactory level using pain rating scale.

- Monitor pain using pain rating scale of 0 to 10.
- Provide medications promptly as ordered *to relieve symptoms.*
- Understand appropriate timing intervals for IV to IM doses of analgesics *as IV analgesics usually have a shorter duration than IM analgesics so that patients do not wait and suffer needlessly.*
- Reposition patient *to promote comfort.*

EVALUATION. Thirty minutes after pain medication is given, patients are asked to rate their pain level. If patients are sleeping at this time, allow them to sleep. When they awaken, ask them to rate their pain level. The goal for pain is met when patients report a decreased level of pain that is satisfactory to them. If the patient does not report satisfactory pain relief, the physician should be promptly notified of the inadequate pain relief.

NURSING CARE TIPS

- For the first dose of an IM analgesic, patients in pain should not have to wait the ordered time interval of the IM dose after an intravenous analgesic dose (i.e., 3 hours if the IM order is morphine 10 mg IM q3h prn). Having to wait when the IV analgesic is no longer effective can cause needless pain.
- Patient controlled analgesia (PCA) may be started in the PACU. The patient's ability to use PCA, the patient's response to the medication, and the relief obtained from it are monitored. If PCA is not effective or if side effects occur, the physician should be notified.
- Comfortable positioning, warming the patient, and relieving a patient's full bladder can also alleviate pain. Attention to environmental factors such as bright overhead lighting, excessive noise or visitors, and extreme room temperatures also helps promote comfort.
- Antiemetics should be given as ordered to relieve the discomfort of nausea and vomiting. If vomiting occurs, patients should be turned onto one side to aid emesis removal and prevent aspiration. A nasogastric tube may be ordered to help control vomiting.

CRITICAL THINKING

Mrs. Wood

■ Mrs. Wood returns to the surgical unit after a hysterectomy. Her postoperative vital signs and assessment findings are normal. Mrs. Wood rates her pain level, and you note that she moans occasionally, repeatedly moves her legs, and pulls at her covers near her abdominal incision. She is drowsy but says it hurts. In the PACU, she received 10 mg of morphine IV 55 minutes ago. Morphine 5 to 10 mg IM is ordered every 3 hours as needed.

1. What nonverbal pain cues does Mrs. Wood display?
2. How should you document Mrs. Wood's pain?
3. What action should you take to relieve Mrs. Wood's pain?
4. When should you next monitor Mrs. Wood's pain level?
5. If Mrs. Wood indicates that her pain is unrelieved after 30 minutes, what action should you take?
6. You are to give Mrs. Wood morphine 8 mg IM now. You have available morphine 10 mg/mL. How many milliliters will you give?

Suggested answers at end of chapter.

Urinary Function

ASSESSMENT/DATA COLLECTION. Monitor the patient's urinary status to ensure normal function is maintained after anesthesia administration. If the patient has a urinary catheter, the amount, color, and consistency of the urine are noted. Otherwise, monitor for the patient's first postoperative voiding to prevent bladder distention. Patients should void within 8 hours of their last voiding. For patients having urinary or gynecological procedures, the patient may need to void within 4 to 6 hours to prevent increased pressure on the surgical site. Catheterization may be necessary if the patient is unable to void. After outpatient surgery, patients may be required to void before being discharged.

If patients report the inability to void, the bladder is palpated for distention or a bladder volume measurement is done, which determines the amount of urine in the bladder. You should be aware that restlessness can be caused by discomfort from a full bladder. A distended bladder requires intervention to empty it. Efforts are made to promote voiding before inserting a urinary catheter because of the risk of infection.

The body's stress response to the surgical experience stimulates the sympathetic nervous system ("fight or flight" response), which saves fluid by reducing urine output. Therefore, initially urine output may be reduced and concentrated. Then it should gradually increase, becoming less concentrated and lighter in color.

NURSING DIAGNOSIS, PLANNING, AND IMPLEMENTATION. Urinary retention related to surgery, pain, anesthesia, altered positioning

EXPECTED OUTCOME: Patient completely and regularly empties her bladder.

- Measure and record output on postoperative patients, especially those undergoing major procedures or urological surgery, older patients, and those with an IV or urinary catheter *to detect urinary elimination problems.*
- Report urinary output less than 30 mL in 1 hour from urinary catheter *as this is minimum acceptable output.*
- Recognize that patients voiding small, frequent amounts (30 to 50 mL every 20 to 30 minutes) or dribble may have retention overflow and may not be emptying their bladder. *This is not normal and may require catheterization to empty the bladder and prevent complications.*
- Patients should be assisted to the bathroom or bedside commode, and men should be allowed to stand or sit to void if possible *to promote voiding.*
- If bedpans are used, they should be warmed *to prevent reflexive sphincter tightening.*
- For patient who is unable to void, techniques to promote voiding should be used before catheterization: running water, pouring warm water over a female patient's perineum, or drinking a hot beverage *may stimulate voiding.*
- Provide privacy after safety is ensured *to promote voiding.*
- Have patients place their feet solidly on the floor *to relax the pelvic muscles to aid voiding.*
- Notify physician if patient is uncomfortable, has a distended bladder, or has not voided within the specified time frame *for treatment orders.*

EVALUATION. The goal for urinary retention is met if the patient is able to void without pain or complications.

Surgical Wound Care   Concern is Bleeding

A wound is a break in the skin. When a wound occurs, it disrupts the integrity of the skin, giving bacteria an entry point into the body. Wounds can be clean or dirty. Clean wounds are surgical wounds that are not infected. Contaminated wounds include accidental wounds or surgical incisions exposed to gastrointestinal (GI) contents or unsterile conditions. Infected wounds and dirty wounds contain microorganisms from trauma, ruptured organs, or infection. Necrotic and infected tissue is removed before infected wounds are closed. This is known as **debridement.**   —Ex. burn patient

An incision is a wound made by a physician with a sharp instrument such as a scalpel. A puncture wound has a small opening and may be made with a scalpel to insert a tube or drain. Incisions are closed with sutures, staples (Fig. 11.12), or surgical glue, which is painless and produces less scarring. As the wound heals, sutures or staples are removed

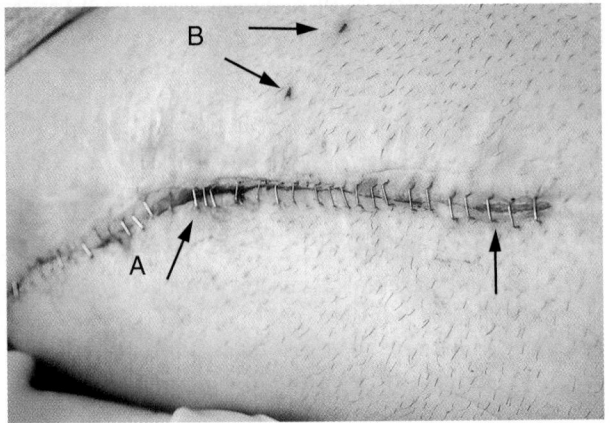

FIGURE 11.12 A stapled incision. *(A)* Note wound edges not approximated at arrows. *(B)* Arrows indicate puncture sites where drains were inserted.

in 7 to 10 days, and Steri-Strips may be applied to continue supporting the wound as it heals.

WOUND HEALING. Wound healing occurs in phases (Table 11.10). Wounds can heal by first intention, second intention, and third intention (Fig. 11.13). The edges of the wound are approximated with staples or sutures with first-intention healing. This usually results in minimal scarring. With healing by second intention, the wound is usually left open and allowed to heal by granulation. Scarring is usually extensive with prolonged healing. With healing by third intention, an infected wound is left open until there is no evidence of infection and the wound is then surgically closed.

WOUND COMPLICATIONS. Wound problems can include hematoma, infection, dehiscence, and **evisceration.** A hematoma occurs from bleeding in the wound and into the tissue around the wound. A clot forms from the bleeding. If the clot is large with swelling, the clot may need to be removed by the physician.

Infected wounds may be warm, reddened, and tender and have **purulent** (pus) drainage. The drainage may have a foul odor. A fever and elevated white blood cell (WBC) count may be present. Antibiotics are used to treat the infection.

Dehiscence and evisceration are serious wound complications (Fig. 11.14). Wound dehiscence is the sudden bursting open of a wound's edges, which may be preceded by an increase in serosanguineous drainage. Evisceration is the viscera spilling out of the abdomen. Dehiscence and evisceration often occur with abdominal incisions in patients who are malnourished, obese, elderly, or who have poor wound healing. Supporting the wound during coughing and other activities that pull on the incision or applying an abdominal binder on patients who are at risk help prevent dehiscence and evisceration. When evisceration occurs, the patient may have pain and vomiting and may report that "something let loose" or "gave way."

If dehiscence or evisceration occurs, place the patient in low Fowler's position with flexed knees. Cover the wound with sterile dressings or towels moistened with warm sterile normal saline. Notify the physician immediately of this surgical emergency. Apply gentle pressure over the wound and keep the patient still and calm. Monitor vital signs for evidence of shock (e.g., tachycardia, tachypnea, dyspnea, hypotension). IV fluids are infused as ordered. Prepare the patient for immediate surgery to close the wound.

For dehisced surgical incisions that resist healing, a newer device, vacuum-assisted closure (VAC), is available to aid in healing the incision. The device can be used on other types of wounds. Wound closure is aided by application of local negative pressure to wound edges by VAC.

ASSESSMENT/DATA COLLECTION. Drains. Drains are inserted into wounds during surgery to prevent accumulation of blood, lymph, or necrotic tissue in wounds that can lead to infection or delayed healing. Drains may work by gravity or suction. Penrose drains are open, soft, flat, rubberlike drains that carry drainage out of the wound. Moderate **serosanguineous** drainage is expected from a Penrose drain and may require frequent dressing changes. Examples of drains that use suction to gently enhance drainage include the Jackson-Pratt, Hemovac, and Mini-Snyder Hemovac. These drains are closed systems that may require periodic emptying and reapplication of the suction by compressing the drain. Output is recorded when the drainage is emptied. The amount of drainage expected varies with the type of surgery. Specialized drainage systems allow the autotransfusion of drainage containing blood back to the patient to maintain hemoglobin levels without the risks associated with blood transfusions, such as transfusion reactions or transmission of infections.

Dressings. Dressings protect the wound, absorb drainage, prevent contamination from body fluids, provide comfort, and apply pressure to reduce swelling or bleeding as in a pressure dressing. The initial dressing is applied in surgery and then is usually removed by the physician approximately 24 hours postoperatively. If drainage appears on the initial

TABLE 11.10   WOUND HEALING PHASES

Phase	Time Frame	Wound Healing	Patient Effect
I	Incision to 2nd postoperative day	Inflammatory response	Fever, malaise
II	Third to 14th postoperative day	Granulation tissue forms	Feeling better
III	3rd to 6th postoperative week	Collagen deposited	Raised scar formed
IV	Months to 1 year	Collagen deposited	Flat, thin scar

---

evisceration: e—out + viscera—body organs

serosanguineous: sero—whey + sanguineous—bloody

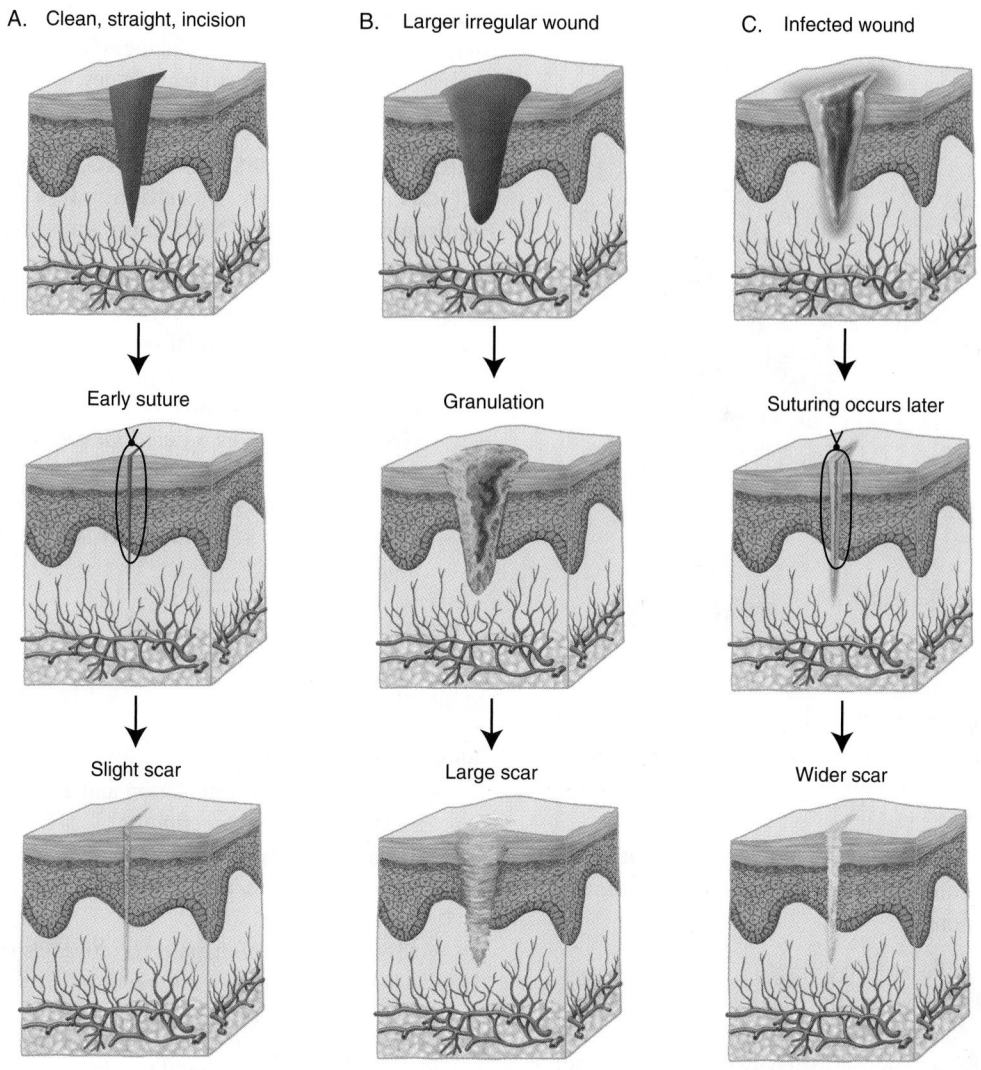

A. Clean, straight, incision
B. Larger irregular wound
C. Infected wound

Early suture
Granulation
Suturing occurs later

Slight scar
Large scar
Wider scar

FIGURE 11.13 Wound Healing. *(A)* Primary intention. Wound healing occurs in a clean wound, such as a surgical wound, whose edges are approximated typically with staples or sutures. Healing occurs quickly with slight scarring. *(B)* Secondary intention. Large irregular or infected wounds are left open to allow healing to occur from the inside out. Pressure ulcers or chronic wounds are often treated this way. Large scarring occurs with lengthy healing time. *(C)* Tertiary intention. Infected or contaminated wound is left open for a brief time period until wound is clean. Granulation tissue fills in for some wound healing and then edges are approximated and closed surgically. Wider scarring occurs.

dressing, reinforce it with another dressing, according to physician orders or institution policy.

After the initial dressing is removed, if the wound is dry and the edges intact (approximated), the physician may not order the dressing to be replaced. This allows easy observation of the wound and avoidance of applying tape to the skin. Draining wounds are dressed with several layers that are changed as needed. When the old dressing is removed, it should be done carefully to prevent dislodging of tubes or drains. The condition of the wound is documented with each dressing change. It is normal for the incision to be puffy and red from the inflammatory response. The surrounding skin should be the patient's normal color and temperature. Correct tape application over the dressing is done by gently laying the tape over the dressing and applying even pressure on each side of the wound. Pressure

should not be applied on top of the wound by pulling on the tape from one side of the wound to the other side.

NURSING DIAGNOSIS, PLANNING, AND IMPLEMENTATION. Impaired skin integrity related to surgical incision

EXPECTED OUTCOME: *Regain skin integrity.*

- Monitor skin color and temperature and report changes.
- Monitor dressings and note drainage color, amount, and consistency. *Surgical wound drainage initially is sanguineous (red) and changes to serosanguineous (pink) and then serous (pale yellow) after a few hours to days.*
- Report drainage that is bright red, remains sanguineous after a few hours, or is profuse promptly

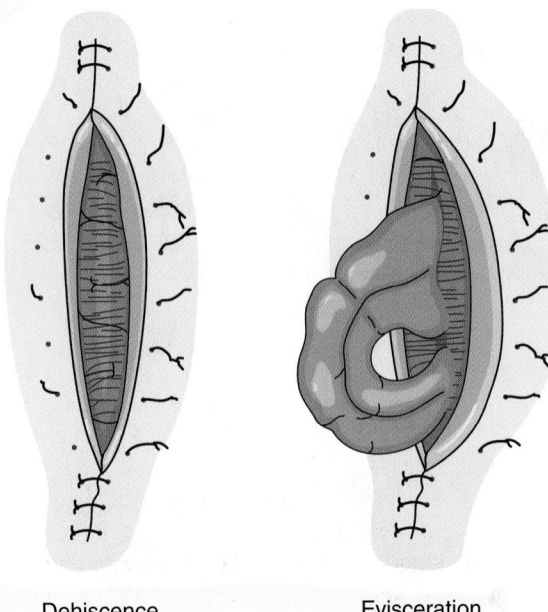

Dehiscence   Evisceration

FIGURE 11.14 *(A)* Wound dehiscence. *(B)* Wound evisceration.

to the physician *because the patient may be hemorrhaging.*

- Use standard precautions when changing dressings *to protect yourself.*

EVALUATION. The goal for impaired skin integrity is met if the patient's wound heals and skin integrity is regained without complications.

Gastrointestinal Function

Nutritional intake and bowel functioning can be affected by surgery and anesthesia. Application of NPO status and undergoing bowel preparation often occur preoperatively. Postoperatively, intestinal handling during surgery, the need to rest the GI tract following a procedure, immobility, lack of peristalsis, and complications such as nausea and vomiting, paralytic ileus (from peristalsis stopping), constipation, or obstruction can interfere with normal GI function.

ASSESSMENT/DATA COLLECTION. Postoperatively, bowel sounds are auscultated every 4 hours. Normally, 5 to 30 bowel sounds are heard per minute. Bowel sounds can be absent, hypoactive, normal, or hyperactive. The abdomen is checked to see if it is soft or firm and flat or distended. When the patient begins passing flatus or stool, document it. Any abnormal findings are reported to the physician.

After abdominal surgery, peristalsis and bowel sounds usually stop for 24 to 72 hours. Flatus is usually absent for 24 to 72 hours postoperatively. Patients do not have bowel movements until peristalsis returns. The patient is kept NPO until flatus and bowel sounds return or as ordered by the physician. The patient's abdominal girth is measured if distention occurs. If a paralytic ileus develops, abdominal distention, absent bowel sounds, and pain may result. As ordered, a nasogastric tube can be used to decompress the GI tract until peristalsis returns. Drainage from the decompression tube is observed for amount, color, and consistency.

Intake and output are measured. Removal of gastric secretions can cause electrolyte imbalances. Signs and symptoms of electrolyte imbalance can include new-onset confusion or weakness, which should be reported.

NURSING DIAGNOSIS, PLANNING, AND IMPLEMENTATION. Imbalanced nutrition: less than body requirements related to NPO, pain, nausea

EXPECTED OUTCOME: *The patient will resume normal dietary intake and maintain weight within normal limits.*

- Maintain IV fluids, total parenteral nutrition, or enteral feedings *until the patient can resume a normal dietary intake* (Box 11.8 Nutrition Notes).
- Give antiemetics as ordered *for nausea and vomiting.*
- Give water and clear liquids at first as ordered, then advance diet to soft and finally solid foods *to promote tolerance.*

Constipation related to decreased peristalsis, immobility, altered diet, narcotic side effect

EXPECTED OUTCOME: *The patient will return to normal bowel elimination patterns and report freedom from gas pains and constipation.*

- Encourage early ambulation and exercise *to promote restoration of GI functioning.*
- If gas pains occur, encourage ambulation, have patient lie prone, and pull the knees up to the chest *to relieve pain.*
- Provide stool softeners or laxatives as ordered.
- Monitor elimination and record.

EVALUATION. The goal for imbalanced nutrition: less than body requirements is met if patients are able to maintain their baseline weight and resume a normal dietary intake. The goal for constipation is met if patients are free from discomfort and establish a regular bowel elimination pattern.

NURSING CARE TIP

Most IV solutions do not provide enough nutrients or calories to prevent malnutrition. The primary purpose of most IV fluids is to provide hydration. A 1000-mL IV solution containing 5% dextrose provides only about 170 calories. This does not meet an adult's daily caloric needs, especially if healing is occurring. You should ensure that early consideration of other nutritional methods is made to meet the patient's dietary needs.

Mobility

ASSESSMENT/DATA COLLECTION. It is important for the patient to move as much as possible to prevent complications and promote healing. Pain, incisions, tubes, drains, dressings, and other equipment may make movement

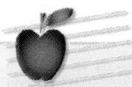

Box 11.8

Nutrition Notes

Nourishing the Postoperative Patient

After surgery, intravenous 5% glucose in water is commonly prescribed. Two liters of this solution contain only 340 calories, which is insufficient to meet the patient's energy needs but enough to prevent ketosis from breakdown of adipose tissue. Previously well-nourished adults generally have nutrient reserves for 3 to 4 days of semistarvation. To prevent excessive muscle protein from being used for energy, adequate nourishment should be delivered to the patient within 3 days. Complete nutrition is available in clear liquid formulations such as Citrotein and Enlive.

To avoid abdominal distension, oral feedings are delayed until peristalsis returns, as evidenced by the patient's passing flatus or the health-care worker's auscultating bowel sounds. Patients usually progress from clear liquids to a regular diet as soon as possible. If "diet as tolerated" is prescribed, the patient should be asked what sounds good. Sometimes a full dinner when the patient doesn't feel well "turns off" the appetite. After gastrointestinal surgery, oral food and fluids are deferred longer than with other surgeries to allow healing. When particular amounts are prescribed, those limits should be strictly implemented to preserve the suture lines. One other precaution is often taken after surgery on the mouth and throat: After tonsillectomy, for example, no red liquids are given so that bleeding can be seen and vomitus is not mistaken for blood.

Specific nutrients necessary for healing are as follows:
- Vitamin C for collagen formation
- Vitamin K for blood clotting
- Zinc for tissue growth, skin integrity, and cell-mediated immunity
- Protein for controlling fluid balance and edema and for manufacturing antibodies and white blood cells, as well as for building scar tissue

difficult. You should determine the patient's ability to move in bed, to get out of bed, and to walk. Pain levels that may interfere with movement are assessed. The patient's tolerance to activity is observed. Understanding of how to perform exercises is noted.

NURSING DIAGNOSIS, PLANNING, AND IMPLEMENTATION. Impaired physical mobility related to surgery, decreased strength, and movement restriction

EXPECTED OUTCOME: The patient's goals are to resume normal physical activity.

- Position patient in bed. Pillows can be used *to support the body in good alignment.*

- Turn at least every 2 hours, alternating from supine to side-to-side if not contraindicated.
- Encourage patients to move themselves *to increase circulation and promote lung expansion.*
- Encourage hourly exercises (deep breathing, range of motion of all joints, and isometric exercises of the abdominal, gluteal, and leg muscles) while awake in bed if ambulation is not possible *to prevent complications.*
- Perform passive joint range of motion *if the patient is unable to do active range of motion.*
- Raise head of the bed slowly *to allow the circulatory system to adjust to the position change.*
- Lower head of bed *if patients report dizziness or feeling faint.*
- Dangle patient on the side of the bed *in preparation for ambulation* (see Fig. 11.10).
- If dangling tolerated, ambulate: Before getting up, patients should pedal their feet to "wake up" the muscles controlling the arteries. To rise, they should keep their eyes forward and move slowly until they feel adjusted to being up. Usually the patient ambulates a short distance the first time and increases the distance as tolerated. One or two health-care workers should assist the patient and use a gait (walking) belt for safety. Walkers with wheels and seats may also be used for support and for resting if the patient becomes dizzy or tired. If patients feel faint or dizzy or their vital signs change, they should be assisted back to bed. A wheelchair may be needed to transport them safely back to their room.

EVALUATION. The goal for impaired physical mobility is met if patients are able to increase ambulation and resume normal activities.

Postoperative Patient Discharge

Discharge planning begins in preadmission testing and continues after admission to ensure that the patient is ready for a timely discharge. When the patient meets discharge criteria, the physician discharges the patient from either the ambulatory setting or the hospital.

Ambulatory Surgery

DISCHARGE CRITERIA. Generally, the patient can be considered a candidate for discharge 1 hour after surgery if clinical discharge criteria or the PACU discharge scoring system are met (see Table 11.9). Clinical discharge criteria include stable vital signs, no bleeding, no nausea or vomiting, and controlled pain that is not severe. Depending on the type of surgical procedure, such as urological, gynecological, or hernia surgery, the patient may be required to void before discharge. The patient should be able to sit up without dizziness before discharge. Patients meeting discharge criteria are discharged by the physician and released to a responsible adult. Patients are not permitted to drive themselves home because of the effects of anesthesia and medications they have received.

DISCHARGE INSTRUCTIONS. Patients and their families are given written discharge instructions before discharge. Elderly patients should have a caregiver participate in the discharge instruction session to understand what observations to make and what to do if complications develop. The instruction form is signed by the patient or an authorized representative to indicate understanding. Prescriptions and a copy of the instructions, to provide a reference for later, are sent with the patient. The patient is encouraged to rest for 24 to 48 hours. The patient is to avoid operating machinery, driving, drinking alcoholic beverages, and making major decisions for 24 hours because the effects of undergoing surgery can alter energy levels and thinking ability. The physician orders any fluid, dietary, activity, or work restrictions.

Patients are taught wound care, medication information (including side effects), and signs and symptoms of complications to report to the physician. Phone numbers for the physician, surgical facility, and emergency care are provided. Patients are informed of the date for their follow up visit to the physician and told to call and make an appointment.

Inpatient Surgery

DISCHARGE CRITERIA. The physician determines the patient's readiness for discharge from the hospital. Postoperative lengths of stay vary based on the surgical procedure and the patient's individual needs. Before discharge, a complete assessment of the patient is performed and documented.

DISCHARGE INSTRUCTIONS. All necessary teaching is completed before discharge (Fig. 11.15). Patients and their families are given prescriptions and a copy of written instructions that are signed by the patient to indicate understanding before discharge. If more teaching or reinforcement is needed, a referral to a home health nurse can be requested.

The physician orders any fluid, dietary, activity, or work restrictions. Patients are taught wound care, medication information (including side effects), and signs and symptoms of complications to report to the physician.

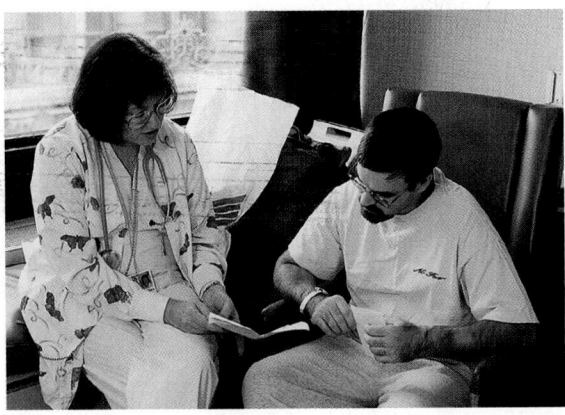

FIGURE 11.15 Nurse providing discharge teaching to patient.

Patients are informed of the date for their follow-up visit to the physician.

Home Health Care

The role of the home health nurse is to assist the patient in the recovery process (Home Health Hints).

A referral to the home health nurse is made when the patient requires the following:

- Continued assistance with skilled nursing interventions, such as wound care, IV medications, or ostomy care
- Additional teaching to be able to perform self-care, such as diabetic teaching for a patient with newly diagnosed diabetes or ostomy care
- Assessment of the recovery process
- Assistance needed because of weakness, lack of social support, or development of complications; care provided in the home is adapted to the patient's resources and environment to facilitate compliance

Home health-care workers can include assistants who help with activities of daily living and household chores, LPNs/LVNs who provide basic nursing care, and registered nurses who perform patient assessments, teaching, and complex nursing care. The frequency of visits is determined by the patient's needs.

Home Health Hints

After a patient comes home from surgery, the home care nurse can help give direction to the family to prepare the room where the patient will be staying:

- It is helpful if the room can be on the same floor with the bathroom, kitchen, and living space.
- If an extended recovery period or illness is expected, the den or living room might be considered as the

primary living space to provide room for equipment and make companionship easier. The patient can see activity in the home and be included in family activity. Also, caregivers can be more attentive to the patient's needs and save countless footsteps.

- Special equipment may be needed, including the following:

- For the patient on bedrest, a hospital bed with full side rails helps with a variety of position changes and better height for the caregiver.
- Draw sheets made of folded twin sheets are needed, as well as extra pillows for positioning.
- A bedside stand is needed for personal and toilet articles.
- A bedside commode can be placed near the bed if the patient cannot walk to the bathroom. A bedpan or urinal may be needed. A functional female urinal is easier to use than a bedpan.
- A flexible tube with a shower head that connects to the bathtub faucet is convenient and allows the patient more independence in bathing.
- Installation of grab bars and tub stools and skid-proofing of a shower or tub are important safety measures to help prevent falls.

- If the patient is eligible for insurance coverage for durable medical equipment, a –physician's order must be obtained.

It is helpful for caregivers to keep a notebook in the hospital and continue it at home. Treatments, medicines, observations, procedures, doctor and nurse visits, instructions, and therapies with dates and times can be recorded. This helps prevent confusion, prepares the next caregiver, and affords better organization of time and resources for everyone. It can also be nice to see who visited the patient.

Families of patients recovering from surgery should provide items to keep the patient occupied and comfortable: talking books, inspirational reading material, pictures, and their favorite pajamas, robe and slippers, and coverlet.

REVIEW QUESTIONS

Multiple response item. Select all that apply.

1. Which of the following nursing actions would reduce surgical risk factors for preoperative patients?
   a. Playing music
   b. Avoiding discussion of fears
   c. Reinforcing pain control methods
   d. Showing use of incentive spirometer
   e. Encouraging smoking cessation 8 hours before surgery

2. Which of the following is the patient care role for the LPN/LVN in the preoperative phase?
   a. Assisting in data collection
   b. Explaining the surgical procedure
   c. Obtaining preoperative orders
   d. Providing informed consent

Multiple response item. Select all that apply.
3. Which of the following is within the LPN/LVN's scope of practice related to the patient providing consent for surgery?
   a. Obtaining informed consent
   b. Providing informed consent
   c. Answering surgical procedure questions
   d. Requesting patient questions be referred to physician
   e. Witnessing the patient's signature on the consent
   f. Reading the consent to a patient prior to signing

4. When teaching the elderly preoperative patient, which of the following is a teaching strategy that improves learning?
   a. Sit near a window with bright sunlight

   b. Use large black-on-white printed materials
   c. Sit beside patient
   d. Use blue and green materials

Multiple response item. Select all that apply.
5. Which of the following interventions would help prevent atelectasis in a postoperative patient?
   a. Coughing and deep breathing
   b. Holding breath while moving
   c. Restricting fluids
   d. Leg exercises
   e. Pain control
   f. Ambulation

6. Which of the following would the nurse evaluate as indicating that the postoperative patient's diet can be resumed, as ordered?
   a. Absence of flatus
   b. Bowel sounds every 8 seconds
   c. Excessive thirst
   d. Absent bowel sounds

7. Which of the following findings would the nurse recognize as being the earliest indicator of hemorrhage or shock that should be reported to the physician?
   a. Tachycardia
   b. Polyuria
   c. Nausea
   d. Fever

8. Which of the following is a criterion the nurse uses to determine patient readiness for discharge from ambulatory surgery?
    a. Ability to drive an automobile
    b. Ability to ambulate 50 feet
    c. Being pain free
    d. Absence of nausea or vomiting

Fill in the blank with the correct answer

9. What is the role of the home health nurse in caring for postoperative patients?

Vitals an help with getting better recovery

References

1. Bruun, LI, et al: Prevalence of malnutrition in surgical patients: Evaluation of nutritional support and documentation. Clin Nutr 18:141, 1999.
2. Kudsk, KA, Tolley EA, DeWitt, RC, et al: Preoperative albumin and surgical site identify surgical risk for major postoperative complications. JPEN J Parenter Enteral Nutr 27:1, 2003.
3. American Society of Anesthesiologists Task Force on Preoperative Fasting: Practice guidelines for preoperative fasting and the use of pharmacologic agents to reduce the risk of pulmonary aspiration: application to healthy patients undergoing elective procedures. Anesthesiology 90:896, 1999.
4. American Society of Anesthesiologists. Anesthesiologists warn: If you're taking herbal products, tell your doctor before surgery. Press release May 26, 1999.
5. JoAnna Briggs Institute: Management of the Day Surgery Patient, Best Practice Supplement 1, 2003, pp 1–4.

SUGGESTED ANSWERS TO

CRITICAL THINKING

■ Mrs. Owens

1. 100 mL per hour. IV pumps are always set to deliver the amount of mililiters per hour. Divide the total volume of 1000 mL × the total time of 10 hours = 100 mL per hour.

2. Intake = 2400 mL.
    To calculate this:
    Remember your conversions:
    30 mL = 1 oz
    1 cup = 8 oz (don't supersize the cup!)
    Calculations:
    1 8-oz ounce cup of coffee = 1 × 8 × 30 = 240 mL
    4 oz orange juice = 4 × 30 = 120 mL
    6 oz of tomato soup = 6 × 30 = 180 mL
    $3/_4$ cup jello = $3/_4$ × 8 × 30 = 180 mL
    2 cups of water = 2 × 8 × 30 = 480 mL
    1200 mL of 0.9 normal saline IV
    The patient's output does not impact the intake total so it is not used for this calculation.

■ Mrs. Wood

1. Moaning occasionally, moving legs restlessly, and pulling covers near abdominal incision are nonverbal pain cues.

2. Document pain levels by actual observations: occasional moaning, restless leg movements, and pulling of covers near abdominal incision. By patient's statement: "It hurts." Because Mrs. Wood is too drowsy to use the pain scale, other data are used. When Mrs. Wood is more awake, explanation of the pain scale should be reinforced and used.

3. Review pain medication orders to determine if analgesics can be given. Noting that an IV analgesic was given 50 minutes ago and the IM analgesic is ordered every 3 hours, you should request that the physician or pharmacist be consulted to determine appropriate time intervals. If the consultation indicates it is time to give the analgesic, verify that vital signs are still stable and then give the analgesic. You should also consider other pain relief measures such as patient warmth, positioning, or environmental issues such as bright lighting, room temperature, and noise.

4. After administration of the analgesic, Mrs. Wood's pain level should be assessed in at least 30 minutes to determine pain relief. If Mrs. Wood is asleep, she should not be awakened unless you determine it is necessary. Nonverbal cues should be observed and respirations counted and documented. If no indication of pain is noted, Mrs. Wood's pain level should be monitored by you at least hourly or as needed.

5. Document pain level on scale of 0 to 10 and have the physician notified of inadequate pain relief. The patient should not have to wait the 3-hour interval in pain. Consider providing other pain relief measures while the physician is being notified.

6. Try unit analysis for solving mathematical calculations. It is easy to understand and our students say it is a great method after they try it.

Unit Analysis Method:

$$\frac{8 \; \text{milligrams} \;|\; 1 \; \text{milliliter}}{|\; 10 \; \text{milligrams}} = \frac{8}{10} = 0.8 \; \text{milliliter}$$

Bibliography

1. Allen, G: Hand hygiene, an essential process in the OR. AORN J 2005 82:561.
2. Hand hygiene guidelines fact sheet: Centers for Disease Control and Prevention, Office of Communication, http://www.cdc.gov/od/oc/media/pressrel/fs021 025.him. Accessed Aug 30, 2005.
3. Barnes, S: Patient preparation: the physical assessment. J Perianesth Nurs 17:1, 2002.
4. Beyea, SC: Antibiotic prophylaxis: What's the fuss? AORN J 82:859–862, 2005.
5. Bond, LM, Flickinger D, Aytes L, et al: Effects of preoperative teaching of the use of a pain scale with patients in the PACU. J Perianesth Nurs 20:333-340, 2005
6. Buss, H, and Melderis, K: PACU pain management algorithm. J Perianesth Nurs 17:1, 2002.
7. Chiravalle, P, McCaffrey, R: Alternative therapy applications for postoperative nausea and vomiting. Holist Nurs Pract 19:207–210, 2005.
8. Dunn. D: Preventing perioperative complications in special populations. Nursing 35:36–43, 2005.
9. Madsen, D, Sebolt T, Cullen L, et al: Listening to bowel sounds: an evidence-based practice project: nurses find that a traditional practice isn't the best indicator of returning gastrointestinal motility in patients who've undergone abdominal surgery. Am J Nurs 105:40–49, 2005.
10. Majasaari, H, Sarajarvi, A, Koskinen, H, et al: Patients' perceptions of emotional support and information provided to family members. AORN J 81:1030–1039, 2005.
11. McNeil, B: Malignant hyperthermia. Br J Perioper Nurs 15:376–377, 379–382, 2005.
12. Power, H: Review: Evidence is lacking that adults given fluids 1.5 to 3 hours preoperatively have greater risks of aspiration or regurgitation than those given a standard fast. Evid Based Nurs 7:44, 2004.
13. Saufl, NM: Preparing the older adult for surgery and anesthesia. J Perianesth Nurs 19:372–378, 2004.
14. Shea, RA, Brooks, JA, Dayhoff, NE, and Keck J: Pain intensity and postoperative pulmonary complications among the elderly after abdominal surgery. Heart Lung 31:440–449, 2002.
15. Wanzer, LJ: Perioperative initiatives for medication safety. AORN J 82:663, 665–666, 2005.
16. Williamson J: Management of postoperative urinary retention. Nurs Times 101:53–54, 2005.

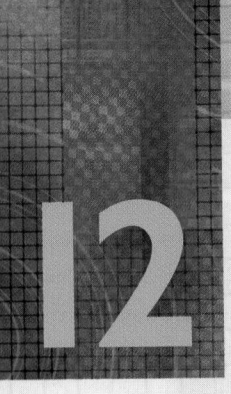

12

Nursing Care of Patients with Emergent Conditions and Disaster/Bioterrorism Response

SUSAN SMITH

KEY TERMS

abrasion (a-BRAY-zhun)
anthrax (an-thur-ax)
amputation (am-pew-TAY-shun)
anaphylactic shock (an-uh-fah-LAK-tik SHAHK)
asphyxia (as-FIX-ee-a)
bioterrorism (bi-o-tear-or-is-um)
botulism (bothch-liz-um)
capillary refill (KAP-ih-lar-ee RE-fill)
cardiac tamponade (KAR-dee-ack tam-pon-AID)
cardiogenic (kar-dee-o-JEN-ick)
distributive (dis-TRIB-u-tive)
flail chest (FLAY-ul chest)
full-thickness burn (FUL-THICK-ness BERN)
gastric lavage (GAS-trick la-VAHJ)
heatstroke (HEET-strohk)
hypovolemic shock (HIGH-poh-voh-LEEM-ik SHAHK)
laceration (lass-ur-A-shun)
obstructive shock (ahb-STRUK-tive SHAHK)
partial-thickness burn (PAR-shul THICK-ness BERN)
plague (play-gah)
shock (SHAHK)
smallpox (small-POX)
tetanus (TET-nus)
triage (TREE-ahj)

QUESTIONS TO GUIDE YOUR READING

1. What are the components of the primary survey?

2. What interventions would you use for a trauma victim?

3. What are the symptoms of inhalation injury?

4. What are the stages of hypothermia and hyperthermia?

5. What are priorities of care for poison overdose?

6. What is your role in crisis situations and psychiatric emergencies?

7. What is your role in identifying a bioterrorist attack or disaster response?

The ability to recognize an emergent condition, prioritize, and provide quick assessments and interventions is essential in nursing. In emergent situations, initial assessment and intervention is guided by the ABCDs of the primary survey. The primary survey of the patient's airway, breathing, and circulation and disability allows recognition, prioritization, and treatment of life-threatening situations. The secondary survey, a rapid head-to-toe assessment, identifies additional serious injuries throughout the body. This chapter presents specific emergent conditions with application of the nursing process.

Upon arrival in the Emergency Department, most patients are triaged by the registered nurse (RN). During the triage process, the RN evaluates the patient's complaint, asks appropriate questions that help to develop a differential diagnosis, and performs a rapid assessment of the patient (Fig. 12.1).

 PRIMARY SURVEY

To recognize life-threatening conditions and determine priorities of care, an initial assessment of the patient's airway, breathing, circulation, and disability is conducted. This process is known as the primary survey. The components of the primary survey are listed in Table 12.1.

A—Airway

The airway is the most important component of the primary survey. The neck should not be hyperextended, flexed, or rotated until spinal injury is ruled out because any movement may worsen an existing cervical spine injury (Fig. 12.2). The airway is inspected for obstruction, including loose teeth, foreign objects, bleeding, and vomitus. Next, any visible airway obstructions are removed using suction.

Airway adjuncts, such as nasopharyngeal or oropharyngeal airways, may be used to keep the airway open.

TABLE 12.1 COMPONENTS OF THE PRIMARY SURVEY

A	Airway
B	Breathing
C	Circulation
D	Disability/Central Nervous System

When additional airway support and mechanical ventilation are required, advanced airway adjuncts, such as endotracheal intubation or cricothyroidotomy, may be performed by specially trained emergency personnel or physicians.

B—Breathing

After the patency of the airway is ensured, the patient is assessed for spontaneous breathing and respiratory rate and depth. The nurse observes whether the patient's chest rises and falls spontaneously and auscultates for breath sounds bilaterally. If the patient is not breathing, interventions are conducted before proceeding. The patient may be ventilated with a mouth-to-face mask or a bag-valve-face mask. Endotracheal intubation is the preferred method of maintaining an airway in an unconscious patient because it ensures airway patency and protects the lungs from aspiration.

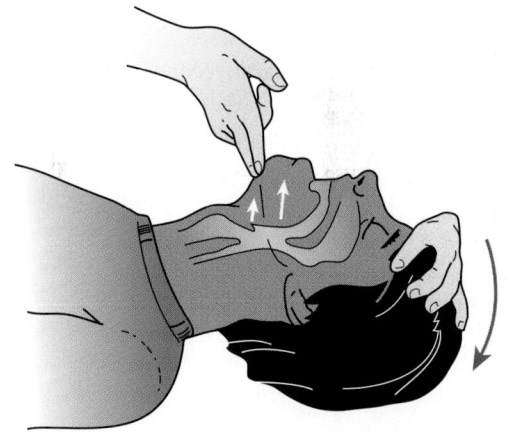

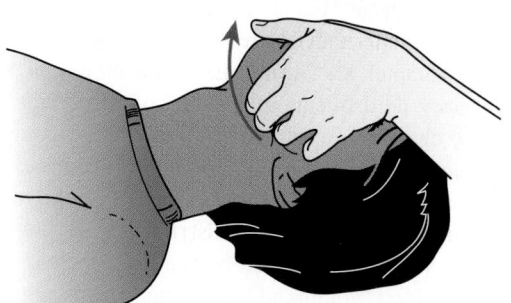

FIGURE 12.2 *(A)* Chin lift maneuver is used to open the airway. *(B)* Jaw thrust maneuver is used to open the airway if the patient may have a head or neck injury.

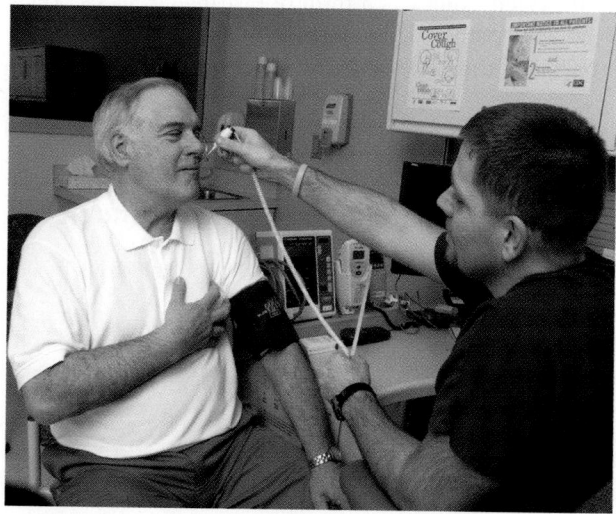

FIGURE 12.1 Triage nurse evaluating patient who has just arrived in emergency room

C—Circulation

The carotid pulse is palpated for quality and rate. The skin is inspected for color and temperature. External bleeding is controlled by external pressure and elevation when possible. Any life-threatening conditions that may compromise circulation are assessed and interventions provided before proceeding. Other conditions that may compromise circulation include internal bleeding, **shock** resulting from hemorrhage, or major burns. Large-gauge intravenous (IV) cannulas (16 or 18 gauge) are initiated for fluid resuscitation. If the patient does not have a pulse, cardiopulmonary resuscitation must be initiated. If a pulse can be palpated, vital signs are taken and recorded.

D—Disability/Central Nervous System

To detect serious central nervous system injury, a brief neurological assessment is conducted to determine the level of consciousness, which may range from alert (A) and responds to verbal stimuli (V) to responds to painful stimuli (P) or unresponsive (U). To assess response to painful stimuli, a painful stimulus is applied, such as rubbing the sternum, pressing a pen against the base of the nail, or applying periorbital pressure. The patient is observed for the response to the pain, and the response is recorded. Movement of all extremities is also assessed.

 SECONDARY SURVEY

For victims of severe trauma, a secondary survey is conducted. This assessment identifies areas of medical or injury problems that are not immediately life threatening but require treatment. Major body areas that may sustain serious injury, such as the head, spine, chest, abdomen, and musculoskeletal system, are quickly examined to detect additional injuries (Table 12.2). To adequately perform a head-to-toe assessment, the patient's clothing is removed. Each major body area is inspected and palpated for deformity, bruising, opens wounds, bleeding, and pain.

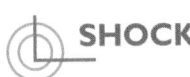 **SHOCK**

Shock is a condition of acute peripheral circulatory failure, causing inadequate and progressively failing tissue perfusion. (See Chapter 8.) During the initial phases of shock, compensatory adjustments allow the body to adapt to the circulatory changes. Eventually, however, these compensatory mechanisms fail and cellular perfusion decreases, causing cell death. There are four types of shock: **hypovolemic, cardiogenic, obstructive,** and **distributive.** Hypovolemic shock signs and symptoms are caused by a decrease in the circulating blood volume. Cardiogenic shock signs and symptoms result from cardiac failure. Obstructive shock caused by a blockage of blood flow in the cardiovascular circuit outside the heart results in signs and symptoms of reduced blood flow and oxygenation. Distributive shock

TABLE 12.2 COMPONENTS OF THE SECONDARY SURVEY

Head	Inspect for lacerations, bleeding from orifices. Check pupil size and response to light. Are pupils equal in size?
Chest	Auscultate for breath sounds in all lung fields. Inspect for lacerations, wounds, foreign bodies.
Abdomen	Auscultate for bowel sounds in all four quadrants. Palpate for areas of tenderness and rigidity. Inspect for lacerations, wounds, foreign bodies.
Extremities	Inspect for lacerations, wounds, and foreign bodies. Inspect for injuries and deformities. Note areas of tenderness. Palpate for pulses. Evaluate temperature and capillary refill and compare the left to the right extremities.

caused by excessive dilation of the venules and arterioles causes signs and symptoms of decreased blood pressure. Therapeutic interventions for shock are listed in Box 12.1 Guiding Principles for Treating Shock.

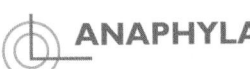 **ANAPHYLAXIS**

Anaphylaxis is a severe allergic reaction. The reaction may occur suddenly after initial contact with an allergen or after any subsequent exposure. Signs and symptoms result from a massive release of chemical mediators from mast cells and basophils throughout the body. Chemical mediators lead to vasodilation and capillary leaking that results in hypotension and eventually vascular collapse. See Box 12.2 Signs and Symptoms of an Allergic Reaction.

Pathophysiology

Anaphylactic shock is a form of distributive shock. There is no loss of blood, but there is excessive vasodilation. Bronchials constrict, and air movement into the lungs

---

Box 12.1

Guiding Principles for Treating Shock

- Maintain an open airway and give oxygen as ordered.
- Control external bleeding by direct pressure.
- Keep the patient supine if possible.
- Accurately record vital signs.
- Give IV fluids as ordered.
- Give the patient nothing to eat or drink until surgery is ruled out.

---

anaphylaxis: an—without + phylaxis—protection

Box 12.2

Signs and Symptoms of an Allergic Reaction

- Generalized itching and burning
- Urticaria (hives)
- Swelling about the lips and tongue
- Dyspnea
- Bronchospasm and wheezing
- Chest tightness and cough
- Anxiety
- Hypotension

becomes increasingly difficult. Increased fluid and mucus are secreted into the bronchial passages. Fluid in the air passages and constricted bronchi cause wheezing. The body is rapidly deprived of needed oxygen by this respiratory system reaction. Signs of severe anaphylaxis include hypotension due to vasodilation, decreased level of consciousness due to decreased oxygenation, and respiratory distress with stridor and cyanosis due to airway constriction and fluid. One of the increasing causes of anaphylactic shock is latex allergy reaction. This type of allergy is on the rise among health-care workers as a result of repeated exposure to health-care products such as latex gloves. Using latex-free products limits exposure and reduces the risk of developing this type of allergy.

Nursing Process for the Patient Experiencing Shock or Anaphylaxis

Assessment/Data Collection

When assessing a patient at risk for shock, be aware of the signs and symptoms common to all types of shock (Box 12.3). It is important to note the patient's initial level of consciousness and monitor the patient for any subsequent changes. A progressive decline in level of consciousness indicates an urgent need for intervention. Pulses indicate the strength of the heart's contractions. Because a pulse is an immediate indicator of the patient's condition, it should be taken frequently during any emergency condition. Changes

Box 12.3

Common Signs and Symptoms of Shock

- Restlessness and anxiety
- Weak, rapid, thready pulse
- Cold and clammy skin
- Pale skin color
- Shallow, rapid, labored breathing
- Gradually and steadily falling blood pressure
- Alteration in consciousness in severe shock state
- Thirst

in blood pressure may also indicate changes in blood volume. Blood pressure changes can occur rapidly but usually not as swiftly as pulse changes.

Skin temperature and color changes may be seen with shock. Severe blood loss activates the "fight-or-flight" response in the sympathetic nervous system, which causes the skin to become cool and clammy. This occurs when peripheral blood vessels constrict to shunt blood to vital organs. Skin color depends on the presence of circulating blood in the vessels of the skin. Pale, white, or ashen skin indicates insufficient circulation. In patients with deeply pigmented skin, color changes may be apparent in the nailbeds, conjunctiva of the eye, or mucous membranes of the mouth.

Capillary refill is checked on nailbeds to evaluate arterial circulation to an extremity. The nailbed is compressed to produce blanching (lighter color change), released, and the seconds counted until color returns to the blanched area. Normally, nail color should return within 3 seconds after the pressure is released. Patients in shock may have delayed or absent capillary refill.

LEARNING TIP

Gently squeeze and release your own nailbed. Do you see the color change? Count the seconds until the color returns. That is your capillary refill time.

Nursing Diagnoses, Planning, and Implementation

Ineffectve tissue perfusion: cerebral and multiple organs related to decreased circulating blood volume secondary to internal and/or external bleeding

EXPECTED OUTCOME: The patient's bleeding will be controlled to maintain vital signs within limits normal for the individual.

- Apply direct pressure to external bleeding site *to stop the flow of blood and allow normal coagulation to occur.*
- Elevate bleeding extremity and combine with direct pressure *to help stop venous bleeding.*
- When direct pressure and elevation do not control hemorrhage, pressure-point control should be attempted (Fig. 12.3). *The chosen artery for pressure-point control must be proximal to the injury site and must be over a bony structure.*
- Monitor vital signs continually, record, and report to the physician *to identify early changes in vital signs indicative of progressing shock.*
- Elevate legs to heart level *to promote venous return to the heart* (contraindicated in cardiogenic shock).
- Use a blanket *to help keep the patient from getting cold; however, the patient also should not be allowed to overheat because this causes peripheral*

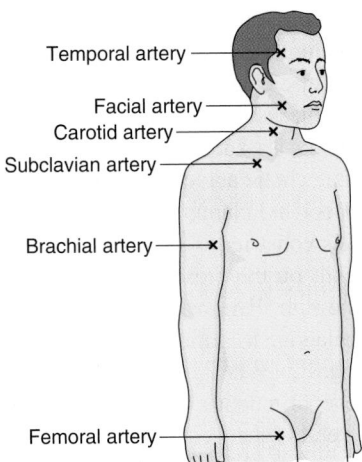

Temporal artery
Facial artery
Carotid artery
Subclavian artery
Brachial artery
Femoral artery

FIGURE 12.3 Arterial pressure points to control bleeding.

blood vessels to dilate, which draws blood away from vital organs.
* Monitor IV fluids as ordered *to increase circulating volume.*

Ineffective breathing pattern related to airway constriction

EXPECTED OUTCOME: The patient will maintain respiratory rate within normal limits and experience improved gas exchange in the lungs and normal arterial blood gases.
* Administer oxygen as ordered using appropriate method which will deliver the maximum amount of oxygen necessary to maintain the pulse oximetry at 92% or greater.
* Administer epinephrine as ordered. *Epinephrine is the drug of choice for treating anaphylaxis and is administered to the adult as a dose of epinephrine 0.2 to 0.5 mg of a 1:1000 solution given subcutaneously. Iinjections can be repeated every 10 to 15 minutes until the desired effect is achieved or significant side effects occur.*
* Give antihistamines as ordered to control the allergic rash and pruritus.
* Steroids are given in gradually tapered doses *to prevent return of symptoms.*

Evaluation

If interventions have been effective, the blood pressure will improve to within normal limits for the individual patient, the patient will demonstrate a strong pulse; warm, dry skin; and be less anxious.

The patient should show an immediate reversal of shock symptoms. Breathing is easy, and blood pressure and pulse return to the normal range. Breath sounds become clear, and hives and pruritus subside.

MAJOR TRAUMA

Major trauma is the fifth leading cause of death in the United States. It mainly affects persons under age 36. Young men

have the highest overall incidence of traumatic injury. Victims of major trauma may receive injury to an isolated vital organ or to multiple body systems.

Mechanism of Injury

When assessing a victim of major trauma, it is important to determine the mechanism of injury (Box 12.4 Geronotological Issues). Injuries are classified as either penetrating or blunt. Penetrating, or open, injuries may be caused by any sharp object, such as broken glass or a knife, or by projectiles traveling at high speed, such as bullets or fragments from an explosion. In blunt, or closed, injuries the skin surface is intact. The injury from blunt trauma usually

---

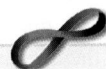

Box 12.4

Gerontological Issues

Injuries and Older Adults

Older adults are at a high risk for falls that put them at risk for bruises, abrasions, cuts, and fractures. Nurses who initially assess older adults with injuries requiring treatment must ask questions and perform assessments that would identify if the patient is a victim of abuse or neglect.

Injuries Caused by Falls Versus Battery or Assault

Any unexplained bruises, burns, abrasions, cuts, fractures, evidence of old injuries or bruises, burns, and cuts that are in different stages of healing suggest abuse. The pattern of an injury can also suggest abuse—for example, cigarette burns in areas covered with clothing; bruises or friction burns in a ring around the neck, ankles, or wrists; welts, burns, or bruises in the outline of a hand or belt buckle; multiple similar injuries in an area, such as whip marks across the buttocks or back of the legs; defensive injury pattern of bruising; and trauma to the hands and forearms.

Injuries related to falls have a predictable injury pattern related to the history and report of the fall. When an older adult falls there is bruising of the hands and knees caused when the person attempts to break the fall. Additional bruising or injuries to the front of the body, arms, and head could be caused by hitting furniture or other items during the fall. Skin tears on the arms are common with a fall. Often, a friend or family member sees the older adult starting to fall and tries to steady the person by grabbing the area, tearing the skin. Ask questions to be sure that the report of the fall incident is consistent with the presenting injuries.

Any form of abuse or suspicion of abuse must be reported to the state agency that investigates reports of suspected abuse. It is not the nurse's responsibility to prove that there has been abuse or neglect, only to report incidents or cases of possible abuse.

extends beyond the point of impact to surrounding and underlying structures. For example, a blow to the chest may cause a fracture of several ribs that in turn may cause blunt trauma (such as a laceration or hematoma) to the spleen.

Damage caused by a gunshot wound and the trajectory of the bullet depends on the projectile mass, the type of tissue struck, the striking velocity, and the range. Entrance wounds are round or oval and may be surrounded by an **abrasion** rim. Powder burns are visible if the firearm was discharged at close range. Documentation of these wounds should include a clear description of their appearance but should not include the words *entry* or *exit*. Patients with gunshot wounds near the level of the diaphragm should be evaluated for both abdominal and thoracic injuries.

Surface Trauma

Surface trauma includes any injury that does not break the skin (closed wound) and any open wound in which the skin surface is broken. Types of closed wounds include contusions (bruising) and hematomas (collection of blood under the skin). Types of open wounds include **abrasions, lacerations,** avulsions, **amputations,** and punctures.

Abrasions are a scratching of the epidermal and dermal layers of the skin. They bleed very little but can be extremely painful because of inflamed nerve endings. Dirt may be ground into abrasions and can increase the risk of infection when large areas of skin are involved.

Puncture wounds result from sharp, narrow objects such as knives, nails, or high-velocity bullets. They can often be deceptive because the entrance wound may be small with little or no bleeding. It is difficult to estimate the extent of damage to underlying organs as a result. Puncture wounds usually do not bleed profusely unless they are located in the chest or abdomen.

Lacerations are open wounds resulting from snagging or tearing of tissue. Skin tissue may be partly or completely torn away. They vary in depth and may be irregular in shape. Lacerations can cause significant bleeding if blood vessels or arteries are involved.

Avulsions involve a full-thickness skin loss in which wound edges cannot be approximated. This type of injury is often seen in machine operators, or in lawn mower and power tool accidents.

An amputation is a partial or complete severing of a body part. In cases of complete amputation, the arteries usually spasm and retract into the tissue, resulting in less bleeding than does a partial amputation, in which the lacerated arteries continue to bleed.

If the patient has sustained an amputation, bleeding is controlled with direct pressure and elevation. A tourniquet is applied only as a last resort. If a tourniquet is necessary, it should be made of wide material such as a blood pressure cuff, which is less damaging to nerves and blood vessels. A dressing is applied to the amputated extremity, which is referred to as the stump. The stump is covered with sterile saline–moistened gauze followed by dry gauze, which is held in place with an elastic bandage for pressure. Amputated parts are taken to the hospital with the patient for possible reattachment. At the hospital, the amputated part is rinsed with saline solution, wrapped in sterile gauze, and placed in a sealed plastic bag, which is then placed in a mixture of ice and ice water.

For a patient with an injury caused by an impaled object, it is imperative that the object not be removed unless it is obstructing the airway. Removing an impaled object may cause additional trauma and uncontrollable internal bleeding. Impaled objects are never cut off, broken off, or shortened unless transportation to the emergency department is otherwise impossible. A bulky dressing is applied around the object to stabilize it and reduce motion.

Tetanus

Tetanus is a disease caused by the bacillus *Clostridium tetani,* which enters the body through an open wound. Tetanus causes seizures, muscle spasms, stiffness of the jaw, coma, and death. Tetanus vaccinations should begin at 2 months of age and be followed by a series of pediatric immunizations until age 15. Thereafter, booster vaccinations are recommended every 10 years in the absence of an open wound.

Head Trauma

Sharp blows to the head can cause shifting of intracranial contents and lead to brain tissue contusion. The pathophysiology of head trauma can be divided into two phases. The first phase is the initial injury that occurs at the time of the accident and cannot be reversed. The second phase involves intracerebral bleeding and edema from the initial injury, which causes increased intracranial pressure (ICP). Management of head trauma is directed at the second phase and involves decreasing ICP. Early and late signs and symptoms are listed in Box 12.5 Signs and Symptoms of Increased Intracranial Pressure.

Box 12.5

Signs and Symptoms of Increased Intracranial Pressure

Early Signs and Symptoms of Increased ICP

- Headache
- Nausea and vomiting
- Amnesia
- Altered level of consciousness
- Changes in speech
- Drowsiness

Late Signs and Symptoms of Increased ICP

- Dilated nonreactive pupils
- Unresponsiveness
- Abnormal posturing
- Widening pulse pressure
- Decreased pulse rate
- Changes in respiratory pattern

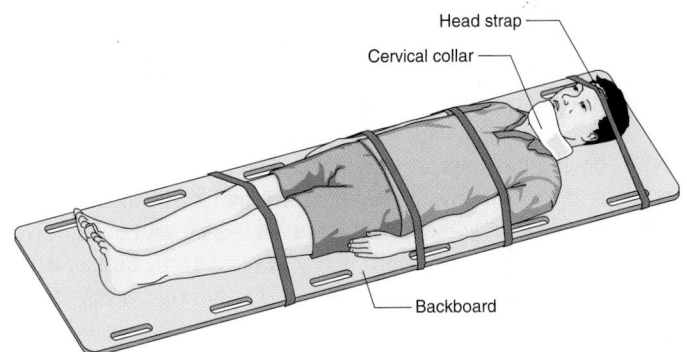

FIGURE 12.4 Immobilization of a patient suspected of having a spinal cord injury using a backboard and cervical collar.

Spinal Trauma

Spinal cord injury most often results from motor vehicle crashes, sports injuries, falls, and assaults, with most cases occurring in men ages 16 to 30. The cervical spine is especially vulnerable to traumatic injury. Patients who have sustained severe multiple injuries should be suspected of having a spinal cord injury, especially when they have signs of head trauma. All trauma patients should be treated as though they have a spinal cord injury until proven otherwise. Moving a patient with a vertebral injury may cause displacement of the injured bones and may increase damage to the spinal cord. Patients should be moved only by qualified people. Stabilization of the neck and back with a cervical collar and backboard is essential until spinal cord injury is ruled out (Fig. 12.4).

SAFETY TIP

Do not move a patient with suspected vertebral or spinal cord injury until sufficient qualified help is available to prevent further injury to the spinal cord.

Chest Trauma

Chest trauma can damage the heart and lungs and cause life-threatening injuries, including pericardial tamponade, hemothorax, tension pneumothorax, and **flail chest**. Potentially life-threatening injuries include pulmonary and myocardial contusion, aortic and tracheobronchial disruption, and diaphragmatic rupture.

Chest trauma can result in laceration of lung tissue and cause a change in the negative intrapleural pressure. Air or blood leaking into the intrapleural space collapses the lung, resulting in a pneumothorax (air) or hemothorax (blood) and ineffective ventilation. In a tension pneumothorax, air is trapped in the pleural space during exhalation, resulting in increased pressure on the unaffected lung. The heart, great vessels, and trachea shift toward the unaffected side of the chest. As a result, blood flow to and from the heart is greatly reduced, causing a decrease in cardiac output. An uncorrected tension pneumothorax is fatal.

Chest trauma can also injure the heart and great vessels

and reduce the amount of circulating blood volume. The heart may be bruised (myocardial contusion) or may sustain direct trauma. **Cardiac tamponade** occurs when blood accumulates in the pericardial sac and increases pressure around the heart. The increased pericardial pressure prevents the heart chambers from filling and contracting effectively. A patient with cardiac tamponade exhibits hypotension, **tachycardia**, and neck vein distention and requires immediate intervention to reduce the pressure in the pericardial sac and restore normal filling and contraction of the heart chambers.

Abdominal Trauma

The organs of the abdomen are vulnerable to injury because there is limited bony protection. Injury to organs such as the spleen and liver, which have a rich blood supply, can result in rapid loss of blood volume and **hypovolemic shock.** Abdominal organs may be injured as a result of severe blunt or penetrating trauma. If hypotension is present, intra-abdominal hemorrhage may exist. If the urinary bladder ruptures, urine leaks into the abdomen and blood may be detected at the urinary meatus or perineum. Penetrating trauma can cause lacerations to abdominal organs, resulting in rapid blood loss and hypovolemic shock.

Orthopedic Trauma

Fractured bones can result in blood loss, compromised circulation, infection, and immobility. Unstable pelvic fractures can cause injury to the genitourinary system or disrupt the veins in the pelvis. Fractures of large bones such as the femur and tibia can cause significant blood loss. For example, a fractured femur can cause up to 1500 mL of blood loss and a fractured tibia or humerus can cause up to 750 mL of blood loss. Joint dislocations can cause neurovascular compromise by applying pressure to the nerves and blood ves-

LEARNING TIP

If an extremity is fractured, splint it as it lies to prevent further damage. If the distal circulation is severely compromised, the patient needs immediate medical intervention.

---

tachycardia: tachy—fast + cardia—heart condition

sels. Delayed fracture reduction (realignment or setting) can cause avascular necrosis, which leads to death of the affected tissue and bone.

Nursing Process for the Patient Experiencing Trauma

Assessment/Data Collection

The mechanism of injury is determined to identify the extent of injury. Loss of consciousness immediately after the injury indicates that a concussion has occurred. The Glasgow Coma Scale (GCS) is used to rate a patient's level of consciousness (Fig. 12.5). The highest score is 15, indicating that the patient is alert and needs only observation. Scores lower than 13 may indicate the need for immediate treatment. Morbidity and mortality are highest for patients with GCS scores of 8 or lower. Pupil size and reaction are monitored and recorded. Dilated or nonreactive pupils indicate increased ICP and a need for immediate intervention.

Spinal nerves are located in the spinal cord and transmit motor and sensory impulses to the body. The higher a traumatic lesion is on the spinal column, the more extensive will be the loss of muscle and sensory function. The patient's muscle functions correlate with the level of spinal injury (Table 12.3). A spinal cord injury at the level of C5 or above interferes with diaphragmatic function and affects respiratory effort, which must be carefully assessed. The patient's level of muscle control and ability to feel each extremity is noted and recorded.

Patients with major chest injuries can have dramatic symptoms. They may exhibit classic signs of shock with

TABLE 12.3 CORRELATING SPINAL INJURY WITH IMPAIRMENT OF MOTOR FUNCTION

Injury Level	Impairment
S3–S5 or above	Patient unable to tighten anus
L4–L5 or above	Patient unable to flex foot and extend toes
L2–L4 or above	Patient unable to extend and flex legs
C5–C7 or above	Patient unable to extend and flex arms

cyanosis, dyspnea, and restlessness. The patient's breathing pattern and effectiveness of respirations are assessed. The rise and fall of the chest is observed, as well as symmetrical chest movement. Any bruising on the chest or upper abdomen is noted. Seat belts and restraint systems can cause significant bruising in high-impact crashes.

Vital signs are taken to detect tachycardia and hypotension from shock. The shape of the abdomen is observed to detect distention from intra-abdominal hemorrhage. Skin color, bruising, open wounds, and penetrating trauma are noted. The abdomen is auscultated for bowel sounds. The perineum is inspected for blood from the urethra.

Vital signs and pain level are assessed to detect orthopedic abnormalities. A respiratory assessment is done to detect a pulmonary embolism as a result of a long bone fracture. The injured extremity is inspected and skin color and capillary refill are noted. Skin integrity, protruding bone, or deformity is noted. Pulses distal to the injury are palpated to assess circulation to the area. Motor function and sensation are assessed to determine the extent of nerve injury.

Nursing Diagnosis, Planning, and Implementation

Acute pain related to tissue trauma

EXPECTED OUTCOME: The patient will experience relief after measures are provided to relieve pain as evidenced by verbal and nonverbal expressions of pain relief.

- Apply ice, elevate, and immobilize the affected area *to decrease swelling and relieve pain.*
- Provide analgesics as ordered *to relieve pain.*

Impaired skin integrity related to trauma

EXPECTED OUTCOME: The patient will demonstrate healing of impaired tissue.

- Apply direct pressure to open wounds *to control bleeding.*
- Irrigate open wounds with sterile saline solution to thoroughly remove dirt and debris and clean exposed tissue *to prevent infection.*

Risk for infection related to tissue trauma

EXPECTED OUTCOME: The patient's wounds will remain free of infection.

GLASGOW COMA SCALE	
Areas of Response	**Points**
Eye Opening	
Eyes open spontaneously	4
Eyes open in response to voice	3
Eyes open in response to pain	2
No eye opening response	1
Best Verbal Response	
Oriented (e.g., to person, place, time)	5
Confused, speaks but is disoriented	4
Inappropriate, but comprehensible words	3
Incomprehensible sounds but no words are spoken	2
None	1
Best Motor Response	
Obeys command to move	6
Localizes painful stimulus	5
Withdraws from painful stimulus	4
Flexion, abnormal decorticate posturing	3
Extension, abnormal decerebrate posturing	2
No movement or posturing	1
Total Possible Points	3–15
Major Head Injury	≤8
Moderate Head Injury	9–12
Minor Head Injury	13–15

FIGURE 12.5 The Glasgow Coma Scale is used to determine level of consciousness.

- With open wounds, give **tetanus** immunization as ordered if it has been more than 5 years since one was last given *to prevent infection.*
- Give antibiotics as ordered *to prevent infection.*

Ineffective tissue perfusion: cerebral, related to cerebral edema

EXPECTED OUTCOME: The patient maintains adequate cerebral homeostasis without cerebral edema as evidenced by a GCS of 14 or greater.

- Give oxygen as ordered *to maintain adequate oxygenation of brain tissues and prevent cellular damage from hypoxia at the cerebral level.*
- If the patient has an altered level of consciousness or deteriorating respiratory effort, anticipate and assist with endotracheal intubation as needed *to provide respiratory support to patient.*
- Elevate the head of the patient's bed 15 to 30 degrees, if possible, *to reduce ICP.*
- Maintain the patient's head position at midline *to ensure unobstructed venous* **drainage** *to help reduce ICP.*
- Maintain intravenous access for fluids to maintain hemodynamic stability and access for medications.
- Monitor mannitol IV, an osmotic diuretic, as ordered *to decrease cerebral edema.*
- If the patient is agitated, calm the patient as *agitation increases ICP.*

Ineffective breathing pattern related to neck injury or unstable chest wall segment or lung collapse

EXPECTED OUTCOME: The patient maintains effective respiratory rate and experiences improved gas exchange in the lungs.

- If the cervical spinal cord has been traumatized, the effectiveness of breathing may be altered. If signs of respiratory distress are present, use the jaw thrust or chin lift maneuver, along with suction and airway adjuncts as needed to maintain patency of the airway.
- Maintain cervical collar and backboard *to prevent further injury.*
- Give oxygen as ordered *to improve tissue oxygenation.* Advanced adjunct airway equipment, including an endotracheal tube, must be readily available.
- Administer supplemental oxygen as ordered *to promote tissue oxygenation.*
- Maintain chest tube drainage system if inserted *to help expand lung.*

Ineffective airway clearance related to neck injury

EXPECTED OUTCOME: The patient will maintain clear lung sounds.

- Suction the oropharynx and nasopharynx *to clear secretions and prevent aspiration of secretions into the airway.*
- If the patient vomits, log roll the patient onto side *to prevent aspiration of emesis.* Use suction as needed.

Impaired physical mobility related to neck injury

EXPECTED OUTCOME: Patient will maintain normal movement of extremities for patient.

- Maintain neck immobility during initial treatment of a patient with head or neck trauma *to prevent serious injury until trauma damage is identified.*

Decreased cardiac output related to compression of heart and great vessels

EXPECTED OUTCOME: The patient will maintain vital signs within baseline limits.

- Report unstable vital signs to physician as *patient may need immediate surgical intervention in the operating room.*
- Explain diagnostic testing to patients with stable vital signs if radiographic studies are ordered *to determine the extent of cardiac or pulmonary injury.*
- Monitor patient's vital signs and oxygen saturation continuously *to detect signs of shock.*

Deficient fluid volume related to hemorrhage or abdominal organ injury

EXPECTED OUTCOME: Patient will maintain vital signs within baseline limits.

- Monitor for signs of shock *to detect hypovolemic shock.*
- Maintain IV fluids as ordered per 18- or 16-gauge IV cannulas *to restore circulating volume.*
- Assist with peritoneal lavage if performed *to detect intra-abdominal hemorrhage.*
- Maintain nasogastric tube if ordered *to decompress the stomach.*
- Cover abdominal wounds with a sterile dressing *to prevent infection.*
- If abdominal organs are exposed, cover with sterile saline-soaked dressings *to prevent tissue necrosis.*
- Assist with blood and blood products administration as ordered per agency policy *to maintain circulating volume and improve tissue oxygenation.*

Impaired physical mobility related to bone injury

EXPECTED OUTCOME: Patient will maintain movement of extremities normal for patient.

- Remove all jewelry before applying a splint *as the extremity may swell after injury.*
- Maintain extremity in splint in the position found unless the distal circulation is severely compromised and keep immobilized if there is severe pain or deformity. *Splinting promotes comfort and prevents further damage to surrounding tissue by preventing movement of broken bone ends.*
- Immobilize the joints above and below the affected area using a folded towel or a pillow *until the patient is evaluated by a physician.*
- Monitor skin color, temperature, distal pulses, capillary refill, movement, and sensation of the extremity after splint application *to detect abnormalities.*

- Elevate and ice extremity *to reduce edema and relieve pain.*

Evaluation

If interventions have been effective the following results will be evident: the patient with trauma reports an acceptable pain level and the patient's wound heals without infection; the patient with spinal injury maintains a regular rate, rhythm, and pattern of breathing, clear lung sounds and maintains intactness of mobility and GCS of 14 to 15; the patient with chest trauma maintains a patent airway and effective breathing pattern; the patient with abdominal trauma has effective circulating volume as evidenced by vital signs within normal limits; patients with orthopedic trauma have strong and palpable pulses, normal blood pressure, normal skin color, skin that is warm and dry, and capillary refill that is less than 3 seconds, pain controlled to a satisfactory level, and normal motor function and sensation in the extremity.

 ## BURNS

The skin protects the body by preventing bacterial or viral invasion, enhancing temperature regulation, and conserving body fluids and electrolytes. These functions are impaired with a burn injury and can lead to multisystem alterations. Burn injuries are acutely painful events that may be dramatic in appearance. Nursing care depends on the extent and depth of the burn injury and the presence of any associated factors such as smoke inhalation, blunt trauma, or fractures. The more extensive the burn injury, the greater the potential for complications and mortality. The patient's age may contribute to the risk of mortality as well. Infants under age 2 and elderly patients over age 60 have the highest mortality rates from major burns. (See Chapter 55 for more on burns.)

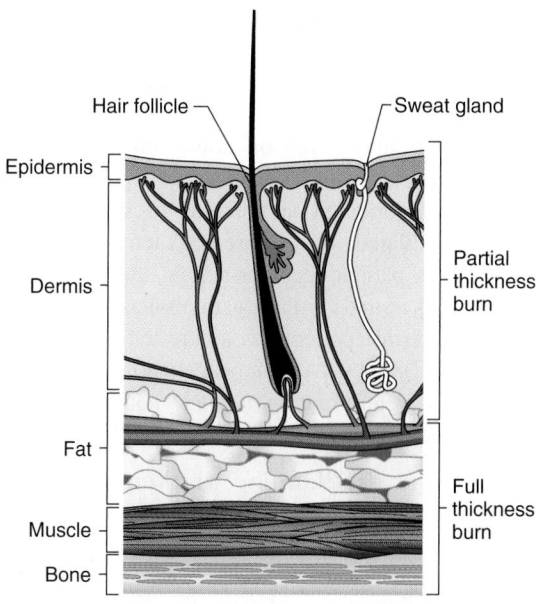

FIGURE 12.6 Partial- and full-thickness burns and structures affected.

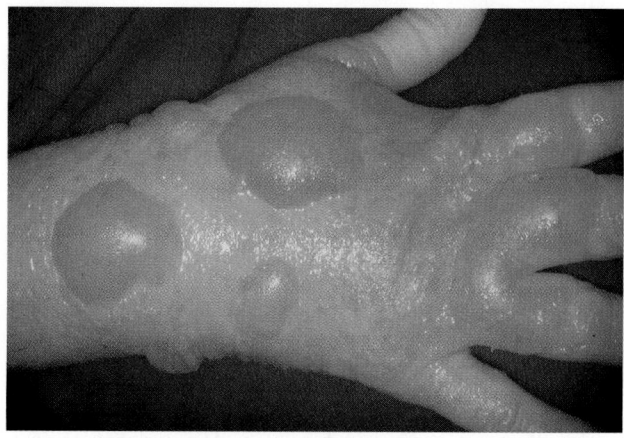

FIGURE 12.7 A blistered partial-thickness thermal burn.

The assessment of the burn patient begins with the ABCDs of the primary survey. The history should include the mechanism and time of the injury and a description of the surrounding environment, including the presence of noxious chemicals and inhalation of smoke in an enclosed space. The greatest threat to life in a patient with a major burn injury is smoke or heat inhalation, which causes edema in the respiratory passages. Continuous assessment of respiratory status is essential when you observe burns or soot on the face, singed nasal hairs, a hoarse voice, coughing, or restlessness.

Burns of the face may swell rapidly and can compromise the airway. Facial burns are treated by elevating the head of the bed to 30 degrees to minimize edema. Oxygen is administered to the patient with potential pulmonary injury. Equipment for endotracheal intubation should be readily available. Because large fluid losses occur in burn injuries, an IV infusion with large-bore cannulas should be started. The patient's weight and the extent of the burn determine fluid resuscitation needs. The patient is kept warm because when skin is lost, a burn victim cannot maintain body heat. IV narcotics are administered for pain.

Burn depth is described as either partial thickness or full thickness (Fig. 12.6). **Partial-thickness burns** are either superficial (epidermis of the skin) or deep (entire epidermal layer and part of the dermis) (Fig. 12.7). **Full-thickness burns** involve all the layers of the skin and the subcutaneous tissue. Partial-thickness burns that involve a small area are cleaned with sterile saline solution, covered with a 1/8-inch layer of an anti-infective cream such as silver sulfadiazine (Silvadene, Flamazine), and covered with dry, bulky, fluffed dressings. Major full-thickness

LEARNING TIP

Over-the-counter ointments, lotions, butter, and antiseptics are never used on a major burn because they may promote infection, retain heat, and cause more pain.

CRITICAL THINKING

Mr. Smith

■ Mr. Smith is a 28-year-old man who was welding close to a natural gas line. The flame of the welder caused the gas line to explode, throwing Mr. Smith 50 feet. He landed on his back. He is brought to the emergency department by the rescue squad. Mr. Smith is awake, alert, and oriented. He has soot around his mouth and nose. He sustained deep partial-thickness burns to his neck, upper chest, and both forearms. He is complaining of pain from his burns and also thoracic back and hip pain. His pulse rate is 100. His blood pressure is 160/90. His respiratory rate is 20.

1. What is the first priority of care for Mr. Smith?
2. Is Mr. Smith at risk for respiratory burns? Why?
3. Are Mr. Smith's vital signs within normal limits?
4. Would wet or dry dressings be preferable for his large areas of deep partial-thickness burns? Why?
5. Mr. Smith is wearing a neck chain and a wedding ring. Should they be removed immediately, or should you wait until Mr. Smith's wife arrives to take them? Why?
6. Mr. Smith continues to complain of hip and back pain. In reviewing his mechanism of injury, what other injuries could Mr. Smith have?

Suggested answers at end of chapter.

TABLE 12.4 DEFINING CHARACTERISTICS AND OUTCOME CRITERIA FOR HYPOTHERMIA

Core Body Temperature	Defining Characteristics
Below 95°F (35°C)	• Skin cold to touch • Lack of coordination • Slurred speech
Below 91.4° F (33°C)	• Cardiac dysrhythmias • Cyanosis
Below 89.6° F (32°C)	• Shivering replaced by muscle rigidity • Hypotension • Dilated pupils
Below 82.4°F (28°C)	• Absent deep tendon reflexes • Hypoventilation (3–4 breaths per minute) • Ventricular fibrillation possible
Below 80.6°F (27°C)	• Coma • Flaccid muscles • Fixed, dilated pupils • Ventricular fibrillation to cardiac standstill • Apnea

Outcome Criteria

• Core body temperature is greater than 95°F (35°C).
• Patient is alert and oriented.
• Cardiac dysrhythmias are absent.
• Acid-base balance is normal.
• Pupils react normally.

wounds are covered with dry, sterile dressings or linen. Patients with major burns are transferred to a specialized burn unit.

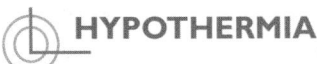

HYPOTHERMIA

Normally the body maintains its temperature in a narrow range on either side of 98.6°F (37°C) to allow chemical reactions to work most efficiently. Body heat escapes to the environment through conduction, convection, radiation, and evaporation. Heat loss is inversely proportional to body size and body fat. Fat insulates because it has less blood flow and consequently has less ability to vasodilate and lose heat.

Hypothermia occurs when the core body temperature falls below 95°F (35°C). As the core temperature falls below 95°F, the body is less able to regulate its temperature and generate body heat, causing progressive loss of body heat to occur.

Nursing Process for the Patient with Hypothermia

Assessment/Data Collection

In cases of mild hypothermia (core temperature between 90°F [32°C] and 95°F [35°C]), the patient is usu-

ally alert, shivering, and may appear clumsy, apathetic, or irritable (Table 12.4). Hypoglycemia can occur because glucose and glycogen stores are depleted by long-term shivering. Respiratory rate, heart rate, and cardiac output decrease.

More severe hypothermia occurs between 85 and 90°F (29.4 and 32.2°C). Shivering stops and muscle activity decreases. Initially, fine muscle coordination ceases. Then, as core body temperature continues to drop, all muscle activity stops and the muscles become rigid. The patient becomes lethargic and less interested in combating the cold environment. The patient's level of consciousness begins to markedly decrease at 89.6°F (32°C); the patient becomes lethargic and disoriented and begins to hallucinate. The pupils become dilated. As the core body temperature falls to 82°F (28°C), the patient becomes apneic, the pulse becomes slower and weaker, and cardiac dysrhythmias occur. The profoundly hypothermic patient has a core temperature of less than 80°F (27°C) and usually appears dead, with no obtainable vital signs. Determination of death should be made only after aggressive core rewarming to at least 90°F (32.2°C).

Nursing Diagnosis, Planning, and Implementation

See Box 12.6 Nursing Care Plan for the Patient with Hypothermia.

Initial treatment of the hypothermic patient consists of rewarming the patient, stabilizing vital functions, and preventing further heat loss. The patient is removed from the cold environment. All wet clothing is removed to prevent

---

Box 12.6   NURSING CARE PLAN for the Patient with Hypothermia

Nursing Diagnosis: Hypothermia related to exposure to cold environment

Expected Outcome Body temperature and vital signs are within normal limits

Evaluation of Outcome Is patient's body temperature greater than 95°F (35°C)? Is patient alert and oriented? Is cardiac rhythm normal?

Intervention	Rationale	Evaluation
Monitor patient's core body temperature.	Abnormal body temperature can be detected and treated.	Is body temperature greater than 95°F (35°C)?
Monitor pulse and electrocardiogram (ECG) rhythm.	Cardiac dysrhythmias may occur at temperatures below 91.4°F (33°C).	Is pulse rate and ECG rhythm normal?
Monitor patient's level of consciousness.	Level of consciousness becomes markedly decreased at temperatures of 32°C (89.6° F).	Is the patient alert?
Institute rewarming passively or actively as ordered.	Rewarming is necessary to return body temperature to desirable range.	Is body core temperature rising to normal range?

---

further heat loss. The patient's core body temperature guides treatment. If the body temperature is above 82.4°F (28°C), passive rewarming is preferred. The room temperature is set to 70 to 75°F (21.1 and 23.8°C). The patient is wrapped in warm, dry blankets. Heat loss from the head is reduced by covering the head with warm towels.

For a patient with a core body temperature below 82.4°F (28°C), active rewarming is needed. A heating blanket (carbon-fiber) and radiant heat lights are used. Warm, humidified oxygen is administered. Warm IV fluids are administered. Body temperature is constantly monitored using a rectal probe. Heated **gastric lavage,** heated peritoneal lavage, or cardiopulmonary bypass may be performed for profound hypothermia. Cardiac drugs are given sparingly because as the body warms, peripheral vasodilation occurs. Drugs that were trapped in the peripheral circulation are then suddenly released during rewarming, leading to a bolus effect that may cause fatal dysrhythmias.

Evaluation

Desired outcome criteria for the patient with hypothermia is a core body temperature higher than 95°F (35°C), no cardiac dysrhythmias, pulse and blood pressure within normal limits, and an alert and oriented status.

FROSTBITE

The extremities are vulnerable to cold injury. Frostnip occurs when exposed parts of the body become very cold but not frozen. This condition usually is not painful. The skin becomes pale and blanched. Contact with a warm object such as someone's hand may be all that is needed to rewarm the part. During rewarming, the affected part may tingle and become red.

Frostbite occurs when body parts become frozen. The extremities are at increased risk because blood shunts away from them to maintain core body temperature. The affected tissue feels hard and frozen. Most frostbitten parts are white, yellow-white, or blue-white. When rewarmed, the skin appears deep red, hot, and dry to touch. The severity of a cold injury is determined by the duration of the exposure, the temperature to which the body part was exposed, and the wind velocity during exposure.

Interventions for frostbite include protecting the affected area from further trauma. To prevent additional damage, the frostbitten part is handled gently and never rubbed. The injured part is loosely covered with a dry, sterile dressing. The patient is not allowed to stand or walk on a frostbitten foot. The affected extremity is elevated to heart level to minimize edema and promote blood flow.

HYPERTHERMIA

Usually the body's heat-regulating mechanisms work very well, allowing people to tolerate significant temperature changes. The body's most efficient mechanisms to decrease body heat are sweating and dilation of blood vessels in the skin. When blood vessels dilate, blood comes to the skin surface to increase the rate of radiation of heat from the body. However, when these mechanisms become overwhelmed, the consequences can be disastrous and irreversible. Those at greatest risk for heat illnesses include children, elderly people, and patients with cardiac disease.

Hyperthermia results when thermoregulation breaks down because of excess heat generation, an inability to dissipate heat, overwhelming environmental heat, or a combination of these factors. Unlike a fever, in which the thermal set point is elevated, in heat illness the thermal set point remains normal and hyperthermia occurs because of an inability to dissipate heat. Antipyretics are of no use in hyperthermia and may contribute to complications.

Nursing Process for the Patient with Hyperthermia

Assessment/Data Collection

Illness from heat exposure can take three forms: heat cramps, heat exhaustion, and **heatstroke** (Box 12.7 Defining Characteristics and Outcome Criteria for Environmental Hyperthermia). As heat illness progresses, circulating blood volume decreases, causing dehydration. Fluid intake is crucial in the prevention of heat illness.

HEAT CRAMPS. Heat cramps, the mildest form of heat illness, involve painful muscle spasms, usually in the legs or abdomen, that occur after strenuous exercise. Large amounts of salt and water can be lost as a result of excessive

sweating, causing stressed muscles to spasm. With adequate rest and fluid replacement, the body adjusts the distribution of electrolytes and the cramps disappear.

HEAT EXHAUSTION. Heat exhaustion occurs when the body loses so much water and electrolytes through heavy sweating that hypovolemia occurs. Heat exhaustion is largely a manifestation of the strain placed on the cardiovascular system attempting to maintain normothermia. Cerebral function is unimpaired, although the patient may show minor irritability and poor judgment. The ability to sweat remains. The skin is usually cold and clammy and the face gray. Sodium and water loss cause the patient to become dehydrated. The body temperature is usually normal or slightly elevated: from 100.4 to 102.2°F (38 to 39°C). The patient may complain of feeling dizzy, weak, or faint, with nausea or a headache. Vomiting and diarrhea may also be present.

HEATSTROKE. If symptoms of heat exhaustion are not treated, heatstroke can develop. Altered mental status and an inability to sweat are key symptoms in heatstroke. Some patients show confusion, irrational behavior, or psychosis; others develop seizures or go into a coma. Because the sweating mechanism has been overwhelmed, many heatstroke victims have hot, dry, flushed skin. The body temperature rises rapidly to 106°F (41°C) or more, and the patient's level of consciousness decreases. If heatstroke is not treated, death results.

Patients suffering from heatstroke are admitted to the intensive care unit because late complications can appear suddenly and require immediate management. Relatively common occurrences include seizures, cerebral ischemia, renal failure, late cardiac decompensation, and gastrointestinal bleeding. Long-term prognosis is variable, depending on the patient's previous state of health and length of time under heat stress.

Nursing Diagnosis, Planning, and Implementation
Hyperthermia related to exposure to hot environment

EXPECTED OUTCOME: The patient will maintain body temperature within normal limits.

- For heat cramps, remove the patient from the hot environment *to allow cooling to begin.*
- Have patient sit or lie down until muscle cramps subside *to prevent further injury.*
- Remove patient from the hot environment, undress patient to allow patient to cool. *Emergency treatment of heatstroke consists of reducing the body temperature and rapidly cooling the victim.*
- Use tepid water as a mist spray over the patient, with a strong continual breeze from electric fans *as evaporative cooling is the most efficient method of cooling.*

Deficient fluid volume related to hypervolemia

EXPECTED OUTCOME: The patient will maintain blood pressure within normal limits of baseline.

Box 12.7

Defining Characteristics and Outcome Criteria for Environmental Hyperthermia

Defining Characteristics

Early signs:
- Core body temperature 100.4 to 102.2°F (38 to 39°C)
- Diaphoresis
- Cool, clammy skin
- Dizziness
- Pulse rate >100

Late signs:
- Increasing body core temperature of 106°F (41°C) or more
- Hot, dry, flushed skin
- Altered mental status
- Coma or seizures possible
- Hypotension

Outcome Criteria
- Core body temperature less than 101°F (38.3°C)
- Patient alert and oriented
- Skin warm and dry to touch

- Give patient oral fluids or water or a diluted (half-strength) balanced electrolyte solution if patient is fully alert *to replace lost fluids.*
- Maintain IV fluids as ordered *to restore volume if patient is hypotensive.*

Evaluation

Interventions have been successful if the hyperthermic patient has a core body temperature below 101°F (38.3°C), warm and dry skin, a strong pulse, blood pressure within normal limits, and is alert and oriented.

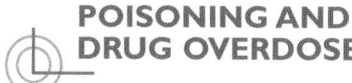

POISONING AND DRUG OVERDOSE

Poisons are introduced into the body by ingestion, inhalation, injection, absorption, or venomous bites. Poisons act by changing cellular metabolism, causing damage to structures, or disturbing function. Many toxins and poisons alter the patient's mental status, making it difficult to obtain an accurate history.

Nursing Process for the Patient with Ingested Poisoning

Assessment/Data Collection

The primary nursing responsibility is to recognize that a poisoning has occurred and then attempt to determine the nature of the poison. The method of exposure is established so that removal or interruption of the toxin can begin. Most ingested poisons are drugs, but about one-third of poisonings are caused by cleaners, soaps, insecticides, acids, or alkalis. Many household plants are poisonous if they are accidentally ingested. Some plants cause local irritation of the skin, and others can affect the circulatory system, gastrointestinal tract, or central nervous system.

Empty medication bottles, scattered pills, or chemicals should be examined by emergency medical personnel at the scene to help establish the identity of the substance. The patient's physical appearance may also give a clue to the type of substance taken. Intravenous needle tracks, burns, erythema, and flushed skin may help identify the poison or toxic exposure. Poison control centers have access to information concerning virtually all poisonous substances, available antidotes, and appropriate emergency treatment.

Nursing Diagnosis, Planning, and Implementation

Risk for injury related to absorption of poisoning agent

EXPECTED OUTCOME: The patient will maintain normal vital signs and be free of injury.

- Administer syrup of ipecac (usual dose of syrup of ipecac is 15 mL for children ages 1 to 5 years and 30 mL for ages 6 years and up) as ordered if patient is fully alert and ingested substance is nonerosive and not petroleum based. Follow with several glasses of water. *Treatment for ingested poisons*

includes rapid removal of poison (vomiting usually occurs within 30 minutes) from gastrointestinal tract with dilution of any remaining poison.

- Repeat syrup of ipecac dose once as ordered *if vomiting does not occur after 30 minutes.*
- Assist with gastric lavage *if indicated to flush ingested poisons from the stomach:* large gastric tube inserted via nose or mouth into patient's stomach; water instilled via tube in 60-mL amounts and withdrawn to evacuate any remaining poison; repeated until 2 L of water has been lavaged or until the gastric return is clear of any pill fragments or substance. Activated charcoal with sorbitol is given *to absorb toxins and facilitate rapid transit of the poison through the intestinal tract.*

LEARNING TIP

Sorbitol and charcoal will cause the patient to have black diarrheal stools.

Evaluation

Interventions have been successful if the patient remains free from injury and has vital signs within normal limits.

Inhaled Poisons

Inhaled poisons include natural gas, pesticides, carbon monoxide, chlorine, and other gases. Carbon monoxide is odorless and can produce profound hypoxia by combining with hemoglobin molecules (and displacing oxygen) in red blood cells. The patient's carboxyhemoglobin levels are monitored to direct appropriate therapy. Inhalation of chlorine is very irritating to the respiratory system and can produce airway obstruction and pulmonary edema.

When an inhalation injury occurs, the patient must be moved into fresh air and away from the toxin. Supplemental oxygen is given as ordered. A patient exposed to prolonged inhalation of a poison may experience lung damage. Respiratory status must be closely monitored to detect complications.

Injected Poisons

Injected poisons pose compelling problems because they are difficult to remove or dilute. Usually they result from drug overdose, but they can also result from the bites and stings of insects or animals. Local swelling and tissue destruction may occur at the injection site. All jewelry is removed because swelling may occur. A cold pack is applied to decrease local pain and swelling around the injection site. The identity of the injected drug or toxin must be established so that adverse effects can be anticipated and managed.

Insects

Insect stings or bites cause anaphylaxis in a small percentage of people; however, symptoms are typically limited to localized pain, swelling, heat, and redness. Potentially dangerous stings or bites may come from bees, wasps, yellow jackets, hornets, certain ants, scorpions, and some spiders. Treatment involves applying ice to the site and elevating the affected part. Cellulitis can occur hours later and may require medical treatment.

When a patient has sustained a bee or wasp sting, examine the area for the stinger and remove it by gently scraping it off the skin. Tweezers or forceps are not used to remove the stinger because squeezing the stinger can inject more venom into the patient. Placing ice over the injury site may help slow the rate of toxin absorption.

Two types of spiders—the black widow and the brown recluse—can inflict serious and sometimes life-threatening bites. Both species are found throughout the United States. Antivenin for treating the toxic effects of both is available. Black widow spiders are glossy black and have a distinctive, bright red-orange marking in the shape of an hourglass on the abdomen. They are found in dry, dim places around buildings, in woodpiles, and among debris. Their venom is neurotoxic and causes systemic symptoms, including cramping of large muscle groups, dyspnea, weakness, sweating, nausea, vomiting, and rash. Death is uncommon, and symptoms generally subside in 48 hours.

The brown recluse spider is dull brown and has a dark violin-shaped mark on its back. It tends to live in dark areas, under rocks, in woodpiles, and in old abandoned buildings. The venom of the brown recluse causes severe local tissue damage. The area becomes red, swollen, and tender and develops a pale, mottled, cyanotic center. A large ulcer can develop within 48 hours if not treated promptly. Systemic symptoms include fever, chills, nausea, vomiting, arthralgia, and weakness.

Snakebites

Only a small percentage of snakebites are caused by poisonous snakes. The most prevalent poisonous snakes are the coral snake and the pit vipers, which include rattlesnakes, copperheads, and cottonmouth moccasins. Envenomation occurs when the snake's hollow fangs puncture the skin and inject venom, which is stored in sacs located at the back of the snake's head. A poisonous snakebite has two small puncture wounds with surrounding discoloration, swelling, and pain. Envenomation by any of the pit viper snakes produces burning pain at the site of the injury. Swelling and discoloration occur within 5 to 10 minutes after the bite.

Interventions are focused on decreasing the circulation of venom throughout the patient's system by keeping the patient calm and immobilizing the affected part. Venous tourniquets placed above and below the fang marks help limit the spread of venom through the veins of the extremity. The tourniquets should not stop arterial flow. The patient's pulse should be palpable below the tourniquets after they are applied. The site of the bite is cleaned with soap and water. The patient is kept calm until antivenin can be given. Medical treatment of the patient with a poisonous snake bite should be directed by an experienced toxicologist.

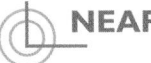

NEAR-DROWNING

Drowning is death from **asphyxia** after submersion in water. Near-drowning is submersion with at least temporary survival of the victim. Life-threatening complications of near-drowning are respiratory failure and ischemic neurological injury from hypoxia and acidosis. When submersion occurs, conscious victims hold their breath until reflex inspiratory efforts override breath holding. As water is aspirated, laryngospasm occurs, producing severe hypoxia. In wet drowning, the laryngospasm is less prolonged and fluid enters the lungs after the vocal cords relax. In dry drowning, cold water causes laryngospasm and vagal stimulation which leads to asphyxiation. Most successfully resuscitated victims experience dry drowning. Risk factors for drowning include inability to swim, diving accidents, use of alcohol and drugs prior to swimming, exhaustion, and hypothermia.

If a person survives submersion, acute respiratory failure may follow. The incidence of serious pulmonary complications is high in this group. Symptoms of impaired gas exchange (known as secondary near-drowning) may be delayed as long as 72 hours after the incident. Contaminants in the water can irritate the pulmonary system and cause inflammatory reactions and impaired surfactant functioning. Metabolic acidosis is usually present, leading to tissue anoxia and dysrhythmias.

Aggressive resuscitative efforts should be used on victims of cold water drowning when submersion time is 1 hour or less. Hypothermia can decrease the metabolic needs of the brain and contribute to neurological recovery after prolonged submersion.

Nursing Process for the Near-Drowning Patient

Assessment/Data Collection

Most near-drowning victims exhibit mild dyspnea, death-like appearance with blue or gray skin color, apnea or **tachypnea**, hypotension, slow heart rate (may be as low as less than 10 beats per minutes), cold skin temperature, dilated pupils, hypothermia, and vomiting. Vital signs are assessed to detect abnormal readings. Respiratory rate and pattern are observed. Any dyspnea or signs of airway obstruction are noted. Skin color or cyanosis is noted. The patient's level of consciousness may be altered due to anoxia.

Nursing Diagnosis, Planning, and Implementation
Ineffective tissue perfusion related to severe anoxia

EXPECTED OUTCOME: The patient will maintain level of

---

tachypnea: tachy—fast + pnea—breathing

consciousness and vital signs within normal range, with clear breath sounds that are equal bilaterally.

- Conduct ABCDs of the primary survey, *which always begin resuscitative efforts.*
- Give supplemental oxygen as ordered *to increase tissue oxygenation.*
- Ensure that adjunct airway equipment is available. *Endotracheal intubation and insertion of a nasogastric tube to decompress the stomach may be needed.*

Evaluation

Factors that influence the outcome of near-drowning include the temperature of the water, length of time submerged, cleanliness of the water, and age of the victim. The younger the patient, the better the chance of survival. Interventions have been successful if the patient has normal respiratory rate and pattern and vital signs, is alert and oriented, and skin that is warm and dry to touch with capillary refill of less than 3 seconds.

 ## PSYCHIATRIC EMERGENCIES

A psychiatric emergency exists when people no longer possess the coping skills necessary to maintain their usual level of functioning. The patient's moods, thoughts, or actions may be so disordered that the patient has the potential to endanger or harm self or others if the situation is not quickly controlled. If acute psychiatric episodes are not managed, they can result in life-threatening, suicidal, violent, or psychologically damaging behavior. If an emotional trauma is not managed successfully, a condition known as posttraumatic stress disorder may result in which tension, anxiety, guilt, and fear concerning the traumatic event produce cognitive, affective, and behavioral responses to memories of the event long after the event has passed.

A crisis occurs when people enter a sudden state of emotional turmoil and are unable to resolve the situation with their own resources. Common emotional or behavioral manifestations of psychiatric crises include responses to stressful events, anxiety, depression, psychosis, and mania. Anxiety may range in severity from mild to panic. Panic evolves into complete disorganization and loss of control. The patient in panic is terrified and needs external controls to avoid harm. Depression is an affective disorder most commonly characterized by physical ailments and somatizations. Antidepressants are used to restore the balance of brain neurochemicals and diminish the symptoms of depression. Psychotic patients experience impaired thought processes and thought content characterized by hallucinations, delusions, ideas of reference, thought broadcasting, and thought insertion. Psychotic thinking and abnormal speech patterns interfere with the patient's attempt to communicate rationally. Manic behavior is most commonly the result of manic-depressive (bipolar) disorder. Manic persons typically exhibit bizarre, extreme, and hyperactive behaviors. Manic persons are also at high risk for injuring themselves or others.

Nursing Process for the Patient with a Psychiatric Emergency

Assessment/Data Collection

Causes of psychiatric emergency symptoms are varied and require thorough assessment of the patient's history and mental status. Information from the patient's medical history may produce possible organic causes contributing to the patient's presenting symptoms. Endocrine dysfunction, electrolyte abnormalities, and head trauma are examples of medical conditions that may cause changes in mental status. A medication history is obtained to determine compliance with medication regimens and any recent changes in medications. Information regarding recent use of alcohol or illicit drugs should be obtained because these substances can heighten psychiatric emergencies. A brief mental status examination is conducted. An assessment of the person's suicide risk is very important. The patient's appearance, behavior, cognitive function, thought content, and thought processes are noted. The nurse determines whether the patient is having problems concentrating, following instructions, or recalling his or her medical history.

Nursing Diagnosis, Planning, and Implementation
Anxiety related to situational stress

EXPECTED OUTCOME: The patient will state reduced anxiety.
- Establish an atmosphere of trust *so the patient feels free to discuss problems.*
- Use active listening *to acknowledge patient's physical and emotional concerns.*
- Speak directly and truthfully to the patient; do not promise unachievable things *to gain patient trust.*
- Trusted supportive members of the patient's family may be involved *to calm the person and encourage cooperation.*
- Do not allow bystanders or adversive family members to visit patient *who could create further upset for the patient.*
- Show respect for the patient *by not laughing or joking.*
- Correct misconceptions, but not in an argumentative manner.

Risk for injury related to impaired judgment
EXPECTED OUTCOME: The patient will remain free from injury.
- Do not threaten, challenge, or argue with a disturbed patient *to prevent injury.*
- Ensure environment is made safe, and external sources of stimulation are reduced *to prevent injury.*
- Be firm but unthreatening *to keep patient safe.*
- Administer antipsychotic medications as ordered and monitor their effect.
- Follow agency policy for use of physical restraint as necessary and ordered. *Restraints should only be used to ensure patient safety with physician order.*
- Document need for restraints and monitor patient and check pulses and capillary refill after restraints

applied. *Restraints must not cause patient harm or restrict circulation.*

- Administer haloperidol (Haldol) as ordered *if patient requires rapid tranquilization.*

Evaluation

Interventions are successful if the patient reports reduced anxiety and remains free from injury.

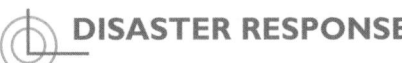

DISASTER RESPONSE

Disaster is defined as any event that overwhelms existing personnel, facilities, equipment, and capabilities of a responding agency, institution, or community. Potential sources of disaster include internal events such as fires and explosions; external events such as floods, storms, fires, earthquakes, and tornados; and created events such as motor vehicle accidents, plane crashes, and acts of terrorism.

External disasters involve a communitywide response of several different agencies, including emergency medical system (EMS) providers, fire agencies, law enforcement, and hospitals. These agencies work together to coordinate search, rescue, transportation, communication, and treatment of multiple victims. Hospitals serve as the major treatment area for victims of a disaster, referred to as casualties. When a disaster occurs, the hospital activates its disaster plan, which outlines specific duties for each nursing unit and the staff for each nonnursing department as well. Typically, each nursing unit prepares for the influx of casualties by calling all available off-duty staff to report to work and by discharging noncritical patients. In a hospital disaster plan, each nursing unit is usually designated to receive specific types of casualties, such as major trauma, burns, medical, pediatric, or psychiatric. The emergency department serves as the **triage** and stabilization area for the casualties. To facilitate the triage (sorting for the purpose of assigning priorities), stabilization, and transportation of numerous causalities, additional emergency department staff may be called in to work. In addition, the hospital disaster plan may require assigning one or more staff from each nursing unit and each nonnursing department to a specific area or task within the emergency department, such as triage, first aid, critical care, burn treatment area, family room, or transportation.

During a disaster, decision making and prioritization of patient care are guided by the resources and personnel available. Patients who are seriously injured and have the greatest chance of full recovery are treated first. Each hospital, as well as each agency involved in responding to a disaster, follows a disaster response plan that outlines the roles and responsibilities of the agency staff and the procedures to follow when interacting with the media, families, other agencies, and casualties. Disaster drills are conducted on a regular basis to evaluate and rework plans. You should be familiar with your agency's disaster plans and policies and know your role and responsibilities in a disaster.

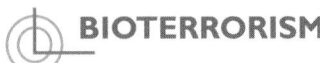

BIOTERRORISM

Well before the 2001 anthrax outbreak, public health and government leaders in the United States recognized the need for increased preparedness to detect and respond to acts of biologic terrorism. The response to a **bioterrorism** attack is in many ways the same as the response to naturally occurring outbreaks of communicable disease. Both situations typically require early identification of ill or exposed persons, rapid implementation of preventive therapy, special infection control considerations, and collaboration or communication with the public health system.

During both bioterrorism attacks and naturally occurring outbreaks, nurses are faced with the challenge of identifying the disease in persons who are worried about potential exposure or who are ill with signs and symptoms similar to those of the outbreak disease. The nurse must have knowledge of the modes of transmission, incubation periods, and communicable periods of these diseases, as well as skill in both clinical evaluation and eliciting an appropriate and thorough history, including relevant occupational, social, and travel information.

Recognition of Potential Bioterrorism Agents

The Centers for Disease Control and Prevention (CDC) evaluates bacteria, viruses, and toxins thought to pose the greatest risk for use in a bioterrorist attack (see http://www. bt.cdc.gov/). Category A agents are thought to pose the highest immediate risk for use as biological weapons; and category B agents, the second highest risk. Category C agents are emerging threat risk agents that pose a potential, but not immediate, risk for use as biological weapons.

As in naturally occurring outbreaks, early recognition of a bioterrorist attack is critical for rapid implementation of preventive measures and treatment. Early recognition can be challenging, however, because patients presenting for medical care after exposure to a biological agent may initially exhibit nonspecific symptoms. One of the most important lessons learned from the 2001 anthrax attack was that clinical illness caused by agents prepared as biological weapons may differ from typical natural infections.

Smallpox/Variola Major

Smallpox is caused by the variola virus, an orthopoxvirus unique to humans. This virus is not known to be transmitted by animals or insects. Smallpox was declared eradicated in 1980, 3 years after the last naturally occurring case was reported. Smallpox is stable and highly infectious in the aerosol form. The risk for a smallpox attack currently is considered low but not zero.

Classification/Variola Major

Smallpox has an average fatality rate of 30%. The incubation period is 7 to 17 days. Symptoms of the initial phase include the acute onset of high fever, malaise, headache, backache, and prostration. Other prominent symptoms include vomiting and abdominal pain.

The characteristic rash occurs 2 to 3 days later, appearing first on the face and forearms. The rash progresses slowly, from macules to papules to vesicles and pustules and finally to scabs, with each stage lasting 1 to 2 days. The lesions are firm, discrete vesicles or pustules (4 to 6 mm in diameter) deeply embedded in the dermis. The patient remains febrile throughout the evolution of the rash, which may become painful as pustules enlarge. A second fever spike 5 to 8 days after onset of the rash may signify a secondary bacterial infection.

Pustules remain for 5 to 8 days, after which crusting occurs. They are more concentrated on the face and distal extremities than on the trunk, and may involve the palms and soles. Scarring occurs with scab separation from destruction of sebaceous glands.

Complications of smallpox include fluid and electrolyte disturbances, extensive skin loss that resembles burns, bronchitis and pneumonitis, blindness from infection of the eye, arthritis, and encephalitis.

Diagnosis

A suspected case of smallpox is a public health emergency. Local and state health authorities, the hospital epidemiologist, and other members of a hospital response team for biological emergencies should be notified immediately.

The differential diagnosis of smallpox includes other illnesses that can cause fever and a rash. Severe varicella (chickenpox) is the disease most likely to be confused with smallpox. However, familiarity with the clinical features of the two diseases, particularly the rash, should help differentiate them. Additional information that may be useful in differentiating smallpox from chickenpox includes a history of exposure to persons with chickenpox, a personal history of chickenpox, a history of vaccination against varicella or smallpox, and the clinical course of illness.

Infection Control and Postexposure Isolation

In the event of a limited outbreak, patients should be admitted to the hospital and confined to rooms that are under negative atmospheric pressure and equipped with high-efficiency particulate air (HEPA) filtration. Standard, contact, and airborne precautions, including use of gloves, gowns, and masks, should be strictly observed. Unvaccinated personnel caring for patients suspected of having smallpox should wear fit-tested N95 or higher quality respirators. Patients should wear a surgical mask and be wrapped in a gown or sheet to cover the rash when they are not in a negative-airflow room. All laundry and waste should be placed in biohazard bags and autoclaved before being laundered or incinerated. Surfaces that may be contaminated with smallpox virus can be decontaminated with disinfectants that are used for standard hospital infection control, such as hypochlorite and quaternary ammonia.

Anthrax

Anthrax is a disease caused by the spore-forming bacterium *Bacillus anthracis*. The organism is found worldwide in soil. Animals become infected through grazing in contaminated areas. Under natural conditions, humans contract the disease after close contact with infected animals or contaminated animal products such as hides, wool, or meat. On exposure to tissues or blood of an animal or an infected human, the spores germinate.

Classification and Epidemiology

Anthrax occurs in three clinical forms in humans: inhalational, cutaneous, and gastrointestinal. In a biological attack, aerosol exposure to anthrax spores would be most likely. Before 2001, exposure to powdered anthrax spores in an envelope or package was not thought to be an efficient means of causing inhalational disease. However, exposure to anthrax spores sent through the U.S. mail in the 2001 anthrax attack resulted in cases of inhalational anthrax and cutaneous disease.

Cutaneous anthrax is the most likely way to develop anthrax. It results from inoculation of spores subcutaneously through a cut or abrasion. Gastrointestinal and oropharyngeal anthrax occur in rural parts of the world where anthrax is endemic. They result from ingestion of meat contaminated with spores.

Inhalational Anthrax

CLINICAL PRESENTATION AND DIAGNOSIS. Clinical symptoms develop rapidly after germination of anthrax spores. The incubation period for inhalational disease is most commonly reported as 1 to 6 days but may be prolonged by antibiotic administration.

Inhalational anthrax has been described as a two-stage disease. The initial stage is a nonspecific, flulike illness lasting from several hours to a few days. The early clinical presentation includes some combination of fever, myalgia, headache, cough, mild chest discomfort, weakness, abdominal pain, and chest pain. Profound malaise, fever, and drenching sweats are prominent symptoms, and nausea and vomiting are frequent. Classically, the initial stage is followed 1 to 3 days later, sometimes after brief improvement, by the rapidly progressive second stage, characterized by fever, dyspnea, diaphoresis, cyanosis, and shock.

There is no rapid screening test to diagnose inhalational anthrax in its early stages. In persons with a compatible clinical illness for whom there is a heightened suspicion of anthrax based on clinical and epidemiological data, the appropriate initial diagnostic tests are a chest x-ray or chest computed tomographic (CT) scan, or both, and culture and smear of peripheral blood. Pleural fluid and cerebrospinal fluid, as well as biopsy specimens taken from the pleura and lung, are also potentially useful for culture and other testing when disease is present in these sites, whereas sputum culture and Gram stain are unlikely to be useful.

THERAPEUTIC INTERVENTION. Early intravenous antibiotic treatment may improve survival in inhalational anthrax. Aggressive supportive care, including attention to fluid, electrolyte, and acid-base disturbances and drainage of pleural effusions, also play an important role in treatment. At present, intravenous ciprofloxacin or doxycycline plus one or two additional antimicrobials are recommended.

Cutaneous Anthrax

After an incubation period of approximately 7 days (range 1 to 12 days), the primary lesion of cutaneous anthrax appears as a nondescript, painless, pruritic papule, usually on an exposed area such as the face, head, neck, or upper extremity. The papule enlarges and develops a central vesicle or bulla with surrounding brawny, nonpitting edema. The central vesicle enlarges and ulcerates over 1 to 2 days, becoming hemorrhagic, depressed, and necrotic and leading to a central black eschar. Satellite vesicles may be present. The eschar dries and falls off over the next 1 to 2 weeks. Tender regional lymphadenopathy, fever, chills, and fatigue may occur. Systemic disease has been reported to have a mortality of 20% if untreated.

INFECTION CONTROL. Person-to-person transmission of anthrax is not known to occur. Patients may be hospitalized in a standard hospital room with standard barrier isolation precautions. No treatment is necessary for contacts of cases.

Plague

Plague is caused by the gram-negative coccobacillus *Yersinia pestis.* Under natural conditions, plague is transmitted to humans by the bite of an infectious flea and, less frequently, by direct contact with infectious body fluids or tissues of an infected animal or by inhaling infectious droplets. Plague has a long history of use and development as a biological weapon. After a biological attack, primary pneumonic plague would be most likely.

Clinical Presentation

Plague is a severe febrile illness. Pneumonic plague, the most fatal form of the infection, can develop from inhalation of plague bacilli (primary pneumonic plague).

The incubation period for pneumonic plague is typically 2 to 4 days (range 1 to 6 days). Presenting symptoms typically include the acute onset of malaise, high fever, chills, headache, chest discomfort, dyspnea, and cough concomitant with or followed rapidly by clinical sepsis. Hemoptysis is a classic sign that should suggest plague in the appropriate clinical context, but sputum may be watery or purulent. Gastrointestinal symptoms may be prominent with pneumonic plague; these include nausea, vomiting, diarrhea, and abdominal pain. A cervical bubo is infrequently present. The disease is rapidly progressive, with increasing dyspnea, stridor, and cyanosis. Rapidly progressive respiratory failure and sepsis within 2 to 4 days of onset of illness is typical of pneumonic plague.

Diagnosis

During a confirmed outbreak of pneumonic plague after a biological attack, a presumptive diagnosis can be made on the basis of symptoms, especially if there is a high index of suspicion. However, other causes of severe pneumonia or rapidly progressive respiratory infection with or without sepsis should be considered.

Laboratory findings are consistent with the systemic inflammatory response syndrome. The leukocyte count is elevated and the differential shows a neutrophil predominance, including immature forms. Platelets may be normal or low. Coagulation abnormalities include prolongation of the international normalized ratio (INR), prothrombin time (PT), and partial thromboplastin time (PTT). Elevated liver function tests and abnormal renal function tests are seen with systemic disease.

Therapeutic Intervention

When plague is suspected, antibiotic treatment should begin before laboratory confirmation of the diagnosis.

Botulism

Botulism is a paralytic illness caused by a potent neurotoxin produced by *Clostridium botulinum,* an anaerobic, spore-forming bacterium. Natural forms of the disease are foodborne botulism, wound botulism, and infant botulism. Foodborne botulism results from ingestion of improperly processed foodstuffs containing preformed toxin produced by *C. botulinum.* Wound botulism results from production of botulinum toxin by *C. botulinum* organisms that contaminate wounds. Infant botulism results from the colonization of the intestinal tract of infants after ingestion of spores. Botulinum toxin has been developed as a biological weapon. An aerosol attack is considered the most likely use of botulinum toxin for bioterrorism.

Botulinum toxin is the most potent lethal toxin known. The estimated toxic dose of type A botulinum toxin is 0.001 μg/kg of body weight. Botulinum toxin acts to block neurotransmission by binding to the presynaptic nerve terminal at the neuromuscular junction and preventing the release of acetylcholine, resulting in skeletal muscle weakness. The toxin is colorless, odorless, and presumably tasteless.

Clinical Presentation

The incubation period for foodborne botulism is 2 hours to 8 days; the typical incubation period is 12 to 72 hours. The incubation period for inhalational botulism is not established. The neurological features of botulism are similar. Although initial symptoms in foodborne botulism may include nausea, vomiting, abdominal cramps, and diarrhea, these symptoms are thought to result from other bacterial metabolites in contaminated food and may not occur in inhalational botulism.

The so-called classic triad of botulism summarizes the clinical presentation: an afebrile patient, symmetrical descending flaccid paralysis with prominent bulbar palsies, and a clear mentation. Patients typically present with difficulty seeing, speaking, or swallowing. Clinical hallmarks include ptosis, blurred vision, and the so-called four Ds: diplopia, dysarthria, dysphonia, and dysphagia.

Anticholinergic symptoms are common, including dry mouth, ileus, constipation, nausea and vomiting, urinary retention, and mydriasis. Other symptoms include dizziness and sore throat. Sensory findings are not present, with the exception of circumoral and peripheral paresthesias secondary to hyperventilation resulting from anxiety. Botulinum toxin does not cross the blood-brain barrier. Cranial nerve dysfunction and facial nerve weakness may make communication difficult; these symptoms may be mistaken for lethargy and signs of central nervous system involvement.

Diagnosis

Initiation of treatment with botulinum antitoxin should be based on the clinical diagnosis and should not await laboratory confirmation. For potential foodborne botulism, samples of stool, gastric aspirate, emesis, and suspect foods should also be submitted.

The possibility of a bioterrorist attack should be considered in any outbreak of botulism. A bioterrorist attack should especially be considered when a cluster of cases occurs, when an outbreak has a common geographical location but there is no common dietary exposure (suggestive of possible aerosol exposure), when there is an outbreak of an unusual botulinum toxin type, or when multiple simultaneous outbreaks occur. A careful dietary and travel history must be taken to help identify the source. Patients should be asked if they know of others with similar symptoms.

Therapeutic Intervention

The mainstay of treatment for botulism is supportive care, including intensive care, mechanical ventilation, and parenteral nutrition. Morbidity and mortality are usually from pulmonary aspiration secondary to loss of the gag reflex and dysphagia leading to inability to control secretions, respiratory failure secondary to inadequate tidal volume from diaphragmatic and accessory respiratory muscle paralysis, and airway obstruction from pharyngeal and upper airway muscle paralysis. Careful and frequent monitoring of the gag and cough reflexes, swallowing, oxygen saturation, vital capacity, and inspiratory force are critical. Airway intubation is indicated for inability to control secretions and impending respiratory failure. Secondary infections are common and should be sought in patients who develop fever.

Trivalent (ABE) equine antitoxin is available from the CDC through state and local health departments and should be administered as soon as possible after clinical diagnosis. Antitoxin can prevent progression of disease caused by subsequent binding of toxin but does not reverse the effects of already bound toxin. For this reason, antitoxin is not useful if the patient is no longer showing progression of disease or is improving from maximum paralysis.

Transmissibility and Infection Control

Botulism is not transmitted from person to person. Botulinum toxin does not penetrate intact skin. Standard infection-control precautions are adequate. Clothes of persons exposed to an aerosol release of botulinum toxin should be removed and washed. Exposed persons should shower with soap and hot water. Exposed environmental surfaces can be decontaminated with 0.1% hypochlorite bleach solution.

REVIEW QUESTIONS

Multiple response item. Select all that apply.

1. Which of the following assessments would the nurse include in a primary survey of a multisystem trauma victim?
   a. Chronic disability
   b. Breathing
   c. Circulation
   d. Airway
   e. Vital signs

2. The nurse is caring for a trauma patient who is hemorrhaging from a puncture wound. Which of the following interventions would the nurse use first to control the arterial bleeding?
   a. Pressure at site
   b. Application of a tourniquet
   c. Pressure point massage
   d. Pressure dressing

3. Which of the following symptoms would alert the nurse to the potential for inhalation injury for a patient who was in a house fire?
   a. Peripheral edema
   b. Singed nasal hairs

   c. Jugular vein distention
   d. Increased capillary refill time

4. Which of the following actions should be taken first for a patient who is found with hyperthermia?
   a. Undress patient
   b. Use tepid water as a mist spray
   c. Remove patient from the hot environment.
   d. Place patient in continual breeze from electric fans

5. A patient who has ingested a poison is to be given activated charcoal with sorbitol by a nasogastric tube. Which of the following does the nurse understand is the purpose for the activated charcoal with sorbitol?
   a. To absorb and expel toxins rapidly through the intestinal tract
   b. To flush and withdraw the poisonous agent from the stomach
   c. To induce vomiting
   d. To coat the esophagus

6. When interacting with a psychotic patient, which of the following interventions is helpful to gain the patient's trust?

a. Play along
b. Make promises
c. Avoid eye contact
d. Show respect

7. Which of the following patients should be treated first in a disaster situation?
   a. 10 year old with a closed fractured leg that is painful
   b. 32 year old with slight bleeding hand laceration
   c. 45 year old with open head injury, no pulse or respirations
   d. 62 year old reporting chest pain and shortness of breath

8. Which one of the following is an immediate threat to life during acute anaphylaxis?
   a. Hypotension
   b. Generalized itching

c. Airway obstruction
d. Tachycardia

9. The nurse is assessing a patient who is hypovolemic. Which of the following signs and symptoms indicate that the patient is experiencing profound shock?
   a. Sacral edema
   b. Jugular vein distention
   c. Decreasing blood pressure
   d. Palpable, bounding pulse

10. The nurse is to give penicillin G 500,000 units IM. The nurse has a 10-mL vial labeled penicillin 400,000 units/mL. How many mililiters should the nurse give?

    _____ mL

Bibliography

1. Danis, DM: Trauma today and tomorrow: recent clinical literature. J Emerg Nurs 31:447–455, 2005.
2. DeBoer, S, and O'Connor, A: Prehospital and emergency department burn care. Crit Care Nurs Clin North Am 16: 61–73, 2004.
3. Fowler, RA, Sanders, GD, Bravata, DM, et al: Cost-effectiveness of defending against bioterrorism: A comparison of vaccination and antibiotic prophylaxis against anthrax. Ann Intern Med 142:601, 2005.
4. Johnson, RM, and Richard R: Partial-thickness burns: identification and management. Adv Wound Skin Care 16:178–187, 2003.
5. Kelley, DM: Hypovolemic shock: An overview. Crit Care Nurs Q 28:2–19, 2005.
6. Mann JJ, Apter, A, Bartolote, J, et al: Suicide prevention strategies: A systematic review. JAMA 294:2064, 2005

7. McGillian, R: Frostbite: case report, practical summary of ED treatment. J Emerg Nurs 31:500–502, 2005.
8. Reading, D:. Managing anaphylaxis. Practice Nurse, 28:28, 2004.
9. Richards, CF, and Mayberry, JC: Initial management of the trauma patient. Crit Care Clin, 20:1–11, 2004.
10. Sheerin, F: Spinal cord injury: acute care management. Emerg Nurse 12:26–34, 2005.
11. Sigillito, RJ, and DeBlieux, PM: Evaluation and initial management of the patient in respiratory distress. Emerg Med Clin North Am 21:239–258, 2003.
12. Travers, D, Waller, A, Bowling, JM et al: Five-level triage system more effective than three-level in tertiary emergency department. J Emerg Nurs 28:395–400, 2002.
13. Weber, DJ, Sickbert-Bennett, E, Gergen, MF, et al: Efficacy of selected hand hygiene agents used to remove *Bacillus atrophaeus* (a surrogate of *Bacillus anthracis*) from contaminated hands. JAMA 289:1274, 2003.

SUGGESTED ANSWERS TO

CRITICAL THINKING

■ *Mr. Smith*

1. The airway is the first priority because edema from inhalation burns can occlude the airway.
2. You know that Mr. Smith is at risk for respiratory burns because of the soot near his mouth and nose. He should be closely monitored. Assessment should include respiratory rate and pattern and the patient's ability to speak without a hoarse voice. Abnormal breathing sounds such as wheezing indicate partial upper airway occlusion.
3. The vital signs are within normal limits.

4. Deep partial-thickness burns should be covered with dry dressings. Because the skin can no longer protect the patient, wet dressings provide a medium for bacterial invasion. Wet dressings can also cause a decrease in body temperature because the skin can no longer maintain thermoregulation.
5. Jewelry should always be immediately removed before edema formation begins.
6. Mr. Smith was involved in an explosive incident and thrown 50 feet. He could have sustained fractures of the pelvis or back. He also may have internal organ injuries from blunt trauma.

unit THREE

UNDERSTANDING LIFE SPAN INFLUENCES ON HEALTH AND ILLNESS

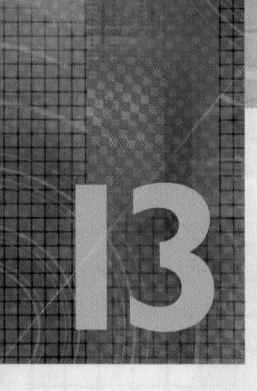

Developmental Considerations in the Nursing Care of Adults

RUTH REMINGTON

KEY TERMS

chronic illness (KRAH-nick ILL-nes)
developmental stage (DEE-vell-up-MEN-tal STAYJ)
hopelessness (HOHP-less-nes)
health (HELLTH)
illness (ILL-ness)
powerlessness (POW-er-less-nes)
respite care (RES-pit CARE)
spirituality (SPIHR-it-u-AL-it-tee)

QUESTIONS TO GUIDE YOUR READING

1. What are the eight developmental stages?

2. What are the effects of chronic illness?

3. What special needs do caregivers have?

4. What are health promotion methods?

5. What nursing interventions would you use in caring for a chronically ill patient?

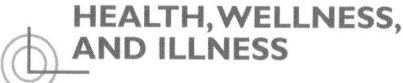

HEALTH, WELLNESS, AND ILLNESS

Health is much more than just the absence of disease. Have you ever known someone with what appears to be a small health problem who considers himself unwell or disabled, or a person with major health problems who sees himself as well? Many things play a role in a person's perception of health. One is the ability to function or perform desired or necessary tasks such as activities of daily living (ADL). Another is the ability to fulfill one's social roles such as student, parent, worker, and so on. The quality of one's life is another component of health. A person's ability to adapt to changes in physical, psychological, social, and spiritual aspects of life needs to be considered when planning health care. *Wellness* is a term that is used to describe a progression toward a higher level of functioning. Even though a person has a disabling illness, he or she can still be seen as achieving a high level of wellness.

NURSING CARE TIP

To foster understanding of how an ill patient, especially an older patient, was once healthy and active, ask family members to bring in photos showing the patient at various ages or engaged in favorite activities. Displaying these photos in the patient's room or on a hallway bulletin board allows caregivers to see the patient in times not associated with illness.

The concept of illness is one of imbalance or disharmony with the environment, resulting from a problem that causes one to be sick. Physical causes of illness are more easily recognized, such as exercise that induces an asthma attack in an asthmatic person or a fall that causes a broken bone. Illness can also result from a psychological, sociological, cultural, or spiritual imbalance. After the loss of a spouse, one may experience loneliness and depression and a loss of balance in the social and psychological aspects of life. A hospitalization may increase disharmony if cultural beliefs and practices are not understood or upheld by health-care providers. A person faced with a terminal diagnosis may lose hope and direction in life, causing anxiety and despair. So rather than being exclusive concepts, **health** and **illness** are dynamic and ever-changing states of being. A health crisis such as a myocardial infarction (MI) overwhelms a patient's ability to maintain a normal level of wellness. Two months after the MI, however, this patient could be enjoying a higher level of wellness than before the MI if he or she has lost weight, is walking daily, and is eating a nutritious low-fat diet.

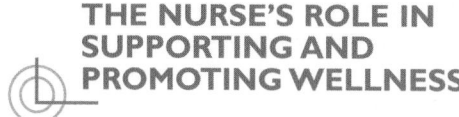

THE NURSE'S ROLE IN SUPPORTING AND PROMOTING WELLNESS

The goal of nursing care can best be defined as helping patients achieve their highest possible level of wellness. To do this, consider the patient's strengths, assets, and resources, as well as weaknesses, liabilities, and disabilities. Encourage the patient to take a personal inventory and recognize what is required to attain wellness. Working together, the patient, family, and members of the health-care team set wellness goals and develop a plan of action that will help meet those goals. The plan of care focuses on the following six main areas:

- Mobilizing resources
- Providing a safe and adaptable environment
- Assisting the patient to learn about his or her health problem and treatment
- Performing and teaching the patient to perform health-care procedures
- Anticipating problems and recognizing potential crises
- Evaluating the plan and progress toward the goals with the patient and family

The emphasis of care is changing from acute hospital care to preventive community-based care. Nurses assume a variety of roles in promoting the health of their patients such as advocate, consultant, caregiver, and educator.

DEVELOPMENTAL STAGES

Understanding the **developmental stage** of the patient can help the nurse accurately assess health and health practices. The developmental stages of life focus on the balance a person must achieve for high-level wellness within that stage. Across the life span at various ages and stages of life there are potential threats to health. Risk factors are related to growth and development, physical attributes, family, behavior, social interactions, environment, lifestyle choices, and ethnic background.

Erik Erikson described eight stages in the psychosocial development of the person. These stages illustrate the acquisition of a sense of trust in self and others and a sense of personal worth. Each stage must be completed before accomplishing the next. The first five stages describe the development of the child and adolescent.[1,2] Developmental stages for the young adult, middle-aged adult, and older adult are discussed here.

The Young Adult

Developing intimacy versus isolation is the sixth psychological development task. The young adult's task is to develop relationships with a spouse, family, or friends that are warm, affectionate, and developed through fondness, understanding, caring, or love. When this stage is not successfully resolved, the individual often experiences isolation from others. This stage encompasses ages 18 to 45. Physically, growth is usually completed by age 20. Socially, young adults begin to move away from their parents to develop their own families. The young adult begins to attempt to develop a place in society through school, work, and social activities. This is the stage in which intimacy or closeness develops with partners and friends. The decision to marry, have children, or have a pet is demonstration of the person's striving for intimacy. Challenges to intimacy are tasks that must be overcome in this stage. Within a marriage, communication, financial issues, and the needs of children must be successfully met to maintain the marriage. Melding one's traditions and customs with the traditions and customs of a spouse, family, or friends is a major responsibility, as is the passing on of culture to children. Values and beliefs, which arise from an individual's culture or conscience, serve as guidelines for behavior.

Common Health Concerns

The lifestyle choices of young adults may place their health at risk. Health promotion for this age group is mainly focused on preventing or limiting possible risk factors. Preventive measures that should be taught at this stage include monthly breast self-examination (BSE) for women and testicular self-examination (TSE) for men. Young adults need to understand the importance of diet and exercise in maintaining health. They are also in the position of teaching these lifelong habits to their children. Positive health practices in young adulthood help prevent long-term complications. Maintaining an aerobic exercise program and following a diet that is low in fat help keep weight down and avoid obesity, as well as promoting cardiovascular health. Blood cholesterol should be kept below 200 mg/dL. Avoiding sun exposure and using sunscreen are important to avoid sunburn and permanent sun damage to the skin. Years of sun exposure may cause skin cancer. Tobacco use started in the teen years is often carried on throughout young adulthood and is linked to chronic bronchitis, emphysema, and oral, throat, and lung cancer in later life.

In the early part of young adulthood, the individual is in the workforce or is preparing for the work world with a college or vocational education. Being a novice in the work world and accepting new independence, freedom, and responsibilities can introduce stressors into the young adult's life. Unfortunately, overeating, alcohol use, drug use, cigarette smoking, and family violence are all negative lifestyle choices and poor coping mechanisms for stress. Young adults need to be aware of their individual stressors and be encouraged to develop positive coping mechanisms for stress. Exercise, support groups, music, and meditation are just a few positive ways to cope with stress.

Although marriage commonly occurs within this age group, this group also has the highest rate of divorce. Trying to make a marriage work is a hard task. The blending of two people into a couple requires a lot of creative communication and loving care. When stressors overwhelm the couple's coping mechanisms or coping strategy, the marriage relationship is in trouble. Sometimes because of the high rate of divorce many couples choose to live together without being married. However, the avoidance of making a commitment may set these relationships up for failure.

If young adults are sexually active with multiple partners, they are at risk for sexually transmitted diseases. Safer sex guidelines and information on birth control should be available for the young adult.

Pregnancy is a common health occurrence for women in this age group. Because research indicates that a mother's health practices directly affect the health of the developing fetus, nutrition, drug and alcohol use, physical health, and effective stress coping mechanisms are lifestyle issues that need to be discussed with every pregnant woman. Prenatal care should be encouraged and readily available to pregnant women.

CRITICAL THINKING

Mrs. Michaels

■ Mrs. Michaels, age 25, and her husband are trying to start a family. She visits her physician, who confirms that she is pregnant. Which information and health practices should Mrs. Michaels and her husband be instructed in during a prenatal health examination?

Suggested answers at end of chapter.

The Middle-Aged Adult

People ages 45 to 65 are considered to be in the middle adult years. The psychological developmental task of this age group is developing generativity versus self-absorption. Generativity includes a sense of productivity and creativity, and is demonstrated by a concern and support for others, along with a vision for future generations. Unresolved conflict could be seen as preoccupation with personal needs or self-absorption. Physically, middle-aged adults start to notice signs of decreased endurance and intolerance for physical exercise if they have not maintained healthy lifestyle choices. Socially, their children are adolescents or young adults who require extra attention and assistance with entering adulthood and launching their own careers and families. The term "empty nest" has been used to describe the middle-aged couple after the children have left the home. This period is often complicated by the challenging demands of caring for aging parents. Middle-aged adults also look over their lives and assess accomplishments versus unrealized goals. Midlife crisis may occur as this self-inspection leads to a desire to change work, social, or family situations to try to meet unrealized goals. Planning for retirement by developing meaningful pastimes and interests outside of work and preparing for financial security is another important task during this period.

Common Health Concerns

Adverse health choices, such as smoking, use of alcohol, drug use, sedentary lifestyle, diet high in saturated fat, and overeating, often have serious consequences for middle adulthood. Hypertension and heart disease are major health concerns, as are chronic bronchitis, emphysema, and lung cancer. Cardiovascular disease and cancer cause most of the deaths in this age group. However, middle adulthood is not too late to begin lifestyle changes that positively affect health. Replacing high-risk habits with lifestyle choices such as regular exercise, healthful eating, weight reduction, and positive stress-coping mechanisms are positive changes. The need for immunizations continue into adulthood. Adults at high risk for hepatitis B (health-care workers, hemophiliacs, people on hemodialysis, intravenous drug users, and foreign travelers) should be vaccinated for hepatitis B if it was not done during childhood. Helping adults recognize the benefits of these lifestyle choices and empowering them to change is the major challenge for health-care professionals for this age group.

CRITICAL THINKING

Mr. Paul

■ Fifty-four-year-old Mr. Paul calls the doctor's office for the fourth time this month complaining of severe indigestion and requesting a medication that will work to fix it. He has refused to have an x-ray examination or other diagnostic tests because he "can't fit them into" his "busy schedule." Mr. Paul has his own insurance business. His wife quit her job to monitor the activities of their 13-year-old son, who was not going to school every day. The couple's twin daughters are both in college out of state.

1. What might be causing Mr. Paul to be experiencing health problems?
2. What is affecting the developmental tasks Mr. Paul needs to perform?

Suggested answers at end of chapter.

The Older Adult

Ageism is a term that describes stereotypical misconceptions about older adults in society. Although they are the most diverse age group, common misconceptions about old people include that they are senile, cranky, disabled, and in nursing homes. More positive attitudes about aging are developing, in part owing to the growing number of older adults. Advances in living conditions and health care have allowed more people to reach old age. People are living productive, fulfilling lives into their 80s, 90s, and even 100s. Many of these older adults are likely to be found working in their gardens, exercising, or socializing (Fig. 13.1).

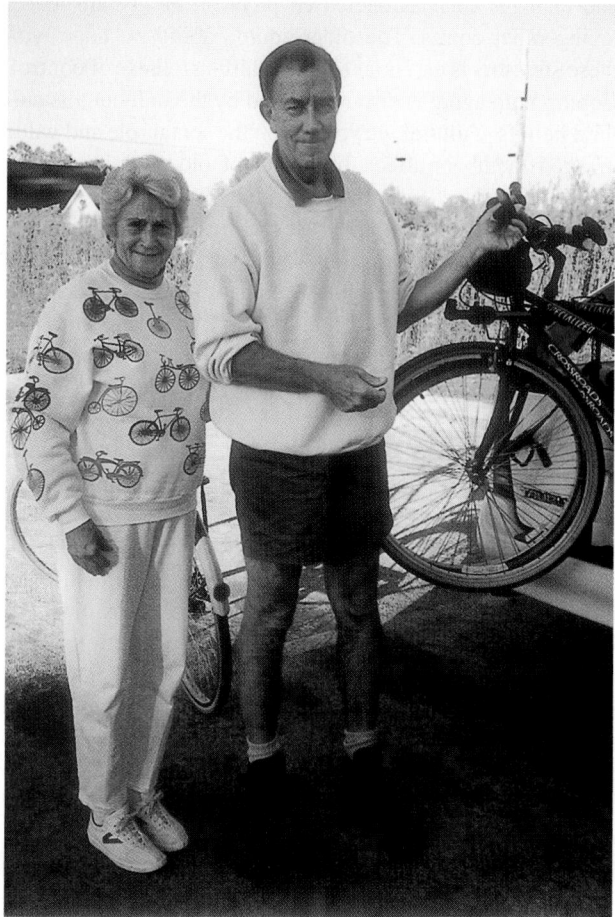

FIGURE 13.1 Socialization helps older adults maintain integrity.

The developmental goal for people age 65 or older is integrity versus despair. In this stage, the older adult looks back and evaluates what has been done with his or her life. *Integrity* refers to accepting responsibility for one's life so far and reflecting on it in a positive way. Reaching this stage is a sign of maturity, while failing to reach this stage is an indication of unsuccessful completion of prior stages, resulting in feelings of despair that life has been lived in vain, and a fear of death. Reminiscence is one way for the nurse to assist the older adult to pass through this stage.

Aging is associated with role changes and transitions. Some roles, such as employee, son, or daughter, are lost because of death or illness, causing sadness or depression. Other roles may arise, such as widow, volunteer, or grandparent. With retirement, household management roles may need to change. If an older adult becomes ill and dependent and needs to be cared for by an adult child, there can be a reversal of the parent-child role.

Health state, environment, relationships, and lifestyle choices influence the diversity found in this group. Physical health is often a concern for older adults. Chronic health problems that require medication and treatment often also require lifestyle changes or adaptations.

Coping with loss is a major challenge for older adults. Life events such as retirement, illness, or death of a spouse and changes such as decreased physical ability are losses facing older adults. The older adult's ability to cope with these stressors is essential for maintaining a sense of control. Coping with aging is also influenced by the individual's cultural beliefs. Cultural viewpoints on the social role and value of aged members affect the health of older adults. Sometimes the greatest loss for older adults is their lack of connection with the world and a lack of being part of a greater purpose. However, being alone is not the same as being lonely. For most older adults, being by oneself for a time allows for reflection to better understand one's situation. Older adults who feel unwanted or unloved are more likely to develop anxiety, depression, and failure to thrive.

Common Health Concerns

The focus of care for the older adult is on assisting them to meet their physical, psychological, cultural, sociological, and spiritual needs. Encouraging the use of community services for seniors and promoting self-care are important. Most older adults continue to live in their own homes or apartments, but impairment in mobility and the ability to carry out instrumental activities of daily living (IADL), such as shopping for groceries, preparing meals, and cleaning and maintaining a home, threaten their independence. Having to ask or pay others to perform tasks that they formerly were able to do themselves is seen as a significant loss by many older adults. Adding the loss of a spouse, the death of friends, or the lack of social contacts may further isolate an older person, leading to depression and **hopelessness**. The accumulation of losses can overwhelm an older adult's resources and coping mechanisms and is related to a high rate of suicide, especially for older men. Suicide is the ultimate expression of hopelessness.

Older adults need to be encouraged to remain active and to continue to pursue interests. Most communities have transportation services such as buses and vans that operate to meet the needs of older adults. Senior centers offer diverse programs and services to older adults. Some senior groups are focused on community service; others mainly plan trips or sponsor activities such as dances or bowling leagues. Older adults also have opportunities to continue to work in areas of interest as volunteers. Schools, hospitals, nursing facilities, parks, museums, zoos, community theaters, and youth groups all welcome older adult volunteers. Colleges and universities offer discounted tuition for senior citizens, and there are elder hostel programs across the country, which are programs especially designed for older adults. Elder hostels offer a variety of programs such as photography, Civil War history, nature survival, bird watching, and painting.

Chronic diseases can limit an older person's ability to be independent in self-care and activities of daily living. Hypertension is common, as are heart disease and strokes in this age group. Managing blood pressure, losing weight, eating a low-fat diet, smoking cessation, enhancing effective stress-coping strategies, and exercising regularly decrease the potential for cardiovascular disease.

One of the most difficult tasks for the nurse in dealing with the older adult is to distinguish normal age-related changes from pathological changes. Changes in mobility and chronic pain may limit an older person's activity and impede an active lifestyle. Falls are a serious concern for older adults, resulting in decreased independence and death. Osteoporosis is a bone disease, common among postmenopausal women and men over 80 years of age, causing bone weakness and fracture risk. Falls and accidents can be prevented by in-home safety assessments and altering the home environment to ensure the safety of the older adult. Bathrooms should be equipped with grab bars and nonskid mats. Bath chairs or benches make getting into a bath or shower safer. Removing clutter, throw rugs, small furniture, and electrical cords decreases the risk of falls.

Hearing and vision losses can affect the physical and psychological health of the older adult. Good sensory function is necessary to protect the individual from accidents, social isolation, and limitations in self-care. One of the most dramatic losses for many older adults is not being able to safely drive a car. This is usually associated with a loss of independence. Sensory impairments can further isolate the patient. Impaired vision can be caused by decreased peripheral vision, macular degeneration, cataracts, or glaucoma. Many older adults continue to drive during the day but not at night because of night vision problems. Decreased hearing is also common in older adults. Loss of high-pitch discrimination and reduced ability to filter background noises cause older adults to hear the background noise more clearly than a one-to-one conversation when in a crowded room. Social stigmas related to memory changes such as forgetfulness, dementia, and senility are a serious worry for many older adults. They often confuse depression with senility and attempt to hide their symptoms rather than seek treatment.

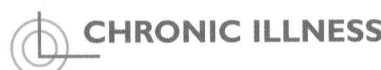 CHRONIC ILLNESS

A major challenge facing health-care providers is the management and prevention of chronic illness. **Chronic illness** is defined as an illness that is long-lasting or that recurs. Chronic illnesses usually interfere with the patient's ability to perform activities of daily living. Chronic illness is never completely cured or prevented. The human body wears out unevenly. The amount of disability depends not only on the kind of condition and its severity but also on the implications they hold for the person. The degree of disability and altered lifestyle relate as much to the persons perception of the disease as to the disease itself. For example, both John F. Kennedy and Franklin D. Roosevelt would have been eligible for 100% disability because of their chronic illnesses, but both managed to serve as presidents. Long-term effects of treatments like radiation therapy become chronic diseases in themselves. Radiation for a tumor can leave the person with persistent diarrhea that may cause the person to be malnourished and exhausted.

CRITICAL THINKING

Mrs. Riccardi

■ Mrs. Riccardi, age 87, lives alone in her small apartment. Her daughter and son are both retired and live in the same community. Mrs. Riccardi had a dizzy spell, so her daughter brought her to the hospital emergency department (ED). Upon admission, Mrs. Riccardi's blood pressure was 208/128 and she had blurred vision in the left eye that resolved after 1 hour in the ED. She was diagnosed with hypertension, which had possibly contributed to a small stroke or transient ischemic attack (TIA). Mrs. Riccardi was started on metoprolol (Lopressor) 100 mg daily. She was discharged to her home with instructions to limit salt in her diet and to begin an exercise program. The plan of care addressed safety issues.

1. Why might Mrs. Riccardi be at increased risk of falling?
2. What nursing interventions would help promote Mrs. Riccardi's independence and safety?
3. The nurse is to give metoprolol 100 mg. Fifty-milligram tablets are available. How many tablets should the nurse give?

Suggested answers at end of chapter.

When caring for those with chronic illness, the goal of nursing care is to maintain and improve the patient's quality of life. A chronic illness also affects the patient's family's quality of life. Therefore, when planning patient care consider the family's needs for adapting to the patient's chronic illness.

Fostering hope is an important intervention that should be a primary foundation of care planning for the chronically ill. A chronic illness may appear to be a hopeless situation if no cure is possible. If recovery from an illness is not possible, it might be thought that nothing can be done for the patient. However, whenever there is life, there is potential for growth in areas such as developmental tasks, health promotion, knowledge, or spirit. Individuals have developmental tasks to perform even as they cope with illness or prepare for a peaceful death.

Incidence of Chronic Illness

The incidence of chronic illness is rising for several reasons. First, people are living longer, in part because of better hygiene, nutrition, vaccinations, antibiotic development, and exercise. Fewer people are dying from acute diseases. As a result, a larger elderly population is living long enough to develop many chronic illnesses. Second, medical advances have resulted in reduced mortality from some chronic illnesses, so that patients live longer with these illnesses. Third, today's technology and modern lifestyles affect the development of some chronic illnesses. Examples

include a sedentary lifestyle; exposure to air and water pollution, chemicals, and carcinogens; substance abuse; and stress.

Some of the most common chronic conditions include chronic sinusitis, arthritis, hypertension, orthopedic dysfunction, decreased hearing, heart disease, bronchitis, asthma, and diabetes. Preventive measures can be taught to reduce the incidence of these conditions.

Types of Chronic Illnesses

There are a variety of chronic illnesses resulting from several different causes (Box 13.1 Examples of Chronic Illnesses by Causes). These illnesses can have varying degrees of severity and can affect length of life. A chronic illness can lead to the development of other illnesses; for example, hypertension that then causes chronic renal failure. Chronic illnesses can have onsets at various ages, but with advancing age, the likelihood of developing a chronic illness increases, and older adults often have several chronic illnesses at one time (Box 13.2 Examples of Chronic Illnesses in the Older Adult).

Gerontological Influence

As people live longer, spouses or older family members are increasingly being called on to care for a chronically ill family member. Children of older adults who themselves are reaching their 60s are being expected to care for their parents. These older caregivers may also be experiencing a chronic illness themselves. The family unit is at great risk

---

Box 13.1

Examples of Chronic Illnesses by Causes

Genetic

Cystic fibrosis
Huntington's disease
Muscular dystrophy
Sickle cell anemia

Congenital

Heart defects
Malabsorption syndromes
Spina bifida

Acquired

Acquired immunodeficiency syndrome (AIDS)
Arthritis
Cancer
Cataracts
Chronic obstructive pulmonary disease
Diabetes
Head or spinal cord injury
Multiple sclerosis
Peripheral vascular disease

Box 13.2

Examples of Chronic Illnesses in the Older adult

Arthritis
Cataracts
Cerebrovascular accident
Chronic lung disease
Diabetes
Hearing impairments
Heart disease
Hypertension
Peripheral vascular disease
Visual impairments

for ineffective coping or further development of health problems. Assess all members of the elderly family to ensure that their health needs are being met.

Older adults are very concerned about becoming dependent on others. They may become depressed and give up hope if they feel that they are a burden to others. Establishing short-term goals or self-care activities that allow them to participate or have small successes are important nursing actions that can increase their self-esteem (Box 13.3 Cultural Considerations).

Barriers to caring for a chronically ill elderly patient include a lack of information about treatments, medications, or special diets and being unfamiliar with supportive services in the community such as meal programs or respite care. You should be aware of these and provide this information, as well as a resource number for questions.

Effects of Chronic Illness

For the patient to live as normally as possible with a chronic illness, many adjustments are usually necessary. Lifelong routines and habits may need to be changed. Daily living patterns are affected by routines that are established to cope with the illness. Treatment needs such as going to therapy sessions, performing peritoneal dialysis exchanges, or monitoring blood sugars can interrupt daily life.

Chronic Sorrow

Chronic sorrow is a normal response felt by those affected by a chronic illness. It is an intermittently occurring sadness in response to the loss caused by a chronic condition. It can be felt by the patient or the patient's significant others. It is a common feeling among those with chronic illness. The nursing diagnosis Chronic Sorrow may apply to those experiencing chronic illness. When this sadness occurs, nursing care should focus on being comforting and supportive. Providing information and assisting with coping strategies such as fostering support systems are great interventions to help those with chronic sorrow.

Spiritual Distress

Patients with chronic illness can experience spiritual distress when faced with the limitations of their illness. Maintaining patients' quality of life includes assisting patients with their spiritual needs. Religious and spiritual needs are important to most people whose lives have been disrupted with new challenges from chronic illness. Patients must be helped to find meaning in the illness and realistic hope. Interventions that address **spirituality** may need to be performed first to allow success of subsequent nursing care.

Develop a comfortable approach in assessing and meeting patients' spiritual needs. Several factors may make one uncomfortable in caring for the patient's spiritual needs. These factors include a lack of training, a lack of understanding of one's own spiritual needs and beliefs, and not recognizing or believing that this is your role. Examine your own spiritual needs to define a personal spiritual view. By doing this, you will develop insight into others' spiritual needs and resources, as well as gain a greater understanding of issues surrounding your patients' spiritual needs.

Many people use spirituality to cope with chronic illness. It helps give them a sense of wholeness, hope, and peace during a time filled with uncertainty and anxiety. Spirituality plays an important role in empowering patients to handle their condition. It is a source of inner strength that allows the patient to experience a sense of unity. Hospital interventions may include use of a meditation room for quiet reflection or prayer, chaplain visits, or worship services. To help meet the patient's spiritual needs, assist the patient with transportation to the meditation room or worship services.

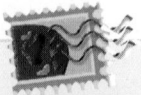

Box 13.3

Cultural Considerations: Traditional Appalachians

Traditional Appalachians believe that disability is natural with aging and is inevitable. This belief discourages the use of rehabilitation as an option. Thus, to promote rehabilitation efforts among Appalachians, the nurse may need to stress self-help and a return to physical function.

NURSING CARE TIP

Spiritual needs should not be thought of in only a religious focus. Spirituality is feeling connected with a higher power. Everyone has spiritual needs that involve hope, peace, and wholeness. Spiritual care goes beyond simply asking the patient's religion. It is assessing patients' perceptions of spirituality and then devising ways to assist them to meet their spiritual needs.

Accreditation agencies require the spiritual needs of patients to be addressed and documented by nurses. Nursing diagnoses related to spiritual needs include Spiritual Distress, Risk for Spiritual Distress, and Readiness for Enhanced Spiritual Well-Being.

Powerlessness

Those with chronic illness may feel powerless because they are uncertain of their ability to control what may happen to them (Fig. 13.2). A chronic illness can take an unknown course in relation to its seriousness and controllability. This leaves the patient vulnerable to the many phases of a chronic illness (the diagnosis, the instability phase, an acute illness or crisis, remissions, and a terminal phase).

Treatments that the patient undergoes can be a new experience that is painful, frightening, and invasive. If patients do not understand what is happening, they can feel overwhelmed and alone. This contributes to a feeling of **powerlessness** because the patient cannot control the outcome. Patients with chronic illness are faced with a lack of control throughout their illness. It influences the reactions of the patient to the illness. The nursing diagnoses of Powerlessness or Risk for Powerlessness may apply to many chronically ill patients.

COPING. Patients can be helped to feel more in control of their illness if you remember to include them in their care; listen to their feelings, values, and goals; and explain all procedures first. Complex medical language should be avoided when talking with patients to increase their understanding and feeling of being included in their care instead of isolated. In addition, coping with a chronic illness can be aided if the patient develops a positive attitude toward the illness. This can be accomplished if the patient gains knowledge, uses a problem-solving approach to difficulties, and becomes motivated to continue adapting to the illness and not succumb to a defeatist attitude.

A variety of coping techniques can be useful. Ask the patient's perception of the illness and identify coping techniques that the patient has previously used successfully. New coping resources may need to be added to effectively deal with the patient-coping tasks that are associated with chronic illness. Support services in the community should be made available to the patient and family. To cope effectively, the patient should become comfortable with the newly defined person he or she is to become. The nursing diagnoses of Ineffective Coping, Compromised Family Coping, Disabled Family Coping, and Readiness for Enhanced Family Coping may apply to those dealing with chronic illness.

HOPE. Before coping resources can be used, hope must be established by the patient. False hope is not beneficial and should be replaced with realistic hope. Providing patients with accurate knowledge regarding their fears helps do this. Hope should not be directed toward a cure that may not be possible but rather at living a quality life with the functional capacity that the patient has. Over the course of the illness, hope needs to be maintained for both the patient and family. Periodically assess if the patient is maintaining hope. Many studies have shown that patients adapt better when hope is high.

Many nursing interventions may increase hope. The use of humor helps patients be lighthearted and hopeful. Patients should be encouraged to live each moment to the fullest and experience the joy of being alive. Awakening the senses to appreciate the environment can bring a feeling of hope and peace. Simple things, such as the smell of baking bread, the clean scent of the air after a rain, or the scent of pine trees, can make one appreciate the beauty of nature and inspire hope. Family members need to be encouraged to help foster hope for the patient. By doing this, family members may gain hope as well. During times of acute illness, the patient needs to maintain as much control as possible and be told that any loss of control related to treatments is usually temporary. This prevents a continual feeling of loss of power. The use of music or inspirational reading material can reduce stress and help the patient find meaning in life. This in turn fosters hope. Hopeful patients are empowered and no longer feel powerless. The nursing diagnosis of hopelessness may apply to the chronically ill.

Sexuality

Chronic illness can affect a patient's sexuality. Sexuality includes femininity or masculinity, as well as sexual activity. Body image changes affect the way patients view them-

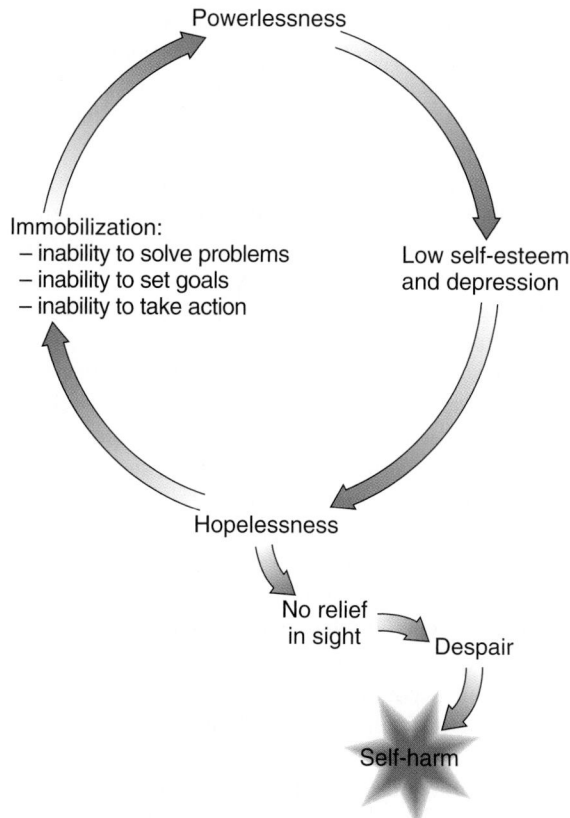

FIGURE 13.2 Powerlessness-hopelessness cycle. *(Modified from Miller, J: Coping with Chronic Illness. Overcoming Powerlessness, ed. 3. F.A. Davis, Philadelphia, 2000, p 526.)*

CRITICAL THINKING

Mr. Soloman

■ Mr. Soloman, age 88, still lives in his own home with his wife of 60 years. He is in good health except for poor vision, which developed slowly over the last 8 years. He cares for his yard, which is his pride and joy, and grows prize-winning tomatoes each year. He plays golf three times a week and walks every day to the neighborhood grocery store or bank. The employees know him and cheerfully assist him with his vision limitations.

Mr. Soloman's wife had always been the home-maker, whereas he was the family provider. Now his wife is in the early stages of Alzheimer's disease, ex-hibiting confusion, fatigue, and paranoia. She is unable to perform activities of daily living, so he has willingly assumed the homemaker and caregiver roles. They complement each other's limitations because she can still see and is helpful to Mr. Soloman when she is not confused.

Over time, Mr. Soloman's wife's health declines and she must be institutionalized. Mr. Soloman remains in his home alone. His family is concerned about him being alone and eventually convinces him to move into a studio apartment in senior housing. He is very reluc-tant to leave his home and does not actively participate in moving and selling his home. Mr. Soloman rarely leaves his apartment, sleeps 14 hours a day, and eats one daily meal. He tries to visit his wife by taking the bus but finds it difficult because of his limited vision, so he rarely goes to see her. Within a year, Mr. Soloman devel-ops pneumonia and after a brief illness dies in his sleep.

1. Why do you think Mr. Soloman behaved the way he did after he moved?
2. What interventions could have been used to empower Mr. Soloman?
3. Why might Mr. Soloman have developed pneumo-nia and died?

Suggested answers at end of chapter.

selves and are viewed by others. If patients have a negative body image perception, they may withdraw and become depressed. When interacting with patients, be aware of your facial expressions, nonverbal cues such as appearing hurried or keeping a distance, use of or lack of touch, and amount of time spent with the patient. When patients believe they have lost their femininity or masculinity, their self-worth decreases. Interventions to enhance sexuality should be used, such as obtaining a wig from the wig bank for patients undergoing chemotherapy.

There are many forms of sexual expression. Sexual intimacy can include touching, hugging, or sharing time together. Provide patients with the opportunity to discuss sexuality concerns or questions. Assume a professional and confidential approach to this topic, which is usually consid-ered a private matter by patients. Chronically ill patients can be referred to sex counselors for information on ways to cope with sexual issues in relation to their illness. Support groups can also be helpful.

Patients in extended-care facilities should be given pri-vate time with their significant other, if appropriate. Older patients need to have their sexuality needs met just as younger patients do. Because sexuality is a part of a person's lifelong identity, ensure that elderly patients' sexuality is addressed in their plans of care. Grooming methods can increase a patient's self-esteem and sexual identity. Women may get their hair and nails done; men can be shaved or get a haircut.

Roles

Chronically ill patients are usually faced with altering their accustomed roles in life. Common roles that may be affected for the adult patient include that of being a spouse, grand-parent, parent, provider, homemaker, or friend. Not only is the patient faced with dealing with these role alterations, the family must also adapt to these changes. Family members may have to take on new roles themselves to compensate for roles the patient is no longer able to perform. The nursing diagnosis of ineffective role performance should be included in the plan of care for the patient and family.

The patient is faced with giving up aspects of old roles at the same time that new roles related to being chronically ill need to be assumed. Grieving accompanies the loss of old roles. If a patient is no longer able to participate in social events such as being a golf team member or a committee member, grief work needs to occur to help the patient accept the loss and maintain dignity. With other roles, only certain aspects of the role may change. For example, in the parent-ing role, patients may still be there as support systems for the child, although they are no longer able to be the disci-plinarian. Whatever the role loss, the patient needs to be allowed to grieve the loss. The nursing diagnosis of Grieving may help in planning care for the patient.

The new roles the patient may have to assume related to chronic illness include dependency, ongoing health-care consumer, and self-care agent, and being chronically ill. Patients need to learn how to cope with these new roles. They need to gather knowledge and be given understanding as they become familiar with these roles. For patients used to being independent before the illness, being dependent on others to meet activities of daily living can cause a loss in self-esteem. Navigating the complex health-care and finan-cial reimbursement systems can be overwhelming. Transportation needs and waiting times for medical appoint-ments can be difficult for the patient who must deal with them on an ongoing basis. Becoming a self-care agent requires assuming responsibility for meeting one's own care needs. Handling chronic illness covers many areas, such as living with pain, having altered mobility, or complying with daily treatments. Deficient knowledge is a nursing diagnosis helpful for fostering learning for these new roles.

As patients live with chronic illness over time, they become experts on their own illness. However, today's health-care system tends to assume control over patients and does not respect the patient's own knowledge. Patients who are not given this respect take charge of caring for themselves by seeking knowledge and trying complementary healing methods. Be sensitive to the patient's knowledge and respect it because respect increases patients' self-esteem.

Family and Caregivers

Families are affected by the chronic illness of a family member in many ways. Chronic illness care is usually provided in the home so that families become involved in the management of the illness (Home Health Hints). Family members may have to take on new family roles or assume the role of caregiver. Decreased socialization, lost income, and increased medical expenses can increase family stress and tension. For more information, visit www.caregiver.org or contact Family Caregiver Alliance, 180 Montogmery St., Suite 1100, San Francisco, CA, 94104, (415) 434-3388 or (800) 445-8106.

Families must learn to cope with the stress of illness and its often unpredictable course. Most families develop ways to cope with the patient's illness the majority of the time and may become closer as a family unit. Children adapt better to a parent's illness when they receive parental support. Families often deal with the illness on a day-by-day basis and take a passive approach for most problems to let them work themselves out. During times of exacerbation or crisis, however, the family may need coping assistance.

Patients are often concerned about being a burden to their families. It is important to determine both the family's and the patient's feelings about the care required by the patient. The family's ability to provide this care adequately must also be considered in care planning. If the family lacks the desire, skills, or resources to adequately care for the patient, alternative care options must be explored such as home health care, adult foster care, or extended-care facilities.

Patients' caregivers often have certain ideas about the care that the patient should receive. This may come into conflict with the views of health-care providers. Caregiver input into the patient's plan of care should be sought so that everyone has a clear understanding of goals and expectations for the patient's care.

Caregivers commonly experience depression, role strain, guilt, powerlessness, and grieving related to caregiving. Be aware of this to detect indications that caregivers are in need of help in dealing with these feelings. Chronic-care coaches are resources available to caregivers who can provide insight, encouragement, and support for caring for the chronically ill. Nursing diagnoses for caregivers include risk for caregiver role strain or caregiver role strain.

RESPITE CARE. When caregivers are required to provide 24-hour care for a patient, they can experience burnout, fatigue, and stress, which, if extreme, in some cases can lead to patient abuse. Caregivers may not be able to leave patients alone even briefly because of wandering behaviors, confusion, or safety issues. They may not ever be able to get a normal night's sleep and suffer from sleep deprivation because of the patient's wandering or around-the-clock treatment needs.

Caregivers must be given periodic relief from their responsibilities of caregiving to reduce the stress of always having to be responsible. Everyone requires private time for reflection or pursuing favorite hobbies. Caregivers may need to get away overnight or for a weekend simply to sleep soundly and be refreshed.

Respite care is designed to provide caregivers with a much-needed break from caregiving by providing someone else to assume the caregiver role. Know your community's respite care services to share with caregivers. Unfortunately, there are often not enough respite care services available to meet the needs of caregivers. Most respite care is provided by volunteers who receive training. As the number of chronically ill persons grows, more respite care programs must be developed to promote the health of the caregiver and in turn the patient.

CRITICAL THINKING

Mrs. Burden

■ Mrs. Burden, age 64, is caring for her husband, who has Alzheimer's disease. He exhibits wandering behaviors. He gets up at night and in freezing winter weather is found walking down the street in only his pajamas. He attempts to cook and burns the pans. He is unable to express his needs. He disrobes frequently and is incontinent. Mrs. Burden quit her job to care for him. She no longer goes to lunch weekly with her friends. Her children live out of town. She places a chair and tin cans in front of the home's doors as an alarm in case her husband tries to open the doors.

1. What indicates that Mrs. Burden is experiencing stress related to caregiving?
2. What nursing diagnoses should be included in a plan of care for Mrs. Burden?
3. What nursing interventions would be beneficial for Mrs. Burden?

Suggested answers at end of chapter.

Finances

Managing a chronic illness can be expensive. Income can be lost if the patient is unable to work or caregivers are forced to stay home. Family savings can quickly be wiped out. If the patient is covered by insurance, it may not cover all the patient's expenses or it may have caps on lifetime coverage amounts. Expenses may involve medications, medical equipment or supplies, therapy, acute care, and home care. Inadequate funds can place a strain on families. This can lead to the nursing diagnoses of Compromised Family

Coping, Disabled Family Coping, or Readiness for Enhanced Family Coping. Nurses may need to refer patients to a social worker or sources of financial aid to help them meet their financial needs.

Health Promotion

Health promotion is possible and necessary at all levels of age or disability. With the increase in the elderly population, it is essential to understand the role of health promotion for older adults who have chronic illness. Patients with chronic illness make daily lifestyle choices that affect their health. For example, the patient with chronic lung disease who smokes can make a choice to smoke or to quit smoking. Patients with degenerative joint disease can choose whether or not to keep their weight within ideal weight ranges to reduce wear and tear on their joints. Arthritic persons can reduce their fatigue levels by pacing their activities and scheduling daily rest periods.

Those with chronic illness consider health promotion important, so encourage health-promotion efforts. Patients need to be assisted to strive toward high-level wellness. This can be achieved by looking at the patient's strengths and weaknesses holistically to develop a plan of care. Determine the patient's risk factors to plan methods of promoting health. Providing patients with knowledge to make informed decisions empowers them to take control of their lives and reach for their greatest potential. The nursing diagnosis of Health-Seeking Behaviors can be used to assist patients in promoting their health.

Nursing Care

Nursing care is primarily devoted to caring for patients with chronic illness. Develop an understanding that the wishes of the patient must be respected even if you do not agree with them. Patients have the right to establish their own goals in partnership with the health-care team. Because of the nature of chronic illness, understand the unique needs of patients and families experiencing chronic illness. These needs differ from acute care as far as depth of knowledge needs and the compounding problems that are usually faced by the patient.

Most chronic illness care occurs in the home and community rather than the acute care setting. Therefore, family members and caregivers, even more so than in acute care, must be assessed and included in the plan of care. As the numbers of those with chronic illness grow, community support for the chronically ill and their caregivers needs to grow. Training programs for caregivers must be available and offered affordably.

A major focus of nursing care for the chronically ill is teaching. These patients and their families have tremendous educational needs if they are to successfully learn to cope

with a long-term illness. The following are primary tasks that the chronically ill need to perform:

- Be willing and able to carry out the medical regimen.
- Understand and control symptoms.
- Prevent and manage crises.
- Reorder time to meet demands caused by the illness, such as treatments, medication schedules, and pacing of activities.
- Adjust to changes in the disease over the course of time, whether positive or negative.
- Prevent social isolation from physical limitations or an altered body image.
- Compensate for symptoms and limitations in order to be treated as normally as possible by others.

Explain individualized interventions to deal with these tasks during teaching sessions. Provide dignity and show respect to these patients (Box 13.4 Patient Perspective). Unique approaches are needed to positively assist chronically ill patients and their families on their long-term journey.

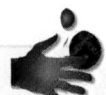

Box 13.4

Patient Perspective

Mr. Lyman

To the nurse caring for me:

- Don't give me a huge glass of water—give me a small glass and don't fill it full. Otherwise when I drink it, it spills all down the front of me.
- Make sure my call light is where I can reach it.
- Make sure my overhead light is working and that I can reach it.
- Ask how I like my blankets, don't just do them the way you do for anyone else.
- Keep a waste basket where I can reach it.
- When you leave my meal tray, make sure I can reach it. Then when you take it away, don't leave a bunch of stuff on my table. There is not much room on those little tables.
- Try to talk quietly in the hallway, instead of being so loud.
- Ask if I need anything before you leave the room.
- Be polite!
- Don't call me sweetie or honey. My name is Mr. Lyman. If I want you to call me by my first name, I'll tell you.

Thank you for preserving my dignity and showing me respect. I appreciate it!

Home Health Hints

- Home care nurses can strengthen a patient's self-care capacity by (1) saying "Let me assist you" instead of "Let me do this for you"; (2) being a partner in caring instead of being a caregiver; (3) empowering the patient instead of doing it all for him or her.
- Using humor can be helpful during a visit, unless the patient is distraught, anxious, or angry. Comics or jokes from magazines can be read. Humor can relieve the patient's and caregiver's stress and humanize the care that must be performed. Keep in mind, however, that humor may be irritating if it is taken as downplaying the seriousness of a situation.
- When patients have the use of only one hand or arm, provide a sponge for personal grooming instead of washcloth; it is easier to use and hold.
- Encourage the family of bed-confined patients to purchase an inexpensive portable intercom (such as a nursery monitor) to give the caregiver freedom to move about the house and hear the patient if help is needed.
- The home health nurse has an opportunity to increase a patient's self-concept by emphasizing the patient's existing abilities, joys, and talents. This can be done by observing the home environment for clues: photographs, trophies, hobby paraphernalia, flowers, or homemade items. Each clue observed can be a springboard to discussing triumphs and losses. It can

help the nurse understand how the patient copes to assist in planning care.
- Being attentive to any of the patient's efforts or accomplishments, such as number of steps taken, shaving without help, interest in a book or TV show, or decisions on fixing up the house or cleaning, provides opportunities to offer support and praise for accomplishments.
- The home health social worker should be informed of any patient concerns regarding cost of medicines or equipment. There are many programs to the assist the chronically ill to obtain resources.
- Always carry a pocket mask for cardiopulmonary resuscitation (CPR).
- Encourage discussion regarding advance directives with the patient and family/caregiver early in the care process. Decisions regarding resuscitation and the use of technology to prolong life are more difficult when the patient is in crisis.
- Refer families to community CPR classes as desired. Families can be empowered and the patient may feel more secure when families are taught CPR.
- Patients and families should be taught that if an ambulance is called they should turn on an outside light, open the door, and move furniture to enable the emergency medical technicians to get to the patient more easily if possible.

REVIEW QUESTIONS

1. The nurse is collecting data regarding a 68-year-old patient's developmental stage and finds that the patient is retired and that the patient's spouse died 4 months ago. The nurse identifies the patient as being in which of the following developmental stages?
   a. Generativity versus self-absorption
   b. Identity versus role confusion
   c. Intimacy versus isolation
   d. Integrity versus despair

2. The nurse is planning care for a patient with diabetes. Which of the following effects does the nurse understand is most likely to occur with a chronic illness?
   a. Powerfulness
   b. Spiritual distress
   c. Increased socialization
   d. Hopefulness

3. A 70-year-old man is the primary caregiver for his wife who has moderately severe Alzheimer's disease. He

becomes angry with her for spilling her dinner on the floor. He later feels guilty and begins to cry. The home health nurse is developing a plan of care. Which of the following would be an appropriate nursing diagnosis for the nurse to include?
   a. Caregiver depression
   b. Caregiver role strain
   c. Ineffective caregiving
   d. Risk for caregiving

4. A 64-year-old woman comes to clinic for a yearly physical. She has a history of hypertension and osteoarthritis. In contributing to the plan of care, which of the following is a priority intervention to promote wellness in this patient?
   a. Teaching her about hypertension and osteoarthritis
   b. Instructing her to take her own blood pressure
   c. Encouraging socialization
   d. Evaluating progress with the patient and family

Multiple Response Item. Select all that apply.

5. The nurse is providing care for a chronically ill patient. Which of the following are appropriate nursing interventions for a chronically ill patient?
   a. Decreasing educational information
   b. Encouraging visits by family members
   c. Including family members in teaching sessions
   d. Setting goals for the patient
   e. Limiting visits from friends
   f. Obtaining patient input on plan of care

References

1. Erikson, EH: Childhood and Society, ed 2. WW Norton, New York, 1963.
2. Erikson, EH: Identity and the Life Cycle. WW Norton, New York, 1980.
3. Kübler-Ross, E: On Death and Dying. Macmillan, New York, 1969.

SUGGESTED ANSWERS TO

CRITICAL THINKING

■ *Mr. Paul*

1. Mr. Paul's physical health is being affected by poor diet choices, excessive stomach acid secretion or other gastrointestinal problems, and stress.
2. It is easy to recognize the psychological stress related to parenting skills when a child is in trouble. Decreased family income with increased family expenses (two children in college) can cause financial strains and more economic pressure on Mr. Paul's business. With family problems or health problems, Mr. Paul may be questioning why things are happening to him and his family, causing him spiritual distress.

■ *Mrs. Michael*

Prenatal education information should be offered to Mrs. Michael and her husband. This education should include an overview of Mrs. Michael's health needs, what to expect during pregnancy, ways Mrs. Michael's husband can be supportive, and information on prenatal classes. Mrs. Michael's physical examination should include a vaginal examination, blood pressure, and blood work. It is important to be aware of any sexually transmitted diseases that may be transferred to the developing fetus or during birth. A rubella titer (a test for immunity to rubella or measles) is important because of potential birth defects if the mother has rubella while pregnant. Elevated blood glucose may be a sign of diabetes, and low red blood cell counts and low hemoglobin are related to anemia. To prepare a woman for pregnancy, prenatal vitamins or vitamins with iron and folic acid (necessary for effective neural tube development in the first 3 months of pregnancy) are recommended. Because of the increased workload of the heart during pregnancy, blood pressure needs to be closely monitored. A balanced diet, maintaining an exercise program, and continuing to develop effective and positive ways to deal with stress are very important for pregnant women. In preparation for pregnancy, Mrs. Michael also needs information on the negative effects that cigarette smoking, alcohol use, and drug use can have on the developing fetus.

■ *Mrs. Riccardi*

1. Falls could be caused by environmental problems, such as throw rugs that may move or cause tripping, clutter, electrical cords in walking paths, lack of hand grips in the bathroom, or lack of nonskid mats in the shower or tub. Poor vision and altered depth perception can result in missing a stair step or obstacles. Weakness or orthostatic hypotension can cause an unsteady gait or fall.
2. It is important for the nurse to instruct the patient and family about home safety. Mrs. Riccardi may even benefit by using a cane or a walker if she is unsteady. Because Mrs. Riccardi lives alone, an emergency alert system, such as a small transmitter that is worn around the neck or wrist with a button that can be activated in emergencies, would be beneficial. When activated, the transmitter alerts an answering service to contact designated individuals to check on the patient. Safety with medications is also an important consideration. Patients who take medications that lower blood pressure must be aware of the potential for orthostatic hypotension. Orthostatic hypotension is a drop in blood pressure that happens when a person moves from a lying to sitting or sitting to standing position. It is often accompanied by dizziness or light-headedness. Some people may even faint, causing a fall.
3. 2 tablets of 50 mg each.

■ *Mr. Soloman*

1. Mr. Soloman had lost control of his world and felt powerless. His environment, both home and outdoors, was shrinking. He had to give up his daily routines and interactions with others. His purpose in life was gone when he was no longer caring for his

wife. He was separated from his loved one. His visual limitations made his new environment unfamiliar and frightening.

2. Options to keep him safely in his home could have been explored with his input. After the move, he should have been thoroughly oriented to his environment. He should have been asked to explain what he wanted his life to be like as he adapted to this new developmental stage. Hobbies and interests should have been continued. Visual support services should have been contacted for ideas. Transportation should have been arranged to allow him to visit his wife. It should have been determined whether phone calls to his wife were possible.

3. He was depressed and slept from a lack of any inter-ests. His lungs were at risk for pneumonia because of his long periods of immobility. He lost hope and gave up on living, which decreased his ability to fight the pneumonia.

■ *Mrs. Burden*

1. Mrs. Burden is at risk for sleep deprivation, fatigue, stress, and burnout.

2. Nursing diagnoses include disturbed sleep pattern, fatigue, social isolation, risk for caregiver role strain, and deficient knowledge.

3. Beneficial nursing interventions would include teaching about Alzheimer's, a chronic care coach, respite care referral, alarm devices for wandering, and stress management techniques.

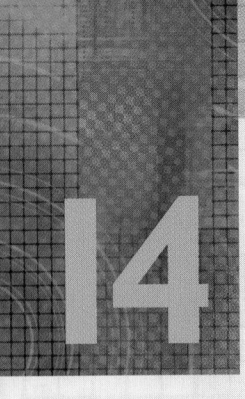

14

Nursing Care of Older Adult Patients

MARYANNE PIETRANIEC-SHANNON

KEY TERMS

activities of daily living (ack-TIV-i-tees of DAY-lee LIV-ing)

arrhythmias (uh-RITH-mee-yahs)

aspiration (ASS-pi-RAY-shun)

cataract (KAT-uh-rackt)

constipation (KON-sti-PAY-shun)

contractures (kon-TRACK-churs)

dementia (dee-MEN-cha)

depression (dee-PRESS-shun)

edema (uh-DEE-muh)

expectorate (eck-SPECK-tuh-RAYT)

extrinsic factors (eks-TRIN-sik FAK-ters)

glaucoma (glaw-KOH-mah)

homeostasis (HOH-mee-oh-STAY-sis)

intrinsic factors (in-TRIN-sik FAK-ters)

macular degeneration (MACK-you-lar dee-JEN-uh-RAY-shun)

nocturia (nock-TYOO-ree-ah)

optimum level of functioning (OP-teh-mum LEV-uhl of FUNK-shun-ing)

osteoporosis (AHS-tee-oh-por-OH-sis)

perception (per-SEP-shun)

pressure ulcer (press-sure ULL-sir)

range of motion (RANJE of MOH-shun)

reality orientation (ree-AL-i-tee OR-ee-en-TAY-shun)

sensory deprivation (SEN-suh-ree DEP-ri-VAY-shun)

sensory overload (SEN-suh-ree OH-ver-lohd)

urinary incontinence (YOOR-i-NAR-ee in-KON-ti-nents)

QUESTIONS TO GUIDE YOUR READING

1. How would you define aging?

2. What are basic physiological changes associated with advancing age?

3. How would you describe psychological and cognitive changes associated with advancing age?

4. What are nursing implications for the physiological and psychological changes associated with advancing age?

5. What nursing practices promote safety for the older patient?

WHAT IS AGING?

Over time it is easy to visually notice changes that occur in the human body. Both physical structures and body functions undergo changes and declines with advancing age. Although there is not one commonly accepted definition or theory to explain these declines, there is an understanding that aging is a universal and normal process that starts at conception and continues until death.

Older adults are increasing in number. In 2000, 34.7 million adults were older than age 65 and by 2025 this number is expected to be 61.9 million.[1] The fastest growing segment within this group is of those older than 84 years of age. Although this group accounted for 4.9 million adults in 2000, this group is expected to grow to 7 million by 2025. For more population data, visit www.census.gov.

In this chapter, aging is defined as a maturational process that creates the need for individual adaptation because of physical and psychological declines that occur during a lifetime. Even though aging truly begins at conception, the focus in this chapter is on the maturational process that is experienced after age 65 (older adult). Those older than age 84 are usually the frailest. The changes discussed do not always occur in the sixth decade of life, so chronological age should not be the basis for determining health issues. For some people, aging effects go unnoticed in their daily functioning; for others these effects cause varying degrees of impairment. Functional age (health, independence, and functional abilities) should be used as the basis of individual care needs. It is important to understand that most older adults function independently in the home and community. Many are still working. With supportive, educative care as needed, these people are able to maintain their independent abilities. This chapter discusses aging changes and resulting disabilities that may require more intensive nursing care than independent, healthy older adults need.

NURSING CARE TIP

Placing older adults into age categories overlooks their unique aging experience. The concept of functional age recognizes that aging is individual and promotes individualized nursing assessment and development of plans of care for the older adult.

Although aging is universal, it remains a unique experience for each individual. Factors that contribute to this process can be grouped into two categories. **Intrinsic factors** focus on genetic theories of aging, such as biological clock theory or programmed aging theory, and some aspects of physiological theories of aging, such as wear-and-tear theory or stress adaptation theory. **Extrinsic factors** focus on environmental influences, such as pollutants, free radical

theory, and stress-adaptation theory. Regardless of which factors have the greatest influence on this process of aging, **perception** and attitude also play key roles in how the changes over time affect the individual. It is through the filter of perception and attitude that the individual identifies, defines, and adapts to the changes that occur in structure and function over time. These factors have implications not only for older patients but also for their families and the healthcare providers working with them.

 PHYSIOLOGICAL CHANGES

Over time, cells change and do not function as efficiently as in earlier years (Table 14.1). The physical changes that are seen when looking at the older patient are slight as compared with the cellular changes that occur. Cellular decline in structure and function increases in severity and extent over time. Although the body works hard to maintain **homeostasis,** it is often unable to fully adapt to many of the declines that result from aging. Cells that die cannot regenerate themselves. As a result, structures are altered, and the body tries to adapt to make the revised structure meet functional demands.

Common Physical Changes in Older Patients and Their Implications for Nursing

Key Changes in the Muscular System with Aging
Key aging-related changes in the muscular system include the following:
- Decrease in muscle mass, so muscles look smaller
- Decrease in muscle tone, so muscles look less toned
- Slower muscle responses, so response time is increased
- Decrease in elasticity of tendons and ligaments, restricting movements

NURSING IMPLICATIONS. Changes in the muscular system have implications for movement, strength, and endurance. Restricted movements are most commonly seen in the arms, legs, and neck of the older patient, who may demonstrate limited **range of motion** (ROM) in these areas. Because muscle response abilities are slowed, it will take longer for the older patient to move. This increased response time has implications on the older individual's confidence level regarding personal ability to perform routine tasks.

Key Changes in the Skeletal System with Aging
Key aging-related changes in the skeletal system include the following:
- Eroding cartilage
- Exaggerated bony prominence
- Joint stiffening and decreased flexibility

---

homeostasis: homios—similar + stasis—standing

TABLE 14.1 PHYSIOLOGICAL AGING CHANGES

Body System	Aging Change	Effect of Change
Cardiovascular	Increased conduction time	Heart rate slows, unable to increase quickly
	Decreased cardiac output	Less oxygen delivered to tissues
	Decreased blood vessel elasticity	Increased blood pressure increases cardiac workload
	Irregular heartbeats	Poor heart oxygenation, decreased cardiac output, heart failure
	Leg veins dilate, valves less efficient	Varicose veins, fluid accumulation in tissues
Endocrine and Metabolism	Basal metabolic rate slows	Possible weight gain
	Altered adrenal hormone production	Decreased ability to respond to stress
	Decreased insulin release	Hyperglycemia
Gastrointestinal	Reduced taste and smell	Appetite may be reduced
	Decreased saliva	Dry mouth, altered taste
	Decreased gag reflex, relaxation of lower esophageal sphincter	Increased aspiration risk
	Delayed gastric emptying	Reduced appetite
	Reduced liver enzymes	Reduced drug metabolism and detoxification
	Decreased peristalsis	Reduced appetite, constipation
Genitourinary	Kidney size decreases	Able to live with 10% renal function
	Decreased bladder size, tone, changes from pear to funnel shaped	Frequency of urination increased
	Muscles weaken	Incontinence
	Decreased concentrating ability	Nocturia
	Less sodium saved	Risk for dehydration
	Reduced renal blood flow	Decreased renal clearance of all medications
Immunological	Decreased function	Infection and cancer risk greater
	Increased autoimmune response	Increased autoimmune diseases
Integumentary	Reduced cell replacement	Healing slower
	Water loss	Dryness of the skin
	Increased pigmentation	Aging spots
	Thinning of skin layers	Skin more fragile
	Decreased subcutaneous fat	Less insulation and protective cushioning
	Decreased sebaceous and sweat glands	Dryness and decreased temperature regulation
	Hard, dry nails	Brittle nails
	Thinning scalp hair	Baldness
	Decreased melanin	Gray hair
	Decreased skin elasticity	Wrinkle development
Musculoskeletal	Decreased muscle mass	Reduced strength
	Decreased muscle tone	Muscles look flabbier
	Decreased elasticity of tendons and ligaments	Movements are restricted
	Muscle responses slowed	Response time increased
	Bone thinning, softening	Decreasing bone density
	Joint stiffening	Decreased flexibility
	Vertebral disk water loss	Decreased height
Neurological		
Central nervous system	Loss of brain cells	Able to maintain function with remaining cells
	Decreased brain blood flow	Short-term memory loss
	Decreased regulation of body temperature	Hypothermia, hyperthermia risk
	Decreased endorphins	Increased depression
Peripheral nervous system	Decreased sensation	Risk for injury, burns
	Increased reaction times	Slow response, injury risk
	Decreased motor coordination	Unsteady, fall risk
Respiratory	Decreased lung capacity	Dyspnea with activity
	Decreased cough and gag reflexes	Aspiration, infection risk
	Reduced lung tissue tone	Shallow, faster respirations
	Reduced lung emptying on exhalation	CO_2 retention
	Decreased fluid and ciliary action	Mucous obstruction, infection risk
Sensory		
Eye	Lens less elastic	Decreased near and peripheral vision
	Lens opaque, yellows	Cataracts
	Cornea more translucent	Blurry vision
	Smaller pupil	Decreased dark adaptation
	Decreased violet, blue, green color vision	See red, orange, yellow colors better
	Arcus senilus—blue or milky lipid ring on iris edge	No effect on vision

Body System	Aging Change	Effect of Change
Ear	Degeneration of auditory nerve	Lose high-frequency tones, deafness
	Excess bone impairs sound conduction	Deafness
Nose	Decreased smell	Decreased ability to smell substances such as smoke, gas causing safety risk; appetite reduced
Sexuality	Availability of partner or privacy decreases	Lack of sexual expression, suppression of desires
	Slower sexual arousal time	Increased time needed for sexual stimulation
Men	Decreased erection, slower ejaculation	Psychologically causes concern
Women	Less vaginal lubrication	Painful intercourse
	Vaginal acidity reduced	Increased vaginal infection risk

- **Osteoporosis,** a thinning and softening of the bone
- Shortening in height caused by water loss in the intervertebral disks of the spinal column, flexion of the spine, and stooped posture

NURSING IMPLICATIONS. Because muscles and bones work together for movement, aging skeletal changes are most obvious when the older patient is moving. **Contractures** of the fingers and hands can limit the individual's ability to perform self-care tasks called **activities of daily living** (ADL). It is important to assist the patient with ROM exercises if help is needed to prevent the long-term disabilities that contractures bring (Fig. 14.1). Performing ROM exercises in warm water helps the patient who experiences discomfort with these exercises. If the individual has arthritis, anti-inflammatory medications should be given so that their action peaks when the exercises begin. Older patients on anti-inflammatory medicines should be monitored closely for gastrointestinal upset or bleeding and taught the symptoms of bleeding to report.

Decreased bone density is influenced by diet and weight-bearing exercise, so balanced diets rich in calcium and vitamin D and safe and sensible exercise programs should be promoted. Patients should be encouraged to ambulate whenever possible, using supportive, sensible shoes with nonskid soles. In addition to making sure the environment is safe for walking, sturdy assistive devices such as handrails, canes, or walkers should be encouraged as needed. When the decreasing density of older bones is considered, it is easy to understand that broken bones do not always result from a fall but may indeed be the reason for the fall in many older patients.

SAFETY TIP

Implement a fall reduction program and evaluate the effectiveness of the program. Involve residents/patients and their families to promote patient safety (2006 National Patient Safety Goals from www.jcaho.org)

Key Changes in the Integumentary System with Aging

Key aging-related changes in the integumentary system include the following:

- Increased dryness of the skin
- Increased pigmentation, causing liver or aging spots
- Thinning in the layers of the skin, which makes the skin more fragile
- Decreased elasticity of the skin, causing wrinkles to develop
- Decreased subcutaneous fat layer of skin, so older patients have less insulation and less protective cushioning
- Hardness and dryness of nails, making them more brittle
- Decrease in nail growth rate and strength
- Thinning of scalp hair (primarily men)
- Increased growth and coarseness of nose, ear, and facial hair

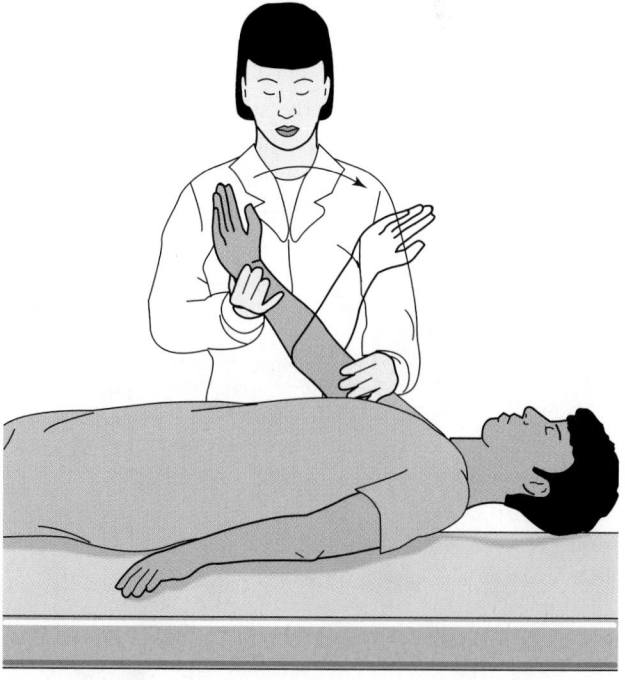

---

osteoporosis: osteon—bone + poros—a passage + osis—condition

FIGURE 14.1 Nurse assists patient in range-of-motion exercises to prevent the development of contractures.

- Decrease in melanin, which results in gray hair
- Decreased sebaceous and sweat glands, which has implications for dryness and decreased temperature regulation

NURSING IMPLICATIONS. The skin, which is the first line of defense against infection and injury, does not work as effectively in older patients (Fig. 14.2). In the older adult, skin injuries take longer to heal, and those longer healing times are usually complicated by the fact that many older patients have multiple chronic diseases, such as diabetes and circulatory ailments.

The older patient with limited mobility is especially prone to developing pressure ulcers (Fig. 14.3). These ulcers usually develop over a bony prominence of the body (e.g., ears, shoulders, elbows, tip of the spine, pelvic bone ridges, knees, heels, or ankles). Pressure ulcers are caused by ischemia that results from continuous pressure on an area of the body. Ischemia from unrelieved pressure can develop in 20 to 40 minutes. Early signs of **pressure ulcer** formation are warmth, redness, tenderness, and a burning sensation at the potential ulcer site. These potential ulcer sites are aggravated by lack of activity and the weight of the body. For this reason it is especially important to take the time to assess skin integrity daily, especially in high risk areas of the body.

SAFETY TIP

Monitor on ongoing basis each resident's/patient's risk for developing a pressure ulcer and implement plan of care for identified risks. (2006 National Patient Safety Goals from www.jcaho.org).

Skin care includes gently stimulating nonreddened intact skin sites with massage, moisturizing with creams regularly, avoiding the use of hot water and a complete daily bath, and limiting the use of soap. If able, patients should be

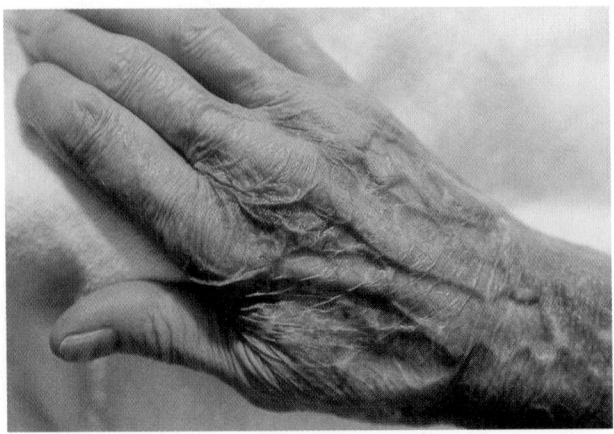

FIGURE 14.2 Thin, fragile skin of older person.

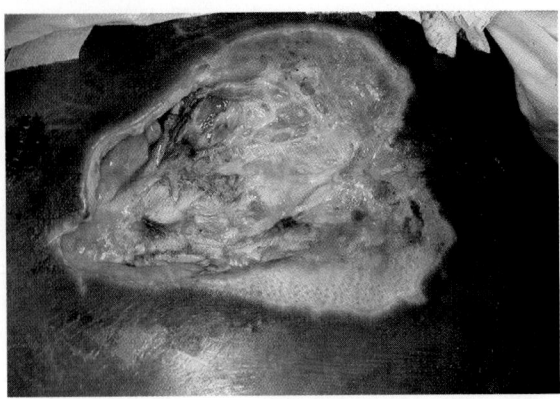

FIGURE 14.3 Pressure ulcer. *(From Goldsmith, LA, Lazarus, GS, and Tharp, MD: Adult and Pediatric Dermatology: A Color Guide to Diagnosis and Treatment. F.A. Davis, Philadelphia, 1997, p 445.)*

taught to shift their weight every 15 minutes when sitting. For immobile patients, consistent repositioning is essential. Ideally, use of pressure-relieving devices or repositioning every 30 minutes as able is the most beneficial for high-risk patients to help prevent pressure ulcer development (see Chapter 54). Keeping bed linens clean, dry, and wrinkle free also aids in the prevention of pressure ulcer formation.

As with care of the skin, nail care is important for older individuals. Soaking in warm water helps soften nails to ease in their trimming while encouraging blood flow to the peripheral areas of the body. Filing the nails with an emery board is safer than cutting the nails. To prevent accidental injury to the feet, patients should be instructed not to walk barefooted. Potential pressure points of the feet should be identified and closely monitored, and the patient should be referred to a podiatrist for treatment should there be any concerns. Diabetics should assess their feet daily because they may have decreased sensation, causing lack of awareness of foot irritation or injury.

Key Changes in the Cardiovascular System with Aging

Key aging-related changes in the cardiovascular system include the following:

- Slowed heart rate
- Decreased cardiac output from less effective functioning of the heart and blood vessels, yielding less oxygen to body tissues
- Decreased elasticity of the blood vessels, so the circulatory system is less efficient
- Reduced ability of the heart to quickly increase its rate in response to an emergency because of thickening of the heart valves, left ventricle, and aorta (when rate finally does increase, the heart takes longer to return to resting rate)
- More irregular heartbeats, **arrhythmias,** which lead to poor oxygenation of the heart
- Commonly, a lack of classic symptoms of cardiac emergencies
- Increased peripheral vascular resistance in blood vessels, yielding increased blood pressure

- More visible superficial blood vessels of the legs
- Less efficient leg vein valves, creating the risk for an accumulation of excess fluids in the leg tissues.

NURSING IMPLICATIONS. Be a good observer when it comes to caring for older patients because many early symptoms related to circulatory problems are subtle. Cardiovascular disease, which is separate from the process of aging, accounts for half of all deaths in people older than 65 years. Older adults must be educated about prevention practices that promote healthy circulation and encouraged to take prescribed medications as ordered and maintain a balanced intake and output of fluids. Older patients receiving intravenous therapy should be monitored closely because fluid overload can occur quickly in older people.

Special care should be taken to maintain good skin integrity and provide appropriate stimulation. If **edema** is present in the legs, they should be elevated to assist the fluid return to the upper body and supportive, nonrestrictive stockings should be worn as ordered. Concerns regarding leg circulation should be identified and reported early to the physician before problems develop. It is important to identify whether the circulation problem is arterial or venous before treatment is ordered.

Because quick changes in body position can make the older patient feel weak and dizzy, it is important to stand next to older patients as they dangle their legs over the side of the bed before rising to stand. Changes in body positioning from lying to sitting to standing need to occur gradually to accommodate the less efficient circulatory systems of older patients. Older patients may find comfort in the security of an ambulatory belt or walker if they fear unsteadiness when in an upright position. Falls continue to rank as a leading cause of accidental death in older patients. Every effort should be made to decrease the risk of falling for the older patient. The fall history of patients should be assessed to identify whether they are at high risk of falling, so that preventive measures can be used.

Key Changes in the Respiratory System with Aging

Key aging-related changes in the respiratory system include the following:

- Decreased lung capacity
- Weaker cough or gag reflex, increasing risk for upper respiratory infections
- Reduced tone of lung tissue, so respirations increase to 16 to 25 per minute and are more shallow
- Reduced tone of the diaphragm muscle
- Less complete emptying of the lungs, with greater CO_2 retention
- Decreased blood flow to the lungs, contributing to cardiac arrhythmias

NURSING IMPLICATIONS. Because the respiratory system is less efficient with advancing age, the older patient has a decreased tolerance for activity in general. Nurses should, therefore, pace activities for older patients instead of letting them confine themselves to bed. It is important to prevent overexertion, so rest periods should be scheduled. However, the rest periods should not outnumber the activity sessions planned throughout the course of the patient's day.

Cough, marked fatigue, and confusion may be early signs of an inadequate oxygen uptake. Respiratory rates greater than 25 per minute may be an early indication of a lower respiratory tract infection. Because overall muscle strength is reduced, the older patient performs the O_2–CO_2 exchange in the less efficient upper lobes of the lung instead of the larger lower lobes specifically designed for this purpose. Because lung recoil strength is decreased, mucus may be more difficult for the older patient to **expectorate.** This situation is compounded by the fact that older individuals also have less effective cough and gag reflexes, which creates greater potential for lung problems. Because of the normal changes in the respiratory system that occur with aging, it is important to include coughing, deep breathing, and position changes in the exercise program designed to stimulate all lobes of the older patient's lungs. At the prevention level, encourage the older individual to receive a pneumonia vaccine and an annual flu shot. This is important because influenza and pneumonia combine to be the fourth leading cause of death in people over age 65. Be aware that lifelong habits, such as smoking and respiratory pollutant exposure in employment settings, second-hand smoke, or paints and glues used in hobbies, are cumulative over time and can contribute to respiratory sensitivity for the older patient. Nurses can help prevent the spread of respiratory illnesses by getting flu shots themselves, hand washing between patients, not exposing patients to own illness, and using universal precautions.

SAFETY TIP

Reduce the risk of influenza and pneumococcal disease in older adults, (2006 National Patinet Safety Goals from www.jcaho.org).

Key Changes in the Gastrointestinal System with Aging

Key aging-related changes in the gastrointestinal system include the following:

- Changes in taste and smell, which affect the enjoyment of eating
- Decreased saliva production
- Decreased gag reflex and relaxation of lower esophageal sphincter, increasing the risk of **aspiration**
- Delayed gastric emptying
- No functional changes in the small intestine

---

edema: oidema—swelling

expectorate: ex—out + pectus—breast

- Decreased tone in external sphincter
- Marked decline in liver enzymes, which affects drug metabolism and detoxification
- Decreased peristalsis from generalized weakness of muscle activity
- Alteration in bowel habits

NURSING IMPLICATIONS. Many factors can alter appetite, ingestion, digestion, and absorption of nutrients in food, regardless of an individual's age. However, the structural and functional changes that occur with advancing age put the older patient at greater risk for not obtaining the nutrients needed to sustain a healthy body (Box 14.1 Nutrition Notes).

There is little that can be done to change the physical alterations in the older body that make getting needed nutrients more difficult. Being knowledgeable and committed to providing the support necessary to meet nutritional goals is important. Patients should be assisted with toileting before helping them eat. An appropriate amount of time for the patient to accomplish the task of eating needs to be provided. If the patient needs assistance with eating, be sensitive to the patient's pace while allowing the patient to have as much control as possible.

Additional forms of support can focus on the need to recognize that for some cultures eating has a strong social component. Encourage the patient to eat out of bed and with others as much as possible, while respecting the patient's right of refusal to eat in a designated social setting. Some patients may not eat as well when seated next to agitated or confused residents in a common dining hall.

Offer continuing support by maintaining a calm and comfortable environment that aids digestion. Certain food combinations enhance nutrient absorption, such as vitamin C foods taken with plant foods high in iron; vitamin C increases the iron's absorption rate. Offer these selections together whenever possible. Family members can be asked to bring in familiar seasonings patients used at home. If acceptable, familiar seasonings in shakers that patients apply themselves can be used to stimulate a lagging appetite. Work closely with the dietitian or nutritionist, who may provide other ideas to promote healthful eating for older patients.

Although many older patients wear dentures or partial plates, it is important not to stereotypically assume that all older individuals wear dentures. Tooth loss is not a normal change of aging. With proper lifelong dental care, teeth should last a lifetime. If the older patient does have dentures, be aware that any significant change in body weight will affect their fit and comfort and the patient's nutritional intake. Because of this, it is important to conduct regular assessments of the mouth when assisting the older patient during oral care.

Medications may cause taste disturbances or problems with dry mouth that may also affect the older patient's ability to meet nutritional needs. Some medications create problems with bowel motility, resulting in **constipation.** Constipation can also result from a change in routine, stress,

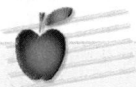

Box 14.1

Nutrition Notes

Older Adult Nutritional Needs

Meeting the Nutritional Needs of the Older Adult

Energy needs decrease 5% for every decade after age 40, partly because a 70-year-old has 40% less skeletal muscle than in younger days. Adipose tissue requires fewer calories to sustain than skeletal muscle does, so special attention must be given to maximizing nutritional content in fewer calories if a healthy weight is to be maintained. A modified food guide pyramid for adults age 70 and older adds eight servings of water to the base of the pyramid, increases milk servings to three, and recommends calcium, vitamin D, and vitamin B_{12} supplements. New recommended daily allowances for vitamin B_{12} specify that fortified foods or supplements furnish most of this vitamin for people over age 50.

Decreased visual acuity and impaired dexterity may make shopping for food and preparing it difficult or even hazardous. Arthritis affects not only mobility, but also jaw movements, so chewing may be problematic. By age 65, about 40% of U.S. residents have lost all their teeth and have to develop skill in the use of dentures. It is recommended that an individual learn to drink with them first, then learn to manipulate soft foods, and lastly learn to bite and chew with the dentures. Older persons produce less saliva than younger people. The sense of taste declines in most but not all aging patients, who as a result may increase their intake of salt and sugar to the detriment of a prescribed diet plan.

Achlorhydria may occur as a result of aging or from chronic ingestion of antacids. In either case, protein digestion and absorption of iron and vitamins B_{12} and C can be impaired by the lack of gastric acid. Although anemia can be caused by poor nutrition, older patients should be evaluated for hidden blood loss just as younger ones are. High-protein supplements should be offered to older individuals with caution, because normal aging reduces kidney function significantly and excretion of nitrogenous products of excessive protein intake could stress the urinary system. In addition, a high-protein intake increases calcium excretion. The vitamin necessary to metabolize calcium, vitamin D, may be deficient in older persons who neither drink milk nor spend time outdoors.

Many mature patients are at increased risk for food, nutrient, and drug interactions. Situations associated with these interactions are the use of many drugs, including alcohol; the need for long-term drug therapy in chronic illness; and poor or marginal nutritional status. Identification of any of these factors should prompt a thorough nutritional assessment or referral to a registered dietician.

and anxiety. To gain a greater understanding of the situation, talk with the patient about previous assistive procedures and establish an expectation baseline for bowel elimination. Educate the older patient about the important relationship between intake of fiber and water and exercise in the promotion of effective bowel evacuation. Enemas, suppositories, and medications should be considered for use only after dietary management is found to be ineffective.

Key Changes in the Endocrine-Metabolic System with Aging

Key aging-related changes in the endocrine-metabolic system include the following:

- Slowing in the basal metabolic rate, requiring a 5% reduction in calorie consumption to maintain weight
- Alteration in hormone production, including changes in estrogen, progesterone, and adrenal secretions
- Decreased pancreatic insulin release and peripheral sensitivity
- Decreased glucose tolerance with advancing age

NURSING IMPLICATIONS. Increased incidence of metabolic disease, such as diabetes, occurs with advancing years. Because of this, older patients should be encouraged to participate in screening programs for early detection of metabolic problems.

Because there is a notable decrease in the effectiveness and interaction of all hormones as one ages, it becomes especially difficult for the older body to respond appropriately to any stressful situations. Nurses should spend time addressing the psychological needs of patients by recognizing and addressing those actual and perceived stressors that affect their care. Preventive care to keep patients free from the stress of illness is also important.

Key Changes in the Genitourinary System with Aging

Key aging-related changes in the genitourinary system include the following:

- Decreased kidney size
- Decreased kidney function, urinary output, and adaptability
- Reduction of blood flow to the kidneys because of decreased cardiac output and increased peripheral resistance
- Diminished kidney filtration rate and tubular function, which cause a decrease in the renal clearance of all medications
- Decreased bladder size and tone
- Increased incidence of urinary tract infection with age, especially in women
- Longer correction times for fluid and electrolyte imbalances

NURSING IMPLICATIONS. Many older people have an urge to urinate at night, which is referred to as **nocturia.**

---

nocturia: nocte—night + ouron—urine

Changes in the kidneys, lack of gravity influence when in the recumbent position, fluid retention, and medication use contribute to nocturia. Approximately 30 minutes after lying down many older people need to urinate because fluid that was held in the legs by gravity is circulated through the kidneys and urine is produced, causing the urge to void. Emptying the bladder becomes more difficult to control from weakening of bladder and perineal muscles and also from a change in brain sensation regarding the need to void. As a result, the older patient may have difficulty controlling urination either knowingly or unknowingly, resulting in **urinary incontinence.**

NURSING CARE TIP

With age, the urge to void is not felt as early as it once was. This aging change combined with other changes in the urinary system, such as the bladder becoming funnel shaped, contributes to the older patient's voiding urgency. If the patient is not assisted to void promptly on request, incontinence can result.

First and foremost, the nurse must plan for safe access for all older patients who utilize the toilet alone or with assistance. Pathways to the toilet must be close and uncluttered. Toilets must be easy to access and clothing must be easy to remove. Incontinence is socially embarrassing and is one of the main reasons older people are placed in nursing care facilities by family members. Urinary incontinence in older men is most often attributed to benign prostate enlargement, while older women are more likely candidates because of short urethras and weakened perineal muscles. Because urinary tract infections are more frequent for older people (and often more dangerous), nurses must closely assess not only the quantity of intake and output for older patients, but also the quality of those measures.

Management of urinary incontinence needs to be tailored to the particular need of the patient. Bladder training programs have been effective when patients are reminded on a regular basis that it is time to urinate. If incontinence results from problems that affect the toileting task itself, such as clothing removal or distance to the bathroom, steps need to be taken to eliminate those obstacles that stand in the way of continence. Clothing with Velcro fasteners can replace buttons or zippers that are difficult for the patient to manipulate. Urinary briefs can help instill confidence in older patients who previously restricted activities because of fear of urine leakage. With use of the supportive incontinence brief, assess for early signs of perineal skin breakdown and proper application of the proper brief to meet individual needs.

Older patients who are aware of their incontinence may try to inappropriately decrease the chance for leakage by severely limiting fluid intake. This approach often results in dehydration, which disturbs the acid-base and electrolyte balance in the body. Over time, dehydrated patients may have problems with vomiting, diarrhea, weakness, and confusion. Because fluid intake needs to be encouraged in older patients, focus educational efforts on topics such as liquid intake timing and beverage selection (e.g., teaching that caffeine and alcoholic beverages should be avoided because they normally increase urinary output).

In addition, review patient medications and personal medication practices, such as taking diuretics late in the day, which then causes nighttime urination. Teaching perineal muscle support exercises and techniques is successful for some. All patients with unexplained urinary incontinence should be referred to a specialist for further evaluation because it is not a normal condition of aging.

CRITICAL THINKING

Mr. Jones

■ Mr. Jones, age 72, lives at home. His home has wood floors with throw rugs. The bathroom is located in the hall outside his bedroom. Mr. Jones has nocturia and is occasionally incontinent from urgency to void. He takes bumetanide (Bumex) 1 milligram orally daily.

1. What additional assessment data should be obtained about Mr. Jones regarding his urinary status and home environment?
2. Are safety concerns present in the home environment?
3. What nursing diagnoses should be included in Mr. Jones's nursing care plan?
4. What should be included in a teaching plan for Mr. Jones?
5. The nurse is to give Bumex 1 milligram orally now. Bumex 0.5-milligram tablets are available. How many tablets will the nurse give?

Suggested answers at end of chapter.

Key Changes in the Immunological System with Aging

Key aging-related changes in the immune system include the following:
- Decreased immune response
- Decreased number and function of T cells, leading to impaired ability to produce antibodies to fight disease

NURSING IMPLICATIONS. Older patients tend to have more chronic diseases that may increasingly depress their immune responses over time. Although older patients have fewer colds, they are at higher risk for influenza and other complications once they get a cold. It takes longer to recover from infections, so patients and their family members need to be told that a prolonged recovery is to be expected. It is also important to screen visitors for illness before they visit a recuperating older patient.

Efforts at prevention should focus on teaching the older patient about the importance of obtaining current immunizations, reducing stress, eating right, exercising, and maintaining a healthful lifestyle. Individuals on medications for conditions that put them at risk for immunosuppression, such as steroids, should be aware of the need to take additional safety precautions around others who are ill. Nurses can help patients help themselves by encouraging techniques such as proper hand washing that support universal precautions.

Key Changes in the Neurological System with Aging

Key aging-related changes in the neurological system include the following:
- Progressive loss of brain cells
- Decreased blood flow and oxygen utilization to the brain
- Decreased protein synthesis
- Decrease in sensitivity and the sensation pathways
- Increased reaction times
- Decreased motor coordination
- Decreased equilibrium
- Decreased ability of the hypothalamus to regulate body temperature
- Change in neurotransmitter secretion levels

NURSING IMPLICATIONS. Changes in the nervous system of the older patient can be seen in both the peripheral and central systems. These changes have significant meaning for the older individual, especially in the area of safety. With normal aging there is a slowed response to stimuli and a marked decrease in the speed of the psychomotor response to that stimuli. Because stronger stimuli are required to elicit any neurological response, the older patient is unable to perceive early signs of danger. To protect from accidental skin burns, the thermostat on water heaters should be lowered and electrical heating devices such as heating pads, electric blankets, and mattress pads should not be used.

Another safety issue of concern focuses on changes in balance. It is more difficult to maintain balance as one ages, especially when musculoskeletal changes are considered. Special caution should be taken to assist older patients with transferring and ambulation activities so optimum levels of safety can be maintained.

Fine tremors of the hand are a normal finding with advancing age and tend to increase when the older patient is cold, excited, hungry, or active. Assistive devices provided by an occupational therapist (such as handle grips or anchored equipment) can help eliminate the unsteadiness created when fine tremors make it more difficult to accomplish activities of daily living (Fig. 14.4). Accompanied by generalized muscle weakness, normal neurological changes that arise with advancing age usually occur on both sides of the body at the same time. One-sided weakness, sensory

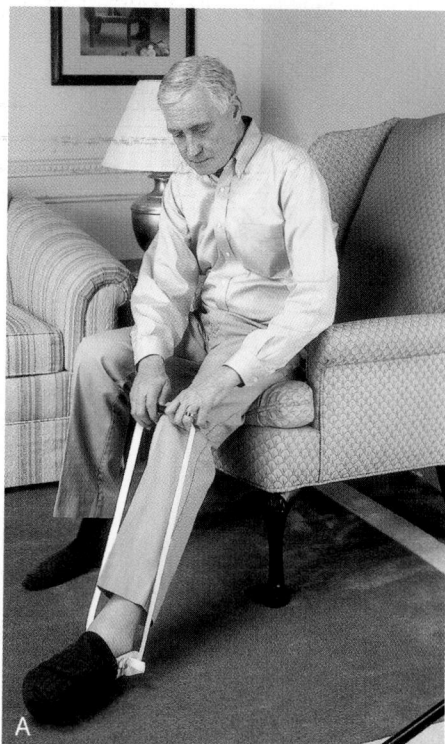

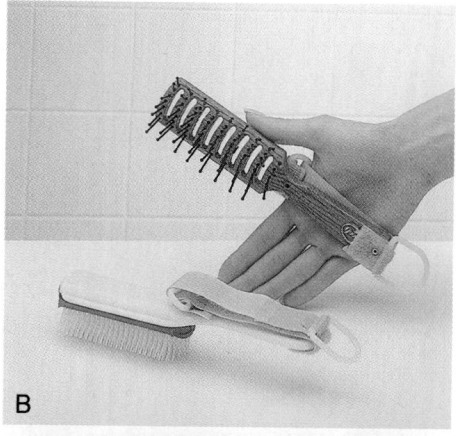

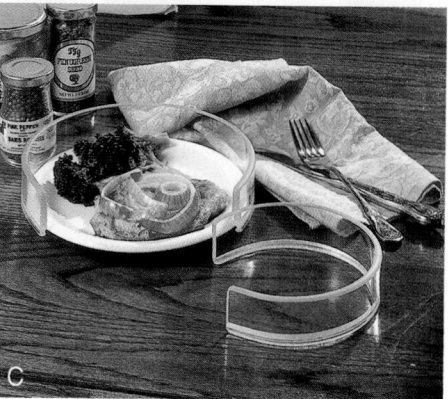

FIGURE 14.4 Assistive devices for activities of daily living. *(A)* Sock and stocking aid. *(B)* Easy-pull hair brush. *(C)* Food guard. *(Courtesy Sammons Preston, Inc., Bollingbrook, Ill.)*

problems, and performance problems should always be referred for further evaluation. Coarse tremors of the finger, forearm, head, eyelids, or tongue that occur when the body part is at rest may be a sign of a neurological problem such as Parkinson's disease. These generally occur on one side of the body first and should always be referred for further evaluation.

Key Changes in the Sensory System with Aging

Key aging-related changes in the sensory system include the following:
- Decreased visual perception
- Decreased elasticity of the eardrum
- Decreased sense of smell
- Decreased taste perception
- Decreased touch sensation

NURSING IMPLICATIONS. Problems that occur with normal changes in the aging sensory system are not inevitable with advancing age. Early identification and prompt referral can minimize sensory loss, which has a strong impact on the older person's psychological health.

Normal aging changes in the eye affect the focus ability of the lens and the maneuverability of the eye muscles to meet the needs of near and far vision. It is especially difficult for older patients to read fine print, although it is usually manageable with reading glasses or a bifocal lens. When caring for patients who wear glasses, it is important to remind patients to consistently wear their glasses as needed and to help the patient keep them clean and in good repair.

When glasses are removed by the patient, keep them accessible and in a protective, labeled case.

The older patient has a more difficult time adjusting to changes between light and dark settings. Seeing in the dark can be enhanced with the use of a red night-light because red lighting is more easily detected by the cones and rods in the older patient's eye. Make every effort to reduce glare from bright sunlight because sensitivity to glare is enhanced with the normal changes that occur in the aging eye (Fig. 14.5). The glare from car headlights may impair vision in older patients and reduce their ability to drive at night.

Several eye disorders can affect the aging eye (see Chapter 52). **Cataracts**, one of the most common pathological problems affecting the aging eye, cloud the lens and impair vision. **Glaucoma** is a chronic disease characterized by increased intraocular pressure that can damage the optic nerve. Another common visual condition that occurs later in life is **macular degeneration**, which results in a loss of central vision. Regardless of the means, any visual loss in older patients puts them at risk for developing psychological problems with disorientation, withdrawal, or self-imposed isolation caused by **sensory deprivation.**

Hearing loss is a common condition found in older individuals. Although the severity of the hearing loss caused by aging is variable, the stigma it carries is the same. For older patients, the first difficult sounds to discriminate are the high-pitched tones. Therefore, it is often more effective to whisper when communicating with the hearing-impaired

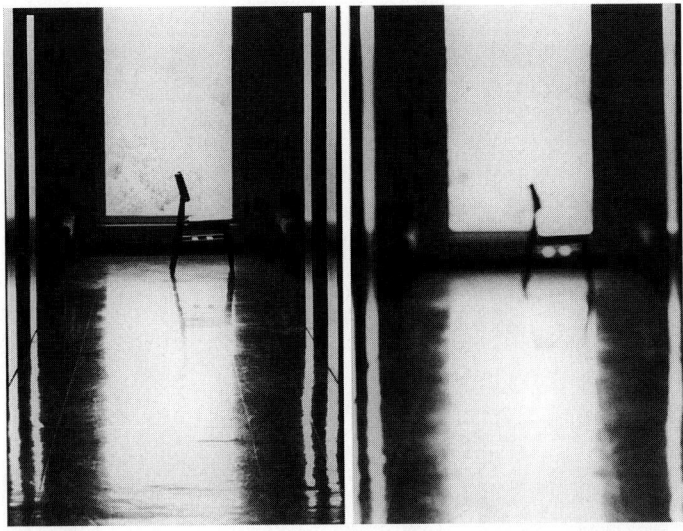

FIGURE 14.5 *(Left)* Normal view. *(Right)* The effects of glare as seen by an older patient. *(From Matteson, MA, and McConnell, ES: Gerontological Nursing. Saunders, Philadelphia, 1988, p 314.)*

individual because whispering decreases the pitch of the sounds. Shouting is not helpful because both volume and pitch are increased. It is best to speak to a hearing-impaired person in a moderate volume and a lower tone. It is also helpful to stand in front of hearing-impaired patients so they can see the speaker's face during communication (Box 14.2 Communicating with Hearing-Impaired Patients).

Two types of hearing loss can occur separately or in combination in the hearing-impaired patient. Conduction loss is due to blockage or damage to the mechanisms that transmit sound to the middle ear, where it is carried by the acoustic nerve to the brain. Conduction hearing loss can be due to a variety of factors, some as simple as ear wax build-up, and in most cases can be successfully managed. The other type of hearing loss, sensorineural loss, is due to damage to the structures in the inner ear and is much more difficult to manage. This type of loss can result from illness, medication use, or long-term abusive noise pollution that damages the sensitive structures involved with sensation and interpretation of sound. It is important to use hearing protection throughout life because damage to the ear is usually not reversible.

New-technology hearing aids can help most people with either type of hearing loss. Patients should be referred to an audiologist for further evaluation if hearing loss is suspected. Hearing aids are not well accepted by all older persons or their family members because they are a visual sign of a loss. Because of this, maintain patient privacy if a referral for further evaluation is made. If the older patient already has a hearing aid, it should be kept accessible to the patient at all times. The hearing aid should be kept clean with soap and water. A cotton swab removes wax build-up in tiny areas of the hearing aid. When not in use, the hearing aid should be stored in a labeled protective container and the battery turned off to conserve it. Extra batteries should be readily available.

As discussed in the gastrointestinal section of this chapter, the senses of taste and smell work closely together. Like other sensory losses, a declining ability to taste is not a problem exclusive to the older individual. Both ill-fitting

dentures and poor oral care can contribute to an alteration in the sense of taste, as can certain medications, tobacco substances, and oral disease.

Although they are often treated together as one sensory loss, the incidence of loss of the sense of smell is more common than the disorder that focuses on the loss of taste. In some cases, the loss of smell may be due to sinus problems, nasal obstruction, or allergies. If olfactory receptors are the primary cause for losing the sense of smell, there is little that can be done to treat the loss. Assess patients' medication charts, as well as their oral cavity, if they report a recent loss of smell or taste sensation.

Nurses also need to be aware of the care environment they provide for the older patient. Overstimulation produced by **sensory overload,** commonly experienced in intensive care hospital settings, can create psychological and physical strains that can make it difficult for the older patient to cope. As a patient advocate, be sensitive to the patient's care environment and changes in the patient's health-care status, identifying and minimizing overload situations early in the recuperation period.

Box 14.2

Communicating with Hearing-Impaired Patients

- Ensure that hearing aids are on with working batteries, if applicable.
- Face patient so the speaker's face is visible to patient.
- Speak toward patient's best side of hearing.
- Speak in a clear, moderate-volume, low-pitched tone.
- Do not shout because this distorts sounds.
- Recognize that high-frequency tones and consonant sounds are lost first—s, z, sh, ch, d, g.
- Eliminate background noise because it can distort sounds.

Key Changes in the Sexuality System with Aging

Key age-related changes in sexuality include the following:

- Chronic illnesses, which may affect sexual functioning
- Functional sexual changes in older men, commonly alteration in ability to obtain or maintain an erection and to ejaculate
- Functional sexual changes in older women, such as decreased vaginal lubrication
- Sexual problems caused by psychological factors, which are more common than physical ones in older adult patients
- Longer sexual arousal time in the older patient
- Increase in sexual activities that focus on non-intercourse intimacy behaviors, including various forms of touch

NURSING IMPLICATIONS. The older patient's sexuality is an important aspect to consider when providing care. It is essential to accept that sexuality is one of the basic physiological needs identified in Maslow's hierarchy for all individuals regardless of age. Be aware of personal attitudes and values about sexuality, sex, and aging, being careful that personal stereotypes and beliefs do not interrupt the older person's attempt to maintain sexual identity. Because privacy remains a common problem for individuals in health-care settings, provide the patient some scheduled private time for sexual expression. As new sexual enhancement treatments become more available to patients, there may be a greater openness to discuss sexual expression in conversations with older patients. Still, there remain many older patients who may have difficulty overcoming barriers to sexual expression because of cultural or religious beliefs, lack of a suitable partner, fear of failure, fear of consequences, illness, side effects of medications, and certain chronic diseases that may alter libido or sexual functional abilities. Because sexual discussions with these patients may be more difficult, it is important to address the sexual history section as sensitively, professionally, and completely as other sections of the patient assessment form (Box 14.3 Nursing Assessment of Sexuality).

COGNITIVE AND PSYCHOLOGICAL CHANGES IN THE OLDER PATIENT

Cognition

In addition to those physiological changes that occur with advancing age, older patients also experience changes that have an effect on cognition. Cognition includes abilities related to intelligence, memory, orientation, judgment, calculation abilities, and learning. Cognition focuses on intake of information and storage, processing, and retrieval of stored information. For the most part, older patients store information without much conscious effort. If dealing with

---

Box 14.3

Nursing Assessment of Sexuality

As with any nursing skill, practice will increase your comfort in collecting sexuality data for the older patient so these needs are not ignored. Assessment of sexuality concerns may lead to the discovery of other health issues and is a valuable part of data collection. As you collect data, be aware of problems (e.g., pain, medication side effects, mobility, dexterity, elimination, angina, surgery) identified in the history that may impact sexual functioning. Also, establish rapport with the patient by collecting other data first and turning to sexuality data at the end of the history. Older patients often respond to sexuality questions but will not initiate the topic.

Naturally, you should use a professional approach and manner, and tell the patient that you will now ask questions about sexuality. Start with questions that are likely to be more comfortable for the patient, as follows:

- Address roles first. For example: What concerns (do you have or has your illness created) in carrying out your roles with your (spouse or sexual partner)?
- Address relationship issues next. For example: What effect on your relationship with your (spouse or sexual partner) has this (illness, symptom, chronic illness) had?
- Address body image. For example: What effect has your (illness, surgery [mastectomy, prostate, ostomy], chronic illness, aging-related changes) had on your self-concept of being a (man or woman)?
- Address sexually transmitted diseases. For example: Do you have any discharge or open sores (vaginal, penile)?

---

information becomes difficult, the older person may begin to worry. Unless this worry is addressed, the patient's concern may result in psychological problems and fears.

Many factors can affect cognition. Sensory changes and diseases associated with age can cause misinterpretation of information being collected. Pain from chronic diseases, such as arthritis, can limit cognition as pain takes over the body and mind. Sleep deprivation caused by worry or fear can make it more difficult to perform routine tasks. Medications that cause drowsiness as a side effect can also impair cognition.

Long-term memory retrieval is easier to accomplish in old age than short-term memory retrieval. Assist the patient having short-term memory problems by using written lists, visual cues, and other memory-enhancing systems to aid in strengthening short-term memory skills.

Intelligence does not decline as one ages if it is measured using an appropriate instrument that focuses on accuracy and not on speed of response. Although cognitive abilities do tend to slow down with advancing age, they are not lost. Most of the subtle declines that do occur with information processing and retrieval do not need to interfere with the older patient's abilities in performing activities of daily living.

Nurses need to assist in the identification of individual problem situations and work with older patients and their families in developing strategies to better address their needs. It is common knowledge that health, good nutrition, and adequate sleep are important factors for brain functioning. These factors should be the cornerstones in planning care for the older patient.

Coping Abilities

How the individual chooses to adapt to a change in functional ability over time has a significant impact on how that individual will work through the entire maturational process called aging. In addition to normal aging changes, many older patients are coping with compounding changes that occur because of chronic disease. Nurses must not lose sight of the fact that in addition to changes caused by some decline in physical and cognitive functioning, older persons simultaneously work to deal with many societal and culturally perceived losses associated with advancing age. Changes in employment status and societal and family roles and shifts from independence to dependence may have a strong psychological impact on both older patients and significant others. With such a combination of "losses," an alteration in the confidence level of the older patient may be seen, requiring encouragement of self-care behaviors.

Personality, attitude, past life experiences, and the desire to adapt to change are all intrinsic influencing factors that assist the older patient in coping with changes brought on by advancing age. Extrinsic factors include things such as financial status, family support, and support provided by those who directly care for the patient. If older patients have the energy, desire, determination, and support of those who care for them, they are better able to optimize use of their cognitive functions toward health.

Depression

There are times when the psychological impact of change is too difficult to cope with, and loneliness, grief, or sadness does not easily allow the older person to cognitively focus on health. When this happens, **depression** can result, with the potential to disable the older individual's mind and body. Depression is the most common psychiatric problem among older adults. This psychological condition, which causes a disturbance in mood, increases the risk for suicide, physical health complaints, and sleep disturbances.

It is important to understand that the frequency and intensity of depression generally increase with advancing age. Depression can result from physical changes in the brain caused by medications or conditions that affect the neurotransmitters in the brain or from psychological changes at an emotional level, such as maladaptive coping from a perceived loss. Regardless of the cause, depression is a condition that has the potential to be reversed with prompt identification and treatment. It is important, therefore, to be sensitive to what the older individual is and is not saying during communications. Patients should be referred for treatment if depression is suspected before maladaptive behaviors occur.

Dementia

Unlike depression, **dementia** involves a more permanent progressive deterioration of mental functioning. Dementia is often characterized by confusion, forgetfulness, impaired judgment, and personality changes. There are two main types of dementia: multi-infarct dementia and Alzheimer's disease.

The multi-infarct classification results from repeated strokes that affect the brain tissue. The onset for this condition can be sudden or gradual, but its course is marked by a cyclical worsening and lessening of signs and symptoms that vary with the intensity and location of the brain damage.

The cause of Alzheimer's disease is unknown, but symptoms gradually begin with impaired memory that progresses to language and motor function losses. The course of this disease is marked by stages that can occur up to 14 years before death. It is only on autopsy of the brain that a definitive diagnosis of Alzheimer's disease can be made. Until then, Alzheimer's is suspected after other types of dementia have been ruled out with testing.

With any dementia, help the older patient maintain an **optimum level of functioning** in an atmosphere that provides for physical and emotional safety. In efforts to help ground the confused patient, incorporate **reality orientation** or validation into all nursing interventions. Sensory overload should be decreased for confused patients. Speak calmly and slowly and provide nonthreatening therapeutic touch if accepted by the patient.

In addition, it is important to address the education and support needs of the patient's family as they learn to deal with changes in behavior demonstrated by the older patient. Refer any patient with confusion for a mental status examination to help in determining whether the person suffers from depression or dementia. It is essential that a sensory status examination be conducted on the older patient before a mental status examination is conducted to help ensure the accuracy of the test results.

Sleep and Rest Patterns

The need for sleep in older adult patients does not decrease with age, but the pattern usually varies from earlier times in their lives. As in any age group, the lack of sleep leads to fatigue, irritability, increased sensitivity to pain, and increased likelihood of accidental behaviors. This is why it is important to obtain a baseline sleep and rest history when the older patient is admitted to the health-care unit. Consider sleep patterns, bedtime rituals, rest and nap patterns, daily exercise patterns, stress level, dietary intake patterns, and lifestyle issues such as caffeine, alcohol, and nicotine intake when completing the sleep and rest assessment of an older patient.

Circulatory problems may disrupt normal sleep patterns for the older person and may be the only clue of an impending health problem. The anxious patient who is unable to sleep may be calmed with back rubs, foot rubs, a warm bath, warm milk, or a glass of wine, if not contraindicated, when patterned bedtime rituals prove to be unsuccessful. Sleep medications should be used only as a last resort because they can affect the quality or depth of the sleep the older person receives and may produce unwanted side effects.

Medication Management

One of the most difficult tasks for older patients, their family members, and the health-care provider caring for them centers around the topic of medication management. Because older patients are more susceptible to drug-induced illness and adverse side effects for a variety of reasons already addressed in this chapter, nurses need to be especially aware of what the older patient is taking, how it is being taken, and what effect it is having.

Older patients use many medicines for various ailments. Most have more than one chronic illness for which they take medications. Sometimes these different medications interact and produce side effects that can be dangerous. Not only do health-care providers need to be concerned about prescribed medicines, they also need to look at the types of over-the-counter medicines older patients take, as well as the self-prescribed extracts, elixirs, herbal teas, cultural healing substances, and other home remedies commonly used by individuals of their age cohort.

Health-care providers not only need to be concerned about overuse and combinations of medications, but also misuse of them. If an older patient crushes a large enteric-coated pill so that it can be taken in food and easily swallowed, it destroys the enteric protection and can inadvertently cause damage to the stomach and intestinal system. Some patients intentionally skip prescribed doses in efforts to save money. When prescribed doses are not being taken as expected, problems do not clear up as quickly and new problems may result. The new Medicare Part D prescription coverage may help with this.

Work closely with older patients and their families on medication education. Patients need to know what each prescribed pill is for, when it should be taken, how it should be taken, and side effects to report. As a patient advocate, work with the pharmacist to remedy administration concerns so that the prescribed dose can be taken as directed. Write down early medication side effects, educating patients or designated care providers to be proactive in their care.

Medication use, abuse, and misuse need to be addressed regularly with older persons. Concerns need to be closely monitored and addressed before they evolve into

SAFETY TIP

- Use two patient identifiers that are not the resident's/patient's room number when giving medications.
- Obtain/document complete list of resident's/patient's current medications upon admission to the organization with involvement of resident/patient. Compare medications the organization provides to those on list.
- Communicate complete list of resident's/patient's medication list to the next provider of service with referral/transfer to another setting, service, practitioner or level of care within or outside the organization. (2006 National Patient Safety Goals from www.jcaho.org)

problem situations. Helping older patients consistently adhere to a prescribed medication routine with visual and verbal supports helps all those involved in the process of their medication management. This method also encourages self-care and supportive independence, as able, making for easier and safer medication use.

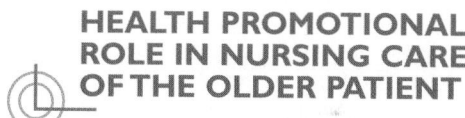

HEALTH PROMOTIONAL ROLE IN NURSING CARE OF THE OLDER PATIENT

Overall, the nurse who works with older patients must recognize the importance of developing strong skills in the areas of listening and observation. With competence in these skill areas, patterns of change can be readily identified and concerns can be addressed before they become problems for the older adult. Although this is important to consider for all patients who receive nursing care, it becomes especially important when working with older patients. This is because older persons often do not present with the typical symptom patterns associated with health problems seen in younger individuals, and early signs of health problems are often not evident in older patients.

By learning about normal changes expected with advancing age, older patients and their families can be helped to recognize commonly held societal myths associated with aging. In efforts to help older patients meet their optimum level of functioning, it is important to assess the older patient holistically, remembering that nursing assessment is an ongoing process. To assist in focusing on health promotion with older patients, look to health education activities, screening efforts for disease detection, immunization programs, and specific safety practices (Table 14.2).

TABLE 14.2 NURSING CARE FOCUS ON SAFETY ALPHABET FOR OLDER PATIENTS

A is for ABILITIES	• Know your abilities. • Know patient's abilities. • Base nursing actions on your abilities. • Seek out assistance when needed.
B is for BODY MECHANICS AND ALIGNMENT	• Use proper body mechanics. • Use appropriate assistive devices. • Ensure patient is in proper body alignment.
C is for COMFORT	• Ensure physical and emotional comfort during care. • Use pain scale during each assessment.
D is for DELIBERATE MOVEMENTS	• Plan ahead and communicate plans to patient. • Demonstrate confidence during care. • Alert patient to planned movements by saying, "Moving on three. One, two, three." • Ensure patient assists with moves as able.
E is for ENVIRONMENT	• Always place call light within reach. • Keep environment uncluttered and safe. • Ask patient's permission before moving items. • Put items back as patient prefers.
F is for FALLS	• Remember falls are a primary concern for older patients. • Use interventions to prevent falls: Assist patients with ambulation, use assistive devices, answer call lights promptly, provide accessible toileting facilities, use night-lights, avoid use of throw rugs.
G is for GIVING YOUR TIME	• Allow more time to perform actions. • Do not rush older patients. • Provide time for listening and observing, so concerns are addressed before becoming problems.
H is for HAND WASHING	• Use correct hand washing protocols to protect yourself and older patients. • Use standard precautions to protect yourself and older patients.

Home Health Hints

• Try to schedule therapy visits and nurse visits on the same day to decrease fatiguing the older patient.

• Because many older patients keep their homes warm, the home health nurse should wear layers of clothing, removing a layer as needed, rather than adjusting the heat in the older patient's home.

• Pagers should be placed on a silent mode if possible to avoid startling or confusing the older patient.

• Nurses should not assume that the older patient remembers them when they answer the door. Nurses should state their name and why they are there. A large-letter name tag should be in clear view.

• To enhance the effectiveness of a visit, the older patient should be asked to visit in a quiet room of the home with the primary caregiver invited in at the appropriate time. This may help the older patient stay more focused, offer privacy, and assist hearing.

• Making a sign for the door of the home giving visitors instructions, such as ringing the doorbell several times, knocking loudly, or using the other door, may be helpful to the older patient. Do not provide information that would inform a stranger that an older patient lives in the home.

• Suggesting that limiting visitors or not allowing persons with colds to visit can be helpful in preventing illness for the older patient.

• Stressors in a patient's life, such as annoying visitors, chastisement by caregivers, and harassment by bill collectors, are often experienced firsthand by the home health nurse. Document and share those with the home care team, so a coordinated approach can be taken.

• When auscultating lungs, ask the older patient to take deep breaths in and out through the mouth. This may stimulate coughing, which is an opportune time to teach deep breathing and coughing exercises.

• If the older patient seems fatigued early in the day, ask about sleeping patterns and things that disturb it, such as barking dogs, traffic noise, and visitors. Recommend ear plugs or changing rooms to obtain a good night's rest. Check medications for insomnia listed as a side effect and suggest dosing of these medications early in the day if appropriate. A 15- to 30-minute nap in the early afternoon can be helpful.

• One of the first signs of infection in the older patient is confusion.

• One of the first signs of dehydration is tachycardia. Instruct the patient regarding adequate hydration.

• Assist patients and/or caregivers with obtaining and setting up a weekly pill dispenser. These can be easily purchased at their local pharmacy. For those patients who are forgetful, a pill dispenser with a timer can be purchased. An audible or visual alarm will go off when it is time for them to take medications. It is important for the home health nurse to assess the patient's ability to follow instructions. During visits check the medication dispenser to ensure that pills are being taken as prescribed. If there is a concern inform the physician.

- Assess the older patient's environment for safety hazards on each visit and promote safety. Patients can easily trip on a scatter rug or fall attempting to navigate around furniture. Encourage the patient and caregiver to dispose of scatter rugs and unnecessary furniture.
  - If the home is a two story, help the patient and caregiver consider how to relocate the bedroom to the first floor. Stairs are difficult to manage especially if patients have a visual disturbance or they use an assistive device.
  - Assist patients in obtaining a medical alert device that can be worn around their neck in case of falls. If they fall emergency medical services can be alerted when they push the button.
- If the older patient has dentures, assess if they are worn for eating. If not, assess why they are not worn (e.g., sores, improper fit from weight loss) and discuss solutions.
- Checking the refrigerator for outdated food is helpful. The older patient is often on a limited budget and has been taught not to waste food. These factors along with a decreased sense of smell and taste can lead to food poisoning in the older patient.
- Encourage the uses of spices and herbs, such as parsley, oregano, lemon, garlic, and basil, instead of salt and sugar. Suggest keeping pared apples and slices of oranges in the refrigerator for snacks.
- If a Meals on Wheels program is available, ask if the older patient would like to be placed on the service.

- Use a warming tray when feeding an older patient who takes a longer time to eat.
- When swallowing is difficult, freezing liquids helps, so they can be eaten with a spoon or like a popsicle. Milkshakes, high-protein drinks, instant breakfast mix, or eggnog are thicker liquids that are easier to swallow.
- If an older person wears perineal pads or adult briefs, ask how many are used in a 24-hour period to assess the degree of incontinency or amount of output. Have the patient keep a voiding diary to further assess the degree of incontinence.
- Suggest a bedside commode when a weakened older patient is on diuretics or has a history of falling or confusion. Placing it next to the bed at night helps reduce the risk of falls and eases the caregiver's burden.
- If the older patient reports constipation, review the diet and make suggestions regarding adequate fluid and fiber. A mixture of equal parts of applesauce, bran, and prune juice is often helpful to prevent or relieve constipation. Discourage the use of mineral oil because it can make vitamins less effective.
- When drawing blood from the hand of an older patient, use the smallest needle possible.
- Hold light pressure for at least 2 minutes after the needle is removed. Do not use a Band-Aid on the fragile skin of the older patient if the bleeding has stopped with pressure.
- When teaching, it is important to acknowledge the patient's knowledge and life experiences. When given a chance, patients tell how they have maintained their health over the years. Use open-ended scenarios for teaching, such as, "What would you do if you were alone and fell?" Teaching should occur with patients, not to them. The nurse is in the patient's home, which is a personal place. Patient dignity should always remain intact during home care visits and teaching sessions.

REVIEW QUESTIONS

1. Which of the following does the nurse understand is considered the definition of aging in planning care for the older adult?
   a. A disease that results in the death of all of a person's body cells
   b. A condition that starts for all people when they reach the age of 65
   c. A maturational process that creates the need for individual adaptations due to physical and psychological changes in the body and mind over time
   d. A state of accelerating and simultaneous decline in body functioning directly related to the death of body and brain cells and the diseases that result

2. The nurse is assessing a patient who says "I am shorter now." The nurse responds based on the understanding that which of the following commonly contributes to individuals becoming shorter with age?
   a. Contractures
   b. Bone degeneration in the legs
   c. Hyperextension of the cervical spine
   d. Water loss from spinal intervertebral disks

3. In teaching an older adult patient who is not cognitively impaired and was recently diagnosed with hypertension about prescribed antihypertensive medication, which of the following is the best approach for the nurse to use to encourage medication compliance?
   a. The nurse looks the patient right in the eye and tells how medicines control the disease. The nurse then says "It is important that you take your BP pill every day." Do you understand this?

b. The nurse talks to the patient about medication management for hypertension. The nurse then gives the patient a grid to record the time each day the BP pill is taken. The nurse then takes out a pencil and says "It's 9:00 a.m. right after you took your BP pill with breakfast, show me how you will write it on this form that you will take to your next doctor's appointment." How do you see this working for you?

c. After talking about the new BP medicine, the nurse asks the patient "Do you have a relative or friend who can call you everyday to remind you to take your BP pill? It is really important that you take it and as you get older it is harder to remember things." Who do you think can help you with this?

d. After the nurse talks about the new BP pill the patient will take home, the nurse says, "If you don't take this pill you will probably have a heart attack or a stroke, so you better figure a way that you don't forget to take it everyday."

4. The nurse contributes to the plan of care for a patient on bed rest based on the understanding that pressure ulcers occur at sites of ischemia which can begin to develop in which of the following time frames?
   a. 5 to 10 minutes
   b. 20 to 40 minutes
   c. 60 minutes
   d. 120 minutes

5. The nurse is planning care for a patient at risk of aspiration. Which of the following does the nurse understand increases the older patient's risk for aspiration?
   a. Increased lung capacity
   b. Decreased lung capacity
   c. Decreased gag reflex
   d. Increased gag reflex

Multiple response item. Select all that apply.
6. Which of the following actions could the nurse institute to help prevent constipation in the older adult patient?
   a. Increasing dietary fiber intake
   b. Decreasing water intake
   c. Encouraging participation in ADLs
   d. Reviewing medication effects
   e. Increasing daily exercise

Reference

1. U.S. Bureau of the Census: Demographic Data, 2000. Retrieved July 13, 2005, from http//:www.census.gov.

SUGGESTED ANSWERS TO

CRITICAL THINKING

■ *Mr. Jones*

1. Does he live alone? Does he have a fall history? If so, does he wear a device to signal for help? What type of night-light is used? How far is it to the bathroom? Does he take his bumetanide early in the day rather than at night? Does he void before going to bed? Does he anticipate needing to void 30 minutes after lying down?

2. Wood floors that are slippery when wet from incontinence are a safety hazard, as well as throw rugs that may slide or cause tripping. An appropriate night-light should be available.

3. Nursing diagnoses include functional incontinence related to distance to bathroom; deficient knowledge related to safety, medication administration, and nocturia; and risk for injury related to slippery floors from incontinence, use of throw rugs, lighting.

4. A teaching plan should include the following:
   • Safety: Place urinal at bedside to prevent incontinence on way to bathroom. Use red night-light to improve vision and prevent falls. Use easily cleaned floor covering that is secure and absorbent to avoid falls. Consider the need for wearing a device that sends a signal for help.
   • Medication administration: Take diuretics early in the day to avoid having to get up frequently at night.
   • Nocturia: Void before lying down. Anticipate need to void after lying down by reclining in chair for 30 minutes before going to bed and then void on way to bed.

5. 2 tablets

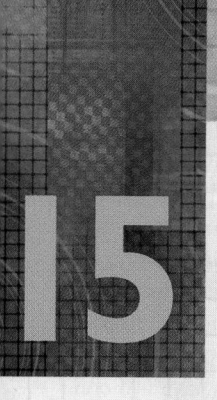

15

Nursing Care of the Patient at Home

KELLY McMANIGLE

KEY TERMS

autonomous (awe-TAHN-ah-mus)
collaborative (cull-AB-or-ah-tiv)
respite (RES-pit)

QUESTIONS TO GUIDE YOUR READING

1. How has the history of home health nursing shaped nursing care of today?

2. Who are the members of the home health team?

3. What needs to be included when documenting information about a home visit with a patient?

4. What are some of the differences between hospital-based nursing and home health nursing?

5. What are some steps the home health nurse can take to ensure infection control?

6. What is the difference between skilled care, hospice care, and private duty care?

INTRODUCTION TO HOME HEALTH NURSING

Home health nursing, as its name implies, is health care conducted in the home by qualified professionals. It is an important component of patient care. A majority of individuals who receive home care are elderly. Because of this, as the "Baby Boomer's" population ages, there will be an increase in the need for nurses to work in home care. The Bureau of Labor Statistics has indicated that there will be increased job demand for licensed practical nurses (LPNs) and licensed vocational nurses (LVNs) in home care.[1]

Also impacting home health care are advances being made in medicine. These advances will make it possible for patients to receive complex care outside the hospital setting. Home health care can offer a cost effective way for patients to receive these advanced medical services. It is important for the LPN/LVN to understand how care is received in the home setting since there are differences between the home and hospital setting that need to be considered. Recognizing these differences will assist LPN/LVNs in their role as part of the home care team.

HISTORY OF HOME HEALTH NURSING

Home care is not a new concept. Nurses have been giving care to patients in the home for hundreds of years. In 1893, Lillian Wald set out to improve the New York community in which she lived. Health care was available only to those who could afford it. Because of limited access to health care and lack of education, the home environment that poor families and immigrants were living in was not conducive to health and wellness. With the help of fellow nurse Mary Brewster, Wald established the Henry Street Settlement in New York City. These services initiated by Wald and Brewster laid the groundwork for establishing home care as a nursing specialty. Because of Lillian Wald and the nurses who worked with her, families were able to receive the necessary care and education in their homes to maintain or improve their health.[2] During the early 20th century nurses took the initiative to develop programs within the community to meet the needs of the patients in their care. Nurses in the 21st century can learn from this and be involved in improving the communities in which they live. Home health nurses can focus not only on the patient but also on the patient's family and the community. In home health, nursing care and its differences from medical care can be truly understood.

HOME HEALTH ELIGIBILITY

Home health care requires skilled nursing care and must be delivered by a licensed professional nurse. Physical therapy and occupational therapy may also be needed, independent of nursing. A patient who is receiving home health nursing is required to be home bound. If patients are able to drive, then it is felt they are able to transport themselves to healthcare services. Patients are allowed to attend special events, go to church, or go to medical appointments and still be considered home bound. If the nurse suspects a patient is driving daily, the nurse needs to reinforce eligibility for home health and suggest alternative options for health care to permit the patient to maintain independence. These options can include activities such as going to a clinic to have a blood pressure reading done, attending an outpatient physical therapy or occupational program, or having skilled needs (such as dressing changes) completed in a day surgery facility. If you have concerns about this, discuss them with the registered nurse who can work to assist the patient in receiving the necessary care.

Home health services are usually ordered for care after discharge from the hospital when there is a need for skilled care in the home. Skilled care includes those skills that patients cannot complete by themselves and that require the interventions of a licensed health-care professional (Box 15.1 Skilled Activities for the Home Health Nurse).

It is not uncommon, though, for a physician's office to request home health services after seeing a patient in the office. The physician might be concerned regarding how the patient is managing his or her care at home. For example, a patient who's having difficulty controlling blood sugars could benefit from having a nurse come to the home to assess how the patient is using a glucometer, what types of food are being purchased, monitoring of blood sugar levels, and to teach the patient appropriate diabetic management. Another example would be patients who cannot easily get to the physician's office to have their blood pressure checked weekly. If the physician has changed the patient's medications, he or she might need to make sure the adjustment is improving the patient's health as demonstrated by stable blood pressure readings. These types of visits are usu-

SAFETY TIP

Accurately and completely reconcile medications across the continuum of care.

Implement a process for obtaining and documenting a complete list of the patient's current medications upon the patient's entry to the organization and with the involvement of the patient. This process includes a comparison of the medications ordered for the patient while under the care of the organization to those on the list. A complete list of the patient's medications is communicated to the next provider of service when a patient is referred or transferred to another setting, service, practitioner, or level of care within or outside the organization (2006 National Safety Goals from www.jcaho.org)

Box 15.1

Skilled Activities for the Home Health Nurse

According to the Center for Medicare & Medicaid, the agency responsible for establishing home health rules and guidelines, a visit is considered skilled and necessary when the patient is unable perform that skill, there is not a family member available to perform the procedure, and the patient's medical issues deem it necessary to have a licensed professional nurse monitor and manage the situation.[3] Examples of activities considered skilled include:

- Dressing changes
- Administration of IV medications.
- Management and assessment of newly inserted feeding tubes and tracheostomies.
- Management and assessment of a new colostomy or urostomy.
- Foley insertion and maintenance.
- Patient and family education.
- Monitoring a patient's status following a change in medications or condition.
- Blood draws only if the patient is receiving *other* home health services. This is not covered as an independent skilled visit.

If a family member is present and able to perform the skill part of the time, the nurse can teach that person how to perform that skill. The nurse is still allowed to complete skilled visits to monitor patient progress and attend to the patient's needs when family is not available. It is important to remember that there needs to be a skill involved, as discussed above. If the patient is able to manage the care either independently or with the help of a family member the services of a home health nurse may not be required.

ally short term with the goal of facilitating independent care by the patient and/or family.

 THE HOME HEALTH CARE TEAM

LPNs and LVNs are an important part of the home care team. Demand for skilled health-care professionals to work in this area is increasing, and as a member of the home health team, licensed practical nurses will be included in this growth pattern. The home care team consists of: the physician, the registered nurse, the home health aide, physical therapy, occupational therapy, speech therapy, social services, assisted living facility staff, LPN/LVNs, and, of course, the patient. It is important to remember that the LPN/LVN is part of the health-care team and that care is **collaborative.** In others words, teamwork and communication play a large

part in ensuring that patients and the families receive the care they need.

The Physician

The physician is considered the team leader. In order for a patient to receive home care, a physician's order is required. The physician works closely with the registered nurse to determine what care the patient needs. Because the physician does not see the patient on a daily basis, he or she relies on the assessment findings of the nurse and communications with the home health agency staff.

The Registered Nurse

The registered nurse (RN) is considered the case manager while the patient is receiving home health. It is the RN who completes the initial assessment, establishes the plan of care, and makes changes as needed. The frequency of nursing and home health visits is established during the admission. After completing the initial assessment a schedule is established and forwarded to the physician for approval (Box 15.2 Scheduling Home Health Care Visits). If it becomes necessary, visits can be increased or decreased based on how the patient is progressing. The registered nurse also works with the physician to adjust treatments such as wound care and medications. These adjustments are based on the

Box 15.2

Scheduling Home Health Care Visits

Home health care is ordered for a 60-day period. The start of care is considered the first day of the visit with the end occurring before day 60. Skilled visits are usually projected during the start of care. Orders are written as follows:

- Skilled nursing care: 3 × wk × 3 weeks, 2 × wk × 3 weeks, 1 × wk × 2 weeks for skilled observation of vital signs and patient response to medication changes and home health aide services; 3 × wk × 8 weeks for assistance with personal care.
- Skilled nursing care: 7 × wk × 4 weeks, 4 × wk × 2 wk, 2 × wk × 2 weeks for wound observation and dressing changes, family education of wound care technique.

Included in the start of care orders are the supplies necessary to complete the ordered skills, such as dressing supplies, urinary catheter supplies, or medical equipment. These need to be authorized and ordered by the physician. Including them with the start of care paperwork ensures all services are ordered by the physician. This function is completed by the Registered Nurse in conjunction with the physician.

Adapted from Centers for Medicare & Medicaid Services: Home Health Agency Manual, 2004.

nurse's assessment of the problem. Remember, the physician is relying on the home health team to be his or her eyes and ears in the home. The nurse's ability to expertly assess a situation is critical to the progress of the patient receiving home health services. The LPN/LVN works closely with the RN collaboratively, or together, in order to help the patient reach the best possible health. The plan of care or treatment plan is certified, or ordered, for 60 days. The treatment plan includes number of skilled visits required, supplies and equipment necessary to complete the care, other services that are required such as a home health aide, and a nursing care plan that establishes goals for discharge. At the end of this period, the patient is either discharged or services are extended or recertified for another 60 days. The registered nurse works closely with all members of the home care team so that the plan of care remains relevant to the patient's situation.

The Home Health Aide

The home health aide assists patients with performing activities of daily living (ADLs). This includes bathing, dressing, grooming, and toileting. The home health aide's frequency of visits is established based on the patient's acuity level and available help within the home. Each case is different. One example would be an alert and oriented patient discharged home following spinal surgery who is widowed and has no assistance in the home. This patient might require frequent visits to ensure ADLs are met. Conversely, there is the patient who is discharged home following open heart surgery who has extensive family available to assist with personal care. Although this patient's acuity is higher, he or she has help available, thus requiring less frequent visits. During visits, the LPN/LVN can assist with identifying if frequencies for care need to be adjusted. Findings can be discussed with the RN who can contact the doctor to adjust the plan of care.

The Physical Therapist

Physical therapists (PTs) are part of the home care team who work autonomously. The physical therapist is responsible for developing a plan of care and visit frequency. Physical therapists work to help the patient regain strength and mobility. They teach the patient and family how to use assistive devices such as walkers and canes and develop exercise regimens that the patient can perform independently. The PT also works with medical supply companies to obtain equipment that is needed. If nurses feel patients might benefit from physical therapy services, such as a patient having difficulty regaining stamina following surgery, they can recommend this service to the physician. The nurse can also reinforce the physical therapy instructions during visits and check to ensure that the activities are being completed as prescribed.

The Occupational Therapist

Occupational therapists (OTs) also function autonomously. Similar to PTs, they establish their own treatment plan and visit frequencies. Occupational therapists' goals are to assist the patient to regain independence with ADLs and improve strength. They teach the patient how to use equipment that improves the patient's independence with daily activities. Nurses can also identify a patient who might benefit from these services. A patient who seems to be having a difficult time performing activities such as bathing, cooking, or cleaning would benefit from the services of an OT. As with the PT, the nurse can review instructions from OT with the patient to ensure they are understood.

The Speech Therapist

Speech therapy (ST) is ordered for patients who require assistance because of swallowing difficulties or speaking difficulties. After assessing the patient, the speech therapist identifies a plan of care and visit frequencies. If the nurse assesses a change in how the patient is swallowing or speaking, he or she can recommend a speech therapy evaluation. Once any new medical concerns have been ruled out, speech therapy can be initiated. As with other therapies, the nurse works closely with the ST and the patient to monitor understanding of instructions.

The Social Worker

Social services visits are usually completed in a shorter period of time. The social worker works closely with many community resources and can assist the patient with obtaining community assistance. Resources the social worker can assist with include things such as obtaining a prescription card, setting up Meals on Wheels, assisting the family with long-term care placement if necessary, identifying private agencies that offer **respite** care and homemaker services, helping the patient create a living will, and helping the patient with financial assistive services. Nurses who work in the patient's home are in a unique position to identify if the patient would benefit from social services. The case manager (RN) can relay the concerns of the home care team to the physician and obtain an order for a social service visit.

CRITICAL THINKING

Mr. Jones

■ Mr. Jones, 75 years old, was just discharged from the hospital following an acute exacerbation of heart failure (HF). You notice that he has little food in his house. It appears that the home has not been cleaned in several weeks, and that the clothes he is wearing are torn and soiled. Talking with him you learn that he lost his wife 6 months ago to cancer and has had a difficult time adjusting.

1. What are some community services that might be available to Mr. Jones?
2. What information would be important to discuss with Mr. Jones's physician?
3. Are there any other services that the home health agency can offer to assist Mr. Jones?

Suggested answers at the end of the chapter.

Assisted Living Facilities

Assisted living facilities (ALFs) become part of the home care team if the nurse has a patient residing in an ALF. Because these homes are not considered skilled nursing facilities, the staff is not able to perform nursing skills. Home health nurses need to understand the facility's policies when visiting a patient in assisted living. Many times the nurse visits several patients in the same location. If appropriate, communicate with staff regarding health-care instructions (e.g., keep the dressing clean and dry). Home health for patients residing in assisted living can be ordered for wound care, blood sugar monitoring, blood pressure monitoring, urinary catheter insertion and maintenance, and patient education.

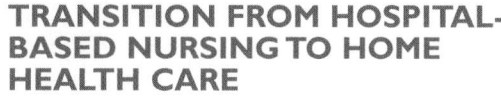

TRANSITION FROM HOSPITAL-BASED NURSING TO HOME HEALTH CARE

When working in the hospital, the nurse has many resources available. There are secretaries, nurses, respiratory therapists, and physicians to name a few. Patients who enter the hospital are leaving behind the comfort of their own homes. They are scared and isolated, not only trying to adjust to an illness, but also to a new environment. The opposite is true in home health nursing. In the patient's home, the nurse is the visitor. There are no support staff to answer questions and the surroundings are not familiar. This can be a difficult adjustment. As your confidence in being a home health nurse grows so too will your comfort level with entering someone else's home. It is important to remember that you have entered *their* home. Cultural issues also need to be recognized and considered (Box 15.3 Cultural Considerations). Do not make quick judgments because the dishes are not done or the bed is not made. People have different values that may not always agree with yours. (See Chapter 3 for further information regarding cultural considerations.) If the home is in such a state that it poses a health or safety risk, then it might be necessary to intervene by talking with the RN.

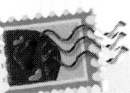

Box 15.3

Cultural Considerations

Within the Hispanic culture, the number of members in a family is typically large while the living space may be small. When the nurse first enters the home, there might be a feeling that the lack of space is unhealthy. It is important, however, to realize that this is part of the Hispanic culture. The nurse must evaluate the overall home environment, not just its appearance. Chapter 3, Cultural Influences on Nursing Care, offers further discussion on understanding transcultural nursing care.

Resources are not always quickly available when working in a patient's home. As such, it is important to have a good understanding of nursing skills. Home health nursing requires an ability to adapt and remain flexible since the home environment, unlike the hospital environment, can be unknown. Because of this, it is necessary to assess both the patient and her or his home setting. Consider the patient who has been referred to home health services following a fall at home and subsequent fracture of an arm. The referral was for initiating physical therapy services, not skilled nursing. During the initial assessment the nurse notes that the patient is lethargic and experiencing extremely low blood pressure readings upon standing. Further data gathering of the home environment leads the nurse to find that the patient's wife has not been administering the patient's heart medications appropriately—actually administering too much. The home health nurse can contact the supervising registered nurse to contact the doctor to obtain the necessary orders to assess the patient's blood levels of this medication. This example demonstrates how nurses in the home need to evaluate the patient's case not just based on the referral diagnosis, but also what can be occurring within the home that could have contributed to that diagnosis, remaining flexible, and adapting to the patient's needs.

Families play a large part in your care of patient's in the home. Do not be surprised to walk into a home and find several anxious family members with a list of questions they would like answered. They too will be very involved during your visits. This can be very intimidating at first. When preparing for a visit, take the time to review and learn about an unfamiliar diagnosis or medication. This will help you feel more comfortable and assist with developing a trusting relationship with your patient and their families.

SAFETY TIP

Encourage the active involvement of patients and their families in the patient's care as a patient safety strategy. Define and communicate the means for patients and their families to report concerns about safety and encourage them to do so (2006 National Patient Safety Goals from www.jcaho.org)

Because of the **autonomous,** or independent, nature of home health, most agencies require at least 1 year of medical surgical nursing experience. This will ensure that you have gained the necessary knowledge to work in home care. Home health agencies also hire nurses in specialty areas; for example, cardiac nursing or wound care. Nurses with a specific specialty will usually work with patients with diagnoses with which they are familiar. See Box 15.4 (Liability Issues to Consider When Working in Home Health) for liability issues.

(Continued on following page)

Always be prepared for the unexpected. Carry extras of common supplies; for example, various sizes of catheters, sterile dressing gauze, different types of tape, and plenty of alcohol wipes.

THE ROLE OF THE LPN/LVN IN HOME HEALTH

The nurse's role in home health is varied and complex. The nurse works closely with all members of the health-care team. Tasks may be similar to those performed in the hospital setting such as wound care or administration of IV medications (Fig. 15.1). The difference is the setting of where these skills are completed. Many factors need to be considered when assisting patients in the home (e.g., having the necessary supplies, infection control, patient education material, documenting, and personal and patient safety).

Box 15.4

Liability Issues to Consider When Working in Home Health Care

When starting in home health care, review your state's Nurse Practice Act and your scope of practice. The National Council of State Boards of Nursing, http://www.NCSBN.org lists all the State Boards of Nursing websites. This is a very useful tool for any nurse. Understanding your scope of practice will ensure that you complete care that follows your state's guidelines. When in patients' homes they might ask you to perform a skill or request something that is outside your scope of practice. It is important that you explain to them that it is outside your scope of practice but still address their concern by contacting your agency immediately to find out how to handle their request. It is important to address their request as it could indicate a change in their status. For example, if a patient asks you if it is "okay" to increase a medication, you should understand that as a nurse you cannot prescribe medications. So if you were to say it was okay, you would be altering the prescribed dose, and thus practicing outside your scope of practice since only a physician or nurse practitioner can prescribe medications.

Always discuss your concerns with your supervisor and review your agency's guidelines, policies, and procedures. Know what you can and cannot do before you start and never be afraid to question something that you feel or know violates your nurse practice act. Remember it is your license so follow your nurse practice act!

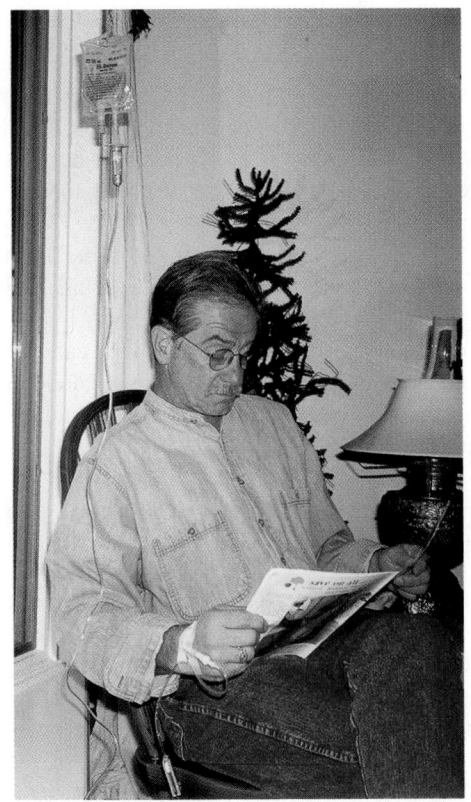

FIGURE 15.1 Patient receiving home IV therapy.

STEPS IN THE HOME HEALTH VISIT

Preparing for the Visit

A typical day for the home nurse consists of six to seven visits. Visits generally last 30 to 45 minutes. Most agencies attempt to arrange visits in the same geographical location for convenience. If your visits are focused on a specialty, such as wound care, you might travel long distances to visit your patients, although your patient assignment would be less than seven visits. Agencies allow for mileage reimbursement, so be sure to keep close track of mileage from house-to-house. The night before your visit, you need to develop a plan of action for how your visits will be structured. Sometimes you will need to be at a certain place at a particular time, so factor this into your planning. Each patient needs to be contacted. Give the patient a 1- to 2-hour window for your arrival time. Remember, you cannot always anticipate what is going to happen during a visit. It is better to let your patients know a time frame range as opposed to an exact time. If you are unsure of how to locate your patient's home, ask while you are arranging the visit time. The agency will usually provide you with an information sheet reviewing the patient's diagnosis, pertinent medical information, and reason for home health. Keep these handy; writing directions to the patient's home on these forms is an easy way to have the information close by. It is important to be organized with this process. If you have too many papers with information on it, it is difficult to manage both your time and the patient's needs, leading to frustration.

LEARNING TIP

The World Wide Web is a great place to find travel information. Mapquest is one such site. The user can type in the beginning and ending address and receive detailed directions on how to get to destinations. The web address is http://www.mapquest.com.

Other things to carry with you are a map and cell phone. Even the best of directions can be confusing once on the road. If for any reason you are going to be late, contact the patient to let him or her know. Remember, these patients are home bound and anxious; arriving late can interfere with developing an effective therapeutic relationship.

Safety Considerations

Home health nurses' travels can take them to dangerous areas. It is important to be vigilant about personal safety. See Box 15.5 (Safety Guidelines for Home Health Nurses) for tips on how to protect yourself before, during, and after a home health visit.

Patient safety is of particular importance in the home. Unlike the hospital, once you leave, there might not be anyone else to visit until you are scheduled to work again. The nurse needs to be alert to things in the home that can pose a hazard to the patient. Box 15.6 (Gerontological Issues) offers some ideas for patient safety consideration in the home.

Remember to consider requesting a referral for physical or occupational therapy. These services can work with the patient to build strength, teach the patient how to use assistive devices, as well as assisting with obtaining those devices. Educating the patient on how to prevent injuries in the home is the best intervention.

Infection Control

Maintaining asepsis in the patient's home may be a challenge. In the hospital, everything is available to ensure infection control. In the home, the nurse is responsible for bringing supplies to ensure safe care. The home health agency will provide information during in-service orientation of their policy and procedures regarding infection control. It is always important to have extras of basic equipment, including:

- Personal safety equipment—disposable gowns, masks, and shoe covers
- Gloves—some latex free
- Red bags of various supplies
- Several biohazard containers

Box 15.5

Safety Guidelines for Home Health Nurses

In general, home health is very safe. Most communities recognize the importance of the role of home health nurses and are receptive to their visits. It is still important to understand how you can protect yourself in case an unsafe situation arises.

Tips for maintaining safety when completing a home health visit:

- Always carry a map, whistle, and cell phone.
- Keep gas tank filled.
- Complete recommended maintenance on your car and have the tires checked regularly.
- If possible, park in the street or road in front of the house. This prevents someone from blocking you in the driveway.
- When entering a home be aware of where the exit doors are and any windows that will allow for safe evacuation from the home.
- Be aware of your outside surroundings. When leaving the home have your supplies packed up and keys out, ready to open the car door.
- If lost in an unknown area, leave and go to a familiar place and contact the patient for directions. Call your agency if concerned about home safety.
- If you need to complete a visit at night, request an escort. Many communities will have a police officer accompany you to and from the home. Discuss this option with your supervisor.
- Never complete a visit if you feel concerned for your safety.

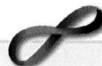 **Box 15.6**

Gerontological Issues

The elderly make up a significant proportion of home health patients. Because of changes in their health, many items in the home can become potential safety hazards. The home health nurse should always assess the patient's safety in the home. Things to look for are:

- Overcrowded spaces
- Scatter/throw rugs
- Bathroom safety
- Adequate lighting
- Access to needed supplies
- Steps to enter the home
- Pets
- Electrical cords

CRITICAL THINKING

Mrs. Smith

■ Mrs. Smith was referred to your home health agency following an appointment with her physician. During that visit it was found that Mrs. Smith was anemic resulting in dizziness, fatigue, and alterations in her blood pressure. The physician requested home health nurses visit for Mrs. Smith to assess her safety and recommend appropriate safety devices.

1. What are some safety devices that can assist Mrs. Smith?
2. What are some hazards in the home the nurse should look for?

Suggested answers at end of chapter.

- Disposable underpads—can be used to provide a clean field for supplies; also good to place one on the floor to put your home health bag on.
- Antibacterial soap
- Sanitizing liquid
- Disinfecting spray to clean your equipment and bag after each visit
- Alcohol wipes for disinfecting thermometers and stethoscopes
- A small chemical spill kit

All these supplies are provided by the home health agency. Periodically go through your supply of this equipment to make sure you have enough. One other important tip to remember is washing your hands. It is important to clean your hands with soap and water prior to beginning and after completing your patient care. If water is not available, use your sanitizing liquid. Do not wash your hands in the patient's kitchen sink, always ask to use the bathroom for your hand washing.

Documentation

Documentation in home health can be challenging. Because of reimbursement guidelines, the nurse needs to document specific things during the visit. Home health agencies receive their income based on a prospective pay system, not per visit payments. On admission, the registered nurse fills out information that is entered into a computer system. This information is called the **O**utcome and **AS**essment Information **S**et, or OASIS. This tool is used to generate information about the home health agency and patient outcomes. It is also used to help develop a plan of care that best meets the patient's problems. The LPN/LVN needs to be familiar with the general function of this form and its relevance to creating a plan of care, although as already stated it generally is the RN who collects this data from the patient.

In order for home health agencies to be reimbursed, they need to demonstrate that a skill was completed. Documenting information is based on the patient's plan of care and the corresponding skill that was completed at the visit. For example, the physician has ordered skilled nursing observation and medication management for a patient. The nurse completing this visit needs to identify when documenting that this skill was completed. Documentation would include:

- Patient's response to a medication—vital signs, level of consciousness, or other potential side effects.
- Patient's current understanding of medication regimen and the action the nurse took to improve that understanding.
- Patient's response to that education and any areas the patient might continue to need assistance.

Home health agencies, like hospitals, have different ways of documenting. The following things are generally included in all home health documentation:

- Arrival and departure times of the nurse
- Assessment findings
- Vital signs
- An area for a narrative note
- Patient's signature verifying the nurse was present in the home

This flow sheet is returned to your facility within an identified time frame (usually within 24 hours of a visit). Nurses who wish to drop off paperwork during times when the office is closed need to find out if their agency has a secure after hours drop box to leave paperwork. If dropping off paperwork after hours, it is necessary to be sure that your forms are neatly organized and papers clipped together.

Information is also kept at the patient's residence. It usually consists of a folder that contains relevant patient information and a communication form that all staff members need to complete at each visit. Similar to hospital charting, this documentation is important to ensure continuity of care, even more so in the home setting because staff members might not cross paths for a verbal report.

 LEARNING TIP

An easy way to ensure you always have the handouts that you need is to organize them into a three-ringed binder. Always have plenty of these handouts when making a visit. Many times families who do not reside with the patient request copies so that they can have them at home. You can organize the information in several different manners; for example, based on the diagnosis or alphabetically.

Patient Education

A primary responsibility of nurses in home health is educating the patient regarding her or his illness and how to effectively manage that illness at home, hopefully decreasing the chance of needing hospitalization. There are many handouts available to offer the patient to help reinforce the verbal instructions you are providing. It is best to utilize forms that are available from your home health agency.

NURSING PROCESS: THE HOME HEALTH PATIENT

Assessment/Data Collection

Monitor and document patient and family's adjustment to change and illness. Perform a complete patient assessment during each visit. Assess the home environment for potential safety hazards and need for devices to assist with care.

Nursing Diagnosis, Planning, and Implementation

Therapeutic regimen management: ineffective related to deficient knowledge, complexity of medical needs, and limited access to social support

EXPECTED OUTCOME: The patient will demonstrate changes in lifestyle necessary to maintain health.

- Work with the patient in developing both short- and long-term goals.
- Recognize small accomplishments positively *to reinforce the progress the patient has made.*
- Educate the patient on management of the health-care regimen.
- Provide educational material in both written and verbal format *to allow for understanding of complex issues with care.*
- Review the plan of care with the patient *to facilitate involvement and eventual independence with care.*
- Identify and work with social support systems.
- Assist the patient with obtaining necessary supplies *to promote wellness.*
- Assess the home environment for hazards and assist the patient with making necessary changes *to promote safety.*
- Assess the patient for changes in health status *that can affect progress.*

Caregiver role strain related to the management of a chronic illness and lack of understanding of resources available

EXPECTED OUTCOME: The caregiver will identify effective ways for dealing with the complexity of a chronic illness.

- Include the caregiver in the plan of care *to help develop an understanding of the management of the illness.*
- Assist the caregiver with identifying community resources available such as respite care, Meals on Wheels, and support groups.
- Enlist the help of a social worker *to facilitate contact with community resources.*
- Assess the caregiver's expectations of the patient's health. *Misconceptions regarding progress can fos-ter anger and frustration toward the patient. Discuss ways to help the caregiver deal effectively with these feelings.*
- Acknowledge the change in roles: for example, child taking care of a parent, and the challenges associated with this change in family roles.

Evaluation

The patient and caregiver will acknowledge acceptance and understanding of the change in health status. This is evidenced by involvement in the plan of care and participation with goal setting, utilization of community resources, maintaining of a safe home environment, and demonstration of ability to manage medical regimen.

OTHER TYPES OF HOME HEALTH NURSING

So far this chapter has focused on Medicare home health that is covered under the Medicare and Medicaid systems. The purpose of this version of home health is to assist the patient with managing health needs on an intermittent basis. There are also other types of home agency service work available for nurses, including private duty nursing and hospice nursing.

Private Duty Nursing

Private duty nursing consists of scheduled care to assist the patient with personnel and homemaking needs. These services have been called home companion services, homemaker services, and private duty care. Many of the services that are offered focus more on companionship and respite care. Families who are taking care of a patient with complex needs, such as an Alzheimer patient, may need time away from the home to complete personal tasks. These agencies provide both licensed and unlicensed assistive personnel (UAP) to help the patient while the family is away. Unlike Medicare home health, these services are considered an out-of-pocket expense, and are not covered by Medicare and Medicaid.

Families can contract with an agency to have a staff member spend 2 to 3 hours a day in the home. The staff can complete homemaking tasks and companion tasks, such as arts and crafts or playing cards. Nurses can work in these agencies in the role of supervisor to unlicensed assistive personnel (UAP). Another role that the nurse can be involved in is assisting the patient with filling weekly medication dispensers. Many nurses enjoy this type of work because of the relationships that are formed with patients and families. They can be involved with the same family for months to years, as opposed to a few months, as is typically seen with Medicare home health patients.

Hospice Nursing

Hospice home agencies work with patients who have a terminal illness with less than 6 months to live. The focus of hospice is not curing the disease but to offer comfort and palliative care for patients who are dying. Hospice nurses are available around the clock, allowing the patient's family to contact them at anytime with questions or when the patient dies. Hospice care also offers bereavement services to the family for up to a year after the patient has died. This service is covered by Medicare. As one can see, hospice can offer many advantages not available through a regular home health agency. A referral to hospice is usually initiated in the hospital. There might, though, come a time when you are working with a patient whose condition declines rapidly. It is important to discuss available options with the home care team before approaching the option of hospice with the patient. Patients need to be ready to accept the fact that they have an incurable illness. Even with that acceptance, sometimes the patient prefers to stay with the agency that they have been working with because of a relationship that has been developed with the staff. Involving social services can help inform the patient of the variations in care they can receive. See Chapter 16, Nursing Care of Patients at the End of Life, Home Health Hint boxes for assistance in understanding how to assist the patient who is dying at home.

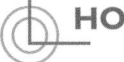 HOME HEALTH NURSING

Home health nursing is a rewarding career path to choose. Nurses who work in the home have the unique opportunity to assist the patient during a time of crisis and be able to experience the results of their interventions. Home health nursing will continue to grow in the 21st century, and the need for qualified professionals will offer many opportunities for the LPN/LVN. Thinking back on the impact that nurses like Lillian Wald had and her ability to change the lives of so many because of her willingness to meet those patients in their homes demonstrates the importance home health nurses have in the successful progression for patients from illness to health and wellness.

REVIEW QUESTIONS

1. What impact did Lillian Wald have on the nursing profession?
   a. Allowed nurses to function as medical care providers
   b. Demonstrated the impact nursing can have on patients' health and wellness
   c. Made it possible for nurses to obtain prescription drugs for patients in the home
   d. Developed the Henry Street Settlement in 1890

Multiple response item. Select all that apply.
2. Which of these are members of the home health team?
   a. LPN/LVN
   b. Physician
   c. Social worker
   d. Home health aide
   e. Lawyer

3. A patient is being seen by home health nurses for monitoring of his weight and vital signs and education about medication changes following an acute exacerbation of heart failure. Documentation for this visit needs to include which of the following?
   a. What the patient ate for breakfast
   b. How far the patient was able to ambulate while working with physical therapy
   c. Education about the role of the home health aide in assisting the patient with personal care
   d. Education about how to keep a log of daily weights and when to contact the physician regarding a potential problem.

4. An LPN/LVN has started working for a local home health agency and is concerned about the transition to home health nursing after working in the hospital for 10 years. What are some recommendations that would ease this transition for the LPN/LVN?
   a. Explain that home health nursing is just like hospital nursing
   b. Instruct him or her to always be prepared, to keep paperwork organized, and spend some time the night before a visit to review patient health information to help her or him gain confidence in the home.
   c. Allow an opportunity for exploring feelings and acknowledging that this is a hard transition.
   d. Let the nurse know it is not possible to completely adjust to home health nursing because of variability in the home.

5. What steps can the home health nurse take to ensure that the patient is not exposed to infectious materials in the home?
   a. Disinfect the home health bag after each patient visit with a germicidal spray supplied by the home health agency.
   b. Wash hands in the kitchen sink rather than the bathroom sink.
   c. Use the same red bag from patient-to-patient for disposing of soiled dressings.
   d. If a chemical spill occurs contact agency to send personnel to clean it up.

6. In reinforcing teaching to a patient about the primary difference between hospice care and home health care, which of the following would the LPN/LVN include in the explanation?
   a. Visits occur weekly in hospice versus daily in home care.
   b. Volunteers provide hospice care but nurses provide home care.
   c. Patients must enter hospice if they are dying.
   d. Palliative care versus managing a return to a functional level of wellness.

References

1. U.S. Department of Labor; Bureau of Labor Statistics, 2005. Retrieved from http://www.bls.gov
2. Friends of Mt. Hope Cemetery. Stories in stone: Famous women in Mt. Hope Cemetery, 2004. Retrieved from http://www.fomh.org/Stories/Wald.htm
3. Centers for Medicare & Medicaid Services. Home Health Agency Manual, Coverage of services, Chapter 11, 2004. Retrieved from http://www.cms.hhs.gov/manuals/11_hha/hh200.asp#_201_1
4. Doenges, ME, Moorhouse, MF, and Murr, AC. Nurse's Pocket Guide: Diagnosis, Interventions, and Rationales, ed. 9. Philadelphia, F.A. Davis, 2004.

SUGGESTED ANSWERS TO

CRITICAL THINKING

■ Mr. Jones

1. The loss of Mr. Jones' wife and his subsequent health problems have impacted his ability to properly care for himself. A proper diet is important for healing and maintenance of health. A referral to Meals on Wheels would be appropriate. This agency will deliver at least one healthy meal each week day (usually lunch). The meal can be adapted to meet the patient's dietary guidelines. Many communities offer elder services to patients at a reduced cost to assist with housekeeping services. Helping the patient set up homemaker services will help him through this difficult time. Offering the patient information about grief counseling services in the community can be beneficial during this time. Once discharged from home health the patient can begin attending counseling services. Other community resources to consider are: neighborhood socials, church services if appropriate, and online communities that match the patient's values.

2. The physician needs to be contacted about the patient's withdrawn demeanor and lack of interest in self care. Mr. Jones may be experiencing a situational depression because of the recent loss of his wife and his own health problems. During this time the physician might decide to prescribe an antidepressant to help.

3. The nurse recognizes that Mr. Jones needs extra help at this time. Consider a referral for social services to assist with community resources and grief counseling. Because heart failure is a chronic disease that can contribute to fatigue, an occupational therapist can work with the patient in developing energy conserving techniques for completing activities of daily living. Also the services of a home health aide can help with personal care and provide additional emotional support.

■ Mrs. Smith

1. Since anemia can cause extreme fatigue it is important for Mrs. Smith to have safety devices in the home to prevent falls. These devices can be obtained from a medical supply store and are usually covered by Medicare. Equipment to consider includes a bath stool for the shower so the patient can sit while bathing, a detachable shower head, hand rails in the shower and hallways, a bedside commode, an over-the-toilet seat, a reacher to assist with obtaining objects at a distance, a medical alert device that can be worn at all times, and if fatigue is severe enough a motorized wheelchair.

2. The home has many hazards. Important things to assess for include: scatter/throw rugs, overcrowded spaces, sharp edges along furniture, inadequate lighting, and stairs. Instruct the patient to keep frequently used kitchen appliances and foods on shelves that are easy to reach. The same is true for the bathroom and bedroom. Assist the patient with setting up a "command center" in the living room so that favorite items are kept in close proximity and the patient does not have to get up so frequently.

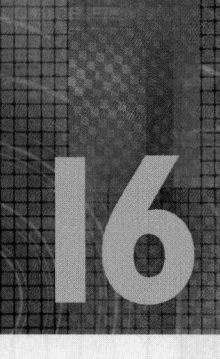

16

Nursing Care of Patients at the End of Life

BETSY MURPHY

KEY TERMS

AdvanceMedical Directive (ad-VANS MED-ik-uhl dur-EK-tiv)
advocate (ADD-voh-kut)
artificial feeding (ART-ih-FISH-uhl FEE-ding)
artificial hydration (ART-ih-FISH-uhl hy-DRAY-shun)
Do Not Resuscitate (DOO not re-SUSS-ih-TATE)
Living Will (LIV-ing WIL)
Durable Medical Power of Attorney (DUR-uh-buhl POW-ur uv uh-TUR-nee)
hospice (HOS-pis)
postmortem care (pohst-MOR-tum KARE)

QUESTIONS TO GUIDE YOUR READING

1. Who is the patient who is approaching the end of life?

2. What are the necessary legal documents for patients with life-limiting illness?

3. What choices are available to patients at the end of life?

4. How do you communicate with dying patients and their families?

5. What are the expected physical changes in the dying process?

6. What are nursing interventions you can provide at the end of life?

7. What is post mortem care?

8. What are nursing interventions you can implement for the grieving patient and family?

9. What is the role of the LPN/LVN in hospice care?

CASE STUDY

Mr. Moran, 89 years old, resides in a nursing home, and has been losing weight and growing weaker for the last 6 months. Despite treatment for depression, he continues to grow weaker and more dependent on his caregivers. As you read this chapter, consider what decisions this family will face and what resources are available to them in their quest to provide appropriate care for him.

A GOOD DEATH

Despite our best efforts, there will become a time that all our patients will die. Death is the expected end to a life well lived. In America, only 10% of us will die suddenly. The remaining 90% will experience a gradual decline over a period of months or years.

In the 21st century, most Americans will die from chronic and acute illnesses from diseases such as cancer, heart disease, stroke, and dementia. We have the technology to prolong life, but sometimes this longer life can carry with it profound disability and reduced quality of life. Our patients sometimes tell us that this is not what they intended for the last phase of their life. The challenge for nurses then is twofold: 1) to help identify patients with life limiting illnesses early, so they and their families have the opportunity to define their goals of care, and 2) to help our patients communicate their wishes to healthcare providers, both orally and in writing, to assure that their wishes are understood.

Perhaps the most important role for nurses is to give our patients support and validation as they move through the series of losses leading to a *good death*. Dying is, after all, the final phase of our growth and development. The developmental tasks associated with this phase involve reflecting on our lives, saying goodbye, saying "I am sorry" and saying "I love you." The goal of having a "good death" is a valid goal.

In a 1999 study, a focus group of terminally ill patients defined what would constitute a *good death* for them. The results fit into 5 categories:

- Adequate pain and symptom management
- Ability to make their own decisions
- Dying that is not prolonged
- Minimal emotional and financial burden on their families
- Ability to use remaining time to strengthen their relationships with their loved ones.

This definition of a good death helps nurses listen to what patients want and to focus on how best to help them achieve their goals. Nurses who choose to provide care for the dying experience personal growth in their own lives. Facing the inevitability of our own mortality can force us to look more deeply at our beliefs, values, and priorities in life. This can result in a richer, more focused life.

IDENTIFYING IMPENDING DEATH

Although most Americans voice that they want to die at home, almost 80% today die in facilities. 20% die in nursing homes, but by the year 2020, it is estimated that 50% will die in nursing homes. Some researchers have found that 1/3 to 1/2 of the patients who enter nursing homes die within a year. Nurses who are working in long-term care and assisted-living facilities will find themselves in a position to both identify patients who are likely to die soon and also to support these patients' families in planning for a good death.

Death can be caused by disease, but some patients simply show weight loss and progressive weakness as indicators that they are in the final months of life. Research has shown that measuring progressive weight loss and increasing dependency can help identify patients who are dying. One research study showed that elderly patients in nursing homes who lose 10% of their body weight in 6 months, have an 85% chance of dying in the next 6 months. Weight loss caused by depression or acute illness can sometimes be reversed with aggressive treatment. But if neither depression nor acute illness is the cause of the patient's decline, he or she may be entering the final months of life.

Experience tells us that elderly patients with gradually increasing weakness and increasing dependence for activities of daily living (ADLs) are declining. Elderly patients who are having trouble swallowing and require treatment for aspiration pneumonia are likely to die within a year. Their decreased respiratory muscle strength, lack of lung elasticity, and poor immune response make recovery unlikely. Elderly patients with poor renal and cardiac functions are at high risk for dying. The final truth is that for some patients with chronic illness, many treatments offer little benefit. This chapter explores some of the choices people have to make at the end of life.

ADVANCE DIRECTIVES, LIVING WILLS, AND DURABLE MEDICAL POWER OF ATTORNEY

The *Patient Self Determination Act* ensures that every patient has the right to accept or refuse any medical treatment that is offered. The Act also requires health-care professionals to ask patients entering a hospital if they have prepared an **Advance Medical Directive**. In preparing an Advance Medical Directive, patients are exercising their rights to make their wishes known regarding specific medical treatments should they become incapacitated. The Directive requires the signatures of two witnesses, neither of whom can be a family member or health-care provider. There are really two parts to an Advance Medical Directive: a **Living Will** and a **Durable Medical Power of Attorney** for Health Care.

Living Wills are documents instructing physicians about patients' preferences (such as to withhold or withdraw life-sustaining procedures) in patients who are unable to communicate, found to be permanently unconscious, and/or have been declared "terminal." A Durable Power of Attorney document specifies who will speak for the patient when he or she cannot speak for himself or herself. Many states have standard forms to use, and may require both a Durable Power of Attorney and Living Will to be legal. An attorney, although not necessary, may be helpful for some families.

Encourage patients to not only fill out the necessary forms, but also to discuss their wishes with all family members. It is estimated that only about 15% of Americans have an Advance Medical Directive. Some patients are reluctant to complete an Advance Directive. They are concerned that they may change their mind about treatments in the future. It can be helpful to talk about advance care planning as a *process*. Treatments we choose to have today may not be wanted tomorrow.

Remind patients that they can revoke an Advance Directive at any time and in any place and institute a new one. What matters most is that they get started and document their wishes today.

 # END OF LIFE CHOICES

Cardiopulmonary Resuscitation

During the 1960s, cardiopulmonary resuscitation (CPR) was developed as a method of rescuing healthy people who suffered a cardiac or respiratory arrest. Some of the early guidelines specified that CPR was not to be used in patients with terminal illnesses. It was intended for healthy patients with reversible conditions. Today, CPR has become standard in both hospitals and nursing homes. All patients will receive CPR unless they have a **Do Not Resuscitate** (DNR) order. There is also a perception that CPR can save most lives. The *real* statistics about CPR are as presented in Table 16.1.

One reason for such low survival rates is that CPR must begin within 3 to 5 minutes of collapse. The most successful cases are ones in which CPR plus AED (automatic external defibrillator) are used within 3 to 5 minutes. Medical researchers reviewed 113 studies on the use of CPR in hospitals over a 33-year period and found some additional reasons for the low survival rate. They found that patients with the lowest chance of survival (less than 2% chance) were those who (1) had more than one or two medical problems, (2) were unable to live independently, and (3) had a terminal illness. All patients living in nursing homes and assisted-living facilities are unable to live independently. Patients with terminal illness would include cancer, dementia, or any progressive illness.

Some patients choose to have CPR because they fear that without CPR they will be deprived of treatments that will benefit them or alleviate their distress. Most patients do not realize that their chance of survival is statistically low and also that after CPR, if they survive, their quality of life may be diminished. A small number of patients actually believe that CPR is a procedure that may improve their overall medical condition. A helpful way of presenting the DNR option is to talk about three issues: (1) the statistics outlined above, (2) that the choice is really whether the patient will receive aggressive comfort care as they are dying or CPR, which may cause distress and will likely prove futile, and (3) even if elderly patients receive successful CPR, their quality of life is usually greatly reduced, not improved.

Do Not Resuscitate Orders

A "No Code" or **Do Not Resuscitate (DNR)** order is written in a hospital or nursing home setting after collaboration with the patient, family, and health-care provider, usually after it has been determined that the patient will not benefit from receiving cardiopulmonary resuscitation (CPR). DNR simply means that CPR will not be done. Patients still must decide whether they want aggressive treatment of their underlying condition, up to but not including CPR, or whether they want only comfort measures without therapeutic treatment. Some hospitals offer several options:

- Do Not Resuscitate, Comfort Care Only
- Do Not Resuscitate, Full Therapeutic Support
- Full Code

Outside of the hospital, at home, or in most nursing facilities, patients will have fewer options for aggressive treatment. Patients can, however, choose to have a DNR order that will be recognized by emergency personnel. Many states have a "Durable DNR" document that, once signed, can be displayed in the patient's home to advise rescue personnel that the patient does not want to receive CPR. These may also be called "out of hospital" or "prehospital" DNR orders.

Many people assume that their documented desire *not* to receive resuscitation in a living will is all that is necessary. In states that have an out of hospital DNR policy, the patient will receive CPR regardless of their stated wishes in their Advance Medical Directive unless they have completed the Durable DNR document.

Some patients fear that in choosing DNR status they will suffer and be alone at the time of their death. It is important to tell patients that DNR does not mean "do not treat." Even patients who have a DNR/Comfort Care order can receive oxygen, medications, and other comfort measures to aggressively manage their symptoms and assure a comfortable death. All DNR orders and discussions with families

TABLE 16.1 SUCCESS OF CPR IN SAVING LIVES

In Hospital: All Patients	10%–15% survival rate
In Hospital : Elderly Patients	Less that 5% survival rate
Out of hospital: All patients	Less than 5% survival rate
Nursing Home Patients	1%–2% survival rate

Box 16.1

Patient Perspective

Anna

My mom, Anna, was diagnosed with cardiomyopathy and congestive heart failure when she was 60 years old. At that time she was still working, and had just remarried. She thought she had many years left in life. She did not have an Advance Directive—Why would she?

Two years later, as her disease progressed, she decided she did not want to "live on machines." So with the help of her doctor and our family, she wrote her Living Will and made her new husband her Durable Power of Attorney, with me as his backup person. Since she was still functioning really well with lots of medications and occasional hospitalization, she chose a DNR status, but with full therapeutic, aggressive interventions. She even took a tour of Europe during this time in her life, knowing she would not be able to do it later.

By the age of 67, she had a lot less energy to do things, and her heart failure really cramped her lifestyle. But she still enjoyed life, and her goal was to see her oldest grandson, my son, graduate from high school. She considered a heart transplant, but her doctor told her she was too old to qualify. She did have a new kind of valve surgery that was supposed to make her feel better, but it didn't help much.

Three months after my son's graduation, she was hospitalized several times with progressively worse outcomes. She weighed barely 100 pounds, and could not eat much. She was only 70 years old, and still looked and acted so young! Finally, she was in a semicoma in the hospital, and our family had to make the difficult decision to withdraw all therapeutic support. She was now a DNR, with Comfort Measures only. We were confident this would be what she wanted because we had talked about it with her.

She was discharged home with hospice care, and died within a week. I moved in for her final days to help out, and between me, her husband, and her hospice nurse (who was a godsend), and frequent visits from family and her minister, she had a really good death. We kept her comfortable with lots of attention and morphine. She was alert and able to converse much of the time. She ate what and when she wanted, which amounted to one-quarter of a cheese and tomato sandwich one day, but she enjoyed it! She could finally enjoy a glass of grapefruit juice, which she had been unable to have for years because it interacted with one of her heart medications.

At the end, she died with me holding her right hand and her husband holding her left. We were telling her we loved her. It was a good death.

CRITICAL THINKING

Mrs. Hart

■ Mrs. Hart has written a living will specifying her wishes should she become incapacitated. Because she has advanced disease, she tells you she would not want to be resuscitated if she has a cardiac arrest. She is currently hospitalized but will be discharged to her home in a few days. What documents does she need to have in place to ensure she will not receive resuscitation?

Suggested answers at end of chapter.

---

should be documented on the patient's chart (Box 16.1 Patient Perspective).

Artificial Feeding and Hydration

When patients can no longer eat or drink, it may happen as a result of three conditions. It may be due to an acute illness, or after a long illness with multiple medical problems, or simply due to the aging process. Otherwise healthy patients who are unable to eat while recovering from an acute illness will probably benefit from tube feeding. Patients who are declining either due to multiple medical problems or the aging process probably will not.

In recent years, there has been important research to help guide the decision to insert a feeding tube. In 1999, a 30-year retrospective review of dementia patients who received feeding tubes revealed the following. These patients did not live longer (than patients who were hand fed), the feeding tube *increased* rather than *decreased* the risk of aspiration pneumonia, the feeding tube did not prevent or reverse weight loss, and it did not heal or prevent decubitus ulcers. As a result of this research, The National Alzheimer's Association recommends that instead of a feeding tube, these patients receive an effective program of hand feeding. It has long been known that although a feeding tube or TPN (total parenteral nutrition) is helpful for cancer patients who are losing weight due to therapeutic treatments such as chemotherapy, it is not helpful for patients who are actively dying from cancer.

There are even some benefits in withholding **artificial feeding** and **artificial hydration** in the final weeks of life in actively dying patients. These benefits are:

- Fewer pharyngeal and lung secretions, which can reduce dyspnea
- Reduced swelling around tumors, which can reduce associated pain
- Less urination, resulting in dryer skin with less breakdown.

It has been theorized that as dehydration occurs, the body produces a form of endorphin, which enhances comfort. As ketone levels rise (from breakdown of body fat), patients experience an anesthetic effect that creates a sense of well-being. Hospices have done comparative research studying patients who received IV hydration and those who did not to understand the effect of hydration on comfort. They surveyed both groups of patients in the days before death, asking about discomfort. They discovered that both groups were comfortable and both voiced only one complaint, having a "dry mouth." Neither group reported complaints of hunger or increased pain. Because both groups experienced dry mouths, it was speculated that the cause of dry mouth was due to the medications used at end of life. When frequent mouth care was added to the care plan, the complaint of dry mouth dissipated.

The issue of feeding is a very emotionally difficult one for families. Often their loved one has been ill a long time. Bringing favorite foods may have been one of the ways they showed love and communicated caring. Families will need support in making decisions about feeding in three important ways: (1) identifying goals of care and evaluating whether artificial feeding will help meet those goals, (2) weighing the benefits and burdens of feeding, and (3) finding new ways (besides feeding) to communicate their love such as skin care, mouth care, or reading to their loved one.

For a different perspective on artificial feeding, see Box 16.2 Ethical Considerations.

Hospitalization

A hospital is where patients go to receive aggressive medical treatment. The goal of care in a hospital is to improve the patient medically and transfer him or her to an appropriate level of care that will better meet individualized needs. There are burdens associated with hospitalization for elderly patients approaching the end of life. These patients may actually decline more rapidly in a hospital setting. Research has shown that *all* elderly patients lose weight in a hospital. Research on dementia patients has shown that patients with dementia lose weight and suffer irreversible cognitive decline with each hospitalization. They enter a foreign environment and are cared for by health-care workers who do not know them. Often the patients are restrained as they become agitated and become fearful away from where they call *home*. Patients who are frail and have poor immunity are also at risk. They often enter the hospital with one infection and are discharged with infections resistant to antibiotics or ones caused by antibiotics, such as *Clostridium difficile* infections.

Patients living in nursing facilities with end-stage dementia who have severe cognitive impairment will benefit from having a "Do Not Hospitalize" order. This will main-

---

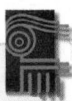

Box 16.2

Ethical Considerations

Euthanasia

Karen has worked in a long-term care facility for the past 9 years. She works very hard in her job as an LPN to ensure that all of her patients receive the best care possible during their stay. Karen values life and has a special interest in palliative care and end of life issues.

Karen has been caring for Adam since he came to the hospice 5 years ago. Adam is a 28-year-old man who has been in a "waking coma" since a car accident. He has made no progress over the time he has been in care. Adam is married and both his wife and parents are actively involved in his care.

Adam occasionally makes indistinguishable sounds, his eyes are open but do not fix upon any object, and he can move his head from side to side. He can't swallow, so he has a gastric feeding tube. Adam is unable to move, and has extensive limb contractures and chronic decubitus ulcers. He is incontinent, so he wears an adult brief and has a urinary catheter. He suffers from frequent bouts of stomatitis, skin and urinary tract infections, and occasionally pneumonia.

Adam's wife believes that Adam will never fully recover or regain any meaningful control over his body. She believes his tube feeding should be discontinued. Should this happen, it seems certain that Adam will die from dehydration soon after. Adam's parents, however, remain hopeful that Adam will eventually recover and regain some normal func-

tion. They are also firm believers in the value of human life, in any condition, and believe it would be wrong to allow him to die. As a result, Adam's wife has petitioned the courts to have his feeding tube stopped. There is tension between the two parties, and they try to avoid each other as much as possible.

Eventually, Adam's wife wins her fight to have the feeding stopped. On the day that this is to happen, Karen is the LPN on duty and it falls to her to discontinue the feeding and clamp the tubing. The tube is left intact in case it is needed to administer medications needed for comfort. Karen is aware that once the feeding is stopped, Adam will not be able to eat or drink by himself and will most likely die in the near future.

What are the important issues here? First, there are two opposing sides. Adam's wife insists that Adam has no viable future and would not have wanted to endure such a state for such a long time. She points out that there has been extensive neurological damage that cannot be reversed, leading to her conclusion that Adam, as he was known, no longer exists. His parents maintain that life, in whatever form and at whatever cost, should be supported and protected. Who is right?

What principles should guide Adam's care?

What is Karen's primary obligation?

Who is protecting Adam's rights?

Should Karen stop the feeding?

tain the patient in an environment that feels "safe" and preserves his or her chosen quality of life.

Hospice Care

Many people think of **hospice** as a "place." It is actually a service. The service is provided in private homes or independent and assisted-living facilities. It can also be provided in hospitals and nursing homes when there is a signed contract between the hospice organization and the facility. In order to qualify for hospice, a patient must have a prognosis of living for 6 months or less.

Some indicators of a 6-month or less prognosis (regardless of diagnosis) are 10% loss of weight in 6 months, functional decline, frequent hospital admissions, and recurrent infections. The goal of hospice care is holistic: to manage symptoms such as pain and nausea, to provide emotional and spiritual counseling for the patient and family, and to support the patient in achieving his or her goals of care. Each patient is assigned a multidisciplinary hospice team (Table 16.2).

Most health insurance companies now provide a hospice benefit. Many are modeled after the Medicare Hospice benefit. The Medicare benefit pays for both routine hospice care at home and inpatient hospice care provided in a hospital or a skilled nursing facility via contract or in a freestanding hospice unit. Medications, medical supplies, oxygen, and durable medical equipment are also covered if they are related to the "terminal" diagnosis.

Hospice care can assist a family to take care of a patient at home, but hospice nurses do not routinely provide 24-hour in home care. Nurses and other team members make regular visits to support the patient and family. (A nurse is "on call" for in home visits 24 hours a day.) If the patient does not have family support for 24-hour care at times of medical crisis, then short-term inpatient hospice services or 24-hour in home continuous nursing care may be provided under some hospice benefits.

COMMUNICATING WITH PATIENTS AND THEIR LOVED ONES

Terminal illness is a family experience. *Family* is defined by the patient and may include blood relatives, friends, significant others, or partners. The primary role of the nurse is to facilitate a comfortable death that honors the choices of the patient and family. The nurse, therefore, becomes the **advocate**, assuring that the patient and family wishes are communicated to other members of the health-care team. In addition, the nurse is often the *professional caregiver* and *educator* of the nonprofessional caregivers and family.

In order to successfully work with dying patients and families, you must demonstrate empathy, unconditional positive regard, trustworthiness, and critical thinking. You are part of an interdisciplinary team. The team consists of the physician; nurse; social worker; chaplain, physical, occupational and speech therapists; and others. Each discipline has expertise and can lend support to the others in providing care. As illustrated in the section on end of life choices, patients and their loved ones need support and evidence-based medical information to make good decisions. All members of the team can assist with this support.

Good communication requires that you take time to listen, answer questions honestly, help to identify choices, and allow verbalization of fears. Eighty percent of communication is nonverbal, such as eye contact, body language, and tone of voice. Take time to identify your own communication barriers that will affect your ability to talk with families. Do you have fears about your own mortality, lack personal experience with death, fear being blamed for decisions, or disagree with decisions that were made? These barriers will affect your ability to sit with patients and families in crisis, sustain eye contact, and support them in their process. Practice attentive listening with patients and families. Encourage them to talk; be silent, don't change the subject, and know that you do not have to have all the answers. Your role can be to help them reflect on what they are trying to communicate and to clarify their goals of care so you may better advocate for them.

Set the stage for communication by sitting down to show you are not in a hurry (Figure 16.1). Maintain eye contact, encourage them to speak, repeat what they said to gain clarification, and reflect on its meaning. Some things to say to facilitate good communication include:

- "Do you feel like talking?"
- "Tell me more about your fears of …."
- Use repetition: "You mentioned you were upset by …."
- Reflect: "So are you saying that ….?"
- "What does this mean to you?"
- "How can I help you?"

TABLE 16.2 THE HOSPICE TEAM

Physician	Works with the patient's primary physician, offering suggestions to improve care. Directs the activities of the team and often will make visits to the patient's home.
Nurse	Makes routine home visits, assessing patient's needs and implementing plan of care. Nurses are available to visit 24 hours per day as needed.
Social worker	Provides emotional counseling and long term planning, assisting patients with insurance issues and helping to identify community resources.
Chaplain or minister	Provides spiritual counseling or coordinates care of spiritual issues with the patient's chosen spiritual counselor. May participate in funeral or memorial service.
Home health aide	Provides personal care, linen changes, light housekeeping.
Volunteers	Give caregivers support by staying with the patient while they get out of the house. May also read to patient, run errands, etc.
Bereavement counselor	Provides counseling for family and significant others for 13 months after the date of the patient's death.

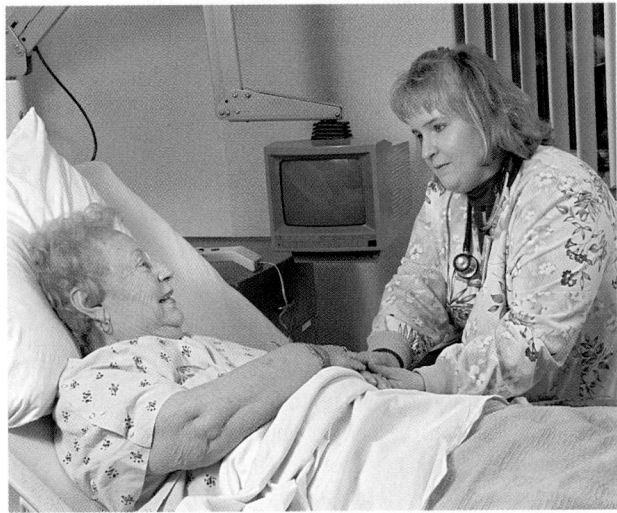

FIGURE 16.1 Nurses can be a comfort to patients and family members.

From the patient's perspective, there are many factors that influence the content and quality of communication with you. Some patients are so afraid they cannot hear what they have been told about their illness. It can be helpful to ask what the doctor has said in order to get baseline information about where they are in understanding their disease.

Patients may use denial as a mechanism to protect themselves from becoming overwhelmed by emotion. The denial is necessary to enable them to survive on a day-by-day basis. It is not necessary for you to remove their denial. Some patients remain in denial throughout the course of their illness. When patients in denial ask you a direct question about their condition, it can be an indicator that they are ready to hear the truth. It is essential that you always answer questions honestly and to the best of your knowledge. Dishonestly destroys trust and credibility.

Patients and their families may also feel angry. Allowing them to express their anger will validate it and enable them to progress emotionally. Comments like, "It is okay to be angry with God and anybody else," will encourage them to continue to talk. Patients who fully understand their prognosis will express sadness and regret. Sitting with patients as they express sadness will allow them to share their feeling and give you an opportunity to offer emotional support.

THE DYING PROCESS

This section discusses the expected changes in the days and hours before death. Assessing the patient for these changes, planning and implementing treatments, and evaluating patient's response to interventions are all important. See Box 16.3 Nursing Care Plan for the Patient at the End of Life for nursing interventions.

Educating caregivers about what to expect is essential. Caregivers who anticipate the expected changes and understand the rationale behind the interventions are more successful in their care giving and have fewer regrets or concerns after the death. See Box 16.3 Nursing Care Plan for the Patient at the End of Life for specific communications that may help caregivers understand what is happening and how they can help.

Eating and Drinking

As bodies move toward death, there is less desire for food and fluids. Patients are conserving energy and often do not feel hunger. The swallowing reflex can be impaired with increased risk of choking. Patients fear choking and may hold their mouth tightly closed when food or fluids are offered. This is normal and the resultant dehydration will enhance comfort due to endorphin production and rising ketone levels.

Changes in Breathing

It is estimated that 50% to 70% of patients have dyspnea at end of life. Dyspnea may be reported by alert patients. Those who are not alert may exhibit tachypnea (respiratory rate >24), facial grimacing, and use of accessory muscles to breathe. Untreated dyspnea will lead to fear and agitation, leading to more dyspnea. Some patients will also have episodes of apnea in the days or hours before they die.

There are many causes of dyspnea. Pneumonia, anemia, congestive heart failure, and pleural effusion can be successfully treated early in the course of illness. Dyspnea that occurs in the final hours of life is not treated by correcting the underlying condition, but can be effectively managed and controlled (see Box 16.3. Nursing Care Plan for the Patient at the End of Life).

Oral Secretions

Saliva that the patient is now unable to swallow may collect in the back of the throat causing a sound sometimes called a "death rattle." This can be disconcerting for the family. See Box 16.3 Nursing Care Plan for the Patient at the End of Life for interventions.

Temperature Changes

As the body loses its ability to control temperature, the patient may become diaphoretic or feel cold all the time. Some patients have experienced fevers as high as 105°F (40.5°C). As death approaches, the feet and legs may become cyanotic and mottled. This is often an indicator that death will occur within hours.

Bowel and Bladder Changes

Most patients will become incontinent of bowel and bladder during the course of the illness. Urine output will decrease as dehydration occurs. Urine will often darken in color and have a strong odor.

(Text continued on page 281)

Box 16.3   NURSING CARE PLAN for the Patient at the End of Life

Nursing Diagnosis: Impaired gas exchange related to dying heart and lungs as evidenced by dyspnea, change in respiratory rate, Sao_2 <90%

Expected Outcomes Patient will state breathing is comfortable; respiratory rate is between 12 and 20 per minute, Sao_2 ≥90%.

Evaluation of Outcomes Is patient's breathing relaxed and rate between 12 and 20? Is Sao_2 ≥90%?

Interventions	Rationale	Evaluation
Monitor respiratory rate and effort.	Increased rate and effort indicate distress.	Is patient in distress? Are further interventions needed?
Administer diuretics or antibiotics as ordered.	Diuretics or antibiotics may be given to treat the dyspnea and promote comfort, not to prolong life.	Do diuretics or antibiotics reduce dyspnea?
Explain to the family the rationale for medical interventions.	Blood transfusions may be given to improve oxygenation and reduce dyspnea; a thoracentesis may promote lung expansion. These are not intended to prolong life, but to promote comfort.	Are additional interventions needed and effective? Does family understand rationale for their use?
Plan activities to conserve energy.	Spacing rest with activity will help reduce oxygen consumption.	Is patient able to tolerate spaced activities?
Place patient upright in a recliner with pillows to 45 degrees.	An upright position allows lung expansion.	Does positioning reduce dyspnea?
Offer alternative comfort measures such as massage and muscle relaxation.	Relaxation reduces anxiety and resulting dyspnea.	Are alternative measures effective?
Administer oxygen as ordered.	Oxygenation raises Sao_2 and reduces dyspnea.	Does oxygen raise Sao_2 and relieve dyspnea?
Place a fan in room if patient desires.	The feeling of breeze may reduce subjective feelings of dyspnea.	Does patient state or appear more comfortable with fan on?
Administer low dose morphine as ordered.	Morphine causes peripheral vasodilation, which can reduce pulmonary edema. It can also reduce anxiety.	Are respirations less labored after morphine?
Explain to patient and family: *This very small dose of morphine will help to slow his breathing down so that he feels more comfortable. It also works on the part of the brain that makes him feel short of breath, to take away the sense of panic.*	The informed patient and family will be able to cooperate and assist with keeping the patient comfortable.	Do patient and family understand reasons for care and feel secure that patient is receiving best possible care?

Nursing Diagnosis: Ineffective airway clearance related to excessive secretions and inability to swallow as evidenced by gurgling sound, "death rattle"

Expected Outcomes The patient's airway will be free of secretions.

Evaluation of Outcomes Is patient's breathing quiet and unlabored?

Interventions	Rationale	Evaluation
Adjust the patient's head to allow secretions to move down the throat.	This will help the patient swallow the secretions and decrease frightening noise.	Is breathing quieter?
Place a humidifier in the room.	Humidified air can liquefy secretions and help the patient to cough.	Is patient able to cough up secretions?

(Continued on following page)

Interventions

If secretions are copious, administer hyoscyamine or scopolamine as ordered.

Administer low dose morphine as ordered.

Suction patient prn.

Teach patient and family *"Because he can no longer swallow saliva, it collects in the back of his throat. This medication will help to reduce the secretions and reduce his feeling of shortness of breath."*

Rationale

These are anticholinergic medications that can dry secretions.

Morphine also has anticholinergic action that can help dry secretions.

If secretions are not controlled by non-invasive measures, suctioning may be necessary.

The informed patient and family will be able to cooperate and assist with keeping the patient comfortable.

Evaluation

Do medications help dry secretions?

Does morphine help quiet breathing and help patient stay calm?

Is suctioning necessary? Is it effective?

Do patient and family understand reasons for care and feel secure that patient is receiving best possible care?

Nursing Diagnosis: Imbalanced nutrition: less than body requirements related to inability to swallow and lack of appetite as evidenced by refusing food, weight loss

Expected Outcomes The patient will state satisfaction with amount and types of food offered. The patient will not aspirate food or fluid.

Evaluation of Outcomes Does patient appear content with foods and fluids offered? Does he or she swallow without aspirating?

Interventions

Allow the patient to choose when and what to eat. Do not force the patient to eat if he does not wish.

Sit the patient upright to eat or drink.

Explain to family as needed: *"He is afraid to swallow now because his swallowing is impaired and it causes him to choke. As he becomes dehydrated, comfort will be enhanced as the body produces endorphins and naturally occurring anesthesia."*

Rationale

The goal is no longer providing adequate nutrition, but keeping the patient comfortable.

This can help the patient swallow and prevent aspiration.

The informed patient and family will be able to cooperate and assist with keeping the patient comfortable.

Evaluation

Is the patient receiving the foods and fluids he wants?

Does patient swallow effectively?

Do patient and family understand reasons for care and feel secure that patient is receiving best possible care?

Nursing Diagnosis: Impaired oral mucous membrane related to dehydration, not eating

Expected Outcomes The patient's mucous membranes will be clean and moist.

Evaluation of Outcomes Are mucous membranes clean and moist? Does patient indicate that his mouth is moist?

Interventions

If alert, offer the patient ice chips or sips of water.

Provide frequent mouth care with sponge tipped toothettes.

Apply lanolin to lips.

Rationale

To keep mucous membranes moist.

This can keep mucous membranes moist when patient is not able to drink adequate fluids.

To keep the mouth and lips from becoming dry and crusty.

Evaluation

Does patient indicate mouth feels comfortable?

Is mouth clean and moist?

Are lips smooth and moist?

Nursing Diagnosis: Impaired comfort (pain, terminal restlessness) related to disease process, dying process, medications

Expected Outcomes The patient will state he or she feels comfortable. If unable to speak, he or she will appear calm and peaceful, not restless or agitated.

Evaluation of Outcomes Is patient comfortable, calm, and peaceful?

Interventions	Rationale	Evaluation
Assess for reversible causes of agitation. • Assess the patient for pain or other discomfort. • Assess for urinary retention or fecal impaction. • Assess for medications that are no longer beneficial. • Assess SaO_2.	Often agitation is a sign of discomfort. Identifying and removing the cause of the discomfort can help calm the patient. Ask the healthcare provider to simplify the medication regimen.	Can causes be identified? Are they removed?
Reposition in bed at least every two hours and prn.	Repositioning frequently can promote comfort and relieve pressure on bony prominences. When other medical interventions are discontinued, the patient still needs to be repositioned regularly to prevent uncomfortable complications.	Does repositioning promote comfort?
If SaO_2 is low, administer oxygen as ordered.	Low SaO_2 causes dyspnea, which is not comfortable.	Is SaO_2 raised to 90%? Is patient's breathing unlabored?
Discuss with the physician discontinuing all uncomfortable procedures, such as blood draws and finger sticks for blood glucose.	Many procedures provide information to the staff but are not beneficial to the patient at the end of life. They should be discontinued.	Are any uncomfortable procedures still being carried out that are not absolutely necessary?
If the cause of the agitation cannot be determined, try medication for pain, dyspnea, or anxiety as ordered.	Medication may need to be administered based on objective observations if the patient is unable to communicate.	Does medication promote comfort?
Keep the patient safe with one on one monitoring and side rails up.	A fall would increase the patient's discomfort.	Is patient safety maintained?
Keep perineal area clean and dry, frequently checking adult briefs.	A wet brief is not comfortable. Unchanged briefs can also lead to skin breakdown, another source of discomfort.	Is patient clean and dry with intact skin?
Teach patient and family *"Restlessness can have many causes. It can be a sign of pain, bowel or bladder problems or due to medication. I will work with the healthcare provider to improve the situation."*	The informed patient and family will be able to cooperate and assist with keeping the patient comfortable.	Do patient and family understand reasons for care and feel secure that patient is receiving best possible care?

(Continued on following page)

Box 16.3 Nursing CARE PLAN for the Patient at the End of Life (Cont'd)

Nursing Diagnosis: Hypothermia or hyperthermia related to dying central nervous system and inability to regulate body temperature

Expected Outcomes The patient's temperature will be maintained as close to normal as possible, and discomfort from temperature extremes will be managed.

Evaluation of Outcomes Is temperature within normal limits (WNL)? If unable to control temperature, does patient appear comfortable?

Interventions	Rationale	Evaluation
Administer acetaminophen suppository as ordered.	Acetaminophen is an antipyretic. It is given by suppository if the patient cannot swallow.	Does acetaminophen reduce fever?
Keep the patient clean and dry. Change gown and bed lines as necessary.	A fever can cause diaphoresis, and lying in damp sheets can be uncomfortable and cause skin breakdown.	Is patient kept dry and comfortable?
If the patient is cold, add blankets as necessary. Do not use an electric blanket or heating pad.	Blankets will warm the patient without risking burns from electric heating devices.	Are blankets helpful?

Nursing Diagnosis: Disturbed thought processes related to neurological changes

Expected Outcomes The family will voice understanding that confusion is not uncommon, and will demonstrate appropriate responses if it occurs.

Evaluation of Outcomes Does the family respond appropriately to patient during times of confusion?

Interventions	Rationale	Evaluation
Assure families that some confusion is common phenomenon.	If they are prepared, it will be less disturbing.	Is family informed? Do they verbalize understanding of what to expect?
Do not correct the patient but instead encourage the patient to talk about what is happening.	Sometimes patients talk about their fears in metaphor. Allowing them to express this fear will promote relaxation and decrease loneliness.	Is the patient less distressed after speaking?
Keep a dim light on in the room and remind the person gently of who is present.	Being able to see clearly helps keep the patient oriented if he awakens during the night.	Is light on? Is patient able to orient himself when he awakens?
Explain to family: *"Many patients make statements that don't make sense at times. It is as if they are in 2 worlds at the same time. He will become less distressed if you allow him to talk about what he is experiencing."*	The family will be less distressed if they understand what is happening.	Does the family respond appropriately to the patient's confused statements?

Nursing Diagnosis: Disturbed sensory perception related to changes in neurological function

Expected Outcomes The patient will be treated as still present and respected, and not as though he is already gone.

Evaluation of Outcomes Is communication respectful toward the patient?

Interventions	Rationale	Evaluation
When providing care, always speak to the patient as if he can hear you. When conversing with family members in the room, remember that the patient also can hear what you are saying.		Are caregivers and family members sensitive to the patient's presence when communicating?
When giving care, explain softly to the patient what you are doing and why.	Knowing what is happening can reduce anxiety and increase cooperation.	Does patient appear calm? Does he respond to your explanations?
Explain to family: *Hearing is the last sense to go. This can be a good time to say the things you have not been able to say. He may still hear you.*	Continued communication can be comforting to both the patient and the family.	Is communication appropriate?

Nursing Diagnosis: Anticipatory grieving related to impending death

Expected Outcomes The patient and family will be able to openly communicate their feelings to each other, and say goodbye.

Evaluation of Outcomes Are patient and family able to communicate effectively and say goodbye to each other?

Interventions	Rationale	Evaluation
Be present with the patient. Just sit quietly and hold his hand for a period of time.	This can help the patient to feel less alone, especially if there are no family members present. Many patients fear dying alone.	Is someone present with the patient as much as possible?
Show appropriate concern.	This will promote trust and empower the family to ask for what they need.	Is the family communicating openly with the providers?
Provide a quiet environment where each loved one can say goodbye in a way that will reflect their cultures and values.	These interactions will serve as valuable memories after the death and provide a feeling that each participant did what they needed to do for their loved one.	Do family members appear satisfied with their participation in the process?
Consult a minister or religious counselor of family's choice.	A minister often has special skills and training in communicating with people during difficult times. Talking about an afterlife may also be comforting to the patient and family.	Does the family appear to benefit from the presence of a minister or religious counselor?
Ask about the family's cultural and religious beliefs and allow time for prayers and ceremonies.	Providing a culturally familiar environment will reduce the patient and family's anxieties and give them more control over the process.	Do family members feel free to carry out cultural and religious beliefs?

Sleeping

In the final weeks of life, patients may be sleeping for most of the day. This is due to a change in metabolism. They also begin to emotionally detach from families as part of their preparation to leave.

Mental Status Changes

As patients progress, they often have confused episodes due to electrolyte imbalance. Some patients will say things like, "I have to catch a train" or "I need my passport." This metaphorical communication is well documented in the hospice literature. It is almost like patients are living in two worlds.

Terminal Restlessness

Terminal restlessness is a syndrome observed in a significant number of patients with various diagnoses during the final days of life. The patient may be unable to concentrate or relax, and may exhibit nonpurposeful motor activities such as picking at the sheets. The patient may hallucinate or try to climb out of bed. Terminal restlessness can have many causes, including hypoxemia, metabolic abnormalities, or hepatic failure. Some physical causes may be reversible so it is important to assess if pain or urinary or fecal impaction is the cause.

Restlessness may also be caused by medications. As kidney and liver functions are reduced, medication levels rise in the body and cause toxicity. Consult with the physician and pharmacist to determine if all the medications the patient is receiving are beneficial or necessary. See Table 16.3 for medications that might be helpful at the end of life.

Unconsciousness

The majority of patients are unconscious for hours or days before they die. Before they lose consciousness, their ability to see may be diminished. Hearing is the final sense to be lost. It is important for you to remember as you are caring for the patient and conversing with the family that your patient likely hears everything you are saying. Encourage the family to continue to talk to the patient.

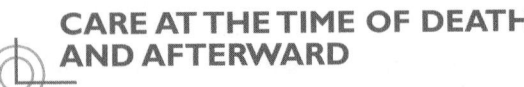

CRITICAL THINKING

Mr. Johnson

■ Mr. Johnson is in the final hours of his life and has become increasingly short of breath throughout the day. With each inspiration, his respirations are moist and noisy. Currently, his respiratory rate is 30 per minute, and you notice he is using his accessory muscles to breathe.

What is the cause of his noisy breathing?

What can be done to lower his respiratory rate and decrease his dyspnea?

Suggested answers at end of chapter

CARE AT THE TIME OF DEATH AND AFTERWARD

Death has occurred when you observe the absence of heartbeat and respirations. The body color becomes pale and waxen, the eyes may remain open, and pupils are fixed. Telling the family that the patient has died should be done with sensitivity, providing small amounts of information according to the family's level of understanding. Be sure to check and adhere to the policies in your setting and state regarding death pronouncement and organ donation. Document the general appearance of the body, including absent pulse and lung sounds. Your goal now is to provide a personal closure experience for the family.

TABLE 16.3 MEDICATIONS TO INCREASE COMFORT AT THE END OF LIFE

Medication Class/Action	Examples	Route	Side Effects	Nursing Implications
Opioids Bind to opioid receptors to reduce pain and dyspnea	Morphine (MS, MS-IR, MS Contin) Hydromorphone (Dilaudid) Fentanyl (Sublimaze, Actiq)	IV, SQ, PO, SL Rectal suppository IV, SQ, PO, SL Patch, IV, SL	Constipation, dry mouth, respiratory depression	Must be given routinely to be effective. Give routinely. Give short-acting analgesia for 24 hours until Fentanyl takes effect.
Anxiolytics Depress central nervous system to reduce anxiety	Lorazepam (Ativan) Diazepam (Valium)	IV, PO, SC	Dry mouth, unsteadiness. Assess for oversedation if used with opioids.	Not first line drugs for treating dyspnea
Neuroleptics Reduce severe agitation, terminal restlessness	Haloperidol (Haldol)	PO, IM	Tardive dyskinesia, Pseudoparkinsonism	Useful in treating anxiety when lorazepam ineffective.
Anticholinergics For treating excessive pharyngeal secretions	Hyoscyamine (Cystospaz) Scopolomine (Transderm-Scop) Glycopyrrolate (Robinul)	SL Patch SQ	Urinary retention, dry mouth	Works faster than scopolamine patch. For early treatment of secretions. Consider if hyoscyamine ineffective.

After death, you provide **postmortem care.** First, remove the tubes, medical supplies, and equipment. Bathing and dressing the patient and making him look presentable for the family shows respect. Some cultures dictate the care of the body after death and who should provide that care. The nurse can assess and advocate for cultural practices requested by the family. Work toward providing a clean, peaceful impression of the deceased. Position the body in proper alignment; replace dentures, place dressings on leaking wounds, and use briefs as necessary. Allow the family time with the body. Embalming is necessary within 12 hours. Do not remove the body until the family is ready. Covering or uncovering the face at removal should be done according to the family's preference. Additional activities, such as contacting the physician or funeral home, should be carried out according to institution policy.

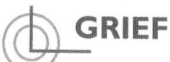 GRIEF

Grief is the emotional response to a loss. Loss is a daily experience in everyone's life. Loss can occur due to divorce, children leaving home, loss of job, loss of possessions, or other losses. People express grief in their own way according to their coping skills, life experiences, and cultural norms. In end of life care, grief is a process that begins before the death of the patient and continues through a series of tasks that the survivors move through to resolve grief. The feelings associated with grief include anger, frustration, regret, guilt, sadness, and many others. This process can be divided into stages (Table 16.4).

Interventions for the grieving patient are addressed in Box 16.4 Nursing Care Plan for the Patient at the End of Life. Nursing process for the grieving family is addressed below.

Nursing Process for the Grieving Family

Assessment/Data Collection

Some things to consider when assessing grief include:

- Where is the family in the grief process?
- Are family members experiencing physical problems such as shortness of breath, sweating, skin color changes?
- Is the stress of grieving exacerbating medical conditions?
- What support systems are available to the family?
- What interventions can I use to facilitate their grief process?

Nursing Diagnosis, Planning, and Implementation

Although many nursing diagnoses may be appropriate, the priority diagnosis is simply Grieving.

Grieving related to impending death or loss of loved one

EXPECTED OUTCOME: The family will be able to express feelings of anger, guilt, or sadness. They will be able to think about the future and perform ADLs as needed.

- Simply be present. *Sitting with the bereaved, without having to have all the answers is very powerful. If you don't know what to say, just be silent.*
- Actively listen, allowing the bereaved to talk about the loved one and their feelings about the loss. Ask open-ended questions to encourage them to continue talking. *One of the greatest needs of the bereaved is to trust someone enough to share their pain.*
- Help family members identify their support systems (church, friends, family) and encourage them to use them. *Support systems can help in practical ways (meals, transportation) as well as lend emotional support.*
- Consider acknowledging the event by attending the memorial service or sending a card. *This simple act of caring is very important to families.*

Evaluation

Healing takes time. If interventions have been effective, however, the family will have the support to function effectively while they grieve.

TABLE 16.4 STAGES OF GRIEF

Stage	Tasks	Characteristics
Stage 1 Shock and disbelief	Acknowledge the reality of the loss. Recognize the loss.	Has difficulty with feelings of numbness, emotional outbursts, poor daily functioning, and avoidance.
Stage 2 Experience the loss	Work through the pain by expressing and experiencing the feelings.	Anger, bargaining, depression. May feel guilt over not preventing the death or not providing enough care. May feel angry at loved one who has "left them behind." May experience insomnia, loss of appetite, apathy, lack of interest in daily life.
Stage 3 Reintegration	Adjust to an environment without the deceased.	Finds hope in the future, participates in social events, feels more energetic.

THE NURSE AND LOSS

Working with dying patients triggers awareness of your own losses and fears about death and mortality. Adapting to the care of the dying requires that you explore and experience your personal feelings toward death. Unresolved losses from your past can resurface and affect your ability to care for dying patients. You may find that you continue to think about patients who have died long after the event. Emotionally continuing to care about deceased patients takes energy away from the daily care you are providing to current patients and your own family. Unresolved grief can lead to symptoms that resemble burnout, such as insomnia, headaches, and fatigue.

If you find yourself distancing and withdrawing from your dying patients, it is an indicator that you need to attend to the care of yourself. Some nurses may find counseling helpful in order to effectively process losses from the past and learn healthy ways to process future losses.

Both formal and informal support systems should be in place to support staff through multiple losses. Informal support can be one-on-one sharing of experiences with coworkers, peers, pastoral counselors, and physicians. Understanding and acknowledging your limitations, asking for help, regular exercise, and relaxation are important components. Some nurses find journal writing a helpful process, where writing down feelings allows you to release them. Formal support systems can be established in many different ways:

- Preplanned gatherings where nurses can express feelings in a safe environment
- Postclinical debriefings after difficult deaths to alleviate anxiety and promote learning
- Ceremonies such as memorial services in facilities

Home Health Hints

- Allow time during your visit to sit quietly with the patient and caregiver. Sitting quietly lets the patient and caregiver know you are there to meet both medical and emotional needs.
- Encourage family involvement with care. Families need reassurance that they are not going to hurt the patient; take the time to teach them how to assist the patient with basic care.
- Prepare the family for what to expect as death approaches.
- When the patient is no longer conscious, encourage the family to spend time at the bedside sharing personal thoughts and memories with the patient. For example, a spouse might talk about when they first met, or family members can play a favorite song.

to allow both staff and residents to recognize and honor the loss of patients

REFLECTIONS ON CASE STUDY

Remember Mr. Moran from the beginning of the chapter? Clearly he is approaching the end of life. Assess what he and his family want to happen in the final months of his life and where he wants to be. What are the goals of care? If comfort is the goal, how can this best be achieved? If keeping him in his familiar and safe environment is the goal, then help his family weigh the benefits and burdens of CPR, hospitalization, artificial feeding, and artificial hydration.

REVIEW QUESTIONS

1. A 94-year-old gentleman is admitted from home to the hospital with pneumonia. What factors lead the nurse to believe he is nearing the end of his life?
   a. His abdomen is distended and his skin tone is yellow.
   b. He has a fever of 101.6°F and a respiratory rate of 28.
   c. He has been having difficulty swallowing and is losing weight.
   d. He has crackles in his lung bases bilaterally.

2. What is a Durable Power of Attorney?
   a. A document that outlines a patient's wishes at the end of life.
   b. A document that gives a patient a "Do Not Resuscitate" status.
   c. A person who will make decisions for a patient once the document is signed.

   d. A person who will make decisions for a patient when the patient is no longer able to speak for himself.

3. A patient's family member says, "I heard someone say my mother could have a 'good death.' What on earth is a good death?" Which response by the nurse is best?
   a. "Some things that can contribute to a good death are allowing patients to make their own decisions at the end of life, and assuring that they die comfortably."
   b. "In reality, no death is a good death, but we do our best to make sure patients are comfortable right up until they die."
   c. "Research has shown that patients can die good deaths if they are kept sedated so they don't really know what is happening during the last days until they die."

d. "A good death occurs when the patient is kept alive as long as possible, so she can take care of all her 'unfinished business' first."

4. A husband whose wife has just died cries, "What am I going to do? She is all I had." What is the best response you can provide?

a. "You are going to go on with your life. You still have your work and your children."

b. "I am sorry you lost your wife, but I know she would not want you to be sad. You have to be strong for her."

c. "I know how you feel. I lost my grandmother recently, and it was really hard."

d. There is no need to say anything. Just be present and listen.

5. A dying patient has excessive secretions that are causing dyspnea. Which medication will best help dry the secretions and increase comfort? Select all that apply.

a. Haloperidol

b. Scopolamine

c. Acetaminophen

d. Diazepam

6. What are nursing interventions the nurse can provide at the end of life? Select all that apply.

a. Position the patient to increase comfort and prevent complications.

b. Provide comfort measures such as massage.

c. Research experimental treatments that may help the patient find a cure.

d. Administer medications to increase comfort.

e. Teach the family CPR for use if the patient dies when the nurse is not present.

f. Sit quietly with the patient and family.

7. A patient has just died, and his family is waiting to see him. What postmortem care is essential first?

a. Document the time and circumstances of the death.

b. Place identification on the body according to hospital policy.

c. Clean the patient up and make him look peaceful.

d. Cover the patient's body and face with a sheet.

8. The wife of a hospitalized patient who died an hour ago is crying and unwilling to leave his hospital room. The rest of the family is in the waiting room. The admitting department just called and wants to have the room cleaned for a new patient. Which action should the nurse take?

a. Allow the wife to stay in the room as long as she likes.

b. Call a taxicab for the wife and gently guide her out of the room.

c. Sit with the wife for a few minutes, then take her to the waiting room.

d. Tell the wife that you are sorry for her loss, but that another patient needs the room.

9. A patient who has been receiving hospice care for 3 months tells the LPN he has decided he wants to return to active treatment of his disease. What should the LPN do?

a. Encourage the patient to discuss his desire with his physician.

b. Tell the patient that he cannot change his goals once hospice care has been initiated.

c. Check his medication supply for any leftover medications he was taking during treatment.

d. Explain to the patient that since he is terminal, treatment will not help the course of his disease.

ETHICAL CONSIDERATIONS

Allowing someone to die, like abortion, generates huge controversy and debate. Each side of the argument can justify its stance using moral and ethical principles. Again, like abortion, religious and secular views may conflict. Both sides put forward strong arguments. For example, those supporting a peaceful death for Adam could state that respect for autonomy would mean that if Adam gave clear indication that he would not want to live in such a progressively worsening condition, his wishes for being allowed to die peacefully should be upheld, regardless of personal or public opinion. Conversely, the opposing side could argue that Adam's autonomy should be protected while he is in this state. He is incapable of making such choices and until the time comes when he can, his right to choose must be protected.

Karen chose to work in a facility where people often die, so she would be familiar with the process. As to whether she could actually participate in an act that would contribute to the death of a patient is the central question. Essentially, Karen must examine her own personal moral values in order to direct her actions. In this case, the ethical principles dictating the interaction between patient and nurse must be weighed carefully against what Karen holds dear. Karen may also want to distinguish between causing someone to die versus allowing someone to die of natural causes after stopping artificial feeding. Beneficence, nonmaleficence, and autonomy have their place in this scenario regardless of opposing sides. It is important to consider Adam's wishes if they are known. Sometimes the person who is the subject of the debate can be forgotten while groups argue about which approach is right.

In the end, the courts decided Adam's outcome. If Karen can't in good conscience discontinue his feeding, she may be able to ask for reassignment during this shift.

References

1. Singer PA, Martin DK, Kelner M: Quality end-of-life care: Patients' perspectives. JAMA 281:163-168, 1995.
2. Murden RA, and Ainslie NK: Recent weight loss is related to short term mortality in nursing homes. J Gen Intern Med, 9:648–650, 1994.
3. Saklayen M, Liss H, and Markert N: In-hospital cardiopulmonary resuscitation: survival in one hospital and literature review. Medicine 74:163–175, 1995.
4. Finucane T, Christmas C, and Travis K: Tube feeding in patients with advanced dementia: A review of the evidence. JAMA 282:1365–1370, 1999.
5. McCann Ñ, Hall W, and Groth-Juncker A: Comfort care for terminally ill patients: The appropriate use of nutrition and hydration. JAMA 272:1263–1266, 1994.
6. Callanan M, and Kelley P: Final Gifts: Understanding the Special Awareness, Needs and Communication of the Dying. Bantam Books, New York, 1992.

Unit Three Bibliography

1. Coke T, Alday R, Biala K, et al: The new role of physical therapy in home care. Home Health Nurse 23:594–599, 2005.
2. Coleman P, and Watson, NM: Oral care provided by certified nursing assistants in nursing homes. J Am Geriatr Soc 54:138–143, 2006.
3. Fakouri, C, and Lyon, B: Perceived health and life satisfaction among older adults: the effects of worry and personal variables. J. Gerontol Nurs 31:17–24, 2005.
4. Goldstein, NE, and Morrison, RS: Treatment of pain in older patients. Crit Rev Oncol Hematol 54:157–164, 2005.
5. Hansen, L, Archibold P; Stewart B, et al: Family caregivers making life-sustaining treatment decisions: factors associated with role strain and ease. J Gerontol Nurs 31:28–35, 2005.
6. Hayes, M: A phenomenological study of chronic sorrow in people with type 1 diabetes. Pract Diabetes Int 18:65, 2001.
7. Hertz, JE, and Anschutz, CA: Relationships among perceived enactment of autonomy, self-care, and holistic health in community-dwelling older adults. J Holist Nurs 20:166–186, 2002.
8. Knestrick, J, and Lohri-Posey, B: Spirituality and health: perceptions of older women in a rural senior high rise. J Gerontol Nurs 31:44–50, 2005.
9. Lach, HW, Langan, JC, and James DC: Disaster planning: are gerontological nurses prepared? J Gerontol Nurs 31:21–27, 2005.
10. Larson, EB, Wang L, Bowen JD, et al: Exercise is associated with reduced risk for incident dementia among persons 65 years of age and older. Ann Intern Med 17:144:73–81, 2006.
11. Lewis, ID, and McBride, M: Anticipatory grief and chronicity: Elders and families in racial/ethnic minority groups. Geriatr Nurs 25:44–47, 2004.
12. Li, H: Hospitalized elders and family caregivers: a typology of family worry. J Clin Nurs 14:3–8, 2005.
13. Lyons, SS: Evidence-based protocol: fall prevention for older adults. J Gerontol Nurs 31:9–14, 2005.
14. Mainarich, K, and Silverstein, P: Is your patient ready for home health care? Nursing. 35:32hn6–32hn7, 2005.
15. Marrelli, TM: Restorative care and home care: new implications for aide and nurse roles? Geriatr Nurs 24:128–129, 2003.
16. McGuire LC, Ahluwalia IB, and Strine TW: Chronic disease-related behaviors in U.S. older women: Behavioral risk factor surveillance system, 2003. J Women's Health (Larchmt) 15:3–7, 2006.
17. McPhaul K. Home care security: nurses can take simple precautions to ensure safety during home visits. Am J Nurs 104:96, 2004.
18. Munroe, DJ: Assisted living issues for nursing practice. Geriatr Nurs 24:99–105, 2003.
19. Nazarko, L: Ageism must be tackled through education. Nurs Times 18–24;101:14, 2005.
20. Piette, JD, and Heisler, M: The relationship between older adults' knowledge of their drug coverage and medication cost problems. J Am Geriatr Soc 54:91–96, 2006.
21. Sparks, M Zehr, D, and Painter, B: Predictors of life satisfaction: perceptions of older community-dwelling adults. J Gerontol Nurs 30:47–53, 2004.
22. Stoker, J: Home Care LPN Utilization. Home Health Nurse 21:85–89, 2003.
23. Timm, SE: Effectively delegating nursing activities in home care. Home Health Nurse 21:260–265, 2003.

SUGGESTED ANSWERS TO

CRITICAL THINKING

■ Mrs. Hart

Mrs. Hart will need both a Do Not Resuscitate order in the hospital setting and when she goes home, she will need an out of hospital, prehospital, or durable DNR, whatever is called for in her state of residence. In addition, her family members should be aware of her wishes.

■ Mr. Johnson

Mr. Johnson's dyspnea is commonly seen in the final hours on life. He may benefit from oxygen. Low-dose morphine will decrease his respiratory rate and improve his oxygenation. Morphine also has a "drying effect" on secretions. If morphine is unsuccessful, the addition of hyoscyamine may be helpful.

unit FOUR

UNDERSTANDING THE IMMUNE SYSTEM

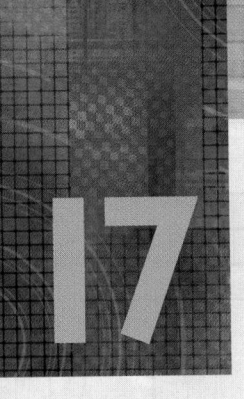

17

Immune System Function, Assessment, and Therapeutic Measures

SHARON M. NOWAK AND
JANICE L. BRADFORD

KEY TERMS

active immunity (AK-tiv im-YOO-ni-tee)
anaphylactic (AN-uh-fi-LAK-tik)
antibody (AN-ti-bod-ee)
antigen (AN-ti-jen)
cell-mediated immunity (SELL ME-dee-ay-ted im-YOO-ni-tee)
humoral immunity (HYOO-mohr-uhl im-YOO-ni-tee)
lymphocyte (LIM-foh-site)
neutrophil (NEW-troh-fil)
passive immunity (PASS-iv im-YOO-ni-tee)
white blood cells (Wight Bluhd Cells)

QUESTIONS TO GUIDE YOUR READING

1. What type of immunity is obtained with a vaccine?

2. How does aging affect the immune system?

3. What subjective data are collected when caring for a patient with a disorder of the immune system?

4. What objective data are collected when caring for a patient with a disorder of the immune system?

5. What nursing care is provided for patients undergoing diagnostic tests for the immune system?

6. What are common therapeutic interventions used for a patient with disorders of the immune system?

NORMAL IMMUNE ANATOMY AND PHYSIOLOGY

Immunity is defined as the ability to destroy pathogens or other foreign material and to prevent further cases of certain infectious diseases. Immunity is most often thought of in terms of the body's response to microorganisms such as bacteria, viruses, and fungi, all of which are foreign to the body. However, immunity also involves processes directed toward other cells or substances that are identified by the body, correctly or incorrectly, as foreign. Malignant cells are foreign in that they have mutated from normal form and are usually destroyed by the immune system before they become malignant. Transplanted organs unfortunately are also perceived as foreign; rejection of a transplanted organ is an immune response. Occasionally, the immune system mistakenly reacts to part of the body itself (autoimmune disease) or to a substance that should be tolerated (allergic reaction).

The immune system consists of lymphoid organs, **lymphocytes** and **other white blood cells**, and the many chemicals produced that are involved in activation of our own cells for the destruction of foreign **antigens** (Fig. 17.1). The lymphatic system consists of lymphatic vessels that help return tissue fluid to the circulatory system; lymph nodes and nodules, which are masses of lymphatic tissue that differ in size and location; the spleen, where macrophages phagocytize pathogens and B and T cells carry out immune functions; and the thymus, which functions primarily in childhood and atrophies with age. Lymph nodes are grouped along lymph vessels to destroy foreign material. Three major

---

lymphocyte: lympho—lymph + kytos—cell
antigen: anti—against + gennan—to produce

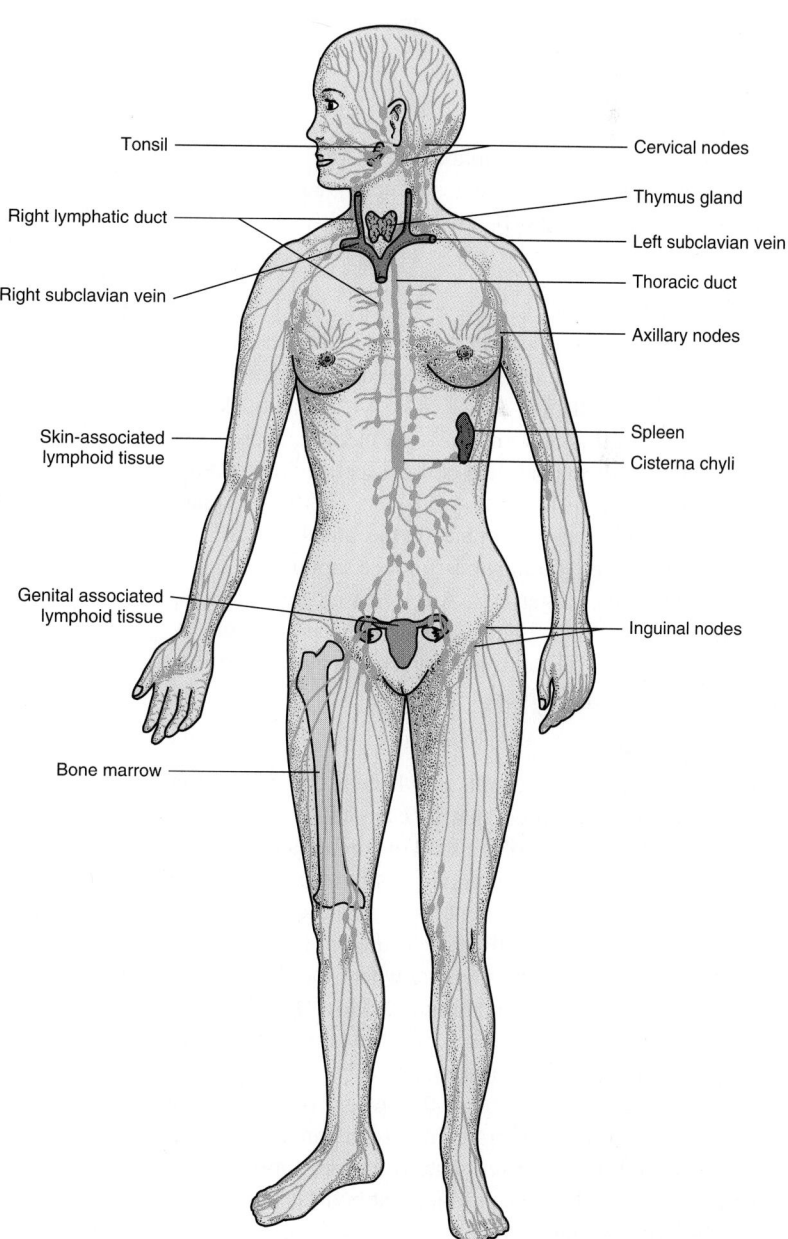

Tonsil

Right lymphatic duct

Right subclavian vein

Skin-associated lymphoid tissue

Genital associated lymphoid tissue

Bone marrow

Cervical nodes

Thymus gland

Left subclavian vein

Thoracic duct

Axillary nodes

Spleen

Cisterna chyli

Inguinal nodes

FIGURE 17.1 Immune system organs, lymph vessels, and major lymph nodes.

groups are the cervical, axillary, and inguinal nodes. Lymph nodules lack encapsulation and are smaller than nodes; lymph nodules are found under the surface of mucous membranes (e.g., tonsils).

Antigens

Antigens are chemical markers that identify cells or molecules. Examples of molecular antigens include bacterial toxins, plant pollens or proteins that trigger allergies, and the protein products of viral activity within cells. Human cells (except red blood cells [RBCs]) have their own self-antigens—thousands of markers that identify the cell as belonging in the body. These are the major histocompatibility complex (MHC) antigens, also called human leukocyte antigens (HLAs), which are genetically determined. The MHC antigens of identical twins are identical. These MHC antigens serve as a comparison for cells of the immune system; the antigens of foreign cells do not "match" MHC antigens and may therefore be recognized as foreign and destroyed in one of several ways.

Lymphocytes

There are three types of lymphocytes: natural killer (NK) cells, thymus-derived lymphocytes (T cells), and bone marrow–derived lymphocytes (B cells), each with very different functions.

Natural Killer Cells

Natural killer cells are found in the blood, red bone marrow, lymph nodes, and spleen and are able to destroy many kinds of infected body cells and tumor cells. NK cells attack any self-cell that displays abnormal plasma membrane proteins. After binding with an abnormal cell, NK cells release toxins in granules, either perforins or granzymes. Perforins create a hole in the plasma membrane of the attacked cell; the result is cytolysis. Granzymes induce apoptosis (self-destruction) of the target cell. Any released microbes are phagocytized by WBCs. The action of NK cells is considered a nonspecific resistance mechanism because it is effective against a variety of foreign antigens.

T Cells and B Cells

The lymphocytes called T cells and B cells are involved in specific immune responses; that is, each cell is genetically programmed to respond to one kind of foreign antigen. It is estimated that the human immune system can respond to hundreds of millions of different foreign antigens.

Both T cells and B cells arise in the red bone marrow. T cells then migrate to the thymus, where the thymic hormones bring about their maturation. Most T cells arise before puberty, but the process continues at a slower pace throughout life. From the thymus, T cells migrate to the lymph nodes and nodules and to the spleen. B cells mature in the bone marrow and migrate directly to lymphatic tissue. When activated during an immune response, some B cells become plasma cells that produce antibodies; meanwhile others become memory cells.

Antibodies

Antibodies are also called immunoglobulins (Ig) or gamma globulins and are proteins produced by plasma cells in response to foreign antigens. Antibodies do not themselves destroy foreign antigens, but rather become attached to such antigens to "label" them for destruction. Each **antibody** is specific for only one antigen, and the B cells (those that become plasma cells) of an individual are capable of producing millions of different antibodies. There are five classes of human antibodies, designated by letter names: IgG, IgM, IgA, IgE, and IgD. Their functions are summarized in Table 17.1.

Mechanisms of Immunity

The two mechanisms of immunity are **cell-mediated immunity,** which involves T cells, and **humoral immunity**, which involves primarily B cells but is assisted by T cells. Although the mechanisms are different, invasion by a pathogen often triggers both.

The first step in the destruction of a foreign antigen is the recognition of it as being foreign. B cells in lymphatic tissue are able to recognize and bind with the foreign antigens to become activated B cells. Their activation is greatly enhanced if the foreign antigen is presented to them by antigen-presenting cells called dendritic cells. T cells have foreign antigen recognition only if subjected to an antigen-presenting cell, such as a dendritic cell, macrophage, or B cell that has previously processed the antigen.

TABLE 17.1 CLASSES OF ANTIBODIES

Immunoglobulin (Ig)	Location	Function
G	Blood, extracellular fluid, lymph	Crosses the placenta to provide passive immunity in newborns
		Provides long-term immunity following a vaccination or illness recovery
A	External secretions (e.g., tears, saliva)	Provides passive immunity for breastfed infants
		Found in secretions of all mucous membranes
M	Blood, lymph	Produced first during an infection (IgG production follows)
D	B cells	Are antigen-specific receptors on B lymphocytes
E	Mast cells or basophils	Important in allergic reactions
		Mast cells release histamine

Source: Scanlon, V, and Sanders, T: Understanding Human Structure and Function. FA Davis, Philadelphia, 2003, p 313.

Cell-Mediated Immunity

This mechanism of immunity does not involve the production of antibodies, but it is effective against intracellular pathogens (such as viruses or fungi), malignant cells, and grafts of foreign tissue. The first step is the recognition of the foreign antigen by helper T cells, assisted by macrophages. The newly activated T cells divide many times and become specialized in one of several ways. Cytotoxic, or killer, T cells (CD8) are able to lyse cells such as cancer cells or those infected by viruses or other intracellular parasites, malignant cells, or transplanted tissues. They also release chemicals that activate phagocytes such as macrophages and **neutrophils**.

Memory T cells remember the specific foreign antigen and quickly activate an immune response should the antigen reappear. Suppressor T cells are believed to inhibit the proliferation of both T cells and B cells, which limits the immune response to just what is needed and no more.

Humoral Immunity

Humoral immunity is also called antibody-mediated immunity and involves antibody production. Again, the first step is the recognition of the antigen as being foreign; this time by B cells. The helper T cells (CD4) that recognize the antigen further stimulate the activated B cells to proliferate and differentiate. Some B cells become plasma cells that produce antibodies specific for this particular antigen. Other B cells become memory B cells that will remember this antigen and initiate a rapid response should it return. Humoral immunity is effective against extracellular pathogens,

which are usually bacteria but can also be viral or fungal infections.

Although B cells are stationary, the antibodies produced by plasma cells circulate throughout the body. The antibodies bond to the antigen, forming an antigen-antibody complex. This immobilizes the bacteria; also the antigen is now "labeled" for phagocytosis by macrophages or neutrophils. The antigen-antibody complex also stimulates the process of complement fixation.

Complement is a group of over 30 plasma proteins that circulate in the blood until activated by an antigen-antibody complex in the classic pathway. (There are two alternative pathways that initiate the complement cascade.) The activation of complement may result in the formation of a protein complex that lyses the cell and brings about its death. Other complement proteins bind to foreign antigens and serve as further labels to attract macrophages.

ANTIBODY RESPONSES

The first exposure to a foreign antigen stimulates antibody production, but the antibodies are produced too slowly to prevent the disease. However, with time, the individual has accumulated antibodies and memory cells that are specific for that pathogen. On a second exposure to the antigen, the memory cells initiate rapid production of large amounts of antibody, often enough to prevent a second occurrence of the illness (Fig. 17.2). This is the basis for the protection given by vaccines. A vaccine contains an antigen that is not pathogenic (e.g., bacterial capsules in the case of the pneumococcal vaccine). The vaccine stimulates the formation of antibodies and memory cells.

---

neutrophil: neutro—neuter + philein—to love

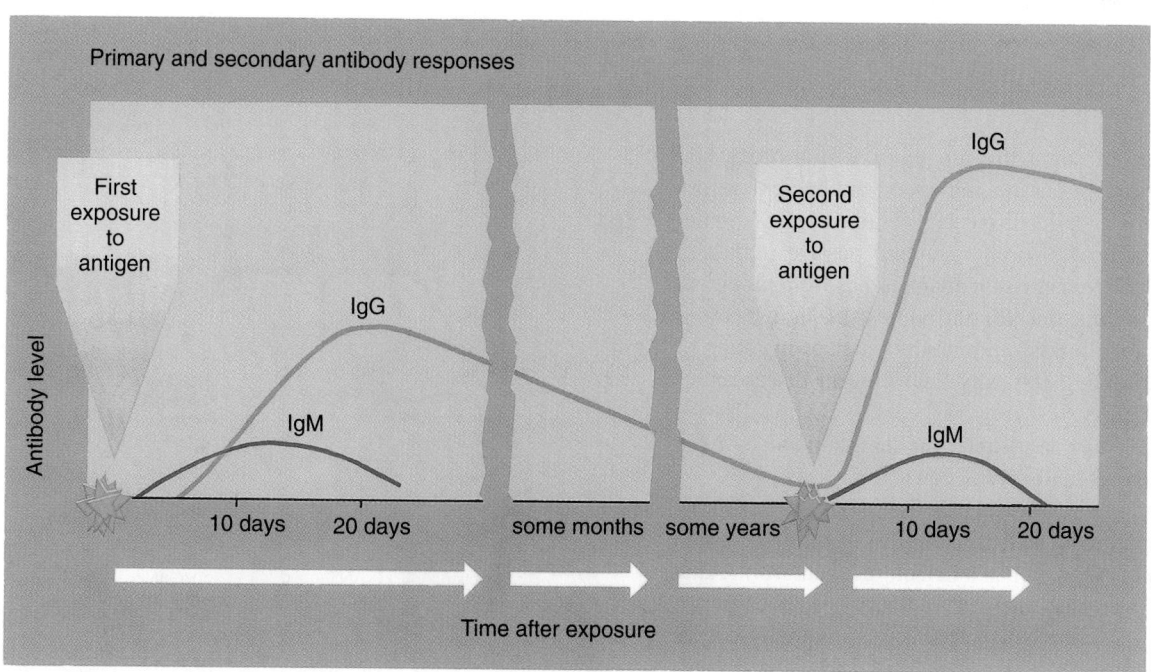

FIGURE 17.2 Antibody responses to a first and then subsequent exposure to a pathogen. *(From Scanlon, V, and Sanders, T: Essentials of Anatomy and Physiology, ed. 4. FA Davis, Philadelphia, 2003, p 317.)*

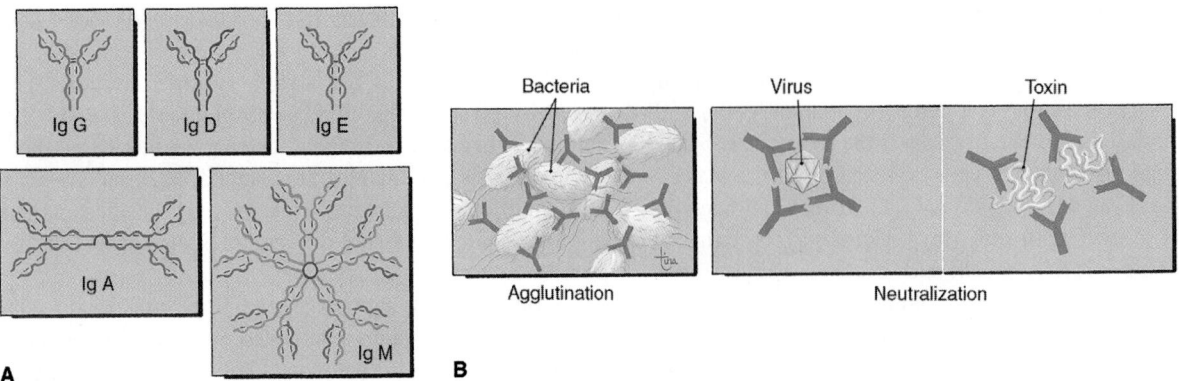

FIGURE 17.3 Antibodies. (A) Structure of the five classes of antibodies. (B) Antibody activity *(Adapted from Scanlon, V and Sanders, T: Essentials of Anatomy and Physiology, ed. 4. FA Davis, Philadelphia, 2003, p 312.)*

Antibodies may also neutralize viruses; that is, they attach to a virus and render it unable to enter a cell (Fig. 17.3). Viruses cannot reproduce outside of living cells, and those coated with antibodies are phagocytized by macrophages. Another aspect of our defenses against viruses is interferon, a chemical produced by cells infected with viruses. Although it does not help the infected cell, interferon protects surrounding cells by enabling them to resist viral replication.

Antibodies are also involved in allergic responses, in which the immune system responds to foreign but harmless antigens (an allergen), such as plant pollen. IgE antibodies bond to mast cells, which break down and release histamine and other chemicals that contribute to inflammation. **Anaphylactic** shock is an allergic reaction, but it is massive in nature. It is characterized by loss of plasma from capillaries (an effect of histamine) and a sudden drop in the intravascular blood volume and blood pressure.

TYPES OF IMMUNITY

Two categories of immunity are **passive immunity** and **active immunity.** In passive immunity, antibodies are not produced by the individual but are obtained from another source. One form of naturally acquired passive immunity includes placental transmission of antibodies from mother to fetus and transmission of antibodies in breast milk. Artificially acquired passive immunity involves injection of preformed antibodies; this may help prevent disease after exposure to a pathogen such as the hepatitis B virus. Passive immunity is always temporary, in that antibodies from another source eventually break down.

Active immunity means that the individual produces his or her own antibodies. An example of naturally acquired active immunity occurs when a person recovers from a disease and then has antibodies and memory cells specific for that pathogen. Artificially acquired active immunity occurs as the result of a vaccine that stimulates production of anti-

bodies and memory cells. The duration of active immunity depends on the particular disease or vaccine; some confer lifelong immunity, but others do not.

AGING AND THE IMMUNE SYSTEM

The efficiency of the immune system decreases with age (Fig. 17.4). As such, older adults are more susceptible to infections and autoimmune disorders (Box 17.1 Gerontological Issues). The incidence of cancer is also higher; malignant cells that might once have been quickly destroyed by the immune system live and proliferate.

IMMUNE SYSTEM ASSESSMENT

Nursing Assessment

Disorders of the immune system can affect every system in the body so it is important to collect head-to-toe data as well as a patient history (Table 17.2).

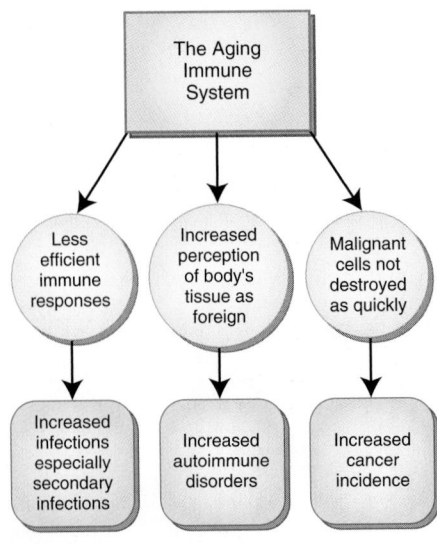

FIGURE 17.4 This concept map shows the effects the aging process has on the immune system.

---

anaphylactic: ana—up + phylaxis—protection

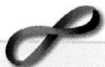

Box 17.1

Gerontological Issues

Significant changes occur in the immune system of the older adult. These changes are known as immune senescence, which refers to a decline in immune system function. Some specific changes include the following:

- Thymus gland decreases in size, increases production of immature T cells, and has a subsequent decline in response to antigens.
- Antibody response to foreign organisms decreases.

Immunizations to support the immune responses of older adults include the following:

- Diphtheria tetanus booster every 10 years
- Pneumovax once in a lifetime (reimmunization or boosters usually not necessary)
- Influenza vaccine yearly (before influenza season), mid October to mid November
- Hepatitis B vaccine if medium to high risk for exposure to hepatitis B.

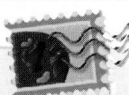

Box 17.2

Cultural Considerations

The Navajo people have a high incidence of severe combined immunodeficiency syndrome (SCIDS) and immunodeficiency syndrome unrelated to acquired immunodeficiency syndrome (AIDS). SCIDS result is a failure of the antibody response and cell-mediated immunity. Infants who survive initially are sent to tertiary care facilities. They must receive gamma globulin on a regular basis until a bone marrow transplant can be performed. Thus far, studies indicate that SCIDS is unique to this Navajo population.

Subjective Data

DEMOGRAPHIC DATA. The patient's gender and ethnicity are important to note because some disease processes tend to be associated with a particular gender or ethnicity. For instance, systemic lupus erythematosus (SLE), an autoimmune disorder, tends to affect women eight times more than men.

HISTORY. Inquiring about the patient's history of past and present medical conditions should also include a family history. Many atopic (allergic) disorders such as allergic rhinitis and asthma or autoimmune disorders such as SLE and ankylosing spondylitis are thought to be either familial or have a genetic predisposition in certain ethnic or cultural groups (Box 17.2 Cultural Considerations).

Patients' previous surgeries may give clues about their current condition or prior health. For example, with thymus gland removal (thymectomy), T-cell production may be altered, which affects the cell-mediated immune response. Or if the spleen was removed (splenectomy), lymphocyte and plasma cell production may be altered, which affects the humoral immune response.

Asking about current medications should specifically include prescription, over-the-counter drugs, and herbal preparations. Corticosteroids and immunosuppressants decrease the immune response, whereas some anti-infectives or antineoplastics depress the bone marrow. This results in decreased production of the cells made in the bone marrow. Bone marrow depression of WBCs can alter cell-mediated and humoral immune responses. The herbal preparation licorice, which is sometimes used for its antiinflammatory and expectorant effects, when taken concurrently with corticosteroids, produces additive effects of corticosteroids.

A patient's lifestyle may influence immune system function and should be assessed. Anaphylactic reactions can be caused by exposure to latex, which may be found in gloves and other medical products that healthcare workers and their patients touch. Be aware of this potentially life-threatening reaction and know the agency's latex allergy protocol. Patients who are allergic to latex should wear a medical alert bracelet and carry an anaphylactic epinephrine kit. Knowing a patient's dietary habits and supplemental vitamins gives insight into the potential reserve of the patient's immune system for fighting infection.

The patient's life stressors, coping behaviors, and support systems should be explored. Stress (environmental, physical, and psychological) can depress the immune system's function. Coping behaviors are essential in keeping stress within manageable limits to maintain an optimum-functioning immune system. Support systems play an important role in coping with stress and should be encouraged and nurtured by nurses.

Current Problem

Use the WHAT'S UP? format to collect data about the current immune system problem. For immune disorders, the patient is asked the following questions:

- **W**here is it? What part of the body is affected?
- **H**ow does it feel? Painful? Itching?
- **A**ggravating and alleviating factors?
- **T**iming. Was there exposure to a pathogen? Did you have a previous infection? Does it occur only in certain settings? Did you have chemotherapy or radiation therapy? How long have symptoms persisted?
- **S**everity. Does it affect activities of daily living (ADLs)? Work? Roles?
- **U**seful data for associated symptoms. Immunosuppression? Family history? Allergies?
- **P**erception of the patient of the problem. What do you think is wrong?

The following are examples of common signs and symptoms that may be found with immune disorders: fever, fatigue, joint pain, swollen glands, weight loss, and skin rash.

TABLE 17.2 SUBJECTIVE ASSESSMENT OF THE IMMUNE SYSTEM

Category	Questions to Ask During History Assessment	Rationale/Significance
Demographic Data	What is your age?	The immune system decreases in functional effectiveness as one ages and a number of immune disorders tend to afflict individuals of particular age ranges.
	Where were you born? What is your ethnic or cultural background?	This information can aid in determining ethnic and cultural background influences. Some immune disorders tend to afflict individuals of particular cultural/ethnic groups more than others.
	Where have you lived? Where do you currently reside?	This information can aid in determining ethnic and cultural background as well as possible environmental influences.
History	Do you have allergies to any medications? Latex? Foods? Insects? Environmental allergens? If yes, have you had a recent exposure to any of these?	This information may lead to a direct cause of current symptoms and provides information regarding the status of the patient's immune system.
	Is there anyone in your family is allergic to medications? Latex? Foods? Insects? Environmental allergens?	If family members (especially immediate) have severe reactions to substances, the patient may be predisposed to immune reactions to the same antigen or in general.
	What medications are you currently taking?	Some medications can mask symptoms or immune responses, others can suppress immune responses.
	What illnesses or conditions are you currently being treated for? Have you been treated for?	May provide clues to patient's current condition or symptoms.
	What surgeries have you had?	Have any immune organs been removed, therefore reducing immune function? May also provide indications to overall health.
	Have you ever had a blood transfusion? If so, why?	Antibodies to various antigen markers on the blood cells may have been formed. Additionally may provide indications to overall health.
	What is your occupation? Have you been exposed to hazardous chemicals, fumes, or radiation?	Many chemicals can produce local reactions, usually skin reactions or systemic immune reactions, and some can lead to bone marrow suppression in which all cell production is reduced.
	Do you engage in any form of risky behavior?	Risky behavior, such as intravenous drug usage and unprotected sex with multiple partners, increases a patient's chances of contracting the human immunodeficiency virus (HIV), which leads to a reduction in the immune system function.
	Describe your overall stress level and life stressors.	Stress is known to suppress the immune system and over prolonged periods can lead to a variety of illnesses.
	What do you do to cope with stress?	Not all coping behaviors and mechanisms are healthy, therefore it's important to assess what the patient's coping behaviors are to see if the patient needs education.
	What sort of support systems do you have?	Support systems can buffer the day-to-day stress as well as during crisis.

Objective Data

PHYSICAL ASSESSMENT. Physical data collection begins by observing the patient's general appearance, color, posture, gait, facial expression, skin, and nailbeds (Table 17.3). Any cyanosis or erythema (redness) is noted. Rashes should be examined for size, shape, location, texture, drainage, and pruritus (itching). Visual and hearing changes can be associated with an immunological disorder. Eye movements are assessed by testing the six cardinal positions of gaze for muscle weakness. (See Chapter 51.)

Adventitious lung sounds, such as wheezing, may indicate asthma or an allergic response. Crackles are often associated with an upper respiratory infection. Crackles heard with a dry cough and labored tachypnea are a sign of *Pneumocystis carinii* pneumonia, a common opportunistic lung infection in patients with HIV. Lymph nodes should be inspected and then gently palpated (often done by the advanced practitioner). (See Fig. 17.1.) Normally, lymph nodes are not palpable in the adult (normally they can be palpated in young children). If on palpation a lymph node is

LEARNING TIP

A normally functioning immune system is required to trigger an inflammatory response that produces the signs of inflammation or infection: fever, redness, pain, swelling, and warmth. If the immune system is suppressed or functioning abnormally, this normal inflammatory response may not occur. Thus the patient may exhibit only a low-grade fever with none of the other signs of inflammation or infection (redness, pain, swelling, and warmth).

Recognize patients with suppressed immune systems so that low-grade fevers are reported to the physician for prompt treatment. This may be the only sign of a life-threatening infection that develops because of the suppressed immune system.

CRITICAL THINKING

Laura Sims

■ Laura is scheduled for a lymph node biopsy and is seen in preadmission testing before surgery. As the licensed practical nurse/licensed vocational nurse (LPN/LVN) prepares to draw blood specimens, he learns that Laura is allergic to latex.
1. Why is this patient allergy information important?
2. What should the LPN/LVN do next?
3. What precautions should the LPN/LVN use for drawing the blood specimen?

Suggested answers at end of chapter.

enlarged, the following characteristics need to be noted: location, size, shape, tenderness, temperature, consistency, mobility, symmetry, pulsation, and if red streaks, redness, or edema are present.

If enlarged, the spleen may be palpable (by the advanced practitioner) in the left upper quadrant of the abdomen with disorders in which there is an overproduction or excessive destruction of red blood cells.

The renal system may also show impairment because of an immunological disorder manifested by a change in urinary output, flank pain, edema, weight gain, or elevated renal function studies.

A general neurological assessment of muscle strength and coordination, changes, or abnormalities is noted. Changes may be an indication of an immunologically

TABLE 17.3 OBJECTIVE ASSESSMENT OF THE IMMUNE SYSTEM

Category	Physical Assessment Findings	Possible Abnormal Findings/Causes
Neurological	Alertness and orientation	Frequently confusion or lethargy seen in later stages of systemic lupus erythematosus (SLE) and acquired immunodeficiency asyndrome (AIDS)
Skin	Warm, dry, smooth, supple, even coloring, nonpruritic	Rashes, urticaria, pruritus, pustules seen with many forms of allergic reactions
		"Butterfly rash" (red rash over bridge of nose and cheek bones) seen in 55%–85% of SLE patients
		Painless purple lesions are seen with Kaposi's sarcoma, which is frequently associated with HIV and AIDS.
	Pink mucous membranes	Pale edematous mucous membranes along with rhinorrhea and "allergic shiners" (dark circles under the eyes) are seen with allergic rhinitis
		Pale conjunctiva is associated with anemia
		Periorbital edema may also be indicative of hypothyroidism
	Nail attached to nailbed	Onycholysis (nail detaches from nailbed) is seen in patient's with Hashimoto's thyroiditis
Heart Sounds	Clear S1 and S2	A pericardial friction rub may be heard with rheumatoid arthritis or in SLE patients owing to inflammation of the connective tissue surrounding the heart (pericardium)
Lung Sounds	Clear throughout	Pleural effusion as evidenced by tachypnea with diminished sounds in bases may be seen in SLE or rheumatoid arthritis patients or a pleural friction rub may occur in these patients.
		Crackles with a dry cough may be indicative of *Pneumocystis carinii* pneumonia (PCP)
Lymph Nodes	Nonpalpable and nontender	Enlarged lymph nodes that are painless, firm, and fixed are associated with cancerous lesions, whereas painful enlarged lymph nodes are associated with inflammation and infection
Gastrointestinal	Appropriate appetite without nausea or vomiting	Anorexia, nausea, and vomiting may be associated with immune disorders.
	Regular pattern of brown, soft, formed stools	Diarrhea frequently occurs in patients with irritable bowel syndrome (IBS)
Renal	An average of 30 mL per hour of clear, yellow/amber urine without presence of protein or pain	Urine output of less than 30 mL per hour, the presence of protein in the urine, and edema are seen in patients with SLE or serum sickness
		Transfusion reactions may cause hematuria, flank pain, or oliguria
		Glomerulonephritis may cause hematuria, flank pain, or oliguria
Musculoskeletal	Painless and nonswollen joints with full range of motion	Swollen, painful joints are seen in rheumatoid arthritis along with limited joint range of motion
	Overall strength, endurance and coordination appropriate for age and physical fitness	Decreased strength and coordination occur with patients with multiple sclerosis
		Patients with myasthenia gravis lose strength and endurance with repetitive movements

based disorder such as multiple sclerosis or myasthenia gravis.

Diagnostic Tests

Presenting signs and symptoms and the patient's history determine which tests and procedures may be ordered. Table 17.4 describes the most common blood tests for patients with allergic, autoimmune, or immune disorders. Table 17.5 presents common noninvasive and invasive procedures for immune disorders.

Gene Testing

Mapping of the human genome has made current and future gene testing and manipulation possible. Scientists are now able to test for numerous diseases, predisposition to diseases, and enzyme deficiencies that can alter immune response.

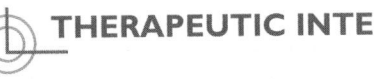

THERAPEUTIC INTERVENTIONS

Allergies

A medical alert bracelet or some sort of readily available identification of an allergy should be worn by the patient. It is important always to be aware of patient allergies. Allergies should be noted before giving any medications or foods. All allergies, including those to food, must be taken seriously.

Food allergies create serious management problems and have caused numerous deaths from anaphylactic shock

TABLE 17.4 DIAGNOSTIC LABORATORY TESTS FOR IMMUNE SYSTEM

Test	Definition/Normal Value	Significance of Abnormal Findings
Red Blood Cells	Number of red blood cells per 1 mm of blood: Adult male: 4.7–6.1 $\times 10^{12}$/L Adult female: 4.2–5.4 $\times 10^{12}$/L	Decreased in all forms of anemia, such as pernicious anemia that develops from the autoimmune form of gastritis or idiopathic autoimmune hemolytic anemia.
Differential	Each of these tests (MCV, MCH, MCHC, RDW) provides information about the RBC size, shape, color, and intracellular structure. MCV: 80–95 mm³ MCH: 27–31 pg MCHC: 32–36 g/dL RDW: 11.0%–14.5 %	Can help determine the cause of anemia. Pernicious anemia can develop because of the autoimmune form of gastritis.
White Blood Cells	Number of white blood cells per 1 mm of blood. Adult: 5–10 $\times 10^9$/L	Increased with immunosuppression and an increase with infection.
Differential	Percentage of type of white blood cells in 1 mm of blood. Or the actual numbers of specific types of WBCs if an absolute count is performed. % Absolute/mm³	Eosinophils elevate with type I hypersensitivity reactions such as allergic rhinitis or anaphylaxis.
• Neutrophils	55–70 2500–8000	
• Lymphocytes	20–40 1000–4000	
• Monocytes	2–8 100–700	
• Eosinophils	1–4 50–500	
• Basophils	0.5–1.0 25–100	
Erythrocyte Sedimentation Rate (ESR)	A nonspecific test for generalized inflammation. Measures the red blood cell descent (in millimeters) in test tube after being in normal saline for 1 hr (Westergren method). Male: up to 15 mm/hr Female: up to 20 mm/hr	There may be a false negative if steroids or nonsteroidal anti-inflammatory drugs (NSAIDs) are being used when test is performed.
Rheumatoid Factor (RF or RA)	An abnormal protein found in serum when IgM reacts with an abnormal IgG; found in 80% of clients with rheumatoid arthritis and other autoimmune disorders. Normal value: negative.	Increased in rheumatoid arthritis, SLE, leukemia, tuberculosis, older age, scleroderma, infectious mononucleosis.

Test	Definition/Normal Value	Significance of Abnormal Findings
Antinuclear Antibody (ANA)	Measures autoantibodies that attack the cell's nucleus. Normal value: negative.	Most commonly present in SLE (with >95% sensitivity), leukemia, scleroderma, rheumatoid arthritis, and myasthenia gravis; many medications influence levels.
Complement	Specific serum proteins that help mediate inflammation. Measures the amount of each of the components in the complement system. Total: 75–160 U/mL C3: 0.55–1.20 g/L C4: 0.2–0.5 g/L	Deficiencies of specific complement proteins are seen with SLE clients.
C-Reactive Protein (CRP)	An abnormal protein found in plasma during acute inflammatory processes; more sensitive than sedimentation rate. <10 mg/L	Increased in rheumatoid arthritis, cancer, SLE. Suppressed by aspirin and steroids.
Radioallergosorbent test (RAST)	Patient serum is mixed with a specific allergen, incubated with radiolabeled anti-IgE antibodies, and then the total amount of the specific IgE antibodies is measured.	A viable alternative to skin testing if the patient does not have multiple allergies.
ELISA	Antibodies in patient's blood are tested for on HIV antigen test plates.	Positive results may indicate HIV infection, but results *MUST* be confirmed by another test, usually the Western blot.
Western Blot	A blood test to detect the presence of any of the four major HIV antigens. Is considered positive when at least two of the four are detected. Used as a confirmation test.	If being used as the confirmation test, positive results indicate HIV infection. False positives do occur in patients who have autoimmune disease, leukemia, lymphoma, or syphilis, and in alcoholics.
Immunoglobulin Assay or Electrophoresis IgG IgM IgA IgE IgD	Antibodies are made up of immunoglobulins, of which there are five different classes. *Normal in milligrams/ deciliter (mg/dL):* 500–1500 50–300 100–490 <100 IU/mL <3 U/mL	IgG. Increase: in all types of infections, liver disease, rheumatoid arthritis, dermatologic disorders. Decrease: agammaglobulinemia, lymphoid aplasia, Bence Jones proteinuria. IgM Increase: malaria, infectious mononucleosis, SLE, rheumatoid arthritis. Decrease: lymphoid aplasia, chronic lymphoblastic leukemia. IgA Increase: during exercise, obstructive jaundice. Decrease: immunosuppressive therapy, benzene exposure, congenital IgE. Increase: allergic reactions, allergic infections. Decrease: agammaglobulinemia.
CD4+ Count	The CD4+ T lymphocytes are counted. Percentage: 60–75 No./µL: 600–1500	Increased in allergy-proven patients. Decreased in cancer, HIV and AIDS, and immunosuppression.
CD8+ Count	The CD8+ T lymphocytes are counted. Percentage: 25–30 No./µL: 300–1000	Increased in viral infections. Decreased in SLE.
CD4+/CD8+ Ratio	The ratio of the CD4+ and CD8+ absolute counts are determined. >1	As HIV and AIDS progresses the CD4+/CD8+ ratio will become smaller as the CD4+ count decreases and the CD8+ count remains relatively unchanged.

MCV = mean corpuscular volume; MCH = mean corpuscular hemoglobin; MCHC = mean corpuscular hemoglobin concentration; RDW = red blood cell distribution width.

TABLE 17.5 DIAGNOSTIC PROCEDURES FOR IMMUNE SYSTEM

Procedure	Definition/Normal Finding (if applicable)	Significance of Abnormal Findings	Nursing Management (if applicable)
		Noninvasive	
Chest X-ray	Radiographic picture to determine size, shape, density of structures within the chest.	Pericarditis, pleuritis, pleural or pericardial effusions or may occur with systemic lupus erythematosus (SLE) or rheumatoid arthritis. Arthritic changes may also be noted on x-ray.	None.
Gene Testing	A sample of DNA which can be taken as an oral or nasal swab is examined and mapped for a variety of genetic disorders.	Abnormal findings may confirm a certain diagnosis or indicate that the patient may develop symptoms or pass a disorder on to offspring.	Assess support systems and for possible counseling referral.
Magnetic Resonance Imagery (MRI)	May be invasive or non-invasive depending upon if an injected contrast dye is used. No radiation is used; rather, magnetic fields are employed. Various body planes can be examined with the MRI. Provides better visualization of the central nervous (CNS) than with the computerized tomography scan.	Destructive bone and joint lesions. Brain lesions, tumors, abscesses, aneurysms, hematomas, and demyelinization of nerves can be visualized.	If dye is used, check for iodine allergy and have the patient's height and weight on record. Patients weighing over 300 lb, are pregnant, requiring continuous monitoring or intravenous equipment, have implanted metal objects (bone pins, screws, pacemakers), are agitated, or are claustrophobic may not be eligible for an MRI.
		Invasive	
Biopsy (of Specific Organ in Question)	Used to confirm a diagnosis, determine a prognosis, or evaluate treatment. May be performed as an inpatient, outpatient, or in a physician's office. The specimen may be obtained through a needle aspiration, incision, excision, or gavage and with or without endoscopy, fluroscopy, stereotaxic, or needle localization.	The biopsy tissue is examined microscopically for diagnosis. Cancers, lymphomas, leukemias, transplant rejections are diagnosed in this manner.	Informed consent must be obtained prior to the procedure. Other preoperative/postoperative care determined by specific organ biopsied. Most organs are quite vascular and there is a high risk for bleeding complications after the biopsy. So vital signs and site monitoring are important.
Computerized Tomography (CT Scan)	This may be invasive or non-invasive depending upon if an injected contrast dye is used.	See MRI above.	If dye is to be used, check for iodine allergy and have patient's height and weight on record.
Skin Testing	Done if immune system is intact. Testing done for *Candida*, tetanus, or tuberculosis (purified protein derivative [PPD] test) or specific allergens such as medications, food, or environmental factors.	If erythema (redness) or induration (firmness) occurs at the site within a prescribed time frame, test is positive. Indicates patient has either been exposed to an organism, has an active infection, or has developed antibodies that stimulate an immune response.	Ask if patients have any allergies and the type of reaction or symptoms that occur.

(Box 17.3 Nutrition Notes). The offending allergen may be present in extremely small amounts. Sometimes a food product is contaminated by a previous batch of food made with the same equipment. Occasionally, the allergen may enter the body not by ingestion but by inhalation or contact with skin or mucous membranes.

Epinephrine is the drug of choice for life-threatening anaphylactic reactions. If possible, treatment should begin immediately with administration of epinephrine until other medical care can be provided.

An EpiPen is often prescribed for patients with allergies to food or insect stings. It is a prepackaged, single-use device that allows the patient to self-inject a physician-ordered dose of epinephrine right through clothing. The patient must carry

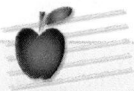

Box 17.3

Nutrition Notes

Respecting Food Allergies

Allergy to food can be fatal. An analysis of 13 anaphylactic reactions to food identifies points along the critical path that had the potential to alter the outcome. Of 13 cases identified, 6 were fatal.

- In all cases, the patient was known to have asthma and to be allergic to some food.
- None of the patients was aware that the allergen was present in the foods consumed (candy, cookies, and pastry).
- Symptoms began soon after ingestion but in some cases abated before becoming severe.
- Of particular significance is the fact that *fewer than half the children had self-injectable epinephrine prescribed and only one of the six children used a dose.* The average delay between ingestion of the allergenic food and receipt of a dose of epinephrine was two and one-half times as long in the fatal cases as in the nonfatal cases.
- More of the fatal cases occurred in public places rather than private homes.

Several recommendations came from this study:

- Epinephrine should be prescribed, kept available, *and used* for patients with IgE-mediated food allergies.
- Children and adolescents who have an allergic reaction to food should be observed for 3 to 4 hours after the reaction at a center capable of dealing with anaphylaxis.
- Parents of such children should be taught to ensure an appropriate, rapid response by schools and other institutions.

Source: Summarized from Sampson AA, Mendelson I, Rosen JP: Fatal and near-fatal anaphylactic reactions to food in children and adolescents. N Engl J Med 327:380, 1992.

the EpiPen at all times when insect stings are possible. The expiration date of the EpiPen must be checked routinely and replaced as necessary. The patient needs to be instructed that the EpiPen does not replace the need for immediate and continued medical attention because the duration of the single dose of epinephrine varies from 1 to 4 hours.

Immunotherapy

To help desensitize a patient with anaphylactic reactions to allergens or with chronic allergic symptoms, immunotherapy involves injecting small amounts of an extract of the allergen. Over time the strength of the allergen injected is increased until the desired hyposensitivity is reached. The subcutaneous injections are given once or twice a week initially, then every few weeks indefinitely for years. It is important that the patient not miss a dose. If this happens, the allergen strength may need to be reduced. This therapy is helpful for insect sting allergies.

When administering the allergen injection, it is important to understand that an anaphylactic reaction can occur. A physician and emergency equipment should be readily available. The patient should be observed following the injection for about 20 to 30 minutes to detect a reaction. The patient and family should be taught that a reaction could occur up to 24 hours after the injection and how to respond if it does occur.

Medications

Medications are one of the primary treatment options for immune disorders. General categories of these medications include epinephrine, corticosteroids, antihistamines, histamine (H_2) blockers, decongestants, mast cell–stabilizing drugs, antivirals, antibiotics, immunosuppressants, interferon, leukotriene antagonists, and hormone therapy. (See Chapter 18.)

Surgical Management

In some cases, splenectomy is necessary to control symptoms of an immunologic disorder.

New Therapies

Monoclonal antibodies can be produced against a variety of antigens. A monoclonal antibody is made by cloning one specific antibody and then growing unlimited amounts of it in tissue cultures. Many uses are being found for these antibodies, such as in dealing with transplant rejections.

Recombinant DNA technology combines genes from one organism with genes from another. This therapy is used for replacing an abnormal or missing gene to produce a normal gene. The normal gene can then be injected into the patient in an attempt to cure the disorder as the patient's body reproduces the normal genes. T-lymphocyte–directed gene transfer for severe combined immune deficiency has been performed successfully. Along these same lines is the research regarding injection of the precursors to all cells, the stem cell, into abnormal areas to produce normal cells. Studies continue in this area for possible uses of gene therapy, and since the completion of the mapping portion of the Human Genome Project, new discoveries in this area occur daily. For additional up-to-date information on these topics, visit the National Institutes of Health at www.nhgri.nih.gov or www.ncbi.nlm.nih.gov.

REVIEW QUESTIONS

1. The nurse who is teaching a patient about vaccines would be correct in teaching that a vaccine provides which of the following types of immunity?
   a. Naturally acquired passive immunity
   b. Artificially acquired passive immunity
   c. Naturally acquired active immunity
   d. Artificially acquired active immunity

2. Which of the following vaccines are recommended annually for the older patient?
   a. Influenza
   b. Pneumovax
   c. Diphtheria tetanus
   d. Polio

3. The nurse is assisting with data collection. Which of the following past surgeries found in the history may influence immune system dysfunction?
   a. Splenectomy
   b. Thyroidectomy
   c. Pneumonectomy
   d. Parathyroidectomy

4. During data collection the patient reports tenderness in the cervical lymph nodes. The nurse recognizes that lymph nodes that are enlarged and tender usually indicate which of the following problems?
   a. Cancer
   b. Degeneration
   c. Inflammation
   d. Arthritis

5. The nurse is caring for a patient with suspected HIV. The nurse anticipates that which of the following is a confirmation test that will be ordered to test for HIV antibodies?
   a. Murex SUDS
   b. Western blot
   c. Enzyme-linked immunosorbent assay
   d. p24 antigen testing

Fill in the blank:

6. Biaxin 200 mg oral suspension is ordered for a patient. The nurse has 125 mg/5 mL available. How many mililiters should the nurse give?

Answer:_____ mL

SUGGESTED ANSWERS TO

CRITICAL THINKING

■ *Laura Sims*
1. The patient can have an anaphylactic reaction if exposed to latex, which may result in death for some patients.
2. The LPN/LVN should follow the agency's latex allergy protocol, enter this information into the patient's medical record, notify surgery scheduling so latex precaution protocols can be planned for surgery, and have the patient's physician informed.
3. Following the agency's protocol, the nurse should wear nonlatex gloves and use nonlatex equipment to draw the specimens.

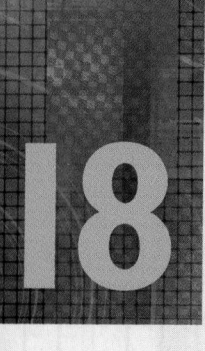

18

Nursing Care of Patients with Immune Disorders

SHARON M. NOWAK

KEY TERMS

anaphylaxis (an-uh-fi-LAK-sis)
angioedema (AN-gee-o-eh-DEE-ma)
ankylosing spondylitis (ANG-ki-LOH-sing SPON-da-LIGHT-is)
histamine (HISS-ta-mean)
urticaria (UR-ti-KAIR-ee-ah)

QUESTIONS TO GUIDE YOUR READING

1. How would you explain the immunological mechanism for the four types of hypersensitivities?

2. How would you explain the pathophysiology of disorders of the immune system?

3. What are the etiologies, signs, and symptoms of immune system disorders?

4. What care would you provide for patients undergoing tests for immune system disorders?

5. What is the current medical treatment for immune system disorders?

6. What data are collected when caring for patients with disorders of the immune system?

7. What factors alter or influence the self-recognition portion of the immune system?

8. What nursing care will you provide for patients with disorders of the immune system?

9. How will you know if your nursing interventions have been effective?

Disorders of the immune system can be divided into three categories. The first category is hypersensitivity reactions, which include conditions such as **anaphylaxis,** hemolytic transfusion reactions, measles, and transplant rejections. Autoimmune disorders (e.g., rheumatoid arthritis, ulcerative colitis, and multiple sclerosis) are the second category. The third category includes the immune deficiencies, such as hypogammaglobulinemia and acquired immunodeficiency syndrome (AIDS). (See Chapter 19.)

HYPERSENSITIVITY REACTIONS

The immune system is an adaptive, protective system of the body. However, there are times when this system causes injury to the body because of its exaggerated response. One of these occasions is when a hypersensitivity reaction occurs.

In the past, these reactions were classified as either immediate or delayed hypersensitivity. Gell and Coombs have developed a more precise classification system, which is used today. This four-division system (types I, II, III, and IV) classifies hypersensitivity reactions according to the way the tissue is injured.

anaphylaxis: ana—up + phylaxis—protection

Type I

A type I reaction, an anaphylactic reaction, is an immediately occurring reaction when exposure to a specific antigen occurs (Fig. 18.1). The reaction can be mild to severe and life threatening. The patient must have had previous exposure (sensitization) to the antigen. During this exposure, immunoglobulin E (IgE) antibodies are made and attach to mast cells throughout the body. When a subsequent exposure occurs, the antigen causes IgE to trigger mast cells to release their contents. One of the substances released is **histamine,** which causes vasodilation, changes in vascular permeability, an increase in mucus production, and contraction of various smooth muscles.

If the second antigen exposure is localized, the reaction is small and remains local. However, if the exposure is systemic, the reaction is massive and widespread. Respiratory allergies, such as allergic rhinitis and allergic asthma, with associated disorders of atopic dermatitis, tend to be reactions of a larger scale. Anaphylaxis, **urticaria,** and **angioedema** are the severest forms of type I reactions.

A type I reaction occurs when the patient has a positive reaction to a scratch test. A scratch test is done to identify specific allergens to which a patient is reactive. Tiny amounts of a variety of common allergens are scratched

angioedema: angeion—vessel + oidema—swelling

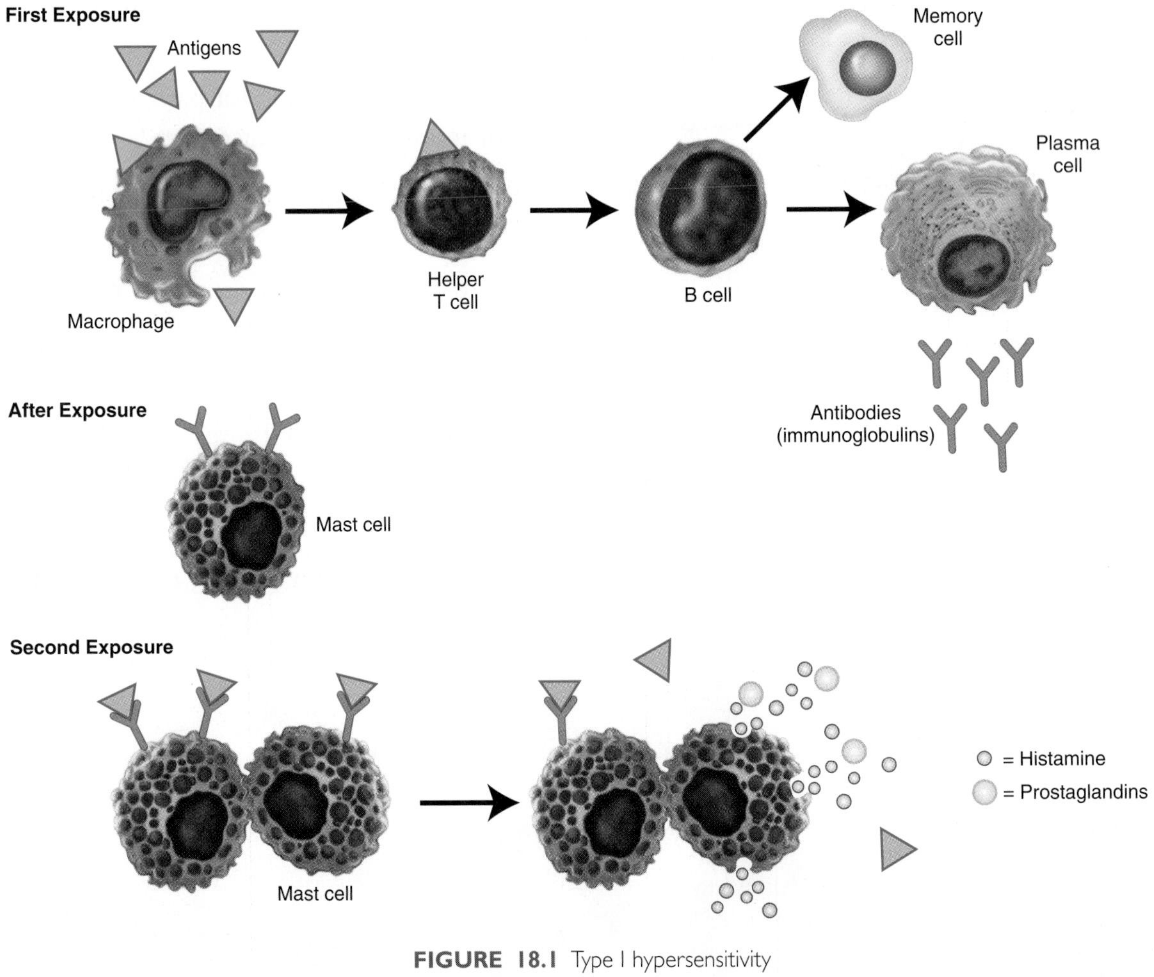

First Exposure

Antigens

Macrophage

Helper T cell

B cell

Memory cell

Plasma cell

Antibodies (immunoglobulins)

After Exposure

Mast cell

Second Exposure

Mast cell

◯ = Histamine

◯ = Prostaglandins

FIGURE 18.1 Type I hypersensitivity

onto the skin, which is then observed for indications of a reaction: redness, edema, and pruritus. If these indicators occur, it is considered to be a local reaction.

Allergic Rhinitis

Allergic rhinitis is the most common form of allergy. When symptoms occur throughout the year, it is called perennial allergic rhinitis. If the symptoms occur seasonally, it is called hay fever. The causative antigens are environmental and airborne.

PATHOPHYSIOLOGY. Allergic rhinitis is the result of an antigen-antibody reaction. Ciliary action decreases and mucous secretions increase. Vasodilation and local tissue edema occur.

SIGNS AND SYMPTOMS. Signs and symptoms vary in intensity and include sneezing, nasal itching, profuse watery rhinorrhea (runny nose), and itchy red eyes. The nasal mucosa is pale, cyanotic, and edematous. Frequently there are dark circles under the eyes, called allergic shiners, caused by venous congestion in the maxillary sinuses.

DIAGNOSTIC TESTS. Sometimes, skin testing is performed to identify the specific offending allergens to allow avoidance of the allergen. However, skin testing is expensive, does not always identify the allergen, and has limited usefulness for allergens that cannot be easily avoided once identified.

THERAPEUTIC INTERVENTIONS. Initial treatment involves eliminating the offending environmental stimuli. Antihistamines and nasal decongestants may be prescribed for symptomatic relief. If the symptoms are severe, corticosteroids via inhalation or nasal spray may also be given.

Rhinophototherapy is a newer treatment that uses light waves to reduce the body's hyperimmune response seen in this disorder. The treatment is usually done three times a week for 3 weeks and relieves symptoms such as sneezing, itching, and runny nose.

Immunotherapy, referred to as allergy shots, is reserved for patients with severe or debilitating symptoms. Immunotherapy involves receiving weekly subcutaneous injections in the allergist's office of tiny amounts of the offending antigen. Once a tolerance to a particular dose is reached, the amount of antigen is slightly increased. This therapy continues until the patient no longer exhibits symptoms when exposed to the environmental antigen. Being alert to signs of anaphylaxis during these procedures is essential for the nurse.

Atopic Dermatitis

Atopic dermatitis, often called eczema, is an inflammatory skin response.

PATHOPHYSIOLOGY. These skin lesions are not typical for a type I hypersensitivity reaction, and there usually is not a specific antigen identified as the cause. However, it is believed that the pathophysiology of atopic dermatitis is a type I hypersensitivity reaction, mediated by IgE antibodies, because it is commonly found in patients with allergic rhinitis or allergic asthma.

SIGNS AND SYMPTOMS. Initially there is pruritus, edema, and extremely dry skin, which is followed by eruptions of tiny vesicles (blisters); these eventually break open, crust over, and scale off. There is decreased sweating in these areas with the skin eventually thickening in the areas of dermatitis.

DIAGNOSTIC TESTS. There are no tests to confirm this diagnosis. A detailed history and physical examination are used to diagnose it. Of course, if there is an infection, culture and sensitivity tests may be ordered to determine the infecting organism and appropriate treatment.

THERAPEUTIC INTERVENTIONS. Treatment focuses on symptoms. Oil-in-water lubricants such as Alpha-Keri oil tend to be the most effective for dryness. Topical corticosteroids may be ordered for their anti-inflammatory properties. Topical calcineurin inhibitors also reduce the inflammatory response and relieve itching and rash when steroids are not effective. If skin lesions become infected, topical or systemic antibiotics are prescribed.

Anaphylaxis

Anaphylaxis is a severe systemic type I hypersensitivity reaction. There are numerous causes of anaphylaxis (Table 18.1).

TABLE 18.1 SUBSTANCES THAT COMMONLY TRIGGER ANAPHYLACTIC REACTIONS

Antibiotics	Foods
Penicillins	Beans
Sulfonamides	Chocolate
Tetracyclines	Eggs
Cephalosporins	Fruits (e.g., strawberries)
Amphotericin B	Grains (e.g., wheat)
Aminoglycosides	Nuts
	Shellfish
Medical Products	
Latex rubber	
Diagnostic Agents	**Pollens**
Contrast dyes	Grass
	Ragweed
Anesthetics/Antiarrhythmics	**Proteins**
Lidocaine	Horse serum
Procaine	Rabbit serum
Other Medications	**Venoms**
Barbiturates	Bees, wasps, hornets
Phenytoin (Dilantin)	Fire ants
Protamine	Snakes
Salicylates	
Diazepam (Valium)	
Food Additives	**Hormones**
Bisulfites	Insulin
Monosodium glutamate (MSG)	Vasopressin
	Estradiol
	Adrenocorticotropic hormone

PATHOPHYSIOLOGY. IgE antibodies produced from previous antigen sensitization are attached to mast cells throughout the body. In this reaction, the antigen is introduced at a systemic level, which causes widespread release of histamine and other chemical mediators contained within the mast cells

The most profound complications of an anaphylactic reaction are respiratory and cardiac arrest. Immediate treatment is necessary to prevent death.

SIGNS AND SYMPTOMS. Anaphylaxis produces sudden and life-threatening signs and symptoms (Table 18.2). Generalized smooth muscle spasms occur, causing bronchial narrowing and creating stridor, wheezing, dyspnea, and laryngeal edema, which can lead to respiratory arrest. Cramping, diarrhea, nausea, and vomiting also result from these spasms. Capillary permeability increases, allowing

fluid to shift from the vessels to the interstitium. This causes hypotension, tachycardia, and an increase in respiratory symptoms. The blood volume within the vessels decreases while the blood vessels dilate, resulting in a further decrease in circulating blood volume. The dilation also causes diffuse erythema (redness) and warmth of the skin. Neurological changes include apprehension, drowsiness, profound restlessness, headache, and possible seizures.

DIAGNOSTIC TESTS. There is no time for tests to be performed during an anaphylactic reaction other than those needed to guide symptom treatment, such as arterial blood gases or electrocardiogram (ECG) monitoring. Anaphylaxis is diagnosed based on physical assessment and history from the patient or significant other. After the patient's recovery, allergen testing may be considered for future prevention.

THERAPEUTIC INTERVENTIONS. Intravenous access is a priority for administration of intravenous epinephrine and vasopressor drugs (dopamine) to increase blood pressure. Oxygen therapy is started. If respiratory symptoms are severe, a tracheostomy or endotracheal intubation may be necessary, with mechanical ventilation. Antihistamines and corticosteroids may also be given orally, by injection, or intravenously.

TABLE 18.2 ANAPHYLAXIS SUMMARY

Signs and Symptoms	Generalized smooth muscle spasms
	- Bronchial narrowing
	  • stridor
	  • wheezing
	  • dyspnea
	  • laryngeal edema
	- Cramping diarrhea
	- Nausea and vomiting
	Increased capillary permeability
	- Fluid shifts from blood vessels to interstitium
	  • hypotension
	  • tachycardia
	  • increased respiratory symptoms
	Blood vessels dilate
	- Further decreasing circulating volume
	- Diffuse erythema (redness)
	- Increased skin temperature
	Apprehension
	Drowsiness
	Profound restlessness
	Headache
	Possible seizures

Diagnostic Tests	Testing to guide treatment • Arterial blood gases • Electrocardiogram (ECG) monitoring History and physical exam After recovery—allergen testing for prevention
Therapeutic Interventions	Intravenous (IV) access Epinephrine IV Vasopressive drugs IV (dopamine) Oxygen Antihistamines (oral, IV, injection) Corticosteroids (oral, IV, injection) If severe respiratory compromise: - Tracheostomy or endotracheal intubation - Mechanical ventilation
Complications Possible Nursing Diagnoses	Respiratory and cardiac arrest Impaired gas exchange Anxiety Ineffective health maintenance

CRITICAL THINKING

Mrs. Barnes

■ Mrs. Barnes, a 32 year old, was brought into the emergency room after having been stung multiple times by bees while gardening. She has numerous red welts over her body which she states are itchy and is very anxious. Her temperature is 99.2°F (37.22°C), blood pressure is 102/58 mm Hg, pulse is 102 bpm, and respiratory rate is 26 per minute.

1. What might be causing Mrs. Barnes's symptoms?
2. What additional information is needed?
3. What should you do to help Mrs. Barnes?

Suggested answers at end of chapter.

Urticaria
PATHOPHYSIOLOGY. Urticaria (hives) is a type I hypersensitivity reaction. The antigen-stimulated reaction of IgE antibodies causing the release of mast cell contents, especially histamine, triggers urticaria.

ETIOLOGY. There are numerous causes of urticaria. In addition to medications and foods, cold, local heat, pressure, and stress can also cause urticaria. Many patients with underlying chronic conditions, such as systemic lupus erythematosus, lymphoma, hyperthyroidism, or cancer, are susceptible to urticaria.

SIGNS AND SYMPTOMS. The lesions of urticaria are raised, pruritic, nontender, and erythematous wheals on the skin. They tend to be concentrated on the trunk and proximal extremities.

DIAGNOSTIC TESTS. Diagnosis is made on the basis of physical examination and history.

THERAPEUTIC INTERVENTIONS. Treatment depends on the degree of symptoms. In the most severe cases, epinephrine may be given to quickly resolve the urticaria. Corticosteroids (orally, topically, or intravenously) may be given. Antihistamines and histamine (H_2) blockers may aid in resolution by blocking the release of histamine.

Angioedema

PATHOPHYSIOLOGY AND ETIOLOGY. Angioedema is a form of urticaria. The pathophysiology and etiology of angioedema are the same as for urticaria. However, angioedema affects submucosal and subcutaneous tissues rather than the skin.

SIGNS AND SYMPTOMS. Angioedema is painless and minimally pruritic, with dermal erythematous and subcutaneous eruptions. There is also skin and mucous membrane edema. The eruptions may last longer than with urticaria.

DIAGNOSTIC TESTS. A comprehensive history and physical examination confirm the diagnosis. Skin testing may be performed to determine the specific antigen.

THERAPEUTIC INTERVENTIONS. The most basic treatment involves avoidance of the antigen. Symptomatic relief may be obtained through the use of antihistamines and corticosteroids. For long-term treatment, immunotherapy for allergen desensitization may be indicated.

NURSING PROCESS: HYPERSENSITIVITY DISORDERS TYPE I. Assessment/Data Collection. Gather information about the patient's signs and symptoms. Immediately report any sudden dyspnea, shortness of breath, anxiety, restlessness, or chest or back pain. Identify any allergies the patient may have as well as the signs and symptoms that occur with exposure to the allergen. Perform a thorough skin assessment and carefully document any lesions or rashes. Note any changes in rashes or lesions or **signs of infection: redness, warmth, drainage.** Assess the patient's knowledge of disease process, **causes, treatment plan, and self-care.** Note responses to treatments.

Nursing Diagnosis, Planning, and Implementation. Impaired gas exchange related to laryngeal edema

EXPECTED OUTCOME: The patient will maintain clear lung fields and remain free of signs of respiratory distress.

- Monitor respiratory rate, depth, and effort such as use of accessory muscles, nasal flaring, or abdominal breathing *to identify problems early.*
- Monitor the patient for restlessness, changes in mentation, level of consciousness, changes in voice, or dysphagia *in order to identify problems and intervene early.*

- Position the patient in a high-Fowler's or semi-Fowler's position *in order to improve ventilation and decrease upper airway edema.*

Anxiety related to dyspnea or pruritus

EXPECTED OUTCOME: The patient will state anxiety is controlled.

- Stay with the patient and speak calmly *to reduce fear or frustration.*
- Teach patient to visualize the absence of anxiety, itching or dyspnea *to decrease anxiety.*
- Provide family with the information needed to distinguish between anxiety or panic versus a serious physiological problem *in order to make informed decisions regarding obtaining emergency medical care.*

Risk for impaired skin integrity related to effects of allergic reaction

EXPECTED OUTCOME: The patient's skin will remain intact.

- Assess and document skin and lesions *to provide a basis for interventions and evaluation.*
- Teach patient to keep fingernails short and clean *to minimize the damage or risk for infection if scratching does occur.*
- Teach patient to apply clean, white cotton clothing over affected area (socks, gloves/mittens, undershirt), especially at bedtime *to minimize scratching while allowing for air movement with minimal irritation from dyes.*
- Teach patient to use gentle rubbing or pressure instead of scratching *to minimize the amount of skin trauma.*

Ineffective health maintenance related to lack of knowledge of methods to decrease inflammation and pruritus and reduce episodes of inflammation

EXPECTED OUTCOME: The patient or caregiver will state understanding and follow the mutually agreed upon plan of care.

- Assess patient's knowledge of disease and its causes *to provide a basis for teaching and evaluation.*
- Assess patient's values and beliefs regarding plan of care *in order to have patient's values and beliefs correspond with the plan of care, thereby improving compliance.*
- Assess barriers to patient's ability to carry out plan of care and plan interventions to decrease barriers *in order to improve the likelihood of the patient implementing the plan of care.*
- Teach patient to wear medical alert identification for allergies *in order for prompt medical attention to be given if the patient is unable to give information.*
- Discuss methods of avoiding allergen with patient such as wearing mask when mowing the lawn or working outdoors, having heating ducts cleaned, covering heat registers with filters, and frequent

home vacuuming and dusting to promote an under-standing *of preventative methods and prevent allergen exposure and anaphylaxis.*

- If antigen is environmental (e.g., insect sting or foods) explain need to obtain prescription for epinephrine pen and teach how to use it. (See Chapter 17.)
- For atopic dermatitis, teaching plan includes signs and symptoms of infection, use of humidification during the winter months *to prevent dryness*, wearing cotton clothing *to minimize irritation*, and cool soaks *to decrease pruritus.*
- For urticaria, some patients may benefit from instruction on stress management and relaxation techniques *to relieve urticaria.* Teach patient to follow therapeutic regimen including prescribed medications and their correct usage *to reduce symptoms.*
- Document teaching and patient understanding.

Evaluation. If interventions have been effective, there will be no signs of respiratory distress and the lung fields will be clear. The patient's posture, facial expressions, gestures, and concentration will reflect no anxiety. The skin will remain intact. If there are lesions, they will be reduced and healing. The patient will express knowledge of disorder and treatment plan. The patient will verbalize no barriers to attaining treatment goals.

Type II

A type II hypersensitivity reaction involves the destruction of a cell or substance that has an antigen attached to its cell membrane, which is sensed by either immunoglobulin G (IgG) or immunoglobulin M (IgM) as being a foreign antigen (Fig. 18.2). When an antigen marker is sensed as foreign, an antibody attaches to the antigen on the cell membrane, causing lysis of the cell or accelerated phagocytosis (engulfing and ingestion). When a cell is foreign, such as a bacterium, this process is beneficial. However, sometimes antigens on the surface of a red blood cell (RBC) can be sensed as foreign for the different ABO blood types, which results in the RBC being destroyed.

Hemolytic Transfusion Reaction

PATHOPHYSIOLOGY. A hemolytic transfusion reaction is a type II hypersensitivity reaction in which incompatible surface antigens on RBCs are transfused. These antigens may be ABO or Rh incompatible. The recipient's antibodies attach to the foreign antigens on the transfused RBCs causing rapid lysis of the RBC. The rapid RBC lysis results in a massive amount of cellular debris that occludes the blood vessels throughout the body. This leads to ischemia and necrosis of tissue and organs and can be life threatening.

ETIOLOGY. Occasionally, antibodies form after a bacterial or viral infection. However, prior sensitization is usually from a previous blood transfusion or past pregnancy. ABO and Rh blood type must be matched for transfusions. The ABO blood types are A, B, AB, and O. People with blood

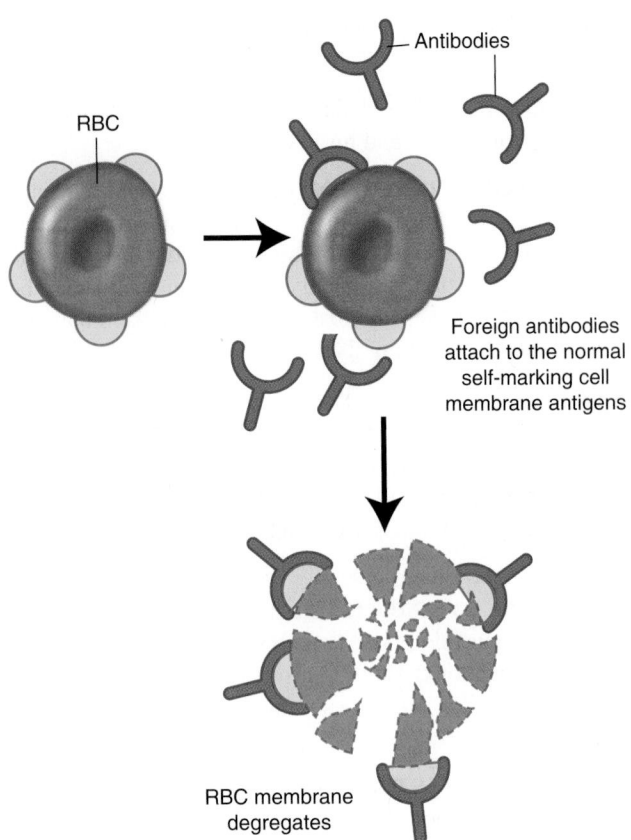

FIGURE 18.2 Type II hypersensitivity

type O are universal donors as they do not have A or B antigens. However, those with type O blood can receive only type O blood. Individuals with type AB blood are universal recipients, as they do not make A or B antibodies. Those with blood types other than AB can not receive AB blood as they have A or B antibodies.

Rh antigens are present in persons who are Rh$^+$. Rh antibodies are present in those who are Rh$^-$. Those who are Rh$^+$ can receive Rh$^-$ blood but those who are Rh$^-$ have antibodies to Rh$^+$ blood. If maternal and fetal blood Rh factors (RBC surface antigens) are different, the mother becomes sensitized by the fetal Rh type, which can affect future fetuses. For example, a Rh$_o$(D)-negative pregnant woman becomes sensitized by a Rh$_o$(D)-positive fetus. As a result, the blood cells of future Rh$_o$(D)-positive fetuses can be destroyed by maternal antibodies crossing the placenta.

CRITICAL THINKING

Blood Types

1. Who is the universal ABO Rh recipient?
2. Who is the universal ABO Rh donor?
3. Can someone with an A Rh$^-$ blood type safely receive O Rh$^+$ blood?

Suggested answers at end of chapter.

SIGNS AND SYMPTOMS. With a hemolytic transfusion reaction, there is usually a rather sudden onset of low back (flank) or chest pain, hypotension, fever rising more than 1.8°F (1°C), chills, tachycardia, tachypnea, wheezing, dyspnea, urticaria, and anxiety (Table 18.3). The patient may also complain of a headache and nausea.

DIAGNOSTIC TESTS. The direct Coombs' test confirms this diagnosis. In the laboratory, a small amount of the patient's RBCs are washed to remove any unattached antibodies. Antihuman globulin is added to see if agglutination (clumping) of the RBCs results. If agglutination occurs, an immune reaction such as a hemolytic transfusion reaction is taking place.

THERAPEUTIC INTERVENTIONS. To prevent production of anti-$Rh_o(D)$ antibodies, a $Rh_o(D)$ immune globulin (RhoGAM) injection is given to Rho(D)-negative patients accidentally given $Rh_o(D)$-positive blood or exposed to Rho(D)-positive fetal blood by delivery, miscarriage, abortion, amniocentesis, or intra-abdominal trauma. When antibodies do not form, then a hemolytic reaction can be prevented.

If a reaction occurs, examples of medications used to treat the reaction are listed in Table 18. 4.

NURSING PROCESS: HEMOLYTIC TRANSFUSION REACTION. Assessment/Data Collection. Prevention of hemolytic reactions is crucial. Following strict institutional guidelines for blood transfusion administration helps ensure the patient's safety. After blood is released from the hospital blood bank, two nurses, designated per institutional policy, double-check specified data. At the bedside, transfusion guidelines include double-checking the patient's name and identification number on the chart, unit of blood, and patient's identification bracelet, as well as checking the patient's blood type in the chart, on the unit of blood, and paperwork with the unit of blood.

Agency policy is followed for taking vital signs during a blood transfusion. Minimally, vital signs are taken before the beginning of the blood transfusion, at 15 minutes into the transfusion and when the transfusion is completed. It takes only a small amount of blood to trigger a hemolytic transfusion reaction, so it is critical to stay with the patient at the bedside during the first 15 minutes of any blood transfusion. This enables detection of a blood transfusion reaction early for quick action to minimize cell destruction and complications, including death.

If symptoms of a reaction are noted, the blood is immediately stopped and agency policy for a suspected transfusion reaction is followed. A normal saline infusion with new tubing is started to keep the vein patent. The physician and blood bank are immediately notified. A nurse remains with the patient for reassurance and monitoring of symptoms and vital signs. If a blood incompatibility is suspected, the unused blood and blood tubing is returned to the blood bank for testing. A series of blood and urine specimens are collected and sent to the laboratory for analysis. The physician's orders are followed to treat the patient's symptoms.

TABLE 18.3 HEMOLYTIC TRANSFUSION REACTION SUMMARY

Signs and Symptoms	Low back or chest pain Hypotension Fever rising more than 1.8°F (1°C) Chills Tachycardia Tachypnea, wheezing, dyspnea Urticaria Anxiety Headache Nausea
Diagnostic Tests	Direct Coombs' test - small amount of patient's RBCs are washed - antihuman globulin is added - if agglutination (clumping) occurs, an immune reaction is occurring
Therapeutic Interventions	Depends on severity of reaction and organs affected Antihistamines Corticosteroids Epinephrine Diuretics, to assist kidneys
Complications	If severe: shock, acute renal failure
Possible Nursing Diagnoses	Fear Ineffective tissue perfusion Risk for injury

 SAFETY TIP

Every unit of blood, even of the same blood type, is unique and can trigger a blood transfusion reaction. Careful monitoring with every transfusion is necessary.

Nursing Diagnosis, Planning, and Implementation. Fear related to serious threat to health status

EXPECTED OUTCOME: The patient will state reduced fear.

- Allow patients to express their concerns *to allow inaccurate information to be corrected.*
- Inform patients about procedures and treatments *to reduce fear.*
- Remain with patient and allow significant others *to offer support.*

Ineffective tissue perfusion: cardiopulmonary, peripheral related to arterial/venous blood flow exchange problems

EXPECTED OUTCOME: The patient demonstrates adequate tissue perfusion AEB palpable peripheral pulses,

TABLE 18.4 MEDICATIONS USED IN HEMOLYTIC TRANSFUSION REACTIONS

Medication Class/Action	Examples	Route	Side Effects	Nursing Implications
Antihistamines Block histamine at histamine₁-receptors therefore preventing or reversing the effects of histamine (capillary permeability, itching, and bronchospasms)	Diphenhydramine (Benadryl)	PO	Significant drowsiness	Take with or without food; avoid ETOH & CNS depressants & OTC antihistamines; avoid prolonged exposure to sunlight; caution with activities requiring mental alertness
	Cetirizine (Zyrtec)	PO	Once a day dosing; nonsedating; highly protein bound	
	Azelastine (Astelin)	Intranasal	Nasal mucosa irritation General side effects: dry mouth; fatigue, pharyngitis, dizziness	
Corticosteroids Hormones with marked anti-inflammatory effects due to inhibition of prostaglandin synthesis and accumulation of macrophages and leukocytes at site.	Dexamethasone (Decadron) Hydrocortisone (Solu-Cortef) Methylprednisone (Solu-Medrol) Prednisolone (Delta-Cortef) Prednisone (Deltasone) Beclomethasone (Beconase)	IM IV PO Topical Ophthalmic Intra-articular	Burning, dryness, stinging, headache, edema, muscle wasting, thrombophlebitis, masking of infections, elevation of blood glucose, gastric irritation	Take PO with food. NEVER stop taking suddenly. Monitor weight. Assess for edema, shortness of breath, jugular vein distention, and signs/symptoms of congestive heart failure. Monitor blood glucoses. Monitor for signs/symptoms of GI bleeding.
Sympathomimetics Marked stimulation of alpha and beta₁&₂ receptors causing vasoconstriction, bronchodilation, and cardiac stimulation	Epinephrine (Adrenalin) (EpiPen)	IM IV SQ Inhalation Topical	Disorientation, panic, anxiety; ventricular fibrillation; cerebral hemorrhage, decreased urine output, urinary retention, angina	Only use 1:1000 solution for IV; 1:100 IV will cause death. Do not expose drug to heat, light, or air. Ophthalmic and nasal preparations may sting. May elevate blood sugar.

urinary output of 30 mL per hour, and no respiratory distress.

- Maintain airway and provide oxygen *to promote oxygenation*.
- Monitor vital signs, intake and output *to detect changes for prompt treatment*.
- Position patient with head elevated if short of breath *to aid breathing*.
- Assess for pain and provide pain relief measures.

Risk for injury related to prolonged shock resulting in multiple organ failure, death

EXPECTED OUTCOME: The patient will remain free of injury.

- Use two methods to identify client before giving blood products *to prevent incorrect identification and administration of blood product*.
- Remain with patient during first 15 minutes of transfusion and then obtain vital signs *to detect signs of reaction*.
- Give medications as ordered *to support affected tissues and organs such as epinephrine or steroids*.

- Give diuretics as ordered *to assist kidney excretion of cellular debris from reaction*.

Deficient knowledge related to lack of exposure to blood transfusions

EXPECTED OUTCOME: The patient will state understanding of blood transfusion options.

- Encourage patient to discuss autologous (self) blood donation option with physician. This may be an option for patients having elective surgery *to avoid a transfusion reaction*.
- After a hemolytic transfusion reaction, tell patients importance of informing future health care providers of reaction, *so that specific blood tests are performed for less common antibodies if the patient is ever typed for a blood transfusion again*.

Evaluation. If interventions have been effective, the patient states reduced fear, shows normal organ and tissue function, and reports understanding of blood transfusion options to prevent transfusion reactions.

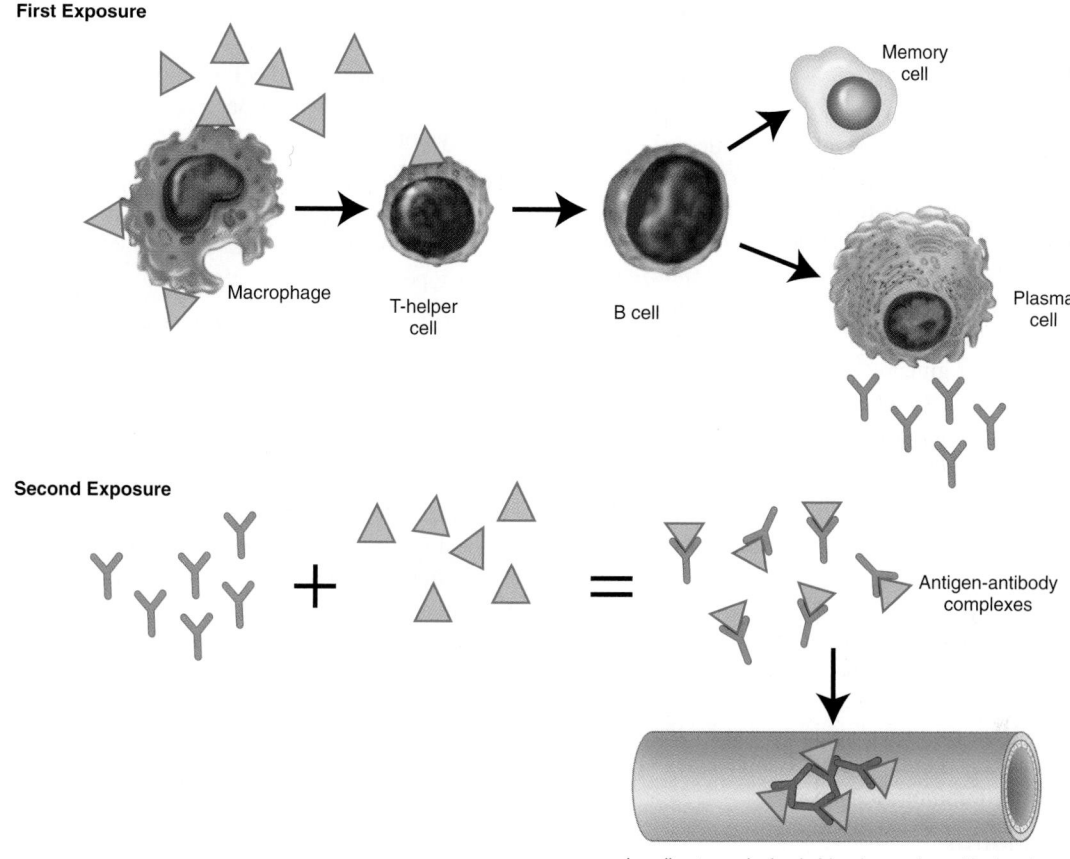

First Exposure

Macrophage   T-helper cell   B cell   Memory cell   Plasma cell

Second Exposure

+ = Antigen-antibody complexes

Leading to occlusion in blood vessels and ischemia

FIGURE 18.3 Type III hypersensitivity

Type III

A type III hypersensitivity reaction involves immune complexes formed by antigens and antibodies, usually of the IgG type (Fig. 18.3). The patient is sensitized with an initial exposure to the antigen, and on a subsequent exposure the reaction occurs. The reaction is localized and evolves over several hours, with symptoms ranging from a red, edematous skin lesion to hemorrhage and necrosis. The process involves the formation of antigen-antibody complexes within the blood vessels as the antigen is absorbed through the vessel wall. Neutrophils are attracted to the area and release enzymes that ultimately lead to blood vessel damage.

Serum Sickness

PATHOPHYSIOLOGY. Serum sickness is a type III hypersensitivity immune reaction in which antigen-antibody complexes are formed and cause symptoms of inflammation.

ETIOLOGY. In the past, serum sickness occurred after inoculation of equine (horse) antiserum for diseases such as tetanus and diphtheria. With the refinement of these vaccines, serum sickness does not usually occur from them. Today, serum sickness is seen occasionally after administration of penicillin and sulfonamide.

SIGNS AND SYMPTOMS. The signs and symptoms usually occur 7 to 10 days after the exposure. The most predominant manifestation is severe urticaria and angioedema. The patient may experience a fever, malaise, muscle sore-

ness, arthralgia, splenomegaly, and occasionally nausea, vomiting, and diarrhea. Lymphadenopathy may occur, especially of the lymph nodes closest to the antigen entry site.

DIAGNOSTIC TESTS. With serum sickness there is often a slight elevation in the white blood cell count and the sedimentation rate, and complement assay decreases.

THERAPEUTIC INTERVENTIONS. Antipyretics may be given for the fever and analgesics for the arthralgia. Antihistamines and epinephrine may be prescribed for the urticaria and angioedema. If the symptoms continue to persist, corticosteroids may be ordered.

NURSING PROCESS: SERUM SICKNESS. Assessment/ Data Collection. Symptoms are noted. Responses to prescribed medications is documented. Identification of the causative agent may be done through the history-taking process and is important for the patient to know to prevent a recurrence of the condition.

Nursing Diagnosis, Planning, and Implementation. Pain related to muscle and joint soreness

EXPECTED OUTCOME: The patient will state pain is reduced to acceptable level.

- Monitor pain using pain rating scale of 0 to 10.
- Provide analgesics as ordered *to relieve symptoms.*

Risk for deficient fluid volume related to fever and gastrointestinal fluid loss

EXPECTED OUTCOME: *The patient will maintain blood pressure, pulse, and urine output within normal limits.*
- Observe for signs of hypovolemia: restlessness, weakness, muscle cramps, headaches, inability to concentrate, irritability and postural hypotension.
- Monitor intake and output *to detect imbalances*.
- Provide antiemetics as ordered *to relieve nausea*.
- Encourage oral replacement therapy with hypotonic glucose-electrolyte solutions such as sports replacement drinks, or ginger ale *as they increase fluid absorption and correct deficient fluid volume.*
- If ordered, maintain IV fluids at ordered rate *to replace lost fluids but avoid fluid overload.*

Evaluation. Goals are met if the patient reports less pain, and if vital signs and urine output are within normal limits.

Type IV

A type IV hypersensitivity reaction, also called a delayed reaction, occurs when a sensitized T lymphocyte comes in contact with the particular antigen to which it is sensitized (Fig. 18.4). The resulting necrosis is caused by the actions of the macrophages and the various T lymphocytes involved in the cell-mediated immune response.

Contact Dermatitis
PATHOPHYSIOLOGY. When a substance or chemical comes in contact with the skin, it is absorbed into the skin and binds with special skin proteins called haptens. With the

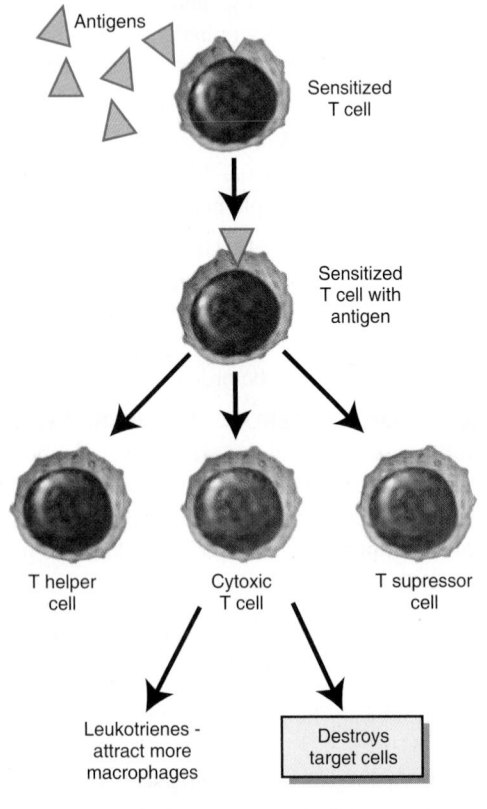

FIGURE 18.4 Type IV hypersensitivity

first contact, there is no reaction or symptoms, but within 7 to 10 days, T memory cells are formed. Therefore, on subsequent exposures, the T memory cells quickly become activated T cells, which secrete the chemicals that may cause symptoms.

ETIOLOGY. Poison ivy and poison oak are the most common irritants causing this reaction. Latex rubber has also been found to be a cause for contact dermatitis and can trigger type I anaphylactic reactions.

Latex Allergy. Latex allergy is a serious problem for health-care workers. Anaphylactic reactions to latex can be fatal. Exposure to latex for health-care workers has increased dramatically since the implementation of universal precautions and the use of latex gloves began in 1987. Many times latex gloves are worn unnecessarily, which increases exposure to the latex protein. Latex-free gloves are available for health-care workers. For patients who are allergic to latex, special protocols are followed using latex-free equipment. For information about latex allergy, visit the American Academy of Allergy, Asthma, and Immunology at www.aaaai.org. Also visit the U.S. Food and Drug Administration at www.fda.gov.

SIGNS AND SYMPTOMS. Within a number of hours from the exposure, the area of contact becomes reddened and pruritic, with fragile vesicles. Secondary infections may develop. (See earlier discussion of atopic dermatitis.)

DIAGNOSTIC TESTS. Diagnosis is made by assessment of the skin and lesions and a detailed patient history.

THERAPEUTIC INTERVENTIONS. Treatment consists of controlling symptoms. Oral or topical antihistamines and topical drying agents may be used. Topical corticosteroids may be used, and if the symptoms are severe, systemic corticosteroids may be prescribed.

NURSING PROCESS: CONTACT DERMATITIS. Assessment/Data Collection. Symptoms are assessed for planning of interventions. Identification of the causative agent is noted in the patient's history. Patient recognition of the cause is important to prevent a recurrence of the condition. Special protocols are used for patients allergic to latex. Some institutions may prepare special latex free kits containing common supplies nurses use to care for patients. Ensure that latex allergy protocols are followed if a patient has a latex allergy to prevent life threatening anaphylaxis that could develop.

Nursing Diagnosis, Planning, and Implementation. See Box 18.1 Nursing Care Plan for the Patient with Contact Dermatitis.

Transplant Rejection
ETIOLOGY AND PATHOPHYSIOLOGY. Any form of transplanted living tissue is sensed as foreign material by the immune system. This is why lifelong immunosuppression is necessary to help prevent transplant rejection, which can occur at any time. Lymphocytes become sensitized during an induction phase immediately after the tissue is trans-

Box 18.1 NURSING CARE PLAN for the Patient with Contact Dermatitis

Nursing Diagnosis: Risk for impaired skin integrity related to effects of allergic reaction and pruritus

Patient Outcomes Patient's skin will remain intact.

Evaluation of Outcome Is patient's skin intact? If not intact, is skin healing? Does patient express a plan for preventing impaired skin integrity?

Interventions	Rationale	Evaluation
Assess and document skin and lesions.	Assessment provides a basis for intervention planning and evaluation of healing.	Are lesions present? Are lesions healing?
Teach patient to keep fingernails short and clean.	Short, clean nails cause less damage or infection if scratching occurs.	Does skin remain intact in spite of scratching?
Teach patient to apply clean, white cotton clothing over affected area (soaks, gloves/mittens, undershirt), especially at bedtime.	Cotton allows air movement. White cloth is less irritating than those with dyes. Scratching is decreased during sleep with the use of gloves/mittens or covering affected area.	Are symptoms of skin irritation reduced?
Teach patient to use gentle rubbing or pressure instead of scratching.	Use of gentle rubbing or pressure instead of scratching causes less skin trauma.	Does skin remain intact in spite of itchy sensation?
Explain tepid baking soda baths, colloidal oatmeal baths (e.g., Aveeno), and cool washcloths or cool baths reduce itching.	These items help dry the vesicle and minimize the pruritus.	Is itching reduced?

Nursing Diagnosis: Ineffective health maintenance related to lack of knowledge of methods to decrease inflammation and reduce episodes of inflammation

Patient Outcomes Patient or caregiver will follow the mutually agreed upon plan of care.

Evaluation of Outcome Can patient express knowledge of etiology, signs and symptoms, and treatment plan? Does patient discuss any emotional, social, financial, or material blocks to attaining treatment goals?

Interventions	Rationale	Evaluation
Assess patient's knowledge of disease and causes.	Assessment provides a basis for the teaching plan.	Does patient state baseline knowledge?
Assess patient's values and beliefs regarding plan of care.	Patients are more compliant if their belief system fits into plan of care.	Does patient's belief system work with plan of care?
Assess barriers to patient's ability to carry out plan of care and plan interventions to decrease barriers.	Barriers can prevent patient from carrying out plan of care.	Are barriers identified? Are solutions to barriers planned?
Teach patient to wear medical alert identification for allergen.	With allergen identification, prompt medical care can be given in case patient is unable to give information.	Does patient agree to use allergen identification?
Discuss methods of avoiding allergen with patient.	Understanding prevention methods can help prevent allergen exposure.	Can patient state methods to help prevent allergen exposure?
Teach patient to wash with a brown soap (e.g., Fels-Naptha) or, if unavailable, any soap when contact with the offending agent is suspected.	This removes offending agent.	Does patient state understanding of need to wash off agent with exposure?
Teach patient not to scratch skin.	Scratching can spread the dermatitis, as well as cause infection.	Does patient avoid scratching?

planted. If immunosuppression is not effective, the sensitized lymphocytes invade the transplanted tissue and destroy it via the release of chemicals and macrophage activity resulting in varying degrees of transplant rejection.

SIGNS AND SYMPTOMS. Various signs and symptoms occur depending on the transplanted tissue or organ that is involved and the severity of the rejection (Table 18.5). Signs and symptoms reflect failure of the organ or tissue, such as renal failure for a rejected kidney.

COMPLICATIONS. A total failure and loss of the transplanted tissue or organ can occur, or the tissue or organ can be damaged from immunological reactions and not function at full capacity. The greatest cause of death following a transplant is from infection. Immunosuppression therapy, which is necessary to prevent tissue rejection following the transplant, is a major contributory factor for severe infection development. Because the immune system is suppressed, it is unable to effectively fight infections.

DIAGNOSTIC TESTS. Biopsy, scans, blood tests, arteriography, and ultrasonography are some tests that may be performed to aid in diagnosing a transplant rejection.

THERAPEUTIC INTERVENTIONS. Depending on the type of transplant, the body's immunological system is prepared before surgery with medications, transfusions, or radiation to minimize the risk of rejection. After the transplant, lifelong immunosuppression is needed. If rejection occurs, medications may be used to attempt to reverse the rejection. Supportive care is provided based on the failing organ such as hemodialysis if a kidney rejection occurs.

TABLE 18.5 TRANSPLANT REJECTION SUMMARY

Signs and Symptoms	Depending on: - the involved transplanted tissue or organ - severity of reaction Reflect failure of the organ or tissue
Diagnostic Tests	Biopsy Scans Blood tests Arteriography Ultrasonography
Therapeutic Interventions	Depends upon the type of transplant Preventative preoperative preparation with medications, transfusions, or radiation to minimize the risk of rejection
Complications	Total failure and loss of transplanted organ or tissue Cause of death is most commonly due to infection with immunosuppression therapy a contributory factor
Possible Nursing Diagnoses	Grieving (actual or anticipatory) Fear Deficient knowledge Others depend upon which organ is failing

NURSING MANAGEMENT. Nursing care depends greatly on the type of transplant performed. Initially the patient is in an intensive care unit under close observation and support. Observing for signs of rejection is a priority throughout the patient's hospitalization. Another consideration for nursing care is the psychological support of the patient and family. Many patients wait on a transplant list a long time before a donor match is found. Once a matching donor is found, there is usually great elation. Yet if a donor's death made the transplant possible, the patient and family may be simultaneously feeling a profound sadness for the donor's family. Patients need time to verbalize feelings and understand that these feelings are normal and diminish with time. Also, the fear of transplant rejection is always present and must be discussed.

Education. Rejection can take place weeks, months, or years following a transplant (with decreasing risk). The patient and family need to be educated about specific signs and symptoms of rejection. Also, because infection is a major complication resulting from long-term immunosuppressive medications, the patient and family need to know signs and symptoms of infection and when to notify the physician of problems. Steroid use may mask the symptoms of infection, so small indicators such as a low-grade fever should be promptly reported. Education regarding prescribed medications is a must because long-term success of a transplant is dependent on compliance with immunosuppressive medication therapy. Avoidance of people with colds or infections is also important to reduce the patient's infection risk due to immunosuppression.

AUTOIMMUNE DISORDERS

In autoimmune disorders, the immune system no longer recognizes the body's normal cells as self and not foreign. Instead the antigens on these normal body cells are recognized as foreign material, and an immune response to destroy them is launched.

A number of factors either cause or influence this breakdown of self-recognition, including viral infections, drugs, and cross-reactive antibodies. Some microbes stimulate the production of antibodies but are so closely related to normal cell antigens that the antibodies also attack some normal cells. Hormones have also been found to influence this breakdown of self-recognition.

Table 18.6 lists additional autoimmune disorders and the chapters in which they are discussed.

Pernicious Anemia

PATHOPHYSIOLOGY. Antibodies that destroy gastric parietal cells lead to decreased production of intrinsic factor. Intrinsic factor plays a role in vitamin B_{12} absorption in the small bowel, so a vitamin B_{12} deficiency may result causing decreased production of RBCs. Intrinsic factor is involved in most vitamin B_{12} absorption, but there is now evidence that

TABLE 18.6 AUTOIMMUNE DISORDERS

Disorder	Refer to
Idiopathic thrombocytopenic purpura	Chapter 28
Multiple sclerosis	Chapter 50
Myasthenia gravis	Chapter 50
Rheumatoid arthritis	Chapter 46
Ulcerative colitis	Chapter 34

there is a route independent of intrinsic factor for some absorption of vitamin B_{12}. This has important treatment implications.

ETIOLOGY. There tends to be a familial tendency toward pernicious anemia in relation to immune causes. Non–immune-related causes of pernicious anemia include any type of gastric or small bowel resections coupled with no or inadequate vitamin B_{12} or intrinsic factor replacement.

SIGNS AND SYMPTOMS. The patient experiences increasing weakness, loss of appetite, glossitis, and pallor. Irritability, confusion, and numbness or tingling in the extremities (peripheral neuropathy) occur because the nervous system is affected.

DIAGNOSTIC TESTS. On microscopic examination of the patient's RBCs, macrocytic (enlarged cells) anemia is diagnosed. Macrocytic anemia and low vitamin B_{12} levels are indicators of pernicious anemia and folic acid deficiency. To determine if the diagnosis is pernicious anemia, intrinsic factor antibodies and parietal cell antibodies can be tested. A Schilling test may be done but is used less today as it is complicated. For the Schilling test, radioactive vitamin B_{12} is administered to the patient. The patient's urine is then collected for 24 hours (48 hours for patients with renal disease), and the amount of radioactive vitamin B_{12} excreted in the urine is measured. If intrinsic factor is decreased, gastric absorption of vitamin B_{12} is also decreased, so that more vitamin B_{12} is excreted in the urine. Gastric secretion analysis is done to measure levels of hydrochloric acid (HCl) because low or absent HCl may be indicative of pernicious anemia.

THERAPEUTIC INTERVENTIONS. Corticosteroids may correct the problem if it is immunologically caused. Otherwise vitamin B_{12} therapy is needed usually for life. It has been found that oral vitamin B_{12} can be effective so that injections may not be needed as was thought in the past.[1, 2]

NURSING MANAGEMENT. Vitamin B_{12} is administered as ordered. Care related to fatigue and safety are important. Ambulation, frequent rest periods, and providing assistance with activities of daily living (ADLs) as indicated by the patient's activity tolerance are helpful for the patient with anemia.

Education. The patient and family need education regarding oral or parenteral medication therapy. If vitamin B_{12} injections are prescribed, they must understand that this is a lifelong need to prevent the return of symptoms. Patients should not miss injections, periodic B_{12} level testing, or follow-up appointments.

Idiopathic Autoimmune Hemolytic Anemia

PATHOPHYSIOLOGY. Autoantibodies, for no known reason, are produced that attach to RBCs and cause them to either lyse or agglutinate (clump). When lysis occurs, fragments of the destroyed RBCs circulate in the blood. If agglutination occurs, occlusions in the small blood vessels followed by tissue ischemia occurs.

SIGNS AND SYMPTOMS. Clinical manifestations vary from mild fatigue and pallor to severe hypotension, dyspnea, palpitations, and jaundice.

DIAGNOSTIC TESTS. The RBC count, hemoglobin (Hgb), and hematocrit (Hct) are low, and microscopic examination reveals fragmented RBCs. Lactate dehydrogenase (LDH) is elevated because of RBC destruction and tissue ischemia.

THERAPEUTIC INTERVENTIONS. Supportive measures such as supplemental oxygen may be initiated. Folic acid may be prescribed to increase production of RBCs. The use of immunosuppressive medications and corticosteroids may be useful in obtaining remission. In more severe cases, blood transfusions and erythrocytapheresis (a process whereby abnormal RBCs are removed and replaced with normal RBCs) may be instituted. A splenectomy may be performed in an attempt to stop the destruction of RBCs for severe cases.

NURSING MANAGEMENT. The patient's signs and symptoms should be monitored and reported as necessary. Frequent rest periods should be planned into the patient's daily routine to prevent fatigue. Blood products are administered as ordered to replace RBCs.

Education. The patient and family are instructed on the medical regimen, and their understanding is verified.

Hashimoto's Thyroiditis

PATHOPHYSIOLOGY. Autoantibodies for thyroid-stimulating hormone (TSH) form in Hashimoto's thyroiditis. However, instead of inactivating TSH, the autoantibodies bind with the hormone receptors on the thyroid gland and stimulate the thyroid gland to secrete thyroid hormones. The thyroid gland enlarges as a result of this overstimulation (hyperthyroidism). It becomes infiltrated with lymphocytes and phagocytes, causing inflammation and further enlargement. Then different autoantibodies appear that destroy thyroid cells, which slows secretion activity, causing hypothyroidism.

ETIOLOGY. The exact cause is unknown, although it occurs in females eight times more often than in males. It is also more common in people 30 to 50 years old and patients with Down's syndrome and Turner's syndrome.

SIGNS AND SYMPTOMS. Initially the manifestations are those of hyperthyroidism, such as restlessness, tremors, chest pain, increased appetite, diarrhea, moist skin, heat intolerance, and weight loss.

These manifestations may go unrecognized and progress quickly into hypothyroidism. At this point, an enlarged thyroid gland (goiter) may be seen. Clinical manifestations may include fatigue, bradycardia, hypotension, dyspnea, anorexia, constipation, dry skin, weight gain, sensitivity to cold, facial puffiness, and a slowing of mental processes.

DIAGNOSTIC TESTS. Immunofluorescent assay, a test that detects antigens on cells using an antibody with a fluorescent tag, detects antithyroid antibodies. Serum thyroid-stimulating hormone levels are elevated, while triiodothyronine (T_3) and thyroxine (T_4) levels are low. A thyroid scan is also done.

THERAPEUTIC INTERVENTIONS. Thyroid hormone replacement therapy of thyroxine is the primary means of treatment. Lifelong thyroid hormone therapy is needed.

NURSING MANAGEMENT. If the patient has a goiter, a soft diet may be necessary for comfort. Frequent rest periods may be necessary, as well as slowly increasing patient activity. Antiembolic stockings may help prevent venous stasis during the low-energy, decreased-activity phase. Daily weights and monitoring intake and output when cardiac status is compromised are important to detect abnormalities such as fluid retention. Because weight gain and facial puffiness alter patients' self-image, they need an opportunity to verbalize their feelings to help them adjust to this disease process.

Education. Patients taking thyroid hormone replacement therapy should avoid foods high in iodine. The diet should also consist of large amounts of fiber to combat constipation. During the hyperthyroidism phase, a diet high in protein and carbohydrates encourages weight gain. Education regarding prescribed medications is also needed.

Lupus Erythematosus

PATHOPHYSIOLOGY. There are three types of lupus: discoid (DLE), drug-induced systemic lupus erythematosus, and systemic lupus erythematosus (SLE) (Table 18.7). The discoid type consists of skin lesions only. Drug-induced SLE develops after use of certain medications (see Table 18.8). SLE is a chronic, inflammatory, multisystem disorder. The body develops antibodies against its own tissue. It is very unpredictable. See Table 18.9 for a list of flare triggers.

Etiology

Systemic lupus erythematosus tends to develop in young women of child-bearing years and occurs in the African American and Hispanic populations more frequently. First-degree relatives of lupus patients also have a greater tendency than the general population to develop SLE.

SIGNS AND SYMPTOMS. Clinical manifestations vary from mild to severe. See Table 18.7 and Figure 18.5.

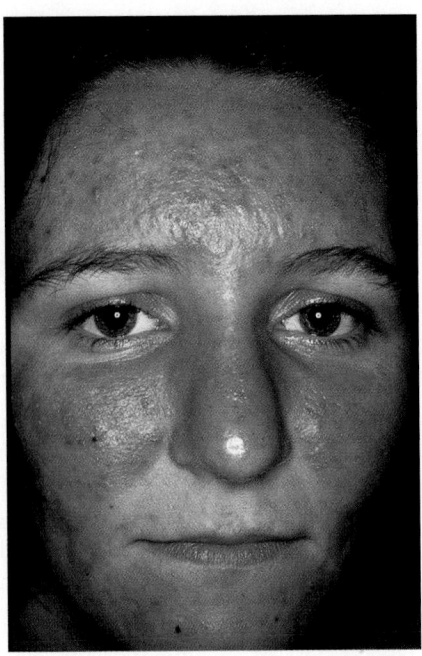

FIGURE 18.5 Lupus erythematosus: red papules and plaques in butterfly pattern on face. *(From Goldsmith, LA, Tharp, M, Lazarus, G, et al: Adult and Pediatric Dermatology. F.A. Davis, Philadelphia, 1997, p. 230.)*

Therapeutic Interventions

Medications used to treat lupus erythematosis are listed in Table 18.10.

NURSING MANAGEMENT. It is vitally important for the patient and family to be aware of and avoid flare triggers. Fatigue during activities of daily living can be minimized through the use of a daily personal schedule. Additionally, a minimum of 8 hours of sleep per night with naps as necessary are important to combat fatigue. Since the majority of patients with SLE develop transitory arthralgia, maintaining fitness and joint range of motion through a regular fitness program while decreasing activity during flares is vital. Warm baths may help with morning stiffness while application of heat and cold compresses, splints, assistive devices, and physical therapy may help soreness. Eating a well-balanced diet will also influence their level of fatigue and weight gain from the corticosteroids which in turn can affect the joint soreness too.

Education. Explain the signs of bleeding and of cardiac and vascular problems, such as myocardial infarction and thrombophlebitis. Encourage the use of a medical alert bracelet. Provide smoking cessation information to those patients who smoke. Since renal disease is a major complication of SLE, patients must learn the signs of impending problems that need to be relayed to the physician immediately. These are such findings as facial puffiness and "foamy" urine or "coke-colored" urine indicative of proteinuria and hematuria, respectively. Explain that regular ophthalmic examinations are necessary for early detection and treatment of the complications that the antimalarials and corticosteroids can produce, such as retinal bleeding, glaucoma, and cataracts.

TABLE 18.7 LUPUS ERYTHEMATOSUS SUMMARY

Signs and Symptoms	Discoid:
	- patchy, crusty, sharply defined skin plaques
	- tend to occur on face or sun-exposed areas
	Drug-induced:
	- pleuropericardial inflammation
	- fever
	- rash
	- arthritis
	Systemic:
	- Early symptoms are vague, then fatigue, fever
	- Dermatologic:
	  • butterfly rash (face), photosensitivity, mucosal ulcers, alopecia, pain, pruritus, bruising
	- Musculoskeletal:
	  • arthralgia, arthritis
	- Hematologic:
	  • anemia, leukocytopenia, elevated ESR, thrombocytopenia, false-positive VDRL
	- Cardiopulmonary:
	  • pericarditis, myocarditis, myocardial infarction, vasculitis, pleurisy, valvular heart disease
	- Renal:
	  • renal failure, urinary tract infections, fluid & electrolyte imbalances
	- Central Nervous System:
	  • cranial neuropathies, cognitive impairment, mental changes, seizures
	- Gastrointestinal:
	  • anorexia, ascites, pancreatitis, intestinal vasculitis
	- Ophthalmologic:
	  • conjunctivitis, dry eyes, glaucoma, cataracts, retinal pigmentation

Diagnostic Tests	CBC Antinuclear antibody (ANA) Anti-Sm (a highly specific immunoglobulin for SLE) Anti-nDNA, + in 60% to 80% of SLE patients Anti-R_o (SSA), an immunoglobulin + in 30% of SLE patients Anti-La (SSB), an immunoglobulin + in 15% of SLE patients. Complement Estimated sedimentation rate (ESR) is nonspecific C-reactive protein (CRP) is nonspecific 24-hour urine creatinine clearance Urinalysis ⎫ Serum creatinine ⎬ If ruling out kidney involvement Kidney biopsy ⎭
Therapeutic Interventions	Symptomatic management Nonsteroidal anti-inflammatory drugs Immunosuppresants Corticosteroids Antimalarials Intravenous immunoglobulin
Complications	Osteonecrosis Renal failure Thrombocytopenia Emboli Myocarditis Vasculitis Mesenteric or intestinal vasculitis leading to obstruction, perforation, or infarction Sepsis
Possible Nursing Diagnoses	Acute pain Disturbed body image Fatigue Ineffective health maintenance

TABLE 18.8 MEDICATIONS ASSOCIATED WITH TRIGGERING LUPUS ERYTHEMATOSUS

Chlorpromazine
Hydralazine
Isoniazid
Methyldopa
Procainamide
Procaine
Other Medications
Barbiturates
Phenytoin (Dilantin)
Protamine
Salicylates
Diazepam (Valium)
Food Additives
Bisulfites
Monosodium glutamate (MSG)

TABLE 18.9 COMMON LUPUS ERYTHEMATOSUS FLARE TRIGGERS

Sunlight (can be reflected off water and snow, emitted from fluorescent and halogen lights; glass does not fully protect)
Stress
Emotional crisis
Overworked
Lack of rest
Infection
Surgery or injuries
Hormones
Pregnancy and postpartum
Stopping medications suddenly
Environmental sensitivities or allergies
Immunizations
Certain prescription drugs
Some over-the-counter drugs such as cough syrups

Finally, but most importantly, the patient's psychological state and support systems need to be addressed. From the onset of symptoms to the diagnosing of lupus is usually costly in time, money, and emotions. Patients may exhibit anger, frustration, and confusion prior to the diagnosis. For many, at diagnosis, there is a sense of relief that may quickly be replaced with feelings of anger, fear, depression, or grief. It is here when empathy, support, hope, and, most importantly, education for the patient, family, and significant others is vital for successful long-term coping skills to be acquired. In addition, local support groups and educational and self-management programs available through the Lupus Foundation of America can provide avenues for attaining more specific knowledge and skills for coping and taking control of their lives.

CRITICAL THINKING

Mr. Ellis

■ Mr. Ellis is suffering from a flare of SLE. The physician has ordered Solu-Cortef 80 mg IM to be given every 8 hours. Solu-Cortef 125 mg per 2 mL is available. How many mLs will the nurse administer per dose?

Suggested answers at end of chapter.

Ankylosing Spondylitis

PATHOPHYSIOLOGY. Ankylosing spondylitis, also called rheumatoid spondylitis, is a chronic progressive inflammatory disease of the sacroiliac, costovertebral, and large peripheral joints. The inflammatory process begins in the lower region of the back and progresses upward. A specific histocompatibility antigen (antigen that identifies self), human leukocyte antigen (HLA) B27, is formed that stimulates an immune response.

ETIOLOGY. There is strong evidence of a familial tendency, but no other specific causes are known. Ankylosing spondylitis tends to afflict men more than women.

SIGNS AND SYMPTOMS. There is an insidious onset of lower back stiffness and pain, which is worse in the morning. As the disease progresses, the pain worsens and there are spasms of the back muscles. The normal curvature of the lower back (lordosis) flattens, and the curvature of the upper back increases (kyphosis). Patients may also experience fatigue, anorexia, and weight loss.

DIAGNOSTIC TESTS. Findings such as a positive family history, radiographs of the joints, a positive HLA-B27 blood test, and negative Rh confirm a diagnosis of ankylosing spondylitis. There are no specific immunological tests to diagnose ankylosing spondylitis.

THERAPEUTIC INTERVENTIONS. Because there is no cure for ankylosing spondylitis, treatment consists of measures to minimize the symptoms. Analgesics for pain relief, anti-inflammatory agents to decrease joint inflammation, and physical therapy to maintain muscle strength and joint range of motion are used. Surgery can be done to replace fused joints. For kyphosis, cervical or lumbar osteotomy can be performed.

NURSING MANAGEMENT. Nursing care focuses on patient education and administration and evaluation of prescribed medications. Pain management, rest periods, and assistance with ADLs are provided.

Education. The patient and family need information about the disease process. Proper posture and range-of-motion exercises are taught and reinforced by nursing staff. The patient should also be instructed not to stay in any one position for any length of time. The patient should sleep on

---

ankylosing spondylitis anayle—stiff joint + osing—condition+
 spondyl—vertebrae + itis—inflammation

TABLE 18.10 MEDICATIONS USED FOR LUPUS ERYTHEMATOSUS

Medication Class/Action	Examples	Route	Side Effects	Nursing Implications
Nonsteroidal Anti-inflammatory Drugs (NSAIDs)	Ibuprofen (Motrin)	PO	Gastric distress Headache Tinnitus Dizziness Rash Pruritus Fluid retention	Take with food Avoid taking with ethyl alcohol Protect from ultraviolet rays. Assess for abnormal bleeding.
	Indomethacin (Indocin) Naproxen (Naprosen)			
Antimalarials Action is not clearly understood but can significantly help reduce inflammation, decreases platelet aggregation while lowering plasma lipid levels	Chloroquine (Aralen)	PO	Gastric distress Anorexia, vomiting Diarrhea Headache Muscle weakness Alopecia Blurred vision Irritability Dry, itchy skin rash	Administer before or after meals at the same time of day. Obtain a thorough assessment for a baseline, including an ophthalmic exam. May take weeks or months for effects to be noticed.
	Hydroxychloroquine sulfate (Plaquenil)	PO		
Corticosteroids Reduces inflammation and suppresses immune response	Dexamethasone (Decadron)	PO IV IM topical inhaled	Increased facial hair, acne Round "moon" face Mood changes Irritability Depression Increased appetite Increased weight Poor wound healing Headache Peptic ulcers Osteoporosis Steroid-induced diabetes	NEVER stop taking suddenly. Don't miss doses. Measures to avoid infection. Take with food or milk. Assess for weight gain >5 pounds, decreased urine output, pulse irregularities, increased blood pressure, edema and temperature. May elevate blood sugar.
	Hydrocortisone (Solu-Cortef)	PO IV IM topical		
	Methylprednisolone (Solu-Medrol)	PO IM IV		
	Prednisone (Deltasone)	PO		
Immunosuppressants Target and damage autoantibody producing cells	Azathioprine (Imuran)	PO IV	Gastric distress Nausea, vomiting Abdominal pain Oral ulcers Dark urine Pale stools Jaundice	Assess joints for range-of-motion, edema, temperature, and erythema. Protect patients from those who may carry infections. Monitor CBC, renal and liver function tests. Give with food if gastrointestinal upset. Monitor for abnormal bleeding.
	Cyclosporine (Sandimmune)	PO IV		
	Methotrexate (Rheumatrex)	PO IM IV		

CRITICAL THINKING

Mr. Beck

■ Mr. Beck, a truck driver who was recently diagnosed with ankylosing spondylitis, verbalizes concern about how this diagnosis will affect his ability to work.

1. How would you answer his questions?
   a. "What is happening to me?"
   b. "Will I have to quit my job driving an interstate truck?"
   c. "Am I eventually going to be in really bad pain?"
   d. "Am I eventually going to be dependent on someone?"
2. Mr. Beck plans to continue driving his truck and therefore has a need upon discharge for specific interventions that will help him maintain his independence. Why is each of the following instructions given to Mr. Beck upon discharge?
   a. Perform range-of-motion exercises daily.
   b. Do not stay in one position too long. You may need to stop and walk around often.
   c. Sleep on a firm mattress without a pillow.
   d. Maintain good posture, even when driving the truck.

Suggested answers at end of chapter.

a mattress that is firm without a pillow to help reduce pain and stiffness.

IMMUNE DEFICIENCIES

Immune deficiencies occur when one or more components of the immune system are either completely absent or deficient in quantities sufficient to elicit or sustain an adequate immune response to combat an infectious agent.

Hypogammaglobulinemia

PATHOPHYSIOLOGY AND ETIOLOGY. This condition is either a hereditary congenital disorder or acquired after childhood from unknown causes. It is characterized by the absence or deficiency of one or more of the five classes of immunoglobulins (IgG, IgM, IgA, IgD, and IgE) from defective B-cell function. The lack of normal function of these antibodies makes the patient prone to infections. The congenital form of this disorder affects males. Patients usually have a normal life span.

SIGNS AND SYMPTOMS. The infant is usually asymptomatic until 6 months of age, when the maternal immunoglobulins are gone. At this time, the infant begins having many recurrent infections, especially from *Staphylococcus* and *Streptococcus* organisms.

DIAGNOSIS. Until the infant is 9 months old, diagnosis is extremely difficult. At 9 months of age, immunoelectrophoresis, which measures the level of each immunoglobulin, can be performed.

THERAPEUTIC INTERVENTIONS. Treatment is aimed at minimizing infections while increasing the immune system through injections of immunoglobulin. These injections mainly contain IgG, so fresh frozen plasma is given to replace IgM. IgA cannot be replaced, increasing the risk for frequent pulmonary infections.

NURSING MANAGEMENT. The infant is monitored for infections. Any break in the skin must be cleansed immediately and monitored for infection development. Genetic counseling may be recommended for parents.

Education. The family is educated about signs and symptoms of a variety of infections and the importance in seeking medical help immediately. They are taught that the infant should not be in crowds and that good nutrition, hydration, and hygiene are important in preventing infections.

Home Health Hints

Atopic Dermatitis

- Instruct patients with atopic dermatitis to use a skin moisturizer daily to help prevent dryness, which can lead to the complications of eczema. Avoid baby lotions or any lotion that contains perfumes since these can be irritating to the skin.
- Use of regular soaps can be drying to the skin. Discuss with your patient and family to only use soaps labeled for sensitive skins.
- Oatmeal baths can be helpful in relieving the skin dryness. Many oatmeal bath products are available over-the-counter. Assist the patient with choosing the correct one.

- Patients and families can be taught to use an ice pack applied to the irritated area to help relieve the itching associated with atopic dermatitis.
- If patients experience a rash anywhere, especially around the torso and abdomen, consider the clothing detergent they are using. Encourage them to switch to a detergent that is mild such as one of those used to wash baby clothes (e.g., Dreft).

Latex Allergy

- Always have on hand latex-free gloves.
- Indwelling catheters are also made from latex. You can obtain a latex-free silicone catheter to use to prevent latex exposure and potential complica-

tions for individuals who have experienced latex sensitivities.

Transplants

• Patients who have had a transplant are required to take medications that turn off their immune system. Because of this, it is important to instruct them to avoid public places such as malls and food stores. If they do go out,

let them know that they should wear a surgical mask to help prevent exposure to illness.

• The importance of taking medications as prescribed needs to be reinforced, especially for immunosuppressive medications for cardiac transplant patients.

• Patients with cardiac transplants should not be exposed to people with illnesses such as colds or the flu. This should be explained to family members and visitors.

REVIEW QUESTIONS

Multiple response item. Select all that apply.

1. The nurse is contributing to the plan of care for a patient with allergic rhinitis. Which of the following interventions should the nurse anticipate will be included in the treatment plan?
   a. Antihistamines
   b. Epinephrine
   c. Gold salts
   d. Steroids
   e. Anticholinergics
   f. Decongestants
   g. Immunotherapy
   h. Avoiding environmental stimuli

2. Which of the following components of a complete blood count with differential would the nurse see elevated in the patient with allergic rhinitis?
   a. Hemoglobin
   b. Eosinophils
   c. RBC Distribution Width (RDW)
   d. Bands

Multiple response item. Select all that apply.

3. A patient who has an allergy to penicillin is receiving preoperative medications, which include ranitidine (Zantac), metoclopramide (Reglan), and cefazolin (Ancef) intravenously. Fifteen minutes after the cefazolin is started, the patient reports an uneasy feeling, as well as feeling very warm. The nurse would appropriately recognize that the patient is experiencing anaphylaxis and perform which of the following?
   a. Offer the patient ice water
   b. Discontinue the IV
   c. Stay with the patient
   d. Turn off the IVPB
   e. Call for assistance
   f. Place the patient in Trendelenberg position
   g. Monitor vital signs

4. The nurse is contributing to the plan of care for a patient with ankylosing spondylitis. Which of the fol-

lowing interventions would be appropriate for the nurse to suggest?
   a. Avoid massage.
   b. Use interferon injections.
   c. Avoid one position for prolonged periods.
   d. Use topical steroids.

5. The nurse is contributing to the plan of care for a patient with an immune system deficiency. Which of the following complications should the nurse consider is most likely to occur when recommending prevention interventions?
   a. Overwhelming infection
   b. Fatal allergic reaction
   c. Asphyxiation
   d. Delayed anaphylactic reaction

6. A patient is admitted with an autoimmune disease and asks the nurse what autoimmune means. Which of the following would be the appropriate response by the nurse?
   a. "Immune cells produce too many antibodies."
   b. "Immune cells grow and multiply too rapidly."
   c. "Immune cells are not produced in sufficient amounts."
   d. "Immune cells are unable to distinguish between 'self' and 'not self.' "

Multiple response item. Select all that apply.

7. The nurse is contributing to the plan of care for a patient with systemic lupus erythematosus. Which of the following would be appropriate for the nurse to suggest?
   a. Take warm showers or baths to relieve the joint stiffness.
   b. Take corticosteroids without food.
   c. Work the pain out of painful or inflamed joints.
   d. If they have stomach upset when taking the corticosteroids they should stop taking it for a few days until the GI symptoms diminish.
   e. Encourage the patient and family members to participate in the planning of care and safety measures for at home.
   f. The patient may eat whatever desired.

8. As a patient is being discharged after being diagnosed with SLE the patient verbalizes that soon they are leaving on a three week tour of the Grand Canyon and white water rafting. Which of the following patient statements conveys to the nurse understanding of the patient's plan of care?
   a. "As long as I wear sunscreen, I'll be fine in the sun."
   b. "I'll need to wear a long-sleeved shirt and pants, hat, and use sunscreen on all exposed skin."
   c. "If I develop a rash, I should avoid the sun."
   d. "I should avoid the sun in the morning."

9. A patient is admitted to the hospital with no allergies to any food, medications or environmental stimuli. The physician orders amoxicillin PO four times a day for the patient. After receiving the second dose of amoxicillin the patient reports itching on the chest, neck and arms, and difficulty swallowing. The nurse notes urticaria on the face, neck, chest and arms of the patient, and the neck and tongue appear to be slightly swollen. The physician is notified and gives orders for Benadryl IM and a change in the antibiotic. The patient asks the nurse how an allergy can develop to a medication that has been taken before without problems. Which of the following is the most appropriate for the nurse to respond?
   a. "It probably is due to your age, because as you age your body becomes more sensitive to environmental stimuli which leads to hypersensitivities."
   b. "What have you eaten in the last 24 hours? Most medications are altered by food thereby producing different effects in the body."
   c. "Viral illnesses, exposure to various chemicals and environmental substances can alter the immune system and its response to previously benign stimuli."
   d. "Patients that have autoimmune disorders such as lupus or arthritis tend to develop sensitivities to common medications."

References

1. Elia, M: Oral or parenteral therapy for B$_{12}$ deficiency. Lancet 352:1721–1722, 1998.

2. Adachi, S, Kawamsoto, T, Otsuka, M, et al: Enteral vitamin B$_{12}$ supplements reverse postgastrectomy B$_{12}$ deficiency. Ann Surg 232:199–201, 2000.

SUGGESTED ANSWERS TO

CRITICAL THINKING

■ *Mrs. Barnes*

Further assessment might include: Identification of any previous allergies to food, medications and environmental stimuli and what reactions occur with any allergies. Thorough respiratory assessment, noting any adventitious sounds, in particular, wheezing. Note any dysphagia or changes in her voice,

Mrs. Barnes is most likely having an anaphylactic reaction to the bee stings with urticaria or even angioedema.

Therapeutic measures to implement: monitoring vital signs, staying with the patient, semi-Fowler's to high-Fowler's position; oxygen at 2 to 3 liters per minute; ensuring a patent intravenous access. Notify the RN and/or physician right away. Anticipate the administration of antihistamines, epinephrine, and fluids.

■ *Blood Types*

1. AB Rh$^+$
2. O Rh$^-$
3. No, they can safely receive only A Rh$^-$ or O Rh$^-$ blood.

■ *Mr. Ellis*

1.28 mL per dose

■ *Mr. Beck*

1. a. "Human leukocyte antigen B27 is formed, stimulating a chronic immune (inflammatory) response specifically in the sacroiliac, costovertebral, and large peripheral joints. This leads to thickening of the joints, joint pain, and stiffness."
   b. "No, you shouldn't have to quite your job, but you may need to alter the way you go about driving your truck."
   c. "No, you may not eventually be in severe pain, with use of medications and exercise."
   d. "No, this disease may not affect your independence, with proper treatment and rehabilitation."
2. a. "Range-of-motion exercises will help maintain joint mobility and a full range of motion and prevent contractures from forming."
   b. "Again, this frequent movement prevents stiffness and joint pain and contractures of joints."
   c. "Sleeping on a firm mattress without a pillow keeps the spine in correct alignment, which in turn helps prevent progressive changes in spine alignment (kyphosis, scoliosis), which affect various major body systems (respiratory, etc)."
   d. "Again, good posture will aid in preventing bone deformities."

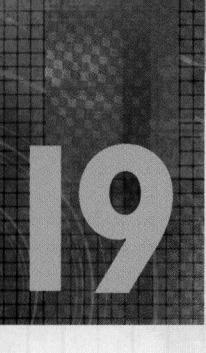

19

Nursing Care of Patients with HIV Disease and AIDS

MARY DILLINGER

KEY TERMS

acquired immunodeficiency syndrome (uh-KWHY-erd im-YOO-noh-de-FISH-en-see SIN-drohm)

cytomegalovirus (sigh-TOW-meg-ul-low-vigh-rus)

human immunodeficiency virus (HYOO-man im-YOO-noh-dee-FISH-en-see VIGH-rus)

Kaposi's sarcoma (ka-POE-sees sar-CO-mah)

personal protective equipment (PUR-sun-al pra-TEK-tiv i-KWIP-mant)

Pneumocystis carinii pneumonia (new-moh-SIS-tis ca-RIN-ee-eye new-MOH-nee-ah)

QUESTIONS TO GUIDE YOUR READING

1. What is human immunodeficiency virus (HIV) and how is it transmitted?

2. How is HIV diagnosed?

3. What is the prognosis for HIV and acquired immunodeficiency syndrome (AIDS)?

4. What would you include in a teaching plan to prevent HIV infection?

5. What are prevention measures to decrease infection and opportunistic diseases for patients with HIV?

6. What would you include in a teaching plan for a patient with HIV receiving highly active antiretroviral therapy?

7. What nursing care will you provide for patients with HIV/AIDS related to medications, coinfection prevention and maintaining nutritional status?

Acquired immunodeficiency syndrome (AIDS) is the final phase of a chronic, progressive immune function disorder. AIDS is caused by the **human immunodeficiency virus** (HIV). Not all HIV-infected people have AIDS. The Centers for Disease Control and Prevention (CDC) defines the diagnosis of AIDS (Box 19.1). There is no cure for AIDS, which may develop after a long period of HIV infection and may eventually be fatal.

LEARNING TIP

HIV disease is no longer characterized as a life-ending illness. With highly active antiretroviral therapy (HAART), HIV disease is a chronic, usually progressive immune disorder.

AIDS, more than any other chronic disease in recent history, is a multidimensional disease that challenges nurses to call into play their physical, emotional, social, and spiritual care skills. As you care for patients who are HIV positive or have AIDS, it is important for you to understand current information. Being informed helps you to provide caring, competent, nonjudgmental care without fear. Knowledge and treatment related to HIV and AIDS rapidly changes with new discoveries. Current information and guidelines can be found at AIDS info, www.hivatis.org or 1-800-HIV-0440 (1-800-448-0440). For other resources, see Table 19.1.

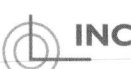

INCIDENCE

The HIV and AIDS epidemic was first reported by the CDC in June 1981 (Table 19.2). A rapid increase in HIV/AIDS was seen through the 1980s, followed by a decrease in the later 1990s. As we move into the third decade of the epidemic, an estimated 40,000 new cases of HIV infection continue to be reported each year in the United States. Increases in HIV infection are occurring fastest in women and men who have sex with men; 65 percent of these infections are in racial and ethnic minority groups. In the United States from 1981 through 2003, 929,985 persons developed AIDS; of these, 524,060 died. The number of persons living today with HIV/AIDS is at its highest level because of treatment with highly active antiretroviral therapy (HAART), which was introduced in 1996. Although any age group can be affected by HIV and AIDS, 85 percent of those diagnosed with HIV/AIDS have been 25 to 44 years old. Given the long latency period between infection with HIV and an AIDS-defining illness, most people diagnosed with HIV disease younger than the age of 30 years were probably infected as adolescents. The number of infections in persons over age 50 has doubled in the past 5 years. Older adults are increasingly contracting HIV and must be educated about prevention. In recent years in the United States, of those with HIV, male-to-male sex has caused the greatest exposure, followed by heterosexual contact, and then by

---

Box 19.1

CDC Conditions in the AIDS Surveillance Case Definition

CD4+ T-lymphocyte count below 200/μL, or a CD4+ T-lymphocyte percentage under 14 of total lymphocytes, or the presence of one of the following specified clinical conditions:
- Candidiasis of bronchi, trachea, or lung
- Candidiasis, esophageal
- Cervical cancer, invasive
- Coccidioidomycosis, disseminated or extrapulmonary
- Cryptococcis, extrapulmonary
- Cryptosporidiosis, chronic intestinal (greater than 1-month duration)
- Cytomegalovirus (CMV) disease (not including liver, spleen, or nodes)
- CMV retinitis with loss of vision
- Encephalopathy, HIV related
- Herpes simplex, chronic ulcers; or bronchitis, pneumonitis, or esophagitis
- Histoplasmosis, disseminated or extrapulmonary
- Isosporiasis, chronic intestinal (greater than 1-month duration)
- Kaposi's sarcoma
- Lymphoma, immunoblastic
- Lymphoma, Burkitt's
- Lymphoma of the brain, primary
- *Mycobacterium avium intracellulare* complex or *Mycobacterium kansasii*, disseminated or extrapulmonary
  Mycobacterium tuberculosis, any site (pulmonary or extrapullmonary)
  Mycobacterium, other species or unidentified species, disseminated or extrapulmonary
- *Pneumocystis carinii* pneumonia
- Pneumonia, recurrent
- Progressive multifocal leukoencephalopathy
- *Salmonella* septicemia, recurrent
- Toxoplasmosis of brain
- Wasting syndrome

Modified from Centers for Disease Control and Prevention: Revised classification system of HIV infection and expanded surveillance case definition for AIDS among adolescents and adults, MMWR 41 (RR17):2, 1992.

---

injected drugs. Current statistics can be found at www.cdc.gov.

Although HIV/AIDS can occur in a person of any age, this chapter focuses on adults with HIV/AIDS.

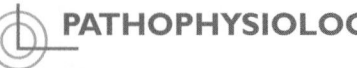

PATHOPHYSIOLOGY

Infection with the HIV virus causes destruction of immune cells. There are two identified subtypes of the HIV virus:

TABLE 19.1 STAYING CURRENT: HIV/AIDS INFORMATION RESOURCES

AIDSinfo	www.aidsinfo.nih.gov
In English and Spanish	(800) 874–2572
Association of Nurses in AIDS Care	www.anacnet.org
	(800) 260–6780
CDC—information in English and Spanish	(800) 342–2437
	([800]-342-AIDS)
CDC National AIDS Hotline TTY service for the deaf	(800) 243–7889
CDC National AIDS Hotline Website	www.cde.gov/ /hiv/hivinfo
CDC National Center for HIV, STD, and TB Prevention	www.cdc.gov/nchstp/od/nchstp.html
CDC National Prevention Information Network in	www.cdcnpin.org
English and Spanish	(800) 458–5231
HIV/AIDS Treatment Information Service	www.hivatis.org
Information available in English and Spanish.	(800) 448–0440
	www.nap.edu/html/hivprevention
	www.ama-assn.org/special/hiv
	(312) 464–2405
National Clinicians' Post-Exposure Prophylaxis Hotline	http://www.ucsf.edu/hivcntr/pepline
	(888) 448–4911
National Library of Medicine	www.nlm.nih.gov
	(888) 346–3656
The BodyPro	www.thebody.com

TABLE 19.2 DATA FOR U.S. ADULTS/ ADOLESCENTS WITH AIDS, 1981–2003

	Since 1981	
Gender		
Male	Declined from 92%–73%	749,887
Female	Increased from 8%–27%	170,679
Years of Age	*Estimated # of AIDS Cases in 2003*	*Cumulative Estimate of AIDS Cases Through 2003*
≤12	59	9419
13–14	59	891
15–24	1991	37,599
25–34	9605	311,137
35–44	17,633	365,432
45–54	10,051	148,347
55–64	2888	43,451
>65	886	13,711
Ethnicity/Race		
White	12,222	376,834
Black	21,304	368,169
Hispanic	8,757	172,993
Asian/Pacific Islander	497	7,166
American Indian/ Alaskan Native	196	3,026
Deceased	18,017	524,060
Estimate of # HIV/AIDS at end of 2003	1,039,000–1,185,000 24%–27% undiagnosed and unaware of their HIV infection	

Source: Data from Centers for Disease Control and Prevention: HIV and AIDS—United States, 1981–2003 2003, http://www.cdc.gov/hiv/stats.htm.

HIV-1 and HIV-2. Both of these subtypes can cause AIDS. HIV-1 is found in Asia, Europe, and the Western Hemisphere. HIV-2 is found in West Africa. Without a normally functioning immune system, infections and cancers may take over. AIDS is the result of this immunodeficiency.

HIV is a retrovirus (which only has ribonucleic acid [RNA] for genetic material). HIV is attracted to immune cells with a surface-attaching site referred to as a CD4 receptor. Cells with CD4 receptors include lymphocytes (called CD4+ T lymphocytes, T4 lymphocytes, or helper T lymphocytes) and macrophages (in which HIV hides). HIV begins its infection by binding to the CD4 receptor of the host cell. The CD4+ T lymphocytes are the primary targets for HIV infection. Because CD4+ T lymphocytes orchestrate all immune functions, HIV's attack on these cells results in progressive impairment of the body's immune response. The CD4+ T lymphocytes do not function normally and are too busy replicating more HIV to perform their own immune function. Recent understanding of how HIV fuses with the cell has been the focus of new developments of treatment for preventing infection by blocking fusion of HIV with its host cell. After fusion with the host cell, the HIV viral particle is taken into a human cell and its covering is destroyed to expose its viral RNA. The retrovirus then uses an enzyme called reverse transcriptase to force the human cell to produce a new piece of deoxyribonucleic acid (DNA) from the viral RNA. The new DNA is integrated into the person's cellular DNA. As a result, the human cell creates more viral particles, which spread through the lymphoid system (Fig. 19.1). Inhibitors of reverse transcriptase were the first anti-HIV medications developed and are still an essential part of current treatment.

Once the genetic material of HIV has been changed to DNA, the enzyme integrase integrates it into the genetic

Normal Immune System

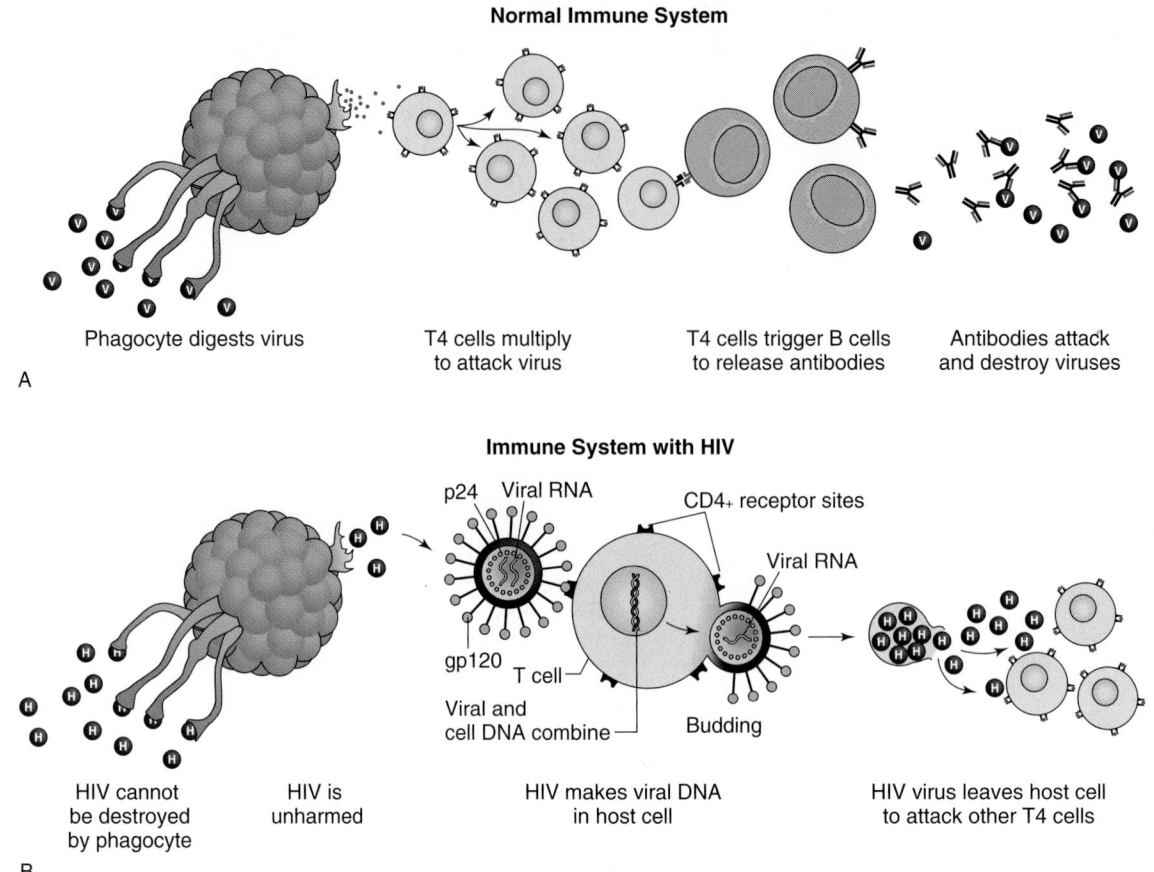

A

Phagocyte digests virus   T4 cells multiply to attack virus   T4 cells trigger B cells to release antibodies   Antibodies attack and destroy viruses

Immune System with HIV

p24   Viral RNA
CD4+ receptor sites
Viral RNA
gp120   T cell
Viral and cell DNA combine
Budding

B

HIV cannot be destroyed by phagocyte   HIV is unharmed   HIV makes viral DNA in host cell   HIV virus leaves host cell to attack other T4 cells

FIGURE 19.1 *(A)* Normal immune system. *(B)* HIV contains several proteins: gp 120 protein around it and viral RNA and p24 protein inside. The gp 120 proteins attach to CD4+ receptors of T lymphocytes; HIV enters the cell and makes viral DNA; the enslaved host cell produces new viruses that bud, which destroys the host cell's membrane, causing cellular death and allowing the virus to leave to attack other CD4+ T-lymphocyte cells.

material of the host cell. The cell is then translated into viral proteins. Among these proteins is HIV protease, which is required to process other HIV proteins into their functional forms. Protease inhibitors, potent types of antiviral medications, act by blocking this critical step. Following development of the cell surface, the virus then buds from the cell and is released to infect another cell. The virus spreads throughout the body unless interrupted by treatment. HIV may persist in a latent state for many years. This makes it very difficult to eradicate or cure HIV. Because of this, currently, patients must remain on antiviral treatment for life. The ultimate challenge is to use knowledge of the HIV life cycle to develop treatments that will eradicate HIV from those who are infected and to create a vaccine that will prevent new infections in the future.

After a person has been infected with HIV, other immune system components form antibodies to fight the HIV. Detection of these antibodies via laboratory testing is the most common way HIV is diagnosed. HIV antibodies typically become present within 3 weeks to 3 months after infection. The time between infection and developing antibodies is called the "window period." Laboratory tests are available that detect the virus directly, rather than antibodies, but these are more costly for routine HIV testing.

 LEARNING TIP

Being HIV positive means that the person has been infected with the HIV virus. It does not mean that the person has AIDS.

Progression

The initial infection is followed by a relatively symptom-free period called the clinical latency stage. The virus remains in the lymph nodes, liver, and spleen and reproduces. If the infection is untreated, a gradual decrease in CD4+ T lymphocytes continues. B lymphocytes also become dysfunctional and dysregulated by the events of HIV progression. B and T cells work together for a normal healthy immune system, so this may further impair the immune system. This period, from infection to the beginning of the symptomatic stage, varies for each person and averages 8 to 12 years. During this stage, the person is considered to be HIV infected. (Many are not aware of their HIV infection until they become symptomatic, and unknowingly pass the virus on to others and do not have the benefit of antiviral treatments to maintain health.) During the early symptomatic stage of HIV disease, symptoms of the weakening immune system are seen. When the immune system is severely weakened, opportunistic infections and cancers may occur. When this occurs, the person is diagnosed with AIDS (Box 19.1 CDC Conditions in the AIDS Surveillance Definition).

LEARNING TIP

Opportunistic diseases are referred to as opportunistic because a normal immune system would prevent them from occurring. With an impaired immune system, invading organisms have the "opportunity" to survive.

PREVENTION

Prevention and education are the best ways to manage the HIV/AIDS epidemic. Education regarding the disease and its transmission should begin with the older school-age child and include the general population, as well as older adults (Box 19.2 Gerontological Issues).

Mode of Transmission

HIV is a fragile virus that is transmitted from human to human only through infected blood, semen, vaginal secretions, or breast milk. HIV is not spread casually. Kissing, hugging, shaking hands, or sharing eating utensils, towels, or bathroom fixtures with an HIV-positive person does not transmit HIV. There is also no evidence that HIV can be transmitted through insect bites or tears, nasal secretions, saliva, sweat, sputum, emesis, urine, or feces unless blood is present. Even then the transmission risk is considered very low. Blood transfusions before 1985 may have been a source for HIV transmission. However, since 1985, donated blood has been tested for HIV.

HIV needs a portal of entry into the body, such as a tear in a mucous membrane or nonintact skin, or access to the bloodstream or lymphatic tissue. Routes of transmission for HIV are as follows:

- Sexual—anal, vaginal, or oral sexual contact of mucous membranes to infected body fluids
- Parenteral—injection by needles contaminated with infected blood, sharing needles, transfusions of contaminated blood products
- Perinatal—infected mother to fetus/infant during pregnancy, childbirth, or breastfeeding

LEARNING TIP

An HIV-infected person can transmit HIV to others within a few days after initial infection and then throughout all stages of the disease. This is thought to be true even when HAART treatment has driven the viral load below detectable levels.

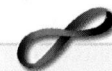

Box 19.2

Gerontological Issues

Nearly 10 percent of diagnosed AIDS cases occur in people age 50 and older. Numbers will continue to rise as the older population increases, yet little attention has been given to this age group. This may be due to an ageist view of the older adult and sexual activity.

It is important to understand that HIV infection can occur at any age. Older adults should be asked about their sexual and drug use history and be given preventive education and information about products that reduce transmission of HIV and sexually transmitted diseases. At-risk people older than age 50 are less likely than younger at-risk adults to use condoms during sex or to be tested for HIV. In this age group, condoms are often thought of as a birth control measure.

HIV/AIDS is thought of as being a disease of young, sexually active people. Older people remain sexually active, and may have multiple partners. Older people are also contracting the virus through homosexual contact.

A decline in the older adult's immune system increases the risk for infection with HIV. Increased vaginal dryness and friability further increases an older woman's susceptibility to HIV infection. Because older adults are not usually taught HIV prevention, the rise in HIV infection among older adults is expected to continue. With AIDS death rates dropping as a result of more effective treatments, the number of older adults living with HIV will increase.

Symptoms of HIV in older adults may be confused with commonly perceived problems of aging, such as fatigue, decreased endurance, and altered cognitive status. The effect of HIV on the brain can be mistaken for Alzheimer's disease, delaying proper treatment.

Counseling

Early knowledge of HIV status aids in reducing the spread of HIV infection. The CDC has recommended guidelines for counseling and testing people at risk for HIV. Counseling should be done by trained workers to help the patient make an informed decision about testing. Education should also be provided that is culturally sensitive and fits the patient's personal risk situation. Posttest counseling is provided to help the patient understand the test results, assist with informing sexual partners and drug needle sharers, risk factor reduction, and care options if needed.

Sexual Transmission

HIV is transmitted more easily to women than men. This is because the vagina has a greater amount of mucous membrane than the penis, as well as the increased amount of virus found in semen as compared with vaginal secretions. Sexual acts that are the riskiest for transmission of HIV are those that promote contact between infected body fluids and mucous membranes or nonintact skin. These risky acts include oral sex or anal sex. Anal sex is the riskiest type of sexual act, for either gender, because it often results in tearing of the mucous membrane that is then exposed to infected semen.

Safer Sex Practices

Abstaining from sexual intercourse is the only sure way to prevent sexual exposure to HIV. A mutually monogamous sexual relationship is considered safe if both partners are not and will not become infected with HIV. Alternative methods of sexual activities can be used that prevent exposure to blood and secretions, such as massage or masturbation. The benefits of limiting sexual partners should be explained. For vaginal or anal intercourse, the use of male or female condoms and safer sex techniques should be discussed (Box 19.3 Patient Education: Condom Use to Prevent HIV Transmission). Latex gloves protect hands during genital or anal contact. Dental dams (latex sheets) should be used as a barrier between the mouth and genitals or anus.

Parenteral Transmission

The best way to prevent parenteral transmission of HIV is to avoid injection drug use. Drug injection equipment should not be shared. If a person who uses injected drugs is unable or unwilling to stop sharing needles, he or she should be carefully taught how to clean the needle and syringe: To optimize the effectiveness of cleaning, soon after use the needle and syringe should be flushed with water until visibly clear of blood. Next, the syringe is filled with full-strength household bleach and shaken for 1 minute. The bleach is flushed through the needle and syringe and they are then rinsed with water. Additionally, sexual activity should be strongly discouraged when judgment is impaired from drug use because protective measures may not be used.

Autologous (one's own) blood transfusion, when possible, is the safest type of transfusion to prevent HIV infection. Screening of blood for HIV antibodies is done on all donated blood in the United States. There is a very small chance of HIV transmission from blood that is infected but has not yet had time to develop antibodies.

Perinatal Transmission

The U.S. Public Health Service guidelines for HIV screening of pregnant women recommend that voluntary HIV pretest counseling and testing be offered during prenatal care for all pregnant women.[1] Pregnant women who know they are HIV positive can reduce the risk of perinatal HIV transmission to less than 4 percent by taking antiretroviral therapy during pregnancy, labor, and delivery. Every effort should be taken during labor and delivery to avoid any procedure such as a scalp monitor or episiotomy that increases the risk of exposure of the infant to the mother's blood. At the time of delivery, pregnant women who have not been tested for HIV or received prophylactic treatment should be offered testing for HIV. After delivery, the infant is given zidovudine (AZT, Retrovir) for 6 weeks.

Health-Care Workers and HIV Prevention

It is essential to understand and use proper infection control practices to protect yourself from exposure and transmission of HIV. Following hand washing protocols, using **personal protective equipment** (gloves, surgical masks, goggles, gowns, and booties) and preventing needle sticks are very important. Personal protective equipment (PPE) to be used is selected and based on the task to be performed and the exposure risk the task presents along with the type of isolation precautions in use. If you are unsure of the appropriate PPE or isolation precautions to use, ask your instructor or the patient's nurse before providing care to the patient.

Needle Sticks

Needle-stick injury is a source of HIV transmission to health-care workers. The Needlestick Safety and Prevention Act is designed to aid health care workers in preventing needle-stick injuries. Careful use of needles—including not recapping needles, use of needless systems, and needle safety devices—can reduce needle-stick injury. Consider an occupational exposure an urgent medical concern and seek medical care immediately. To prevent HIV after a needle stick or other forms of exposure to patient body fluids, the CDC has developed postexposure prophylaxis guidelines (Table 19.3).

Standard Precautions

All those at risk of contacting blood and body fluids and substances must follow CDC standard precautions to reduce their risk of HIV exposure as well as other bloodborne pathogens. (See Chapter 7.) Health-care workers should

---

Box 19.3

Patient Education: Condom Use to Prevent HIV Transmission

Condoms should be:
- New for each intercourse act.
- Latex (or polyurethane if allergic to latex) because other materials have large pores that allow HIV to pass.
- Nondamaged, current (not past expiration date).
- Applied before partner is touched. (Tip of condom is held while unrolled over erect penis, allowing room at tip for semen collection.)
- Used with adequate amounts of only water-soluble lubricants. (Petroleum or oil-based lubricants such as petroleum jelly, cooking oil, shortening, or lotions can damage latex condoms.)
- Replaced if broken. (If ejaculation occurs before replacement, immediate use of a spermicide may give some protection.)
- Withdrawn from partner by holding condom against base of erect penis to avoid semen leakage.

TABLE 19.3 OCCUPATIONAL HIV EXPOSURE: POSTEXPOSURE PROPHYLAXIS

Consider occupational exposure an urgent medical condition.

Immediate care	Wash exposure site with soap and water.
	For mucous membrane exposure, flush with water.
Consider exposure risk	What is the type of fluid person was exposed to?
	What is the type of exposure?
Test exposure source	Assess risk of infection and test known sources for HIV antibody.
Postexposure prophylaxis	Start treatment within hours of exposure for 4 weeks.
	Consider pregnancy test if of childbearing age.
	Basic prophylaxis regimen or alternate basic prophylaxis regimen available: zidovudine (Retrovir, ZDV, AZT) 300 bid and lamivudine (Epivir, 3TC) 150 mg bid; or as combination tablet of both drugs: Combivir one tablet bid.
	Expanded prophylaxis regimen (basic prophylaxis regimen and one of the following): indinavir (Crixivan, IDV) 800 mg q8h; nelfinavir (Viracept, NFV) 750 mg tid or 1250 mg bid; efavirenz (Sustiva, EFV) 600 mg qh; or abacavir (Ziagen, ABC) 300 mg bid. Trizivir, a combination of ZDV, 3TC, and ABC, may be used.
Follow-up testing and counseling	HIV-antibody testing at baseline, 6 weeks, 3 months, and 6 months after exposure or if a retroviral syndrome–type illness occurs.
	During postexposure care, exposed person should use precautions to prevent secondary transmission of HIV, including abstaining from sex or using condoms; no donation of blood, plasma, organs, or semen; if breastfeeding, consider stopping.

Source: CDC: Basic and Expanded HIV Postexposure Prophylaxis Regimens. MMWR 50(RR11):47, 2001.

always use these precautions for all patients to protect themselves and other patients. Additionally, to protect patients, HIV-infected health-care workers with open lesions or weeping dermatitis should avoid direct patient care.

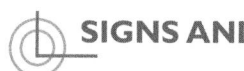 **SIGNS AND SYMPTOMS**

Initially after HIV infection, the patient may have no symptoms or may develop mononucleosis-like symptoms (called an acute retroviral syndrome), such as extreme fatigue, headache, fever, lymphadenopathy (enlarged lymph nodes in two different sites other than inguinal nodes), diarrhea, or a sore throat (Fig. 19.2 and Box 19.4 HIV/AIDS Summary). Symptoms generally develop 6 to 12 weeks after HIV transmission and may last a few days to weeks. These symptoms are usually mild and not attributed to an HIV infection.

Each patient's response to HIV is unique. After an extended asymptomatic phase, untreated HIV infection usually progresses to a symptomatic stage when the virus has greatly impaired the immune system. The patient may exhibit shortness of breath, fever, weight loss, fatigue, night sweats, persistent diarrhea, oral or vaginal candidiasis ulcers, dry skin, skin lesions, peripheral neuropathy,

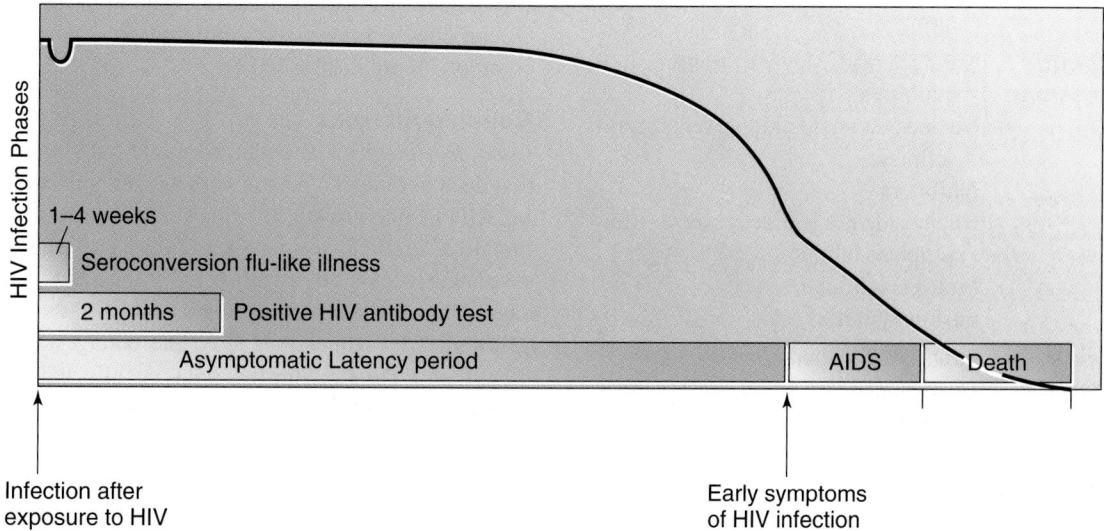

FIGURE 19.2 Typical phases of HIV infection, AIDS development, and CD4+ T-lymphocyte counts without treatment. Length of latency period varies but is usually many years. As CD4+ T-lymphocyte counts drop, symptoms, AIDS, and then death result.

shingles (varicella zoster virus reactivation), seizures, or dementia. In the final stage of HIV infection, AIDS is diagnosed when the CD4+ T-lymphocyte count is below 200 or opportunistic infections and diseases, with their specific signs and symptoms, occur. (See Box 19.1 CDC Conditions in the Aids Surveillance Definition.)

 ## COMPLICATIONS

Many complications are seen with HIV/AIDS that vary from patient to patient. Some of the common complications are discussed next.

Box 19.4

HIV/AIDS Summary

Signs and symptoms	Initially vary: None or acute retroviral syndrome Asymptomatic phase Immune system impairment: dyspnea, fever, weight loss, fatigue, night sweats, persistent diarrhea, oral or vaginal candidiasis ulcers, dry skin, skin lesions, peripheral neuropathy, shingles, seizures, or dementia AIDS diagnosed when CD4+ T-lymphocyte count below 200 or opportunistic infections and diseases occur.
Diagnostic tests	HIV antibody tests Complete blood cell count/lymphocyte count CD4+/CD8+ T-lymphocyte count Viral load testing Viral culture Genotyping
Therapeutic Interventions	Nonnucleoside reverse transcriptase inhibitors Nucleoside/nucleotide reverse transcriptase Inhibitors Nucleoside/nucleotide reverse transcriptase inhibitors Protease inhibitors Fusion inhibitors
Complications	AIDS wasting syndrome Opportunistic infection and cancer AIDS dementia complex
Possible Nursing Diagnoses	Risk for infection Acute or chronic pain Fatigue Imbalanced nutrition Ineffective individual coping

---

AIDS Wasting Syndrome

AIDS wasting syndrome occurs in most patients with AIDS. The syndrome is defined by the occurrence of the following:
- Involuntary baseline body weight loss of more than 10 percent
- Chronic weakness or fever for more than 30 days or chronic diarrhea of two loose stools daily for more than 30 days

Several factors contribute to this syndrome: decreased appetite, oral lesions, altered metabolism, malabsorption, gastrointestinal (GI) infections, diarrhea, medication side effects, and cognitive impairment. The progressive weight loss impairs function of all body systems from malnourishment. Careful intervention, planning, and education of the patient when HIV is first diagnosed can help maintain body weight.

 ## NURSING CARE TIP

AIDS wasting syndrome is challenging. Do not give up! Be creative in developing interventions to help increase the patient's appetite and caloric intake.

Opportunistic Infection and Cancer

Opportunistic infections (OI) are a primary complication of HIV/AIDS because the person with HIV/AIDS has a very impaired immune system. Other types of infections that occur even with a healthy immune system are seen as well, such as tuberculosis. OI are not spread to those with healthy immune systems, but other types of infections can be. Certain kinds of cancer incidence also rise when the immune system is impaired. Opportunistic infections can be viral, bacterial or mycobacterial, fungal, protozoal, or parasitic. They can affect many different areas of the body. Some OI can now be prevented by prophylactic treatments. Some common OI are discussed here.

Candida Albicans
Candida albicans is a fungus normally found in the GI tract that does not infect a person with a healthy immune system. In AIDS, overgrowth of this fungus occurs from the impaired immune system. Candidiasis of the mouth or esophagus occurs often with AIDS. Signs and symptoms of candidiasis include oral or esophageal pain, dysphagia, and yellow-white plaques that look like cottage cheese in the mouth and throat. Nutrition can be affected by oral or esophageal candidiasis. Recurrent vaginal candidiasis is more common in women with AIDS. Severe itching and a white discharge occur.

Cytomegalovirus
Cytomegalovirus (CMV) is a common viral infection that can affect many areas of the body. The eye is a common site (cytomegalovirus retinitis). Vision impairment ranges from

little impairment to total blindness. Prompt diagnosis and treatment can minimize the loss of vision. A variety of symptoms are seen when other areas are involved, such as fever, fatigue, diarrhea, GI upset, and hepatitis, to name a few.

Pneumocystis Carinii Pneumonia

Pneumocystis carinii pneumonia (PCP) is caused by a fungus (formerly thought to be a protozoa) that produces shortness of breath, fever, nonproductive cough, and fatigue. PCP is the most common opportunistic infection in HIV/AIDS. To prevent PCP, oral trimethoprim-sulfamethoxazole (Septra) is given prophylactically. Other treatments for those who cannot tolerate Septra are available, including dapsone, Mepron, and pentamidine isethionate (Pentam) inhalation therapy to prevent PCP when CD4+ T-lymphocyte counts fall below 200/µL. PCP may be treated with oxygen, oral or intravenous trimethoprim-sulfamethoxazole, or parenteral pentamidine isethionate. Steroids may also be given to reduce lung inflammation.

Tuberculosis

Tuberculosis is a bacterial infection and may occur in up to 10 percent of those with AIDS. Symptoms include dyspnea, cough, chest pain, fever, night sweats, and weight loss. A purified protein derivative (PPD) skin test should be performed at least annually in patients with HIV infection. Induration of 5 mm or more is defined as a positive result in patients with HIV infection. (See Chapter 31.)

NURSING CARE TIP

When assessing the results of a PPD test, only the raised area (if present) is measured and recorded in millimeters. (If there is no induration, it is recorded as 0 mm.)

Viral Infections

Herpes simplex virus infections may be found in the oral, genital, or rectal area of those with AIDS. Symptoms include blister-like lesions that rupture and leave ulcerations, fever, pain, or bleeding. Varicella zoster virus infection is usually the result of the virus being present from a prior episode of the chickenpox. The virus remains present in the nerve ganglia. With depressed immune function, the virus can cause shingles.

Neoplasms

Kaposi's sarcoma (KS) is the most common cancer associated with AIDS. Painless, small purple-blue lesions on the skin occur. The lesions may scale, ulcerate, and bleed. KS may occur anywhere on the body in patients with HIV. HAART has affected the incidence of KS, decreasing it by approximately 60 percent since 1996. Cervical neoplasia is more common in women with HIV. Non-Hodgkin's lymphoma is more likely to occur in persons with substantial immunosuppression.

AIDS Dementia Complex

HIV infection of the brain or other parts of the central nervous system results in AIDS dementia complex (ADC). Symptoms range from mild to severe and may include memory impairment, personality changes, hallucinations, leg weakness, loss of balance, and slower responses. ADC is a common complication of HIV/AIDS. With ADC, safety is an important consideration for the patient and caregiver. The only treatment for AIDS dementia is optimal viral suppression from antiviral treatment.

 DIAGNOSIS

Finger-stick blood, oral fluid, and urine and serum specimens are used for HIV testing. Rapid HIV testing provides results the same day. Home sample collection devices can be purchased; the sample is sent in for HIV testing, with the person calling for results, counseling, and referral if needed.

HIV Antibody Tests

After HIV infection, antibodies may not be formed for 3 weeks to 3 months or longer in some cases. The typical HIV antibody testing pattern is as follows:

- Enzyme-linked immunosorbent assay (ELISA) test is done to detect antibodies in the patient's blood to HIV antigen on test plates.
- If positive, the ELISA test is repeated because false positives may occur (0.1 percent).
- If the ELISA test is again positive, the Western blot test is done to detect the presence of antibodies to four major HIV antigens. The test is positive if two antibodies are present.
- If all test results are positive, the patient is HIV-antibody positive.
- (If the test is negative, the patient is said to be in the window period or HIV negative.)
- Other tests can be used, especially if initial test results are not conclusive such as viral cultures to confirm HIV status.

Complete Blood Cell Count/Lymphocyte Count

Because patients with HIV are susceptible to leukopenia, lymphopenia, anemia, and thrombocytopenia related to HIV infection and as a complication of antiretroviral therapy, a complete blood cell count (CBC) including a lymphocyte count should be obtained. The CBC should be repeated at 3- to 4-month intervals or more often if there is a change in therapy or the patient's clinical course is unstable.

CD4+/CD8+ T-Lymphocyte Count

The count of CD4+ and CD8+ (cytotoxic cells) T lymphocytes is essential for evaluating the status of the immune system. In healthy adults, CD4+ levels average 500 to 1600 cells per mm^3. In HIV/AIDS, CD4+ cell levels drop but

CD8+ cell levels do not. A low ratio of CD4+ cells to CD8+ cells is seen as HIV/AIDS progresses. It is recommended that CD4+/CD8+ T-lymphocyte counts be performed at 3-month intervals for most patients.

Viral Load Testing

Viral load testing measures the amount of HIV RNA in plasma and is extremely important for determining prognosis and monitoring the response to antiretroviral therapy. Combination antiretroviral regimens usually produce a 50 percent decrease in total-body HIV levels within just a few days. Viral loads should be performed 1 month after initiation of new treatments and at 3-month intervals thereafter.

Genotyping

Genotyping measures resistance to current antiviral treatments. This information guides medical providers in choosing treatment regimens that will most likely be effective against that individual's virus.

General Tests

Standard serological testing for syphilis is recommended annually in patients who are sexually active. Hepatitis A, B, and C serologies and liver chemistry panels are indicated in the early evaluation of most patients because of the high incidence of concurrent hepatitis for HIV-positive patients.

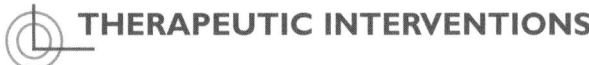

THERAPEUTIC INTERVENTIONS

Because there is no cure for HIV/AIDS, the goal of therapy is to prevent or delay development of opportunistic diseases. There is some inconsistency in the recommendations of when to start an antiretroviral regimen. The 2005 Guidelines for Use of Antiretroviral Agents in HIV-1 Infected Adults and Adolescents are clear that they should be started before the CD4 cell count falls below 200 cells/mm³, but there are inconsistent data on the value of starting when the CD4+ T-lymphocyte cell count falls below 350 cells per cubic milliliter (Table 19.4). To increase life expectancy and treatment cost effectiveness, it may be recommended that patients be prophylactically treated for opportunistic infections, especially hepatitis A and hepatitis B viruses, herpes simplex virus, *Mycorobacterium avium* complex, and *Pneumocystis carinii* pneumonia (Table 19.5). Other opportunistic infections are treated with appropriate medications if they occur.

Antiretroviral drugs that inhibit reproduction of the virus (but do not kill it) are used to treat HIV infection. These antiretroviral agents have been developed to act predominantly on processes specific to the viral particle to keep the integrity of the host cell. Several potential strategies specifically aimed at interruption of the viral life cycle have been defined, including the following:

(Text continued on page 333)

TABLE 19.4 MEDICATIONS FOR HIV INFECTION

Medication Class/Action	Examples	Route	Side Effects	Nursing Implications
Nonnucleoside reverse transcriptase inhibitors (NNRTIs) Block active site of HIV reverse transcriptase	delavirdine (Rescriptor)	PO: 200 mg, 2 tid. Take with/without food.	Rash, headache	Monitor WBC count, liver tests, especially with history of hepatitis B or C. Do not give within 1 hour of antacids or didanosine (ddI, Videx).
	efavirenz (Sustiva)	PO: 600 mg daily. Take on an empty stomach, preferable at bedtime.	Rash, vivid dreams, CNS symptoms False-positive cannabinoid test	Monitor for rash (especially during first month); may be severe and life threatening. Teach patient to report rash.
	nevirapine (Viramune)	PO: 200 mg daily for 7 days, then 200 mg bid. Take with/without food.	Rash	Monitor for rash (especially first month); may be life threatening and require stopping drug immediately. Teach patient to report rash immediately. Stevens-Johnson syndrome may occur. Monitor liver tests. For contraception advise a nonhormonal contraceptive during therapy.

Medication Class/Action	Examples	Route	Side Effects	Nursing Implications
Nucleoside/Nucleotide Reverse Transcriptase Inhibitors (NRTIs) Inhibit production of reverse transcriptase and viral replication.	combivir (lamivudine, [3TC] and zidovudine [AZT])	150 mg of lamivudine and 300 mg of zidovudine PO: bid. With/without food	Peripheral neuropathy	Monitor for peripheral neuropathy and report
	emtriva (Emtricitabine or FTC)	PO: 200 mg daily. Take with/without food.	Minimal side effects Lactic acidosis rare	Monitor for symptoms of lactic acidosis.
	epivir (Lamivudine, 3TC)	PO: 150 mg bid or 300 mg daily. Take with/without food	Peripheral neuropathy	Monitor for peripheral neuropathy and report.
	epizicom (abacavir sulfate and lamivudine)	PO: abacavir 600 mg + lamivudine 300 mg daily. With/without food	See sections for the two meds in this drug.	See sections for the two meds in this drug.
	hivid (Zalcitabine, ddC)	PO: 0.75 mg q8h. With/ without food	Peripheral neuropathy	Monitor for peripheral neuropathy and report.
	zidovudine (Retrovir, AZT, ZDV)	PO: 300 mg bid. With/ without food	Nausea, vomiting, dizziness. Decrease in bone marrow function and liver and kidney toxicity.	Monitor CBC for anemia. Use strategies to decrease nausea and vomiting. Monitor labs for kidney and liver function.
	trizivir (Abacavir + lamivudine + zidovudine)	PO: Abacavir 600 mg, lamivudine 150 mg, zidovudine 300 mg bid With/without food	See sections for the each of the three meds.	See sections for each of the three meds.
	truvada (emtricitabine + tenofovir)	PO: Emtricitabine 200 mg + Tenofovir 300 mg daily With/without food	See sections for the two meds in this drug,	See sections for the two meds in this drug.
	videx (Didanosine, ddI)	PO: 200 mg bid on an empty stomach. Chew or dissolve in water. (Take at least 30 minutes before or 2 hours after a meal.)	Peripheral neuropathy, pancreatitis, nausea, diarrhea	Monitor for peripheral neuropathy. Monitor CBC for bone marrow suppression.
	videx EC (Didanosine, ddI)	PO: 400 mg if >60 kg. Also comes in 250 mg.	Peripheral neuropathy, pancreatitis, nausea, diarrhea	Monitor for peripheral neuropathy. Monitor CBC for bone marrow suppression.
	viread (tenofovir)	PO: 300 mg daily With/without food	Nausea, vomiting, diarrhea, headaches, flatulence	Monitor for hepatomegaly with steatosis for lactic acidosis, which can be fatal, especially in women. Take 2 hours before or 1 hour after didanosine.
	zerit (Stavudine, d4T)	PO: 40 mg bid. With/without food.	Peripheral neuropathy, lactic acidosis (which can be fatal)	Monitor for peripheral neuropathy and report. Monitor liver function and report.
	ziagen (Abacavire sulfate)	PO: 300 mg bid or 300 mg daily With/without food	Fever, rash, nausea, vomiting, malaise or fatigue, loss of appetite, respiratory symptoms such as sore throat, cough, shortness of breath (Hypersensitivity reaction, which can be fatal)	Flulike symptoms indicate need to discontinue drug or life-threatening condition may develop. Report immediately.

(Continued on following page)

TABLE 19.4 MEDICATIONS FOR HIV INFECTION *(Continued)*

Medication Class/Action	Examples	Route	Side Effects	Nursing Implications
Protease Inhibitors (PIs) Bind to active site of HIV protease enzyme, which cuts reproduced HIV strands. Interrupt formation of mature viral particles and reduce viral replication. Rapid resistance development if not taken as directed	agenerase (Amprenavir)	PO: 8- to150-mg caps bid or 8- to 150-mg caps +100 mg Norvir daily With/without food	Nausea, vomiting, diarrhea Rash, oral parasthesias hyperglycemia, transaminase elevation, lipodystrophy and lipid abnormalities	Care for GI intolerance, Report rash. Monitor labs. Watch for increased bleeding in patient with hemophilia.
	crixivan (Indinavir)	PO: 800 mg q8h on an empty stomach	Nephrolithiasis, GI intolerance, headaches, asthenia, blurred vision, dizziness, rash, metallic taste, thrombocytopenia, alopecia, hemolytic anemia, hyperglycemia, lipodystrophy, elevated lipids	Teach about importance of hydration. Manage GI symptoms. Monitor labs.
	fortovase (Saquinavir)	PO: 6- to 200-mg caps tid with food	Nausea, diarrhea, abdominal pain, headache, dyspepsia, hyperglycemia, lipodystrophy, elevated lipids, elevated transaminases	Manage GI intolerance. Monitor labs. Watch for increased bleeding if patient has hemophilia.
	invirase (Saquinavir)	PO: 5- to 200- mg caps + 100 mg Ritonavir bid with food	GI intolerance, headache, hyperglycemia, lipodystrophy, elevated lipids, elevated transaminases	Same as fortovase
	kaletra (Lopinavir/ ritonavir)	PO: 3 caps bid with food	GI intolerance, asthenia, hyperglycemia, lipodystrophy, elevated lipids, elevated transaminases	Refrigerate caps. Manage GI symptoms. Monitor labs. Watch for increased bleeding in patients with hemophilia.
	lexiva (Fosamprenavir)	PO: 2- to 700-mg tabs bid OR 2- to 700-mg tabs + 200 mg Ritonavir daily OR 700 mg+100 Norvir bid with/without food	Skin rash, GI intolerance, headache, hyperglycemia, transaminase elevation, lipodystrophy, elevated lipids, elevated transaminases	Manage GI symptoms. Report rash. Watch for increased bleeding in patients with hemophilia.
	novir (Ritonavir)	PO: 6- to 100-mg caps bid. With food. Dose is titrated up slowly. (Mainly used in small doses to boost other PIs.)	GI intolerance, paresthesias, hepatitis, pancreatitis, asthenia, taste perversion, elevated lipids, hyperglycemia, lipodystrophy	Manage GI symptoms. Monitor labs. Monitor side effects. Watch for bleeding episodes in patients with hemophilia.
	reyataz (Atazanavir)	PO: 2- to 200-mg caps daily or 300 mg with 100 mg Norvir daily with food.	Indirect hyperbilirubinemia, hyperglycemia, lipodystrophy	Watch for jaundice and report. Monitor labs. Watch for bleeding episodes in patients with hemophilia.
	viracept (Nelfinavir)	PO: 5- to 250-mg caps bid or two 625-mg tabs bid with food	Diarrhea, asthenia, hyperglycemia, lipodystrophy, elevated lipids, elevated transaminase	Manage diarrhea. Monitor labs. Watch for increased bleeding in hemophilia patients.
Fusion Inhibitors Blocks HIV-1 fusion with the CD4+ cell membrane to prevent cell entry.	enfuvirtide (Fuzeon) www.fuzeon. com	SC: 90 mg (1 mL) bid. Mix with 1.1 mL sterile water for injections. Rotate sites: upper arm, abdomen, upper thigh.	Local injection site reactions. Hypersensitivity reaction (rash, fever, nausea, vomiting, chills, rigor, hypotension), diarrhea, nausea, fatigue, bacterial pneumonia	Teach: Does not cure HIV. Must continue other HIV meds. Drug resistance can develop if used alone. Use aseptic technique for administering injections. If dizzy, do not drive.

CBC = complete blood count; CNS = central nervous system; GI = gastrointestinal.

TABLE 19.5 TREATMENT FOR AIDS-RELATED CONDITIONS

Opportunistic Infection/Complication	Treatment
Candidiasis	Nystatin, ketoconazole (Nizoral), fluconazole (Diflucan), amphotericin B (Fungizone)
Cytomegalovirus retinitis	Ganciclovir (Cytovene)
Hepatitis B virus	Hepatitis B virus vaccine when HIV infection diagnosed, unless already infected with hepatitis B
Hepatitis C virus	Interferon, lamivudine, tenofovir for infection; pegylated interferon and ribavirin
Herpes simplex, herpes zoster, varicella zoster	Acyclovir (Zovirax) therapy, valacyclovir, famciclovir, foscarnet
Influenza	Annual influenza vaccine
Mycobacterium avium complex	Azithromycin, clarithromycin, ethambutol
Pneumococcal pneumonia	Pneumococcal vaccine when HIV infection diagnosed
Pneumocystis carinii pneumonia	Trimethoprim-sulfamethoxazole (Bactrim, Septra), dapsone, atovaquone, pentamidine isethionate
Tuberculosis	PPd testing; drug therapy per CDC guidelines: pyrazinamide, isoniazid (Laniazid, Isotamine), ethambutol (Myambutol)
HIV wasting	Patient education: Eat three high-calorie and high-protein meals with snacks daily. Drink liquids before meals. Eat low-residue diet for diarrhea control. Control odors. Develop easy meal plan: favorite foods, meal programs, frozen dinners, cold food to control nausea. Use antiemetics, appetite stimulants, and/or testosterone. Rest, listen to music. Numb painful oral sores with ice, popsicles, or topical analgesic; avoid spicy foods. Use artificial saliva for dry mouth. Use nutritional supplements. Use food stamps, community food pantries, or free meal programs as needed. Exercise to increase muscle mass. Take medications prescribed to treat HIV wasting.

- Preventing the virus from attaching to the CD4+ receptor of the T-4 lymphocyte
- Interfering with "uncoating" of the virus within the cell, the first essential step in allowing the virus to integrate into the cell's DNA
- Inhibiting reverse transcriptase (RT), a viral enzyme specific to retroviruses, which enables the virus to make a DNA copy from single-stranded viral RNA prior to integration into cellular DNA
- Blocking viral regulatory and transactivating proteins, which are involved in the transcription and translation of viral RNA proteins from proviral DNA as the virus goes from the quiet, integrated state to active replication
- Inhibiting protease, a viral enzyme responsible for the adherence of viral proteins both before proviral integration and as the viral particles recombine into functional proteins needed for viral maturation
- Preventing viral assembly and budding out of the cell

For more information, visit the Medscape quick reference guide to antiretrovirals at www.medscape.com.

Highly Active Antiretroviral Therapy (HAART)

Aggressive treatment with multiple-drug therapy, aimed at reducing the viral load to an undetectable amount, is the most effective line of treatment for HIV. (See Table 19.4.) "Cocktails" of multiple antiretroviral drugs (i.e., HAART) have reduced viral loads in the bloodstream and increased CD4+ T-lymphocyte counts, resulting in prolonged survival. HAART, in use since 1996, has made monotherapy (using one drug) an outdated concept except for some cases involving pregnant women. Many combination drug regimens can be used. The use of HAART is important to help reduce drug resistance, which is a common cause of treatment failure. The major cause of drug resistance occurs when HAART is not taken as directed. "Adherence" is the word used to describe taking medications exactly as directed.

Many anti-HIV drugs have side effects. If they occur, the drug regimen may be changed or interventions may be used to help control side effects. The patient should be taught always to report side effects immediately, especially rashes (such as with trimethoprim-sulfamethoxazole) and abdominal pain (such as with zidovudine [AZT, Retrovir]); they could be serious and potentially life threatening.

Fusion Inhibitors

Fusion inhibitors (also referred to as entry inhibitors) are the newest class of antiretroviral agents. (See Table 19.4.) This is the first treatment to work outside the CD4+ cell by blocking HIV fusion with the CD4+ cell membrane and preventing cell entry. This prevents infection of healthy CD4 cells if HIV is not able to gain entry into the cell. This type of medication is used in combination therapy with other anti-HIV medications. Fusion inhibitors reduce the viral load (amount of HIV present in the blood) and increase CD4 cell levels. This type of drug can be helpful to those who have become resistant to other medications since it works in a different way than other medications. One drug, enfuvirtide (Fuzeon), has been approved by the Food and Drug Administration (FDA) for use while several others are in development. These drugs are given either by injection or intravenously.

Integrase Inhibitors

Integrase inhibitors, which block the third HIV enzyme integrase (protease and reverse transcriptase are the other two HIV enzymes), are a new class of drugs in development for the treatment of HIV.

Blocking integrase prevents the integration of the virus's DNA into the cell's chromosome. If this occurs, then the cell cannot be infected with HIV. Look for more information on the development of these drugs as it becomes available.

 NURSING MANAGEMENT

Nursing Process: The Adult Patient with HIV/AIDS

Assessment/Data Collection

Ongoing assessment is important for the patient with HIV/AIDS to detect problems early. Health history information is obtained (Box 19.5 Assessment: Health History Information for HIV/AIDS). Determining patient understanding of HIV/AIDS information is necessary for planning and teaching. A physical assessment provides data on the effects of HIV/AIDS and antiviral treatments. Assessing the patient's pain level is ongoing. It is helpful to have patients use standardized pain rating scales such as the Wong Baker faces scale. (See Chapter 9.) As the disease

progresses, patients may have more pain but reduced cognitive ability to express the pain level. Several types of standardized pain rating scales allow assessment of pain with reduced cognitive ability. Signs and symptoms of opportunistic diseases are noted.

Nursing Diagnosis

Nursing care is individualized to the patient's presenting symptoms. Primary nursing diagnoses for HIV/AIDS include:

- Risk for infection related to decreased immune function
- Impaired gas exchange related to respiratory infection
- Acute or chronic pain related to neuropathy, cancer, infection, or dyspnea
- Fatigue related to HIV infection and/or side effects of treatments
- Imbalanced nutrition: less than body requirements related to anorexia, nausea and vomiting, increased caloric need, diarrhea, dysphagia, oral lesions
- Impaired oral mucous membranes related to decreased immune function
- Diarrhea related to infection, medications

Box 19.5

Assessment: Health History Information for HIV/AIDS

Demographic data: Gender, age, marital status, occupation, residence
Date of diagnosis of HIV/AIDS
Past medical history and surgeries
Current health status and concerns
Allergies
Medications history of antivirals used with reason for discontinuing
Current medications, dose and frequency (including over-the-counter medication and supplements)
Immunizations
Family history
Height/weight: weight loss
Infections/cancers (see Box 19.1, CDC Conditions in the AIS Surveillance Case Definition)
Sexually transmitted diseases and treatments
Social history, sexual practices, risk behaviors, safe sex practices
Needle and blood exposure, injection drug use, blood transfusions/treatment for hemophilia
Tobacco use
Drug and alcohol use
Exercise and sleep
Pets
Occupational history
Nutrition history
Women's health, last Pap, ob/gyn

 LEARNING TIP

Key points to remember:
- HIV and AIDS are disease labels, not people labels.
- Each person reacts to an HIV or AIDS diagnosis differently.
- It is not HIV that ultimately causes death; it is compromised immunity and the invasion of an opportunistic infection or disease that the patient's body is unable to successfully fight off even with medical intervention.
- With today's current successful antiretroviral treatments, HIV has changed from being a life-ending infection to more of a chronic disease requiring constant management.

- Impaired skin integrity related to infection, cancer, immobility, incontinence
- Social isolation related to fear of disclosure of status, infection control, transmission of virus
- Risk for situational low self-esteem related to body image changes
- Deficient knowledge related to lack of prior experience with HIV/AIDS and treatment

Additional diagnoses may include:

- Anticipatory grieving related to loss of function or death
- Disturbed thought processes related to AIDS dementia
- Disabled family coping related to chronic, progressive disease
- Ineffective coping related to chronic progressive disease
- Ineffective sexuality pattern related to disease transmission
- Risk for injury related to weakness, fatigue, sedation, neurological impairment

See Box 19.6 Nursing Care Plan for the Patient with AIDS.

Implementation

HIV/AIDS affects every system of the body and every aspect of a person's life. Nurses have the opportunity to positively influence the patient's experience with HIV/AIDS with a nonjudgmental approach, empathy, and psychological support.

Box 19.6 NURSING CARE PLAN for the Patient with AIDS

Nursing Diagnosis: Risk for infection, nosocomial related to weakened immune system, skin breakdown, intravenous therapy, and possible invasive procedures

Expected Outcomes Patient will remain free of nosocomial infections. Patient will describe measures to maintain skin integrity and avoid infections.

Evaluation of Outcomes Is patient free of nosocomial infections? Can patient explain and demonstrate skin maintenance techniques?

Interventions	Rationale	Evaluation
Assess patient's risk factors, such as skin condition, laboratory results, portals of entry for infections, and presence of any infections.	Status of these assessment factors determines plan for care.	Does patient have intact skin or nonreddened, nonpurulent sites of interrupted integrity?
Caregivers should use standard precautions and strict aseptic technique for *all* patients and procedures.	Transmission of microorganisms can occur in both directions. Many patients with HIV are not aware of their HIV status	Do all caregivers use standard precautions?
Instruct visitors about techniques to avoid transmission of infection, such as hand washing and not visiting when they have an infection. The nurse with an infection, especially respiratory infection, should not care for patient with AIDS. (If must care for patient, wear a mask and explain why you are wearing mask.)	The immune system is damaged by HIV. Ability to combat infections may be severely compromised. A minor infection for most people may kill a person who has AIDS.	Do those with infections avoid contact with patient until their infection is resolved? Do laboratory tests indicate that patient is so immunocompromised that reverse isolation may be necessary?
Promote skin integrity by frequent turning, optimum mobilization, protective mattress and chair pads, application of emollient to dry areas, and prompt treatment of any injuries.	Skin is the body's first line of defense.	Does patient's skin remain intact and infection free?
Teach strategies for skin care and avoidance of infection to patient.	Self-care offers a measure of control in frequently uncontrollable situation.	Does patient satisfactorily explain or demonstrate good skin care and knowledge of how to avoid infection?

(Continued on following page)

Box 19.6   NURSING CARE PLAN **for the Patient with AIDS** *(Continued)*

Nursing Diagnosis: Risk for injury related to impaired mobility, weakness, fatigue, possible electrolyte imbalances, neurological impairment, and sedative effects of pain medications

Expected Outcomes Care and mobility needs will be met without injury.

Evaluation of Outcomes Does patient remain free from injury?

Interventions	Rationale	Evaluation
Assess patient's abilities and disabilities.	Particular disabilities may increase danger to patient.	Does patient have deficits?
Look for potential hazards in environment (hospital or home) and eliminate as many hazards as possible.	Awareness of hazards is necessary to decrease occurrence of accidents and injuries.	Are there any hazards in the environment presently?
Instruct patient about how to avoid hazards (if cognitively and physically able to comply).	Patients can help avoidance of injury if they understand hazards.	Is patient effectively avoiding hazards, or is patient a danger to self?
Encourage self-care as much as is feasible without tiring patient.	Self-care promotes feelings of self-efficacy and can combat depression.	Does patient evidence satisfaction with self-care efforts?
Assist with care activities as needed.	Varying levels of assistance with care are necessary due to the potentially debilitating nature of disease.	Are patient's care and mobility needs being met satisfactorily without injury?
Institute safety measures as required, such as close observation, frequent reorientation, two staff members for ambulation, use of side rails, bed motion alarm, or room near nurse's station.	Protection of patient against inadvertent removal of tubes or equipment, falls, and other injuries may require extraordinary measures due to neurological damage.	Are safety measures effective for patient? Does patient respond negatively to the protective measures? Can these be modified to be less offensive?

Nursing Diagnosis: Ineffective individual coping related to terminal disease and progressive debility

Expected Outcome Patient will show use of effective coping skills.

Evaluation of Outcome Does patient show use of effective coping skills?

Interventions	Rationale	Evaluation
Establish and maintain open and trusting therapeutic relationship.	Effective communication is based on trust—assurance of confidentiality is essential.	Does patient talk about concerns with nurse?
Allow grieving to take place (keeping a journal has been effective for some patients who have AIDS).	AIDS brings about losses of health, strength, employment, and in many cases friends and threatens one's sense of security and reasonableness of life. Healthy grieving is a natural coping response.	Is grief being expressed? Is patient finishing things that matter to him or her?
Encourage patient to express feelings and concerns. Contact counselor, chaplain, or AIDS support worker if patient so desires.	Talking about feelings and concerns helps defuse anger, clarify needs, and relieve tension.	How are family members, friends, and support persons interacting with patient? How is patient responding to family members, friends, and support persons?
Provide patient with desired information or refer to others who can supply information.	Knowledge dispels unreasonable fears and helps patient prepare adequately to cope with stressors.	Does patient evidence enough understanding of disease to be able to cope effectively?
Ask if patient would like information about support group and arrange such.	Social support can help patient cope.	Does patient show satisfaction with coping resources?

Source: Linda Hopper Cook.

RISK FOR INFECTION. To reduce infection risk, the patient should be taught to wash hands frequently, especially before eating and after toileting; bathe regularly; avoid sharing personal grooming items (e.g., toothbrush, toothpaste, razor); cleanse toothbrush; and wash all dishes between uses (Table 19.6). In addition, the patient is taught signs of infection to report to health-care provider immediately (Box 19.7 Patient Teaching: Signs and Symptoms of Oppotunistic Infections to Report). Treatment of opportunistic infections is most effective when begun early.

IMPAIRED GAS EXCHANGE. If a patient develops a con-

TABLE 19.6 PATIENT TEACHING: PREVENTING OPPORTUNISTIC INFECTIONS

Precaution Category	Reducing Exposure Risk	To Protect From
Environmental/ Occupational	Consider risk for exposure to infectious agents from the following: health-care setting, correctional facilities, homeless shelters.	Tuberculosis
	Child care settings: wash hands after diaper changing/body fluid contact.	CMV, cryptosporidiosis, hepatitis A, giardiasis
	Animal contact: exposure possible from veterinary work, pet stores, farms.	Cryptosporidiosis, toxoplasmosis, salmonellosis, campylobacteriosis
	Gardening/soil contact: avoid gardening/houseplant care/bird-roosting site, soil, cleaning chicken coops. Wear gloves and mask and wash hands after soil contact.	Cryptosporidiosis, toxoplasmosis, histoplasmosis, coccidioidomycosis
Food/water	General measures for home or restaurants include the following:	Foodborne and waterborne infections caused by bacterial, viral, protozoal, or parasitic pathogens
	Food handlers should practice good hand washing and hygiene.	
	Discard food past expiration date, dented or swollen cans.	
	Maintain adequate refrigeration and cooking temperatures.	
	Control insects and rodents to prevent food contamination.	
	Foods to avoid:	
	Raw/undercooked eggs and foods with raw eggs, such as hollandaise sauce, caesar dressing, mayonnaise, uncooked batters, ice cream, eggnog.	
	Raw/undercooked poultry, meat, seafood.	
	Unpasteurized milk/dairy products and fruit juice, raw seed sprouts.	
	Soft cheeses, which may harbor bacteria: fera, Brie, Camembert, blue veined, queso fresco.	
	Wash produce and avoid unwashed produce on salad bars.	
	Avoid cross contamination of foods with uncooked meat.	
	Cook meat until internal temperature is 180°F (82.2°C) for poultry, 165°F (73.8°C) for red meats, with no trace of pink.	
	Foods to avoid or cook until steaming hot: leftovers, ready-to-eat, delicatessen foods, refrigerated pates, and meat spreads.	Cryptosporidiosis, giardiasis
	Water safety:	
	Avoid public drinking fountains.	
	Avoid drinking or swallowing water directly from lakes or rivers.	
	Use safe water supply or boil water 1 minute when unsure.	
	Avoid beverages made from tap water in public places.	
	Drink bottled water purified from reverse osmosis, filtration through absolute 1-μm filter, or distillation (only safe methods). For information, contact www.bottledwater.org.	
	Bottled or canned carbonated soft drinks, commercially packaged nonrefrigerated beverages, pasteurized beverages, and beers are safe.	
Sexual	Always use latex condom for every sex act.	STDs, herpes simplex virus, cytomegalovirus, human papillomavirus, resistant HIV strain

(Continued on following page)

TABLE 19.6 PATIENT TEACHING: PREVENTING OPPORTUNISTIC INFECTIONS *(Cont'd)*

Precaution Category	Reducing Exposure Risk	To Protect From
	Avoid oral-anal contact or use dental dams; use latex gloves for hand-anal contact; wash hands and genitals with warm soapy water after contact.	Intestinal infections: amebiasis, hepatitis A, cryptosporidiosis, shigellosis, campylobacteriosis, giardiasis
	Get hepatitis A vaccine.	Hepatitis A
	Get hepatitis B vaccine	Hepatitis B
Injection drug use	Get hepatitis A and B vaccines.	Hepatitis A, hepatitis B, hepatitis C, resistant HIV strain
	Stop using injection drugs and enter substance abuse treatment.	
	If unable to stop, never reuse or share syringes, needles, water, or drug preparation equipment.	
	If shared, use bleach and water to clean equipment.	
	Use sterile syringes from pharmacies or community syringe exchange programs and dispose of safely.	
	Use clean water and equipment and new alcohol swab.	
Pet-related	Avoid pet feces/diarrhea; seek veterinary treatment for pet's illness.	*Cryptosporidium, Salmonella, Campylobacter* spp. infection
	Counsel on pet contact risks but recognize emotional benefits of pets. Pets should have up-to-date immunizations.	For new pet, avoid those younger than 6 months old (and cats younger than 1 year old); obtain pets from known sanitary source; avoid strays; wash hands after handling pets.
	Avoid exotic pets.	
	Cat ownership increases risk from litter box cleaning, scratches, bites, licking, fleas. If must clean litter box, wear mask and gloves and wash hands well afterward. Efforts should be made to keep cats indoors to avoid contact with infected prey.	Toxoplasmosis, *Bartonella* spp. infection, salmonellosis, campylobacteriosis
	Unhealthy birds may transmit infectious organisms.	*Cryptococcus neoformans, Mycobacterium avium, Histoplasma capsulatum* infection
	Avoid reptiles, turtles, chicks, and ducklings.	Salmonellosis
	Wear gloves for cleaning aquariums.	*Mycobacterium marinum* infection
Travel	Consult health-care providers on travel to developing countries.	Opportunistic pathogens, foodborne and waterborne infections
	Traveler's diarrhea prophylaxis is not recommended. Carry supply of antimicrobial agent to take for diarrhea.	
	Consider prophylaxis for other types of exposures.	
	Avoid raw fruits, vegetables, raw/undercooked seafood or meat, tap water, ice from tap water, unpasteurized milk/dairy products, items from street vendors.	
	Safe items include steaming-hot foods, self-peeled fruits, bottled (especially carbonated) beverages, hot coffee/tea, beer, wine, and water boiled 1 minute.	
	Avoid soil/sand contact by wearing shoes, using beach towels.	

CMV = cytomegalovirus; STD = sexually transmitted disease.

Source: Data from U.S. Department of Health and Human Services: 2001 USPHS/IDSA Guidelines for the Prevention of Opportunistic Infections in Persons Infected with Human Immunodeficiency Virus. http://hivatis. org, November 28, 2001.

dition that interferes with respiration, the goal is to maintain oxygenation within normal limits and reduce dyspnea. PCP is a respiratory infection with AIDS. (See Table 19.5.) Monitoring the patient's vital signs, including respiratory rate, depth, and rhythm and oxygen saturation, is important. Medications and oxygen therapy are given as ordered. Positioning the patient for comfort is often done by raising the head of the bed. Assisting with activities helps reduce fatigue.

PAIN. Pain may occur from a variety of causes. Treatment is focused on the cause to achieve pain control and relief. Medications may be given as ordered. Timing medication administration prior to planned activities is helpful in increasing ability to function. Complementary therapy may be used by patients. (See Chapter 4.) Measures such as heat or cold, massage, and frequent position changes may be helpful.

FATIGUE. Many patients with HIV experience fatigue. Other causes of fatigue include infections, medications, anemia, dehydration, depression, and poor nutrition. The patient can help manage fatigue by alternating periods of activity and rest. Tasks that use more energy should be planned at times when the patient is most energetic. Helping a patient prioritize activities is important in planning the best use of the energy available.

Box 19.7

Patient Teaching: Signs and Symptoms of Opportunistic Infections to Report

Instruct patient to monitor temperature daily and to report the following symptoms to a health care provider immediately:

New fever higher than 100°F (38.5°C) or a change in fever pattern if low-grade fevers are commonly present

Cough, shortness of breath, fever, or chest tightness, which may be signs of early pneumonia

Signs of central nervous system infection, such as severe headache; stiff neck; visual changes; problems with balance, walking, or speech; weakness of an arm or leg; and changes in moods or memory

Foul-smelling drainage or pus

Cloudy or foul-smelling urine

Signs of dehydration, such as a dry mouth, dark concentrated urine, or dizziness when standing

Diarrhea lasting longer than 48 hours; more than six stools a day; watery, mucous, or bloody stools

Rashes (possible side effect of medication)

Sore mouth or tongue, difficulty swallowing, white patches on tongue or back of mouth

Worsening fatigue

Change in vision and if floaters develop

IMBALANCED NUTRITION: LESS THAN BODY REQUIREMENTS. Maintaining general health and nutrition is important for a healthy immune system. For patients with HIV, maintaining health is vital. Patients with AIDS often have difficulty maintaining adequate nutrition and preventing weight loss. Many factors interfere with nutrition in HIV/AIDS (e.g., anorexia, oral lesions, nausea and vomiting, diarrhea, or wasting syndrome). The cause needs to be identified for appropriate intervention planning.

The patient's baseline weight is obtained. Then ongoing monitoring of the patient's weight, calorie intake, and intake and output is done. A dietitian is consulted to help plan nutritious and affordable meals. The patient should be on a high-calorie, high-protein diet. Small, frequent meals may be helpful. Vitamins, nutritional supplements, tube feedings, or parenteral nutrition (partial parenteral nutrition [PPN] or total parenteral nutrition [TPN]) may be needed to maintain adequate nutrition. Antiemetics are used to control nausea and vomiting. Medications that help stimulate appetite may be helpful. Easy to prepare meals are helpful when energy is limited. Creative interventions and resources may be needed to ensure the patient receives adequate nutrition. (See Table 19.5.) Along with adequate nutrition, exercise helps maintain muscle mass, promotes relaxation, aids sleep, and gives an individual a sense of control and well-being. An effective exercise program includes exercises that increase strength, flexibility, and endurance. Becoming physically fit is a lifestyle change that requires dedication.

IMPAIRED ORAL MUCOUS MEMBRANES. Oral or esophageal candidiasis is common. The painful lesions interfere with swallowing and nutrition. In patients with AIDS who smoke there is an increased incidence of oral thrush (candidiasis). Therefore, patients should be encouraged to quit smoking. Antifungal medication is given. Mouth care is very important. A soft toothbrush promotes comfort. Viscous lidocaine can be given to decrease pain during eating.

DIARRHEA. Diarrhea often occurs in the patient with HIV. Diarrhea can be caused by HIV infection, opportunistic infections, or antiretroviral treatments. An antimotility agent (diphenoxylate/atropine [Lomotil]) may be prescribed (except in salmonellosis). Consulting the dietitian may be helpful in making dietary changes that reduce diarrhea (e.g., low-residue diet, no dairy products, no spicy foods, no caffeine or alcohol). Sitz baths may be soothing. Thorough cleansing of the rectal area after each stool is a must. Ointments may be applied to protect and soothe the anal area from excoriation.

IMPAIRED SKIN INTEGRITY. There are many skin conditions that can occur with HIV infection. Medications can cause skin infections that can be life threatening and must be reported immediately. A dermatologist may need to be consulted to help diagnose and treat skin infections.

SOCIAL ISOLATION. Many patients with HIV/AIDS face discrimination, rejection, and isolation. The Americans with Disabilities Act (ADA) makes discrimination toward patients with HIV illegal. Relatives, friends, and others sometimes avoid or refuse to have anything to do with the person with HIV (Box 19.8 Ethical Considerations). Misunderstanding and fear lead to misuse of infection control procedures and increase a patient's isolation. Being knowledgeable about the transmission of HIV allows interaction with the patient to reduce feelings of isolation. Providing patient education to reduce fear of HIV transmission also decreases isolation. Care to maintain confidentiality is essential. Many patients with HIV do not share their diagnosis with family or friends who may visit when they are hospitalized.

RISK FOR SITUATIONAL LOW SELF-ESTEEM. Changes in self-esteem and self-concept occur from several of the effects of HIV infection. Patients often experience changes in their relationships with others and in day-to-day activities such as work. Major weight loss and changes in fat distribution from antiviral treatments, called lipodystrophy, may cause dramatic changes in appearance that alter body image and reduce self-esteem. Nurses can assist patients in maintaining self-esteem and self-concept by ensuring a climate of acceptance and promoting a trusting relationship. Patients should be encouraged to express feelings if ready and to identify positive aspects of self. Emotional and spiritual support of the patient can help improve self-esteem.

Stress impacts health. Having others to talk with and provide support is essential to stress management.

Box 19.8

Ethical Considerations

Caring for a Patient with AIDS

Edward Klee, 28, is hospitalized in a large research hospital in California. He is in the terminal stages of AIDS, with widespread metastatic cancer and lung infections. He wants to see his parents before he dies as he has not seen them for nearly 10 years when he was leaving for college. Edward grew up in a middle-class household deep in the heart of the Bible Belt of Oklahoma. His homosexuality was hidden from his friends, his schoolmates, and especially his family.

Even though he is dying, with no hope of another remission, Edward does not want his parents to know about his homosexuality or that he has a disease that still carries such a stigma. He feels that their rigid religious beliefs may push them towards disowning him. In addition, Edward is terrified of any scene they may make, and he was fearful that such an incident could influence his care. In order to prepare for their visit, Edward asks the licensed practical nurse/licensed vocational nurse (LPN/LVN) who is assigned to care for him to answer any of his parents' questions about his illness by telling them he has leukemia, pneumonia, or another rare disease that they would know nothing about. After the third day of visiting their severely ill son, Edward's parents approached the LPN/LVN, and with a stern tone asked, "Does our son have AIDS?"

• How should the LPN/LVN respond?
• To whom does the LPN/LVN owe the greatest obligation, the patient or his family?
• What principles are in conflict?
• What virtues play a role in this situation?

Use the decision-making model and determine several possible solutions for this situation.

Identifying and maintaining social networks is important. Patients should be taught a variety of relaxation strategies and techniques to reduce stress. Relaxation strategies can range from working on a favorite hobby to talking with friends. Relaxation techniques include progressive muscle relaxation and imagery to aid in relaxation. Stress management techniques are most effective when used every day, not just during times of stress.

DEFICIENT KNOWLEDGE. Extensive teaching is needed for patients to understand this chronic, life-threatening disease that alters everything in their lives. (See also the Prevention section.) Teaching needs to be evaluated for understanding and done as the patient is ready. Adherence to treatment and medication regimens is necessary to prevent infection and prolong the time before AIDS occurs.

MEDICATIONS. It is vital that medication doses not be missed; this must be stressed during patient teaching.

Teaching aids to assist patients in remembering to take their medications is very important. Encourage the patient to take medications exactly as instructed. If a dose is missed, it should be taken as soon as possible unless it is very close to the time of the next dose. Doses should not be doubled. Missing doses of medication could cause therapy failure because viral loads can increase and resistance develops. Tell the patient to consult the physician with any questions or side effects promptly. Many of these medications can cause severe reactions.

FOOD AND WATER SAFETY. Food and water safety is vital to an immunocompromised patient. Bacterial, viral, protozoal, or parasitic pathogens can cause foodborne and waterborne infections. The patient must be taught methods to prevent foodborne and waterborne infections for all phases of handling. (See Table 19.6.) Kitchen counters and food preparation appliances (e.g., cutting boards, can openers) should be disinfected. Freezing does not kill bacteria in foods. Foods should not be thawed at room temperature. Dating and using the oldest foods first is helpful. If symptoms of foodborne or waterborne infection develop (e.g., diarrhea, nausea, vomiting, abdominal cramps, headache, fever), teach patient to report them immediately. In certain areas of the country tap water is not safe. Patients may need to be taught to boil water for drinking and making ice cubes or to drink bottled water.

RESOURCES. Financial resources may need to be addressed so that food and medications can be obtained. Treatment can be expensive and the patient may be unable to work. However, with the new combination antiretroviral therapies, many individuals are now able to continue working longer. Referrals to financial resources and support groups can be important.

COMMUNITY AND HOME HEALTH CARE. During the course of HIV infection, the patient will be primarily at home and in the community. Hospitalization may be needed intermittently for acute illness. If the disease progresses, the patient may require more care from caregivers and home health nurses. The home health nurse provides physical care, establishes a therapeutic relationship with patients with AIDS and their significant others and family/friends, and coordinates care with other health-care team members (Home Health Hints). Caregivers should be assessed for caregiver role strain. Support services should be identified, such as community AIDS organizations, Meals on Wheels, respite care services, community mental health, and Internet support groups. Respite care provides the caregiver time away from the caregiver role to reduce stress. When a patient is terminal, comfort care and emotional support for the family are essential. Hospice care may be used at this time.

Evaluation

Patient goals are met if the patient remains free from infection and maintains desired quality of life and activities as long as possible. As the disease progresses, goals are met if the patient's needs are met and the patient's dignity is maintained.

CRITICAL THINKING

Zoe Sampson

■ Zoe, 22, is diagnosed as HIV positive. She is tearful and asks many questions.

1. How would you answer her questions?
   a. "Am I going to die?"
   b. "How is AIDS diagnosed?"
   c. "Can my boyfriend get it?"

2. What food and water safety methods would you teach her?

3. Years later Zoe loses weight and becomes malnourished. What interventions can you use to promote adequate nutrition?

Suggested answers at end of chapter.

Home Health Hints

- When providing patient care, wash hands frequently, follow standard precautions, and use plastic bags to contain soiled items or clothing.
- Teach patients with AIDS and their families how to properly clean and disinfect the home to prevent infections. The recommended disinfectant is a diluted bleach mixture that contains 1 part household bleach to 10 parts water.

- Wearing gloves, clean body fluid spills with soap and water.
- Flush body fluids, solid waste, and contaminated solutions down toilet.
- Use disinfectant to (a) disinfect spill areas; (b) clean toilet seats and bathroom fixtures; (c) clean inside the refrigerator to avoid mold growth.
- Rinse clothing and then wash separately from other clothes with 1 cup of bleach if soiled with blood, urine, feces, or semen.
- Patients with AIDS do not require separate sets of dishes or silverware. Dishes and silverware are washed in hot, soapy water and rinsed thoroughly or placed in dishwasher.
- Dispose of sharps (e.g., needles, razors) in a rigid labeled container (such as a tin can with a sealable lid). Add 1:10 bleach solution to disinfect. Tape the lid. Place in a bag and dispose of in the trash.
- Contaminated articles are disposed of by bagging in plastic and placing in the trash.
- Teach the family of a patient with AIDS which signs and symptoms to report to the physician or nurse immediately: fever; increased dyspnea; pain; change in sputum production; upper respiratory tract infection; pneumonia; respiratory distress syndrome; diarrhea five times a day or more for 5 days; uncontrolled weight loss greater than 10 pounds in the last month; persistent headaches; falling; seizures; mental status changes, including memory loss and personality changes; rashes and skin changes; difficulty swallowing; and problems with urination.

REVIEW QUESTIONS

1. The nurse would evaluate the patient as understanding modes of HIV transmission if the patient stated that the modes of HIV transmission include which of the following?
   a. Saliva, tears, fecal-oral contamination
   b. Close physical contact involving skin surfaces, mosquito bites
   c. Sharing towels, sharing eating utensils, skin contact
   d. Unprotected sex with HIV-infected partner, contact with infected blood/products

2. The nurse is teaching a patient about HIV testing. Place HIV diagnostic tests in the sequential order that they are performed.
   a. Western blot test
   b. Enzyme-linked immunosorbent assay (ELISA) test
   c. ELISA test is repeated

3. A patient who is newly diagnosed with HIV infection asks what his future health status will be. The best response for the nurse to give is based on the understanding that HIV disease and AIDS are now characterized as which of the following?
   a. An acute disease
   b. A life-ending disease
   c. A chronically managed disease
   d. A disease with remissions and exacerbations

Multiple response item. Select all that apply.
4. What should the nurse include in a teaching plan to prevent HIV infection?
   a. Caregiver may recap used needles
   b. Abstain from sexual intercourse
   c. Avoid injection drug use
   d. Avoid use of male or female condoms
   e. Autologous blood transfusion
   f. Test for HIV at time of labor

Multiple response item. Select all that apply.

5. Which of the following should the patient with HIV be taught to do to decrease risk of infections?
   a. Wash hands before eating
   b. Wash toothbrush
   c. Reuse dishes
   d. Buy prepared deli foods
   e. Report signs of infection
   f. May share razor with no visible blood

6. The nurse would recognize that the patient needs further reinforcement of knowledge if the patient stated that one of the goals of highly active antiretroviral therapy is which of the following?
   a. Reduce the viral load
   b. Improve survival rates
   c. Decrease CD4+ T lymphocytes
   d. Delay the progression of HIV disease

7. The nurse would recognize that the patient is having a reaction to zidovudine (AZT) if which of the following occurred?
   a. Rash
   b. Edema
   c. Abdominal pain
   d. Blurred vision

8. The nurse is to give lamivudine (3TC) 150 mg PO now and has available a 10 mg/mL oral solution. How many milliliters should the nurse give?
   _____mL

References

1. Centers for Disease Control and Prevention: Revised U.S. Public Health Service Recommendations for HIV Screening of Pregnant Women. MMWR, 50(RR19), 2001.

2. Centers for Disease Control and Prevention: Basic and Expanded HIV Postexposure Prophylaxis Regimens. MMWR 50(RR11), 2001.

Unit Four Bibliography

1. Arbuckle, MR, et al: Development of autoantibodies before the clinical onset of systemic lupus erythematosus. N Engl J Med 349:1526, 2003.
2. Fernandez, M, et al: Systemic lupus erythematosus in a multiethnic US cohort (LUMINA): XXI. Disease activity, damage accrual, and vascular events in pre- and postmenopausal women. Arthritis Rheum 52;1655–1664, 2005.
3. Hultsch, T, et al: Immunodulation and safty of topical calcineurin inhibitors for the treatment of atopic dermatitis. Dermatology 211:174–187, 2005.
4. Justesen, US: Therapeutic Drug Monitoring and Human Immunodeficiency Virus (HIV) Antiretroviral Therapy. Basic Clin Pharmacol Toxicol 98:20–31, 2006.
5. Koreck, A, et al: Intranasal phototherapy for the treatment of allergic rhinitis. Orv Hetil 146:965–969, 2005.
6. Kylma, J. Dynamics of hope in adults living with HIV/AIDS: a substantive theory. J Adv Nurs 52:620–630, 2005.
7. Kylma, J, et al: Dynamics of hope in HIV/AIDS affected people: an exploration of significant others' experiences. Res Theory Nurs Pract 17:191–205, 2003.
8. Lalezari JP, et al. A Phase II clinical study of the long-term safety and antiviral activity of enfuvirtide-based antiretroviral therapy. AIDS 17:691–698, 2003.
9. Lalezari JP, et al. Enfuvirtide, an HIV-1 fusion inhibitor, for drug-resistant HIV infection in North and South America. N Engl J Med 348:2175–2185, 2003.
10. Lawrence, D: Researchers discover susceptibility gene for lupus. Lancet 360:1399, 2002.
11. Mrus, JM, et al: Health values of patients coinfected with HIV/hepatitis C: are two viruses worse than one? Med Care 44:158–166, 2006.
12. National Institute of Arthritis and Musculoskeletal and Skin Diseases. Lupus: a patient careguide for nurses and other health professionals. NIH Publication No. 98-4262. Bethesda, MD, 2001.
13. O'Brien, K, et al: Progressive resistive exercise interventions for adults living with HIV/AIDS. Cochrane Database Syst Rev 18:CD004248, 2004.
14. Robin, BH, et al: Clinical significance of fever in the systemic lupus erythematosus patient receiving steroid therapy. Kidney Int 68:747–759, 2005.
15. Shmerling, RH: Autoantibodies in systemic lupus erythematosus—there before you know it. N Engl J Med 349:1499, 2003.
16. Shoenfeld, Y, and Katz, U: IVIg therapy in autoimmunity and related disorders: our experience with a large cohort of patients. Autoimmunity 38:123–137, 2000.
17. Stampley, CD, et al: HIV/AIDS among midlife African American women: an integrated review of literature. Res Nurs Health 28:295–305, 2005.
18. Vyse, TJ, et al: Mapping autoimmune disease genes in humans: lessons from IBD and SLE. Novartis Found Symp 267:94–107, 2005.
19. Werth, VP: Clinical manifestations of cutaneous lupus erythematosus. Autoimmune Rev 4:296–302, 2005.
20. Willemot P, and Klein MB. Prevention of HIV-associated opportunistic infections and diseases in the age of highly active antiretroviral therapy. Expert Rev Anti Infect Ther 2:521–32, 2004.
21. Wolosin RJ: HIV/AIDS patient satisfaction with hospitalization in the era of highly active antiretroviral therapy. J Assoc Nurses AIDS Care 16:16–25, 2005.
22. Wraith, DC, et al: Vaccination and autoimmune disease: what is the evidence? Lancey 362:1659, 2003.

SUGGESTED ANSWERS TO

CRITICAL THINKING

■ *Zoe Sampson*

1. a. There currently is no cure for HIV/AIDS; however, medications are available that slow the disease's progression and make HIV a manageable chronic illness. Research continues on finding improved treatments and search for a cure.

   b. AIDS is diagnosed when CD4+ T-lymphocyte counts are below 200 cells per microliter or CD4+ T-lymphocyte percentage is under 14 of total lymphocytes and an opportunistic clinical disease, as defined by the CDC, is present in an HIV-infected person.

   c. Yes, your boyfriend could become infected through exposure to your blood or vaginal secretions. You need to learn about preventive measures and discuss them with him. If you have had unprotected sex, he should be tested.

2. Food handlers must maintain good hand washing and hygiene practices. Discard food past the expiration date and dented or swollen cans. Ensure adequate refrigeration and cooking. Control insects and rodents to prevent food contamination. Avoid public drinking fountains. Drink purified bottled water if you live in areas of unsafe drinking water. Use a safe water supply or boil water 1 minute when unsure. Avoid unpasteurized milk, other dairy products, and fruit juice and raw seed sprouts. Avoid raw and undercooked eggs, meats, and seafood.

3. Eat three high-calorie, high-protein meals and snacks daily. Drink liquids before meals. Eat a low-residue diet for diarrhea control. Develop easy meal plan. Use antiemetics. Numb painful oral sores. Avoid spicy foods. Refer for food stamps/free meal programs if necessary. Engage in regular exercise.

unit FIVE

UNDERSTANDING THE CARDIOVASCULAR SYSTEM

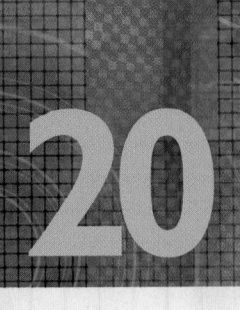

20

Cardiovascular System Function, Assessment, and Therapeutic Measures

LINDA S. WILLIAMS AND JANICE L. BRADFORD

KEY TERMS

atherosclerosis (ATH-er-oh-skle-ROH-sis)
bruit (brew-E)
cardioplegia (KAR-dee-oh-PLEE-jee-ah)
claudication (KLAW-di-KAY-shun)
clubbing (KLUB-ing)
dysrhythmias (dis-RITH-mee-yahs)
Homans' sign (HOH-manz SIGHN)
ischemic (iss-KEY-mik)
murmur (MUR-mur)
pericardial friction rub (PER-ee-KAR-dee-uhl FRIK-shun RUB)
poikilothermy (POY-ki-loh-THER-mee)
point of maximum impulse (POYNT OF MAKS-i-muhm IM-puls)
preload (PREE-lohd)
pulse deficit (PULS DEF-i-sit)
sternotomy (stir-NAH-tuh-mee)
thrill (THRILL)

QUESTIONS TO GUIDE YOUR READING

1. What is the normal anatomy of the cardiovascular system?

2. What is the normal function of the cardiovascular system?

3. What data should you collect when caring for a patient with a disorder of the cardiovascular system?

4. What are the diagnostic tests commonly performed to diagnose disorders of the cardiovascular system?

5. What nursing care should you provide for patients undergoing each of the diagnostic tests?

6. What are common therapeutic measures used for patients with disorders of the cardiovascular system?

7. What are the preoperative and postoperative routines and procedures for cardiac surgery?

REVIEW OF NORMAL ANATOMY AND PHYSIOLOGY

The cardiovascular system consists of the heart, blood, and blood vessels (including arteries, capillaries, and veins). Its function is to pump and distribute the blood throughout the body.

Heart

Cardiac Location and Pericardial Membranes

The heart is located in the mediastinum, the area between the lungs in the thoracic cavity. It is enclosed by three pericardial membranes that make up the pericardial sac. The outermost of these membranes is the fibrous pericardium, which forms a loose-fitting sac around the heart. The second, or middle, layer is the parietal pericardium, a serous membrane that lines the fibrous layer. The third and innermost layer, the visceral pericardium or epicardium, is a serous membrane on the surface of the heart muscle. Between the parietal and visceral layers is serous fluid, which prevents friction as the heart beats.

Cardiac Structure and Vessels

The walls of the four chambers of the heart are made of cardiac muscle (myocardium) and are lined with endocardium, which is smooth epithelial tissue that prevents abnormal clotting. The endocardium also covers the valves of the heart and continues into blood vessels as the lining. The coronary vessels include the arteries and capillaries that circulate oxygenated blood throughout the myocardium and the veins that return deoxygenated blood to the heart's interior chambers. The two main coronary arteries are the first branches of the ascending aorta, just outside the left ventricle (Fig. 20.1).

The upper chambers of the heart are the thin-walled right atrium and left atrium, which are separated by the interatrial septum. The lower chambers are the thicker walled right and left ventricles, which are separated by the interventricular septum. Each septum is made of myocardium that forms a common wall between the two chambers.

The right atrium receives deoxygenated blood from the upper body by way of the superior vena cava and from the lower body by way of the inferior vena cava. (See Fig. 20.1.) This blood flows from the right atrium through the tricuspid valve into the right ventricle. Backflow during ventricular systole (contraction and emptying) is prevented by the tricuspid, or right, atrioventricular (AV) valve (Fig. 20.2). The right ventricle pumps blood through the pulmonary semilunar valve to the lungs by way of the pulmonary artery. The pulmonary semilunar valve prevents backflow of blood into the right ventricle during ventricular diastole (relaxation and filling).

The left atrium receives oxygenated blood from the lungs by way of the four pulmonary veins. This blood flows through the mitral, or left, AV valve (also called the bicuspid valve) into the left ventricle. The mitral valve prevents backflow of blood into the left atrium during ventricular systole. The left ventricle pumps blood through the aortic semilunar valve to the body by way of the aorta. The aortic valve prevents backflow of blood into the left ventricle during ventricular diastole.

The tricuspid and mitral valves consist of three and two cusps, respectively. These cusps, or flaps, are connective tissue covered by endocardium and are anchored to the floor of the ventricle by the chordae tendineae and papillary muscles. The papillary muscles are columns of myocardium that contract along with the rest of the ventricular myocardium.

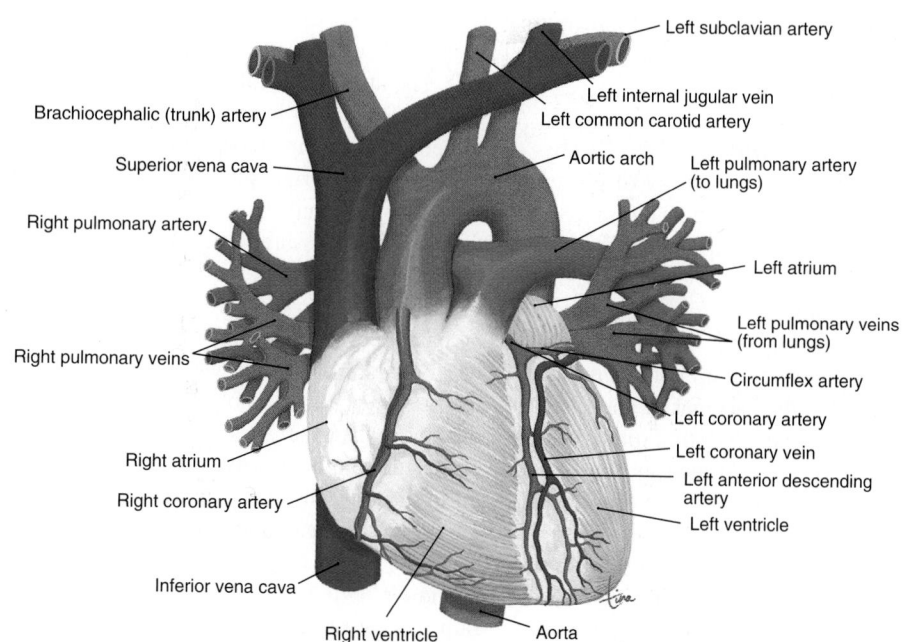

FIGURE 20.1 Anterior view of the heart and major blood vessels. *(From Scanlon, V, Sanders, T: Essentials of Anatomy and Physiology, ed 5. F.A. Davis, Philadelphia, 2007, p 276.)*

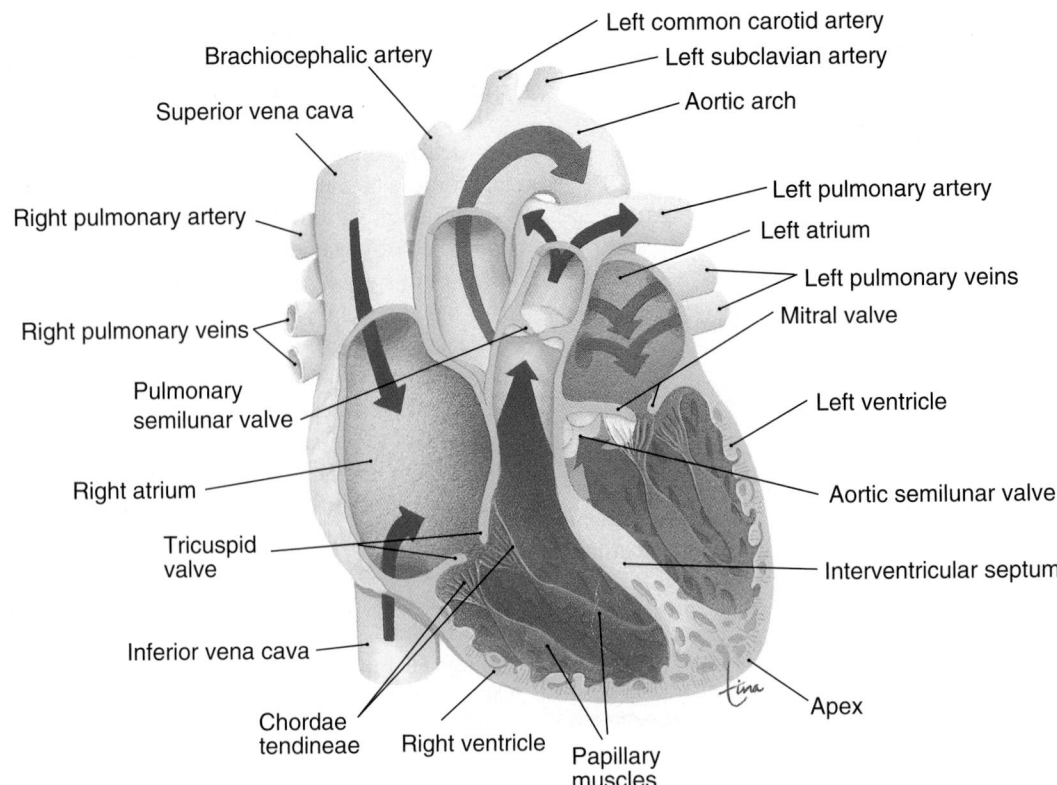

FIGURE 20.2 Frontal section of the heart showing internal structures and cardiac blood flow. *(From Scanlon, V, Sanders, T: Essentials of Anatomy and Physiology, ed 5. F.A. Davis, Philadelphia, 2007, p 276.)*

This contraction pulls on the chordae tendineae and prevents inversion of the AV valves during ventricular systole. (See Fig. 20.2.)

Although each ventricle pumps the same amount of blood, the much thicker walls of the left ventricle pump with approximately six times the force of the right ventricle to distribute the blood throughout the body. This difference in force is reflected in the great difference between systemic and pulmonary blood pressure.

Cardiac Conduction Pathway and Cardiac Cycle

The cardiac conduction pathway is the pathway of electrical impulses that generates a heartbeat. The sinoatrial (SA) node in the wall of the right atrium is a specialized mass of cardiac muscle that depolarizes rhythmically and most rapidly, about 100 times per minute, and therefore initiates each heartbeat. (While at rest, parasympathetic fibers dominate and slow the SA node to about 75 bpm.) For this reason, the SA node is sometimes called the pacemaker, and a normal heartbeat is called a normal sinus rhythm. From the SA node, impulses travel to the AV node located in the lower interatrial septum, to the atrioventricular bundle (bundle of His) in the upper interventricular septum, to the right and left bundle branches in the septum, and to the Purkinje fibers in the rest of the ventricular myocardium. If the SA node becomes nonfunctional, the AV node can initiate each heartbeat, but at a slower rate of 40 to 60 beats per minute. The bundle of His is capable of generating the beat of the ven-

tricles, but at the much slower rate of 20 to 35 beats per minute.

A cardiac cycle is the sequence of mechanical events during one heartbeat. Simply stated, the two atria contract simultaneously, followed a fraction of a second later by the simultaneous contraction of the two ventricles. The contraction, or systole, of each set of chambers is followed by relaxation, or diastole, of the same set of chambers.

The atria in diastole continually receive blood from the veins. As pressure in the atria increases, the AV valves are forced open, causing most of the blood to flow passively into the ventricles. Atrial systole pumps the remaining blood into the ventricles, and then the atria relax. Ventricular systole follows. The pressure in the ventricles causes the AV valves to close and forces the semilunar valves to open. Blood is then pumped into the aorta and pulmonary artery. There is no passive blood flow. Any blood leaving the ventricles must be pumped. Toward the very end of ventricular systole, as the pressure drops, the blood tends to flow backward within the two exiting arteries. It is this backflow of blood that closes the semilunar valves. The ventricles and atria are then all in diastole; the atria continue to fill until pressure opens the AV valves again, and the cycle is repeated.

The events of the cardiac cycle create the normal heart sounds. The first of the two major sounds (the lubb of lubb-dupp) is caused by the closure of the AV valves during ventricular systole. The second sound is created by the closure of the aortic and pulmonary semilunar valves.

Cardiac Output

Cardiac output is the amount of blood ejected from the left ventricle in 1 minute (the right ventricle pumps a similar amount). It is determined by multiplying stroke volume by heart rate. Stroke volume is the amount of blood ejected by a ventricle in one contraction and averages 60 to 80 mL/beat. With an average resting heart rate of 75 beats per minute, an average resting cardiac output is 5 to 6 L (approximately the total blood volume of an individual that is pumped within 1 minute). During exercise, venous return increases and stretches the ventricular myocardium, which in response contracts more forcefully. This is known as Starling's law of the heart, and the result is an increase in stroke volume. More blood is pumped with each beat, and at the same time, the heart rate increases, causing cardiac output to increase to as much as four times the resting level, and even more for athletes.

The ejection fraction is a measure of ventricular efficiency and is usually about 60%. It is the stroke volume divided by total blood in the ventricle (also known as the end-diastolic volume, which is approximately 120 to 130 mL). Lower values indicate that the ventricle is not pumping as forcefully and that more blood remains in the ventricle at the end of systole. The normal end-systolic volume is about 50 to 60 mL.

Regulation of Heart Rate

The heart generates its own electrical impulse, which begins at the SA node. The nervous system, however, can change the heart rate in response to environmental circumstances (Fig. 20.3). In the brain, the medulla contains the cardiovascular centers: the accelerator center and the inhibitory center. Sympathetic nerve impulses—along sympathetic nerves from the thoracic spinal cord to the SA node, AV node, and most of the myocardium—increase rate and force of contraction. Parasympathetic impulses—along the vagus nerve to the SA node, AV node, and atrial myocardium—decrease heart rate.

The information for changes necessary in the heart rate comes to the medulla from proprioceptors and from baroreceptors and chemoreceptors located in the internal carotid arteries and the aortic arch. The baroreceptors, specialized cells in the carotid and aortic sinuses, detect changes in blood pressure. The chemoreceptors are located in the carotid and aortic bodies and are cells specialized to detect changes in the oxygen content of the blood (as well as changes in carbon dioxide and hydrogen ion content). In response to either a drop in blood pressure or a decrease in blood oxygen level, the heart receives sympathetic impulses and beats faster in an attempt to provide sufficient oxygenation for tissues.

Hormones and the Heart

The hormone epinephrine, secreted by the adrenal medulla in stressful situations, is sympathomimetic in that it increases the heart rate and force of contraction and it dilates the coronary vessels. This in turn increases cardiac output and systolic blood pressure.

Aldosterone, a hormone produced by the adrenal cortex, is important for cardiac function because it helps regulate blood levels of sodium and potassium, both of which are needed for the electrical activity of the myocardium. The

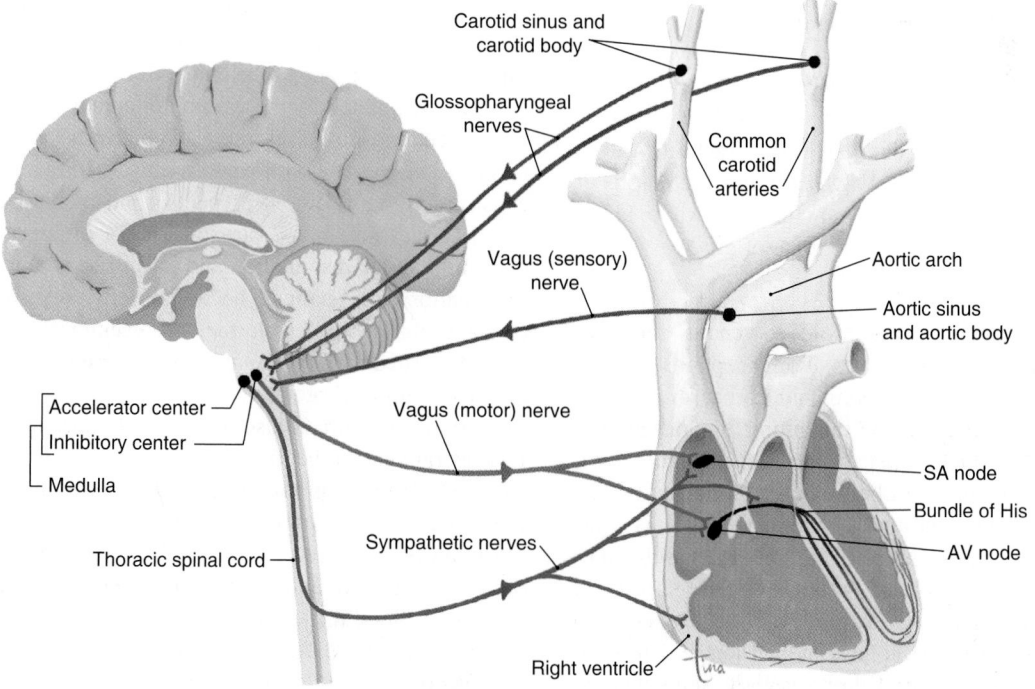

FIGURE 20.3 Nervous system regulation of the heart. *(From Scanlon, V, Sanders, T: Essentials of Anatomy and Physiology, ed 5. F.A. Davis, Philadelphia, 2007, p 285.)*

blood level of potassium is especially critical because even a small deficiency or excess impairs the rhythmic contractions of the heart.

The atria of the heart secrete a hormone of their own called atrial natriuretic peptide (ANP) or atrial natriuretic hormone (ANH). As its name suggests, ANP increases the excretion of sodium by the kidneys, by inhibiting secretion of aldosterone by the adrenal cortex. Atrial natriuretic peptide is secreted when a higher blood pressure or greater blood volume stretches the walls of the atria. The loss of sodium is accompanied by the loss of more water in urine, which decreases blood volume and therefore blood pressure as well.

Blood Vessels

Arteries and Veins

Arteries and arterioles carry blood from the heart to capillaries. Their walls are relatively thick and consist of three layers. Arteries carry blood under high pressure, and the outer layer of fibrous connective tissue prevents rupture of the artery. The middle layer of smooth muscle and elastic connective tissue contributes to the maintenance of normal blood pressure (BP), especially diastolic BP, by changing the diameter of the artery. The diameter of arteries is regulated primarily by the sympathetic division of the autonomic nervous system. By use of the smooth muscle, the arteries can also alter where the greatest volume of blood is directed. The lining is simple squamous epithelium, called endothelium, which is very smooth to prevent abnormal clotting.

Veins and venules carry blood from capillaries to the heart. Their walls are relatively thin because there is less smooth muscle (veins do not have as important a role in the maintenance of BP as arteries). Sympathetic impulses can bring about extensive constriction of veins, however, and this becomes important in situations such as severe hemorrhage. The lining of veins is, again, endothelium that prevents abnormal clotting; at intervals it is folded into valves to prevent backflow of blood. Valves are most numerous in the veins of the extremities, especially the legs, where blood must return to the heart against the force of gravity.

Capillaries

Capillaries carry blood from arterioles to venules and form extensive networks in most tissues. The exceptions are cartilage, the epidermis, and the lens and cornea of the eye. Their walls, a continuation of the lining of arteries and veins, are one cell thick to permit the exchanges of gases, nutrients, and waste products between the blood and tissues (Fig. 20.4). Blood flow through a capillary network is regulated by a precapillary sphincter, a smooth muscle fiber ring that contracts or relaxes in response to tissue needs. In an active tissue such as exercising skeletal muscle, for example, the rapid oxygen uptake and carbon dioxide production causes dilation of the precapillary sphincters to increase blood flow. At the same time, precapillary sphincters in less active tissues constrict to reduce blood flow. This is important because there is not enough blood in the body to fill all the capillaries at once; the fixed volume must constantly be shunted or redirected to where it is needed most.

The blood pressure in capillaries is 30 to 35 mm Hg at the arterial end of the network, and it drops to about 15 mm Hg at the venous end. This pressure is low enough to prevent rupture of the capillaries but high enough to permit filtration. Tissue fluid is formed from the plasma in capillaries by the process of filtration. Because capillary blood pressure is higher than the pressure of the surrounding tissue fluid, plasma and dissolved materials such as nutrients are forced through the capillary walls to become tissue fluid. Some of this tissue fluid returns to the capillaries, and some is collected in lymph capillaries. Now called lymph, it too is returned to the blood by the system of lymph vessels. Should blood pressure within the capillaries increase, more tissue fluid than usual is formed, which is too much for the lymph vessels to collect. This is called edema.

Blood Pressure

Blood pressure is the force of the blood against the walls of the blood vessels and is measured in millimeters of mercury (mm Hg), systolic over diastolic. The normal range of systemic arterial pressure is 90 to 135/60 to 85 mm Hg. Blood pressure decreases in the arterioles and capillaries, and the systolic and diastolic pressures merge into one pressure. As blood enters the veins, BP decreases further and approaches zero as it flows into the right ventricle. As mentioned previously, the blood pressure in the capillaries is of great importance, and normal blood pressure is high enough to permit filtration for nourishment of tissues but low enough to prevent rupture.

The arteries and veins are usually in a state of slight constriction that helps to maintain normal blood pressure, especially diastolic pressure. This is called peripheral resistance; it is regulated by the vasomotor center in the medulla, which generates impulses along sympathetic vasoconstrictor nerves to all vessels with smooth muscle to maintain slight constriction. More impulses per second increase vasoconstriction and raise blood pressure; fewer impulses per second bring about vasodilation and lower blood pressure. The information for changes needed in the vessel diameter comes to the medulla from the baroreceptors and chemoreceptors located in the internal carotid arteries and aortic arch and from proprioceptors.

Blood pressure is also affected by many other factors. If heart rate and force increase, blood pressure increases to a limit. If the heart is beating very fast, the ventricles are not filled before they contract, cardiac output decreases, and blood pressure drops. The strength of the heart's contractions depends on adequate venous return, which is the amount of blood that flows into the atria. Decreased venous return results in weaker contractions.

Venous return depends on several factors: constriction of the veins so that blood does not pool in them, the skeletal muscle pumping to squeeze the deep veins of the legs, and the muscles of respiration compressing the veins in the chest

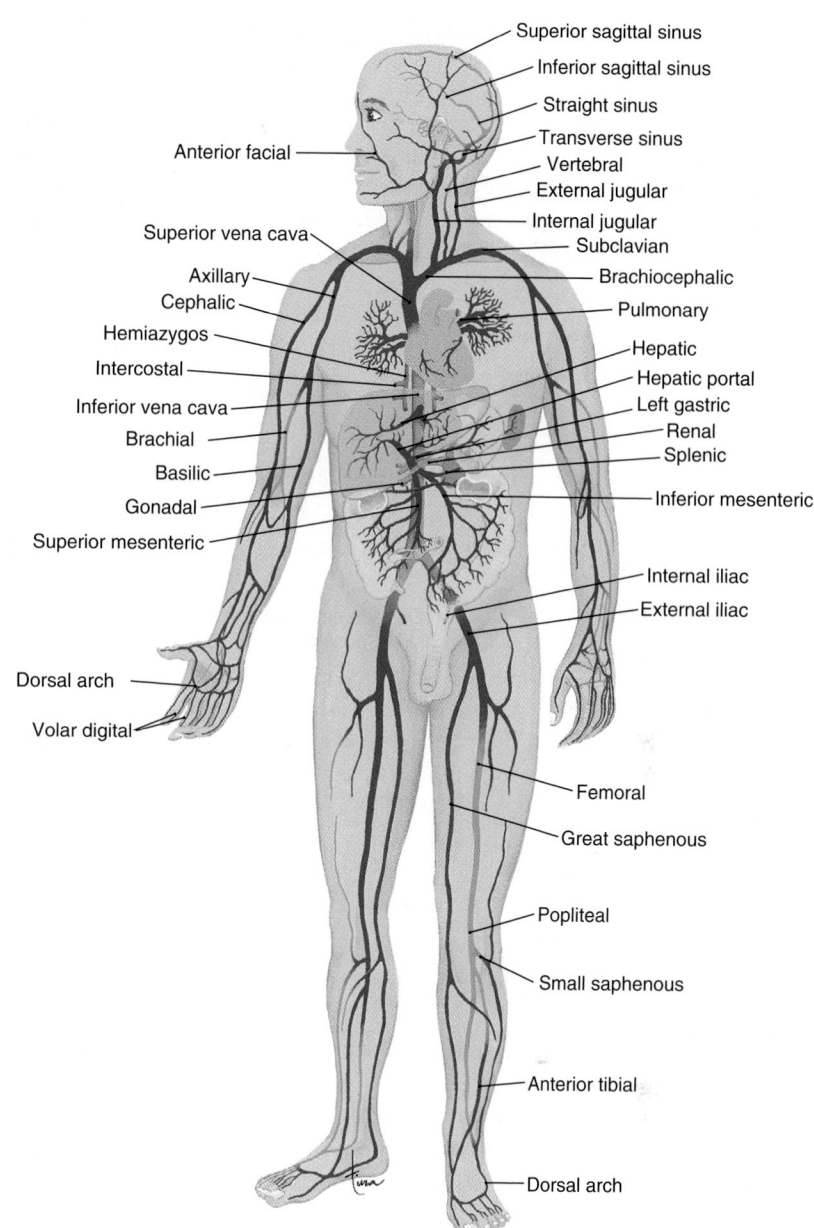

FIGURE 20.4 Systemic veins shown in anterior view. *(From Scanlon, V, Sanders, T: Essentials of Anatomy and Physiology, ed 5. F.A. Davis, Philadelphia, 2007, p 298.)*

cavity. The valves in the veins prevent backflow of blood and thus contribute to the return of blood to the heart.

The elasticity of the large arteries also contributes to normal blood pressure. When the left ventricle contracts, the blood stretches the elastic walls of the large arteries, which absorb some of the force. When the left ventricle relaxes, the arterial walls recoil or snap back and put pressure on the blood. Normal elasticity, therefore, lowers systolic pressure, raises diastolic pressure, and maintains normal pulse pressure. Pulse pressure is the difference between the systolic and diastolic pressures. The usual ratio of systolic to diastolic to pulse pressure is 3:2:1.

Renin-Angiotensin-Aldosterone Mechanism

The kidneys are of great importance in the regulation of blood pressure. If blood flow through the kidneys decreases, renal filtration decreases and urinary output decreases to preserve blood volume. Decreased blood pressure stimulates the kidneys to secrete renin, which initiates the renin-angiotensin-aldosterone mechanism (Fig. 20.5). Renin splits the plasma protein angiotensinogen (from the liver) to form angiotensin I, which is changed to angiotensin II by a converting enzyme found primarily in lung tissue. Angiotensin II causes arteriole vasoconstriction and stimulates secretion of aldosterone, both of which raise blood pressure.

Aldosterone, secreted by the adrenal cortex, increases the reabsorption of sodium ions by the kidneys. Water follows the sodium back to the blood; this increases blood volume and blood pressure. Other hormones that affect BP include those of the adrenal medulla: norepinephrine, which causes vasoconstriction throughout the body, and epinephrine, which increases cardiac output and causes vasoconstriction in skin and viscera. Antidiuretic hormone (ADH), from the posterior pituitary, directly increases water reab-

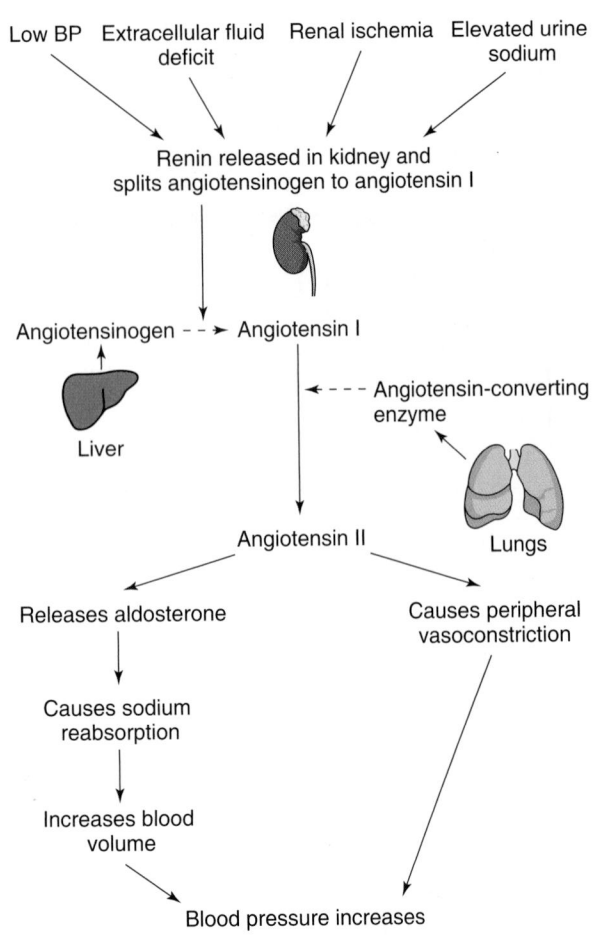

Low BP   Extracellular fluid   Renal ischemia   Elevated urine
                deficit   sodium

Renin released in kidney and
splits angiotensinogen to angiotensin I

Angiotensinogen - - ▶ Angiotensin I

                              ◀ - - - Angiotensin-converting
                                              enzyme

Liver

Angiotensin II   Lungs

Releases aldosterone   Causes peripheral
                                          vasoconstriction

Causes sodium
reabsorption

Increases blood
volume

Blood pressure increases

FIGURE 20.5 The renin-angiotensin-aldosterone mechanism.

sorption by the kidneys, thus increasing blood volume and blood pressure. Atrial natriuretic peptide, secreted by the atria of the heart, inhibits aldosterone secretion and thereby increases renal excretion of sodium ions and water, which decreases blood volume and subsequently blood pressure.

Pathways of Circulation

The two pathways of circulation are pulmonary and systemic (see Fig. 20.2). Pulmonary circulation begins at the right ventricle, which pumps deoxygenated blood into the pulmonary artery. The pulmonary artery branches into two arteries, one to each lung. The pulmonary capillaries around the alveoli of the lungs are the site of gas exchange. Oxygenated blood returns to the left atrium by way of the pulmonary veins. The blood pressure in the pulmonary circulation is always low because the right ventricle pumps with only about one-sixth the force of the left ventricle. The pulmonary arterial pressure is approximately 20 to 25 over 8 to 10 mm Hg, and the pulmonary capillary pressure is lower still. This is important to prevent filtration in pulmonary capillaries, which keeps tissue fluid from accumulating in the alveoli of the lungs, causing pulmonary edema.

Systemic circulation begins in the left ventricle, which pumps oxygenated blood into the aorta, the many branches

of which eventually give rise to capillaries within the tissues. Deoxygenated blood returns to the right atrium by way of the superior and inferior vena cava and the coronary sinus. The hepatic portal circulation is a special part of the systemic circulation in which blood from the capillaries of the digestive organs and spleen flows through the portal vein and into the capillaries (sinusoids) in the liver before returning to the heart. This pathway permits the liver to regulate the blood levels of nutrients such as glucose, amino acids, and iron and to remove potential toxins such as alcohol or medications from circulation.

Aging and the Cardiovascular System

It is believed that the "aging" of blood vessels, especially arteries, begins in childhood, although the effects are not apparent until later in life (Fig. 20.6). **Atherosclerosis** is the deposition of lipids in the walls of arteries over a period of years, which can narrow their lumens and form rough surfaces that may stimulate intravascular clot formation. Atherosclerosis decreases blood flow to the affected organ: cerebral flow can diminish by 20% and renal flow by 50% by age 80.[1] With age, the heart muscle becomes less efficient, and there is a decrease in both maximum cardiac output and heart rate, although resting levels may be more than sufficient (Box 20.1 Gerontological Issues). Valves may become thickened by fibrosis, leading to heart **murmur.**

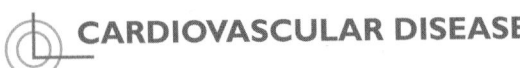 CARDIOVASCULAR DISEASE

According to statistics of the American Heart Association, cardiovascular disease is still the number one killer of people in the United States, being responsible for 1.0 of every 2.6 U.S. deaths.[2] In 2002, the single leading cause of death in America was coronary heart disease.[2] About 335,000 people a year die of cardiovascular disease either in the emergency room or without ever reaching the hospital, usually due to a heart attack and ventricular fibrillation or tachycardia.[2]

In women, the greatest cause of death is cardiovascular disease. The effect of cardiovascular disease in women has been understudied, but more attention is now being focused n this. There is a movement called Go Red for Women to give women encouragement and tools to prevent cardiovascular disease and live healthy. For more information on Go Red for Women, visit www.americanheart.org. Women can further reduce their risk for cardiovascular disease through the American Heart Association's free program Simple Solutions at www.americanheart.org/simplesolutions.

Lifestyle plays a major role in risk factors for cardiovascular disease. Smoking contributes to approximately one in five cardiovascular disease deaths. Dietary fat intake

---

atherosclerosis: athere—porridge + sklerosis—hardness

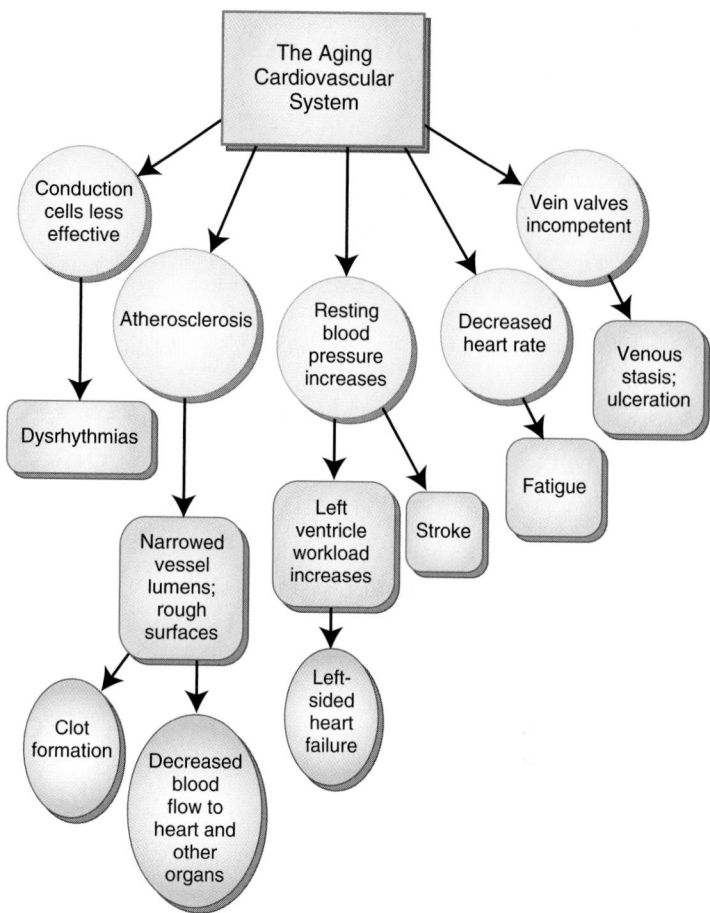

FIGURE 20.6 Aging and the cardiovascular system. This concept map shows the effects the aging process has on the cardiovascular system

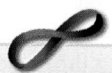

Box 20.1

Gerontological Issues

The older adult is at increased risk for developing orthostatic hypotension, which could precipitate a fall. This is often due to a combination of age related changes, immobility, chronic illnesses, and medications.

accounts for approximately 34% of the American diet, which increases cholesterol. Eating two servings weekly of oily fish like tuna or salmon is recommend by the American Heart Association. Exercise needs to be promoted for all, including children, as Americans continue to be sedentary. For more information on cardiovascular disease statistics, visit www.americanheart.org.

NURSING ASSESSMENT OF THE CARDIOVASCULAR SYSTEM

Nursing assessment of the cardiovascular system includes a patient health history and physical examination (Box 20.2 Gerontological Issues). If the patient is experiencing an acute problem, focus on the most serious signs and symptoms and physical assessment data until the patient is stabi-

lized (Table 20.1). An in-depth nursing assessment can be completed when the patient is stable. For stable or chronic cardiac conditions, a complete nursing assessment is done on admission.

Subjective Data

To understand the patient's cardiovascular problems, ask about past and current symptoms, use of prescribed and over-the-counter medications, use of recreational drugs, surgeries, treatments, and such risk factors as diet, activity, tobacco use, and recent stressors. Assessment of symptoms includes asking questions for WHAT'S UP?: where it is, how it feels, aggravating and alleviating factors, timing, severity, useful data for associated symptoms, and perception by the patient of the problem.

Box 20.2

Gerontological Issues

Older adults commonly have signs and symptoms that are not typical of a disorder. For example, the only symptom of myocardial infarction in an older patient may be dyspnea. Chest pain, a typical symptom, may not be present.

TABLE 20.1 ACUTE CARDIOVASCULAR NURSING ASSESSMENT

History	Significance
Allergies	For medication administration, diagnostic dyes
Smoking history	Risk factor for cardiovascular disorders
Medications	Toxic levels; influencing symptoms
Pain	Location—chest, calf; radiation—arms, jaw, neck; description—pressure, indigestion, tightness, burning, angina, myocardial infarction, thrombus, embolism
Dyspnea	Left-sided heart failure; pulmonary edema or embolism
Fatigue	Decreased cardiac output
Palpitations	Dysrhythmias
Dizziness	Dysrhythmias
Weight gain	Right-sided heart failure
Physical Assessment	**Possible Abnormal Findings**
Vital signs	Bradycardia, tachycardia, hypotension, hypertension, tachypnea, apnea, shock
Heart rhythm	Dysrhythmias
Edema	Right-sided heart failure
Jugular vein distention	Right-sided heart failure
Breath sounds	Crackles, wheezes with left-sided heart failure
Cough, sputum	Acute heart failure—dry cough, pink frothy sputum

Health History

All body systems can be affected by cardiovascular problems. Some symptoms can occur due to more than one cause. For example, shortness of breath can be the result of either heart failure or chronic obstructive pulmonary disease. The health history helps determine the cause of the symptom. For cardiovascular problems, the assessment focuses on the areas listed in Table 20.2.

MEDICAL HISTORY. If previous medical records are available, they can provide objective patient data that can be supplemented with patient responses. If medical records are not available, the patient is asked about previous conditions that could affect the cardiovascular system. A history of childhood illnesses that can lead to heart disease, such as rheumatic fever or scarlet fever, is noted. Other conditions include pulmonary disease, hypertension, kidney disease, cerebral vascular accident or brain attack, transient **ischemic** attack, renal disease, anemia, streptococcal sore throat, congenital heart disease, thrombophlebitis, and alcoholism. Patient allergies, previous hospitalizations, and surgeries are documented. Baseline diagnostic tests are helpful for comparison with current tests. Functional limitations that are related to cardiovascular problems, such as performing activities of daily living (ADLs), walking,

---

ischemic: ischein—hold back + haima—blood

---

climbing stairs, or completing household tasks, are also assessed.

MEDICATIONS. Medication use is noted. This includes prescription drugs, over-the-counter medications such as aspirin that can prolong clotting time, and recreational drugs. The medication history includes the patient's understanding of the medication and the medication name, dosage, reason for taking, last dose, and length of use.

FAMILY HISTORY. A family history of cardiovascular conditions is assessed because many cardiac problems are hereditary. Health histories of close relatives, such as parents, siblings, and grandparents, are the most significant. For example, those who have had a parent die of sudden cardiac death prior to age 60 are at increased risk for sudden cardiac death.

HEALTH PROMOTION. Risk factors such as diet, activity, tobacco use, and recent stressors for the patient are assessed in the health history. The patient's health promotion activities are noted, especially for risk factors that are modifiable through changes in lifestyle.

Objective Data

Physical Assessment

The patient's general appearance is observed. The patient's level of consciousness, which is an indicator of oxygenation of the brain, is assessed. Height and weight are recorded. Vital signs are measured.

BLOOD PRESSURE. For accurate measurement, the correct size cuff for the patient is used. Normal blood pressure is considered less than 120/80 (see Chapter 21). Readings in both arms are done for comparison. A difference in the readings is reported to the physician. The arm with the higher reading is used for ongoing measurements. If necessary, blood pressure may be measured in the leg using a larger blood pressure cuff. The reading in the leg is normally 10 mm Hg higher than in the arm.

Blood pressure measurements are done with the patient lying, sitting, and standing to detect abnormal variations with postural changes. When the patient sits or stands, a drop in the systolic pressure of up to 15 mm Hg and either a drop or slight increase in the diastolic pressure of 3 to 10 mm Hg is normal. In response to the drop in blood pressure, the pulse increases 15 to 20 beats per minute to maintain cardiac output. Orthostatic hypotension, also referred to as postural hypotension, is a greater than normal change in these pressures and indicates a problem that should be investigated by the physician (Box 20.3). The patient may experience dizziness when changing positions, so fall prevention methods should be used during blood pressure measurement.

PULSES. The apical pulse is auscultated for 1 minute to assess rate and rhythm. Normal heart rate is 60 to 100 beats per minute. In athletic people, the heart rate is often slower, around 50 beats per minute, because the well-conditioned

TABLE 20.2 CARDIOVASCULAR HISTORY ASSESSMENT

Question	Rationale
	Pain: WHAT'S UP? Format
• Where is pain? Does it radiate?	• Cardiac pain may radiate to shoulders, neck, jaw, arms, or back. Vascular disorders cause extremity pain.
• How does it feel? Discomfort, burning, aching, indigestion, squeezing, pressure, tightness, heaviness, numbness in chest area? Fullness, heaviness, sharpness, throbbing in legs?	• Pain can be associated with angina or MI. The quality of pain varies. Venous pain is a fullness or heaviness. Sharpness or throbbing is arterial pain.
• Aggravating/alleviating factors that increase/relieve the pain?	• Activity may cause or increase angina. Rest or medications may relieve angina. Leg activity pain, intermittent claudication, results from decreased perfusion that is aggravated by activity. Rest pain, from severe arterial occlusion, increases when lying. Dangling reduces the pain because blood flow is increased by gravity.
• Timing of pain: onset, duration, frequency?	• Pain may be continuous, intermittent, acute, or chronic. Arterial occlusion causes acute pain.
• Severity of pain?	• Rate pain on a scale of 0 to 10.
• Useful data for associated symptoms?	• Accompanying symptoms and their characteristics guide diagnosis and treatment.
• Perception of patient about problem?	• Patient's insight to problem is helpful in planning care.
	Level of Consciousness (LOC)
• What is your name? What is the month? Year? Where are you now?	• A lack of oxygen caused by cardiac disease can decrease LOC.
	Dyspnea
• Are you short of breath? What increases your shortness of breath? What relieves your shortness of breath?	• Dyspnea can be present with heart failure that reduces cardiac output, on exertion in angina pectoris or from a pulmonary embolus resulting from thrombophlebitis, heart failure, or dysrhythmias.
	Palpitations
• Are you having palpitations or irregular heartbeat? Does your heart ever race, skip beats, or pound?	• Palpitations can occur from dysrhythmias resulting from ischemia, electrolyte imbalance, or stress. Dizziness can be associated with dysrhythmias.
	Fatigue
• Have you noticed a change in your energy level?	• Fatigue occurs from reduced cardiac output resulting from heart failure.
• Are you able to perform activities that you would like to?	• Functional abilities can be limited from fatigue.
	Edema
• Have you had any swelling in your feet, legs, or hands?	• Right-sided heart failure can cause fluid accumulation in the tissues.
• Have you gained weight?	• Fluid retention causes weight gain.
	Paresthesia/Paralysis
• Any numbness, tingling, or other abnormal sensations in extremities?	• Numbers and tingling, pins and needles, and crawling sensations are paresthesia.
• Can you move your extremity?	• Paralysis is inability to move extremity. Reduced nerve conduction from decreased oxygen supply causes paresthesia and paralysis.

heart pumps more efficiently. Apical pulse rhythm is documented as regular or irregular. The apical rate can be compared with the radial rate to assess equality. If there are fewer radial beats than apical beats, a **pulse deficit** exists and should be reported to the physician.

Arterial pulses are palpated for volume and pressure quality. They are palpated bilaterally and compared for equality. A normal vessel feels soft and springy. A sclerotic vessel feels stiff. The quality of the pulses is described on a 4-point scale as follows: 0 is absent; 1+ is weak, thready; 2+ is normal; and 3+ is bounding. An absent pulse is not palpable. A thready pulse is one that disappears when slight pressure is applied and returns when the pressure is removed. The normal pulse is easily palpable. The bounding pulse is strong and present even when slight pressure is applied. When the normal vessel is palpated, a tapping is felt. In the abnormal vessel that has a bulging or narrowed wall, a vibration is felt, which is called a **thrill.** When aus-

SAFETY TIP

Anticipate potential drops in blood pressure with position changes. Orthostatic, or postural, hypotension is a drop in systolic blood pressure greater than 15 mm Hg, a drop or slight increase in the diastolic blood pressure greater than 10 mm Hg, and an increase in heart rate greater than 20 beats per minute in response to the drop in blood pressure. It can be found in patients of any age but is most commonly found in the older patient. The patient often reports light-headedness or syncope because the drop in pressure decreases the amount of oxygen-rich blood traveling to the brain. The change from a lying to a sitting or a sitting to a standing position may cause the drop in pressure. This blood pressure drop increases the risk of fainting and falling. Factors that can contribute to orthostatic hypotension include fluid volume deficit, diuretics, analgesics, and pain. Use fall precautions for patients at risk of or with orthostatic hypotension.

cultating an abnormal vessel, a humming is heard that is caused by the turbulent blood flow through the vessel. This is referred to as a **bruit.**

RESPIRATIONS. The rate and ease of respirations are observed. Breath sounds are auscultated. Sputum characteristics such as amount, color, and consistency are noted. Pink, frothy sputum is an indicator of acute heart failure. A dry cough can occur from the irritation caused by the lung congestion resulting from heart failure.

INSPECTION. During the health history, inspection begins by noting any shortness of breath when the patient speaks or moves. The patient's skin is noted for oxygenation status through the color of skin, mucous membranes, lips, ear lobes, and nailbeds. Pallor may indicate anemia or lack of arterial blood flow. Cyanosis shows an oxygen distribution deficiency. A reddish brown discoloration (rubor) found in the lower extremities occurs from decreased arterial blood flow. A brown discoloration and cyanosis when the extremity is dependent may be seen in the presence of venous blood flow problems. Hair distribution on the extremities is observed. Decreased hair distribution, thick, brittle nails, and shiny, taut, dry skin occur from reduced arterial blood flow. Venous blood return is assessed by inspecting extremities for varicose veins, stasis ulcers, or scars around the ankles and signs of thrombophlebitis such as swelling, redness, or a hard, tender vein.

The internal and external jugular neck veins are observed for distention. Normally, in the upright position, the veins are not visible. Distention of the veins in an upright position of 45 to 90 degrees indicates an increase in the

Box 20.3

Orthostatic Hypotension Assessment

To assess orthostatic hypotension:

1. Use correct size blood pressure cuff.
2. Explain procedure to patient; determine if patient can safely stand.
3. Have patient lie flat in bed at least 5 minutes prior to readings.
4. Patient should not eat or smoke 30 minutes before readings; patient should not talk during readings and should sit up with legs uncrossed while sitting.
5. Take patient's lying blood pressure and heart rate.
6. Assist patient to sitting position. Ask if dizzy or light-headed with each position change. If yes, ensure safety from fainting or falling. A gait or walking belt can be used. With any position change, if patient experiences additional symptoms with the dizziness and decreased blood pressure and increased heart rate, assist the patient to lie down, take blood pressure, and notify the physician. Consider the possible cause of the orthostatic hypotension (hemorrhaging, dehydration, diuretics) to plan patient care.
7. Wait 3 minutes, and then take patient's sitting blood pressure and heart rate. If patient is dizzy or light-headed, continue sitting position for 5 minutes if tolerated. Do not attempt to bring the patient to standing. Repeat sitting blood pressure. If blood pressure has increased and patient is no longer dizzy, assist patient to stand.
8. Assist patient to stand and take blood pressure and pulse immediately. Then take again in 3 minutes. If blood pressure drops and patient is dizzy or light-headed, do not attempt to ambulate patient.
9. Document all heart rate and blood pressure measurements, including extremity used and patient position when reading was obtained (e.g., right arm lying 132/78, sitting 118/68, standing 110/60). Also document patient tolerance, symptoms, and nursing interventions if symptomatic.
10. Report abnormal findings to physician.

venous volume. This is most commonly caused by right-sided heart failure. To observe for this, the patient is gradually elevated to a 45- to 90-degree position and any distention noted.

Capillary refill time assesses arterial blood flow to the extremities. The patient's nailbed is briefly squeezed, causing blanching, and then released. The amount of time that it takes for the color to return to the nailbed after release of the squeezing pressure is the capillary refill time. Normal capillary refill time is 3 seconds or less. Longer

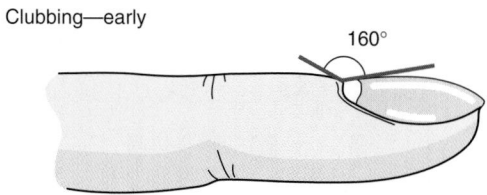

Clubbing—early

160°

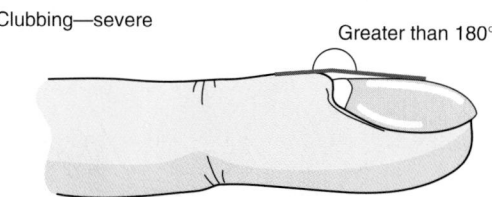

Clubbing—severe

Greater than 180°

FIGURE 20.7 Clubbing of the fingers.

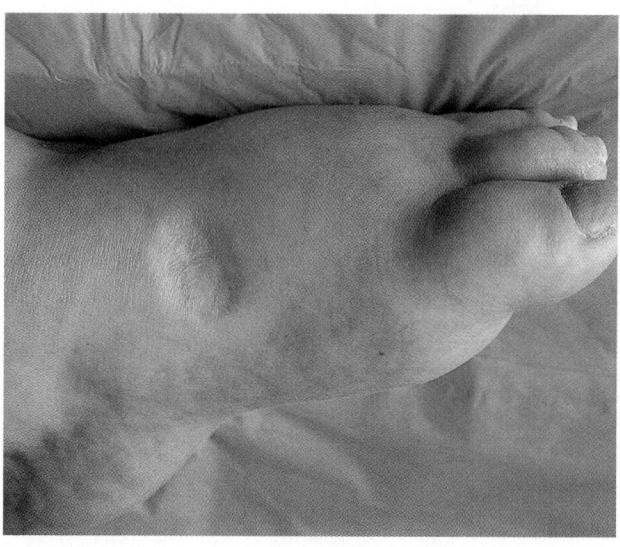

FIGURE 20.8 Pitting edema. Application of pressure over a bony area displaces the excess fluid, leaving an indentation or pit.

times indicate anemia or a decrease in blood flow to the extremity.

Clubbing of the nailbeds occurs from oxygen deficiency over time. It is often caused by congenital heart defects or the long-term use of tobacco. The distal ends of the fingers and toes swell and appear clublike. With clubbing, the normal 160-degree angle formed between the base of the nail and the skin is lost, causing the nail to be flat (Fig. 20.7). Later, the nail base elevates, the angle exceeds 180 degrees, and the nail feels spongy when squeezed.

LEARNING TIP

Six Ps characterize peripheral vascular disease:

- Pain
- Poikilothermia
- Pulselessness
- Pallor
- Paralysis
- Paresthesia (decreased sensation)

PALPATION. In addition to palpating the arteries, the thorax can be palpated at the **point of maximum impulse** (PMI). The PMI is palpated by placing the right hand over the apex of the heart. If palpable, a thrust is felt when the ventricle contracts. An enlarged heart may shift the PMI to the left of the midclavicular line.

The temperature of the extremities is palpated bilaterally for comparison. Palpation begins proximally and moves distally along the extremity. In areas of decreased arterial blood flow, the ischemic area feels cooler than the rest of the body because it is blood that warms the body. In the absence of sufficient arterial blood flow, the area becomes the temperature of the environment. This is called **poikilothermy.**

---

poikilothermy: poikilos—varied + therme—heat

A warm or hot extremity indicates a venous blood flow problem.

Edema is palpated in the extremities and dependent areas such as the sacrum for the supine patient (Fig. 20.8). Edema can occur from right-sided heart failure, gravity, or altered venous blood return. The nurse assesses the severity of the edema by pressing with a finger for 5 seconds over a bone, the medial malleolus or tibia, in the area of edema. If the finger imprint or indentation remains, the edema is pitting. Measuring the leg circumference is an accurate method for monitoring the edema.

Homans' sign is an assessment for venous thrombosis; however, in less than 50% of patients with thrombosis, the test is not positive. A positive Homans' sign is pain in the patient's calf or behind the knee when the foot is quickly dorsiflexed with the knee in a slightly flexed position (Fig. 20.9). Homans' sign should not be performed if a positive diagnosis of thrombosis has been made.

PERCUSSION. Percussion is performed by a physician to detect cardiac enlargement. Usually only the left border of the heart can be percussed. The heart is heard as dullness, which is in contrast to the resonance heard over the lungs.

AUSCULTATION. The normal heart sounds heard with a stethoscope placed on the wall of the chest are produced by the closing of the heart valves. These areas indicate where the sounds are best heard because sound in blood-flowing vessels is transmitted in the direction of the blood flow. The first heart sound (S1) is heard at the beginning of systole as "lubb" when the tricuspid and mitral (AV) valves close (Fig. 20.10). The second heart sound (S2) is heard at the start of diastole as "dupp" when the aortic and pulmonic semilunar valves close. The diaphragm of the stethoscope is used to hear the high-pitched sounds of S1 and S2. Extra heart sounds, usually indicating a pathological condition, may be heard with practice. Normally no other sounds are heard between S1 and S2. With the bell of the stethoscope placed

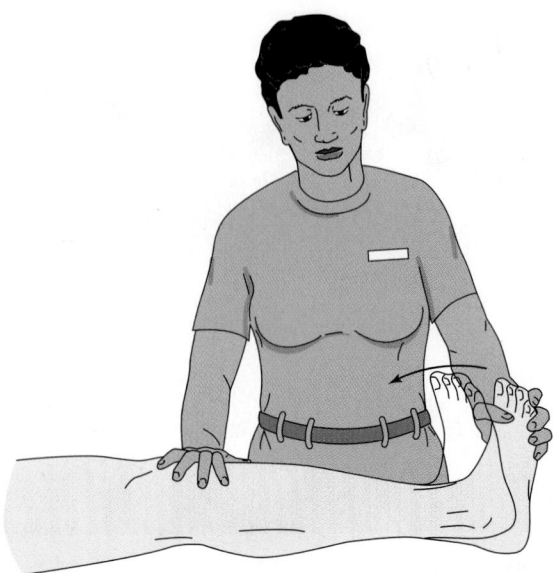

FIGURE 20.9 Assessment of Homans' sign for venous thrombosis. The foot is quickly dorsiflexed with the knee flexed. Calf or knee pain is noted. This assessment should not be performed if a positive diagnosis of thrombosis has been made.

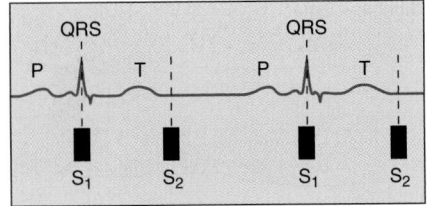

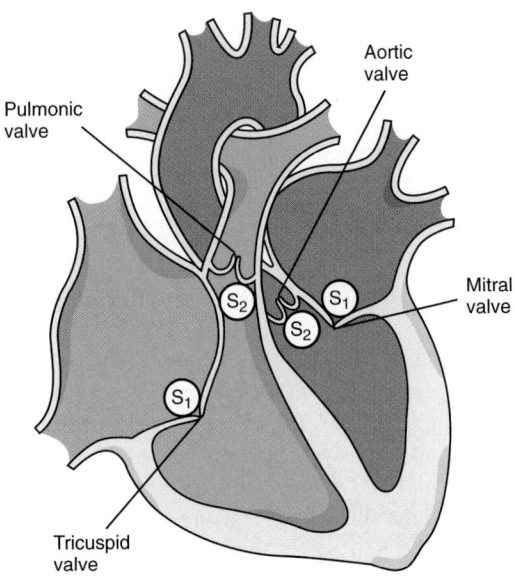

FIGURE 20.10 Heart sounds shown on electrocardiogram. S1 is heard at the beginning of systole, and S2 is heard at the beginning of diastole.

at the apex, a third heart sound (S3) or a fourth heart sound (S4) may be heard. Having patients lean forward or lie on their left side can make the heart sounds easier to hear by bringing the area of the heart where the sound may be heard closer to the chest wall. S3 is normal for children and younger adults. It sounds like a gallop and is a low-pitched sound heard early in diastole. S3 may be heard with left-sided heart failure, fluid volume overload, and mitral valve regurgitation. S4 is also a low-pitched sound, similar to a gallop but heard late in diastole. It occurs with hypertension, coronary artery disease, and pulmonary stenosis.

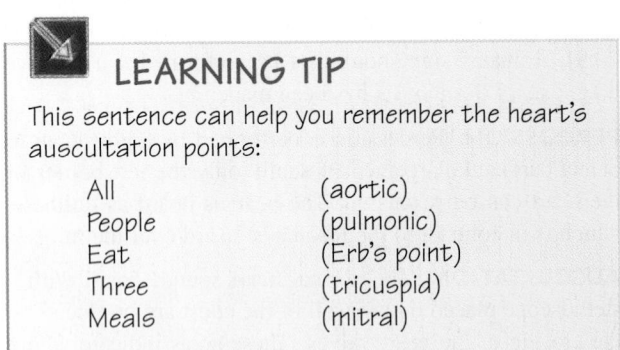

LEARNING TIP

This sentence can help you remember the heart's auscultation points:

All	(aortic)
People	(pulmonic)
Eat	(Erb's point)
Three	(tricuspid)
Meals	(mitral)

Murmurs are caused by turbulent blood flow through the heart and major blood vessels. A murmur is a prolonged sound caused by a narrowed valve opening or a valve that does not close tightly. A swishing sound that ranges in intensity from faint to very loud is produced. The intensity of the murmur is graded by the physician on a scale of 1 to 6. The timing of the murmur in relationship to the cardiac cycle of systole or diastole is also documented by the physician.

A **pericardial friction rub** occurs from inflammation of the pericardium. The intensity of a rub can range from soft and faint to loud enough to be audible without a stethoscope. A rub has a grating sound like sandpaper being rubbed together that occurs when the pericardial surfaces rub together during the cardiac cycle. (See the Learning Tip on pericardial friction rub in Chapter 22.) Having the patient sit and lean forward allows a rub to be heard more clearly. The rub is best heard to the left of the sternum using the diaphragm of the stethoscope. A pericardial friction rub may occur after a myocardial infarction or chest trauma.

Diagnostic Studies

Diagnostic test results provide valuable assessment information for the nurse (Table 20.3). These data are combined with the health history and physical assessment to plan care for the patient.

NONINVASIVE STUDIES. Chest X-ray Examination. A chest x-ray examination shows the size, position, contour, and structures of the heart (Fig. 20.11). It shows heart enlargement, calcifications, and fluid around the heart. Heart failure can be confirmed with a chest x-ray examination. Correct placement of pacemaker leads and pulmonary artery catheters in the heart can be confirmed.

Fluoroscopy uses a luminescent x-ray screen to show cardiac structures and pulsations. It is used as a guide when placing cardiac catheters or pacemaker leads.

CRITICAL THINKING

Mrs. Smith

■ Mrs. Smith, age 78, baseline weight 162 pounds, is admitted to the hospital with shortness of breath. Initial assessment findings are BP 152/88, pulse 104, respirations 26, temperature 99.4°F (37.2°C), shortness of breath at rest, shortness of breath increases with activity, ankles swollen, heart tones sound far away, nailbeds are very light pink, no pain, has not eaten well for 2 weeks, 6-pound weight gain in 1 week, sleeps on three pillows, veins in neck are visible on both sides. A diagnosis of acute myocardial infarction with heart failure is made by a physician.

1. Why is Mrs. Smith not having chest pain with a diagnosis of acute myocardial infarction?
2. How should swollen ankles be assessed to provide complete and measurable data?
3. What should be documented for the assessment performed on the swollen ankles?
4. How should the assessment findings for the swollen ankles be documented?
5. How should the assessment findings be documented for the additional symptoms Mrs. Smith has?
6. What is Mrs. Smith's weight in kilograms?

Suggested answers at end of chapter.

SAFETY TIP

Improve the accuracy of patient identification.

Use at least two patient identifiers (neither to be the patient's location) whenever collecting laboratory samples or administering medications or blood products, and use two identifiers to label sample collection containers in the presence of the patient. Processes are established to maintain samples' identities throughout the preanalytical, analytical, and postanalytical processes.

Immediately prior to the start of any invasive procedure, conduct a final verification process to confirm the correct patient, procedure, site, and availability of appropriate documents. This verification process uses active—not passive—communication techniques. The patient's identity is reestablished if the practitioner leaves the patient's location prior to initiating the procedure. Marking the site is required unless the practitioner is in continuous attendance from the time of the decision to do the procedure and patient consent to the initiation of the procedure (e.g., bone marrow collection or fine-needle aspiration). (2006 National Patient Safety Goals from www.jcaho.org)

Cardiac Calcium Scan. A computed tomographic (CT) scan using x-rays shows areas with plaque or calcification (the body deposits calcium to harden plaques, which are not normally found in the coronary arteries). Plaque indicates CAD. Calcium scoring is done to diagnose CAD and determine its severity. This screening test is not routinely done, especially for younger people. Scoring: 0 = no evidence of plaque, low heart attack risk; 1 to 10 10% CAD risk, low risk; 11 to 100 mild hardening, moderate risk; 101 to 400 CAD with possible coronary artery blockage, moderate-high risk, >400 90% chance plaque blocking artery, high risk. Patients are told to avoid caffeine and smoking for 4 hours before the test.

Magnetic Resonance Imaging. A three-dimensional image of the heart is produced by magnetic resonance imaging (MRI). Patients such as those with pacemakers or metal implants, metal shavings, or shrapnel are not candidates for this test. MRI use is currently limited for the heart owing to difficulties in imaging moving parts such as in the heart. Research is ongoing to overcome these obstacles. Cardiac MRI will likely be more common in a few years for things such as diagnosis of a heart attack as it is occurring, which will save valuable time or allow viewing types of plaque formations.

Electrocardiogram. The electrocardiogram (ECG) assesses the electrical activity of the heart from different views. The ECG shows abnormalities related to conduction, rate, rhythm, heart chamber enlargement, myocardial ischemia, myocardial infarction, and electrolyte imbalances. Abnormalities in cardiac function can be detected and the area of abnormality pinpointed with the aid of the different views on the ECG.

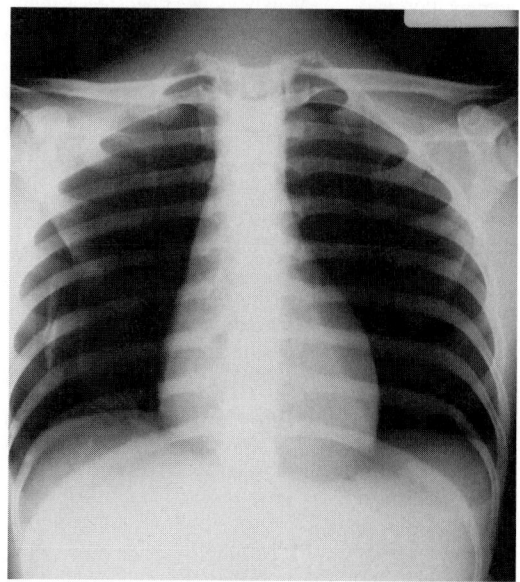

FIGURE 20.11 Normal chest x-ray film. Note white outline of heart borders in center. *(From McKinnis, LN: Fundamentals of Orthopedic Radiology. F.A. Davis, Philadelphia, 1997, p 15.)*

(Text continued on page 363)

TABLE 20.3 DIAGNOSTIC TESTS AND PROCEDURES FOR CARDIOVASCULAR SYSTEM

Procedure	Definition/Normal Finding (if applicable)	Significance of Abnormal Findings	Nursing Management
	Noninvasive		
Chest x-ray film	Anterior-posterior and left lateral views of chest taken to show heart size and contour and lungs.	Heart enlargement; calcifications; fluid around heart	Assess x-ray history and whether pregnant, Remove metal items. Teaching—no discomfort.
Magnetic resonance imaging (MRI)	Three-dimensional image of heart. Mainly used in research.	Cardiac abnormalities	Assess for metallic items and claustrophobia. Give antianxiety medication as ordered before MRI. Teaching—must lie still in long, small cylinder with loud, pounding sounds. Can talk to technician, listen to music.
Electrocardiogram (ECG)	Electrodes on skin carry electrical activity of heart from different views to show rhythm of heart, size of chambers, and heart damage. Normal: Normal Sinus Rhythm.	Dysrhythmias; enlarged heart chamber size; myocardial ischemia or infarction; electrolyte imbalances.	Teaching—no discomfort. Explain procedure.
Holter monitor	Recording of ECG for up to 48 hours to match abnormalities with symptoms recorded in patient's diary. Normal: Normal sinus rhythm.	Dysrhythmias; myocardial ischemia occurring less often.	Apply electrodes and leads. Teaching—keep accurate diary; push event button for symptoms. No showers or baths. Return visit.
Transtelephonic event recorder	Records ECG events infrequently occurring for transmission over phone to interpreting center for analysis. Pacemaker checks done.	Dysrhythmias; pacemaker malfunction	Teaching—explain use of recorder and how to transmit. Ensure good skin contact for best ECG tracing.
Pressure measurement	Blood pressures taken at several sites along extremity.	Shows area of occlusion or decreased blood flow at rest and with exercise.	Teaching—no discomfort. Explain procedure.
Exercise treadmill test (ETT)	Evaluates effects of exercise on heart and vascular circulation; ECG and vital signs are continuously monitored. Test stopped if symptoms develop.	Dysrhythmias; ischemia	Monitor vital signs and ECG before, during, and after test until stable. Teaching—explain procedure, wear walking shoes and comfortable clothes.
Echocardiogram	Transducer transmits sound waves that bounce off heart to produce heart images and show blood flow. Provides audio and graphic data.	Heart enlargement, coronary artery disease, valvular abnormalities, thickened cardiac walls or septum, pericardial effusion	May be done at bedside. Patient lies on left side. Teaching—no discomfort, gel applied.
Transesophageal echocardiogram	Probe with transducer on end inserted into esophagus, depth and angle directed by physician. Shows clearer images of heart because no lung or rib tissue is crossed. Dye injected for blood flow study.	Heart enlargement, coronary artery disease, valvular abnormalities, thickened cardiac walls or septum, pericardial effusion	Monitor vital signs and oxygen saturation. Encourage patient to relax. Suction continually during procedure. Teaching—NPO 6 hours before test. Sedation and local throat anesthetic given.
	Radioisotopes		
	IV injection of radioactive isotopes, which are taken up by heart and scanned with scintillation camera to show cardiac contractility, injury, and perfusion.		Assist patient to lie supine with arms over head for about 30 minutes Teaching—explain procedure, inform that radioactivity is small and gone within a few hours.

Procedure	Definition/Normal Finding (if applicable)	Significance of Abnormal Findings	Nursing Management
Thallium Imaging	IV injection of thallium 201 to evaluate cardiac blood flow. With exercise, thallium given 1 minute before end of test to circulate thallium. Scan done within 10 minutes and repeated in 2 to 4 hours for comparison.	If thallium not delivered to cardiac cells by good blood flow then see "cold spots" that show ischemia initially or infarcted areas later.	Teaching—explain procedure, inform that radioactivity is small and gone within a few hours. Light meal only between scans.
Dipyridamole thallium imaging	Dipyridamole (Persantine) IV is a vasodilator given to increase blood flow to coronary arteries; test is same as thallium imaging.	If thallium not delivered to cardiac cells by good blood flow then see "cold spots" that show ischemia initially or infarcted areas later.	Teaching—explain procedure, instruct no caffeine or aminophylline 12 hours before. Same as thallium imaging.
Technetium pyrophosphate imaging	Technetium 99m pyrophosphate IV given. Scanned 2 hours later.	Shows hot spot in heart injury area.	Teaching—explain procedure, inform that radioactivity is small and gone within a few hours.
Blood pool imaging	Technetium 99m pertechnetate IV. Serial studies are done over several hours. May be done at bedside.	Studies effects of drugs, recent MI, and congestive heart failure.	Teaching—explain procedure.
Positron emission tomography (PET)	Nitrogen 13–ammonia IV given and scanned for cardiac perfusion. Then fluoro-18-deoxyglucose IV given and scanned for cardiac metabolic function. Exercise may also be used.	In normal heart, scans match; in injured heart, they differ.	Patient's blood glucose must be 60 to 140 mg/dL for accuracy. Teaching—explain procedure. Must lie still during scan. If exercise used, NPO and no tobacco use.
Doppler ultrasound	Sound waves bounce off moving blood, producing recordings. Evaluates PVD.	Decreased blood flow in PVD	Teaching—explain procedure.
Plethysmography	After the leg being tested is raised 30 degrees with the patient supine, a pressure cuff is inflated on the leg to distend the veins. Blood flow is measured with electrodes. Cuff is then rapidly deflated and venous volume changes recorded.	Thrombi detected by less venous volume	Teaching—explain procedure. No discomfort. Takes 30 to 45 minutes.
Technetium 99m sestamibi	Technetium 99m sestamibi is given IV and scanned 1.5 to 2 hours later.	Areas of myocardial cell damage take up the radioisotope; when scanned, these areas appear as hot spots.	Explain procedure.
Serum Tests			
Creatine kinase (CK)	Heart, brain, skeletal muscle contain CK enzymes. Normal: male 5 to 55 U/mL; female 5 to 25 U/mL.	Damaged cells release CK. With MI, CK elevates in 6 hours and returns to baseline in 48–72 hours.	Avoid IM injections and take baseline CK before inserting IVs to avoid elevating CK from muscle cell damage. Serial sampling done.
CK-MB	Only heart muscle contains MB isoenzyme. Normal: 0 to 7 IU/L.	Rises with MI in 6 hours and returns to baseline in 72 hours.	Same as CK.
Myoglobin	Protein found in cardiac cells. 99% indicative of MI. Normal: 250 to 450 ng/mL.	Rises in 1 hour after MI and peaks in 4 to 12 hours so must be drawn within 18 hours of chest pain onset.	No special care.
Cardiac troponin I or T	Cardiac cell protein. Normal: Varies by lab; very low levels.	Elevated levels sensitive indicator of MI. Levels elevated up to 7 days.	No special care.

(Continued on following page)

Procedure	Definition/Normal Finding (if applicable)	Significance of Abnormal Findings	Nursing Management
C-reactive protein	CRP levels can indicate low-grade inflammation in coronary vessels. Low cardiovascular disease risk: <1 mg/L; average risk 10 mg/L–3 mg/L; high risk >3 mg/L	Elevated levels indicate heart attack risk.	No special care
Serum Lipids			
Cholesterol	Measures CAD risk. Normal: 140 to 200 mg/dL.	>200 increased CAD risk.	Fasting not required.
Triglycerides	Elevated in cardiovascular disease. Normal: <150 mg/dL	CAD risk	Eat normal diet for 2 weeks before test. Fasting required for 12 hours. Water allowed but no alcohol.
Phospholipids	May elevate in cardiovascular disease. Normal: 125 to 380 mg/dL.	CAD risk	Same as triglycerides.
Lipoproteins	Electrophoresis done to separate lipoproteins: VLDL, LDL, HDL. HDL protects against CAD; Normal lipoproteins: 400 to 800 mg/dL. Desirable: LDL less than HDL (values vary with age).	Elevated LDL increases CAD risk. LDL <100 desirable; HDL >60	Same as triglycerides.
Invasive			
Angiography	Dye injected into vessels to make them visible on x-rays. Coronary—coronary arteries via cardiac catheter. Peripheral—peripheral arteries or veins.	Assesses vessel patency, injury, or aneurysm.	Precare: Informed consent required. NPO 4 to 18 hours before test. Assess dye allergies.
			Teaching—sedative and local anesthesia may be used; burning sensation from dye; monitored continuously. Postcare: assess vital signs, circulation mobility sensation, catheter insertion site, or puncture site for hemorrhage, hematoma every 15 minutes for 1 hour, then every 30 minutes to 1 hour. Apply insertion site pressure (dressing, sandbag) as needed. Immobilize extremity for several hours as ordered.
Cardiac catheterization	Catheter inserted into heart for data on oxygen saturation and chamber pressures. Dye may be injected to visualize structures.	Cardiac disease	Same as angiography.
			Sensory teaching—table is hard, cool cleansing solution used, sting felt from local anesthetic, hear monitor beeping, feel pressure of catheter insertion, dye warm, burning feeling, headache, chest pain briefly, hear camera, feel table move.

Procedure	Definition/Normal Finding (if applicable)	Significance of Abnormal Findings	Nursing Management
Hemodynamic monitoring	Continuous readings of arterial BP, cardiac and pulmonary pressures, CO and Svo obtained with catheter attached to transducer and monitor to diagnose and guide treatment. Normal: BP less than 120/80; right atrial pressure 2 to 6 mm Hg; pulmonary artery systolic pressure/pulmonary artery diastolic pressure 20 to 30/0 to 10; pulmonary artery wedge pressure 4 to 12 mm Hg; CO 4 to 8 L/min; Svo_2 60% to 80%.	Blood pressure, cardiac and pulmonary pressure abnormalities.	Informed consent signed for insertion. Continuous assessment to ensure proper placement of catheter is maintained and a permanent catheter wedge does not go undetected. Recording of readings and monitoring of insertion site for signs of infection.
Central venous pressure (CVP)	Catheter inserted into a vein and threaded into vena cava. Normal: 2 to 6 mm Hg.	Monitors CVP, which reflects fluid volume status.	Informed consent signed for insertion. Recording of readings and monitoring of insertion site for signs of infection.

When an ECG is requested, information that aids in its interpretation is provided, including the patient's sex, age, height, weight, blood pressure, and cardiac medications. The patient requires no special preparation but is given an explanation of the procedure and told that the ECG is painless.

To obtain an ECG, electrodes are placed on the skin to transmit electrical impulses to the ECG machine for recording. The electrical impulses from the heart appear as waves on graph paper. One electrode is placed on each limb and several across the chest. The right leg is a ground electrode. One view of the heart using a combination of the electrodes to obtain the view is called a lead. The standard 12-lead ECG, using a combination of the electrodes, provides 12 views of the heart. Eighteen-lead ECGs may also be done.

Signal-averaged ECG. The signal-averaged ECG is used to diagnose whether a patient is at risk of developing ventricular tachycardia and possible sudden death. A computer records low-level signals not detected by a regular ECG. These electrical signals, referred to as late potentials, occur at the end of the QRS wave and into the ST segment. Late potentials place the patient at risk for ventricular **dysrhythmias**.

Ambulatory Electrocardiogram Monitoring. Continuous monitoring of the ambulatory patient is possible with the use of tape recorders.

Holter Monitoring. A Holter monitor, which weighs 2 pounds, continuously records one lead for up to 48 hours. The patient wears loose-fitting clothing and may only sponge bathe while wearing the monitor. The patient records a diary of activities and symptoms and pushes the event button if symptoms occur. Symptoms are documented for later correlation with the ECG recordings. Dysrhythmias or myocardial ischemia that occurs infrequently can be de-

tected. Recordings are scanned by a computer and interpreted by a physician.

Transtelephonic Event Recorders. This recorder is used for dysrhythmic events that occur so infrequently that they would not likely be captured in 48 hours, or for follow-up evaluation of permanent pacemakers. With this recorder the patient has greater flexibility because the device is worn when needed or when symptoms occur. The disadvantage is that if the event is brief, it may be missed before the recorder is on. When an event is recorded, the patient can transmit it at a convenient time over the telephone for printout and analysis. The telephone mouthpiece is placed over the signal transmitter box for transmission. After transmission, the recording can be erased and the recorder reused.

Pressure Measurement. Pressure readings are done to assess areas of occlusion or narrowing in vessels. Blood pressure readings are taken at intervals along the extremity. Reduced readings are found in areas with blood flow problems.

Tilt Table Test. The tilt table test is used to help diagnose the cause of syncope ("fainting spells"). Heart rate and blood pressure are monitored during a change in position from lying down to standing up.

Exercise Tolerance Testing. The exercise tolerance test, or stress test, measures cardiac function or peripheral vascular disease during a defined exercise protocol (Fig. 20.12). Before the test, patients are given an explanation of the test and told not to smoke, eat, or drink for 2 to 4 hours before the test. They are also instructed to wear comfortable walking shoes, a loose top, and for women a supportive bra. After the test, patients should rest and wait to eat. They should also avoid eating or drinking stimulants such as caffeine and temperature extremes such as going out into cold weather for a few hours after the test.

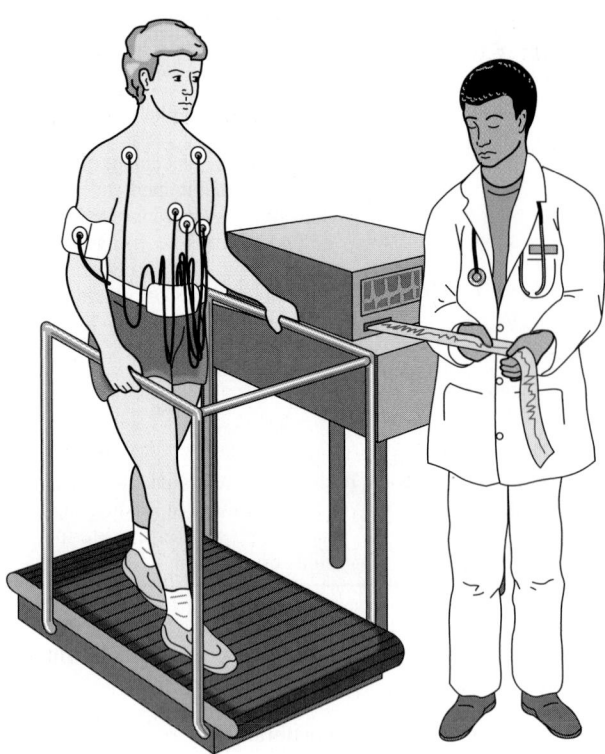

FIGURE 20.12 Performance of stress test.

Cardiac Stress Test. This test simulates sympathetic nervous system (fight or flight) stimulation. It shows the heart's response to increased oxygen needs. Before the test, baseline vital signs are obtained. Then, while the patient exercises on a treadmill, on a stationary bicycle, or by climbing stairs, vital signs, oxygen saturation, skin temperature, physical appearance, chest pain, and ECG are monitored to help ensure patient safety. The test is completed when the patient reaches peak heart rate (patient's age subtracted from 220), experiences chest pain, is unable to exercise further, or develops vital sign or ECG changes. Vital signs and ECG continue to be monitored after the test until they return to baseline.

The cardiac stress test is used to evaluate coronary artery disease. It aids in diagnosing ischemic heart disease, the cause of chest pain and dysrhythmias. The functional capacity of the heart can also be measured after a cardiac event or to plan a physical fitness or rehabilitation program.

Peripheral Vascular Stress Test. The patient walks for 5 minutes at 1.5 miles per hour on the treadmill. At certain intervals, pulse volume measurements are taken, including baseline resting, during the test, and final resting after the test. This test assesses response to activity. If **claudication** occurs, the test is stopped.

Echocardiogram. An echocardiogram is an ultrasound test that records the motion of the heart structures, including the valves, as well as the heart size, shape, and position. No

claudication: claudicare—to limp

preparation is required for a cardiac ultrasound. This test transmits ultrasonic sound waves into the heart so that the returned echoes can be recorded on videotape as audio and visual information. An ECG is recorded at the same time for comparison purposes. Abnormalities that may be seen on the echocardiogram include heart enlargement, valvular abnormalities, thickened cardiac walls or septum, and pericardial effusion.

Exercise echocardiography diagnoses CAD during exercise-induced cardiac ischemia by detecting cardiac wall motion abnormalities.

Transesophageal Echocardiogram. Transesophageal echocardiogram provides a clearer picture than transthoracic echocardiography. It produces images by using a transducer on a probe that is placed in the esophagus. The images are clearer because lung and rib tissue does not have to be penetrated by the sound waves. The physician controls the position of the probe and takes pictures as it travels within the esophagus. Patients take nothing by mouth (NPO) for about 6 hours before the test, receive a sedative, and have their throat locally anesthetized. After the procedure, patients remain NPO until the nurse has verified (touching the back of the throat with a cotton tip swab) that their gag reflex has returned.

Radioisotope Imaging. For this type of imaging, small amounts of radioisotopes are given intravenously. The patient is then scanned with a gamma camera and a radionuclide image is produced. Radiation exposure is similar to that of other x-ray examinations. These tests can provide information about myocardial ischemia or infarction, cardiac blood flow, and ventricle size and motion.

Thallium Imaging. Thallium 201, a radioactive analog of potassium, is used to detect impaired myocardial perfusion. It is injected intravenously (IV), and muscle cells absorb it. After 10 to 15 minutes the heart is scanned to see where the thallium has concentrated. Four hours later the scan is repeated to look for changes. Healthy myocardial cells with good blood flow take up the thallium. Areas in which the thallium is not seen are referred to as cold spots and indicate ischemia or infarction. The patency of a coronary artery graft may also be assessed with this test. This test is used often because the short half-life of thallium results in lower radiation exposure.

Exercise testing may be combined with thallium injection to detect blood flow changes with activity and after rest. The patient exercises and about 2 minutes before stopping is given thallium. Scans are taken immediately and again in 2 to 4 hours. Cold spots on initial images indicate ischemia. If the cold spots are gone in later images, it indicates exercise-induced ischemia. If the cold spots are still present in later images, they show scarred areas.

If patients are unable to participate in exercise for the thallium stress test, dipyridamole (Persantine) or adenosine, coronary vasodilators, can be given. These drugs simulate the increased blood flow to healthy myocardial cells that occurs with exercise.

Technetium Pyrophosphate Scan. Technetium 99m pyrophosphate is injected for this test. Areas of ischemia or myocardial cell damage take up the radioisotope, and when scanned these areas appear as hot spots. Acute myocardial infarction (MI) size and location can be detected, but old MIs cannot be detected.

Technetium 99m Sestamibi. Technetium 99m sestamibi is given IV and the patient is scanned 1.5 to 2 hours later. Areas of myocardial cell damage take up the radioisotope, and when scanned these areas appear as hot spots.

Blood Pool Imaging. Technetium 99m pertechnetate is injected IV and remains in the bloodstream; it is not taken up by myocardial cells. A camera follows the flow of the radioactivity, which shows ventricular function and wall motion and the ejection fraction of the heart.

Positron Emission Tomography. Positron emission tomography (PET) shows myocardial perfusion and viability with three-dimensional images. Nitrogen 13–ammonia is injected IV first and then scanned to show myocardial perfusion. Next, fluoro-18-deoxyglucose is given intravenously and then scanned to show myocardial metabolic function. If there is ischemia or heart damage, the two scans are different. For example, in ischemia of viable cells, blood flow is decreased but metabolism elevated. Treatment to increase blood flow improves cardiac function in this case. Before the test the patient's blood glucose should be normal, and caffeine and tobacco should be avoided for 4 hours before the test.

Doppler Ultrasound. In this test, sound waves are transmitted to an artery or vein to assess blood flow problems. The sound waves bounce off moving blood cells and return a sound frequency in relationship to the amount of blood flow. With decreased blood flow the sounds are reduced. This test requires no patient preparation, takes about 20 minutes to complete, and is painless.

Plethysmography. With this test, blood volume and changes in blood flow are measured to diagnose deep vein thrombosis and pulmonary emboli and to screen patients for peripheral vascular disease. The leg being tested is raised 30 degrees with the patient supine. A pressure cuff is then inflated on the leg to distend the veins. Blood flow is measured with electrodes, and the cuff is then rapidly deflated and venous volume changes are recorded. Thrombi are detected by reduction in venous volume.

Arterial Stiffness Index (ASI). A newer test measures stiffness of the brachial artery to determine arteriosclerosis and cardiovascular disease risk. The brachial artery correlates with the coronary arteries in regard to the extent of atherosclerosis. The test is done with a device with a blood pressure cuff hooked to a computer. The waveforms during the blood pressure reading are mapped in the computer to provide information on the artery stiffness.

BLOOD STUDIES. Homocysteine. In recent years, homocysteine has been used to predict risk for cardio-vascular disease when elevated. Homocysteine is an amino acid made in the body that can irritate blood vessels, leading to blockages or clots. Normal levels are 12 mmol/L or less. Often folate, vitamin B_6, and vitamin B_{12} are not adequate in the diet. Homocysteine levels can be reduced with green leafy vegetables or prescribed folate (folic acid) supplements. For more information, visit http://www.homo cysteine.net.

C-reactive Protein (CRP). C-reactive protein is a newer test for assessing cardiac disease risk. Elevated cardiac CRP levels can indicate low-grade inflammation in coronary vessels. This can signal increased long-term heart disease risk. CRP is found in small amounts in healthy people. Negative emotions and stress can elevate CRP, increasing cardiac disease risk. Elevated levels indicate risk for myocardial infarction and allow nurses the chance to help patients understand and reduce cardiac risk factors. This test is often done along with cholesterol screening.

Myeloperoxidase Antigen (MPO). Myeloperoxidase antigen (MPO), a leukocyte enzyme, is made when inflammation is present in arteries. Levels are higher in ruptured plaques and can lead to heart attack. Risk of heart attack up to 6 months in advance may be predicted with elevated MPO levels (without the presence of myocardial necrosis) for patients with chest pain. This test may be more predictive than CRP of cardiac risk, especially for use in emergency departments when troponin levels are normal.

Cardiac Troponin. Cardiac muscle contains proteins called troponins, which control the muscle fibers that contract or squeeze the heart muscle. Troponin I and troponin T are highly sensitive indicators of myocardial damage, which is helpful in diagnosing MI. They are proteins found only in cardiac cells. When injured or dead, cardiac cells release these proteins, which results in elevated levels within 4 to 6 hours of damage. These levels peak in 10 to 24 hours and remain elevated for up to 7 days after injury. Troponin T appears slightly earlier than troponin I after cardiac damage. Troponin T is better at showing slight cardiac damage and predicting 30-day mortality for cardiac patients.

Troponin I can also be used to monitor critically ill patients in the critical care setting. Heart damage may be occurring undetected that is delaying recovery. Studies are being done to see if troponin may be useful for ongoing monitoring of cardiac injury so that medications can be given.

Cardiac Enzymes. When heart cells are damaged or die, they rupture and release enzymes into the bloodstream. Levels of these enzymes rise in the serum as a result. A common cardiac enzyme test is creatine kinase (CK), also referred to as creatine phosphokinase (CPK). It is often ordered with troponin tests. Lactic dehydrogenase (LDH), a nonspecific enzyme test, is rarely used today as troponin has basically replaced it. CK enzymes are also found in body cells other than the heart, so a more organ-specific test in which the enzyme's isoenzymes (or different forms) are measured is used.

Creatine Kinase. Creatine kinase (CK) is found in three types of tissue: brain, skeletal muscle, and heart muscle. Isoenzymes of CK contained in these tissues are CK-BB (brain), CK-MM (skeletal muscle), and CK-MB (heart muscle). Levels of CK-MB rise within 4 to 6 hours after cardiac cells are damaged, peak in 12 to 24 hours, and return to normal in 48 to 72 hours. Serial CK levels are drawn at intervals to track trends. It is important to avoid invasive procedures such as IV and intramuscular (IM) injections before drawing the first CK to prevent elevation in the CK levels from cell trauma caused by the procedure. Then medications are often given IV rather than IM to prevent contributing to this elevation.

Myoglobin. Myoglobin is a protein found in skeletal and cardiac muscle and is released into the bloodstream when cell damage occurs. Because myoglobin is not site specific, it can only provide an estimate of damage and is used with other more specific tests such as troponin to diagnosis an MI. Myoglobin levels elevate within 1 hour of an acute MI. Peak levels are reached 4 to 12 hours after an MI, and levels return to normal within 18 hours after the onset of chest pain, so it is a test that must be done early when MI is suspected.

Blood Lipids. Lipids include triglycerides, cholesterol, and phospholipids. Lipoproteins carry these lipids attached to proteins. Triglycerides are found in very low-density lipoproteins (VLDLs). Cholesterol is mainly found in low-density lipoproteins (LDLs). High-density lipoproteins (HDLs) are a mixture of one-half protein and one-half phospholipids and cholesterol.

A lipid profile can screen for increased risk for coronary artery disease. For more information, visit http://www.nhlbi.nih.gov/guidelines/cholesterol/atglance.pdf. Patients must fast for 12 hours before the test, and although water is not withheld, alcohol is restricted for 24 hours before the test. High levels of LDLs are linked to an increase in CAD because they circulate cholesterol in the arteries. High-density lipoproteins play a protective role against CAD because they carry cholesterol to the liver to be metabolized. Controlling lipids is very important in reducing CAD (Box 20.4 Cultural Considerations).

INVASIVE STUDIES. Angiography. Arteriography and venography are the two types of angiography (Fig. 20.13).

SAFETY TIP

Improve the effectiveness of communication among caregivers.

For verbal or telephone orders or for telephonic reporting of critical test results, verify the complete order or test result by having the person receiving the order or test result "read back" the complete order or test result. (2006 National Patient Safety Goals from www.jcaho.org)

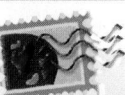

Box 20.4
Cultural Considerations

Among French Canadians, familial chylomicronemia (hyperlipoproteinemia type I), an autosomal recessive disorder, occurs with the highest frequency worldwide. Familial hypercholesterolemia can lead to coronary thrombosis. Thus, the nurse can improve the health of French Canadians by encouraging early diagnostic workups for familial chylomicronemia and encouraging healthful lifestyles.

Arteriography examines arteries. Venography studies veins. Angiography uses dye injected into the vascular system to visualize the vessels on radiographs. This test is used to assess blood clot formation, to assess peripheral vascular disease (PVD), and to test vessels for potential grafting use.

The patient must be assessed for allergies, give informed consent, be NPO for about 4 hours before the test, and be informed that the dye produces a hot, burning feeling when injected. After the procedure the patient is assessed for several hours. Vital signs, allergic reaction signs, hemorrhage at the injection site, and pulses are monitored.

Cardiac Catheterization. Cardiac catheterization allows the study of the heart's anatomy and physiology. It is an invasive diagnostic procedure that measures pressures in the heart chambers, great blood vessels, and coronary arteries and provides information on cardiac output and oxygen saturation. Fluoroscopy is used, and dye can be injected once the catheter is in place to visualize the heart chambers and vessels. This procedure is often done before heart surgery.

An informed consent must be obtained. The patient is assessed for allergies to iodine, and procedure dyes and kept NPO before the procedure. Patients should be told that during the test they are awake and a warm, flushing sensation

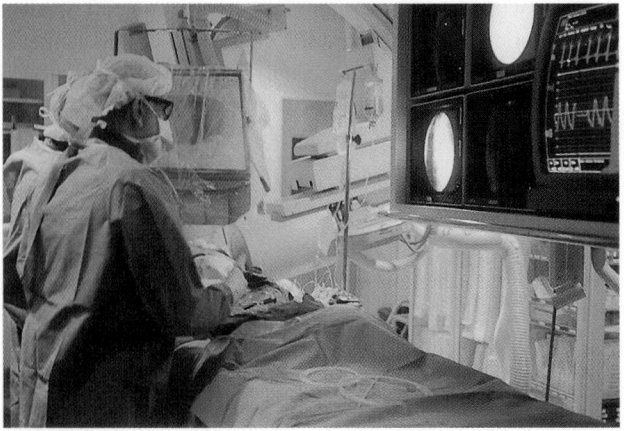

FIGURE 20.13 Coronary angiography and cardiac catheterization.

Box 20.5

Nutrition Notes

CYP Enzymes and Fruit Juices

Cytochrome P450 (CYP450) is a superfamily of enzymes found mainly in the liver but also in the gastrointestinal tract, lungs, and kidneys. The isoenzyme CYP3A4, the main form in the small intestine, is estimated to participate in the metabolism of more than 50% of all pharmaceutical agents, a function that may have evolved to protect the body from toxins. After uptake by the intestinal epithelial cells, many substances are metabolized by CYP3A4 or returned to the intestinal lumen by a transporter protein[3], thus limiting the amount of the substance available for absorption into the bloodstream. Individuals show a wide variation in the amount of CYP3A4 in the liver and the intestine due to genetic, physiological, and environmental effects so that persons with more of the isoenzyme show greater effects to its inhibition than those with lesser amounts of intestinal CYP3A4.[3, 4]

Grapefruit juice appears to inhibit intestinal CYP3A4 so that the oral bioavailability of affected drugs is increased dramatically, in some cases sufficient to cause drug toxicity or treatment failure. A single glass (240 mL) of grapefruit juice is enough to produce measurable effects for 24 hours, presumably until the body manufactures more of the enzyme. Applying this knowledge to clinical practice is complicated by the fact that even within a given class of drugs, not all agents are metabolized by CYP3A4. For instance, felodipine (Plendil), diazepam (Valium), and simvastatin (Zocor) interact with grapefruit juice, whereas nifedipine (Procardia), alprazolam (Xanax), and pravastatin (Pravachol) are thought by some to show little or no interaction. Likewise, cyclosporine, an immunosuppressive agent used to prevent transplant rejection, is metabolized by intestinal CYP3A4, and elevated blood levels have occurred when administered with grapefruit juice.[5]

Other fruits may have this same effect which is being studied. Fruits that could have this effect include Seville oranges, lime juice, and tangelos, which are from a form of grapefruit. Other citrus fruit should be safe: lemons, sweet oranges, tangerines, and citrons.

A similar mechanism but a different isoenzyme is proposed to explain an interaction between warfarin (Coumadin) and cranberry juice. Warfarin is mainly metabolized by the cytochrome P450 isoenzyme CYP2C9, and cranberry juice contains flavonoids known to inhibit P450 enzymes. Bleeding problems and hemorrhage have been attributed to this interaction.[6,7]

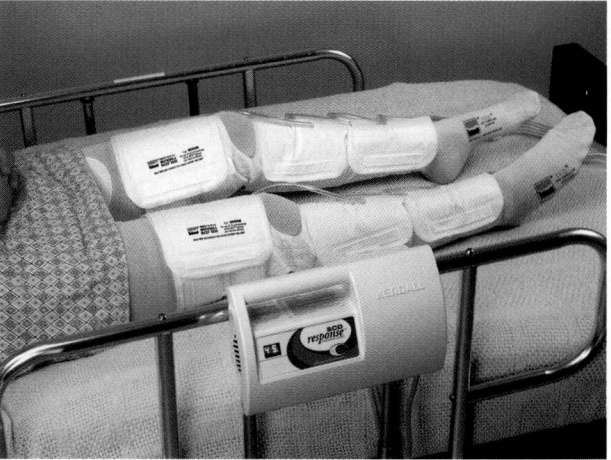

FIGURE 20.16 The Kendall SCD Response Compression system provides sequential personalized compression cycles that minimize stasis and maximize blood flow to prevent thrombosis and pulmonary embolus development. *(Courtesy Kendall, Mansfield, MA.)*

standing habits are difficult to change. Support groups can offer encouragement that is helpful in promoting a healthy lifestyle. Patients should be referred to community support groups as needed.

Patients recovering from cardiac disorders are often anxious about resuming sexual activity but are embarrassed to discuss it. This is an area that is often overlooked when caring for patients. Sexual counseling should be offered to patients and their partners. Patients often have misconceptions that are unfounded but interfere with resuming their sexual activity. If patients have angina, nitroglycerin can be taken prophylactically before sexual activity. After a myocardial infarction, sexual activity can be resumed in 1 to 2 months or when the patient can climb two flights of stairs without symptoms, as ordered by the physician. Sexual activity is a form of physical activity. Patients should be given information to make an informed decision on when they are ready to resume this activity.

Cardiac Surgery

As heart disease symptoms increase in severity and frequency or the disease process worsens, cardiac surgery may be used as treatment. Although cardiac surgery has become commonplace, it is still a major surgery with numerous complications, as well as physical, emotional, and social stressors.

Preparation for Surgery

For elective heart surgery, patients may be admitted to the hospital on the morning of surgery or 1 to 3 days before the surgery based on their medical history. A nursing assessment is important to provide baseline data that can be used for postoperative comparison and early discharge planning. In addition to routine admission testing, patients with chronic obstructive pulmonary disease (COPD) may have pulmonary function tests and baseline arterial blood gases (ABGs) done (Box 20.6). Patients with carotid bruits have

Box 20.6

Routine Admission Testing

12-lead electrocardiogram (ECG)
Chest x-ray exam
Complete blood cell count (CBC)
Coagulation studies
Chemistry profile
Crossmatched for blood

carotid studies to determine the amount of occlusion in the carotid artery. If the occlusion is significant, a carotid endarterectomy, which removes the plaque on the lining of the blocked or diseased carotid artery, is performed, usually several weeks before having cardiac surgery.

Medications that may increase bleeding or reduce fluid volume may be ordered by the physician to be held before surgery. Drugs that increase bleeding include aspirin, often stopped 3 to 7 days preoperatively; warfarin (Coumadin), often stopped 4 to 5 days preoperatively; and heparin, stopped 4 hours preoperatively. During surgery fluid volume and blood pressure may be decreased by blood loss or medications. Therefore, diuretics, which could further reduce fluid volume and blood pressure, are withheld up to 2 days before surgery. Because the patient takes nothing by mouth (NPO) 8 to 12 hours before surgery, insulin and oral hypoglycemic agents are reduced or withheld the morning of surgery.

Patients recover more quickly and have less postoperative stress when they have thorough preoperative teaching. Explanations of pain management, endotracheal tube (ETT), methods of communicating, ventilator, chest tubes, coughing and deep breathing exercises, intravenous (IV) lines, urinary catheter, incision care, and various equipment alarms are provided to the patient and family. It should be emphasized that patients are not able to talk while the ETT is in place.

Additionally, a preoperative family tour of the patient's initial postoperative unit and the waiting area helps prepare them for the surgical experience. A referral to pastoral care, if desired, can be comforting to the patient and family.

The anesthesiologist assesses the patient before surgery and orders preoperative medications. An antiseptic scrub shower is taken the night before and the morning of surgery. The patient is NPO after midnight the night before surgery.

Cardiopulmonary Bypass

The majority of cardiac surgeries use a cardiopulmonary bypass (CPB) pump in which blood is temporarily diverted away from the heart and lungs to the special pump (Fig. 20.17). This diversion allows for a bloodless and motionless surgical field while the function of the heart and lungs is maintained by the pump. After the **sternotomy** is made, the vena cava and ascending aorta are cannulated (a small tube with multiple holes is placed into each of them). The aorta is cross-clamped between the heart and the cannula by clamping two large hemostats over the aorta in opposite directions. The cannulas are then attached to the pump tubing. Blood then flows from the body through the vena cava cannula to the CPB pump for oxygenation. After the pump oxygenates and removes carbon dioxide from the blood, the blood is returned to the body. The blood flows through the cannula into the ascending aorta, where it then circulates through the body (Fig. 20.18).

Using the CPB pump can have a unique set of complications. Before going on the pump, the patient is anticoagulated with heparin until the partial thromboplastin time (PTT) is five to six times greater than normal. Immediately before the patient comes off the pump, the effects of the heparin are reversed with protamine sulfate (antidote for heparin). Heparin is absorbed and stored in organs and tissue and can be sporadically released hours after surgery. As a result, the patient may have excessive bleeding. The risk of

---

sternotomy: stern—sternum + otomy—incision into

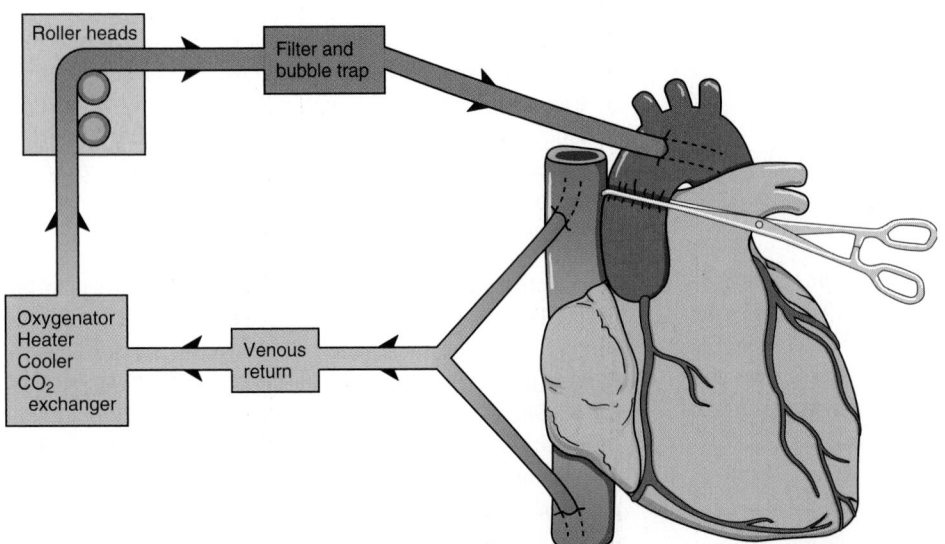

FIGURE 20.17 Cardiopulmonary bypass pump components.

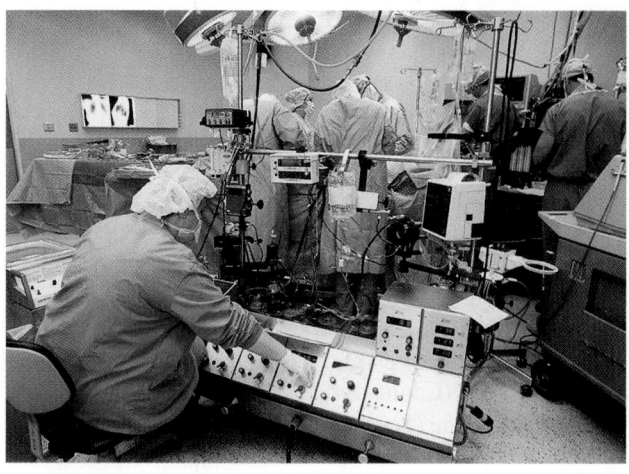

FIGURE 20.18 Cardiopulmonary bypass pump in use.

an air embolism is minimized by priming the pump with lactated Ringer's solution and maintaining careful observation. The priming solution increases circulating volume, which then results in a shifting of fluid into the interstitial tissue and edema formation. These fluid shifts can continue up to 6 hours after surgery and can cause hypotension.

Methods for providing closed-chest cardiopulmonary bypass and **cardioplegia** are being studied. Instead of opening the chest, small incisions are made in the chest and a

_____

cardioplegia: cardio—heart + plegia—paralysis

video-assisted thoracoscope is inserted and used to perform the entire surgery. This technique of closed-chest surgery, with or without CPB, is termed minimally invasive direct coronary artery bypass (MIDCAB) surgery. When CPB is not used, mechanical devices are used to stabilize the portion of the heart being bypassed while the remainder of the heart continues to beat. Risk for complications associated with MIDCAB are much lower than with the traditional CABG procedure, and the recovery time is often weeks less.

General Procedure for Cardiac Surgery

After the patient is placed on CPB, a cardioplegic solution is infused into the aortic root along with iced saline. This solution is placed around the heart to cause cardiac standstill. When the surgery is completed, the patient's blood is warmed in the CPB circuit and the patient is slowly weaned from CPB. The heart starts beating again after it is warmed and defibrillated. Temporary pacing wires are attached to the heart before the CPB pump is discontinued, so an external temporary pacemaker can be used if bradycardia develops. Once the heart is beating, CPB is stopped. Mediastinal chest tubes are placed to drain remaining blood and fluid from the chest. The sternotomy is closed with wires through the sternum and then sutures for the layers of tissue and skin. While still under anesthesia, the patient is transferred to an intensive care unit (ICU). Patients usually stay in ICU for 1 to 2 days, although those undergoing MIDCAB may not need an ICU stay.

REVIEW QUESTIONS

1. The mitral and tricuspid valves prevent backflow of blood from which of the following?
   a. Ventricles to atria when the ventricles contract
   b. Atria to ventricles when the ventricles relax
   c. Ventricles to atria when the atria contract
   d. Atria to ventricles when the atria contract

2. Which of the following describes the purpose of the endocardium of the heart?
   a. Covers the heart muscle and prevents friction.
   b. Supports the coronary blood vessels.
   c. Lines the chambers of the heart and prevents abnormal clotting.
   d. Prevents backflow of blood from atria to ventricles.

3. The function of the coronary blood vessels is to do which of the following?
   a. Prevent abnormal clotting within the heart.
   b. Bring oxygenated blood to the myocardium.
   c. Carry deoxygenated blood to the lungs.
   d. Carry oxygenated blood to the lungs.

4. Which of the following is where the location of the cardiac centers in the nervous system is found?
   a. Cerebrum

   b. Hypothalamus
   c. Spinal cord
   d. Medulla

5. The functions of angiotensin II are to increase which of the following?
   a. Vasodilation and ADH secretion
   b. Vasoconstriction and aldosterone secretion
   c. Heart rate and vasodilation
   d. Heart rate and ADH secretion

6. The increase of resting blood pressure with age may contribute to which of the following?
   a. Dysrhythmias
   b. Thrombus formation
   c. Left-sided heart failure
   d. Peripheral edema

7. Which of the following is a modifiable cardiovascular risk factor that should be noted during patient data collection?
   a. Age
   b. Gender
   c. Ethnic origin
   d. Tobacco use

8. If it takes longer than 3 seconds for the color to return when assessing capillary refill, it may indicate which of the following?
   a. Decreased arterial flow to the extremity
   b. Increased arterial flow to the extremity
   c. Decreased venous flow from the extremity
   d. Increased venous flow from the extremity

9. Which of the following is an important safety intervention that should be used while assessing a patient for orthostatic hypotension?
   a. Reality orientation
   b. Gait or walking belt
   c. Liquids at bedside
   d. Standing patient quickly

10. In which area should the nurse assess a patient who is on bedrest for the presence of edema?
    a. Arms
    b. Ankles
    c. Sternum
    d. Sacrum

Multiple response item. Select all that apply.

11. Which of the following should be included in patient teaching for coronary angiography with femoral catheter insertion site?
    a. Dye injection causes hot, flushing sensation.
    b. General anesthesia is administered.
    c. Claustrophobia may be experienced.
    d. Ambulation is not possible immediately after procedure.
    e. Allergies are assessed prior to testing.

12. A high-fiber diet for cardiac patients is recommended for which of the following purposes?
    a. Increase absorption of nutrients
    b. Reduce cardiac workload
    c. Reduce edema development
    d. Reduce appetite

13. A patient is scheduled for vascular surgery. The patient is taking digoxin (Lanoxin), furosemide (Lasix), potassium, warfarin (Coumadin) and famotidine (Pepcid). Which medication may be stopped by the physician several days before surgery?
    a. Digoxin (Lanoxin)
    b. Furosemide (Lasix)
    c. Warfarin (Coumadin)
    d. Famotidine (Pepcid)

References

1. The values of cerebral blood flow being cut by 20% and renal by 50% by age 80 are from Tortora and Derrickson, Principles of Anatomy and Physiology, ed 11. New York, Wiley, 2005, p 796.
2. Accessed at www.American Heart Association.org on September 20, 2005. American Heart Association: 2005 Cardiovascular Disease Statistical Update. American Heart Association, Dallas, 2005.
3. Kane, GC, and Lipsky, JJ: Drug-grapefruit juice interactions. Mayo Clin Proc 75:933, 2000.
4. Anderson, GD: Sex differences in drug metabolism: Cytochrome P-450 and uridine diphosphate glucoronosyltransferase. J Gender Specific Med 5:25, 2002.
5. Dahan, A, and Altman, H: Food-drug interaction: Grapefruit juice augments drug bioavailability—mechanism, extent and relevance. Eur J Clin Nutr 58:1, 2004.
6. Grant, P: Warfarin and cranberry juice: An interaction? J Heart Valve Dis 13:25, 2004.
7. Suvarna, R, Pirmohamed, M, and Henderson, L: Possible interaction between warfarin and cranberry juice. BMJ 327:1454, 2003.

SUGGESTED ANSWERS TO

CRITICAL THINKING

■ Mrs. Smith

1. An older patient commonly does not experience typical disorder symptoms. Chest pain is often not present because of reduced nerve sensitivity with aging for an MI. Dyspnea is the classic symptom of MI in the older patient.

2. Inspect both legs to determine edematous areas. Determine location and severity of edema by pressing finger for 5 seconds over the medial malleolus and moving up the leg along the tibia until no edema is found. Assess bilaterally. Measure leg circumference.

3. Document location of edema and whether edema is nonpitting or pitting. Document findings for both legs.

4. Documentation should state "Bilateral pitting ankle edema" with leg circumference measurement number.

5. Additional symptoms should be documented as follows: Dyspnea at rest that increases with exertion, heart tones clear and distant, nailbeds pale, pain free, poor appetite for 2 weeks, 6-pound weight gain in 1 week, three-pillow orthopnea, bilateral jugular vein distention.

6. Unit Analysis Method:

$$\frac{162 \text{ pounds}}{} \; \Big| \; \frac{1 \text{ kilogram}}{2.2 \text{ pounds}} = 73.6 \text{ kilograms}$$

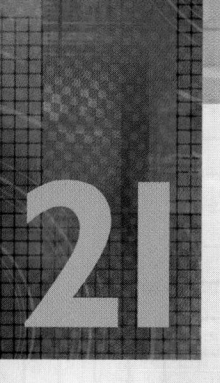

21

Nursing Care of Patients with Hypertension

BRENDA ANDERSON

KEY TERMS

cardiac output (KAR-dee-yak OWT-put)

diastolic blood pressure (dye-ah-STAH-lik BLUHD PRE-shure)

essential hypertension (e-SEN-shul HIGH-per-TEN-shun)

hypertension (HIGH-per-TEN-shun)

hypertensive emergency (HIGH-per-TEN-siv e-MERGE-n-see)

hypertensive urgency (HIGH-per-TEN-siv UR-gen-see)

hypertrophy (high-PER-truh-fee)

isolated systolic hypertension (EYE-suh-lay-ted sis-TAL-lik HIGH-per-TEN-shun)

normotensive (nor-mo-TEN-siv)

peripheral vascular resistance (puh-RIFF-uh-ruhl VAS-kyoo-lar ree-ZIS-tense)

plaque (PLAK)

primary hypertension (PRY-mare-ee HIGH-per-TEN-shun)

secondary hypertension (SEK-un-DAR-ee HIGH-per-TEN-shun)

systolic blood pressure (sis-TAL-ik BLUHD PRE-shure)

viscosity (vis-KAH-si-tee)

QUESTIONS TO GUIDE YOUR READING

1. How would you explain the pathophysiology of hypertension?

2. What are the causes and risk factors for hypertension?

3. What are the signs and symptoms of hypertension?

4. What are the current therapeutic interventions for hypertension?

5. What are the classifications of hypertension in adults and recommendations for treatment?

6. How would you classify hypertensive emergency?

7. What are common complications of hypertension?

8. What nursing care will you provide for patients with hypertension?

9. How will you know if your nursing interventions have been effective?

The seventh report of the Joint National Committee on Prevention, Detection, Evaluation and Treatment of High Blood Pressure (JNC 7)[1] has redefined normal and abnormal blood pressures for adults age 18 years and older, and treatment guidelines for physicians, clinicians, nurses, and community programs to follow (Table 21.1). For more information on the JNC7 guidelines, visit www.nhlbi.nih.gov. More people are now considered hypertensive as well as prehypertensive under these new guidelines. It is important to stay aware of new changes in this area to best serve your patients.

To have a normal blood pressure (BP) both the systolic and diastolic readings taken in a seated position must be below 120/80 (Box 21.1). If either the **systolic blood pressure** is above 119 mm Hg or the **diastolic blood pressure** is above 79 mm Hg, patients are classified in the prehypertensive or hypertensive category that matches their highest reading. **Hypertension,** also known as high blood pressure, is a condition in which the average of at least two or more readings on different dates is above prehypertensive levels of either 120 to 139 over 80 to 89. As we age, the incidence of hypertension increases. Therefore, we can expect to see more cases of hypertension as the population ages and life spans increase. For more information on hypertension, visit www.americanheart.org.

PATHOPHYSIOLOGY OF HYPERTENSION

Normally the heart pumps blood through the body to meet the cells' needs for oxygen and nutrients. As it pumps, the heart forces blood through the blood vessels. The pressure exerted by blood on the walls of the blood vessels is meas-

---

systolic: systole—concentration
diastolic: diastole—expansion
hypertension: hyper—excessive + tensio—tension

Box 21.1

Taking Accurate Blood Pressure Measurements

- Use auscultatory method with properly calibrated and validated blood pressure instrument.
- Seat patient quietly for at least 5 minutes in a chair (not on examination table) with feet on the floor and arm supported at heart level.
- Use appropriate-sized cuff in which cuff bladder encircles at least 80% of arm.
- Take at least two blood pressure measurements.
  - SBP = first of two or more sounds heard
  - DBP = disappearance of sounds
- Provide patients, verbally and in writing, their specific BP reading.

Adapted from JNC 7, 2004.

---

ured as blood pressure. Blood pressure is determined by **cardiac output** (CO), **peripheral vascular resistance** (PVR; the ability of the vessels to stretch), the **viscosity** (thickness) of the blood, and the amount of circulating blood volume. Decreased stretching ability of blood vessels, increased blood viscosity, and/or increased fluid volume may cause an increase in blood pressure.

Several processes influence blood pressure. These processes include nervous system regulation, arterial baroreceptors and chemoreceptors, the renin-angiotensin-aldosterone mechanism, and balancing of body fluids. One way blood pressure is influenced is through adjustment of the CO, which is the amount of blood that the heart pumps out each minute. The heart rate rises to increase CO in

---

viscosity: viscous—sticky

TABLE 21.1 BLOOD PRESSURE CATEGORIES AND THERAPEUTIC INTERVENTIONS*

BP Category	Systolic Blood Pressure (mm Hg)	Diastolic Blood Pressure (mm Hg)	Recommended Follow-up	Lifestyle Modification	Drug Therapy Without Other Indicators
Normal	<120	<80	2 years	Encourage	None
Pre-hypertension	120–139	80–89	1 year	Yes	None
Stage 1 Hypertension	140–159	90–99	2 months	Yes	Thiazide-type diuretics. Consider ACEI, ARB, BB, CCB, or combination.
Stage 2 Hypertension	≥160	≥100	1 month For BP >180/110 evaluate and seek treatment immediately; then 1 week as needed	Yes	Two-drug combination (usually thiazide-type diuretic and ACEI or ARB, or BB or CCB).

*Treatment is based on highest BP category.

Drug abbreviations: ACEI, angiotensin-converting enzyme inhibitor; ARB, angiotensin receptor blocker; BB, beta blocker; CCB, calcium channel blocker.

Adapted from JNC 7, 2004.

response to either physical or emotional activities that require more oxygen for the organs and tissues. PVR also influences blood pressure; it is the opposition that blood encounters as it flows through vessels. Anything causing blood vessels to become narrower causes an increased PVR. Any time PVR is increased, more pressure is needed to push the blood through the vessel, so blood pressure increases as a result. If PVR is decreased, less pressure is needed. Increased arteriolar PVR is the main mechanism that elevates blood pressure in hypertension.

Factors that impair normal regulation of blood pressure may lead to hypertension. Many of these factors are not well understood. Sympathetic nervous system overstimulation, which causes vasoconstriction, can contribute to hypertension. Alterations in baroreceptors and chemoreceptors may also influence the development of hypertension. For example, baroreceptors may become less sensitive from prolonged increases in vessel pressure and subsequently fail to stimulate vasodilation through vessel stretching. Additionally, increases in hormones that cause sodium retention, such as aldosterone, lead to increased fluid retention. Changes in kidney function that alter the excretion of fluid also result in an increase in overall body fluid that may contribute to hypertension.

Primary Hypertension

Primary, or **essential, hypertension** is the chronic elevation of blood pressure from an unknown cause.

Secondary Hypertension

Secondary hypertension has a known cause. In other words, it is a sign of another problem, such as a kidney abnormality, a tumor of the adrenal gland, or a congenital defect of the aorta. When the cause of secondary hypertension is treated before permanent structural changes occur, blood pressure usually returns to normal.

Isolated Systolic Hypertension

Isolated systolic hypertension (ISH) is a systolic pressure of 140 mm Hg or greater and a diastolic pressure of 90 mm Hg or less. This type of hypertension occurs mainly in the elderly, although it can occur at any age (Box 21.2 Gerontological Issues). For people with a systolic pressure higher than 140 mm Hg and a diastolic pressure under

90 mm Hg found on two separate readings, a referral to a physician for further evaluation is recommended. Treatment of ISH is recommended to decrease cardiovascular disease, especially heart failure episodes and risk of stroke. Lifestyle modifications are usually tried first if the systolic elevation is not too severe. If lifestyle modifications fail to reduce the systolic pressure, antihypertensive medication is added.

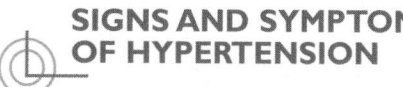

SIGNS AND SYMPTOMS OF HYPERTENSION

Often hypertension causes no signs or symptoms other than elevated blood pressure readings. As a result, hypertension is referred to as the "silent killer." Patients with hypertension are often first diagnosed when seeking health care for reasons unrelated to hypertension. In a small number of cases, a patient with hypertension may complain of a headache, bloody nose, severe anxiety, or shortness of breath, although it is usually impossible for a patient to correlate the absence or presence of symptoms with the degree of blood pressure elevation (Box 21.3 Hypertension Summary).

Most signs and symptoms of hypertension stem from long-term damaging effects on the large and small blood vessels of the heart, kidneys, brain, and eyes. These effects are known as target organ disease.

 ## DIAGNOSIS OF HYPERTENSION

Diagnosis of hypertension considers a patient's risk factors for hypertension, a previous diagnosis of hypertension, presence of signs and symptoms, history of kidney or heart disease, and current use of medications. When the average of

---

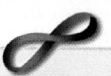 ### Box 21.2

Gerontological Issues

In the past, it was thought that diastolic pressure was the most important part of blood pressure to control. However, it is now known that after age 55, diastolic pressure falls while systolic pressure continues to rise with age. This means that it is important to control systolic blood pressure, not just diastolic pressure in older adults to prevent heart disease and stroke.

Box 21.3

Hypertension Summary

Signs and Symptoms	Often none
	Increased blood pressure
	Headache, bloody nose, severe anxiety, or shortness of breath.
Diagnosis	Prehypertension is greater than systolic of 120 and diastolic of 80.
	Hypertension is the average blood pressure, for two or more readings on different dates, greater than systolic of 139 and diasolic of 89.
Therapeutic Interventions	Lifestyle modification
	Antihypertensive medications
Complications	Heart failure, myocardial infarction, stroke, renal failure
Nursing diagnoses	Deficient knowledge
	Potential ineffective therapeutic regimen management

seated blood pressure is above prehypertensive levels of either 120 to 139 or 80 to 89 on two or more occasions, then hypertension is diagnosed (see Table 21.1). Research has shown that the most effective method for predicting risk for stroke and heart attack are self blood pressure monitoring twice a day for a week.[2]

Diagnostic Tests

The JNC7 recommends physicians order various routine tests before beginning therapy for high blood pressure to identify damage to organs or blood vessels. Tests recommended by JNC7 include ECG, blood glucose, hematocrit, serum potassium, calcium, lipoprotein profile, high-density and low-density lipoprotein cholesterol (HDL-C and LDL-C, respectively), and triglyceride levels. These tests help determine if target-organ damage has been caused by elevated blood pressure. An example of this is testing for kidney damage with a urinalysis or serum creatinine level.

RISK FACTORS FOR HYPERTENSION

A combination of genetic (nonmodifiable) and environmental (modifiable) risk factors are thought to be responsible for the development of hypertension, although the cause remains unknown. Nonmodifiable risk factors—those that cannot be changed—include a family history of hypertension, age, ethnicity, and diabetes mellitus. Modifiable risk factors—those that can be changed—include blood glucose levels, activity levels, smoking, and salt and alcohol intake. Smoking cessation; reduced salt, caffeine and alcohol intake; weight reduction; improved meal planning; increased physical activity; and managing stress can all help to decrease blood pressure.

Nonmodifiable Risk Factors

Family History of Hypertension

Hypertension is seen more commonly among people with a family history of hypertension. Indeed, people with a family history have almost twice the risk of developing hypertension as those with no family history. People with a family history of hypertension should be encouraged to have their blood pressure checked regularly.

Age

People age differently because of their genetic and environmental risk factors and lifestyle habits. Thus, the results of the aging process may be reflected in wide variations of blood pressure among elderly people. As a person ages, **plaque** builds up in the arteries and the blood vessels become stiffer and less elastic, causing the heart to work harder to force blood through the vessels. These vessel changes increase the amount of work required by the heart to maintain blood flow into the circulation and subsequently blood pressure increases.

Race and Ethnicity

Box 21.4 (Cultural Considerations) discusses hypertension among various ethnic groups.

Diabetes Mellitus

Many adults who have diabetes mellitus also have hypertension. The risk of developing hypertension with a family history of diabetes and obesity is greater than when there is no family history. Lifestyle modifications and adherence to therapy are crucial to prevent the heart attacks, strokes, blindness, and kidney failure associated with high blood glucose and blood pressure levels.

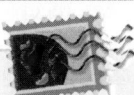

Box 21.4

Cultural Considerations

Hypertension continues to be the most serious health problem for African Americans in the United States. More than 5 million of the 26 million African Americans living in the United States are hypertensive. They suffer higher mortality and morbidity rates related to hypertension and at an earlier age. African Americans from lower socioeconomic backgrounds have higher blood pressure than African Americans from higher socioeconomic backgrounds. Additionally, African Americans are 3.2 times more likely to develop kidney failure related to hypertension than European Americans.

Hypertension among African Americans is usually caused by increased renin activity resulting in greater sodium and fluid retention. Thus, African Americans respond better to diuretics such as furosemide (Lasix) and hydrochlorothiazide (HydroDIURIL) than to beta blockers such as propranolol (Inderal). Hypertension among European-Americans is more often caused by chemical imbalances; thus they respond better to beta blockers.

Chinese people are more sensitive than Caucasians to the effects of propranolol on heart rate and blood pressure, requiring only half the blood level of European Americans to achieve a therapeutic effect. Propranolol is eliminated from the bodies of many Chinese persons at double the rate of European Americans. They are more likely to suffer fatigue as a side effect. Thus, the nurse must carefully monitor the Chinese patient for therapeutic and side effects.

Hypertension among Japanese Americans is primarily related to the high sodium content of the Japanese diet, stress, and a high rate of cigarette smoking.

High rates of hypertension among Koreans and Filipinos are due to the stress of immigration, preserving foods in salt, and using condiments high in sodium.

Modifiable Risk Factors

The JNC7 suggests advising patients with hypertension to use lifestyle modifications. These modifications include weight reduction; adoption of the Dietary Approaches to Stop Hypertension (DASH) eating plan; moderation of dietary sodium, caffeine, and alcohol intake; increased physical activity; and smoking cessation (Box 21.5 Lifestyle Modifications for Hypertension). Lifestyle modifications are often used with antihypertensive drugs to control hypertension and enhance the drug effects (Box 21.6 Nutrition Notes).

Weight Reduction

There is a strong relationship between excess body weight and increased blood pressure. Weight reduction is one of the most important lifestyle modifications to lower blood pressure. The health-care provider and dietitian should be consulted to help the patient develop a weight-reduction plan.

Meal Planning

SALT INTAKE. High blood pressure is associated with a diet high in salt. Patients whose blood pressure can be lowered by restricting dietary sodium are called salt sensitive. This sensitivity is particularly common among African Americans, elderly persons, and patients with diabetes and obesity. Patients with hypertension should be instructed not to add salt while cooking and/or table salt to their food. Processed foods and foods in which salt can be easily tasted (e.g., canned soups, ham, bacon, salted nuts) should also be avoided.

CAFFEINE. Intake of caffeine should be limited as it can increase aortic stiffness. This raises the risk of cardiovascular disease for those with high blood pressure.

INTAKE OF POTASSIUM, MAGNESIUM, AND CALCIUM. The JNC7 recommends a balanced diet that

---

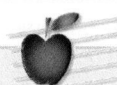

Box 21.6

Nutrition Notes

Reducing Blood Pressure with Diet

The Dietary Approaches to Stop Hypertension (DASH) diet reduced blood pressure significantly in **normotensive** people and produced even greater reductions in hypertensive people in the eight week trial. Rather than emphasizing restriction of foods, the DASH diet increases the intake of certain commonly available, not specialty, foods. So that weight loss would not confound the results, participants were given additional calories if they began to lose weight. All the tested diets contained about 3 grams of sodium. Also, everyone was instructed to consume no more than three caffeinated beverages and no more than two standard alcoholic beverages per day to minimize the effects of those substances on the results. On a 2000-calorie diet, an individual following the DASH diet would consume the following:

7 to 8 servings of grains, equivalent to 7 to 8 slices of bread

4 to 5 servings of vegetables, equivalent to 4 to 5 cups of raw, leafy or 2 to 2 $\frac{1}{2}$ cups cooked

4 to 5 servings of fruits, equivalent to 4 to 5 medium fresh fruits or 1 to 1 $\frac{1}{4}$ cups dried fruit

2 to 3 servings of low-fat or nonfat dairy foods, equivalent to 16 to 24 ounces of milk

2 or fewer servings of lean meats, poultry, and fish, equivalent to 6 ounces or less per day

4 to 5 servings *per week* of nuts, seeds, and legumes, equivalent to 1 1/3 to 1 2/3 cups nuts or 2 to 2 $\frac{1}{2}$ cups cooked legumes

2.5 servings of fats and oils, equivalent to 2 $\frac{1}{2}$ teaspoons, preferably monounsaturated oils (canola, olive, peanut oils)

---

ensures adequate intake of these nutrients. Low levels of these nutrients can contribute to cardiovascular events. Foods rich in potassium include oranges, bananas, and broccoli. Magnesium is found in green vegetables such as spinach, nuts, seeds, and some whole grains. Milk, yogurt, and spinach are rich in calcium. Whenever possible, fresh or frozen foods should be selected rather than canned foods to increase intake of these nutrients.

Alcohol Consumption

The regular consumption of three or more drinks per day can increase the risk of hypertension and cause resistance to antihypertensive therapy. The nurse should counsel hypertensive patients who drink alcohol to consume no more than 1 oz of alcohol per day for men (two drinks) and no more than 1/2 oz per day for women (one drink). One drink should be considered 12 oz of beer, 1.5 oz of 80-

---

Box 21.5

Lifestyle Modifications for Hypertension

- Lose weight.
- Limit alcohol intake.
- Get regular aerobic exercise.
- Decrease amount of salt intake.
- Include daily allowances of potassium and calcium.
- Stop smoking.
- Reduce dietary saturated fat and cholesterol.

See Nutrition Notes, Box 21.6

Adapted from The Seventh Report of the Joint National Committee on Prevention, Detection, Evaluation, and Treatment of High Blood Pressure.

proof liquor, or 5 oz of wine (JNC7). Blood pressure may decrease or return to normal when alcohol consumption is modified.

Exercise

People with sedentary lifestyles have an increased risk of hypertension. Exercise helps prevent and control hypertension by reducing weight, decreasing peripheral resistance, and decreasing body fat. Anyone who is able should participate in regular aerobic physical activity, such as brisk walking, for at least 30 minutes per day on most days of the week. Patients with hypertension should be evaluated by a health-care provider before starting an exercise program.

Smoking

Smoking is a major risk factor for cardiovascular disease. Blood pressure may increase because nicotine constricts the blood vessels. Nurses should counsel patients with hypertension to quit smoking for overall cardiovascular risk reduction benefits. A referral to a smoking cessation program can be helpful in reaching this goal.

CRITICAL THINKING

Mrs. Miller

■ Mrs. Miller, age 54, visits a health clinic because she has a headache every morning. The nurse collects data on Mrs. Miller and finds that she is an office manager, smokes a pack of cigarettes a day, eats fast food for lunch at her desk, has two adult children, is recently divorced, and has two to three alcoholic drinks every evening. Mrs. Miller has been in good health and takes two aspirin tablets for her headaches daily.

1. What are Mrs. Miller's risk factors for hypertension?
2. What is the most significant patient information identified? Why?
3. Why is hypertension referred to as the silent killer?
4. Why should Mrs. Miller be told of the need for lifelong therapy if she is diagnosed with hypertension?

Suggested answers at end of chapter.

THERAPEUTIC INTERVENTIONS

The JNC7 provides guidelines for selecting therapy based on the patient's blood pressure, severity of blood pressure risk factors, and the presence of target-organ disease or cardiovascular disease. The no- or low-risk hypertensive patient's therapy begins with lifestyle modifications. If lifestyle modifications alone do not result in obtaining a blood pressure at the target goal, then drug therapy is recommended. For patients with severe hypertension, high-risk factors, or target-organ disease, drug therapy is started

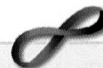

Box 21.7

Gerontological Issues

Managing Antihypertensive Therapy

For safety, teach older adults who take antihypertensive drugs to rise slowly to prevent the effects of orthostatic hypotension. Dizziness may result, increasing the risk of falling. Deficiencies in fluid volume can be a common problem for older adults as well, and diuretics can contribute to fluid volume deficiencies. Careful fluid balance assessment is important to prevent dehydration. Older adults may be more sensitive to medications, so monitor them carefully for adverse effects. Older patients may need lower dosages of medications.

immediately along with lifestyle modifications. Safe administration of medications is important, especially for the older person (Box 21.7 Gerontological Issues).

Goals of therapeutic interventions are less than 140/90 mm Hg, or less than 130/80 mm Hg for those with diabetes or chronic kidney disease. For most patients with hypertension, initial drug therapy should be thiazide-type diuretics. If the response is inadequate to achieve the blood pressure goal, the dosage may be increased or a second drug from a different class may be added. There are eight categories of medications to treat hypertension: diuretics, alpha-adrenergic blockers, beta blockers, calcium channel blockers, angiotensin-converting enzyme (ACE) inhibitors, angiotensin II antagonists (ARB), central acting agents, adrenergic neuron blockers (peripherally acting), and vasodilators. Examples of these medications are given in Table 21.2.

The treatment plan of lifestyle modifications and medications is effective only when patients are motivated to accept the diagnosis of hypertension and include lifelong treatment in their daily routine. Empathy and trust can increase patient motivation. Patients should be instructed that antihypertensive therapy must usually be continued for the rest of their lives. Patients should be reminded that although they may be feeling better with the modifications and medications, the hypertension is still present even if it is well controlled. Patients should be told not to stop taking their medications unless instructed to do so by their health-care provider.

Antihypertensive medications can have unpleasant side effects. Patients should be told what these side effects are and to report them if they do occur, so that medication alterations can be made if possible. Erectile dysfunction can be one of the side effects of these medications. Male patients may be reluctant to discuss this side effect and instead choose to stop the medication. The nurse should be proactive and inform male patients about this side effect so they will understand that if it occurs and is reported, the physician can make adjustments in the medication regimen.

TABLE 21.2 ANTIHYPERTENSIVE MEDICATIONS

Medication Class/Action	Examples	Route	Side Effects	Nursing Implications
Diuretics Increase urine output by inhibiting sodium and water reabsorption by the kidney. Several types.				Take with food to prevent GI upset. Monitor I&O and weight to determine fluid loss. Assess for improvement of edema in patients with HF and reduced BP in hypertension. Electrolyte imbalances may occur quickly. Teach patient to take during awake hours to prevent excessive urination during sleeping hours.
Thiazide and thiazide-like diuretics Increase urine output by promoting sodium, chloride and water excretion; not immediate effect, most effective in normal renal function; causes loss of sodium potassium, magnesium, calcium saved.	Thiazide: hydrochlorothiazide (HydroDIURIL) chlorothiazide (Diuril) bendroflumethiazide (Naturetin) benzthiazide (Exna) hydroflumethiazide (Saluron, Diucardin) methyclothiazide (Aquatensen, Enduron) polythiazide (Renese-R). Thiazide-like: chlorthalidone (Hygroton) indapamide (Lozol) metolazone (Zaroxolyn, Mykrox) quinethazone (Hydromax)	PO IV form available for chlorothiazide.	Dizziness, fatigue, weakness, hypokalemia, hypercalemia, nausea, vomiting, anorexia, hyperglycemia, rash	Blood sugar may increase in diabetics. Teach patient to wear sunscreen and protective clothing to prevent photo-sensitivity. Hypercalcemia could be hazardous to patient on digoxin.
Loop diuretics Act on ascending loop of Henle in kidney to cause sodium and water loss; also causes loss of potassium, magnesium, and calcium.	bumetanide (Bumex) furosemide (Lasix) ethacrynic acid (if allergic to sulfonamides) torsemide (Demadex)	PO/IV/IM	Hyperkalemia, rash, nausea, hypoglycemia, tinnitus, rash, increased uric acid levels.	Contraindicated if allergic to sulfonamides. Teach to use sunscreen to prevent photo-sensitivity. Take with food or milk to prevent GI upset.
Potassium-sparing diuretics Mild diuretic, can be used as combination therapy; promote sodium and water excretion and potassium retention by the kidney.	amiloride (Midamor) triamterene (Dyrenium) spironolactone (Aldactone)	PO	Hyperkalemia, headache, nausea, vomiting, anorexia, diarrhea, rash, itching	Avoid foods rich in potassium such as oranges, bananas, salt substitutes, dried fruits. Triamterene -take after meals for GI upset -may turn urine blue
Sympatholytics: **Beta Blockers** Decrease sympathtetic nervous system resulting in decreased blood pressure, heart rate, contractility, cardiac output, and renin activity.	acebutolol (Sectral) atenolol (Tenormin) betaxolol HCL (Kerlone) carteolol HCL (Cartrol) metoprolol (Lopressor) metoprolol extended release (Toprol XL)	PO IV form available for atenolol, metoprolol, and propranolol	Orthostatic hypotension, decreased heart rate, diarrhea, nausea, vomiting, bronchospasm, blood dyscrasias, and HF	Daily I & O and weight. Check heart rate and blood pressure before administration. Teach patient not to stop drug abruptly to avoid rebound hypertension, angina or dysrhythmias.

(Continued on following page)

TABLE **21.2** **ANTIHYPERTENSIVE MEDICATIONS** *(Continued)*

Medication Class/Action	Examples	Route	Side Effects	Nursing Implications
	nadolol (Corgard) penbutolol (Levatol) propranolol (Inderal) propranolol long acting (Inderal LA) timolol maleate (Blocadren)			**High Alert:** IV vasoactive medications are inherently dangerous. Oral and parenteral doses of propranolol are not interchangeable; IV dose is 1/10 the oral dose. Patient harm or fatalities have occurred when switching from oral to IV route.
Alpha₁ blockers Block effects of sympathetic nervous system on smooth muscle of blood vessels resulting in vasodilation and decreased blood pressure.	prazosin (Minipress) terazosin (Hytrin)	PO	Hypotension, increased heart rate, nasal stuffiness, nausea, vomiting, diarrhea	Monitor for hypotension. Teach to make position changes slowly.
Combined alpha and beta blockers Block alpha-adrenergic receptors causing vasodilation and reduced blood pressure; Decrease sympathetic nervous system resulting in decreased heart rate, and contractility.	carvedilol (Coreg) carteolol HCl (Cartol) labetalol (Normodyne)	PO IV form available for labetalol	Dizziness, diarrhea, nausea, vomiting, tinnitus, bradycardia, postural hypotension, sexual dysfunction, high blood sugar	Daily I&O and weight, Assess heart rate prior to administration. Assess edema, neck vein distention, lung sounds. Teach patient not to stop drug abruptly.
Central acting alpha₂ agonists Block effects of sympathetic nervous system centrally.	clonidine* (Catapres) guanabenz acetate (Wytensin) guanfacine HCl (Tenex) methylodopa (Aldomet)	PO Transdermal patch available for clonidine IV methylodopa	Drowsiness, sedation, headache, fatigue, nausea, vomiting, malaise, dry mouth, rash, postural hypotension, palpitations	Assess for edema and/or decreased BP. Suggest gum or hard candy for dry mouth. Teach not to stop drug abruptly.
Adrenergic neuron blockers (peripherally acting) Block norepinephrine release resulting in reduced blood pressure for severe hypertension control.	guanethidine (Ismelin) reserpine (Serpalan)	PO	dizziness, GI upset, edema, headache, dry mouth, orthostatic hypotension, chest pain, bradycardia, dyspnea, muscle pain, depression, difficulty sleeping, sexual dysfunction.	Teach to rise slowly to prevent falls. Teach to chew gum or use hard candy for dry mouth. Reserpine can cause nightmares and suicidal intent.
Angiotension-converting enzyme (ACE) inhibitors Blocks production of angiotension II, a potent vasoconstrictor; Reduces peripheral arterial resistance and blood pressure.	benzepril HCl (Lotensin) captopril (Capoten) enalapril (Vasotec) fosinopril (Monopril) lisinopril ((Prinavil, Zestril) moexipril (Univasc) perindopril (Aceon) quinapril (Accupril) ramipril (altace) trandolapril (Mavik)	PO IV form available for enalapril	Hypotension, increased heart rate, dyspnea, cough, angioedema	Monitor patient for edema with HF and decreased BP with hypertension. Teach patient that sensitivity to sunlight may occur and not to stop agent abruptly.

Medication Class/Action	Examples	Route	Side Effects	Nursing Implications
Angiotensin II Receptor antagonists (ARB) Block angiotension II receptors causing vasodilation and reduction in blood pressure.	candesartan (Atacand) eprosartan (Teveten) irbesartan (Avapro) losartan (Cozaar) olmesartan (Benicar) telmisartan (Micardais) valsartan (Diovan)	PO	Dizziness, insomnia, diarrhea, cough	Monitor patient for edema with HF and decreased BP with hypertension. Teach patient sensitivity to sunlight may occur.
Aldosterone receptor antagonist Blocks binding of aldosterone at receptor site to reduce sodium reabsorption and then blood pressure.	eplerenone (Inspra)	PO	Headache, dizziness, angina, hyperkalemia, increased creatinine	Monitor potassium before and during therapy.
Calcium channel blockers Prevent movement of extracellular calcium into the cell which vasodilates.	amlodipine (Norvasc) diltiazem (Cardizem) felodipine (Plendil) isradipine (DynaCirc) nicardipine HCl (Cardene, Cardene SR) nifedipine (Procardia) nisoldipine (Sular, Nisocor) verapamil (CalanSR, Isoptin SR)	PO IV form available for diltiazem, verapamil, nicardipine	Dysrhythmias, edema, headache, fatigue, drowsiness, flushing	Take pulse prior to administration, assess for decreased BP, heart rate dysrhythmias, angina. May increase blood levels of digoxin.
Direct vasodilators Relax smooth muscles of blood vessels causing vasodilation and decreased blood pressure.	hydralazine (Apresoline) minoxidil (Loniten)	PO/IV/IM	Headache, nausea, hypotension or hypertension and changes in heart rhythm	Treat headache with acetaminophen. Monitor for increasing heart rate. Often given with diuretic to reduce edema resulting from water and sodium retention.

HF = heart failure; I&O = input and output; PO = oral; IV = intravenous; IM = intramuscular.
*Clonidine and clonazepam have been identified as potential problematic drug names. (*www.jcaho.org, 2006*)

LEARNING TIP

Hypertension lifestyle modifications:

L—Limit salt, caffeine, and alcohol.
I—Include daily potassium and calcium.
F—Fight fat and cholesterol.
E—Exercise regularly.
S—Stay on your blood pressure regimen.
T—Try to quit smoking.
Y—Your medications are to be taken daily.
L—Lose weight.
E—End-stage complications will be avoided!

COMPLICATIONS OF HYPERTENSION

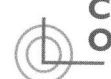

Common complications of hypertension include coronary artery disease, atherosclerosis, myocardial infarction (MI), heart failure (HF), stroke, and kidney or eye damage. The severity and duration of the increase in blood pressure determine the extent of the vascular changes causing organ damage. High blood pressure levels may also result in an increase in the size of the left ventricle, referred to as **hypertrophy.** Elevated blood pressure damages the small vessels of the heart, brain, kidneys, and retina. The results are a progressive functional impairment of these organs, known as target-organ disease.

SPECIAL CONSIDERATIONS

Blood pressure should be well controlled before any invasive procedure. Hypertensive patients are at greater risk for strokes, MI, HF, kidney failure, and pulmonary edema. These patients should be instructed to continue their blood pressure medications until the time of the procedure, unless otherwise directed by their physician or health-care provider. Antihypertensive medications should be resumed as soon as possible after the procedure as directed by the physician.

CRITICAL THINKING

Mrs. Bell

■ Mrs. Bell, 80 years old, is seen in the physician's office. She lives a sedentary lifestyle alone in her own home with a bathroom down the hall from the bedroom. Mrs. Bell's son lives in the same city and visits her often. She has wood floors with throw rugs in the hall and a tile floor in the bathroom. She wears glasses and has a cataract. She has an unsteady gait and nocturia. She is 40 pounds overweight and has a 10-year history of hypertension for which she is taking chlorothiazide (Diuril) and propranolol (Inderal) when she remembers them.

1. What are Mrs. Bell's modifiable and nonmodifiable risk factors for hypertension?
2. Why is Mrs. Bell taking clorothiazide and propranolol to treat her hypertension?
3. What teaching methods could be used to help ensure that Mrs. Bell will understand and follow her treatment plan?
4. Why should patient safety needs be addressed in the nursing care plan?
5. What safety interventions should the patient and family be taught?
6. Inderal 20 mg PO is ordered now as Mrs. Bell forgot to take her medication. The nurse has on hand Inderal 10-mg tablets. How many tablets should the nurse give?

Suggested answers at end of chapter.

 ## HYPERTENSIVE EMERGENCY

Hypertensive emergency is a severe type of hypertension characterized by elevations in SBP greater than 180 mm Hg and DBP greater than 120 that are complicated by risk for or progression of target-organ dysfunction (examples include MI, HF, and dissecting aortic aneurysm). Patients who are untreated, fail to comply with antihypertensive therapy, or stop their medication abruptly are at risk for hypertensive emergency. These patients require immediate reduction of BP to prevent or limit damage to target organs. It is recommended that patients with hypertensive crises be admitted to the critical care unit. In some cases, the blood pressure may need to be reduced 25% within 1 hour to prevent organ damage. If the patient is stable, blood pressure is then decreased to 160/100 to 110 in the next 2 to 6 hours. Gradual reduction of the BP is desired to prevent decreased blood flow to the kidneys, heart, and/or brain. An intravenous medication such as nitroprusside (Nipride)

may be given to quickly reduce blood pressure during this crisis.

 ## HYPERTENSIVE URGENCY

The JNC7 considers **hypertensive urgency** to occur in situations when there is severe elevation of BP as in hypertensive emergency but without target-organ dysfunction progression. The patient with hypertensive urgency may experience severe headaches, nosebleeds, shortness of breath, and severe anxiety. Patients experiencing hypertensive urgency can usually be treated with combination oral medication and scheduled for a follow-up visit within several days.

NURSING PROCESS

Nursing Assessment/Data Collection

Assessment of a patient with hypertension includes the patient's health history, blood pressure measurements, medications, and physical assessment (Fig. 21.1). Assessing what hypertensive patients and their families know about hypertension and associated risk factors is essential for planning patient and family education and subsequent lifelong lifestyle modification needs.

Nursing Diagnosis, Planning, Interventions, and Evaluation

Possible nursing diagnosis, planning, interventions, and evaluation must be agreed upon by the patient and the health care team. See Box 21.8 Nursing Care Plan for the Patient with Hypertension.

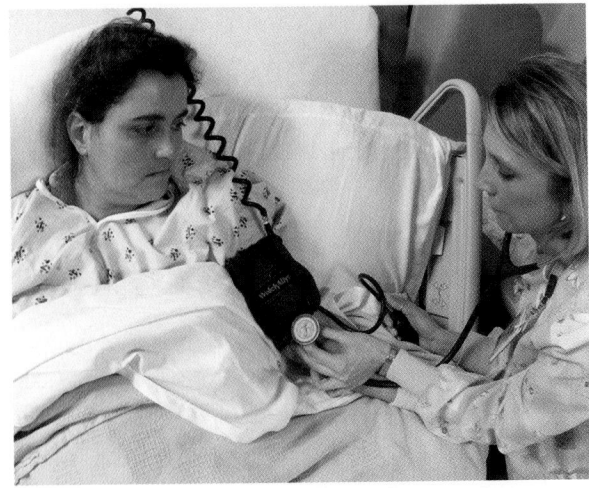

FIGURE 21.1 Nurse obtaining blood pressure measurement. Correct size cuff use is essential for accurate reading.

Box 21.8 NURSING CARE PLAN **for the Patient with Hypertension**

Nursing Diagnosis: Deficient Knowledge related to disease process and treatment regimen

Expected Outcomes Verbalizes knowledge of disease process and treatment regimen.

Evaluation of Outcomes Is Patient Able to Discuss and Explain Hypertension Disease Process Including its Risk Factors, Complications and Treatment Regimen?

Intervention	Rationale	Evaluation
Identify patient's readiness and ability to learn.	Patient must accept ownership of hypertension diagnosis and be able to receive and understand information given. Determine patient's preferred method of learning.	Does patient verbalize acceptance of hypertension diagnosis? Does patient demonstrate ability to read, write and retain information?
Provide patient with information concerning disease process including risk factors, complications, and treatment regimen	Patient will be more willing to participate in treatment regimen when able to understand need for changes in behavior.	Is patient able to participate in discussion concerning hypertension disease process including risk factors, complications and treatment regimen?

Nursing Diagnosis: Potential for ineffective therapeutic regimen management related to complexity of therapy, cost of medications, lack of symptoms, side effects of medications, need to alter long-term lifestyle habits, normal blood pressure controlled by therapy.

Expected Outcomes The patient verbalizes ability and willingness to comply with treatment.

Evaluation of Outcomes Is patient able to state how lifestyle will include therapy? Does patient identify and problem solve barriers for therapy?

Intervention	Rationale	Evaluation
Identify patient's modifiable risk factors and lifestyle modification needs.	Identifying risk factors is the first step in planning therapy. Patient must understand the relationship of these risk factors with hypertension and complication development.	Can patient state rationale for modifying risk factors to prevent complication development?
Identify factors that are barriers to patient complying with therapy.	Factors such as finances, transportation, aging changes, patient motivation, habits, and reading and educational level can be barriers for therapy.	Are barriers present for patient?
Develop plan to overcome barriers. Make referrals as needed.	Identified barriers can be overcome with planning and intervention, such as referral to support groups or for financial assistance or prescription delivery service and instructions provided at level of patient's learning ability.	Have barriers been eliminated?
		Is patient willing to use referrals?

(Continued on following page)

Box 21.8   NURSING CARE PLAN for the Patient with Hypertension (Continued)

Geriatric

Intervention	Rationale	Evaluation
Assess ability to take medications daily: financially, obtaining refills, understanding directions.	Elderly patients may be on a fixed income, lack transportation, or lack ability to take several medications several times a day. Simplifying this process, to one medication if possible, can increase compliance.	Is patient able to obtain medications? Can patient self-administer medications accurately on daily basis?
Teach patient to take medications as prescribed and not to skip dosages.	Elderly patients may skip dosages to save money, reduce side effects, or reduce need to void.	Does patient take dosages as prescribed?
		Does patient express concern over cost, side effects, or frequent voiding?
Teach patient to change positions slowly to prevent falls.	Antihypertensive medications can cause hypotension, resulting in dizziness and weakness and possibly leading to falls.	Does patient understand how to change positions slowly?
		Does patient experience dizziness or weakness?

Home Health Hints

- For meal planning, most patients eat fast foods occasionally. Assist them in choosing foods that are low in fat, sugar, and salt (e.g., choose chicken salads with low-fat dressing or fajitas without sour cream and guacamole).
- Instruct patients and caregivers to avoid frozen dinners and deli meats since many of these are high in sodium.
- Because medication and electrolyte interaction can occur with a salt substitute, which often contains potassium, the physician should be consulted before the patient uses it.
- Teach patients how to read labels for fat and salt content. If patients are on a 2- to 3-g sodium diet, instruct them about eating breads or cereals that contain 200 mg or less of sodium per serving or canned vegetables of 150 mg of sodium per serving. Fresh vegetables are better, but cost and storage must be considered. Providing written suggestions for the caregiver who does the grocery shopping increases compliance with diet therapy.
- Home exercise using weights can be improvised using canned goods and bags of sugar as weights. The amount of weight being used is easily identified for documentation by the labeling on the food item.

- The following suggestions may help a patient decrease or stop smoking: Use cinnamon mouthwash on arising; put away all ashtrays but one and keep it in a place not normally used for smoking; find ways to keep hands busy at times when usually holding cigarette, such as when drinking coffee or alcohol.
- Encourage patients to put "No Smoking" signs on their door to avoid passive smoking.
- Medication compliance can be a challenge for the elderly hypertensive patient. Instruct patients to take medication as prescribed even if they are feeling well or if side effects, which they should report, are present. If the medicines are too expensive for the patient, check with the physician and pharmacist for less expensive alternatives.
- During home visits count the amount of pills in a bottle to assess compliance. Remind the patient to get refills and keep physician appointments by writing them on the calendar.
- Advise patients who are leaving home for the weekend or holidays to refill medicines ahead of time to ensure that they do not run out. The physician can write a prescription for the patient to have for emergency refills.

- Because many of the antihypertensive medicines can cause bradycardia, teach the patient or caregiver to take the patient's pulse and to call the nurse if it is below 60 or the parameters defined by the physician or agency.
- Monitor carefully for symptoms of congestive heart failure when the patient is on beta blockers. This is a side effect that needs to be caught early and reported to the physician.
- Encourage the patient to obtain a home blood pressure monitoring device. Instruct the patient caregiver on proper use and logging the date, time, and reading obtained. The home health nurse should review the log on each visit.
- Patients should be instructed to weigh themselves every morning after voiding, to wear the same amount of clothing each time, and to keep a log for the nurse to review.

REVIEW QUESTIONS

1. Which of the following does the nurse understand as a cause of primary hypertension to plan care for a patient with hypertension?
   a. It is caused by a tumor of the adrenal gland.
   b. It is caused by renal artery stenosis.
   c. It is caused by coarctation of the aorta.
   d. There is no known cause.

2. Which of the following is the most important lifestyle modification for the hypertensive patient who is obese?
   a. Reduce weight.
   b. Restrict salt intake.
   c. Increase potassium intake.
   d. Decrease alcohol intake.

3. Which of the following does the nurse understand is often the only sign of hypertension?
   a. Sacral edema
   b. Elevated blood pressure
   c. Tachycardia
   d. Jugular vein distention

Multiple response item. Select all that apply.
4. Which of the following instructions would be included in dietary education for a patient with high blood pressure?
   a. Canned fruit and vegetables are best to eat.
   b. Add salt to food during cooking and just before eating.
   c. Increase foods high in saturated fat.
   d. Chose fresh or frozen fruits and vegetables.
   e. Read food labels.
   f. Watch for potassium in salt substitutes.

5. For which of the following blood pressure readings should a 1-year follow-up visit be recommended?
   a. 108/66
   b. 116/76
   c. 138/84
   d. 142/90

6. During a health screening a patient's blood pressure is confirmed by two nurses to be 210/120 mmHg. Which of the following interventions should be recommended?
   a. The patient takes off the rest of the day and rests.
   b. The patient rest quietly while the nurses calls 911 to request an ambulance.
   c. The patient should take two doses of blood pressure medication right now.
   d. The patient may return to work and have blood pressure rechecked in two days.

7. Which of the following would the nurse expect to find in a patient experiencing the complication of heart failure from hypertension?
   a. Abnormal hair growth pattern on face.
   b. Distended jugular veins in semi-Fowler's position.
   c. Pain in the right hand when writing.
   d. Depression from taking blood pressure medication.

8. The nurse should give which of the following instructions to a patient receiving a diuretic?
   a. Eliminate salt in your diet.
   b. Change positions slowly.
   c. Take your medication before bed.
   d. Empty your bladder after taking the first dose.

9. At a follow-up visit for a patient with hypertension, which of the following data best indicates that the patient's blood pressure therapy is successful?
   a. Weight decreased 3 pounds.
   b. Diary of dietary intake within suggested diet
   c. BP less than 120/80 mmHg.
   d. Patient reports walking 30 to 40 minutes daily.

References

1. United States Department of Health and Human Services (2004). The Seventh Report of the Joint National Committee on Prevention, Detection, Evaluation, and Treatment of High Blood Pressure.Retrieved August 12, 2005 from http://www. nhlbi.nih.gov/guidelines/hypertension/jnc7full.htm
2. Clement DI, De Buyzere ML, De Bacquer DA: Office versus ambulatory pressure study investigators. Prognostic value of ambulatory blood pressure recordings in patients with treated hypertension. N Engl J Med 348:2407–2415, 2003.
3. Joint Commission on Accreditation of Healthcare Organizations. National Patient Safety Goals for 2006. National Patient Safety Goal-Identify and, at a minimum annually review a list of look-alike/sound-alike drugs used in the organization, and take action to prevent errors involving the interchange of these drugs. Retreived on August 12, 2005 from, http://www.jcaho.org/accredited+organizations/patient+ safety/npsg.htm

SUGGESTED ANSWERS TO

CRITICAL THINKING

■ *Mrs. Miller*

1. Risk factors include gender; age; smoking; a diet high in fat, salt, and calories; consumption of two to three alcoholic drinks per evening; and possibly her morning headaches.
2. Morning headaches. Mrs. Miller may be experiencing an episode of hypertensive urgency and should be evaluated immediately by a health-care provider.
3. "Silent killer" refers to the fact that there are often no signs or symptoms associated with hypertension.
4. Lifelong therapy is required because there is no cure for hypertension and complications need to be prevented.

■ *Mrs. Bell*

1. Nonmodifiable risk factors include age, gender, and history of hypertension. Modifiable risk factors include weight and compliance with antihypertensive therapy.
2. Thiazide diuretics are first-line drugs. Diuretics remove excess salt and water to decrease blood volume and lower blood pressure. Beta blockers stop the beta receptors from receiving the message from the brain for the heart to work harder. Therefore, the heart rate and blood pressure decrease.
3. Assess patient's reading level and primary language.

Provide patient with written instructions in large letters about medications. Include family members and enlist their support in reinforcing the importance of adhering to the treatment plan.

4. Patient is 80 years old, makes frequent trips to the bathroom related to diuretics, has vision problems, and a side effect of propranolol is weakness and fatigue.
5. Make arrangements for a bedside commode to reduce the distance and urgency to get to the bathroom. Encourage the patient and family to place night-lights in the bedroom, hall, and bathroom. Explain that throw rugs increase the risk of falling and that wood or tile floors can be slippery when wet and hard if a fall occurs. Encourage removal of throw rugs, and suggest carpeting these areas if possible. Suggest the use of safety bars in hall and bathroom for support or other walking aids as needed. If incontinence is a concern, suggest wearing an adult brief to prevent a wet, slippery floor. Suggest discussing with the physician an exercise program to increase strength, such as lifting small, lightweight objects (e.g., soup can), squeezing a rubber ball, or riding an exercise bike if able. These exercises can be done while sitting so they are not a fall-risk activity.
6. Unit Analysis Method:

$$\frac{20 \text{ mg} \quad | \quad 1 \text{ tablet}}{| \quad 10 \text{ mg}} = 2 \text{ tablets}$$

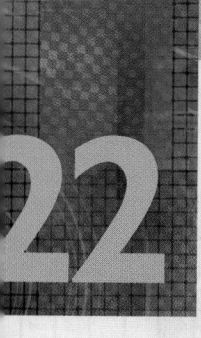

22

Nursing Care of Patients with Inflammatory and Infectious Cardiovascular Disorders

LINDA S. WILLIAMS

KEY TERMS

beta-hemolytic streptococci (BAY-tuh-HEE-moh-LIT-ick STREP-toh-KOCK-sigh)

cardiac tamponade (KAR-dee-yak TAM-pon-AYD)

cardiomegaly (KAR-dee-oh-MEG-ah-lee)

cardiomyopathy (KAR-dee-oh-my-AH-pah-thee)

chorea (kaw-REE-ah)

Dressler's syndrome (DRESS-lers SIN-drohm)

emboli (EM-boh-li)

infective endocarditis (in-FECK-tive EN-doh-kar-DYE-tis)

international normalized ratio (IN-ter-NASH-uh-nul NOR-muh-lized RAY-she-oh)

myectomy (my-ECK-tuh-mee)

myocarditis (MY-oh-kar-DYE-tis)

pericardial effusion (PER-ee-KAR-dee-uhl ee-FYOO-zhun)

pericardial friction rub (PER-ee-KAR-dee-uhl FRICK-shun RUB)

pericardiectomy (PER-ee-kar-dee-ECK-tuh-mee)

pericardiocentesis (PER-ee-KAR-dee-oh-sen-TEE-sis)

pericarditis (PER-ee-kar-DYE-tis)

petechiae (pe-TEE-kee-ee)

rheumatic carditis (roo-MAT-ick kar-DYE-tis)

rheumatic fever (roo-MAT-ick FEE-ver)

stenosis (ste-NOH-sis)

thrombophlebitis (THROM-boh-fle-BYE-tis)

QUESTIONS TO GUIDE YOUR READING

1. What are the pathophysiology, etiology, signs and symptoms, diagnostic tests, therapeutic interventions, and nursing care for rheumatic carditis, infective endocarditis, myocarditis, and pericarditis?

2. What are the pathophysiology, etiology, signs and symptoms, complications, diagnostic tests, therapeutic interventions, and nursing care for dilated, hypertrophic, and restrictive cardiomyopathy?

3. What are the pathophysiology, etiology, signs and symptoms, complications, diagnostic tests, and therapeutic interventions for thrombophlebitis?

4. What are risk factors, prevention measures, and nursing care for thrombophlebitis?

INFLAMMATORY AND INFECTIOUS CARDIAC DISORDERS

The entire heart (**rheumatic carditis**) or layers of the heart (endocarditis, **myocarditis,** and **pericarditis**) can become inflamed or infected (Fig. 22.1).

Rheumatic Carditis

Pathophysiology and Etiology

A serious complication of **rheumatic fever** is rheumatic carditis. The incidence of rheumatic carditis has dropped greatly likely due to antibiotic availability. Rheumatic fever occurs as an autoimmune reaction to an upper respiratory (throat) group A **beta-hemolytic streptococci** infection (Table 22.1). Two to 3 weeks after the streptococcal infection, rheumatic fever occurs. Although rheumatic fever can occur at any age, it typically occurs between ages 5 and 15, and can recur along with rheumatic carditis.

With carditis from rheumatic fever, all layers of the heart become inflamed. Pericardial layers are covered with an exudate and become thickened. As healing takes place, the pericardial sac can be damaged or destroyed by fibrosis. Nodules (Aschoff's bodies) form in myocardial tissue that become scar tissue over time. The endocardium, specifically the mitral valve, is the most seriously affected. Tiny,

---

myocarditis: myo—muscle kardia—heart + itis—inflammation
pericarditis: peri—around kardia—heart + itis—inflammation

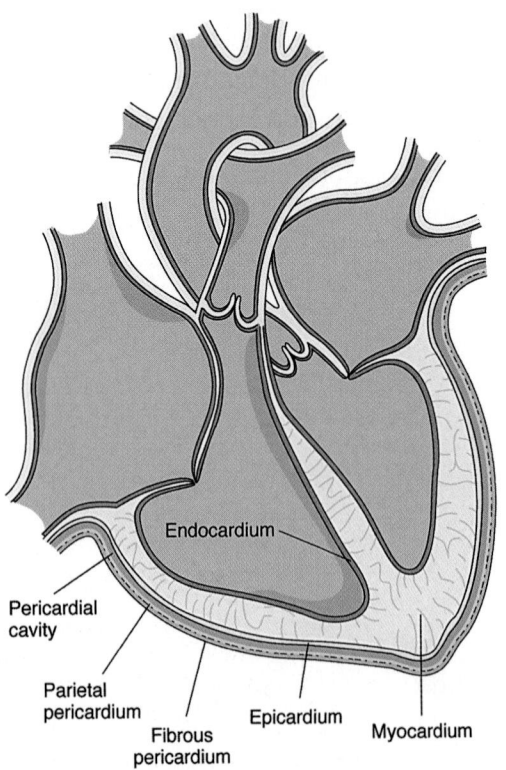

FIGURE 22.1 Layers of the heart.

TABLE 22.1 RHEUMATIC FEVER SUMMARY

Signs and Symptoms	Fever Polyarthritis Subcutaneous nodules **Chorea** with rapid, uncontrolled movements Rheumatic carditis Arthralgia Pneumonitis
Diagnostic Tests	Throat culture (identifies streptococcal infection) Antistreptolysin O titer level greater than 250 IU/mL. Elevated ESR and WBC
Therapeutic Interventions	Antimicrobial medication Anti-inflammatory medication Control of symptoms Prophylactic antibiotics
Possible Nursing Diagnoses	Acute pain related to joint or cardiac inflammation Anxiety related to disease process Decreased cardiac output related to valvular damage and carditis

ESR = erythrocyte sedimentation rate.

pinhead-size vegetations from blood and fibrin form on the valve leaflets. This can lead to thickening, fibrosis, and calcification of the valve leaflets and support structures. If the valve leaflets do not close completely, regurgitation of blood can occur. If the valve leaflets do not open fully (valvular stenosis), blood movement is impaired and severe heart failure may result.

Signs and Symptoms

Rheumatic carditis signs and symptoms include tachycardia, heart murmur, **pericardial friction rub,** mild to moderate chest pain, heart enlargement, electrocardiographic changes (e.g., PR interval lengthening), and evidence of heart failure.

Prevention

Preventing rheumatic fever by detecting and treating streptococcal infections promptly with penicillin (or erythromycin [Erythromid] for a patient with a penicillin allergy) is important to prevent rheumatic carditis.

Therapeutic Interventions

Activity is limited based on the severity of cardiac involvement. Other treatment for cardiac involvement is based on symptoms.

Nursing Management

A history of recent illnesses (e.g., sore throat, streptococcal infection, or scarlet fever) is obtained from the patient, including past episodes of rheumatic fever, heart disease, joint pain, and current medications. A physical assessment detects murmurs, pericardial friction rub, and heart failure signs (e.g., jugular vein distension, edema, dyspnea, crackles, cough, and fatigue). Vital signs are documented, noting fever and tachycardia.

Nursing care focuses on relieving the patient's pain and anxiety, maintaining normal cardiac function, and educating the patient about the disease. Pain is relieved with analgesics, aspirin, or corticosteroids as ordered. Vital signs are monitored and symptoms of heart failure are reported to the physician. An explanation of the disease and its treatment is provided to promote understanding of acute and lifelong prophylactic treatment. A patient statement of willingness to maintain health supports goal achievement.

Infective Endocarditis

Infective endocarditis (IE) is an infection of the endocardium. Males develop IE more often than females. There is a higher incidence of IE in the older adult. Even with antibiotic treatment, this infection can be fatal related to end-organ failure and other disease processes.

Pathophysiology

Cardiac defects result in turbulent blood flow that erodes the normally infection-resistant endocardium. Infective endocarditis begins when the invading organism (most commonly a bacteria, or maybe fungi) attaches to eroded endocardium where platelets and fibrin deposits have formed a vegetative lesion. Then more platelets and fibrin cover the multiplying organism. This covering protects the microbes, reducing the ability to destroy them. Damage to valve leaflets occurs as the vegetations grow. As blood flows through the heart, these vegetations may break off and become **emboli.**

With bacteremia, bacteria attach mainly to the valves of the heart, although any heart endothelial surface can be infected. Damaged valves from conditions such as mitral valve prolapse with regurgitation, rheumatic heart disease, congenital defects, and valve replacements are especially prone to bacterial invasion. The mitral valve is the valve most commonly infected, with the aortic valve being the second most commonly infected. Heart failure may result from valve damage, especially of the aortic valve.

Etiology

Portals of entry for organisms into the bloodstream result from intravenous (IV) drug use, surgery, dental or invasive procedures, and infections of the skin and gastrointestinal or genitourinary tract. Risk factors include the following:
- IV drug use
- Compromised immune system
- Congenital or valvular heart disease (e.g., mitral valve prolapse with regurgitation, valvular replacement surgery, or rheumatic carditis)
- Gingival gum disease

Prevention

Because dental disease is thought to be a common cause of IE, oral care is an important preventative measure. Additionally, antibiotic therapy before invasive or dental procedures is recommended for high-risk patients with cardiac disease or prior endocarditis.[1] It is important that these patients be taught to inform health-care team members (including their dentists) of their history before a procedure, so that prophylactic therapy can be given if needed.

Signs and Symptoms

Fever (99°F to 103°F [37.2°C to 39.4°C]) is a common sign, although the older adult may be afebrile (Table 22.2). A new murmur is usually heard as valvular damage occurs. Splinter hemorrhages may be seen in the distal nailbed (black or red-brown longitudinal short lines). **Petechiae** (tiny red flat spots) resulting from microembolization of the vegetation may occur on mucous membranes, conjunctivae, or skin (Fig. 22.2). Janeway lesions (small, painless red-blue lesions on palms and soles) are an acute finding. Osler's nodes (small, painful nodes on fingers and toes) from cardiac emboli are a late finding (Fig. 22.3).

Complications

Vegetative emboli can be a major complication of IE. If organ embolization occurs, signs and symptoms that reflect the organ that was affected by the emboli are seen. Brain emboli may produce changes in level of consciousness or

petechiae: petecchia—skin spot

TABLE 22.2 INFECTIVE ENDOCARDITIS SUMMARY

Signs and Symptoms	Fever
	Murmur
	Night sweats
	Fatigue
	Weight loss
	Weakness
	Pain in abdomen, joints, muscles, back
	Nailbed splinter hemorrhages
	Petechiae
Diagnostic Tests and Findings	Blood cultures (identify causative organism)
	Transesophageal echocardiography (identifies vegetations on heart valves)
	WBC count with differential (identifies elevation)
Therapeutic Interventions	*Acute therapy:*
	IV antimicrobial medications such as penicillin, vancomycin, amphotericin B (to cure infection)
	Antipyretics (to reduce fever)
	Rest (to decrease cardiac workload)
	Surgical valve replacement (to restore normal valve function)
	Prophylactic antibiotic therapy (to prevent infection)
Complications	Emboli
	Heart failure
Possible Nursing Diagnoses	Acute pain related to fever from cardiac infection
	Activity intolerance related to reduced oxygen delivery from decreased cardiac output
	Decreased cardiac output related to impaired valvular function or heart failure
	Deficient diversional activity related to restricted mobility from prolonged IV therapy
	Ineffective tissue perfusion related to emboli

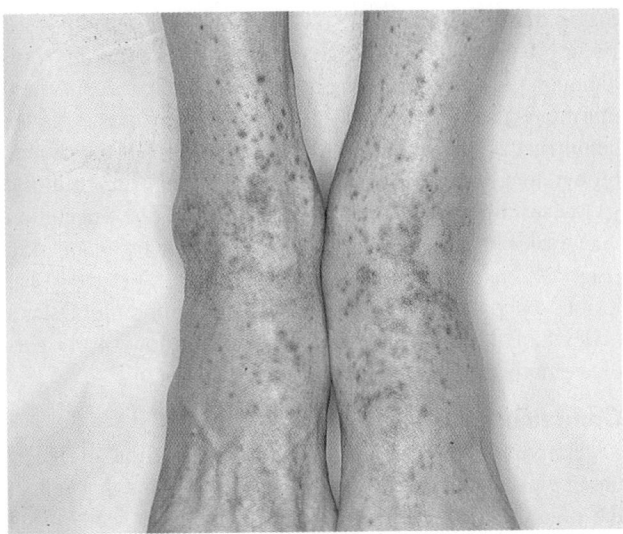

FIGURE 22.2 Petechiae. *(From Goldsmith, L: Adult & Pediatric Dermatology. F.A. Davis, Philadelphia, 1997, p 61.)*

stroke. Kidney emboli cause pain in the flank area, hematuria, or renal failure. Emboli in the spleen cause abdominal pain. Emboli in the small blood vessels can impair circulation in the extremities. Pulmonary emboli result in sudden dyspnea, cough, and chest pain.

Heart structures can be damaged or destroyed by IE. **Stenosis** (valve narrowing) or regurgitation (valve leakage) of a heart valve may also result. As the infection progresses and causes more damage to heart structures, heart failure may occur. (See Chapter 26.)

Diagnostic Tests
Table 22.2 shows diagnostic tests for IE. Positive blood cultures identify the causative organism of IE, and echocardiography shows cardiac effects.

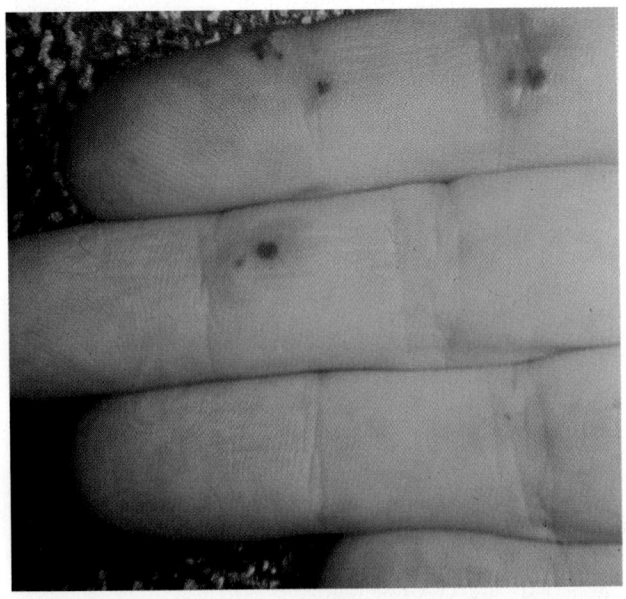

FIGURE 22.3 Osler's nodes. *(From Goldsmith, L: Adult & Pediatric Dermatology. Philadelphia, F.A. Davis, 1997, p 188.)*

Therapeutic Interventions
Initial treatment begins with hospitalization. An antimicrobial drug is selected that will destroy the organism identified by the blood culture. For bacterial infections, penicillin (or vancomycin for those allergic to penicillin) is commonly used. These medications are given intravenously over a period of 4 to 6 weeks, often once a day. A lengthy course of high-dose antibiotics is needed to penetrate the vegetations to reach all the microbes inside to kill them. Rest and supportive symptom care are also used. If afebrile and without complications, the patient is discharged to continue IV antibiotic therapy at home. The patient's response to the drug is monitored via the home care nurse and through laboratory testing. Changes in antibiotics may be made in response to side effects, allergies, organism resistance to the drug, or relapses.

Surgical replacement or repair of valves is usually required for patients with severely damaged heart valves, prosthetic valve infection, recurrent infection, multiple emboli from damaged valves, or heart failure. (See Chapter 24.) Recovery from the disease can be greatly improved with surgery. Antimicrobial therapy continues after surgery.

Nursing Process for the Patient with Infectious Endocarditis
ASSESSMENT/DATA COLLECTION. A patient history is obtained that includes risk factors for IE and recent infections or invasive procedures (Table 22.3). Vital signs are measured and recorded, and heart sounds are auscultated to detect murmurs. Signs of heart failure and emboli are noted. The physician is notified immediately if circulatory impairment, such as cold skin, decreased capillary refill, cyanosis, or absent peripheral pulses in an extremity, or symptoms of organ-related emboli are detected.

NURSING DIAGNOSIS, PLANNING, IMPLEMENTATION, AND EVALUATION. See Box 22.1 Nursing Care Plan for the Patient with Infective Endocarditis. Teaching about the disease and its treatment provides patients and families with the ability to provide IV antibiotics at home and promotes health maintenance to prevent IE. Good hygiene including dental care is essential. Skin care includes bathing, using proper hand washing technique with soap, avoiding nail biting, not popping pimples or lancing boils, and washing and applying antibiotic ointment to cuts. Brushing with a soft-bristle toothbrush (prevents gum trauma) twice a day reduces plaque formation, which traps bacteria. Twice yearly dental cleaning using prophylactic antibiotics, if indicated, is important. It is essential that patients understand the need to request and take prophylactic antibiotics as needed before invasive procedures. Patients are also taught symptom recognition (e.g., fever, chills, sweats) and seeking of prompt medical care. The patient is educated on the importance of having blood cultures drawn before antibiotics are started. The patient's statement of understanding and a willingness to follow lifestyle changes supports goal achievement.

TABLE 22.3 NURSING ASSESSMENT/DATA COLLECTION FOR PATIENTS WITH INFECTIVE ENDOCARDITIS

Subjective Data

Health History
Infections (rheumatic fever, previous endocarditis, streptococcal or staphylococcal, syphilis)?
Cardiac disease (valvular surgery, congenital)?
Childbirth?
Invasive procedures (surgery, dental, catheterization, IV therapy, cystoscopy, gynecologic)?
Malaise?
Anorexia?

Medications
Steroids, immunosuppressants, prolonged antibiotic therapy, IV drug use, alcohol abuse?

Respiratory
Dyspnea on exertion or when lying (orthopnea)?
Cough?

Cardiovascular
Palpitations, chest pain, fatigue, or activity intolerance?

Musculoskeletal
Weakness, arthralgia, myalgia?

Knowledge of Condition

Objective Data

Fever, Diaphoresis

Respiratory
Crackles, tachypnea

Cardiovascular
Murmurs, tachycardia, dysrhythmias, edema, headache

Integumentary
Nailbed splinter hemorrhages, petechiae on lips, mouth, conjunctivae, feet, or antecubital area

Renal
Hematuria

Diagnostic Test Findings
Anemia, elevated WBC count, elevated ESR, positive blood cultures, ECG showing conduction problems, echocardiogram showing valvular dysfunction and vegetations, chest x-ray exam showing heart enlargement (cardiomegaly) and lung congestion

ECG = electrocardiogram; ESR = erythrocyte sedimentation rate; WBC = white blood cell.

Pericarditis

Pathophysiology and Etiology

Pericarditis is an acute or chronic inflammation of the pericardium (the sac surrounding the heart). The inflammation creates a problem for the heart as it tries to expand and fill. As a result, ventricular filling is reduced, which then decreases cardiac output and blood pressure. Acute pericarditis can be caused by a variety of factors, including the following:

- Infections: viruses, bacteria, fungi, or Lyme disease
- Drug reactions
- Connective tissue disorders: systemic lupus erythematosus, rheumatic fever, or rheumatoid arthritis
- Neoplastic disease
- Postpericardiotomy (e.g., after cardiac surgery)

CRITICAL THINKING

Mrs. Jones

■ Mrs. Jones, 28 years old, is admitted to the hospital with a fever of 100°F (37°C), chills, fatigue, anorexia, and pain in her joints. A physical assessment reveals splinter hemorrhages in left index finger nailbed and petechiae on her chest. She is diagnosed with a heart murmur and infective endocarditis.

1. Why is a heart murmur heard with endocarditis?
2. What do splinter hemorrhages look like?
3. What do petechiae indicate?
4. How would you document Mrs. Jones's assessment findings?
5. What type of medication would you expect to be ordered to treat the infection?
6. Why does Mrs. Jones have chills if her temperature is elevated?
7. What signs and symptoms might occur if the complications of heart failure develop?
8. Why does Mrs. Jones need to be taught that she needs prophylactic antibiotics before dental or invasive procedures?
9. Tylenol 650 mg q 6 hours for pain is ordered. It comes as 325-mg tablets. How many tablets would be given per dose?

Suggested answers at end of chapter.

- Postmyocardial infarction, 1 to 12 weeks (**Dressler's syndrome**)
- Renal disease or uremia
- Trauma from chest injury or invasive thoracic procedures

Acute pericarditis resolves usually in less than 6 weeks. Recurrence is possible.

Chronic constrictive pericarditis is the result of fibrous scarring of the pericardium. The heart becomes surrounded by a thickened, stiff sac that limits the stretching ability of the heart's chambers for filling. Heart failure may result. Chronic constrictive pericarditis results from neoplastic disease and metastasis, radiation, or tuberculosis.

Signs and Symptoms

Chest pain is the most common symptom of pericarditis (Table 22.4). The pain is located substernally and over the heart and may radiate to the clavicle, neck, left scapula, or epigastric area. The intense, sharp, creaky, grating pain increases with deep inspiration, coughing, moving the trunk, or lying flat. The pain may be relieved by sitting up and leaning forward. Other symptoms depend on the cause of the pericarditis and may include dyspnea, low-grade fever, and cough. Dyspnea occurs as a result of decreased cardiac output and reduced oxygenation.

The classic sign of pericarditis is a pericardial friction rub, a grating, scratchy, high-pitched sound that is heard

Box 22.1 NURSING CARE PLAN for the Patient with Infective Endocarditis

Nursing Diagnosis: Decreased cardiac output related to impaired valvular function or heart failure

Expected Outcome Has adequate cardiac output as evidenced by vital signs within normal limits, no dyspnea or fatigue.

Evaluation of Outcomes Are patient's vital signs within normal limits with no dyspnea or fatigue?

Interventions	Rationale	Evaluation
Assess vital signs, murmurs, dyspnea, and fatigue.	Vital signs, dyspnea, and fatigue are indicators of cardiac output decline.	Are vital signs within normal limits with no dyspnea or fatigue?
Give oxygen as ordered.	Supplemental oxygen provides more oxygen to the heart.	Are breathing pattern and oxygen saturation within normal limits?
Provide rest as ordered.	Cardiac workload and oxygen needs are reduced with rest.	Are vital signs within normal limits and no fatigue reported?
Elevate head of bed 45 degrees.	Venous return to heart is reduced and chest expansion improved.	Are vital signs within normal limits and respirations easy?

Nursing Diagnosis: Activity intolerance related to reduced oxygen delivery from decreased cardiac output

Expected Outcomes Patient will state less fatigue in response to activity.

Evaluation of Outcomes Does patient report less fatigue? Is patient able to participate in desired activities?

Interventions	Rationale	Evaluation
Assist with activities of daily living (ADLs) prn.	Assistance conserves energy.	Are ADLs completed?
Provide rest and space activities.	Cardiac workload and oxygen needs are reduced with rest.	Does patient report less fatigue?

Nursing Diagnosis: Deficient diversional activity related to restricted mobility from prolonged intravenous therapy

Expected Outcomes States participation in satisfying diversional activities.

Evaluation of Outcomes Does patient participate in diversional activities? Does patient state satisfaction with activities?

Interventions	Rationale	Evaluation
Assess patient's preferred activities and hobbies.	Activity preference should be known to plan satisfactory diversional activities.	Are patient's preferred activities known?
Plan patient's schedule around relaxing and fun activities.	Self-esteem is fostered with increased patient control.	Does patient offer input into scheduled care? Is input followed?
Use pet therapy.	Individuals who can interact with pets live longer and healthier.	Does patient state enjoyment of pet therapy?
Provide a mix of physical, mental, and social activities on a rotating schedule.	Rotating stimulating activities and visitors will keep patient interested and avoid fatigue.	Does patient state satisfaction in activities with no fatigue?

TABLE 22.4 PERICARDITIS SUMMARY

Signs and Symptoms	Chest pain Dyspnea Low-grade fever Cough Pericardial friction rub
Diagnostic Tests	Complete blood cell count Electrocardiogram Echocardiogram MRI CT
Therapeutic Interventions	Anti-inflammatory medication Corticosteroids Pericardiocentesis Pericardial window
Complications	Pericardial effusion Cardiac tamponade
Possible Nursing Diagnoses	Acute pain related to inflammation of pericardium Anxiety related to disease process Decreased cardiac output related to cardiac constriction

when a rub is present. The rub is a result of friction from the inflamed pericardial and epicardial layers rubbing together as the heart fills and contracts. Depending on the severity of the pericarditis, the rub may be faint when auscultated or loud enough to be audible without auscultation. The rub may be heard intermittently or continuously. It is usually heard over the lower left sternal border of the chest during each heartbeat. It is present in approximately 50% of those with pericarditis.

Chronic constrictive pericarditis produces the signs and symptoms of right-sided heart failure. Atrial fibrillation may also be seen in some patients with chronic constrictive pericarditis.

LEARNING TIP

To simulate the sound of a pericardial friction rub, hold the diaphragm of a stethoscope against the palm of one hand; listen through the stethoscope as you rub the index finger of the opposite hand over the knuckles of the hand holding the diaphragm. The sound you hear is similar to that of a pericardial friction rub.

Diagnostic Tests

Table 22.4 lists diagnostic tests for pericarditis. The electrocardiogram reveals ST-T wave elevation in all leads. Echocardiogram results show **pericardial effusions**. Serum laboratory tests focus on causes of the pericarditis, such as an elevated white blood cell (WBC) count, indicating a bacterial or viral infection, or elevated blood urea nitrogen or creatinine levels, indicating uremia. Fluid obtained during

pericardiocentesis is examined to diagnose the cause. In chronic constrictive pericarditis, computed tomography (CT) or magnetic resonance imaging (MRI) may show a thickened pericardium.

Therapeutic Interventions

If the patient is unstable, prompt intervention is required, such as an emergency pericardiocentesis. When the patient's blood pressure and heart rate are stable and adequate, the cause is determined so that appropriate treatment can be administered, such as antibiotics for bacterial infections. Bedrest is used to reduce the heart's workload during acute symptoms. Nonsteroidal anti-inflammatory drugs (NSAIDs) such as indomethacin (Indocin) are given to resolve inflammation and reduce pain. Corticosteroids may be used when NSAIDs are not effective. Hemodialysis is used to treat uremic pericarditis.

Chronic effusive pericarditis can be treated with a pericardial window to allow continuous drainage of pericardial fluid into the pleural space. A pericardial window is created surgically by removing a portion of the outer pericardial layer.

Chronic constrictive pericarditis is treated with **pericardiectomy,** which is the surgical removal of the entire tough, calcified pericardium. Pericardiectomy relieves constriction of the heart and allows normal filling of the ventricles.

Complications

A pericardial effusion (build-up of fluid in pericardial space) is the most common complication of pericarditis. A rapidly developing effusion, such as one occurring from trauma, can produce symptoms at smaller amounts of fluid than slowly developing effusions, such as pericarditis from tuberculosis, with larger amounts of fluid. The increasing fluid presses on nearby tissue. Pressure on lung tissue can produce dyspnea, cough, and tachypnea. The heartbeat sounds distant. The body's compensatory mechanisms attempt to maintain blood pressure.

As the fluid accumulation grows, **cardiac tamponade,** another complication of pericarditis, can occur. Cardiac tamponade is a life-threatening compression of the heart by fluid accumulated in the pericardial sac. Cardiac output drops and to compensate, heart rate increases. Then blood pressure falls as compensatory mechanisms fail. The patient shows symptoms of decreased cardiac output, such as restlessness, confusion, tachycardia, and tachypnea. Jugular vein distention is present from increased venous pressure, and heart sounds are distant. Cardiac tamponade requires immediate treatment with pericardiocentesis to puncture the pericardium with a 16-gauge needle and remove the excess fluid in the pericardial sac (Fig. 22.4). After the procedure, the patient is monitored for complications, such as dys-

---

pericardiocentesis: peri—around + kardia—heart + centesis—puncture

cardiac tamponade: kardia—heart + tamponade—plug

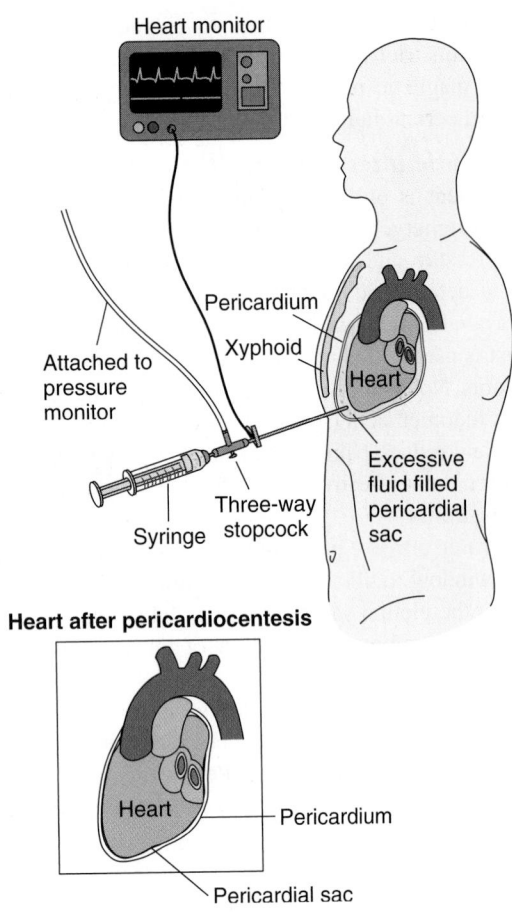

Heart monitor

Attached to
pressure
monitor

Pericardium

Xyphoid

Heart

Syringe   Three-way
stopcock

Excessive
fluid filled
pericardial
sac

Heart after pericardiocentesis

Heart   —— Pericardium

—— Pericardial sac

FIGURE 22.4 Pericardiocentesis.

rhythmias, laceration of a coronary artery, or laceration of the myocardium or pneumothorax.

Nursing Management

A patient history is obtained that includes any cardiac disease, recent infections, and current medications. Chest pain, pericardial friction rub, heart sounds, and signs of heart failure are noted. Vital signs are documented, noting fever and tachycardia.

Nursing care focuses on relieving the patient's pain and anxiety and maintaining normal cardiac function. Symptoms are monitored to detect complications. Pain, which may be severe, is relieved by giving NSAIDs or corticosteroids as ordered. Allowing the patient to assume a position of comfort by sitting up and leaning forward also relieves pain. Maintenance of normal cardiac function includes monitoring vital signs and observing for the presence of symptoms of cardiac tamponade or heart failure. The detection of these symptoms is immediately reported to the physician. Teaching the patient about pericarditis and its treatment relieves anxiety and allows a feeling of control by allowing the patient to make knowledgeable health-care decisions.

Myocarditis

Pathophysiology and Etiology

In myocarditis, inflammation of the myocardium occurs. The amount of muscle destruction and necrosis that occurs

as a result of myocarditis determines the extent of damage to the heart. The heart may enlarge in response to the damaged muscle fibers, although most cases of myocarditis are benign, with few signs or symptoms.

Myocarditis is a rare condition that most commonly develops following a viral infection. Other causes are bacteria, parasites, fungi, rickettsiae, spirochetes, medications, lead toxicity, autoimmune factors, human immunodeficiency virus (HIV), rheumatic fever, systemic lupus erythematosus, pericarditis or infective endocarditis, or cardiac transplant rejection.

Signs and Symptoms

Signs and symptoms of myocarditis vary from none to severe cardiac manifestations. Fatigue, fever, pharyngitis, malaise, dyspnea, palpitations, muscle aches, gastrointestinal (GI) discomfort, and enlarged lymph nodes may occur early from a viral infection. Cardiac manifestations such as chest discomfort, pain, or tachycardia may occur about 2 weeks after a viral infection. Occasionally, sudden death may occur.

Diagnostic Tests

A percutaneous endomyocardial biopsy during the first 6 weeks of inflammation is the preferred diagnostic test for myocarditis, although it is positive only about 30% of the time. MRI and gallium-67 scanning are helpful. An electrocardiogram (ECG) shows dysrhythmias, commonly sinus tachycardia.

Therapeutic Interventions

Interventions to reduce the heart's workload are essential and include bedrest and limited activity. Administration of oxygen treats hypoxia. Exercise increases myocardial inflammation and mortality and should be avoided until symptoms improve and inflammation is gone. Treatment is aimed at the cause, if known, such as antibiotics for bacterial infections. The use of alcohol and tobacco should be avoided. Heart failure is treated with medication to strengthen the heart's contractility and slow the heart's rate, which reduces the heart's workload and oxygen needs. With myocarditis, the heart is sensitive to digoxin, which may be used to treat heart failure, and toxicity may occur even with small doses. The patient should be monitored closely for signs of digoxin toxicity, which may include anorexia, nausea, vomiting, bradycardia, dysrhythmias, or malaise. The use of immunosuppressive therapy is being investigated and may result in new treatment options in the future.

Nursing Management

Recent illnesses, toxin exposure, cardiac diseases, activity tolerance, and current medications are documented. Vital signs and signs of heart failure, such as jugular vein distention, peripheral edema, crackles, and dyspnea are noted.

Nursing care is aimed at the patient's maintenance of normal cardiac function by monitoring vital signs and symptoms and administering medications as ordered. Interventions to reduce fatigue include providing assistance as needed, having frequent rest periods, and teaching energy conservation methods. Reducing the patient's anxiety and increasing the patient's knowledge can be achieved through teaching about the disease. Determining diversional activities with the patient for times when activity is restricted further reduces anxiety.

Cardiac Trauma

Two types of cardiac trauma can occur: nonpenetrating and penetrating. Nonpenetrating injuries, or contusions, occur from blunt trauma such as motor vehicle accidents or contact sports in which direct compression or force is applied to the upper torso. Contusions may vary from small bruises to hemorrhage.

There may be few or no external injuries indicating traumatic cardiac injury. The patient may be asymptomatic or exhibit signs and symptoms identical to a myocardial infarction. In severe contusions, laboratory results may show elevated creatine kinase MB (CK-MB) or troponin-I levels.

If bleeding occurs into the pericardial sac, cardiac tamponade (compression of the heart from the blood collecting in the sac) may occur (discussed above). If signs of shock occur, a pericardiocentesis must be performed. With its own pressure, the tamponade may seal the area of bleeding, so no cardiac decompensation occurs. In this case, only bedrest and observation are required. There are no long-term effects with most contusions. With severe contusions, however, scarring and necrosis of the myocardium may decrease cardiac output and increase the risk for cardiac rupture.

Penetrating traumas may be an external injury to the chest, such as a stab or gunshot wound, or an internal injury, such as invasive lines that penetrate the cardiac muscle. Complications vary depending on the size, location, and cause of injury. Tamponade occurs from bleeding into the pericardial sac if the pericardium is sealed off by clot formation. A hemothorax develops if blood drains into the pleural space in the chest. A pneumothorax occurs if air collects in the pleural space. Signs and symptoms of hemorrhage and myocardial ischemia may be noted. Cardiac trauma treatment usually requires surgery to repair the damage so that hemostasis can be regained.

Cardiomyopathy

Cardiomyopathy is an enlargement of the heart muscle. There are three types of cardiac structure and function abnormalities in cardiomyopathy: (1) dilated, (2) hypertrophic, and (3) restrictive (Fig. 22.5). A consequence of all types of cardiomyopathy can be heart failure (Fig. 22.6), myocardial ischemia, and myocardial infarction due to reduced cardiac output. There is currently no cure for cardiomyopathy. The greatest advancement for the cardiomyopathies has been in genetic research that has identified potential causes of these diseases. This research will help lead to better diagnosis and treatment in the future.

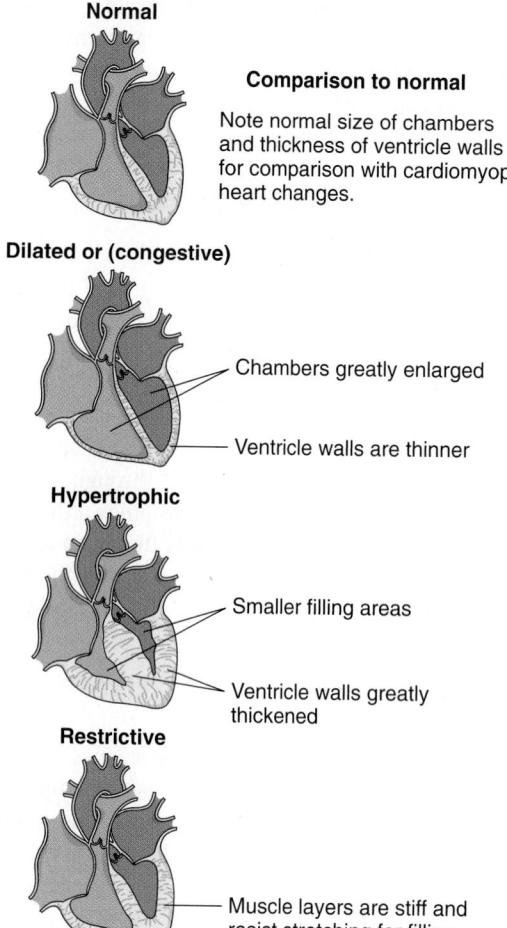

Normal

Comparison to normal

Note normal size of chambers and thickness of ventricle walls for comparison with cardiomyopic heart changes.

Dilated or (congestive)

— Chambers greatly enlarged

— Ventricle walls are thinner

Hypertrophic

— Smaller filling areas

— Ventricle walls greatly thickened

Restrictive

— Muscle layers are stiff and resist stretching for filling.

FIGURE 22.5 Comparison of the normal heart structure with each type of the cardiomyopic heart structure.

Dilated Cardiomyopathy

In dilated cardiomyopathy, the size of the ventricular cavity enlarges with reduced cardiac output. Contractile function decreases as the myocardial tissue is destroyed. Blood

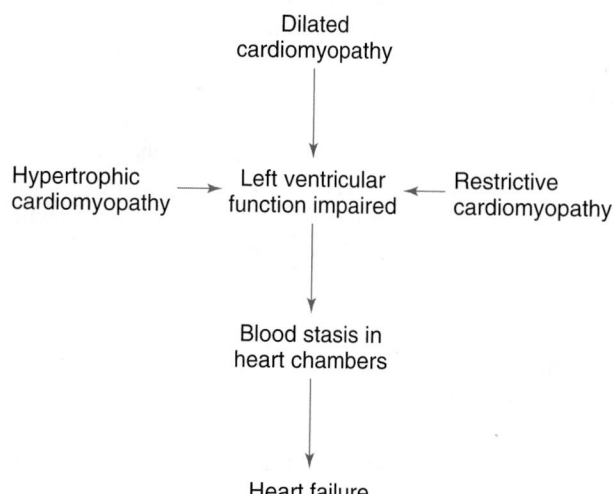

Dilated cardiomyopathy

↓

Hypertrophic cardiomyopathy → Left ventricular function impaired ← Restrictive cardiomyopathy

↓

Blood stasis in heart chambers

↓

Heart failure

FIGURE 22.6 All types of cardiomyopathies can lead to heart failure.

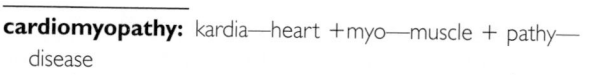

cardiomyopathy: kardia—heart +myo—muscle + pathy— disease

moves more slowly through the left ventricle, which often results in blood clot formation. Dilated cardiomyopathy is the most frequent type of cardiomyopathy and one of the most frequent causes of heart failure. Dilated cardiomyopathy may be hereditary, follow infectious myocarditis, or be caused by chronic alcohol or cocaine use, HIV, thiamine or zinc deficiencies, infections, or other causes.

Hypertrophic Cardiomyopathy

Hypertrophic cardiomyopathy is enlargement of the cardiac muscle wall, often of the septum and left ventricle. The hypertrophy may occur asymmetrically. It can be a hereditary disorder that is transmitted as a dominant trait. Hypertrophic cardiomyopathy causes the ventricular wall to be rigid, which decreases ventricular filling. If an enlarged septum obstructs the outflow of blood through the aortic valve, it is known as obstructive hypertrophic cardiomyopathy. Death occurs suddenly and is likely due to an abnormal heart rhythm. Genetic research is focusing on the mutant genes associated with the disease, which will guide future diagnosis and therapy.

Restrictive Cardiomyopathy

Restrictive cardiomyopathy impairs ventricular stretch and limits ventricular filling. Cardiac muscle stiffness is present with no ventricular dilation, although systolic emptying of the ventricle remains normal. Restrictive cardiomyopathy is the rarest form of cardiomyopathy. It may be caused by infiltrative diseases such as amyloidosis that deposit the protein amyloid within the myocardial cells, making the muscle stiff and resistant to stretching for easy ventricular filling. Treating the underlying cause may help reduce heart damage. Visit the American Heart Association at www. americanheart.org for more cardiac information.

Signs and Symptoms

Manifestation of cardiomyopathy depends on the type of abnormality. Most patients show varying degrees of signs and symptoms of heart failure (Table 22.5). With dilated cardiomyopathy, left ventricular and then right-sided heart failure with a poor prognosis are seen. Dyspnea on exertion, orthopnea, fatigue, and sometimes atrial fibrillation occur. In hypertrophic cardiomyopathy, exertional dyspnea related to the obstruction of cardiac output is the most common symptom. Angina is not common, but atypical chest pain that occurs at rest and is not relieved with nitrates may occur. With restrictive cardiomyopathy, heart failure symptoms (Chapter 26) result from the ventricles' inability to fill during diastole. Syncope, arrhythmias, and thrombi may occur.

Diagnostic Tests

Cardiomegaly is seen on a chest x-ray examination. Echocardiography shows muscle thickness and chamber size to differentiate between the types of cardiomyopathy. Changes related to enlarged chamber size, tachycardia, and dysrhythmias can be seen on the ECG. Cardiac catheterization with angiocardiography may also be useful. Cardiovascular magnetic resonance is a newer tool that is being used that has greater accuracy in diagnosing cardiomyopathy.

Therapeutic Interventions

Treatment is palliative and aimed at managing heart failure and the underlying cause if known for both dilated and restrictive cardiomyopathies (see Chapter 26). In dilated cardiomyopathy, treatment focuses on the symptoms of heart failure seen. Angiotensin-converting enzyme (ACE) inhibitors, beta blockers, diuretics, and digoxin may be given to increase cardiac output. Biventricular pacing and implantable defibrillators may be used. Therapy is not very useful for restrictive cardiomyopathy. Diuretics or nitrates may be used to relieve venous congestion that occurs due to heart failure. However, a fine balance is needed when using these drugs so that preload is not reduced too greatly, which would worsen symptoms. Anticoagulants are given to prevent emboli formation in patients with atrial fibrillation. Antidysrhythmics or cardioversion are used for dyrhythmias.

For obstructive hypertrophic cardiomyopathy, beta blockers (propranolol) and calcium channel blockers (Calan) are given to slow the heart rate to allow more filling time and lessen the strength of the heart's contraction. An antiarrhythmic agent such as disopyramide (Norpace) may be used. Patients must remain hydrated at all times to maintain cardiac output.

In obstructive hypertrophic cardiomyopathy, digoxin and vasodilators are avoided because they can increase the

TABLE 22.5 CARDIOMYOPATHY SUMMARY

Signs and Symptoms	Angina
	Arrhythmias
	Dyspnea
	Fatigue
	Syncope
Diagnostic Tests	ECG
	Chest x-ray
	Cardiac catheterization
	Cardiac magnetic resonance imaging
	Echocardiography
Therapeutic Interventions	Anticoagulants
	Antidysrhythmics
	Dilated cardiomyopathy: vasodilators, cardiac glycosides, cardiomyoplasty, heart transplant
	Hypertrophic cardiomyopathy: beta blockers, calcium channel blockers, myectomy, septal ablation
	Restrictive cardiomyopathy: vasodilators, heart transplant
Complication	Heart failure
Possible Nursing Diagnoses	Decreased cardiac output related to impaired myocardial function
	Activity intolerance related to cardiac insufficiency
	Anxiety related to disease process

---

cardiomegaly: kardia—heart + mega—large

obstruction. Strenuous exercise and athletic sports are restricted to prevent sudden death. Lower levels of exercise may be allowed. For patients in whom medical therapy is not effective, atrioventricular (AV) sequential pacemakers, implantable automatic defibrillators, or invasive procedures are considered. For those without obstruction, fewer treatment options exist. Diuretics are used to reduce elevated pressures along with beta blockers and calcium channel blockers.

If medical therapy is not successful, surgery is considered. For hypertrophied muscle, surgery to remove part of the ventricular septum (**myectomy**) is done to allow greater outflow of blood. Another option especially for those who are not candidates for surgery is septal ablation. In septal ablation, alcohol is delivered via a catheter to necrose and reduce septal heart wall thickness. The CorCap™ Cardiac Support Device, an investigational device, is a polyester mesh stocking that is pulled over the bottom portion of the heart through a surgical chest incision (Acorn Cardiovascular, St. Paul, Minn.). It becomes part of the heart as tissue grows around it. The stocking provides support for the heart and also reshapes the heart to its more normal shape and size, which reduces heart failure symptoms. Cardiomyoplasty is an experimental surgical approach for dilated cardiomyopathy when heart transplant is not an option (see Fig. 26.6). The heart's contraction strength is aided by the patient's latissimus dorsi muscle, which has been wrapped around the heart. For severe heart failure, primarily in those with dilated cardiomyopathy, a heart transplant may be the only hope for survival. A ventricular assist device may be used until a donor is found. Many patients die while waiting for a donated heart because donated organs are limited.

Nursing Management

A patient history is obtained that includes signs and symptoms and assessment of family support systems because of the chronic nature of the disease. A physical assessment is done, noting vital signs and any signs or symptoms of heart failure.

Nursing care focuses on maintaining normal cardiac function, increasing activity tolerance, relieving anxiety, and educating the patient about the disease and its treatment. Patients with cardiomyopathy can be very ill. Careful monitoring is done to detect complications, such as heart failure, emboli, or dysrhythmias. The physician is immediately notified of problems. Home health care is often used for these patients to maintain their functional ability and reduce hospitalizations.

Maintenance of normal cardiac function includes monitoring vital signs and symptoms of heart failure. Increasing activity tolerance includes planning rest periods, scheduling activities in small amounts, avoiding tiring activities, and providing small meals that require less energy to digest than large meals. Patients are taught to avoid alcohol because it decreases cardiac function.

Reducing anxiety is important and can be accomplished by providing explanations for procedures, as well as educating the patient about the disease and its treatment. This may allow patients to feel in control of their lives by being able to make knowledgeable decisions about their health care. Methods to incorporate necessary lifestyle changes such as avoiding fatigue and scheduling rest periods can be helpful. Emotional support is greatly needed by these patients and their families because of the chronic nature of this disease.

Patient and Significant Other Education

Patients need to be taught the importance of medication compliance to prevent heart failure. The patient and family should have emergency telephone numbers readily available. Families should learn cardiopulmonary resuscitation (CPR). In terminal stages of the disease, the patient and family should be informed about the availability of hospice care and be emotionally supported during the grieving process.

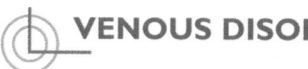 VENOUS DISORDERS

Thrombophlebitis

Thrombophlebitis is the formation of a clot and inflammation within a vein. The clot usually forms first and then inflammation occurs. Thrombophlebitis is the most common disorder of veins, with the legs being most often affected. Any superficial or deep vein in the body can be involved. Deep vein thrombosis (DVT) is the most serious form of thrombophlebitis because pulmonary emboli can result if the thrombus detaches. (See Chapter 28.)

Pathophysiology

A venous thrombus is made up of platelets, red blood cells, white blood cells, and fibrin. Platelets attach to a vein wall and then a tail forms as more blood cells and fibrin collect. As the tail grows, it drifts in the blood flowing past it. The turbulence of the blood flow can cause parts of the drifting thrombus to break off and become emboli that travel to the lungs.

Etiology

Three factors, Virchow's triangle, are involved in the formation of a thrombus: stasis of blood flow, damage to the lining of the vein wall, and increased blood coagulation (Table 22.6). Venous stasis occurs when blood flow is reduced, veins are dilated, muscle contractions are decreased, or vein valves are faulty. When the wall of a vein is damaged, it provides a site for a thrombus to form. Intravenous therapy and venipuncture cause trauma to the vein, and IV catheters in place longer than 48 to 72 hours increase the risk of inflammation and thrombus. Increased coagulation of the blood promotes thrombus formation. Patients on oral anticoagu-

---

myectomy: myo—muscle + ectomy—cutting out

thrombophlebitis: thromb—lump (clot) + phleb—vein + itis—inflammation

TABLE 22.6 PREDISPOSING CONDITIONS FOR THROMBOPHLEBITIS (VIRCHOW'S TRIANGLE)

Condition	Type	Example
Venous Stasis	Reduction of blood flow	Shock, heart failure, myocardial infarction, atrial fibrillation
	Dilated veins	Vasodilators
	Decreased muscle contractions	Immobility, sitting for long periods as in traveling, fractured hip, paralysis, anesthesia, surgery, obesity, advanced age
	Faulty valves	Varicose veins, venous insufficiency
Venous Wall Injury		Venipuncture, venous cannulation at same site for >48 hours, venous catheterization, surgery, trauma, burns, fractures, dislocation, IV medications (potassium, chemotherapy drugs, antibiotics, IV hypertonic solutions), contrast agents, diabetes, cerebrovascular disease
Increased Coagulation of Blood		Anemia, malignancy, antithrombin III deficiency, oral contraceptives, estrogen therapy, smoking, discontinuance of anticoagulant therapy, dehydration, malnutrition, polycythemia, leukocytosis, thrombocytosis, sepsis, pregnancy

lants that are abruptly stopped experience increased clotting of the blood. Smoking, oral contraceptive use, and estrogen therapy also increase blood coagulation. Hematological disorders can also lead to altered blood coagulation and increased risk of thrombus formation.

Prevention

Identification of risk factors for thrombosis (Table 22.6) and patient education promote the use of interventions (discussed below) to prevent thrombosis. Because the elderly are at increased risk for thrombus formation, a family member should be instructed along with the elderly person in techniques that may be difficult for the elderly person to perform. Dehydration, which is common in the elderly population, should be avoided to reduce thrombus risk.

IMMOBILITY. People with sedentary jobs that require long periods of sitting, standing, or traveling long distances should change positions, perform knee and ankle flexion exercises, or walk at regular intervals to prevent stasis of blood. Patients on bedrest should have legs elevated above the level of the heart if possible and turn every 2 hours to prevent pooling of blood. Postoperatively or in times of bedrest, active or passive range-of-motion exercises should be done to increase blood flow. Postoperatively, early ambulation is a major preventive technique for thrombosis. Patients' pain should be controlled to facilitate their ability to participate in early ambulation. Deep breathing aids in improving blood flow in the large thoracic veins. Smoking should be avoided because nicotine causes vasoconstriction.

PROPHYLACTIC ANTIEMBOLISM DEVICES. Patients with peripheral vascular disease, those on bedrest, and those who have had surgery or trauma may use antiembolism devices to improve blood flow. Knee- or thigh-length elastic stockings apply pressure to the leg. They must be applied correctly to avoid a tourniquet effect. Older patients with decreased manual dexterity may need assistance. The skin should be inspected daily for irritation under the stockings as ordered. Sequential compression devices (SCD) fill

intermittently with air to move venous blood in the legs by simulating contraction of the leg muscles. They may be used in combination with elastic stockings. Research that compares the various preventive measures for DVT and rates of DVT in surgical patients has shown that the lowest incidence of DVT occurs with elastic stockings and SCDs used together.

PROPHYLACTIC MEDICATION. Low molecular weight heparin (LMWH) is given postoperatively to prevent thrombosis (e.g., enoxaparin [Lovenox] subcutaneously [Table 22.7]). LMWH is more effective for orthopedic patients. Anticoagulation tests are not monitored with LMWH due to the predictability of its dose related response. Subcutaneous heparin may also be used postoperatively to prevent thrombosis. Platelet counts must be monitored with either LMWH or heparin to detect heparin induced thrombocytopenia.

Oral anticoagulants such as warfarin (Coumadin) can be used in the high-risk patient to decrease thrombosis. The **international normalized ratio** (INR) measures the effectiveness of warfarin therapy. The INR uses a standardized testing reagent. This means that it can be used around the world with no variation in results as occurs with prothrombin time (PT). Prothrombin time was previously the most commonly used test; however, PT control values can vary from laboratory to laboratory. INR is reported along with the prothrombin time. These values should correspond in meaning (i.e., normal, subtherapeutic, therapeutic, toxic). INR should be used; however, some practitioners still order PT, so a discussion of how to interpret the PT is presented for your understanding. For more information on these medications, visit www.fda.gov/cder/drug/default.htm.

INTRAVENOUS THERAPY. Monitoring of venous IV sites should be performed according to institutional policy time frames to detect signs of thrombophlebitis. Venous cannula sites should be changed regularly according to institutional guidelines (e.g., every 48 to 72 hours) to prevent thrombus formation.

TABLE 22.7 ANTICOAGULANT MEDICATIONS

Medication Class/Action	Examples	Route	Side Effects	Nursing Implications
Anticoagulants Inhibit clot formation to prevent new clot formation.				
Coumarins Inhibit liver synthesis of vitamin K dependent clotting factors: II, XII, IX, X.	dicumarol (Bishydroxy-coumarin) warfarin (Coumadin)	PO	Hemorrhage or bleeding. Risk increased with NSAIDs.	Monitor PT/INR regularly. Acetaminophen (Tylenol) used instead of aspirin during therapy. Antidote: Oral or parental vitamin K.
Heparins Bind to antithrombin III, which then inhibits fibrin formation.	heparin sodium (Lipo-Hepin)	IV SubQ	Itching, burning, bleeding, hemorrhage, ecchymosis, severe hypotension.	Antidote: Protamine sulfate. Do not give IM due to pain and hematoma. Monitor PTT: 1.5–2 times control. Monitor platelet count as may decrease. Monitor for bleeding. Teach patient to report bleeding.
Low Molecular weight heparins (LMWH) Bind with antithrombin III inhibiting making of factor Xa and the formation of thrombin.	ardeparin (Normiflo) dalteparin sodium (Fragmin) enoxaparin (Lovenox) www.lovenox.com	SubQ	Bleeding rare.	Monitoring of aPTT not needed. Teach patient to give injection (prefilled syringes available) typically in abdomen. Treatment is usually 7–14 days.
Thrombolytics Promote fibrinolysis to break down fibrin in blood clot.	tissue plasminogen activator (t-PA, alteplase) streptokinase (Streptase, Kabikinase) urokinase (Abbokinase)	IV	Allergic reaction (especially streptokinase), hemorrhage, hypotension (streptokinase)	Monitor for bleeding, vital signs, signs of allergic reaction. Use bleeding precautions (avoid needle sticks). Teach patient to report side effects. Avoid use of ASA, NSAIDs. Aminocarproic acid (Amicar) is antidote.

LEARNING TIP

Before administering anticoagulants, laboratory values must be assessed to ensure patient safety. INR normal and desired therapeutic values for the patient's disorder are provided on the laboratory report. These INR values do not require calculation of a therapeutic range because the values are given on the report. Compare the patient's INR value with the desired INR value to determine if it is safe to give the warfarin.

Understanding that INR is the preferred test for warfarin effectiveness, you may still want to know how to calculate a therapeutic range for prothrombin time. Prothrombin times are measured in seconds. The normal value range gives the seconds required for a fibrin clot to form during the test. If a patient is on warfarin, the purpose is to increase the time (seconds) it takes the blood to clot. It is therefore expected that the prothrombin time will be elevated by warfarin therapy.

Because a therapy, warfarin, is being given, a prothrombin time range that safely considers the expected effects of the warfarin is needed. This is called the therapeutic range (i.e., a low and a high value). Warfarin's therapeutic range is 1.5 to 2 times the normal prothrombin time range. To monitor the patient's therapeutic prothrombin time, compare the patient's result with the therapeutic range that you calculate. For example:

Patient's value on warfarin: 16 seconds (sec.)
Normal prothrombin time range: 9 to 12 seconds

To calculate therapeutic range,
multiply

$$1.5 \qquad 2$$
$$\times 9 \text{ sec.} \qquad \times 12 \text{ sec.}$$

The therapeutic range is: 13.5 sec. to   24 sec.

Compare the patient's value of 16 seconds with the therapeutic range of 13.5 to 24 seconds to determine that the patient is safely within the therapeutic range.

TABLE 22.8 THROMBOPHLEBITIS SUMMARY

Signs and Symptoms	Superficial veins: redness, warmth, swelling, and tenderness
	Deep veins: swelling, edema, pain, warmth, venous distention, and tenderness
Diagnostic Tests	Venous duplex ultrasound
	Magnetic resonance venography
Therapeutic Interventions	Superficial veins: warm, moist heat; analgesics; NSAIDs; compression stockings
	Deep veins: LMWH; heparin; warfarin; bedrest with extremity elevation above the level of the heart for 5–7 days; warm, moist heat; compression stocking therapy; thrombolytic therapy; thrombectomy; vena cava filter
Complications	Pulmonary embolism
	Chronic venous insufficiency
	Varicose veins
	Recurrent deep vein thrombosis
Possible Nursing Diagnoses	Acute pain related to inflammation of vein
	Impaired skin integrity related to venous stasis
	Anxiety related to uncertain prognosis of disease

Signs and Symptoms

Up to 50% of patients have no symptoms with thrombophlebitis in the legs. For others, the symptoms vary according to the size and location of the thrombus (Table 22.8). If adequate collateral circulation is present near the involved area, symptoms may be reduced. For some patients a pulmonary embolus is the only evidence of a DVT.

SUPERFICIAL VEINS. Thrombophlebitis in a superficial vein may produce redness, warmth, swelling, and tenderness in the area around the site of the thrombus. The vein feels like a firm cord, which is referred to as induration. The saphenous vein is the most commonly affected vein in the leg. Varicosity of the vein is usually the cause. In the arm, IV therapy is the most common cause.

DEEP VEINS. In a deep vein thrombus of the leg (femoral vein), swelling, edema, pain, warmth, venous distention, and tenderness with palpation of the calf may be present in the affected leg. Obstruction of blood flow from the leg causes edema and varies with the location of the thrombus. An elevated temperature may also be present. Pain in the calf with sharp dorsiflexion of the foot, a classic indication known as a positive Homans' sign, is present in less than 50% of those with thrombophlebitis and is not specific to DVT. Once a DVT is positively diagnosed, it is important to avoid performing Homans' sign because it may cause the clot to become dislodged. Cyanosis and edema may occur if the large veins such as the vena cava are involved.

Complications

The most serious complication of deep vein thrombophlebitis is pulmonary embolism, which is a life-threatening emergency (see Chapter 28). Another complication, chronic venous insufficiency, results from damage to the valves in the vein and causes venous stasis. Signs and symptoms from venous insufficiency that may appear years after a thrombus include edema, pain, brownish discoloration and ulceration of the medial ankle, venous distention, and dependent cyanosis of the leg. This condition can be difficult to treat.

Therapeutic Interventions

Diagnostic tests are done to guide treatment, with venous duplex ultrasound being the primary test used (see Table 22.8). The goals of treatment are to relieve pain and prevent pulmonary emboli, thrombus enlargement, and further thrombus development. Superficial thrombophlebitis is treated with warm, moist heat, analgesics, NSAIDs, and compression stockings.

Patients with a proximal DVT may be treated at home if they do not have pulmonary embolism, cardiovascular or pulmonary disease, obesity, or renal failure and are able to comply with follow-up care. A LMWH (e.g., enoxaparin, dalteparin, or ardeparin) is given subcutaneously daily or twice a day while oral warfarin is started (see Table 22.7). Both are taken until the INR is within therapeutic range (about 5 days); the LMWH is then stopped.

For some DVTs, a hospital stay may be required. Treatment includes bedrest with leg elevation above heart level for 5 to 7 days, warm, moist heat, elastic stocking (initially on unaffected leg only until acute symptoms are gone on affected leg), and anticoagulants. A continuous heparin IV infusion is usually started for up to 10 days to prevent further enlargement of the thrombus and development of new thrombi; it has little effect on the existing clot, which the body dissolves over time. An oral anticoagulant, warfarin, is begun 4 to 5 days before the heparin is stopped. When the therapeutic INR goal is reached, the heparin is stopped. Warfarin is continued for several months. For second DVT episodes, lifelong warfarin therapy is used. In some cases of massive DVT, thrombolytic therapy (tissue plasminogen activator, streptokinase) may be used to dissolve the clot, but there is a high risk of bleeding with these drugs. New research is looking at an oral thrombin inhibitor which will have fewer side effects than warfarin.

Surgical treatment is used to prevent pulmonary emboli or chronic venous insufficiency when anticoagulant therapy cannot be used or the risk of pulmonary emboli is great. Venous thrombectomy removes the clot through a venous incision. In some cases, a vena cava filter is placed into the inferior vena cava through the femoral or right internal jugular vein (Fig. 22.7). Once in place, it is opened and attaches to the vein wall. The filter traps clots traveling toward the lungs without hindering blood flow.

Nursing Process for the Patient with Thrombophlebitis

ASSESSMENT/DATA COLLECTION. A patient history is obtained that includes recent IV therapy or use of contrast dyes, surgery, extremity trauma, childbirth, bedrest, recent long trip, cardiac disease, recent infections, and current

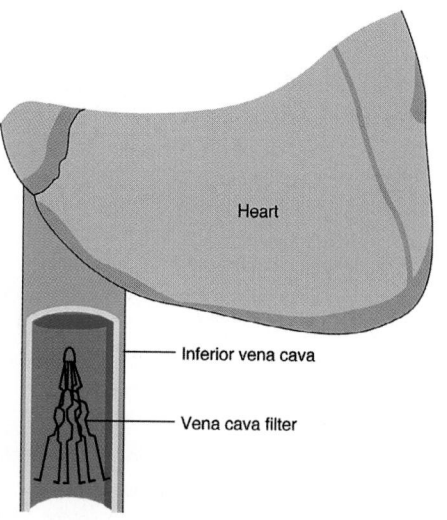

FIGURE 22.7 Vena cava filter placed in the inferior vena cava to prevent emboli from reaching the lungs.

medications. A physical assessment is done noting pain, fever, tenderness, positive Homans' sign, redness, warmth, swelling, edema, and a firm, cordlike vein in the affected extremity. Daily measurements are taken of bilateral thighs and calves and recorded to monitor swelling. Coagulation tests are monitored. Signs of a pulmonary embolism, such as dyspnea, tachycardia, tachypnea, blood-tinged sputum, chest pain, or changes in level of consciousness are immediately reported to the physician.

NURSING DIAGNOSIS, PLANNING, INTERVENTIONS, AND EVALUATION. See Box 22.2 Nursing Care Plan for the Patient with Thrombophlebitis for specific nursing interventions. Teaching the patient about the disease and treatment is important to reduce anxiety about complications and to enhance compliance with treatment to prevent complications (Box 22.3 Education for Patients Receiving Anticoagulant Therapy).

Box 22.2   NURSING CARE PLAN for the Patient with Thrombophlebitis

Nursing Diagnosis: Acute pain related to inflammation of vein

Expected Outcome Reports satisfactory pain relief.

Evaluation of Outcome Does patient report satisfactory pain relief?

Interventions	Rationale	Evaluation
Assess pain using rating scale such as 0–10.	Self-report is the most reliable indicator of pain.	Does patient report pain using scale?
Provide analgesics and NSAIDS as ordered.	Pain is reduced when inflammation is decreased.	Is patient's rating of pain lower after medication?
Apply warm, moist soaks.	Heat relieves pain and vasodilates, which increases circulation to reduce swelling. Moist heat penetrates more deeply.	Does patient report increased comfort with warm, moist soaks? Is swelling reduced?
Maintain bedrest with leg elevation above heart level.	Elevation decrease swelling, which reduces pain.	Is swelling reduced?

Nursing Diagnosis: Impaired skin integrity related to venous stasis

Expected Outcome Skin remains intact without edema.

Evaluation of Outcome Does patient's skin remain intact? Is edema present?

Interventions	Rationale	Evaluation
Assess skin for edema, skin color changes, and ulcers. Measure extremities.	Assessment will detect signs of skin integrity impairment and extremity swelling.	Are skin changes seen? Do daily measurements show a change in swelling?
Elevate legs.	Elevation decreases swelling.	Is swelling reduced?
Fit and apply elastic stockings after edema reduced as ordered.	Elastic stockings are fitted after edema is reduced to avoid constriction. They increase venous blood flow to reduce swelling.	Is swelling reduced?
Teach patient to avoid crossing legs or wearing constricting clothes.	Crossing legs and constrictive clothes impair venous return.	Does patient state understanding of teaching?

Box 22.3

Education for Patients Receiving Anticoagulant Therapy

Anticoagulants prolong the time it takes blood to clot, so it is important to prevent injury and to recognize and report signs of bleeding to the physician.

To Prevent Injury

- Wear shoes or slippers; avoid going barefoot.
- Use an electric razor to shave.
- Use a soft toothbrush.

Signs of Bleeding to Report to Physician

- Easy bruising
- Nosebleeds
- Bleeding that does not stop
- Blood in urine
- Blood in sputum
- Blood in stools or black stools

Additional Instructions

- Avoid use of aspirin/NSAIDS because they further prolong clotting time.
- Have your lab work done as prescribed by your physician to monitor your clotting time and medication dosage.

Home Health Hints

- Encourage the patient to move frequently since immobility can contribute to thrombophlebitis.
- If the patient is bed bound, instruct both the patient and caregiver on simple active and passive ROM. If necessary, consider involving occupational and physical therapy. Working collaboratively with therapy, an appropriate activity program can be planned.
- On admission, measure the patients mid calves so you have a baseline size. Reassess measurements during each visit. Subtle changes in measurement can indicate a potential problem.
- Following cardiovascular surgeries, patients are at a high risk for the development of thrombophlebitis. They are also at risk for developing an incisional infection, pneumonia, or pulmonary emboli. Report any abnormal findings.
- Home health nurses can assist patients to develop energy-conserving techniques by being observant of their lifestyles. For instance, notice the room and chair that they spend most of the day in. Television trays and baskets can be used to hold items they may need or want, such as water pitcher and glass, TV remote, reading material, paper and pen, mail, medicines, telephone and phone book, snacks, washcloth, or tissues. Answering the door should be done by the caregiver. When the patient is alone, a note can be placed on the door with instructions; however, the instructions should not convey that the patient is alone.
- Other techniques to conserve energy are putting a carrying pouch on the front bar of a walker to carry items such as a portable phone or tissues and, if the house has stairs, putting a chair at the top and bottom of the stairs so the patient can rest.
- When a patient with venous circulation problems is sitting in a recliner with the leg rest up, the nurse should note whether pressure is being applied on the popliteal area or calf muscle. The angle of the recliner and the patient's height affect the position of the pressure. A small, flat pillow is placed underneath the knees and lower legs to open the angle and relieve the pressure.

REVIEW QUESTIONS

1. The nurse evaluates the patient as understanding how to prevent rheumatic fever if the patient states that rheumatic fever can be prevented by treating streptococcal infections with which of the following?
   a. Penicillin
   b. Prednisone
   c. Cortisone
   d. Cyclosporine

2. For patients recovering from infective endocarditis, discharge teaching to prevent recurrence should include which of the following?

   a. Proper use of isolation techniques
   b. Keeping vaccinations up to date
   c. Need to obtain annual flu injection
   d. Need for antibiotics before invasive procedures

3. The nurse is planning care for a patient with cardiomyopathy. For which of the following complications of cardiomyopathy should the nurse collect data?
   a. Thrombophlebitis
   b. Heart failure
   c. Rheumatic fever
   d. Pulmonary embolism

Multiple response item. Select all that apply.

4. Which of the following signs and symptoms indicates to the nurse the presence of a deep vein thrombus in the patient's leg?
   a. Calf swelling
   b. Crackles
   c. Jugular vein distention
   d. Positive Homans' sign
   e. Warmth

5. The nurse is to give warfarin (Coumadin). Which of the following laboratory tests should the nurse review before giving the medication?
   a. International normalized ratio
   b. Partial thromboplastin time
   c. Plasma fibrinogen level
   d. Bleeding time

Reference

1. Dajani, A, Taubert KA, Wilson W, et al: Prevention of bacterial endocarditis: Recommendations by the American Heart Association. JAMA 277:1794, 1997.

SUGGESTED ANSWERS TO

CRITICAL THINKING

■ Mrs. Jones

1. A heart murmur is heard from damaged heart valves.

2. Splinter hemorrhages appear as black or red lines in the nails.

3. Petechiae indicate that tiny pieces of a lesion on the endocardium or valves have broken off and become microemboli.

4. Subjective assessment findings might include patient statements such as, "I have pain in my joints and am chilled" or "I am fatigued and have no appetite." Objective findings are as follows: temperature 100°F (37°C), red splinter hemorrhages in left index finger nailbed, many petechiae on chest.

5. Expected medications include IV antibiotics.

6. Removing blankets to decrease fever results in chills and shivering, which further increases body temperature from the heat generated by muscular activity during shivering. Therefore, Mrs. Jones should be kept covered to prevent chills.

7. For left-sided heart failure, crackles, wheezes, cough, or dyspnea might be seen. In right-sided heart failure, peripheral edema or jugular vein distention could be present.

8. Prophylactic antibiotics are needed to prevent another episode of infective endocarditis, which can result from bacteria entering the circulation during the invasive procedure, attaching to areas of the endocardium damaged from the current infection, and growing.

9. 2 tablets

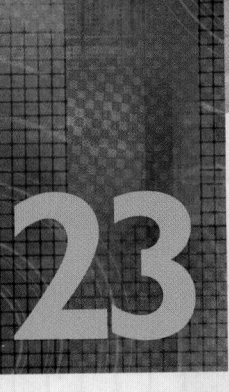

23
Nursing Care of Patients with Occlusive Cardiovascular Disorders

MAUREEN McDONALD

KEY TERMS

acute coronary syndromes (a-CUTE KOR-uh-na-ree sin-dr-OMEs)
anastomosed (an-AST-ta-most)
aneurysm (AN-yur-izm)
angina pectoris (an-JIGH-nah PEK-tuh-riss)
arteriosclerosis (ar-TIR-ee-oh-skle-ROH-sis)
atherosclerosis (ATH-er-oh-skle-ROH-sis)
atheroma (ATH-er-OMA)
collateral circulation (koh-LA-ter-al SIR-kew-LAY-shun)
coronary artery disease (KOR-uh-na-ree AR-tuh-ree di-ZEEZ)
embolism (EM-buh-lizm)
high-density lipoprotein (HIGH DEN-si-tee LIP-oh-PROH-teen)
hyperlipidemia (HIGH-per-LIP-i-DEE-mee-ah)
intermittent claudication (IN-ter-MIT-ent KLAW-di-KAY-shun)
lymphangitis (lim-FAN-je-EYE-tis)
myocardial infarction (MY-oh-KAR-dee-yuhl in-FARK-shun)
peripheral arterial disease (puh-RIFF-uh-ruhl ar-TIR-ee-uhl di-ZEEZ)
plaque (PLAK)
Raynaud's disease (ra-NOHZ di-ZEEZ)
thrombosis (throm-BOH-sis)
varicose veins (VAR-i-kohz VAINS)
venous stasis ulcers (VEE-nus STAY-sis UL-sers)

QUESTIONS TO GUIDE YOUR READING

1. What are the etiologies, signs, symptoms, and therapeutic interventions of coronary artery disease, angina pectoris, and myocardial infarction?

2. What data should you collect and what nursing care will you provide for patients with coronary artery disease, angina pectoris, or myocardial infarction?

3. What are therapeutic interventions for coronary artery disease, angina pectoris, and myocardial infarction?

4. What are the etiologies, signs, and symptoms for each of the peripheral vascular disorders?

5. What are therapeutic interventions for each peripheral vascular disorder?

6. What nursing care will you provide for patients with each peripheral vascular disorder?

Cardiovascular disorders are the leading cause of disability and death in the United States. Diseases of the heart and peripheral vessels can affect quality of life and alter the ability of the individual to perform tasks of everyday living. Long-term disability can place a burden on families and businesses and can create high insurance costs. Many factors leading to cardiovascular diseases can be controlled or modified. Education is important in preventing and treating occlusive cardiovascular diseases.

According to the American Heart Association, in 2003 6,500,000 people had angina with 400,000 new cases of stable angina and 150,000 cases of unstable angina occurring each year.[1] Seven million two hundred thousand people have had heart attacks. One in three adults has cardiovascular disease (CVD). Two of three women develop CVD, which occurs about 10 years later than in men, often after menopause. CVD is the number one killer in the United States and the leading killer of women, with 500,000 women dying each year.

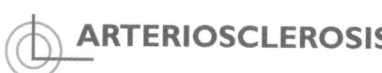

ARTERIOSCLEROSIS

Arteriosclerosis is part of the aging process in which the intimal lining of the artery wall looses elasticity and weakens. This weakening is due to the high pressure that carries blood within arteries. Arteriosclerosis may be called hardening of the arteries, although the arteries are actually weakened.

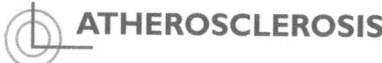

ATHEROSCLEROSIS

Atherosclerosis is the formation of **plaque** within the arterial wall. Arteriosclerosis and **atherosclerosis** are conditions that may begin in early childhood and progress without symptoms through adult life.

Pathophysiology

Atherosclerosis is a multistep process that affects the inner lining of the artery (Fig. 23.1). The first step in the development of atherosclerosis is injury to the endothelial cells that line the walls of the arteries. This injury causes inflammation and immune reactions. Damage to the endothelium stimulates the growth of smooth muscle cells. These cells secrete collagen and fibrous proteins. Lipids, platelets, and other clotting factors accumulate. Scar tissue replaces some of the arterial wall. An early indication of injury is a fatty streak on the lining of the artery. This build-up of fatty deposits is known as plaque. Plaque is composed of smooth muscle cells, fibrous proteins, and cholesterol-laden foam cells. Plaque has irregular, jagged edges that allow blood cells and other material to adhere to the wall of the artery. The portion of the plaque that faces the bloodstream develops a fibrous cap, a firm shell that often contains calcium.

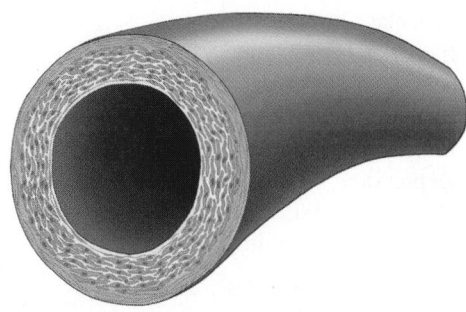

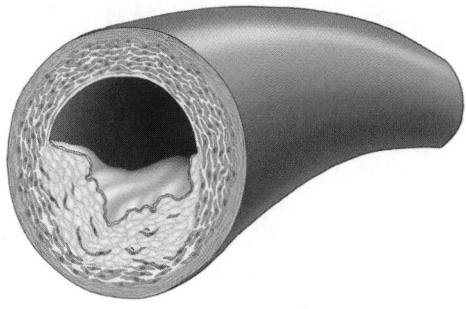

FIGURE 23.1 (*Top*) Cross-section of normal coronary artery. (*Bottom*) Coronary artery with atherosclerosis narrowing the lumen.

Over time this build-up becomes calcified and hardened, causing turbulence that damages cells and increases the build-up within the vessel. Sometimes the plaque's fibrous cap tears or ruptures and a blood clot forms. This blood clot can completely block the coronary artery, or it may break loose and lodge within a smaller artery leading to the heart. The vessel may also become stenosed (narrowed) by plaque build-up. This build-up of plaque may cause partial or total occlusion of the artery resulting in reduced blood flow. The area distal to the occlusion may become ischemic as a result. Atherosclerosis often progresses asymptomatically through adult life. However, it is often noted when the patient has symptoms of ischemic coronary syndromes, stroke, transient ischemic attack (TIA), and peripheral artery disease.

Causes

Risk factors for atherosclerosis can be divided into two categories: those that can be modified and those that cannot. Nonmodifiable risk factors include:
- Age
- Gender
- Ethnicity
- Genetics: predisposition for **hyperlipidemia**
Modifiable risk factors include:
- Diabetes mellitus
- Hypertension
- Smoking
- Obesity

---

arteriosclerosis: arterio—artery + sklerosis—hardness

hyperlipidemia: hyper—above + lipos—fat + emia—blood

- Sedentary lifestyle
- Increased serum homocysteine levels (an amino acid)
- Increased serum iron levels
- Infection
- Depression
- Hyperlipidemia
- Excessive alcohol intake

Signs and Symptoms

Atherosclerosis is not usually symptomatic until later stages of development, often when a major portion of the lumen of a blood vessel is occluded (Box 23.1). If symptoms do occur, they may include chest pain or dizziness caused by decreased blood supply and oxygen to the heart. Other symptoms noted may include diaphoresis, shortness of breath, nausea, weakness, and fatigue. Reduced blood flow in the extremities is reflected by pallor in the nailbeds, a reddish purple color in the lower extremities, thickened nails, dry skin, or loss of hair on the extremities. Peripheral pulses may be diminished or absent. Skin temperature in the extremities is cooler, and there is prolonged capillary refill (greater than 3 seconds). A carotid bruit (abnormal sound on auscultation) indicates atherosclerosis in the carotid artery. Sometimes symptoms occur only with exertion. In some people, symptoms occur at rest.

Diagnostic Tests

Cholesterol and triglycerides are often elevated in patients with atherosclerosis. (See Table 20.3.) Total cholesterol levels above 200 mg/dL increase risk of myocardial infarction. Low-density lipoproteins (LDLs) increase **coronary artery disease** (CAD) risks, but **high-density lipoproteins** (HDL) are protective against CAD. A premature risk factor is a high Lp(a) cholesterol (a genetic variation of plasma LDL). C-reactive protein can indicate low-grade inflammation in coronary vessels and long-term heart disease risk. (See Chapter 20.)

Blood glucose levels should also be checked because elevated levels may increase the risk for atherosclerosis. Radiological studies of the arteries can be performed to show narrowed or occluded vessels. (See Chapter 20.)

Therapeutic Interventions

A healthy lifestyle that includes good nutrition and exercise, cholesterol screening, frequent check-ups, and medications are helpful in controlling arteriosclerosis and atherosclerosis.

Diet

Saturated fats are the primary cause of increased cholesterol levels, which promote arteriosclerosis and atherosclerosis. Because the formation of plaque within arteries is primarily caused by fatty deposits, an adherence to a low-fat diet is recommended (Box 23.2 Nutrition Notes). The liver is capable of producing cholesterol from saturated fats even when the dietary intake of fats is low. The American Heart Association has complete guidelines and diets for decreasing fat and cholesterol intake. For more information, visit http://www.americanheart.org.

Smoking

The risk of developing CAD is two to six times higher in cigarette smokers than in nonsmokers. Risk is proportionate to the number of cigarettes smoked. Smoking contributes to a loss of high-density lipoproteins (HDLs). These proteins are considered the best cholesterol to have in the body to decrease the risk of cardiovascular disorders. The rate of progressive damage to blood vessels is increased with smoking. Smoking also causes vasoconstriction, which leads to **angina pectoris** and cardiac dysrhythmias. The benefits of smoking cessation are dramatic and almost immediate. Education about the risks of smoking and exposure to second-hand smoke should be presented to patients. The American Cancer Society has many programs to help patients quit smoking. For more smoking cessation information, visit http://www.cancer.org.

---

angina pectoris: angina—to choke + pectora—chest

Box 23.1

Atherosclerosis Summary

Signs and Symptoms	Asymptomatic until later stages
	Vascular
	Capillary refill greater than 3 seconds
	Diminished peripheral pulses
	Dry skin
	Loss of hair on extremities
	Pallor in nail beds
	Thickened nails
	Leg cramps
	Cardiac
	Chest pain
	Diaphoresis
	Dizziness
	Fatigue
	Nausea
	Shortness of breath
	Weakness
	Arterial bruits
Diagnostic Tests	Cholesterol
	Triglycerides
	Arteriogram
Therapeutic Interventions	Diet—low fat, low cholesterol
	Smoking cessation
	Increased exercise—walk 30 minutes daily
Nursing Diagnoses	Deficient knowledge related to self-care and health promotion
	Pain related to reduced vascular or coronary artery blood flow

Box 23.2

Nutrition Notes
Controlling Blood Cholesterol with Diet

Two-thirds of the body's cholesterol is produced by the liver and intestines. Most people can produce less cholesterol or increase its excretion in response to high levels of dietary cholesterol, but others respond weakly, a phenomenon that may be genetically based. Although only foods of animal origin contain cholesterol, some vegetable oil products contain *trans* fats, potent risk factors for cardiovascular disease. About 63% to 75% of *trans* fat intake comes from baked goods, fried fast foods, and other prepared foods rather than from margarines (Ascherio, Katan, and Stampfer, 1999). *Trans* fats are on labels beginning 2006.

Manufacturers of certain foods may make health claims that the food *as part of a diet low in saturated fat and cholesterol* may reduce the risk of heart disease. The Food and Drug Administration has approved such health claims for omega-3 fatty acids (salmon, lake trout, tuna, and herring), psyllium (e.g., Kellogg's Bran Buds), and soy protein.

The National Cholesterol Education Program therapeutic lifestyle changes (TLC) diet for individuals at increased risk of heart disease is based on the following:

Saturated fat and *trans* fats	Less than 7% of total calories
Dietary cholesterol	Less than 200 milligrams per day
Moderate physical activity	To use 200 calories per day

For patients with diabetes or metabolic syndrome, unsaturated fats may be prescribed as follows:

Monounsaturated fat	Up to 20% of total calories
Polyunsaturated fat	Up to 10% of total calories

After 6 weeks on the above program, the following may be added:

Fiber	20 to 30 grams per day
Plant stanols/sterols*	2 grams per day

After another 6 weeks, cholesterol-lowering medication may be prescribed.

---

*These compounds in plants, which structurally resemble cholesterol but are not absorbed in the human body to any extent, actually inhibit the absorption of cholesterol. Table spreads and salad dressings containing plant sterols are commercially available. In a rare autosomal recessive disorder called sitosterolemia, both cholesterol and plant sterols are absorbed at a high rate and are not removed effectively by the liver, resulting in accelerated atherosclerosis and premature coronary artery disease (Lee, Lu, and Patel, 2001).

Exercise

Increased activity raises HDL levels (the desirable cholesterol). Increasing physical activity may also lower insulin resistance and facilitate weight loss. Over time, exercise also leads to the development of **collateral circulation,** which allows blood to flow around occluded sites. Before beginning an exercise program, the patient should consult a physician.

Medications

Lowering lipid levels is the major treatment for atherosclerosis (Table 23.1). When dietary control is not effective, medication is also used. It may take 4 to 6 weeks before lipid levels respond to drug therapy. If one drug does not control the lipids, another drug can be added. High doses of statins, which lower lipid levels, are being researched to see if they significantly reduce the risk of heart attack.

Complications

Complications of atherosclerosis include CAD, MI (discussed below), and TIA or stroke (see Chapter 49).

CORONARY ARTERY DISEASE AND ACUTE CORONARY SYNDROME

Coronary artery disease is a term applied to obstructed blood flow through the coronary arteries to the heart muscle. The primary cause of coronary artery disease is atherosclerosis. The term *acute coronary syndrome (ACS)* is used to encompass the continuum of coronary artery disease. ACS describes the manifestations of coronary artery disease, such as unstable angina, non-ST elevation myocardial infarction, and ST elevation. (See Chapter 25 for ST definition.) If blood flow reduction resulting from CAD is severe and prolonged, a **myocardial infarction** (MI, heart attack) can occur, causing irreversible damage.

Pathophysiology and Etiology

As discussed in the sections on atherosclerosis and arteriosclerosis, an accumulation of fatty deposits and minerals in the coronary arteries, called an **atheroma** or plaque, leads to stenosis and eventually occlusion of the artery. In CAD, blood flow to the myocardium is reduced. The arteries are unable to dilate to meet increased metabolic needs. When myocardial oxygen demands are not met, ischemia results, which can cause chest pain. The pain associated with CAD occurs from a lack of oxygen to the myocardium from CAD and is called angina pectoris.

Prevention

Risk factors for CAD are listed in Table 23.2. If coronary artery disease is not prevented or treated early, it can progress to more serious cardiac disorders. These include angina, myocardial infarction, heart failure, cardiac dysrhythmias, and even sudden death. The appropriate management of risk factors can prevent, modify, or retard the progression of atherosclerosis and coronary artery disease.

TABLE 23.1 LIPID-LOWERING DRUGS

Medication Class/Action	Examples	Route	Side Effects	Nursing Implications
Statins First-line drugs to reduce low-density lipoprotein by reducing cholesterol synthesis	Atorvastatin (Lipitor) Fluvastatin (Lescol XL)	PO	Impaired liver function Rhabdomyolysis— Lethal breakdown of skeletal muscle	Tell patient to take in the evening when cholesterol synthesis is highest. Teach patient to report any muscle pain. Monitor liver function studies.
	Lovastatin (Mevacor) Pravastatin (Pravachol) Simvastatin (Zocor)	PO PO		
Fibrates Reduce triglycerides	Fenofibrate (Tricor) Clofibrate (Atromid) Gemfibrozil (Lopid)	PO	Heartburn Gallstones	Tell patient to take 30 minutes before morning and evening meal. May increase the effects of anticoagulants and hypoglycemia.
Bile Acid Sequestrants Lower cholesterol by binding bile acids, so stored cholesterol is used to make more bile acids	Colestipol (Colestid)	PO		
	Colesevelam HCl (WelChol, Sankyo)	PO	Headache, heartburn, constipation, gas	Fruits and vegetables high in fiber should be added to diet to reduce constipation and other GI effects noted with bile acid sequestrants. May interfere with absorption of digoxin, thiazides, and beta blockers.
	Cholestyramine (Questran)	PO		
Niacin Prevents conversion of fats into very-low-density lipoproteins. First antilipid agent used	Niacin (nicotinic acid) Niaspan (extended-release niacin)	PO	Gastritis Gout Flushing	Take aspirin 30 minutes prior to taking drug to reduce flushing.
	Zetia (Ezetimibe) (intestinal cholesterol absorption inhibitor)			Tell patient to take with liquids and meals and to take other drugs 1 hour before or 4 hours after. Tell patient to take with meals or milk to avoid GI upset. Used with diet, exercise, and smoking cessation therapy to lower lipids.

Therapeutic Interventions

Most risk factors for heart disease are related to lifestyle and environmental factors. The guidelines for prevention of heart disease by the American Heart Association target the risk factors that have the potential for change. Educating patients on cessation of smoking, dietary changes, controlling hypertension, maintaining weight, and diabetes can decrease their risk of CAD. Dietary changes are made to reduce saturated fats to less than 10% of daily food intake. Cholesterol intake on the Step 1 diet is less than 300 mg per day and less than 200 mg per day on the step 2 diet. Medication may be given to reduce cholesterol levels. Low-dose aspirin and anticoagulants are used to prevent the formation of a thrombus.

Percutaneous Transluminal Coronary Angioplasty

Percutaneous transluminal coronary angioplasty (PTCA) is a minimally invasive procedure that helps reduce symptoms of CAD (Fig. 23.2). In a cardiac catheterization laboratory, a catheter with a balloon tip is inserted usually via the femoral artery and advanced into the heart. However, the radial artery has also been used with fewer complications like bleeding. Once the blocked coronary artery is entered, the balloon on the catheter is inflated and the atherosclerotic plaque is compressed. This results in a dilated vessel being able to deliver more oxygen-rich blood to the myocardium. The patency of the vessel is restored. The symptoms of CAD are usually reduced, but the underlying progression of ath-

TABLE 23.2 RISK FACTORS FOR CORONARY ARTERY DISEASE

Risk Factors that Cannot Be Changed	
Heredity	CAD risk factors can run in families.
Ethnicity	African Americans have a higher incidence of atherosclerosis.
Gender	Men have more risk factors and higher incidence of CAD.
Age	Men have increased incidence after age 50. Women have increased incidence after menopause.
Risk Factors that Can Be Changed or Controlled	
Smoking	Causes vasoconstriction and increases myocardial oxygen demand. Decreases HDL.
Hypertension	Vasoconstriction increases myocardial oxygen demand.
Elevated serum cholesterol	Level above 240 mg/dL increases the risk of developing CAD.
Diabetes	Increases the risk of hypertension, obesity, and elevated blood lipids.
Obesity	Increases heart workload and risk of hypertension, diabetes, glucose intolerance, hyperlipidemia.
Stress	Increases heart workload and risk for hypertension.
Elevated serum homocysteine	Increases CAD risk. Foods that contain folic acid (fruits, green leafy vegetables) reduce homocysteine levels.
Sedentary lifestyle	Increases obesity, hypertension, hyperlipidemia.
Excessive alcohol use	Raises blood pressure leading to heart failure, increase triglycerides, cause irregular heart beats.

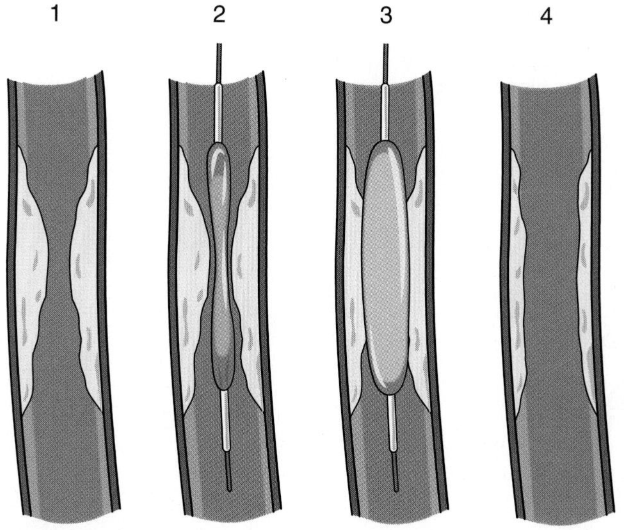

erosclerosis continues. Reocclusion of the artery often occurs within a few months. Over time, PTCA may need to be repeated. Angioplasty can be done with or without the placement of stents (discussed below), but it is often more successful when stents are used.

Coronary Atherectomy

Coronary atherectomy is used to cut and remove plaque from atherosclerotic coronary arteries. The catheter has a central rotating blade that shaves off the plaque and contains it for removal and pathological analysis. Calcium channel blockers are given before the procedure to prevent vasospasms from the vibrating cutter. To prevent clot formation, an antiplatelet agent is given after the procedure.

Coronary Artery Stents

Coronary artery stents are used to prevent closure of a coronary artery from an atherosclerotic lesion. Stents are put in place during an angioplasty. A stent is an expandable metal mesh tube that is implanted at the site of blockage in the coronary artery. A stent provides support to a coronary artery wall at the area of stenosis to keep blood flowing through the artery. Different types of materials, such as bioabsorbable materials or stainless steel mesh, and designs, such as self-expanding or balloon expandable, are used to make stents (Fig. 23.3). Complications associated with stent placement include **thrombosis,** bleeding from anticoagulation, stent occlusion, or coronary artery dissection. Some stents are coated with medication (drug-eluting stents) that can be released at the implantation site to reduce the risk of restenosis. After the procedure, medications are given to help prevent clot formation. Antiplatelets (such as aspirin, clopidogrel bisulfate [Plavix], ticlopidine [Ticlid], or enoxa-

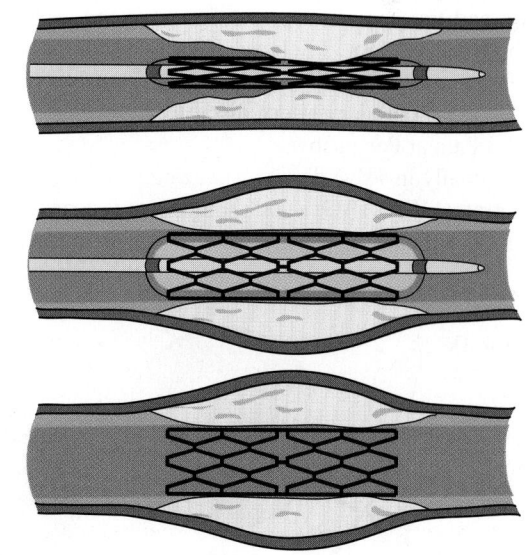

FIGURE 23.3 Insertion of a coronary artery stent: (A) A balloon catheter with a collapsed stent is advanced to the location of a coronary artery lesion. (B) The balloon is inflated, which expands the stent and compresses the lesion to increase the artery opening. (C) The balloon is then deflated and removed, leaving the expanded stent in place to prevent the artery from closing.

1   2   3   4

FIGURE 23.2 Percutaneous coronary angioplasty opens narrowed coronary arteries.

parin [Lovenox]) and anticoagulants (warfarin [Coumadin]) may be used. Aspirin can be used long term, but the other medications may only need to be used for several weeks until the stent is covered with tissue and the risk of clot formation is over. Fondaparinux (Arixtra) is a new anticoagulant that inhibits factor Xa only. A daily subcutaneous injection of 2.5 mg is given.

Myocardial Revascularization–Coronary Artery Bypass Graft

Coronary artery bypass graft (CABG) surgery is a procedure used to increase blood flow and oxygen to the myocardium and alleviate anginal symptoms. During bypass surgery, a blood vessel from the leg or chest is used to reroute blood around a segment of a coronary artery that is narrowed by atherosclerosis. Significant occlusions in the coronary arteries are bypassed with vein or artery grafts (Fig. 23.4). One or more vessel bypasses can be performed during the procedure. The saphenous vein from the leg or an internal mammary artery from the chest wall is generally used. The right gastroepiploic artery (RGEA), a branch of the gastro duodenal artery, and the inferior epigastric artery (IEA) have also been used for repeat CABG operations.

While the sternotomy is made, the vein graft is being removed from the body. The graft is flushed with a heparinized solution to check for leaks, and then set aside for use during the surgery. The patient is then placed on cardiopulmonary bypass (CPB) (see Chapter 20). After cardiac standstill occurs, one end of the graft is **anastomosed** (joined) to the coronary artery distal to the occlusion while the proximal end of the graft is anastomosed, usually to the ascending aorta.

Resecting the mammary arteries for grafting is more difficult and time consuming than resecting the saphenous vein, but their patency is longer. The proximal end of the artery is left attached to its origin, and the distal end is anastomosed to the coronary artery distal to the occlusion. See Box 23.3 Patient Perspective.

Minimally invasive direct visualization coronary artery bypass graft (MIDCABG) is a technique that is done without the use of cardiopulmonary bypass. Several small incisions are used to access the coronary arteries instead of a sternotomy. This technique uses a thoracoscope to mobilize the internal mammary artery (IMA) or the left internal mammary artery (LIMA). Single-vessel disease patients may take advantage of this new technique. The main disadvantage of MIDCAB is that it cannot be used to treat several diseased vessels, especially if arteries on both the left and right sides of the heart are blocked. The limited number of small incisions made using MIDCAB makes it difficult to treat more than two coronary arteries during the same surgery.

Transmyocardial Laser Revascularization

Transmyocardial laser revascularization is an option for patients who are not candidates for angioplasty or coronary

---

CRITICAL THINKING

Mr. Jones

■ Mr. Jones is transferred to the nursing unit 12 hours after a quadruple CABG. Preoperative vital signs were blood pressure 164/88, apical pulse 62 regular, respiratory rate 8, temperature 98.4°F (36.9°C). Assessment findings are blood pressure 100/56, apical pulse 105 and irregular, respiratory rate 28 and shallow, temperature 99.8°F (37.7°C), lung sounds diminished with crackles in bilateral bases, pedal pulses weak bilaterally, chest and leg dressings dry and intact, and no urinary catheter. Mr. Jones is being monitored for first postoperative voiding.

1. Which findings may indicate pulmonary problems?
2. List four nursing interventions for the altered pulmonary status.
3. What are three reasons why the apical pulse could be elevated?
4. What are two reasons why the blood pressure could be low?

Suggested answers at end of chapter.

---

transmyocardial: trans—across + myo—muscle + cardial—heart

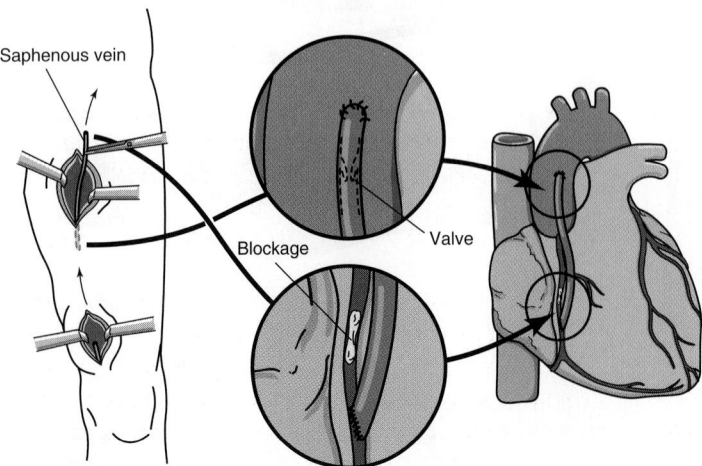

FIGURE 23.4 Myocardial revascularization: coronary artery bypass graft surgery.

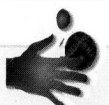

Box 23.3

Patient Perspective

Keith: Coronary Artery Bypass Graft

I was 72 when I had coronary artery bypass surgery. I had some very minor symptoms, and a heart catheterization showed significant coronary artery blockage. I ended up having five bypass grafts performed. It was a long surgery. I felt disoriented for several days afterward—mostly while I was in the intensive care unit.

I felt absolutely no pain of any type after surgery. However, I have had a strange sensation in my legs at the incision sites ever since surgery, but not pain! I also have experienced no depression and have assumed an attitude that I am in better condition than before surgery, so why should I worry?

I was provided with excellent care at home after discharge from the hospital. The nursing and rehab personnel were outstanding. I had a capable visiting nurse, physical therapist, or occupational therapist practically every day. Physical therapy was difficult at first but shortly became routine and easy.

My experience during cardiac rehab was outstanding. I had three sessions per week for 12 weeks. I have always exercised a lot, so I had no problems attaining the exercise levels suggested. It was a very positive experience, and I enjoyed the association with others in the same situation. We even staged a graduation when we finished. I wore a tuxedo jacket with my gym shorts! Since completing my rehab, I have religiously maintained a minimum 40-minute exercise schedule three times per week. I do this because I want to stay healthy for a long time.

The only negative aspect I experienced was a minor stroke during surgery. As a result, my balance is not as good as I would like. I need to be more careful, particularly when running or bike riding. Perhaps this is just older age, but it started just after surgery, so that is the reason I assume it is due to the minor stroke.

The impact on my life and family has been minimal. The primary change is being more conscious of my diet and an emphasis on exercise. Otherwise, I live pretty much the same as before.

artery bypass surgery. Carbon dioxide laser revascularization uses a high-powered carbon dioxide laser to create approximately 40 transmural channels directly in the myocardium. The laser is synchronized to fire on the R wave of the electrocardiogram (ECG). This minimizes dysrhythmias and ensures that the ventricle is at rest and full of blood. The channels created allow blood to flow into the ischemic areas. This enables oxygen-rich blood to flow directly into ischemic myocardium. Optimal results are seen in about 3 to 12 months after the procedure. Over time the ischemic myocardial tissue is reperfused as a new system of circulation develops. Anginal pain is decreased and cardiac function may be improved.

Nursing Process: The Patient with Atherosclerosis and Coronary Artery Disease

Assessment/Data Collection

A health history is obtained regarding the patient's risk for athersclerosis and coronary artery disease. Data collected would include nonmodifiable risk factors such as age, race, gender, ethnicity, and family history and modifiable risk factors such as smoking, diabetes, hypertension, obesity, physical inactivity, infection, depression, drug use, alcohol use, and cocaine use. A history of chest pain, fatigue, or activity intolerance is noted. Current medications, including over-the-counter and prescription drugs are documented as well as allergies to medications. Height, weight, and diet history as well as laboratory values for lipids and cholesterol are recorded.

Nursing Diagnosis, Planning, and Implementation
Deficient knowledge related to ineffective management of regimen for atherosclerosis or coronary artery disease

EXPECTED OUTCOME: The patient will report understanding and management of atherosclerosis and coronary artery disease.

- Identify cognitive or physical impairments *that would interfere with the patient's ability to learn desired information.*
- Include significant other as appropriate *to support patient during learning.*
- Collect data on the patient's present understanding of atherosclerosis and CAD *to determine baseline knowledge.*
- Collect data on the patient's readiness to learn and desired learning needs and feelings about incorporating lifestyle changes into daily routine *to prioritize teaching topics.*
- Determine cultural beliefs *as they may influence learning.*
- Provide for the physical comfort of the patient during teaching *to increase learning.*
- Use appropriate teaching tools to meet individual learning needs of the patient *such as pamphlets, diagrams, or other written materials in simple language.*
- Use an interpreter as needed and provide written materials in the patient's native language *to facilitate understanding.*
- Explain pathophysiology of atherosclerosis and CAD to patient.
- Explain to patient how to control risk factors and manage symptoms of CAD including the following as appropriate: weight reduction plans, stress management, smoking cessation, cardiovascular fitness, low-fat diet, smoking cessation, increasing activity level, hypertension, and diabetes management.

- Explain action, side effects, and importance of taking medications as prescribed *to prevent complications*.
- Teach to consult health-care provider prior to taking over-the-counter preparations *that may interfere with desired effects of medication regimen*.
- Provide information about community resources *that can assist in making life-style changes such as weight loss, smoking cessation, stress management, and exercise*.
- Teach to monitor blood pressure and heart rate as appropriate and to report chest pain or dyspnea, *which may point to the presence of complications from CAD*.
- Assist the learner to plan how to incorporate information into daily life *to increase likelihood change will occur*.
- Encourage questions and allow the patient the opportunity to verbalize new information and skills *to enhance learning*.
- Document teaching and evaluation of patient knowledge.

See Box 23.4 Nursing Care Plan for the Patient Undergoing Cardiac Surgery for additional nursing care.

Evaluation

Interventions are successful if the patient has an increased understanding of atherosclerosis, CAD, and their management and states he or she will modify risk factors of CAD.

ACUTE CORONARY SYNDROMES

Acute coronary syndromes are a group of conditions that are caused by a lack of oxygen to the heart muscle. These conditions may include unstable angina, non–Q wave myocardial infarction, and ST-segment elevation myocardial infarction. Patients with acute coronary syndromes are at high risk for myocardial infarction and death.

Angina Pectoris

Pathophysiology

Angina pectoris (chest pain) is a symptom of ischemia and is the primary symptom of coronary artery disease and heart attack. When an increased workload is placed on the heart, as in exercise or strenuous activity, there is an increased demand for oxygen. Normally, when the heart needs more oxygen, the coronary arteries dilate to carry more blood. However, with CAD, the narrowed vessels are unable to dilate and supply the heart with this extra blood and oxygen. This inability to supply more blood and oxygen causes myocardial ischemia and chest pain. Chest pain results from the ischemia but usually lasts only for a few minutes, especially if activity is stopped. If adequate blood supply to the myocardium is restored with rest, no myocardial damage usually occurs.

LEARNING TIP

Angina pectoris is not a disease. It is a symptom of coronary artery disease. Ischemia results from a lack of oxygen and blood flow to the heart muscle. Ischemia = pain or angina.

Signs and Symptoms

Anginal pain manifests itself in several ways. Patients often describe the pain as heaviness, tightness, squeezing, vise-like, or crushing pain in the center of the chest. The pain can radiate down one or both arms, with pain in the left arm being more common, into the shoulder, neck, jaw, or back. Patients may also describe heaviness in their arms or a feeling of impending doom. During the episode of pain, the patient may be pale, diaphoretic, or dyspneic. The pain is usually brought on by exertion and subsides with rest. It can be relieved with a vasodilator medication such as nitroglycerin (NTG). Episodes of chest pain may increase in frequency and severity over time. If patients do not heed this warning to stop their activity and rest, they may be at risk for a myocardial infarction or sudden death. Any event that increases oxygen demand can cause an anginal attack. Most often precipitating events include large meals, exercise, cold, stimulant drugs such as cocaine or amphetamines, and emotional tension. Often angina may occur in the morning hours between 6:00 a.m. and noon when the patient arises and the heart experiences increased workload. Women often exhibit atypical symptoms that should be recognized as being cardiac related so that treatment is sought.

Types

STABLE ANGINA. Stable angina is chest pain that occurs with moderate exertion in a pattern that is familiar to the patient. The pain is predictable and can usually be managed with nitroglycerin and rest. The atherosclerotic arteries cannot dilate to increase blood flow to the myocardium. When increased physical activity and stress place an added demand on the heart, the patient develops midsternal chest pain. The pain of stable angina usually subsides when the activity is stopped.

VARIANT ANGINA (PRINZMETAL'S ANGINA). The pain of variant angina is similar to the pain in stable angina except it has a longer duration and may occur at rest. The pattern of occurrence is often cyclical, with the pain presenting about the same time each day. This type of angina is often caused by coronary artery spasms and usually does not cause damage to the myocardium. Accelerating or "crescendo" pattern of chest pain lasts longer than in stable angina.

UNSTABLE ANGINA. Unstable angina occurs in patients with worsening CAD and is noted by its changing pattern. Rest does not decrease the chest pain of unstable angina. This pain may even occur when the patient is at rest. The

Box 23.4   NURSING CARE PLAN for the Patient Undergoing Cardiac Surgery

Nursing Diagnosis: Acute Pain Related To Sternotomy, Leg Incisions, Internal Mammary Artery Resection, Or Pericarditis

Expected Outcomes Patient will state pain is relieved or tolerable. Patient is able to rest and perform respiratory treatments.

Evaluation of Outcomes Does patient state pain is within acceptable levels? Is patient able to rest and perform respiratory therapies?

Interventions	Rationale	Evaluation
• Assess characteristics of pain with each episode.	A thorough description is needed to determine cause and plan actions.	Does patient describe pain on scale of 0 to 10?
• Splint chest incision with all movement and coughing and deep breathing.	Stabilizes sternum and incision to increase comfort.	Can patient splint chest incision independently?
• Encourage patient to report pain even when pain is mild.	It is easier to keep pain under control when mild.	Does patient report pain when mild?
• Turn, reposition every 2 hours.	Changes muscle position, relieving stiffness.	Is patient comfortable without stiffness?
• Offer back rubs frequently.	Relaxes tense muscles retracted during operation.	Is patient able to rest comfortably?
• Instruct patient to take a deep breath before movement and exhale slowly during movement.	Keeps muscles relaxed, minimizing tension with guarding and pain.	Can patient perform coughing and deep breathing techniques as instructed?

Nursing Diagnosis: Decreased cardiac output related to myocardial depression, hypothermia, bleeding, unstable dysrhythmias, or hypoxemia

Expected Outcomes Patient will remain free of major side effects of pharmacological support. Patient will maintain vital signs within normal limits (WNL), palpable peripheral pulses, urine output greater than 30 mL/hr, and normal sinus rhythm.

Evaluation of Outcomes Is patient free of major side effects? Are vital signs WNL?

Interventions	Rationale	Evaluation
• Monitor vital signs.	Trends reflect problems.	Are vital signs WNL?
• Check peripheral circulation.	Mottling or weak pulses may indicate poor cardiac output (CO).	Do peripheral pulses remain strong with normal skin color, temperature, capillary refill?
• Monitor intake and output.	Fluid deficit or excess can alter CO.	Does total intake equal output?
• Listen to lung sounds and note character of sputum.	Wet lung sounds may indicate heart failure or pulmonary edema.	Are lungs clear?
• Monitor temperature closely while rewarming the patient.	Febrile state increases heart rate and myocardial oxygen consumption.	Does temperature remain less than or equal to 98.6°F (37°C)?
• Note shivering.	Shivering increases the blood pressure, decreasing CO and increasing risk for bleeding.	Is patient's shivering controlled?
• Monitor chest tube drainage for increase or sudden decrease.	Drainage >200 mL/hr may lead to hypovolemia and a decrease in CO.	Is patient free from cardiac tamponade and hypovolemia?
• Monitor ECG.	Premature ventricular contractions and atrial fibrillation decrease CO.	Does patient remain in normal sinus rhythm or controlled dysrhythmia?

(Continued on following page)

Box 23.4   NURSING CARE PLAN for the Patient Undergoing Cardiac Surgery (Continued)

Interventions	Rationale	Evaluation
• Monitor electrolytes.	Low calcium and magnesium and high potassium decrease contractility and CO.	Are electrolytes WNL?
• Monitor ABGs.	Acidosis decreases heart function, and a low CO may lead to further acidosis.	Are ABGs WNL?

Nursing Diagnosis: Risk for infection related to inadequate primary defenses from surgical wound

Expected Outcomes Patient will remain free from infection.

Evaluation of Outcomes Does patient remain free from infection?

Interventions	Rationale	Evaluation
• Observe incision for signs and symptoms of infection.	Redness, warmth, fever, and swelling indicate infection.	Are signs and symptoms of infection present?
• Monitor drainage and maintain drains.	Drains remove fluid from the surgical site to prevent infection development.	Are drainage amount and color normal for procedure? Are drains functioning?
• Maintain sterile technique for dressing changes.	Sterile technique reduces infection development.	Is incision free of signs and symptoms of infection?
• Monitor and report abnormal findings for temperature, lung sounds, sputum, and urine consistency.	Low-grade or high-grade fever, crackles, yellow-green sputum color, or cloudy urine can indicate infection.	Is the patient's temperature WNL and are lung sounds, sputum, and urine clear?
• Encourage coughing and deep breathing and incentive spirometer use.	Lung infections can be prevented with lung expansion and secretion removal.	Does patient perform coughing and deep breathing and use incentive spirometer?

episodes of chest pain with unstable angina increase in frequency and severity, placing the patient at risk for myocardial damage or sudden death. Symptoms of angina usually occur when an artery is narrowed by at least 60% to 70%. Women may experience anginal pain as chest pain, jaw pain, or heartburn or have symptoms different than those thought of as being typical of angina. These symptoms include fatigue, nausea, and breathlessness.

SILENT ISCHEMIA. Many people may have myocardial ischemia without chest pain or symptoms of angina. This is called silent ischemia. Ischemia with or without pain usually has the same prognosis. The older adult and people with hypertension or diabetes are most often noted to have silent ischemia.

Diagnostic Tests

Diagnostic tests of cardiovascular system function are discussed in Chapter 20. Tests commonly done for acute coronary syndromes include electrocardiogram, exercise electrocardiogram, graded exercise testing, stress echocar-

diography, chemical stress testing, radioisotope imaging, and coronary angiography (see Table 20.3).

BIOLOGICAL MARKERS. When cardiac cells become damaged they release enzymes and other molecules into the blood stream that can be measured: troponin, creatine kinase, myoglobin (see Table 20.3). C-reactive protein levels are elevated in the presence of inflammation. Myeloperoxidase is an enzyme produced by activated white blood cells. Myeloperoxidase levels are elevated in the presence of unstable atherosclerotic plaque. Elevated levels of these markers can help detect a heart attack in patients with severe chest pain. Often these markers identify individuals who may have otherwise been misdiagnosed such as the elderly and women.

New marker tests are being developed that may in the future benefit the patient with acute coronary syndrome. One test on the horizon is the albumin cobalt–binding test. This test can be used with ECG findings and troponin levels to increase the accuracy of cardiac disease diagnosis.

Therapeutic Interventions

Treatment for angina is directed at relieving and preventing anginal episodes that could lead to a myocardial infarction. The risk factors identified for the patient determine the course of treatment. Weight reduction; a low-fat, low-cholesterol diet; and stress reduction may help slow disease progression. Most patients with angina are placed on medication that reduces oxygen demand and increases oxygen supply to the myocardium. The three major groups of medication used for angina are vasodilators, calcium channel blockers, and beta blockers (Table 23.3).

For those with unstable angina, taking the Fab Four of cardiac drugs has been shown to be beneficial for heart health.[2] The Fab Four include antiplatelets, statins, ACEIs, and beta blockers. A drug from each of these drug classes should be taken by patients. These drugs when taken together have a synergistic effect in fighting plaque, which means they have a greater positive result for the patient. Generic drugs are available in these drug classes, making the four-drug combination affordable with remarkable benefits. However, research has shown that not all eligible patients are prescribed each of these medications. Patient teaching can include the need to ask the health-care provider about these drug classes to ensure they receive the ones for which they are eligible.

VASODILATORS. Nitroglycerin (a nitrate) is the drug of choice for acute anginal attacks. Nitrates dilate coronary arteries to increase oxygen to the myocardium, and dilate peripheral vessels so the heart does not have to work so hard to pump blood into them. NTG can be administered sublingually, orally, transdermally, intravenously, or as a lingual spray. When administered sublingually, NTG may relieve chest pain within 1 to 2 minutes (Box 23.5 Key Points for Using Sublingual Nitroglycerin). Newer guidelines tell people at home to call 911 immediately if after one tablet and 5 minutes the pain is not relieved *and* symptoms of a myocardial infarction are occurring.

Long-acting nitrates are used to prevent chest pain rather than treat acute pain, and can be given orally, in ointment, or by transdermal patches. A problem with long-acting nitrates is the development of a tolerance to the drug. To prevent tolerance, the patch or ointment is usually removed at bedtime and reapplied in the morning, giving the patient an 8- to 12-hour nitrate-free period. Headaches may be experienced when nitrates are first begun. This side effect usually subsides after a week or two.

CALCIUM CHANNEL BLOCKERS. Calcium is required for electrical excitability of cardiac cells and contraction of the myocardium and vascular smooth muscle. Calcium channel blockers relax vascular smooth muscle, which leads to decreased peripheral vascular resistance (afterload) and decreased myocardial oxygen demand. These drugs dilate main coronary arteries, increasing the myocardial oxygen supply. Nifedipine (Procardia) and verapamil (Calan, Isoptin) are potent inhibitors of coronary artery spasms and are used to treat variant (Prinzmetal's) angina.

SAFETY TIP

Those who take nitrates should not use drugs such as sildenafil (Viagra), tadalafil (Cialis), or vardenafil (Levitra) for erectile dysfunction because these types of drugs dilate blood vessels and may cause a significant drop in blood pressure if used together.

Calcium channel blockers are also used to decrease systolic and diastolic blood pressures and to slow the heart rate. These drugs are commonly given in conjunction with other vasodilators and beta blockers. Because these drugs are slow acting, they are ineffective in relieving acute anginal attacks. Side effects of calcium channel blockers are usually mild and include constipation, fluid retention, headache, and dizziness.

Beta Blockers. Beta blockers decrease heart rate, lower blood pressure, and prevent release of rennin. This results in decreased workload on the heart to help prevent anginal attacks. Because of these decreased effects, beta blockers should be used with caution in patients with any degree of heart failure because it makes heart failure worse. There are nonselective and selective types of beta-adrenergic blockers. People with asthma or chronic obstructive pulmonary disease (emphysema, bronchitis, and bronchiectasis) should avoid nonselective beta-adrenergic blockers because they cause bronchoconstriction. Metoprolol and atenolol are more cardioselective and can be used in patients with asthma and chronic obstructive pulmonary disease (COPD). Beta blockers are not effective for coronary artery spasms.

LEARNING TIP

To help you identify beta blockers, remember that their generic names end with -olol.

Angiotensin-Converting Enzyme Inhibitors (ACEIs). ACEIs block production of angiotension II, which is a potent vasoconstrictor. This action reduces peripheral arterial resistance, which lowers blood pressure. Some patients taking an ACEI may develop a cough. If this occurs, they should inform their health care provider so that the medication can be changed.

Statins. Cholesterol and inflammation in artery walls are involved in atherosclerosis development. Statins lower cholesterol levels by reducing cholesterol production in the liver (see Table 23.1). They also reduce inflammation and CRP levels, which improves patient outcomes in CAD. Statins are used to prevent and treat atherosclerosis and the disorders caused by it.

(Text continued on page 418)

TABLE 23.3 PHARMACOLOGICAL TREATMENT FOR ANGINA PECTORIS

Medication Class/Action	Examples	Route	Side Effects	Nursing Implications
Antiplatelets Inhibit platelet activation, adhesion, or pro-coagulant activity	Aspirin	PO	Increased risk of bleeding including hemorrhagic stroke	Enteric coated may be given for daily dosing.
Statins See Table 23.1				
Nitrates: Vasodilators Relax smooth muscle in blood vessel walls. Produces vasodilation, which relieves cardiac workload. Prelaod and afterload reduction. Reduces oxygen consumption of myocardium.	Nitrates/nitroglycerin (Nitrostat, NitroQuick)	Sublingual	Hypotension Headache Contraindicated in head trauma, hypotension, uncorrected hypovolemia	Take apical pulse the AP and BP pre and post administration. Caution patient to rise slowly because of orthostatic hypotension, especially with sublingual nitroglycerin. Document onset, type, radiation, location, and duration of chest pain. Place tablet in buccal pouch to lessen burning sensation under the tongue. If chest pain is not relieved call the physician, or emergency medical assistance. Tablets should be replaced every 3 to 6 months. Check expiration date. Do not remove tablets from bottle. Vasodilators become inactive when exposed to light, air, heat, and moisture. Tell the patient a burning or tingling sensation may be felt under the tongue with sublingual nitroglycerin.
	Isosorbide dinitrate (Isordil), Isosorbide monitrate (ISMO)	Oral or Sublingual	Hypotension Transient flushing of face and neck Dizziness if standing Orthostatic hypotension Nausea Vomiting Restlessness	Tolerance may occur with repeated prolonged therapy. High dose may produce severe headache. Elderly may be more sensitive to drug dosing. Instruct the patient to rise slowly from a lying position. Caution against using one brand of drug to another. Avoid alcohol during therapy. Alcohol intensifies the drug's hypotensive effect.
	Nitroglycerin (Transderm Nitro, Nitro-Bid) Nitroglycerin patch (Nitro-Dur, Nitrek)	Transdermal	Hypotension Transient flushing of face and neck Dizziness if standing Orthostatic hypotension Nausea Vomiting Restlessness	Remove patch before defibrillation. Rotate application sites. Apply the patch to a clean, dry, hairless area. Tolerance may develop.
Angiotensin-Converting Enzyme Inhibitors Block the production of angiotension II, a potent vasoconstrictor. Reduces peripheral arterial resistance, pulmonary capillary wedge pressure, improves cardiac output and exercise tolerance.	captopril (Capoten), lisinopril (Prinivil, Zestril), ramipril (Altace)	PO	Persistent cough may develop in 20% of patients. Hyperkalemia may develop in patients with diabetes mellitus or renal impairment.	Angioedema, swelling of the face and lips may occur. Agranulocytosis and neutropenia may be noted in patients with concurrent collagen vascular disease including scleroderma and systemic lupus erythematosus, and impaired renal function. Take baseline blood pressure before each dose. Give 1 hour before meals; food delays absorption.

(Continued on following page)

Medication Class/Action	Examples	Route	Side Effects	Nursing Implications
Calcium Channel Blockers Prevent the movement of extracellular calcium into the cell. The result is dilation of peripheral arteries, decreased myocardial contractility, and depressed conduction system. The result is decreased workload of the heart. In variant angina these drugs reduce coronary artery spasm.	Diltiazem (Cardizem, Dilacor XR), amlodipine (Norvasc)	Oral	Headache Peripheral edema Dysrhythmias Flushing Dizziness Atrioventricular blocks Nausea Constipation	Assess apical pulse and blood pressure prior to administration. If blood pressure is less than 90 systolic or heart rate is less than 50, call the physician. Assess liver and renal function tests during therapy. Administer before meals and at bedtime.
	Nifedipine (Procardia)	Oral	Headache Peripheral edema Dysrhythmias Flushing Dizziness Atrioventricular blocks Abdominal discomfort	Grapefruit juice may alter absorption. Take apical pulse and blood pressure prior to administration. Monitor liver and renal function tests during therapy.
	Verapamil (Calan, Isoptin, Covera-HS)	Oral IV	Headache Peripheral edema Dysrhythmias Flushing Dizziness Atrioventricular blocks	Not removed by hemodialysis. Monitor heart rate and blood pressure. Monitor for constipation. If blood pressure is less than 90 systolic or heart rate is less than 50, call the physician.
Beta Blockers Cause a decrease in heart rate, blood pressure, cardiac output, and suppress renin activity. They decrease myocardial contractility and oxygen demand. Decreases the risk of sudden death and may reduce ventricular remodeling.	Propranolol (Inderal)	Oral		
	Metoprolol succinate (Lopressor, Toprol XL)	Oral, IV		
	Atenolol (Tenormin)	Oral	Cold extremities, constipation, diarrhea, diaphoresis, dizziness, fatigue, and nausea. Abrupt withdrawal may result in diaphoresis, palpitations, headache, and tremors. May precipitate thyroid storm in persons with thyrotoxicosis. Hypoglycemia may occur in patients with previously controlled diabetes. Thrombocytopenia.	Warn the patient not to get up quickly. Avoid salt and alcohol. Take the apical pulse and blood pressure immediately prior to administration. If pulse is less than 60 beats per minute, or blood pressure less than systolic 90 mm Hg, withhold the medication and notify the physician. Use cautiously in patients with diabetes. Beta blockers are contraindicated in patients with asthma, heart block, bradycardia, or pulmonary conditions with bronchoconstriction. Do not stop abruptly.
Anti-Ischemic Agent New class of antianginal agent for use as combination therapy for those not responding to other antianginal agents. Action not fully known.	Ranolazine (Ranexa)	PO	Prolongs QT interval. Dizzy, headache, constipation, nausea.	May not be as effective in women.

Box 23.5

Key Points for Using Sublingual Nitroglycerin (NTG)

- Carry NTG at all times.
- Keep NTG tightly sealed in the original container.
- Replace NTG every 6 months for maximum effect.
- Take NTG before an activity known to cause chest pain.
- Sit or lie down when taking NTG if possible
- Take one NTG tablet and repeat every 5 minutes up to three doses if pain is not relieved. If pain is unrelieved after one dose and other symptoms of myocardial infarction are present, call 911 for emergency medical care.
- Tingling should be felt under the tongue when NTG is used.
- NTG may cause a headache.
- NTG may cause light-headedness; rise slowly to prevent falls.

Antiplatelets. Aspirin, clopridogrel (Plavix), and ticlodipine (Ticlid) are commonly used antiplatelets that help prevent cardiovascular events. Aspirin is the one most often prescribed and may be used in combination with another antiplatelet. Patients with unstable angina, stent placement, or heart attack are given antiplatelets.

Nursing Process for the Patient with Angina

ASSESSMENT/DATA COLLECTION. Assess the patient's description of pain. Note the type, location, and pain radiation to other areas of the body. Note skin color and temperature. Note any factors that may make the pain worse or better. This will provide information to determine improvement or lack of improvement in pain. Ask how long the patient has had angina, triggering activities, and how the pain has been relieved in the past. Note the presence of dyspnea, labored respirations, diaphoresis, or nausea. Obtain vital signs, blood pressure, apical pulse, respiration, and oxygen saturation to provide a baseline of the patient status.

NURSING DIAGNOSIS, PLANNING, AND IMPLEMENTATION. Acute pain related to reduced coronary artery blood flow and increased myocardial oxygen needs causing an imbalance between oxygen supply and demand

EXPECTED OUTCOME: The patient reports an absence of pain.

- Ensure vascular access established. *Intravenous access may be necessary to use to administer drugs for pain relief.*
- Consult physician for pain management.
- Obtain a 12-lead ECG as ordered *to determine ischemia or injury of the myocardium with evaluation of the ST segment.*
- Administer analgesics or aspirin as prescribed *to provide pain relief.*
- Administer oxygen as ordered via nasal cannula *to increase oxygen availability to myocardium.*
- Administer sublingual NTG as ordered. *Notify the physician if pain is unrelieved after three doses of nitroglycerin or as prescribed, or vital signs change.*
- Remain with the patient and reassess the pain in 5 minutes after the administration of medication. *A patient who is experiencing chest pain should never be left alone.*
- *Chest pain unrelieved by nitrates may represent unstable angina or myocardial infarction.*
- Notify physician of ECG changes. *ST segment changes may indicate a myocardial infarction.*
- Offer the patient assurance and emotional support *to decrease anxiety. Emotional support is important because patients and their families are often afraid that the patient may die.*
- Promote rest and decrease anxiety for the patient with chest pain.
- Document patient data in the medical record *to communicate patient's problem and outcome.*

Evaluation

Interventions are successful if the patient is pain free.

Myocardial Infarction

A myocardial infarction (MI), commonly known as a heart attack, results in the death of heart muscle. The affected myocardial cells in the heart are permanently destroyed. An MI occurs from a partial or complete blockage of a coronary artery, which decreases the blood supply to the cells of the heart supplied by the blocked coronary artery. The extent of the cardiac damage varies depending on the location and amount of blockage in the coronary artery. This is a potentially devastating condition. The ability of the heart to contract, relax, and propel blood throughout the body requires healthy cardiac muscle. When the patient has an MI, part of the heart muscle no longer functions as it should. Cardiac conduction, blood flow, and function can be dramatically altered by an MI.

Those with MIs are typically men over 40 with atherosclerosis development. Although MIs can occur at any age in men or women, women who smoke and use oral contraceptives are at greater risk for MI.

Pathophysiology

Myocardial infarction does not happen immediately. Ischemic injury evolves over several hours before complete necrosis and infarction take place. The ischemic process affects the subendocardial layer, which is most sensitive to hypoxia. This process leads to depressed myocardial contractility. The body's attempt to compensate for decreased cardiac function triggers the sympathetic nervous system to increase heart rate. The change in heart rate increases myocardial oxygen demand, further depressing the myocardium.

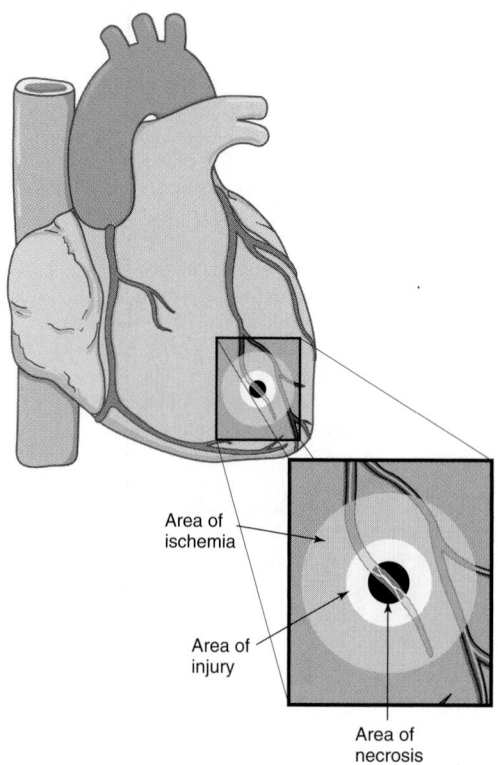

FIGURE 23.5 Myocardial infarction. Areas of ischemia, injury, and necrosis caused by a blockage in the left anterior coronary artery.

Prolonged ischemia can produce severe cellular damage and necrosis of cardiac muscle. Once necrosis takes place, the contractile function of the muscle is permanently lost. The heart has a zone of ischemia and injury around the necrotic area (Fig. 23.5). The zone of injury is next to the necrotic area and is susceptible to becoming necrosed. If treatment is initiated within the first hour of symptoms of the MI, the area of damage can be minimized. Around the injury zone is an area of ischemia and viable tissue. If the heart responds to treatment, this area can rebuild and maintain collateral circulation. If prolonged ischemia takes place, the size of the infarction can be quite large. The size of the infarction depends on how quickly the blood supply from the blocked artery can be restored.

The area that is affected by an MI depends on the coronary artery involved and the extent of occlusive coronary disease (Fig. 23.6). Being familiar with the anatomy of the heart and the area of the MI helps the nurse anticipate dysrhythmias, conduction disturbances, and heart failure, which are the major complications of MIs (Table 23.4).

The anterior interventricular branch of the left coronary artery is the area that feeds the anterior wall of the heart, which also includes most of the left ventricle. An occlusion in this area causes an anterior wall MI. When the left ventricle is affected, there can be severe loss of left ventricular function, leading to severe changes in the hemodynamic status of the patient.

The right coronary artery (RCA) feeds the inferior wall and parts of the atrioventricular node and the sinoatrial node. An occlusion of the RCA leads to an inferior MI and abnormalities in impulse formation and conduction. Serious dysrhythmias can occur early in an inferior MI that may be life threatening.

The left circumflex coronary artery feeds the lateral wall of the heart and part of the posterior wall of the heart. A lesion in the circumflex leads to a lateral wall infarction of the left ventricle.

Signs and Symptoms

Chest pain is a classic symptom of an MI. The pain begins suddenly and continues without relief with rest or NTG. The pain in the center of the chest is usually described as crushing, viselike, or as if an elephant is standing on the chest. The pain may radiate to the back, one or both arms and shoulders, neck, or jaw. The pain can imitate indigestion or a gallbladder attack with abdominal pain and vomiting. Other classic MI symptoms include shortness of breath, dizziness, nausea, and sweating (Box 23.6 Myocardial Infarction Summary). When listening to lung sounds, crackles or wheezing may be heard. The pulse may be rapid or irregular, and an extra heart sound (referred to as S3 or S4) may be present. The presence of an extra heart sound can mean ventricular failure is imminent.

People often deny or fail to recognize that they are having an MI because they experience atypical MI symptoms or their symptoms are similar to other mild conditions such as

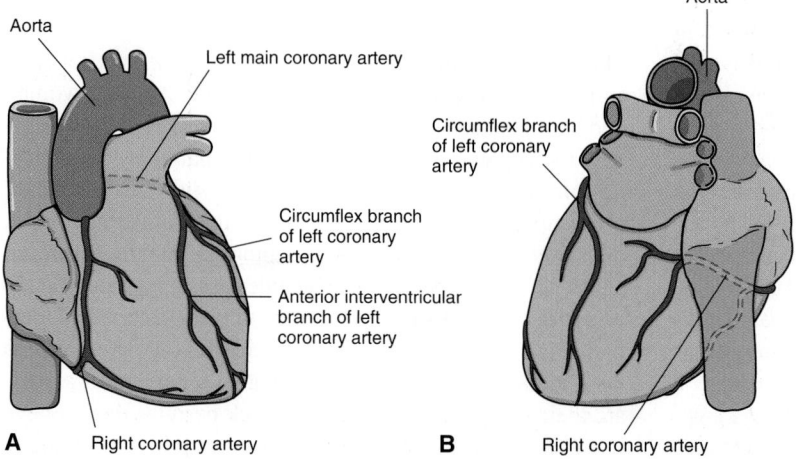

FIGURE 23.6 (A) Coronary arteries, frontal view. (B) Coronary arteries, posterior view.

TABLE 23.4 COMPLICATIONS OF MYOCARDIAL INFARCTION

Complication	Types or Symptoms	Interventions
Dysrhythmias	Premature ventricular contractions, ventricular tachycardia, ventricular fibrillation, heart block	Continuous cardiac monitoring Protocols for treatment of dysrhythmias (see Chapter 25)
Cardiogenic shock	Decreased blood pressure; increased heart rate; diaphoresis; cold, clammy, gray skin	Immediate initiation of treatment to decrease infarct size, control pain and dysrhythmias Thrombolytic therapy Dopamine and dobutamine
Heart failure/pulmonary edema	Dizziness, orthopnea, weight gain, edema, enlarged liver, jugular venous distention, crackles	Correct underlying cause, relieve symptoms, increase cardiac contractility, administer furosemide (Lasix) and digoxin
Emboli	Dependent on location of emboli.	Anticoagulants to prevent; supportive symptom treatment.
Ventricular aneurysms, rupture of muscles or valves of the heart, septal rupture Pseudoaneurysm	Signs of cardiogenic shock, death	Mortality rate high; immediate treatment of MI to limit extent of damage
Pericarditis (inflammation of the heart muscle)	Chest pain, increased with movement, deep inspiration, or cough; pericardial friction rub (fine grating sound)	Relieved when sits up and leans forward Anti-inflammatory drugs (aspirin, indomethacin [Indocin])

LEARNING TIP

To remember what coronary artery occlusion results in a specific MI location, use coast-to-coast U.S. location initials such as those given below. You can personalize the locations with initials of landmarks familiar to you.

Location	Coronary Artery	Resulting MI Location
Los Angeles	Left anterior descending	Anterior
Cedar Point	Circumflex	Posterior
Rhode Island	Right	Inferior

indigestion. Patients have reported that the symptoms of an MI that they experienced were not what they expected. If people expect to have the dramatic heart attack symptoms seen on television (which are usually not the same as those in real life) and they do not, they are likely to wait to seek treatment. People often wait 2 to 24 hours before seeking medical care, yet the first hour after symptom onset is crucial for seeking the newer reperfusion treatments that restore blood flow, minimize tissue damage, and save lives.

Because so few patients arrive at the emergency room quickly enough to benefit from newer treatments, the National Heart, Lung, and Blood Institute (NHLBI) and the American Heart Association launched a major new heart attack education campaign on 9-11-01 called "Act in Time to Heart Attack Signs." The purpose of this campaign is to educate people on the importance of recognizing heart attack symptoms, working with a physician to create a heart attack survival plan, and calling 911 as soon as symptoms begin. For more information on the Act in Time to

Heart Attack Signs, visit http://www.nhlbi.nih.gov/actintime/, http://www.4woman.gov/faq/h-attack.htm, and www.americanheart.org.

The National Heart Attack Alert Program (NHAAP) is another public education program developed by the NHLBI. The message of this program is symptom recognition and "60 minutes to treatment" to improve survival and reduce tissue damage. For more information, visit http://www.nhlbi.nih.gov/about/nhaap.

Women and Heart Health
Heart disease remains the leading cause of death in women in the United States. American women are six times more likely to die of heart disease than breast cancer. Heart disease kills more women than all cancers combined in the over 65-year-old group. Ethnicity is also a factor among women. African American women are more likely than Caucasian women to develop heart disease. Women tend to have an acute myocardial infarction at an older age than men. Women also have a higher mortality rate and are more likely to have complications such as ventricular fibrillation and heart failure than men.

Women often have classic chest pain but they are also likely to have other symptoms as well that men do not typically have. Research is focusing on understanding women and cardiac disease. Atypical symptoms reported by women may include extreme fatigue, epigastric pain, jaw pain, indigestion, nausea and vomiting, dyspnea, shortness of breath, or cramping in the chest. A high percentage of women (more than 50%) noted prodromal symptoms a month before an acute MI. These symptoms include unusual fatigue, sleep disturbances, and shortness of breath. Less than 30% complained of chest discomfort. Delay in seeking care has also been identified in women. Women also often do not associate their symptoms with a heart attack because they believe it is a male disease. Women with atypical symptoms usually

Box 23.6

Myocardial Infarction Summary

Signs and Symptoms	*Classic*
	Crushing, viselike chest pain with radiation to arm, shoulder, neck, jaw, or back
	Shortness of breath
	Dizziness
	Nausea
	Sweating
	Atypical
	Absence of chest pain
	Fatigue
	Cramping in chest
	Anxiety
	Feeling of impending doom
	Falling
Symptoms More Common in Women	Epigastric or abdominal pain
	Chest discomfort, pressure, burning.
	Arm, shoulder, neck, jaw, or back pain.
	Discomfort/pain between shoulder blades
	Shortness of breath
	Fatigue
	Indigestion or gas pain
	Nausea or vomiting
Diagnostic Tests	ECG
	CBC
	Serum cardiac troponin I or T
	Serum myoglobin
	Serum CK-MB
	Serum magnesium and potassium
	Vital signs, oxygen saturation, intake and output
Therapeutic Interventions	Medications
	Oxygen
	Fab Four cardiac medications—aspirin, statin, ACEI, beta blocker
	Platelet aggregation inhibitor (Plavix)
	Morphine sulfate
	Thrombolytics
	Anticoagulants
	Antidysrhythmics
	Nitrates
	Vasodilators
	Fluid restriction
	Low-sodium diet advanced to diet as tolerated; no caffeine
	Bedrest with bedside commode/bathroom privileges
	Daily weights
	Cardiac rehabilitation
	Percutaneous coronary interventions
	Intracoronary stents
	Myocardial revascularization–CABG
Complications	Dysrhythmias
	Heart failure
	Cardiogenic shock
	Valvular insufficiency
Possible Nursing Diagnoses	Acute pain
	Anxiety
	Decreased cardiac output
	Deficient knowledge

delay treatment, and when treated have less aggressive management which leads to increased mortality.

Gerontological Implications

With age the heart has decreased elasticity and decreased ability to respond to changes in pressure. This causes increases in the resistance to its pumping action and therefore increases the workload of the myocardium to perfuse the body. Elderly patients should be taught never to neglect symptoms of shortness of breath, fatigue, fast or slow heartbeats, or chest discomfort. Some myocardial infarctions occur without the presence of pain. This is referred to as a silent MI and occurs most often in the older adult. It may also occur in those with diabetes regardless of age. When pain is not present, the only symptom may be a sudden onset of shortness of breath or fainting, restlessness, or a fall experienced by the patient. Atypical presentation of MI symptoms is normal in the elderly patient, especially in those older than age 85. Because the older adult has had more time to develop collateral circulation than younger people, they often do not have as many complications with an MI.

In the elderly, revascularization therapies such as angioplasty and bypass surgery seem to be superior in improving quality of life without increasing mortality risk. Statin therapy has also shown to reduce mortality in those over 80 years of age.

Diagnostic Tests

Patients with a strong familial history of MI should be considered at risk until an MI is ruled out. The most useful indicators of an MI are patient history, ECG, and serum cardiac troponin I or T, myoglobin, and CK-MB levels. (See Chapter 20.) Magnesium levels are also checked, especially for those on diuretic therapy. Before thrombolytic or heparin therapy, prothrombin time (PT) and partial thromboplastin time (PTT) are determined. The ECG usually shows the area that has infarcted, as well as the ischemic areas of the heart. Myocardial damage is seen as ST-segment elevation, the presence of a Q wave, or T-wave abnormalities (Fig. 23.7). Serial ECGs are done to monitor changes indicating damage or ischemia.

Therapeutic Interventions

Treatment should be sought within 5 minutes for any unrelieved chest pain. The American Heart Association recommends chewing one uncoated adult aspirin at the onset of chest pain. Delays in seeking care can limit treatment options and result in more cardiac damage (Box 23.7 Preventing Delays in Myocardial Infarction Treatment). Patients need to be educated that "time is muscle." As time passes during an MI, more muscle is lost. Patients should not drive themselves to the hospital if they are having chest pain. Emergency medical care (911 or local emergency services number) should be called.

The presence of chest pain indicates a lack of oxygen to the myocardium. Patients reporting chest pain are treated as if they have an MI until it has been proven otherwise

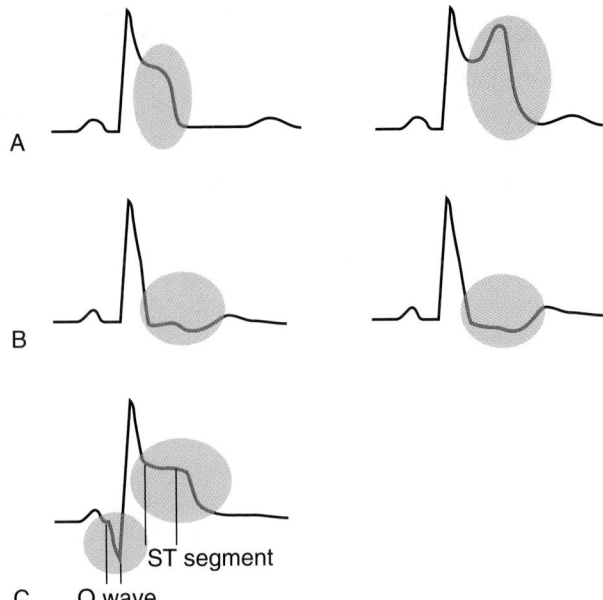

FIGURE 23.7 ECG changes during myocardial infarction. *(A)* Injury: ST-segment elevation. *(B)* Ischemia: ST-segment inversion. *(C)* Necrosis: large Q wave and ST- segment elevation.

through testing. Treatment is given to increase oxygen supply to the heart muscle.

OXYGEN. Oxygen is administered immediately, usually at 2 L per minute via nasal cannula. Oxygen therapy may be limited to the first 6 hours in stable patients. Too much oxygen may lead to systemic vasoconstriction, which may increase myocardial workload. Arterial blood gases (ABGs) are drawn to determine the patient's oxygen needs. Oxygen saturation should be monitored and kept above 94%. Oxygen can be administered via mask if higher concentrations are needed. Mechanical ventilation can be provided when indicated by ABGs.

MEDICATION. Table 23.5 summarizes pharmacological treatment of myocardial infarction. The Fab Four cardiac

---

Box 23.7

Preventing Delays in Myocardial Infarction Treatment

- Understand symptoms and "time is muscle" principle.
- Develop an action plan and rehearse it.
- Understand normal emotional responses of anxiety, denial, or embarrassment.
- Educate family to follow action plan.
- Establish protocols in workplaces for employees experiencing myocardial infarction.
- Establish emergency room policies that reduce delays, such as having equipment and medication readily available.

TABLE 23.5 PHARMACOLOGICAL TREATMENT FOR MYOCARDIAL INFARCTION

Medication Class/Action	Examples	Route	Side Effects	Nursing Implications
Antiplatelets Inhibit platelet activation, adhesion, or procoagulant activity	Aspirin	PO Chew if MI symptoms.	Increased risk of bleeding including hemorrhagic stroke	Should be given as soon as ACS or MI is suspected. Enteric coated may be given for daily dosing.
	Ticlopidine (Ticlid)	PO	May cause diarrhea and other gastrointestinal distress.	Teach patient to take drug with food. Also report any unusually bleeding or bruising.
	Clopidogrel (Plavix)	PO	May cause diarrhea and other gastrointestinal distress.	Teach patient to take drug with food. Also report any unusually bleeding or bruising.
Analgesics Opioids that bind with opioid receptors in the central nervous system	Morphine sulfate	IV push	Use cautiously in patients with COPD. May cause respiratory depression, hypotension, and bradycardia. May cause constipation.	Reduces preload and afterload. Decreases anxiety. Slows respiratory rate. Decreases myocardial oxygen demand. Monitor RR, HR, and BP prior to and after administration. Monitor vital signs for 10 minutes after IV administration.
Nitrates: **Vasodilators** Relax smooth muscle in blood vessel walls. Produce vasodilation, which relieves cardiac workload. Preload and afterload reduction. Reduce oxygen consumption of myocardium.	Nitroglycerin (Nitro-stat, Nitro Quick)	Sublingual	Hypotension Headache Contraindicated in head trauma, hypotension, uncorrected hypovolemia	Assess the AP and BP before and after administration. Document onset, type, radiation, location, and duration of chest pain. Place tablet in buccal pouch to lessen burning sensation under the tongue. Tablets should be replaced every 3 to 4 months. Check expiration date.
	Nitrolingual translingual spray	Sublingual spray	Hypotension Headache Contraindicated in head trauma, hypotension, uncorrected hypovolemia	Do not shake aerosol canister prior to administration of lingual spray.
	Isosorbide dinitrate (Isordil, Iso-Bid)	Sublingually PO	Hypotension Transient flushing of face and neck Dizziness if standing Orthostatic hypotension Nausea Vomiting Restlessness	Tolerance may occur with repeated prolonged therapy. High dose may produce severe headache. Elderly may be more sensitive to drug dosing. Instruct the patient to rise slowly from a lying position. Avoid alcohol during therapy. Alcohol intensifies the drug's hypotensive effect.
	Isosorbide mononitrate (Imdur)	PO	Hypotension Transient flushing of face and neck Dizziness if standing Orthostatic hypotension Nausea Vomiting Restlessness	Tolerance may occur with repeated prolonged therapy. High dose may produce severe headache. Elderly may be more sensitive to drug dosing. Instruct the patient to rise slowly from a lying position.

(Continued on following page)

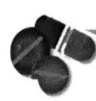

TABLE 23.5 PHARMACOLOGICAL TREATMENT FOR MYOCARDIAL INFARCTION *(Continued)*

Medication Class/Action	Examples	Route	Side Effects	Nursing Implications
	Nitroglycerin patch (Nitro-Dur, Nitrek)	Transdermal	Hypotension Transient flushing of face and neck Dizziness if standing Orthostatic hypotension Nausea Vomiting Restlessness	Caution against using one brand of drug to another. Avoid alcohol during therapy. Alcohol intensifies the drug's hypotensive effect. Remove patch before defibrillation. Rotate application sites. Apply the patch to a clean, dry, hairless area. Tolerance may develop.
Thrombolytics Dissolve blood clots in blood vessels or in catheters in the body such as dialysis catheters.	alteplase (Ativase, tissue plasminogen activator [t-PA]), anistreplase (Eminase), reteplase (Retavase), streptokinase (Streptase)	IV	Bleeding, stroke, dysrhythmias may occur when blood flow is reestablished.	Thrombolytic drugs are most effective when administered within 6 hours of coronary event. Indicated when a patient has unrelieved chest pain for 30 minutes with nitrates, and ischemia on ECG. Prior to use INR, aPTT, platelet count and fibrinogen levels should be checked. Avoid venipunctures after administration.
Anticoagulants Heparin inactivates clotting factors IX, X, XI, and XII. It inhibits the conversion of prothrombin to thrombin to prevent thrombus formation. Low doses of heparin are given to prevent DVT and pulmonary embolism.	Heparin sodium: dose regulated by activated partial thromboplastin time (aPTT). aPTT should be 1.5 to 2.5 times the control or baseline value. Normal control is 25 to 35 seconds. enoxaparin (Lovenox): aPTT is not necessary for low molecular weight heparins.	IV, SC		Contraindicated in peptic ulcer disease, blood dyscrasias, recent eye surgery. Low molecular weight heparins cannot be used unit for unit as regular heparin. They can be used to prevent embolus and may be used in out patient settings. Platelets counts should be monitored.
Beta blockers Decrease heart rate, blood pressure, cardiac output, and suppress renin activity. They decrease myocardial contractility and oxygen demand. Decrease the risk of sudden death and may reduce ventricular remodeling.	atenolol (Tenormin), metoprolol (Lopressor, Toprol XL), propranolol (Inderal)	IV or PO	Diminished sexual activity, fatigue, weakness, difficulty sleeping, bradycardia, depression, hypotension, nasal congestion, nausea.	Take the apical pulse and blood pressure immediately prior to administration. If pulse is less than 60 beats per minute, or blood pressure less than systolic 90 mm Hg, withhold the medication and notify the physician. Use cautiously in patients with diabetes. Beta blockers are contraindicated in patients with asthma, heart block, bradycardia, or pulmonary conditions with bronchoconstriction. Do not stop abruptly.

Medication Class/Action	Examples	Route	Side Effects	Nursing Implications
Angiotensin-converting enzyme inhibitors Block the production of Angiotension II, a potent vasoconstrictor. Reduce peripheral arterial resistance, pulmonary capillary wedge pressure. Improve cardiac output and exercise tolerance.	captopril (Capoten), lisinopril (Prinivil, Zestril), ramipril (Altace)	PO	Persistent cough may develop in 20% of patients. Hyperkalemia may develop in patients with diabetes mellitus or renal impairment.	Angioedema, swelling of the face and lips may occur. Agranulocytosis and neutropenia may be noted in patients with concurrent collagen vascular disease including scleroderma and systemic lupus erythematosus, and impaired renal function. Obtain baseline blood pressure before each dose. Give 1 hour before meals; food delays absorption.
Statins See Table 23.1				
Antidysrhythmics bolus or infusion Inhibit ventricular arrhythmias. Depolarization, automaticity, and excitability of the ventricle during diastole is decreased by direct action.	lidocaine (Xylocaine)	IV	High doses can produce cardiac depression. Potential exists for malignant hyperthermia. CNS toxicity may occur. Seizures, respiratory depression, and somnolence may occur.	Obtain baseline vital signs, ECG, and serum electrolytes. Elderly more sensitive to side effects. Therapeutic serum level is 1.5 to 6 μg/mL. Monitor level of consciousness. Drowsiness may signal high lidocaine blood levels.
Additional Medications as needed: **Antiemetics** **Anxiolytics** **Antacids** **Stool softeners**	Specific for drugs given	PO/IV	May be drug specific.	Controls nausea/vomiting, anxiety, gastric upset, and constipation.

drugs—antiplatelets, statins, ACEIs, and beta blockers—should be considered for use as discussed in the section on angina to improve patient outcomes.

Analgesics. Analgesics are given for relief of chest pain. Morphine sulfate is the most commonly used narcotic for several reasons. It is usually give in increments of 2 to 8 mg intravenously every 5 to 15 minutes until pain is relieved. The patients should be monitored for hypotension, respiratory depression, oversedation, and morphine sensitivity. In addition to pain relief, morphine helps decrease anxiety, opens bronchioles, and reduces preload and afterload, which can help increase blood supply and oxygen to the myocardium.

Vasodilators. NTG sublingually, topically, or by intravenous (IV) drip can be administered for vasodilation to supply more blood to the myocardium to reduce pain and the workload of the heart. In the acute phase, the IV route is usually used. Nitrates should not be given if the patient has a systolic blood pressure less than 90 mm Hg or 30 mm Hg or more below baseline, severe bradycardia less than 50 beats per minute, or if the patient has taken a phosphodiesterase inhibitor for erectile dysfunction. Catastrophic hypotension may result.

Thrombolytics. Thrombolytic therapy is used to dissolve a blood clot that is occluding a coronary artery. Many communities allow initiation of thrombolytic therapy by paramedics in the field. Studies have revealed a decreased incidence of mortality and morbidity and less extensive tissue damage when thrombolytic treatment is used. Thrombolytic therapy must be started within a specified time range from the onset of symptoms, usually within 1 to 6 hours, before necrosis results. Aim for a "door to needle" interval of under 30 minutes for patients who are candidates of thrombolytic therapy.

Glycoprotein 11b/111a inhibitors (abciximab, tirofiban) may be used as an adjunct to thrombolysis or PTCA in patients with acute myocardial infarction. These drugs work by inhibiting platelet aggregation.

ACTIVITY. Initially patients are kept on bedrest with a bedside commode for bowel movements to decrease myocardial oxygen demand. Then activity is advanced gradually as tolerated.

GLUCOSE CONTROL. Recent research indicates that maintaining blood glucose levels within a range of 70 to 100 mg/dL significantly reduces mortality for critically ill patients. Protocols to regulate blood sugar are determined by the institution. Insulin infusions may be given until the patient's blood glucose is within the targeted range.

DIET AND WEIGHT LOSS. During the acute phase of an MI, small, easily digested meals are served. Caffeine is restricted because it increases heart rate and causes vasoconstriction. Fluids may be restricted if the patient is in heart failure as well. Initially a low-sodium clear liquid diet may be ordered. Then a low-fat, low-cholesterol, and low-sodium diet may be ordered. The number of grams of sodium is prescribed by the physician. If the patient is obese, weight loss is desirable to reduce cardiac workload. A dietitian can work with the patient and family to devise a weight-loss diet for the patient.

SMOKING. Smoking should be avoided, and patients are instructed on the hazards of continuing to smoke. Referral to a tobacco cessation program can be made. The nurse needs to work with patients to help them understand and accept lifestyle changes.

VENTRICULAR ANEURYSM REPAIR. Ventricular aneurysms may occur after an MI. Indications that a ventricular aneurysm requires surgery include persistent angina, symptoms of heart failure, large aneurysms impeding the function of the heart, left ventricular failure, or tachydysrhythmias. Once the patient is on CPB, an incision is made exposing the heart and then the aneurysm is resected (cut out), leaving a fibrous border (Fig. 23.8). The ventricle is wiped clean and irrigated to ensure all thrombi are removed. The opening is then closed with sutures or patched with a graft. Air that entered the ventricle while it was open is aspirated, and the surgery continues as described in the general surgery procedure section.

Nursing Process for the
Patient Experiencing Myocardial Infarction
ASSESSMENT/DATA COLLECTION. A thorough history is obtained to identify risk factors that may contribute to a myocardial infarction. All patients admitted with chest pain are treated as having a possible MI until it has been ruled out. Continuous cardiac monitoring, serial ECGs, and laboratory values help identify life-threatening dysrhythmias and determine the degree of cardiac damage. Controlling chest pain immediately helps diminish anxiety and the negative physiological effects pain has on the body.

NURSING DIAGNOSIS, PLANNING, IMPLEMENTATION, AND EVALUATION. See Box 23.8 Nursing Care Plan for the Patient with Myocardial Infarction.

Patient Education
Teaching about the therapeutic regimen includes information about the disease, medications, diet, activity, and rehabilitation needs that may require lifestyle changes. Diet, stress reduction, a regular exercise program, cessation of smoking if necessary, and following a medication schedule require extensive patient and family teaching. This disease can affect all aspects of a patient's lifestyle. Issues about

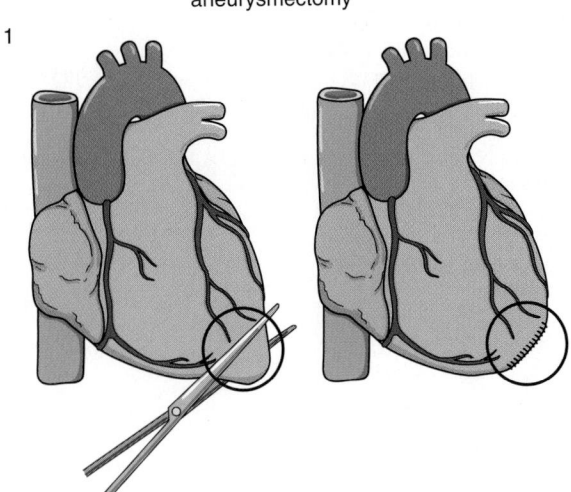

Ventricular
aneurysmectomy

1

Ventricular
aneurysmorrhaphy
Dacron patch

2

1: Aneurysm is cut and closed.
2: Patch inserted inside incision, then closed.

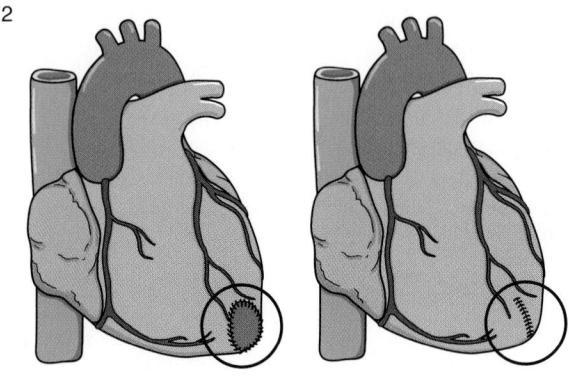

FIGURE 23.8 Ventricular aneurysm repair.

family and job roles and sexual activities need to be addressed. Patients need time to understand information that has been presented and should be encouraged to express any questions, needs, or fears.

Cardiac Rehabilitation and Exercise
Cardiac rehabilitation is begun when the patient's acute symptoms are relieved. The purpose of cardiac rehabilitation is to improve cardiac function and assist the patient to return to as normal a life as possible. Cardiac rehabilitation protocols are used in many institutions. The first two phases of rehabilitation occur in the hospital. Activities for each hospital day, such as types and amounts of self-care and activity, are specified in protocols. The third phase begins with hospital discharge and focuses on returning to prior levels of activity and function. Outpatient programs are often ordered for patients in this phase. In this phase, patients are encouraged to maintain optimum physical fitness and to continue healthy lifestyles that include exercise and losing weight to maintain an ideal body weight.

(Text continued on page 430)

Box 23.8 Nursing Care Plan for the Patient with Myocardial Infarction

Nursing Diagnosis: Acute pain related to decreased coronary blood flow causing myocardial ischemia

Expected Outcomes Patient will exhibit signs of decreased pain. Patient will exhibit signs of relaxation.

Evaluation of Outcomes Does patient state pain is reduced?

Interventions	Rationale	Evaluation
• Monitor location, duration, intensity, and radiation of pain; use a scale of 0 to 10.	Identifies type and severity of pain.	What is pain level, location, duration, intensity, and radiation?
• Monitor blood pressure, pulse, and respiration.	Vital signs may elevate with episodes of pain.	Are vital signs within normal limits?
• Obtain ECG as ordered.	Identifies location of infarction or ischemia.	Is ECG normal?
• Administer oxygen as ordered.	Helps prevent hypoxia.	Are ABGs within normal limits? Is oxygen saturation greater than 90%?
• Instruct patient to report pain at first onset.	Helps control pain quickly to prevent further ischemia.	Does patient report pain?
• Instruct patient to rest during pain.	Activity increases oxygen demand and can increase chest pain.	Does patient remain quiet and relaxed?
• Remain with patient during chest pain until it is relieved.	Provides comfort and reassurance to decrease anxiety and fear.	Are anxiety and fear decreased?
• Assist with alternative pain relief measures: related to positioning, diversional activities, relaxation techniques.	These measures help decrease painful stimuli, allowing the patient to focus on other things.	Does patient express relief and decreased stress?
• Medicate as ordered.	Helps eliminate pain.	Is pain relieved?
Geriatric		
• Monitor and ensure that older patient's pain is relieved.	Pain is not an expected part of the aging process as many believe.	Does patient report pain is relieved?

Nursing Diagnosis: Decreased cardiac output related to ischemia or infarction, changes in heart rate and rhythm, and decreased contractility

Expected Outcomes Patient will maintain adequate cardiac output and tissue perfusion. Patient will exhibit signs of improved cardiac output and tissue perfusion.

Evaluation of Outcomes Does patient have heart rate greater than 60 and less than 100, blood pressure greater than 90/60 and less than 140/90, and urine output greater than 30 mL/hr?

Interventions	Rationale	Evaluation
• Monitor blood pressure, heart rate, and urine output.	Indirect indicators of cardiac output.	Are indicators within normal limits?
• Listen to lung sounds.	Crackles indicate heart failure.	Are lungs clear?
• Monitor peripheral circulation, pulses, capillary refill, edema, color, and temperature.	Indicators of adequate tissue perfusion.	Does patient have strong peripheral pulses, capillary refill less than 3 seconds, no edema, warm skin, pink nailbeds?
• Monitor ECG.	Identifies dysrhythmias.	Is patient's ECG within normal limits?

(Continued on following page)

Box 23.8 NURSING CARE PLAN for the Patient with Myocardial Infarction (Continued)

Interventions	Rationale	Evaluation
• Administer medications as ordered by physician, such as vasodilators, beta blockers, calcium channel blockers, and cardiac glycosides.	Helps improve contractility, cardiac output, and tissue perfusion.	Does patient show signs of improved contractility, increased cardiac output, and tissue perfusion?
• Promote and provide for adequate rest, quiet environment, bedrest; place in semi-Fowler's position.	Decreases cardiac workload and stress and allows for improved breathing.	Is patient relaxed?

Geriatric

Interventions	Rationale	Evaluation
• Observe for atypical pain such as jaw pain or no pain with dyspnea or fatigue.	In acute MI older adults may have not had typical chest pain or have a silent MI.	Does patient have atypical symptoms of MI?
• Observe patient carefully for side effects of medications.	Older patients are more likely to have medication toxicity owing to reduced renal and hepatic function.	Does patient exhibit toxic side effects of medications?

Nursing Diagnosis: Fear related to threat of death, changes in lifestyle, chest pain, and procedures

Expected Outcome Patient verbalizes reduced fear. Patient demonstrates effective coping mechanisms.

Evaluation of Outcomes Does patient verbalize reduced fear?

Interventions	Rationale	Evaluation
• Assess level of fear and note non-verbal communication.	Controlling anxiety will reduce sympathetic activity that may intensify condition.	Does patient report fear or have signs of being fearful?
• Ask the patient's usual coping pattern.	This allows building on patient's strengths.	What are patient's coping techniques?
• Orient the patient and family to surroundings and equipment, oxygen, cardiac monitoring, IVs, and explain procedures.	Information may promote trust and reduce emotional stress.	Does patient state understanding of environment and equipment?
• Assure patient he/she will be closely monitored.	Assurance of detection for prompt treatment of any complications will reduce fear.	Does patient state less fear due to continuous monitoring?
• Allow patient to verbalize fear of dying.	Ventilation helps identify and reduce fear.	Is patient able to verbalize fears?
• Provide diversional materials such as newspapers, music, and television.	Diversion can be relaxing and prevent feelings of isolation.	Does patient report that use of diversional activities reduces fear?
• Offer family support.	Significant others often ignore their own needs, experience anxiety and need support, including ongoing information and explanations, being allowed to stay with the patient, and being involved in the patient's care. Nurses need to help spouses or significant others meet their own needs, so that they are better able to support the patient.	Does family verbalize ability to offer support to patient without anxiety?

Provide protective, safe environment with consistent caregivers	Older adults adapt to change with more difficulty during illness that younger adults	Is continuity of care provided? Does patient report less fear?

Nursing Diagnosis: Activity intolerance related to imbalance between oxygen supply and demand, weakness, and fatigue.

Expected Outcomes Patient tolerates progressive activity as evidenced by heart rate, blood pressure, pulse oximetry, and respiratory rate within normal limits.

Evaluation of Outcomes Is patient's heart rate, blood pressure, pulse oximetry, and respiratory rate within normal limits with progressive activity?

Interventions	Rationale	Evaluation
Obtain patient's vital signs before activity.	Identifies baseline data comparison with activity.	What are vital signs?
Observe patient during and after activity and document abnormal responses to activity which include: increased heart rate over 120 beats per minute or 20 beats over resting heart rate, increased blood pressure over 20 mm Hg systolic during activity, chest pain, dizziness, skin color changes, diaphoresis, dyspnea, dysrhythmias, excessive fatigue, and ST segment changes on ECG.	Observation allows detection of abnormal responses to stop activity.	Are vital signs within normal limits? Is activity tolerated without symptoms?
Position patient for comfort and ease in breathing.	Semi-Fowler's position is usually preferred by patients having respiratory distress. When patients are sitting upright in bed, supporting their arms on pillows reduces the workload of the heart by eliminating the force of gravity on unsupported arms.	Is patient able to breathe easily?
Maintain progression of activities as ordered by physician or cardiac rehabilitation program.	The patient should have increasing activity to condition the myocardium.	Is patient able to progress activity?
Stage One activities—ADLs, dangle at bedside for 15 minutes, use commode with assistance		
Stage Two activities—Out of bed to chair for 30 to 60 minutes, partial bath, ROM.		

Geriatric

Slow the pace of care.	Allow patient extra time to complete activity to reduce cardiac demand and fatigue.	Is patient able to complete care without symptoms or fatigue?
Refer patient to cardiac rehabilitation as able.	Older adults with CAD in exercise programs benefit comparably with younger persons in similar situations.	Does patient participate in cardiac rehab?
Encourage families to allow patient to be independent in activities.	Families may believe being sedentary is helpful to the patient.	Do families encourage patient to be as active as able?

429

CRITICAL THINKING

Mrs. Sims

■ Mrs. Sims, age 43, is admitted to the intensive care unit with a diagnosis of atypical chest pain. She has a history of midsternal chest cramping. The pain is radiating to her left and right shoulders and down her left arm. Her pain increases with activity and decreases with rest. She smokes one and a half packs of cigarettes per day and is 50 pounds overweight. The cardiac monitor shows normal sinus rhythm without dysrhythmias. She has NTG sublingual ordered prn for chest pain.

One hour after admission, Mrs. Sims reports midsternal chest pain radiating to left neck and jaw. The cardiac monitor shows sinus tachycardia with occasional premature ventricular contractions (PVCs). Her blood pressure is 100/70, respirations are 20 and unlabored, and skin is warm and dry.

1. What actions should you take?
2. What is happening to Mrs. Sims?
3. How is angina differentiated from an MI?
4. What are four indicators of an MI?
5. What medical interventions can be used for an MI?
6. What education is indicated for Mrs. Sims?

Suggested answers at end of chapter.

 PERIPHERAL VASCULAR SYSTEM

Peripheral vascular disease (PVD) may be either arterial or venous in origin. PVD is very common in people who are older or diabetic. It is important for the nurse to understand if the origin of the problem is arterial or venous to prevent serious complications from occurring.

Arterial Thrombosis and Embolism

Pathophysiology

Acute arterial occlusions are often sudden and dramatic. Occlusions are most common in the lower extremity; but may occur in the upper extremity as well. A thrombus (blood clot) adheres to the vessel wall. Acute arterial thrombi occur where there is injury to an arterial wall, sluggish flow, or plaque formation secondary to atherosclerotic changes. Other causes of arterial thrombosis are polycythemia, dehydration, and repeated arterial needle sticks. If a thrombus breaks off and travels, it becomes an **embolism** that occludes an arterial vessel that is too small to allow it to pass. Some of the causes of an arterial embolism are dysrhythmias, prosthetic heart valves, and rheumatic heart disease.

Signs and Symptoms

Usually there is an abrupt onset of symptoms with acute arterial occlusion. If a patient also has chronic arterial insufficiency, the symptoms may not occur as rapidly because collateral circulation has developed and can supply some blood to the occluded area. Symptoms depend on the artery occluded, the tissue supplied by that artery, and whether collateral circulation is present.

There are six clinical signs of acute arterial occlusion, known as the six Ps: pain, pallor, pulselessness, paresthesia (numbness), paralysis, and poikilothermia (temperature). The patient experiences pain, numbness, and decreased movement in the extremity, which is pale and without pulses distal to the occlusion. The extremity feels cold because blood normally provides warmth. If treatment is not initiated immediately, ischemia occurs and can progress to tissue necrosis and gangrene development within hours.

Therapeutic Interventions

Early treatment is necessary to protect and save the affected limb. Anticoagulant therapy is started immediately. Intravenous heparin is the treatment of choice to prevent further clotting. Heparin has no effect on existing clots. An initial IV bolus of heparin, usually 5000 IU, is given. An IV infusion is then started as ordered. The patient remains on heparin therapy for several days. Daily PTTs are monitored to maintain therapeutic heparin levels. After 3 to 7 days, warfarin (Coumadin) is added. Warfarin, an oral anticoagulant, takes 3 to 5 days to reach therapeutic levels. The heparin is continued until a therapeutic warfarin level is reached. To monitor warfarin's effects, international normalized ratios (INRs) and PTs are done daily, and adjustments in warfarin doses are made based on the results.

For patients with severe occlusions, especially if the risk of limb loss is imminent, surgery or thrombolytic agents are used to save the extremity. During an emergency embolectomy or thrombectomy, the artery is cut open, the emboli or thrombus is removed, and the vessel is sutured closed. Thrombolytic agents dissolve the thrombus or emblus.

Peripheral Arterial Disease

Peripheral arterial disease (PAD) is a disorder of the arterial circulation usually caused by chronic, progressive narrowing of arterial vessels that lead to obstruction or occlusion. PAD usually affects the lower extremities. Peripheral arterial disease is sometimes referred to as lower extremity arterial disease (LEAD). Atherosclerosis is the leading cause of occlusive disease. Peripheral arterial disease can be described as organic or functional. Organic disease is caused by structural changes from plaque or inflammation in the blood vessels. Functional disease is a short-term localized spasm in the blood vessel as noted in Raynaud's disease. It is estimated that eight to 12 million people have PAD.

Pathophysiology

The purpose of the arterial system is to delivery oxygen-rich blood to the vascular beds. Anything that impedes this flow causes an imbalance in supply and demand for oxygen. Decreased nutrition, cellular waste accumulation, and the development of ischemia occur at the area distal to the

CRITICAL THINKING

Mrs. May

■ Mrs. May is admitted with severe rheumatoid arthritis, which has left her immobile for 7 months. She is returning to her room following a whirlpool treatment when she suddenly reports severe pain in her left groin.

1. What is your first action?
2. After assessing Mrs. May, what action should be taken next?
3. What are the possible causes of these sudden symptoms?
4. How would you document Mrs. May's symptoms?
5. What would the immediate interventions be?
6. What medical interventions would you anticipate?
7. What surgical procedure may need to be done if the risk of losing the limb is imminent?

Suggested answers at end of chapter.

obstruction. With the increased debris and sluggish flow, thrombosis and embolism become major problems.

The body has several mechanisms to attempt to compensate for reduced blood flow, including peripheral vasodilation, anaerobic metabolism, and development of collateral circulation. However, these mechanisms are not intended to meet the ongoing blood supply needs of the body. It takes time for collateral circulation to develop, blood vessels eventually reach their limit of dilation, and anaerobic metabolism is only a very short-term compensatory mechanism. Eventually this lack of blood supply produces signs of ischemia, and if not corrected, ulceration, gangrene, and necrosis of the extremity occur; amputation of the limb may then become necessary.

Signs and Symptoms

Many people with PAD, especially women, have no symptoms. Symptoms often occur late in the course of PAD when diminished blood flow begins to produce changes in the extremities that symptoms occur. Pain in the calves of the lower extremities associated with activity or exercise, called **intermittent claudication,** is a common symptom of arterial occlusive disease. When blood supply to the muscles is decreased, the muscles are unable to receive adequate oxygen and ischemia develops. As ischemia increases, the muscle develops a cramping-type pain that usually subsides when the activity is stopped. As PAD progresses, the pain is present even at rest, thus indicating severe arterial occlusion.

Skin color changes are associated with decreased blood supply. The extremity is pale when the leg is elevated. If the leg is in a dependent position, it becomes reddish purple or cyanotic. The extremity is cool to touch even in warm environments. There may be hair loss on the lower calf, ankle, and foot. Other findings include dry, flaky, scaly, pale, or mottled skin. The toenails may be thickened. As occlusion

Therapeutic Interventions

Conservative treatment is initiated with mild to moderate occlusive disease. This includes patients who experience pain on activity that ceases with rest. This type of patient usually receives medication for vasodilation and diet management if necessary. Surgical intervention is used for the patient who experiences pain at rest or who has leg ulcers that do not heal. Surgical treatment includes endarterectomy to remove atherosclerotic lesions or grafting to bypass the occluded area. See vascular surgery section later in this chapter.

DIET. To help control atherosclerosis development, the diet should be low fat, low cholesterol, and low calorie if the patient is overweight. Teaching the patient to avoid red meats, fried foods, whole milk, and cheese is important. Avoiding high-cholesterol foods, such as egg yolks, organ meats, animal fats, and shellfish, helps lower lipid levels.

MEDICATIONS. Drug therapy is geared toward the symptoms and causes of the occlusive disease. The same drugs used to decrease cholesterol and lipid levels in atherosclerosis are used with occlusive disease. Vasodilators can be used, but their effectiveness is not the same for all patients. Pentoxifylline (Trental) or cilostazol (Pletal) is used for patients with occlusive disorders who experience intermittent claudication. This drug makes red blood cells more flexible to improve perfusion. The major side effect is gastrointestinal upset, so it should be taken with meals. Thrombolytic therapy is used when an occlusion is caused by a thrombus or an embolus.

INVASIVE THERAPIES. Percutaneous transluminal angioplasty (PTA) can be used to dilate a narrowed peripheral vessel. It is similar to PTCA, which was discussed earlier. Complications that can occur with this procedure are a ruptured artery as a result of the stretching caused by the balloon and clot formation. Peripheral atherectomy is

...ve plaque from
...ts can also be used
...fter stent placement,
...on inhibitors.

...e causing ischemia from expo-
...s known as **Raynaud's disease**. It
... women who live in cold climates.
... primarily affects the hands but can also
...et, ears, or nose. To be diagnosed with
...ease, the patient must experience intermittent
...ischemia for at least 2 years.

...physiology

...naud's disease is characterized by spasms of small arter-
...es in the digits. These spasms prevent arterial blood from
perfusing the fingertips and sometimes the toes. The spasms
can occur unilaterally and in one or two digits, but most
often they occur bilaterally and in all digits. Raynaud's disease may be seen with collagen diseases such as rheumatoid
arthritis, scleroderma, and systemic lupus erythematosis.

Signs and Symptoms

The hands, when exposed to cold, exhibit vascular spasms
and a marked decrease in blood flow to the tissues. The
resulting effect in the tissues is ischemic pain. After several
minutes of ischemia, hyperemia occurs. Hyperemia is
intense reddening of the hands from dilation of all the vessels of the hands. Pain becomes more intense at this time.
Patients with Raynaud's disease go through various phases
which include blanching of the skin, pain, and reddening of
the skin. This disease can progress over time; the vessels
remain constricted and the severe decrease in blood flow can
lead to fingers becoming gangrenous and necrotic.

Therapeutic Interventions

Conservative treatment is attempted first. The patient is
instructed to keep the hands warm. Gloves should be worn
when going outside, cleaning a refrigerator, or preparing
cold foods. Patients are instructed in the importance of protecting the hands from injury and avoiding things that contribute to vasoconstriction, such as smoking, alcohol, and
caffeine. Reducing stress levels can also help prevent vasoconstriction. Immersing the hands in warm water may
decrease the vasospasm. Vasodilators are sometimes prescribed to help the patient avoid peripheral vasoconstriction.
Low doses of nifedipine or long-acting nitrates can be used.

To treat Raynaud's disease surgically, the sympathetic
reflex must be blocked. This is accomplished by interrupting
the sympathetic nerve impulses from the spinal cord to the
hand, which is known as sympathectomy.

Nursing Management

Education is the primary goal for patients with Raynaud's
disease. Teaching the patient to protect the hands is very
important. Stressing the use of gloves in cold climates,
reducing vasoconstrictive activity, and decreasing stress levels helps reduce the number and severity of attacks.

Thromboangiitis Obliterans (Buerger's Disease)

Buerger's disease is a recurring inflammation of small and
medium arteries and veins of the lower extremities. The disease is usually the result of occlusion of the vessels by
thrombus formation. The cause is unknown, but heavy cigarette smoking is a major contributing factor. Some studies
indicate an autoimmune response to tobacco products as a
possible cause. The disorder is more prevalent in young men
between the ages of 25 and 40 years.

The inflammation and irritation of the vessels contribute to the development of vasospasms. These vasospasms
lead to an obstruction in blood flow. The tissues become
hypoxic, and the development of ischemic pain can occur.
Left untreated, this ischemia can lead to ulceration and
gangrene.

Intermittent claudication and other symptoms of occlusive disease are common in patients with Buerger's disease.
Other symptoms include numbness or decreased sensation
and cool extremities. Lower extremities can be red or cyanotic when in a dependent position, and pulses may be diminished. Depending on the degree of ischemia, ulceration or
gangrene may be present.

Because the primary contributing factor is smoking,
there is an urgency in helping the patient to cease smoking.
The patient must be made aware of the effect smoking has
on the body and that the disease will progress and further
damage other vessels. Therapy and nursing care for
Buerger's disease is the same as those used for other arterial
occlusive diseases. The use of calcium channel blockers
such as diltiazem (Cardizem) promotes vasodilation and
may help with intermittent claudication. Careful inspection
of the lower extremities for signs of breakdown is important,
so early treatment can begin.

Nursing Process: The Patient with Peripheral Arterial Disorders

ASSESSMENT/DATA COLLECTION. When dealing with
patients having arterial occlusive disorders, monitoring
peripheral circulation is most important. Careful assessment
of pulses, capillary refill, temperature, color, and presence of
edema helps identify patients at risk for complications.
Absent pulses are reported immediately. Skin that is shiny
and hairless points to chronic diminished blood flow to the
extremity. Laboratory blood testing is not necessary to test
for peripheral arterial disease; but a lipid panel, and serum
glucose can identify diabetes which is a significant risk
factor for PAD. The presence of any skin lesions and
ulcerations is noted.

**NURSING DIAGNOSIS, PLANNING, IMPLEMENTA-
TION, AND EVALUATION.** See Box 23.9 Nursing Care
Plan for the Patient with Peripheral Arterial Occlusive
Disorders.

Aneurysms

An **aneurysm** is a bulging, ballooning, or dilation at a weakened point of an artery. The artery diameter is often

Box 23.9 NURSING CARE PLAN for the Patient with Peripheral Arterial Occlusive Disorders

Nursing Diagnosis: Acute pain related to impaired circulation to extremities causing intermittent or continuous pain

Expected Outcomes Patient will report that pain is controlled at acceptable level.

Evaluation of Outcomes Does patient report relief from pain by nonpharmacological or pharmacological methods?

Interventions	Rationale	Evaluation
• Note peripheral circulation, pulses, color, temperature, presence of edema, and skin breakdown.	Determines the degree of tissue perfusion and complications.	Does patient have pulses, warm skin, capillary refill less than 3 seconds, no evidence of skin breakdown?
• Monitor for intermittent claudication or pain at rest.	Helps determine degree of occlusive disease. Pain at rest is an indicator that the arterial occlusion is becoming worse.	Does patient have pain during activity or at rest?
• Administer medication as ordered:		Does patient show signs of increased circulation and relief of pain following administration of medications?
• Analgesics	Relieves chronic or acute pain.	
• Vasodilators	Increases blood flow to extremities.	
• Calcium channel blockers	Decrease vasospastic episodes.	
• Encourage rest if pain is present.	Rest decreases muscle contraction and prevents further ischemia in extremities.	Is patient able to rest?
• Position lower extremities below heart level.	Increases arterial flow to lower extremities.	Are pulses strong, capillary refill less than 3 seconds, extremities pink and warm?
• Protect extremities from cold or trauma.	Extremities with decreased circulation have decreased sensation, which increases risk of injury.	Are extremities injury free?
• Teach the patient importance and use of relaxation techniques.	Relaxation will decrease the stress response and vasoconstriction related to catecholamine release.	Does patient demonstrate use of relaxation techniques?

Nursing Diagnosis: Ineffective tissue perfusion related to interruption of arterial flow in arms and legs

Expected Outcomes Patient will exhibit signs of increased arterial blood flow and tissue perfusion.

Evaluation of Outcomes Does patient have strong peripheral pulses, capillary refill less than 3 seconds, warm skin, absence of edema?

Interventions	Rationale	Evaluation
• Check peripheral pulses, capillary refill, color, temperature, and presence of edema every 4 hours.	Indication of adequate tissue perfusion.	Are peripheral pulses strong, nailbeds pink, capillary refill less than 3 seconds with no edema noted?
• Report absent or diminished pulses immediately.	Indication of inadequate tissue perfusion requiring immediate treatment.	Are peripheral pulses present and strong?

(Continued on following page)

Interventions

- Check skin for intactness, healed areas, signs of ulceration or infection.
- Place extremities lower than heart, feet on floor in sitting position, head of bed elevated on blocks.
- Avoid bending knees, pillows under knees, prolonged sitting, or crossing legs.
- Inspect lower extremities frequently. Clean feet with mild soap; dry carefully. Protect from injury.
- Encourage use of well fitting shoes.
- Refer to progressive activity program.
- Keep extremity warm using socks and blankets.

Rationale

Chronic arterial occlusion leads to decreased blood flow, resulting in tissue damage and poor wound healing.

Dependent position increases blood flow to the legs and feet.

These activities impede blood flow to extremities.

Cleaning prevents trauma to feet, protecting feet from things that can lead to ulcerations.

Prevents irritation and tissue breakdown leading to ulcer.

Gradual progressive exercise promotes collateral circulation.

Prevents vasoconstriction and promotes comfort.

Evaluation

Is skin intact?

Does patient have adequate tissue perfusion signs?

Does patient exhibit understanding of improving blood flow?

Is patient free from trauma or breaks in skin of the lower extremities?

Does patient verbalize shoes fit well?

Does patient participate in exercise program?

Are extremities warm?

Nursing Diagnosis: Activity intolerance related to activity pain and diminished blood flow

Expected Outcomes Patient will report that pain is relieved during desired activities.

Evaluation of Outcomes Does patient participate in activities without pain?

Interventions

- Begin walking program:
  Start on flat surface.
  Walk 30 minutes per day.
- Walk every day increasing the distance in small increments until experiencing claudication. Walk one half city block after pain begins per physician order. Stop and rest until pain subsides.

Rationale

Promotes collateral circulation without greatly increasing oxygen demand.

Walking through the pain will promote collateral circulation. Pain should subside with rest.

Evaluation

Does patient participate in walking program?

Does patient increase distance with claudication?

Does pain stop with rest?

Nursing Diagnosis: Deficient knowledge: peripheral arterial disease related to complications, medications, or postoperative care.

Expected Outcomes Patient and family will verbalize self care measures to control disease and prevent complications.

Evaluation of Outcomes Does patient and family verbalize understanding of teaching?

Interventions

- Ask patient's and family's knowledge of the physiology of the disease, and treatment and preventive techniques.

Rationale

This will determine educational topics.

Evaluation

What is patient's and family's baseline knowledge of PAD?

Interventions	Rationale	Evaluation
• Describe peripheral arterial disease, symptoms, diagnosis, treatment, complications to patient and his family.	The patient should understand PAD to help control disorder.	Does patient and family verbalize understanding of PAD?
• Teach healthy lifestyle and risk factor control: Smoking cessation, low fat diet, walking programs, hyperlipidemia, diabetes and hypertension control.	Healthy lifestyle promotes circulation and decreases functional impairment and pain.	Is patient willing and able to incorporated healthy lifestyle into daily routine?
Explain daily foot care: • Inspect feet for ingrown toenails, redness, sores, or blisters, wash feet with warm soap and water, dry with gentle patting, lubricate skin to prevent cracking, wear clean socks.	Daily foot care and reporting problems promptly can help prevent complications of PAD.	Does patient state will perform daily foot care and verbalize understanding?
Do not walk barefoot and inspect inside of footwear for foreign objects before inserting foot.	Ulceration of the toes may follow trauma if foreign object is walked on, which can result in infection.	Does patient verbalize understanding of need to protect feet?
Explain prescribed drug treatment protocols.	Medication explanation can help patient comply with therapy.	Does patient verbalize understanding of medications?

increased by 50 percent. The cause is unknown, but anything that weakens the artery wall or causes loss of elasticity in the artery can cause an aneurysm. Atherosclerosis, hypertension, smoking, trauma, and congenital abnormalities are risk factors for an aneurysm. Heredity may also play a role. Aneurysms can occur in any artery in the body but are common in the abdominal aorta, which is the focus of the rest of this discussion.

An abdominal aortic aneurysm (AAA) is often silent if it is less than 4 cm. Most people do not even know that they have an AAA. Men older than age 50 are at the highest risk of death from an AAA. The incidence of AAA increases with age. Survival improves with elective surgery rather than emergency surgery after the aneurysm ruptures.

Types

There are different types of aneurysms (Fig. 23.9). A fusiform aneurysm is the dilation of the entire circumference of the artery. A saccular aneurysm is a bulging on only one side of the artery wall. A dissecting aneurysm occurs when a cavity is formed from a tear in the artery wall, usually the intimal (inner) layer. The layers of the artery are then separated as blood is pumped into the tear with each heartbeat, expanding the cavity, which is then prone to rupturing.

Signs and Symptoms

Usually there are few if any symptoms (Box 23.10 Aneurysm Summary). As the AAA grows, symptoms may develop. Back or flank pain is the classic symptom; the pain is caused by the aneurysm pressing against nerves of the vertebrae. Depending on the location and size of the

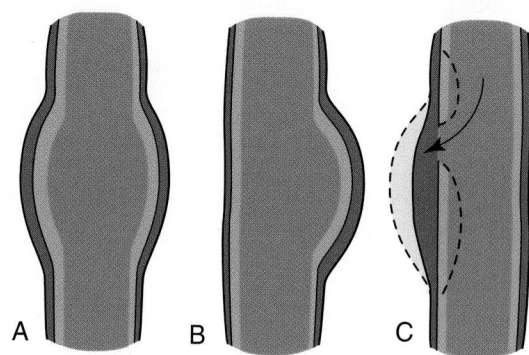

FIGURE 23.9 Types of aneurysms. (A) *Fusiform.* The entire circumference of the artery is dilated. (B) *Saccular.* One side of artiery is dilated. (C) *Dissecting.* A tear in the inner layer causes a cavity to form between the layers of the artery and fill with blood. The cavity expands with each heartbeat.

aneurysm, there may be complaints of abdominal pain, a feeling of fullness, or nausea caused by pressure on the intestines. The pain may mimic pain associated with any abdominal or back disorder. Changing positions may temporarily relieve the symptoms. Because the symptoms are vague, they are often not associated with an AAA. There may be a pulsating mass in the abdomen caused by an AAA that is discovered only during routine physical or x-ray examination.

Severe, sudden back, flank, or abdominal pain and a pulsating abdominal mass can indicate that the aneurysm may be about to rupture. With rupture, the patient's blood pressure may drop and signs of shock may be present.

Box 23.10

Aneurysm Summary

Signs and Symptoms	Back pain
	Flank pain
	Abdominal fullness
	Nausea
	Pulsating mass in abdomen
	Severe sudden back pain with rupture
	Shock from blood loss
Diagnostic Tests	Ultrasound
	Chest x-ray
	MRI
	CT scan
	Aortography
Therapeutic Interventions	Observe for growth of aneurysm
	Maintain blood pressure
	Surgical repair and graft
Complications	Rupture
	Shock
	Hemorrhage
Possible Nursing Diagnoses	Acute pain
	Risk for deficient fluid volume
	Risk for ineffective tissue perfusion

Immediate surgery is needed for a ruptured AAA. The mortality rate is high with a ruptured aneurysm.

Diagnostic Tests

Computed tomography (CT) and abdominal ultrasound are the most common diagnostic tools used to confirm the presence of an aneurysm. Small aneurysms may be watched over time to see if they enlarge. Aortography can be performed when surgical intervention is considered to identify the size and exact location of the aneurysm.

Therapeutic Interventions

Medical treatment consists of medication to maintain lower blood pressures because patients with aneurysms often have hypertension. If the blood pressure is allowed to get too high, it can cause the arterial wall to rupture. Surgical treatment—a bypass graft—is performed when the patient is experiencing pain or showing signs of circulatory compromise. An aneurysm that is larger than 5 cm requires surgery. The risk of rupture is greatest when the aneurysm reaches 5 cm or greater.

A conventional open surgical repair or newer endovascular grafting may be done for an AAA. Endovascular grafting involves the transluminal placement (through the femoral artery) and attachment of a sutureless aortic endograft or stent-graft prosthesis at the site of the AAA. In the endograft procedure, a balloon catheter positions and opens the graft. The graft remains attached to the inner wall of the aorta when the catheter is withdrawn. Blood flow continues through the aorta, bypassing the aneurysm. Another method uses a stent-graft that opens to fit the diameter of the aorta to reduce pressure on the aneurysm. Endovascular surgery requires less hospitalization time and a quicker recovery.

Nursing Process

ASSESSMENT/DATA COLLECTION. Careful monitoring of a patient with an AAA is necessary. Understanding must be assessed so patients know their medications and the importance of taking antihypertensives as prescribed. Stress may be a risk factor that should be addressed. Lifting heavy objects can increase pressure within the artery and may be restricted even in the individual being treated with more conservative measures. Postoperatively, the patient should avoid lifting heavy objects (see Home Health Hints).

NURSING DIAGNOSIS, PLANNING, IMPLEMENTATION, AND EVALUATION. See Box 23.11 Nursing Care Plan for the Patient After Vascular Surgery (page 439).

Varicose Veins

Varicose veins are elongated, tortuous, dilated veins. The exact cause is unknown. The condition tends to be familial. Varicose veins are divided into primary and secondary varicosities.

Pathophysiology

Primary varicosities are believed to be caused by a structural defect in the vessel wall. Along with the defect, the dilation of the vessel can lead to incompetent venous valves. The valves help prevent blood from refluxing. If reflux occurs, it can cause further dilation of the vessel. The superficial veins are the vessels most often involved in primary varicosities.

Secondary varicosities are caused by an acquired or congenital pathological condition of the deep venous system. This produces dilation of collateral and superficial veins. As a result, there is an interference of blood return to the heart, which leads to stasis, or pooling, of the blood in the deep venous system. This increases the pressure within the system, pushing blood into the collateral vessels and producing varicosities in the superficial veins.

Causes

A number of factors can lead to varicose veins. The wall defects have been identified as a familial tendency and may be inherited. Any factor that may contribute to increasing hydrostatic pressure within the leg, such as prolonged standing, pregnancy, and obesity, may promote venous dilation. Incompetent valves within the veins can cause blockage of blood flow and lead to dilated veins.

Signs and Symptoms

The most common manifestation is the disfigurement of the lower extremity with primary varicosities. There may be dull pain, especially after prolonged standing. This usually can be relieved by walking or elevating the extremity. With secondary varicosities, the pain and disfigurement may be more severe. There can be development of edema or ulceration if circulation is severely compromised.

Therapeutic Interventions

The primary goals are to improve circulation, relieve pain, and avoid complications. Treatment is usually not indicated if the problem is only cosmetic. Conservative treatment is geared to reduction of factors that contribute to varicose veins. Elastic compression stockings should be used as ordered. Injection sclerotherapy or lasers treat superficial varicosities. Surgical intervention is radiofrequency ablation stripping the vein to remove incompetent valves. Surgery is performed when venous insufficiency cannot be controlled or prevented with conservative treatment.

Venous Insufficiency

Venous insufficiency is a chronic condition. Damaged or aging valves within the veins interfere with blood return to the heart, causing pooling of blood in the lower extremities. Chronic venous insufficiency can lead to venous stasis ulcers.

Venous Stasis Ulcers

PATHOPHYSIOLOGY. Venous stasis ulcers are the end result of chronic venous insufficiency. Dysfunctional valves in the venous system prevent or reduce venous blood return. As venous pressure increases, venous stasis occurs. Over time the congestion and decreased venous circulation lead to changes in the lower extremities. There may be edema and a brownish discoloration of the leg and foot, with the surrounding skin hardened and leathery in appearance. The brown color occurs when veins rupture, releasing red blood cells into the tissues; the red blood cells then break down and stain the tissue brown.

Stasis ulcers develop from the increased pressure and rupture of small veins. Signs of skin breakdown are most commonly seen at the medial malleolus of the ankle. Stasis ulcers are a serious complication of venous insufficiency that are difficult to cure and can affect the patient's quality of life.

THERAPEUTIC INTERVENTIONS. The focus of treatment is to decrease edema and heal skin ulcerations. Compression wraps such as elastic stockings or bandage wraps are necessary to decrease edema. Elastic wraps should be started at the foot, with greater tension applied there, and wrapped up the leg. Rewrapping the elastic bandage twice a day is necessary. It is important to ensure that the wraps are not too tight at the top, which prevents return of blood to the heart.

Bedrest and elevation of legs and feet above the heart are important to assist with drainage of lower extremities. Patients are advised not to keep legs dependent and to avoid long periods of standing or sitting to prevent increased pressure and pain. The foot of the bed should be elevated 5 to 6 inches. Additionally, patients should be encouraged to exercise and walk often during nonacute episodes. Patients should be taught not to cross their legs or wear constrictive clothing that would decrease venous blood return to the heart.

Skin ulcers are usually cultured and treated with topical antibiotics if needed. Wound care can be chronic and challenging. (See Chapter 54.) An Unna boot, which is a gauze dressing coated with zinc oxide, calamine, and glycerin, may be used to promote healing in severe ulcers. Zinc promotes wound healing and can be soothing. The Unna boot is applied snugly and provides compression therapy as well. It is changed every 2 to 7 days. Skin grafting may be necessary if ulcerations are severe or do not heal.

NURSING PROCESS: THE PATIENT WITH A VENOUS DISORDER. Assessment/Data Collection. Risk factors for varicose veins are identified. Symptoms and concerns about body image are noted. Leg appearance, presence of edema, and ulcerations are noted. Patient-coping skills are assessed to determine patient's ability to cope with chronic ulcers that may affect quality of life. Baseline knowledge of contributing factors for venous disorders is determined for teaching plans.

Nursing Diagnosis, Planning, and Implementation. Acute pain related to edema and increased pressure

EXPECTED OUTCOME: *The patient reports pain is at a tolerable level.*

- Use rating scale such as 0 to 10 to identify pain level *to provide consistency in pain reporting.*
- Elevate legs above heart level (such as in a reclining chair) and avoid long periods of standing *to reduce pooling of fluid.*
- Apply compression therapy as ordered *to promote drainage and reduce edema.*
- Administer analgesics as prescribed *to provide pain relief.*

Impaired tissue integrity related to chronic venous congestion

EXPECTED OUTCOME: *The patient has intact tissue integrity.*

- Assess and document size, shape, and depth of wound *to evaluate healing of wound over time.*
- Provide a comprehensive plan for wound care including methods of pressure relief from edema, treatments, and nutrition as ordered *to ensure that quality wound care is provided.*
- Provide wound care as ordered.

Ineffective health maintenance related to deficient knowledge of venous disease

EXPECTED OUTCOME: *The patient will report understanding and management of his or her venous disorder.*

- Assess the patient's present understanding of the disease *to determine baseline knowledge.*
- Explain to patient how to control risk factors and prevention of varicose veins: weight reduction, elevation of the extremities, walking, and exercise *help increase muscle strength and contraction.*
- Explain tight-fitting clothes at tops of legs or waist should not be worn *to prevent venous occlusion.*

- Encourage to wear support hose with varicose veins *to assist blood flow return to the heart.*
- Explain need to avoid heating devices *because of decreased sensitivity and risk of burns.*
- Encourage questions and allow the patient the opportunity to verbalize new information and skills *to enhance learning.*
- Document teaching and evaluation of patient knowledge.

See also Box 23.11 Nursing Care Plan for the Patient After Vascular Surgery.

Evaluation. Interventions are successful if the patient reports understanding of venous disease and prevention. Interventions are successful if the patient reports pain is at acceptable level.

Vascular Surgery

Vascular impairments requiring surgery may be acute or chronic and involve arteries, veins, or lymphatic vessels. When intermittent claudication becomes severe or disabling or when the limb is at risk for amputation, then surgical vascular grafting may be done.

Nursing Process: Preoperative Vascular Surgery

ASSESSMENT/DATA COLLECTION. A baseline assessment is important for postoperative comparison and discharge planning. Pain control needs and circulatory status are assessed. Diagnostic test (CBC, electrolytes, PT, PTT, and bleeding time) results are reviewed and typing and crossmatching of blood to be placed on hold is performed.

NURSING DIAGNOSES. The nursing diagnoses for preoperative vascular surgery may include:

- Acute or chronic pain related to ischemia of tissue distal to occlusion or aneurysm
- Anxiety related to unknown outcome, pain, powerlessness, or threat of death
- Deficient knowledge: preoperative and postoperative procedures related to unfamiliar process.

See Chapter 11 for further preoperative nursing process information.

Embolectomy and Thrombectomy

When an artery becomes completely occluded by an embolus or thrombus, it is considered a surgical emergency. Emergency embolectomy is the procedure of choice only if the affected extremity is viable.

Surgical removal to restore blood flow and oxygenation to the tissue distal to the occlusion is imperative to decrease ischemia and necrosis. Fogarty catheters (long narrow catheters with an inflatable balloon tip) are used to remove the thrombus or embolus. A small incision is made in the blood vessel near the occlusion, and the catheter tip is inserted past the occlusion. The balloon is inflated, and the catheter with the occlusive material is drawn back through the incision. The blood vessel and wound are sutured as circulation is assessed.

Vascular Bypasses and Grafts

Vascular bypass surgery involves the use of either autografts, such as the patient's own saphenous vein, or a synthetic graft material. The graft is anastomosed to the artery proximal to the occlusion and tunneled past the occlusion, where the distal end of the graft is anastomosed to the artery (Fig. 23.10). The graft is assessed for hemostasis and function, and then the wound is sutured closed.

Repair of a diseased area of a blood vessel, such as an aortic abdominal aneurysm, is performed with resection of the diseased area and replacement with a graft (aortic aneurysmectomy). This is usually an elective procedure. However, if an aneurysm is dissecting or ruptures, it is a surgical emergency.

Newer techniques are being used for bypass surgery. One technique uses video-assisted aortofemoral bypass without laparotomy. This method reduces length of hospital stay and patient recovery times.

Endarterectomy

Arteriosclerotic plaques are dissected from the lining of the arterial wall and removed in a procedure called an **endarterectomy**. This is most commonly performed on the carotid artery but may be done on peripheral arterial vessels as well. To control blood flow, the artery is clamped on both sides of the occlusion, and an incision is made into the artery. The plaque within the artery is removed with forceps. The artery is irrigated to remove any further debris and then closed with sutures. The clamps are removed, and the skin

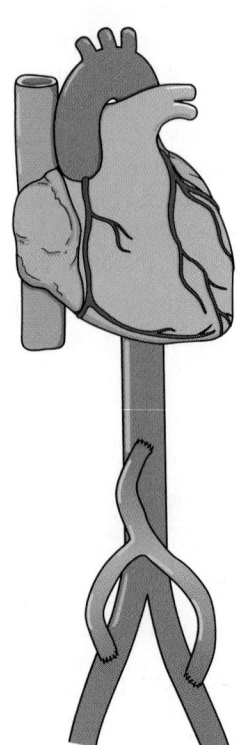

FIGURE 23.10 Aortic-femoral bypass.

---

endarterectomy: end—inside + arter—artery + ectomy—excision

Box 23.11   NURSING CARE PLAN for the Patient After Vascular Surgery

Nursing Diagnosis: Acute pain related to surgical incision and reperfusion of tissue

Expected Outcomes Patient will state that the pain is relieved or is tolerable. Patient will rest comfortably, perform respiratory treatments as necessary, and perform activities of daily living (ADLs).

Evaluation of Outcomes Does patient state pain is relieved or acceptable? Is patient able to rest and participate in respiratory treatments and ADLs?

Interventions	Rationale	Evaluation
• Ask severity of pain, as well as all other qualities.	Peripheral vascular surgery pain is usually mild, and severe pain may indicate reocclusion. Major vascular surgery pain is severe.	Does patient state pain is at a tolerable level with a patent vessel?
• Ask patient to rate pain after analgesic is given.	Pain relief is individualized.	Does patient state pain is controlled at a tolerable level?
• Notify physician if pain is unrelieved.	Different analgesic may be needed to give relief.	Are patient's pain relief needs met?

Geriatric

Interventions	Rationale	Evaluation
• Ensure that older patient's pain is relieved.	Pain is not a normal part of aging, and elderly patients need and are entitled to adequate pain relief.	Does patient rate pain as none or at a tolerable level using a scale of 0 to 10?
• Use opioid pain medications cautiously. Consider reducing frail older patient's first opioid dose by 25%–50%, and increase as safe and needed and as ordered.	Older patients are more susceptible to peak effects and duration of analgesia of opioids.	Are patient's vital signs and sedation levels within normal limits (WNL)?

Nursing Diagnosis: Ineffective tissue perfusion related to hypotension, hypothermia, emboli, vascular spasm, or reocclusion

Expected Outcomes Patient will have palpable peripheral pulses: adequate capillary refill; and normal color, temperature, motor, and sensory function of extremities. Patient will have reactive pupils and baseline cognitive function.

Evaluation of Outcomes Is patient's circulatory status WNL? Does patient have reactive pupils and baseline cognitive function intact?

Interventions	Rationale	Evaluation
• Monitor circulation, movement, and sensation to extremities every 1 to 4 hours.	Early detection of spasm or reocclusion minimizes risk of ischemia and necrosis.	Does graft or vessel remain patent?
• Mark location of pulses on affected extremity.	Allows for quick location of pulses.	Are pulses located easily?
• Perform neurological checks every 2 to 4 hours (carotid).	Allows early detection of complications.	Are major neurological or circulatory problems detected?
• Perform circulation or neurological check between nurses when changing caregiver.	Subtle changes can be detected and new caregiver has baseline for comparison.	Is baseline assessment done?
• Measure abdominal girth every shift (abdominal aortic surgery).	Increasing girths may indicate bleeding into abdomen.	Does abdominal girth remain unchanged?

(Continued on following page)

439

Box 23.11   NURSING CARE PLAN for the Patient After Vascular Surgery (Continued)

Interventions	Rationale	Evaluation
• Take temperature every 4 hours.	May indicate infection or hypothermia with need for further warming.	Does patient remain normothermic?
• Monitor CBC as ordered.	RBC count, hemoglobin, and hematocrit decrease with insidious bleeding into abdomen or significant hematoma formations.	Is CBC WNL?
• Avoid constricting measures on affected extremity: knee gatch of bed, adhesive tape, tight dressings.	Prevent further decrease in blood flow to compromised extremity.	Is blood flow to affected extremity maintained?
• Auscultate AV shunts and grafts for bruits and palpate for thrills.	Any decrease or cessation of bruit or thrill indicates occlusion.	Does AV shunt or fistula remain patent?

incision is closed. A drain may be placed to help prevent hematoma formation.

Angioplasty

Minimally invasive techniques can also be used to open plaque-blocked arteries. These techniques include balloon or laser angioplasty. A flexible laser-tipped catheter is inserted into an artery and advanced to the site of the blockage. The laser sends out pulsating beams of light, which vaporize the plaque. This procedure is used for patients with smaller occlusions in the distal superficial femoral, proximal popliteal, and common iliac arteries.

Stents

Stents are placed inside an artery to provide support to the artery walls and keep them open. Stents are placed in a procedure similar to percutaneous transluminal coronary angioplasty (PTCA) discussed earlier. Stents may also be used in combination with other procedures such as angioplasty.

Complications of Vascular Surgery

Bleeding and hemorrhage can occur with all vascular surgeries. Drainage can be expected with most surgeries. Drainage is usually small when peripheral vessels are involved. But with involvement of the great vessels, drainage is usually heavier and drains are often placed to prevent swelling and hematoma formation. If hemorrhage occurs, manual pressure is applied to the site of bleeding and the physician notified immediately.

Reocclusion is possible with any vascular surgery. If thrombi or emboli develop and block blood flow, it is a surgical emergency. Extensive surgeries may also result in significant blood loss, leading to fluid volume deficit or shock.

Postoperative Therapeutic Intervention

Frequent assessments are ordered postoperatively. Neurovascular checks of extremities every 1 to 4 hours are usually ordered. The incisional area is monitored for hematoma formation. Abdominal girth measurements (for aortic aneurysm repair) are ordered. An increase in abdominal girth may indicate hemorrhage. Any abnormal change is reported immediately to the physician. A loss of a pulse can indicate that circulation has been impaired in the vessel. The patient's need to return to surgery is anticipated if signs of impaired circulation are found.

CBC, INR, PT, PTT, and electrolytes may be ordered daily. Intake and output monitoring may be initially ordered hourly, then every 4 to 8 hours. Imbalances in fluid status should be reported. IV crystalloid solutions, volume expanders, or blood may be ordered for fluid deficits.

Nursing Process: The Patient After Vascular Surgery

ASSESSMENT/DATA COLLECTION. On transfer postoperatively to either the ICU or surgical unit, the patient is positioned comfortably and a head-to-toe assessment is performed and documented. Abnormal findings are reported to the physician. Once a patent airway is ensured, vital signs are monitored according to institutional policy or more frequently if they are unstable. The patient's pain level is rated on a scale of 0 to 10. All IVs and drains are monitored. Measurement of intake and output is usually done hourly. Laboratory tests are also monitored.

Initially, neurovascular checks are performed hourly for aortic or extremity vascular surgery. Neurovascular checks include extremity movement and sensation, presence of numbness or tingling, pulses, temperature, color, and capillary refill (less than 3 seconds normally). Peripheral pulses are palpated, or assessed with Doppler ultrasound if not palpable, marked, and compared with the unaffected extremity to detect deficits. If a pulse is absent or weak or the extremity is cool or dusky, the physician is notified immediately. A return to surgery for an embolectomy or other procedure is anticipated.

NURSING DIAGNOSIS, PLANNING, IMPLEMENTATION, AND EVALUATION. See Box 23.11 Nursing Care Plan for the Patient After Vascular Surgery.

NURSING CARE TIP

Neurovascular checks refer to the assessment of an extremity. (Neurological checks refer to assessment of the central nervous system.) The following are areas to examine on an extremity when doing neurovascular checks. They are identified under the category for which they provide information:

Neurological	Vascular
Movement	Pulses
Sensation	Capillary refill
Numbness	Color (nailbed or skin)
Tingling	Temperature

CRITICAL THINKING

Mr. Jangles

■ You are caring for Mr. Jangles, age 63, who has just returned from surgery after an embolectomy of the right lower leg. He has a history of insulin-dependent diabetes mellitus, hypertension, renal insufficiency, and a myocardial infarction 2 weeks ago. He is 6 feet tall and weighs 316 pounds.

1. What are four priority assessment areas for you to perform for Mr. Jangles?
2. What other information might you want to know regarding Mr. Jangles's medical history?
3. List three priority nursing diagnoses for Mr. Jangles.
4. State one outcome for each nursing diagnosis.
5. What are nursing interventions for each nursing diagnosis that you will perform?

Suggested answers at end of chapter.

 LYMPHATIC SYSTEM

The lymphatic system returns fluid from other tissues in the body to the bloodstream. It is a pumpless system with one-way valves that return the fluid to the heart. Any interruption in the flow of lymph results in edema.

Lymphangitis

Lymphangitis is a bacterial infection of the lymphatic channels. The infection can occur in the arms or legs and is commonly caused by *Staphylococcus* or *Streptococcus* bacteria. It is a serious infection that can cause sepsis and be fatal.

Signs and Symptoms

Symptoms include painful red streaks in the extremity. Fever and chills may be present. Lymph nodes in the area of infection can be enlarged and painful.

Therapeutic Interventions

Therapy is initiated with a broad-spectrum antibiotic as the drug of choice. The use of heat on the extremity, as well as elevating it, can help improve circulation. Physicians may order the use of pneumatic pressure devices to help alleviate congestion.

Nursing Process: Lymphangitis

ASSESSMENT/DATA COLLECTION. Frequent monitoring of the affected area for edema and skin breakdown is needed to prevent complications from edema. The nurse monitors the size of the extremity and notifies the physician of any increase in size or possible spread of infection. Pain level and fever are monitored.

Nursing Diagnosis, Planning, and Implementation

Acute pain related to tissue damage and edema from infection

EXPECTED OUTCOME: The patient reports an absence or acceptable level of pain.

- Explain and have patient use pain rating *to report pain level for consistency.*
- Administer analgesics as prescribed *to provide pain relief.*
- Re-check pain level 30 to 60 minutes after analgesic given.
- Position extremity for comfort and elevate *to reduce edema, which can cause pressure and pain.*

Risk for excess fluid volume related to congested lymph nodes from infection

EXPECTED OUTCOME: The patient has no evidence of edema.

- Apply heat on the extremity as ordered *to increase circulation and reduce edema.*
- Elevate extremity *to help improve circulation and prevent edema.*

EVALUATION. Interventions are successful if the patient reports pain is at acceptable level and no edema is present.

Home Health Hints

Cardiac

- Both patients and caregivers can experience stress and frustration related to cardiovascular disease. Patients who have undergone open heart surgery may experience feelings of powerlessness, depression, and anger. The home health nurse can be instrumental in helping the family deal with these life changing illnesses. Appropriate interventions include:
  - Have a home health social worker visit a postsurgical cardiac patient. This can be useful to help the patient and family plan for lifestyle changes to reduce anxiety and environmental stress.
  - The ability of the patient caregiver to provide necessary care should be assessed. The support and resources available to the caregiver should be explored to prevent caregiver role strain.
  - The need for caregiver respite care should be assessed, especially over time. If respite care is needed, assist the caregiver in identifying respite care resources in the family or community.
  - Assist the caregiver to identify a plan to distribute the care workload among family members, if possible.
  - Teach the caregiver stress management techniques to use. This can include deep breathing exercises, reading a book, meditation, massage therapy, guided imagery, exercise, socializing with friends, and/or working on a favorite hobby.

- After open heart surgery, many patients suffer from depression. If your patient appears withdrawn, offers limited eye contact during interaction, and seems uninterested with following through on postoperative instructions, discuss with the patient how they feel they have changed since having surgery. Report concerns to the patient's physicians; antidepressants might be helpful during this time. Also identify community resources that are available such as a support group and offer that information to your patient.
- Chest pain from esophageal reflux can mimic cardiovascular symptoms. The home health nurse should ask if the pain is related to consuming large meals, lying down, or bending over, or if it is relieved with antacids or food. Inform the physician of these findings.

Vascular

- Instruct the patient that if pain develops in the lower extremities during exercise to stop and rest.
- It is important to monitor peripheral pulses and capillary refill to ensure adequate tissue perfusion. Report absence pulses or sluggish capillary refill to the patient's physician.
- Patients with peripheral vascular disorders are at a high risk for developing lower extremity wounds that are often slow to heal. Instruct the patient to report changes in skin color, insect bites, and/or rashes to his or her physician.

References

1. Ascherio, A, Katan, MB, and Stampfer, MJ: Trans fatty acids and coronary heart disease N Eng J Med 340:1994, 1999.
2. 2006 heart and stroke statistical update. Dallas, American Heart Association, 2005.
3. Lee, MH, LW, K, and Patel, SB: Genetic basis of sitosterolemia, Curr Opin Lipidol 12:141, 2001.
4. Mukherjee, D, Fang, J, Chetcuti, S, et al. Impact of Combination Evidence-Based Medical Therapy on Mortality in Patients With Acute Coronary Syndromes. Circulation 109:745-749, 2004.

REVIEW QUESTIONS

1. Which of the following is a risk factor that can be controlled to prevent the development of cardiovascular disease?
   a. Family history of cardiovascular disease
   b. Hypertension
   c. Ethnicity
   d. Family history of diabetes mellitus

2. Which of these assessment findings is an atypical symptom of a myocardial infarction when chest pain is not present?
   a. Fatigue
   b. Dizziness
   c. Sweating
   d. Nausea

3. Which of the following is the purpose of CABG surgery?
   a. Cure coronary artery disease
   b. Increase blood flow to the myocardium
   c. Prevent spasms of the coronary arteries
   d. Decrease blood flow to the coronary arteries

4. Which of the following is a classic symptom of peripheral arterial occlusive disease?
   a. Angina
   b. Edema

c. Intermittent claudication

d. Stasis ulcers

5. The nurse is caring for a patient who has peripheral arterial disease. Which of the following statements by the patient indicates understanding of how to manage the pain of peripheral arterial disease?
   a. "I will lie down frequently."
   b. "I will use a reclining chair."
   c. "I will sit with my legs down."
   d. "I will do knee flexion exercises."

6. A patient who had a myocardial infarction is to receive aspirin, 5 grains PO, now. How many milligrams of aspirin will the nurse give?
   _____mg

SUGGESTED ANSWERS TO

CRITICAL THINKING

■ *Mrs. Sims*

1. Place on bedrest, administer oxygen via nasal cannula at 2 L per minute, assess blood pressure and pulse, administer nitroglycerin sublingual as ordered, obtain ECG, and notify physician.
2. She may be having an anginal attack versus acute MI.
3. Nitroglycerin usually stops chest pain associated with angina. Rest may also alleviate chest pain. Neither nitroglycerin nor rest will relieve the pain of an acute MI.
4. Indicators of an MI include patient history, ECG changes with ST segment elevation, elevated troponin I, and CK-MB elevation.
5. Medical interventions may include nitroglycerin drip, morphine, anticoagulant therapy (heparin), and thrombolytic agents to dissolve the clot. A cardiac catheterization can determine which coronary artery is blocked. Angioplasty or a coronary artery bypass graft may be done to reroute blood.
6. Educate Mrs. Sims about the risks of smoking and being overweight.

■ *Mrs. May*

1. Monitor the patient's left leg for color, temperature, capillary refill, and pulses: femoral, popliteal, dorsalis pedis, and posterior tibial. Compare findings with findings in the right leg.
2. If unable to palpate pulses, use a Doppler ultrasound that enhances sound to locate pulses.
3. The patient's symptoms could be caused by an embolism above left femoral artery.
4. To document finding, you would obtain more assessment data. A sample of SOAP charting for your additional findings is given:

   S: "I have a severe pain in my left groin that just started. It is at 9."

   O: Grimacing, moaning, and holding left upper leg. Left leg cool, color pale, nail beds pale, capillary refill 10 seconds, unable to palpate pulses. Faint femoral and popliteal pulse, no dorsalis pedis or posterior tibial pulse heard with Doppler. Right leg warm, pink, capillary refill 3 seconds, with all pulses palpable.

   A: Ineffective tissue perfusion

   P: Notify physician stat.

5. Immediate interventions include complete bedrest, protecting the leg, and notifying the physician.
6. Medical interventions could include medication for pain and use of an anticoagulant, such as heparin. If no pulses are present, a thrombolytic agent, such as streptokinase or tissue plasminogen activator, which dissolves already formed clots, may be ordered. Surgery is possible.
7. Thrombolectomy or embolectomy may be necessary to save the limb.

■ *Mr. Jangles*

1. Priority assessments include respiratory status, circulatory status of right leg and foot, vital signs, and pain level.
2. A medical history should include Mr. Jangles's usual blood sugar values, insulin dose, ambulation aids, gait, knowledge base regarding his various disease processes, and what led to this hospitalization.
3. (a) Priority nursing diagnoses include pain related to surgery of right lower leg; (b) ineffective tissue perfusion related to embolectomy of right lower leg, renal insufficiency; (c) risk for injury related to leg surgery, diabetes, obesity.
4. Outcomes include (a) verbalizes relief of pain; (b) maintains adequate tissue perfusion as evidenced by palpable peripheral (pedal) pulses, warm and dry skin; (c) remains free from injury.
5. Nursing interventions include the following: (a) Position (especially right leg) for comfort; keep the right leg slightly elevated; educate the patient regarding the need to ask for pain medication before pain is too severe; educate the patient regarding the need to take pain medication to minimize the negative physiological effects of pain; monitor pain on a pain scale; evaluate the effectiveness of medication using the same pain scale, report ineffective pain measures. (b) Check pedal pulses, surgical dressing, pedal sensation and movement, and color, initially and every hour; report changes; check capillary refill; monitor for pain in extremities; monitor for edema in extremities; keep leg elevated slightly. (c) Make sure the nursing call light is within reach; provide assistance with ambulation; use walking aids.

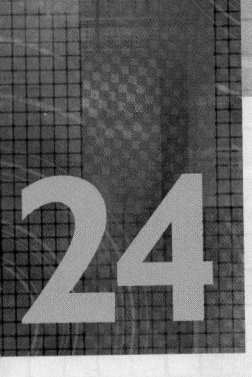

24

Nursing Care of Patients with Cardiac Valvular Disorders

LINDA S. WILLIAMS

KEY TERMS

annuloplasty (AN-yoo-loh-PLAS-tee)
commissurotomy (KOM-i-shur-AHT-oh-mee)
insufficiency (IN-suh-FISH-en-see)
murmur (MUR-mur)
regurgitation (ree-GUR-ji-TAY-shun)
stenosis (ste-NOH-sis)
valvotomy (val-VAH-tuh-mee)
valvuloplasty (VAL-vyoo-loh-PLAS-tee)

QUESTIONS TO GUIDE YOUR READING

1. What is the pathophysiology, etiology, signs and symptoms, and diagnostic tests for each of the valvular disorders?

2. What nursing care would you provide for a patient with a valvular disorder?

3. Why are prophylactic antibiotics prescribed for some patients with valvular disorders?

4. What are the differences between commissurotomy, annuloplasty, and valve replacement?

5. What postoperative complications can occur for the two types of cardiac valve replacements?

In the normal heart, blood flows in one direction because of the presence of heart valves. There are four valves in the heart: mitral, tricuspid, pulmonic, and aortic (see Fig. 20.2). The chordae tendineae and papillary muscles are attachment structures for both the mitral and tricuspid valves. They ensure that the valves close tightly. The pulmonic and aortic valves do not have these attachment structures.

Damage to the valves or their surrounding structures can result in abnormal valvular functioning (Fig. 24.1). The valves of the left side of the heart are most commonly affected and are discussed in this chapter. Forward blood flow can be hindered if the valve is narrowed, or stenosed, and does not open completely. If the valve does not close completely, blood backs up, which is referred to as **regurgitation** or **insufficiency.** The abnormal blood flow increases the workload of the heart and increases the pressures in the affected heart chamber.

Valvular damage may occur from congenital defects, rheumatic fever, or infections. Congenital defects occur mainly in children, and rheumatic heart disease occurs mainly in adults. Prophylactic antibiotic therapy helps prevent rheumatic fever and subsequent rheumatic heart disease and is recommended to prevent valvular disease.

VALVULAR DISORDERS

Mitral Valve Prolapse

Pathophysiology

During ventricular systole, when pressure in the left ventricle rises, the flaps of the mitral valve normally remain closed and stay within the atrioventricular junction. In mitral valve prolapse (MVP), however, one or both flaps bulge backward into the left atrium during systole. This is due to one flap

---

regurgitation: re—again + gurgitare—to flood
insufficiency: in—not + sufficiens—sufficient

LEARNING TIP

The opening of a stenosed valve and an insufficient valve look very similar, and the results of extra blood building up in a chamber are the same (see Fig. 24.1). However, the problem is different. Remember what the defect is in each disorder to understand why the blood is building up in a chamber.

A valve that does not open fully (stenosed) does not allow a chamber to empty normally. Blood builds up in that chamber as a result. For example, mitral **stenosis** does not allow the left atrium to empty easily, so blood builds up in the left atrium.

A valve that does not close fully (insufficient) allows blood to flow back into the chamber that emptied. Blood builds up in that chamber as a result. For example, mitral insufficiency allows blood to backflow from the left ventricle into the left atrium after the left atrium has emptied, so blood builds up in the left atrium.

being too large or a defect in the chordae tendineae that secures the valve to the heart wall. If the bulging flaps do not fit together, mitral regurgitation can occur with varying degrees of severity. Increased pressure on the papillary muscles results in ischemia within the muscle, causing further dysfunction of the mitral valve.

Etiology

In some people, MVP is a hereditary collagen tissue disorder, although the cause is unknown. Infections that damage the mitral valve, ischemic heart disease, or cardiomyopathy

---

stenosis: stenos—narrow

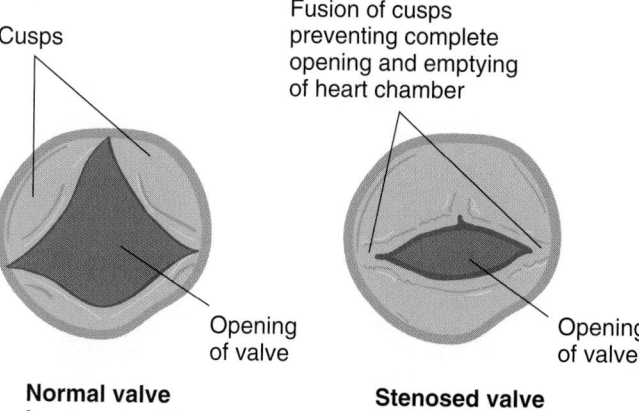

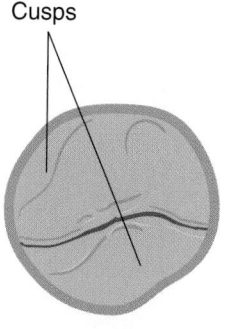

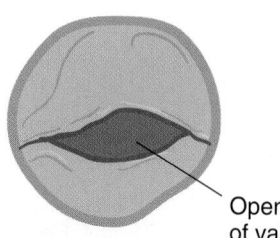

Cusps

Fusion of cusps preventing complete opening and emptying of heart chamber

Opening of valve

Opening of valve

Normal valve in open position

Stenosed valve in open position

Cusps

Opening of valve

Normal valve in closed position

Insufficient valve in closed position allowing backflow of blood through the valve

FIGURE 24.1 Openings of stenosed and insufficient valves compared with a normal valve.

may cause it. MVP is the most common form of valvular heart disease. It typically occurs in women mainly from 15 to 30 years of age who are thin and have slight chest deformities. Over age 50, males are frequently affected with more severe effects.

Signs and Symptoms

Most patients with MVP do not have symptoms and prognosis is very good (Table 24.1). The degree of MVP severity ranges from a **murmur** to chordae tendineae rupture with mitral regurgitation. The murmur, which is best heard at the apex, begins midsystolic and becomes more intense until the end of systole. If symptoms do occur, they may include atypical chest pain not related to exertion, dysrhythmias such as premature ventricular contractions causing palpitations, dizziness or syncope, fatigue, dyspnea, or anxiety. Emboli and infective endocarditis with mitral regurgitation are concerns.

TABLE 24.1 CARDIAC VALVULAR DISORDERS SUMMARY

Valve Disorder	Signs and Symptoms	Diagnostic Tests	Complications	Therapeutic Interventions	Nursing Interventions
Mitral Valve Prolapse	None Murmur Chest pain Palpitations Dizziness Syncope Fatigue Dyspnea	Echocardiography Cardiac catheterization	Emboli Infective endocarditis	None Beta blockers Antidysrhythmics Valvuloplasty Valve replacement	Activity intolerance Decreased cardiac output
Mitral Regurgitation	None Murmur Chest pain Palpitations Fatigue Exertional dyspnea Cough Hemoptysis Acute: Pulmonary edema Shock	ECG Chest x-ray Echocardiography Doppler ultrasound TEE Cardiac MRI Cardiac catheterization	Emboli Heart failure	None Antibiotic prophylaxsis ACEI Anticoagulants Valvuloplasty Valve replacement	Activity intolerance Decreased cardiac output
Mitral Stenosis	None Murmur Chest pain Palpitations Fatigue Exertional dyspnea Cough Hemoptysis	ECG Chest x-ray Echocardiography Doppler ultrasound TEE Cardiac catheterization	Emboli Heart failure	None Antibiotic prophylaxsis Anticoagulants PBV Valvuloplasty Valve replacement	Activity intolerance Decreased cardiac output
Aortic Stenosis	None Angina Murmur Syncope Heart failure	ECG Chest x-ray Echocardiography Serial echocardiogram Cardiac catheterization	Heart failure	Valve replacement	Activity intolerance Decreased cardiac output
Aortic Regurgitation	None Forceful pulse Murmur Chest pain Palpitations Fatigue Exertional dyspnea Corrigan's pulse Diaphoresis	ECG Chest x-ray Echocardiography Cardiac catheterization	Heart failure	Antibiotic prophylaxsis Valve replacement Digitalis (Lanoxin) Diuretics ACEI Nifedipine (Procardia)	Activity intolerance Decreased cardiac output

ECG = electocardiogram; TEE = transesophageal endoscopy; PBV = percutaneous balloon valvuloplasty.

Box 24.1

Diagnostic Tests for Cardiac Valvular Disorders

History and physical examination
Electrocardiogram
Chest x-ray examination
Echocardiography
Cardiac catheterization

Diagnostic Tests

Auscultation for a click or murmur, caused by the stress on the chordae tendineae or valve leaflets when they prolapse, is the first diagnostic step for MVP. Other diagnostic tests are used when MVP is suspected (Box 24.1 Diagnostic Tests for Cardiac Valvular Disorders). A normal electrocardiogram (ECG) is usually seen with MVP, although inverted T waves may be seen. A two-dimensional echocardiogram can show valve abnormalities and Doppler echocardiogram identifies mitral regurgitation from MVP. For more severe cases, cardiac catheterization, an invasive test, can show the bulging flaps of the mitral valve on a coronary angiogram.

Therapeutic Interventions

Unless patients have severe mitral regurgitation, MVP is a benign disorder. No treatment is needed unless symptoms are present (Box 24.2 Therapeutic Interventions for Cardiac Valvular Disorders). The severity of MVP and symptoms produced determine the treatment used. A healthy lifestyle, including a good diet, exercise, stress management, and avoidance of stimulants and caffeine, can be important to prevent symptoms. Beta blockers for those with rapid heart rates reduce heart rate and may relieve chest pain. Antidysrhythmic agents may need to be considered. Surgical repair or replacement of the valve can be done for severe cases of MVP (Box 24.2 Therapeutic Interventions for Cardiac Valvular Disorders and the section on Surgical Interventions).

Complications

Rare complications include dilation of the left side of the heart, heart failure, infective endocarditis, and emboli. Preventive antibiotic therapy before invasive procedures may be needed for some patients with thickened mitral valves to prevent endocarditis.[1] Aspirin or anticoagulants may be ordered to help prevent emboli.

CRITICAL THINKING

Mrs. Tepley

■ Mrs. Tepley, age 32, has mitral valve prolapse and reports palpitations whenever she experiences stress. She drinks three cups of coffee daily. Today, she is admitted for an outpatient cystoscopy.
1. What might you hear when auscultating Mrs. Tepley's heart sounds?
2. Why does Mrs. Tepley experience palpitations?
3. What medication might you expect to be ordered preoperatively for Mrs. Tepley?
4. Why does Mrs. Tepley need to be informed that she may need prophylactic antibiotics before invasive procedures?
5. What other information does Mrs. Tepley need to manage her MVP?

Suggested answers at end of chapter.

Box 24.2

Therapeutic Interventions for Cardiac Valvular Disorders

Rheumatic fever prophylaxis
Prophylactic antibiotic therapy considered
Anticoagulant therapy
Medication therapy
  Digitalis
  Diuretics
  ACEIs
  Beta blockers
  Antidysrhythmics
Percutaneous balloon valvuloplasty
Surgical:
  Valvuloplasty
  Closed commissurotomy
  Open commissurotomy
  Annuloplasty
  Valve replacement

Mitral Stenosis

Pathophysiology

Mitral stenosis results from thickening of the mitral valve flaps and shortening of the chordae tendineae, causing narrowing of the valve opening. Older patients with mitral stenosis usually have calcification and fibrosis of the mitral valve flaps. The narrowed opening obstructs blood flow from the left atrium into the left ventricle. The left atrium enlarges to hold the extra blood volume caused by the obstruction. As a result of this increased blood volume, pressure rises in the left atrium. Pressures then rise in the pulmonary circulation and the right ventricle as blood volume backs up from the left atrium. The right ventricle dilates to handle the increased volume. Eventually the right ventricle fails from this excessive workload, reducing the blood volume delivered to the left ventricle and subsequently decreasing cardiac output.

Etiology

The major cause of mitral stenosis is rheumatic fever, with symptoms often taking two to four decades to appear after the illness. It is a continuous and progressive disease. Since rheumatic fever is declining in developed nations less mitral stenosis is being seen in those countries. It is still a problem in underdeveloped areas where rheumatic fever still occurs. Less common causes include congenital defects of the mitral valve, tumors, rheumatoid arthritis, systemic lupus erythematosus, calcium deposits, and rheumatic endocarditis.

Signs and Symptoms

At first, patients may be asymptomatic (see Table 24.1). A click or low-pitched murmur may be heard. The murmur presents as a rumbling sound over the apex during diastole and is more pronounced right before systole. Then mild symptoms progressing to more severe symptoms develop. Pulmonary symptoms are most commonly seen. Exertional dyspnea, cough, and hemoptysis are the major symptoms. Fatigue and intolerance to activity result from decreased cardiac output. Palpitations from atrial flutter or fibrillation caused by atrial enlargement and chest pain from decreased cardiac output may be experienced. Complications from emboli formed from the stasis of blood in the left atrium include stroke and seizures. If the right ventricle fails, symptoms related to heart failure are seen (see Chapter 26).

Diagnostic Tests

Mitral stenosis is diagnosed with data from the patient history and physical examination and findings from diagnostic tests (see Box 24.1 Diagnostic Tests for Cardiac Valvular Disorders). The ECG shows enlargement of the left atrium and right ventricle and changes in the P waveform. Atrial flutter or fibrillation may be seen. A chest x-ray examination confirms enlargement of the affected heart chambers. Transthoracic two-dimensional color flow Doppler echocardiography and Doppler ultrasound are the noninvasive gold standard for evaluation of valvular disease. They show the narrowed mitral valve opening and decreased motion of the valve. Transesophageal echocardiography can be used if transthoracic images are not effective. A cardiac catheterization is typically done only if needed to validate unclear echocardiography results for preoperative evaluation or postprocedure for symptom recurrence.

Therapeutic Interventions

Individualized prophylactic antibiotic therapy may be given to prevent endocarditis.[1] Anticoagulants are given to patients with atrial fibrillation to prevent development of emboli from stasis of blood in the atrium. If heart failure develops, symptoms are treated with medications such as digitalis and diuretics and other therapies used for heart failure (see Chapter 26).

For less severe cases, percutaneous balloon **valvuloplasty,** which uses a balloon to dilate the stenosed heart valve, is done in a cardiac catheterization laboratory (Fig. 24.2). One approach for valvoplasty is to insert a balloon catheter via the venous circulation into the right atrium. Then the catheter is threaded through a small hole pierced into the right atrial septum that emerges into the left atrium and is then passed through the mitral valve. Inflation of the balloon within the mitral valve opens the stenosed valve flaps. Complications may include dysrhythmias, emboli,

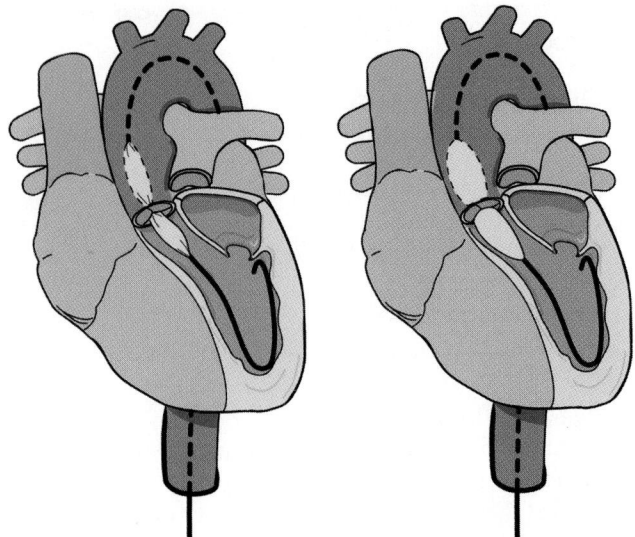

FIGURE 24.2 Percutaneous balloon valvuloplasty.

hemorrhage, and cardiac tamponade. There are fewer complications with balloon valvuloplasty than with surgery.

Surgical treatment can include **commissurotomy** or **annuloplasty,** both forms of valvular repair (valvuloplasty) or valve replacement (see Box 24.2 Therapeutic Interventions for Cardiac Valvular Disorders and the discussion on Surgical Interventions). Mitral valve replacement is used for more severe cases and when symptoms of ventricular failure develop. These procedures may require the use of cardiopulmonary bypass. In commissurotomy, the valve flaps that have adhered to each other and closed the opening between them, known as the commissure, are separated to enlarge the valve opening. Annuloplasty is the repair or reconstruction of the valve flaps or annulus. It may involve the use of prosthetic rings. Valve replacement with prosthetic valves has been done since 1952. Valve replacement uses mechanical or biological valves from animal or human tissue (Fig. 24.3).

Mitral Regurgitation

Pathophysiology

Mitral regurgitation, or insufficiency, is the incomplete closure of the mitral valve leaflets. It allows backflow of blood into the left atrium with each contraction of the left ventricle. This blood is then extra volume that is added to the incoming blood from the lungs. With chronic mitral regurgitation, the increase in blood volume dilates and increases pressure in the left atrium. In response to the extra blood volume delivered by the left atrium, the left ventricle compensates by dilating. If the compensatory mechanism of dilation is inadequate, pressures rise in the pulmonary circulation and then in the right ventricle as blood vol-

---

commissurotomy: commissura—joining together + tome—incision
annuloplasty: annulus—ring + plasty—formed

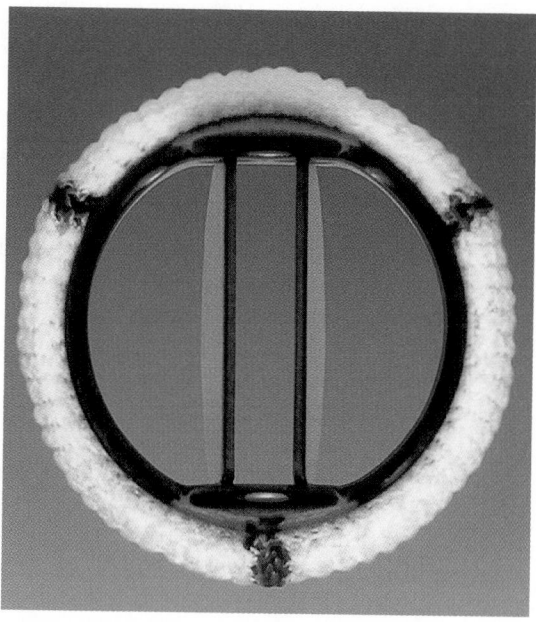

FIGURE 24.3 Valve prosthesis. An SJM Masters Series valve. *(Courtesy St. Jude Medical, Inc., St. Paul, MN.)*

ume backs up from the left atrium. The left ventricle and eventually the right ventricle may fail from this increased strain.

Etiology

The major cause of mitral regurgitation is rheumatic heart disease. Other causes include endocarditis, rupture or dysfunction of the chordae tendineae or papillary muscle, MVP, cardiomyopathy, annulus calcification, or congenital defects.

Signs and Symptoms

Initially, patients may be asymptomatic (see Table 24.1). The symptoms of chronic mitral regurgitation are similar to those of mitral stenosis. The murmur begins with S1 (first heart sound) and continues during systole up to S2 (second heart sound). Exertional dyspnea and fatigue occur slowly. Palpitations and an irregular pulse due to atrial fibrillation may result. Weakness from decreased cardiac output occurs if the left ventricle begins to fail.

If acute mitral regurgitation develops, such as in papillary muscle rupture following myocardial infarction, pulmonary edema and shock symptoms will be exhibited.

Diagnostic Tests

The ECG shows enlargement of the left atrium and left ventricle and changes in the P waveform. Atrial flutter or fibrillation may be seen. A chest x-ray examination confirms hypertrophy of the affected heart chambers. Two-dimensional or Doppler echocardiography shows left atrial enlargement and regurgitation of blood. Transesophageal echocardiography can also be used to identify causes. Cardiac MRI may be used for some people to determine treatment approaches. Cardiac catheterization further identifies regurgitation effects.

Therapeutic Interventions

Without symptoms, there is no general medical treatment. Prophylactic antibiotic therapy may be given to prevent infectious endocarditis before invasive procedures.[1] Angiotensin-converting enzyme (ACE) inhibitors are often used to reduce afterload. If atrial fibrillation with rapid heart rate is present, it can be controlled with digitalis, calcium channel blockers, or beta blockers. Emboli occur less frequently, but anticoagulation is still prescribed. Symptoms of heart failure are treated with therapies for heart failure (see Chapter 26). When symptoms develop or surgery is indicated to prevent further left ventricular dysfunction, mitral valve repair or replacement is done (Fig. 24.4). For acute mitral regurgitation, emergency surgery may be needed (see Box 24.2 Therapeutic Interventions for Cardiac Valvular Disorders and the discussion on Surgical Interventions).

Aortic Stenosis

Pathophysiology

Blood flow from the left ventricle into the aorta is obstructed through the stenosed aortic valve. The opening of the aortic valve may be narrowed from thickening, scarring, calcification, or fusing of the valve's flaps. To compensate for the difficulty in ejecting blood into the aorta, the left ventricle contracts more forcefully. In chronic stenosis, the left ventricle hypertrophies to maintain normal cardiac output. With increased narrowing of the valve opening, the compensatory mechanisms are unable to continue and the left ventricle fails to move blood forward. This results in decreased cardiac output and heart failure.

Etiology

The major causes of aortic stenosis are congenital defects or rheumatic heart disease. Mitral valve stenosis is often also

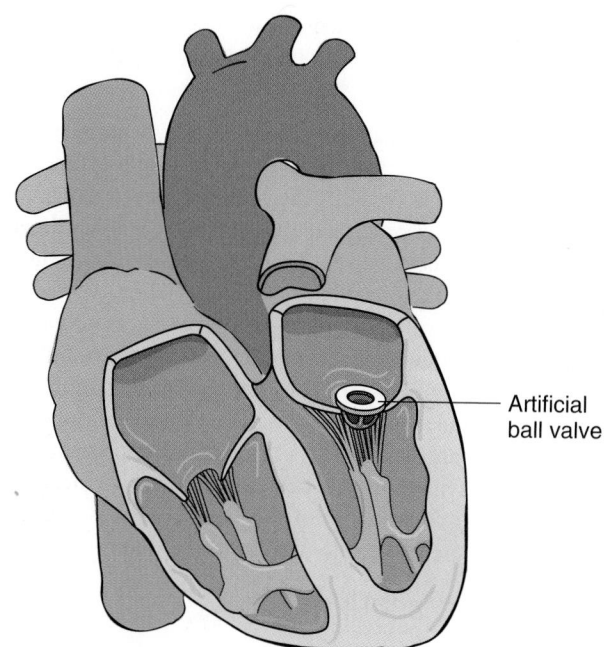

Artificial ball valve

FIGURE 24.4 Mitral valve replacement with ball valve prosthesis.

present when the cause is rheumatic heart disease. Calcification of the aortic valve can be related to aging and is seen after the age of 50.

Signs and Symptoms

It may take many years or decades before signs or symptoms of aortic stenosis are observed (see Table 24.1). When symptoms do occur, evaluation is essential because the disease can progress dramatically. If the mitral valve is also diseased, signs and symptoms may appear earlier.

Angina pectoris is a primary symptom that occurs as a result of the increased oxygen needs of the hypertrophied myocardium. The extra workload of the left ventricle and the hypertrophy of the cardiac muscle require more oxygen. Angina results if these oxygen needs are not met. In the young patient, angina indicates severe obstruction.

Other signs and symptoms include a murmur, syncope from dysrhythmias or decreased cardiac output, and heart failure signs and symptoms. The murmur is a systolic murmur that begins just after the first heart sound, increasing in intensity till midsystole, then decreasing and ending right before the second heart sound. Orthopnea, dyspnea on exertion, and fatigue are indicators of left ventricular failure. Progressive heart failure can result in pulmonary edema and right-sided heart failure.

Diagnostic Tests

ECG usually shows enlargement of the left ventricle and left atrium. A chest x-ray examination confirms hypertrophy of the left ventricle and calcification of the aortic valve. Left atrial enlargement may be seen but occurs primarily when mitral stenosis is also present. Two-dimensional and Doppler echocardiography show thickening of the left ventricular wall, impaired movement of the aortic valve, and the severity of the disease. Serial echocardiography (e.g., annually or less often) may be recommended for those with moderate or severe disease. Cardiac catheterization will show elevated left ventricular pressure and decreased cardiac output.

Therapeutic Interventions

Generally, the treatment of choice is valve replacement because of the risk of sudden death when severe symptoms are present (see Box 24.2 Therapeutic Interventions for Cardiac Valvular Disorders and the section on Surgical Intervention). Mechanical valves are often chosen for middle-aged adults and require lifelong anticoagulation. For older adults, biological valves (porcine or bovine) are usually used as they do not require anticoagulation therapy and last about 12 years. **Valvotomy** may be considered for young adults but is not used for older adults due to early restenosis. Prophylactic antibiotics are considered before invasive procedures.[1] Heart failure symptoms are treated carefully. Medications that reduce the contractility of the heart and subsequently cardiac output are avoided to prevent further failure.

Aortic Regurgitation

Pathophysiology

The aortic valve cusps may be scarred, thickened, or shortened in chronic aortic regurgitation. A backflow of blood

---

CRITICAL THINKING

Mrs. Hesche

■ Mrs. Hesche, age 72, has aortic stenosis and is admitted to the hospital with angina. She had an episode of syncope 2 days ago. She reports that she tires easily.

1. Mrs. Hesche asks what aortic stenosis is. What will you tell her and how will you document it?
2. Why might Mrs. Hesche be experiencing angina?
3. What nursing care related to safety needs are important to include in Mrs. Hesche's plan of care?
4. What nursing diagnosis and care are relevant for Mrs. Hesche's report of being tired?
5. Digoxin (Lanoxin) 0.25 mg is prescribed for Mrs. Hesche. It is time to give her digoxin and you have available digoxin 0.125 mg tablets. How many tablets will you give?

Suggested answers at end of chapter.

---

from the aorta into the left ventricle occurs if the aortic valve cusps do not close completely. The left ventricle's blood volume increases with this backflow of blood that is in addition to the normal flow of blood from the left atrium. To handle the increased volume, the left ventricle compensates with dilation and hypertrophy to deliver a stronger contraction. This stronger contraction ejects more blood volume with each beat to maintain cardiac output. Over time the heart's contraction is not effective and the left ventricle fails, causing a cardiac output drop and pulmonary edema.

Etiology

Rheumatic heart disease (which is becoming less common) is the usual cause of aortic regurgitation. Other causes include congenital defects, syphilis, severe hypertension, and rheumatoid arthritis. An acute cause of aortic regurgitation may be endocarditis or aortic dissection.

Signs and Symptoms

No symptoms may be apparent for many years with chronic aortic regurgitation (see Table 24.1). Initially, the patient may report feeling a forceful heartbeat which is more pronounced lying down. Also, palpitations and pounding in the head may be experienced. Then exertional dyspnea, fatigue, and worsening levels of dyspnea (orthopnea, paroxysmal noctural dyspnea) occur after years of progressive valvular dysfunction. A murmur is heard during diastolic after the second heart sound. The palpated pulse is forceful and then quickly collapses (Corrigan's pulse). The diastolic blood pressure decreases to widen the pulse pressure. This compensates for an increase in systolic blood pressure. Angina pectoris may occur late. The angina is atypical, often happening at rest or at night along with diaphoresis, when a lower pulse rate results in delivery of less oxygen to the myocardium. Eventually heart failure symptoms develop if the left ventricle fails.

In acute dysfunction, profound symptoms of pulmonary distress, chest pain, and shock symptoms occur. The prognosis is poor.

Diagnostic Tests

The ECG shows left ventricle hypertrophy, ST segment depression, and T wave inversion in some leads (see Chapter 25). A chest x-ray confirms hypertrophy of the left ventricle and aorta. With severe regurgitation, left atrial enlargement may also be seen. An echocardiogram and Doppler echocardiography show an enlarged left ventricle and severity of aortic regurgitation. Cardiac catheterization reveals elevated left ventricular diastolic pressure and, with dye injection, shows the regurgitation of blood into the left ventricle.

Therapeutic Interventions

Surgical valve replacement is the treatment of choice prior to heart failure development (see Box 24.2 Therapeutic Interventions for Cardiac Valvular Disorders and the Surgical Interventions section). Treatment with digitalis, diuretics, and vasodilator therapy such as ACE inhibitors and nifedipine (Procardia) may be useful for some patients to reduce systolic blood pressure and subsequently cardiac workload until surgery is needed. Prophylactic antibiotic therapy may be given before invasive procedures.[1] If dysrhythmias develop, they are promptly treated. Acute aortic regurgitation requires immediate surgery.

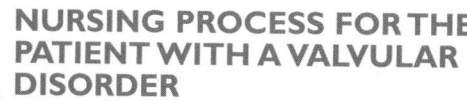

NURSING PROCESS FOR THE PATIENT WITH A VALVULAR DISORDER

Nursing Assessment/Data Collection

A history that includes information presented in Table 24.2 is obtained. Vital signs are measured and recorded. Heart sounds are auscultated to detect murmurs. Any signs and symptoms of heart failure are noted (see Chapter 26).

Nursing Diagnoses, Planning, Interventions, and Evaluation

The major nursing diagnoses for all valvular disorders are the same and include those for heart failure as well if heart failure symptoms are present. See Box 24.3 Nursing Care Plan for the Patient with Cardiac Valvular Disorders.

Patient Education

Education, an important nursing intervention, promotes understanding of the valvular disorder, health maintenance, prevention of complications, and early recognition of symptoms, so medical care can be sought. For older adult patients, it is important to include caregivers or family members in teaching sessions to assist with understanding of the information being taught. Teaching is provided for medications the patient is taking. If the patient is on anticoagulants for atrial fibrillation or mechanical valve replacement, a Medic Alert identification should be used and monthly appointments to check international normalized ratio (INR) values should be kept.

Information on endocarditis prevention is essential for patients with most valvular problems. Damaged cardiac valves are prone to developing infection from organisms such as *Streptococcus viridans* or *Staphylococcus epidermidis*. During invasive procedures in which bleeding is possible, these organisms can enter the circulation, attach to damaged valves, and multiply. Patients should be taught the possible need for prophylactic antibiotics before invasive procedures, including dental work or surgery, to prevent endocarditis.[1] Patients should consult their physician about the need for prophylactic antibiotics.

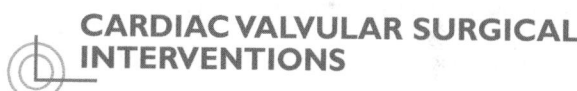

CARDIAC VALVULAR SURGICAL INTERVENTIONS

There are several types of heart valve repairs and replacements. Technological advances have created less invasive

TABLE 24.2 NURSING ASSESSMENT FOR PATIENTS WITH CARDIAC VALVULAR DISORDERS

	Subjective Data
Health History	Infections—rheumatic fever, endocarditis, streptococcal or staphylococcal, syphilis
	Congenital defects
	Cardiac disease—myocardial infarction, cardiomyopathy
Respiratory	Dyspnea at rest, on exertion, when lying, or that awakens patient?
	Cough or hemoptysis?
Cardiovascular	Any palpitations, chest pain, dizziness, fatigue, activity intolerance?
Medications	
Knowledge of Condition	
Coping skills	
	Objective Data
Respiratory	Crackles, wheezes, tachypnea
Cardiovascular	Murmurs, extra heart sounds, dysrhythmias, edema, jugular vein distention, Corrigan's pulse, increased or decreased pulse pressure
Integumentary	Clubbing; cyanosis; diaphoresis; cold, clammy skin; pallor
Diagnostic Test Findings	

Box 24.3 NURSING CARE PLAN for the Patient with Cardiac Valvular Disorders

Nursing Diagnosis: Decreased cardiac output related to valvular stenosis or insufficiency or heart failure

Expected Outcomes Patient has adequate cardiac output as evidenced by vital signs within normal limits (WNL), no dyspnea or fatigue.

Evaluation of Outcomes Does patient have vital signs WNL with no dyspnea or fatigue?

Interventions	Rationale	Evaluation
Assess vital signs, chest pain, and fatigue.	Vital signs, chest pain, and fatigue are indicators of cardiac output decline.	Are vital signs WNL with no chest pain or fatigue?
Give oxygen as ordered.	Supplemental oxygen provides more oxygen to the heart.	Is breathing pattern normal?
Provide bedrest or rest periods as ordered.	Cardiac workload and oxygen needs are reduced with rest.	Are vital signs WNL and no fatigue reported?
Elevate head of bed 45 degrees.	Venous return to heart is reduced and chest expansion improved.	Are vital signs WNL and respirations easy?

Geriatric

Interventions	Rationale	Evaluation
Assess for cardiac medication side effects and teach patient side effects to report.	Toxic side effects are more common owing to altered metabolism and excretion of medications in the elderly.	Are side effects present for medications patient is taking?
		Does patient understand side effects to report?

Nursing Diagnosis: Activity intolerance related to decreased oxygen delivery from decreased cardiac output

Expected Outcomes Patient will show normal changes in vital signs with less fatigue in response to activity.

Evaluation of Outcomes Does patient have normal changes in vital signs with activity? Does patient report decreased fatigue with activity?

Interventions	Rationale	Evaluation
Assist as needed with activities of daily living(ADLs).	Energy is consered with ADL assistance.	Are all ADLs completed?
Provide rest and space activites.	Cardiac workload and oxygen needs are reduced with rest.	Are vital signs WNL with activity?
		Is patient able to perform activities when allowed extra time?

Geriatric

Interventions	Rationale	Evaluation
Slow pace of care and allow patient extra time to perform activities.	Elderly patients can often perform activities if allowed time to slowly perform them and rest at intervals.	Does blood pressure remain WNL when changing position?
Ensure safety when mobilizing elderly patient.	Orthostatic hypertension is common in the elderly.	Does patient ambulate without injury?

options than the traditional open cardiac surgery with cardiopulmonary bypass (CPB) for valve repair and replacement. New percutaneous approaches are being researched such as a transseptal stitch repair and coronary sinus tucking that reduces mitral annular size. A minithoracotomy can be used to repair or replace valves such as the mitral valve. Robotic devices are being trialed that can reduce incision size even more. Less invasive surgery means a quicker recovery, less pain and healing time. It is a good surgical option for older adults who meet the criteria.

Heart Valve Repairs

A **commissurotomy** is a heart valve repair for a stenosed valve. For commissurotomy, the patient is placed on CPB and an atriotomy (incision into the atrium) is made to expose the valve (see Chapter 20). The valve cusps are either incised with a knife or broken apart with a dilator. The atrium is sewn closed, CPB is discontinued, and surgery continues as described in the general surgery procedure section. Commissurotomy is most commonly performed on the mitral valve.

A balloon valvotomy is a procedure that repairs a stenosed heart valve. The balloon catheter is inserted through a diseased valve and then inflated to open the stenosed valve.

Another type of valve repair is **annuloplasty,** which repairs the annulus of a valve. The mitral valve is the most common valve repaired in this way. Sutures or a ring may be placed in the valve annulus to improve closure of the leaflets. Similar procedures are used on the tricuspid valve; however, the aortic valve is not readily repaired in this manner.

Heart Valve Replacement

Valves used for cardiac valve replacement may be either mechanical or biological. There are three types of mechanical valves: caged ball, monoleaflet, and bileaflet (Fig. 24.5). Mechanical valves are durable but create turbulent blood flow. The turbulent flow can lead to clot formation, requiring lifelong anticoagulant therapy. Biological (tissue) valves come from three sources: porcine (pig), bovine (cow), or allograft (human donor) (Box 24.4 Cultural Considerations). Allografts are available in limited numbers because they rely on donors. Visit www.lifenet.org for more information on allografts and www.sjm.com to view heart valves. Tissue valves have a very low incidence of thrombus formation and do not require lifelong anticoagulant therapy, but do not last as long as mechanical valves. Selecting the type of valves to use depends on several factors. If anticoagulation is a concern, then biologic valves may be preferred especially for the older adult or women considering pregnancy.

For mitral valve replacement (MVR), a left atriotomy is made after the patient is on CPB. For an aortic valve replacement (AVR), an incision is made above the right coronary artery in the aorta. Then in either valvular procedure, the diseased valve is excised and the new valve sutured

A. Caged ball valve

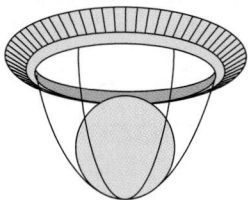

B. Monoleaflet

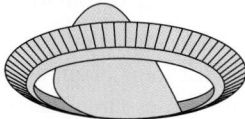

C. Bileaflet

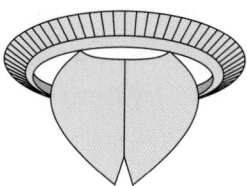

FIGURE 24.5 Types of mechanical heart valves.

in place. The incision is closed, and surgery then continues as described in the general surgery procedure section.

Valve Replacement Complications

In tissue valves, degenerative changes and calcification can occur, leading to valve failure. For mechanical valves, the most common complication is thrombus formation. An embolism can occur when thrombi form on the mechanical valve and then break off. Embolism rarely occurs with tissue valves and is prevented with anticoagulant therapy for mechanical valves. When the patient is on warfarin, ongoing monitoring of international normalized ratio (INR) is important. The general target for INR with certain aortic valve replacements is 2.0 to 3.0, and 2.5 to 3.5 with mitral or aortic valve replacement along with thromboembolitic risks.

Other complications include anemia and endocarditis. Anemia is due to hemolysis of red blood cells (RBCs) as they come in contact with mechanical valve structures. In

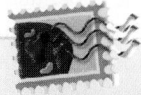

Box 24.4

Cultural Considerations

Cardiac Valves

Because the pig is considered a dirty animal to religious Jews and Muslims, only bovine, synthetic, or human valves should be used for these patients. Likewise, because the cow is sacred among Hindus, only porcine, synthetic, or human valves should be used for Hindu patients.

endocarditis, microorganisms tend to grow on the valve leaflets or the sewing ring of mechanical valves. These growths can make valves incompetent or break off to become emboli.

NURSING PROCESS FOR THE PREOPERATIVE CARDIAC SURGERY PATIENT

Assessment/Data Collection

A baseline assessment is important for postoperative comparison and to begin discharge planning. Pain control needs and circulatory status are essential items. Results of diagnostic laboratory tests, x-ray examinations, and other studies are reported if abnormal. Typing and crossmatching of ordered units of blood is done and placed on hold.

Nursing Diagnoses, Planning, Interventions, and Evaluation

See Nursing Process for Preoperative Patients in Chapter 11.

NURSING PROCESS FOR THE POSTOPERATIVE CARDIAC SURGERY PATIENT

After cardiac surgery, the patient goes to the intensive care unit (ICU) for about 1 to 2 days for close observation and cardiac monitoring. Tubes are removed as the patient's status allows. Then the patient is transferred to a stepdown or general surgical unit for continued cardiac monitoring as recovery continues.

Assessment/Data Collection

The patient is accompanied to the ICU by the anesthesiologist, who gives the nurse a report of the procedure, complications, and hemodynamic and ventilatory management of the patient. The patient is connected to a cardiac monitor and mechanical ventilator. The mechanical ventilator is used for 4 to 24 hours. The patient is placed under a warming device, such as a light or blanket. A head-to-toe assessment of the patient, including dressings, tubes, and IV lines, is performed. The patient may have several tubes that require monitoring including a chest tube, nasogastric tube, and a urinary catheter. Of importance are signs of awakening, shivering, pain, lung and heart sounds, and palpation of the entire chest and neck to detect crepitus (air in the subcutaneous tissue from opening the chest). Trends in the patient's cardiac output are monitored. Body temperature is continuously monitored until warming measures are discontinued, which occurs when the core body temperature nears 37°C (98.6°F). While patients are being rewarmed, they are assessed for shivering, which may be felt as a fine vibration at the mandibular angle of the jaw. Shivering greatly increases cardiac oxygen needs. Paralyzing agents given with narcotics eliminate shivering. Blood is drawn for a CBC, electrolytes, coagulation studies, and arterial blood gases.

After the initial transfer assessment, vital signs, oxygen saturation, and cardiac pressures are monitored and recorded every 15 to 30 minutes, with decreasing frequency as the patient stabilizes. Body temperature is monitored continuously while warming measures are used. The patient is warmed slowly to avoid peripheral vasodilation and onset of signs and symptoms of shock. Intake and output are measured and vital signs are checked. A 12-lead electrocardiogram (ECG) is done to detect perioperative myocardial infarction. A chest x-ray examination is done to check central line and endotracheal tube placement and to detect a pneumothorax or hemothorax, diaphragm elevation, or mediastinal widening from bleeding. At this point, the family may see the patient, and patient care is explained.

Awakening with many questions, strange auditory and tactile sensations, and the inability to speak are very frightening and frustrating to the patient. Keeping eye contact with the patient and using touch appropriately can be very soothing to the patient. If lip reading is unsuccessful, use simple closed-ended questions, nonverbal gestures, communication boards, and magic slates. Give explanations regarding procedures in simple terms.

After cardiac surgery, pain is monitored in relation to the patient's preoperative anginal or infarction-associated pain. Chest pain after surgery can be frightening for patients. Knowing that chest pain can occur from the surgical incision rather than the heart is important to the patient. Otherwise the patient may not associate surgical chest pain with the incision and instead think the pain is anginal or myocardial infarction pain.

Nursing Diagnoses, Planning, Interventions, and Evaluation

Nursing diagnoses for postoperative cardiac surgery are discussed in Box 24.5 Nursing Care Plan for the Postoperative Patient Undergoing Cardiac Surgery. Additional general postoperative nursing care is discussed in Chapter 11.

BOX 24.5   NURSING CARE PLAN for the Postoperative Patient Undergoing Cardiac Surgery

Nursing Diagnosis: Pain related to sternotomy, or pericarditis

Expected Outcomes Patient will state pain is relieved or tolerable. Patient is able to rest and perform respiratory treatments.

Evaluation of Outcomes Does patient state pain is within acceptable levels? Is patient able to rest and perform respiratory therapies?

Interventions	Rationale	Evaluation
• Ask about characteristics of pain with each episode.	A thorough description is needed to determine cause and plan actions.	Does patient describe pain on scale of 0 to 10?
• Splint chest incision with all movement and coughing and deep breathing.	Stabilizes sternum and incision to increase comfort.	Can patient splint chest incision independently?
• Encourage patient to report pain even when pain is mild.	It is easier to keep pain under control when mild.	Does patient report pain when mild?
• Turn, reposition every 2 hours.	Changes muscle position, relieving stiffness.	Is patient comfortable without stiffness?
• Offer back rubs frequently.	Relaxes tense muscles retracted during operation.	Is patient able to rest in comfort?
• Instruct patient to take a deep breath before movement and exhale slowly during movement.	Keeps muscles relaxed, minimizing tension with guarding and pain.	Can patient perform coughing and deep breathing techniques as instructed?

Nursing Diagnosis: Decreased cardiac output related to myocardial depression, hypothermia, bleeding, unstable dysrhythmias, or hypoxemia

Expected Outcomes Patient will remain free of major side effects of pharmacological support. Patient will maintain vital signs within normal limits (WNL), palpable peripheral pulses, urine output greater than 30 mL/h, and normal sinus rhythm.

Evaluation of Outcomes Is patient free of major side effects? Are vital signs WNL?

Interventions	Rationale	Evaluation
• Monitor vital signs.	Trends reflect problems.	Are vital signs WNL?
• Monitor peripheral circulation.	Mottling or weak pulses may indicate poor cardiac output (CO).	Do peripheral pulses remain strong with normal skin color, temperature, capillary refill?
• Monitor intake and output.	Fluid deficit or excess can alter CO.	Does total intake equal output?
• Listen to lung sounds and note character of sputum.	Wet lung sounds may indicate heart failure or pulmonary edema.	Are lungs clear?
• Monitor temperature closely while rewarming the patient.	Febrile state increases heart rate and myocardial oxygen consumption.	Does temperature remain less than or equal to 98.6°F (37°C)?
• Monitor for shivering.	Shivering increases the blood pressure, decreasing CO and increasing risk for bleeding.	Is patient's shivering controlled?
• Monitor chest tube drainage for increase or sudden decrease.	Drainage >200 mL/hr may lead to hypovolemia and a decrease in CO.	Is patient free from cardiac tamponade and hypovolemia?
• Monitor ECG.	Premature ventricular contractions and atrial fibrillation decrease CO.	Does patient remain in normal sinus rhythm or controlled dysrhythmia?
• Monitor electrolytes.	Low calcium and magnesium and high potassium decrease contractility and CO.	Are electrolytes WNL?
• Monitor ABGs.	Acidosis decreases heart function, and a low CO may lead to further acidosis.	Are ABGs WNL?

(Continued on following page)

BOX 24.5   NURSING CARE PLAN **for the Postoperative Patient Undergoing Cardiac Surgery** (*Continued*)

Nursing Diagnosis: Risk for infection related to inadequate primary defenses from surgical wound

Expected Outcomes Patient will remain free from infection.

Evaluation of Outcomes Does patient remain free from infection?

Interventions	Rationale	Evaluation
• Use good hand hygiene and cleanse stethoscope with alcohol between patients.	Hands and stethoscopes can carry infectious agents.	Are infectious preventive techniques used? Does patient remain free from infection?
• Observe incision for signs and symptoms of infection.	Redness, warmth, fever, and swelling indicate infection.	Are signs and symptoms of infection present?
• Monitor drainage and maintain drains.	Drains remove fluid from the surgical site to prevent infection development.	Are drainage amount and color normal for procedure? Are drains functioning?
• Maintain sterile technique for dressing changes.	Sterile technique reduces infection development.	Is incision free of signs and symptoms of infection?
• Monitor and report abnormal findings for temperature, lung sounds, sputum, and urine consistency.	Low-grade (immunosuppressed) or high-grade fever, crackles, yellow-green sputum color, or cloudy urine can indicate infection.	Is the patient's temperature WNL and are lung sounds, sputum, and urine clear?

REVIEW QUESTIONS

1. The nurse is evaluating patient teaching for mitral valve prolapse. The patient shows understanding of the prognosis of MVP by stating which of the following?
   a. "The prognosis is poor."
   b. "There are often no symptoms."
   c. "Heart failure often occurs."
   d. "Symptoms then quickly progress."

2. Which of the following symptoms would the nurse identify as a priority to report for a patient with aortic stenosis?
   a. Angina
   b. Peripheral edema
   c. Headache
   d. Weight loss

3. A patient just diagnosed with aortic regurgitation asks what this means. Which of the following is the nurse's best response for describing what occurs in aortic regurgitation?
   a. "Backflow of blood into the right ventricle."
   b. "Backflow of blood into the left ventricle."
   c. "Impaired emptying of the right ventricle."
   d. "Impaired emptying of the left ventricle."

4. A patient with mitral stenosis develops atrial fibrillation. Which of the following medications does the nurse understand is given to the patient to prevent embolitic complications from atrial fibrillation?
   a. Bumetanide (Bumex)
   b. Furosemide (Lasix)
   c. Penicillin (Bicillin)
   d. Warfarin (Coumadin)

5. A patient is scheduled for cardiac valve testing. Which of the following tests would the nurse explain will show the cardiac valves and how they function?
   a. ECG
   b. Chest x-ray examination
   c. Echocardiogram
   d. Cardiac catheterization

6. The nurse is planning care for a patient having a cardiac valve replacement. With which type of valve will the patient be on anticoagulant therapy to prevent thrombus formation?
   a. Mechanical valve
   b. Porcine valve
   c. Allograft valve
   d. Bovine valve

Multiple response item. Select all that apply.

7. A patient with mitral regurgitation receives antibiotic prophylaxis. Which of these patient statements would indicate the need for further explanation by the nurse?
   a. "I am at less risk for developing endocarditis."
   b. "The antibiotics I take prevent further heart valve damage."
   c. "The antibiotics I am taking are to prevent a heart infection."
   d. "Invasive procedures put me at risk of endocarditis which the antibiotics are to prevent."
   e. "The antibiotics I take are to prevent a cold."

References

1. Dajani, A, Taubert, KA, Wilson, W, et al: Prevention of bacterial endocarditis: recommendations by the American Heart Association. JAMA 277:1794, 1997.

SUGGESTED ANSWERS TO

CRITICAL THINKING

■ Mrs. Tepley

1. You might hear a murmur.
2. Stress and caffeine increase the occurrence of palpitations.
3. Prophylactic antibiotics might be ordered preoperatively.
4. She might need prophylactic antibiotics to prevent infective endocarditis, which can result from bacteria entering the circulation during invasive procedures, attaching to the damaged valve, and growing.
5. To help manage her condition, Mrs. Tepley needs a definition of MVP, stress management techniques, to know she should reduce caffeine intake (e.g., with decaffeinated coffee), and to understand symptoms of endocarditis to report to her physician.

■ Mrs. Hesche

1. In aortic stenosis, the valve is narrowed, which makes it more difficult for blood to leave the left ventricle and go into the aorta. This means there can be less blood flow to the body.

Documentation: S: "What is aortic stenosis?" O: Listened attentively during explanation that in aortic stenosis the valve is narrowed making it more difficult for blood to leave left ventricle to go to aorta. This means there can be less blood flow to the body. A: Interested in learning more about diagnosis. P: Provide more information

2. Angina results if the heart's oxygen needs are not met because of reduced cardiac output.
3. Nursing care should include fall precautions due to syncope and fatigue.
4. Diagnoses and care include the following: Self-care deficits related to fatigue, so plan for meeting ADL needs. Activity intolerance related to fatigue, so plan rest periods between activity and monitor vital signs with activity.
5. You should give 2 tablets. An example of solving this problem is:
   Unit Analysis Method

$$\frac{0.25 \text{ milligrams}}{} \cdot \frac{1 \text{ tablet}}{0.125 \text{ milligrams}} = 2 \text{ tablets}$$

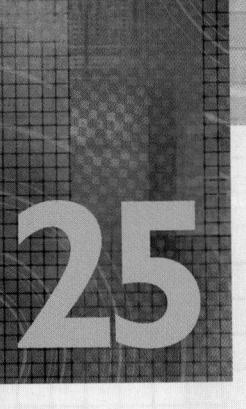

25

Nursing Care of Patients with Cardiac Dysrhythmias

LINDA S. WILLIAMS

KEY TERMS

ablation (uh-BLAY-shun)

atrial depolarization (AY-tree-uhl DE-poh-lahr-i-ZAY-shun)

atrial systole (AY-tree-uhl SIS-tuh-lee)

atrioventricular node (AY-tree-oh-ven-TRICK-yoo-lar NOHD)

bigeminy (bye-JEM-i-nee)

bradycardia (BRAY-dee-KAR-dee-yah)

bundle of His (BUN-duhl of HISS)

cardioversion (KAR-de-oh-VER-zhun)

defibrillation (dee-FIB-ri-lay-shun)

dysrhythmia (dis-RITH-mee-yah)

electrocardiogram (ee-LECK-troh-KAR-dee-oh-GRAM)

fluoroscopy (fluh-RAHS-kuh-pee)

hyperkalemia (HIGH-per-kuh-LEE-mee-ah)

hypomagnesemia (HIGH-poh-MAG-nuh-ZEE-mee-ah)

isoelectric line (EYE-so-e-LECK-trick LINE)

multifocal (MUHL-tee-FOH-kuhl)

nodal or junctional rhythm (NOHD-uhl or JUNGK-shun-uhl RITH-uhm)

sinoatrial node (SIGH-noh-AY-tree-al NOHD)

trigeminy (try-JEM-i-nee)

unifocal (YOO-ni-FOH-kuhl)

ventricular diastole (ven-TRICK-yoo-lar dye-AS-tuh-lee)

ventricular escape rhythm (ven-TRICK-yoo-lar es-KAYP RITH-uhm)

ventricular repolarization (ven-TRICK-yoo-lar RE-pol-lahr-i-ZAY-shun)

ventricular systole (ven-TRICK-yoo-lar SIS-tuh-lee)

ventricular tachycardia (ven-TRICK-yoo-lar TACK-ee-KAR-dee-yah)

QUESTIONS TO GUIDE YOUR READING

1. How does electrical activity flow through the heart?

2. What are the five steps used for dysrhythmia interpretation?

3. What are current medical treatments for each of the cardiac dysrhythmias?

4. What are types and uses of cardiac pacemakers?

5. What nursing care would you provide for patients with dysrhythmias or a pacemaker?

⬡ CARDIAC CONDUCTION SYSTEM

The heart's electrical conduction system initiates an impulse whose purpose is to stimulate the cardiac muscle to contract (Fig. 25.1). This electrical activity can be viewed on a cardiac monitor or recorded on an **electrocardiogram** (ECG) tracing. The activity seen on the ECG does not necessarily mean that the heart has contracted in response to the electrical impulse. The patient's vital signs and pulses verify that contraction occurs.

Located in the upper posterior wall of the right atrium is the **sinoatrial** (SA) **node.** The SA node is the primary pacemaker of the heart. It normally fires at a rate of 60 to 100 beats per minute (bpm). As a protective mechanism if the SA node does not function properly, other areas of the heart can initiate impulses to keep the heart beating. If the SA node fails, the **atrioventricular** (AV) **node** initiates an impulse at 40 to 60 bpm. This is referred to as a **nodal or junctional rhythm.** The body can usually function adequately with this rhythm. If the AV node is unable to initiate an impulse, then the ventricles take over at 20 to 40 bpm. When the ventricles initiate the impulse, the heart's rhythm is third-degree or complete heart block, or **ventricular escape rhythm.** Ventricular rhythms are the heart's last attempt to compensate for loss of SA and AV node impulse initiation. The ventricular rate of 20 to 40 bpm is not adequate to meet the body's oxygen needs, so the patient begins to show signs of inadequate cardiac output such as dyspnea, abnormal vital signs, and changes in level of consciousness. Treatment is usually necessary to reestablish a normal heart rate as soon as possible.

Normally after the SA node fires, the impulse travels across both atria, stimulating them to contract. This is known as **atrial systole.** This atrial contraction propels blood out of the atria and into the relaxed ventricles during **ventricular diastole.** The impulse then travels down the atria to the AV node where it is delayed briefly. Next it travels down the **bundle of His,** which divides into right and left bundle branches. From there the impulse quickly travels through the Purkinje fibers, stimulating both ventricles to contract. This contraction is known as **ventricular systole.**

Cardiac Cycle

A cardiac cycle is the period from the beginning of one heartbeat to the beginning of the next. The cardiac cycle is the electrical representation of the impulse that stimulates contraction and then relaxation of the atria and ventricles. Within the normal cardiac cycle, there is a P wave, a QRS complex, and a T wave (Fig. 25.2).

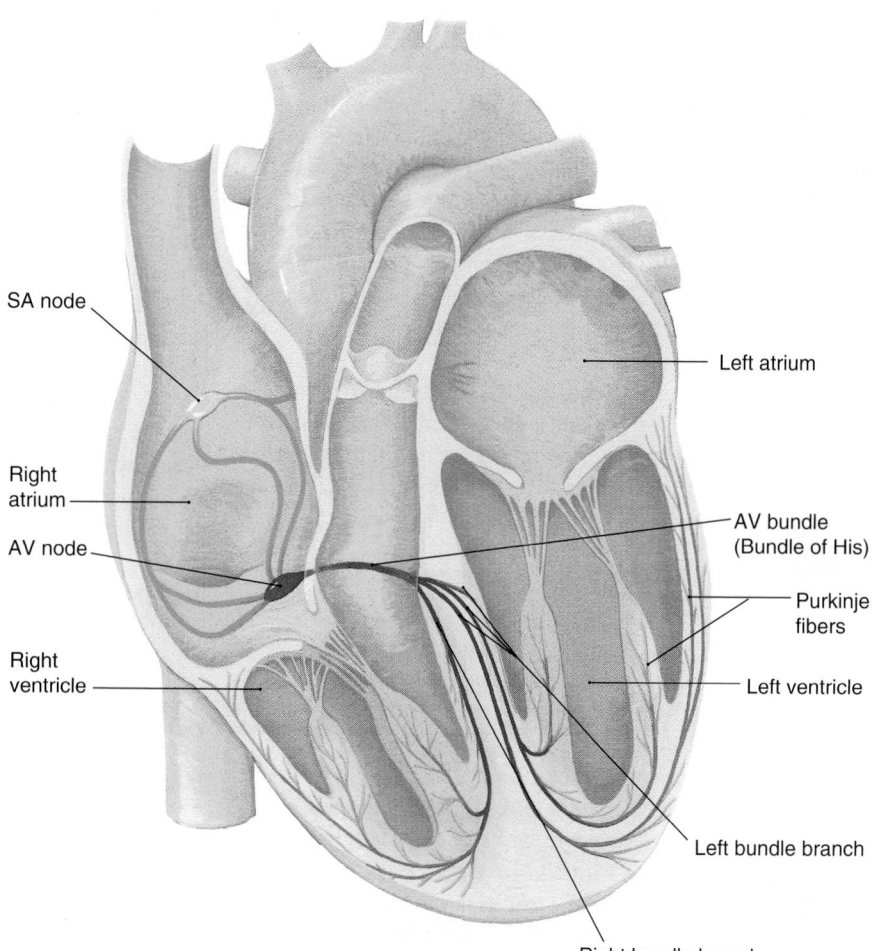

FIGURE 25.1 Conduction pathway of the heart. (*From Scanlon, V, and Sanders, T: Essentials of Anatomy and Physiology, ed. 5. F.A. Davis, Philadelphia, 2007.*)

SA node

Right atrium

AV node

Right ventricle

Left atrium

AV bundle (Bundle of His)

Purkinje fibers

Left ventricle

Left bundle branch

Right bundle branch

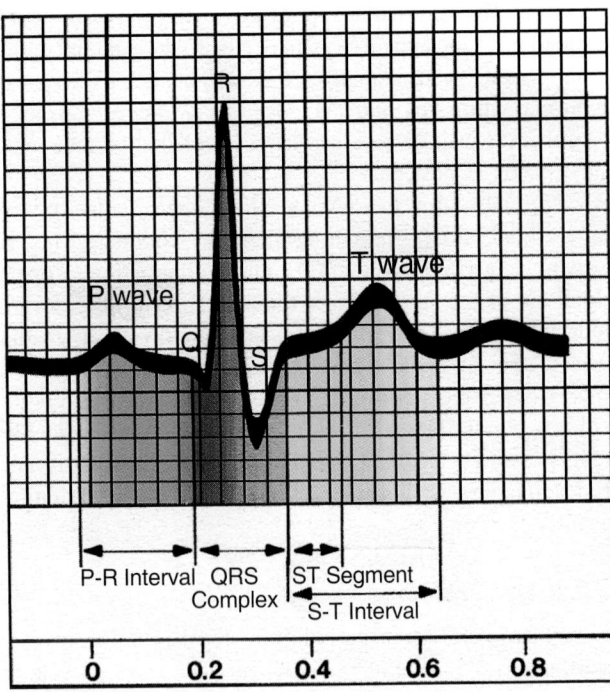

FIGURE 25.2 Components of the cardiac cycle. *(From Scanlon, V, and Sanders, T: Essentials of Anatomy and Physiology, ed. 5. F.A. Davis, Philadelphia, 2007.)*

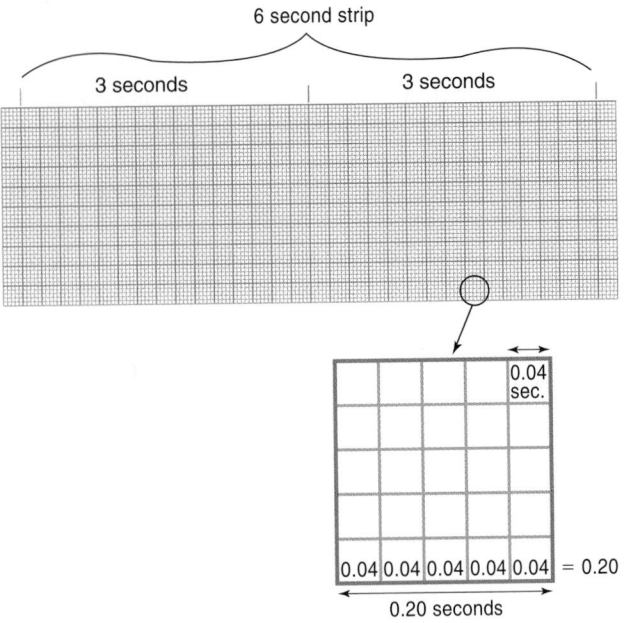

FIGURE 25.3 Electrocardiogram recording paper time intervals.

 ELECTROCARDIOGRAM

The electrical activity of the heart can be viewed with ongoing cardiac monitoring or by obtaining an ECG reflecting the activity just at that moment. Leads placed on the patient allow different views of the heart to be seen. A 12-lead ECG provides 12 different perspectives of the heart, while an 18-lead ECG allows 18 views. Waveforms change in appearance in the different leads. For continuous monitoring, lead II is the most commonly used. In lead II, the waveforms can be expected to be upright.

Specialized training usually by physicians is required to interpret ECGs for normal and abnormal function. By learning characteristics of a normal heart rhythm and rules

for common **dysrhythmias,** you will be able to report rhythm changes to your supervisor or physician.

Electrocardiogram Graph Paper

The intervals of each of the components of a cardiac cycle can be measured on the ECG graph paper on which the rhythm is recorded. The graph paper is calibrated in a grid with small squares divided into heavy lined blocks of 25 (five squares wide and five squares high; Fig. 25.3). Each small box is 0.04 seconds wide. There are five small squares, which equal 0.20 seconds of time, between two horizontally heavy vertical black lines (see Fig. 25.3). The height of waveforms (amplitude) is measured vertically. Each small square is 1 mm. Ten millimeters is the standard height that the ECG uses to measure patient waveforms.

When the ECG is on but there is no electrical activity detected, a straight line is produced. This **isoelectric line** occurs when there are no positive or negative electrical wave deflections. Cardiac cycle impulses (seen as waves), depending on how they travel through the heart, are either upright (positive) or downward (negative) from the isoelectric line on the ECG graph paper.

LEARNING TIP

Think of a 12- or 18-lead ECG as if you had a camera that you were using to take pictures or views of an object such as an apple. To obtain views that showed you all the sides of the apple—front, side, back, side—you would take a picture and then move the camera a little to get the view next to the one you had just taken. You would continue moving the camera until you had worked your way around the apple. This would then give you a complete view of the entire apple. This is what an ECG does for viewing the heart.

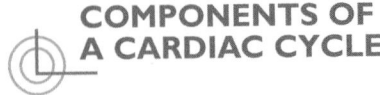 **COMPONENTS OF A CARDIAC CYCLE**

P Wave

The P wave is the first wave of the cardiac cycle and represents **atrial depolarization.** When the SA node fires, the P wave normally appears rounded and symmetrical. There is

---

dysrhythmia: dys—difficult or abnormal + rhythm—rhythm

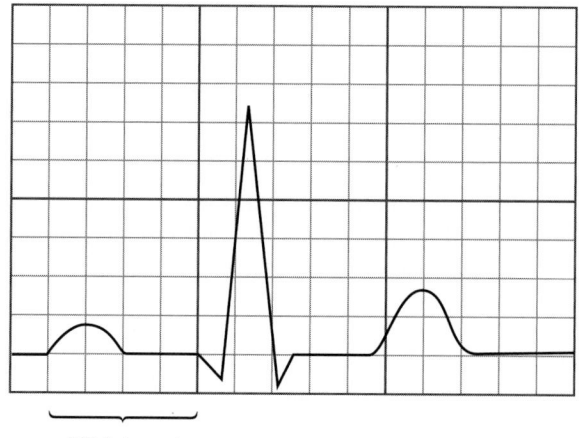

PR interval

FIGURE 25.4 PR interval.

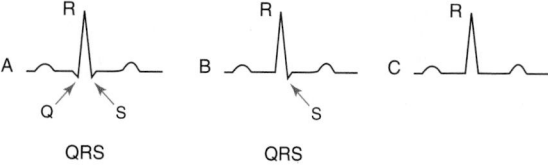

FIGURE 25.5 *(A)* QRS complex with a Q wave. *(B)* QRS complex without a Q wave. *(C)* QRS complex without a Q or an S wave.

to the isoelectric line (this is why locating the isoelectric line is helpful when first learning to identify waves). It is important to note that all three waves are not always present in every QRS complex. Even with absent waves, the QRS is still referred to as the QRS complex and can be considered normal (Fig. 25.5).

Atrial repolarization occurs during the interval of the QRS but is not seen because of the more powerful ventricular activity. The presence of the P wave in the following cardiac cycle indicates that atrial repolarization has occurred.

QRS Interval

To measure the QRS interval, count the number of boxes from the wave that begins the QRS complex to the end of the wave that completes the QRS complex. For example, when a Q, R, and S are present, measure from the beginning of the Q wave to the end of the S wave (Fig. 25.6). If there is only an R present, measure from the beginning of the R to the end of the R. The normal QRS interval is <0.12 seconds.

T Wave

The T wave represents **ventricular repolarization,** the resting state of the heart, when the ventricles are filling with blood and preparing to receive the next impulse. The T wave starts at the next upward (positive) deflection, after the QRS complex, and ends with a return to the isoelectric line. The T wave can be a downward deflection after the QRS complex in some ECG leads, or it can indicate ischemia of the heart (Fig. 25.7).

LEARNING TIP

To make measuring waves easier:
- Identify the isoelectric line as you measure waveform tracings to help you determine the type of wave. Use a straight edge resting below the line to see any waves above the line; then rest the straight edge above the line to see any waves that fall below the line.
- Try to find a wave that starts at the beginning of one small box (Fig. 25.4). If the wave starts or ends in the middle of a box, count it as one-half of a box, which is 0.02 seconds.

one P wave in a normal cardiac cycle. Disorders that change atrial size cause alterations in P wave shape and size.

PR Interval

The PR interval represents the time it takes the electrical impulse to travel down the atrium to the AV node. It starts at the beginning of the P wave and ends at the beginning of the QRS complex. Counting the number of small boxes horizontally that the interval covers determines the length of the PR interval (see Fig. 25.4). The normal PR interval is 0.12 to 0.20 second.

QRS Complex

The QRS complex represents ventricular depolarization and is composed of three waves, the Q, R, and S. The Q wave is the first downward deflection after the P wave but before the R wave. The R wave is the first upward deflection after the P wave. The last part of the QRS complex is the S wave, which is the second negative deflection after the P wave when a Q wave is present or the first negative deflection after the R wave (see Fig. 25.2). The S wave ends when it returns

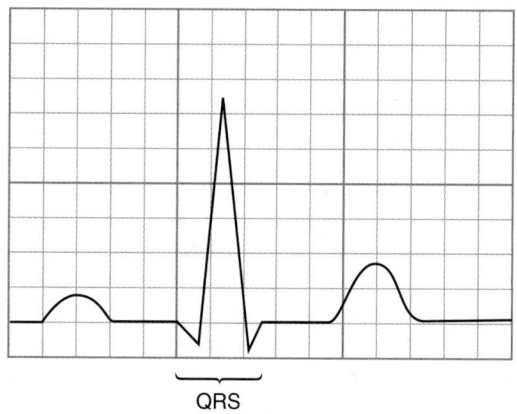

QRS

FIGURE 25.6 QRS interval. This QRS interval covers two and one-half boxes. Each full box is 0.04 seconds. One-half box is 0.02 seconds; 2.5 × 0.04 = 0.10 seconds.

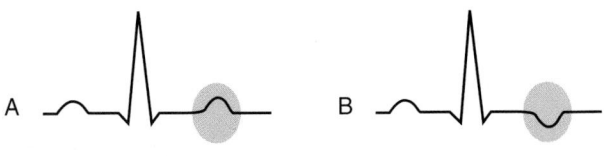

FIGURE 25.7 *(A)* T wave with positive deflection. *(B)* T wave with inverted, negative inflection, indicating ischemia.

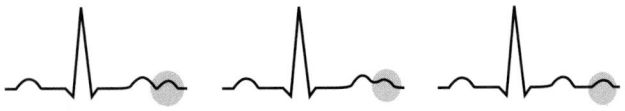

FIGURE 25.8 Various locations where U waves may appear.

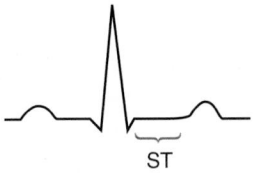

FIGURE 25.9 ST segment.

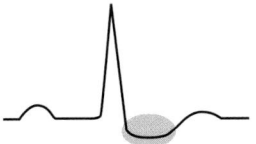

FIGURE 25.10 ST segment inverted or depressed.

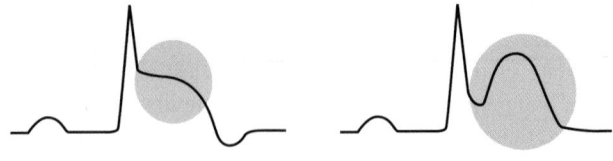

FIGURE 25.11 ST segment elevated.

U Wave

The U waveform is usually not present. It is seen in patients with hypokalemia, which is a low serum potassium level. It occurs shortly after the T wave and can distort the configuration of the T wave (Fig. 25.8).

ST Segment

The ST segment reflects the time from completion of a contraction (depolarization) to recovery (repolarization) of myocardial muscle for the next impulse. The ST segment starts at the end of the QRS and ends at the beginning of the T wave (Fig. 25.9). The ST segment is examined for patients experiencing chest pain. Changes in the ST segment can indicate the presence of ischemia or an injury pattern suggestive of myocardial damage. If a patient has ischemia, the ST segment can be inverted or depressed (Fig. 25.10). With cardiac injury, the ST segment elevates from the isoelectric line (Fig. 25.11).

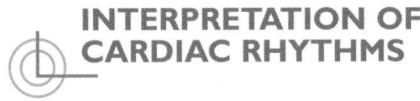

INTERPRETATION OF CARDIAC RHYTHMS

Five-Step Process for Dysrhythmia Interpretation

An orderly, systematic method for interpreting ECG rhythms should be used to increase understanding of items to examine and ensure nothing is overlooked. Five steps are examined in this process (Table 25.1). The findings of these five steps allow interpretation of the ECG rhythm according to the rules for each dysrhythmia. A 6-second ECG strip is used when interpreting rhythms. (See Fig. 25.3.)

Step 1. Regularity of the Rhythm

The regularity or rhythm of the heartbeat can be determined by looking at the R-R interval on the ECG (Fig. 25.12). The same spacing between each R-R interval, with a variation of no greater than two small boxes, is seen in a normal rhythm. To determine the regularity of a rhythm, count the number of small boxes between every R wave, which normally should remain the same, or use a caliper to measure the R-R interval.

A caliper is a small, two-sided, movable metal instrument with a sharp point at the end of each side. It is V-shaped when spread apart to measure distances. To use a caliper for measuring, one point is placed at the top of an R wave and the other point is spread apart until it rests on the top of the next R wave. Then, without changing the distance between the caliper points, the caliper is moved from one R wave to the next across the ECG tracing (also known as a strip) to see if the distance remains the same for each R-R interval. If the distance is the same, the rhythm is regular. If the distance changes, the rhythm is irregular. An irregular rhythm can be regularly irregular, which means it has a predictable pattern of irregularity, or irregularly irregular, without any pattern of irregularity.

LEARNING TIP

If a caliper is not available, a piece of paper can be placed on the ECG strip. A mark can be made on the paper at the top of one R wave and another mark made on the paper at the top of the next R wave. The marks on the paper can then be moved across the R-R intervals on the strip (just as caliper points would be) to determine whether the rhythm is regular or irregular.

Step 2. Heart Rate

After the rhythm regularity is determined, the heart rate is counted. One of the two following methods may be used.

1. Six-second method: The 6-second method is used for irregular rhythms. It may also be used when a rapid estimate of a regular rhythm is needed,

although it is not the most accurate method for regular rhythms. At the top of ECG graph paper there are vertical marks at 3-second intervals (see Fig. 25.3). Count the number of R waves in a 6-second strip and multiply the total by 10 (the number of 6 seconds in a minute) to obtain the beats per minute (6 seconds × 10 = 60 seconds or 1 minute) (Fig. 25.13).

2. Count the number of small (0.04-second) boxes between two R waves and divide that number into 1500. This gives the bpm, because 1500 small boxes equal 1 minute (Fig. 25.14). This method is used only for regular rhythms and is very accurate.

Step 3. P Wave

The P waves on the ECG strip are examined to see if (1) there is one P wave in front of every QRS, (2) the P waves are regular, and (3) the P waves all look alike. (See Fig. 25.1.) If all the P waves meet these criteria, they are considered normal. If they do not, further examination of the strip is necessary to determine the dysrhythmia.

Step 4. PR Interval

All PR intervals are measured to determine whether they are normal and constant. If the PR is found to vary, it is important to note whether there is a pattern to the variation.

Step 5. QRS Complex

The QRS intervals are measured to determine whether they are all normal and constant. Then the QRS complexes are examined to see if they all look alike.

TABLE 25.1 FIVE-STEP PROCESS FOR DYSRHYTHMIA INTERPRETATION

After answering the questions listed here, you should be able to name the patient's dysrhythmia.

Step	Topic	Assessment Questions
1	Regularity of rhythm	• Is the rhythm regular? Irregular?
2	Heart rate	• Is there a pattern to the irregularity?
3	P waves	• What is the heart rate?
		• Is there one P wave for every QRS complex?
		• Are the P waves regular and constant?
		• Do the P waves look alike?
		• Are the P waves upright and in front of every QRS complex?
4	PR interval	• Is the PR interval normal?
		• Is the PR interval constant or varying?
5	QRS interval	• Is the QRS interval normal?
		• Is the QRS interval constant?
		• Do the QRS complexes all look alike?

NORMAL SINUS RHYTHM

Description

Normal sinus rhythm is the normal cardiac rhythm (Fig. 25.15). It begins in the SA node and has complete, regular cardiac cycles.

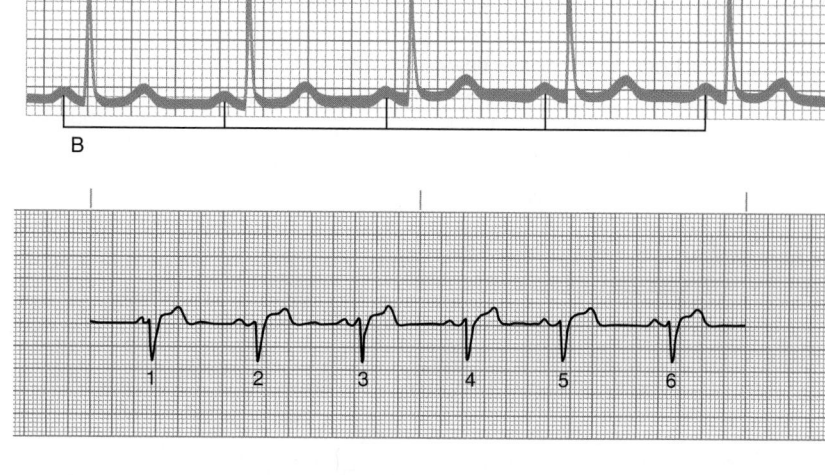

FIGURE 25.12 Normal cardiac waves are equal distances apart. *(A)* R-R waves. *(B)* P-P waves.

FIGURE 25.13 Counting R waves in a 6-second strip. There are six R waves in this 6-second strip, and 6 × 10 = 60 beats per minute.

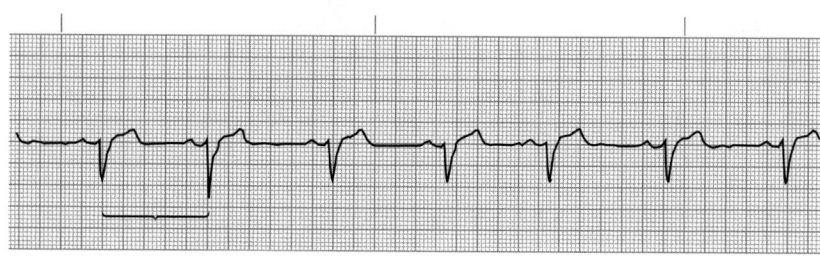

FIGURE 25.14 Heart rate. Count small boxes and divide by 1500 or count large boxes and divide by 300. Count number of large boxes between two R waves and divide into 300; five large boxes, 300/5 = 60 beats per minute.

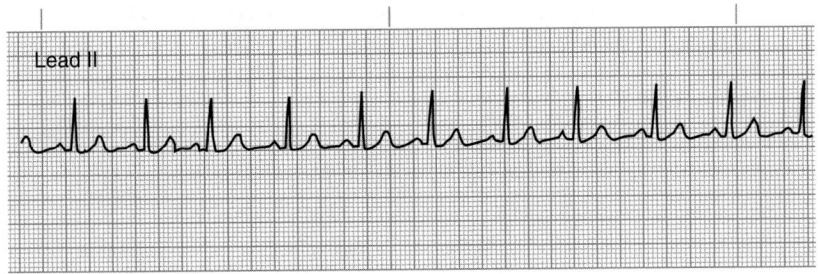

FIGURE 25.15 Normal sinus rhythm.

Normal Sinus Rhythm Rules

1. Rhythm: regular
2. Heart rate: 60 to 100 bpm
3. P waves: rounded, precede each QRS complex, alike
4. PR interval: 0.12 to 0.20 seconds
5. QRS interval: <0.12 seconds

 DYSRHYTHMIAS

Two terms are used for rhythm disturbances: *arrhythmia* and *dysrhythmia*. An arrhythmia is an irregularity or loss of rhythm of the heartbeat, and a dysrhythmia is an abnormal, disordered, or disturbed rhythm. These two terms are used interchangeably, but dysrhythmia is the most accurate term for the discussion of abnormal rhythms. For more information about cardiac care for dysrhythmias, visit the American Heart Association website at www.americanheart.org.

Several mechanisms can cause irregularity or dysrhythmia. Two examples of these mechanisms are a disturbance in the formation of an impulse and a disturbance in the conduction of the impulse. When impulse formation is disturbed, the impulse may arise from the atria, the AV node, or the ventricles. This disturbance can be seen as an increased or decreased heart rate, early or late beats, or atrial or ventricular fibrillation. With a disturbance in conduction there may be normal formation of the impulse, but it becomes blocked within the electrical conduction system, resulting in abnormal conduction (as in heart block or bundle branch blocks).

Dysrhythmias Originating in the Sinoatrial Node

Rhythms arising from the SA node are referred to as sinus rhythms. The SA node, being the pacemaker of the heart, fires normally at 60 to 100 bpm. Disturbances in conduction from the SA node can cause irregular rhythms or abnormal heart rates. Dysrhythmias arising from the SA node are rarely dangerous. Patients, especially those with heart, lung, or kidney disease, who cannot tolerate a rapid or slow heart rate may require treatment.

LEARNING TIP

The origin and type of a problem are used to name a dysrhythmia. Let us name a slow dysrhythmia that originates in the SA node. The origin is sinus and the type of problem (slow) is bradycardia = sinus bradycardia. The term *normal* is not used since there is a problem. So what would a fast dysrhythmia originating in the SA node be called? Yes, it is *sinus tachycardia*.

Sinus Bradycardia

DESCRIPTION. **Bradycardia** is a slower than normal heart rate. Sinus bradycardia has the same cardiac cycle components as a normal sinus rhythm. The only difference between the two is a slower heart rate caused by fewer impulses originating from the SA node (Fig. 25.16). Can you see that the name *sinus bradycardia* tells you this difference? The name says the impulse is coming from the sinus node (sinus) but at a slower rate than normal (bradycardia). See, it is easy to understand what is happening in the dysrhythmia when you look at what the name tells you.

CAUSES. Medications such as digoxin (Lanoxin), myocardial infarction (MI), and electrolyte imbalances can cause bradycardia. Well-conditioned athletes also can have slower heart rates because their hearts work more efficiently.

---

bradycardia: bradys—slow + kardia—heart

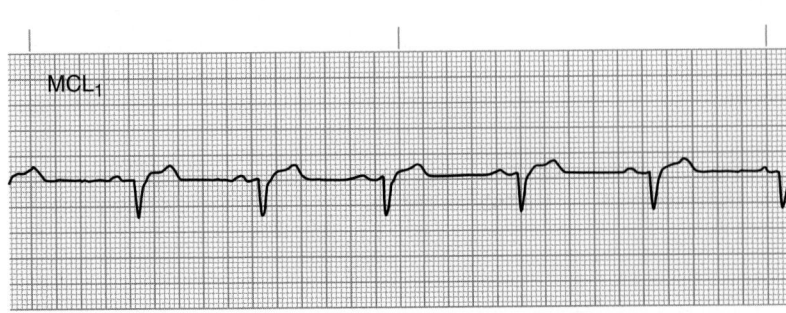

FIGURE 25.16 Sinus bradycardia.

SINUS BRADYCARDIA RULES

1. Rhythm: regular
2. Heart rate: less than 60 bpm
3. P waves: smoothly rounded, precede each QRS complex, alike
4. PR interval: 0.12 to 0.20 seconds
5. QRS interval: <0.12 seconds

SIGNS AND SYMPTOMS. Sinus bradycardia rarely produces symptoms unless it is so slow that it reduces cardiac output. Symptoms consist of fatigue or fainting episodes.

THERAPEUTIC INTERVENTIONS. Treatment is usually not required if the patient is asymptomatic. The patient is observed for symptoms, and the underlying cause is determined for correction. Oxygen and intravenous (IV) access may be started. If bradycardia is due to a heart block dysrhythmia, insertion of a cardiac pacemaker may be required. If the patient is symptomatic, therapeutic interventions may include atropine sulfate, transcutaneous pacing, dopamine, epinephrine, or isoproterenol. Medications are given IV by a registered nurse for immediate effect. The treatments increase the heart rate for a short time until a cause can be determined and treated.

Sinus Tachycardia

DESCRIPTION. Tachycardia is defined as a heart rate greater than 100 beats per minute. Sinus tachycardia has the same components as a normal sinus rhythm except the heart rate is faster (Fig. 25.17). More impulses originating from the SA node than normal cause this.

CAUSES. Sinus tachycardia causes include physical activity; hemorrhage; shock; medications such as epinephrine, atropine, or nitrates; dehydration; fever; MI; electrolyte imbalance; fear; and anxiety. Tachycardia occurs as a compensatory mechanism for hypoxia when more cardiac output is needed to deliver oxygen to organs and tissues.

SINUS TACHYCARDIA RULES

1. Rhythm: regular
2. Heart rate: 101 to 180 bpm
3. P waves: rounded, precede each QRS complex, alike
4. PR interval: 0.12 to 0.20 seconds
5. QRS interval: <0.12 seconds

SIGNS AND SYMPTOMS. Sinus tachycardia may not produce symptoms. If the heart rate is very rapid and sustained for long periods, the patient may experience angina or dyspnea. Older patients may become symptomatic more rapidly than younger patients (Box 25.1 Geronotological Issues). Patients with MI may not tolerate a rapid heart rate and have more severe symptoms since cardiac workload is increased.

THERAPEUTIC INTERVENTIONS. Treatment depends on the cause and symptoms. Medications such as digoxin, calcium channel blockers (verapamil [Calan]), or beta blockers (propranolol [Inderal]) may be used to slow the heart rate. Oxygen may also be prescribed to ensure an

adequate supply for the heart. The treatment goal is to decrease the heart's workload and resolve the cause, which then usually corrects the tachycardia. For example, if the patient is hemorrhaging, immediate intervention is needed to stop the bleeding and restore normal blood volume. Once normal blood volume is restored, the heart rate should return to normal.

LEARNING TIP

Tachycardia is often the first sign of hemorrhage. It is a compensatory mechanism to maintain cardiac output. If a patient develops sudden tachycardia, consider whether hemorrhage could be the cause, such as in postoperative patients, patients with gastrointestinal bleeding or cancer, or trauma patients. The bleeding may be external, or it may be internal and therefore not visible. Apply pressure to the site if the bleeding is obvious. Monitor the patient and report the tachycardia and any obvious bleeding promptly.

Dysrhythmias Originating in the Atria

As previously discussed, all areas of the heart can initiate an impulse. The SA node is the primary pacemaker, but if the atria initiate impulses faster than the SA node, they become the primary pacemaker. Atrial rhythms are usually faster than 100 bpm and can exceed 200 bpm. When an impulse originates outside the SA node, the P waves produced look different from the rounded P waves from the SA node (flatter, notched, or peaked), which indicates that the SA node is not controlling the heart rate. These atrial impulses travel to the ventricles to initiate a normal QRS complex after each P wave.

LEARNING TIP

- If a QRS complex measures less than 0.12 seconds and there is a dysrhythmia present, the problem originated above the ventricles. This is known as a supraventricular (above the ventricle) dysrhythmia.
- Ventricular originating dysrhythmias produce wide QRS complexes that are greater than 0.11 seconds.

Premature Atrial Contractions

DESCRIPTION. The term *premature* refers to an "early" beat. When the atria fire an impulse before the SA node fires, a premature beat results. If the underlying rhythm is sinus rhythm, the distance between R waves is the same

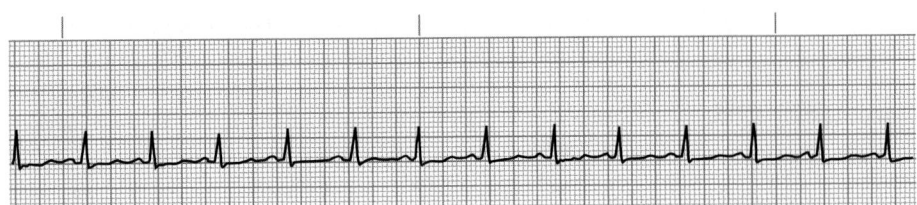

FIGURE 25.17 Sinus tachycardia.

except where the early beat occurs. When looking at the ECG strip, a shortened R-R interval is seen where the premature beat occurs. The R wave preceding the premature atrial contraction (PAC) and the PAC's R wave are close together, followed by a pause, with the next beat being regular (Fig. 25.18).

CAUSES. Causes of PACs include hypoxia, smoking, stress, myocardial ischemia, enlarged atria in valvular disorders, medications (such as digoxin), electrolyte imbalances, atrial fibrillation onset, and heart failure.

PREMATURE ATRIAL CONTRACTIONS RULES

1. Rhythm: premature beat interrupts underlying rhythm where it occurs
2. Heart rate: depends on the underlying rhythm; if normal sinus rhythm (NSR), 60 to 100 bpm
3. P waves: early beat is abnormally shaped
4. PR interval: usually appears normal, but premature beat could have shortened or prolonged PR interval
5. QRS interval: <0.12 seconds (indicates normal conduction to ventricles)

SIGNS AND SYMPTOMS. Premature atrial contractions can occur in healthy individuals, as well as in the patient with a diseased heart. No symptoms are usually present. If many PACs occur in succession, the patient may report the sensation of palpitations.

THERAPEUTIC INTERVENTIONS. PACs are usually not dangerous, and often no treatment is required other than correcting the cause. Frequent PACs indicate atrial irritability, which may worsen into other atrial dysrhythmias. Quinidine or procainamide can be given to a patient having frequent PACs to slow the heart rate.

Atrial Flutter

DESCRIPTION. In atrial flutter, the atria contract, or flutter, at a rate of 250 to 350 bpm. The very rapid P waves appear as flutter, or F waves, on ECG and appear in a saw-toothed pattern. Some of the impulses get through the AV node and reach the ventricles, resulting in normal QRS complexes. There can be from two to four F waves between QRS complexes. If impulses pass through the AV node at a consistent rate, the rhythm is regular (Fig. 25.19). The classic characteristics of atrial flutter are more than one P wave before a QRS complex, a saw-toothed pattern of P waves, and an atrial rate of 250 to 350 bpm.

CAUSES. Causes of atrial flutter include rheumatic or ischemic heart diseases, congestive heart failure (CHF), hypertension, pericarditis, pulmonary embolism, and post-operative coronary artery bypass surgery. Many medications can also cause this dysrhythmia.

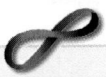

Box 25.1

Gerontological Issues

Dysrhythmia Risk

Factors that increase the risk of dysrhythmias in older adults include the following:
- Digitalis toxicity (most common)
- Hypokalemia
- Acute infection
- Hemorrhage
- Angina
- Coronary insufficiency (exercise, stress)

   Dysrhythmias that occur most often in older adults include the following:
- Atrial fibrillation (atria beating 400 to 700 times per minute)
- Sick sinus syndrome (alternating episodes of bradycardia, normal sinus rhythm, tachycardia, and periods of long sinus pause)

- Heart block (delayed or blocked impulses to the atria or ventricles)

   Age-related effects of dysrhythmias include the following:
- Weakness
- Fatigue
- Forgetfulness
- Palpitations
- Dizziness
- Hypotension
- Bradycardia
- Syncope

   Older adults are especially sensitive to changes in heart rate that increase the heart's workload. Whenever the heart works harder, as in tachycardia, the cardiac cells require more oxygen to function properly. Older patients have less ability to adapt to sudden changes or stressors, and they may not be able to tolerate tachycardia for very long. Any new-onset tachycardia in an older patient should be reported promptly.

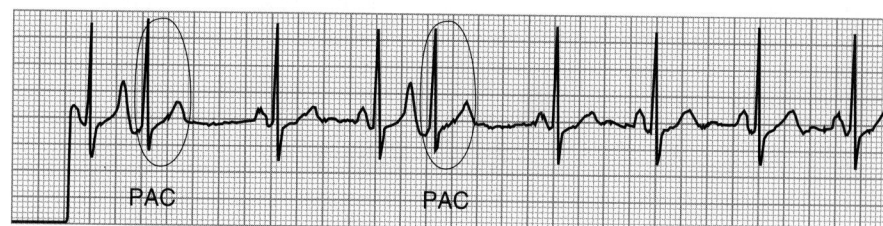

FIGURE 25.18 Premature atrial contractions (PAC).

ATRIAL FLUTTER RULES

1. Rhythm: atrial rhythm regular; ventricular rhythm regular or irregular depending on consistency of AV conduction of impulses
2. Heart rate: ventricular rate varies
3. P waves: flutter or F waves with saw-toothed pattern
4. PR interval: none measurable
5. QRS complex: <0.12 seconds

SIGNS AND SYMPTOMS. The presence of symptoms in atrial flutter depends on the ventricular rate. If the ventricular rate is normal, usually no symptoms are present. If the rate is rapid, the patient may experience palpitations, angina, or dyspnea.

THERAPEUTIC INTERVENTIONS. The ventricular rate and cardiac output guide treatment. The goal is to control the ventricular rate and convert the rhythm. A rapid ventricular rate or symptoms of decreased cardiac output require **cardioversion** (electrical shock). If the rate is greater than 150 bpm, immediate cardioversion is needed. Medications that may be used to control the rate include calcium channel blockers and beta blockers. For rhythm conversion, digoxin can be used to slow conduction through the AV node and increase cardiac contractility. Other medications, such as quinidine, procainamide, or propranolol, can also be used to slow the heart rate.

Atrial Fibrillation

DESCRIPTION. In atrial fibrillation, the atrial rate is extremely rapid and chaotic. An atrial rate of 350 to 600 bpm can occur. However, the AV node blocks most of the impulses, so the ventricular rate is much lower than the atrial rate. There are no definable P waves because the atria are fibrillating, or quivering, rather than beating effectively. No P waves can be seen or measured. A wavy pattern is produced on the ECG. Because the atrial rate is so irregular and only a few of the atrial impulses are allowed to pass through the AV

node, the R waves are irregular. The ventricular rate varies from normal to rapid.

Atrial fibrillation can be self-limiting, persistent, or permanent. A complication of this dysrhythmia is an increased risk of thrombus formation in the atria from blood stasis caused by poor emptying of blood from the quivering atria (Fig. 25.20). This can result in stroke or pulmonary emboli.

CAUSES. Causes of atrial fibrillation include aging, rheumatic or ischemic heart diseases, heart failure, hypertension, pericarditis, pulmonary embolism, and postoperative coronary artery bypass surgery. Medications can also cause this dysrhythmia.

ATRIAL FIBRILLATION RULES

1. Rhythm: irregularly irregular
2. Heart rate: atrial rate not measurable; ventricular rate under 100 is controlled response; greater than 100 is rapid ventricular response
3. P waves: no identifiable P waves
4. PR interval: none can be measured because no P waves are seen
5. QRS complex: 0.06 to 0.10 seconds

LEARNING TIP

Atrial fibrillation is easy to identify based on its two classic characteristics: a lack of identifiable P waves and an irregularly irregular rhythm (R waves).

SYMPTOMS. With atrial fibrillation, most patients feel the irregular rhythm. Many describe it as palpitations or a skipping heartbeat. When checking a patient's radial pulse, it may be faint because of a decreased stroke volume (volume of blood ejected with each contraction). If the ventricular rhythm is rapid and sustained, the patient can go into left ventricular failure.

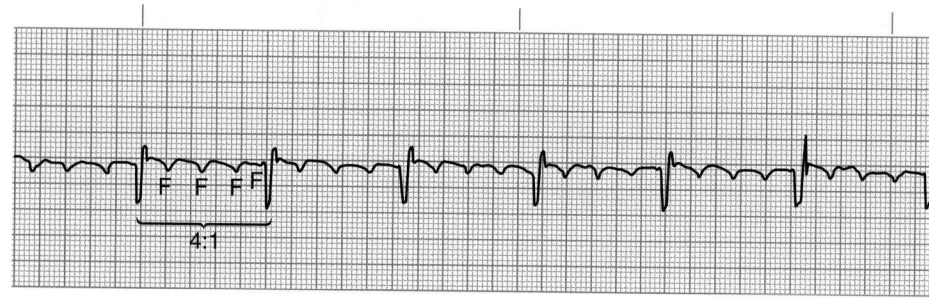

FIGURE 25.19 Atrial flutter.

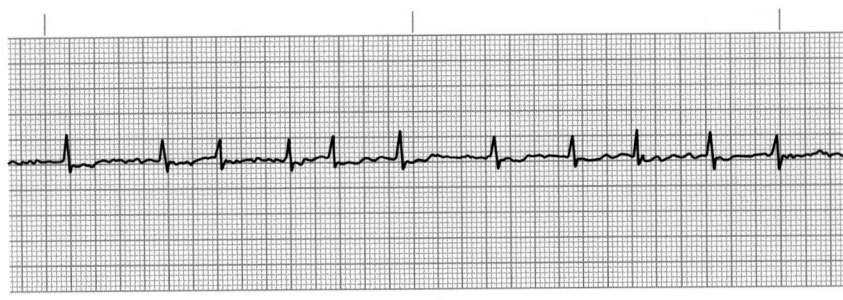

FIGURE 25.20 Atrial fibrillation.

THERAPEUTIC INTERVENTIONS. Treatment is based on the patient's stability. If the patient is unstable, cardioversion is done immediately to try to return the heart to normal sinus rhythm. If the patient is stable, medications to restore and maintain a normal sinus rhythm and control the ventricular rate may be used. The ventricular rate may be controlled with such medications as digoxin, beta blockers, or calcium channel blockers. Medications approved by the Food and Drug Administration to convert atrial fibrillation and maintain a normal sinus rhythm include dofetilide, quinidine, flecainide, propafenone, and ibutilide IV. Anticoagulant therapy (aspirin for low-risk patients, warfarin for those at high risk), which can be long term or lifelong, is given to reduce thrombi. International normalized ratio (INR) and prothrombin time levels must be carefully monitored for patients on warfarin. Chemical or electrical cardioversion may be performed to convert the rhythm after sufficient anticoagulation (about 3 weeks). If known, the underlying cause of the atrial fibrillation should also be treated.

Dual-chamber pacing for those with sinus node problems or biatrial pacing, as well as pacemaker recognition of atrial fibrillation, helps to prevent this dysrhythmia. Implantable cardioverter defibrillators (ICDs) can deliver a shock activated by the physician or patient to end the atrial fibrillation. Because this is a planned event, medications for comfort can be taken by the patient before the shock.

For patients with atrial fibrillation who do not respond to medications, **ablation** procedures may be performed

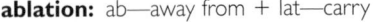

ablation: ab—away from + lat—carry

(discussed later). A surgical procedure can be performed if other treatments fail. The maze procedure was first done as open heart surgery, but a percutaneous, nonsurgical catheter maze procedure may be used to eliminate the risks of open heart surgery. In the open heart maze procedure, incisions are made in the atria that create a "maze," or route, for electrical impulses to travel through to the AV node. These impulses cannot go off course because scar tissue surrounds the incision sites. In many cases, this cures atrial fibrillation. However, some patients may need continued medications or a pacemaker following this procedure.

Ventricular Dysrhythmias
Premature Ventricular Contractions

DESCRIPTION. Premature ventricular contractions (PVCs) originate in the ventricles from an ectopic focus (a site other than the SA node). The ventricles are irritable and fire prematurely, before the SA node. When the ventricles fire first, the impulses are not conducted normally through the electrical pathway. This results in a wide (greater than 0.11 seconds), bizarre QRS complex on an ECG (Fig. 25.21).

PVCs can occur in different shapes. The shape of the PVC is referred to as **unifocal** (one focus) if all the PVCs look the same because they come from the same irritable ventricular area. **Multifocal** PVCs do not all look the same because they are originating from several irritable areas in the ventricle. There can be several repetitive cycles or patterns of PVCs:

- **Bigeminy** is a PVC that occurs every other beat (a normal beat and then a PVC) (Fig. 25.22).

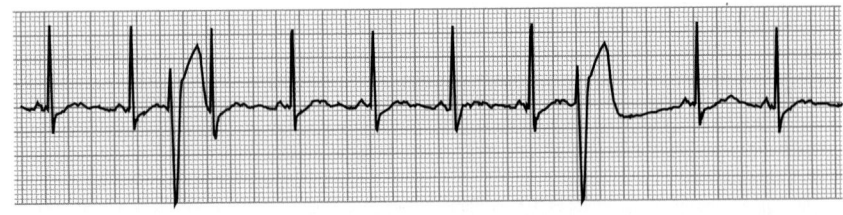

A

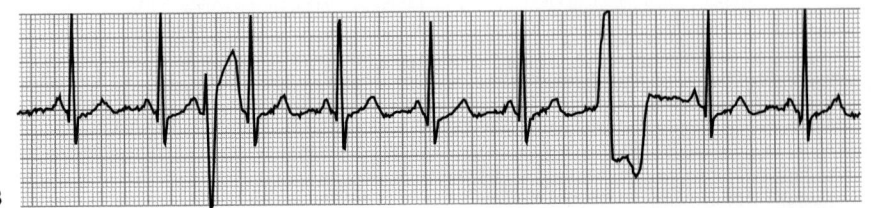

B

FIGURE 25.21 Premature ventricular contractions. (A) Unifocal PVCs arise from one area and look the same. (B) Multifocal PVCs arise from different foci and may look different.

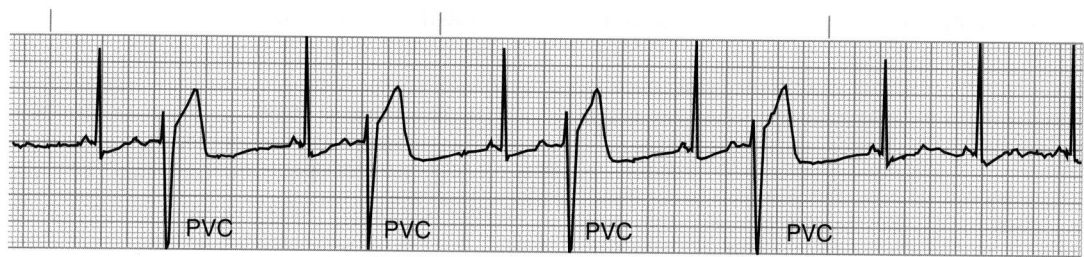

FIGURE 25.22 Bigeminal premature ventricular contractions.

- **Trigeminy** is a PVC that occurs every third beat (two normal beats and then a PVC).
- Quadrigeminy is a PVC that occurs every fourth beat (three normal beats and then a PVC).
- When two PVCs occur together, they are referred to as a couplet (pair).
- If three or more PVCs occur in a row, it is referred to as a run of PVCs or ventricular tachycardia.

CAUSES. Use of caffeine or alcohol, anxiety, hypokalemia, cardiomyopathy, ischemia, and MI are common causes of PVCs.

PREMATURE VENTRICULAR CONTRACTION RULES
1. Rhythm: depends on the underlying rhythm; PVC usually interrupts rhythm
2. Heart rate: depends on underlying rhythm
3. P waves: absent before PVC QRS complex
4. PR interval: none for PVC
5. QRS complex: if PVC, is greater than 0.11 seconds; T wave is in the opposite direction of QRS complex (i.e., QRS upright, T downward or QRS downward, T upright)

SIGNS AND SYMPTOMS. PVCs may be felt by the patient and are described as a skipped beat or palpitations. With frequent PVCs, cardiac output can be decreased, leading to fatigue, dizziness, or more severe dysrhythmias.

THERAPEUTIC INTERVENTIONS. Treatment depends on the type and number of PVCs and whether symptoms are produced. A few PVCs do not usually require treatment. However, if the PVCs are more than six per minute, regularly occurring, multifocal, falling on the T wave (known as "R-on-T phenomenon," which can trigger life-threatening dysrhythmias), or caused by an acute MI, they can be dangerous. Antidysrhythmic drugs that depress myocardial activity are used to treat PVCs. Examples of drugs that may

be given intravenously by the registered nurse and then followed by a continuous IV drip are procainamide (Procan) and lidocaine (Xylocaine).

Ventricular Tachycardia

DESCRIPTION. The occurrence of three or more PVCs in a row is referred to as **ventricular tachycardia** (VT) (Fig. 25.23). VT results from the continuous firing of an ectopic

---

CRITICAL THINKING

Mrs. Mae

■ Mrs. Mae, age 70, is 5 days post-MI without complications. You assist her back to bed at 1400 hours after she ambulates. Her oxygen is on at 2 L/min via nasal cannula. Her vital signs are 126/78, 82, 18. She has no pain and says she feels good after walking. The cardiac monitor shows normal sinus rhythm. Five minutes later, you see that the monitor shows sinus rhythm with PVCs of less than six per minute. Her vital signs are now 132/84, apical 92 irregular, 22. She reports no pain but says, "I can feel my heart skipping, it takes my breath away." You call the RN while staying with the patient for reassurance.

1. What should you do first?
2. What should you do regarding the dysrhythmia?
3. What might be some of the causes for this dysrhythmia?
4. What symptoms, if any, would you expect to be present?
5. What would you do if symptoms were present?
6. What type of orders would you anticipate from the physician?
7. How would you document your findings?

Suggested answers at end of chapter.

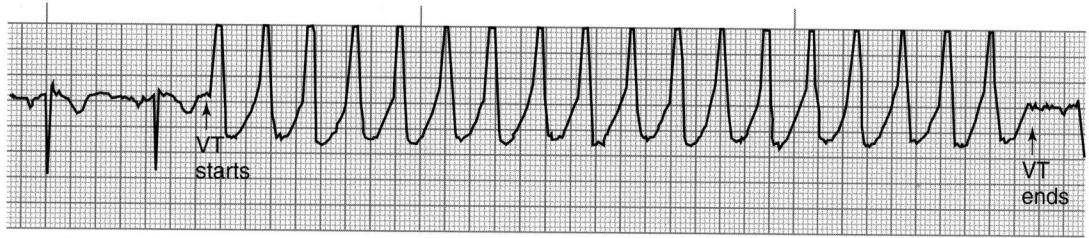

FIGURE 25.23 Ventricular tachycardia.

ventricular focus. During VT, the ventricles rather than the SA node become the pacemaker of the heart. The pathway of the ventricular impulses is different from normal conduction, producing a wide (greater than 0.11 seconds), bizarre QRS complex.

CAUSES. Myocardial irritability, MI, and cardiomyopathy are common causes of VT. Respiratory acidosis, hypokalemia, digoxin toxicity, cardiac catheters, and pacing wires can also produce VT.

VENTRICULAR TACHYCARDIA RULES
1. Rhythm: usually regular, may have some irregularity
2. Heart rate: 150 to 250 ventricular bpm; slow VT is below 150 bpm
3. P waves: absent
4. PR interval: none
5. QRS complex: greater than 0.11 seconds

SIGNS AND SYMPTOMS. The seriousness of ventricular tachycardia is determined by the duration of the dysrhythmia. Sustained VT compromises cardiac output. Patients are aware of a sudden onset of rapid heart rate and can experience dyspnea, palpitations, and light-headedness. Angina commonly occurs. The severity of symptoms can increase rapidly if the left ventricle fails and complete cardiac arrest results.

THERAPEUTIC INTERVENTIONS. If the patient is pulseless or not breathing, cardiopulmonary resuscitation (CPR) and immediate defibrillation are required. Current advanced cardiac life support (ACLS) protocols for VT treatment should follow.

If the patient is stable, medications can be tried first, such as amiodarone, procainamide, sotalol, lidocaine, phenytoin, or beta blockers following ACLS protocols. Magnesium can be used to help stabilize ventricular muscle excitability if the patient's magnesium level is low.

Ventricular Fibrillation
DESCRIPTION. Ventricular fibrillation occurs when many ectopic ventricular foci fire at the same time. Ventricular activity is chaotic with no discernible waves (Fig. 25.24). The ventricle quivers and is unable to initiate a contraction. There is a complete loss of cardiac output. If this rhythm is not terminated immediately, death ensues.

CAUSES. Hyperkalemia, hypomagnesemia, electrocution, coronary artery disease, and MI are all possible causes of ventricular fibrillation. Placement of intracardiac catheters and cardiac pacing wires can also lead to ventricular irritability and then ventricular fibrillation.

VENTRICULAR FIBRILLATION RULES
1. Rhythm: chaotic and extremely irregular
2. Heart rate: not measurable
3. P waves: none
4. PR interval: none
5. QRS complex: none

SIGNS AND SYMPTOMS. Patients experiencing ventricular fibrillation lose consciousness immediately. There are no heart sounds, peripheral pulses, or blood pressure. These are all indicative of circulatory collapse. Additionally, respiratory arrest, cyanosis, and pupil dilation occur.

THERAPEUTIC INTERVENTIONS. Immediate defibrillation is the very best treatment for terminating ventricular fibrillation. Each minute that passes without defibrillation reduces survival. CPR is started until the defibrillator is available. Automatic external defibrillators (AEDs) provide quick access to easily used technology for defibrillation (see defibrillation section). Endotracheal intubation and ventilation support respiratory function. Medications are given

---

hyperkalemia: hyper—above + kalium—potassium + emia—blood

hypomagnesemia: hypo—below + magnes—magnesium + emia—blood

> ### CRITICAL THINKING
>
> #### Mrs. Parker
>
> ■ You are caring for Mrs. Parker, age 66, on the cardiac medical unit. She had an MI and several episodes of ventricular tachycardia while she was in the ICU before transferring to your unit. At 1600 hours you find her unresponsive, with no palpable pulses and shallow respirations and in VT on the ECG. Vital signs are BP 80/40, P 150, R 6.
> 1. Why are there no palpable pulses?
> 2. What is occurring to the heart when it is in VT?
> 3. What action should you take?
> 4. How will you document your findings?
> *Suggested answers at end of chapter.*

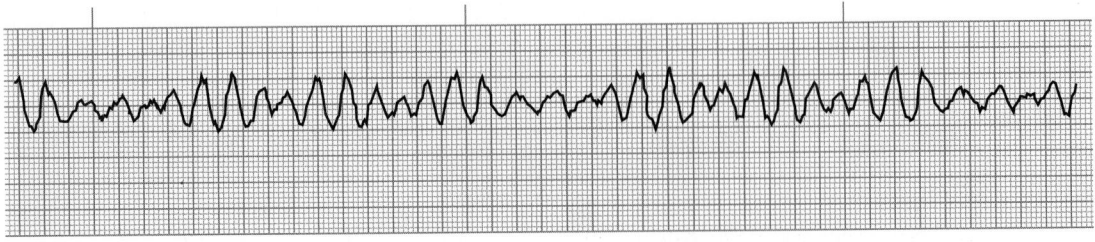

FIGURE 25.24 Ventricular fibrillation.

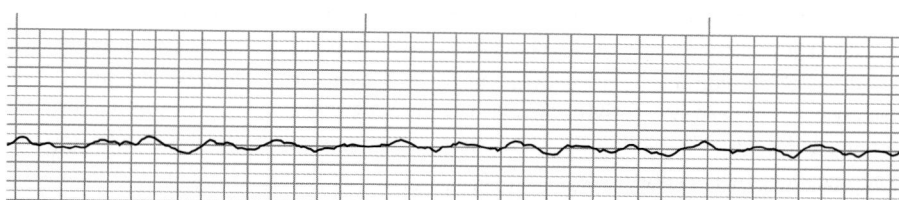

FIGURE 25.25 Asystole.

according to ACLS protocols and may include epinephrine, vasopressin, amiodarone, lidocaine, magnesium, and procainamide.

Asystole

DESCRIPTION. Asystole (the silent heart) is the absence of electrical activity in the cardiac muscle. It is referred to as cardiac arrest. A straight line appears on an ECG strip (Fig. 25.25). Ventricular fibrillation usually precedes this rhythm and must be reversed immediately to help prevent asystole.

CAUSES. Ventricular fibrillation and a loss of a majority of functional cardiac muscle due to an MI are common causes of asystole. Hyperkalemia is another cause of asystole.

ASYSTOLE RULES
1. Rhythm: none
2. Heart rate: none
3. P waves: none
4. PR interval: none
5. QRS complex: none

THERAPEUTIC INTERVENTIONS. CPR is started immediately. ACLS protocols for asystole are used. Endotracheal intubation to support respirations is performed. Transcutaneous pacing is considered, then epinephrine and atropine are administered.

CRITICAL THINKING

Mr. Peet

■ You are making rounds. When you enter Mr. Peet's room, you note that he is having difficulty breathing and is unresponsive.
1. What are your initial actions?
2. What should you do after assessing and finding no pulse or respirations?
3. What is your responsibility during a cardiac/respiratory arrest code?

Suggested answers at end of chapter.

CARDIAC PACEMAKERS

Pacemakers can be external and temporary or internal and permanent (Fig. 25.26). They are used to override dysrhythmias or to generate an impulse when the heart is beating too

slowly. Transcutaneous pacemakers are used in emergency situations because they are quick and easy to apply. Impulses are delivered to the heart through the skin from the external generator via electrodes that are attached to the chest and back.

Temporary pacemakers are used for bradycardias or tachycardias that do not respond to medications or cardioversion. They may also be used after an MI to allow the heart time to heal when the diseased myocardium is unable to respond to or is not receiving electrical conduction because of damage within the system. The temporary pacemaker becomes the electrical conduction system and stimulates the atria and ventricles to contract to maintain cardiac output. Temporary pacemakers can be inserted during valve or open heart surgery or in the cardiac catheterization laboratory or critical care unit at the bedside as emergency treatment until surgery can be scheduled to insert a permanent pacemaker.

Permanent pacemaker insertion is a surgical procedure in which **fluoroscopy,** a screen that shows an image similar to a radiograph, is used. The pacemaker generator is implanted subcutaneously and attached to one or two leads (insulated conducting wires) that are inserted via a vein into the heart. The lead can then deliver the impulse directly to the heart wall. A single-lead pacemaker paces either the right atrium or right ventricle depending on its chamber placement. Dual-chamber pacemakers have two leads, with one in the right atrium and the other in the right ventricle.

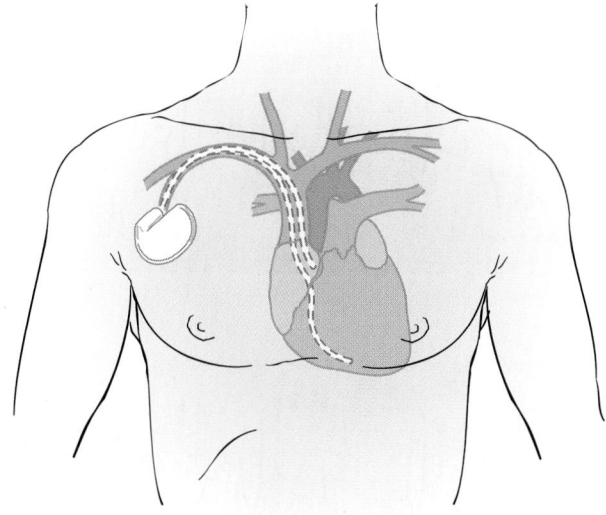

FIGURE 25.26 Insertion of dual-chamber permanent pacemaker.

This allows pacing of both chambers. Usually pacemakers are set at a prescribed rate of 72 bpm. Activity-responsive pacemakers provide a rate range (e.g., 60 to 115 bpm) in response to a person's activity level. This provides the patient with greater flexibility for increasing cardiac output when needed, such as during exercise.

When a patient is in a paced rhythm, a small spike is seen on the ECG before the paced beat. This spike is the electrical stimulus. It can precede the P wave, QRS complex, or both depending on what is being paced (Fig. 25.27). Patients may have all paced beats (100% paced), a mixture of their own beats and paced beats, or all of their own beats. Pacemakers should not fire when patients have their own beats.

Problems that can occur with pacemakers include the following:

- Failure to sense the patient's own beat
- Failure to pace because of a malfunction of the pulse generator
- Failure to capture, which is a lack of depolarization

Nursing Care for Patients with Pacemakers

Patients are placed on a cardiac monitor and rest for several hours after insertion of a pacemaker. The patient's apical pulse is monitored frequently to detect changes in the heart rhythm. Irregular heart rhythms or a rate slower than the pacemaker's set rate can indicate pacemaker malfunction. The dressing at the pacemaker insertion site is monitored every 2 to 4 hours for signs of bleeding. Any change in heart rhythm, complaints of chest pain, or changes in vital signs must be reported immediately. Patients may have a sling on the operative side arm for 24 to 48 hours to help prevent dislodgement of the pacemaker lead from the cardiac wall. The patient may remain in the hospital for a short stay.

Patient education for pacemaker care before discharge includes the following:

- Incision care. The patient should check the incision daily and report evidence of inflammation or infection (redness, swelling, warmth, tenderness, pain, fever, or discharge) to a physician. A hard ridge may form over the incision that will disappear with healing.
- Methods for taking a radial pulse. The patient should call a physician if the pulse is slower than the pacemaker's set rate.
- The patient should report symptoms of dizziness, fainting, irregular heartbeats, or palpitations.
- The patient should understand the importance of wearing medical alert jewelry and carrying a pacemaker information card.
- The patient should avoid radiation, magnetic fields (e.g., magnetic resonance imaging [MRI], industrial

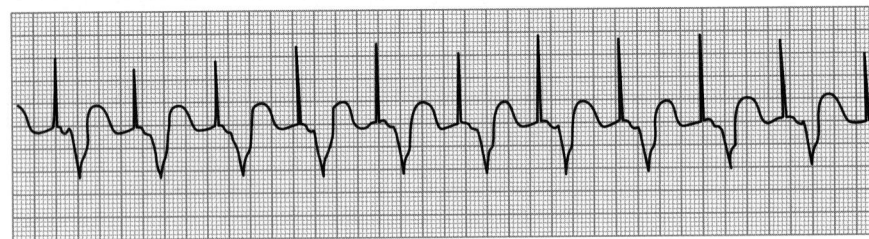

A

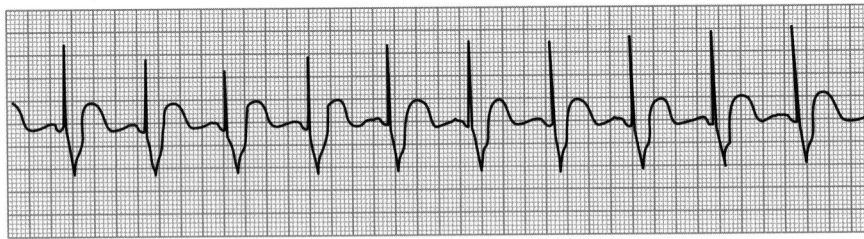

B

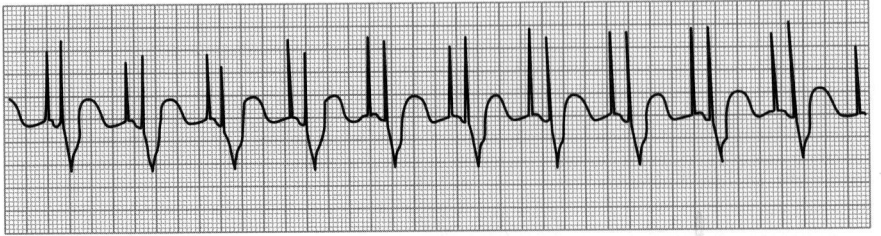

C

FIGURE 25.27 (A) Atrial-only pacemaker. (B) Ventricular-only pacemaker. (C) AV sequential pacemaker that paces both atrial and ventricular chambers.

magnets), high voltage (e.g., power plant, arc welding, high-tension wires), antitheft devices, and large running motors (e.g., distributor coil of running engine).

- The patient will need to tell airport security about the pacemaker, because it may trigger metal detectors (they do not harm the pacemaker).
- Grounded appliances (usually includes microwave ovens) and office equipment are safe to use.
- The patient must avoid lifting more than 10 pounds, making major arm movements, or participating in contact sports for 6 weeks after surgery. Normal activity is usually resumed after 6 weeks.
- The patient must keep scheduled appointments with the physician. Periodic pacemaker checks will be done by the physician or over the telephone. Reprogramming of the pacemaker can be done by the physician if needed.

CRITICAL THINKING

Mr. Treacher

■ Mr. Treacher, age 58, underwent pacemaker placement 6 days ago and is being transferred to the medical floor. After transfer, his vital signs are 138/72, 72 bpm, and 100% paced rhythm. Thirty minutes later, he says that he feels weak and tired. His vital signs are now 100/60, 60 bpm, and irregular.
1. What is your first action?
2. What actions should be taken next?
3. What might be happening to Mr. Treacher?
4. What interventions should you anticipate next?

Suggested answers at end of chapter.

DEFIBRILLATION

Defibrillation is a lifesaving procedure used for lethal dysrhythmias. It delivers an electrical shock to reset the heart's rhythm. It is used to terminate pulseless ventricular tachycardia or ventricular fibrillation. Self-adhesive pads, conductive jelly, or saline pads are placed on the patient's chest to prevent electrical burns from the defibrillator and promote conduction of the electrical charge. After the defibrillator is charged, the paddles are pressed firmly and evenly against the chest wall at the second intercostal space, right of the sternum and on the anterior axillary line at the fifth intercostal space (Fig. 25.28).

If the paddles are not pressed firmly against the chest wall during defibrillation, burns or electrical arcing can result when the shock is delivered. For safety, the person defibrillating must announce "clear." The phrase "One. I'm

defibrillation: de—from + fibrillation—quivering fibers

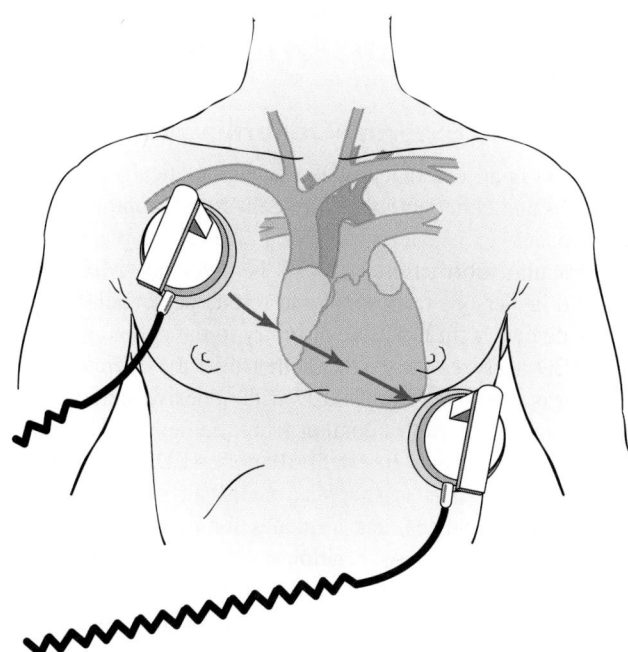

FIGURE 25.28 Placement of defibrillator paddles on chest.

clear. Two. You're clear. Three. All clear" is suggested. No one, including the person defibrillating, should touch the bed or patient during this time to avoid also being shocked. ACLS protocols specify guidelines for resuscitation. If the first shock is unsuccessful, a total of three shocks can be given initially, at increasing energy levels (200, 300, 360 joules).

A defibrillator may have a synchronization mode that allows R waves, if present, to be sensed so that an electrical shock can be delivered at an appropriate time in the cardiac cycle. This timing is important to prevent a more life-threatening dysrhythmia from developing. When defibrillation of a pulseless ventricular dysrhythmia is desired, the synchronize mode must be off (unsynchronized cardioversion). In this mode the charge is immediately released when the trigger is pressed. In the synchronized mode (synchronized cardioversion) there is a delay in the release of the charge while the R wave is sensed for appropriate timing.

After successful defibrillation, the patient is assessed for a pulse and adequate tissue perfusion. Vital signs, peripheral pulses, and level of consciousness should be noted. The patient is treated in the critical care unit after successful resuscitation.

Emotional support for the patient having experienced cardiac arrest and defibrillation is a very important aspect of nursing care. This can be an extremely frightening event for the patient. It is important to explain what happened to the patient and to listen and allow the patient to express any concerns. The patient is reassured that continuous monitoring is done in the critical care unit. Families also require emotional support during resuscitation of a loved one.

OTHER METHODS TO CORRECT DYSRHYTHMIAS

Automatic External Defibrillators

An AED is an external device that automatically analyzes rhythms and either automatically delivers or prompts operators to deliver an electrical shock if a shockable rhythm (ventricular fibrillation or VT) is detected. Minimally trained laypersons or hospital and rescue personnel can use these devices with little risk of injury to the patient because the AED analyzes the rhythm rather than the operator. The patient is connected to the AED with adhesive sternal-apex pads attached to cables coming from the device. This connection allows hands-free defibrillation. AEDs are found in public places such as shopping malls, airports, stadiums, casinos, golf courses, and airplanes for immediate access. The American Heart Association encourages increasing the availability of AEDs because defibrillation attempts must occur within minutes of cardiac arrest to increase chance of survival. AEDs are available for home use. They are recommended for people at high risk of sudden cardiac arrest, and for those at risk with rescue access that will take longer than 4 minutes such as those in rural areas, gated communities or secured access buildings. (Visit the Internet and search for AED to view more information and photographs on AEDs.)

Implantable Cardioverter Defibrillator

An implanted ICD is surgically placed during a minor procedure into the chest of a patient who experiences life-threatening dysrhythmias or is at risk for sudden cardiac death (Fig. 25.29). ICDs have decreased the number of deaths from these dysrhythmias by analyzing and treating these heart rhythms. When an abnormal rhythm is detected that could cause death (ventricular fibrillation), it automatically delivers an electrical shock. If the dysrhythmia does not convert on the initial shock, more shocks are delivered sequentially.

If the device detects VT, it cardioverts the rhythm using lower energy. ICDs also have antitachycardia pacing ability if a tachycardic rhythm is detected. Battery life depends on usage, but a battery may last up to 7 years. A physician can tell when the battery is getting low and that the entire unit needs to be changed within a few months.

Patients with ICDs are extremely anxious about having another cardiac arrest and receiving shocks from the ICD. Defibrillator or cardioversion shocks may feel like a kick in the chest. Reinforcement of patient and family education is very important in preparing the patient for discharge. Those with ICDs should take precautions to prevent problems with the ICD by taking the following precautions:
- Avoiding MRIs
- Avoiding metal detectors and standing near security gates or store entrances
- Avoiding equipment with strong electrical or magnetic fields (e.g., amusement rides, slot machines, remote-control toys, stereo speakers)
- Keeping cell phones 6 inches from the ICD

The nurse provides emotional support, answers all questions, and ensures that any misunderstood information is corrected before discharge.

Cardioversion

Elective cardioversion is used for dysrhythmias such as atrial fibrillation, atrial flutter, and supraventricular tachycardias that are not responsive to drug therapy. Conscious sedation is often used. The patient is given a sedative and monitored by anesthesia personnel during the procedure. Cardioversion is performed with a defibrillator set in the synchronize mode. The defibrillator is attached to the patient by electrode wires, which enables the ECG to be viewed on a screen. On the defibrillator there is a switch labeled "synchronize," which is on during cardioversion. When the defibrillator is in the synchronized mode, it marks a highlighted area on the patient's R waves, which must be recognized to deliver a shock.

The number of joules delivered with each shock is determined by a physician but usually ranges from 25 to 50 joules. Self-adhesive pads or conduction jelly is placed on the chest. The paddles must be firmly and evenly pressed against the pads or jelly on the chest until the shock is delivered to prevent skin burns and electrical arcing. When the discharge trigger is pressed, the shock is released when the machine senses it is safe to do so. The cardiac monitor screen is observed to see the discharge of the shock and to note the patient's ECG response. The patient's pulse and vital signs are checked.

If cardioversion is successful, there should be a return to normal sinus rhythm. If the rhythm does not immediately convert, more cardioversion attempts can be made as determined by the physician. After the procedure, the patient is monitored for skin burns, rhythm disturbances,

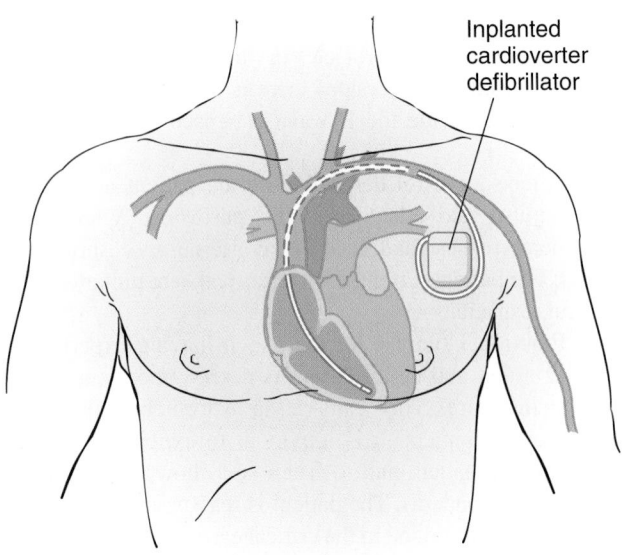

Inplanted cardioverter defibrillator

FIGURE 25.29 An implanted cardioverter defibrillator in place.

respiratory problems, hypotension, and changes in the ST segment.

Ablation

When medications or other treatments are not successful in treating a dysrhythmia, ablation of cardiac conduction pathways may be used to stop the dysrhythmia. Intracardiac echocardiography and intracardiac mapping are done before ablation to determine the area of the heart requiring treatment.

Forms of ablation include mechanical, chemical, and radio frequency. Mechanical ablation destroys the involved tissue with cryosurgery or through surgical removal. Chemical ablation inserts alcohol or phenol through an angioplasty catheter into the area of the heart producing the unwanted beats. Radio frequency ablation delivers high-frequency energy via a catheter to necrose selected conduction pathway areas. Following any of these ablation procedures, a temporary or permanent pacemaker may be needed if normal conduction tissue is damaged. Postprocedural care is similar to postangioplasty or postcardiac catheterization care (see Chapter 20).

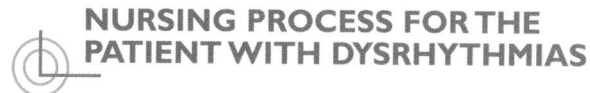

NURSING PROCESS FOR THE PATIENT WITH DYSRHYTHMIAS

Assessment/Data Collection

Assessment of the cardiac system, respiratory rate, breath sounds, and urinary output is important. Monitoring apical and radial pulses at frequent intervals helps detect dysrhythmias. Most dysrhythmias are not life threatening. Patients at risk for dysrhythmias require careful monitoring so that any dysrhythmias are detected and treated. A patient's complaints of dizziness, chest pain, or palpitations should always be reported to the physician.

Nursing Diagnoses, Planning and Implementation, and Evaluation

See Box 25.2 Nursing Care Plan for the Patient with Dysrhythmias.

To implement the plan of care, the patient and family should be included. Assist them in understanding the plan and the reasons for the prescribed interventions and allow them to express their needs and fears.

Box 25.2   Nursing Care Plan for the Patient with Dysrhythmias

Nursing Diagnosis: Decreased cardiac output related to dysrhythmias

Expected Outcomes (1) Patient cardiac status stabilizes. (2) Patient tolerates activities of daily living (ADL).

Evaluation of Outcomes (1) There is an absence of dysrhythmias. (2) Patient is able to perform ADL without tachycardia, chest pain, or weakness.

Interventions	Rationale	Evaluation
Take apical and radial pulses every 2 to 4 hours. Monitor blood pressure and urinary output.	Monitors for dysrhythmias, impending cardiac arrest, or shock. Blood pressure, pulse, and urinary output are indicators of cardiac output.	Is the patient free of dysrhythmias with vital signs within normal limits?
Monitor mental status every 2 to 4 hours.	Dizziness, confusion, and restlessness may indicate decreased cerebral blood flow.	Does patient show signs of decreased cerebral perfusion, such as confusion?
Listen to lung sounds every 2 to 4 hours.	Dysrhythmias can cause heart failure.	Are lungs clear with no report of dyspnea?
Administer O$_2$ as ordered.	Increases oxygenation to the heart and brain.	Is patient free of chest pain, confusion, and light-headedness?
Ensure that patient gets adequate rest and does not exceed activity tolerance.	Reduces dyspnea and decreases O$_2$ demand on the myocardium.	Does patient rest and tolerate activity without dyspnea or chest pain?

Geriatric

Administer medications as ordered and observe for adverse reactions.	Older patients may have decreased renal and liver function that may lead to rapid development of toxicity.	Does patient have signs of toxicity?

(Continued on following page)

BOX 25.2   NURSING CARE PLAN for the Patient with Dysrhythmias *(Cont'd)*

Nursing Diagnosis: Anxiety related to situational crisis

Expected Outcomes (1) Patient is able to effectively manage anxiety. (2) Patient will report decreased anxiety.

Evaluation of Outcomes (1) Patient uses effective coping mechanisms to manage anxiety. (2) Patient expresses decreased anxiety.

Interventions	Rationale	Evaluation
Ask about level of anxiety.	Establishes a baseline.	What is patient's level of anxiety?
Encourage patient and family to verbalize fears.	Helps correct and clarify their concerns.	What are patient's feelings or fears?
Explain procedures to patient and family.	Lack of knowledge increases anxiety. Also will help with compliance of therapy.	Does patient express understanding of therapy with decreased anxiety?
Identify and reduce as many environmental stressors as possible.	Anxiety often results from lack of trust in the environment.	Can patient describe two situations that increase tension?
Teach patient relaxation techniques to be performed every 4 to 6 hours, such as guided imagery, muscle relaxation, and meditation.	These measures can restore psychological and physical equilibrium and help decrease anxiety.	Is patient successful in demonstrating relaxation methods?
Medicate with antianxiety agents as ordered.	Aids the patient in decreasing anxiety.	Does patient show decreased anxiety?

Family members should be taught CPR or given information on local CPR classes. This training gives the patient and family a sense of control and hope. In the event the patient requires CPR, the family can take action instead of simply standing by and feeling helpless. The patient will feel more secure in knowing that immediate help from family members is available at home until medical help arrives.

Home Health Hints

- The nurse should have a pocket mask for CPR available at all times.
- A car phone or portable phone affords a home health nurse safety, convenience, and efficiency, especially if emergency help is needed, because some patients do not have phones.
- Patients prone to dysrhythmias should avoid straining with bowel movements. If the patient reports strain-

ing, request a laxative or stool softener order from the physician.
- Patients who come home with a pacemaker should be instructed to wear loose tops. Women should not wear tight bras.
- Symptoms of infection to watch for after a pacemaker is implanted are redness, swelling, warmth, and pain at the site.
- Instruct patients with a pacemaker to take their pulse once a day, in the morning, for a full minute. Assist them in setting up a log to record date, time, and pulse reading. Instruct them to call if the pulse varies outside parameters set by the physician.
- Patients on beta blockers need to know how to take their pulse, because bradycardia is a major side effect. For pulse below 50, call the nurse or physician.
- Advise patients who are leaving home for weekend or holidays to refill medicines ahead of time. Also, the physician may write a prescription for patients to keep in their wallet for emergencies.

REVIEW QUESTIONS

1. Which of the following is the correct sequence for normal electrical impulse movement through the cardiac conduction system?
   a. Vena cavae, right atrium, right ventricle, pulmonary artery
   b. SA node, AV node, bundle of His, Purkinje fibers
   c. Pulmonary veins, left atrium, left ventricle, aorta
   d. Purkinje fibers, AV node, bundle of His, SA node

2. Why is it most important for the nurse to use a systematic method for analyzing hearth rhythm tracings?
   a. So abnormalities are not missed
   b. To save time
   c. To develop a routine for examining tracings
   d. To increase memory of the steps

3. If a patient is in pulseless ventricular tachycardia, which of the following is the first choice of treatment?
   a. Synchronized cardioversion
   b. Pacemaker
   c. Defibrillation
   d. Antiarrhythmic medication

4. Which of the following instructions should the nurse give the patient regarding pacemaker care?
   a. "Avoid microwaves."
   b. "You may have an MRI."
   c. "Take your radial pulse daily."
   d. "You will need to be on bedrest for 48 hours."

5. The nurse is ambulating a patient who is recovering from an MI and the patient develops chest pain with an irregular pulse. What is the safest way to return the patient to bed?
   a. Ambulate to room with one assistant
   b. With assistance by stretcher
   c. With assistance by a wheelchair
   d. After completion of ambulation

6. A patient has a radial pulse of 58 bpm. Which of the following is the appropriate term for documenting this rhythm?
   a. Normal
   b. Bradycardia
   c. Tachycardia
   d. Asystole

7. The nurse is to give a patient amiodarone 800 mg/day PO in two divided doses. The nurse has available 200-mg tablets. How many tablets should the nurse give for each dose?

   _____ tablets

SUGGESTED ANSWERS TO

CRITICAL THINKING

■ Mrs. Mae

1. Assess the patient's vital signs and heart sounds; note symptoms; obtain an ECG per agency protocol.
2. Report the patient findings to the RN or physician.
3. Possible causes include hypokalemia or ischemia leading to irritability of the heart.
4. Symptoms might include light-headedness, feeling of heart skipping, chest pain, or fatigue.
5. To alleviate symptoms, elevate head of bed to comfort, monitor vital signs, and maintain oxygen at 2 L/min via nasal cannula per agency protocol. Remain with the patient to help alleviate anxiety. Notify the RN.
6. Orders might include ECG, oxygen, potassium, or electrolytes.
7. Documentation should include the following:
   1400: Ambulated 20 feet with one assist. Vital signs stable. Stated "feel good. Pain zero."
   Tolerated well. Assisted to bed. Oxygen at 2 L/min via nasal cannula.
   1405: See ECG strip with intermittent PVCs. Vital signs: 132/84, apical 92 irregular, 22.
   "Pain zero. I can feel my heart skipping, it takes my breath away." RN notified.

■ Mrs. Parker

1. A heart in VT has an ectopic focus firing. The heart is unable to maintain adequate cardiac output with such a rapid heart rate. The rapid and irregular heart rhythm does not allow the heart chambers time to adequately fill and empty, thereby reducing the blood volume with each beat. This in turn affects the peripheral circulation, causing the absence of palpable pulses.
2. In VT, one or more sites in the ventricle may be initiating impulses. The rapid rate of VT overrides the normal pacemaker of the heart. The rhythm can be regular or irregular. The inability of the heart to conduct impulses along normal pathways prevents the chambers from emptying and filling properly. This leads to a decreased cardiac output and can lead to cardiac arrest if the rhythm is not converted.

3. Call a code and begin CPR. Report findings to code team upon their arrival.
4. Documentation should include the following: 1600: Patient found in bed unresponsive to verbal and tactile stimuli. Respirations shallow. No palpable pulses. BP 80/40, P 150, R 6. Monitor shows VT (see strip). Code called from room. CPR started. Code team arrived at 1602. Report given to code team leader.

Mr. Peet

1. Initially you should assess responsiveness and the presence of a carotid pulse. Check for breathing.
2. Open the airway. Call for assistance or use the patient's phone to report a cardiac arrest. Initiate CPR until help arrives.
3. Once help or the code team arrives, the licensed practical nurse/licensed vocational nurse (LPN/LVN) reports the patient's status. The code team leader delegates responsibilities. Many facilities have protocols for each team member in a code. The LPN/LVN assists in the code as delegated by the RN in charge.

Mr. Treacher

1. Your first actions should be to obtain an ECG per agency protocol and to notify the RN and physician.
2. You should keep the head of the bed elevated and administer oxygen at 2 L/min via nasal cannula per protocol. Turn the patient onto his side because this may help float the pacemaker wire to the chamber wall for better contact. Monitor the patient's ECG, vital signs, and symptoms, and remain with patient to provide emotional support.
3. Mr. Treacher could be experiencing pacemaker malfunction.
4. Interventions could include transfer to a step-down unit or intensive care unit (ICU), reprogramming of the pacemaker, or a return to surgery for manipulation or replacement of the pacemaker wires.

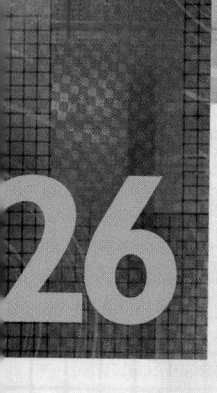

26

Nursing Care of Patients with Heart Failure

LINDA S. WILLIAMS

KEY TERMS

afterload (AFF-ter-lohd)
cor pulmonale (KOR PUL-mah-NAH-lee)
cyanosis (SIGH-an-NOH-sis)
hepatomegaly (HEP-uh-toh-MEG-ah-lee)
orthopnea (or-THOP-knee-a)
paroxysmal nocturnal dyspnea (PEAR-ox-IS-mall knock-TURN-al DISP-knee-a)
peripheral vascular resistance (puh-RIFF-uh-ruhl VAS-kyoo-lar ree-ZIS-tense)
preload (PREE-lohd)
pulmonary edema (PULL-muh-NAIR-ee uh-DEE-muh)
splenomegaly (SPLEE-noh-MEG-ah-lee)

QUESTIONS TO GUIDE YOUR READING

1. How would you describe the pathophysiology of left- and right-sided heart failure?

2. What is acute heart failure?

3. What are causes of acute and chronic heart failure?

4. What are signs and symptoms of acute and chronic heart failure?

5. What nursing care would you provide for diagnostic tests for heart failure?

6. What is the medical treatment for acute and chronic heart failure?

7. What nursing care would you provide for acute and chronic heart failure?

8. What would you include in your teaching plan for patients with heart failure and their families?

HEART FAILURE

Heart failure (HF) is a clinical syndrome that occurs as a result of the inability of the ventricle(s) to fill or pump enough blood to meet the body's oxygen and nutrient needs. It may cause dyspnea, fatigue, and fluid volume overload in the intravascular and interstitial spaces, resulting in reduced quality and length of life. Causes of HF are varied and may include coronary artery disease (most often), myocardial infarction, cardiomyopathy, heart valve problems, and hypertension. Any heart problem may potentially lead to HF. In the elderly, the most common cause of HF is cardiac ischemia. It may develop rapidly (acute), as with cardiogenic shock and **pulmonary edema,** or over time (chronic) as a result of another disorder, such as hypertension or pulmonary disease.

The incidence of HF is growing as the older adult population and patient survival rates increase. According to the American Heart Association, 5 million people have HF with over 550,000 new cases each year. Heart failure is the most common reason for hospital admission in the older adult. The patient may experience many functional limitations and symptoms, and there is a high mortality rate. Quality of life is often impaired. Readmission rates to hospitals soon after discharge for heart failure treatment are high and pose a challenge for health-care providers. For more information, visit the American Heart Association at www.american-heart.org.

Congestive Heart Failure

Congestive heart failure is the older term for heart failure. It is still used interchangeably by some to indicate heart failure in general. The new term of *heart failure* is preferred since volume overload or "congestion" either in the lungs or periphery is not present in everyone with heart failure or at all times.[1]

Pathophysiology

The heart is divided into two separate pumping systems. The right side of the heart forms one pump. The left side of the heart forms the other pump. Normally these pumps work together to ensure that equal amounts of blood enter and leave the heart.

Normally, blood flow through the heart begins in the right atrium (see Chapter 20). Unoxygenated blood from the body's venous system enters the right atrium from the inferior and superior venae cavae. Next the blood enters the right ventricle to be pumped into the pulmonary artery and into the lungs for oxygenation. After receiving oxygen in the lungs, the blood is returned to the left atrium via the four pulmonary veins. The oxygenated blood then enters the left ventricle and is pumped out into the aorta and the systemic circulation.

Proper cardiac functioning requires each ventricle to pump out equal amounts of blood over time. If the amount of blood returned to the heart becomes more than either ventricle can handle, the heart can no longer be an effective pump. Conditions that cause heart failure may affect one or both of the heart's pumping systems. Therefore, heart failure can be classified as right-sided heart failure, left-sided heart failure, or biventricular heart failure. The ventricle is the area of the heart's pumping system that commonly fails. Of the two ventricles, the left ventricle is typically the one to weaken first because it has the greatest workload. The right and left sides of the heart's pumping system work together in a closed system to continuously move blood forward, so failure of one side eventually leads to failure of the other side.

LEARNING TIP

To visualize and understand the effects of heart failure, trace the flow of blood backward from each ventricle. Along the backward path from the failing ventricle, congestion develops and produces the signs and symptoms seen in heart failure. If you understand the backward path of congestion, you can identify the signs and symptoms specifically associated with right- or left-sided heart failure.

LEARNING TIP

To understand heart failure, compare it to a dam in a river:

In a river without a dam, the water flows freely; in the normal circulatory system, blood flows freely.

- In a river with a dam, the water is blocked by the dam and builds up behind it; in heart failure, the failing ventricle acts like the dam in the river, causing blood to back up behind it.
- When the dam on the river malfunctions, too much water builds up behind it and the riverbanks flood; in heart failure, if too much blood builds up behind the failing ventricle, the lungs or peripheral tissues are flooded (edema).
- Heart failure can be the result of systolic (contractile) dysfunction, diastolic (relaxation) dysfunction, or a mixed systolic and diastolic dysfunction. Systolic dysfunction is a contractile problem in which the ventricle is unable to generate enough force to pump blood from the ventricle. Diastolic dysfunction is a problem with the ventricle's ability to relax and fill. Mixed systolic and diastolic dysfunction is a combination of the two defects.

Left-Sided Heart Failure

A certain amount of force must be generated by the left ventricle during a contraction to eject blood into the aorta through the aortic valve. This force is referred to as **afterload.** The pressure within the aorta and arteries influences the force needed to open the aortic valve to pump blood into the aorta. This pressure is called **peripheral vascular resistance** (PVR).

Hypertension is one of the major causes of left-sided heart failure because it increases the pressure within arteries. Increased pressure in the aorta makes the left ventricle work harder to pump blood into the aorta. Over time the strain caused by the increased workload causes the left ventricle to weaken and fail. Other conditions that can lead to left-sided heart failure are described in Table 26.1. Among these conditions are disorders that (1) restrict the outflow of blood from the left ventricle, as in aortic valve stenosis or coarctation of the aorta, which is a malformation causing narrowing; (2) impair contractility of the heart, as in myocardial infarction or cardiomyopathy; and (3) allow blood to flow backward into the left atrium, as in valvular disorders.

With left-sided heart failure, blood backs up from the left ventricle into the left atrium and then into the four pulmonary veins and lungs (Fig. 26.1). This increases pulmonary pressure, causing movement of fluid first into the interstitium and then the alveoli. Alveolar edema is more serious because it reduces gas exchange across the alveolar capillary membrane. Shortness of breath and **cyanosis** may result from the decreased oxygenation of the blood leaving the lungs. If the fluid build-up is severe, pulmonary edema occurs, which requires immediate medical treatment.

Right-Sided Heart Failure

Causes of right-sided heart failure are described in Table 26.2. The major cause of right-sided heart failure is left-sided heart failure. When the left side fails, fluid backs up into the lungs and pulmonary pressure is increased. The right ventricle must continually pump blood against this

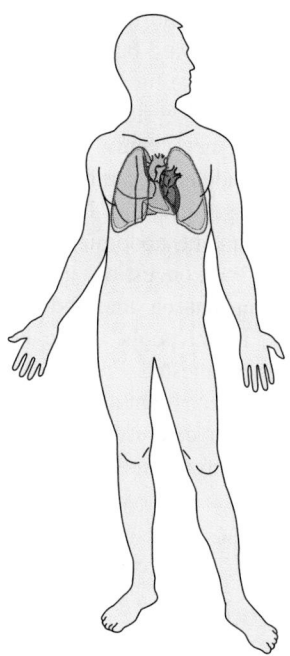

FIGURE 26.1 Left-sided heart failure. Shaded areas indicate areas of congestion from blood back-up caused by the failing left side of the heart.

increased fluid and pressure in the pulmonary artery and lungs. Over time this additional strain eventually causes it to fail.

Conditions causing right-sided heart failure increase the work of the right ventricle. They increase the amount of contractile force needed or they require pumping of excess blood volume (**preload**). Among these conditions are disorders that (1) increase pulmonary pressures, such as emphysema or congenital heart defects; (2) restrict the outflow of blood from the right ventricle, as in pulmonary valve stenosis; and (3) allow left atrial blood to flow into the right atrium, thereby increasing blood volume in the right ventricle, as in septal defects. When the right ventricle hypertrophies or fails because of increased pulmonary pressures, it is referred to as **cor pulmonale.**

cor pulmonale: cor—heart + pulm—lung

TABLE 26.1 EXAMPLES OF CAUSES OF LEFT-SIDED HEART FAILURE

Cause	Primary Effect on Left Ventricular Workload
Aortic Stenosis	Increased volume to pump
Cardiomyopathy	Increased workload from poor contractility
Coarctation of the Aorta	Resistance increased from elevated pressure
Hypertension	Resistance increased from elevated pressure
Heart Muscle Infections	Increased workload from damaged myocardium
Myocardial Infarction	Increased workload from poor contractility
Mitral Regurgitation	Increased volume to pump

TABLE 26.2 CAUSES OF RIGHT-SIDED HEART FAILURE

Cause	Primary Right Ventricular Workload Effect
Atrial Septal Defect	Increased volume to pump
Cor Pulmonale	Resistance increased from elevated pressure
Left-Sided Heart Failure	Resistance increased from backup of fluid and elevated pressures
Pulmonary Hypertension	Resistance increased from elevated pressure
Pulmonary Stenosis	Increased volume to pump

When the right ventricle fails, it does not empty normally and there is a backward build-up of blood in the systemic blood vessels. As the blood backs up from the right ventricle, right atrial and systemic venous blood volume increases. The jugular neck veins, which are not normally visible, become distended and can be seen when the person is in a 45-degree upright position. Edema may occur in the peripheral tissues, and the abdominal organs can become engorged (Fig. 26.2). Congestion in the gastrointestinal tract causes anorexia, nausea, and abdominal pain. As the failure progresses, blood pools in the hepatic veins and the liver becomes congested, known as **hepatomegaly.** Pain in the right upper quadrant and impaired liver function are caused by this liver congestion. Systemic venous congestion also leads to engorgement of the spleen, known as **splenomegaly.**

LEARNING TIP

To understand the signs and symptoms of left-sided versus right-sided heart failure, remember that left-sided signs and symptoms are found in the lungs. Left begins with L, as does Lung: Left = Lungs, L = L.

Any signs and symptoms not related to the lungs (L) are caused by right-sided failure.

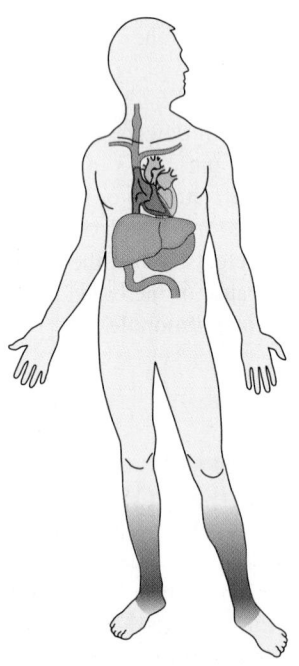

FIGURE 26.2 Right-sided heart failure. Shaded areas indicate areas of congestion from blood back-up due to the failing right side of the heart.

hepatomegaly: hep—liver + mega—large
splenomegaly: splen—spleen + mega—large

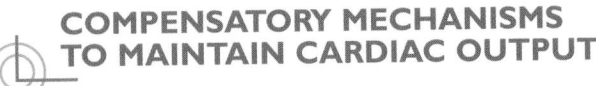

COMPENSATORY MECHANISMS TO MAINTAIN CARDIAC OUTPUT

Compensatory mechanisms help ensure that an adequate amount of blood is being pumped out of the heart. Although these mechanisms are designed to maintain cardiac output, they contribute to a cycle that instead of being helpful leads to further heart failure.

When the sympathetic nervous system detects low cardiac output, it speeds up the heart rate by releasing epinephrine and norepinephrine. Although this raises cardiac output (cardiac output = heart rate × stroke volume), the increased heart rate also increases the oxygen needs of the heart. In response to low renal blood flow, the kidneys activate the renin-angiotensin-aldosterone system, and antidiuretic hormone is released from the pituitary gland to conserve water, causing decreased urine output. This adds to the fluid retention problem already found in heart failure.

Over time the heart responds to the increased workload by enlarging its chambers (dilation) and increasing its muscle mass (hypertrophy), referred to as remodeling. In dilation, the heart muscle fibers stretch to increase the force of myocardial contractions, which is known as the Frank-Starling phenomenon. In hypertrophy, the muscle mass of the heart increases, creating more contractile force. Both of these compensatory mechanisms increase the heart's oxygen needs, which further contributes to heart failure. Additionally, the heart walls stiffen, which further reduces pumping ability.

PULMONARY EDEMA (ACUTE HEART FAILURE)

Pulmonary edema, also known as acute heart failure, is severe fluid congestion in the alveoli of the lungs and is life threatening. Pulmonary edema occurs in an acute event such as a myocardial infarction (MI) or when the heart is severely stressed, causing the left ventricle to fail. Complications of pulmonary edema include dysrhythmias and cardiac arrest.

Pathophysiology

First, pressure rises in the lung's venous blood vessels and blood builds up. As pressures continue to rise, fluid moves into the interstitial spaces. Then, with continued pressure increases, fluid containing red blood cells moves into the alveoli. Finally, the alveoli and airways become filled with fluid, reducing gas exchange and oxygen levels.

Signs and Symptoms

Signs and symptoms of pulmonary edema are listed in Table 26.3. Pink, frothy sputum is a classic symptom of pulmonary edema caused by the increased lung congestion and pressures that allow leaking of fluid into the alveoli. Compensatory mechanisms increase the heart rate and blood

TABLE 26.3 ACUTE HEART FAILURE SUMMARY

Signs and Symptoms	Rapid respirations with accessory muscle use
	Severe dyspnea, orthopnea
	Crackles and wheezes
	Coughing
	Pink, frothy sputum
	Anxiety, restlessness
	Pale skin and mucous membranes
	Clammy, cold skin
Diagnostic Tests	Chest x-ray examination
	Arterial blood gases
	Electrocardiogram
	Hemodynamic monitoring
Therapeutic Interventions	Oxygen via cannula, mask, or mechanical ventilation
	Positioning in high or semi-Fowler's position
	Bedrest
	IV Drugs: morphine, diuretics, inotropic agents, vasodilators, human B-type natriuretic peptide (Neseritide)
	Frequent vital signs, urinary output
	Pulmonary pressures
	Daily weights
	Treatment of underlying cause
Nursing Diagnoses	Impaired gas exchange
	Decreased cardiac output
	Excess fluid volume

IV = intravenous.

pressure; however, as pulmonary edema worsens, the blood pressure may fall.

Diagnosis

Diagnostic studies are listed in Table 26.3. The congested pulmonary system can be seen on x-ray examination. Arterial blood gases (ABGs) will show a decrease in PaO_2 that continues as the edema worsens and an increase in $PaCO_2$, causing respiratory acidosis (pH = 7.35). The pulmonary artery catheter will show elevated pulmonary pressures and a decreased cardiac output.

Therapeutic Interventions

Immediate treatment is necessary to prevent patients from drowning in their own secretions (see Table 26.3). The goal of therapy is to reduce the workload of the left ventricle in order to improve cardiac output and reduce the patient's anxiety. Care for the patient is usually provided in an intensive care unit. Treatment for the underlying cause occurs at the same time that the patient is being treated for the pulmonary edema.

Treatment includes positioning the patient upright to make breathing easier. In Fowler's position, the lungs can more easily expand. Ask the patient what position is preferred. Oxygen is given usually by mask to provide higher

amounts. In severe cases of pulmonary edema, endotracheal intubation and mechanical ventilation may be necessary. Medications are given intravenously to reduce anxiety, relax airways, and increase peripheral blood pooling to decrease preload (morphine); reduce fluid congestion; reduce preload; strengthen heart contractions; reduce arterial pressure and sodium and water retention to relieve dyspnea (nesiritide [Natrecor]). Nesiritide belongs to a newer drug class called human B-type natriuretic peptide (hBNP). hBNP is normally secreted by the ventricular myocardium in response to heart failure. It has been found to reduce symptoms of acute HF.

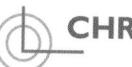 ## CHRONIC HEART FAILURE

Signs and Symptoms

The signs and symptoms of chronic heart failure are influenced by the patient's age, the underlying cause and severity of the heart disease, and the ventricle that is failing. Chronic heart failure is a progressive disorder, so signs and symptoms may worsen over time. Signs and symptoms caused by a specific failing ventricle are listed in Table 26.4.

Fatigue and Weakness

Fatigue and weakness are the earliest symptoms of heart failure. They occur from the decreased amount of oxygen reaching the tissues. Throughout the day the fatigue worsens, especially with activity.

Dyspnea

A failing left ventricle produces prominent respiratory effects. Dyspnea is a common symptom of left-sided heart failure. It occurs from the pulmonary congestion that impairs gas exchange between the alveoli and capillaries. Dyspnea stimulates compensatory mechanisms that produce short, rapid respirations. Dyspnea is classified in several ways:

- Exertional dyspnea is shortness of breath that increases with activity.
- **Orthopnea** is dyspnea that increases when lying flat. In an upright position, gravity holds fluid in the lower extremities. In a supine position, gravitational forces are removed, allowing fluid to move from the legs to the heart, which overwhelms the already congested pulmonary system. When orthopnea is present, two or more pillows are often used for sleeping, and the documentation should state the number of pillows used. For example, use of three pillows would be three-pillow orthopnea.
- **Paroxysmal nocturnal dyspnea** (PND) is sudden shortness of breath that occurs after lying flat for a time. PND results from excess fluid accumulation in the lungs. The sleeping person awakens with feelings of suffocation and anxiety. Relief is obtained

orthopnea: orth—straight + pnea—to breathe

TABLE 26.4 CHRONIC HEART FAILURE SUMMARY

Signs and Symptoms

Right-Sided Heart Failure
Jugular vein distention
Dependent peripheral edema
Ascites
Weight gain
Splenomegaly
Hepatomegaly
GI pain, anorexia, nausea
Fatigue, weakness
Tachycardia
Nocturia

Left-Sided Heart Failure
Dyspnea on exertion
Dry hacky cough, especially supine
Crackles, wheezing
Orthopnea
Paroxysmal nocturnal dyspnea
Cheyne-Stokes respirations
Cyanosis
Tachypnea, tachycardia
Nocturia

Diagnostic Tests
History and physical
    examination
Electrocardiogram
Chest x-ray examination
Exercise stress test,
    pharmacological stress test
Nuclear imaging studies
Echocardiography, TEE
Coronary angiography
Cardiac catheterization
Serum laboratory tests:
    ABGs, CBC, ProBNP,
    electrolytes, liver enzymes,
    BUN, creatinine,
    thyroid function
Urinalysis
Hemodynamic monitoring

Complications
Hepatomegaly
Splenomegaly
Pleural effusion
Left ventricular throm-
    bus and emboli
Cardiogenic shock

Therapeutic Interventions
Noninvasive
Treat underlying cause
Oxygen by cannula or mask
Drug therapy: See Table 26.5
Individualized activity plan
Dietary sodium restriction
Fluid restriction
Daily weights
Invasive
Resynchronization therapy
ICD
Mechanical assistive devices
    Intra-aortic balloon pump
    Left ventricular assist device
    Total artificial heart
Valvuloplasty
Heart valve replacement
Cardiac transplant

Nursing Diagnoses
Impaired gas exchange
Decreased cardiac output
Excess fluid volume

ABGs = arterial blood gases; ACE = angiotensin-converting enzyme; BUN = blood urea nitrogen; CBC = complete blood count; ICD = implantable internal cardiac defibrillator; TEE = transesophageal echocardiography.

by sitting upright for a short time, which reduces the amount of fluid returning to the heart.

Cough

A chronic, dry cough is common in heart failure. The coughing increases when lying down from increased irritation of the lung mucosa. This irritation is due to the increase in pulmonary congestion that occurs when gravity no longer keeps fluid in the legs and more fluid returns to the heart and lungs.

Crackles and Wheezes

Pulmonary congestion causes abnormal breath sounds such as crackles and wheezes. These sounds indicate the presence of increased fluid in the lungs. Crackles are produced from fluid build-up in the alveoli resulting from increased pressure in the pulmonary capillaries. Wheezes occur from bronchiolar constriction caused by the increased fluid.

Tachycardia

The sympathetic nervous system compensates for the decreased cardiac output in heart failure by releasing epinephrine and norepinephrine to increase the heart rate. Normally, this is helpful because the increased heart rate

LEARNING TIP

To simulate the sound of crackles, open a piece of Velcro or rub hair together next to your ear. These sounds are similar to the sound of crackles heard with a stethoscope.

increases the amount of blood ejected by the heart to maintain an adequate cardiac output. However, whenever the heart works faster, it also requires more oxygen, which a failing heart finds it difficult to supply.

Chest Pain

Chest pain may occur from ischemia in the patient with heart failure. Decreased cardiac output results in decreased oxygen delivery to the heart itself via the coronary arteries. Compensatory mechanisms designed to maintain cardiac output increase the workload and oxygen needs of the heart and are counterproductive in heart failure. Tachycardia increases the oxygen needs of the heart. The kidneys compensate by retaining sodium and fluid, which increases the fluid volume returning to the heart (preload) and therefore the heart's workload and oxygen needs. Pain also increases oxygen requirements, adding further to the cycle of heart failure.

Cheyne-Stokes Respiration

A breathing pattern of shallow respirations building to deep breaths followed by a period of apnea characterizes Cheyne-Stokes breathing. The apneic period occurs because the deep breathing causes carbon dioxide levels to drop to a level that does not stimulate the respiratory center. This apnea may last up to 30 seconds and is then followed by the shallow to deeper respiratory pattern of Cheyne-Stokes as carbon dioxide levels rise again.

Edema

Edema occurs in heart failure as a result of (1) systemic blood vessel congestion and (2) sympathetic compensatory mechanisms that cause the kidneys to activate the renin-angiotensin-aldosterone system, in which antidiuretic hormone is released from the pituitary gland, causing sodium and water to be retained. Systemic or pulmonary edema can occur in heart failure. The effect of backward build-up of pressure in the systemic blood vessels is seen with distention of the jugular veins, swelling of the legs and feet, sacral edema in the individual on bedrest, and increased fluid within the abdominal cavity and organs. An acute build-up of fluid in the lungs produces pulmonary edema.

Anemia

Many patients with heart failure are anemic due to decreased angiotension-converting enzyme (ACE) action. This reduced ACE action decreases production of red blood cells, resulting in anemia and decreased hemoglobin levels.

Nocturia

Nocturia is an increase in urine output at night. After lying down, fluid in the lower legs returns to the circulatory system. Renal blood flow and filtration is increased, resulting in greater urine production and the need to urinate frequently during the night. Nocturia may occur up to six times per night, contributing to the patient's fatigue from lack of sleep.

Cyanosis

The skin, nailbeds, or mucous membranes may appear blue, or cyanotic, from decreased oxygenation of the blood.

NURSING CARE TIP

Patients often have to get up to void shortly after going to bed. This is due to fluid in the legs returning to the heart and then the kidneys for filtering after a person lies down. To help patients get as much undisturbed rest as possible, teach them to recline with legs at or above heart level for at least 30 minutes before going to bed. Then they can void before going to bed, instead of soon after going to bed.

Cyanosis is a late sign of heart failure. It is associated primarily with left-sided heart failure.

Altered Mental Status

Less cardiac output decreases the amount of oxygen delivered to the brain. As a result, restlessness, insomnia, confusion, and impaired memory may occur. A decrease in level of consciousness may occur.

Malnutrition

Several factors contribute to malnutrition in the person with chronic heart failure. Altered mental status, dyspnea, and fatigue interfere with the ability to eat. Anorexia and gastrointestinal (GI) upset occur from pressure exerted by excess fluid surrounding the GI structures. Absorption of food may also be impaired by this pressure.

CRITICAL THINKING

Mr. Shepard (1)

■ Mr. Shepard, age 66, has a family history of cardiac disease. He has been hypertensive for 10 years and takes captopril daily. His baseline vital signs are blood pressure 122/78, pulse 80, respiration 18, height 66 in, and weight 170 lb. During a visit to his physician, he states that he has been short of breath during his daily 2-mile walk and has been using two pillows at night for sleep. As he talks, the physician notes that he has an intermittent dry cough. His physical examination shows blood pressure 140/86, pulse 106, respiration 24, weight 178 lb, and bilateral crackles in the lung bases.

1. What signs and symptoms of heart failure does Mr. Shepard have?
2. Do the signs and symptoms reflect right- or left-sided heart failure?
3. Why are each of the signs and symptoms occurring?
4. Why is Mr. Shepard using two pillows for sleeping?

Suggested answers at end of chapter.

Complications of Heart Failure

Complications of heart failure are listed in Table 26.4. The liver and spleen enlarge from the fluid congestion, which causes impaired function, cellular death, and scarring. Pleural effusion, a leakage of fluid from the capillaries of the lung into the pleural space, can occur. The elevated pressures in the capillaries of the lung cause this leakage. Thrombosis and emboli can occur as a result of poor emptying of the ventricles, which leads to stasis of blood. Aspirin or anticoagulants are often prescribed to prevent thrombus formation in patients with heart failure. Cardiogenic shock, often caused by a myocardial infarction that damages the left ventricle, occurs when the left ventricle is unable to supply the tissues with enough oxygen and nutrients to meet their needs. Cardiogenic shock is a life-threatening condition that requires immediate treatment (see Chapter 8).

Diagnostic Tests

Diagnostic tests are done to identify the cause of the failure and determine the degree of failure present (see Table 26.4):

- A chest x-ray examination shows the size, shape, and enlargement of the heart and congestion in the pulmonary vessels.
- Echocardiography measures the size of the heart chambers to detect enlargement and assess valvular function and motion of the ventricles.
- Cardiac dysrhythmias that precipitate and contribute to heart failure can be diagnosed with electrocardiogram (ECG; see Chapter 20). Chamber enlargement in the atrium from heart failure is shown by P-wave changes and in the left ventricle by increased voltage and deeper S waves in some V leads.
- Exercise stress testing and nuclear imaging studies provide information on activity tolerance, which is usually limited in heart failure.
- Cardiac catheterization and angiography are used to detect underlying heart disease that may be the cause of heart failure.
- Direct assessment of the heart's pressures is done with hemodynamic monitoring. A catheter is inserted into the heart and pulmonary artery to transmit pressures to a cardiac monitor. These cardiac and pulmonary pressures are then used to guide medical therapy.
- Serum laboratory tests may show elevated serum blood urea nitrogen (BUN) and elevated serum creatinine from renal failure and elevated liver enzymes from liver damage.

CRITICAL THINKING

Mr. Shepard (2)

■ Mr. Shepard's chest x-ray examination shows an enlarged heart (cardiomegaly).
1. Why is Mr. Shepard's heart enlarged?
2. What is the significance of an enlarged heart?
Suggested answers at end of chapter.

Therapeutic Interventions

The overall goal of medical treatment for chronic heart failure is to improve the heart's pumping ability and decrease the heart's oxygen demands. Treatment of heart failure focuses on (1) identifying and correcting the underlying cause, (2) increasing the strength of the heart's contraction, (3) maintaining optimum water and sodium balance, and (4) decreasing the heart's workload. Heart failure management requires a team approach that may involve physicians, case

managers, nurses, dietitians, physical therapists, occupational therapists, pharmacists, social workers, and clergy. Heart failure critical pathways (treatment guidelines), as well as heart failure clinics, are being used to ensure quality-based outcomes while reducing treatment costs.

The severity of heart failure determines the individualized therapy selected. Noninvasive approaches are usually tried first. If noninvasive treatment is not effective, invasive approaches may be used.

Oxygen Therapy

One of the major problems caused by heart failure is a reduction in oxygen delivered to the tissues. The heart failure signs and symptoms of this are fatigue, dyspnea, altered mental status, and cyanosis. Oxygen therapy assists in supplying the oxygen needs of the tissues. In mild heart failure, oxygen may be delivered via nasal cannula. For more severe cases, arterial blood gas values guide oxygen delivery, either via masks that provide high concentrations of oxygen or with mechanical ventilation.

Activity

Activity tolerance depends on the severity of heart failure signs and symptoms. Severe symptoms may require bedrest with restricted activity until treatment reduces the symptoms. For stable heart failure, a regular exercise program can be helpful in improving cardiac function and reducing heart failure effects. Patients should be encouraged to stay as active as possible within the parameters the physician has prescribed. An individualized walking program that increases activity over time is often prescribed. Patients should be taught how to exercise safely without causing symptoms and to understand that overexertion can produce fatigue the next day. Referral to a cardiac rehabilitation program can be helpful.

Nutrition

Dietary sodium is often restricted to decrease fluid retention. Restricting sodium is challenging. Compliance is often low because low-sodium foods are not very appealing. A referral to a dietitian is important. Diet counseling helps the patient and family understand the need for dietary compliance and the need to provide menus that are appealing and easy to use. Salt substitutes often use potassium in place of sodium, so the patient and physician should discuss their use. Spices, herbs, and lemon juice may be suggested to flavor unsalted

---

 NURSING CARE TIP

In severe heart failure with abdominal discomfort present, malnutrition is a concern. The patient can be anorexic, but the weight gain that occurs with fluid retention can mask the weight loss occurring from the anorexia. Monitor food intake to ensure weight gain from fluid retention does not allow malnutrition to be undetected.

foods. Eating should remain pleasurable for the patient to avoid malnutrition. Focus on showing patients the foods that they like and can still have rather than talking about only the foods they cannot have.

Drug Therapy

Current guidelines generally recommend the use of three drug combination therapy for those with HF. These drug categories include angiotensin-converting enzyme inhibitors (ACEIs), or angiotensin receptor blockers (ARBs), diuretics, and beta blockers. Digoxin can be used as a fourth drug for symptom control. The major classifications of oral drugs used to treat heart failure are listed in Table 26.5. Potassium supplements, anticoagulants, and antidysrhythmics may be used as needed to prevent complications on an individualized basis.

ANGIOTENSIN-CONVERTING ENZYME INHIBITORS (ACEIs). ACEIs are considered the first-choice drug over angiotensin receptor blockers (ARBs). They are used for vasodilation. They also offer additional benefit by preventing remodeling. These remodeling changes lead to progressive cardiac deterioration, so inhibiting these changes is of great benefit. They decrease progression of chronic heart failure and hospitalization and improve survival.

LEARNING TIP

To help you identify ACE inhibitors, remember that their generic names end with -pril.

TABLE 26.5 ORAL MEDICATIONS FOR HEART FAILURE

Class	Drugs	Side Effects	Nursing Implications
ACE Inhibitor plus a Diuretic			
First-line therapy to decrease afterload. Decreases cardiac hypertrophy.	Captopril (Capoten) Enalapril (Vasotec) Fosinopril (Monopril) Lisinopril (Prinivil, Zestril) Moexipril (Univasc) Perindopril (Aceon) Quinapril (Accupril) Ramipril (Altace) Trandolapril (Mavik)	Cough, hypotension, altered taste, rash, proteinuria, hyperkalemia, angioedema (dyspnea, facial swelling), neutropenia (with captopril) Teach patient to change positions slowly to reduce orthostatic hypotension.	Check blood pressure before giving. Monitor WBC with captopril. Take captopril and moexipril on an empty stomach (1 hour before or 2 hours after meals). Teach to report development of cough, so drug can be changed Teach to check blood pressure weekly and report changes to physician. Teach to report rash, sore throat/ mouth, fever, swelling of hands/feet/face/ tongue, difficulty breathing/swallowing, chest pain or irregular heartbeat.
Angiotensin II Receptor Inhibitor			
Decreases cardiac hypertrophy and apoptosis. May be used if ACE inhibitor not tolerated.	Candesartan (Atacand) Irbesartan (Avapro) Losartan (Cozaar) Valsartan (Diovan)	Headache, dizziness, angioedema (dyspnea, facial swelling)	Take blood pressure and pulse before giving. Correct dehydration before initiating therapy. Teach to change positions slowly to reduce orthostatic hypotension. Teach to report rash, sore throat/ mouth, fever, swelling of hands/ feet/face/tongue, difficulty breathing/swallowing, chest pain or irregular heartbeat.
Diuretics			
Loop diuretics			
Decrease fluid overload. *Potassium wasting*	Bumetanide (Bumex) Furosemide (Lasix) Torsemide (Demadex)	Hypokalemia, hypochloremia, hypomagnesemia, hyponatremia, dehydration, hypotension	Do not give loop or thiazide diuretics to sulfa-allergic patients. Take blood pressure and pulse before giving. Monitor electrolyte levels (especially potassium level and for those on digitalis), and fluid status (daily weight, intake, output, thirst, dry mouth, weakness, oliguria) throughout therapy. Administer per patient lifestyle (usually in AM) to avoid nocturia.

(Continued on following page)

TABLE 26.5 ORAL MEDICATIONS FOR HEART FAILURE (Continued)

Class	Drugs	Side Effects	Nursing Implications
Potassium-sparing	Spironolactone (Aldactone)	Hyperkalemia, nausea, vomiting, anorexia, diarrhea, headache, clumsiness, gynecomastia	Do not give potassium sparing diuretic if hyperkalemic. Teach to report signs of hyperkalemia: weakness, fatigue, confusion, dyspnea, arrhythmias, confusion. Older patients are at higher risk for electrolyte imbalances.
Thiazide diuretics *Potassium wasting* Decrease fluid overload.	Chlorothiazide (Diuril) Chlorthalidone (Hygroton, Thalitone) Hydrochlorothiazide (Hydro DIURIL, HCTZ, Microzide) Metolazone (Zaroxolyn)	Hypokalemia, dizziness, hypotension, photosensitivity	Teach about potassium supplements and, if on digitalis, about increased risk of toxicity with hypokalemia. Teach to monitor weight daily and report changes. Teach use of sunscreen to prevent photosensitivity reaction.
Beta Blockers Reduce sympathetic nervous system input, reduce cardiac remodeling, improve cardiac output, reduce symptoms, reduce disease progression and sudden death.	Bisoprolol (Zebeta) Carvedilol (Coreg), specific for heart failure, contains beta blocker plus antioxidant, effective in slowing progression of heart failure Metoprolol tartrate (Toprol XL, Lopressor)	Dizziness, hypotension, hyperglycemia, fluid retention, diarrhea, bradycardia, heart blocks, impotence, bronchospasm (carvedilol)	Avoid carvedilol in patients with asthma (causes bronchospasm). Check apical heart rate and blood pressure. If heart rate is below 50 or blood pressure below 100 systolic, contact physician before giving. Teach to take pulse daily and blood pressure biweekly and to contact physician before taking drug if pulse rate is below 60. Teach to change positions slowly to reduce orthostatic hypotension. Diabetic patients should closely monitor blood sugar. Teach to monitor for worsening of heart failure symptoms.
Inotropes—Cardiac Glycoside (positive inotrope and negative chronotrope) Increase the force and contraction of the myocardium, which increases cardiac output. Slows heart rate to reduce workload of heart and controls atrial fibrillation if present.	Digoxin (Lanoxicaps, Lanoxin)	Fatigue, nausea, vomiting, anorexia, headache, bradycardia, cardiac arrhythmias Toxicity: abdominal pain, anorexia, nausea, vomiting, visual changes (blurred, yellow-green halos, photophobia, diplopia) bradycardia, dysrhythmias	Take apical pulse for 1 minute; if below 60, contact physician before giving. Instruct patient to take medication exactly as directed, at the same time each day. Teach patient to take pulse and to contact health care professional before taking medication if pulse rate is below 60 or above 100. Therapeutic digoxin levels: 0.5 to 2 mg/mL. Older patients are more susceptible to toxicity. Teach signs and symptoms of digitalis toxicity to patient and family. Periodically monitor drug level and electrolytes (hypokalemia, hypomagnesemia, hypercalcemia make patients more susceptible to toxicity). Antidote for toxicity is digoxin immune FAB (Digibind).

Class	Drugs	Side Effects	Nursing Implications
Vasodilators Decrease after-load, which increases cardiac output and reduces cardiac work-load. Used for patients who cannot take ACE inhibitors.	Isosorbide dinitrate (ISDN, Isorbid, Isordil, Isonate) Hydralazine (Apresoline)	Headache, dizziness, hypotension, tachy-cardia	Take blood pressure and pulse before giving. Teach to change positions slowly to reduce orthostatic hypotension. Isosorbide dinitrate: Administer 1 hour before or 2 hours after meals for faster absorption. Chewable tablets should be chewed well before swallowing and held in the mouth for 2 minutes. Extended-release tablets and capsules should be swallowed whole. Do not chew, crush, or break. Sublingual tablets should be held under tongue until dissolved; no eating, drinking, or smoking until tablet is dissolved; replace sublingual tab if swallowed. Headache is common initially and is treated with aspirin. Hydralazine: Take with meals to enhance absorption. Teach to avoid sudden changes in position to avoid orthostatic hypotension. Teach to immediately report fatigue, fever, aching, rash, chest pain, sore throat, numbness, tingling, or weakness of hands/feet.

ACE = angiotensin-converting enzyme; WBC = white blood cell.

ANGIOTENSIN RECEPTOR BLOCKERS (ARBs). ARBs are an alternative to ACEIs for inhibiting the renin-angiotensin-aldosterone system. Several ARBs are available. They should be used carefully if ACEIs are also used as hyperkalemia and renal dysfunction risks increase.

DIURETICS. Diuretics are used to reduce fluid volume and decrease pulmonary venous pressure, so the heart does not have to work so hard. Since they are given to help prevent edema, edema does not need to be present for their use. Diuretics act on various areas of the kidneys to promote the excretion of edema fluid. A combination of diuretics may be used to achieve the desired effect. Electrolytes (especially potassium levels to prevent hypokalemia) and fluid balance (to prevent dehydration) should be carefully monitored during therapy. Potassium supplements are often given with potassium-wasting diuretics.

A potassium-sparing diuretic, spironolactone (Aldactone), blocks the effects of aldosterone and has a positive effect on sodium and potassium balance. Potassium must be monitored carefully, as spironolactone is a potassium-sparing agent and the risk of hyperkalemia increases if ACEIs or ARBs are also used.

BETA BLOCKERS. Initially the sympathetic nervous system (SNS) acts to compensate for HF. Long-term

NURSING CARE TIP
Always check potassium levels before giving a potassium-wasting diuretic such as loop diuretics furosemide (Lasix), bumetanide (Bumex), or torsemide (Demadex) or before giving a potassium supplement, which the patient may be taking due to diuretic therapy. Do not give a diuretic if the potassium level is low or a potassium supplement if the potassium level is high.

sympathetic effects, however, are not helpful in heart failure. Beta blockers block the adverse effects of the SNS. Improved cardiac output, reduced symptoms, reduced disease progression and reduced sudden death are benefits of this therapy.

LEARNING TIP
To help you identify beta blockers, remember that their generic names end with -ol.

INOTROPIC AGENTS. Inotropic drugs strengthen ventricular contraction to increase cardiac output. Inotropic agents include the cardiac glycosides (digitalis, digoxin), sympathomimetics (dopamine, dobutamine), and phosphodiesterase inhibitors (amrinone, milrinone). The sympathomimetics and phosphodiesterase inhibitors are usually used short term.

Digitalis. In addition to improving contraction strength, digitalis preparations decrease conduction time within the heart, which slows the heart rate to allow more complete emptying of the ventricles. Digitalis may increase myocardial oxygen needs, so it is used cautiously. Monitoring of serum drug levels is necessary to detect toxic levels of the drug. If toxic levels are present, the drug is stopped to allow digitalis levels to decrease over time. If life-threatening dysrhythmias occur, a digoxin antibody, digoxin immune FAB (Digibind), can be administered.

CRITICAL THINKING

Mr. Shepard (3)

■ During Mr. Shepard's visit, the physician tells him to continue the ACE inhibitor, the diuretic, and a 2-g sodium diet.
1. Why is the ACE inhibitor continued?
2. Will the ACE inhibitor affect preload or afterload?
3. Why is the diuretic ordered?
4. Why is a 2-g sodium diet ordered?
5. What is the overall goal of the ordered treatment?

Suggested answers at end of chapter.

Cardiac Resynchronization Therapy

Cardiac resynchronization therapy (CRT) is an option for some patients with heart failure and ventricular dyssynchrony. In heart failure, the ventricles do not always beat together. This ventricular dyssynchrony results in less effective pumping by the ventricles and reduced stroke volume. Cardiac resynchronization therapy restores normal contraction timing of both ventricles. Resetting the heartbeat reduces symptoms and improves quality of life. Cardiac resynchronization therapy uses a biventricular cardiac pacing system. An atrial lead senses or paces the atria as needed. A right and left ventricular lead stimulates the ventricles to synchronize their contractions in response to the atrial event. Left ventricular filling is then improved. Several types of CRT devices are available. CRT therapy is available with an implantable cardiac defibrillator therapy (CRT-D). One newer type of CRT device is also able to monitor fluid status within the thorax (chest). For more information and pictures of the InSync CRT devices, visit www.medtronic.com.

Mechanical Assistive Devices

Newer technology is improving treatment options for the failing heart. Mechanical assistive devices can provide temporary support to patients in cardiogenic shock or be a bridge to transplantation or a long-term solution when other options are not available for the failing heart. These devices increase the cardiac output of the patient. They are used primarily in critical care settings and include the intra-aortic balloon pump, ventricular assist devices, and artificial heart. Technology in this area is continually being updated. For current information and to see pictures of artificial hearts and ventricular assist devices, visit the National Institutes of Health or a manufacturer's website at the following addresses:

http://www.nlm.nih.gov/medlineplus/
www.abiomed.com
www.syncardia.com
www.thoratec.com
www.worldheart.com

INTRA-AORTIC BALLOON PUMP. The purpose of using an intra-aortic balloon pump (IABP) is to increase circulation to the coronary arteries and reduce the work of the heart. The IABP catheter is inserted into the femoral artery and positioned in the descending aortic arch (Fig. 26.3). Then the IABP is attached to a computer that senses ventricular contraction and controls the balloon. While the heart is relaxed (diastole), the balloon is inflated, which sends more blood into the coronary arteries without having the heart work harder. Just before the heart contracts (systole), the balloon deflates to allow blood to flow past it. The deflation of the balloon also reduces pressure in the aorta which allows the blood to flow more easily from the

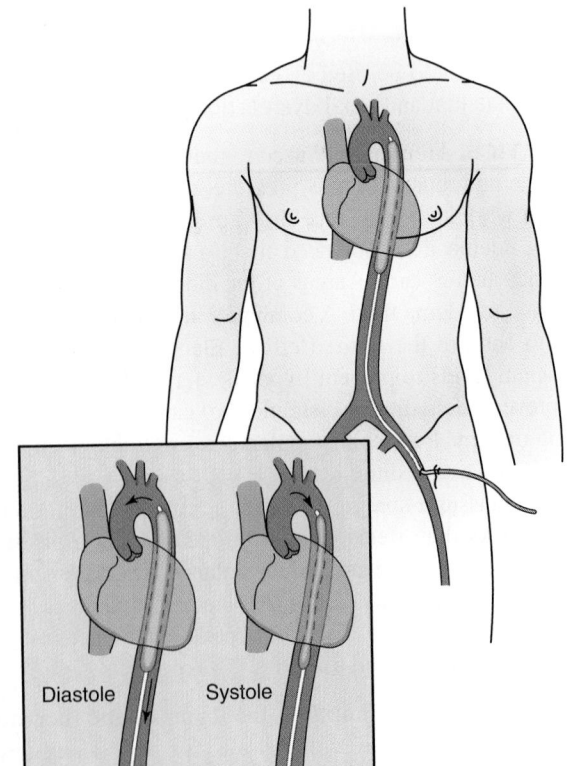

Diastole   Systole

FIGURE 26.3 Intra-aortic balloon pump.

heart. The IABP is inserted in a cardiac catheterization laboratory, critical care unit, or surgery and is used short term for several days.

VENTRICULAR ASSIST DEVICES. Ventricular assist devices (VADs) are implanted mechanical devices that assist cardiac pumping. These devices maintain cardiac output and allow the failing ventricle to rest. VADs are used temporarily as a bridge to transplantation (while awaiting a donor heart), bridge to recovery (for hearts that potentially can recover), or as permanent, long-term therapy referred to as destination therapy for those who are not candidates for heart transplant. They may also be referred to as left ventricular assist devices (LVADs) if used in the left ventricle only, right ventricular assist devices (RVADs) if used in the right ventricle only, or bi-VADs (biventricular assist devices) if used in both ventricles. The types of VADs are shown in Figure 26.4. VADs can pump blood directly from either the right atrium to the pulmonary artery (right ventricular failure) or the left atrium to the aorta (left ventricular failure). Two devices can be used for biventricular failure.

Autologous Adult Stem Cell Therapy

Autologous adult stem cell therapy is a treatment option for some with heart failure that is available in other countries. The stem cells taken from a person's own blood are later injected or implanted into a coronary artery or the heart. These stem cells then stimulate the growth of new blood vessels or heart muscle to improve blood flow or cardiac function. For more information on stem cells, visit http://stemcells.nih.gov/info/basics/. For information on an example of this therapy, visit http://www.vescell.com/index.php.

Surgical Management

Many conditions can cause heart failure. Many of these causes may be treated surgically. Examples of surgical procedures include coronary artery bypass for coronary artery disease or valve replacement for valvular disease. Once these conditions are treated, heart failure symptoms should resolve.

LEFT VENTRICULAR RECONSTRUCTIVE SURGERY (DOR PROCEDURE). Left ventricular reconstructive surgery is done to remove areas of dead heart tissue or ventricular aneurysm. This returns the ventricle to a more normal shape to improve heart failure symptoms.

Ventricular Aneurysm Repair. Indications that a ventricular aneurysm requires surgery include persistent angina, symptoms of heart failure, large aneurysms impeding the function of the heart, left ventricular failure, or tachy-dysrhythmias. Once the patient is on CPB, an incision is made exposing the heart and then the aneurysm is resected (cut out), leaving a fibrous border (Fig. 26.5). The ventricle is wiped clean and irrigated to ensure all thrombi are removed. The opening is then closed with sutures or patched with a graft. Air that entered the ventricle while it was open is aspirated, and the surgery continues as described in the general surgery procedure section.

Treatments Being Researched

Several treatments are being studied for potential use in treating heart failure. Medications include oral phosphodiesterase III inhibitors, vasopressin receptor antagonists, and intermittent nesiritide infusions. Other therapies being studied include implantable hemodynamic monitors, external counterpulsation, internal cardiac support devices, stem cell transplantation, intravascular volume reduction, and surgical ventricular restoration.

HEART RESIZING PROCEDURES. Newer often minimally invasive surgical treatments are being explored to help reshape the heart so that it can function more normally as a

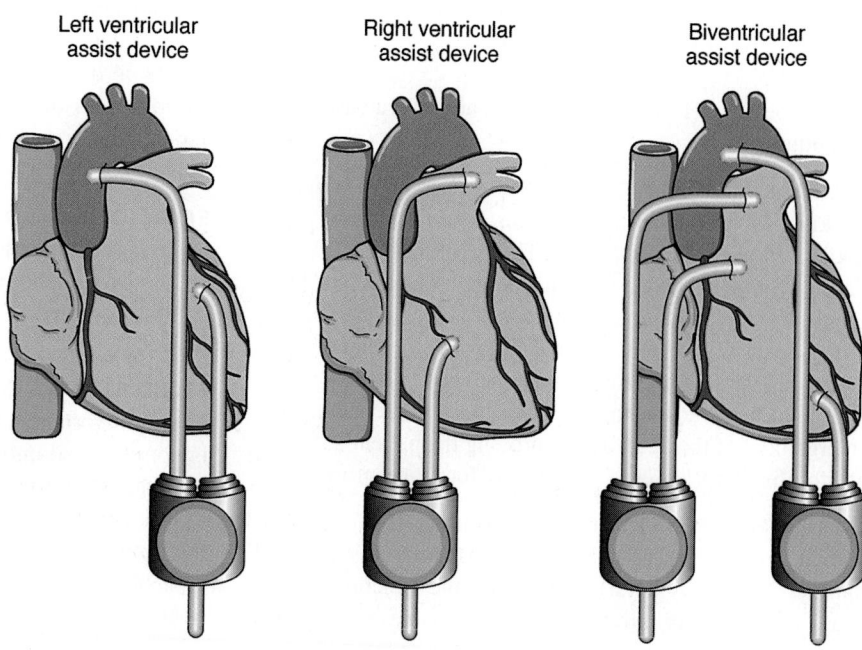

FIGURE 26.4 Different types of ventricular assist devices. *(Modified from Ruppert, S, Kernicki, J, and Dolan, J: Dolan's Critical Care Nursing. F.A. Davis, Philadelphia, 1996, p 336.)*

Left ventricular
assist device

Right ventricular
assist device

Biventricular
assist device

Ventricular
aneurysmectomy

1

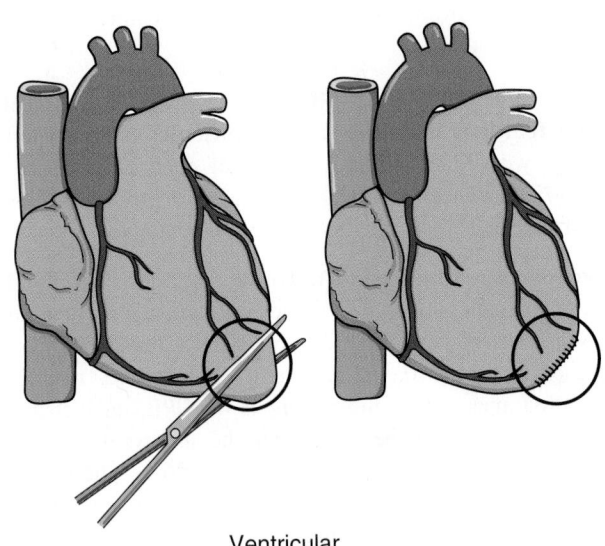

Ventricular
aneurysmorrhaphy
Dacron patch

2

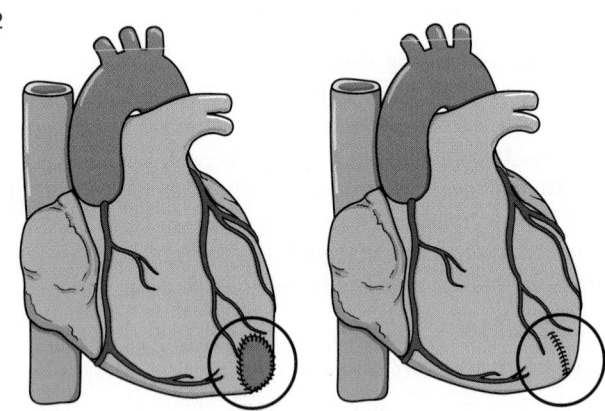

1: Aneurysm is cut and closed.
2: Patch inserted inside incision, then closed.

FIGURE 26.5 Ventricular aneurysm repair.

pump. The STICH trial began in 2002 and is evaluating this technique.

CARDIAC SUPPORT DEVICE. A meshlike support stocking for the heart is available in Europe and being studied in the United States. The stocking, the Corcap Cardiac Support Device (Acorn Cardiovascular A; St. Paul, Minn.), is implanted during surgery. It gives gentle support to the heart and permits normal function. In heart failure, increasing cardiac pressures dilate the heart. The stocking's goal is to help reduce this pressure thereby preventing the enlargement of the heart and improving the patient's quality of life. Visit http://www.acorncv.com/ for more information.

CARDIOMYOPLASTY. Cardiomyoplasty is an experimental surgical procedure using the patient's own skeletal muscle (latissimus dorsi) to enhance the function of the heart and improve circulation. The muscle is wrapped

around the aorta or heart, and a cardiomyostimulator is implanted to stimulate muscle contraction. Cardiomyoplasty may reduce the need for heart transplantation by delaying or preventing end-stage heart failure.

Nursing Process for Chronic Heart Failure

Nursing Assessment/Data Collection
While obtaining data for the patient with heart failure, focus on areas that might indicate the presence of heart failure (Table 26.6).

Nursing Diagnosis, Planning, Interventions, and Evaluation
See Box 26.1 Nursing Care Plan for the Patient with Chronic Heart Failure for common nursing diagnoses.

The major focus of nursing care for chronic heart failure patients is to improve oxygenation and decrease the body's need for oxygen with rest, positioning, medications, fluid balance, and oxygen consumption control.

OXYGEN. Oxygen therapy is ordered by the physician and guided by blood gas analysis. Before starting oxygen therapy, explain the therapy to the patient. For chronic heart failure, oxygen is administered at 2 to 6 L/min via nasal cannula. The effects of the oxygen should be monitored carefully. Oxygen should be used cautiously in all patients, so that their stimulus to breathe is not diminished (especially if the patient has chronic obstructive pulmonary disease [COPD]).

Home Oxygen Therapy. If a patient will be using home oxygen therapy, instructions must be given on the proper use of the oxygen and safety precautions for oxygen use. The family must also understand oxygen safety precautions and be willing to comply with them. Smoking is prohibited when oxygen is in use.

REST AND ACTIVITY. Reduction of the body's oxygen demands decreases the workload of the heart. A balance of rest and activity that does not produce signs or symptoms of oxygen deprivation is essential. The activity level of the patient is determined by the severity of the heart failure. During times of exertion, monitor the patient's vital signs and respiratory effort for oxygen deprivation. If activity intolerance develops, the activity should be stopped.

POSITIONING. Semi-Fowler's or high-Fowler's position makes breathing easier. In upright positions, the lungs are able to expand more fully and gravity decreases the amount of fluid returned to the heart, thereby reducing the heart's workload.

FLUID RETENTION. Monitoring daily weights for weight gain is important in detecting fluid retention. Edema usually is not observed until there are 5 to 10 pounds of extra fluid present. A baseline weight should be obtained when heart failure is diagnosed. Daily weights should be measured on the same scale, at the same time of day, and with the same type of clothing worn to ensure accuracy. A good time to obtain a daily weight is in the morning after the bladder is

TABLE 26.6 NURSING ASSESSMENT FOR THE PATIENT WITH CHRONIC HEART FAILURE

Subjective Data	Objective Data
History	**Respiratory**
Respiratory	Tachypnea, crackles, wheezing, respiratory effort, dyspnea with exertion
Lung disease?	**Cardiovascular**
How many flights of stairs can be climbed without dyspnea?	Tachycardia, dysrhythmias, jugular vein distention, peripheral edema—degree of pitting
How many pillows used for sleeping?	**Gastrointestinal**
Dyspnea at rest or that awakens from sleeping?	Abdominal distention, ascites, hepatomegaly, splenomegaly
Cardiovascular	**Neurological**
Any cardiac disease history: hypertension, myocardial infarction, valvular problem, anemia, dysrhythmias, palpitations	Confusion, decreased level of consciousness, restlessness, impaired memory
Chest pain—precipitating factors, severity, relieving factors	**Integumentary**
Can activities of daily living be performed?	Cold, clammy skin; pallor; cyanosis
Can activities performed 6 months, 4 months, 2 months, 2 weeks ago still be done?	**General**
Any dizziness (vertigo) or fainting (syncope)?	Weight
Fluid retention	**Diagnostic test findings**
Daily sodium intake?	
Weight gain?	
Are shoes tight? Do ankles swell?	
Gastrointestinal	
Is appetite good?	
Any nausea, vomiting, or abdominal pain?	
Urinary	
Decrease in daytime urine output?	
How often does patient go to the bathroom at night (nocturia)?	
Neurological	
Any change in behavior?	
Medications	
Knowledge of condition	
Coping skills	

emptied. Documentation of daily weights should include the date and time of the weight, the scale used, the clothing worn, and the weight measurement. A weight journal can be kept by the patient. Tell patients to report weight gains of 2 to 3 lb over 1 to 2 days.

OXYGEN CONSUMPTION. Increased oxygen consumption by the heart should be avoided. Tachycardia increases the oxygen needs of the heart and should be reported promptly to the physician for treatment. Older patients are especially vulnerable to the effects of tachycardia because of their decreased reserves. Constipation should be prevented because straining during defecation, Valsalva's maneuver, increases the heart's workload by increasing venous return to the heart. Stool softeners should be administered, as ordered, to prevent straining.

Patients should be taught methods of saving energy while performing activities of daily living (ADL). Activities should be alternated with periods of rest. Fatigue should be avoided. A referral to occupational therapy and physical therapy can be helpful in developing techniques that allow the patient to conserve energy during self-care. Some suggestions for conserving energy include placing frequently used objects at waist level to avoid reaching overhead, planning bathing activities to include rest periods, and using Velcro fasteners to make dressing easier.

MEDICATIONS. Because heart failure is a progressive, chronic condition, patients may require lifetime medications. Combination drug therapy is often needed. Taking many pills each day can be challenging. Financial resources, compliance, and ongoing monitoring are issues that must be considered.

Diuretics require monitoring of the patient's potassium levels and blood pressure. To prevent hypokalemia, potassium supplements may be prescribed during diuretic therapy, and a diet with high-potassium foods is encouraged. If too much fluid is removed, the patient may become hypotensive and orthostatic hypotension can develop. The patient may then be dizzy and at risk of falling. Caution the patient to change positions slowly to prevent falls during diuretic therapy.

Box 26.1 NURSING CARE PLAN for the Patient with Chronic Heart Failure

Nursing Diagnosis: Activity intolerance related to fatigue caused by oxygen imbalance

Expected Outcomes Patient will show increased activity tolerance with vital signs within normal limits (WNL) in response to activity.

Evaluation of Outcomes Does the patient participate in activities and maintain vital signs WNL?

Interventions	Rationale	Evaluation
Provide rest, space activities, and conserve energy.	Myocardial oxygen need is decreased with rest and energy conservation.	Does patient participate in activity with no pulse rate or ECG changes?
Assist as needed with activities of daily living (ADLs).	Conserve energy by assisting with ADLs.	Are patient's ADLs met?
Teach use of assistive devices and lifestyle changes.	Assistive devices can overcome limitations to increase activity.	Does patient incorporate assistive devices into lifestyle changes?

Geriatric

Interventions	Rationale	Evaluation
Increase time allowed to complete activities.	Independence and participation are increased if extra time is allowed for tasks.	Does patient report greater ability to complete activities with fewer symptoms?

Nursing Diagnosis: Excess fluid volume related to heart failure and the secondary reduction in renal blood flow for filtration

Expected Outcomes Patient remains free from edema and dyspnea, has clear lung sounds, and maintains baseline weight.

Evaluation of Outcomes Does patient have clear lung sounds with baseline weight maintained?

Interventions	Rationale	Evaluation
Monitor for edema, weight gain, jugular vein distention (JVD), lung crackles.	Excess fluid is indicated by edema, sudden weight gain, JVD, and crackles in the lungs.	Is edema, weight gain, JVD, or crackles present?
Decrease sodium intake as ordered.	Sodium retains fluid.	Does patient restrict sodium intake?
Administer diuretics or inotropics as ordered.	Diuretics promote fluid excretion. Inotropics increase cardiac contraction strength.	Is output increased and edema or dyspnea reduced?
Monitor intake and output.	Intake and output will show imbalances.	Are intake and output balanced for 24 hours?

Nursing Diagnosis: Disturbed sleep pattern related to nocturia and inability to lie down and sleep comfortably

Expected Outcomes Patient awakens refreshed and is less fatigued during the day.

Evaluation of Outcomes Does patient wake up less frequently during the night and feel more refreshed with less fatigue during the day?

Interventions	Rationale	Evaluation
Identify barriers to sleep.	Anxiety, nocturia, diuretics, orthopnea, or paroxysmal nocturnal dyspnea can make sleep difficult.	Does patient identify sleep barriers?
Assist patient in identifying positions of comfort for sleeping.	Use of pillows or a recliner can decrease orthopnea.	Can patient identify a position of comfort?

Interventions	Rationale	Evaluation
Teach patient cause of dyspnea at night.	Anxiety about falling asleep and waking up short of breath is reduced.	Can patient explain cause of dyspnea?
Encourage patient to recline for 30 to 60 minutes before bedlime.	Reclining before bedtime redistributes fluid and increases voiding that can occur before going to sleep instead of after going to sleep.	Is patient awakened to void after going to bed less often?
Geriatric		
Encourage patient to take diuretics early in the day.	Nocturia is reduced if diuretics are taken earlier in the day.	Does patient take diuretics early and report less nocturia?

Inotropic agents such as digitalis strengthen heart contractions and slow the heart rate. Before administration of a digitalis drug, the patient's apical pulse should be counted for 1 minute. If the pulse is below 60 beats per minute, notify the physician to determine if the drug should be given. Some patients are given digitalis even if their heart rates are between 50 and 60 beats per minute, as long as their heart's conduction system is normal or if it is due to other medications such as a beta blocker. When giving digitalis, be aware that hypokalemia increases the heart's sensitivity to digitalis. A patient can become toxic on a normal dose of digitalis when hypokalemia is present. This is important to note because many people on digitalis also take diuretics, which may lower potassium levels. Monitoring for signs and symptoms of digitalis toxicity should be done routinely during patient assessment. Early symptoms of digitalis toxicity are anorexia, nausea, and vomiting. Other signs and symptoms include bradycardia or other dysrhythmias, visual problems, and mental changes. The elderly are especially prone to toxic effects of this drug and may exhibit confusion when levels are toxic.

Medications with vasodilating effects reduce the heart's workload by decreasing vascular pressure. Blood pressure is monitored when administering vasodilators.

Medication Teaching. Patients and their families are taught the purpose, side effects, and precautions for prescribed medications. Teach them to report side effects to the physician. If dizziness occurs from drugs that reduce blood pressure, the drugs can be staggered so that they are not all taken at the same time. Patients taking a digitalis preparation should be taught to take their pulse. They should hold the medication and call their physician if their heart rate is less than 60 beats per minute or below the lower-limit heart rate set by their physician. Patients on diuretics should be taught the following:

- Take them during the day before 4 p.m. to decrease being awakened at night to void (if desired).

- Have a readily available and obstacle-free bathroom or commode to prevent incontinence and falls.
- Eat high-potassium foods if taking a potassium-wasting diuretic.
- Weigh themselves daily and report weight gains.

Patients should understand the importance of taking their medication as prescribed, even if they do not have symptoms. A schedule should be developed so patients remember to take their medications.

LOW-SODIUM DIET AND WEIGHT CONTROL. A diet assessment should include patient's food likes and dislikes, cultural influences, economic status, and food preparation resources (e.g., shopping ability, storage, refrigeration, and cooking equipment). It is helpful to include a dietitian in the planning process, as well as the food preparer or a support person, to increase diet compliance.

For overweight patients, weight reduction may help eliminate the underlying cause of heart failure. Diet counseling and support should be given to the obese patient to encourage weight loss. The body mass index (BMI) should guide weight loss. If anorexia occurs in the later stages of heart failure, the patient's intake should be evaluated. Several small meals rather than three large meals will decrease the heart's workload. If the patient's nutritional needs are not being met, the physician should be informed for a referral to a dietitian.

Patients should be taught to read food labels; foods that are high and low in sodium content and that salt substitutes may contain potassium. With this knowledge, patients can help design a daily meal plan using low-sodium foods that are appealing to them. Food preparers should be taught not to salt food during cooking, and table salt should be eliminated. Explaining seasoning alternatives such as spices, herbs, and lemon juice is helpful in making food taste better.

EDUCATION. Chronic management of heart failure requires patient and family understanding of the disease process, management of home oxygen therapy, diet and weight control, need for immunizations such as the annual flu shot, and medications (see Home Health Hints). The patient and family must recognize the importance of each of these factors in order to foster a productive life for the patient with chronic heart failure. A discussion of heart failure and signs and symptoms to report to the physician using simple terms should be included in the teaching plan (Box 26.2 Patient and Family Education).

COPING. Living with a chronic illness can be frustrating for both patients and their families. An assessment of coping skills used by patients and their families can be used to develop a plan for coping with this current illness. Available support systems are explained to patients. Referrals to social workers, sexual counselors, telehealth management, and nurse-managed clinics can be helpful in providing resources that may make living with heart failure easier. Providing patients options for traveling can help maintain quality of life. Understanding the chronic nature of heart failure is important for patients, families, and caregivers to positively deal with the emotions and feelings that can result. Nurse-managed heart failure clinics have been shown to decrease hospitalization rates and increase effective management of the therapeutic regimen.

CRITICAL THINKING

Mr. Shepard (4)

■ The nurse meets with Mr. Shepard after the physician orders the ACE inhibitor to be continued, a diuretic, and 2-g sodium diet.

1. What information should the nurse teach Mr. Shepard based on the prescribed treatment?
2. What types of foods should be included in Mr. Shepard's diet?
3. Why does the nurse instruct Mr. Shepard to weigh himself daily?
4. Why does the nurse tell Mr. Shepard to weigh himself at the same time of day, on the same scale, and with the same type of clothing?

Suggested answers at end of chapter.

CARDIAC TRANSPLANTATION

Cardiac transplantation is reserved for patients with end-stage cardiac disease. Strict criteria for the selection of recipients and donors are applied to optimize survival (Box 26.3 Cardiac Transplant Criteria). Preoperative teaching is done once the recipient is accepted into the transplant program. For more information on heart transplantation, visit http://www.nlm.nih.gov/medlineplus/hearttransplantation.html.

Box 26.2

Patient and Family Education

Heart Failure Signs and Symptoms to Report to the Physician

Shortness of breath
Fatigue
Dry cough
Shortness of breath when lying down (orthopnea)
Episodes of sudden awakening with shortness of breath (PND)
Weight gain of 2 to 3 lb over 1 to 2 days
Ankle or foot edema
Nocturia
Anorexia

Surgical Procedure

Once a donor heart is found, the recipient is notified, admitted to the hospital, and immediately prepared for surgery. The general procedures for this surgery are similar to those described in the cardiac surgery section. Two types of cardiac transplant procedures are performed: orthotopic and heterotopic. In the orthotopic procedure, once the patient is on CPB, the recipient's diseased heart is removed, leaving the posterior wall of the atria, superior vena cava and inferior vena cava, and pulmonary vein (Fig. 26.6). The aorta and pulmonary artery are cut. The donor's atria, aorta, and pulmonary artery are then anastomosed to the recipient's atria, aorta, and pulmonary artery. Surgery then continues as previously described. The heterotopic procedure joins the

---

Box 26.3

Cardiac Transplant Criteria

Donor Criteria	Recipient Criteria
Younger than 40 years of age	Younger than 55 years of age
No significant cardiac or malignant disease	Class IV cardiac disease (not treatable with other medical or surgical treatment, less than 6–12 months survival)
No active infections	No irreversible pulmonary hypertension
No severe hypertension or diabetes mellitus	No unresolved pulmonary infarcts
Only ± 20 lb difference in weight between donor and recipient	No systemic disease limiting survival
	No drug addiction or peptic ulcer disease

donor heart and vessels to the recipient's heart and vessels without removing the recipient's heart. The donor heart rests in the right side of the chest.

Immunosuppressive therapy begins preoperatively with high loading doses of cyclosporine (Neoral, Sandimmune), azathioprine (Imuran), steroids, or other medications. The risk for rejection is highest immediately after surgery and decreases with time, so doses of immunosuppressive medication are also highest initially after surgery and decrease with time (Box 26.4 Nutrition Notes). Lifelong antirejection therapy is required.

Complications

Heart transplantation complications may include all those stated for cardiac surgery, as well as heart rejection, which is the major cause of death within the first year. Immunosuppressive therapy is required to prevent rejection of the heart. To detect rejection, biopsies of cardiac muscle are commonly performed weekly during the first 3 to 6 weeks

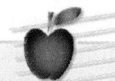

Box 26.4
Nutrition Notes

The potency of antirejection medications may be reduced if patients drink grapefruit juice with them. Grapefruit increases body metabolism.

Individuals who drink wine may not get the desired therapeutic effects of certain immunosuppressive medications.

after surgery, then every 3 months for 1 year, and then yearly. If a biopsy shows damaged cells, indicating rejection, antirejection drug therapy may be changed.

In addition, infection and malignancies may occur as a result of the immunosuppressive therapy. The medications used for immunosuppressive therapy also may cause adverse reactions. Cyclosporine is nephrotoxic and hepato-

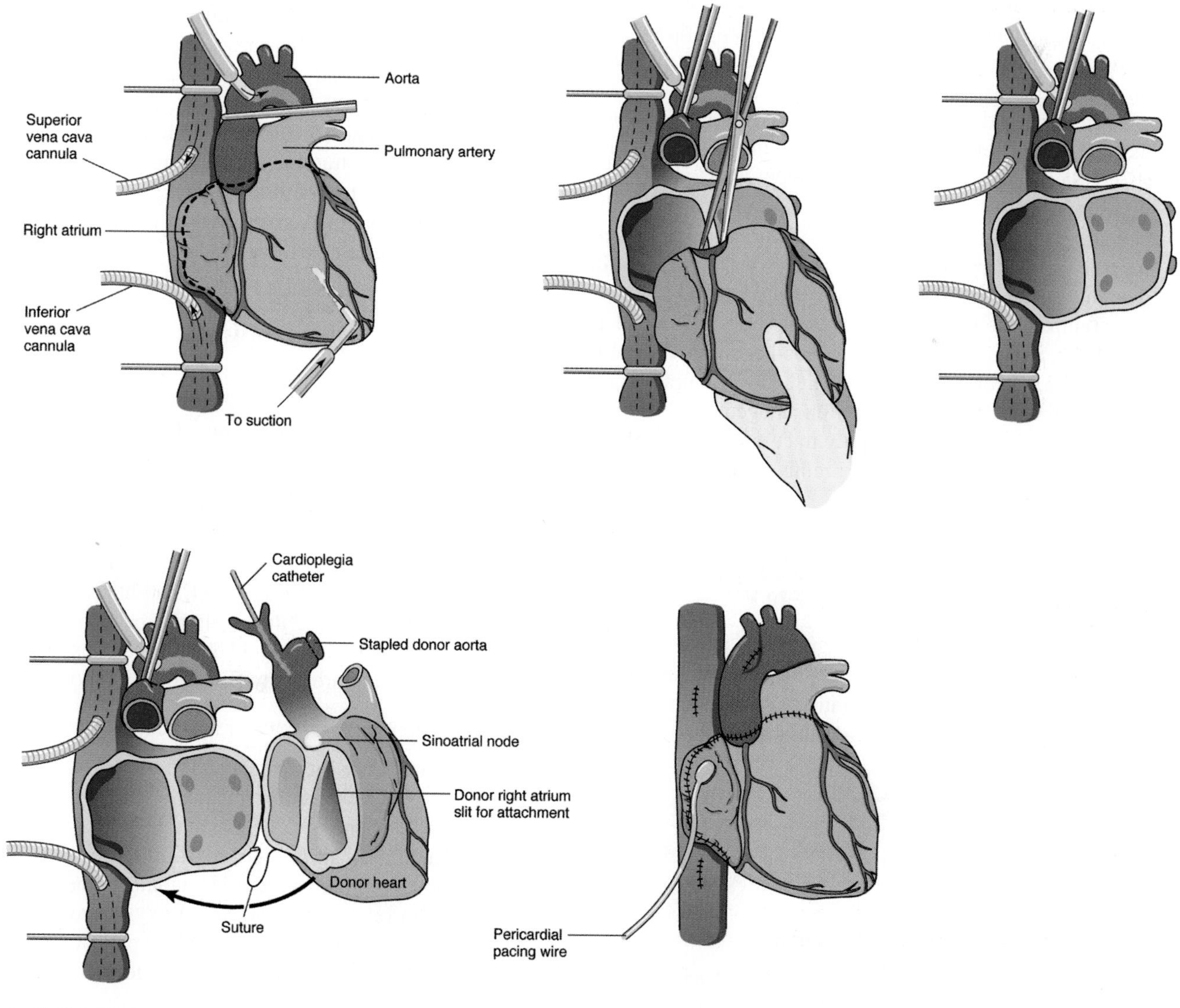

FIGURE 26.6 Heart transplantation.

toxic. Azathioprine is also hepatotoxic and may cause bone marrow depression or skin sensitivity to the sun. Steroids can cause osteoporosis, hyperglycemia, sodium and water retention, gastritis, hypertension, and cataract formation. Muromonab-CD3 (Orthoclone OKT3), used to treat rejection reactions in spite of immunosuppressive therapy, can cause fever, malaise, and headaches.

Therapeutic Interventions

The patient receives a diuretic when CPB is stopped to aid in excretion of excessive circulating fluid. Intake and output are monitored hourly, and the patient is observed for fluid overload. Lung sounds are monitored frequently for crackle, and weight and electrolyte levels are checked daily.

Postcardiotomy syndrome (PCS) may occur from days 2 to 5 after surgery and last a few weeks. Patients may arouse normally and be oriented but exhibit mild confusion or psychosis. Pupillary reaction and motor response are assessed. The safety of the patient is maintained with side rails up, bed in low position, and nursing call light within reach. The patient is given as much rest and as little sensory stimulation as possible. The family is kept informed and involved in the patient's recovery.

Sleeping is difficult because of postoperative pain and the continuous level of activity in the intensive care unit (ICU). Sleep is promoted in 90-minute intervals by dimming lights and decreasing all sensory stimulation near the patient. Additionally, listening to a favorite soothing tape recording with earphones or the use of ordered narcotics for pain may also help sedate and relax the patient.

Temperature is monitored every 4 hours and complete blood cell count (CBC) and white blood cell (WBC) results are monitored for indications of infection. If oral thrush (white patches) develops, an antifungal agent is ordered. A urine culture to diagnose a urinary tract infection is ordered if cloudy urine or urinary tract burning occurs.

NURSING PROCESS FOR THE PREOPERATIVE CARDIAC TRANSPLANT PATIENT

General preoperative and postoperative surgical care is discussed in Chapter 11. Postoperative needs for the patient undergoing cardiac surgery are discussed here.

NURSING PROCESS FOR THE POSTOPERATIVE CARDIAC TRANSPLANT PATIENT

Assessment/Data Collection

The patient is accompanied to the ICU by the anesthesiologist, who gives the nurse a report of the procedure, compli-cations, and hemodynamic and ventilatory management of the patient. The patient is connected to a cardiac monitor and mechanical ventilator. The mechanical ventilator is used for 4 to 24 hours. A temporary pacemaker is connected to the epicardial pacing wires if they were placed during surgery as a precaution to treat bradycardia. The patient is placed under a warming device, such as a light or blanket. The chest tubes are monitored, the nasogastric tube is placed to suction, and the urinary catheter is placed for gravity drainage. A head-to-toe assessment of the patient, including dressings, tubes, and IV lines, is performed. Of importance are signs of awakening, shivering, pain, lung and heart sounds, and palpation of the entire chest and neck to detect crepitus (air in the subcutaneous tissue from opening the chest). Blood is drawn for a CBC, electrolytes, coagulation studies, and arterial blood gases. Cardiac transplant patients may be in isolation for their own protection, depending on the agency's policy.

After the initial transfer assessment, vital signs, oxygen saturation, and cardiac pressures are monitored and recorded every 15 to 30 minutes, with decreasing frequency as the patient stabilizes. Body temperature is monitored continuously while warming measures are used. Intake and output are measured and vital signs are checked. An electrocardiogram (ECG) is done to detect perioperative myocardial infarction. A chest x-ray examination is done to check central line and endotracheal tube placement and to detect a pneumothorax or hemothorax, diaphragm elevation, or mediastinal widening from bleeding. At this point, the family may see the patient, and patient care is explained.

Nursing Diagnosis, Planning, Interventions, and Evaluation

Nursing diagnoses for postoperative cardiac surgery or transplant are discussed in Box 26.5 Nursing Care Plan for the Postoperative Patient Undergoing Cardiac or Transplant Surgery.

Coping with Cardiac Transplant

Cardiac transplant patients may have feelings of sadness and grief for the donor and his family. These feelings may be offset by great elation, relief, and hope after a long wait for the transplant. Patients should be told that these feelings are normal. They should be allowed to express their feelings when they are ready. Emotional support may be needed.

Transplant rejection is a possible complication of this surgery. Patients need to understand the importance of following instructions regarding medications and testing that are related to preventing or detecting rejection.

Cardiac transplant patients are followed in an exercise rehabilitation program that closely monitors their activity progression in relation to myocardial oxygen consumption and signs of activity intolerance. Most patients reach an activity level allowing them to participate in many recreational sports.

CRITICAL THINKING

Mrs. Eden

■ Mrs. Eden, age 45, a single mother of two, is transferred to a surgical unit 5 days after a cardiac transplant. She is withdrawn and has a poor appetite. Her vital signs are stable. However, on ambulating to the bathroom, she is very weak, requiring two nurses to help her. Her respiratory rate increases from 20 to 32 and is slightly labored, and her apical pulse increases from 88 to 103.

1. Is Mrs. Eden tolerating this activity? Why or why not?
2. List four reasons why Mrs. Eden has a poor appetite.
3. Give four nursing interventions for Mrs. Eden's poor appetite.
4. Give three reasons why Mrs. Eden is withdrawn.

Suggested answers at end of chapter.

Box 26.5   NURSING CARE PLAN for the Postoperative Patient Undergoing Cardiac or Transplant Surgery

Nursing Diagnosis: Acute pain related to sternotomy, leg incisions, internal mammary artery resection, or pericarditis

Expected Outcomes Patient will state pain is relieved or tolerable. Patient is able to rest and perform respiratory treatments.

Evaluation of Outcomes Does patient state pain is within acceptable levels? Is patient able to rest and perform respiratory therapies?

Interventions	Rationale	Evaluation
• Obtain characteristics of pain with each episode.	A thorough description is needed to determine cause and plan actions.	Does patient describe pain on scale of 0 to 10?
• Splint chest incision with all movement and coughing and deep breathing.	Stabilizes sternum and incision to increase comfort.	Can patient splint chest incision independently?
• Encourage patient to report pain even when pain is mild.	It is easier to keep pain under control when mild.	Does patient report pain when mild?
• Turn, reposition every 2 hours.	Changes muscle position, relieving stiffness.	Is patient comfortable without stiffness?
• Offer back rubs frequently.	Relaxes tense muscles retracted during operation.	Is patient able to rest in comfort?
• Instruct patient to take a deep breath before movement and exhale slowly during movement.	Keeps muscles relaxed, minimizing tension with guarding and pain.	Can patient perform coughing and deep breathing techniques as instructed?
• Explain that chest pain can occur from the surgical incision rather than the heart.	Chest pain after surgery can be frightening for patients as they may not associate surgical chest pain with the incision and instead think the pain is anginal or infarction pain.	Does patient state understanding of pain sources?

(Continued on following page)

Nursing Diagnosis: Decreased cardiac output related to myocardial depression, hypothermia, bleeding, unstable dysrhythmias, or hypoxemia

Expected Outcomes Patient will remain free of major side effects of pharmacological support. Patient will maintain vital signs within normal limits (WNL), palpable peripheral pulses, urine output greater than 30 mL/hr, and normal sinus rhythm.

Evaluation of Outcomes Is patient free of major side effects? Are vital signs WNL?

Interventions	Rationale	Evaluation
• Monitor vital signs.	Trends reflect problems.	Are vital signs WNL?
• Monitor peripheral circulation.	Mottling or weak pulses may indicate poor cardiac output (CO).	Do peripheral pulses remain strong with normal skin color, temperature, capillary refill?
• Monitor intake and output.	Fluid deficit or excess can alter CO.	Does total intake equal output?
• Listen to lung sounds and note character of sputum.	Wet lung sounds may indicate heart failure or pulmonary edema.	Are lungs clear?
• Monitor temperature closely while rewarming the patient.	Febrile state increases heart rate and myocardial oxygen consumption.	Does temperature remain less than or equal to 98.6°F (37°C)?
• Monitor for shivering.	Shivering increases the blood pressure, decreasing CO and increasing risk for bleeding.	Is patient's shivering controlled?
• Monitor chest tube drainage for increase or sudden decrease.	Drainage >200 mL/hr may lead to hypovolemia and a decrease in CO.	Is patient free from cardiac tamponade and hypovolemia?
• Monitor ECG.	Premature ventricular contractions and atrial fibrillation decrease CO.	Does patient remain in normal sinus rhythm or controlled dysrhythmia?
• Monitor electrolytes.	Low calcium and magnesium and high potassium decrease contractility and CO.	Are electrolytes WNL?
• Monitor ABGs.	Acidosis decreases heart function, and a low CO may lead to further acidosis.	Are ABGs WNL?

Nursing Diagnosis: Risk for infection related to inadequate primary defenses from surgical wound or immunosuppression (transplants)

Expected Outcomes Patient will remain free from infection.

Evaluation of Outcomes Does patient remain free from infection?

Interventions	Rationale	Evaluation
• Observe incision for signs and symptoms of infection.	Redness, warmth, fever, and swelling indicate infection.	Are signs and symptoms of infection present?
• Monitor drainage and maintain drains.	Drains remove fluid from the surgical site to prevent infection development.	Are drainage amount and color normal for procedure? Are drains functioning?

Interventions	Rationale	Evaluation
• Maintain sterile technique for dressing changes.	Sterile technique reduces infection development.	Is incision free of signs and symptoms of infection?
• Monitor and report abnormal findings for temperature, lung sounds, sputum, and urine consistency.	Low-grade (immunosuppressed) or high-grade fever, crackles, yellow-green sputum color, or cloudy urine can indicate infection.	Is the patient's temperature WNL and are lung sounds, sputum, and urine clear?
• Encourage coughing and deep breathing and incentive spirometer use.	Lung infections can be prevented with lung expansion and secretion removal.	Does patient perform coughing and deep breathing and use incentive spirometer?

Nursing Diagnosis: Deficient knowledge related to lack of prior experience with transplant.

Expected Outcomes Patient will demonstrate understanding of care post cardiac transplant.

Evaluation of Outcomes Does patient state understanding and ability to carry out care post cardiac transplant?

Interventions	Rationale	Evaluation
Give information in small increments and use written materials and audiotapes.	Cardiac transplant patients commonly have memory deficits, cognitive dysfunction, and short attention spans resulting from long-term decreased cerebral perfusion.	Does patient state understanding of information?
Include families in teaching sessions and encourage them to promote self-care by the patient.	Family involvement in teaching sessions is important to promote understanding and retention.	Does family participate and state understanding of teaching sessions?
Address or refer sexual functioning questions with patients and their partners.	Patients usually have questions regarding sexual functioning. Referrals can be made to sexual conselors.	Does patient state questions have been addressed?
Discharge teaching includes treatment, complications, activity, medications, enhancing quality of life.	Patients need comprehensive information to comply with post transplant care.	Does patient state understanding of discharge care?

Home Health Hints

- Some patients may not have a scale in their home. It may be necessary to assist them in obtaining one or to leave an agency scale in the home for daily weights.
- The most objective way to document edema is to use a tape measure on the abdominal girth, thigh, calf, and ankle in centimeters. Measure at the same place each visit, such as measuring the girth of the calf at a specified distance above the medial malleolus. Edema may be present if the patient's waistband is getting tighter or shoes and socks feel tighter.

- The sacrum, back, and sides of a bedridden patient should be checked to note edema. These are dependent areas in the bedridden patient, so fluid accumulates in these areas instead of the ankles.
- Blood drawn for potassium levels needs to be transported to the laboratory within 1 hour. Ice should not be put directly on the tube because this can cause destruction of the cells and a false elevation in the potassium level.
- Blood drawn for digoxin levels should be taken to the lab within 2 to 3 hours.

(Continued on following page)

Home Health Hints *(Continued)*

- Patients should use no salt added canned vegetables. Patients on sodium-restricted diets who already have canned vegetables in their home can still use them even though they are not the low-sodium type. They should be instructed to pour off the liquid and rinse the vegetables before heating them for serving. The use of herbs and spices helps make them more flavorful.
- For the patient on a low-sodium diet, an effective diet teaching technique is to have the patient name the foods highest in sodium. Asking the patient to rename the list on each visit helps knowledge retention and compliance.
- If patients have a poor appetite, ask their caregiver if they eat well when eating with others. Anorexia could be a sign of loneliness and depression if they eat well with others instead of an effect from the heart failure.
- Assist patients in taking medications at times that fit their lifestyle. A morning dose of a diuretic may limit what they can do for the next few hours. An afternoon dose might encourage compliance. Lack of compliance is a major factor in the rehospitalization of patients with heart failure. A dose of diuretic too late in the day may cause frequent awakenings during the night to void.
- The home health nurse should periodically check the contents of medicine bottles. If pills have been cut in half, ask about this. Often it is an attempt by the patient to "stretch" the medicine to decrease expenses. There are community or drug company programs that help purchase medicines for patients with financial need. Eligible Medicaid patients can apply for medication cards. The new Medicare Part D prescription program may be helpful, as well.

- Visual disturbances can occur from digitalis toxicity. If the patient sees halos around lights or red-green tinting on everything, report this to the physician.
- Troublesome side effects of an ACE inhibitor such as captopril (Capoten) are an intractable cough and hypotension. It should be noted how the patient is coughing. Teach the patient to report the cough.
- Oxygen concentrators are widely used in home care. Long tubing allows the patient ease in moving about the home. Patients need to be cautioned about keeping the tubing out of their way and not kinking it. If the patient also has chronic obstructive pulmonary disease (COPD), the oxygen flow rate is generally limited to 2 L/min, so the patient's drive to breathe is not decreased. A note stating this should be placed near the gauge as a reminder to the patients.
- As the home health nurse becomes acquainted with the patient, it is easier to pick up on signs of oxygen deprivation and hypoxia, such as confusion, combativeness, or unusual expressions of anger.
- For patients with orthopnea, a foam wedge can be obtained from a medical equipment company to use under their head when sleeping instead of pillows.
- As patients with heart failure feel better, they may go back to the old habits that cause an increase in fluid. The home health nurse can help by providing information about the disease and help patients foster their own independence and ways of coping with the condition. Each home health visit is a teaching opportunity that empowers patients with a knowledge base to help them to take control of their health.

REVIEW QUESTIONS

1. A patient asks the nurse what heart failure is. Which of the following is the nurse's best response?
   a. "In heart failure the heart pumps too much blood into the pulmonary veins."
   b. "In heart failure the heart is unable to pump enough blood for the body's oxygen needs."
   c. "Heart failure is a buildup of blood in the aorta from the heart's left ventricle."
   d. "With a failing heart, the heart stops beating, so blood is not pumped out."

2. Which of the following does the nurse understand is a major cause of left-sided heart failure?

   a. Hypertension
   b. Congenital heart defects
   c. Pulmonary valve stenosis
   d. Septal defects

3. A patient who has been treated for heart failure is being discharged from the hospital on 20 mg furosemide (Lasix) daily. Which of the following statements by the patient would indicate understanding of instructions for this medication?
   a. "I will take the Lasix in the morning."
   b. "I will take the Lasix at bedtime."

c. "I will drink lots of fluids with the Lasix."

d. "I will take it with meals."

4. The nurse is caring for a patient receiving bumetanide (Bumex) to reduce preload for heart failure. While assessing the patient the nurse notes the patient has less ankle edema and jugular vein distention than earlier. The next dose of bumetanide is scheduled in 1 hour. Which of the following actions should the nurse take next?

a. Notify the physician.

b. Hold the bumetanide.

c. Give the bumetanide as scheduled.

d. Give the bumetanide early.

5. Which of the following assessments should the nurse teach the patient to perform to monitor fluid status at home?

a. Weigh daily.

b. Weigh weekly.

c. Weigh biweekly.

d. Weigh monthly.

6. A 160-lb patient is to receive cyclosporine (Neoral) 12.5 mg/kg daily in two divided doses. How many mg will the patient receive with each dose?

_____ mg

Reference

1. Hunt, SA, Abraham, WT, Chin, MH, et al: ACC/AHA 2005 guideline update for the diagnosis and management of chronic heart failure in the adult: a report of the American College of Cardiology/American Heart Association Task Force on Practice Guidelines (Writing Committee to Update the 2001 Guidelines for the Evaluation and Management of Heart Failure). American College of Cardiology Web Site. Accessed 1/23/06 at http://www.acc.org/clinical/guidelines/failure/update/index.pdf

Unit 5 Bibliography

1. ACCP Conference on Antithrombotic and Thrombotic Therapy. Chest 126(Suppl):S457–S482.

2. Allen, J. (2005) Gender, ethnicity, and cardiovascular disease. J Cardiovasc Nurs 20:1–6.

3. American Heart Association: Step I, Step II, and TLC diets. Accessed September 1, 2004 at http://www.americanheart.org/presenter.jhtml?identifier=4764.

4. Anderson, C, Deepak, BV, Amoateng-Adjepong Y, and Zarich, S: Benefits of comprehensive inpatient education and discharge planning combined with outpatient support in elderly patients with congestive heart failure. Congest Heart Fail 11:315–321, 2005.

5. Ascherio, A, Katan, MB, and Stampfer, MJ: "Trans" fatty acids and coronary heart disease. N Engl Med 340:1994, 1999.

6. Aurigemma, GP, Zile, MR, and Gaasch, WH: Contractile behavior of the left ventricle in diastolic heart failure. Circulation 113:296–304, 2006.

7. Badhwar, V et al: Mitral valve surgery: when is it appropriate? Congest Heart Fail 8:210, 2002.

8. Baicu, CF, Zile, MR, Aurigemma, GP, and Gaasch, WH: Left ventricular systolic performance, function, and contractility in patients with diastolic heart failure. Circulation 111:2306–2312, 2005.

9. Beese-Bjurstrom, S: Aortic aneurysms & dissections. Nursing 2004 34:36–41, 2004.

10. Best, D, and Grainger, P: Treating acute coronary syndromes with enoxaparin. Nursing 2004 34(5):32cc1–2, 2004.

11. Block, PC: Percutaneous mitral valve repair for mitral regurgitation. J Interv Cardiol 16:93, 2003.

12. Breddin, HK, Hoch-Wunderlee V, Nakov, R, et al: Effects of a low-molecular-weight heparin on thrombus regression and recurrent thromboembolism in patients with deep-vein thrombosis. N Engl J Med 344:626, 2001.

13. Carabello B: Clinical practice. Aortic stenosis. N Engl J Med 346:677, 2002.

14. Carter, T: Pericarditis inflammation or infarction? J Cardiovasc Nurs 20:239–244, 2005.

15. Chant, T: Peripheral vascular disease. Primary Health Care 14:29–34, 2004.

16. Chang, SM, Nagueh, SF, Spencer, WH, et al: Complete heart block: Determinants and clinical impact in patients with hypertrophic obstructive cardiomyopathy undergoing nonsurgical septal reduction therapy. J Am Coll Cardiol 42:296, 2003.

17. Cilliers, AM, Mangemba, J, Saloojee, H, et al: Anti-inflammatory treatment for carditis in acute rheumatic fever. Cochrane Database Syst Rev 2:CD003176, 2003.

18. Chen-Scarabelli, C: Beating-heart coronary artery bypass surgery: Indications, advantages, and limitations. Crit Care Nurse 22:44–58, 2002.

19. Cho, GY, Song, JK, Park, WJ, et al: Mechanical dysschrony assessed by tissue Doppler imaging is a powerful predictor of mortality in congestive heart failure with normal QRS duration. J Am Coll Cardiol 46:2237–2243, 2005.

20. Chojnowski, D: Peripheral arterial disease danger! Slow blood flow ahead. Nursing Made Incredibly Easy 3:4–18, 2005.

21. Cleland, JG, Daubert, JC, Erdmann, E, et al and Cardiac Resynchronization-Heart Failure (CARE-HF) Study Investigators: The effect of cardiac resynchronization on morbidity and mortality in heart failure. N Engl J Med 352:1539–1549, 2005.

22. Copeland, JG, Smith, RG, Arabia, FA, et al: Cardiac replacement with a total artificial heart as a bridge to transplantation. N Engl J Med 351:859–867, 2004.

23. Copeland, JG, Smith, RG, Arabia, FA, et al: Total artificial heart bridge to transplantation: a 9-year experience with 62 patients. J Heart Lung Transplant 23:823–831, 2004.

24. Craig, K: Take charge with an automated external defibrillator. Nursing 2005 35:50–52, 2005.

25. Garren Corona, G: Is my patient having an acute myocardial infarction?. Nursing Management 36(9):72E–72F, 2005.

26. De Von, H, and Ryan, C: Chest pain and associated symptoms of acute coronary syndromes. J Cardiovasc Nurs 20:232–238, 2005.

27. Donohue, M: Evidence based care for acute myocardial infarction. Nurs Management 36(8):23–27, 2005.

28. Douglas, JG, Bakris, GL, Epstein, M, et al: Management of high blood pressure in African Americans. Consensus statement of the Hypertension in African-Americans Working

Group of the International Society on Hypertension in Blacks. Arch Intern Med 163:525–541, 2003.

29. Efre, A: Gender bias in acute myocardial infarction. Nurse Practitioner 29:42–55, 2004.

30. El-Ahdab, F, Benjamin DK, Wang, A, et al: Risk of endocarditis among patients with prosthetic valves and *Staphylococcus aureus* bacteremia. Am J Med 118:225, 2005.

31. Expert Panel on Detection, Evaluation and Treatment of High Blood Cholesterol in Adults: Executive summary of the third report of the Expert Panel on Detection, Evaluation and Treatment of High Blood Cholesterol in Adults (Adult Treatment Panel III). JAMA 285:2486, 2001.

32. Firoozi, S, Elliott, PM, Sharma, S, et al: Septal myotomy-myectomy and transcoronary septal alcohol ablation in hypertrophic obstructive cardiomyopathy. A comparison of clinical, haemodynamic and exercise outcomes. Eur Heart 23:1617–1624, 2002.

33. Forster, A, Wells, P, et al: Tissue plasminogen activator for the treatment of deep venous thrombosis of the lower extremity: a systematic review. Chest 19:572, 2001.

34. Frazier, OH, Rose, EA, Oz, MC, et al: Multicenter clinical evaluation of the HeartMate vented electric left ventricular assist system in patient awaiting heart transplantation. J Thorac Cardiovasc Surg 22:1186–1195, 2001.

35. Frazier, OH, Myers, TJ, Gregoric, 10, et al: Initial clinical experience with the Jarvik 2000 implantable axial-flow left ventricular assist system. Circulation 105:2855–2860, 2002.

36. Goldstein, JA: Cardiac tamponade, constrictive pericarditis and restrictive cardiomyopathy. Current Problems in Cardiology 29:503–567, 2004.

37. Ezekowitz, JA, McAlister, FA, and Armstrong, PW: Anemia is common in heart failure and is associated with poor outcomes: insights from a cohort of 12, 065 patients with new-onset heart failure. Circulation 107:223–225, 2003.

38. Fox, CH, Mahoney, MC, Ramsoomair, D, et al: Magnesium deficiency in African Americans: does it contribute to increased cardiovascular risk? J Natl Med Assoc 95: 257–262, 2003.

39. Freed, LA, Benjamin, EJ, Levy, D, et al: Mitral valve prolapse in the general population: the benign nature of echocardiographic features in the Framingham Heart Study. J Am Coll Cardiol 40:1298, 2002.

40. Gendreau-Webb, R: Is it a kidney stone or an abdominal aortic aneurysm? Nursing 36(5) 22–24, 2006.

41. Goldrick, G: Myocardial infarction: Getting in line with the new guidelines. Nursing 2005 35(9): 99, 2005.

42. Hering, D, Piper, C, and Horstkotte D: Drug insight: an overview of current anticoagulation therapy after heart valve replacement. Nature 2:8:415–422, 2005.

43. Holman, J: Peripheral arterial disease: tips of diagnosis and management. Consultant January:101–108, 2004.

44. Horvath, K: Mechanisms and results of transmyocardial laser revascularization. Cardiology 101:37–47, 2004.

45. Hoq, S, Chen, W, Srinivasan, SR, et al: Childhood blood pressure predicts adult microalbuminuria in African Americans but not in Whites: the Bogalusa Heart Study. Am J Hypertens 15:1036–1041, 2002.

46. Iakovou I, Schmidt T, Bonizzoni E, et al: Incidence, predictors, and outcome of thrombosis after successful implantation of drug-eluting stents. JAMA 293:2126–2130, 2005.

47. Isselbacher, E: Thoracic and abdominal aortic aneurysms. Circulation 111:816–828, 2005.

48. Johnson, P, and Manson, J: How to make sure the beat goes on protecting a woman's heart. Circulation 111:28–33, 2005.

49. Khaldoun, G: Myocardial viability testing and the effect of early intervention in patients with advanced left ventricular systolic dysfunction. Circulation 113:230-237, 2006. Accessed at http://circ.ahajournals.org/cgi/content/abstract/CIRCULATIONAHA.105.541664v1 on 1/15/06.

50. Klein, LW: Are drug-eluting stents the preferred treatment for multivessel coronary artery disease? J Am Coll Cardiol 47:22–26, 2006.

51. Krauss, R, Eckel, RH, Howard, B, et al: AHA dietary guidelines Revision 2000: A statement for healthcare professionals from the nutrition committee of the American Heart Association. Circulation 102:2296–2311, 2005.

52. Krauss, RM, Eckel, RH, Howard, B, et al: AHA dietary guidelines. Circulation 102:(18)2284, 2000.

53. Lee, MH, Lu, K, and Patel, SB: Genetic basis of sitosterolemia. Curr Opin Lipidol 12:141, 2001.

54. Leprince, P, Bonnet, N, Rama, A, et al: Bridge to transplantation with the Jarvik-7 (CardioWest™) total artificial heart: a single-center 15-year experience. J Heart Lung Transplant 22(12):1296–303, 2003.

55. Leya FS, Arab D, Joyal D, et al: The efficacy of brain natriuretic peptide levels in differentiating constrictive pericarditis from restrictive cardiomyopathy. J Am Coll Cardiol 45:1900–1902, 2005.

56. Lindsay, M: Transmyocardial laser revascularization revisited. Crit Care Nurs Q 26:69–75, 2003.

57. Lord, C: Preventing surgical-site infections after coronary artery bypass graft: a guide for the home health nurse. Home Healthcare Nurse. 24:28–35, 2006.

58. Masip, J, Roque, M, Sanchaz, B, et al: Noninvasive ventilation in acute cardiogenic pulmonary edema: systematic review and meta-analysis. JAMA 28:294:3124–3130, 2005.

59. McDermott, M, Liu, K, Ferrucci, L, et al: Physical performance in peripheral arterial disease: a slower rate of decline in patients who walk more. Ann Intern Med 3:144:10–20, 2006.

60. McDonald, M, Currie, BJ, Carapetis, JR, et al: Acute rheumatic fever: a chink in the chain that links the heart to the throat? Lancet Infect Dis 4:240, 2004.

61. McMurray, JJ, Ostergren, J, Swedberg, K, et al. for the CHARM Investigators and Committees: Effects of candesartan in patients with chronic heart failure and reduced left-ventricular systolic function taking angiotensin-converting-enzyme inhibitors: the CHARM-Added trial. Lancet 362:767–771, 2003.

62. Morgan, E: When critical limb ischemia strikes. Nursing 2005 35(8): 32cc 1–4, 2005.

63. Morgan, TO, and Anderson, A: Different drug classes have variable effects on blood pressure depending on the time of day. Am J Hypertens 16:46–50, 2003.

64. Morris, M: Peripheral arterial disease detection and nonsurgical management. Clin Rev 15:46–52, 2005.

65. Mohty, D, Enriquez-Sarano, M et al: The long-term outcome of mitral valve repair for mitral valve prolapse. Curr Cardiol Rep 4:104, 2002.

66. Mozaffarian, D, Nye R, and Levy, WC: Anemia predicts mortality in severe heart failure: the Prospective Randomized Amlodipine Survival Evaluation (PRAISE). J Am Coll Cardiol 41:1933–1939, 2003.

67. Nagueh, SF, Ommen, SR, Lakhis, NM, et al: Comparison of ethanol septal reduction therapy with surgical myectomy for the treatment of hypertrophic obstructive cardiomyopathy. J Am Coll Cardiol 38:1701, 2001.

68. Narula, J, Chandrasekhar, Y, and Rahimtoola, S: Diagnosis of

acute rheumatic carditis: the echoes of change. Circulation 100:1576, 1999.

69. Oliver, B, Sharma, SK, and Ayello, E: How drug-eluting stents keep coronary blood flowing. Nursing 2005 35(2):36–41, 2005.

70. Otto, CM: Timing of surgery in mitral regurgitation. Heart 89:100, 2003.

71. Rathore, SS, Curtis, JP, Wang, Y, et al: Association of serum digoxin concentration and outcomes in patients with heart failure. JAMA 289:871–878, 2003.

72. Review: multidisciplinary interventions reduce hospital admission and all cause mortality in heart failure Simon Stewart (commentator). Evid Based Nurs 9:23, 2006. doi:10.1136/ebn.9.1.23.

73. Rice, K: How to measure ankle/brachial index. Nursing 2005 35:56–57, 2005.

74. Ridker, P, Goldhaber, S, Samuelson, P, et al: Long-term, low-intensity warfarin therapy for the prevention of recurrent venous thromboembolism. N Engl J Med 349:398–400, 2003.

75. Rodriguez, AE, Mieres, J, Fernandez-Pereira, C, et al: Coronary stent thrombosis in current drug-eluting stent erainsights from ERACI III trial. J Am Coll Cardiol 47:205–207, 2006.

76. The PREPIC Study Group: Eight-Year Follow-Up of Patients with Permanent Vena Cava Filters in the Prevention of Pulmonary Embolism: The PREPIC (Prevention du Risque d'Embolie Pulmonaire par Interruption Cave) Randomized Study. Circulation 112: 416–422, 2005.

77. Salem, DN et al: Antithrombotic therapy in valvular heart disease—native and prosthetic. The Seventh ACCP Conference on Antithrombotic and Thrombolytic Therapy. Chest 126(suppl 3): 457S–482S, 2004.

78. Samuels, LE, and Dowling, R: Total artificial heart: destination therapy. Cardiol Clin 21:115–118, 2003.

79. Nishimura, R, Ommen, S, and Tajik, A: Hypertrophic cardiomyopathy: a patient perspective. Circulation 108;133–135, 2003.

80. Schmitt JP, Kamisago M, Asahi M, et al: Dilated cardiomyopathy and heart failure caused by a mutation in phospholamban. Science 299:1410–1413, 2003.

81. Stern, S, Behar, S, and Gottlieb, S: Aging and diseases of the heart. Circulation 108:99–101, 2003.

82. Thuny, F, Disalvo, G, Belliard, O, et al: Risk of embolism and death in infective endocarditis: prognostic value of echocardiography; a prospective multicenter study. Circulation 112:69–75, 2005.

83. Tough, J: Assessment and treatment of chest pain. Nurs Stand 18:45–53, 2005.

84. Tough, J: Thrombolytic therapy in acute myocardial infarction. Nurs Stand 19:55–64, 2005.

85. van der Meer, P, Lipsic, E, Westinbrink, BD, et al: Levels of hematopoiesis N-acetyl-seryl-aspartyl-lysyl-proline partially explain the occurrence of anemia in heart failure. Circulation 112:1743–1747, 2005.

86. Viles-Gonzalez, J, Anand, S, Valdiorezo, C, et al: Update of atherothrombotic disease. Mt Sinai J Med 71:197–208, 2004.

87. Vlachopoulos, C, Hirata, K, Stefandis, C, et al: Caffeine increases aortic stiffness in hypertensive patient. Am J Hypertens 16:63–66, 2003.

88. Vlasic, W: An evidence-based approach to reducing bed rest in the invasive cardiology patient population. Evid Based Nurs 7:100–101, 2004.

89. Waggoner, AD, Faddis, MN, Gleva, MJ, et al: Improvements in left ventricular diastolic function after cardiac resynchronization therapy are coupled to response in systolic performance. J Am Coll Cardiol 46:2244–2249, 2005.

90. Chaitman, BR, Pepine, CJ, and Parker, JO: Effects of ranolazine with atenolol, amlodipine, or diltiazem on exercise tolerance and angina frequency in patients with severe chronic angina. A randomized controlled trial. JAMA 291:309–316, 2004.

91. White, HD, Aylward, PE, Huang, Z, et al: Mortality and morbidity remain high despite captopril and/or valsartan therapy in elderly patients with left ventricular systolic dysfunction, heart failure, or both after acute myocardial infarction. Circulation 112:3391–3399, 2005.

92. Willenheimer, R, van Veldhuisen, DJ, Silke, B, et al: Effect on survival and hospitalization of initiating treatment for chronic heart failure with bisoprolol followed by enalapril, as compared with opposite sequence. Circulation 112:2426–2435, 2005.

93. Woo, A, Williams, WG, Choi, R, et al. Clinical and echocardiographic determinants of long-term survival after surgical myectomy in obstructive hypertropic cardiomyopathy. Circulation 111:2033–2041, 2005.

94. Young, JB, Dunlap, ME, Pfeffer, MA, et al: Candesartan in Heart failure Assessment of Reduction in Mortality and morbidity (CHARM) Investigators and Committees. Mortality and morbidity reduction with candesartan in patients with chronic heart failure and left ventricular systolic dysfunction: results of the CHARM low-left ventricular ejection fraction trials. Circulation 110:2618–2626, 2004.

SUGGESTED ANSWERS TO

CRITICAL THINKING

■ *Mr. Shepard (1)*

1. Signs and symptoms of heart failure include shortness of breath, two-pillow orthopnea, dry cough, tachycardia (pulse 106), tachypnea (respiration 24), and bilateral crackles.

2. Left-sided heart failure is indicated by the findings.

3. Shortness of breath: fluid in the lungs impairs gas exchange; orthopnea: lying flat increases fluid accumulation in the lungs, causing dyspnea; dry cough: fluid in the lungs irritates the mucosal lining of the lungs; tachycardia: sympathetic compensation to increase cardiac output; tachypnea: sympathetic compensation to increase blood oxygenation; bilateral crackles: fluid trapped in the lungs.

4. The two pillows help prevent orthopnea by using a more upright position, which allows gravity to decrease fluid accumulation in the lungs.

■ *Mr. Shepard (2)*

1. Mr. Shepard's heart is enlarged to compensate for the strain caused by increased peripheral vascular resistance from hypertension in order to maintain an adequate cardiac output.
2. An enlarged heart requires more oxygen, which often cannot be supplied in heart failure.

■ *Mr. Shepard (3)*

1. The ACE inhibitor is needed for vasodilation, which reduces peripheral vascular resistance and decreases the heart's workload, to prevent cardiac remodeling and improve functioning.
2. The ACE inhibitor will affect afterload.
3. The diuretic is ordered to decrease fluid volume, which reduces preload and decreases the heart's workload.
4. The diet is ordered to reduce water retention, which decreases preload and decreases the heart's workload.
5. The goal is to decrease the heart's workload and increase its efficiency by reducing preload and peripheral vascular resistance and to decrease progression of chronic heart failure and improve survival.

■ *Mr. Shepard (4)*

1. After assessment of Mr. Shepard's knowledge base, medication teaching should be given on the ACE inhibitor and diuretic that includes their purpose, side effects, and precautions. A schedule for taking the medications can be planned. An explanation of the purpose of a low-sodium diet and menu planning based on Mr. Shepard's likes and dislikes should be done.
2. Low-sodium foods should be selected to prevent fluid retention, and high-potassium foods should be included to prevent hypokalemia from the diuretic if appropriate. Read food labels. Low-sodium foods include puffed rice, wheat cereals, fruits, chicken, beef, eggs, and potatoes. High-sodium foods include tomato juice, sauerkraut, softened water, buttermilk, cheese, smoked meats, canned tuna, canned soup, pickles, instant rice, and instant potatoes. High-potassium foods include salt substitutes, bran products, avocado, bananas, prunes, oranges, baked potato, sweet potato, spinach (cooked), chocolate, nuts, and molasses.
3. Daily weighing is necessary to detect a rapid weight gain that indicates fluid retention (2 lb in 24 hours) and to measure weight loss resulting from the diuretic.
4. These instructions ensure accuracy of the weight so that comparison to the baseline weight detects a weight gain or loss.

■ *Mrs. Eden*

1. No, Mrs. Eden is not tolerating this activity, as evidenced by her increased respiratory rate and apical rate.
2. Steroids, immunosuppressive therapy, depression, and fatigue could be causing her poor appetite.
3. Nursing interventions related to Mrs. Eden's poor appetite could include the following: offering small, frequent meals; having family bring favorite foods from home; allowing the patient to rest before meals; providing oral hygiene before meals; administering antiemetics before meals; giving a high-calorie meal at peak appetite.
4. Mrs. Eden could be withdrawn because of changes in her lifestyle as a result of her transplant, extreme fatigue and concerns regarding how she will raise her children, grieving for the donor, and fear that she will reject her new heart.

unit SIX

UNDERSTANDING THE HEMATOPOIETIC AND LYMPHATIC SYSTEMS

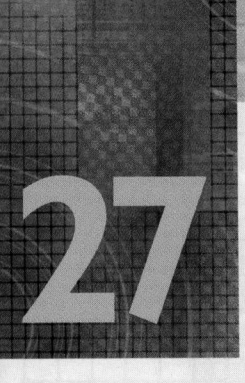

27

Hematopoietic and Lymphatic System Function, Assessment, and Therapeutic Measures

JANICE L. BRADFORD AND
LUCY L. COLO

KEY TERMS

ecchymoses (ECK-ih-MOH-sis)
lymphedema (LIMPF-uh-DEE-mah)
petechiae (puh-TEE-kee-eye)
purpura (PUR-pur-uh)

QUESTIONS TO GUIDE YOUR READING

1. What are the components of blood?

2. How are changes in the blood or blood-producing processes manifested as disease processes?

3. What is the sequence of events in the process of blood clotting?

4. What data should you collect when caring for a patient with a disorder of the hematological or lymphatic system?

5. What laboratory and diagnostic studies are used when evaluating the hematological and lymphatic systems?

6. What nursing care should you provide for patients undergoing each of the diagnostic tests?

7. What are common therapeutic measures for patients with hematological and lymphatic disorders?

8. What is the role of the licensed practical vocational nurse (LVN) in administering blood products?

NORMAL ANATOMY AND PHYSIOLOGY

Blood

The hematologic system comprises the bone marrow, blood, and blood components. The lymphatic system includes the lymph nodes and nodules that destroy pathogens, and lymph vessels that return lymph back to the blood.

The general functions of blood are transportation of oxygen, nutrients, and cellular waste products; regulation of body temperature, pH, and fluid balance; and production of cells that offer the body protection. Specific aspects of these functions are discussed further with the particular part of the blood that is responsible for each.

A human body holds 4 to 6 L of blood; 46 to 63 percent is plasma and the remainder is formed elements. The blood cells are the red blood cells (RBCs or erythrocytes) and white blood cells (WBCs or leukocytes); platelets (thrombocytes) are cell fragments. All of these formed elements are produced by the red bone marrow (RBM), a hematopoietic (blood-producing) tissue found in flat bones, irregular bones, and the epiphyses of long bones. The red bone marrow contains the undifferentiated stem cells that are the precursor cells for all blood cells. Final maturation and differentiation of T lymphocytes occur in the thymus. Table 27.1 shows normal blood cell counts.

Plasma

Plasma is the liquid portion of the blood and is about 91 percent water. It is the transporting medium for nutrients, wastes, hormones, enzymes, electrolytes, and gases. Plasma proteins include clotting factors, albumin, and globulins. Clotting factors such as prothrombin and fibrinogen are synthesized by the liver and circulate until activated in the clotting mechanism. Albumin, also synthesized by the liver, helps maintain blood volume and blood pressure by pulling tissue fluid into the venous ends of the capillary networks. Alpha and beta globulins are synthesized by the liver to be carrier molecules for substances such as fats, and gamma globulins are the antibodies produced by lymphocytes.

Plasma is also important in maintaining body temperature because blood carries heat. The water of plasma is warmed by passage through active organs, such as the liver or skeletal muscles, and this heat is distributed as blood circulates throughout the body. This process may be visible in people with light skin. The flush of fever or vigorous exercise is caused by vasodilation in the dermis, allowing blood to circulate near the body surface and lose heat. A person in a cold environment may be pale, as vasoconstriction in the dermis keeps blood circulating in the core of the body to preserve heat.

The normal pH range of blood is 7.35 to 7.45, which is slightly alkaline. Chemical buffer systems in the blood prevent sudden fluctuations in pH and contribute to the body's acid-base balance.

Red Blood Cells

Mature RBCs are biconcave disks without nuclei; they carry oxygen bonded to the iron in hemoglobin (Hgb). Oxyhemoglobin is formed in the pulmonary capillaries where the hemoglobin combines with the oxygen in the lungs. Once hemoglobin gives up its oxygen to the cells of the body, it becomes reduced hemoglobin. The amount of hemoglobin

TABLE 27.1   REVIEW OF BLOOD CELL VALUES AND DISORDERS

Test	Normal Value	Significance of Abnormal Findings
	Red Blood Cells	
Red blood cells (RBCs)	Male: 4.6–6.2 million/mm^3 Female: 4.2–5.4 million/mm^3	Increased in chronic hypoxia; decreased in anemia or blood loss
Hematocrit (cellular portion of blood)	Male: 40%–54% Female: 38%–47%	Increased in dehydration or chronic hypoxia; decreased in anemia or blood loss
Hemoglobin (reflects oxygen carrying capacity of blood)	Male: 13.5–18.0 g/100 mL Female: 12–16 g/100 mL	Increased in chronic hypoxia; decreased in blood loss or anemia
Reticulocytes (number of circulating immature RBCs)	0%–1.5%	Increased in hypoxia or anemia; decreased in RBC maturation defect
	White Blood Cells	
White blood cells (WBCs)	5000–10,000/mm^3	Increased in infection
Neutrophils	54%–75%	Increased in infection
Eosinophils	1%–4%	Increased in allergic response, some leukemias
Basophils	0.5%–1.0%	Increased in hyperthyroidism, some bone marrow disorders, ulcerative colitis
Lymphocytes	25%–40%	Increased in viral infections, chronic bacterial infection, some leukemias
Monocytes	2%–8%	Increased in chronic inflammatory disorders, some leukemias
	Platelets	
Thrombocytes/Platelets	150,000–450,000/mm^3	Increased from trauma; decreased with blood disorders; low platelet count causes risk for bleeding.

in RBCs, the amount of iron in that hemoglobin, and the number of RBCs are the determining factors for the amount of oxygen the blood can carry. A lack of iron, hemoglobin, or RBCs can cause anemia, which results in symptoms such as shortness of breath and weakness.

The rate of RBC production by the red bone marrow is most influenced by the blood oxygen level. Hypoxia stimulates the kidneys to secrete erythropoietin, which increases the rate of RBC production and thus the oxygen-carrying capacity of the blood. At such times, immature RBCs (reticulocytes) may be found in greater abundance in peripheral blood. A reticulocyte becomes a mature RBC when it ejects its nucleus. This causes the characteristic biconcave disk shape. Reticulocytes usually remain in the red bone marrow until they mature; their presence in large numbers in peripheral blood indicates an insufficient amount of mature RBCs to meet the oxygen demands of the body.

Sufficient dietary intake of protein and iron to synthesize hemoglobin is also required for normal production of RBCs. The vitamins folic acid and vitamin B_{12} are necessary for DNA synthesis in the stem cells of the red bone marrow. The continuous mitosis of these cells depends on their ability to produce new sets of chromosomes. Vitamin B_{12} is also called *extrinsic factor* because it comes from an extrinsic source: food. The parietal cells of the stomach lining produce *intrinsic factor*, which is a chemical that combines with vitamin B_{12} to promote its absorption in the small intestine.

Red blood cells live for about 120 days and then become fragile and are phagocytized by fixed macrophages in the liver, spleen, and red bone marrow. The iron is returned to the red bone marrow for synthesis of new hemoglobin or is stored in the liver. The heme portion of the hemoglobin is converted to bilirubin, a bile pigment that the liver excretes into bile for elimination in the feces. Diseases such as malaria and sickle cell anemia cause an accelerated destruction of red blood cells. This hemoglobin release may cause the blood level of bilirubin to rise. When the bilirubin level is elevated, it discolors the sclerae, skin, and mucous membranes bright yellow to dark orange, depending on the bilirubin levels. This is known as jaundice.

Each person has a hereditary blood type, which refers to the antigens present on the RBCs. The two most important type categories are the ABO group and the Rh factor. The ABO type (A, B, O, or AB) indicates the antigens present (or not present, as in the case of type O) on the RBCs. In the plasma are antibodies for antigens that are not present in the blood. These antibodies can interact with antigens in transfused blood if the donor's blood does not match the recipient's blood (Table 27.2). To be Rh positive means that the D antigen is present on the RBCs; Rh negative means that the antigen is not present. Rh-negative people do not have natural antibodies to the D antigen but will produce them if given Rh-positive blood.

White Blood Cells

White blood cells are larger than RBCs and have nuclei when mature. The granular WBCs (neutrophils, eosinophils, and basophils) are produced only in the red bone marrow.

TABLE 27.2 ABO BLOOD TYPES

Type	Antigens Present on RBCs	Antibodies Present in Plasma
A	A	Anti-B
B	B	Anti-A
AB	Both A and B	Neither anti-A nor anti-B
O	Neither A nor B	Both anti-A and anti-B

The agranular WBCs (lymphocytes and monocytes) are also produced in the red bone marrow; however the T lymphocytes complete their development in the thymus. The T lymphocytes and B lymphocytes become activated, proliferate, and differentiate in the lymph nodes, spleen, and lymphatic nodules. Table 27.1 shows normal values and percentages for each type of WBC in a differential count. WBCs carry out their functions in tissue fluid, as well as the blood, and all are involved in the immunity or inflammatory response to injury.

Monocytes become macrophages, which phagocytize pathogens and dead tissue; neutrophils are more numerous but phagocytize only pathogens. Eosinophils combat the effects of histamine, detoxify foreign proteins during allergic reactions, and respond to parasitic infections. Basophils release histamine as part of inflammatory reactions. There are two groups of lymphocytes: T cells and B cells. T cells may be helper, suppressor, killer, or memory T cells. B cells become plasma cells, which produce antibodies to foreign antigens and also become memory cells.

Platelets

Platelets are formed in the red bone marrow; they are fragments of large cells called megakaryocytes. Platelets are involved in all mechanisms of hemostasis: vascular spasm, platelet plugs, and chemical clotting.

When a blood vessel is damaged, platelets release serotonin, which promotes contraction of smooth muscle and thereby vasoconstriction of an artery or a vein. Such constriction makes the break smaller; perhaps small enough to be covered by a clot. Constriction also allows the clot to adhere and stop any continued bleeding because it has to cover a smaller area. Capillaries have no smooth muscle and cannot constrict but are so small that breaks can be closed by platelet plugs. Platelets become sticky, adhering to the rough edges of the broken capillary and to one another, eventually forming a platelet plug that stops the bleeding.

Platelets also produce platelet factors, chemicals whose release is stimulated by contact of blood with a rough surface such as a broken or damaged vessel lining. Platelet factors are necessary for the first of the three stages of chemical clotting. In stage 1, platelet factors, clotting factors from the liver, tissue factor (thromboplastin), and calcium ions react to form prothrombinase (also called prothrombin activator). In stage 2, prothrombinase converts prothrombin (synthesized by the liver) into thrombin. In stage 3, thrombin converts soluble fibrinogen (also from the liver) to insoluble fibrin, strands which form the clot. Calcium ions are also required for stages 2 and 3.

Excessive clotting in the vascular system is prevented in several ways. The very smooth endothelial lining of blood vessels repels platelets so that they do not stick to intact vessel walls. Heparin produced by mast cells inhibits the clotting mechanism. Antithrombin (synthesized by the liver) inactivates excess thrombin to prevent the clotting mechanism from becoming a vicious cycle.

Lymphatic System

The lymphatic system consists of lymph, the system of lymph vessels, the lymph nodes and nodules, the spleen, and the thymus. Functions of the lymph system are to return tissue fluid to maintain blood volume and to protect the body against pathogens and other foreign material. (Immunity is covered in Unit 4).

Lymphatic Vessels

Lymph is tissue fluid that has entered lymph capillaries. Lymph must be returned to the blood to maintain blood volume and blood pressure. Lymph capillaries are found in most tissue spaces; they anastomose, forming larger and larger lymph vessels, which have valves to prevent backflow of lymph. Lymph from areas below the diaphragm and the upper left quadrant enters the thoracic duct (in front of the vertebral column) and is returned to the blood in the left subclavian vein (Fig. 27.1). Lymph from the upper right quad-

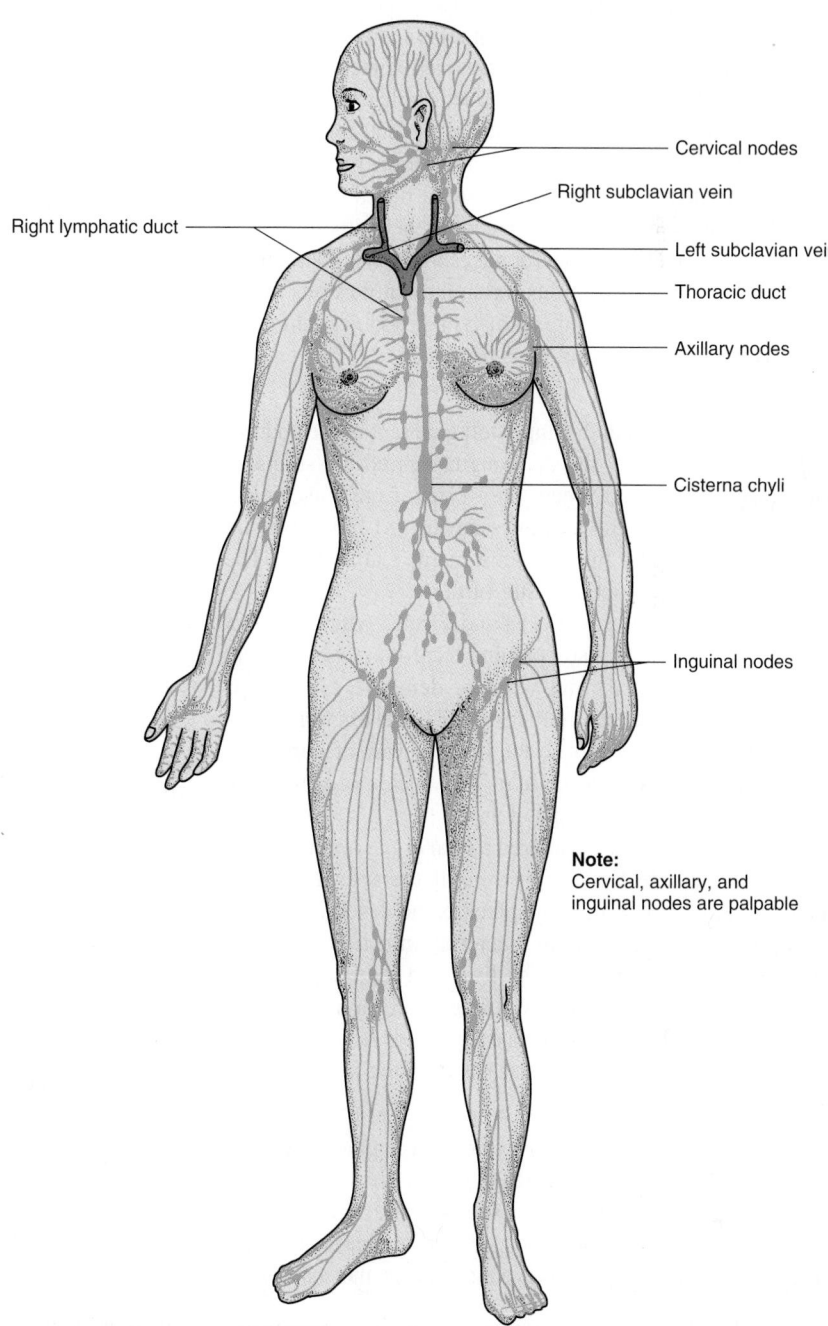

Cervical nodes

Right subclavian vein

Right lymphatic duct

Left subclavian vein

Thoracic duct

Axillary nodes

Cisterna chyli

Inguinal nodes

Note:
Cervical, axillary, and inguinal nodes are palpable

FIGURE 27.1 System of lymph vessels and major groups of lymph nodes. *(From Scanlon, V, Sanders, T: Essentials of Anatomy and Physiology, ed 5. FA Davis, Philadelphia, 2007.)*

rant enters the right lymphatic duct and is returned to the blood in the right subclavian vein.

Lymph Nodes and Nodules

Lymph nodes are masses of lymphatic tissue along the pathways of the lymph vessels. They form activated lymphocytes and monocytes. Nodes are scattered both superficially and deep. As lymph flows through the nodes, the WBCs enter the lymph. Foreign materials are phagocytized by fixed macrophages, and fixed plasma cells produce antibodies to foreign antigens. The major paired groups of lymph nodes are the cervical, axillary, and inguinal nodes. These areas are located at the junction of the head (cervical) and extremities (axillary and inguinal) with the trunk to remove pathogens in the lymph from the extremities before the lymph is returned to the blood.

Lymph nodules are small masses of lymphatic tissue found just beneath the epithelium of all mucous membranes. They are often referred to as mucosa-associated lymphatic tissue (MALT). The body tracts lined with mucous membranes are those that have openings to the environment: the respiratory, digestive, urinary, and reproductive systems. Any natural body opening is a potential portal of entry for pathogens; any pathogens that penetrate the epithelium usually are destroyed by the macrophages in the lymph nodules. The tonsils, which protect the oral and nasal portions of the pharynx, are familiar examples of lymph nodules, although most lymph nodules do not have names.

Spleen

The spleen is located in the upper left quadrant of the abdominal cavity, just below the diaphragm, behind the stomach. The lower rib cage protects the spleen from mechanical injury. In the fetus, the spleen produces red blood cells, a function assumed by the red bone marrow after birth. The spleen has several functions after birth.

The spleen contains B cells and T cells, which conduct immune responses. It also contains fixed macrophages that phagocytize pathogens and worn or defective blood cells and platelets. The heme unit from RBC destruction forms bilirubin. Bilirubin is sent to the liver by way of portal circulation for excretion in the bile. The spleen also stores up to one-third of the body's platelets.

The spleen is not considered a vital organ because other organs compensate for its functions if the spleen must be removed. A person without a spleen is, however, somewhat more susceptible to certain bacterial infections such as pneumonia and meningitis. The liver and red bone marrow remove worn RBCs from the circulation, and the many lymph nodes and nodules produce lymphocytes and monocytes and phagocytize pathogens (as does the liver).

Thymus

The thymus is located inferior to the thyroid gland and anterior to the trachea. With increasing age, the thymus atrophies; relatively little thymic tissue is found in adults. The thymus contains T lymphocytes, or T cells, that mature and proliferate. Thymic hormones contribute to the maturation of the T cells. (Immunity is covered in Unit 4.)

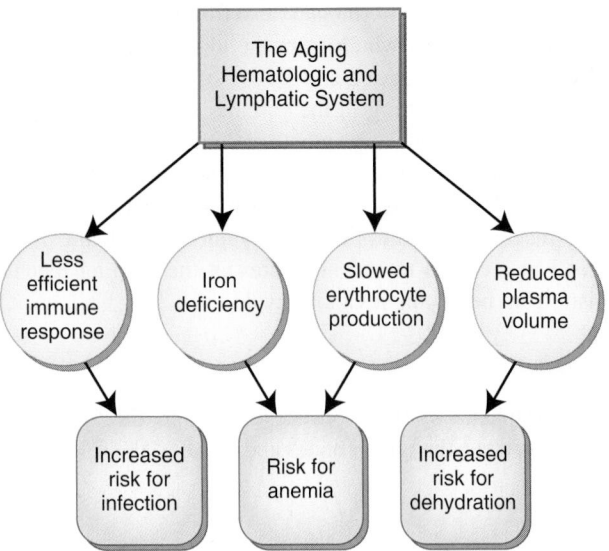

FIGURE 27.2 Effects of aging on the hematologic and lymphatic systems.

Aging and the Hematopoietic and Lymphatic Systems

Older people undergo a number of changes in the hematological and lymphatic systems (Fig. 27.2).

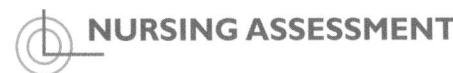

NURSING ASSESSMENT

History

A thorough nursing assessment starts with an in-depth patient history (Table 27.3). Specific problems that might be seen in patients with hematological disorders include abnormal bleeding, **petechiae** (small purplish hemorrhagic spots under the skin), **ecchymoses** (larger areas of discoloration from hemorrhage under the skin), and **purpura** (hemorrhage into the skin, mucous membranes, and organs), as well as fatigue, weakness, shortness of breath, and fever. Fatigue, malaise, and weight loss can accompany cancers of the lymphatic system.

Begin by obtaining the patient's biographical data, marital status, occupation, religion, age, sex, and ethnic background. This information can give you valuable clues to risk factors. For example, even though hemophilia almost always occurs in males, females may carry the gene. Sickle cell anemia occurs mostly in African Americans but also affects people of Mediterranean or Asian ancestry. Pernicious anemia occurs most often in people of northern European ancestry. By carefully collecting this information, you may be obtaining important clues that will help pinpoint the patient's problem. Finally, focus on the assessment of symptoms by using the WHAT'S UP? format presented in Chapter 1.

A complete review of past illnesses and family history is always indicated and can provide some valuable information. The social history is also useful. After developing good

TABLE 27.3 SUBJECTIVE ASSESSMENT OF THE HEMATOLOGIC AND LYMPHATIC SYSTEMS

Category	Questions to Ask During History/Assessment	Rationale/Significance
Reason for seeking health care	• Why are you seeking health care? • What has brought you in to see the doctor today?	Signs and symptoms of hematological/lymphatic disorders may be nonspecific. Any body system can be involved.
Family History	• How is the health of your blood relatives? • Does anyone in your family have any blood-related diseases?	Some blood and immune disorders are hereditary.
Diet History	• Describe your usual diet.	Dietary deficiencies can lead to anemia or altered immune responses.
Medications/Supplements	• What medications do you take? • What herbs or alternative therapies do you use? • How much alcohol do you drink each day?	Herbs and drugs can cause adverse reactions in the blood and immune system. Excess alcohol intake can lead to folic acid– deficiency anemia.
Occupational/Exposure History	• What is your occupational history? • What is your military history?	Exposure to certain hazardous substances can lead to leukemias, other cancers, or anemias.
Fatigue	• Have you noticed any change in your energy level?	Anemia and many cancers are associated with fatigue.
Bleeding Tendency	• Have you experienced nosebleeds or any other unusual bleeding? • Have you had bloody or black bowel movements?	Bleeding may indicate low platelet levels or a clotting factor deficiency.
Respiratory	• Do you experience shortness of breath or faintness?	These are symptoms of anemia.
Integumentary	• Have you noticed any changes in your skin?	Bleeding into the skin or mucous membranes can indicate a bleeding disorder.
Lymphadenopathy	• Have you noticed swelling in your neck, armpits, or groin?	Swollen lymph nodes may indicate inflammation, infection, or some cancers.

rapport with the patient, explore dietary and alcohol intake habits, any drug use or abuse, and sexual habits, all of which may cause changes in the hematological system.

An occupational review may reveal exposure to some hazardous substances that can cause bone marrow dysfunction. Certain occupations, such as working in a paint factory, tool and dye processing, and even dry cleaning can be related to the formation of some hematological cancers. Military information may also reveal sources of exposure that can help during the diagnostic phase for hematological and lymphatic disorders.

Physical Examination

Hematological and lymphatic disorders can involve almost every body system, so each system must be carefully assessed. First, assess vital signs, which can reveal important clues. For example, frequent fevers indicate a poorly functioning immune system. Markedly subnormal temperatures may indicate an overwhelming gram-negative infection when combined with other abnormal assessment data. Heart and respiratory rate abnormalities may indicate decreased blood volume or decreased oxygen supply. Finally, check the level of consciousness; changes may occur with hypoxia, fever, and intracranial bleeding.

An inspection of physical structures most relevant to the blood and lymph systems includes the skin, mucous membranes, fingernails, eyes, lymph nodes, liver, and spleen.

Observe the patient's skin color, noting pallor (indicating anemia), cyanosis (indicating poor oxygenation of RBCs), or jaundice (indicating liver disease or hemolysis). Observe the face, neck, and hands for areas of local inflammation, enlargements, or obvious sites of infection. Check the entire skin surface for purpura or other signs of bleeding, and examine the oral mucosa for color changes and petechiae or ecchymoses. These findings may indicate a bleeding disorder. Other important findings can be obtained with careful examination of the skin to look for dryness and coarseness, which can indicate anemia. Inquire about itching, which may also indicate blood or lymph disorders.

Fingernails can give important clues about the patient's health. For instance, long striations (lines) on the nails or spoon-shaped nails may indicate anemia. Clubbed fingertips and raised nailbeds may indicate long-term hypoxia, which can be caused by anemia or heart disease.

Abdominal assessment should include the use of auscultation, or listening with the stethoscope. Listen intently and try to identify high-pitched, tinkling sounds, which might indicate intestinal obstruction, versus the regular, gurgling, and lower pitched noises normally heard in the intestines. In some cases, you will measure the abdominal girth and record the measurement in the nurse's notes. This baseline measurement might be useful if the patient begins to exhibit abdominal enlargement secondary to ascites or bleeding.

Next, progress to palpation, making sure that the patient is comfortable and that the patient's privacy is protected. Make sure to warm your hands. You can start with an examination of the lymph nodes, although this is more commonly done by a primary care practitioner. The nodes of the neck can be gently palpated with one or two fingers while the patient is sitting. When examining the axillary nodes, the patient may lie down. Nodes that are palpable, with or without **lymphedema,** are not usually normal. Occasionally, normal superficial nodes of 1 cm or less may be palpable. Note the location, size, tenderness, texture, and fixation of the node groups. Enlarged or tender nodes indicate current or previous inflammation. Sternal tenderness may or may not be present. If present, this finding indicates that the bone marrow may be "packed" with an abnormal number and type of cells.

NURSING CARE TIP

If abdominal girth must be monitored for changes, use a marker to identify the site where you measure so it can be measured at the same spot each time.

DIAGNOSTIC TESTS

A number of diagnostic tests can help rule out or confirm a suspected diagnosis based on the analysis of the formed elements of the blood and the bone marrow. Specific studies include a complete blood cell count (CBC), coagulation studies, agglutination studies, bone marrow aspiration, and needle biopsy.

Blood Tests

Examples of laboratory studies routinely done for patients with hematological disorders include CBC, total hemoglobin concentration (Hgb), hematocrit levels (Hct), and platelet levels. (See normal values in Table 27.1.)

Coagulation Tests

Tests in this category include bleeding times, capillary fragility test, prothrombin time (PT), international normalized ratio (INR), partial thromboplastin time (PTT), and thrombin clotting time (TCT) (Table 27.4). Agglutination tests include ABO blood typing, Rh typing, cross matching blood samples, and direct antiglobulin tests (also known as a Coombs' test).

Bone Marrow Biopsy

Biopsy information may be obtained through removal of a small amount of bone marrow with a needle, which in most

---

lymphedema: lymph—fluid found in lymphatic vessels + edema—swelling

LEARNING TIP

When a patient has a bacterial infection, the neutrophils, which are one type of WBC, rise in number to help fight it. There are two forms of neutrophils: segmented (mature) and bands (immature). Initially the number of segmented neutrophils goes up. Then, as the infection becomes more severe, the number of immature bands begins to rise.

An easy way to remember this is that the WBCs are part of the body's defenses, just like the military is part of a country's defenses. When needed, sergeants who are fully trained or mature are called to battle first. If they are unable to fight off the invading enemy, new recruits being trained in boot camp are called in to help.

So segmented neutrophils (**S**egs) are like the **S**ergeants, fully mature and ready to fight. The **B**ands are like **B**oot camp recruits, immature and not fully trained. However, in an acute infection, bands are necessary to prevent the body from being overwhelmed by the infection and losing the battle.

As you look at the differential WBC count, if the segs are elevated but the bands are normal, it is probably a new infection. If the bands are also elevated, the infection is worsening. The more elevated they are, the more severe the infection.

Lymphocytes fight viral infections and are elevated during a virus. A common pattern in the WBCs is produced for either a bacterial or viral infection. If the infection is acute bacterial:

Segs ↑ Bands ↑ Lymphocytes ↓

If the infection is viral:

Segs ↓ Bands ↓ Lymphocytes ↑

This can be remembered as the bone marrow producing the cells most needed during the time of viral infection and reducing production of those cells least needed. When the infection is resolved, all the cells should return to their normal production levels.

states must be obtained by a physician. Aspiration of liquid and biopsy of the solid portion of the bone marrow is done to obtain a specimen that can be viewed under the microscope. Purposes of this test include the diagnosis of hematological disorders; monitoring the course of treatment; discovery of other disorders, such as primary and metastatic tumors, infectious diseases, and certain granulomas; and isolation of bacteria and other pathogens by culture.

TABLE 27.4 COAGULATION STUDIES

Test	Normal Value	Significance of Abnormal Findings
Prothrombin time (PT) (affected by activity of clotting factors V, VII, X, prothrombin, and fibrinogen)	Men 9.6–11.8 seconds Women 9.5–11.3 seconds Therapeutic range 1.5–2.0 times normal for patient on warfarin (Coumadin) therapy.	Abnormalities in these values when the patient is not receiving anticoagulant therapy can indicate liver malfunction and bleeding tendency.
International normalized ratio (standardized test adopted by World Health Organization)	<1.3 Therapeutic range 2.0–3.0 for patient on warfarin (Coumadin) (3.0–4.5 for recurrent problems).	
Partial thromboplastin time (PTT) (affected by activity of clotting factors, prothrombin, and fibrinogen)	30–45 seconds Therapeutic range 1.5–2.0 times normal for patient on heparin therapy	
Thrombin clotting time (TCT) (measures time for fibrin clot to form after addition of thrombin)	10–15 seconds Therapeutic range 1.5–2.0 times normal for patient on heparin therapy.	Prolonged TCT indicates fibrinogen deficiency.
Bleeding time (measures time for small puncture wound to stop bleeding)	2.5–9.5 minutes	Prolonged bleeding time indicates a platelet disorder.
Capillary fragility test	Fewer than 10 petechiae appearing in a 2-inch circle after application of a blood pressure cuff at 100 mm Hg for 5 minutes	Tests ability of capillaries to resist rupture under pressure. More than 10 petechiae could be related to fragile capillaries or thrombocytopenia.

CRITICAL THINKING

Mrs. Brown

■ Mrs. Brown is on warfarin (Coumadin) therapy because of a blood clot in her leg. She has a PT drawn at the lab, and the result is 12 seconds. Will the physician most likely increase her daily dose of warfarin, decrease it, or leave it the same? (Use Table 27.4 to figure out the answer.)

Suggested answer at end of chapter.

An accurate bone marrow specimen in an adult can be obtained from the sternum, the spinous processes of the vertebrae, or the anterior or posterior iliac crest. Bone marrow biopsy is considered a minor surgical procedure, and is carried out under aseptic conditions. For iliac crest aspiration, the patient is placed comfortably on the side with the back slightly flexed. The posterior iliac crest is cleansed and covered with antiseptic solution. The skin, the subcutaneous tissue, and the periosteum are anesthetized using 1 or 2 percent lidocaine (Xylocaine). A 2- to 3-mm incision is made to facilitate penetration with a 14-gauge, 2- to 4-cm bone marrow needle. The incision is made to avoid introducing a skin plug into the marrow cavity, which can cause infection.

The nurse's role in bone marrow biopsy is multifaceted. You may need to help coordinate between the laboratory and the physician, establishing a time to do the procedure and determining who obtains the supplies, such as the disposable bone marrow aspiration tray and specialized needles, from the central supply department. Be sure to obtain an order for an analgesic and administer it before the procedure. You may also help position the patient before and during the procedure, help the patient maintain the necessary position, and observe the aspiration site for bleeding and infection. You can also provide emotional support to the patient before, during, and after the procedure.

 SAFETY TIP

Prior to the start of any invasive procedure, conduct a final verification process to confirm the correct patient, procedure, site, and availability of appropriate documents. This verification process uses active, not passive, communication techniques (2006 National Safety Goals from www.jcaho.org).

Lymphangiography

Disorders of the lymph system can be evaluated using lymphangiography. This procedure involves injection of a dye into the lymphatic vessels of the hand or foot. Various x-ray views are then taken to determine lymph flow or blockages. X-ray examinations are repeated in 24 hours to assess lymph node involvement.

Following the procedure, the physician may order a pressure dressing and immobilization of the injected limb to prevent leakage at the site. Continue to monitor the limb for swelling, circulatory status, and changes in sensation. Warn the patient that the skin, urine, or feces may be blue tinged from the dye for about 2 days.

Lymph Node Biopsy

If a lymph node is enlarged, it may be biopsied to determine whether the cause is infection or malignancy. A biopsy may be done with a needle aspiration or surgical incision. A small dressing or Band-Aid is applied to the site. Following the procedure, review with the patient signs of bleeding and infection that should be reported to the physician.

 ## THERAPEUTIC MEASURES

Blood Administration

Blood may be administered by a registered nurse (RN) or licensed practical/vocational nurse (LPN/LVN), depending on the state in which you practice. Some states require that only RNs administer blood. As an LPN/LVN, you may be called on to assist with proper identification procedures and monitoring of vital signs during the transfusion. Table 27.5 lists blood components that may be ordered. The main goal is to administer them safely and avoid mistakes. Make sure to use proper identifying information to ensure that the right patient is receiving the right blood products. A careful system most often used in health care institutions is outlined next.

Safety Steps

BASELINE ASSESSMENT. Prior to the blood transfusion, it is important to assess the patient's vital signs and history of transfusions or transfusion reactions. Vital signs provide baseline data. If the patient has had a reaction in the past, be sure to alert the physician and the lab before proceeding.

IDENTIFICATION. Safety is the first priority. This includes checking and double checking the patient's identity. Great care is taken in the blood bank to match the donor's blood type with the recipient's blood type. After obtaining the unit of blood from the blood bank but before hanging the unit,

two nurses (according to the state's guidelines) will check the following information at the patient's bedside (Fig. 27.3). Do not take this identification step for granted, because if you make an error and accidentally transfuse blood that does not match the patient's blood type, the results can be fatal.

- Ask the patient to state his or her name and birth date aloud if alert and able to speak.
- Use the patient's identification band to confirm the identity and compare it with the information on the paperwork obtained from the blood bank.
- Examine the blood bag and verify that the patient information and any other information, such as the ABO type, Rh type, and unit number, all match.
- Finally, check the expiration date on the blood bag.

Do not give the unit of blood if any of the information does not match. Notify the blood bank immediately of any discrepancies, and delay the transfusion until the differences are cleared up. Remember, there is no room for error when transfusing blood products.

 ### SAFETY TIP

Use at least two patient identifiers (neither to be the patient's room number) whenever administering medications or blood products (2006 National Safety Goals www.jcaho.org).

FILTERING. Filters are used with blood administration tubing to prevent potentially harmful particles from entering the patient. Most often, the filter that comes with the transfusion tubing is sufficient for each unit of packed RBCs. In some situations, special filters may be needed to remove leukocytes or microaggregates. The blood bank can advise in these situations.

WASHED OR LEUKOCYTE–DEPLETED BLOOD. There are instances when packed RBCs (PRBCs) are ordered as "washed"; often arriving from the blood bank in a round bag.

TABLE 27.5 BLOOD PRODUCTS

Product	Use
Packed red blood cells	Severe anemia or blood loss
Frozen red blood cells	Autotransfusion (blood taken from patient and saved for future surgery), prevention of febrile reactions
Platelets	Bleeding caused by thrombocytopenia
Albumin	Hypovolemia caused by hypoalbuminemia
Fresh frozen plasma	Provides clotting factors for bleeding disorders; occasionally used for volume replacement
Cryoprecipitates	Bleeding caused by specific missing clotting factors

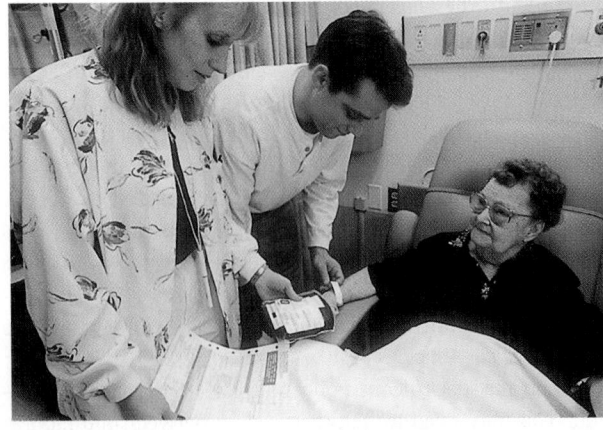

FIGURE 27.3 Two nurses check a patient's identification before administering a unit of blood.

The washing process removes almost all the plasma and can decrease the risk or severity of a febrile reaction. In addition, leukocyte filters may be used to completely remove all WBCs. This removal process is used in cases in which many transfusions are anticipated, and decreases the chance of antigen sensitization. It can also reduce transmission of certain viruses, such as cytomegalovirus.

WARMED BLOOD. If the patient has had a severe bleeding episode and the nurses are helping to give replacement therapy through rapid, multiple transfusions, the physician may consider ordering a blood warmer. It works just as the name implies, warming the cold blood from the blood bank to the standard body temperature of 98.6° F (37.0°C). This warming helps prevent hypothermia, which can cause heart dysrhythmias, or shivering, which can destroy blood cells and platelets.

Administration

GUIDELINES. It is important to use the correct intravenous needle size to infuse blood. The best sizes are 18- and 20-gauge catheters to prevent hemolysis of red blood cells. Make sure to use only normal saline solution to help dilute the blood and to flush the intravenous lines before and after the transfusions. Any other type of fluid or medication may cause the blood product to clump, clot, or not infuse at all. Generally, 2 hours is a good time frame to transfuse each unit of packed cells. If it must transfuse more slowly because of the patient's condition, make sure that the unit does not hang longer than 4 hours to prevent deterioration and bacterial proliferation.

MONITORING. Carefully monitor the patient's response to the transfusion to prevent complications or to detect and treat them quickly if they occur. Stay with the patient for the first 15 minutes of the blood transfusion to assess for any immediate reactions. The 15 minutes begins when the blood enters the vein. If saline is in the tubing, it may take several minutes before the blood reaches the patient. Check and document vital signs before starting the transfusion, after the blood has begun to infuse, and after the infusion is complete. Some institutions require vital sign monitoring every 15 to 30 minutes during the earliest part of the transfusion and then slightly less often for the duration of the infusion. Always follow institution guidelines. During the transfusion, assess the patient for signs and symptoms of transfusion reactions.

Complications

Quick detection of complications may be lifesaving. It is easy to think of transfusing blood components as a routine procedure because it is a common activity. Do not be fooled. It is a serious procedure that can be life threatening if errors occur. Complications include febrile reactions, hypersensitivities, hemolytic reactions, anaphylaxis, circulatory overload, and even death. Regular monitoring according to institution policy can help detect complications early when treatment is most effective.

FEBRILE REACTION. By far the most common reaction is fever (febrile reaction); occurring up to 2 percent of the time. The risk of a febrile reaction goes up with each unit of blood product given to the patient. Many times, febrile reactions occur after the transfusion is completed, but they can occur at any time. This is the reason for obtaining a set of baseline vital signs, including the patient's temperature. Once a febrile reaction begins, the most common signs are an increasing fever and shaking chills, which can be severe. Other symptoms may include headache and back pain. If febrile symptoms occur, stop the transfusion and notify the physician. Acetaminophen may be ordered. If a hemolytic reaction is not suspected, the physician may order the transfusion to continue once the patient is more comfortable. Make sure that the 4-hour hang rule is not violated. Future febrile reactions can usually be prevented by administering leukocyte-depleted blood as described previously.

URTICARIAL REACTION. Urticarial (hive) reactions are considered to be minor allergic reactions and are usually associated with antigens in the plasma accompanying the transfusion. There may be a fever, but the cardinal sign is the appearance of urticaria, a hive-like rash. On discovery of this reaction, stop the transfusion and notify the physician immediately. Expect that the patient will be given a dose of an antihistamine such as diphenhydramine (Benadryl). If the transfusion is restarted, continue to monitor the patient closely. Again, make sure the 4-hour hang rule is not violated.

HEMOLYTIC REACTION. The most deadly and, fortunately, the rarest of the possible reactions is an acute hemolytic reaction. The cause of this reaction is transfusion of incompatible blood. The result is hemolysis (destruction) of RBCs. Generally, this type of serious reaction is noticed within minutes of starting the transfusion. The patient may report back pain, chest pain, chills, fever, shortness of breath, nausea, vomiting, or a feeling of impending doom. As the reaction progresses, the patient begins to show signs of shock, hypotension, oliguria, and decreased consciousness. Late signs and symptoms include those associated with disseminated intravascular coagulation: uncontrollable bleeding from many different sites at the same time, usually ending in death. At the first sign of this type of reaction, immediately stop the transfusion and stay with the patient. Institute emergency procedures to notify the charge nurse, the physician, and the blood bank. The vein is kept open with normal saline using a new administration set (ensuring that no more incompatible blood is administered) so that emergency drugs can be administered. High volumes of fluids are administered to decrease shock and hypotension, and high doses of diuretics are given to promote urine flow because the kidneys are the most likely organs to be damaged. Dialysis may be instituted.

ANAPHYLACTIC REACTION. Anaphylactic reactions are not common but may be seen more often in patients who have received many transfusions or have had many pregnancies. Usually the source of the anaphylaxis is from sensitization to immune globulins passed from the donor's unit of blood product. In this type of reaction the very first milliliters of blood containing the allergens to pass into the patient's system may be enough to cause the patient to develop respiratory or cardiovascular collapse. Other more common symptoms include severe gastrointestinal cramping, instant vomiting, and uncontrollable diarrhea. If the patient exhibits these signs and symptoms, stop the transfusion at once and stay with the patient. Have someone else notify the registered nurse and the physician, using institutional emergency procedures. Emergency resuscitation measures, including cardiopulmonary resuscitation if necessary, must be instituted until the code team arrives. Expect the patient to be intubated and receive oxygen, steroids, and other drugs as needed for life support. After the emergency has passed, this patient will likely need to receive transfusions from frozen, deglycerolized blood cells.

CIRCULATORY OVERLOAD. Circulatory overload is caused by rapid transfusion in a short period, particularly in older and debilitated patients. Usual signs and symptoms

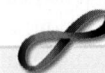

Box 27.1

Gerontological Issues

Older patients have less cardiac and renal ability to adapt to changes in blood volume, so they have a much higher risk of fluid overload when receiving blood transfusions. Carefully monitor lung sounds and vital signs both before and during a transfusion. New onset of dyspnea, crackles, hypertension, or bounding pulse should be reported to the registered nurse or physician immediately.

include chest pain, cough, frothy sputum, distended neck veins, crackles and wheezes in the lung fields, and increased heart rate. If symptoms occur, stop the transfusion and notify the physician. Anticipate administration of diuretics, which help get rid of the excess fluid. The transfusion may be restarted later at a slower rate (Box 27.1 Gerontological Issues).

REVIEW QUESTIONS

1. Clotting factors such as prothrombin are produced by which structure?
   a. Red bone marrow
   b. Liver
   c. Spleen
   d. Lymph nodes

2. Which of the following best describes the function of erythropoietin?
   a. Increase production of platelets to promote clotting
   b. Decrease production of platelets to prevent abnormal clotting
   c. Increase RBC production to correct hypoxia
   d. Decrease RBC production to prevent hypoxia

3. Why is the return of tissue fluid to the blood important?
   a. To maintain blood clotting
   b. To maintain blood volume
   c. To promote white blood cell formation
   d. To promote red blood cell formation

4. Which of the following is the portion of the blood in which cellular elements are suspended?
   a. Cytoplasm
   b. Platelets
   c. Plasma
   d. Hemoglobin

5. Which of the following actions should the nurse take when caring for a patient with a platelet count of 23,000/mm^3?
   a. Request an order for an anticoagulant.
   b. Protect the patient from injury.

   c. Encourage the patient to drink plenty of fluids.
   d. No action is necessary. This is a normal level.

6. The nurse is assessing a patient and finds small red-purple dots over most of his skin surfaces. The patient says that he has not noticed them before. Which action should the nurse take first?
   a. Report the findings immediately to the registered nurse or physician.
   b. Document the findings objectively in the medical record.
   c. Assist the patient to apply lotion.
   d. Administer an antihistamine as needed.

7. Which of the following checks should be done prior to initiating a blood transfusion? Choose all that apply.
   a. Ask the patient to state his or her name.
   b. Verify the correct room number.
   c. Check the patient's arm band.
   d. Check the identifying information on the unit of blood.

8. The nurse is monitoring a patient during a blood transfusion. After the blood has been hanging for 30 minutes, the patient's temperature rises from 98.6°F (37.0°C) at baseline to 101.0°F (38.3°C). The patient also complains of severe chills. Which action should the nurse take first?
   a. Document the vital signs in the medical record.
   b. Administer acetaminophen for the fever.
   c. Notify the physician of the change.
   d. Stop the transfusion and hang normal saline.

SUGGESTED ANSWERS TO

CRITICAL THINKING

■ *Mrs. Brown*

The physician will most likely increase Mrs. Brown's warfarin dose. Note in Table 23.4 that the PT for a patient on warfarin should be 1.5 to 2.0 times normal.

That is the reason the warfarin is ordered—to prolong the time it takes for blood to clot. If a normal PT is 9.5 to 11.3 seconds, a therapeutic PT for Mrs. Brown would be 14.25 seconds (9.5 × 1.5) to 22.6 (11.3 × 2.0). Her result of 12 seconds is not therapeutic.

28

Nursing Care of Patients with Hematological and Lymphatic Disorders

LUCY L. COLO

KEY TERMS

anemia (uh-NEE-mee-yah)
aplastic (ay-PLAS-tik)
disseminated intravascular coagulation (dis-SEM-i-NAY-ted IN-trah-VAS-kyoo-lar koh-AG-yoo-LAY-shun)
glossitis (gloss-SIGH-tis)
hemarthrosis (HEEM-ar-THROH-sis)
hemolysis (he-MAHL-e-sis)
hemolytic (he-moh-LIT-ik)
hemophilia (HEE-moh-FILL-ee-ah)
idiopathic thrombocytopenic purpura (ID-ee-oh-PATH-ik THROMB-boh-SIGH-toh-PEE-nik PUR-pew-rah)
leukemia (loo-KEE-mee-ah)
lymphoma (lim-FOH-mah)
pancytopenia (PAN-sigh-toh-PEE-nee-ah)
panmyelosis (PAN-my-e-LOH-sis)
pathological fracture (PATH-uh-LAH-jik-uhl FRAK-chur)
phlebotomy (fle-BAH-tuh-mee)
polycythemia (PAH-lee-sigh-THEE-mee-ah)
splenectomy (sple-NEK-tuh-mee)
splenomegaly (SPLEE-noh-MEG-ah-lee)
thrombocytopenia (THROM-boh-SIGH-toh-PEE-nee-ah)

QUESTIONS TO GUIDE YOUR READING

1. What is the pathophysiology of each of the disorders discussed in this chapter?

2. What are the etiologies, signs, and symptoms of each disorder?

3. What are current therapeutic interventions for each disorder?

4. What data should you collect when caring for patients with disorders of the hematological or lymphatic systems?

5. What nursing care will you provide for patients with hematological disorders?

6. What nursing care will you provide for patients with lymphatic disorders?

7. How will you know if your nursing interventions have been effective?

8. What precautions should you institute to prevent bleeding in patients with clotting disorders?

9. What nursing care and teaching will you provide for patients undergoing a splenectomy?

HEMATOLOGICAL DISORDERS

Patients with hematological disorders have problems related to their blood. Some problems are caused by too many cells, others by too few or defective cells. When red blood cells (RBCs) are affected, oxygen transport is also affected, causing symptoms of poor oxygenation. When white blood cells (WBCs) are affected, the patient is unable to effectively fight infections. If platelets or clotting factors are affected, bleeding disorders occur.

DISORDERS OF RED BLOOD CELLS

Anemias

The term **anemia** describes a condition in which there is a deficiency of RBCs, hemoglobin, or both, in the circulating blood. Because hemoglobin carries oxygen, this results in a reduced capacity to deliver oxygen to the tissues, producing symptoms such as weakness and shortness of breath, which lead the patient to seek medical help.

Pathophysiology

A decrease in the numbers of RBCs can be traced to three different conditions: (1) impaired production of RBCs, as in **aplastic** anemia and nutrition deficiencies; (2) increased destruction of RBCs, as in **hemolytic** or sickle cell anemia; or (3) massive or chronic blood loss. Some anemias are related to genetic problems in certain cultures (Box 28.1 Cultural Considerations). It is important to remember that the general term *anemia* refers to a symptom or a condition secondary to another problem and is not a diagnosis in itself. Different types of anemia are discussed later in this chapter.

Etiologies

DIETARY DEFICIENCIES. Iron, folic acid, and vitamin B_{12} are all essential to production of healthy RBCs. A deficiency of any of these nutrients can cause anemia. Pernicious anemia is associated with a lack of intrinsic factor in stomach secretions, which is necessary for absorption of vitamin B_{12}. See Box 28.2 Nutrition Notes for more information.

HEMOLYSIS. Hemolysis is the destruction, or lysis, of RBCs. Destruction of RBCs leads to a type of anemia called hemolytic anemia. This may be a congenital disorder or it may be caused by exposure to certain toxins.

OTHER CAUSES. Thalassemia anemia is a hereditary anemia found in persons from Southeast Asia, Africa, Italy, and the Mediterranean islands. Individuals with thalassemia do not synthesize hemoglobin normally. Individuals with

---

anemia: a—not + emia—blood
aplastic: a—not + plastic—develop
hemolytic: heme—blood + lytic—break down
hemolysis: heme—blood + lysis—dissolution

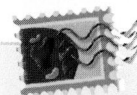

Box 28.1

Cultural Considerations

In the past, Iranian cross-cousin marriages have resulted in an increased incidence of several forms of anemia and hemophilia. These marriages are now being addressed through genetic counseling and premarital screening for carriers.

A sex-linked genetic disease common in the Chinese is glucose-6-phosphate dehydrogenase (G6PD) deficiency, an enzyme deficiency affecting the person's red blood cells and resulting in anemia. Mediterranean G6PD is common, causing a hemolytic crisis when fava beans are eaten, when aspirin or certain other drugs are taken, or in acidotic or hypoxemic states. Mediterranean-type G6PD deficiency is an inherited disorder most fully expressed in males, with a carrier state in females.

Among Asian Indians, sickle cell disease is highly prevalent; the gene is detected in 16.5 percent of selected populations. Sickle cell anemia is the most common genetic disorder among African American populations. Sickle cell anemia also is found in individuals who live in areas where malaria is endemic, such as the Caribbean, the Middle East, the Mediterranean region, and Asia.

---

chronic disease also develop anemia (Box 28.3 Gerontological Issues). Additional causes of anemia are discussed under the separate headings of aplastic and sickle cell anemias.

Signs and Symptoms

Symptoms of anemia include pallor, tachycardia, tachypnea, irritability, fatigue, and shortness of breath (Table 28.1). In addition to these symptoms, the patient with pernicious (vitamin B_{12}) anemia may experience numbness of the hands or feet and weakness because vitamin B_{12} is necessary for normal neurological function. Pernicious anemia is also associated with a sore, beefy red tongue. Patients with iron deficiency may have fissures at the corners of the mouth, an inflamed tongue (**glossitis**), and spoon-shaped fingernails.

Diagnostic Tests

A complete blood cell count (CBC) is done to determine the number of RBCs and WBCs per cubic millimeter. The size, color, and shape of the blood cells are determined by microscopic examination. Hemoglobin and hematocrit are below normal in anemia. Serum iron, ferritin, and total iron-binding capacity measurements are done to diagnose iron deficiency anemia. Serum folate is measured if folic acid deficiency is suspected. A bone marrow biopsy and analysis may also be done.

---

glossitis: glos—tongue + itis—inflammation

Box 28.2

Nutrition Notes

Understanding Common Nutritional Anemias

Nutritional deficiencies can produce some forms of anemia. Nutrients vital to the construction of red blood cells include iron, folic acid, and vitamin B_{12}. Even if the cause of the anemia is dietary, other therapies may be employed in addition to nutritional interventions.

MICROCYTIC ANEMIA. Iron deficiency anemia, the most common nutrient deficiency in the world, is characterized by smaller than normal RBCs. Insufficient intake of iron, excessive blood loss, or lack of stomach acid can lead to iron deficiency anemia. Individuals at greatest risk of iron deficiency are women of childbearing age and young children. Even before frank anemia is seen, cognitive abilities can be impaired. In early iron deficiency, serum transferrin, a blood protein that carries iron, rises in an attempt to increase iron-carrying capacity. Later the hemoglobin and hematocrit levels drop.

Relatively good sources of iron that are commonly included in Western diets are red meat; dark green leafy vegetables; dried fruits; and enriched, fortified, or whole grain products. Foods rich in vitamin C can be used to enhance absorption of iron from nonmeat sources. Likewise, stewing acidic foods such as tomatoes in iron cookware increases their iron content. If iron supplements are given to treat iron deficiency, they should be continued for several months after hemoglobin and hematocrit levels return to normal to enable the body to rebuild iron stores.

MACROCYTIC ANEMIA. Folic acid or vitamin B_{12} deficiencies produce anemias characterized by larger than normal RBCs. Both these vitamins are necessary for normal RBC production. Folic acid aids in the formation of DNA and heme, the iron-containing portion of hemoglobin. Conditions that increase the metabolic rate increase the need for folic acid. Many drugs, including alcohol, anticonvulsants, and oral contraceptives, interfere with its absorption, metabolism, or excretion and can lead to anemia. Good food sources of folic acid include liver, green leafy vegetables, legumes, and enriched grain products. Because folic acid markedly decreases the occurrence of fetal neural tube defects such as spina bifida, women capable of becoming pregnant are advised to consume 400 µg of synthetic folic acid from fortified foods or supplements in addition to the folic acid furnished by a varied, balanced diet.

Vitamin B_{12} is essential for the manufacture of RBCs and for synthesis and maintenance of myelin, the fatty covering of nerves that facilitates rapid transmission of impulses. Vitamin B_{12} requires a highly specific protein-binding factor called intrinsic factor, secreted by glands in the stomach, to be absorbed. Intrinsic factor and vitamin B_{12} (also called extrinsic factor) combine in the proximal small intestine to form a complex to transport vitamin B_{12} to the ileum, where it is absorbed. Extrinsic factor (vitamin B_{12}) is found in foods from animal sources such as meat, fish, shellfish, poultry, and milk. A healthy person eating these foods regularly is not at risk of vitamin B_{12} deficiency, but strict vegetarians are at risk. Because the deficiency here is dietary, a dietary supplement is the treatment.

In contrast, pernicious anemia is a disease caused by lack of intrinsic factor. Pernicious anemia occurs more frequently in older persons and is attributed to antibodies against gastric parietal cells and intrinsic factor. Extensive gastric resection surgery can also result in insufficient intrinsic factor. Because the deficiency is not dietary, neither is the treatment. Pharmaceutical vitamin B_{12} is usually given by injection to circumvent the absorption problem. Symptoms of vitamin B_{12} deficiency are, in usual order of appearance, numbness and tingling in hands and feet followed by RBC changes. Moodiness, confusion, depression, delusions, and overt psychosis appear next. Finally, irreparable nerve damage occurs and eventually death occurs. Because of the neurological damage, vitamin B_{12} deficiency should be considered in a person being evaluated for dementia.

Patients with pernicious anemia have low gastric acid levels, and many have antibodies to intrinsic factor. Both abnormalities are associated with poor absorption of vitamin B_{12}. If blood loss is suspected, additional tests are done to determine the source of bleeding.

Therapeutic Interventions

Treatment begins with elimination of contributing causes. Intake of the deficient nutrient can sometimes be increased in the diet or administered as a supplement. Changing cooking habits, taking dietary supplements, decreasing alcohol intake, and controlling chronic diarrhea can help correct folic acid deficiency. If symptoms of anemia are acute, a blood transfusion may be necessary.

Nursing Process for the Patient with Anemia

ASSESSMENT/DATA COLLECTION. Monitor hemoglobin and hematocrit levels and other laboratory studies as ordered and report any downward trend. Monitor responses to therapy. Assess the patient's fatigue level and ability to ambulate safely and perform activities of daily living (ADLs). Monitor degree of dyspnea. Assess for pallor in the skin and conjunctivae.

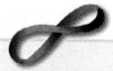

Box 28.3

Gerontological Issues

Anemia of chronic disease is often diagnosed in an older patient who has an underlying medical condition that causes altered iron metabolism, deficiency of erythropoietin, or shortened life span of red blood cells. Unfortunately, anemia of chronic disease is often mistaken for iron deficiency anemia. Nutritional deficiencies and blood loss are common causes of iron deficiency anemia.

NURSING DIAGNOSIS, PLANNING, AND IMPLEMENTATION. Possible nursing diagnoses are listed below with outcomes and interventions.

Activity intolerance related to tissue hypoxia and dyspnea

EXPECTED OUTCOME: The patient will be able to complete ADLs with minimal assistance.

EXPECTED OUTCOME: The patient will have knowledge about conserving energy.

- Monitor vital signs to evaluate tolerance to activity. *The patient experiencing activity intolerance may have tachycardia, increased respiratory rate, and decreased blood pressure with activity.*
- If the pulse or respiratory rate increases more than 20 percent from baseline during activity, reduce the activity level. *This is evidence that the activity is too strenuous and will result in increased hypoxia and dyspnea.*
- Plan care to conserve energy after periods of activity. *Balancing activities and rest periods assists the patient to conserve energy.*
- Assist the patient with self-care activities as needed. *Assisting with ADLs helps to decrease the amount of energy expended by the patient.*
- Place articles within easy reach of the patient *to reduce physiological demands on the body.*
- Encourage the patient to limit visitors, telephone calls, and unnecessary interruptions *to conserve energy.*
- Administer oxygen as ordered to relieve dyspnea. *The anemic patient does not have enough hemoglobin to carry oxygen to vital organs.*
- Assist with blood transfusion as ordered if hemoglobin levels are very low or symptoms are severe. *A blood transfusion is a quick way to raise hemoglobin levels and to correct severe symptoms.*

Imbalanced nutrition: less than body requirements related to disease, treatment, or lack of knowledge of adequate nutrition

EXPECTED OUTCOME: The patient will be able to appropriately select foods that will meet nutritional requirements.

- Consult a dietitian *to provide diet instruction if the anemia is caused by a dietary deficiency.*
- Teach the patient with folic acid deficiency that daily requirements can be met by including foods from each food group at every meal. *A balanced diet includes adequate amounts of folic acid.*
- Include foods high in iron for the patient with iron deficiency and to consume iron-rich foods with vitamin C *to enhance absorption* (see Box 28.2 Nutrition Notes).
- Administer supplements as ordered *when dietary intake alone is not sufficient.*

TABLE 28.1 CLINICAL MANIFESTATIONS OF ANEMIA

Body System	Mild (Hgb = 10–14 g/dL)	Moderate (Hgb = 6–10 g/dL)	Severe (Hgb <6 g/dL)
Skin	None	None	Pallor, jaundice, pruritus
Eyes	None	None	Jaundiced conjunctivae and sclerae, retinal hemorrhages, blurred vision
Mouth	None	None	Glossitis, smooth tongue
Cardiovascular	Palpitations	Increased palpitations	Tachycardia, increased pulse pressure, systolic murmurs, angina, congestive heart failure, myocardial infarction
Lungs	Exertional dyspnea	Frank dyspnea	Tachypnea, orthopnea, dyspnea at rest
Neurological	None	None	Headache, vertigo, irritability, depression, impaired thought processes
Gastrointestinal	None	None	Anorexia, hepatomegaly, splenomegaly
Musculoskeletal	None	None	Bone pain
General	None	Fatigue	Sensitivity to cold, weight loss, lethargy

- Instruct the patient to take the supplements as ordered by the physician. *The patient should not stop taking the medication until the physician advises him or her to do so.*
- Instruct the patient that vitamin B$_{12}$ injections are given for lifetime with pernicious anemia *since it is a chronic disease.*
- Instruct the patient with iron deficiency on the correct use of an iron supplement. *An iron supplement should be taken with vitamin C to enhance absorption.*
- Instruct the patient to notify the physician of any side effects related to iron supplements *such as nausea, diarrhea, constipation, and dark stools.*
- Administer intramuscular iron injections by the Z-track method *to avoid staining the injection site.*
- Administer liquid supplements with a drinking straw *to avoid staining the teeth.*

Risk for injury: falls related to weakness and dizziness

EXPECTED OUTCOME: The patient will be safe from injury related to fall.

- Assess the patient at risk for falls using a fall risk assessment tool *to determine risks.*
- Assist the patient to change positions slowly *to decrease dizziness and risk of falls.*
- Assist the patient with ambulation *to prevent a fall.*
- Protect the patient with pernicious anemia from injuries resulting from decreased sensation; i.e., take special care with heating pads and turning and positioning *since the ability to sense pain may be impaired.*

Impaired oral mucous membranes related to altered dietary status

EXPECTED OUTCOME: The patient will have intact oral mucous membranes.

- Provide good oral hygiene *to keep the oral cavity clean and prevent infection.*
- Encourage soft, bland foods, *which are more tolerable until healing can occur.*
- Instruct the patient to use a soft toothbrush for oral care *because it is more gentle until the healing can occur.*

EVALUATION. When successfully treated, the patient will tolerate a normal level of activity without shortness of breath or excess fatigue. The patient should be able to explain the correct treatment plan and therapeutic measures for long-term prevention including dietary choices and supplements as well as self-care measures. The patient will remain free from injury, and oral mucosa will be intact.

Aplastic Anemia

PATHOPHYSIOLOGY. Aplastic anemia differs from other types of anemia in that the bone marrow becomes fatty and incapable of production of the necessary numbers of RBCs. Also known as hypoplastic anemia, the cells that are produced are normal in size and shape, but there are not enough of them to sustain life. The resulting **pancytopenia** (reduced numbers of all the formed elements from the bone marrow—RBCs, platelets, and WBCs) is the indicator that something is wrong with the bone marrow. Left untreated, aplastic anemia is almost always fatal.

CAUSES. Aplastic anemia may be congenital—that is, the person is born with bone marrow incapable of producing the correct number of cells. Or it may be due to exposure to toxic substances such as industrial chemicals (e.g., benzenes and insecticides), chemotherapy medications, or use of cardiopulmonary bypass during surgery. Other causes include certain bacterial and viral infections, such as tuberculosis and hepatitis.

SIGNS AND SYMPTOMS. The clinical features of aplastic anemia vary with the severity of the bone marrow failure. As with other anemias, early symptoms include progressive weakness, fatigue, pallor, shortness of breath, and headaches. As the disease progresses and the anemia and pancytopenia worsen, other symptoms, such as tachycardia and heart failure, may appear. Ecchymoses and petechiae appear on the skin surface because of the reduced platelet count (Fig. 28.1; also see Fig. 28.5). Blood may ooze from mucous membranes. Puncture sites may progress from oozing to frank bleeding. Often there is overt bleeding into vital organs. Infection occurs owing to reduced WBCs. When aplastic anemia is left untreated, most patients die from infection or bleeding.

DIAGNOSTIC TESTS. The diagnosis of aplastic anemia begins with a CBC. Usually all values are reported as being very low, with the occasional exception of the red blood cell count, in part because of the longer life span of RBCs.

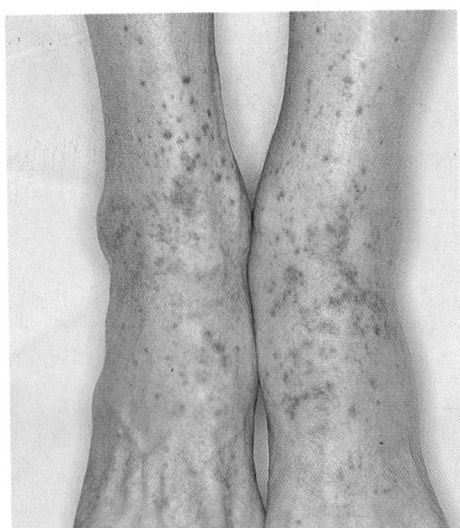

FIGURE 28.1 Petechiae on the skin from thrombocytopenia. *(From Goldsmith, LA, et al: Adult and Pediatric Dermatology. FA Davis, Philadelphia, 1997, p 61, with permission.)*

pancytopenia: pan—all + cyto—cell + penia—poverty

Eventually the RBCs are also depleted. If the patient is having gross bleeding internally or externally, the RBC level can drop rapidly and dramatically. The most definitive test is the bone marrow biopsy. Because the bone marrow is essentially dead, the result is often described as a "dry tap," in which pale, fatty, yellow, fibrous bone marrow is extracted instead of the red, gelatinous bone marrow normally seen. Not surprising, the more fatty and pale the marrow is, the more dysfunctional it is. Other diagnostic tests include total iron-binding capacity (TIBC) and serum iron level. It is common to find both these levels elevated because the RBCs are not being produced to use up the stores of iron in the production of hemoglobin.

TREATMENT. Early identification of the cause of the anemia and correction of the underlying problem are important to survival. Unfortunately, it is often difficult to determine the cause, and there is no way to reverse the damage already done. Aggressive supportive measures may be the only treatment. Most of these measures are aimed at prevention of infection and bleeding.

Today the most effective treatment for aplastic anemia is bone marrow transplantation (Box 28.4 Patient Perspective). Another common therapy is the administration of steroids to stimulate production of cells in the weakened bone marrow. Occasionally the administration of hormones may work to increase the viability of the marrow. Steroid and other hormone treatments may be tried before attempting a bone marrow transplant.

A new line of therapy is also available. In many treatment institutions, limited success is being obtained with the use of colony-stimulating factors, natural elements now being produced synthetically (Table 28.2). For example, erythropoietin (Epogen) stimulates the production of RBCs and filgrastim (granulocyte colony stimulator [Neupogen]) stimulates the production of WBCs. The major drawback to this type of therapy is the high cost. Many of the pharmaceutical manufacturers have patient access programs that help with the costs of these medications.

NURSING INTERVENTIONS. Nursing care of patients with symptoms related to reduced RBCs was presented earlier under Nursing Process for the Patient with Anemia. If the patient's platelet count is low (usually less than 20,000), the patient is placed on bleeding precautions (Box 28.5 Interventions to Prevent Bleeding in the Patient with Thrombocytopenia). If the white count is low, the patient must be protected from infection (Box 28.6 Interventions for the Patient at Risk for Infection).

Sickle Cell Anemia

PATHOPHYSIOLOGY. Sickle cell anemia is an inherited anemia in which the RBCs have a specific mutation that makes the hemoglobin in the red cells very sensitive to oxygen changes. Any time a decrease in the oxygen tension is sensed, the cells begin an observable physical change process from their usual spherical shape to a sickle or crescent shape (Fig. 28.2). Sickled cells are very rigid and

Box 28.4

Patient Perspective

Bone Marrow Transplant

In June 2002, I took my daughter to the doctor for her sports physical. Later that day, I received a call telling me to take her to the university hospital immediately because she had a serious life-threatening illness. I kept telling myself and my husband that our small-town hospital must have made some sort of error. As it turned out, they had not. My daughter was diagnosed with aplastic anemia and needed a bone marrow transplant. I became obsessed with the illness, poring over every tidbit of medical information I could find. Sometimes I found myself out in the car unable to remember where I was going; sometimes I had to pull over because my eyes were filled with tears and I could no longer see.

My daughter was 16 at the time of her illness, yet it is the parents who sign consent forms and make the choices in care. When the chemotherapy was started and running through the IV tubing, I felt like grabbing the tubing and pinching it off, yelling, "I need more time to think about this decision," but time was running out. Without a bone marrow transplant, she had about 8 months to live.

After transplantation, my daughter was in an isolation room for a month. I stayed with her every day, and at night I stayed at the inn that was attached to the hospital. If I was needed, I wanted to be no more than a minute away. I was one of the luckier parents because I had the financial means to manage this process. I thought about how horrible it would be if I had other children at home. Sometimes I would have such an urge to run away and escape from it all. I attended support groups that were held on the hospital unit. I got to know a lot of other parents with sick kids, and it became very upsetting to me at times. One day parents told me how well their child was doing; the next day I saw the child's room empty and thought he must have gone home, only to find out later that he had died during the night. I wondered if my daughter would be next.

I look at my daughter now, 4 years later, alive and perfectly healthy, and I tell myself that I made the right choices for her. But she tells me that, if it happens again, she will not go through chemotherapy. I wonder, is chemo worse than death?

easily cracked and broken. The abnormal shape also causes the cells to become tangled in the blood vessels and organs. The result is congestion, clumping, and clotting.

As red cells are broken, the cellular contents spill out into the general circulation. The resulting increase in the bilirubin level causes jaundice. Gallstones (cholelithiasis) may develop because of the increased amounts of bile pig-

TABLE 28.2 HEMATOPOIETIC GROWTH FACTORS FOR CANCER THERAPY SUPPORT

Medication Class/Action	Example	Route	Side Effects	Nursing Implications
Colony-Stimulating Factors are hormones that stimulate the bone marrow to produce blood cells. They are synthetically produced for specific functions such as proliferation of white blood cells, red blood cells, and platelets.	Filgrastim (Neupogen) Pegfilgrastim (Neulasta) Target production of neutrophils so the patient has a better chance of recovery prior to the next cycle of chemotherapy	IV, subcutaneous Subcutaneous	Bone pain, leukocytosis	The patient may use acetaminophen for the bone pain. Monitor WBC counts until the desired level is achieved. The drug is discontinued once the absolute neutrophil count reaches 10,000/mm^3.
	Epoetin alfa (Epogen, Procrit) Targets production of red blood cells	IV, Subcutaneous	Hypertension	Monitor the hematocrit and hemoglobin levels. Monitor blood chemistry. It may take up to 8 weeks to see a response to the medication. After 8 weeks, the dose may be increased. Given three times a week.
	Oprelvekin (Neumega) Targets production of platelets. Given for chemotherapy-induced thrombocytopenia to reduce the need for platelet transfusions.	Subcutaneous	Fluid retention, tachycardia, atrial fibrillation, atrial flutter	Monitor complete blood counts including platelet count; fluid and electrolyte status.

ments. The spleen and liver may enlarge because of the increase in retained cells and cellular materials.

Because the cells are fragile, there is a significant decrease in the life span of the RBCs in patients with sickle cell anemia. Normal red cells live about 120 days. Sickled cells survive only about 15 to 20 days, an 80 to 90 percent decrease in cell survival.

ETIOLOGY. Sickle cell disease is an autosomal recessive hereditary disorder. This means that if both parents pass on the abnormal hemoglobin, the child will have the disease. If only one parent passes on the abnormal hemoglobin, the child will have the sickle cell trait and will be able to pass the trait (or the disease if the other parent is also affected) on to his or her child.

In the United States, sickle cell anemia is most often found in those of African or Eastern Mediterranean heritage. Worldwide, many persons residing in Asia, the Caribbean, the Middle East, and Central America are affected. Nearly 10 percent of African Americans have the sickle cell trait; 1 of every 400 African American infants born has inherited the two sets of abnormal genes necessary to have the disease. Symptoms do not appear in infants until after the age of 6 months because up to that age the infant is using hemoglobin manufactured during fetal life, which is not affected by the sickling process.

SIGNS AND SYMPTOMS. The sickling changes just described are a daily occurrence. The rapid return of the oxygen level to normal usually returns the cells to their normal shape.

Occasionally, the sickling process cannot be reversed and the problem continues unabated. This sudden and severe sickling is called a *sickle cell crisis.* As more and more sickling occurs, the blood becomes sluggish and does not flow easily. It tends to collect in the capillaries and veins of the organs of the chest and abdomen, as well as joints and bones, and can cause infarction (tissue necrosis resulting from lack of blood supply). Tissue necrosis results in pain, fever, and swelling.

Factors that contribute to the development of a sickle cell crisis include those related to decreased oxygenation. Some examples include pneumonia with hypoxia, exposure to cold, diabetic acidosis, and severe infection. Sickle cell anemia presents problems for the patient who needs surgery. Anesthesia and blood loss during surgery and postoperative dehydration can trigger a crisis.

Common symptoms produced during sickle cell crises include severe pain and swelling in the joints, especially of the elbows and knees, as the sickled cells impede circulation. Abdominal pain is common with swelling of the spleen and engorgement of the vital organs. Hypoxia occurs as fever and pain increase, causing the patient to breathe rap-

Box 28.5

Interventions to Prevent Bleeding in the Patient with Thrombocytopenia

- Use an electric razor instead of a safety razor for shaving.
- Use a soft toothbrush or gauze to clean the teeth. Avoid flossing.
- Avoid invasive procedures as much as possible, including enemas, douches, suppositories, and rectal temperatures.
- Avoid intramuscular injections.
- To avoid injury when checking blood pressure, pump cuff up only until pulse is obliterated.
- Avoid blood draws whenever possible. Use established access sites or group draws into once daily.
- Maintain pressure on intravenous (IV), blood draw, and other puncture sites for 5 minutes.
- Encourage use of shoes or slippers when out of bed.
- Keep area clutter free to prevent bumps and bruises.
- Avoid use of drugs that interfere with platelet function, such as aspirin products and nonsteroidal anti-inflammatory drugs.
- Administer stool softeners as ordered to prevent straining to have a bowel movement.
- Move and turn patient gently to avoid bruising.
- Instruct patient to avoid blowing the nose.

Box 28.6

Interventions for the Patient at Risk for Infection

- Place the patient in a private room.
- Assure that all personnel and visitors wash hands before entering the room.
- Teach the patient to wash hands before and after using the toilet and before and after eating.
- Teach the patient and family to wash hands before touching.
- Prevent staff or visitors with known infections from entering the patient's room.
- Teach the patient to not handle flowers or plants brought into the room.
- Teach the patient to avoid raw fruits, vegetables, and milk products.
- Avoid use of Foley catheters and other invasive devices.
- Use strict aseptic technique if invasive procedures are necessary.
- Use acetaminophen if an antipyretic is necessary; aspirin may induce bleeding.

idly. The male patient may have a continuous, painful erection (priapism) from impaired blood flow through the penis. Symptoms of renal failure are common as circulation is slowed and the kidneys become clogged with cellular debris.

Repeated crises and infarctions lead to chronic manifestations such as hand-foot syndrome, an unequal growth of fingers and toes from infarction of the small bones in the hands and feet (Fig. 28.3). Additional manifestations of sickle cell disease are shown in Figure 28.4.

The patient with sickle cell anemia has impaired quality of life. Often, strenuous exercise or more exotic activities, such as scuba diving, are impossible because of the risk of crisis. Dehydration exacerbates the symptoms of sickle cell disease. Crises may occur without any apparent cause. In general, crises last from 4 to 6 days. They may occur in cycles close together for a time and then may become dormant for months to years. The cause of death in patients with sickle cell anemia is usually infection, stroke, or organ involvement.

DIAGNOSTIC TESTS. The most telling feature of sickle cell disease is a blood smear that shows sickle-shaped RBCs in circulation. The Sickledex test is a screening test that shows sickling of RBCs when oxygen tension is low.

Hemoglobin electrophoresis is a test used to determine the presence of hemoglobin (Hgb) S, the abnormal form of hemoglobin. Also, there is a decreased amount of hemoglobin, a lowered RBC count, an elevated WBC count, and a decreased erythrocyte sedimentation rate.

TREATMENT. No cure is available for sickle cell anemia. Treatment is aimed at patient education to prevent crises and supportive care when crises occur. Some patients may be placed on low-dose oral penicillin to help prevent infections, decreasing the risk of crises.

During acute crises, the patient is admitted to the hospital for 5 to 7 days. The nurse can anticipate that the patient will require sedation and analgesia for severe pain and blood transfusions to replace the sickled red cells lost by their being caught, crushed, and destroyed. Oxygen therapy decreases the dyspnea caused by the anemia, and large

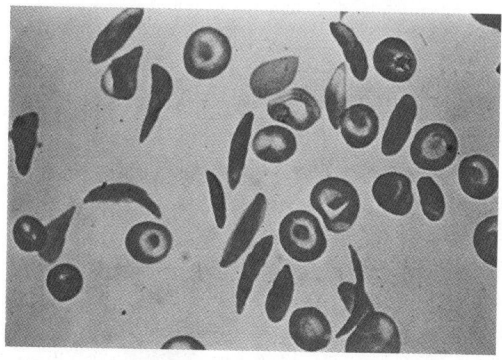

FIGURE 28.2 Sickled cells in sickle cell disease.

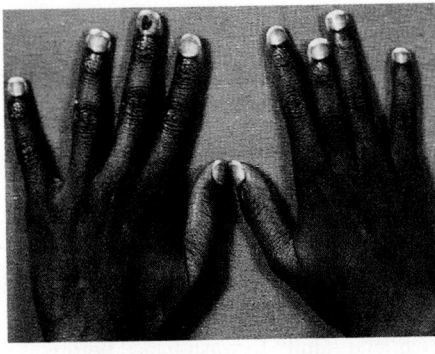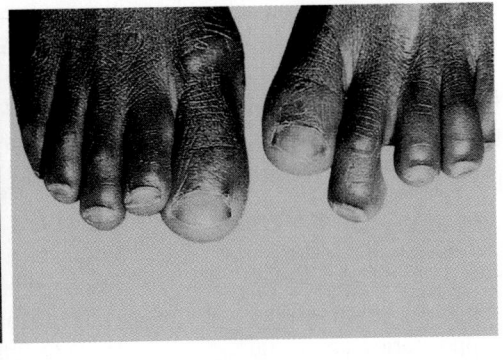

FIGURE 28.3 Hand-foot syndrome. Note different lengths of fingers and toes. *(Courtesy Sandoz Pharmaceutical Corp., East Hanover, NJ)*

amounts of oral and intravenous fluids are given to flush the kidneys of the by-products of the many broken cells' debris. Antibiotics are used to treat infection that may have triggered the crisis.

New treatments are being developed to treat sickle cell disease. Frequent blood transfusions, often monthly, are one of the newest treatment recommendations. Hydroxyurea (Droxia) is a drug that has been shown to decrease crises, but it can cause life-threatening side effects; it should also be used with caution in female patients of childbearing years because of the risk of birth defects. Corticosteroids may reduce the need for analgesics and oxygen. Bone marrow transplantation is also being investigated as a potential cure.

NURSING PROCESS: SICKLE CELL ANEMIA. Assessment/Data Collection. In the patient in crisis, assess circulation in the extremities every 2 hours, including pulse oximetry, capillary refill, peripheral pulses, and temperature. Frequent pain assessment is also necessary.

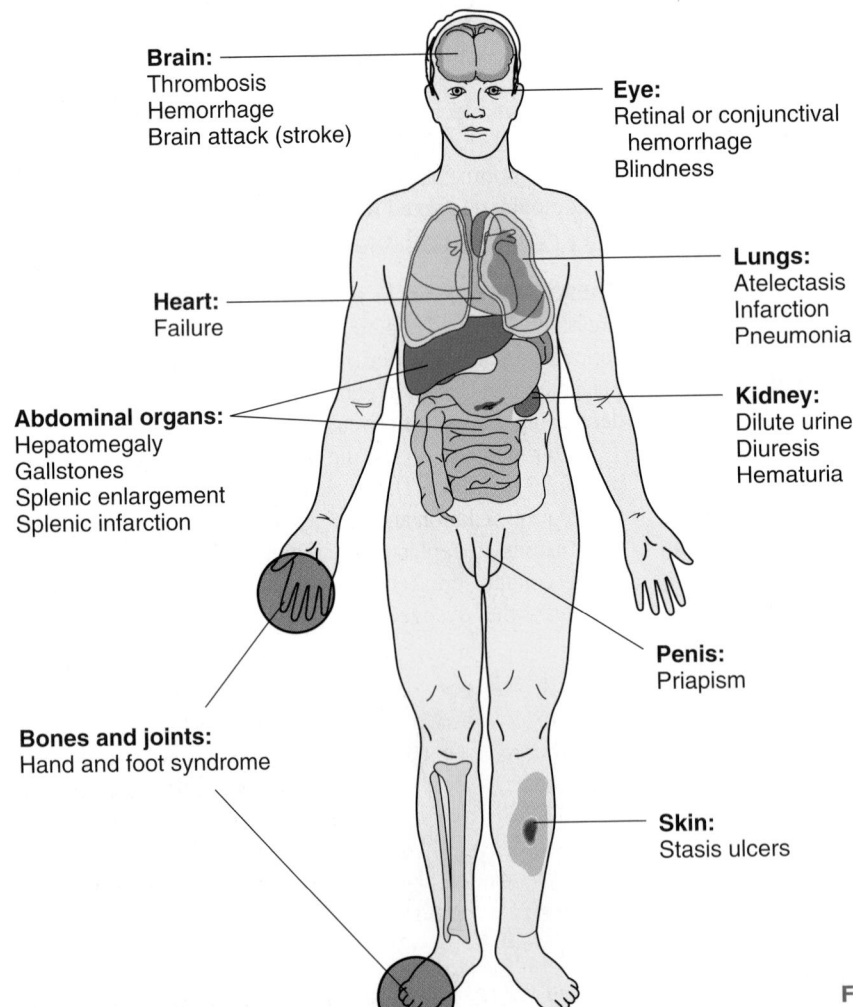

Brain:
Thrombosis
Hemorrhage
Brain attack (stroke)

Eye:
Retinal or conjunctival
  hemorrhage
Blindness

Heart:
Failure

Lungs:
Atelectasis
Infarction
Pneumonia

Abdominal organs:
Hepatomegaly
Gallstones
Splenic enlargement
Splenic infarction

Kidney:
Dilute urine
Diuresis
Hematuria

Penis:
Priapism

Bones and joints:
Hand and foot syndrome

Skin:
Stasis ulcers

FIGURE 28.4 Clinical manifestations of sickle cell anemia.

Nursing Diagnosis, Planning, and Implementation
Risk for ineffective tissue perfusion related to sickled cells and infarction

EXPECTED OUTCOME: *Patient will have adequate tissue perfusion as evidenced by presence of peripheral pulses, warm extremities, urine output within normal limits, and capillary refill less than 3 seconds.*

- Encourage oral fluids, and assist the registered nurse (RN) to monitor intravenous (IV) fluids *to dilute and aid in elimination of cell debris.*
- Apply warm compresses as ordered to the painful areas, cover the patient with a blanket, and keep the room temperature above 72°F (~22°C) *to reduce the vasoconstricting effects of cold.*
- Avoid cold compresses *because they decrease circulation and increase the number of sickled cells caught in a painful area.*
- Avoid restrictive clothing and raising the knee gatch of the bed. *These can restrict circulation.*

Acute pain related to tissue infarction

EXPECTED OUTCOME: *Patient will state pain is controlled at acceptable level.*

- Administer opioid analgesics such as morphine as ordered *for acute pain.* (Analgesics may be given intravenously by the RN or by use of patient-controlled analgesia.)
- Administer acetaminophen (Tylenol) *to control fever.*
- Avoid giving aspirin *because it may increase acidosis, which can worsen the crisis.*
- Encourage bedrest during the acute phase of the crisis *to reduce oxygen demand.*

Evaluation. If nursing care has been effective, the patient will state that he or she is comfortable, and will not exhibit signs of poor circulation.

PATIENT TEACHING. During remission, teach the patient how to prevent acute episodes. Advise the patient to avoid tight-fitting clothing that restricts circulation. Also encourage the patient to avoid strenuous exercise, which increases oxygen demand, and cold temperatures and smoking, which cause vasoconstriction. Alcoholic beverages can also trigger a crisis and should be avoided. Patients should never fly in unpressurized aircraft or undertake mountain climbing or other sports that can cause hypoxia. Encourage patients to get a pneumococcal vaccine and

yearly flu vaccine. Encourage fluids to maintain hydration and reduce blood viscosity. Genetic counseling is important to prevent passing on the trait or disease to children. For more information, visit www.sicklecelldisease.org.

Polycythemia
Pathophysiology and Etiology

Polycythemia is really two separate disorders that are easily recognizable by similar characteristic changes in the RBC count. In both forms of polycythemia, the blood becomes so thick with an overabundance of RBCs that it closely resembles sludge. This thickness does not allow the blood to circulate easily. Laboratory tests show a hemoglobin level greater than 18 mg/dL, the RBC mass greater than 6 million, and a hematocrit more than 55 percent.

Polycythemia vera (PV) is known as primary polycythemia. Its cause is unknown. In PV, the RBCs, platelets, and WBCs are all overproduced, and the bone marrow becomes packed with too many cells. As this overabundance of cells spills out into the general circulation, the organs become congested with cells and the tissues become packed with blood. The skin takes on a plethoric (dark, flushed) appearance from the build-up of red cells. The thick blood and excess platelets can cause thrombosis and occlusion of vessels. PV is usually found in patients over age 50.

In contrast, secondary polycythemia is the result of long-term hypoxia. Common coexisting conditions that may predispose a patient to develop secondary polycythemia include pulmonary diseases such as chronic obstructive pulmonary disease (COPD), cardiovascular problems such as chronic heart failure, living in high altitudes, and smoking. The body makes more red cells in response to the low oxygenation associated with these conditions. Secondary polycythemia is a compensatory mechanism rather than an actual disorder.

Signs and Symptoms

The patient with PV commonly presents with hypertension, visual changes, headache, vertigo, dizziness, and ringing in the ears (tinnitus). Laboratory results show an increased level of all the bone marrow components (RBCs, WBCs, platelets), which is called **panmyelosis.** The patient may exhibit nosebleeds and bleeding gums, retinal hemorrhages, exertional dyspnea, and chest pains because of the increased pressure exerted by the excess cells. The patient with PV usually has a dark, flushed complexion. Intense itching is related to excess mast cells (and, therefore, histamine) in the skin. Abdominal pain with an early feeling of fullness with meals occurs because of the enlarged liver and spleen. Nearly all the symptoms in PV are due to the major problems of hypervolemia, hyperviscosity, and engorgement of capillary beds. Without treatment, patients with PV die of thrombosis or hemorrhage.

Treatment

Treatment of PV takes place in two stages. The first stage is to decrease the hyperviscosity problem. The most common

SAFETY TIP

Develop and implement a protocol for administration and documentation of the flu and pneumococcal vaccines (2006 National Patient Safety Goals from www.jcaho.org).

first-line treatment is therapeutic **phlebotomy.** Phlebotomy involves withdrawal of blood, which is then discarded. From 350 to 500 mL of blood are removed each time on an every-other-day basis, with the goal being a hematocrit of about 45 percent. This reduces the RBC levels, and the patient usually feels more comfortable quickly. Repeated phlebotomies eventually cause iron deficiency anemia, which in turn stabilizes RBC production; phlebotomies can then be reduced to every 2 to 3 months.

The problem that remains is the increased white blood cell and platelet counts because phlebotomy does very little to correct these overloads. Chemotherapeutic agents or radiation therapy, including radioactive phosphorus, may be used to suppress production of blood cells in some patients. **Leukemia** is a side effect of this therapy, so it is used only if the benefits outweigh the risks.

Nursing Care

Explain the phlebotomy procedure and reassure the patient that the treatment will relieve the most distressing symptoms. The procedure is the same as that used for donating blood. The patient should be active and ambulatory to help prevent thrombus formation. When bedrest is necessary, passive and active range-of-motion exercises should be implemented. Monitor the patient for complications such as hypovolemia and bleeding. Advise the patient to report any signs or symptoms of bleeding immediately.

If the patient has more advanced manifestations, such as an enlarged liver or spleen, offer several small meals each day so that the patient will be more comfortable while still receiving adequate nutrition. A dietitian can be consulted to discuss ways to maintain good nutrition. If the patient is on drug therapy, monitor CBC and platelet counts.

Patient Education

Instruct the patient to drink at least 3 L of water daily to reduce blood viscosity. Encourage avoidance of tight or restrictive clothing and elevation of feet when resting to prevent impairment of circulation. Use of support hose when active also promotes circulation. If anticoagulants or antiplatelet agents are ordered, instruct the patient about side effects to watch for and the importance of routine laboratory tests. Routine bleeding precautions are implemented (see Box 28.5 Interventions to Prevent Bleeding in the Patient with Thrombocytopenia). Warn the patient to stop activities at the first sign of chest pains. Instruct the patient to report chest pain, increased joint pain, decreased activity tolerance, or fever, as well as signs of iron deficiency anemia, such as pallor, weight loss, and dyspnea.

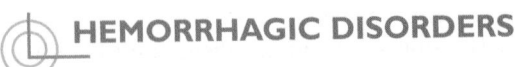

HEMORRHAGIC DISORDERS

Disseminated Intravascular Coagulation

Pathophysiology

Disseminated intravascular coagulation (DIC) involves a series of events that result in hemorrhage.

As its name implies, this syndrome is a catastrophic, overwhelming state of accelerated clotting throughout the peripheral blood vessels. In a short period, all the clotting factors and platelet supplies are exhausted and clots can no longer be formed. This results in bleeding from nearly every bodily route possible. DIC is not a disease but is a syndrome that develops secondary to some other severe physical problem. Once this deadly syndrome develops, the progression of symptoms is rapid.

Massive clotting in blood vessels leads to organ and limb necrosis. Organs most often affected include the kidneys and the brain, but other blood-engorged organs, such as the lungs, the pituitary and adrenal glands, and the gastrointestinal mucosa, are commonly involved. DIC is usually acute in onset, although in some patients it becomes a chronic condition. The prognosis depends on early diagnosis and intervention and the severity of the hemorrhaging. DIC has a very high mortality rate.

Etiology

DIC can develop after any condition in which the body has sustained major trauma. The sources of trauma are varied and can include an overwhelming infection; obstetric complications such as abruptio placentae, amniotic fluid embolism, or a retained dead fetus; or cancer-related causes such as acute leukemia or lung cancer. Massive tissue necrosis found in severe crush or burn injuries may increase the risk for development of DIC. Tissue necrosis secondary to extensive abdominal surgery with leakage of the intestinal contents can be related to DIC onset. Rarer causes of this condition have included heat stroke, shock, and poisonous snakebites, as well as fat embolism secondary to broken long bones.

Signs and Symptoms

Abnormal bleeding without a history of a serious hemorrhagic disorder is a cardinal sign of DIC. Early signs of bleeding include petechiae, ecchymoses (Fig. 28.5), and bleeding from venipuncture sites. Bleeding may progress to IV sites, skin tears, surgical sites, incisions, and the gastrointestinal tract and oral mucosa. Pain and enlargement of joints develop if bleeding into the joints occurs. All these signs and symptoms may occur at the same time. Massive bleeding may also be accompanied by nausea, vomiting, dyspnea, oliguria, convulsions, coma, shock, major organ system failure, and severe muscle, back, and abdominal pain.

Diagnostic Tests

Initial laboratory findings in DIC include a prolonged prothrombin time (PT) and partial thromboplastin time (PTT), decreased platelet count, and increased evidence of fibrin degradation products. A decrease in hemoglobin is the result of spilled hemoglobin from the increased numbers of broken red cells. Blood urea nitrogen (BUN) and serum creatinine levels may also be increased. See Table 28.3 for laboratory findings specific for DIC.

Therapeutic Interventions

Effective treatment of DIC depends on early recognition of the condition. Treatment is first aimed at correcting the

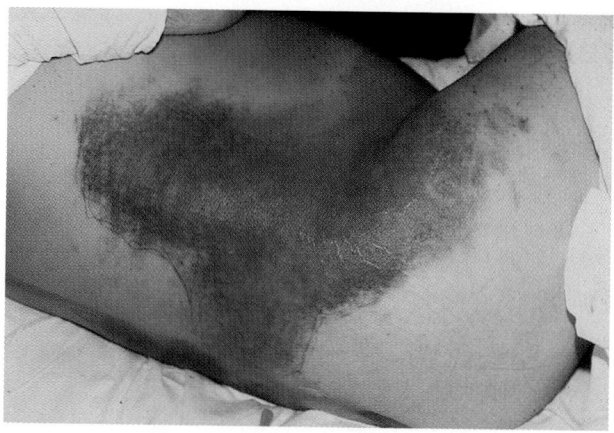

FIGURE 28.5 Extensive hemorrhage into the skin in DIC. Note how the area is outlined in pen so the nurse can assess if the area is spreading. *(From Harmening, DM: Clinical Hematology and Fundamentals of Hemostasis, ed 3. FA Davis, Philadelphia, 1997, p 520, with permission.)*

underlying cause. Additional treatment consists of supportive interventions, including administration of blood, fresh frozen plasma, and platelets and the infusion of cryoprecipitate (containing clotting factors) to support hemostasis. Some health-care organizations include the use of intravenous heparin to help prevent the initial microembolization, but this practice is controversial. Additional therapies are being investigated.

Nursing Care

Care of the patient with DIC is a nursing challenge. Early intervention requires early recognition and reporting of signs of bleeding. In addition to supportive care, focus on the prevention of further bleeding episodes. Care should be taken to avoid any trauma that might cause bleeding. Be careful not to dislodge clots from any site because another clot may not form and the patient will hemorrhage. See Box

TABLE 28.3 LABORATORY ABNORMALITIES IN DISSEMINATED INTRAVASCULAR COAGULATION

Screening Test	Finding
Prothrombin time (PT)	Prolonged
Partial thromboplastin time (PTT)	Prolonged
Activated partial thromboplastin time (APTT)	Prolonged
Thrombin time (TT)	Prolonged
Fibrinogen	Reduced
Platelets	Reduced
Fibrin split products (FSP; also known as fibrin degradation products [FDP])	Elevated
Protamine sulfate	Strongly positive
Dimers (cross-linked fibrin fragments)	Elevated
Antithrombin III	Reduced
Factor assays (for factors V, VII, VIII, X, and XIII)	Reduced

28.5 (Interventions to Prevent Bleeding in the Patient with Thrombocytopenia) for bleeding precautions.

SAFETY TIP

Measure, assess and, if appropriate, take action to improve the timeliness of reporting, and the timeliness of receipt by the responsible licensed caregiver, of critical test results and values (2006 National Patient Safety Goals from www.jcaho.org).

Patient Teaching

Because a patient with DIC is often cared for in the intensive care unit, there are many chances for patient and family teaching. Explain all diagnostic tests to the patient if he or she is alert. If not, keep the family informed. A large part of family education is preparing the family for what the patient may look like in terms of bleeding and bruising, as well as specific equipment that may be in place, such as IV lines, a nasogastric (NG) tube, and a Foley catheter. It may be helpful to enlist the aid of social workers, chaplains, and other members of the health-care team to help support the family.

CRITICAL THINKING

Mrs. Johns

■ Mrs. Johns is admitted to your unit with DIC following the difficult delivery of her new baby.
1. What will you assess as you care for Mrs. Johns?
2. What treatment do you anticipate?
3. What concerns is Mrs. Johns likely to have?
4. Mrs. Johns is to receive IV fresh frozen plasma 300 mL over 30 minutes. How many milliliters per hour should be set on the IV controller?

Suggested answers at end of chapter.

Idiopathic Thrombocytopenic Purpura

Pathophysiology and Etiology

Acute **idiopathic thrombocytopenic purpura** (ITP) results from increased platelet destruction by the immune system. Any time platelet numbers are reduced, the risk for bleeding increases. Acute ITP usually affects children between the ages of 2 and 6, whereas chronic ITP mainly affects adults younger than age 50. The population most affected is women between ages 20 and 40.

Acute ITP usually occurs after an acute viral illness such as rubella or chickenpox. It may also be drug induced

---

idiopathic thrombocytopenic purpura: idio—unknown + pathic—disease + thrombo—clot + cyto—cell + penic—lack + purpura—hemorrhage in the skin

or associated with pregnancy. ITP is generally thought to be related to an immune system dysfunction. Antibodies responsible for platelet destruction have been found in nearly all diagnosed patients.

Signs and Symptoms

ITP produces clinical changes that are common to all forms of **thrombocytopenia**: petechiae, ecchymoses, and bleeding from the mouth, nose, or gastrointestinal (GI) tract. Bleeding may occur in vital organs, such as the brain, which may prove fatal. In the acute type, onset may be sudden and without warning, causing easy bruising, nosebleeds, and bleeding gums. Onset of chronic ITP is usually insidious.

Diagnostic Tests

A platelet count of less than 20,000/mm³ and a prolonged bleeding time suggest ITP. The greatly decreased platelet level places the patient at serious risk for hemorrhage. Examination of the platelets under the microscope shows them to be small and immature. Anemia may be present if there has been a bleeding episode. If a bone marrow aspiration is performed, the results show an adequate amount of the precursor cells for platelets, the megakaryocytes. However, instead of the 7- to 10-day life span that platelets usually have, these immature platelets have a life span of just a few hours.

Treatment

Most cases of acute ITP resolve spontaneously without treatment. Initial treatment, if necessary, is often the administration of steroids. The purpose of the steroids is to prolong the life of the platelets and strengthen the capillaries, making them less likely to break and cause bleeding. Some physicians order the use of chemotherapeutic drugs. The spleen may be removed because it is the primary site involved in platelet destruction. Often the patient undergoing splenectomy has tried all other courses of treatment unsuccessfully and may be experiencing bleeding episodes. Acute bleeding episodes are treated with transfusions of blood, platelets, and vitamin K.

Nursing Interventions

Care for the patient with ITP is the same as any patient with a bleeding disorder. See Box 28.5 (Interventions to Prevent Bleeding in the Patient with Thrombocytopenia) for bleeding precautions. Teach the patient to watch for and report signs and symptoms of bruising and bleeding (Box 28.7 Patient Teaching: Signs and Symptoms of Bleeding). The patient should avoid trauma and restrict activity during severe episodes.

Hemophilia

Hemophilia is a group of hereditary bleeding disorders that result from a severe lack of specific clotting factors. The two most common are hemophilia A (classic hemophilia) and

---

Box 28.7

Patient Teaching: Signs and Symptoms of Bleeding

Notify your health care provider if the following occur:
- Easy bruising of skin
- Petechiae (small red spots on skin)
- Blood in urine
- Black tarry stools
- Bleeding from nose or gums
- New onset of painful joints

---

hemophilia B (Christmas disease). Von Willebrand's disease is another related bleeding disorder, but it represents a minority of cases and is not discussed in this chapter.

Pathophysiology

Recall that many different clotting factors make up the clotting mechanism. Hemophilia A accounts for 80 percent of all types of hemophilia and results from a deficiency of factor VIII. Hemophilia B is a factor IX deficiency; approximately 15 percent of persons with hemophilia have this type. The severity and prognosis of hemophilia depend on the degree of deficiency of the specific clotting factors. Mild hemophilia has the best prognosis because it does not cause spontaneous bleeding and joint deformities as severe hemophilia can.

After an injury, the person with hemophilia forms a platelet plug (which differs from a clot) at the site of an injury as would normally be expected, but the clotting factor deficiency keeps the patient from forming a stable fibrin clot. Continued bleeding washes away the platelet plug that initially formed. Contrary to popular myths, people with hemophilia do not bleed "faster" and are not at risk from small scratches.

Etiology

Hemophilia A and B are inherited as X-linked recessive traits. This means that the female carrier (daughter of an affected father) has a 50 percent chance of transmitting the gene to each son or daughter. Daughters who receive the gene are carriers, and sons who receive the gene are born with hemophilia. It is technically possible for daughters to be affected with hemophilia, although it is very rare.

Signs and Symptoms

Bleeding occurs as a result of injury or, in severe cases, spontaneously (unprovoked by injury). Bleeding into the muscles and joints (**hemarthrosis**) is common. Severe and repeated episodes of joint hemorrhage cause joint deformities, especially in the elbows, knees, and ankles, which decrease the patient's range of motion and ability to walk.

In mild hemophilia, excessive bleeding is usually associated only with surgery or significant trauma. However,

---

thrombocytopenia: thrombocyte—platelet + penia—lack
hemophilia: hemo—blood + philia—to love

hemarthrosis: hem—bleeding + arthr—joint + osis—condition

once a person with mild hemophilia begins to bleed, the bleeding can be just as serious as that of the patient with a more severe form.

The patient with moderate hemophilia has an occasional bout of spontaneous bleeding. In severe hemophilia, spontaneous bleeding occurs more frequently. It would be possible for the patient to develop hemarthrosis or bleeding into the brain without any precipitating trauma. Severe episodes can produce large subcutaneous and deep intramuscular hematomas. Major trauma can cause bleeding so severe that it becomes life threatening.

Another unfortunate problem related to hemophilia treatment is the frequent need to replace clotting factors and other blood products. Before 1986, blood banks and other centers did not routinely test for human immunodeficiency virus (HIV) antibodies. Depending on the patient's age and frequency of treatment, many patients may have been exposed to HIV or hepatitis. Blood banks and pharmacies have checked their blood supplies for the presence of HIV since 1986. Today, the plasma proteins are artificially created or thoroughly cleansed to prevent transmission of disease.

Diagnostic Tests

Laboratory data reveal a prolonged PTT. The various factor levels are measured to determine which is missing. Once the missing factor is identified, the type of hemophilia is determined and necessary treatments can be implemented.

Therapeutic Interventions

Hemophilia is not curable. However, treatment advances have improved outcomes and many patients can now live a normal life span. Treatment is aimed at the prevention of crippling deformities and at increasing life expectancy. Treatment involves stopping bleeding episodes by administering the missing clotting factors. Hemophilia A is treated with factor VIII; hemophilia B is treated with factor IX. Each is available in a freeze-dried powder that is reconstituted with water and administered intravenously. The newest treatment employs factors made using recombinant DNA technology without the use of any human blood products. Blood transfusions are uncommon but may be necessary after severe trauma or surgery.

Complications related to therapy usually occur when therapy is started too late. Minor trauma generally needs to be treated with at least 72 hours of added clotting factors; major traumas and surgeries may require up to 14 days of added factors to prevent sudden bleeding. Health-care workers should pay careful attention to the patient who says that bleeding is starting even when no outward signs are evident. The patient usually knows from experience if bleeding is starting. If treatment is delayed at this time, the results can be disastrous. Some patients with severe disease are treated prophylactically to prevent bleeding.

Nursing Process: Hemophilia

ASSESSMENT/DATA COLLECTION. Because one goal is prevention of bleeding episodes, assess the patient and family for knowledge of the disease and its treatment and understanding of preventive measures. Most patients care for themselves at home, starting their own IVs and administering treatment independently. Hospitalization is necessary only for surgery or major trauma. During an acute episode of bleeding, the hemoglobin and hematocrit are carefully monitored. Factor VIII or IX levels are monitored to determine if factor replacement has reached adequate levels. Vital signs are monitored for falling blood pressure and rising pulse rate, which are signs of hypovolemic shock. All body systems are assessed for signs of bleeding (see Box 28.7 Patient Teaching: Signs and Symptoms of Bleeding). A pain assessment is done using the WHAT'S UP? format.

NURSING DIAGNOSIS, PLANNING, AND IMPLEMENTATION. Pain related to bleeding into tissues

EXPECTED OUTCOMES: *The patient will verbalize that pain is relieved to a satisfactory level..*

- Have the patient report the location, intensity, and quality of the pain. *Assessment of the pain provides the caregiver with data for treatment plan.*
- Administer opioids as prescribed including patient-controlled analgesia. *Analgesics are the primary way to manage moderate to severe pain.*
- Avoid the administration of intramuscular injections *because of the risk of bleeding into the muscle, which would cause more pain.*
- Reassess the level of pain within 1 hour after administration of analgesia *to determine the effectiveness of the treatment ordered.*
- Monitor sedation and respiratory status of the patient receiving opioids for pain. *Opioids depress the respiratory center of the brain.*

Ineffective protection: Risk for bleeding related to factor deficiencies

EXPECTED OUTCOMES: *The patient will not have evidence of bleeding. The patient will verbalize understanding of bleeding precautions.*

- Instruct the patient on bleeding precautions noted in Box 28.5 (Interventions to Prevent Bleeding in the Patient with Thrombocytopenia). *Identification of signs of bleeding will promote early intervention to prevent injury.*
- Assist with administration of factor concentrates, fresh frozen plasma, cryoprecipitate, blood, or a combination of these as ordered *to treat acute episodes of bleeding. See Chapter 27 for transfusion of blood products.*
- Apply ice or pressure on bleeding sites *to help slow bleeding.*
- Avoid intramuscular, subcutaneous, or rectal medications. *These routes can cause bleeding into tissues.*
- Instruct the patient that preventive care will be needed if surgery or dental procedures are needed. *These invasive procedures can be life-threatening events for the patient with hemophilia.*

Risk for ineffective management of therapeutic regimen related to knowledge deficit

EXPECTED OUTCOME: *The patient will be able to discuss hemophilia and the treatment regimen required.*

- Assess knowledge base and determine readiness to learn and incorporate new information. *Each patient is unique in the way that they learn new information.*
- Instruct the patient on ways to prevent bleeding and recognition of signs and symptoms of bleeding (Boxes 28.5 Interventions to Prevent Bleeding in the Patient with Thrombocytopenia and 28.7 Patient Teaching: Signs and Symptoms of Bleeding). *Identification of signs of bleeding will promote early intervention to prevent injury.*
- Instruct the patient to obtain emergency care in the event that bleeding occurs. *Intervention is critical for survival for acute bleeding.*
- Instruct the patient to administer factor treatments at home. *Treatment can often be administered at home and can be given more promptly if a trip to the emergency department is not necessary.*
- Instruct patients and families on the community services and hemophilia treatment centers available to the patient. *These centers are nationwide and coordinate care for patients with hemophilia.*
- Instruct the patient that the approach to care is multidisciplinary in nature and includes social services, dental, rehabilitation, nursing, financial, and medical needs. *These are all areas that impact the care of the patient with hemophilia.*

EVALUATION. If interventions have been effective, the patient will be comfortable and bleeding will be prevented or complications minimized. The patient and family will be able to state appropriate measures to prevent and treat bleeding episodes. The patient will be knowledgeable about the resources available to cope with the diagnosis of hemophilia.

SAFETY TIP

Encourage the active involvement of patients and their families in the patient's care as a patient safety strategy (2006 National Patient Safety Goals www.jcaho.org).

DISORDERS OF WHITE BLOOD CELLS

Leukemia

The term *leukemia* literally means "white blood." It was first identified in 1845 when the blood of victims was examined and found to have an excess of "colorless" cells.

Pathophysiology

Leukemia is a malignant disease of the WBCs that affects all age groups. The immature WBCs (blast cells) generate in an explosive fashion in the bone marrow, lymph tissue, and spleen. The cells are abnormal and unable to effectively fight infection. There are so many abnormal cells developed and dumped into the peripheral circulation that they tend to collect in the body tissues and organs, especially where circulation is sluggish. Areas especially prone to infiltration with immature WBCs are the oral mucosa, anus, sinuses, and lungs. At the time of diagnosis, these areas are often inflamed, painful, and infected. It is common for patients to be diagnosed only after suffering with an infection that does not clear up easily.

As the disease progresses, the bone marrow continues to produce large numbers of the useless cells, the peripheral circulation is filled with them, and the bone marrow is packed with blast cells. Because so many of the blood stem cells are being used to make defective white cells, production of most other normal cells is impossible. The patient becomes anemic because of the lack of RBC production, and bleeding becomes a problem as fewer and fewer platelets are manufactured. But most importantly, even though the WBC count is very high, there are very few normal, mature, and active white cells with which to fight infection. Thus, the patient often begins to have raging infections that do not respond to antibiotics. Without treatment, leukemia leaves the patient unable to fight infection, unable to control bleeding, and in a downward spiral of fatigue and anorexia. Untreated leukemia is almost always fatal.

Classifications

Leukemias are classified as either acute or chronic and either lymphoid or myeloid. Symptoms of the acute leukemias begin very suddenly and the patient is very sick, whereas chronic leukemias develop very slowly and patients can be surprised by the diagnosis because they feel well. Lymphoid leukemias affect the lymphocytes. Myeloid leukemias originate in the stem cells of the bone marrow that develop into monocytes, granulocytes, erythrocytes, and platelets. The most common leukemias are discussed next.

ACUTE LEUKEMIAS. Acute lymphocytic leukemia (ALL) commonly affects children younger than age 15 and involves abnormal growth of the lymphocyte precursors (lymphoblasts). Acute myelogenous (myeloblastic) leukemia (AML) usually affects persons older than age 20 and has a poor prognosis. The patient with acute leukemia may present with sudden onset of high fever, abnormal bleeding from the mucous membranes, petechiae, ecchymoses, and easy bruising after minor trauma. Death usually results from infection.

CHRONIC LEUKEMIAS. Chronic lymphocytic leukemia (CLL) predominantly affects the B and T lymphocytes and usually occurs in adults older than age 40. Chronic myelogenous leukemia (CML) is characterized by the Philadelphia chromosome and occurs most often between the ages of 40 and 45.

Chronic leukemia usually develops in a three-stage process. First is the insidious phase, characterized by anemia and mild bleeding abnormalities. During this stage, the patient often feels well and is not even aware that he or she is sick. After a time, generally years, the disease progresses to the accelerated and acute phases, in which the scenarios are similar to the events seen in acute leukemias. Chronic leukemia is almost always fatal; the average survival time is 3 to 4 years after onset of the chronic phase and 3 to 6 months after onset of the acute phase. With advances in treatments, it is not uncommon to encounter patients who have been living with chronic leukemia for 10 years or more.

Etiology

The cause of leukemia is unknown. Risk factors are thought to include certain viruses because remnants of viruses have been found in leukemic cells. Often there are genetic and immunological factors involved. For example, persons with Down syndrome are more likely to develop leukemia. Other authorities point to exposure to radiation, in part because radiologists have been found to have a higher than average development of leukemia. Some patients have developed leukemia after being treated for another unrelated malignancy using radiation or chemotherapy. Researchers have noted the higher occurrence rate in persons who lived through the Hiroshima and Nagasaki atomic bombings during World War II. Water polluted with benzenes and other chemicals may be a factor. There is no single clear-cut cause for the development of leukemia.

Signs and Symptoms

Symptoms are similar for all types of leukemia and include low-grade fever caused by infection and pallor, weakness, lassitude, shortness of breath, and malaise caused by anemia. These symptoms may be present weeks or months before the appearance of other symptoms. The patient may also have fatigue, tachycardia, palpitations, and abdominal pain. Sternal pain and rib tenderness may result from crowding of bone marrow. If the leukemia has invaded the central nervous system, the patient may experience confusion, headaches, and personality changes. During the acute phase the patient may exhibit high fevers from infection. Ecchymosis or petechiae may result from thrombocytopenia.

Diagnostic Tests

Although a simple CBC often points toward the diagnosis, only bone marrow aspiration can show the degree of proliferation of the malignant WBCs and confirm the diagnosis of leukemia. The complete blood cell count may also show a decrease in the numbers of platelets, RBCs, and mature WBCs. A lumbar puncture helps determine if the central nervous system is involved. Genetic analysis of the peripheral blood and bone marrow components may show the presence of the Philadelphia chromosome in patients with CML.

Therapeutic Interventions

CHEMOTHERAPY. Systemic chemotherapy aims to eradicate the leukemic cells and induce a remission. Remission means that the bone marrow is free to produce normally occurring cells in normal proportions without production of the immature WBCs. Chemotherapy types vary with the types of leukemia and the level of involvement. Radiation therapy is also sometimes used for initial treatment of leukemia.

The overall goal of the first treatments is to get the patient to a state of remission. Occasionally, partial remission is achieved when everything looks good except for an occasional leukemic cell seen in the bone marrow. Remission is not the same as cure.

There are four phases to the treatment of leukemia: induction, intensification, consolidation, and maintenance. Induction is the period in which an attempt to get the patient into remission is made. This first phase is difficult because chemotherapy is given in extremely high doses and on an aggressive timetable. Often the patient becomes quite ill from complications of the treatment. The patient may become depressed because the treatment seems worse than the disease at this stage. The nurse must help the patient deal with the side effects of anemia, thrombocytopenia, and leukopenia (See Box 28.8 Leukemia Summary, Box 28.6 Interventions for the Patient at Risk for Infection, and Chapter 10 Nursing Care of Patients with Cancer.)

If the first remission is accomplished, the other phases of treatment are begun. Intensification is similar to the initial induction phase, using the same drugs at even higher doses. The next phase, consolidation, is used to ensure that all leukemic cells have been eradicated from the body. Finally, the patient graduates to maintenance therapy in which the patient is kept free of leukemic cells (and in remission) for a period of years (and hopefully a lifetime). This requires years of continued chemotherapy treatments, often on a monthly basis. Radiation therapy may be used throughout this course of treatment to decrease the size of the liver or spleen or to decrease the numbers of leukemic cells in the central nervous system.

BONE MARROW TRANSPLANT. Bone marrow transplant (BMT) is sometimes used to treat leukemia. Preparation for BMT includes high-dose chemotherapy and/or total body irradiation. The goal is to destroy all the patient's malignant bone marrow and then, at the last possible moment, replace it with a donor's clean and healthy bone marrow (allogenic transplant). Another type of bone marrow transplant, known as an autologous transplant, uses the patient's own diseased bone marrow, which is harvested, chemically treated and cleaned, stored, and later reinfused. Transplanted bone marrow is given to the patient like a blood transfusion; generally through a central line placed in the chest. Once infused into the bloodstream, the new marrow travels to the bones, where, ideally, it will begin to grow and function normally. Bone marrow transplants are being performed at more and more centers across the United States.

A new and promising treatment for leukemia is peripheral blood stem cell transplantation. Hematopoietic stem cells can be collected from the patient during remission and

Box 28.8

Leukemia Summary

Signs and symptoms	Fever (related to infection)
	Pallor
	Weakness, malaise
	Tachycardia
	Dyspnea
	Bone pain
	Headaches, confusion
Diagnostic tests	CBC
	Bone marrow aspiration
	Lumbar puncture
Therapeutic interventions	Chemotherapy
	Radiation therapy
	Bone marrow transplant
Priority nursing diagnoses	Risk for bleeding related to thrombocytopenia (see Boxes 28.5 Interventions to Prevent Bleeding in the Patient with Thrombocytopenia and 28.7 Patient Teaching: Signs and Symptoms of Bleeding)
	Risk for infection related to altered immune response (see Chapter 10 and Box 28.6 Interventions for The Patient At Risk For Infection)
	Fatigue related to decreased tissue oxygenation (see Chapter 10)

then reinfused at a later time. Donor stem cells are also sometimes used if a good match can be found.

Nursing Process

The patient with leukemia is at risk for many problems, including fatigue, bleeding, infection, and other complications of the disease and its treatment. The patient must understand the disease process and treatment regimen in order to participate in self-care. See Box 28–9 (Nursing Care Plan for the Patient with Leukemia) for interventions to deal with these problems. Additional diagnoses include knowledge deficit and anxiety. The following Web sites provide resources for patients and families with leukemia. See also Chapter 10 for general care of the patient with cancer.

For more information, visit the following Web sites:

American Cancer Society at www.cancer.org.

Leukemia and Lymphoma Society at www.leukemia.org.

National Cancer Institute at www.nci.nih.gov.

MULTIPLE MYELOMA

Multiple myeloma is a deadly cancer of the plasma cells in the bone marrow. When the disease is caught in its early

stages, treatment can prolong life by 3 to 5 years. More important, early detection can decrease the amount of pain and disability due to bony destruction and **pathological fractures.** Unfortunately, almost half the patients die within the first 3 months after diagnosis because of the silent and deadly nature of the disease. Another 40 percent of patients die within 2 years after diagnosis. Because early diagnosis is not often made, only 10 percent of patients can expect to live to the 5-year mark. Multiple myeloma most often affects men ages 50 to 70.

Pathophysiology

In this disorder, cancerous plasma cells in the bone marrow begin reproducing uncontrollably. These cells infiltrate bone tissue all over the body and produce hundreds of tumors that begin to devour the bone tissue. X-ray examination may show holes in the bones forming a Swiss cheese pattern (Fig. 28.6). As more and more of these holes are formed, the bone integrity becomes compromised and weak. Multiple myeloma usually affects the bones of the skull, pelvis, ribs, and vertebrae.

As the disease continues, the plasma cells infiltrate the major organs, including the liver, spleen, lymph nodes, lungs, adrenal glands, kidneys, skin, and GI tract. Because the diagnosis is usually made only after widespread invasion of the bones is well underway, the prognosis for patients with this disease is poor. Although the overall result of the disease is the devastating destruction of the bone and widespread osteoporosis, death is often from sepsis.

Etiology

The cause of multiple myeloma is unknown, although it is being researched. Some authorities believe this disease to be related to chronic allergies and hypersensitivity reactions. This line of thought stems from the fact that plasma cells are the first line of defense and are the producers of the immunoglobulins that help fight foreign bodies. For some reason, these defenders get out of control and begin to attack the host as well as foreign invaders. People who work in rubber, leather, farming, and petroleum industries are more likely to develop multiple myeloma. Radiation and chemical exposure may also be factors.

Box 28.9 NURSING CARE PLAN for the Patient with Leukemia

Nursing Diagnosis: Risk for injury from infection or bleeding related to pancytopenia

Expected Outcomes The patient is free from infection and bleeding. Signs and symptoms of infection or bleeding are reported promptly.

Evaluation of Outcomes Is the patient free from infection and bleeding, or are problems reported so that quick intervention can prevent further complications?

Interventions	Rationale	Evaluation
Monitor vital signs every 4 hours and as needed.	Elevated temperature is a sign of infection. Falling blood pressure and elevated pulse rate may indicate sepsis or blood loss.	Are vital signs stable?
Monitor for swelling, redness, purulent drainage.	These are signs of infection and should be reported promptly.	Are signs of infection present?
Protect patient from sources of infection (see Box 28.6 Interventions for the Patient at Risk for Infection).	Patient is at risk for infection because of ineffective WBCs.	Are precautions being observed to prevent infection?
Observe for tarry stools, petechiae, ecchymosis (see Box 28.7 Patient Teaching: Signs and Symptoms of Bleeding).	These are signs of bleeding and should be reported promptly.	Are signs of bleeding present?
Protect patient from injury that could cause bleeding (see Box 28.5 Interventions to Prevent Bleeding in the Patient with Thrombocytopenia).	Patient is at risk for bleeding because of reduced platelet count.	Are precautions being observed to prevent injury and bleeding?

Nursing Diagnosis: Fatigue related to decreased red cell count and oxygenation and effects of treatments

Expected Outcomes Patient is able to participate in activities that are important to him or her.

Evaluation of Outcomes Is patient able to identify and participate in activities that are important to him or her?

Interventions	Rationale	Evaluation
Assess fatigue using the WHAT'S UP? format.	A good assessment establishes a baseline and aids in planning.	Is fatigue present? To what degree?
Assist patient to identify activities that are important to him or her (e.g., activities of daily living [ADLs], attending a child's wedding, taking a trip). Assist in setting goals to work toward the desired activity.	If the patient cannot do everything he or she wishes, it may help to focus on the most important things.	Can patient identify important activities? What are they? How can the nurse assist the patient to reach activity goals?
Encourage a balanced diet. Contact dietitian as needed.	Poor nutrition contributes to fatigue.	Is patient eating a balanced diet? Is weight stable?
Allow periods of rest between activities.	Any activity (ADL, x-rays, even talking) can increase fatigue.	Is patient able to rest?
Ensure adequate sleep. Obtain order for sleeping aid if indicated.	Lack of sleep worsens fatigue.	Does patient state feeling rested on awakening? Is medication needed?
Provide for ADLs when patient is unable to do so independently.	Extreme fatigue may prevent the patient from participating in self-care.	Does patient need total assistance?

(Continued on following page)

Box 28.9   NURSING CARE PLAN for the Patient with Leukemia *(Cont'd)*

Nursing Diagnosis: Impaired oral mucous membranes related to chemotherapy and pancytopenia

Expected Outcomes The patient's oral mucous membranes will remain intact.

Evaluation of Outcomes Are oral mucous membranes intact, without lesions?

Interventions	Rationale	Evaluation
Assess mouth daily for redness, edema, and lesions.	Routine assessment helps identify problems early so treatment can be implemented.	Are mucous membranes intact?
Encourage adequate nutrition and fluids.	Poor nutrition and dehydration increase the risk of oral lesions.	Is patient eating and drinking?
Encourage patient to brush teeth after meals with a soft toothbrush. If irritation is severe or if the patient is at risk for bleeding, use swabs or sponge Toothettes instead of a toothbrush.	Brushing the teeth controls tooth and gum disease; a toothbrush may be too harsh if the patient is at risk for bleeding.	Is mouth care being provided after meals? Is mouth care irritating? Are alternative methods needed?
Avoid use of lemon-glycerin swabs for mouth care.	Lemon-glycerin swabs are drying to oral mucosa.	Are products used appropriate?
Obtain an order for a mouthwash containing diphenhydramine (Benadryl). Obtain an order for a topical anesthetic if mouth is very inflamed and painful.	Diphenhydramine reduces inflammation; anesthetics reduce pain.	Does mouthwash soothe pain?
Encourage the patient to avoid smoking, alcohol, acidic food or drinks, extremely hot or cold foods and drinks, and commercial mouthwash.	These things can be irritating to the mucosa.	Does patient state understanding of things to avoid?
Geriatric		
Advise patient to remove dentures for cleaning and at bedtime.	Dentures left in for long periods can impair circulation and increase risk of lesions.	Are oral mucous membranes intact?

Signs and Symptoms

Skeletal pain is the most common complaint. The patient may describe the pain as constant severe back pain that increases with exercise or movement. The patient may complain about pain in the ribs. Other signs and symptoms include achiness of the long bones, joint swelling and tenderness, low-grade fever, and general malaise. Sometimes there is evidence of early peripheral neuropathy secondary to vertebral collapse and mild spinal cord compression. The patient may be unable to feel the true temperature of bath water and be burned or may be unable to feel wounds and infections on the feet. In more severe cases of cord compression, the patient may lose control of bladder and bowels. This is a true oncological emergency. Prompt emergency treatment is necessary to keep the patient from becoming paralyzed.

Occasionally, the patient will have pathological fractures of the long bones. These are fractures that occur with no trauma, such as the person who breaks a leg just turning over in bed or breaks a rib while sneezing. In advanced disease there is anemia, weight loss, thoracic spinal deformities from multiple rib destruction, and a loss of height because of pathological fractures and compacting of the vertebrae.

Because calcium is mobilized from the bones and into the blood, the patient is at risk for hypercalcemia. Signs and symptoms of hypercalcemia include anorexia, nausea, vomiting, mental changes (especially confusion), seizures, and weakness and fatigue. Kidney stones may result as the excess calcium passes through the kidneys.

Patients are susceptible to infection because of compromised immune function. Pneumonia is a common finding in patients with multiple myeloma. They may develop

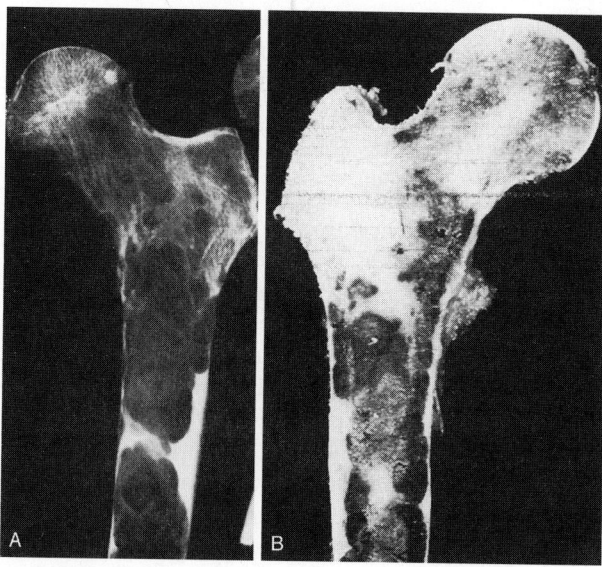

FIGURE 28.6 X-ray of bone destruction in multiple myeloma. *(From Huether, SE, and McCance, KL: Understanding Pathophysiology. Mosby, St Louis, 1996, p 548, with permission.)*

anemia because of bone marrow dysfunction and reduced erythropoietin formation by diseased kidneys.

Patients often develop kidney failure as the filtering capacity of the kidney is blocked with calcium. Other factors include recurrent infections and deposits of myeloma cells in the kidneys.

Diagnostic Tests

A CBC shows moderate to severe anemia. Examination of the WBC count may show an increase in the number of white cells secondary to infection. X-ray examinations may show changes in the lungs and diffuse osteoporosis in the bones not already riddled with holes. Urine studies are positive for M-type globulins (Bence-Jones proteins) in 40 percent of patients. Bone marrow biopsy is done to confirm the diagnosis and determine the disease's stage.

Blood chemistries often show an increased amount of calcium in the blood. Hypercalciuria results as the calcium released out of the bones is flushed out in the urine. An intravenous pyelogram may be done to see how much calcium is collecting in the kidneys. A 24-hour urine collection is done to evaluate protein excretion.

Therapeutic Interventions

Long-term treatment of multiple myeloma consists of a two-pronged approach: (1) managing the disease and (2) managing the symptoms. To manage the disease, high-dose steroids (prednisone) and oral or intravenous chemotherapy agents are given. Another drug that is showing encouraging results for slowing progression of the disease is thalidomide. The goal of drug therapy is to suppress the plasma cell proliferation, which then helps decrease the amount and speed of bone destruction.

The second approach is control of symptoms. The nurse monitors the patient for signs and symptoms of hypercalcemia, hyperuricemia, dehydration, respiratory infection, renal problems, and pain. The physician may order the administration of intravenous bisphosphonate agents such as pamidronate (Aredia). This class of drugs inhibits bone resorption and is used to help keep serum calcium levels controlled. Oral compounds are also available to help keep the calcium within normal limits. The goal is to get the serum calcium level below 10 mg/dL. If hypercalcemia occurs, the physician will order an IV of normal saline to infuse at a high rate followed by regular administration of diuretics.

External beam irradiation may be given to especially painful areas of bone involvement. Fortunately, this treatment is quite effective, usually decreasing pain intensity in just a few days. The patient can expect to have a daily (or perhaps a twice-daily) therapy treatment over a course of 10 to 14 days that is delivered directly to the painful bony areas. Vigorous attention to administering pain medications during the early course of treatment greatly reduces the patient's pain levels.

The patient may need a laminectomy if vertebral collapse occurs. Because of demineralization of the bone, with resulting large amounts of calcium in the blood and urine, surgery for kidney stones and eventual dialysis for acute or chronic kidney failure may be necessary.

A newer treatment involves high-dose chemotherapy combined with stem cell transplantation. The patient's own peripheral stem cells can be removed and reinfused. These stem cells can then differentiate into new, healthy cells. Methods of cleaning the cells to prevent contamination with malignant cells are being researched.

Nursing Process: Multiple Myeloma

Assessment/Data Collection

Assess for fever or malaise that can signal the onset of infection. Other conditions to be alert for include anemia, hypercalcemia, fractures, and renal complications. Monitor intake and output, and strain urine for stones. Elevated BUN and creatinine levels will alert you to possible renal failure. Report back pain, leg weakness, sensory loss, or loss of bowel or bladder function because these can indicate spinal cord compression.

Nursing Diagnosis, Planning, and Implementation
Risk for infection related to compromised immune function

EXPECTED OUTCOME: *Patient will remain free from infection as evidenced by temperature within normal limits, lungs clear*

- See Box 24.6 Interventions for the Patient at Risk for Infection
- Encourage deep breathing, and keep patient active *to decrease the risk of respiratory complications.*

Risk for injury: fracture related to weakened bones; complications of immobility; complications due to hypercalcemia

EXPECTED OUTCOME: Patient will remain free from injury as evidenced by no fracture, and no complications related to immobility or hypercalcemia.

- Keep the patient mobile. Consult physical and occupational therapy as needed. *Bones in use are strongest, so the patient should remain up and moving as much as possible to help stimulate calcium resorption and decrease demineralization.*
- Assist the patient with walking *to reduce the risk of pathological fractures of the long bones.*
- If the patient is unsteady, use a walker or a support belt *to reduce the risk of falls.*
- If the patient is bedridden, reposition him or her every 2 hours *to prevent complications related to immobility.*
- Use a lift sheet to move the patient gently in bed *to decrease the risk of skin damage and pathological fractures.*
- Provide passive range-of-motion exercises *to maintain mobility if the patient is unable to be independently mobile.*
- Administer fluids so that daily output is never less than 1500 mL *to flush kidneys and reduce the risk of kidney stones.*
- Teach the patient the importance of good hydration at all times to *minimize complications of hypercalcemia.* Depending on time of year and the type and level of patient activities, the patient may need to have an intake of more than 4 L daily.

Evaluation

If nursing care has been effective, the patient will be free of infection or infection will be recognized and treated promptly. The patient will avoid injury, with no fracture, skin breakdown, or complications related to hypercalcemia. See Home Health Hints at the end of this chapter for additional suggestions for patients being cared for at home.

 LYMPHATIC DISORDERS

Lymphatic disorders include Hodgkin's disease and the non-Hodgkin's **lymphomas.** Because the spleen is part of the lymph system, this section also discusses **splenectomy.**

Hodgkin's Disease

Despite its name, Hodgkin's disease (HD) is a lymphoma, which is a cancer of the lymph system. Its distinguishing feature is the presence of Reed-Sternberg cells, which make it different from all the other forms of lymphoma. HD is more prevalent in men than in women and occurs most often in young adults ages 15 to 40. After a decrease in incidence in persons ages 40 to 55, the incidence peaks again in adults older than age 55. Of all the lymphomas, HD is the most curable type even when the disease is widely spread at the time of diagnosis.

Pathophysiology

Lymph nodes are made of tightly bound fibers and cells that serve as filtering devices for the body's immune system. Most often, HD begins as a single changed lymph node, usually in the cervical lymph nodes of the neck. As the disease progresses, the cancer invades the lymph node chains node by node. The path of cancer infiltration is usually the same as the path for lymph fluid flow. Left untreated, other lymphoid tissues such as the spleen become infiltrated with HD. The major organs eventually become involved with Hodgkin's disease. Common complaints of patients with organ involvement may include shortness of breath, feelings of fullness, weakness, and malaise. These organ-related symptoms usually motivate the patient to seek medical help.

A tentative diagnosis of HD is based on one or more painlessly enlarged nodes in the cervical, axillary, or inguinal areas. A biopsy of several of the enlarged nodes is performed to search for the presence of Reed-Sternberg cells, which confirms the diagnosis.

Etiology

The exact cause of HD is unknown. A possible viral origin has been proposed; it is more common in people who have had mononucleosis. Sometimes it occurs in families, suggesting a genetic link. Patients with impaired immune function, such as those with acquired immunodeficiency syndrome (AIDS) or those taking immunosuppressive drugs after organ transplant are also at higher risk.

Signs and Symptoms

Painless swelling in one or more of the common lymph node chains is a usual presentation (Fig. 28.7). Swelling can range from barely perceptible to the size of a softball, occasionally even larger. The patient may complain of generalized pruritus. One other curious event, alcohol-induced pain, is occasionally present. With just a few sips of any type of alcohol-containing beverage (beer, wine, or liquor), the patient may complain of intense pain at the site of disease. Because the lymph nodes in the upper chest and neck are often involved, the patient may have symptoms of obstruction, such as cough, dysphagia, or stridor.

Other common symptoms may include persistent low-grade fever, night sweats, fatigue, weight loss, and malaise. When these additional symptoms are present, the prognosis is worse. In older adults, there may be no enlarged lymph nodes visible, and these secondary symptoms may be the only presenting symptoms. Other symptoms associated with late-stage disease include edema of the neck and face, possible jaundice, nerve pain, enlargement of the retroperitoneal nodes, and infiltration of the spleen; liver and bones may also be involved.

Diagnostic Tests and Staging

Diagnosis usually begins with a lymph node biopsy of the easiest lymph node to access. Lymph node biopsies are done

---

lymphoma: lymph—fluid found in lymphatic vessels + oma—tumor

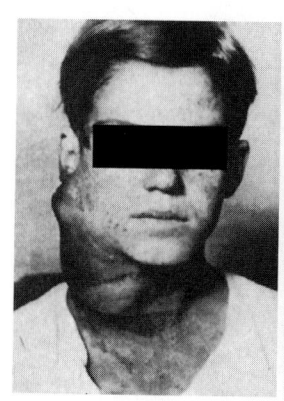 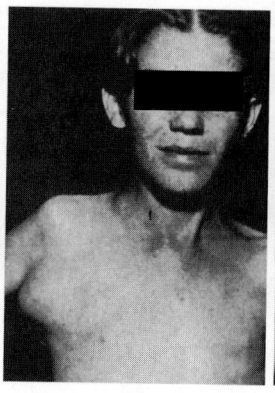 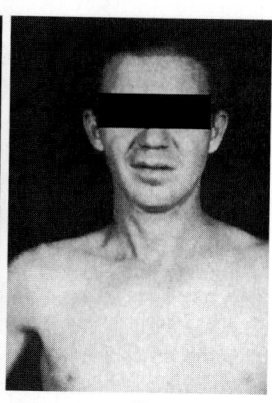

A   B   C

FIGURE 28.7 Cervical Hodgkin's disease. (A) Young boy with extensive cervical Hodgkin's disease. (B) Appearance several years later, when axillary manifestation developed. (C) Appearance 23 years after initial treatment with radiation. (From del Regato, JA, Spjut, HJ, and Cox, JD: Cancer: Diagnosis, Treatment, and Prognosis, ed 6. Mosby, St Louis, 1985, with permission.)

to check for abnormal histiocyte proliferation, nodular fibrosis, and necrosis. Other tests include bone marrow biopsy and aspiration, liver and spleen biopsies, routine chest x-ray examination, abdominal computed tomography (CT) scan to check for the presence of disease in the liver and spleen, lung scan, and bone scan. In some larger cancer centers, lymphangiography may be performed to view the flow of lymph in the lymph network. This test is accomplished by a skilled physician injecting dye into the lymph tracts located between the toes. The dye is observed as it migrates up the lymph chains, signaling blockages where present.

Hematological tests (e.g., complete blood cell count [CBC]) may show wide variability of red blood cells, indicating mild to severe anemia. The white blood cell (WBC) count is often abnormal and extreme (either very high or very low) because of bone marrow infiltration by disease.

These same tests are used for staging. HD is staged based on the Ann Arbor Clinical Staging Classification and is as follows:

- Stage I disease is limited to a single lymph node or site.
- Stage II disease occurs when two or more nodes are involved on the same side of the diaphragm. Limited organ involvement may or may not be present.
- Stage III disease is characterized by nodes on both sides of the diaphragm with or without organ involvement.
- Stage IV, the most serious form of the disease and the least curable, includes widely disseminated disease in several organs or tissues with or without associated lymph node involvement.

Therapeutic Interventions

Appropriate therapy includes the use of radiation and chemotherapy and depends on the stage of the disease. Radiation therapy, administered on an outpatient basis over a 4- to 6-week period, can cure most patients with stage I or stage II disease. Combinations of chemotherapy and radiation therapy are used for patients with stage III and stage IV disease. Results vary depending on the location and the stage of disease.

Nursing Care

Most nursing interventions are aimed at symptom management. If the patient is experiencing pruritus or night sweats,

nursing interventions are aimed at alleviation of discomfort. These may include changing the gown and bed linens several times a night and helping the patient remain clean and dry. Keeping the patient and family involved in the plan of care may relieve anxiety.

Later, nursing interventions are tailored to alleviate problems that arise secondary to chemotherapy and radiation therapy. See Chapter 10 for nursing interventions for these problems. Also see Box 28.9 Nursing Care Plan for the Patient with Leukemia.

Patient Teaching

In addition to the teaching needs outlined above, make sure that the patient and the family know about local chapters of the American Cancer Society and the Leukemia and Lymphoma Society. Both of these organizations have information, financial assistance, and counseling referral sources, which most patients find valuable. Another source for chemotherapy and radiation therapy information is the National Cancer Institute (NCI). The NCI can send as much information as the patient requests regarding all aspects of treatment at no charge. For more information about Hodgkin's lymphoma, visit www.cancer.org. Or visit the Leukemia and Lymphoma Society at www.leukemia.org or the National Cancer Institute at www.nci.nih.gov.

CRITICAL THINKING

Jeanine

■ Jeanine is a 60-year-od nurse diagnosed with stage II Hodgkin's disease. She wishes to continue working at her job on a respiratory unit at the local hospital while she undergoes treatment. What concerns do you have about this?

Suggested answers at end of chapter.

Non-Hodgkin's Lymphomas

All of the other types of lymphomas are clumped into a diverse classification known as the non-Hodgkin's lymphomas (NHLs). It is possible to sort these other types of

TABLE 28.4 HODGKIN'S DISEASE VERSUS NON-HODGKIN'S LYMPHOMA

	Hodgkin's Disease	Non-Hodgkin's Lymphomas
Age	Younger	Older
Degree of debilitation (overall)	Less	More
Presence of fever, night sweats (indicating more advanced disease)	More likely	Less likely
Spread to other areas at time of diagnosis	Local to regional area of spread	Advanced cancer—may have spread to many different areas
Types	Just one	Many different types

lymphomas into different categories based on the degree of malignancy. Non-Hodgkin's lymphomas arise in the lymphoid tissues of the body, just as Hodgkin's disease does, but they differ in several ways (Table 28.4).

Pathophysiology

The most distinguishing difference is the absence of the Reed-Sternberg cells in non-Hodgkin's lymphomas. Instead, many of these lymphomas arise from the B cells and T cells. The B cells are involved in recognizing and destroying specific antigens. Cells specifically involved include the memory B cells and the plasma cells. The T cells also are involved in registering antigens, but there are many more kinds of T cells. These include the amplifier T cells, helper T cells, suppressor T cells, memory T cells, cytotoxic T cells, and delayed hypersensitivity T cells. An abnormality in any of these cells can result in a type of NHL. Most cases of NHL are of B-cell origin.

Etiology

The cause of non-Hodgkin's lymphomas is unclear, but some viruses, such as the Epstein-Barr virus and herpesvirus, are thought to play a role in their development. Genetics also plays a role. Immune problems such as AIDS increase risk. Exposure to nuclear waste and some toxic chemicals may also increase risk.

Signs and Symptoms

Clinical features of malignant lymphomas include enlarged, painless, rubbery nodes in the cervical and supraclavicular areas, enlarged tonsils and adenoids, and occasional symptoms of dyspnea and cough. As the disease progresses, the patient may report fatigue, malaise, weight loss, and night sweats similar to Hodgkin's disease. NHL usually progresses more rapidly than HD.

Diagnostic Tests

Diagnosis is confirmed by histological evaluation of biopsied lymph nodes, tonsils, bone marrow, liver, bowel, skin, or other affected tissues. Other relevant tests include bone

Box 28.10

Lymphoma Summary

Signs and Symptoms	Swollen lymph nodes
	Fatigue
	Low-grade fever
	Night sweats
Diagnostic tests	CBC
	Lymph node biopsy
	Lymphangiography
	CT Scan
Therapeutic Interventions	Chemotherapy
	Radiation
	Bone marrow or stem cell transplant
Priority Nursing Diagnoses	Activity Intolerance
	Risk for Infection
	Risk for Ineffective Coping

scans, chest x-ray examination, lymphangiography, liver and spleen scans, CT of the abdomen, and intravenous pyelogram to determine the extent of the disease. Laboratory tests include a CBC, which often indicates anemia, serum uric acid level, and liver function studies. Serum calcium level may be elevated if bone lesions are present.

Therapeutic Interventions

Treatment usually involves multimodal therapy, including the use of chemotherapy and radiation therapy given in combination. Chemotherapy treatments are given on a set schedule of approximately once every month for about 6 months. These treatments may be performed on an inpatient or an outpatient basis. Radiation therapy is given to affected areas in advanced stages of NHL. Stem cell transplant may be tried in patients with advanced disease.

Nursing Care

You can provide emotional support by keeping the patient and family informed during the testing phase. Symptoms such as night sweats can be managed with frequent linen and gown changes. Help the patient maintain nutrition with attractively prepared meals. Spend time listening to the patient's concerns; involve the hospital chaplain in the patient's care if the patient desires. Refer the patient and family to the resources listed earlier for more information. See Box 28.10 Lymphoma Summary and Box 28.11 Nursing Care Plan for the Patient with Lymphoma for more information.

 SPLENIC DISORDERS

The spleen is involved in a number of disorders, including cancers of the blood, lymph, and bone marrow; hereditary conditions such as sickle cell disease; and acquired problems such as idiopathic thrombocytopenia. Under normal

Box 28.11 NURSING CARE PLAN for the Patient with Lymphoma

Nursing Diagnosis: Activity intolerance related to fatigue and anemia

Expected Outcomes Patient will have activities of daily living (ADLs) needs met by self or caregiver.

Evaluation of Outcomes Is patient able to carry out ADLs or are ADL needs met by a caregiver?

Interventions	Rationale	Evaluation
Assess amount of activity that causes fatigue.	Assessment helps guide plan of care.	How much can patient do before becoming fatigued?
Assist patient with activities as necessary.	The patient may need assistance with ADLs if fatigue is extreme.	Does the patient need assistance? Can family members assist?
Provide oxygen therapy as ordered.	Oxygen therapy can increase oxygen levels and activity tolerance.	Does patient tolerate activity better with oxygen therapy?
Instruct patient to space rest with activities.	Rest periods decrease oxygen needs and allow patient to conserve energy for next activity.	Is patient able to tolerate activity better after a rest period?

Nursing Diagnosis: Risk for infection related to bone marrow involvement and side effects of treatment

Expected Outcomes Patient will have no signs or symptoms of infection.

Evaluation of Outcomes Are signs and symptoms of infection absent? Is temperature within normal limits?

Interventions	Rationale	Evaluation
Assess patient for risk factors for infection.	The WBC count may be very high or very low, placing the patient at risk for infection.	Is the patient at risk? Are additional interventions indicated?
Monitor patient for signs and symptoms of infection, such as cough, fever, malaise, erythema, pain, or drainage and report immediately.	Early detection and treatment of infection provides the best results.	Are signs and symptoms of infection present?
Teach patient and significant other signs and symptoms of infection to watch for and report.	The patient must be involved in monitoring for infection when at home.	Does patient verbalize understanding of signs and symptoms of infection and importance of reporting?
Teach the patient to avoid exposure to others with influenza or other infections.	Exposure increases risk for infection, especially with compromised immune function.	Does patient verbalize understanding of sources of infection to avoid?
Teach patient proper hand washing and good oral and personal hygiene.	These activities reduce risk of infection.	Does patient demonstrate proper hand washing and hygiene?

Nursing Diagnosis: Risk for ineffective coping related to new diagnosis and potential lifestyle changes to accommodate treatments

Expected Outcomes The patient states ability to manage lifestyle changes and medical management of condition.

Evaluation of Outcomes Does patient carry out self-care necessary to manage treatment?

Interventions	Rationale	Evaluation
Assess patient's level of distress related to uncertainty of the future, bothersome symptoms, changes in self-concept, and past coping mechanisms.	Obtaining information regarding past experiences helps the nurse identify and correct misconceptions. The nurse can support effective coping mechanisms that worked in the past.	Is patient able to identify sources of anxiety?

(Continued on following page)

Box 28.11 NURSING CARE PLAN for the Patient with Lymphoma (Cont'd)

Interventions	Rationale	Evaluation
		Are past coping mechanisms effective?
Assess for signs of maladaptive behaviors that interfere with responsible health practices, such as missed appointments or failure to attend to symptoms.	Long-term survival depends on keeping therapy schedule. The ability to manage and report symptoms early keeps the patient out of the hospital and in control of his or her own life.	Does the patient keep appointments? Does the patient participate in self-care activities and report symptoms promptly?
Assist the patient to identify support systems and resources. Refer to social worker or other community resources as needed.	Resources can assist with participation in treatment plan, home care, or financial assistance.	Are resources identified and helpful?
Refer patient and family to a cancer survivors' support group.	Others who have been through treatment themselves can be a good support for patients with cancer.	Does the patient state that the support group is helpful?

circumstances, the spleen is not paid much attention; it generally performs its functions without much fanfare.

If the spleen enlarges markedly, the condition is referred to as **splenomegaly.** Other times, the spleen may or may not be enlarged, but the function is out of control so that too many red blood cells and platelets are removed from the peripheral circulation. Sometimes the spleen is not able to perform its job because of bleeding into the pulp of the organ, which renders it useless. Bleeding into the spleen can occur from various illnesses or from trauma. Regardless of the nature of the malfunction, one treatment option may be splenectomy.

Splenectomy

Splenectomy is the surgical removal of the spleen. This is sometimes used to treat selective hematological disorders and is also used, under different circumstances, to stage (or determine spread in) lymphomas. Splenectomy is performed fairly often in the United States, but, like any surgery, it is not without risk.

Patient Teaching

Explain to patients that this surgery removes the spleen, usually under general anesthesia. Inform patients that they can live a normal life after the surgery but that they may be more prone to infection, and that they should receive the influenza vaccine each year, preferably in the early fall.

Preoperative Care

Before the surgery, ensure that the CBC and coagulation profile are completed and reported to the physician. Blood transfusion may be ordered to correct the underlying anemia and to prepare for the loss of a great deal of blood stored in the spleen. Vitamin K is often ordered to correct clotting factor deficiencies.

Take the patient's vital signs and perform a baseline respiratory assessment. Note especially any signs of respiratory infections such as fever, chills, crackles, wheezes, or cough. If any of these are noted, make sure that the physician is aware of them because surgery may need to be delayed. Teach the patient routine coughing and deep breathing techniques to help prevent postoperative respiratory complications.

Postoperative Care

During the early postoperative period, watch carefully for bleeding, either external or internal. Be prepared to administer narcotics for pain, usually on an around-the-clock schedule so the patient is comfortable enough to deep breathe, cough, and ambulate. After narcotic administration, be sure to observe for side effects, which may include incomplete pain relief or hypoventilation. Monitor for fever every 4 hours, and expect a mild, low-grade, transient fever postoperatively. A persistent fever may indicate abscess or hematoma formation.

If the surgery was performed to decrease the numbers of cells being removed from the peripheral circulation, monitor the platelet count. Often the count begins to rise in just a few days, but it may take up to 2 weeks for the platelets to normalize.

Complications

A splenectomy can cause complications such as bleeding, pneumonia, and atelectasis. Respiratory problems occur because of the spleen's position close to the diaphragm. This placement requires the need for a high surgical incision that is very painful. Often the patient tries to restrict lung expansion after surgery to keep from hurting, but this splinting behavior may leave the patient at risk for pneumonia and respiratory problems. In addition, splenectomy patients are usually more vulnerable to infection, especially influenza, because the spleen's role in the immune response is no longer filled.

Other possible complications from splenectomy include

the development of pancreatitis and fistula formation. This is due to the fact that the tail of the pancreas is very close to the spleen, and irritation may have occurred.

Another serious complication is that of overwhelming postsplenectomy infection (OPSI). The causative agents in OPSI include streptococci, *Neisseria* spp., and influenza bacteria (as opposed to a flu virus). Patients at greatest risk of OPSI may include patients who had a splenectomy secondary to a cancer condition or during childhood.

Early symptoms of OPSI include fever and malaise that seem unremarkable. However, the infection may progress within a few hours to sepsis and death. Unfortunately, OPSI has a mortality rate as high as 70 percent. Be sure to include the signs and symptoms of OPSI in presplenectomy patient education. Also, stress the need to promptly obtain medical attention for the patient at the first signs and symptoms of OPSI. The patient should be directed to continue to receive lifetime vaccinations against these bacteria.

Home Health Hints

- Patients who are at risk for infection can place a sign on the front door of their homes to limit visitors or ask persons with colds to come back when they are well. The patient may appreciate the home nurse giving permission to be assertive in such circumstances.
- To prevent bruising, have the patient cut the feet off of white sport socks and wear them on the arms. They can be hidden under long-sleeve shirts and blouses and provide a cushion when doing housework.
- Patients with sickle cell anemia usually have lower blood pressures. It is important to report even mild hypertension in these patients.

REVIEW QUESTIONS

1. Which assessment finding would you expect to find in the patient who has anemia?
   a. Pain
   b. Dyspnea
   c. Vision changes
   d. Skin rash

2. Which of the following activities is contraindicated for the patient with sickle cell anemia?
   a. Riding in an elevator
   b. Taking a long car trip
   c. Running in a marathon
   d. Listening to a concert

3. Which explanation for bleeding should you give to the family member of a patient with DIC?
   a. "He is bleeding because he does not have enough RBCs."
   b. "He is bleeding because his white cells are depleted."
   c. "He is bleeding because his blood pressure is so high that it forces blood from mucous membranes."
   d. "He is bleeding because his body's clotting factors have all been used up."

4. Which instruction will help the mother of a child with hemophilia prevent bleeding episodes?
   a. "Your son should avoid contact sports."
   b. "Your son will have to avoid all potentially irritating foods."
   c. "Your son must never shave."
   d. "Your son should always live near a major hospital system."

5. Which family member should not be permitted to visit a patient with newly diagnosed leukemia?

   a. The one who has a new baby at home.
   b. The one who has a history of asthma.
   c. The one who has received recent radiation treatment for cancer.
   d. The one who has a runny nose.

6. Which assessment finding is most frequently encountered in patients with multiple myeloma?
   a. Pathological fractures
   b. Mental status changes
   c. Raging infections
   d. Bleeding tendencies

7. Which of the following nursing interventions are appropriate for a patient with thrombocytopenia? Choose all correct answers.
   a. Avoid intramuscular injections.
   b. Keep visitors who are ill away from the patient.
   c. Encourage 4 L of fluid daily.
   d. Avoid use of aspirin and NSAIDs.
   e. Allow rest between activities.
   f. Encourage use of shoes or slippers.

8. A patient with hypercalcemia needs to drink at least 3 L of fluid per day. Today, he has had 1 measuring cup of coffee, 1 L of water, a can of soda that says it has 355 mL, and a half cup of juice. How many mililiters has he had so far today?
   _____ mL

9. Stage III Hodgkin's disease is defined as which of the following?
   a. Lymphatic involvement on both sides of the diaphragm

b. Localized involvement of more than two adjacent or nonadjacent regions on one side of the diaphragm

c. Diffuse involvement of one or more extralymphatic organs or tissues such as the bone marrow or liver

d. Localized involvement of a single lymph node site, usually located in the cervical or supraclavicular area

10. Which circumstance places the patient at most risk for respiratory complications following a splenectomy?

a. Disturbance of clotting factors
b. Nothing by mouth (NPO) status
c. Need for frequent dressing changes
d. Location of surgical incision

Unit Six Bibliography

1. Atassi, KA, and Harris, ML: Actionstat: Disseminated intravascular coagulation. Nursing 2001 31:64, 2001.
2. Barrick, MC, and Mitchell, SA: Multiple myeloma: Recent advances for this common plasma cell disorder. Am J Nurs Apr, Suppl:6–12, 2001.
3. Cavanaugh, BM: Nurse's manual of Laboratory and Diagnostic Tests, ed 4. F.A. Davis, Philadelphia, 2003.
4. Cole, S, and Dunne, K: Hodgkin's lymphoma. Nurs Stand 18:46, 2004.
5. Curry, H: Bleeding disorder basics. Pediatr Nurs 30:402–407, 2004.
6. D'Antonio, J: You can lessen leukemia's toll. Nursing 34:32, 2004.
7. Dharmarajan, TS, Pais, W, and Norkus, EP: Does anemia matter? Anemia, morbidity, and mortality in older adults: Need for greater recognition. Geriatrics 60:22–28, 2005.
8. Gutaj, DA: Oncology today: Lymphoma. RN 63:32–38, 2000.
9. Holcomb, SS: Anemia: Pointing the way to a deeper problem. Nursing 2001 31:36–43, 2001.
10. Lehne, RA: Pharmacology for Nursing Care, ed 5. Saunders, St. Louis, 2004.
11. Lutz, CA, and Przytulski, KR: Nutrition and Diet Therapy, ed 4, F.A. Davis, Philadelphia, 2006.
12. Maxson, JH: Management of disseminated intravascular coagulation. Crit Care Nurs Clin North Am 12:341–352, 2000.
13. Medoff, E: Oncology today: New horizons. Leukemia. RN 63:42–50, 2000.
14. Murphy-Ende K, and Chernecky, C: Assessing adults with leukemia. Nurse Practit 27:49–56, 2002.
15. Sulton, LL: What's wrong with this patient? Idiopathic thrombocytopenic purpura. RN 61:35–39, 1998.
16. Held-Warmkessel, J: Test your knowledge: Assessment of febrile neutropenic patients. Clin J Oncol Nurs 4:182 and 184, 2000.

SUGGESTED ANSWERS TO

CRITICAL THINKING

■ *Mrs. Johns*

1. Monitor Mrs. Johns's vital signs and report falling blood pressure and rising pulse immediately. Inspect her skin for petechiae and ecchymoses. Outline ecchymotic areas with an ink pen in order to see if the area is increasing in size. Monitor urine for signs of blood. Test stools for occult blood. Monitor vaginal discharge for increasing bleeding. Report any changes promptly.

2. Anticipate assisting the RN with administration of blood or blood products. Instruct Mrs. Johns in the importance of preventing injury that could cause further bleeding. Other care will be supportive.

3. Mrs. Johns will be concerned for her new baby, who is most likely on another unit or already discharged home. Allow Mrs. Johns to talk about her concerns. Arrange visits with her family and baby if permitted by her condition and her physician.

4.

$$\frac{300 \text{ mL}}{30 \text{ min}} \, \Big| \, \frac{60 \text{ min}}{1 \text{ hour}} = 600 \text{ mL per hour}$$

■ *Mr. Washington*

1. Because of his leukemia and his treatment, Mr. Washington is at risk for infection. If he develops an infection, he will have great difficulty getting over it. With so many visitors in the room, it is likely that one or more has a cold or virus. They may not be aware of the risk this poses to Mr. Washington. Mr. Washington is probably also fatigued because of his disease and treatment, and visiting requires energy.

2. You should kindly explain that while family visits are very important, Mr. Washington is very susceptible to catching colds or other illnesses and that it would be best to limit visitors to one or two at a time. Point out that persons with symptoms of colds or flu should not enter the room at all. Visits should also be brief to prevent overtiring the patient.

■ *Jeanine*

Jeanine will probably be fatigued from her disease, and fatigue may increase further from side effects of treatment. Staff nursing jobs can be tiring even for healthy nurses. In addition, she will be around patients with respiratory diseases, many of whom are contagious. Because of risk for infection secondary to the disease process and the treatment regimen, Jeanine might want to take a leave of absence during treatment or ask to be reassigned to a different area that is less demanding and away from direct patient care until her treatments have been completed.

unit SEVEN

UNDERSTANDING THE RESPIRATORY SYSTEM

29

Respiratory System Function, Assessment, and Therapeutic Measures

PAULA D. HOPPER

QUESTIONS TO GUIDE YOUR READING

1. What are the structures of the respiratory system, and what is the function of each?

2. How does aging affect the respiratory system?

3. What questions should you ask when you take a history from a patient with a respiratory problem?

4. What findings do you expect when you inspect, palpate, percuss, and auscultate the chest?

5. What are the common diagnostic tests performed to diagnose disorders of the respiratory system?

6. What nursing care should you provide for patients undergoing each of these diagnostic tests?

7. What are common therapeutic measures used for patients with respiratory disorders?

NORMAL ANATOMY AND PHYSIOLOGY

The respiratory system consists of the nose, nasal cavities, pharynx, larynx, trachea, bronchial tree, lungs, and respiratory muscles. The parts superior to the chest cavity are collectively called the upper respiratory system, and those within the chest cavity make up the lower respiratory system (Fig. 29.1). The alveoli of the lungs are the site of gas exchange between the air and the blood; the rest of the system moves air into and out of the lungs.

Nose and Nasal Cavities

The nose is made predominantly of bone and cartilage covered with muscle and epithelium. Hairs inside the nostrils block the entry of dust and other particles. The two nasal cavities are inside the skull and are separated by the nasal septum, which is made of the vomer, ethmoid, and septal cartilage. The nasal mucosa is ciliated epithelium that is highly vascular; it warms and moistens inhaled air. Dust and microorganisms become trapped on mucus produced by goblet cells and are swept backward and down into the pharynx by the cilia. See Table 29.1 for a summary of protective mechanisms in the respiratory system.

The paranasal sinuses are air cavities in the maxillae and the frontal, sphenoid, and ethmoid bones that open into the nasal cavities. They too are lined with ciliated epithe-lium. The mucus produced usually drains into the nasal cavities. The sinuses lessen the weight of the skull and provide resonance for the voice.

Pharynx

The pharynx is posterior to the nasal and oral cavities. It has three parts: nasopharynx, oropharynx, and laryngopharynx. The nasopharynx is an air passage above the level of the soft palate. The soft palate and uvula rise to block the nasopharynx during swallowing. The eustachian tubes from the middle ear cavities open into the nasopharynx; the adenoid (pharyngeal tonsil) is a lymph nodule on its posterior wall. The oropharynx is posterior to the oral cavity and is both an air and a food passage. The palatine tonsils are on the lateral

TABLE 29.1 PROTECTIVE MECHANISMS IN THE RESPIRATORY SYSTEM

Nasal hairs and turbinates	Trap dust and microorganisms
Mucous membranes	Warm and moisten inhaled air; trap inhaled particles
Cilia	Move particles toward pharynx to be swallowed or coughed out
Irritant receptors in nose and airways	Trigger sneeze and cough to remove foreign debris
Alveolar macrophages	Phagocytize foreign particles and bacteria

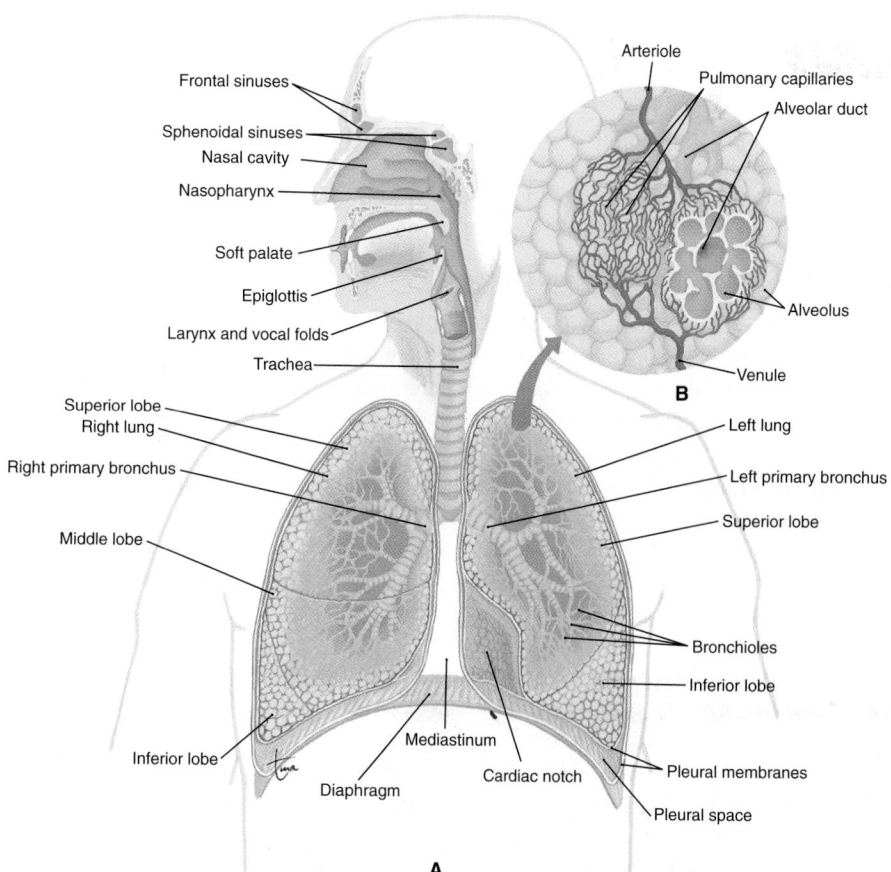

FIGURE 29.1 Respiratory system, anterior view, with microscopic view of alveoli and pulmonary capillaries. *(Modified from Scanlon, VC, Sanders, T: Essentials of Anatomy and Physiology, ed 5. F.A. Davis, Philadelphia, 2007.)*

walls. Together with the lingual tonsils on the base of the tongue and the adenoid, the palatine tonsils form a ring of lymphatic tissue around the pharynx and destroy pathogens that penetrate the mucosa. The laryngopharynx is both an air and a food passage; it opens anteriorly into the larynx and posteriorly into the esophagus.

Larynx

The larynx is the voice box and the airway between the pharynx and trachea. It is made of nine pieces of cartilage, yielding a firm yet flexible tissue that keeps the airway open. It is lined with ciliated epithelium. The thyroid cartilage, commonly called the Adam's apple, is the largest of these cartilage pieces and is palpable on the front of the neck. The epiglottis is the uppermost cartilage and covers the larynx like a flap when the larynx is elevated during swallowing. The vocal cords are on either side of the rima glottidis (the airway opening). When pulled together across the rima glottidis and vibrated by exhaled air, the vocal cords produce sounds that may be turned into speech. The vagus and accessory cranial nerves are the motor nerves to the larynx.

Trachea and Bronchial Tree

The trachea is a tube, 4 to 5 inches in length, that extends from the larynx to the primary bronchi. **C**-shaped pieces of cartilage in the wall keep the trachea open. The mucosa is ciliated epithelium; mucus with trapped dust and microorganisms is swept upward toward the pharynx and is usually swallowed.

The bronchial tree is the series of air passages within the lungs, a succession of progressively smaller tubes that terminate in the alveoli. The right and left primary bronchi are branches of the trachea. Each gives rise to secondary bronchi: their structure is like that of the trachea. The bronchioles, however, have no cartilage in the walls to maintain patency, and they may be closed completely by contraction of their smooth muscle.

Lungs and Pleural Membranes

The lungs occupy the chest cavity on either side of the heart, extending from the clavicles to the diaphragm. On the medial (mediastinal) surface of each lung is an indentation called the hilus, where the primary bronchus and the pulmonary artery and veins enter the lung.

The pleural membranes are the serous membranes of the thoracic cavity. The visceral pleura is the membrane that covers the lungs; the parietal pleura lines the chest cavity. A small amount of serous fluid between these membranes prevents friction and keeps the membranes adhered together during breathing.

The functional units of the lung are the millions of alveoli, the air sacs that are the site of gas exchange. Both the alveoli and the surrounding alveolar capillaries are made of simple squamous epithelium; that is, their walls are only one cell in thickness to permit diffusion of gases (see Fig. 29.1).

Each alveolus is lined with a thin layer of tissue fluid that is essential for the diffusion of gases, but the surface tension of the fluid tends to make the walls of an alveolus stick together internally. Certain alveolar cells secrete pulmonary surfactant, a lipoprotein that mixes with the tissue fluid and decreases surface tension to permit inflation. Also in the alveoli are the alveolar macrophages, which phagocytize pathogens or fine dust particles and debris that have not been trapped and swept out by the cilia.

Between clusters of alveoli is elastic connective tissue; it is capable of recoil when stretched (during inhalation) and contributes significantly to normal exhalation. The recoil of this tissue ensures that normal exhalation during quiet breathing is a passive process that does not require the expenditure of energy.

Mechanism of Breathing

Ventilation is the term for the movement of air into and out of the alveoli. Air moves from high-pressure to low-pressure areas, some of which are created by the respiratory muscles that are controlled by the nervous system. The respiratory centers are in the medulla oblongata and pons. The main respiratory muscles are the diaphragm inferior to the lungs and the external and internal intercostal muscles between the ribs. Accessory muscles of respiration are used during exercise and times of respiratory distress; these include the sternocleidomastoid, scalene muscles, and abdominal musculature.

Pressures important to breathing include atmospheric pressure, intrapleural pressure, and intrapulmonic (alveolar) pressure. Atmospheric pressure is the pressure of the air around us, which at sea level is 760 mm Hg; atmospheric pressure decreases as altitude increases. Intrapleural pressure is in the potential pleural space between the pleural membranes. Serous fluid causes the two membranes to adhere to each other, and because the elastic lungs are always tending to collapse and pull the visceral pleura away from the parietal pleura, the pressure in this potential space is always below atmospheric pressure (about 756 mm Hg). This is called a negative pressure. Intrapulmonic (alveolar) pressure is the pressure inside the alveoli and bronchial tree. This pressure fluctuates below and above atmospheric pressure during each cycle of breathing.

Inhalation

Inhalation, also called inspiration, occurs when motor impulses from the medulla cause contraction of the respiratory muscles. Impulses along the phrenic nerves cause the dome-shaped diaphragm to contract and flatten downward. Impulses along the intercostal nerves cause the external intercostal muscles to pull the ribcage upward and outward, expanding the chest cavity in the anteroposterior dimension. This then expands the pleural membranes. Intrapleural pressure becomes even more negative, but the serous fluid keeps the membranes together and the lungs expand as well. As the lungs expand, alveolar pressure falls below atmospheric pressure and air enters the nose and respiratory passages. Entry of air continues until alveolar pressure equals atmospheric pressure; this is a normal inhalation. A deeper inhalation requires a more forceful contraction of the respiratory muscles (including accessory inspiratory muscles) to expand the chest cavity and lungs even further and permit the entry of more air.

Exhalation

Normal exhalation is a passive process that begins when motor impulses from the medulla decrease and the diaphragm and external intercostal muscles relax. The lungs are compressed as the chest cavity becomes smaller and the recoil of the elastic lung tissue compresses the alveoli. Alveolar pressure rises above atmospheric pressure, and air is forced out of the lungs until the two pressures are again equal. Under normal circumstances, energy is not required for exhalation (as it is for inhalation) because the elasticity of the lungs causes recoil and forces air out. A forced exhalation beyond the normal amount is an active process that requires contraction of the internal intercostal muscles to pull the rib cage downward and inward and contraction of the abdominal muscles to force the dome of the diaphragm upward, increasing compression of the lungs.

Transport of Gases in the Blood

Oxygen is carried in the blood by iron in the hemoglobin (Hgb) of red blood cells (RBCs). The iron-oxygen bond is formed in the lungs, where the partial pressure of oxygen (Po_2) is high. In tissues where the Po_2 is low, hemoglobin releases much of its oxygen.

Most carbon dioxide is carried in the blood in the form of bicarbonate ions in the plasma. These ions are formed when carbon dioxide enters RBCs and is converted to carbonic acid (H_2CO_3), which ionizes to bicarbonate ions (HCO_3^-) and hydrogen ions (H^+). The bicarbonate ions leave the RBCs for the plasma, and the remaining hydrogen ions are buffered by the hemoglobin in the RBCs. When the blood reaches the lungs, an area of lower partial pressure of carbon dioxide (Pco_2), these reactions are reversed—carbon dioxide is re-formed and diffuses into the alveoli to be exhaled.

Regulation of Respiration

Respiration is regulated by both nervous and chemical mechanisms. The medulla oblongata contains an inspiratory center and an expiratory center. The inspiratory center generates impulses that bring about contraction of the respiratory muscles, resulting in inhalation. When the impulses stop, exhalation occurs. If the lungs are overinflated, bronchi and bronchiole baroreceptors are stretched. The stretching inhibits the inspiratory center (and apneustic center) and exhalation follows. This protective mechanism is called the Hering-Breuer inflation reflex. In the pons, the apneustic center prolongs inhalation and the pneumotaxic center helps bring about exhalation. These centers provide a normal breathing rhythm, 12 to 20 breaths per minute with exhalation slightly longer than inhalation. When there is a need for more forceful exhalations, the inspiratory center activates the expiratory center, which brings about contraction of the internal intercostal muscles.

Normal breathing is essentially a reflex, but because the respiratory muscles are skeletal (or voluntary) muscles, it is possible to make changes. The cerebral cortex may override the medulla to permit voluntary changes in breathing, such as faster or slower breathing, holding one's breath, or singing. Eventually, the medulla resumes control and breathing is again a reflex.

Chemical regulation of respiration involves the blood levels of oxygen and carbon dioxide. Decreased blood oxygen is detected by chemoreceptors in the carotid body and aortic body; the response by the medulla is to increase respiration to take more air into the lungs. Increased blood carbon dioxide or a decrease in pH is detected by central chemoreceptors in the medulla and peripheral chemoreceptors; the response is increased respiration to exhale more carbon dioxide, which raises the pH back toward normal.

Carbon dioxide is usually the major regulator of respiration because even small changes in its blood level change the pH. Fluctuations in the oxygen level have no effect on pH, and an adequate oxygen level in the blood can be maintained even if breathing ceases for a few minutes. Residual air in the lungs is a contributing factor, as is the fact that air contains much more oxygen than we typcially use (exhaled air is 16 percent oxygen). Oxygen becomes the major regulator only when its blood level is very low, as may occur with severe, chronic pulmonary disease.

Respiration and Acid-Base Balance

Because of its role in regulating the amount of carbon dioxide in body fluids, the respiratory system is important in the maintenance of acid-base balance, measured by blood pH. Any decrease in the rate or efficiency of respiration permits excess carbon dioxide to accumulate in the blood. The resultant accumulation of excess hydrogen ions lowers pH. This is called respiratory acidosis and can occur as a consequence of pulmonary disease or any impairment of gas exchange in the lungs.

Respiratory alkalosis occurs when the rate of respiration increases, eliminating exhaled carbon dioxide very rapidly. Less carbon dioxide in the blood means that fewer hydrogen ions are formed and the pH rises. Although not a common condition, respiratory alkalosis may occur during states of anxiety accompanied by hyperventilation or when accommodating to a high altitude, before RBC production increases to provide sufficient oxygenation of tissues.

The respiratory system may also help compensate for pH changes that are said to be metabolic; that is, of any cause other than respiratory. Metabolic acidosis occurs when the concentration of hydrogen ions in body fluids is above normal due to lowered HCO_3^- buffer. Common causes include kidney disease, uncontrolled diabetes mellitus, and severe diarrhea. Respiratory compensation involves an increase in the rate and depth of respiration to exhale more carbon dioxide, which decreases hydrogen ion formation and raises the pH toward normal. Metabolic alkalosis may be caused by overingestion of antacid medications or by vomiting of gastric contents high in hydrochloric acid. Respiratory compensation involves a decrease in the breathing rate to retain carbon dioxide in the body, increasing the formation of hydrogen ions, which lowers the pH toward normal.

Respiratory compensation for an ongoing metabolic pH imbalance (such as kidney failure) cannot be complete because the amount of carbon dioxide that may be exhaled or retained is limited. At most, respiratory compensation is only about 75 percent effective.

Acid-base balance is discussed further in Chapter 5.

Effects of Aging on the Respiratory System

See Figure 29.2 for the effects of aging on respiration.

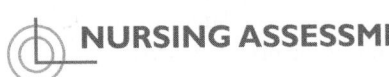

NURSING ASSESSMENT

Health History

Many factors in a patient's personal and family history affect respiratory function. Questions to ask while assessing the patient with a history of respiratory dysfunction are presented in Table 29.2. If at any time while you are taking the history the patient relates a specific symptom, redirect the line of questioning to further assess that symptom. One such line of questioning, as presented in Chapter 1, is the WHAT'S UP? format. For example, if the patient admits to shortness of breath (SOB), respond with the following questions (*Where is it?* doesn't apply to shortness of breath, so it may be skipped.):

- **H**ow does it feel? Does breathing feel tight, gasping, suffocating?
- **A**ggravating and alleviating factors? How much activity causes the SOB? Does anything else aggravate it? What do you do to lessen your SOB?
- **T**iming? When did you first experience SOB? Does it happen more at any particular time of day or year?
- **S**everity? Rate your SOB on a scale of 0 to 10, with 0 being easy breathing and 10 being the worst shortness of breath you can imagine.
- **U**seful other data? Do you have any other symptoms that occur along with the shortness of breath?
- **P**atient's perception? What do you think is causing your shortness of breath?

Because smoking is such a major risk factor for many types of lung disease, it is essential to ask about smoking history and encourage cessation (see Therapeutic Measures). Document smoking history in terms of *pack-years*. For example, if a patient has smoked two packs of cigarettes per day for 20 years, he has a 40 pack-year smoking history ($2 \times 20 = 40$ pack-years). It is also important to be aware of cultural influences on the patient's respiratory health (Box 29.1 Cultural Considerations).

Physical Assessment

Inspection

Inspection begins during the nursing history and continues during the physical assessment. Start with the nose, observing for symmetry, swelling, or other abnormalities. Note

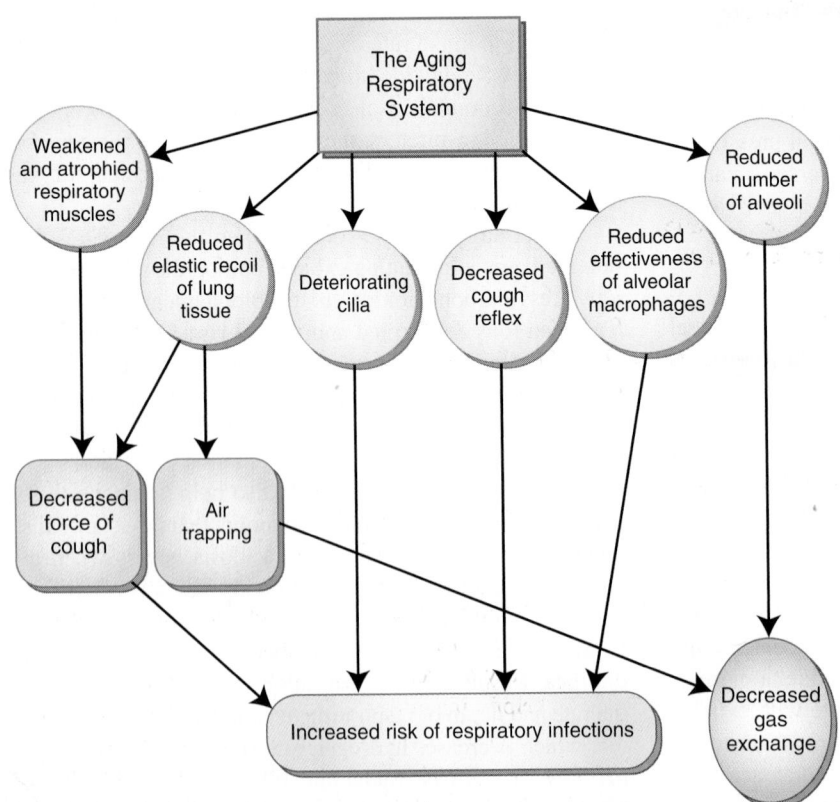

FIGURE 29.2 Effects of aging on respiration.

TABLE 29.2 QUESTIONS ASKED DURING NURSING ASSESSMENT OF THE RESPIRATORY SYSTEM

Category	Questions to ask	Rationale/Significance
Upper respiratory tract	Do you often have headaches or sinus tenderness?	These may indicate sinusitis.
	Do you often experience nosebleeds?	A history of nosebleeds may indicate an abnormality that can predispose to future nosebleeds.
	Has your voice changed?	A voice change may indicate a variety of disorders of the nose or throat, including cancer. Further investigation is necessary.
Lower respiratory tract	Do you ever feel short of breath, like you can't get enough air?	Many respiratory and cardiac problems result in shortness of breath.
	Do you have a cough? Is it productive?	A cough indicates respiratory irritation or excessive secretions.
	What does the sputum look like?	Yellow or green sputum may accompany an infection. Blood in the sputum may occur with tuberculosis, pulmonary embolism, or cancer.
	Have you recently experienced night sweats, chills, fever?	These are symptoms of tuberculosis.
	Do you ever feel confused, light-headed, or restless?	These symptoms might indicate a low P_{O_2}, reducing oxygen to the brain.
	Have you had any chest surgeries?	This may reveal problem areas the patient has not yet mentioned.
Exposures	Do you have any allergies that cause respiratory symptoms? How do you treat them?	The patient may take over-the-counter medications for allergies that affect respiratory function or interact with prescribed medications.
	Do you smoke? How many packs per day? For how many years? Are you exposed to secondhand smoke?	Many respiratory disorders are caused or aggravated by exposure to tobacco smoke.
	Are you or have you been exposed to airborne pollutants at work?	Pollutants such as asbestos, coal dust, or chemicals can cause lung disease.
Treatments	Do you take any medications or use inhalers (prescribed or over-the-counter) for your respiratory problems?	Information about medications gives further information about disorders, severity, and treatment. You should also consider drug interactions and side effects.
	Do you use home oxygen or other home respiratory treatments?	This helps determine the severity of disease and the severity of disease and the treatment.
Family history	Do any of your blood relatives have emphysema, asthma, or tuberculosis?	Some respiratory disorders have a hereditary tendency. Tuberculosis is contagious.

whether the patient is short of breath (dyspneic) while speaking or moving. If the patient is very dyspneic, he or she may speak in short sentences.

Observe the patient for use of accessory muscles of breathing (Figure 29.3). Use of the sternocleidomastoid muscles causes the shoulders to rise during labored inspiration. During forced expiration, the abdominal and intercostal muscles contract. The use of accessory muscles for breathing indicates respiratory distress. Retraction of the chest wall between the ribs can indicate serious distress.

Note the color of the skin, lips, mucous membranes, and nailbeds. A bluish color is called **cyanosis** and is a late sign of oxygen deprivation. Observe the trachea and chest for symmetry. Count the number of respirations per minute, noting depth and rhythm. Irregular respirations, or periods of **apnea** (absence of respirations), can indicate a patholog-

ical condition and are described in Figure 29.4. Observe the shape of the chest. Normally the chest is about twice as wide (side to side) as it is deep (front to back). If it is more rounded, it is called a barrel chest, which is associated with air trapping. See Table 29.3 for a summary of objective assessment data.

Palpation

Palpate the frontal and maxillary sinuses if sinus inflammation is suspected (Fig. 29.5). Use your thumbs to palpate gently below the eyebrows and below each cheekbone. Tenderness may indicate sinus inflammation or infection.

Respiratory excursion can also be palpated. This is a rough measurement of chest expansion on inspiration. It is not necessary to palpate expansion on every patient, but it may be helpful if hypoventilation or asymmetry is suspected. See Figure 29.6 for how to palpate respiratory excursion. You can palpate for **crepitus** (also called subcutaneous emphysema) if indicated. Crepitus feels like Rice Krispies under the

---

cyanosis: cyan—dark blue + osis—condition
apnea: a—not + pnea—breath

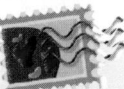

Box 29.1

Cultural Considerations

Pulmonary diseases associated with Japanese people include asthma related to dust mites in the straw mats that cover floors in Japanese homes and air pollution from living in urban areas. The nurse should encourage patients who have straw mats and who wish to keep them to have them sterilized.

Patients from Poland, Ireland, or other countries where mining is a primary occupation may have an increased incidence of respiratory disease. It is essential that health-care providers carefully screen Polish and Irish immigrants for respiratory conditions.

Health care practitioners should be aware of the variations among ethnic peoples of color when assessing for cyanosis. Cyanosis and decreased blood hemoglobin levels in darker skinned individuals gives the skin an ashen color instead of a bluish color. Thus, the nurse must examine the sclerae, conjunctivae, buccal mucosa, tongue, lips, nailbeds, and palms and soles of the feet to assess for lowered oxygen levels.

Smoking is deeply ingrained in the Arab American culture. Offering cigarettes is a rite of Arab hospitality. Arabs may have difficulty stopping smoking because of these cultural rituals.

Populations living in inner cities are at increased risk for respiratory diseases related to pollution. Strategies to increase the effectiveness of smoking cessation in African Americans include working with community and church groups in African American communities.

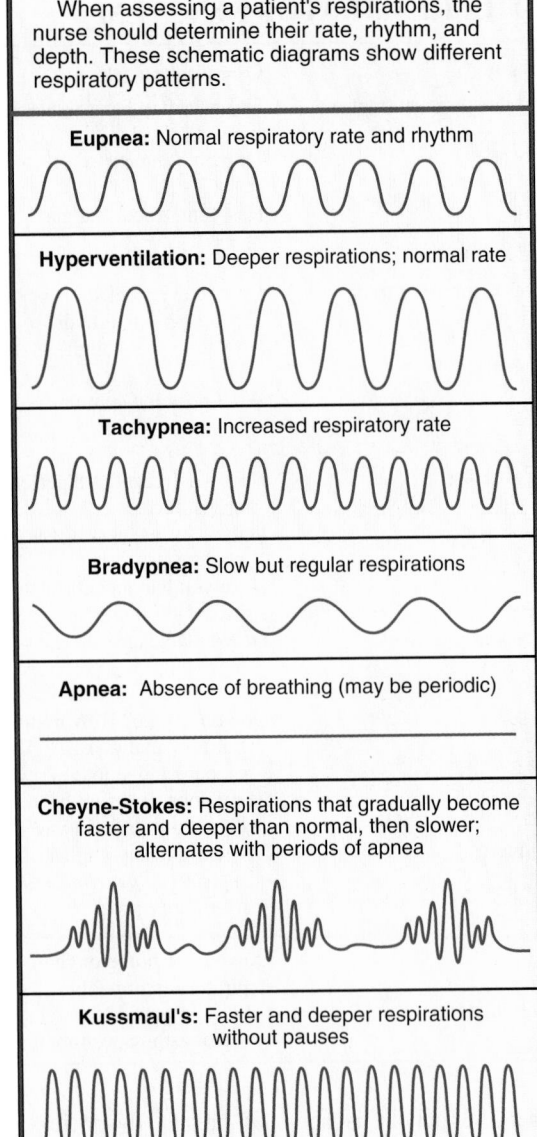

Respiratory patterns

When assessing a patient's respirations, the nurse should determine their rate, rhythm, and depth. These schematic diagrams show different respiratory patterns.

Eupnea: Normal respiratory rate and rhythm

Hyperventilation: Deeper respirations; normal rate

Tachypnea: Increased respiratory rate

Bradypnea: Slow but regular respirations

Apnea: Absence of breathing (may be periodic)

Cheyne-Stokes: Respirations that gradually become faster and deeper than normal, then slower; alternates with periods of apnea

Kussmaul's: Faster and deeper respirations without pauses

FIGURE 29.4 Abnormal respiratory patterns.

skin when felt with the fingers. It occurs when air leaks into subcutaneous tissues because of pneumothorax or a leaking chest tube site. Palpation for crepitus is not done routinely, but rather when the possibility of an air leak exists.

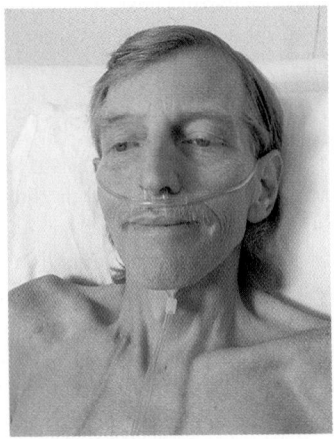

FIGURE 29.3 Accessory muscles of breathing. Note the prominent sternocleidomastoid muscles.

Percussion

Percussion is done by the experienced nurse. It involves tapping on the anterior and posterior chest, in each intercostal space, and comparing sounds from side to side. A normal chest sounds resonant and is the same on both the right and left sides except over the heart. If other percussion notes are heard, they may indicate a pathological condition and should be reported.

Auscultation

Auscultation provides valuable information about respiratory status. Use the diaphragm of your stethoscope to listen to the anterior and posterior chest during an entire inspiration and expiration at each interspace (Fig. 29.7). Auscultation of the posterior chest is easiest if the patient is sitting,

TABLE 29.3 OBJECTIVE ASSESSMENT OF THE RESPIRATORY SYSTEM

Category	Abnormal Findings	Possible Causes
Respiratory	Respiratory Rate <12	Respiratory depression, possibly from opioid or sedative use
	Respiratory Rate >24	Respiratory distress from underlying disorder
	Use of accessory muscles	Restrictive or obstructive disorders
	Barrel chest	Air trapping from obstructive disorder (COPD)
	Adventitious sounds	See Table 29.4
	Cough	Airway irritation or secretions
	Sputum	Green, yellow, or tan sputum may indicate infection. Blood in sputum can indicate tuberculosis, cancer, or pulmonary embolism.
Integumentary	Cyanosis	Tissue hypoxia
	Nail clubbing	Chronic tissue hypoxia
Neurological	Confusion	Lack of oxygen to the brain
Gastrointestinal	Weight loss	Dyspnea interfering with eating; use of calories for breathing

but if necessary, it may be done with the patient in a side-lying position. Asking the patient to breathe deeply through the mouth can help enhance the sounds. Allow the patient to rest at intervals to prevent hyperventilation. Regular and frequent practice helps you learn to distinguish normal from abnormal breath sounds. Abnormal extra sounds (another term is **adventitious**) indicate a pathological condition and are described in Table 29.4.

LEARNING TIP

Listen to breath sounds on all your friends and family members. Assuming they are normal, this will give you a good baseline so when you hear an abnormal or adventitious sound on a patient, you will recognize it as "not normal"!

CRITICAL THINKING

Timothy

■ Timothy is a 16 year old brought into the emergency room by his mother because of an asthma attack. He says he feels short of breath, but when you listen to his lungs you hear no wheezing.
1. Does Timothy really need to be in the emergency room?
2. What should you do?
3. What do you think could be happening?
Suggested answers at end of chapter.

DIAGNOSTIC TESTS

Laboratory Tests

Blood Tests

COMPLETE BLOOD COUNT. Measurement of red blood cells and hemoglobin can give information about the oxygen-carrying capacity of the blood. **Dyspnea** can be

dyspnea: dys—bad + pnea—breathing

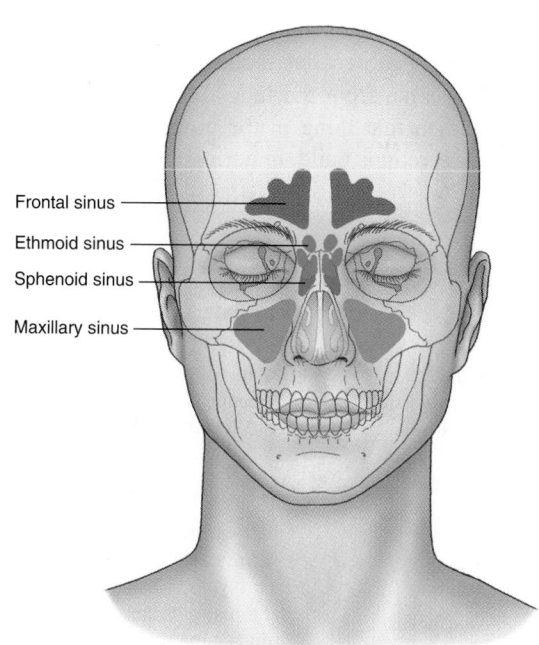

FIGURE 29.5 Paranasal sinuses.

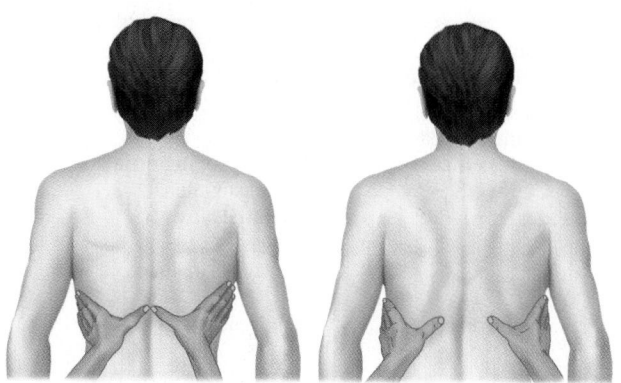

FIGURE 29.6 Palpation of respiratory excursion.

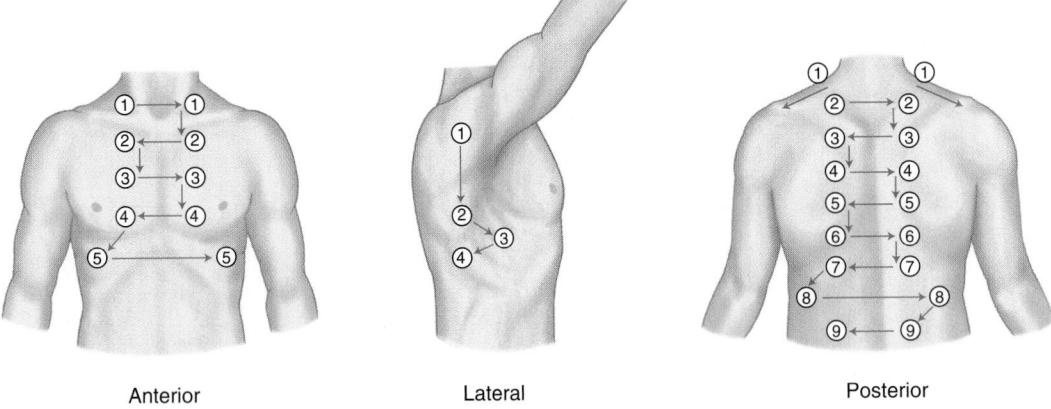

Anterior Lateral Posterior

FIGURE 29.7 Auscultation of the chest. Use a systematic approach to auscultate the chest, comparing sounds from side to side.

COPD Respiratory Aicdosis

caused by a reduction in RBCs or Hgb. See Table 29.5 for normal values.

ARTERIAL BLOOD GAS ANALYSIS. Arterial blood gases (ABGs) are measured to determine the effectiveness of gas exchange. The "Pa" portion of the ABG results refer to the partial pressure of the gas in arterial blood. See Table 29.6 for a basic interpretation of ABGs. The blood sample is usually taken from the radial artery in the wrist by a physician or laboratory technician specially trained to do this. This can be painful for the patient. Place pressure on the site for 5 minutes after the test to prevent bleeding.

D-DIMER. This blood test measures fibrin degradation products, which are present if there is a blood clot in the body. It helps diagnose the presence of a pulmonary embolism.

LEARNING TIP

If you remember that a normal blood pH is 7.35 to 7.45, then it is easy to remember a normal $Paco_2$ is 35 to 45 mm Hg.

LEARNING TIP

Remember 50. If the Pao_2 falls below 50 and the $Paco_2$ is above 50, the patient is in trouble and the physician should be notified. This is a crude analysis, but it is helpful when a quick assessment is needed.

Sputum Culture and Sensitivity

A sputum culture identifies pathogens present in the sputum. The sensitivity test determines which antibiotics will be effective against those pathogens. To obtain a sputum specimen, first obtain a sterile container. Some institutions have special containers for sputum that help prevent transmission of infection to the health-care worker (Fig. 29.8). Instruct the patient to take several deep breaths and then cough sputum into the sputum container. It is important that the patient not simply spit saliva or sinus drainage into the cup. The specimen must come from the lungs. It may be easiest to obtain a specimen first thing in the morning (after mouth care) because secretions build up during the night. Send the

TABLE 29.4 ABNORMAL LUNG SOUNDS

Abnormal (Adventitious) Sound	Cause of Sound	Description	Associated Disorders
Coarse crackles (sometime called rales)	Fluid in airways	Moist bubbling sound, heard on inspiration or expiration	Pulmonary edema, bronchitis, pneumonia
Fine crackles (rales)	Alveoli popping open on inspiration	Velcro being torn apart, heard at end of inspiration	Heart failure, atelectasis
Wheezes	Narrowed airways	Fine high-pitched violins mostly on expiration	Asthma
Stridor	Airway obstruction	Loud crowing noise heard without sterhoscope	Obstruction from tumor or foreign body
Pleural friction rub	Pleura rubbing together	Sound of leather rubbing together, grating	Pleurisy, lung cancer, pneumonia, pleural irritation
Diminished	Decreased air movement	Faint lung sounds	Emphysema, hypoventilation, obesity, muscular chest wall
Absent	No air movement	No sounds heard	Pneumothorax, pneumectomy

TABLE 29.5 COMMON LABORATORY TESTS

Test	Normal Values	Associated Conditions
Red blood cell count	Male: 4.5–6.2 million Female: 4.2–5.4 million cells/ mm^3 venous blood	↑ in chronic lung disease, dehydration ↓ in anemia, hemorrhage, overhydration with intravenous fluids
Hemoglobin	Male: 13.5–18 g/dL Female: 12–16 g/dL	Same as RBC count
White blood cell count	5000–10,000 cells/ mm^3 venous blood	↑ in infection

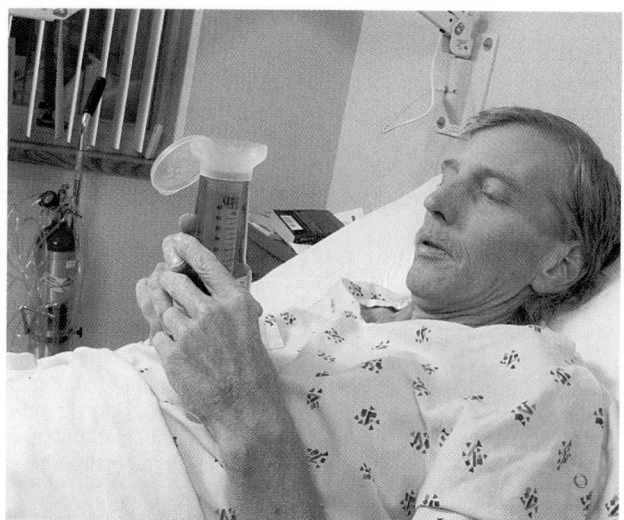

FIGURE 29.8 A special container that helps prevent transmission of infection is often used to collect sputum for culture.

specimen to the laboratory immediately. If the patient is unable to cough up sputum, extra fluids or a bedside humidifier may help. A respiratory therapist (RT) may be able to help obtain a specimen with a nebulized mist treatment or with a special suction catheter with a sputum trap. A physician order may be needed for these procedures.

Throat Culture

A throat culture is done to determine the presence of viral or bacterial pathogens in the pharynx. Use a swab to reach into the pharynx (without touching the patient's mouth) and rub the red area or lesions. Use a tongue blade to help hold the tongue down while obtaining the culture. Warn the patient that a gag reflex may be triggered. Once the culture is obtained, place it in a sterile tube with culture medium, according to package instructions. Send it immediately to the laboratory for analysis.

Oxygen Saturation

The oxygen saturation test (also called pulse oximetry, O_2 sat, and SaO_2) is simple and noninvasive. A sensor is placed on the patient's finger or ear that measures the percentage of hemoglobin that is saturated with oxygen. Oxygen saturation can be measured at rest or while the patient is walking to determine the patient's exercise tolerance. It is also often done with and without supplemental oxygen to determine the patient's need for oxygen supplementation at home. See Table 29.6 for normal values. An SaO_2 value below 95 percent should be reported to the RN or physician. If the SaO_2 is less than 75 percent, prepare for emergency intervention.

PATIENT CARE TIP

If the physician orders a "sputum for AFB," tuberculosis is suspected, which is caused by an acid-fast bacillus. Ask whether the patient should be isolated while waiting for test results.

TABLE 29.6 ARTERIAL BLOOD GAS ANALYSIS

Normal Values	Interpretation	
PaO_2	75–100 mm Hg	↑ in hyperventilation ↓ in impaired respiratory function
$PaCO_2$	35–45 mm Hg	↑ in impaired gas exchange ↓ in hyperventilation
pH	7.35–7.45	↑ in respiratory alkalosis with low $PaCO_2$ ↓ in respiratory acidosis with high $PaCO_2$
HCO_3	22–26	↑ to buffer $PaCO_2$ in acidosis ↓ to buffer $PaCO_2$ in alkalosis
Oxygen saturation	95%–100%	↑ in hyperventilation ↓ in impaired respiratory function

Other Tests

Chest X-ray Examination

A chest x-ray examination may be ordered to help diagnose a variety of pulmonary disorders. Usually, posterior-anterior (PA) and side views (lateral) are taken. If a hospitalized patient is too ill to go to the radiology department, a portable chest x-ray machine can be used at the bedside to obtain a PA view.

Ventilation-Perfusion Scan

During a ventilation-perfusion scan (also called a lung scan or VQ scan), a radioactive substance is injected intravenously and a scan is done to view blood flow to the lungs (perfusion). Another radioactive substance is inhaled, and scanning shows how well oxygen is distributed in the lungs

TABLE 29.7 PULMONARY FUNCTION VALUES

Test	Definition	Normal Values*
Tidal volume (TV)	Air inspired and expired in one breath	400–600 mL at rest
Residual volume (RV)	Air remaining in lungs after maximum exhalation	1000–1500 mL
Functional residual capacity (FRC)	Air remaining in lungs after normal expiration	2300 mL
Inspiratory reserve	Amount of air beyond tidal volume that can be taken in with the deepest possible inhalation	2000–3000 mL
Expiratory reserve	Amount of air beyond tidal volume in the most forceful exhalation	1000–1500 mL
Forced vital capacity (FVC)	Maximum amount of air expired forcefully after maximum inspiration	3000–5000 mL
Forced expiratory volume in one second (FEV$_1$)	Amount of air expired in first second of forced exhalation, expressed as percent of FVC	65%–85% of the FVC
Peak expiatory flow rate (PEFR)	Maximum flow of air expired during FVC (this is a rate rather than a volume)	450 L/min

*Normal values are approximate—normal values are individualized based on patient's sex, height, and age.

(ventilation). If an area of the lungs is well ventilated but has no blood supply, a pulmonary embolism is suspected. Chronic lung disease may cause poor ventilation and perfusion.

Pulmonary Function Studies

Pulmonary function studies are a series of tests done to determine lung volume, capacity, and flow rates. These are commonly used to help diagnose and monitor restrictive or obstructive lung disease. The patient is asked to use a special mouthpiece to blow into a cylinder that is connected to a computer. A computer printout is generated to show the results. See Table 29.7 for normal values. Some patients use handheld peak expiratory flow rate (PEFR) meters at home to monitor asthma symptoms. They might notice changes in PEFR before symptoms occur, allowing them to begin treatment before the problem becomes more serious.

Pulmonary Angiography

Pulmonary angiography involves an x-ray examination of the pulmonary vessels after intravenous (IV) administration of a radiopaque dye. A catheter is inserted into the femoral, brachial, or jugular vein and threaded through the heart to the pulmonary artery, where the dye is injected. Pulmonary angiography is used to help diagnose pulmonary embolism or other pulmonary vessel disorders. Patients receive nothing by mouth (NPO) for 4 to 8 hours before the procedure. Question the patient about allergies to x-ray dyes before scheduling the test. As with any procedure involving dye, inform the patient that the dye may cause a warm feeling when injected. Make sure a signed consent form is obtained before any invasive procedure is performed. Medications may be administered before or during the test for patient comfort.

After angiography, place the patient flat in bed for 3 to 8 hours, as ordered by the physician. Monitor vital signs and observe the injection site for bleeding. A sandbag may be used to place pressure on the site. Encourage fluid intake to promote excretion of the dye.

Bronchoscopy

Bronchoscopy involves the use of a flexible endoscope to examine the larynx, trachea, and bronchial tree. Bronchoscopy can be used diagnostically for visualization or to obtain a biopsy specimen for examination. It can also be used therapeutically to remove an obstruction, foreign body, or thick secretions. Instruct the patient the he or she will be able to breathe through the nose and that oxygen can be administered through the tube if necessary. A signed consent form is necessary for this invasive procedure.

The patient is NPO for 6 to 8 hours before the procedure. Be prepared to administer a sedative, and commonly an injection of atropine to dry excess secretions, before the procedure. An anesthetic spray may be used to numb the throat. After the test, monitor vital signs and watch for signs of laryngeal edema. Sputum may be blood tinged. The patient is NPO until the gag reflex returns. Check for the gag reflex by touching the pharynx with a cotton swab. After the gag reflex returns, ask the patient to swallow a sip of water before offering foods or fluids. A sore throat may be relieved with lozenges once the patient is able to swallow.

THERAPEUTIC MEASURES

Smoking Cessation

Probably the most important intervention for preventing and treating respiratory disease is smoking cessation. Many respiratory disorders are caused or aggravated by smoking, and stopping can prevent disease from occurring or slow its progression significantly. See Table 29.8 for interventions used to help patients stop smoking. Remind patients that if they have tried quitting before and failed, that does not mean that they will never be able to quit. Many patients try several times before quitting successfully. Formal smoking cessation programs and support groups can be helpful.

Many internet sites have information to help people stop smoking. Among these are the American Lung

TABLE 29.8 INTERVENTIONS TO STOP SMOKING

Intervention	Rationale
Behavior modification	If the patient can identify situations that are associated with smoking, such as eating a meal or experiencing stress, he can substitute other healthier behaviors, such as going for a walk.
Counseling	Counseling by a health care worker alone can result in a 3%–5% quit rate.
Setting a quit date	The cold turkey method is more effective than slow tapering, although the patient may choose to taper before the quit date.
Nicotine replacement therapy	Nicotine gum, patches, nasal sprays, and inhalers can reduce withdrawal symptoms.
Drug therapy (bupropion [Zyban], buspirone [BuSpar])	Better success rates are achieved with a combination of nicotine and bupropion.
Hypnosis	Hypnosis can help reduce the stress and anxiety associated with smoking cessation.

Association site at www.lungusa.org and the National Lung Health Education Program at www.nlhep.org. Or simply type *smoking cessation* into any search engine. The American Lung Association has a free online smoking cessation program that can be accessed at http://www.ffsonline.org. Alternatively, individuals can call 1-800-QUIT NOW to speak with a representative who will assist with cessation strategies.

Deep Breathing and Coughing

Effective coughing can keep the airways clear of secretions. An ineffective cough is exhausting and fails to bring up secretions. Instruct the patient to take two or three deep breaths, using the diaphragm. This helps get the air behind the secretions. After the third deep inhalation, tell the patient to hold the breath and cough forcefully. This is repeated as necessary. Good hydration can facilitate this process.

Huff Coughing

Patients with chronic obstructive pulmonary disease (COPD) typically have a weak cough and airways that collapse easily. Huff coughing may work better for them. To do this, instruct the patient to exhale deeply to remove as much trapped air as possible, then take a deep breath in to get air behind the secretions. Instead of closing the glottis to generate a forceful cough, the patient should keep the glottis and mouth open, and use the abdominal muscles to create a series of forced expirations, moving air and mucus up the bronchial tree. This creates "huff" sounds. Finally, the patient should take one more controlled inhalation and a final huff cough to expel the mucus.

Breathing Exercises

Breathing exercises are essential for patients with chronic lung disease. Diaphragmatic and pursed-lip breathing increase the effectiveness of breathing and help reduce panic when dyspnea occurs.

Diaphragmatic Breathing

The diaphragm is the major muscle of breathing, but patients often use less efficient accessory muscles when they are short of breath. Conscious use of the diaphragm during breathing can be relaxing and conserves energy. With practice, the patient should be able to use diaphragmatic breathing all the time without thinking about it. Teach the patient to do the following:

1. Place one hand on the abdomen and the other on the chest.
2. Concentrate on pushing out the abdomen during inspiration and relaxing the abdomen on expiration. The chest should move very little.

Pursed-Lip Breathing

This technique can be used any time the patient feels short of breath. It helps keep airways open during exhalation, which promotes carbon dioxide excretion. It should be done with diaphragmatic breathing. Counting during breathing also distracts the patient, reducing panic. Teach the patient to do the following:

1. Inhale slowly through the nose to the count of two.
2. Exhale slowly through pursed lips to the count of four.

Positioning

The patient who is short of breath should be positioned to conserve energy while allowing for maximum lung expansion. The patient in bed can use a Fowler's or semi-Fowler's position to keep abdominal contents from crowding the lungs. Most respiratory patients do not tolerate lying flat. Some patients prefer to sit in a chair while leaning forward and placing their elbows on their knees or an over-bed table with a pillow on it.

Patients with unilateral (one-sided) lung disease can benefit from the "good lung down" lateral position. This is a side-lying position with the good lung in the dependent position. Gravity causes greater blood flow to the dependent, "good" lung, thereby increasing oxygen saturation.

Oxygen Therapy   92% receive oxygen

Oxygen therapy is ordered by the physician when the patient is unable to maintain oxygenation. Many patients are placed on supplemental oxygen when their oxygen saturation is less than 90 percent on room air. The physician's order should include the method of administration and the flow rate. A variety of delivery methods are described in the following sections. The role of the nurse in oxygen therapy includes monitoring the flow rate, ensuring that the cannula and tubing or other device remain properly placed, and monitoring the patient's response to treatment. If the patient becomes short of breath while on oxygen therapy, an RT or a physician should be notified. Instruct the patient to avoid smoking, using electrical equipment, and performing other activities that can cause fire in the presence of oxygen. The RT is knowledgeable about oxygen therapy and is an excellent resource when questions arise.

PATIENT CARE TIP

If a patient suddenly becomes confused, check the oxygen delivery system. The patient may have taken off the cannula, or the tubing may be kinked or disconnected, resulting in hypoxia and confusion.

Low-Flow Devices

NASAL CANNULA. The nasal cannula is the most common method of oxygen administration. Oxygen is delivered through a flexible catheter that has two short nasal prongs (Fig. 29.9). For the nasal cannula to be most effective, the patient must breathe through his or her nose. The cannula allows the patient to eat and talk, and it is generally more comfortable than other methods of administration. If the nasal mucous membranes become dry, an RT can place a water source on the system to humidify the oxygen. Oxygen can be delivered at 1 to 6 L/minute via a nasal cannula, according to the physician's order.

MASKS. Masks are used when a higher oxygen concentration is needed (Fig. 29.10). A disadvantage to masks is that they make some patients feel claustrophobic. Also, a mask must be replaced by a cannula for eating.

SIMPLE FACE MASK. A rate of 5 to 10 L/minute can deliver oxygen concentrations from 40 to 60 percent with a simple face mask.

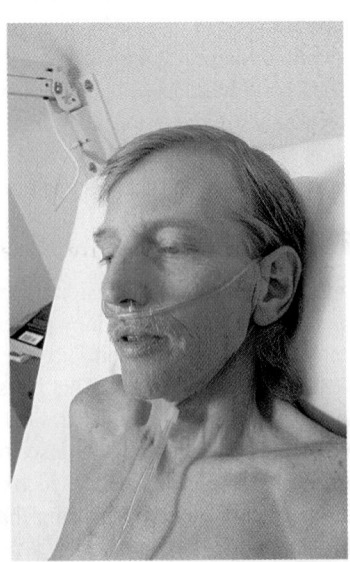

FIGURE 29.9 Nasal cannula for oxygen delivery.

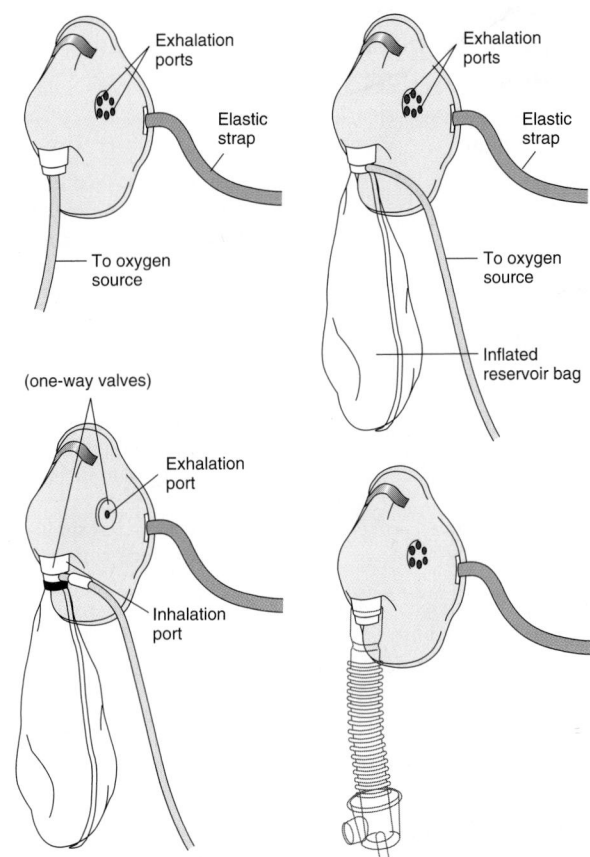

FIGURE 29.10 Oxygen masks. *(A)* Simple mask. *(B)* Partial rebreather mask. *(C)* Nonrebreathing mask. *(D)* Venturi mask.

PARTIAL REBREATHER MASK. A partial rebreather mask uses a reservoir to capture some exhaled gas for rebreathing. Vents on the sides of the mask allow room air to mix with oxygen. It can deliver oxygen concentrations of 50 percent or greater.

NONREBREATHER MASK. A nonrebreather mask has one or both side vents closed to limit the mixing of room air with oxygen. The vents open to allow expiration but remain closed on inspiration. The reservoir bag has a valve to store oxygen for inspiration but does not allow entry of exhaled air. It is used to deliver oxygen concentrations of 70 to 100 percent.

When a patient is using a partial rebreather or nonbreather mask, ensure that the reservoir is never allowed to collapse to less than half full.

High-Flow Devices

VENTURI MASK. A Venturi mask is used for the patient who requires precise percentages of oxygen, such as the patient with chronic lung disease with CO_2 retention. A combination of valves and specified flow rates determines oxygen concentration.

Transtracheal Catheter

A transtracheal catheter is a small tube that is surgically placed through the base of the neck directly into the trachea to deliver oxygen (Fig. 29.11). This is an attractive alternative for some patients who are on long-term oxygen therapy

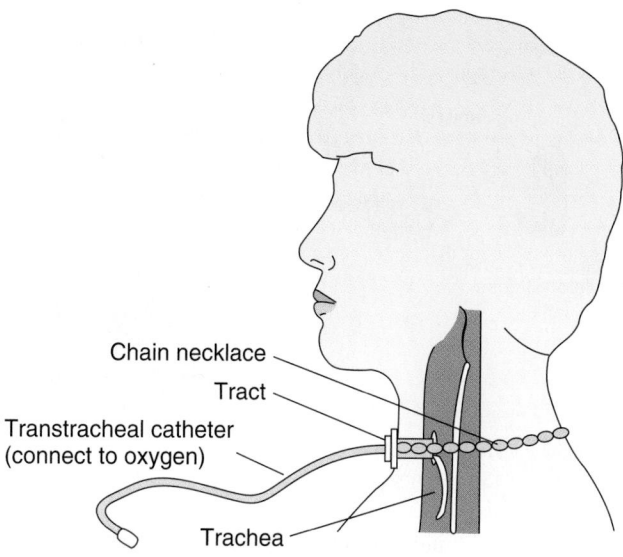

FIGURE 29.11 Transtracheal oxygen catheter.

Labels in figure:
Chain necklace
Tract
Transtracheal catheter (connect to oxygen)
Trachea

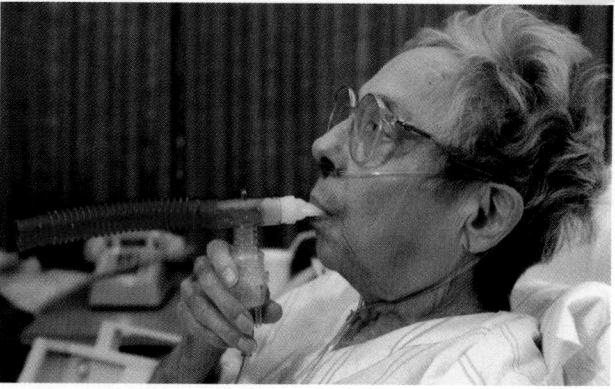

FIGURE 29.12 Patient receiving nebulized mist treatment.

at home because it does not obstruct the nose or mouth and can be easily covered with a loose scarf or collar. The patient is taught to remove and clean the catheter two or three times a day to prevent mucus obstruction. Check institution policy and procedure and the respiratory care department for specific care instructions.

Risks of Oxygen Therapy

Patients with chronic obstructive pulmonary disease (COPD) have chronically high $Paco_2$ levels. Therefore, they depend on low Pao_2 levels to stimulate breathing, and high supplemental oxygen flow rates can depress respirations. Patients with COPD should be maintained on no more than 1 to 2 L of oxygen per minute. Occasionally, hospitalized patients receive higher flow rates, but they must be carefully monitored.

In addition, any patient can suffer lung damage from high oxygen concentrations delivered for more than 24 hours. If a patient exhibits symptoms of dry cough, chest pain, numbness in the extremities, lethargy, or nausea, the physician should be contacted. A Pao_2 greater than 100 mm Hg should also be reported.

Nebulized Mist Treatments

Nebulized mist treatments (NMTs) use a nebulizer to deliver medication directly into the lungs (Fig. 29.12). Such topical use of medication reduces systemic side effects. Bronchodilators such as albuterol or metaproterenol, mixed with normal saline solution and sometimes with supplemental oxygen, are most commonly administered. Other medications, including corticosteroids, mucolytics, and antibiotics, may also be given. An RT or a specially trained nurse administers the NMT. The patient uses a hand-held reservoir with tubing and a mouthpiece to breathe in the medication. NMTs are commonly ordered every 4 to 6 hours and as needed. You may call for an NMT as needed (prn) when a patient with chronic pulmonary disease becomes acutely

dyspneic. Some patients are taught to administer their own NMTs at home.

Inhalers

Inhalers are another way to administer topical medication directly into the lungs, minimizing systemic side effects. Medications that can be inhaled include corticosteroids, bronchodilators, and mast cell inhibitors (cromolyn sodium). Metered-dose inhalers (MDI) use propellants to deliver medication. Figure 29.13 shows one way to use an MDI. Use of a spacer can increase the amount of medication that gets to the lungs (Fig. 29.14). Many MDIs use a chlorofluorocarbon (CFC) as a propellant, but CFC damages the ozone, so new ways to deliver inhaled medications are being developed. Many new models of inhalers (especially dry powder inhalers that do not use any propellants) are now available. It is important to carefully read the instructions for use before assisting a patient with any inhaler.

The RT or nurse must carefully instruct the patient because improper use can reduce the effectiveness of the medication. It is also important to teach the patient to avoid overuse of adrenergic bronchodilator inhalers. Patients with chronic lung disease may tend to use extra puffs when they feel short of breath. Adrenergic bronchodilators, when used too often, can cause severe rebound bronchoconstriction and even death.

Incentive Spirometry

Incentive spirometers are devices used to encourage deep breathing in patients at risk for collapse of lung tissue, a condition called atelectasis (Fig. 29.15). These devices are commonly ordered for postoperative patients. Patients are instructed to use the spirometer 10 times each hour they are awake. Because a variety of spirometers are available, consult with an RT and read package inserts for specific directions for use.

Chest Physiotherapy

Chest physiotherapy (CPT), which includes postural drainage, percussion, and vibration, helps move secretions from deep inside the lungs (Fig. 29.16). It is indicated for the patient who has a weak or ineffective cough and is therefore at risk for retaining secretions. Patients with COPD,

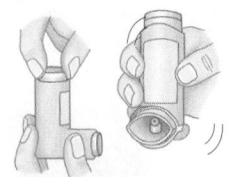

1. Gently twist the canister into the inhaler unit. Shake the inhaler, and remove the cap.

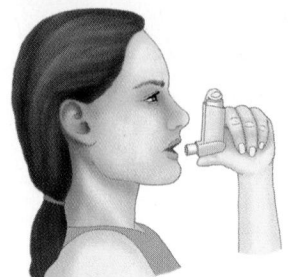

2. Exhale.

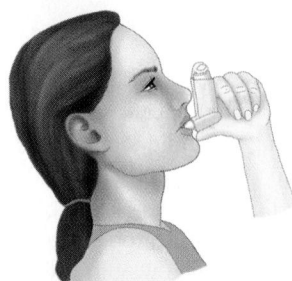

3. Place the inhaler mouthpiece in your mouth.

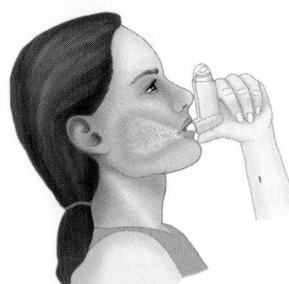

4. Press the canister down to actuate a dose of medication. As you do so, breathe in slowly and deeply. Time the dose and breath so the medication goes into the lungs, and not onto the tongue.

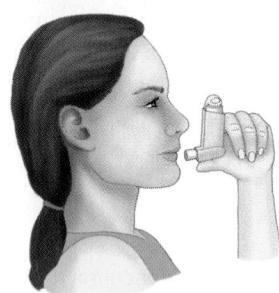

5. Hold your breath for 5 – 10 seconds. Repeat steps 2 – 4 if two puffs are ordered.

FIGURE 29.13 Instructions for use of a metered dose inhaler. See package inserts for specific instructions, since there are many types of inhalers available.

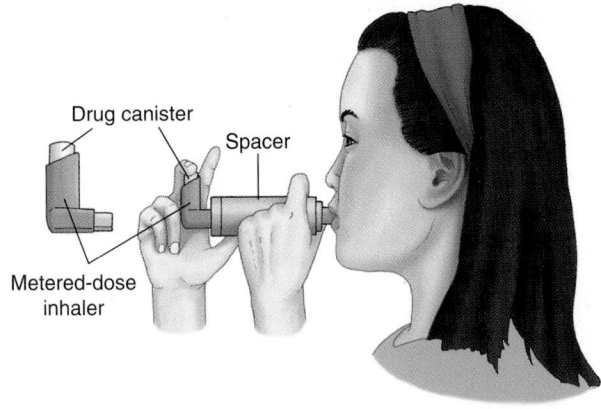

Drug canister   Spacer

Metered-dose inhaler

FIGURE 29.14 Use of a spacer increases the amount of medication that gets to the lungs.

transmitted through the chest, loosening secretions. The therapist may also apply vibration to the patient's chest, using the hands or a vibrator, to loosen secretions. A nebulizer treatment should be given before CPT to humidify secretions. The patient is instructed to cough and deep breathe at intervals during and after the treatment.

Flutter Mucus Clearance Device

An alternative to chest physiotherapy is a small hand-held device called the Flutter mucus clearance device (Fig. 29.17). When the patient blows into the mouthpiece, it makes a heavy steel ball inside bounce around in its chamber, which then sends vibrations back into the airways. This helps to loosen mucus and open the airways.

Thoracentesis

Thoracentesis involves the insertion of a needle into the pleural space. It is commonly done to aspirate fluid in patients with pleural effusion (fluid trapped in the pleural space). The procedure may be diagnostic, to determine the source of fluid, or therapeutic, to remove fluid and reduce respiratory distress. It may also be performed to aspirate blood or air or to inject medication.

When assisting a physician with a thoracentesis, first verify that the patient understands the procedure and that written consent has been obtained if required by institution policy. Have the patient void before the procedure. The patient should be aware that a sensation of pressure may be felt, but that severe pain is rare. Administer an analgesic if ordered before the procedure. Obtain a special procedure tray that has the equipment needed by the physician. Place the patient in a sitting position, bending over a bedside table, or in a side-lying position if unable to sit. You can position yourself in front of the patient and encourage relaxation during the procedure. If you are asked to hand equipment to the physician, be sure to keep everything sterile. The physician uses a local anesthetic before inserting a needle into the

cystic fibrosis, or bronchiectasis and patients on ventilators benefit from CPT.

CPT is performed by an RT or specially trained nurse. For postural drainage, the patient is placed in various positions (head down to help drain secretions) and turned periodically during the treatment so all lobes of the lungs are drained. The therapist uses cupped hands to strike the chest repeatedly (percussion), producing sound waves that are

---

thoracentesis: thoraco—chest + centesis—puncture

Box 29.2

Care of the Patient with a Chest Drainage System

Assess the patient according to institution policy. Start with the patient and move toward the drainage system.

1. Observe respiratory rate, effort, and symmetry.
2. Assess shortness of breath, pain, or other discomforts.
3. Auscultate lung sounds (lung sounds may initially be muffled or absent on the side of a collapsed lung but should gradually return to normal as the lung reinflates).
4. Confirm that dressing is intact; observe for drainage. If necessary, reinforce the dressing and notify the physician. Do *not* change the dressing.
5. Palpate around insertion sites for crepitus.
6. Check all tubing for kinds, breaks, or broken connections. Verify that all connections are securely taped.
7. Ensure that there are no dependent loops of tubing. Excess tubing should be coiled on the bed.
8. Verify that drainage system is below level of patient's chest at all times.
9. Check drainage system or bottles for cracks or leaks.
10. Check water seal chamber for correct water level and for tidaling (unless lung reinflated). Add water if evaporation has decreased level. If continuous bubbling is present, check entire system for leaks and notify physician.
11. Check suction control chamber for gentle bubbling (or open to air). Confirm correct amount of water if indicated. Add water if needed.
12. Check and mark amount of drainage in collection chamber every 8 hours and prn or as ordered. Report any marked increase in bloody drainage. Record drainage as output.
13. Document findings.

Notify RN or physician if
- *The patient suddenly complains of increasing dyspnea.*
- *The drainage chamber is full and needs to be changed.*

If a chest tube is accidentally pulled out before the pneumothorax is resolved, air can reenter the pleural space. Some physicians want an occlusive dressing placed over the site to prevent air from reentering. However, an occlusive dressing increases the risk of trapped air building up and placing pressure on the heart. You should be aware of the preferences of the patient's physician.

Stripping and Milking

In the past, it was routine to strip and milk the tubing from the patient to the drainage system to dislodge clots and maintain patency. Stripping is done by holding the proximal end of the tubing and using the other hand to squeeze the tubing between two fingers while sliding the fingers toward the drainage system. This is repeated on small sections of tubing until all have been stripped. It is now known, however, that this process can create negative pressure at the openings in the tubing that are within the pleural space, which can suck lung tissue in and cause damage. Stripping should be done only if it is ordered by the physician.

Milking is done by gently squeezing portions of tubing from the patient to the system without any sliding motion. This is somewhat safer for the patient but is still not done routinely. If tubing appears to be occluded, consult with the physician for specific orders.

Removal of Chest Tube

When the reason for the chest tube is resolved, the physician removes it and places petroleum jelly gauze and a sterile occlusive dressing over the site. Continue to watch for development of crepitus and to monitor the dressing site and respiratory status.

CRITICAL THINKING

Miss Israel

■ Miss Israel has a chest tube in place for a spontaneous pneumothorax. You note that the water seal chamber is bubbling vigorously. (1) What could cause bubbling in the water seal chamber? What should you do? (2) You are totaling intake and output for your 8-hour shift. There is 240 mL of serous fluid in the drainage chamber of the drainage system at 10 p.m. At 2 p.m., there was 190 mL. How much output should you record?

Suggested answers at end of chapter.

specific assessment and care. If permitted by the physician, patients can be free to move around with the chest tube and drainage system. The drainage system must always be kept upright and below the level of the chest. If the patient must be transported, the drainage system is transported with the patient. Ask the physician if the patient can be safely transported without suction. The suction control chamber is then left open to allow air to escape. Tubing is not clamped for transport.

Tracheostomy

A **tracheotomy** is a surgical opening through the base of the neck into the trachea. It is called a **tracheostomy** when it is more permanent and has a tube inserted into the opening to maintain patency (Fig. 29.19). The patient breathes

---

tracheotomy: trach—trachea + otomy—incision
tracheostomy: trache—trachea + ostomy—opening or mouth

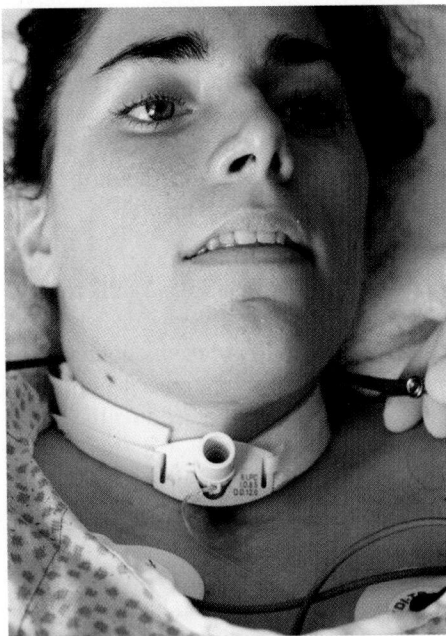

FIGURE 29.19 Patient with tracheostomy.

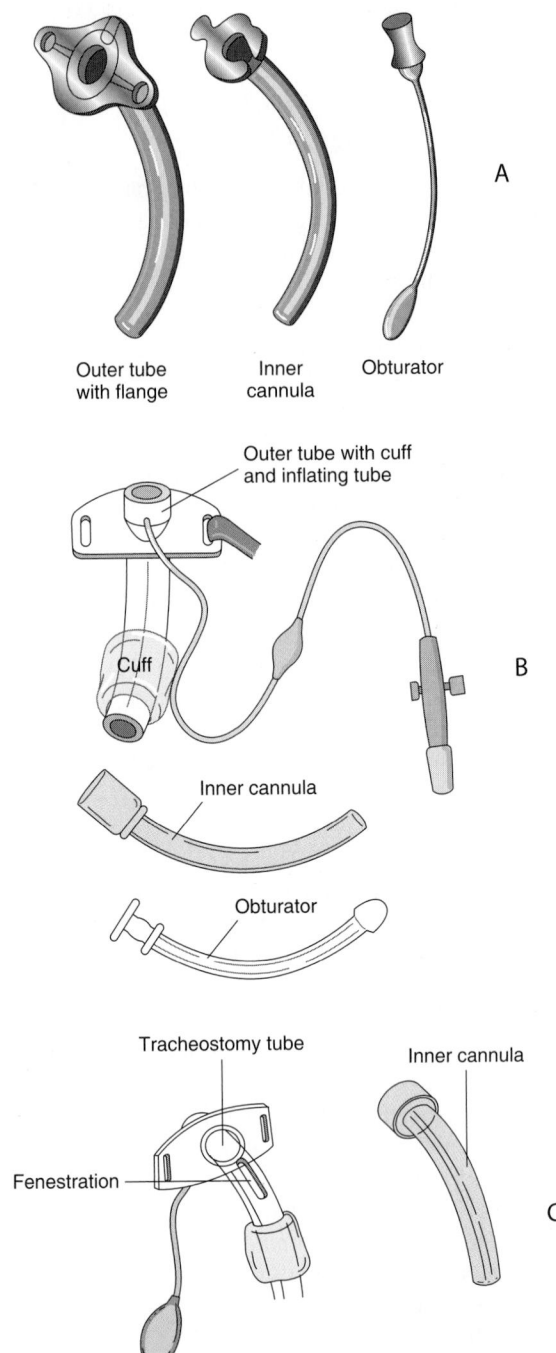

FIGURE 29.20 Tracheostomy tube. *(A)* Metal tube. *(B)* Cuffed plastic tube. *(C)* Fenestrated tube.

through this opening, bypassing the upper airways. A tracheostomy is performed for a variety of reasons, such as in patients who have had a cancerous larynx removed, patients with airway obstruction caused by trauma or tumor, patients who have difficulty clearing secretions from the airway, and patients who need prolonged mechanical ventilation.

The tracheostomy tube consists of three parts: an outer cannula, an inner cannula, and an obturator (Fig. 29.20). The obturator is a guide that is used only during insertion of the tube. After insertion, the obturator is immediately removed and kept at the bedside (commonly taped to the wall above the bed) for emergency use if the tracheostomy tube is accidentally removed. The outer cannula remains in place at all times and is secured by ties to prevent dislodging. The inner cannula is removed at intervals; usually every 8 hours and as needed for cleaning. Some newer tracheostomy tubes eliminate the need for an inner cannula. The tube may be metal or plastic. Plastic tubes generally have disposable inner cannulas, which can be replaced rather than cleaned. Plastic tubes may also have balloonlike cuffs that are inflated to prevent air escape during mechanical ventilation and to prevent aspiration of food or secretions. Institution policy may dictate that cuffs be deflated routinely to prevent tissue damage. See Box 29.3 Tracheostomy Cleaning Procedure for routine tracheostomy cleaning.

Communication is problematic for the patient with a tracheostomy tube because air is diverted out the tube rather than past the vocal cords and out the mouth. Fenestrated tubes are tubes with openings (fenestra) in the cannula to allow air to flow up into the larynx for speaking (see Fig. 29.20). The patient can be taught to plug the opening of the tube while speaking to divert air through the fenestra. Another option is a valve such as the Passy-Muir Tracheostomy and Ventilator Swallowing and Speaking Valve (Fig.

29.21). This is a special valve that allows air into the tracheostomy during inspiration but closes and redirects air up through the vocal cords and out the nose and mouth on expiration, allowing the patient to speak. For the valve to work, the tracheostomy tube must be small enough for air to flow around it or it must be fenestrated to allow air to flow up through the vocal cords. If cuffed, the cuff must be completely deflated.

Some tracheostomies are permanent. However, some patients can be weaned from the tracheostomy tube when

Box 29.3

Tracheostomy Cleaning Procedure

1. Assemble equipment: tracheostomy care kit, sterile water or saline, suction equipment, hydrogen peroxide.
2. Explain the procedure to the patient.
3. Suction inner cannula if necessary. See Box 29.6 Suctioning Procedure for the Patient with a Tracheostomy.
4. Open and prepare the kit, keeping all equipment sterile. Fill one side of basin with half peroxide and half saline and the other with saline.
5. Don clean gloves.
6. Remove old tracheostomy dressing.
7. Remove inner cannula from tracheostomy tube and place it in peroxide solution.
8. While inner cannula is removed, the patient may be suctioned if necessary.
9. Don sterile gloves.
10. Use brush and pipe cleaners to clean inner cannula. Place in water or saline to rinse. Dry inside of cannula with pipe cleaner. Reinsert into tracheostomy tube.
11. Use cotton swab and sterile gauze with sterile peroxide and saline to clean around tracheostomy site. Rinse with saline to prevent skin irritation.
12. Replace ties. Remove old ties after new ties are securely in place.
13. Apply sterile tracheostomy dressing (drain sponge or "trach pants"). Use precut or folded dressing. Cutting gauze creates fibers that can enter the tracheostomy.
    NOTE: A procedure manual should be consulted for more detailed instruction.

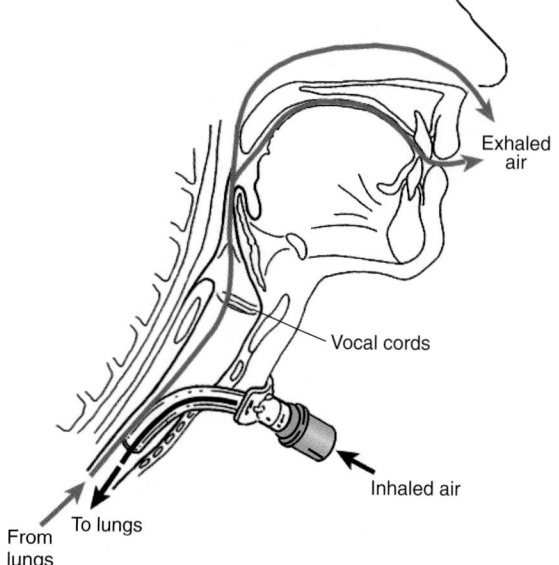

FIGURE 29.21 The Passy-Muir Tracheostomy Speaking Valve allows air into the tracheostomy during inspiration but closes and redirects air up through the vocal cords and out the nose and mouth on expiration, allowing the patient to speak *(Courtesy of Passy-Muir, Inc., Irvine, CA).*

CRITICAL THINKING

Mr. Smith

■ Mr. Smith had a plastic cuffed tracheostomy tube that was small enough to allow airflow around it for talking when the cuff was deflated. The cuff was inflated for lunch to prevent him from aspirating. A friend stopped by for a chat and assisted Mr. Smith to plug his tracheostomy so he could talk. Mr. Smith's face turned dark red, and his expression showed extreme anxiety.
1. What happened?
2. How could you help prevent this in the future?
3. How would you document this occurrence?
Suggested answers at end of chapter.

their condition has improved enough to allow breathing without it. The physician may replace the tube with a smaller tube to prepare the patient for its removal. This allows a plug to be inserted into the tracheostomy tube at intervals to force the patient to breathe around the tube through the nose and mouth. When the tracheostomy tube has been removed, the opening may be taped shut and covered with gauze until it is healed. The gauze often becomes saturated with secretions and is changed as needed.

Nursing Process for the Patient with a Tracheostomy

See Box 29.4 Nursing Care Plan for the Patient with a Tracheostomy.

Suctioning

Suctioning involves the use of a flexible catheter to remove secretions from the respiratory tract of a patient who is unable to cough effectively. This may be a patient with overwhelming secretions or a patient with a tracheostomy or endotracheal tube.

The procedures for suctioning are presented in Boxes 29.5 and 29.6. A procedure manual should be consulted for more detailed instruction. Remember that suctioning is both frightening and uncomfortable for a patient. Patients sometimes feel as though oxygen is being "vacuumed" from their lungs. Suctioning can cause hypoxia, vagal stimulation with resulting bradycardia, and even cardiac arrest. It is done only when necessary rather than on a routine basis. Coughing is the most effective way to clear secretions and should be encouraged if the patient is capable. Signs that suctioning is needed include crackles or wheezes heard with or without a stethoscope or a dropping oxygen saturation.

(Text continued on page 570)

Box 29.4   NURSING CARE PLAN for the Patient with a Tracheostomy

Nursing Diagnosis: Risk for ineffective airway clearance related to increase in secretions

Expected Outcomes Airway is free of secretions as evidenced by no audible crackles or wheezes in airway, inner cannula clear.

Evaluation of Outcome Is airway free of secretions?

Intervention	Rationale	Evaluation
Assess lung sounds every 4 hours and pm.	Coarse crackles or wheezes may indicate secretions in airways.	Are coarse crackles or wheezes present?
Encourage patient to deep breathe and cough as able.	Patients may be able to clear own secretions without suctioning.	Is patient able to cough up secretions effectively?
Encourage fluids if not contraindicated.	Fluids help hydrate secretions, making them easier to cough up.	Is patient taking adequate fluids? Are secretions thin?
Encourage ambulation as able, or turn every 2 hours.	Movement helps mobilize secretions.	Is patient mobilized as much as possible?
Clean tracheostomy according to agency policy. (See Box 29.3 Tracheostomy Cleaning Procedure.)	Cleaning helps remove excess mucus and keeps airway clear.	Does cleaning help maintain an open airway?
Suction patient using sterile technique pm (Box 29.6 Suctioning Procedure for the Pathient with a Tracheostomy). Suction only when necessary.	Suctioning clears secretions from airways. Unnecessary suctioning irritates airways.	Is suction necessary? Is airway free of secretions after suctioning?
Monitor and document amount, color, and character of secretions. Report increase in secretions accompanied by fever.	Purulent sputum accompanied by fever may indicate pneumonia.	Is sputum clear or white, and scant in amount? Was purulent sputum reported?

Nursing Diagnosis: Risk for infection related to bypass of normal respiratory defense mechanisms

Expected Outcomes Patient is free of infection, as evidenced by vital signs within normal limits, clear secretions.

Evaluation of Outcome Is patient free from symptoms of infection?

Intervention	Rationale	Evaluation
Use good hand-washing practice.	Hand-washing is important in preventing infection.	Do all caregivers use good hand-washing technique?
Monitor and report signs and symptoms of infection: fever, increased respiratory rate, purulent sputum, elevated white blood cell (WBC) count.	Early recognition and treatment of infection enhances outcome.	Are signs of infection present?
Protect tracheostomy opening from foreign material: food, sprays, powders.	Foreign materials in the tracheostomy may cause pneumonia.	Is tracheostomy adequately protected?
Use meticulous sterile technique for all tracheostomy care and suctioning.	Use of nonsterile technique may introduce microorganisms into the respiratory tract.	Is sterile technique used by all caregivers?
Encourage a well-balanced diet. Consult dietitian prn.	A well-balanced diet enhances immune function.	Is patient eating a balanced diet or receiving adequate supplementation?
Take measures to prevent aspiration of food or secretions.	Aspiration can cause pneumonia.	Is there evidence that the patient is aspirating?

Nursing Diagnosis: Impaired verbal communication related to presence of tracheostomy tube

Expected Outcomes Patient uses alternate methods of communication effectively. Patient expresses satisfaction with ability to communicate needs.

Evaluation of Outcome Is patient able to use alternative methods to express needs? Does patient express satisfaction with ability to do so?

Intervention	Rationale	Evaluation
Take time to allow patient to communicate needs.	Communication takes time; patient may become frustrated if hurried.	Does patient feel he or she is given adequate time for communication of needs?
Watch for patient's nonverbal cues.	Gestures and facial expression can provide valuable cues.	Is the patient attempting to communicate with nonverbal cues?
Offer pen and paper or magic slate (if patient is literate).	The patient may be able to write out his or her needs/concerns.	Is patient able to write out needs?
Use picture board (available from Speech Therapy Department).	The patient can point to a picture (water, toileting) that indicates his or her need.	Is patient able to point appropriately to needs?
Teach patient with fenestrated or small tracheostomy tube how to cover opening with a plug or clean finger in order to talk.	Covering opening diverts air into larynx and allows speech.	Is patient able to communicate in this manner?
Consult with speech therapist.	Speech therapist may have additional methods for communicating with patient.	Did speech therapist provide alternative communication techniques?

Nursing Diagnosis: Disturbed body image related to presence of tracheostomy

Expected Outcomes Patient verbalizes acceptance of tracheostomy. Patient is willing to participate in tracheostomy care.

Evaluation of Outcomes Does patient verbalize acceptance of tracheostomy? Does patient participate in learning to care for tracheostomy?

Intervention	Rationale	Evaluation
Assess patient's feelings about tracheostomy.	Assessment provides basis for care.	Are the patient's feelings within an expected range for such a change in body image?
Approach patient with an accepting attitude.	The patient will be aware of the nurse's nonverbal body language.	Does the patient indicate a feeling of acceptance from the nurse?
Allow patient opportunity to verbalize concerns about tracheostomy.	Verbalizing concerns helps the patient to sort out feelings and problem solve.	Does the patient verbalize feelings as needed? (Note: Some patients do not wish to share feelings and should not be forced to do so.)
Refer patient to support group if available.	The patient may benefit from talking with others with tracheostomies.	Is patient receptive to a support group referral?
Assist patient in finding attractive ways to conceal tracheostomy if desired.	Loose scarves or collars can help conceal and protect the tracheostomy.	Is patient satisfied with appearance of tracheostomy?

(Continued on following page)

Box 29.4   NURSING CARE PLAN for the Patient with a Tracheostomy (Continued)

Nursing Diagnosis: Deficient knowledge related to care of new tracheostomy

Expected Outcomes Patient and significant other will verbalize understanding of self-care, demonstrate tracheostomy self-care procedures, and state resources for help after discharge.

Evaluation of Outcomes Are patient and significant other able to verbalize self-care actions and rationale? Are patient and significant other able to correctly demonstrate care procedures? Is patient able to state how to obtain help after discharge?

Intervention	Rationale	Evaluation
Assess patient's and significant other's baseline knowledge of self-care.	Teaching should only be initiated if a knowledge deficit exists.	Does patient exhibit knowledge of self-care?
Instruct patient and significant other in the following (see text for specific instruction): • Tracheostomy cleaning • Deep breathing and coughing • Suctioning • Prevention of infection and symptoms to report to health care provider • Protection of tracheostomy from pollutants, water (no swimming, careful showering)	The patient will need to care for self after discharge.	Does patient verbalize understanding of self-care and demonstrate all procedures correctly?
Provide follow-up with home health nurse after discharge.	A home health nurse can provide reinforcement of instruction at home.	Is patient receptive to having a home health nurse assist?

Each step should be explained to the patient during suctioning even if he or she is unresponsive.

Intubation

Some patients are unable to breathe effectively and maintain adequate oxygenation because of airway obstruction or respiratory failure. These patients are intubated with a special endotracheal (ET) tube through the nose or mouth and into the trachea (Fig. 29.22). Patients in cardiopulmonary arrest are intubated during advanced cardiac life support, and patients undergoing general anesthesia during surgery are intubated and mechanically ventilated. Most intubated patients are also mechanically ventilated. Some patients have advance directives that indicate that they do not wish to be intubated. You should be familiar with the patient's wishes and bring them to the attention of the physician if necessary.

Because intubation can damage the vocal cords and surrounding tissues, it is usually a short-term intervention. Patients who need long-term ventilatory support have a tracheostomy tube placed.

NURSING CARE. Nursing care of the intubated patient includes regular assessment of the patient's respiratory status and tube placement. Lung sounds are auscultated bilaterally to ensure that the tube has not been displaced into one bronchus. The tube is carefully secured with tape or a Velcro holder to avoid dislodging. Oral tubes are repositioned and resecured to the opposite side of the mouth every 24 hours or according to institution policy to prevent tissue damage. An adhesive skin barrier should be applied under the tape to protect the skin. If the patient is alert, he or she is instructed to be careful not to pull on the tube. You may need to obtain an order for soft wrist restraints if absolutely necessary for the confused patient. Restraints can be avoided if a family member is available to sit with the patient. Some nursing interventions for the patient with a tracheostomy are also appropriate for the intubated patient. (See Box 29.4 Nursing Care Plan for the Patient with a Tracheostomy.)

Endotracheal tubes have a cuff (a balloonlike area around the tube) to help maintain proper placement and to prevent leakage of air around the tube. An RT usually inflates

Box 29.5

Oropharyngeal or Nasopharyngeal Suction Procedure

1. Gather equipment: sterile suction catheter, sterile gloves, sterile container (these items may be found in a single "cath and glove" kit); sterile water or saline, suction machine with tubing.
2. Explain procedure to patient.
3. Connect catheter to suction tubing, keeping catheter inside sterile sleeve. Turn on suction to level specified by institution policy (usually 80–120 mm Hg for wall suction).
4. Pour saline into sterile container.
5. Put on sterile gloves. Keep dominant hand sterile at all times.
6. Suction small amount of saline into catheter to rinse catheter and test suction.
7. Have patient take several deep breaths.
8. With thumb control uncovered to stop suction, insert suction catheter through mouth or nose into the trachea until resistance is met or patient coughs.
9. Slowly withdraw catheter, suctioning intermittently while rotating it. The entire procedure should take no more than 10 to 15 seconds.
10. After allowing patient to rest, repeat steps 6 through 9 two more times if needed.
    NOTE: A procedure manual should be consulted for more detailed instruction.

Box 29.6

Suctioning Procedure for the Patient with a Tracheostomy

1. Gather equipment: sterile suction catheter, sterile gloves, sterile container (these items may be found in a single "cath and glove" kit); sterile water or saline, suction machine with tubing, manual resuscitation bag.
2. Explain procedure to patient.
3. Connect catheter to suction tubing, keeping catheter inside sterile sleeve. Turn on suction to level specified by institution policy (usually 80 to 120 mm Hg for wall suction). Connect oxygen source to manual resuscitation bag.
4. Pour saline into sterile container.
5. Put on sterile gloves. Keep dominant hand sterile at all times.
6. Suction small amount of saline into catheter.
7. Oxygenate patient with three ventilations using a manual resuscitation bag connected to an oxygen source, using the nonsterile hand. If the patient is mechanically ventilated, use manual sigh.
8. With thumb control uncovered to stop suction, insert suction catheter through tracheostomy tube until patient coughs or resistance is met.
9. Slowly withdraw catheter, suctioning intermittently while rotating it. The entire procedure should take no more than 15 seconds.
10. Allow patient to rest.
11. Repeat steps 6 through 10 two more times if needed. Some older sources recommend instilling sterile saline into the tracheostomy to loosen secretions. *This should be avoided.* It is now known that this procedure is not effective and may actually cause a drop in the patient's SaO_2
    NOTE: A procedure manual should be consulted for more detailed instruction.

the cuff and maintains a specific cuff pressure and should be consulted for assistance with this activity.

Patients with ET tubes may need suctioning if they are unable to cough effectively. Visible secretions in the tube, crackles or wheezes heard with or without the stethoscope, or a drop in SaO_2 without another obvious cause are signs that suctioning is necessary. The ET tube suctioning procedure is sterile and is the same as suctioning a tracheostomy tube. Some institutions have in-line suctioning devices, which are connected to the ET tube within a sterile sleeve. This maintains sterility, protects the nurse, and simplifies the suctioning procedure. Oral suction keeps the mouth free of secretions.

The intubated patient is often extremely anxious, especially if she or he is alert. Explain the purpose of all care activities. Suctioning is particularly anxiety-producing and should be explained carefully even if the patient is unresponsive.

Intubated patients are at risk of developing ventilator-associated pneumonia (VAP) because normal respiratory defense mechanisms are bypassed. Good hand washing and frequent mouth care to reduce risk of aspirating oral microorganisms can help prevent VAP.

Because the ET tube passes between the vocal cords, the patient is unable to speak. Provide paper and pencil or a picture board for communication. Yes/no questions can be answered by a nod or shake of the head.

Monitor arterial blood gas and oxygen saturation values and notify the physician of changes. If oxygen values drop or the patient becomes confused or agitated, the patient should be immediately inspected for a disconnected oxygen source or excessive secretions.

If the physician determines that the patient can breathe effectively without the tube, the tube will be removed. The patient will be slowly weaned from the ventilator first. Prior

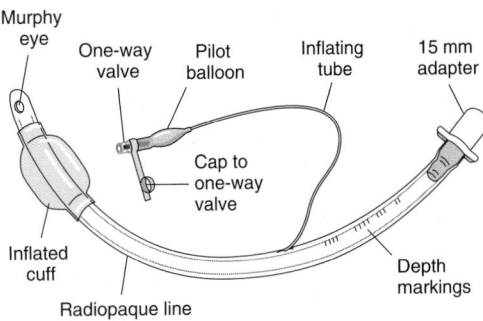

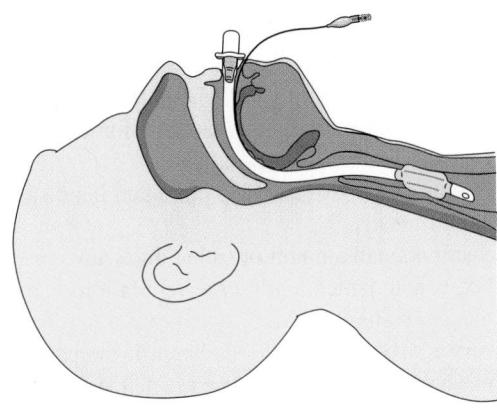

Placement of tube in airway

FIGURE 29.22 Endotracheal tube. *(Modified from Barnes, TA: Respiratory Care Principles. F.A. Davis, Philadelphia, 1991, p 425.)*

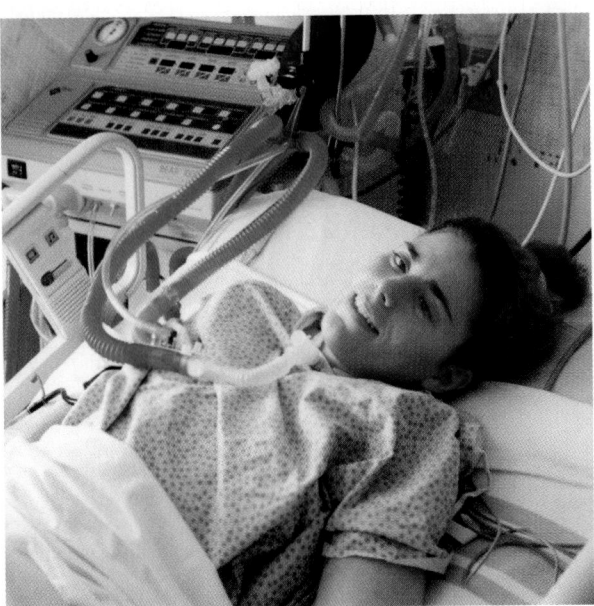

FIGURE 29.23 Patient on ventilator.

in the system. This can be caused by disconnected tubing, leaks in tubing or around the ET tube, or an underinflated cuff. A low-pressure alarm may also sound if the patient has attempted to remove the tube.

High-pressure alarms sound for higher than normal resistance to airflow. This might occur if the patient needs to be suctioned; if the patient is biting on the tube, coughing, or trying to talk; if tubing is kinked or otherwise obstructed; or if worsening respiratory disease causes decreased lung

to tube removal, the patient's mouth and tube are suctioned and the cuff is deflated. After removal, the patient is observed closely for laryngeal edema or respiratory distress. The patient is maintained in high Fowler's position to maximize chest expansion.

Mechanical Ventilation

Ventilators are devices that provide ventilation (respirations) for patients who are unable to breathe effectively on their own (Fig. 29.23). Ventilators use positive pressure to push oxygenated air via a cuffed ET or tracheostomy tube into the lungs at preset intervals. Patients may need mechanical ventilation after some surgeries, after cardiac or respiratory arrest, for declining arterial blood gases related to worsening respiratory disease, or for neuromuscular disease or injury that affects the muscles of respiration.

Ventilator Modes

Ventilators can control ventilation or assist the patient's own respirations. See Table 29.9 for terms that aid understanding of ventilator function. There are many types and models of ventilators. Consult with the respiratory care department for an explanation of a patient's ventilator and how to troubleshoot alarms that may sound.

Ventilator Alarms

Several types of alarms are found on ventilators. Low-pressure alarms sound if the ventilator senses reduced pressure

TABLE 29.9 VENTILATOR TERMINOLOGY

FIO_2	Fraction of inspired oxygen.
Tidal volume	Amount of air delivered with each breath.
Rate	Frequency of breaths delivered.
Assist control mode (AC; also called continuous mechanical ventilation, or CMV)	Ventilator delivers a breath each time patient begins to inspire. If patient does not breathe, the machine continues to deliver a preset number of breaths per minute.
Synchronized intermittent mandatory ventilation (SIMV)	Allows patient to breathe independently but delivers a minimum number of ventilations per minute as necessary. Synchronized to patient's own respiratory pattern.
Pressure support (PS)	Provides positive pressure on inspiration to decrease the work of breathing.
Continuous positive airway pressure (CPAP)	Provides positive pressure on inspiration and expiration to keep alveoli open in a spontaneously breathing patient.
Positive end-expiratory pressure (PEEP)	Provides positive pressure on expiration to help keep small airways open.

compliance. In addition, the high-pressure alarm may be triggered if the patient is anxious and is unable to time his or her breaths with those of the ventilator. Water in the tubing might also cause a high-pressure alarm. Consult with the respiratory care department for guidance in draining the tubing.

A loss of power alarm may signal a power failure or a disconnected plug. Be aware of emergency power sources and be prepared to manually ventilate if necessary. Volume and frequency alarms sound when tidal volume or number of breaths per minute fall outside preset parameters.

When an alarm sounds, always check the patient first. If the patient is stable, the machine may then be checked. Determine why the alarm is sounding and correct the problem quickly. If no cause can be found, disconnect the patient from the ventilator and call for help. Use a manual resuscitation bag until an RT arrives.

NURSING RESPONSIBILITIES. Before initiating mechanical ventilation, it is important that the health-care team be aware of advance directives and consult with the patient and family because many patients do not wish to be intubated and mechanically ventilated. Some patients accept mechanical ventilation if it is a temporary measure but not if it might be a permanent intervention.

Until recently, ventilators were used only in intensive care units. Now ventilators are seen on medical-surgical units, in nursing homes, and even in patients' homes. It is important that a team approach be used when caring for a mechanically ventilated patient. The social worker; RT; physical, occupational, and speech therapists; dietitian; nurse; and physician all work together to provide the comprehensive care needed by the patient. Respiratory therapists usually take responsibility for routine monitoring and equipment maintenance. The nurse is responsible for monitoring the patient, ensuring that ventilator settings are maintained as prescribed, providing initial response to alarms, keeping tubing free from water accumulation, and keeping the patient's airway free from secretions. In addition, the nurse keeps a manual resuscitation bag at the bedside for emergencies.

Good nursing care is essential for preventing ventilator-associated complications, especially pneumonia. Keep the head of the bed at a 45-degree angle to reduce the risk of aspiration. Oral care including toothbrushing every 12 hours and sponge Toothettes every 2 to 4 hours helps keep oral bacteria under control. Regular suctioning helps keep the airway clear.[1] Good nutrition is also essential, and has been shown to be related to eventual successful weaning.

Patients who are mechanically ventilated are unable to talk and can become very uncomfortable and anxious with no easy way to communicate. See Box 29.7 Tips for Caring for Mechanically Ventilated Patients for one nurse's tips for making ventilated patients feel more secure. These tips were developed after the author interviewed 12 patients who had been intubated. They shared their fears, anxieties, and physical discomforts.

Box 29.7

Tips for Caring for Mechanically Ventilated Patients

- Introduce yourself to the patient each time you enter the room. Make sure he or she can see you.
- Explain everything you are about to do.
- Check ventilator settings regularly.
- Give sedatives or antianxiety drugs as ordered. Request an order if necessary. Find out cause of unexplained anxiety (patient may be hypoxemic).
- Reassure the patient that anxiety is normal and that relaxing will help the ventilator to work with him or her.
- Assess for comfort and reposition at regular intervals. Be careful not to pull on the ventilator tubing. (Pulling hurts.)
- Suction quickly and smoothly, without jabbing. Avoid the use of saline with suctioning.
- Provide good oral care, moistening the lips with a cool washcloth and water-based lubricant. (Patients get thirsty.)
- Use restraints only as a last resort.
- Take the time to communicate with the patient. Talk to him or her, and provide a magic slate or pen and paper for the patient to talk to you. Make sure the call light is within reach at all times.
- Answer patient's call light and ventilator alarms promptly.

Source: Modified from Jablonski, RAS: If ventilator patients could talk. RN, 58:2:32, 1995.

Noninvasive Positive-Pressure Ventilation

Noninvasive positive-pressure ventilation (NIPPV) is an alternative to intubation and mechanical ventilation for patients who are able to breathe on their own but are unable to maintain normal blood gases. Patients with severe respiratory disease, sleep apnea, or neuromuscular diseases such as amyotrophic lateral sclerosis (ALS) that weaken respiratory muscles can benefit from this treatment. Instead of the invasive endotracheal or tracheostomy tube, NIPPV uses an external masklike device that fits over the nose or mouth and nose (Fig. 29.24). It can be successful in patients who are alert, able to cooperate, do not have excessive secretions, and are able to breathe on their own for periods of time. It can be used with or without supplemental oxygen. In an acutely ill patient, oxygen saturations are monitored.

Two basic types of NIPPV are available: continuous positive airway pressure (CPAP) and bilevel positive airway pressure (BiPAP, Respironics, Inc. Murrysville, PA). In CPAP, the same amount of positive pressure is maintained throughout inspiration and expiration to prevent airway col-

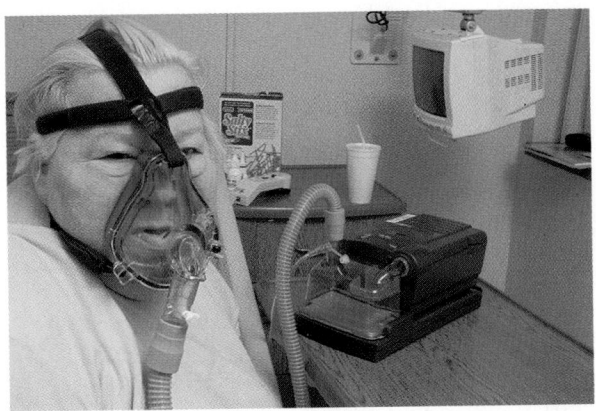

FIGURE 29.24 Noninvasive positive-pressure ventilation. Note round face from steroid use.

lapse. In BiPAP, a different level of positive pressure is used on inspiration and expiration.

Problems to be alert for in patients receiving NIPPV include skin irritation from the mask and gastric distention from swallowing air. Apply an adhesive skin barrier to the areas that come in contact with the mask to prevent irritation. To prevent gastric distention, place the patient in semi-Fowler's position and consult with the RT to adjust air delivery pressure if necessary. Topical saline or a special humidifier on the machine can reduce nose and mouth dryness. An air leak around the mask can cause air to blow in the patient's eyes, which can be irritating. If this happens, remove the mask and reposition it. Another problem is patient acceptance of NIPPV. Many patients do not like the tight mask covering their nose or mouth. Be patient in explaining the reason for this treatment and check the patient frequently to help control anxiety. Be sure to assess the patient's goals for therapy. Some patients may choose not to use NIPPV, but they must be fully aware of possible consequences.

Patients can use NIPPV nearly continuously, removing it to eat or use the bathroom. Other patients use it only when they are sleeping and are able to breathe effectively on their own during the day. Some use it for a few days until an acute exacerbation of disease is resolved, and others continue its use indefinitely at home.

REVIEW QUESTIONS

1. During inhalation, which of the following muscle contractions takes place to enlarge the chest cavity from top to bottom?
   a. Diaphragm moves down.
   b. External intercostal muscles move down.
   c. Diaphragm moves up.
   d. Internal intercostal muscles move up.

2. Deteriorating cilia in the respiratory tract predispose the elderly to which of the following?
   a. Chronic hypoxia
   b. Pulmonary hypertension
   c. Respiratory infection
   d. Decreased ventilation

3. How should the nurse record smoking history on a patient who has smoked 2.5 packs of cigarettes per day for 10 years?
   a. Patient has smoked cigarettes for 10 years.
   b. Patient smokes 2.5 packs of cigarettes per day.
   c. Patient has a 12.5 pack-year smoking history.
   d. Patient has a 25 pack-year smoking history.

4. Which of the following terms is used to describe violin-like sounds heard on chest auscultation?
   a. Crackles
   b. Wheezes
   c. Friction rub
   d. Stridor

5. Which of the following is a normal value for oxygen saturation?
   a. Less than 60 percent
   b. 61 to 85 percent
   c. 86 to 95 percent
   d. More than 95 percent

6. Place the following steps in the correct sequential order for obtaining a sputum specimen for culture.
   a. Have the patient cough deeply from the lungs.
   b. Teach the patient to inhale deeply several times.
   c. Check the order for the test.
   d. Send the specimen immediately to the laboratory.
   e. Obtain the appropriate container.

7. Which instruction is correct when teaching a patient how to use a metered-dose inhaler?
   a. "Inhale deeply, place canister in mouth, depress top of canister, exhale."
   b. "Exhale, place canister in mouth, depress canister and inhale at the same time."
   c. "Cough, place canister in mouth, inhale deeply, cough again."
   d. "Exhale, depress canister, place in mouth, inhale deeply."

Reference

1. Lindgren, VA, and Ames, NJ: Caring for Patients on Mechanical Ventilation. AJN, 105:5, 2005.

SUGGESTED ANSWERS TO

CRITICAL THINKING

■ *Timothy*

1. There is no way to know whether Timothy needs to be in the emergency room without further assessment. Remember that shortness of breath is very subjective and must be evaluated before discharge.
2. Collect further data. Have Timothy rate his shortness of breath. Look at his color and use of accessory muscles. Check his vital signs, peak expiratory flow rate, and oxygen saturation.
3. If Timothy is having an asthma attack, one explanation for the absence of wheezing on auscultation is that he is not moving enough air to generate the wheezing sound. If his airways are extremely tight, breath sounds may be so diminished that wheezing is not heard. This is a bad sign rather than a good one. If you suspect that this is happening, call for help. The physician may want to begin treatment quickly before further evaluation is done.

■ *Miss Israel*

(1) Bubbling in the water seal chamber indicates a leak in the system. Vigorous bubbling may indicate a large leak, and the physician should be contacted immedi-ately. After you check the patient, check the entire system for cracks or leaks and correct any problems discovered. (2) 50 mL.

■ *Mr. Smith*

1. Mr. Smith plugged his tracheostomy while the cuff was still inflated, so no air could get to his lungs. If the plug is not removed immediately, he will be totally unable to breathe. Whenever the plug is in place, air must be able to travel around the tracheostomy tube or through the opening of a fenestrated tube for the patient to breathe.
2. To prevent this from happening in the future, Mr. Smith should be taught how his tracheostomy tube works and how to care for it.
3. "Trach tube cuff inflated for lunch as ordered. Answered call for help at 1230, found patient dark red in color, unable to breathe, trach plugged. Trach unplugged, respirations restored, vital signs stable. Patient stated he plugged trach so he could talk to his friend. Function of trach cuff explained to patient and friend. Both verbalize understanding to only plug trach when cuff is deflated or to call for nurse if unsure."

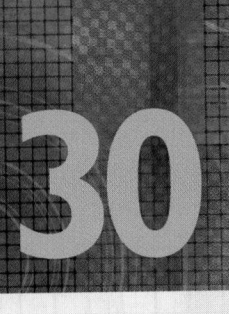

30

Nursing Care of Patients with Upper Respiratory Tract Disorders

PAULA D. HOPPER

KEY TERMS

dysphagia (dis-FAYJ-ee-ah)
epistaxis (EP-iss-TAX-iss)
exudate (EKS-yoo-dayt)
laryngectomee (lare-in-JEK-tah-mee)
laryngitis (lare-in-JIGH-tiss)
myalgia (my-AL-jee-ah)
nasoseptoplasty (NAY-zoh-SEP-toh-plass-tee)
pharyngitis (fair-in-JIGH-tiss)
rhinitis (rye-NIGH-tiss)
rhinoplasty (RYE-noh-plass-tee)
sinusitis (SINE-u-SIGH-tiss)

QUESTIONS TO GUIDE YOUR READING

1. What are the pathophysiologies of the disorders of the upper respiratory tract?

2. What are the etiologies, signs, and symptoms of disorders of the upper respiratory tract?

3. What are current therapeutic interventions for disorders of the upper respiratory tract?

4. What nursing care should you be prepared to provide for the patient with an upper respiratory disorder?

5. How will you know if your care has been effective?

6. What are the special needs of the patient who has undergone a laryngectomy?

Disorders of the upper respiratory tract include problems occurring in the nose, sinuses, pharynx, larynx, and trachea. Many of these problems are minor illnesses that can be cared for at home. Others can become serious if they are not recognized and treated in a timely manner.

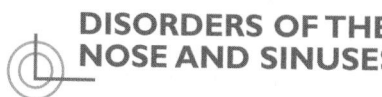

DISORDERS OF THE NOSE AND SINUSES

Epistaxis

Pathophysiology

Epistaxis is more commonly known as a nosebleed. The nose can bleed either from the anterior or posterior region. Anterior bleeds are much more common and originate from a group of vessels called the Kiesselbach plexus. Anterior bleeds are easier to locate and treat than posterior bleeds because the blood vessels of the posterior nose are larger and bleeding can be severe and difficult to control.

Etiology

The most common cause of epistaxis is dry, cracked mucous membranes. Trauma, forceful nose blowing, nose picking, and increased pressure on fragile capillaries from hypertension are also factors. Anything that reduces the blood's ability to clot, such as hemophilia or leukemia, regular aspirin use, anticoagulant therapy, or chemotherapy, can also predispose a patient to nosebleeds. Cocaine use can also cause epistaxis.

Therapeutic Interventions

Instruct the patient with a nosebleed to sit in a chair and lean forward slightly to avoid aspirating or swallowing blood. If the patient swallows blood, it will be difficult to assess the extent of bleeding, and it might cause nausea and vomiting. Be sure to wear gloves and follow standard precautions. Place pressure on the nares for 5 to 10 minutes to stop bleeding. However, avoid placing pressure on the nose if a fracture is suspected to avoid further trauma. Ice packs to the nose and eye area may be used to constrict the bleeding vessels.

If first aid measures are ineffective in stopping bleeding, a physician may attempt more invasive treatment. Local application of a vasoconstrictive agent might be used to constrict the bleeding vessels. If the bleeding vessel can be located, the physician may cauterize it by use of an electrical cauterizing device, or by application of silver nitrate.

Gauze may be used to pack the anterior or posterior nasal cavity. The anterior cavity is packed firmly but gently, usually with half-inch petroleum gauze. To pack the posterior cavity, the physician must use a catheter and string via the nose to draw the packing through the mouth and into the posterior nasal cavity (Fig. 30.1). The strings are then brought out the mouth and taped to the patient's face so they can be used 2 to 4 days later to remove the packing. Placement and removal of packing can be very uncomfortable for the patient. If there is time, administration of an analgesic before the procedure is helpful. Petroleum jelly on the packing helps prevent gauze from adhering to the nasal

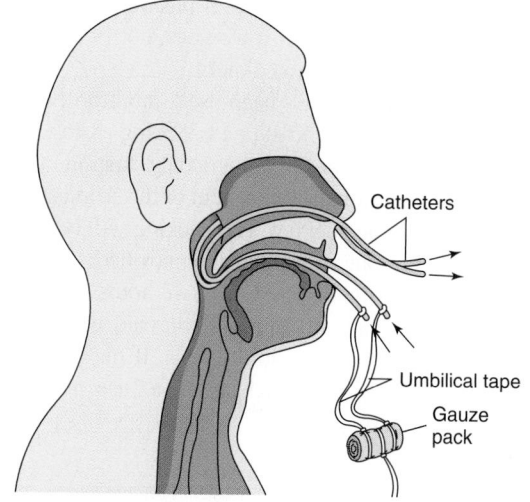

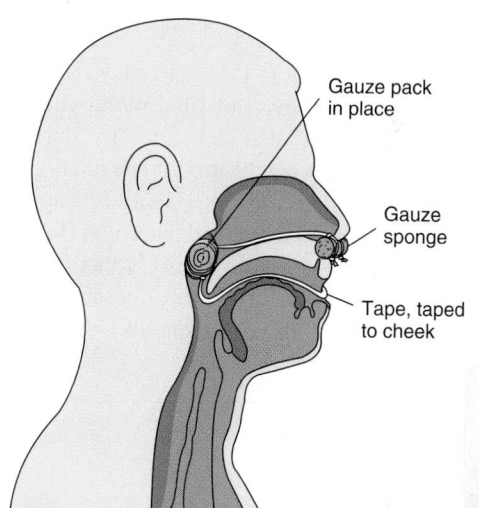

FIGURE 30.1 Nasal packing. *(A)* Catheters are used to pull packing into place. *(B)* Nasal packing in place.

mucosa. If the packing is to remain in place for a prolonged period, it is coated with an antibiotic ointment to reduce the risk of infection.

Additional products such as compressed sponges and nasal tampons are also available to pack the nose. A nasal balloon catheter employs a catheter with a balloon on the end (a specially made catheter, or a Foley catheter) that is inflated after placing it near the bleeding vessels in the nasal cavity. The inflated balloon places pressure on the bleeding vessels to stop the bleeding.

If the patient has lost a significant amount of blood, a transfusion may be necessary. Nosebleeds rarely cause death because blood loss lowers blood pressure, which in turn slows the bleeding. Ultimately the cause of the epistaxis is determined and corrected if possible.

Nursing Care

Monitor bleeding, noting the amount and color of drainage. Monitor vital signs and hemoglobin level for signs of excessive blood loss. If the patient swallows repeatedly, inspect the back of the throat for bleeding. If bleeding does not stop within 10 to 15 minutes, or if it worsens, notify a registered nurse (RN) or physician immediately.

If posterior packing has been used, monitor the patient for airway obstruction from slipped packing. Know how to remove the packing in case of emergency. Institute comfort measures, and maintain the placement of the strings that will be used to remove the packing. The packing will be removed by the physician. Once bleeding is controlled, caution the patient not to blow the nose for up to 48 hours and to avoid nose picking. The patient should also avoid bending over, which can increase pressure in the nose. If the cause of the bleeding is dryness, teach the patient to use nasal saline spray or a room humidifier.

CRITICAL THINKING

Mr. Jondahl

■ Mr. Jondahl is brought to the emergency room with a nosebleed. His vital signs are BP 140/90, pulse 92, respirations 20. He states that he has never had a nosebleed before. He denies any history of coagulation disorders. His current medications include captopril (Capoten), furosemide (Lasix), and ibuprofen (Motrin). What are two areas you should assess further in trying to determine a cause? (Hint: If you are not familiar with Mr. Jondahl's medications, look them up.)

Suggested answers at end of chapter.

Nasal Polyps

Pathophysiology and Etiology
Polyps are grapelike clusters of mucosa in the nasal passages. They are usually benign, but they can obstruct the nasal passages. Although the exact cause is unknown, they are related to chronic inflammation, and people with allergies are prone to developing them. Some patients with nasal polyps also have asthma and are allergic to aspirin. This is called aspirin triad disease because the three components often occur together.

Therapeutic Interventions
Control of allergy symptoms may help control polyp development. Oral antihistamines or nasal corticosteroid sprays can help control inflammation. If polyps obstruct breathing, they can be removed. This is done as an outpatient procedure under local anesthesia, using laser or endoscopic surgery. Patients are taught to avoid aspirin products following surgery because they increase the risk of postoperative bleeding and recurrence of the polyps.

Deviated Septum

Pathophysiology and Etiology
The septum dividing the nasal passages is slightly deviated in most adults. This may result from nasal trauma but often

has no cause. Some septa may be so deviated that they block sinus drainage or interfere with breathing.

Signs and Symptoms
The patient may complain of a chronically stuffy nose or discomfort from blocked sinus drainage. Some patients experience headaches and nosebleeds.

Therapeutic Interventions
If the deviated septum is causing chronic discomfort, a submucous resection (SMR), or **nasoseptoplasty,** can be done. This surgery involves making an incision through the mucous membrane covering the septum and revising or removing the deviated portion. Nasal packing is then placed to reduce bleeding. This is generally done as an outpatient surgical procedure, under local anesthetic.

Nursing Care
Monitor vital signs and bleeding until the patient is stable following surgery. Excessive swallowing should alert you to check for blood running down the back of the throat. The patient will have nasal packing and a "mustache dressing" of folded gauze under the nose to catch drainage.

Most patients are discharged home once they are stable, so teaching is important. The patient should maintain a semi-Fowler's position as much as possible and avoid anything that might increase pressure and cause bleeding, such as sneezing, coughing, or straining to move the bowels. Stool softeners and cough suppressants may be ordered by the physician if necessary. Aspirin and related medications are avoided because they increase the risk of bleeding. Antibiotics may be ordered if packing is in place because of the risk of infection from nasal bacteria. The physician should be contacted for specific orders if the patient is on anticoagulant therapy at home. Ice can be used to reduce swelling and bruising. Instruct the patient to contact the physician if fever, excessive pain, swelling, or bleeding occurs and to return in 24 to 48 hours for removal of nasal packing. See Box 30.1 Patient Teaching After Nasal Surgery.

Rhinoplasty

Rhinoplasty is the surgical reconstruction of the nose, usually for cosmetic purposes. It may also be done to correct deformity caused by trauma. Nursing care is similar to that for the patient after nasoseptoplasty, described previously and in Box 30.1 Patient Teaching After Nasal Surgery.

Sinusitis

Pathophysiology and Etiology
Sinusitis is inflammation of the mucosa of one or more sinuses. It can be either acute or chronic. Chronic sinusitis is diagnosed if symptoms are present for more than 2 months and are unresponsive to treatment. The maxillary and eth-

---

nasoseptoplasty: naso—nose + septo—septum + plasty—plastic surgery

rhinoplasty: rhin—nose + plasty—to mold

sinusitis: sinu—sinus + itis—inflammation

Box 30.1

Patient Teaching After Nasal Surgery

1. Your nose will feel stuffy and may drain. Change the moustache dressing as often as needed. Do *not* blow your nose. If you must sneeze, do so with your mouth open.
2. Drink plenty of fluids unless your physician advises otherwise.
3. Use a cool mist vaporizer to humidify air and prevent nasal drying.
4. Keep your head elevated on two pillows or sleep in a recliner chair.
5. An ice pack on your face may help reduce swelling.
6. Take pain medication as prescribed.
7. Call your physician if you have a fever higher than 101°F.
8. Return to see your physician in _____ days.

moid sinuses are the most commonly affected. The inflammation is often the result of a bacterial infection and may follow a viral upper respiratory illness. Because the mucous lining of the nose and sinuses is continuous, nasal organisms easily travel to the sinuses. When the infected mucous lining of the sinuses swells, drainage is blocked. Bacteria that normally reside in the sinuses multiply in the retained secretions. The most common infecting organisms are *Streptococcus pneumoniae* and *Haemophilus influenzae*. Other causes of sinusitis include swelling caused by allergies, fungal infection, or intubation with a nasotracheal or nasogastric tube.

Signs and Symptoms
The patient usually has pain over the region of the affected sinuses and purulent nasal discharge. If a maxillary sinus is affected, the patient experiences pain over the cheek and upper teeth. In ethmoid sinusitis, pain occurs between and behind the eyes. Pain in the forehead typically indicates frontal sinusitis. Fever may be present in acute infection, with or without generalized fatigue and foul breath.

Complications
The patient who has received inadequate treatment, or who has not complied with treatment, is at risk for complications. Uncontrolled sinusitis may spread to surrounding areas, causing osteomyelitis, cellulitis of the orbit (infection of the soft tissues around the eye), abscess, or meningitis.

Diagnostic Tests
Uncomplicated sinusitis may be diagnosed based on symptoms alone. If repeated episodes occur, x-ray examination, a computed tomographic (CT) scan, or magnetic resonance imaging (MRI) may be done to confirm the diagnosis and determine the cause. Nasal discharge may be cultured to determine appropriate antibiotic therapy.

Therapeutic Interventions
Treatment is aimed at relieving pain and promoting sinus drainage. Adrenergic nasal sprays such as oxymetazoline (Afrin, Dristan) constrict blood vessels and therefore reduce swelling, but they should be used cautiously by patients with heart disease or hypertension because vasoconstriction increases blood pressure. Sprays may be used for up to 3 days; longer use may cause rebound congestion. Hot moist packs over the affected sinus for 1 to 2 hours twice a day may help decrease inflammation. Nasal irrigation with normal saline solution and a bulb syringe has helped some sufferers of chronic sinusitis. Acetaminophen or ibuprofen is given for pain and fever. Codeine or meperidine may be used if pain is severe. Expectorants such as guaifenesin (Robitussin), fluids, and a room humidifier can help liquefy secretions. Antihistamines dry and thicken secretions and are generally avoided. Antibiotics are used only if bacterial infection is suspected, as in the patient with purulent drainage and fever. If conservative treatment does not relieve symptoms, the physician may surgically drain the affected sinus and irrigate it with normal saline or an antibiotic solution.

One drainage procedure is the Caldwell-Luc procedure. The surgeon enters the maxillary sinus above the upper teeth, under the upper lip. The infected mucosa and bone are removed, and a new, larger opening is made to drain the sinus. Newer procedures use endoscopy to open and drain a chronically infected sinus.

Nursing Care
Patients with uncomplicated sinusitis are cared for at home. Instruct the patient to increase water intake to 8 to 10 glasses per day unless contraindicated. Excess water might be contraindicated in patients with fluid overload, such as those with cardiovascular compromise or kidney disease. Pressure may be relieved if the patient maintains a semi-Fowler's position, as in a reclining chair. Explain use of hot moist packs, analgesics, and prescribed medications. Instruct the patient to finish the antibiotic prescription even if he or she is feeling better before it is completed and to call the physician if pain becomes severe or if signs of complications such as a change in level of consciousness occur.

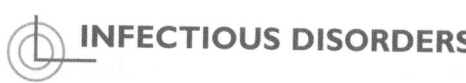

INFECTIOUS DISORDERS

Rhinitis/Common Cold
Pathophysiology and Etiology
Rhinitis (also called coryza) is inflammation of the nasal mucous membranes. The release of histamine and other substances causes vasodilation and edema, which result in symptoms. It may occur as a reaction to allergens (sometimes called hay fever) such as pollen, dust, molds, or some foods, or it may be caused by viral or bacterial infection. Viral rhinitis is another name for the common cold.

---

rhinitis: rhin—nose + itis—inflammation

TABLE 30.1 DIFFERENTIATING RESPIRATORY TRACT INFECTIONS

Signs and Symptoms	Cold	Influenza	Bacterial Infection
Onset	Slow	Sudden	Usually slow
Fever	None or low grade	Common, may be >101°F (38.3°C)	Common, may be >101°F (38.3°C)
Headache	Rare	Common	Less common
Muscle aches	Less common	Common, may be severe	Less common
Cough	Present	Present, usually dry	Present, may be dry or productive
Chest pain	Absent	Common	Common
Fatigue	Slight	Common, prolonged, may be severe	Common
Runny nose	Common	Less common	Less common
Sore throat	Common	Less common	Less common
Complications	Rare	Pneumonia	Pneumonia
Treatment	Rest and fluids	Rest and fluids, antiviral agents in some cases	Antibiotics

Signs and Symptoms

Common symptoms include nasal congestion, localized itching, sneezing, and nasal discharge. Viral or bacterial rhinitis may also be accompanied by fever and malaise. Sometimes it is difficult to differentiate between a cold and the flu. See Table 30.1 for signs and symptoms of each.

Diagnostic Tests

If allergic rhinitis is suspected, skin testing may be done to determine the offending allergens. A blood test for IgE antbodies may also be done to determine if allergies are the cause.

Therapeutic Interventions

Treatment of viral rhinitis is symptomatic. Because most colds are caused by viruses, antibiotics are not effective. In one study, however, researchers found that 60% of patients who visited their physician for cold symptoms received a prescription for an antibiotic.[1] This practice is not only expensive, it also increases the risk of developing strains of bacteria that are resistant to antibiotics. Explain to the patient that requesting antibiotics for a viral infection is not only ineffective but potentially dangerous. Teach the patient that rest and fluids are the most effective treatment (Box 30.2 Nursing Care Plan for the Patient with an Upper Respiratory Infection).

Box 30.2 NURSING CARE PLAN for the Patient with an Upper Respiratory Infection

Nursing Diagnosis: Acute pain related to infectious process

Expected Outcomes Patient will be comfortable as evidenced by (1) statement of increased comfort and (2) ability to sleep at night.

Evaluation of Outcomes (1) Does patient express comfort? (2) Is patient able to sleep?

Interventions	Rationale	Evaluation
• Assess for cause of discomfort: malaise, muscle aches, fever.	Knowing cause of discomfort helps guide intervention.	Can interventions be directed toward specific symptoms?
• Offer acetaminophen or other analgesic/antipyretics as ordered.	Analgesics relieve pain. Antipyretics relieve fever, which may contribute to discomfort.	Do analgesics/antipyretics relieve discomfort?
• Offer throat lozenges and salt-water gargles as ordered for irritated throat.	Lozenges soothe irritated mucous membranes. Saltwater gargles may reduce swelling.	Do measures relieve throat irritation?
• Encourage rest.	Physical stress increases need for sleep. Rest boosts immune function.	Is patient resting comfortably?

Nursing Diagnosis: Hyperthermia related to infectious process

Expected Outcomes (1) Temperature lower than 103°F (39.4°C). (2) No signs/symptoms of dehydration.

Evaluation of Outcomes (1) Is fever controlled at safe level? (2) Is patient well hydrated?

Interventions	Rationale	Evaluation
• Monitor temperature daily; every 4 hours if fever present.	Screening helps detect temperature changes early.	Is patient febrile?
• If patient begins chilling, recheck temperature when chilling subsides.	Chilling indicates rising temperature.	Is chilling present? Should temperature be checked more often?
• Monitor for signs of dehydration: dry skin and mucous membranes, thirst, weakness, hypotension.	Fever causes loss of body fluids.	Are signs of dehydration present?
• Encourage oral fluids if not contraindicated.	Fluids prevent or treat dehydration.	Is patient taking fluids well?
• Administer antipyretic such as acetaminophen if fever is higher than 102.5°F (39°C) or for discomfort.	Antipyretics reduce fever. Fever enhances immune function, so should only be treated if very high, if patient has a history of febrile seizures, or if patient is uncomfortable.	Is fever higher than 102.5°F (39°C)? Are antipyretics indicated? Are they effective?

Nursing Diagnosis: Risk for infection: transmission to others related to presence of infectious disease

Expected Outcomes Risk for infection of others is reduced, as evidenced by the following: (1) Patient states measures to prevent transmission. (2) Patient takes precautions against spread.

Evaluation of Outcomes Is transmission to others prevented?

Interventions	Rationale	Evaluation
• Assess patient's understanding of infection transmission.	Understanding of mode of transmission is essential to prevention.	Does patient understand how infection is transmitted?
• Based on patient's previous knowledge, teach patient and all caregivers the importance of good handwashing after contact with patient or patient's belongings, covering nose and mouth when coughing or sneezing, and not sharing eating or drinking utensils.	The nurse should build on patient's previous understanding and not repeat information. Hand washing prevents spread of infection. Covering nose and mouth prevents spread of infectious droplets. Many infections are transmitted via contaminated objects.	Does patient take precautions to prevent spread of infection?

Acetaminophen can be used for generalized discomfort. Antihistamines may help control symptoms by inhibiting the histamine response. Decongestants cause vasoconstriction, which reduces swelling and congestion. Any drugs that cause vasoconstriction should be used cautiously in patients with heart disease or hypertension. Severe allergies may be treated with desensitization ("allergy shots").

Pharyngitis

Pathophysiology and Etiology

Pharyngitis, or inflammation of the pharynx, is usually related to bacterial or viral infection. It may also occur as a result of trauma to the tissues. The most common bacterial infection is caused by beta-hemolytic streptococci, commonly referred to as strep throat. If strep throat is not treated with antibiotics, it can lead to rheumatic fever, glomerulonephritis, or other serious complications.

Signs and Symptoms

The most common symptom of pharyngitis is a sore throat. Some patients may also experience **dysphagia** (difficulty swallowing). The throat appears red and swollen, and **exudate** (drainage or pus) may be present. Exudate usually signifies bacterial infection and may be accompanied by fever, chills, headache, and generalized malaise.

Diagnostic Tests

A physician may order a throat culture and sensitivity test (explained in Chapter 29) to identify the causative organism and determine which antibiotic will be effective.

Therapeutic Interventions

If the pharyngitis is bacterial, antibiotics are ordered. Acetaminophen or throat lozenges may be used to relieve discomfort. Saltwater gargles help reduce swelling, and increased fluids (if not contraindicated) and rest are encouraged. (See Box 30.2 Nursing Care Plan for the Patient with an Upper Respiratory Infection.)

Laryngitis

Pathophysiology and Etiology

Laryngitis is an inflammation of the mucous membrane lining the larynx (voice box). It can be caused by irritation from smoking, alcohol, or chemical exposure or a viral, fungal, or bacterial infection. If often follows an upper respiratory infection.

Signs and Symptoms

The most common symptom is hoarseness. Cough, dysphagia, or fever may also be present.

Diagnostic Tests

A physician may use a laryngeal mirror to view the larynx. If hoarseness persists for more than 2 weeks, a laryngoscopy may be done to rule out cancer of the larynx.

Therapeutic Interventions

Treatment includes rest, fluids, humidified air, and aspirin (in adults) or acetaminophen. Antibiotics are used if bacterial infection is present. Encourage the patient to avoid speaking to rest the voice. Obtain a "magic slate" (from the speech therapy department) or paper and pen to help the patient communicate. Throat lozenges may help increase comfort. Help the patient to identify and avoid causative factors. (See Box 30.2 Nursing Care Plan for the Patient with an Upper Respiratory Infection.)

Tonsillitis/Adenoiditis

Pathophysiology and Etiology

The tonsils are masses of lymphoid tissue that lie on each side of the oropharynx. They filter microorganisms to protect the lungs from infection. Tonsillitis occurs when the filtering function becomes overwhelmed with a virus or bacteria and infection results. The adenoids, a mass of lymphoid tissue located at the back of the nasopharynx, can also become involved. Tonsillitis is more common in children, but it is more serious when it occurs in adults. The most common organisms causing tonsillitis are *Streptococcus* species, *Staphylococcus aureus, Haemophilus influenzae,* and *Pneumococcus* species.

Signs and Symptoms

Tonsillitis usually begins suddenly with a sore throat, fever, chills, and pain on swallowing. Generalized symptoms include headache, malaise, and **myalgia.** On examination, the tonsils appear red and swollen and may have yellow or white exudate on them. The patient's voice may sound like the patient has a hot potato in his or her mouth. If the adenoids are involved, the patient may have complaints of snoring, nasal obstruction, and a nasal tone to the voice.

Diagnostic Tests

A throat culture is done to discover the causative organism and determine effective treatment. A white blood cell count helps identify whether the infection is viral or bacterial. A chest x-ray examination may be done if respiratory symptoms are present.

Therapeutic Interventions

Antibiotics are prescribed for bacterial infection. Acetaminophen, lozenges, and saline gargles help promote comfort. For care of the patient who is not having a tonsillectomy, see Box 30.2 Nursing Care Plan for the Patient with an Upper Respiratory Infection.

TONSILLECTOMY. If tonsillitis becomes chronic, or if breathing or swallowing is affected, a tonsillectomy may be considered, although this is not a common procedure in an adult. An adenoidectomy may be performed at the same time. After the tonsillectomy, the patient is maintained in a semi-Fowler's position to reduce swelling and promote drainage. Monitor the patient for bleeding and airway

---

pharyngitis: pharyng—pharynx + itis—inflammation
dysphagia: dys—bad + phagia—to swallow
exudate: to sweat out
laryngitis: laryng—larynx + itis—inflammation

---

myalgia: myo—muscle + algia—pain

patency, and provide comfort measures. Encourage fluids for hydration; cold fluids may help reduce pain and bleeding. Red-colored drinks are avoided because they interfere with observation for bleeding. A room humidifier helps prevent drying. Keep suction equipment available for emergencies.

CRITICAL THINKING

Mrs. Hiler

■ You are assessing Mrs. Hiler after a tonsillectomy. She is sleeping, but you notice that she swallows every few seconds. She has an intravenous (IV) line of normal saline solution running at 100 mL per hour. How do you respond? How many drops per minute do you set on her IV if the tubing has a drop factor of 15?

Suggested answers at end of chapter.

Influenza

Pathophysiology and Etiology

Influenza, commonly referred to as the flu, is a viral infection of the respiratory tract. Many different flu viruses have been identified, and new strains appear each year. Influenza is the cause of millions of lost work days each year. The elderly are at particular risk for complications and even death from influenza because of preexisting chronic disease and compromised immune function.

Influenza is easily transmitted via droplets from coughs and sneezes of infected individuals, or it may be transmitted by physical contact with a person or object that harbors the virus. The incubation period from time of exposure to onset of symptoms is 1 to 3 days.

Prevention

Yearly immunization is recommended for prevention of influenza. The Centers for Disease Control and Prevention (CDC) updates specific recommendations yearly based on research and availability of vaccine. For the 2005 to 2006 flu season, the CDC recommended priority influenza vaccination for the following high-risk groups:

- Persons aged ≥65 years with comorbid conditions
- Residents of long-term care facilities
- Persons aged 2 to 64 years with comorbid conditions
- Persons aged ≥65 years without comorbid conditions
- Children aged 6 to 23 months
- Pregnant women
- Health-care personnel who provide direct patient care
- Household contacts and out-of-home caregivers of children aged <6 months[2]

Although Medicare covers the cost of a flu shot, many elders do not get one. Stress that they will not get the flu from the shot because it does not contain any live virus. Once the shot has been administered, it takes about 2 weeks

for antibodies to develop; it is then effective for about 4 months. Other preventive measures include hand washing and avoidance of individuals with influenza.

SAFETY TIP

In assisted living and long-term care facilities, develop and implement a protocol for administration and documentation of the flu and pneumococcus vaccines. Develop and implement a protocol to identify new cases of influenza and to manage an outbreak (2000 National Patient Safety Goals from www.jcaho.org).

Signs and Symptoms

Symptoms of flu include abrupt onset of fever, chills, myalgia, sore throat, cough, general malaise, and headache. It can last for 2 to 5 days, with malaise lasting up to several weeks.

Complications

The most common complication of influenza is pneumonia, which may be caused by the same virus as the flu or by a secondary bacterial infection. This should be considered if the patient experiences persistent fever and shortness of breath or if the lungs develop crackles or wheezes.

Diagnostic Tests

Viral cultures of throat or nasal swabbings can be done to identify influenza, but results may take 5 to 10 days. Rapid tests can identify the presence of flu virus in less than 30 minutes in an office setting, but are less reliable than cultures. Cultures may also be done to rule out bacterial infection. Once influenza has been identified in a geographical area, practitioners will test less often, and treat based on symptoms.

Therapeutic Interventions

Treatment is primarily symptomatic. Acetaminophen is given for fever, headache, and myalgia. Aspirin is avoided in children because it increases the risk for Reye's syndrome. Rest and fluids are essential. Antibiotics are used only if a secondary bacterial infection is present.

Antiviral drugs such as zanamivir (Relenza) and oseltamivir (Tamiflu) may be helpful for high-risk patients if given within 48 hours of exposure. These drugs may reduce the severity and duration of symptoms. Amantadine (Symmetrel) may also be given prophylactically to high-risk people who have not been immunized, and is recommended for use in nursing home residents where an outbreak of flu has occurred.

Nursing Care

Elderly or other high-risk patients may be hospitalized for treatment of influenza. These patients are closely monitored for signs of complications. Assess lung sounds and vital signs every 4 hours, and monitor for dehydration. Report changes to an RN or physician. Encourage rest and fluids (if not contraindicated), and provide comfort measures. Educate patients about avoiding aspirin to treat influenza symptoms in children under 18 to prevent Reye's syndrome (see Box 30.2 Nursing Care Plan for the Patient with an Upper Respiratory Infection).

CRITICAL THINKING

Murdie

■ Murdie is a 97-year-old nursing home resident who develops flu symptoms. She is lethargic, confused, and feverish. Because of her mental status changes, you want to send her to the hospital, but her son asks you to please keep her where she is. She has a history of chronic obstructive pulmonary disease (COPD) and diabetes.

1. How could Murdie have caught the flu?
2. How could it have been prevented?
3. What can be done now to prevent her from developing complications that could lead to pneumonia or even death?
4. What other concerns do you have?

Suggested answers at end of chapter.

Other Viral Infections

In recent years, new viruses have become a worldwide concern. Three of these are described below. Continuous research is being conducted to learn more about the spread, prevention, and treatment of new viral infections.

Bird Flu

Avian influenza, more commonly known as bird flu, has been identified in Asia, Canada, and the Netherlands, and is a growing concern. Humans can contract it from contact with infected birds (often poultry) or their secretions or excrement. Transmission from human to human is rare, but is also a potential concern. Symptoms of bird flu are similar to influenza symptoms described above, but complications can be more severe and deadly. Conventional vaccines are not effective in preventing bird flu. Oseltamivir (Tamiflu) may be useful in treatment, along with supportive measures.

SARS

Severe acute respiratory syndrome (SARS) is another new virus that has influenzalike symptoms. It first appeared in China in 2002. SARS in a concern because it also can progress to deadly pneumonia and respiratory failure, even in previously healthy individuals. Transmission of SARS is believed to occur from contact with a contaminated person or object, or through the air. Antiviral medications used to treat HIV infection are currently being researched for treatment of SARS.

West Nile Virus

A third new virus, West Nile virus, is less deadly then bird flu or SARS, but can still cause serious complications. West Nile virus is transmitted from birds to humans by mosquitoes, and causes either no symptoms or flulike symptoms. However, in a few people, especially the elderly, it can progress to encephalitis (inflammation of the brain) and meningitis (inflammation of the covering of the brain and spinal cord). There is no specific treatment for West Nile virus. If patients develop complications, they are hospitalized for supportive care.

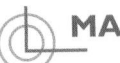 MALIGNANT DISORDERS

Cancer of the Larynx

Pathophysiology

Cancer of the larynx (the voice box) usually develops in the mucosal epithelium. It is evaluated based on the tumor-node-metastasis (TNM) staging system described in Chapter 10. It is usually a primary cancer and can spread to the lungs, liver, or lymph nodes. The prognosis for a patient with laryngeal cancer is often poor because metastasis (spread) may occur before the patient seeks help.

Etiology

Risk factors for cancer of the larynx include a history of alcohol and tobacco use. Exposure to industrial chemicals, hardwood dust, and chronic overuse of the voice are also factors. Men are five times as likely to be affected as women.

Prevention

Prevention begins with education; you can help educate patients about the relationship between cancer of the larynx and use of alcohol and tobacco. It is also important to teach patients to seek help when symptoms first occur because a delayed diagnosis may mean metastasis of the cancer and a poor prognosis. Teach that any hoarseness that lasts longer than 2 weeks should be investigated by a physician.

Signs and Symptoms

The most common symptom is persistent hoarseness because the vocal cords are located in the larynx (Box 30.3 Laryngeal Cancer Summary). The patient may also have throat or ear pain, shortness of breath, a chronic cough, and difficulty swallowing. Stridor may indicate a tumor obstructing the airway. Late signs include weight loss and halitosis (foul breath).

Diagnostic Tests

The larynx can be examined with a laryngeal mirror. Laryngoscopic examination and biopsy are used to diagnose and determine the stage of laryngeal cancer. A CT scan, magnetic resonance Imaging (MRI), or other diagnostic tests may be done to determine the presence or extent of metastasis.

Box 30.3

Laryngeal Cancer Summary

Signs and Symptoms

Hoarse voice
Pain
Cough
Shortness of breath
Difficulty swallowing
Weight loss
Foul breath

Diagnostic Tests

Examination with laryngeal mirror
Laryngoscopy with biopsy
Additional blood and radiographic studies to detect
  metastasis

Therapeutic Interventions

Radiation therapy
Chemotherapy (adjunct to radiation or surgery)
Endoscopic laser surgery to destroy tumor
Partial laryngectomy (preserves some voice)
Radical neck dissection with total laryngectomy (loss
  of voice)

Nursing Diagnoses

Risk for ineffective airway clearance
Acute pain
Impaired verbal communication
Risk for imbalanced nutrition

Therapeutic Interventions

If laryngeal cancer is diagnosed early in the disease, it may be treatable with radiation therapy; this treatment can preserve the patient's voice. Chemotherapy may be used with radiation or surgery, but it is not usually used alone. In more advanced cases, surgical intervention is necessary. The larynx will be either partially or completely removed (Fig. 30.2). If cancer has spread beyond the larynx, a radical neck dissection, which removes adjacent muscle, lymph nodes, and tissue, may be done. Surgery can be done using laser technology, endoscopy, or traditional methods.

After a partial laryngectomy, the patient may have a permanently hoarse voice. If a total laryngectomy is done, the patient will have a permanent tracheostomy (in this case called a laryngectomy) tube in place and no voice. Alternative methods of communication must be employed. A person who has had a total laryngectomy is sometimes referred to as a **laryngectomee.**

---

laryngectomee: larng—larynx + ectome—excision (person who has undergone laryngectomy)

Several alternatives for long-term speech exist:
- Esophageal speech involves swallowing air and forming words as the air is regurgitated back up the esophagus.
- Electronic devices are also available, which the patient places next to the neck or mouth. These devices use sound vibrations to help the patient form words. UltraVoice (Ultravoice Ltd) is a new electronic device that is placed inside an upper denture or retainer, and the patient speaks into a small microphone (Fig. 30.3A).
- Another alternative is a tracheoesophageal puncture (TEP), such as the Blom-Singer Voice Prosthesis (InHealth Technologies), which uses a surgically implanted voice prosthesis that creates a valve between the trachea and esophagus. If the patient holds a finger over the laryngectomy, air is diverted into the esophagus and the patient forms words as the air exits via the mouth (Fig. 30.3B).

All these devices take time to adjust to, and the patient will need support after discharge to continue to develop communication skills.

LEARNING TIP

Did you or your child ever "burp the ABCs"? If not, ask most any child to demonstrate! This is the same idea as esophageal speech.

Nursing Process: The Patient Undergoing Total Laryngectomy

PREOPERATIVE CARE. In addition to routine preoperative teaching, the patient undergoing laryngectomy surgery must be prepared for the loss of ability to breathe through the mouth and nose and the loss of the ability to speak. Initial instruction in communication techniques should take place before surgery to prevent the patient from feeling panicky after surgery when he or she is unable to communicate needs. A variety of techniques and devices are available. Consult the speech therapist before surgery to provide a picture board, magic slate, or paper and pencil. (See Chapter 49.) The patient is instructed to point to the picture that corresponds with the need or to write out his or her concern. A dietary consult is also important before surgery if the patient has been undernourished.

POSTOPERATIVE CARE. Assessment/Data Collection. Assessment of physical and psychosocial status, comfort, nutritional status, and ability to swallow is important both before and after surgery. After surgery, assessment of airway patency and respiratory function takes priority. Monitor lung sounds, oxygen saturation, and arterial blood gases. In addition, be sure to assess the patient's understanding of the disease process and self-care needs after surgery. It is important to evaluate the patient's support systems and

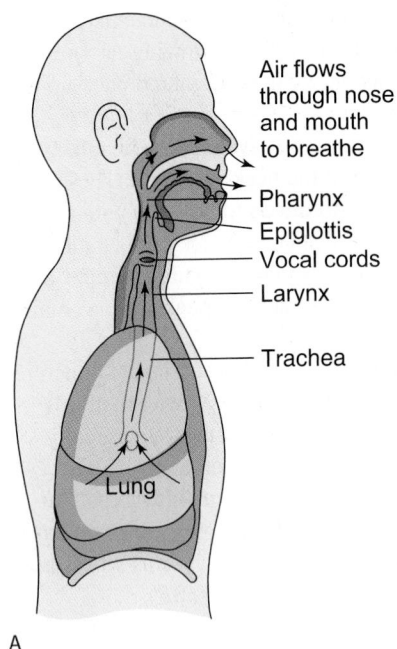

Air flows
through nose
and mouth
to breathe

Pharynx
Epiglottis
Vocal cords
Larynx

Trachea

Lung

A

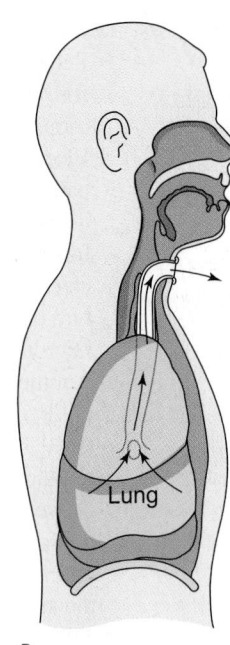

Patient breathes
through opening
in neck. There is
no connection
between nose and
mouth, and lungs.

Lung

B

FIGURE 30.2 Laryngectomy. *(A)* Before laryngectomy. *(B)* After laryngectomy.

ability to cope with the partial or total loss of voice after surgery. Continued alcohol and tobacco use will increase the patient's risk of recurrence.

Nursing Diagnosis, Planning, and Implementation Risk for ineffective airway clearance related to excessive secretions and new tracheostomy

EXPECTED OUTCOME: The patient will maintain a clear airway as evidenced by clear lung sounds and ability to cough up secretions.

- Monitor and record amount, color, and consistency of secretions; vital signs; oxygen saturation; lung sounds; and signs of respiratory distress. *Visible secretions, a drop in Sao₂, or an increase in crackles may indicate a need for suctioning.*

A change in amount or color of secretions, an increased temperature, or presence of adventitious sounds can indicate infection and should be reported to the physician immediately.

- Provide tracheostomy care and suctioning according to agency policy (see Chapter 29). *This keeps the airway clear.*
- Maintain strict sterile technique. *Prevention of infection is essential, since the airway no longer has the protection of normal upper airway defense mechanisms.*

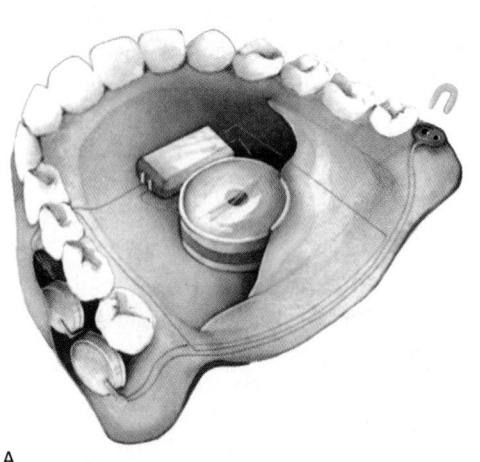

A

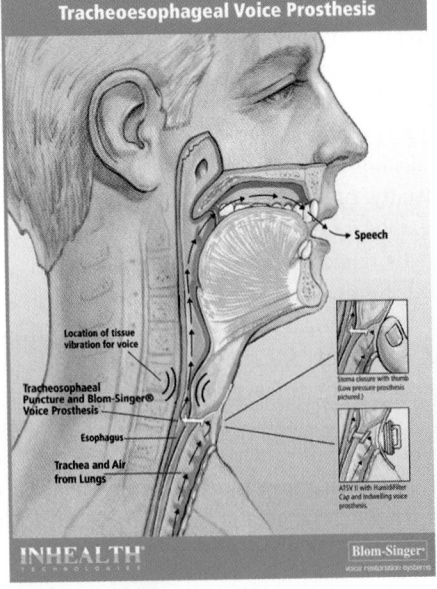

Tracheoesophageal Voice Prosthesis

Speech

Location of tissue
vibration for voice

Tracheosophaeal
Puncture and Blom-Singer®
Voice Prosthesis

Esophagus

Trachea and Air
from Lungs

INHEALTH

Blom-Singer

B

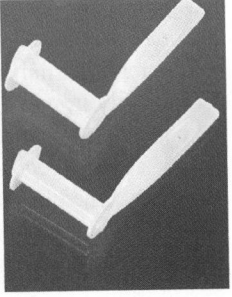

FIGURE 30.3 Devices to aid speech in the laryngectomy patient. *(A)* UltraVoice is an electronic device that is placed inside a denture or retainer; the patient speaks into a small microphone. *(Courtesy of UltraVoice Ltd.)* (B) The Blom-Singer Voice Prosthesis diverts air into the esophagus and out the mouth to form tracheoesophageal speech. *(Courtesy of by InHealth Technologies.)*

- Place the patient in semi-Fowler's position *to allow for lung expansion and more effective coughing.*
- Encourage the patient to deep breathe and cough every hour *to keep airway free of secretions.*
- Administer oxygen as ordered. A special tracheostomy collar may be used to provide oxygen and humidification. *Humidification can help keep secretions mobile.*
- Avoid use of powders, sprays, or other airborne materials near the patient. *These can cause irritation or infection if they enter the laryngectomy.*

Acute pain related to surgical procedure

EXPECTED OUTCOME: *The patient will state his pain level is acceptable.*

- Assess pain level every 4 hours and prn. *A good assessment must guide treatment.*
- Assess sedation and respiratory status frequently. *Opioids are given carefully because they may reduce respiratory rate and cough reflex, which is vital to clearing the airway.*
- Include nonpharmacological pain control interventions (see Chapter 9). *Interventions such as distraction and relaxation may help with pain control and reduce (not eliminate) the need for opioids.*
- Administer analgesics as ordered, on an around-the-clock basis or via a patient-controlled pump, for the first few days after surgery. If the liver has been damaged from alcohol abuse, dosages are adjusted by the physician. *The patient who is pain free will be better able to participate in care and take measures to prevent complications, such as coughing and ambulating.*

Impaired verbal communication related to loss of vocal cords

EXPECTED OUTCOME: *The patient will be able to communicate his or her needs.*

- Use a picture board or paper and pencil *so the patient can communicate without speaking.*
- Make sure the patient has a call light or bell nearby at all times. *Patients can become panicky if they have a need and no way to summon a nurse.*
- Work with the speech therapist and physician to provide the patient with a method of communication that best fits his or her needs (Fig. 30.3). *Different patients prefer different long-term communication methods.*

Risk for imbalanced nutrition, less than body requirements related to absence of oral feeding

EXPECTED OUTCOME: *The patient's weight and serum albumin levels will be within normal limits for height and age.*

- Monitor weight and albumin levels. *Weight loss or low albumin levels reflect inadequate nutrition.*
- Monitor parenteral nutrition or tube feedings after

surgery until the neck has begun to heal and swallowing can be evaluated. *Nutrition must be maintained to support healing.*
- Consult a dietitian for nutrition guidance. *If the patient has a history of alcohol abuse, he or she may have been undernourished before surgery. You may need to advocate for the patient and ensure that he or she is receiving adequate calories for healing. A dietitian can assist with specific recommendations.*

Impaired swallowing related to edema or laryngectomy tube

EXPECTED OUTCOME: *The patient will be able to swallow effectively.*

- Consult a speech therapist to assist with a swallowing assessment and recommendations. *Speech therapists are trained to assess and treat swallowing disorders.*
- Assure the patient that aspiration will not occur *because there is no longer a connection between the mouth and the lungs.*
- Place the patient in high-Fowler's position *to make swallowing easier.*
- Stay with the patient during the first attempts to eat *to help alleviate anxiety.*

Grieving related to loss of voice

EXPECTED OUTCOME: *Patient will express feelings of loss, and begin to plan for the future.*

- Assess patient's feelings of loss. *Inability to speak is a loss that cannot be overemphasized. The patient may also be facing a career change if job-related exposure contributed to the disease or if loss of voice prevents returning to a previously held job.*
- Actively listen to the patient *to show your support and validate his feelings.*
- Assess and involve support systems. *Family support is important to the patient's long-term adjustment to his laryngectomy.*
- Contact the patient's clergy if he or she wishes. *A religious counselor can help with grief and spiritual distress.*

Disturbed body image related to change in body structure and function

EXPECTED OUTCOME: *The patient will verbalize acceptance of new laryngectomy, and participate in self-care.*

- Portray an accepting attitude. *Patients are very aware of nurses' nonverbal behavior, and looks of distaste can be very disturbing.*
- Allow the patient to share his or her feelings if he indicates a need to do so. *This may help the patient to work through feelings about the changes to his body image.*
- With the patient's permission, contact a local support group that may have names of people who have had similar experiences who are willing to visit

with the patient. *Visitors can provide firsthand information and support.*

- Assist the patient to find ways to camouflage the change, such as scarves or necklines that conceal but do not obstruct the airway. *Camouflage can help the patient feel less conspicuous, and also protect the airway.*

Evaluation. When evaluating the patient's progress toward goals, ask the following questions:

Is the airway clear, without signs of infection?

Does the patient verbalize an acceptable level of comfort?

Do the patient and significant others demonstrate understanding of self-care at home or have referrals to continue learning self-care at home?

Does the patient indicate satisfaction with the level and quality of communication?

Are nutritional needs met, as evidenced by albumin levels greater than 3.0 and stable weight?

Is the patient able to swallow if taking oral nutrition? Is the patient able to grieve appropriately?

Does the patient have someone to talk to if he or she wishes?

Does the patient show acceptance of the laryngectomy by learning to look at it and care for it?

It should be noted that many of these evaluative criteria are long term and may not be seen while the patient is hospitalized, so follow-up by a home care nurse is essential.

Patient Education. After assessing the patient's readiness to learn, the patient is taught self-care measures for his or her laryngectomy, including how to perform cleaning and suctioning. (See Chapter 29.) Involve the significant other or family whenever possible.

The patient must also be instructed to perform gentle range-of-motion exercises of the neck. Some patients may avoid extending the neck because of the location of the incision, causing muscle contracture and eventual inability to do so.

Referral to home nursing after discharge will provide assessment of the home environment, as well as follow-up instruction. A social service referral may be made for financial or psychosocial concerns if needed. Consult with the physician or check the local phone directory for laryngectomee support groups, and refer the patient to them if appropriate. The local branch of the American Cancer Society may also be able to provide information.

To find additional information for laryngectomees, visit the National Cancer Institute website www.cancer.gov. Many other websites can be found by using a search engine and searching the term "laryngectomy."

REVIEW QUESTIONS

1. Which is the best explanation by a nurse for why a physician did not prescribe antibiotics for influenza?
   a. "Most cases of influenza are caused by antibiotic-resistant bacteria."
   b. "Influenza is caused by viruses."
   c. "Antibiotics have too many serious side effects."
   d. "Antibiotics can interact with other medications used for influenza."

2. After a laryngectomy, which of the following assessments takes priority?
   a. Airway patency
   b. Nutritional status
   c. Lung sounds
   d. Patient acceptance of surgery

3. Which of the following responses is correct when a patient asks why her physician didn't order a new antiviral drug for her flu?
   a. "Antiviral drugs are for AIDS, not the flu."
   b. "The side effects of the antiviral drugs are worse than having the flu."
   c. "Antiviral drugs are only for children."
   d. "These drugs work only if you start them within 48 hours after flu symptoms start."

4. Which of the following positions is recommended for a patient experiencing a nosebleed?
   a. Lying down with feet elevated
   b. Sitting up with neck fully extended
   c. Lying down with a small pillow under the head
   d. Sitting up leaning slightly forward

5. The nurse knows that the patient understands teaching related to prevention of influenza transmission when the patient demonstrates which behaviors? Choose all responses that are correct.
   a. Washing hands frequently
   b. Covering the nose and mouth during coughing or sneezing
   c. Taking acetaminophen as ordered
   d. Drinking extra fluids
   e. Avoiding sharing eating utensils with others

6. Which of the following communication methods will not work for the patient with a laryngectomy?
   a. Placing a finger over the stoma
   b. Providing a special valve that diverts air into the esophagus
   c. Obtaining a picture board
   d. Teaching the patient esophageal speech

References

1. Mainous, AG, Hueston, WJ, Clark, JR, et al: Antibiotics and upper respiratory infection. J Fam Pract 42:4, 1996.

2. http://www.cdc.gov/flu/professionals/vaccination/ accessed January 8, 2006.

SUGGESTED ANSWERS TO

CRITICAL THINKING

■ Mr. Jondahl

Consider the possibility of hypertension as a contributing factor. Mr. Jondahl's blood pressure is currently 140/90, which may be lower than normal for him because he has been bleeding. He is also on an antihypertensive drug and a diuretic. Explore the amount of ibuprofen being taken daily, because nonsteroidal anti-inflammatory drugs can interfere with platelet aggregation.

■ Mrs. Hiler

Mrs. Hiler may be swallowing blood. Examine the back of her throat with a flashlight. Check vital signs for evidence of impending shock. Notify a physician if bleeding is confirmed.

Use this formula to determine drops per minute:

$$\frac{100\ mL}{1\ hour} \cdot \frac{1\ hour}{60\ minutes} \cdot \frac{15\ gtt}{mL} = \frac{25\ gtt}{mL}$$

■ Murdie

1. Murdie may have contracted the flu from a visitor or a staff person at the nursing home. She is susceptible because of her age and comorbid conditions (COPD, diabetes).
2. Murdie's flu could probably have been prevented with a flu vaccination, but her son refused it because he believed it could cause her to get the flu.
3. If it is within 48 hours of symptom onset, a physician can prescribe an antiviral agent to help reduce her symptoms and shorten the course of her illness. In addition, you can provide fluids, acetaminophen, and comfort measures. You should also monitor her closely for evidence of bacterial infection or pneumonia, and report signs or symptoms immediately to a physician.
4. A major concern is that Murdie could transmit the flu to other residents or staff. Hopefully, they have all been vaccinated. In addition, you must decide whether or not to send Murdie to the hospital. Check her advance directives, and talk to her son about goals for her care. If necessary, educate him about differences in nursing home and hospital care.

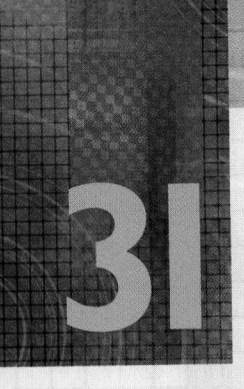

31

Nursing Care of Patients with Lower Respiratory Tract Disorders

PAULA D. HOPPER

KEY TERMS

adjuvant (ad-JOO-vant)
anergy (AN-er-jee)
antitussive (AN-tee-TUSS-iv)
atelectasis (AT-e-LEK-tah-sis)
atypical (ay-TIP-i-kuhl)
bleb (BLEB)
bronchiectasis (BRONG-key-EK-tah-sis)
bronchitis (brong-KIGH-tis)
bronchodilator (BRONG-koh-DYE-lay-ter)
bronchospasm (BRONG-koh-spazm)
bulla (BUHL-ah)
compliance (kom-PLIGH-ens)
ectopic (ek-TOP-ik)
embolism (EM-boh-lizm)
emphysema (EM-fi-SEE-mah)
empyema (EM-pigh-EE-mah)
exacerbation (egg- ZASS-er-BAY-shun)
expectorant (ek-SPEK-tuh-rant)
exudate (EKS-yoo-dayt)
hemoptysis (hee-MOP-ti-sis)
hemothorax (HEE-moh-THOR-aks)
hypostatic (HIGH-poh-STAT-ik)
immunocompromised (IM-yoo-noh-KOM-prah-mized)
induration (IN-dyoo-RAY-shun)
lobectomy (loh-BEK-tuh-mee)
mucolytic (MYOO-koh-LIT-ik)
paradoxical respiration (PAR-uh-DOK-si-kuhl RES-pi-RAY-shun)
pleurodesis (PLOO-roh-DEE-sis)
pneumonectomy (NOO-moh-NEK-tuh-mee)
pneumothorax (NOO-moh-THOR-aks)
polycythemia (PAH-lee-sigh-THEE-mee-ah)
status asthmaticus (STAT-us az-MAT-i-kus)
tachypnea (TAK-ip-NEE-uh)
thoracotomy (THOR-ah-KOT-ah-mee)

QUESTIONS TO GUIDE YOUR READING

1. What is the pathophysiology of each of the disorders of the lower respiratory tract?

2. What are the etiologies, signs, and symptoms of each of the disorders?

3. What tests are useful for diagnosis of each of the disorders?

4. What are therapeutic interventions for disorders of the lower respiratory tract?

5. What data should you collect when caring for patients with disorders of the lower respiratory tract?

6. What nursing care will you provide for patients with disorders of the lower respiratory tract?

7. What specific nursing care can you provide for patients experiencing impaired gas exchange, ineffective airway clearance, or ineffective breathing pattern?

8. How will you know if your nursing interventions have been effective?

Disorders of the lower respiratory tract include problems of the lower portion of the trachea, bronchi, bronchioles, and alveoli. These disorders may be related to infection, noninfectious alterations in function, neoplasm (cancer), or trauma. Any pathological condition of the lower respiratory tract can seriously impair carbon dioxide and oxygen exchange.

INFECTIOUS DISORDERS

Acute Bronchitis

Bronchitis is an inflammation of the bronchial tree, which includes the right and left bronchi, secondary bronchi, and bronchioles. When the mucous membranes lining the bronchial tree become irritated and inflamed, excessive mucus is produced. The result is congested airways. Acute bronchitis is usually an isolated episode. If it occurs more than 3 months out of the year for 2 consecutive years, chronic bronchitis is diagnosed. See discussion of chronic bronchitis later in this chapter for more information that applies to both the acute and chronic forms.

Bronchiectasis

Pathophysiology

Bronchiectasis is a dilation of the bronchial airways (Fig. 31.1). The dilated areas form sacs that can remain localized or spread throughout the lungs. Secretions pool in these sacs and frequently become infected.

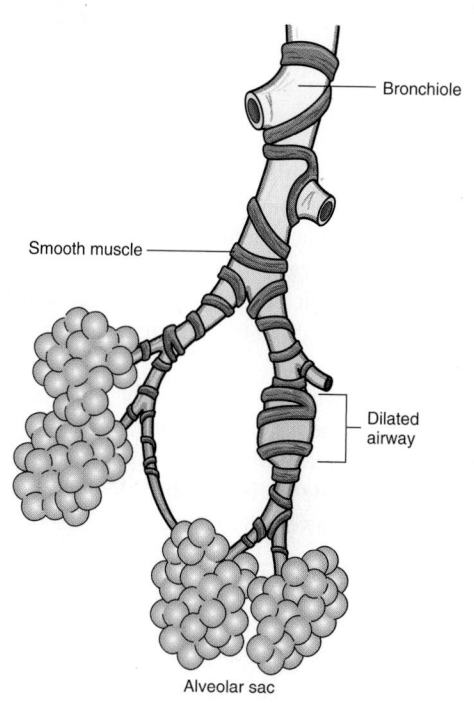

Bronchiole

Smooth muscle

Dilated airway

Alveolar sac

FIGURE 31.1 Bronchiectasis. Note dilated airway.

Etiology

Bronchiectasis usually occurs secondary to another chronic respiratory disorder, such as cystic fibrosis, asthma, tuberculosis, bronchitis, or exposure to a toxin. Airway obstruction from a tumor or foreign body can also be a predisposing factor. Infection and inflammation of the airways weakens the bronchial walls and reduces ciliary function. Airway obstruction from excessive secretions then predisposes the patient to development of bronchiectasis.

Signs and Symptoms

The patient with bronchiectasis has recurrent lower respiratory infections. Sputum is copious and purulent and pools in the dilated airways. The accompanying cough can produce as much as 200 mL of thick, foul-smelling sputum in a single episode of coughing. Extreme airway inflammation may cause sputum to be bloody. If bronchiectasis is widespread throughout the lungs, the patient may experience dyspnea even with minimal exertion. Wheezes and crackles may be auscultated. Fever is present during active infection. Cor pulmonale (right-sided heart failure; covered in Chapter 26) and clubbing of the fingers may develop with chronic disease.

Diagnostic Tests

A chest x-ray examination may be done, but it may not show early disease. A computed tomographic (CT) scan provides a better view of the dilated airways. Sputum cultures determine infecting organisms and guide antibiotic therapy. Additional testing is done to determine the cause of bronchiectasis.

Therapeutic Interventions

Treatment is aimed at keeping the airways clear of secretions, controlling infection, and correcting the underlying problem. Antibiotics may be used intermittently or for prolonged periods. Measures to prevent infection, including vaccinations for flu and pneumonia, should be taken. **Bronchodilators** improve airway obstruction. **Mucolytic** agents help thin secretions, and chest physiotherapy helps mobilize secretions so they can be more effectively expectorated. Oxygen is used if hypoxemia is present. If the affected area of the lung is localized and symptoms are severe, surgery may be considered to remove the diseased area. Lung transplant may be considered in severe cases.

Pneumonia

Pneumonia is the cause of more than 10% of hospital admissions each year and is the most common cause of death from infection.

Pathophysiology

Pneumonia is an acute infection of the lungs that occurs when an infectious agent enters and multiplies in the lungs of a susceptible person. Infectious particles can be transmitted by the cough of an infected individual, from contaminated respiratory therapy equipment, from infections in other parts of the body, or from aspiration of bacteria from

---

bronchitis: bronch—airway + itis—inflammation
bronchiectasis: bronch—airway + ectasis—dilation or expansion

bronchodilator: broncho—airway + dilator—to expand
mucolytic: muco—mucus + lytic—break up

the mouth, pharynx, or stomach. Organisms from the mouth and pharynx may be related to poor oral hygiene or may be present because of a cold or influenza virus. When pathogens enter the body of a healthy person, normal respiratory defense mechanisms and the immune system prevent the development of infection. In a person who is **immunocompromised,** however, even microorganisms that are normally present in the oropharynx can cause an infection. Persons at risk for pneumonia are the very young, the elderly, and those who are immunocompromised, such as people with acquired immunodeficiency syndrome (AIDS) or another chronic illness.

When the microorganisms multiply, they release toxins that induce inflammation in the lung tissue, causing damage to mucous and alveolar membranes. This leads to the development of edema and **exudate,** which fills the alveoli and reduces the surface area available for exchange of carbon dioxide and oxygen. Some bacteria also cause necrosis of lung tissue.

Pneumonia may be confined to one lobe, or it may be scattered throughout the lungs. If it affects only one lobe, it is called lobar pneumonia. Generalized pneumonia is much more serious and is called bronchopneumonia. Bronchopneumonia occurs more often as a nosocomial (hospital-acquired) infection in hospitalized patients, the very young, or the very old.

Etiology

Pneumonia has a variety of causes, which are listed next.

BACTERIAL PNEUMONIA. The most common cause of community-acquired bacterial pneumonia, is *Streptococcus pneumoniae;* also called pneumococcal pneumonia. This organism accounts for approximately 90% of all bacterial pneumonias. Other community-acquired infections are caused by *Staphylococcus aureus* and *Mycoplasma pneumoniae.* Hospital-acquired pneumonias are often more serious and may be caused by *Escherichia coli, Haemophilus influenzae,* and *Pseudomonas aeruginosa,* among others.

VIRAL PNEUMONIA. Influenza viruses are the most common cause of viral pneumonia. The presence of viral pneumonia increases the patient's susceptibility to a secondary bacterial pneumonia. Generally, patients are less

SAFETY TIP

In assisted living and long-term care facilities, develop and implement a protocol for administration and documentation of the flu and pneumococcus vaccines. Develop and implement a protocol to identify new cases of influenza and to manage an outbreak (2006 National Patient Safety Goals www.jcaho.org).

ill with viral pneumonia than with bacterial pneumonia, but they may be ill for a longer period because antibiotics are ineffective against viruses.

FUNGAL PNEUMONIA. *Candida* and *Aspergillus* are two types of fungi that can cause pneumonia. *Pneumocystis carinii* is a fungus that typically causes pneumonia in patients with AIDS.

ASPIRATION PNEUMONIA. Some pneumonias are caused by aspiration of foreign substances. This most often occurs in patients with decreased levels of consciousness or an impaired cough or gag reflex. These conditions can occur with alcohol ingestion, stroke, general anesthesia, seizures, or other serious illness. Aspiration pneumonia increases the risk for subsequent bacterial pneumonia.

VENTILATOR–ASSOCIATED PNEUMONIA. A type of aspiration pneumonia, ventilator-associated pneumonia (VAP), develops in patients who are intubated and mechanically ventilated. The endotracheal tube keeps the glottis open, so secretions can be aspirated in to the lungs.

HYPOSTATIC PNEUMONIA. Patients who hypoventilate because of bedrest, immobility, or shallow respirations are at risk for **hypostatic** pneumonia. Secretions pool in dependent areas of the lungs and can lead to inflammation and infection.

CHEMICAL PNEUMONIA. Inhalation of toxic chemicals can cause inflammation and tissue damage, which can lead to chemical pneumonia.

CRITICAL THINKING

Mr. Smith

■ Mr. Smith is an 86-year-old man who was watching television when he couldn't sleep one night. After seeing a commercial for toilet cleaner, he decided his own toilet could use some attention. He used bleach and ammonia "to get it really clean." The combination created toxic fumes, which caused a severe chemical pneumonia. He was brought to the emergency room in acute respiratory distress.

1. As his nurse, what questions might you ask as you further assess the cause of his pneumonia?
2. What will you teach Mr. Smith related to prevention of similar episodes in the future?

Suggested answers at end of chapter.

Prevention

A vaccine is available to help prevent *Streptococcus pneumoniae* pneumonias in high-risk patients and people older than age 65. It is effective about 80% to 90% of the time and requires only a one-time injection. Some individuals may require a repeat vaccination after 5 years. Yearly influenza vaccination is also recommended for high-risk individuals.

---

immunocompromised: immune—referring to immune system + compromised—lacks resistance

exudate: to sweat out

hypostatic: hypo—below + static—standing

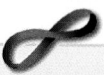

Box 31.1

Gerontological Issues

Advanced age is a significant risk factor for serious complications from respiratory infections such as influenza and pneumococcal pneumonia. Therefore, it is recommended that people over the age of 65 and individuals with chronic disease have yearly influenza vaccines and a once-in-a-lifetime pneumococcal vaccine.

Nursing care plays an important role in the prevention of nosocomial pneumonia. Regular coughing, deep breathing, and position changes for patients on bedrest or after surgery, prevention of aspiration for patients at risk, and good hand washing practices by both patients and health-care personnel can help prevent many cases (Box 31.1 Gerontological Issues). Ventilator-associated pneumonia risk can be reduced with frequent mouth care and use of a special endotracheal tube that allows continuous suctioning of secretions.

SAFETY TIP

To reduce the risk of health care–associated infections, comply with current Centers for Disease Control and Prevention (CDC) hand hygiene guidelines, found at www.cdc.gov/handhygiene (2006 National Patient Safety Goals from www.jcaho.org).

Signs and Symptoms

Patients with pneumonia present with fever, shaking chills, chest pain, dyspnea, and a productive cough. Sputum is purulent or may be rust colored or blood tinged. Crackles and wheezes may be heard on lung auscultation because of the secretions in the avleoli and airways.

Some bacterial and many viral pneumonias cause **atypical** symptoms. The patient may experience fatigue, sore throat, dry cough, or nausea and vomiting.

Elderly patients may not exhibit expected symptoms of pneumonia. New-onset confusion or lethargy in an elderly patient can indicate reduced oxygenation and should alert you to look for other symptoms or request further testing. New onset of fever or dyspnea should also cause suspicion of possible pneumonia in the elderly.

Complications

Complications from pneumonia most commonly occur in patients with other underlying chronic diseases. Pleurisy and pleural effusion (discussed later in this chapter) are two of the most common complications and generally resolve within 1 to 2 weeks. **Atelectasis** (collapsed alveoli) can

occur as a result of trapped secretions and may be resolved with efforts to keep the airways clear. Other complications result from spread of infection to other parts of the body, causing septicemia, meningitis, septic arthritis, pericarditis, or endocarditis. Treatment for each of these is antibiotics. Although antibiotics have greatly reduced the incidence of death related to pneumonia, it is still a common cause of death in the elderly.

Diagnostic Tests

A chest x-ray examination is done to identify the presence of pulmonary infiltrate, which is fluid leakage into the alveoli from inflammation (Fig. 31.2). In addition, sputum and blood cultures are obtained to identify the organism causing the pneumonia and determine appropriate treatment. Cultures should be obtained before antibiotics are started to avoid altering culture results. If the patient is unable to produce a sputum specimen, a nebulized mist treatment may be ordered to promote sputum expectoration. If this is unsuccessful, a bronchoscopy may be done to obtain a specimen from a very ill patient.

Therapeutic Interventions

Broad-spectrum antibiotics are initiated before culture results are completed (be sure to obtain the specimen before starting the antibiotics). Once the culture and sensitivity report is available, specific antibiotics are ordered if the cause is bacterial. Many patients can be treated with oral antibiotics as outpatients, but hospitalization and intravenous (IV) therapy may be necessary in the elderly, chronically ill, or acutely ill individual. If the pneumonia is caused by a virus, rest and fluids are recommended. Occasionally, antiviral medications are used.

Expectorants, bronchodilators, and analgesics may be given for comfort and symptom relief. Nebulized mist treatments or metered-dose inhalers may be used to deliver bron-

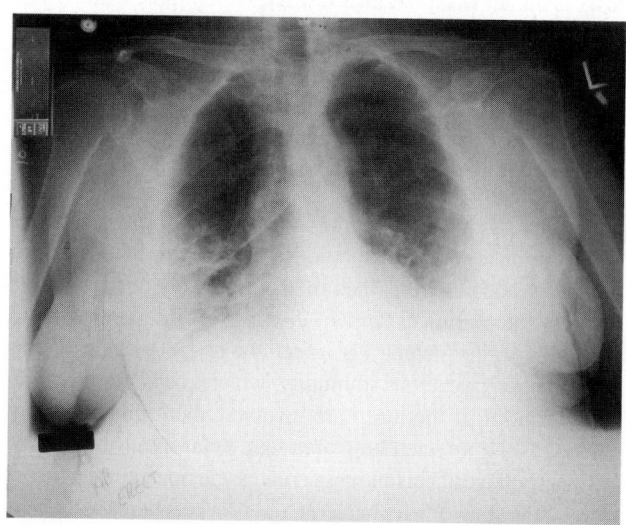

FIGURE 31.2 Chest x-ray examination showing infiltrates in pneumonia.

---

atypical: a—not + typical—usual
atelectasis: atel—imperfect + ectasis—expansion

expectorant: ex—out + pect—breast

Box 31.2

Pneumonia Summary

Signs and Symptoms	Fever, chills
	Chest pain
	Dyspnea
	Productive cough
	Crackles and wheezes
Diagnostic Tests	Chest x-ray
	Sputum cultures
Therapeutic Interventions	Antibiotics
	Supplemental oxygen
	Bronchodilators, expectorants
	Rest, fluids
Complications	Pleurisy, pleural effusion
	Atelectasis
Priority Nursing Diagnoses	Impaired gas exchange
	Ineffective airway clearance
	Activity intolerance

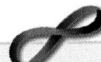

Box 31.3

Gerontological Issues

The age-related decline in immune system function can decrease the effectiveness of the tuberculosis antibodies in someone who previously had latent infection. The tuberculosis bacilli can be activated, causing active disease. Because of the risk of false negative tuberculin test results, a two-step test is recommended, with the second test done 1 to 3 weeks after the first.

bacteria can become active, causing active disease. Only 5% to 10% of infected individuals in the United States actually develop the disease, and even then it may not occur for many years (Box 31.3 Gerontological Issues).

NURSING CARE TIP

If the physician orders "sputum culture for AFB," tuberculosis is suspected. Ask whether isolation precautions should be taken while waiting for culture results.

chodilators. Supplemental oxygen via nasal cannula or mask is used as necessary.

See Box 31.2 Pneumonia Summary.

Tuberculosis

Pathophysiology

Tuberculosis (TB) is an infectious disease caused by the bacterium *Mycobacterium tuberculosis.* TB primarily affects the lungs, although other areas, such as the kidneys, liver, brain, and bone, may be affected as well. *M. tuberculosis* is an acid-fast bacillus (AFB), which means that when it is stained in the laboratory and then washed with an acid, the stain remains, or stays "fast." *M. tuberculosis* can live in dark places in dried sputum for months, but a few hours in direct sunlight kills it. It is spread by inhalation of the tuberculosis bacilli from respiratory droplets (droplet nuclei) of an infected person.

Once the bacilli enter the lungs, they multiply and begin to disseminate to the lymph nodes and then to other parts of the body. The patient is then infected but may or may not go on to develop clinical (active) disease. TB infection without disease is called latent TB infection, or LTBI. During this time the body develops immunity, which keeps the infection under control. If the lungs are involved, the immune system surrounds the infected lung area with neutrophils and alveolar macrophages. This process creates a lesion called a tubercle, which seals off the bacteria and prevents spread. Similar processes take place in other affected areas of the body. The bacteria within the tubercle die or become dormant, and the patient is no longer infectious. If the patient's immune system becomes compromised, however, some of the dormant

Etiology

Crowded or poorly ventilated living conditions place people at risk for becoming infected with tuberculosis. Although tuberculosis can infect any age group, the elderly are especially at risk. Elders may have contracted the disease many years before, but it reactivates as the aging process diminishes immune function. Patients with AIDS and chronic alcohol abuse have a very high risk because of their compromised immune function. In the United States, tuberculosis is also prevalent among the urban poor and minority groups.

Before 1985 the incidence of TB was steadily decreasing. Now it is again on the rise, in part because of the prevalence of AIDS, the development of antibiotic-resistant strains of the TB bacillus, and ineffective treatment programs. TB kills 8000 people each day worldwide, and is the world's biggest killer of young people and adults.[1]

Prevention

Clean, well-ventilated living areas are essential to the health of all people. If a hospitalized patient is known or suspected to have tuberculosis, he or she is placed in respiratory isolation to prevent spread to staff or other patients. Special isolation rooms are ventilated to the outside. Staff should wear special high-efficiency filtration masks when in the patient's room. A regular surgical mask is *not* effective against TB. Verify with the institution's infection control department that the masks provided are effective for use with TB patients. If the patient must travel through the hallway for tests or other activities, the patient must wear a mask. Additional protective barriers, such as gowns, gloves, or goggles, are used when contact with sputum is likely.

A vaccine against tuberculosis is available and is used in areas where TB is prevalent. It is safe, but its effectiveness has been questioned. It is not used routinely in the United States. Individuals who have had the vaccine will have a positive skin test for TB, so alternative methods for screening must be used.

Ultimately prevention will come from adequate treatment of patients with TB. A current concern is the development of antibiotic-resistant strains of the tuberculosis bacillus, which can develop when patients are noncompliant with drug therapy. When antibiotics are taken intermittently or discontinued early, the more virulent (stronger) bacteria survive and multiply, and are resistant to the drugs being used. This multi–drug-resistant TB (MDR-TB) can then be passed on to someone else. It is therefore vital to teach all patients the importance of strict compliance with drug therapy. Patients who are at risk for noncompliance with drug therapy must have a visiting nurse or other health professional observe each dose of antibiotic taken. This is called directly observed therapy (DOT) or directly observed therapy–short course (DOTS). DOT transfers responsibility for making sure the drugs are taken from the patient to the health-care worker. The World Health Organization reports the highest treatment success rates with DOT(S).

Signs and Symptoms

Active tuberculosis is characterized by a chronic productive cough, blood-tinged sputum, and drenching night sweats. A low-grade fever may be present. If effective treatment is not initiated, a downhill course occurs, with pulmonary fibrosis, **hemoptysis,** and progressive weight loss.

Complications

Spread of the tuberculosis bacilli throughout the body can result in pleurisy, pericarditis, peritonitis, meningitis, bone and joint infections, genitourinary or gastrointestinal infection, or infection of many other organs.

Diagnostic Tests

Routine screening for tuberculosis infection is usually done with a purified protein derivative (PPD) skin test. The PPD is injected intradermally; the test is considered positive if a raised area of **induration** occurs within 48 to 72 hours. If there is a red area around the induration, this is not measured. The size of induration that indicates a positive test varies based on the individual's history (Table 31.1). A red area without induration is not considered a positive result. A positive result indicates that a person has been exposed; it does not mean that active TB disease is present.

In 2004, a new test was approved by the Food and Drug Administration (FDA) that may be more specific and reliable than the PPD test. The QuantiFERON-TB Gold (QFT-G) test is a blood test that detects the cell-mediated immune response to TB bacteria in blood. Unlike the PPD skin test, the QFT-G is valid in individuals who have been vaccinated against TB.

---

hemoptysis: hem—blood + ptysis—to spit
induration: in—in + durus—hard

TABLE 31.1 CLASSIFYING A TUBERCULIN SKIN TEST REACTION

Size of Induration	Considered Positive for
5 mm or more	• People with HIV infection • Close contacts • People who have had TB disease before • People who inject illicit drugs and whose HIV status is unknown
10 mm or more	• Foreign-born persons • HIV-negative persons who inject illicit drugs • Low-income groups • People who live in residential facilities • People with certain medical conditions • Children younger than age 4 • People in other groups, as identified by local public health officials
15 mm or more	• People with no risk factors for TB

HIV = human immunodeficiency virus.
Source: Retrieved August 5, 2002, from Centers for Disease Control and Prevention: Diagnosis of tuberculosis infection and disease. www.phppo.cdc.gov.

 (handwritten note: make sure you see them take the medication)

NURSING CARE TIP

You have probably had a PPD skin test so you can do your clinical practice for school. When you have it checked, the clinician should touch your arm. Just looking at it is not adequate to judge whether there is a raised area of induration.

Some health care institutions use a two-step process for baseline testing of employees and residents. If an individual has a negative test, he or she is retested in 1 to 3 weeks. This is because someone who was exposed many years ago may not react to the first test. The first test acts as a "reminder" to the immune system to react. The second test will then be positive in the person with a past TB infection.

A chest x-ray examination is used as a screening tool in someone with a known positive test. Diagnosis is made based on sputum culture results.

Therapeutic Interventions

Treatment consists of specific antibiotic therapy. First-line drugs have the fewest adverse effects (Box 31.4). However, these drugs can be toxic to the liver and nervous system, as well as have other side effects. Second-line drugs are more toxic and are reserved for cases that do not respond to first-line drug therapy. Generally, two or three antibiotics are given simultaneously to allow lower doses of each individual drug, reduce the incidence of serious side effects, and reduce the risk of developing resistant bacteria. Drugs must be taken for 6 months, or up to 2 years for MDR-TB. Because of the

Box 31.4

Antibiotics Used to Treat Tuberculosis

First-Line Drugs	Second Line Drugs
Isoniazid *INH*	Rifabutin
Rifampin ~red urine	Rifapentine
Ethambutol	
Pyrazinamide	

[handwritten: Less Side effects]
[handwritten: Harsher]
[handwritten: PZT]

NURSING CARE TIP

Some institutions use a *Candida* or mumps skin test along with a PPD skin test. This does not mean the patient is being tested for *Candida* or mumps because everyone generally reacts to these. Rather the patient is being tested for **anergy,** or the inability of the immune system to react to an antigen. If a *Candida* or mumps test produces positive results, the TB results are considered to be reliable.

The *Candida* or mumps test is administered in the same way as the PPD test. If more than one test is administered, use an indelible marker to identify which test is which, and clearly document (draw a picture) of where each test was placed. Check institution policy; it may direct where the tests are administered—PPD in the right arm and *Candida* in the left, for example.

length of therapy and the incidence of side effects, you must anticipate that compliance may be a problem.

Additional treatment is supportive. Rest and good nutrition are important for aiding the patient's own immune system to work. Patients must be isolated until their sputum no longer contains bacteria.

Patients with latent TB infection do not need to be treated, but some health departments recommend treatment to reduce the risk of progression to active disease and subsequent spread to others.

The Centers for Disease Control and Prevention has an excellent website with lots of information about tuberculosis at www.cdc.gov. Simply type "tuberculosis" into the search window.

Nursing Process

ASSESSMENT/DATA COLLECTION. Perform thorough respiratory and psychosocial assessments of the patient with TB. The severity of the disease determines the impact on the patient's lifestyle. It is also imperative to determine the patient's knowledge of the disease and treatment and his or her compliance with drug treatment.

NURSING DIAGNOSES, PLANNING, AND IMPLEMENTATION. Nursing interventions for impaired gas exchange,

ineffective airway clearance, ineffective breathing pattern, and activity intolerance are found in Box 31.5 Nursing Care Plan for the Patient with a Lower Respiratory Tract Disorder. Additional nursing diagnoses for the patient with TB follow.

Risk for ineffective management of therapeutic regimen related to knowledge deficit

EXPECTED OUTCOME: *Patient will follow treatment regimen and infection will be cured.*

- Assess patient's and family's ability and intent to follow treatment regimen. *It is essential that patients are diligent about taking their drugs in order to eradicate the infection and to prevent spread to others.*
- Teach patient and family that drugs must be taken as scheduled for the entire course (6 months or longer) or a drug-resistant form of disease may develop. *Patients may be more likely to comply if they understand the rationale for taking their medications.*
- Forwarn the patient that rifampin turns urine and other body fluids red. *This might frighten the patient from taking drugs if he or she is unprepared.*
- Teach patient to report side effects of medications. *If side effects can be managed, the patient is more likely to comply with therapy.*
- Request an order for a visiting nurse. *A visiting nurse can monitor compliance. Directly observed therapy (DOT) has been found to increase compliance with medications.*

Risk for infection transmission related to knowledge deficit about how infection is spread, or noncompliance with control measures

EXPECTED OUTCOME: *Patient will verbalize understanding of and employ measures to prevent spreading infection.*

- Assess patient's understanding of how TB is spread. *Teaching should build on patient's current knowledge.*
- Teach the patient how TB is spread and the importance of following measures to avoid spread. *The patient will be more likely to comply if he understands the rationale for his actions.*
- Teach the patient to use a tissue to cover the mouth and nose when coughing or sneezing. *TB is spread by droplet nuclei that can be contained with a tissue.*
- Teach patient to flush tissues down the toilet or dispose of carefully in the trash. *TB bacteria can live in dried sputum for months, so careful disposal is essential.*
- Teach all family members the importance of careful hand washing. *Hand washing is an important measure in preventing all kinds of infections.*
- Instruct the patient in the importance of compliance with follow-up sputum cultures. *Once sputum cultures are negative, the patient is no longer contagious.*

Box 31.5 NURSING CARE PLAN for the Patient with a Lower Respiratory Tract Disorder

Note: The most commonly used nursing diagnoses related to respiratory disorders are presented in the following care plan. This is not a care plan for any one respiratory disorder. Rather, use it as a reference for use when one of the nursing diagnoses applies to the patient, based on a thorough respiratory assessment.

Nursing Diagnosis: Impaired gas exchange related to decreased ventilation or perfusion

Expected Outcomes The patient will experience improved gas exchange, as evidenced by (1) improving arterial blood gases or pulse oximetry and (2) statement of acceptable level of dyspnea.

Evaluation of Outcomes (1) Are blood gases or Sao_2 improving? (2) Does patient state that dyspnea is gone or controlled at an acceptable level?

Interventions	Rationale	Evaluation
• Assess lung sounds, respiratory rate and effort, use of accessory muscles.	Respiratory rate less than 12 or more than 24 or use of accessory muscles indicates distress. Diminished lung sounds indicate possible poor air movement and impaired gas exchange.	Are lung sounds clear and audible? Is respiratory rate 12 to 20 per minute and unlabored?
• Observe skin and mucous membranes for cyanosis.	Cyanosis indicates poor oxygenation. Oral mucous membrane cyanosis indicates serious hypoxia.	Are skin and mucous membranes pink?
• Assess degree of dyspnea on a scale of 0 to 10, 0 = no dyspnea, 10 = worst dyspnea.	The patient's subjective report is the best measure of dyspnea.	Is patient's degree of dyspnea within parameters that are acceptable to patient?
• Monitor for confusion or changes in mental status.	Changes in mental status can signal impaired gas exchange.	Is patient alert and oriented? If not, could poor gas exchange be the reason?
• Monitor arterial blood gas values and pulse oximetry as ordered.	Pao_2 < 80 mm Hg, $Paco_2$ >45 mm Hg, or Sao_2 <90 indicate impaired gas exchange.	Are values within patient's baseline values?
• Elevate head of bed or help patient to lean on overbed table.	Upright positioning promotes lung expansion.	Did change of position relieve some distress?
• Position with good lung dependent ("good lung down").	This position allows the healthier lung to be better perfused and increases gas exchange.	Is Sao_2 improved in this position?
• Administer supplemental oxygen at <2 L/min unless ordered otherwise.	Supplemental oxygen decreases hypoxia. Rates more than 2 L/min may depress hypoxic drive.	Is oxygen placed properly on patient? Does it provide relief from dyspnea?
• Place a fan in the patient's room.	The feeling of a breeze on the patient's face may make the patient feel he is getting more air.	Is a fan available to the patient and does it help?
• Teach patient relaxation exercises.	Relaxation exercises decrease perceived dyspnea.	Does patient use relaxation effectively?
• For chronic disease, teach patient diaphragmatic and pursed-lip breathing. (See Chapter 29.)	Breathing exercises promote relaxation and increase CO_2 excretion.	Does patient use breathing exercises correctly? Do they help?
• Encourage patient to stop smoking if patient is a current smoker.	Smoking is damaging to lungs and respiratory function.	Is patient receptive to smoking cessation? Are resources available?
• For severe dyspnea, ask physician about an order for intravenous morphine sulfate.	Low doses of IV morphine cause vasodilation, which helps relieve pulmonary edema and anxiety.	Does morphine provide relief from dyspnea?

(Continued on following page)

Box 31.5   NURSING CARE PLAN for the Patient with a Lower Respiratory Tract Disorder (Continued)

Nursing Diagnosis: Ineffective airway clearance related to excessive secretions

Expected Outcomes The patient will have improved airway clearance as evidenced by (1) clear breath sounds and (2) ability to cough up secretions.

Evaluation of Outcomes (1) Are breath sounds clear? (2) Is patient able to effectively cough up and expectorate secretions?

Interventions	Rationale	Evaluation
• Assess lung sounds q4th and prn.	Crackles and wheezes may indicate excess secretions in airways.	Do lung sounds indicate retained secretions?
• Monitor amount, color, and consistency of sputum.	Thick, purulent sputum indicates infection and should be reported to the physician.	Does sputum indicate infection?
• Encourage oral fluids; use cool steam room humidifier.	Hydration decreases viscosity of secretions and aids expectoration.	Is patient able to take oral fluids? Are secretions thin and easily expectorated?
• Turn patient q2h or encourage to ambulate if able.	Movement mobilizes secretions.	Is patient mobile?
• Encourage patient to cough and deep breathe every hour and prn.	Controlled coughing following deep breaths is more effective.	Does patient cough and deep breathe effectively?
• Administer expectorants as ordered.	Expectorants help liquefy secretions and trigger the cough reflex.	Are expectorants effective?
• If patient is unable to cough up secretions, suction per institution policy.	Suctioning is necessary to remove secretions when the patient is unable to cough effectively.	Is suctioning necessary? Does it help remove secretions?
• Obtain order for chest physiotherapy or flutter valve if indicated.	Percussion and postural drainage help mobilize secretions.	Is chest physiotherapy effective and well tolerated by the patient?

Nursing Diagnosis: Ineffective breathing pattern related to anxiety or pain

Expected Outcomes The patient will maintain an effective breathing pattern as evidenced by (1) respiratory rate between 12 and 20 per minute, even, and unlabored; and (2) arterial blood gas and oxygen saturation results within patient's normal range.

Evaluation of Outcomes (1) Is patient's respiratory rate within normal limits and unlabored? (2) Does breathing pattern support normal blood gas and Sao_2 values?

Interventions	Rationale	Evaluation
• Assess respiratory rate, depth, and effort q4h and prn.	Respirations less than 12 or more than 20 may indicate an ineffective pattern.	Is respiratory pattern ineffective?
• Monitor blood gas and oxygen saturation values.	An ineffective breathing pattern will not maintain oxygenation.	Is breathing pattern adversely affecting oxygenation?
• Determine and treat the cause of ineffective breathing pattern.	Pain or anxiety can cause a patient to change the breathing pattern, and should be treated.	Is a contributing factor identifiable and correctable?
• Place patient in Fowler's or semi-Fowler's position.	This allows for maximum chest expansion.	Is the patient in a comfortable position that enables adequate expansion?
• Teach patient to use diaphragmatic breathing, with a regular 2 second in, 4 second out pattern.	Breathing exercises promote relaxation and increase CO_2 excretion.	Is the patient able to demonstrate an effective breathing pattern?

Nursing Diagnosis: Activity intolerance related to imbalance between oxygen supply and demand

Expected Outcomes Patient will receive assistance with self-care until he or she is able to carry out own ADLs.
Patient will space rest and activity in order to provide as much self-care as possible.

Evaluation of Outcomes Are patient's care needs met by self or caregiver?

Interventions	Rationale	Evaluation
• Assess amount of activity the patient can tolerate without becoming short of breath.	Patients should be encouraged to do as much as they can for themselves, to avoid becoming deconditioned.	What is patient able to do?
• Monitor vital signs and oxygen saturation with activities.	Respiratory rate will rise and Sao_2 will drop if activity is not tolerated.	Are vital signs and Sao_2 stable?
• Allow patient to rest between activities. Bedrest may be necessary during acute dyspnea.	Even talking or eating can be exhausting to a patient who is dyspneic.	Is patient able to catch his or her breath between activities?
• Obtain bedside commode, shower chair, handheld showerhead, if needed.	Assistive devices can help the patient conserve energy.	Do assistive devices allow patient more independence?
• Obtain portable oxygen if patient is able to ambulate.	Portable oxygen may enable the patient to ambulate and prevent deconditioning.	Is patient able to ambulate and maintain Sao_2 WNL with portable oxygen?
• Allow uninterrupted rest at night as much as possible.	Lack of sleep can contribute to activity intolerance.	Is patient able to sleep uninterrupted? Can interferences be delayed till morning?
• Slowly increase activity as able.	Increasing activity helps maintain muscle tone and endurance.	Is patient able to increase a little each day? Is this a realistic goal for patient?
• Refer patient with chronic lung disease to a pulmonary rehabilitation program.	Pulmonary rehabilitation programs can help patient increase exercise tolerance.	Is patient willing to participate in a rehabilitation program?

EVALUATION. If nursing care has been effective, the patient will understand his or her disease and the importance of taking care of himself or herself. The patient will take medications and receive follow-up care as ordered. He or she will take measures to protect others from catching TB. Additional evaluation is found in Box 31.5 Nursing Care Plan for the Patient with Lower Respiratory Tract Disorder.

CRITICAL THINKING

Mr. Woo

■ Mr. Woo is being tested for tuberculosis. You check his skin tests, and find that the PPD test in his left forearm is negative, with no redness or induration. You also find that the *Candida* test in his right forearm is negative, with no redness or induration. How do you document these results? How do you interpret them?

Suggested answers at end of chapter.

NURSING PROCESS FOR THE PATIENT WITH A LOWER RESPIRATORY INFECTION

Priority nursing diagnoses and interventions for patients with lower respiratory infections are presented in Box 31.5 Nursing Care Plan for the Patient with a Lower Respiratory Tract Disorder.

RESTRICTIVE DISORDERS

Restrictive disorders are those problems that limit the ability of the patient to expand his or her lungs. These are caused by a decrease in the **compliance** (or elasticity) of the lungs or chest wall.

Pleurisy (Pleuritis)

Pathophysiology

Recall that the visceral and parietal pleurae are the membranes that surround the lungs. Between these membranes is

CRITICAL THINKING

Jim

■ Jim is a 36-year-old accountant with bronchiectasis secondary to cystic fibrosis. You enter his room during an episode of uncontrollable coughing and offer him support. You observe his sputum as you dispose of it—a whole Styrofoam coffee cup full of thick, bright yellow sputum; the smell makes you nauseous. Even after coughing, his lungs sound congested from retained secretions. You offer him mouth care before you leave his room.

1. What questions can you ask Jim to assess his cough?
2. What nursing diagnosis is most appropriate for Jim?
3. What nursing care can you provide to enhance secretion removal?
4. You have an order for guaifenesin 300 mg q4h prn. It is supplied as 200 mg per 5 mL. How much will you administer?
5. How would you document this episode of coughing?

Suggested answers at end of chapter.

a small amount of serous fluid that prevents friction as the pleurae slide over each other during respiration. If the membranes become inflamed for any reason, they do not slide as easily. Instead of sliding, one membrane may "catch" on the other, causing it to stretch as the patient attempts to take a breath. This causes the characteristic sharp pain on inspiration. The irritation causes an increase in the formation of pleural fluid, which in turn reduces friction and decreases pain.

Etiology

Pleurisy is usually related to another underlying respiratory disorder, such as pneumonia, tuberculosis, tumor, or trauma. Nonrespiratory disorders such as pancreatitis or certain autoimmune disorders can also result in pleurisy.

Signs and Symptoms

Pleurisy causes a sharp pain in the chest on inspiration. Pain also occurs during coughing or sneezing. Breathing may be shallow and rapid because deep breathing increases pain. The patient may also exhibit fever, chills, and an elevated white blood cell count if the cause is infectious. A pleural friction rub is heard on auscultation.

Complications

As pleural membranes become more inflamed, serous fluid production increases, which may result in pleural effusion (see next section). If pleuritic pain is not controlled, patients have difficulty breathing deeply and coughing, which may lead to atelectasis. If infection goes untreated, **empyema** can result.

If fluid is pus

Diagnostic Tests

Diagnosis is based on signs and symptoms, including auscultation of a pleural friction rub. A chest x-ray examination

and complete blood cell count (CBC) may be done. FVC (forced vital capacity) is reduced more than FEV_1 (forced expiratory volume in one minute) since expansion is limited by the restrictive disorder; airways and FEV_1 may be normal. Additional testing is done to determine the underlying cause.

Therapeutic Interventions

Treatment is aimed at correcting the underlying cause. Nonsteroidal anti-inflammatory drugs (NSAIDs) or opioids are given to control pain and facilitate deep breathing and coughing. The physician may perform a nerve block by injecting anesthetic near the intercostal nerves to block pain transmission.

Pleural Effusion

Pathophysiology

When excess fluid collects in the pleural space, it is called a pleural effusion. Fluid normally enters the pleural space from surrounding capillaries and is reabsorbed by the lymphatic system. When a pathological condition causes an increase in fluid production or inadequate reabsorption of fluid, excess fluid collects. A normal amount of pleural fluid around each lung is 1 to 15 mL. More than 25 mL of fluid is considered abnormal; as much as several liters of fluid can collect at one time. The effusion can be either transudative, forming a watery fluid from the capillaries, or exudative, with fluid containing white blood cells and protein from an inflammatory process.

Etiology

Like pleurisy, pleural effusion is generally caused by another lung disorder. It is a symptom rather than a disease. Transudative effusions may result from heart failure, liver disorders, or kidney disorders. Exudative effusions more commonly occur with lung cancer, infection, or inflammation.

Signs and Symptoms

Symptoms depend on the amount of fluid in the pleural space. The patient may or may not experience pleuritic pain. Increasing shortness of breath occurs because of the decreasing space for lung expansion. Cough and **tachypnea** may be present. A dull sound is heard when the affected area is percussed. Lung sounds are decreased or absent over the effusion, and a friction rub may be auscultated.

Diagnostic Tests

A chest x-ray examination is done to determine whether pleural effusion is present. If a thoracentesis is done, fluid samples are sent to the laboratory for culture and sensitivity and cytological examination. Further tests may be done to determine the cause of the effusion.

Therapeutic Interventions

Bedrest is recommended to enhance spontaneous resolution of the effusion. If symptoms are severe, a therapeutic thoracentesis is done to remove the excess fluid from the pleural space and relieve the patient of dyspnea. See Chapter 29 for

---

tachypnea: tachy—rapid + pnea—breathing

how to assist with a thoracentesis. The physician will use x-ray examinations and percussion, or sometimes ultrasound, to determine where to insert the needle to obtain the fluid. If the fluid accumulation is large or recurring, a chest tube might be placed to continuously drain the pleural space. Occasionally talc or another irritating agent will be instilled via the chest tube to cause the pleural membranes to adhere to each other, eliminating the pleural space and preventing future episodes of pleural effusion. Treatment of the underlying cause of the effusion is necessary to prevent recurrence.

Empyema

Empyema is the collection of pus in the pleural space. It is a pleural effusion that is infected. Empyema is usually a complication of pneumonia, tuberculosis, or lung abscess.

Symptoms, diagnosis, therapeutic interventions, and nursing care are the same as the care of the patient with a pleural effusion, with an added emphasis on resolving the infection. A chest tube or surgery may be necessary to drain the area.

Pulmonary Fibrosis

Pathophysiology

Pulmonary fibrosis (PF), sometimes called interstitial lung disease, is a group of disorders that cause scarring and fibrosis of lung tissue. PF may evolve from injury to the alveoli, causing chronic inflammation; inflamed tissues are gradually replaced by fibrous connective tissue. Alveoli become thick and scarred, and gas exchange becomes difficult.

Etiology

A variety of factors are linked with pulmonary fibrosis, including heredity, exposure to certain viral illnesses, wood and metal dust exposure, medications, and smoking. It may also be associated with some autoimmune disorders such as lupus erythematosus or rheumatoid arthritis. Chronic GERD (gastroesophageal reflux disease) may play a role. Often PF is called idiopathic PF because no specific cause can be found.

Signs and Symptoms

Patients with PF experience progressive shortness of breath. Inspiratory crackles and chronic cough are present. Some experience flulike symptoms. Fatigue is common. Clubbing of fingers may be present. Patients usually follow a downhill course.

Diagnostic Tests

A chest x-ray may show lung infiltrates. A CT scan may be done. Spirometry is done to verify that the condition is restrictive. ABGs may show reduced Pao_2. A bronchoscopy and lung biopsy can help rule out other causes of the patient's symptoms, and can show inflammation and fibrosis. A blood test (ANA titer) may show whether an autoimmune response is involved.

Therapeutic Interventions

Glucocorticoids (steroids) are used to reduce inflammation. Drugs to suppress the immune system may reduce autoimmune activity. Patients should be encouraged to stop smoking. Oxygen is used if needed to maintain blood gasses. Patients should receive flu and pneumococcus vaccines. Younger patients may be considered for a lung transplant. Pulmonary rehabilitation helps patients maintain optimum activity tolerance.

Atelectasis

Atelectasis is the collapse of alveoli. It most commonly occurs in postsurgical patients who do not cough and deep breathe effectively, although it can be caused by anything that causes hypoventilation. Areas of the lungs that are not well aerated become plugged with mucus, which prevents inflation of alveoli. As a result, alveoli collapse. Compression of lung tissue from effusion or a tumor can also cause atelectasis. The focus of nursing care is on prevention. Patients should be taught the importance of coughing and deep breathing whenever there is the risk for hypoventilation. Frequent position changes and ambulation are also important.

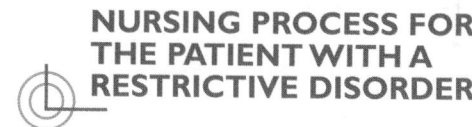

NURSING PROCESS FOR THE PATIENT WITH A RESTRICTIVE DISORDER

Assessment/Data Collection

Perform a routine respiratory assessment. Monitor lung sounds for friction rub or decreasing breath sounds in any of the lobes. Assess pain level. Promptly report any increase in dyspnea, changes in vital signs or pulse oximetry, or increased white blood cell count or temperature.

Nursing Diagnosis, Planning, and Implementation

Priority nursing diagnoses are similar to other respiratory disorders, and are addressed in Box 31.5 Nursing Care Plan for the Patient with a Lower Respiratory Tract Disorder. In addition, it is essential to address pain if present since pain can prevent the patient from breathing effectively.

Acute pain

EXPECTED OUTCOME: *Patient will be comfortable enough to breathe deeply and cough; respiratory rate 12 to 20.*

- Position patient for comfort. *Sometimes laying on the affected side for short periods will help reduce chest wall movement and pain.*
- Administer pain medication as ordered, preferably around-the-clock, to prevent pain from becoming severe. *Pain must be controlled so patient can breathe deeply and prevent further complications. NSAIDs or acetaminophen is usually tried first since they will not suppress cough and respirations.*
- If opioids are required to control pain, carefully monitor respirations and cough. *Opioids can suppress respirations and cough, which can further complicate the underlying disorder.*

- Teach patient the importance of deep breathing and coughing. *This can help prevent further complications, but may be difficult if associated with pain or suppressed by opioids.*

Evaluation

If interventions have been effective, the patient should report a decrease in dyspnea and anxiety. Pain will be controlled so that the patient is able to take deep breaths and cough effectively, and the patient will be free of signs and symptoms of infection.

OBSTRUCTIVE DISORDERS

Chronic Obstructive Pulmonary Disease/Chronic Airflow Limitation

Chronic obstructive pulmonary disease (COPD) is the fourth leading cause of death in the United States, and is expected to move to third place by 2020. Approximately 12.1 million adults have been diagnosed with COPD.[2] In the past, it was more common in men, but the incidence in women is rising due to more women smoking. The death rate from COPD in women nearly tripled between 1980 and 2000.

Pathophysiology

Chronic obstructive pulmonary disease is a group of pulmonary disorders characterized by difficulty exhaling because of airways that are narrowed or blocked by inflammation and mucus. More effort is required to push air out through obstructed airways (Fig. 31.3). **Emphysema, chronic bronchitis, and asthma are disorders that limit airflow.** A patient with COPD often has some degree of both emphysema and chronic bronchitis, although usually bronchitis is the dominant disorder. Asthma may also be present, but it differs somewhat because the airway constriction in asthma is usually reversible. A patient with asthma that is unremitting is treated as having COPD. Airflow limitation in emphysema and bronchitis is progressive and minimally reversible (Fig. 31.4).

COPD may also be referred to as chronic airflow limitation (CAL) or chronic obstructive lung disease (COLD). COPD develops over at least 30 years before symptoms become evident and may be advanced by the time the patient seeks treatment. It is characterized by periods of relative stability and **exacerbation**s (acute worsening of symptoms), which may be triggered by respiratory infection or another stressor. See Box 31.6 COPD Summary.

>
> ## LEARNING TIP
>
> Restrictive disorders cause difficulty with inhalation and lung expansion. Obstructive disorders are associated with difficulty exhaling.

---

emphysema: to inflate

AIR TRAPPING IN CHRONIC AIRFLOW LIMITATION

A. Air trapping from excess mucous

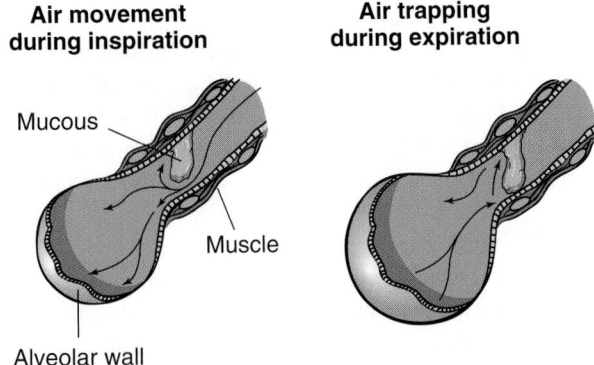

B. Air trapping from decreased elastic recoil and narrowed airways

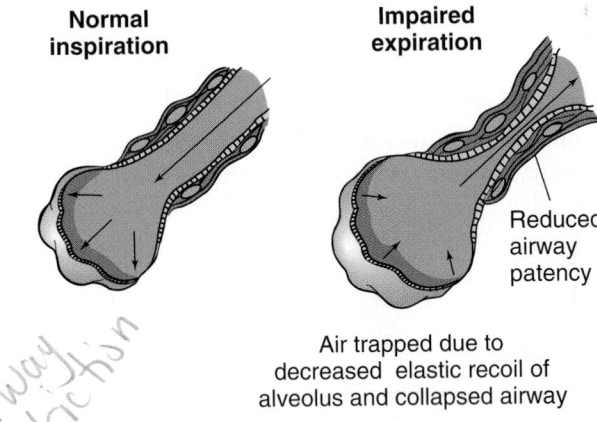

Air trapped due to decreased elastic recoil of alveolus and collapsed airway

FIGURE 31.3 Air trapping in COPD.

CHRONIC BRONCHITIS PATHOPHYSIOLOGY. Chronic bronchitis is similar to acute bronchitis, with symptoms occurring for at least 3 months of the year for 2 consecutive years. Patients may have multiple exacerbations, each lasting 2 weeks or more. The bronchial tree becomes inflamed from inhaled irritants, and impaired ciliary function reduces the ability to remove the irritants. The mucus-producing glands in the airways become hypertrophied, producing excessive thick, tenacious mucus, which obstructs airways and traps air (Fig. 31.5). These changes lead to chronic low-grade infection.

EMPHYSEMA PATHOPHYSIOLOGY. Emphysema affects the alveolar membranes, causing destruction of the alveolar walls and loss of elastic recoil. This also causes damage to adjacent pulmonary capillaries. Because of the loss of elastic recoil, passive expiration is impaired and air is trapped in the alveoli. Reduction in pulmonary capillaries reduces gas exchange. Emphysema can occur primarily in the respiratory bronchioles (centrilobular emphysema), with delayed alveolar damage, or in the respiratory bronchioles and alveoli (panlobular emphysema) (Fig. 31.6).

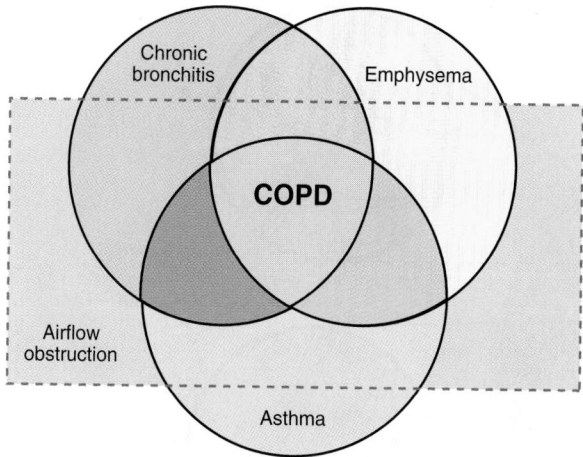

FIGURE 31.4 Chronic bronchitis and emphysema are the primary underlying disorders in COPD. Asthma may also play a role.

Etiology

Smoking is the single most important risk factor for COPD. Other factors include passive (secondhand) smoking, air pollution, and exposure to industrial chemicals. Some familial predisposition to chronic bronchitis has been demonstrated. A small number of individuals have an inherited deficiency of the enzyme alpha-antitrypsin (α_1AT), which causes a predisposition to the development of emphysema. Patients with this inherited tendency who also smoke have a very high risk of developing the disease. Children of smoking parents are at higher risk because of secondhand smoke exposure.

Prevention

Prevention is important because no cure for COPD is currently available. Avoidance of smoking and other inhaled irritants is vital, especially in those individuals with parents or siblings with COPD. According to the Global Initiative for Chronic Obstructive Lung Disease (GOLD) guidelines, "smoking cessation is the single most effective- and cost-effective intervention to reduce the risk of developing COPD and slow its progression."[3]

NURSING CARE TIP

This is a self-care tip. If you are a smoker, now is a good time to quit. COPD is deadly. Check Chapter 29 for ways to quit smoking. Good luck!

Signs and Symptoms

Classic symptoms of COPD are cough, sputum production, and dyspnea. Patients exhibit prolonged expiration because of obstructed air passages. Air trapping causes the lungs to become hyperinflated, which in turn leads to the classic barrel-shaped chest. The patient with chronic bronchitis has a chronic productive cough, shortness of breath, and activity

---

Box 31.6

COPD Summary

Signs and Symptoms

Cough
Chronic sputum production
Dyspnea that occurs every day, worse with exercise
Activity intolerance
Crackles, wheezes, diminished breath sounds
Barrel chest
Use of accessory muscles

Diagnostic Tests

Chest x-ray examination, CT scan
Arterial blood gas analysis
CBC
Sputum analysis
Spirometry
α_1AT level if hereditary deficiency suspected

Therapeutic Management

Smoking cessation
Bronchodilators (PO, NMT, MDI)
Corticosteroids, expectorants
Flu and pneumonia vaccinations
Supplemental oxygen
Breathing exercises
Chest physiotherapy
Pulmonary rehabilitation

Priority Nursing Diagnoses

Impaired gas exchange
Ineffective airway clearance
Activity intolerance

MDI = metered-dose inhaler; NMT = nebulized mist treatment; PO = by mouth.

---

intolerance. Symptoms may initially be worse in the winter months. Crackles and wheezing are often noted on auscultation and may improve after coughing.

The most characteristic symptom of emphysema is progressive shortness of breath, accompanied by activity intolerance. Use of accessory muscles is evident. Auscultation reveals diminished breath sounds. Remember that many patients have symptoms of both chronic bronchitis and emphysema.

Arterial blood gases (ABGs) may be checked during an acute exacerbation of COPD and may show an increase in $Paco_2$ and often a low Pao_2. The patient develops **polycythemia** in response to reduced oxygenation, which results in a ruddy skin color. Cyanosis may also be present.

---

polycythemia: poly—many + cyt—cells = emia—in the blood.

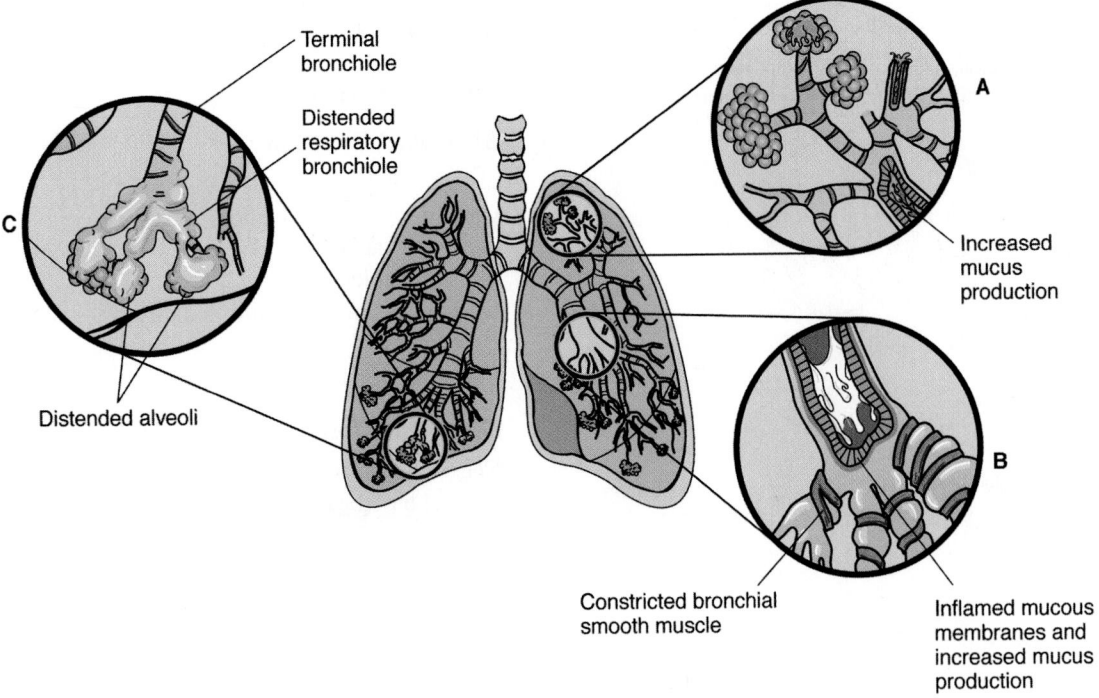

Terminal bronchiole

Distended respiratory bronchiole

C

Distended alveoli

A

Increased mucus production

B

Constricted bronchial smooth muscle

Inflamed mucous membranes and increased mucus production

FIGURE 31.5 *(A)* Chronic bronchitis. Note inflamed airways and excessive mucus. *(B)* Asthma. Note narrowed bronchial tubes and swollen mucous membranes. *(C)* Emphysema. Note distended respiratory bronchioles and alveoli.

In late stages of COPD, patients may lose weight and become malnourished. They have difficulty eating because of severe dyspnea, and the increased work of breathing expends more calories. Chronic hypoxemia causes release of certain chemicals that may also lead to weight loss.

Complications

Some patients with emphysema develop large air spaces within the lung tissue (**bullae**) or adjacent to the pleurae (**blebs**). These are like blisters that can rupture and cause the lung to collapse. Right-sided heart failure may develop because the heart has to work harder to pump blood to the diseased lungs. (See the section on cor pulmonale in Chapter 26.) Death usually results from respiratory infection or respiratory failure.

Diagnostic Tests

Information from a chest x-ray examination, CT scan, blood gas analysis, CBC, and sputum analysis is correlated with the history and physical examination to diagnose COPD. Spirometry can help differentiate an obstructive versus a restrictive disorder: FEV_1 is reduced more than FVC in COPD: lung volume may be relatively normal, but forced expiration is reduced because of the obstruction. An α_1AT level is checked if deficiency is suspected, especially in patients with a family history of COPD.

COPD is classified according to spirometry results and symptoms (Box 31.7 COPD Stages).

Therapeutic Interventions

The goals of COPD treatment, according to the GOLD guidelines, are to:

- Prevent disease progression
- Relieve symptoms
- Improve exercise tolerance
- Improve health status
- Prevent and treat complications
- Prevent and treat exacerbations
- Reduce mortality
- Prevent or minimize side effects from treatment

In addition, cessation of cigarette smoking should be included as a goal throughout any management program.[3]

SMOKING CESSATION. Even late in the disease process, stopping smoking can slow disease progression and prolong life. Exposure to other respiratory contaminants should also be minimized. Hair spray, body powder, and other household aerosols should be avoided. Figure 31.7 shows the benefit of smoking cessation and impact on the length of time to disability and death. Box 31.8 Patient Perspective is a personal account from one woman who understood too late the importance of smoking cessation.

OXYGEN. Oxygen therapy is usually delayed until stage IV disease, and then is used to keep Sao_2 at or above 90%. It is generally ordered at a flow rate of 1 to 2 L/minute. Higher flow rates may suppress the hypoxic drive in patients who are chronic CO_2 retainers, although this is uncommon. Higher flow rates may be used during acute exacerbations in a monitored setting. Patients with chronic oxygen saturation levels of less than 88% should be placed on home oxygen.

A **Normal lungs**

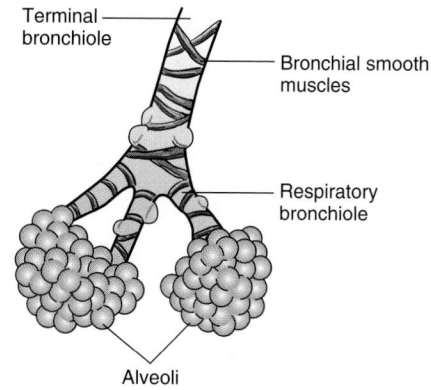

B **Centrilobular emphysema**

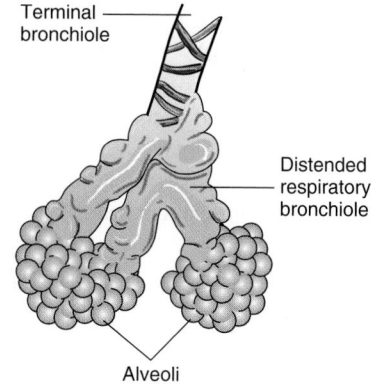

C **Panlobular emphysema**

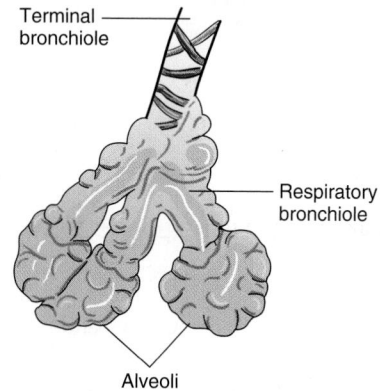

FIGURE 31.6 Types of emphysema. (A) Normal lungs. (B) Centrilobular emphysema. (C) Panlobular emphysema.

MEDICATIONS. Medications commonly used include adrenergic and anticholinergic MDIs (inhalers) or NMTs (nebulized mist treatments) to open airways, corticosteroid inhalers to control inflammation, expectorants, and, intermittently when needed, antibiotics. Much focus is now placed on a combination of long-acting adrenergic agents and corticosteroids (Advair, Symbicort) and a new long-acting anticholinergic agent (tiopropium/Spiriva), all of which may reduce exacerbations and prolong survival.

Box 31.7

COPD Stages

Stage 0—At Risk. Patient has cough and sputum production, but lung function is normal.

Stage 1—Mild COPD. Mild airflow limitation, with cough and sputum. Patient may not realize his lung function is abnormal.

Stage 2—Moderate COPD. Airflow limitation worsening, patient begins to feel short of breath on exertion.

Stage 3—Severe COPD. Increasing airflow limitation and shortness of breath. Patient experiences decreased quality of life.

Stage 4—Very Severe COPD. Severe airflow limitation; exacerbations may be life-threatening.

Adapted from GOLD Guidelines, 2005.[3]

Antitussives should be avoided in patients with COPD because they need to be able to cough up secretions.

Oral theophylline bronchodilators are sometimes used, but have a lot of side effects so are avoided if possible. Oral corticosteroids may be used late in the disease to increase reduction in airway inflammation, but should ideally be reserved for acute exacerbations. A newer treatment is

---

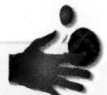

Box 31.8

Patient Perspective

Sarah

At the age of 17, I started the habit which would change my life. I started to smoke.

At first it was just a few cigarettes, but as time passed I smoked more and more until I reached two packs a day. This habit continued for 42 years, disregarding all the warnings about what could happen. I was sure this would never happen to me.

Now at age 75, I must do three breathing treatments a day, and carry an inhaler with me at all times. I have a cough that cannot be controlled. I can no longer ride a bike with my grandchildren, play badminton, or even bowl. My lungs won't let me. Going shopping is no longer fun—it's a chore. I have to walk slowly or I can't breathe.

All the things I enjoyed most I've given up because for 42 years I was a slave to cigarettes. If any of you smoke, stop now. Smell the coffee and roses without coughing.

---

antitussive: anti—against + tussive—cough

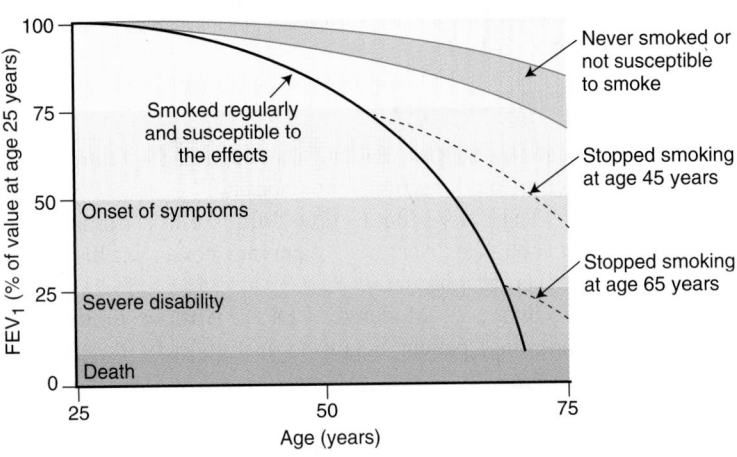

FIGURE 31.7 Fletcher and Peto Chart.
(Fletcher C, Peto R: The natural history of chronic airflow obstruction. BMJ 1:1645–1648, 1977.)

replacement of $\alpha_1 AT$ in those patients who are deficient. See Table 31.2 for a more detailed list of medications used in the treatment of COPD.

Patients with COPD should also be assessed for depression. Depression is common with chronic illness, and often goes undiagnosed. Patients may not complain of feeling depressed, but may experience more physical symptoms. Antidepressant medications, if indicated, can increase quality of life for COPD patients.

SUPPORTIVE CARE. A pneumococcal vaccination and yearly influenza vaccinations are recommended to reduce the risk of respiratory infection. Avoidance of crowds and exposure to people with respiratory infections is advised.

Good hydration and a cool mist humidifier help keep secretions loose. Chest physiotherapy may be used to help the patient remove excessive secretions. A dietitian consultation is helpful for the patient who is unable to maintain a

TABLE 31.2 SELECTED MEDICATIONS USED FOR LOWER RESPIRATORY TRACT DISORDERS

Drug Class/Action	Examples	Route	Side Effects	Nursing Implications
Adrenergic bronchodilators Stimulate beta receptors to dilate bronchioles	Albuterol (Ventolin, Proventil)	PO, Inhaled	Increased heart rate, tremor, anxiety	Use with care in patients with cardiac disease. Overuse can cause rebound bronchospasm. Albuterol, metaproterenol, and pirbuterol are short acting; used as rescue inhalers. Serevent and Foradil are long acting, used bid to prevent symptoms.
	Metaproterenol (Alupent, Metaprel)	PO, Inhaled		
	Pirbuterol (Maxair)	Inhaled		
	Salmeterol (Serevent)	Inhaled		
	Formoterol (Foradil)	Inhaled		
Anticholinergic agents Block parasympathetic response, causing bronchodilation	Ipratropium (Atrovent)	Inhaled	Dry mouth	Caution in narrow-angle glaucoma and prostatic hypertrophy
	Tiopropium (Spiriva)	Inhaled		
Methylxanthines Relax bronchial smooth muscle to dilate airways	Theophylline (Theovent, Theolair, Uniphyl)	PO	Tremor, anxiety, tachycardia, nausea, vomiting	Can become toxic. Therapeutic theophylline level 10–20 $\mu g/mL$.
	Aminophylline	PO, IV		
Corticosteroids Reduce inflammation in airways	Methylprednisolone (Medrol, Solu-Medrol)	PO, IV	Cushingoid side effects with prolonged use: moon face, sodium and water retention, buffalo hump, osteoporosis, hyperglycemia. Fewer side effects with inhaled route.	Must be used regularly to prevent symptoms. Never discontinue abruptly. Monitor blood glucose while on high doses. Rinse mouth following use to prevent local infection. If using glucocorticoid and adrenergic MDIs together, use adrenergic inhaler first to open airways.
	Prednisone	PO		
	Triamcinolone acetonide (Azmacort)	Inhaled		
	Beclomethasone (Beclovent)	Inhaled		
	Fluticasone (Flovent)	Inhaled		
	Budesonide (Pulmicort)	Inhaled		

(Handwritten margin notes: "cause dilation", "relaxing", "must be weaned", "elevated blood sugar", "healing poor", "off")

Drug Class/Action	Examples	Route	Side Effects	Nursing Implications
Combination Agents	Albuterol and ipratropium (Combivent)	Inhaled	See individual agents	See individual agents
	Fluticasone and salmeterol (Advair)	Inhaled		
	Budesonide and formoterol (Symbicort)	Inhaled		
		Inhaled		
Mast Cell Inhibitors				
Stabilize mast cells to reduce histamine release	Cromolyn sodium (Intal)	Inhaled	Few side effects.	⟨Effective for allergic asthma.⟩ May be used prophylactically before exercise or allergen exposure.
	Nedocromyl (Tilade)	Inhaled		
Expectorants *make you cough up*				
Liquefy secretions and stimulate cough	Guaifenesin (Robitussin, Mucinex)	PO	Few side effects.	Encourage fluids.
Antileukotrienes				
Inhibit leukotriene synthesis or activity, a mediator of inflammation in asthma	Zafirlukast (Accolate) Montelukast (Singulair) Zileuron (Zyflo)	PO PO PO	Headache *Asthma*	Must be taken regularly to prevent symptoms. Monitor for elevation of liver enzymes.
Antitussives				
Suppress cough reflex *not cough* *make you*	Codeine	PO	Related to opioids; may be sedating at high doses.	Avoid giving to patient who has secretions that need to be expectorated.
	Dextromethorphan (DM suffix in cough preparations)	PO		

NOTE: This table is an overview. A drug guide should be consulted for complete administration guidelines.
    PO = by mouth; IV = intravenous; MDI = metered-dose inhaler.

desirable weight. Breathing exercises help improve oxygenation and reduce anxiety. (See Chapter 29.)

REHABILITATION. Pulmonary rehabilitation programs can help patients increase exercise tolerance and maintain a sense of well-being (Fig. 31.8). Patients exercise in a monitored environment, and benefit from the support of other patients with similar problems. Some groups of pulmonary rehabilitation patients have even formed harmonica clubs! Playing their harmonicas mimics pursed lip breathing and may strengthen the diaphragm, the major muscle of breathing.

SURGERY. A newer treatment for emphysema is the surgical removal of some of the diseased lung tissue (called lung volume reduction surgery, or LVRS). This increases the space available for good lung tissue to expand, reducing dyspnea and increasing exercise tolerance. This is a high-risk procedure, but it has allowed some patients to return to a more normal activity level and increase quality of life. It does not lead to longer survival in most patients. Lung transplant may be an option in select patients.

MECHANICAL VENTILATION. If arterial blood gases worsen despite treatment, intubation and mechanical ventilation may be considered, depending on the patient's Advance Directive. Unfortunately, mechanical ventilation will not make a patient's disease better, and weaning may be

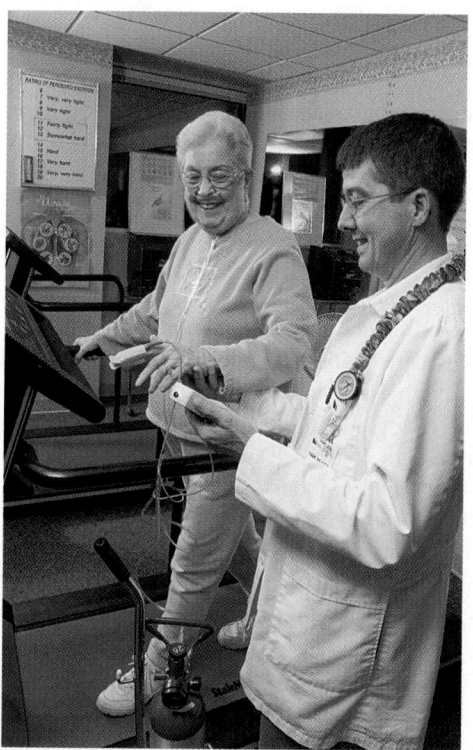

FIGURE 31.8 Patients build exercise tolerance in pulmonary rehabilitation programs. Note therapist monitoring oxygen saturation.

difficult or impossible once it is initiated. Use of noninvasive positive pressure ventilation (NIPPV; see Chapter 29) may be a good alternative for many patients.

END-OF-LIFE PLANNING. It is important to assess whether the patient has a Living Will or Durable Power of Attorney (DPOA) for Healthcare (see Chapter 16). COPD is a progressive disease, and patients can increase the quality of their life and death by making decisions in advance. Patients should make decisions about whether they would want to be intubated and mechanically ventilated, or have CPR in event of a cardiac arrest. CPR is rarely successful in a patient with end-stage COPD. Patients should be made aware of palliative care options, and assured they will be kept as comfortable as possible.

Research is ongoing to determine which treatments will alter long-term outcomes of the disease. Check the American Lung Association website for more information at www.lungusa.org.

Nursing Process

See Nursing Process for the Patient with an Obstructive Disorder, following the section on cystic fibrosis, and Box 31.5 Nursing Care Plan for the Patient with a Lower Respiratory Tract Disorder. Priority nursing diagnoses for the patient with COPD include Impaired Gas Exchange, Ineffective Airway Clearance, and Activity Intolerance.

Asthma

The incidence of asthma is on the rise. Nearly 20 million people in the United States have asthma, and 5000 people die from asthma each year.[4] It is more prevalent in African Americans than in whites. Asthma deaths are more prevalent in lower socioeconomic groups, presumably because of lack of compliance with treatment regimens. With careful monitoring and treatment, however, patients with asthma can control their symptoms and lead normal lives.

Pathophysiology and Etiology

Asthma is characterized by inflammation of the mucosal lining of the bronchial tree and spasm of the bronchial smooth muscles (**bronchospasm**). This causes narrowed airways and air trapping, which is why it is considered an obstructive disorder (see Fig. 31.5). Inflammation occurs in part because asthma triggers cause release of inflammatory substances such as histamine and leukotrienes. Symptoms are intermittent and generally reversible, with periods of normal airway function. About 50% of asthmatics develop the disorder in childhood, and many outgrow it. However, a significant number develop symptoms again later in life. Children with asthma should be counseled that smoking can increase the risk of recurrence in adulthood.

The tendency to develop asthma is inherited. Some sources classify asthma as either allergic or idiosyncratic (unusual). Allergic asthma is triggered by allergens such as

---

bronchospasm: broncho—airway + spasm—convulsion, narrowing

pollen, foods, medications, animal dander, air pollution, molds, or dust mites. It is commonly seasonal. Individuals who developed asthma as children tend to have allergic asthma. Idiosyncratic asthma is generally diagnosed in adults and is related to environmental or other nonallergic factors, such as environmental irritants, smoking, and respiratory or sinus infection.

Emotional upset and exercise can also trigger symptoms in some persons with asthma. Gastroesophageal reflux disease (GERD) can also trigger symptoms. It is believed that stomach acid may reflux into the esophagus and then be aspirated, triggering asthma. This occurs especially at night. GERD and its treatment are discussed in Chapter 33. Asthma frequently complicates chronic bronchitis or emphysema.

Prevention

Although asthma cannot be prevented at this time, research is ongoing to determine factors associated with its development. Exposures to allergens and respiratory syncytial virus (RVS) in infancy are believed to play a role. Smoking may be associated with recurrence of asthma that started in childhood. It is important that the patient identify triggers of asthma symptoms and avoid them whenever possible. Compliance with prophylactic and maintenance therapy is also important.

Signs and Symptoms

Asthma symptoms are intermittent and are often referred to as "attacks," which may last from minutes to days. The patient complains of chest tightness, dyspnea, and difficulty moving air in and out of the lungs. Once initial symptoms are controlled, airways may remain hypersensitive and prone to asthma symptoms for many weeks.

On examination, you will note an increased respiratory rate as the patient attempts to compensate for narrowed airways. Inspiratory and expiratory wheezing is heard because of turbulent airflow through swollen airways with thick secretions and may sometimes be audible even without a stethoscope. Air is trapped in the lungs, and expiration is prolonged. A cough is common and may produce thick, clear sputum. Use of accessory muscles to breathe is a sign that the attack is severe and warrants immediate attention.

Be aware that an absence of audible wheezing may not signal improvement but rather may be an ominous sign that the patient is not moving enough air to make a sound. If wheezing is not heard, use of accessory muscles and peak expiratory flow rate values must be carefully evaluated. Once treatment begins to be effective and the patient is moving more air, wheezing may become audible.

Asthma is classified according to frequency of symptoms (Table 31.3).

nothing you are giving isn't working

Complications

Status asthmaticus occurs if bronchospasm is not controlled and symptoms are prolonged. As the patient increases the respiratory rate to compensate for narrowed airways, a lot of carbon dioxide is blown off and respiratory

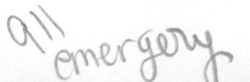 *911 emergency*

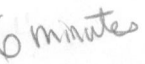 *6 minutes*

TABLE 31.3 CLASSIFICATION OF ASTHMA

Mild Intermittent	Asthma symptoms twice a week or less, night symptoms twice a month or less.
Mild persistent	Asthma symptoms more than twice a week, but no more than once a day; symptoms at night more than twice a month. Asthma attacks affect activity.
Moderate persistent	Asthma symptoms every day; nighttime symptoms more than once a week. May affect activity.
Severe persistent	Symptoms throughout the day on most days; nighttime symptoms often. Physical activity likely limited.

From the National Heart, Blood, and Lung Institute, http://www.nhlbi.nih.gov, July 2005.

alkalosis occurs. If the attack is not resolved and the patient begins to tire, the patient will no longer be able to compensate and $PaCO_2$ will rise, resulting in respiratory acidosis. This can lead to respiratory failure and death if untreated.

Diagnostic Tests

Diagnosis is based on the patient's report of symptoms, physical examination, and spirometry. Peak expiratory flow rate and forced expiratory volume in one second (FEV_1) are reduced during symptomatic periods. Asthma can be differentiated from COPD during spirometry testing by administering an adrenergic agonist (such as an albutrol inhaler) and then retesting. Asthma symptoms can generally be reversed with the medication, while COPD cannot. Allergy skin test-

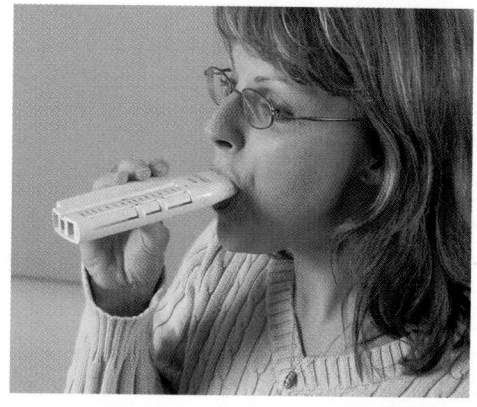

FIGURE 31.9 Patient with asthma using a peak flowmeter to monitor peak expiratory flow rate.

ing and increased serum IgE and eosinophil levels indicate allergic involvement and may help determine treatment.

During a severe attack, arterial blood gases may initially show decreased $PaCO_2$. Late in the course of an attack, PaO_2 decreases and $PaCO_2$ increases.

Therapeutic Interventions

Patients must learn to manage their asthma at home. The better they can monitor and manage their symptoms, the fewer acute episodes and hospitalizations will be required.

MONITORING. Some patients monitor their peak expiratory flow rate (PEFR) at home (Fig. 31.9). This is a measure of the amount of air the patient can blow into a peak flowmeter from fully inflated lungs and is measured in liters per minute. The patient determines his or her normal PEFR during symptom-free times. Readings can be charted to keep track of progress (Fig. 31.10). If the PEFR begins to

FIGURE 31.10 Peak flow chart. The green zone is 80% to 100% of the patient's normal peak flow rate. The yellow zone is 50% to 80% of normal. The red zone is less than 50% of normal. The patient works with the physician to determine which actions to take when readings fall in the yellow or red zones.

Name														
Green zone _____ Yellow zone _____ Red zone _____														
Date														
	AM	PM	AM	PM	AM	PM	AM	PM	AM	PM	AM	PM	AM	PM
800														
750														
700														
650														
600														
550														
500														
450														
400														
350														
300														
250														
200														
150														
100														
Notes														

Asthma Action Plan for _____ Doctor's Name _____ Date _____

Doctor's Phone Number _____ Hospital/ Emergency Room Phone Number _____

GREEN ZONE: Doing Well

- No cough, wheeze, chest tightness, or shortness of breath during the day or night
- Can do usual activities

And, if a peak flow meter is used,

Peak flow: more than _____
(80% or more of my best peak flow)

My best peak flow is: _____

Take These Long-Term-Control medicines Each Day (include an anti-inflammatory)

Medicine	How much to take	When to take it

Before exercise ☐ _____ ☐ 2 or ☐ 4 puffs 5 to 60 minutes before exercise

YELLOW ZONE: Asthma is Getting Worse

- Cough, wheeze, chest tightness, or shortness of breath, or
- Waking at night due to asthma, or
- Can do some, but not all, usual activities

-Or-

Peak flow: _____ to _____
(50% – 80% of my best peak flow)

First ⟩ **Add: Quick-Relief Medicine – and keep taking your GREEN ZONE medicine**

_____ ☐ 2 or ☐ 4 puffs, every 20 minutes up to 1 hour
(short-acting beta₂-antagonist) ☐ Nebulizer, once

Second ⟩ **If your symptoms (and peak flow, if used) return to GREEN ZONE after 1 hour of above treatment**

☐ Take the quick-relief medicine every 4 hours for 1 to 2 days
☐ Double the dose of your inhaled steroid for _____ (7-10) days
-Or-
If your symptoms (and peak flow, if used) do not return to GREEN ZONE after 1 hour of above treatment
☐ Take: _____ ☐ 2 or ☐ 4 puffs or ☐ Nebulizer
(short-acting beta₂-antagonist)
☐ Add: _____ mg/day For _____ (3-10) days
(oral steroid)
☐ Call the doctor before/ ☐ within _____ hours after taking the oral steroid.

RED ZONE: Medical Alert!

- Very short of breath, or
- Quick-relief medicines have not helped, or
- Cannot do usual activities, or
- Symptoms are same or get worse after 24 hours in Yellow Zone

-Or-

Peak flow: less than _____
(50% of my best peak flow)

Take this Medicine

☐ _____ ☐ 4 or ☐ 6 puffs or ☐ Nebulizer
(short-acting beta₂-antagonist)
☐ _____ mg
(oral steroid)

Then call your doctor NOW. Go to the hospital or call for an ambulance if:
✔ You are still in the red zone after 15 minutes AND
✔ You have not reached your doctor

DANGER SIGNS
- **Trouble walking and talking due to shortness of breath**
- **Lips or fingernails are blue**

⟹ ✔ Take ☐ 4 or ☐ 6 puffs of your quick-relief medicine AND
✔ Go to the hospital or call for an ambulance (_____) NOW!

WHITE – PATIENT COPY   YELLOW – WORK/SCHOOL COPY   PINK – PROVIDER COPY

FIGURE 31.11 Asthma action plan.

fall below the patient's personal norm, treatment that has been predetermined with the health-care provider should be initiated (Fig. 31.11). PEFR results may indicate the onset of asthma before the patient experiences any symptoms.

AVOIDANCE OF TRIGGERS. The patient is instructed to identify and avoid asthma triggers. If triggers cannot be avoided, the patient can use bronchodilator or mast cell inhibitor inhalers as prescribed before exposure. Inhalers can be especially useful before exercise. Recent studies have shown that a high-salt diet may worsen exercise-induced airway inflammation. Animal dander and foods that cause symptoms are best avoided when possible. Eliminating carpets and curtains in bedrooms, using vinyl mattress and pillow covers, and installing a portable or central air filter can reduce dust mite exposure. Maintenance of indoor humidity between 40% and 50% can reduce mold growth. If cold air triggers symptoms, the patient should keep the nose and mouth covered when outside in cold weather. Smoking and exposure to secondary smoke are strongly discouraged.

Aspirin and nonsteroidal anti-inflammatory drugs can cause asthma symptoms in some individuals. Beta-blocking medications (propranolol, metoprolol), used commonly for hypertension, block beta receptors in the lungs, preventing the sympathetic nervous system from promoting bronchodilation. These drugs should be avoided if they make symptoms worse.

MEDICATIONS. Medications for asthma treatment may be intermittent or continuous, depending on the chronicity of symptoms. See Table 31.2 for a summary of medications used in the treatment of lower respiratory disorders.

For patients with only occasional symptoms, adrenergic bronchodilators such as albuterol (Proventil, Ventolin) are used. They may be administered via MDI when symptoms occur, or before exercise or other events that trigger asthma. Long-acting bronchodilators (Serevent, Foradil) can help prevent symptoms.

If the patient needs to use an adrenergic MDI more than three times a week, an inhaled corticosteroid (Pulmicort, Flovent) may be added. Because they are used topically, side effects are minimal. Inhaled corticosteroids are important in maintenance therapy to prevent symptoms. Instruct the patient that corticosteroids must be used regularly to prevent

NURSING CARE TIP

If separate bronchodilator and corticosteroid inhalers are used at the same time, instruct the patient to use the bronchodilator first. This opens the airways and allows the corticosteroid to be better distributed in the lungs.

symptoms and they do not provide immediate symptom relief during an acute attack. Combined corticosteroids and long-acting adrenergic bronchodilators (Advair, Symbicort) in one inhaler have been shown to be very effective in controlling asthma symptoms.

Mast cell inhibitors (Intal, Tilade) may help prevent symptoms, but are often not useful. Some patients use mast cell inhibitors 10 to 15 minutes before exposure to allergens or exercise to reduce symptoms.

If inhaled medications do not control symptoms, or if the patient has nocturnal symptoms, oral antileukotrienes may be tried; theophylline bronchodilators are generally used as a last resort because of their many side effects. Immunotherapy (allergy shots) may be used for some patients with allergic asthma.

An acute asthma attack may be treated with an inhaled (MDI or NMT) or subcutaneous adrenergic bronchodilator or, rarely, intravenous aminophylline. Intravenous or oral corticosteroids (methylprednisolone, prednisone) are potent anti-inflammatory agents that are useful in an acute episode but are avoided for long-term therapy if possible because of their cushingoid side effects. (See the section on Cushing's syndrome in Chapter 39.) Corticosteroids must be tapered before discontinuing to prevent withdrawal symptoms. (See the section on addisonian crisis in Chapter 39.)

Medications that are used routinely are called maintenance medications. Short-acting adrenergic inhalers such as albuterol are used for acute attacks and are called rescue medications. It is important that patients understand the difference between maintenance and rescue medications and use them appropriately.

Oxygen is generally not necessary because many patients hyperventilate during an acute attack. If the attack is prolonged and the patient becomes cyanotic or Pao_2 levels begin to fall, oxygen therapy will be used.

NURSING CARE TIP

Instruct the patient to contact the health-care provider if using more than two adrenergic MDI canisters per month. This has been associated with an increased risk of death.

Nursing Process

See Nursing Process for the Patient with an Obstructive Disorder, following cystic fibrosis section in this chapter.

Box 31.9

Asthma Summary

Signs and Symptoms	Chest tightness, dyspnea Wheezing
Diagnostic Tests	Spirometry ABGs in acute attack
Therapeutic Interventions	Identification and avoidance of triggers Inhaled corticosteroids Inhaled bronchodilators Oral bronchodilators and steroids if inhaled ineffective
Complications	Status asthmaticus
Priority Nursing Diagnoses	Impaired gas exchange Ineffective airway clearance Anxiety

Primary nursing diagnoses include Impaired Gas Exchange, Ineffective Airway Clearance, and Anxiety.

See Box 31.9 Asthma Summary.

Cystic Fibrosis

In the past, cystic fibrosis (CF) was thought to be just a childhood disease because most affected children did not survive past puberty. However, with new treatments, patients with CF are living longer and more productive lives. Some CF patients now marry, have careers, and live well into their 30s.

Pathophysiology

CF is a disorder of the exocrine glands that affects primarily the lungs, gastrointestinal (GI) tract, and sweat glands. The disease varies in severity; some patients have no GI involvement. Abnormal sodium and chloride transport across cell membranes, causing thick, tenacious secretions, is responsible for many of the characteristic symptoms. Thick, sticky respiratory secretions that are difficult to remove cause airway obstruction, resulting in air trapping and frequent respiratory infections.

Similar abnormalities in the pancreas cause blocked ducts and retained digestive enzymes. These retained enzymes digest and destroy the exocrine pancreas. The absence of digestive enzymes in the intestines causes malabsorption of essential nutrient, frequent foul-smelling, fatty stools, and excess flatus.

Patients with CF secrete sweat that is high in sodium and chloride because these electrolytes are not reabsorbed as they pass through the sweat ducts.

Etiology

CF is a genetic disorder. Both parents must be carriers of the defective gene for CF to be present in a child. Patients who marry are counseled on the risk of potential offspring having the disease.

Signs and Symptoms

Symptoms usually first appear in infancy or childhood, although a few individuals are not diagnosed until adulthood. Respiratory symptoms are often the first visible manifestation of the disease and range from chronic sinusitis to production of thick, tenacious sputum. Patients with CF are at risk for frequent respiratory infections, manifested by an increase in cough and purulent sputum. Finger clubbing is common. Late in the disease, hemoptysis may occur related to damaged blood vessels within the lungs. Over time, bouts of infection become more frequent, with eventual loss of lung function and respiratory failure. Antibiotic-resistant bacteria are a threat to life in these individuals.

Frequent foul-smelling stools result from the lack of enzymes in the small intestine. Inability to absorb fat-soluble vitamins and poor appetite due to respiratory disease result in malnutrition. Bowel obstruction, cirrhosis, cholecystitis, and cholelithiasis are associated findings.

Chronic disease causes delayed sexual maturation in both males and females, and infertility is common.

Complications

Patients with CF are at risk for a variety of complications, including bronchiectasis, pneumothorax, cor pulmonale, and respiratory failure. Bowel obstructions can occur as a result of thick mucus binding with poorly digested fecal matter. Diabetes from pancreatic islet cell involvement may be present late in the disease. Death is usually the result of pulmonary complications, especially antibiotic-resistant infection.

Diagnostic Tests

Because so many different gene mutations can occur in CF, genetic testing may be used to confirm a suspicion of CF but not for screening. The standard diagnostic test is the sweat chloride test. If respiratory symptoms are accompanied by excessive amounts of sodium chloride in sweat, CF is diagnosed. You may recall public health campaigns that advise parents to kiss their babies and report any salty taste to their physicians. Chest x-ray and spirometry may also be done.

Therapeutic Interventions

Because there is no cure for CF, treatment is aimed at controlling infection and relieving symptoms. Removal of thick sputum is promoted with hydration, use of the Flutter mucous clearance device, and chest physiotherapy up to four times a day. Regular exercise also helps mobilize secretions. A hot shower may be an easy occasional alternative to loosen secretions. Nebulized mist treatments using saline or mucolytic medications may be used before chest physiotherapy. Medications to decrease the viscosity of secretions have not yet been entirely successful, but new drugs are constantly being tested. Inhaled bronchodilators and corticosteroids are sometimes useful. High doses of ibuprofen (Motrin) may slow lung deterioration. Breathing exercises, incentive spirometry, and effective coughing techniques are also helpful. Lung transplant is a potentially promising treatment.

Prevention of infection is vital to slowing progression of lung damage. Patients should receive a yearly flu vacci-

nation. Antibiotics must be administered as soon as signs of infection occur. Prophylactic antibiotic therapy may be used. Some patients use home intravenous antibiotic therapy. Antibiotic-resistant infections are a deadly threat to the CF patient.

Pancreatic enzyme replacement (Pancrease, Viokase) helps reduce symptoms related to malabsorption and improve nutritional status. An increase in calorie requirements necessitates a high-calorie, nutrient-dense diet. For more information, visit the Cystic Fibrosis Foundation at www.cff.org.

Nursing Process

See Nursing Process: The Patient with an Obstructive Disorder below. Also, be sure to remember the special needs of the adolescent patient with this chronic, debilitating disease. Not only are normal physical growth and development delayed, but psychosocial development is also affected by repeated hospitalizations and the necessity of routine daily medication and treatments.

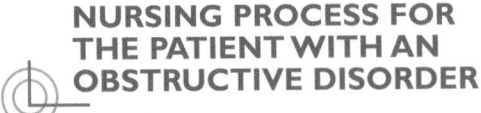

NURSING PROCESS FOR THE PATIENT WITH AN OBSTRUCTIVE DISORDER

Assessment/Data Collection

Perform a complete respiratory assessment as presented in Chapter 29. Frequency of assessment is dictated by the severity of the patient's condition. Note level of consciousness; poor gas exchange can cause confusion and lethargy. Assess respiratory rate and effort. Observe skin and mucous membranes for cyanosis. Auscultate lung sounds for adventitious sounds. Monitor cough and color and amount of sputum. Note exercise tolerance, and measure degree of dyspnea on a scale of 0 to 10. Monitor oxygen saturation or arterial blood gases. Careful documentation of findings allows you to monitor and report trends in the patient's progress.

Nursing Diagnosis, Planning, and Implementation

A number of nursing diagnoses are appropriate for the patient with an obstructive disorder. As always, choose diagnoses based on defining characteristics and the patient's individual assessment findings.

Impaired Gas Exchange, Ineffective Airway Clearance, Ineffective Breathing Pattern, and Activity Intolerance

These are priority problems for most chronic respiratory patients. Interventions for these diagnoses are presented in Box 31.5 Nursing Care for the Patient with a Lower Respiratory Tract Disorder.

Imbalanced nutrition related to poor appetite and increased calorie expenditure

EXPECTED OUTCOME: The patient's weight will be stable at desired weight for height.

- Monitor food intake and weekly weight. *Regular monitoring can help identify nutrition problems before they are severe.*
- If the patient is too dyspneic to eat, schedule rest periods and bronchodilator treatments before meals. *Eating takes a lot of energy, and resting can help conserve energy before a meal. Bronchodilators can reduce dyspnea while eating.*
- Create a pleasant eating environment. *Unpleasant views or odors can spoil an appetite.*
- Provide smaller, more frequent meals of the patient's favorite foods. *Eating a lot at one time can fill up the stomach and reduce room for lung expansion.*
- Encourage family members to bring favorite foods from home for the hospitalized patient. *A large tray of unappetizing food may be more than a patient can handle, and may spoil the appetite. Be sure to note sodium or other restrictions; although the patient with end-stage disease may be allowed a more lenient diet, excess sodium can cause fluid retention and increase dyspnea.*
- Consult a dietitian for liquid supplements recommendations. *A specialized supplement such as Pulmocare provides less carbon dioxide when metabolized and may be used for patients with respiratory disease*
- *See also Box 31.10 Nutrition Notes.*

Anxiety related to acute dyspnea

EXPECTED OUTCOME: The patient will state that anxiety is controlled; the patient will be able to use techniques to control dyspnea and anxiety when they occur.

- Remain with the patient who is acutely dyspneic and anxious. *Feeling alone during episodes of dyspnea can increase anxiety.*
- Calmly remind the patient to breathe slowly in through the nose and out through pursed lips. *During acute episodes of dyspnea, the patient may forget that breathing exercises can help.*
- Teach relaxation exercises during times when anxiety is minimal, and remind the patient to use them during acute anxiety. *Relaxation can help reduce muscle tension and distract the patient.*
- Administer antianxiety medications as ordered. *Medications can reduce anxiety but can also depress respirations, so should be used with caution.*
- Contact RN to administer intravenous morphine. *Morphine helps acute dyspnea and anxiety in patients with end-stage disease.*

Evaluation

If interventions have been effective, the patient will learn techniques to make breathing as comfortable as possible, and will be able to cough up secretions and maintain a clear airway. He or she will be able to manage anxiety symptoms and complete ADLs or other desired activity without dysp-

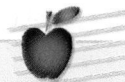

Box 31.10

Nutrition Notes

Optimizing Nutrition in Patients with Respiratory Disease

Many factors affect nutrition in a patient with respiratory disease. For example, patients commonly have an inadequate food intake because of anorexia, shortness of breath, gastrointestinal (GI) distress, or a combination of these problems.

Caloric requirements are frequently increased in patients with pulmonary disease. The caloric cost of breathing ranges from 36 to 72 calories each day in normal people, but it increases to 430 to 720 calories each day in patients with chronic obstructive pulmonary disease (COPD). Both decreased food intake and increased energy requirements may contribute to the weight loss often seen in these patients. When caloric intake is decreased, the body begins to break down muscle stores, including the respiratory muscles, which only exacerbates the problem.

The GI distress common in respiratory patients may be related to malnutrition of the GI tract. Malnutrition and the resulting decrease in antibody production lower the patient's resistance to infection. Also, the malnourished patient's lungs produce less pulmonary phospholipid, a fatlike substance that assists in lubricating lung tissue and helps to protect the lungs from inhaled pathogens.

To some extent, all the respiratory muscles atrophy from inactivity when a machine does the work for the patient. Nutrition support improves the likelihood of successful weaning in patients receiving mechanical ventilation.

Many patients with COPD have carbon dioxide retention and oxygen depletion. The medical goal for these patients is to decrease the level of carbon dioxide in their blood. Because fat calories produce less carbon dioxide when metabolized than carbohydrate calories, a diet with as much as 50% of the calories from fat may be prescribed. Several companies produce complete nutritional supplements with higher fat content formulated for patients with respiratory disease. Medical opinion is not unanimous on this issue because some evidence has related a high fat intake to immunosuppression in some patients.

Nursing Intervention

Many respiratory patients are breathless and lack the energy to eat. Offer small frequent feedings of nutrient-dense foods. Select foods that require little or no chewing. To lessen abdominal pressure on the diaphragm, discourage gaseous foods.

nea. The patient's intake should be adequate to maintain a stable weight. If any of the patient's goals have not been met, the plan of care should be revised.

Patient Education

The patient must be aware of the contributing factors to the disease and eliminate them if at all possible. The patient who is a smoker should not simply be told to quit smoking; he or she should be referred to a smoking cessation program and be provided with medication, nicotine patches, or other resources and support as necessary to quit. (See Chapter 29.) Techniques for effective breathing and anxiety control should also be taught.

PULMONARY VASCULAR DISORDERS

Pulmonary Embolism

Pathophysiology

An **embolism** is a foreign object that travels through the bloodstream. It may be a blood clot, air, or fat. A pulmonary embolism (PE), sometimes called pulmonary thromboembolism (PTE), is usually a blood clot that has traveled into a pulmonary artery (Fig. 31.12). Resulting obstruction of blood flow causes a ventilation-perfusion mismatch, which

in this case means that an area of the lung is well ventilated with air but has no blood flow, or perfusion. Because reduced or no blood supply is available to pick up the oxygen in the affected portion of the lung, it becomes pulmonary "dead space," causing seriously impaired gas exchange.

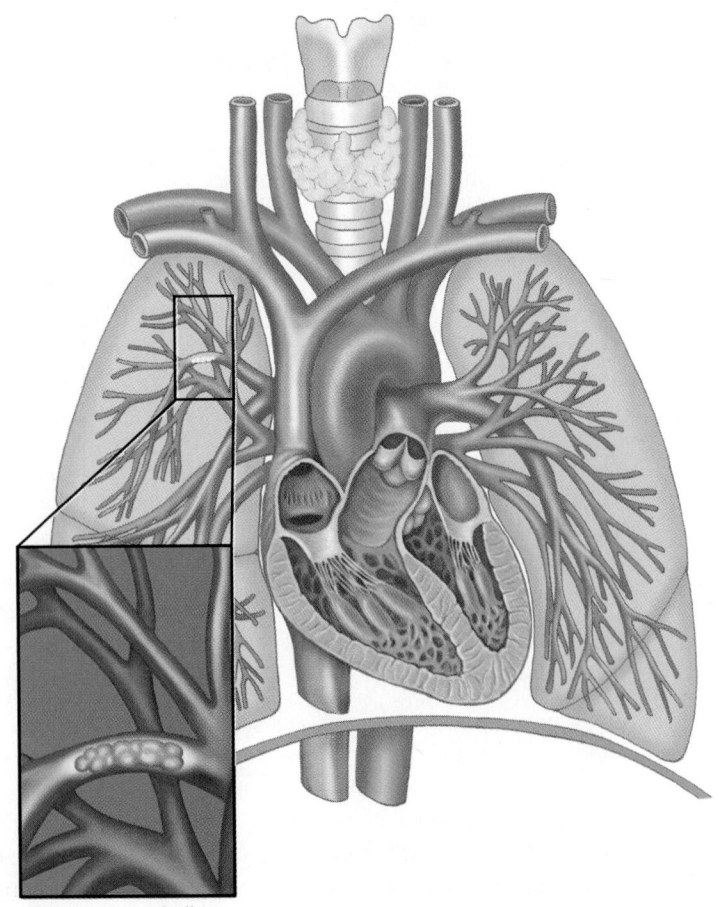

Pulmonary embolism

FIGURE 31.12 Pulmonary embolism.

Occasionally damage occurs to a portion of the lung because of lack of oxygen. This is called lung infarction, and it is not common because oxygen is delivered to lung tissue not only from the pulmonary arteries but also via the bronchial arteries and the airways.

Etiology

Most pulmonary emboli originate in the deep veins of the lower extremities (deep vein thrombosis, or DVT). Some risk factors of DVT, and therefore PE, include surgical procedures done under general anesthesia, heart failure, fractures of the lower extremities, immobility, obesity, oral contraceptive use, smoking, and a previous history of DVT or PE. Less common causes of PE include fat emboli from compound fractures, amniotic fluid embolism during labor and delivery, and air embolism from entry of air into the bloodstream.

Prevention

Prevention of thrombi in the deep veins of the legs is the most important factor in the prevention of a pulmonary embolism. Regular ambulation is advised if the patient is able. If a patient is at risk for DVT or PE, low-dose heparin, enoxaparin, warfarin (Coumadin), or intermittent compression stockings are used to prevent thrombus formation. If a DVT is diagnosed, prompt treatment is essential to prevent PE.

Signs and Symptoms

The most common symptom of PE is a sudden onset of dyspnea for no apparent reason. The patient may be gasping for breath and appear anxious. Tachycardia, tachypnea, and cough may be present. Auscultation may reveal crackles or a friction rub. If lung infarction has occurred, hemoptysis and pleuritic chest pain may also be present. Some patients have no symptoms at all. Be alert to the presence of risk factors and obtain immediate assistance if the cause of dyspnea might be PE. Death can occur if treatment is not quick and effective.

Complications

High blood pressure within the pulmonary circulation (pulmonary hypertension) may result from arterial occlusion and lead to right ventricular failure. This occurs because the right ventricle is unable to push blood into the occluded artery. As a result, the contraction becomes weak, cardiac output falls, and the patient becomes hypotensive.

Diagnostic Tests

A spiral CT scan is a new and fast type of CT scan that is noninvasive and can diagnose PE quickly. If this is not available, a lung scan (ventilation-perfusion scan) is done to assess the degree of ventilation of lung tissue and the areas of blood perfusion. If an area is well ventilated but poorly perfused (i.e., a mismatch), PE is suspected.

A pulmonary angiogram can outline the pulmonary vessels with a radiopaque dye injected via a cardiac catheter. This can show where blood flow is diminished or absent, suggesting an embolism.

Chest x-ray examination, electrocardiogram (ECG), arterial blood gas analysis, or magnetic resonance imaging (MRI) may also be done. However, many of these show changes only in the presence of a very large embolism or infarction.

A blood test called D-dimer can be helpful to rule out PE. Results can be obtained in less than an hour. D-dimer is a fibrin fragment that is found in the blood after any thrombus formation. It can be present in a number of disorders, but if it is negative, PE can be eliminated as a possible cause of the patient's symptoms.

Therapeutic Interventions

The body naturally dissolves clots in 7 to 10 days. However, if the embolism is large, a thrombolytic agent might be used. These agents, such as streptokinase, urokinase, reteplase and tissue plasminogen activator (t-PA), dissolve clots and are very effective. However, they must be used within 4 to 6 hours of the clot's occurrence and are associated with a risk for hemorrhage.

If a thrombolytic agent is not used, treatment is aimed at preventing extension of the clot and the formation of additional clots. Heparin, a potent anticoagulant medication, is administered via continuous intravenous infusion. Sometimes an intermittent IV or subcutaneous route is used. Heparin is never given intramuscularly because of the risk of hematoma development. Clotting studies (partial thromboplastin time [PTT]) is monitored and maintained at 1.5 to 2 times the control value. Sometimes heparin therapy is initiated even before a diagnosis of PE is made. It is believed that it is safer to begin therapy and then stop if PE is not confirmed than to wait until all test results are available.

Oxygen is administered as ordered. Intubation and mechanical ventilation may be required in some cases.

Warfarin sodium (Coumadin), an oral anticoagulant, is used for at least 3 to 6 months following PE to prevent recurrence. It can also be used for long-term prevention of repeated clots in patients who have risk factors that cannot be resolved. Warfarin therapy can be initiated 2 to 3 days after the initiation of heparin therapy. Because it has a slow onset of action, it may require several days for the full anticoagulant effect to occur. The patient will be on both anticoagulants for a time. Warfarin therapy is monitored regularly with prothrombin time (PT) and international normalized ratio (INR). See Chapter 22 for nursing care of patients on anticoagulant therapy.

If clots are a recurring problem, a filter may be placed into the inferior vena cava via the jugular or femoral vein. One filter that is commonly used is the Greenfield filter, which filters out clots traveling from the lower extremities toward the heart and lungs.

In patients with life-threatening symptoms, a surgical embolectomy can be performed. This is a rare procedure that is reserved for emergency situations.

Nursing Process

ASSESSMENT/DATA COLLECTION. Assess the patient for respiratory distress, including respiratory rate and effort, cyanosis, confusion, and subjective feelings of dyspnea and anxiety. Auscultate lung sounds. Note sputum color and amount, watching especially for hemoptysis. Monitor arterial blood gases and oxygen saturation. Monitor heart sounds and peripheral edema for signs of heart failure. Contributing factors, such as calf pain, should be noted. Remember, any sudden onset of dyspnea should be taken seriously and reported quickly.

NURSING DIAGNOSIS, PLANNING, AND IMPLEMENTATION. The priority nursing diagnosis for a patient with a pulmonary embolism is impaired gas exchange (see Box 31.5 Nursing Care Plan for the Patient with Lower Respiratory Tract Disorder for interventions for impaired gas exchange). Because of the impaired perfusion of the affected area of the lung, oxygen and carbon dioxide exchange are limited. Anxiety occurs related to dyspnea. Risk for injury related to anticoagulant therapy is a concern once treatment is initiated (see Chapter 22).

Risk for injury (bleeding) related to anticoagulant therapy

EXPECTED OUTCOME: The patient will have no evidence of bleeding related to anticoagulant therapy. The patient will verbalize understanding of self care measures.

- Monitor coagulation studies and report results to the physician. *Anticoagulant therapy may be adjusted as often as every 6 hours based on laboratory results.*
- Protect the patient from injury *so that excessive bleeding does not occur.*
- Encourage the patient to wear shoes or slippers when ambulating *to protect from injury.*
- Teach patient to use a soft toothbrush and an electric razor *to prevent injury.*
- Avoid use of IM injections. *IM injection can result in hematoma in an anticoagulated patient.*
- Instruct the patient to report any signs of bleeding, such as hematuria or easy bruising. *Bleeding may be associated with excessively prolonged clotting, and may require a change in anticoagulant dosing or administration of an antidote.*

EVALUATION. The patient should state that dyspnea and anxiety are controlled, and verbalize understanding of anticoagulant therapy and precautions.

See Box 31.11 Pulmonary Embolism Summary.

Pulmonary Arterial Hypertension

Pathophysiology and Etiology

Primary pulmonary arterial hypertension (PAH) occurs when the arteries that carry deoxygenated blood from the heart to the lungs become narrowed as a result of changes in the lining and smooth muscle of the vessels. The result is elevated pressure in the pulmonary arteries, causing the right ventricle to work harder to push blood into them. Eventually the right ventricle fails (cor pulmonale). The reason for these vascular changes is not known. Primary PAH is more common in women between ages 20 and 40 and has a hereditary tendency.

Box 31.11

Pulmonary Embolism Summary

Signs and Symptoms	Sudden-onset dyspnea, tachypnea Tachycardia Hemoptysis Crackles History of blood clot
Diagnostic Tests	D-dimer CT scan Ventilation perfusion lung scan Angiogram
Therapeutic Interventions	Thrombolytic therapy Anticoagulants Oxygen
Complications	Pulmonary hypertension
Priority Nursing Diagnoses	Impaired gas exchange Anxiety Risk for injury from anticoagulant therapy

Secondary PAH results from other disorders, such as coronary artery disease or mitral valve disease, both of which increase pressures in the left side of the heart. Liver disease, systemic lupus erythematosus, and scleroderma are also associated with PAH, as is capillary destruction related to alveolar damage in COPD. Right ventricular failure eventually occurs as the heart works to push blood against high pulmonary arterial pressures.

PAH has also been caused by use of the appetite suppressants fenfluramine (Fen-Phen) and dexenfluramine. Both of these drugs have been removed from the U.S. market by the FDA.

Signs and Symptoms

The most common symptoms include dyspnea and fatigue, which worsen over time. Crackles and decreased breath sounds are heard on auscultation. Cyanosis and tachypnea are noted. If heart failure is present, peripheral edema and distended jugular veins are seen. Angina may result from right ventricular ischemia. Death used to occur within 2 to 3 years of diagnosis, but newer treatments can extend life for up to 15 or 20 years.

Diagnostic Tests

Arterial blood gases commonly show hypoxemia and hypocapnia. Cardiac catheterization can be done to determine high pulmonary arterial pressures. An ECG may show right ventricular hypertrophy. A chest x-ray examination, spirometry, lung scan, and pulmonary angiogram may be done to determine underlying causes in secondary PAH.

Therapeutic Interventions

No cure is available for pulmonary hypertension except for lung or heart-lung transplant. In secondary pulmonary hypertension, the underlying disorder is treated. Supportive care includes a low-sodium diet and diuretics to reduce blood volume (and therefore pressure), oxygen, and cardiac monitoring. Vasodilators such as calcium channel blockers or angiotensin-converting enzyme (ACE) inhibitors may be used to reduce pulmonary artery pressure. Warfarin may be used to prevent clotting. Epoprostenol (Flolan) is a vasodilator that may reverse some of the vascular changes and prolong survival, but has many serious side effects, and must be continuously administered IV via an implanted pump. Bosentan (Tracleer) is a new oral drug that blocks endothelin, a substance that causes blood vessels to constrict. Silfenadil (Viagra) is being tested for possible use in PAH.

Nursing care is collaborative and focuses primarily on patient assessment. Fowler's or high-Fowler's position may help reduce dyspnea, and rest and comfort measures are helpful in treating fatigue and anxiety.

TRAUMA

Pneumothorax

The term **pneumothorax** literally means "air in the chest" and is used to describe conditions in which air has entered the pleural space outside the lungs. If the pneumothorax occurs without an associated injury, it is called a spontaneous pneumothorax. A secondary spontaneous pneumothorax may occur due to underlying lung disease. Traumatic pneumothorax results from a penetrating chest injury.

Pathophysiology and Etiology

Recall that the pleural cavity has visceral and parietal pleurae. These membranes normally are separated only by a thin layer of pleural fluid. Each time a breath is taken in, the diaphragm descends, creating negative pressure in the thorax. This negative pressure pulls air into the lungs via the nose and mouth. If either the visceral pleura or the chest wall and parietal pleura are perforated, air enters the pleural space, negative pressure is lost, and the lung on the affected side collapses (Fig. 31.13). Each time the patient takes a breath, the temporary increase in negative pressure draws air into the pleural space via the perforation. During expiration, air may or may not be able to escape through the perforation.

SPONTANEOUS PNEUMOTHORAX. If no injury is present, the pneumothorax is considered spontaneous. This occurs mostly in tall, thin individuals and in smokers. Patients who have had one spontaneous pneumothorax are at greater risk for a recurrence. Patients with underlying lung disease (especially emphysema) may have blisterlike defects in lung tissue, called bullae or blebs, that can rupture, allowing air into the pleural space. Weakened lung tissue from lung cancer can also lead to pneumothorax.

TRAUMATIC PNEUMOTHORAX. Penetrating trauma to the chest wall and parietal pleura allows air to enter the

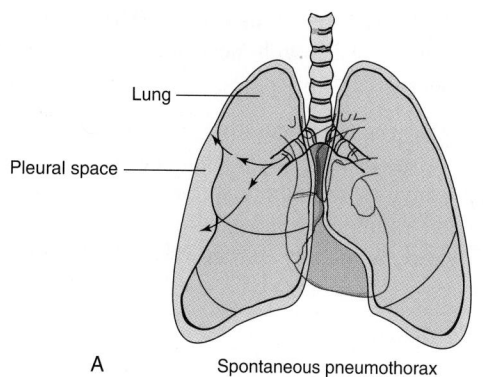
A   Spontaneous pneumothorax

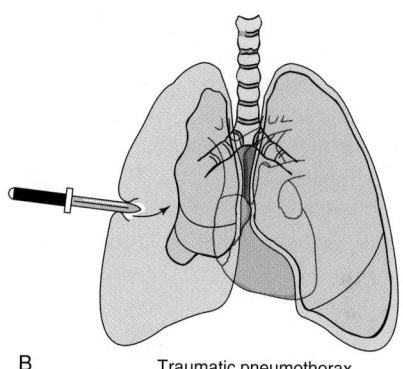
B   Traumatic pneumothorax

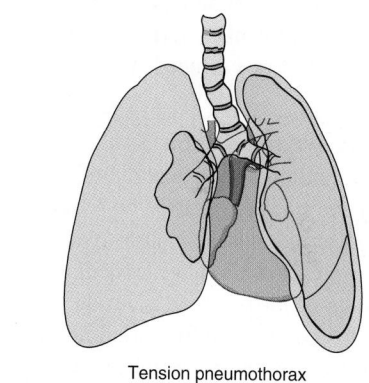
C   Tension pneumothorax

FIGURE 31.13 Types of pneumothorax. (A) Spontaneous pneumothorax. (B) Traumatic pneumothorax. (C) Tension pneumothorax with mediastinal shift.

pleural space. This can occur as a result of a knife or gunshot wound or from protruding broken ribs.

OPEN PNEUMOTHORAX. If air can enter and escape through the opening in the pleural space, it is considered an open pneumothorax.

CLOSED PNEUMOTHORAX. If air collects in the space and is unable to escape, a closed pneumothorax exists.

TENSION PNEUMOTHORAX. If a pneumothorax is closed, air, and therefore tension, builds up in the pleural space. As tension increases, pressure is placed on the heart and great vessels, pushing them away from the affected side of the chest. This is called a mediastinal shift. When the heart and vessels are compressed, venous return to the heart is impaired, resulting in reduced cardiac output and

---

pneumothorax: pneumo—air + thorax—chest

symptoms of shock. Tension pneumothorax is often related to the high pressures present with mechanical ventilation. It is a medical emergency.

HEMOTHORAX. The term **hemothorax** refers to the presence of blood in the pleural space. This can occur with or without accompanying pneumothorax (hemopneumothorax) and is often the result of traumatic injury. Other causes include lung cancer, pulmonary embolism, and anticoagulant use.

Signs and Symptoms
Sudden dyspnea, chest pain, tachypnea, tachycardia, restlessness, and anxiety occur with pneumothorax. On examination, asymmetrical chest expansion on inspiration may be noted. Breath sounds may be absent or diminished on the affected side. In a "sucking" chest wound, air can be heard as it enters and leaves the wound.

If tension pneumothorax develops, the patient becomes hypoxemic and hypotensive as well. The trachea may deviate to the unaffected side. Heart sounds may be muffled. Bradycardia and shock occur if emergency intervention is not provided.

Diagnostic Tests
History, physical examination, and chest x-ray examination are used to diagnose pneumothorax. Chest x-ray examinations are repeated to monitor the resolution of the pneumothorax with treatment. Arterial blood gases and oxygen saturation are monitored as needed throughout the course of treatment.

Therapeutic Interventions
A small pneumothorax may absorb with no treatment other than rest, or the trapped air may be removed with a small-bore needle inserted into the pleural space. Chest tubes connected to a water seal drainage system are used to remove larger amounts of air or blood from the pleural space. See Chapter 29 for complete information about chest drainage. Smaller devices that have special one-way valves to allow air to escape but not reenter the chest may be used for some patients who are treated at home. Some injuries require surgical repair before the pneumothorax can be resolved.

If the pneumothorax is recurrent, other treatments can be used to prevent additional episodes. Sterile talc or certain antibiotics (such as tetracycline) can be injected into the pleural space via thoracentesis, irritating the pleural membranes and making them stick together. This is called **pleurodesis,** or sclerosis, and prevents recurrent pneumothorax. Pleurodesis is painful; prepare the patient with an analgesic before the procedure.

Nursing Care
Nursing care of the patient with a pneumothorax involves close monitoring of the condition. A frequent and thorough assessment should be done, including level of consciousness, skin and mucous membrane color, vital signs, respiratory

rate and depth, and presence of dyspnea, chest pain, restlessness, or anxiety. Regular auscultation of lung sounds provides information about reinflation of the affected lung. Any signs of increasing or tension pneumothorax are reported to the physician immediately. See Chapter 29 for care of the patient with a chest tube and water seal drainage system.

See Box 31.12 Pneumothorax Summary.

Rib Fractures

Etiology and Signs and Symptoms
Chest trauma is often accompanied by fractured ribs. Uncontrolled coughing, especially in the presence of osteoporosis or cancer can also fracture ribs. The fourth through ninth ribs are the most commonly affected. Broken ribs can be very painful, and often prevent the patient from breathing deeply or coughing effectively, which can result in atelectasis or pneumonia. Displaced ribs can also damage abdominal organs or lung tissue, causing pneumothorax.

Treatment
In the past, elastic rib belts were used to stabilize the ribs while healing took place. These are no longer used because it further restricts deep breathing. Pain control is the most important treatment. Keeping the patient comfortable allows coughing and deep breathing, which in turn prevents complications such as pneumonia and atelectasis. If traditional pain control measures such as NSAIDs or opioids are ineffective, intercostal nerve blocks may be used. Ribs generally heal in about 6 weeks.

Flail Chest

Pathophysiology and Etiology
When multiple ribs are fractured, the structural support of the chest is impaired. As a result, the affected part of the

---

Box 31.12

Pneumothorax Summary

Signs and Symptoms	Sudden-onset dyspnea, chest pain, tachypnea Asymmetrical chest expansion Diminished or absent breath sounds on affected side
Diagnostic Tests	Chest x-ray ABGs
Therapeutic Interventions	Chest tube and water seal drainage Pleurodesis for recurrent pneumothorax
Complications	Tension pneumothorax Shock
Priority Nursing Diagnoses	Impaired gas exchange Acute pain Anxiety

---

hemothorax: hem—blood + thorax—chest

pleurodesis: pleur—pleural membrane + desis—binding

chest collapses with inspiration and bulges with expiration. This is called **paradoxical respiration,** which is ineffective in ventilating the lungs and results in hypoxia.

Signs and Symptoms

The patient with a flail chest exhibits chest movement that is opposite to that usually seen with respiration. The patient is dyspneic, anxious, tachypneic, and tachycardic.

Treatment

The patient is given supplemental oxygen. Intubation and mechanical ventilation may be necessary. If lung damage has occurred, chest tubes may be necessary for reinflation.

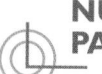

NURSING PROCESS FOR THE PATIENT WITH CHEST TRAUMA

The following nursing process is based on the stabilized patient. For emergency care of the trauma patient, see Chapter 12.

Assessment/Data Collection

When caring for the patient following chest trauma, it is important to monitor respiratory status continuously. Any sign of worsening status should be reported to the physician immediately, such as a change in vital signs or lung sounds; change in respiratory rate; increase in dyspnea, chest pain, pallor, or cyanosis; development of tracheal deviation; or new onset of anxiety or restlessness. Pain is monitored. If a chest wound is present, it is cared for and closely monitored. Additional assessment may be necessary depending on the type of injury sustained.

Nursing Diagnosis, Planning, and Implementation

Priority nursing diagnoses for the patient with chest trauma include Impaired Gas Exchange, Ineffective Breathing Pattern, and AcutePain. Additional diagnoses may be appropriate depending on the individual patient's assessment. See Box 31.5 Nursing Care Plan for the Patient with a Lower Respiratory Tract Disorder for interventions for impaired gas exchange and ineffective breathing pattern.

Acute pain related to chest trauma

EXPECTED OUTCOME: *Patient will state pain is controlled, and will be able to cough and deep breathe.*
- Administer NSAIDs or opioids as ordered. *Pain must be controlled so the patient is able to breathe deeply and prevent atelectasis and pneumonia.*
- If opioids are used, monitor for depressed respirations and reduced cough reflex. *Depressed respirations and cough increase the risk of atelectasis and pneumonia.*
- Teach the patient to splint the chest for coughing. *This may help reduce chest movement and pain during coughing.*

Evaluation

Are pain, anxiety, and dyspnea controlled? Is the respiratory rate within normal limits? Are vital signs stable? Frequent evaluation is essential, so that failure to progress can be quickly reported.

RESPIRATORY FAILURE

Acute Respiratory Failure

Pathophysiology

Acute respiratory failure is diagnosed when the patient is unable to maintain adequate blood gas values. Hypoxemia may result from inadequate ventilation (air movement in and out of lungs) or poor oxygenation (adequate ventilation but inability to get the oxygen into the blood and therefore the cells) or both.

Etiology

An acute respiratory infection in a patient with chronic airway obstruction is often the precipitating factor in acute respiratory failure. Other causes include central nervous system disorders that affect breathing, such as a stroke or myasthenia gravis, inhalation of toxic substances, opioid overdose, and aspiration.

Prevention

Avoidance of respiratory infections in patients with chronic respiratory disease is important. Patients should be instructed to notify their physician immediately if sputum becomes purulent so treatment can be initiated.

Sedatives and narcotics should be used carefully or avoided in patients with chronic respiratory disease because these are respiratory depressants and can precipitate failure.

Signs and Symptoms

The patient with impending respiratory failure may become restless, confused, agitated, or sleepy. Arterial blood gases show decreasing PaO_2 and pH and increasing $PaCO_2$, which lead to respiratory acidosis. The patient is cyanotic and dyspneic, and respiratory rate becomes rapid and deep in an effort to blow off excess CO_2.

Diagnostic Tests

Respiratory failure is diagnosed when PaO_2 falls below 60 mm Hg or $PaCO_2$ is elevated above 50 mm Hg. Some patients with chronic respiratory disease have adapted to impaired gas exchange. In these patients a drop in PaO_2 of 10 to 15 mm Hg is considered acute failure. Sputum cultures or chest x-ray examinations may be used to determine the cause and guide treatment. Pulse oximetry is used to continuously monitor oxygen saturation.

Therapeutic Interventions

Carefully assess the patient and report significant findings to the physician immediately. It is easy to mistakenly treat symptoms of agitation or confusion with sedatives, which will speed the onset of respiratory failure. Oxygen therapy via nasal cannula or mask is provided. If the patient has a chronically high PaCO$_2$, oxygen is administered at a flow rate of 1 to 2 L to prevent interference with the hypoxic drive. Antibiotics or other treatments are ordered to correct the underlying cause of the failure. Bronchodilators promote ventilation and secretion removal. The patient is instructed to cough and deep breathe if able. Suctioning is indicated if the patient is unable to cough effectively. Mechanical ventilation via endoctracheal tube or noninvasive positive pressure ventilation (NIPPV) may be required. Before invasive ventilation is initiated, it is important to check the patient's advance directives.

Acute Respiratory Distress Syndrome/Acute Lung Injury

Acute respiratory distress syndrome (ARDS), also called adult respiratory distress syndrome, is a group of disorders that has diverse causes but similar pathophysiology, symptoms, and treatment.

Pathophysiology and Etiology

ARDS occurs because of acute lung injury (ALI). The most common cause of injury is sepsis. Other causes include pneumonia, trauma, shock, narcotic overdose, inhalation of irritants, burns, pancreatitis, and aspiration, among others. Each of these causes begins a chain of events leading to alveolocapillary damage and noncardiac pulmonary edema (pulmonary edema that is not caused by heart failure). ARDS usually affects patients without a previous history of lung disease.

The alveolocapillary membranes become inflamed and damaged either by direct contact with an inhaled irritant or by chemical mediators that are released when systemic injury occurs. The membranes become leaky, so that proteins, blood cells, and fluid move from the capillaries into the interstitial space and then into the alveoli. Surfactant, a substance that reduces surface tension in the alveoli, is reduced. Alveoli collapse (atelectasis) and fibrotic changes take place. These changes cause the lungs to become stiff, or less compliant, making the patient work very hard to inspire. Blood supply to the alveoli may be adequate, but collapsed, wet alveoli are unable to oxygenate it. In other areas of the lungs, vasoconstriction reduces the ability of the vessels to pick up oxygen from functioning alveoli. Tired respiratory muscles, in combination with edema and atelectasis, reduce gas exchange and result in hypoxia. As the condition progresses, atelectasis and edema worsen and the lungs may hemorrhage. A chest x-ray examination appears white because of the excessive fluid in the lungs. These changes explain some of the older names for what is now known as ARDS: wet lung, white lung, shock lung, and stiff lung.

Prevention

Early recognition and treatment of underlying disorders is important in prevention of ARDS. Good nursing care can help reduce aspiration and some types of pneumonia.

Signs and Symptoms

Initially the patient may experience dyspnea and an increase in respiratory rate. Respiratory alkalosis results from hyperventilation. Fine inspiratory crackles may be auscultated. As the condition worsens, breathing becomes more rapid and labored and the patient becomes cyanotic. The patient is no longer able to oxygenate the blood and get rid of carbon dioxide, and respiratory acidosis occurs. Oxygen therapy does not reverse the hypoxemia. If ARDS is not reversed, eventually hypoxemia leads to decreased cardiac output, shock, and death.

Complications

Complications that can result from ARDS include heart failure, pneumothorax related to mechanical ventilation, infection, and disseminated intravascular coagulation (DIC). The death rate for ARDS in the past was 100%. With newer treatments, it is now closer to 70%. Most patients who survive ARDS recover completely.

Diagnostic Tests

Diagnosis is made based on history of a causative injury, physical examination, chest x-ray examination, and blood gas analysis. An ECG is done to rule out a cardiac-related cause.

Therapeutic Interventions

The patient with ARDS is cared for in an intensive care unit. Treatment begins with oxygen therapy that is adjusted based on repeated ABG results. Intubation and mechanical ventilation are necessary in most cases, with the use of positive end-expiratory pressure (PEEP) to keep the airways open. Diuretics may be used to reduce pulmonary edema, but care must be taken to prevent fluid depletion. IV fluids are administered if blood pressure or urine output is low. A pulmonary artery catheter may be used to monitor hemodynamic status. If infection is the underlying cause, antibiotics are administered. Parenteral nutrition may be given to maintain nutritional status while the patient is acutely ill. Positioning the patient with the less involved lung in the dependent position ("good lung down") allows the better lung to be well perfused with blood and may increase PaO$_2$. Prone positioning has also been shown to increase oxygenation in patients with ARDS.

NURSING PROCESS FOR THE PATIENT EXPERIENCING RESPIRATORY FAILURE

Assessment/Data Collection

Assess the patient's degree of dyspnea on a scale of 0 to 10 if the patient is able to participate. Respiratory rate, effort, and use of accessory muscles are noted. Arterial blood gases and oxygen saturation values are monitored as ordered. The presence of cyanosis is noted.

Mental status, including restlessness, confusion, and level of consciousness, is also assessed, because reduced oxygenation can produce central nervous system (CNS) symptoms. Symptoms of the underlying cause of respiratory failure are monitored. If the cause is infectious, sputum amount and color, temperature, and white blood cell counts are monitored.

All assessment findings should be compared with earlier data. Even subtle changes in the assessment findings can be significant and should be reported.

Nursing Diagnosis, Planning, and Implementation

Priority nursing diagnoses include Impaired Gas Exchange, Ineffective Airway Clearance, and Ineffective Breathing Pattern (see Box 31.5 Nursing Care Plan for the Patient with a Lower Respiratory Tract Disorder). Related diagnoses include Activity Intolerance, Anxiety, Disturbed Thought Processes, and Self-Care Deficit.

NURSING CARE TIP

The good lung down position can help increase oxygenation in patients with lung disease. Gravity results in more blood in the dependent lung, where it can receive oxygen from the healthier lung tissue. If both lungs are diseased, the right lung down position may be beneficial, because the right lung has a larger surface area.[6]

Evaluation

If interventions have been effective, the patient will state that dyspnea is controlled. Mental status will be normal for the patient. Airways will be kept clear at all times, and the patient's respiratory rate will be regular and within normal limits.

LUNG CANCER

Lung cancer is the leading cause of cancer death in the United States. More men and women die from lung cancer each year than any other type of cancer. An estimated 172,570 new cases and 163,510 deaths are predicted for the United States in 2005.[6] The 5-year survival rate for lung cancer ranges from 1% to 47% depending on the type of lung cancer and on how early in the course of the disease it is diagnosed. The incidence of lung cancer among men is slowly decreasing. The incidence in women was steadily rising for years because of increasing numbers of women who smoke, but now appears to have leveled off.

Pathophysiology

Lung cancers originate in the respiratory tract epithelium; most originate in the lining of the bronchi (Fig. 31.14). The four major types of lung cancer are identified by the type of cells that are affected. These include small cell lung cancer (SCLC), large cell carcinoma, adenocarcinoma, and squamous cell carcinoma. The latter three types are classified as non–small cell lung cancer (NSCLC).

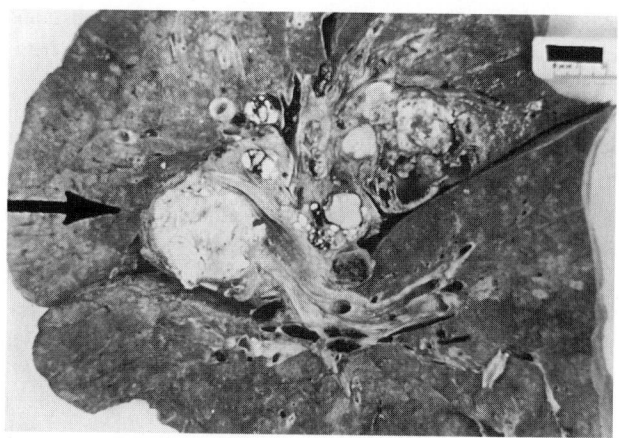

FIGURE 31.14 Lung cancer. The black arrow marks the tumor site. *(Photograph courtesy Dinesh Patel, MD, Medical Oncology, Internal Medicine, Zanesville, Ohio.)*

About 13% of lung cancers are SCLC (sometimes called oat cell carcinoma). SCLC grows rapidly and often has metastasized by the time of diagnosis. It is usually caused by smoking and is most often found centrally, near the bronchi. The patient with small cell carcinoma has a poor prognosis, with survival time averaging less than 1 year.

The remaining 87% of lung cancers are classified as non–small cell. Large cell carcinoma is a rapidly growing cancer that can occur anywhere in the lungs. It metastasizes early in the disease, so these patients also have a poor prognosis.

Adenocarcinoma occurs more often in women, and most often in the peripheral lung fields. It is slow growing but often is not diagnosed until metastasis has occurred. It is less closely linked with smoking. Prognosis may be better than other lung cancer types.

Squamous cell carcinomas usually originate near the bronchi and metastasize late in the disease. They are associated with a history of smoking. The prognosis for individuals with squamous cell carcinoma may also be better than for some other lung cancers.

Etiology

The most common cause of lung cancer is tobacco smoke. Cigarettes contain chemicals that cause DNA to mutate, creating changes in cells and development of tumors. Smokers have an approximately 13 times greater risk for developing lung cancer than nonsmokers. If a patient stops smoking, the risk of lung cancer decreases significantly. Unfortunately, even with all this information, 25.2% of men and 20.7% of women in the United States continue to smoke.[7] Twenty-eight percent of high school teens smoke; 90% of adults who smoke started as teens.[8]

Environmental tobacco smoke (ETS) has also been shown to cause lung cancer. A study by the American Cancer Society showed that women who were married to smokers but who had never smoked themselves were 20% more likely to die of lung cancer.[9] Other factors that contribute to increased lung cancer risk are exposure to asbestos, radon, or arsenic; air pollution; diesel exhaust; and radiation. Genetic predisposition and a diet poor in fruits and vegetables may also be factors.

Prevention

The single most important way to prevent lung cancer is to reduce smoking. Many programs educate schoolchildren about the dangers of smoking. Smoking cessation programs are available for people who desire to quit. Contact your local American Cancer Society chapter for smoking cessation programs that can be recommended to patients. See Chapter 29 for more information on smoking cessation.

Signs and Symptoms

Manifestations of lung cancer depend on the location of the tumor. Commonly, patients exhibit a cough with sputum production. These symptoms may be ignored by the patient because they are also associated with smoking and other chronic respiratory disorders. Repeated respiratory infections may occur, producing thick, purulent sputum. Sputum may become bloody (hemoptysis). The patient may experience dyspnea. If the airway becomes obstructed by the tumor, wheezing or stridor may be heard. Late signs include chest pain, weight loss, anemia, and anorexia.

Complications

Pleural Effusion

Fifty percent of patients with lung cancer develop pleural effusion. Pleural fluid collects in the pleural space as a result of irritation or obstruction of lymphatic or venous drainage by the tumor.

Superior Vena Cava Syndrome

If the tumor obstructs the superior vena cava, blood flow is interrupted, causing distention of the jugular veins and swelling of the chest, face, and neck. Diuretics may help relieve the fluid build-up. Radiation may be used to shrink the obstruction.

Ectopic Hormone Production

Some lung cancers produce **ectopic** hormones that mimic the body's own hormones. Ectopic production of antidiuretic hormone (ADH) can produce syndrome of inappropriate ADH production (SAIDH), which is associated with fluid retention. Ectopic production of adrenocorticotropic hormone (ACTH) can cause Cushing's syndrome. These disorders are discussed in Chapter 39.

Atelectasis and Pneumonia

Atelectasis occurs when tumor growth prevents ventilation of areas of the lung. Patients with lung cancer also have a greater risk for pneumonia.

Metastasis

Common sites of lung cancer metastasis include the brain, bones, opposite lung, liver, adrenal gland, and lymph nodes.

Diagnostic Tests

A complete medical history and physical examination are done to look for symptoms and risk factors for lung cancer. A chest x-ray examination is done to identify a mass. However, all tumors may not show up on a radiograph. A CT scan and lung scan may be done to provide more specific information about the size and location of a tumor. Sputum is analyzed for abnormal cells. Brain and bone scans are done to find metastatic lesions.

Diagnosis is confirmed with a biopsy of the lesion. A biopsy specimen may be obtained via bronchoscopy, percutaneous biopsy (a needle through the skin guided by radiograph), or mediastinoscopy (use of an endoscope into the mediastinum to look for changes in mediastinal lymph nodes).

Therapeutic Interventions

Tumors are staged based on the tumor-node-metastasis (TNM) staging system. (See Chapter 10.) Staging helps determine appropriate treatment (Table 31.4). If NSCLC is localized and in an early stage, it may be cured with surgical removal of the tumor. This can be accomplished with a segmental or wedge resection, which removes only the affected lung segment. A **lobectomy** (removal of a lobe) or removal of an entire lung may be done in more advanced cases (Fig. 31.15). Surgery is contraindicated if the cancer has spread to the other lung or has metastasized to distant areas.

Chemotherapy is the treatment of choice in SCLC, because usually it has metastasized by the time of diagnosis. New types of chemotherapy that target only cancer cells may be effective in some people. Radiation may be used in combination with chemotherapy. Surgery is not indicated in SCLC; the goal of treatment is not cure but rather palliation of symptoms.

TABLE 31.4 STAGES OF LUNG CANCER

Cancer Type	Stage	Characteristics
Non–small cell lung cancer	I	No metastasis to lymph nodes. Atelectasis or pneumonia may be present.
	II	Cancer has spread to local lymph nodes.
	III	Cancer has invaded chest wall and usually has spread to lymph nodes.
	IV	Tumor has metastasized to distant organs and lymph nodes.
Small cell lung cancer	Limited	Cancer is limited to one side of the chest.
	Extensive	Cancer cells are found outside one side of the chest or in pleural fluid.

---

ectopic: displaced

lobectomy: lobe—lobe (of lung) + ectomy—excision

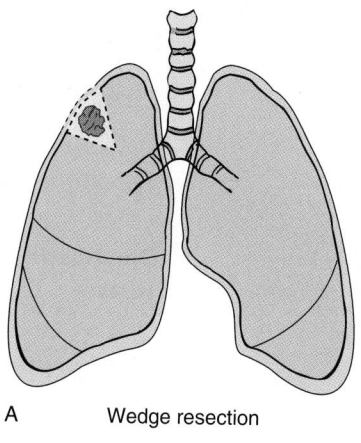

A   Wedge resection

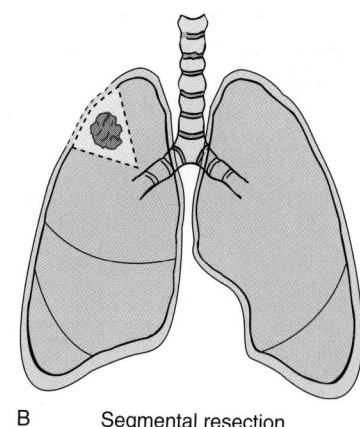

B   Segmental resection

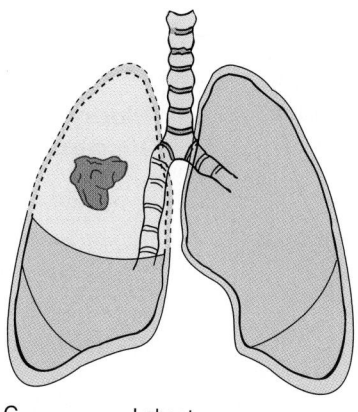

C   Lobectomy

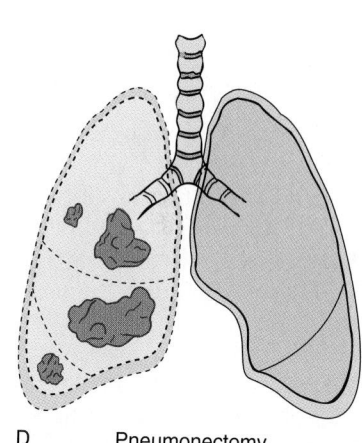

D   Pneumonectomy

FIGURE 31.15 Types of surgeries for lung cancer. (A) Wedge resection. (B) Segmental resection. (C) Lobectomy. (D) Pneumonectomy.

Radiation may be used to shrink a tumor to reduce symptoms in patients who are unable to undergo surgery. Both radiation and chemotherapy may be used before or after surgery as **adjuvant** treatments. For more information about cancer treatments and nursing care, see Chapter 10. For more on lung cancer, visit the American Cancer Society website at www.cancer.org.

NURSING PROCESS FOR THE PATIENT WITH LUNG CANCER

Assessment/Data Collection

Perform a complete biopsychosocial assessment of the patient with lung cancer. Assess and document respiratory rate and depth, skin and mucous membrane color, lung sounds, cough, and sputum amount and character. Ask the patient to rate the degree of pain and dyspnea on appropriate scales. Ask about appetite and weight loss, as well as symptoms of other complications. Note activity tolerance and fatigue.

The patient will likely be grieving about his or her illness and its prognosis. Assessment of the patient's coping strategies and support systems will help you plan care for psychosocial needs. When you recall the prognosis for patients with some types of lung cancer, the need to consider

planning for terminal care becomes obvious (Box 31.13 Ethical Considerations). The presence of a Living Will or Durable Power of Attorney should be noted (see Chapter 16).

Nursing Diagnosis, Planning, and Implementation

Possible diagnoses that may be experienced by the patient with lung cancer include Impaired Gas Exchange, Ineffective Airway Clearance, Imbalanced Nutrition: Less Than Body Requirements, Pain, Constipation Related to Opioid Use, Anticipatory Grieving, and Activity Intolerance, among others. See Box 31.5 Nursing Care Plan for the Patient with a Lower Respiratory Tract Disorder for care of patients with respiratory diagnoses. See Chapter 10 Nursing Care of Patients with Cancer for interventions related to cancer diagnoses.

Evaluation

Carefully consider the patient's individual goals when evaluating care. Is the patient comfortable and free from unnecessary dyspnea? Is the airway clear, and is nutrition maintained? Are medication side effects manageable? Have patients with terminal conditions come to terms with their impending death, and have they been able to do those things most important to them before their death?

See Box 31.14 Lung Cancer Summary.

Box 31.13

Ethical Considerations

Truth Telling

Mr. David Hammill, 88 years old, is admitted to a room on the surgical unit following a thoracotomy. He has been diagnosed with a metastatic tumor of the lung but does not yet know the diagnosis. His son has power of attorney, so Dr. Lester told the son and family the diagnosis. Dr. Lester decided not to tell Mr. Hammill the diagnosis because he believes that Mr. Hamill would become upset and depressed. Dr. Lester has written an order saying that the patient should not be told his diagnosis.

Mr. Hammill has been asking the nurses, staff, and his family what the physician found in surgery and what the results of the pathology reports were. Dr. Lester has visited Mr. Hammill several times but has avoided talking about the diagnosis by saying that not all the laboratory tests are back yet. The family has been avoiding visiting the patient so that he will not ask them about the diagnosis. The family often asks the nurse when Mr. Hammill will be told his diagnosis. They believe the physician should tell him. Some questions to consider are:

- If the patient is continually asking for information, should the nurse tell him?
- What degree of "truth" is required?
- What about partial truths and white lies?
- Can it ever be beneficial to withhold the truth?
- Would it be different if the patient and family were not asking for information?
- What does *paternalism* mean, and why might the physician be taking such a position with this patient?
- Does the hospital have an ethics committee? Could such a committee help?
- What options are available to the nurse or for the nurse to suggest to the family?

 ## THORACIC SURGERY

A surgical incision made into the chest wall is called a **thoracotomy**. A thoracotomy may be performed for a number of reasons, including biopsy; removal of tumors, lesions, or foreign objects; to repair trauma following penetrating or crushing injuries; or to repair or revise structural problems.

Types

Pneumonectomy

A **pneumonectomy** is the surgical removal of a lung. This is usually done to treat lung cancer. It may also be used to treat severe cases of tuberculosis, bronchiectasis, or lung

---

pneumonectomy: pneum—lung + ectomy—exicision

Box 31.14

Lung Cancer Summary

Signs and Symptoms	Cough, hemoptysis Dyspnea, wheezing Repeat respiratory infections
Diagnostic Tests	Chest x ray CT scan Biopsy
Therapeutic Interventions	Resection Chemotherapy Radiation
Complications	Pleural effusion, superior vena cava syndrome, ectopic hormone production, atelectasis, metastasis
Priority Nursing Diagnoses	Impaired gas exchange Ineffective airway clearance Activity intolerance

abscesses. Chest drainage is not usually used following a pneumonectomy because once the lung is removed, the air in the thoracic cavity is absorbed and the cavity fills with serosanguineous fluid. At about 6 months after surgery, the fluid is coagulated and the thoracic cavity is stabilized.

Lobectomy

Lobectomy is the surgical removal of one lobe. This also may be done for lung cancer, tuberculosis, or another localized problem.

Resection

Resection refers to removal of a smaller amount of lung tissue; that is, less than one lobe. A segmental resection is the removal of one segment of a lobe; a wedge resection is removal of a small wedge of lung tissue. See Figure 31.15.

Video-Assisted Thorascopic Surgery

Video-assisted thorascopic surgery (VATS) is a new technique that uses a specialized endoscope to perform surgery. It can be done with two or three small incisions, so is much less invasive than traditional thoracotomy that requires opening the chest. It can be used for staging and treatment of some tumors.

Lung Transplantation

Lung transplant can benefit patients with a variety of serious pulmonary disorders, including pulmonary hypertension, emphysema, cystic fibrosis, and bronchiectasis. Either a single lung, both lungs, or heart and lungs have been successfully transplanted. Better criteria for selecting patients and donors, as well as advancements in surgical techniques, have improved outcomes for these patients.

NURSING PROCESS FOR THE PATIENT UNDERGOING THORACIC SURGERY

Preoperative Nursing Care

Perform a thorough assessment before surgery, with a focus on the respiratory system. This gives a baseline against which to judge changes postoperatively. Routine preoperative teaching is done by the nurse in conjunction with the physician and health team. The patient should understand that he or she will wake up in an intensive care environment. If at all possible, it is helpful to have the patient and family tour the intensive care unit before the surgery to decrease anxiety postoperatively. Prepare the patient for waking up after surgery with an endotracheal tube connected to a ventilator, oxygen, chest tubes, intravenous fluids, cardiac monitor, Foley catheter, and possibly an epidural catheter for pain control. Let the patient know he or she will not be able to talk while the ET tube is in, and explain the use of the call light, picture board, or alternate communication techniques. Consult the surgeon for specific plans.

Advise the patient that position changes and early ambulation help prevent complications following surgery. Also instruct the patient in the use of an incentive spirometer and coughing and deep breathing techniques.

Postoperative Nursing Care

Assessment/Data Collection

Following thoracic surgery, patients initially are in an intensive care unit. Larger hospitals have special intensive care units specifically for surgical or thoracic patients. Here patients can be closely monitored for signs of complications. Frequent assessment of vital signs and hemodynamic stability; respiratory rate, depth, and effort; and lung sounds is performed. Remember that lung sounds are absent on the side of a pneumonectomy. An increase in pulse rate or a falling blood pressure may indicate internal bleeding and should be reported immediately. Oxygen saturation is monitored continuously. Often patients report an immediate improvement in breathing because the pulmonary blood supply is no longer being routed to diseased lung tissue.

Assessment for tracheal deviation alerts you to the possible complication of mediastinal shift. The trachea is normally positioned straight above the sternal notch. If the trachea deviates from the midline position, the surgeon should be notified immediately. Secretions are monitored and reported to the physician if they become thick, yellow or green, or foul smelling. Arterial blood gases are monitored closely. Chest tubes are usually present (except following pneumonectomy) and are monitored as explained in Chapter 29. Pain is assessed using a pain rating scale, and incision sites are monitored for redness, edema, or drainage. If the patient is mechanically ventilated, additional assessment of the endotracheal tube and ventilator settings will be necessary.

Nursing Diagnosis, Planning, and Implementation

See Box 31.5 Nursing Care Plan for the Patient with a Lower Respiratory Tract Disorder for basic interventions. Following are some additional interventions specific to the patient following thoracic surgery.

Ineffective airway clearance related to presence of ventilator, inability to cough, sedation

EXPECTED OUTCOME: Patient will have a clear airway as evidenced by clear lung sounds, and absence of airway noise and high pressure ventilator alarms.

- Suction according to agency policy. *The airway must remain free of secretions to prevent ventilator-associated pneumonia and dyspnea. Continuous suction may be possible with some ET tubes.*
- Once extubated, remind the patient to cough and deep breathe regularly. *This helps clear the airway.*
- Administer analgesics as ordered. *Postoperative pain must be controlled for the patient to be able to cough effectively.*

Impaired gas exchange related to surgical intervention, opioid use, and removal of lung tissue

EXPECTED OUTCOME: Sao$_2$ will be ≥90%.

- Monitor Sao$_2$. *Interventions should maintain Sao$_2$ at or greater than 90%.*
- Reposition patient every 1 to 2 hours. Consult surgeon for specific positioning orders. *Some surgeons want patients positioned with the operative side up, others with the operative side down. Fowler's position allows room for lung expansion and helps prevent aspiration.*
- Encourage use of an incentive spirometer as ordered following extubation *to encourage the patient to deep breathe and maximize oxygenation.*
- Monitor chest tube and water seal drainage system, if used. *This helps reexpand the lung and must remain intact at all times.*
- Administer oxygen and bronchodilators as ordered *to maintain oxygenation.*

Acute pain related to surgical procedure

EXPECTED OUTCOME: Patient will state or indicate that pain is controlled. If unable to communicate, objective signs of acute pain (increase in vital signs, restlessness) are absent.

- Administer analgesics as ordered, around the clock. *Pain control is important for the patient to be able to ambulate and deep breathe and cough effectively.*
- Monitor respiratory rate and effort if not mechanically ventilated. *Opioids depress respirations.*
- Teach the patient to splint the incision while coughing. *This can stabilize the site and reduce pain, increasing the likelihood of effective coughing.*

Impaired physical mobility related to discomfort at surgical site

EXPECTED OUTCOME: Patient will maintain mobility.

- Perform range-of-motion exercises, passively at first, then actively when the patient is able. *This helps prevent contracture of the arm and shoulder on the affected side.*
- Assist the patient to ambulate as tolerated on first or second postoperative day as ordered. *Ambulation helps maintain mobility and prevent postoperative complications.*

Risk for infection related to surgical incision and stress of major surgery

EXPECTED OUTCOME: Patient will be free of signs of infection as evidenced by clean and dry incision, temperature and WBC count WNL, clear sputum, and clear urine.

- Monitor temperature, WBC count, incision, sputum, and urine for signs of infection *so infection can be identified and treated quickly.*
- Use meticulous sterile technique for all invasive procedures: suctioning, dressing changes, catheter insertion. *This prevents introduction of pathogens.*

- Use standard infection control precautions, including careful hand washing *because the patient is at increased risk for infection.*
- Monitor nutritional intake. Consult dietitian for recommendations. *Adequate nutrients are essential for wound healing and immune function.*
- Maintain head of bed at minimum 30 degrees elevation *to help prevent aspiration of gastric contents.*
- Provide frequent oral care *to reduce risk of aspiration of oral bacteria.*
- Assist with ventilator weaning and extubation as soon as possible. *Mechanical ventilation is associated with increased risk of pneumonia.*

Evaluation

The patient's airway should remain clear, and secretions should be easily coughed up. The patient should report an acceptable comfort level and be able to cough, deep breathe, and ambulate without excessive discomfort. The patient's breathing should be unlabored, with a respiratory rate of 12 to 20 per minute. The patient's affected arm and shoulder should maintain full range of motion. Signs of infection should be absent.

Home Health Hints

- When a patient is using oxygen by nasal cannula, the area around the ears can become irritated or excoriated. A small sponge-type hair roller can be placed around the tubing to protect the ears.
- When a home health patient has a metered-dose inhaler (MDI), the nurse should not assume he or she is using it correctly. The patient should be observed using it.
- When a patient requires more than one MDI, the canisters can be numbered in the order they are to be taken.
- Read inhaler package inserts to find how many puffs are in an inhaler, and help the patient devise a system for keeping track of how many puffs are used so he does not run out. Manufacturers no longer recommend seeing if canisters float or sink in water to determine if they are empty—this can be unreliable.
- To help the COPD patient conserve energy, he or she can be encouraged to sit on a stool when cooking at the stove or doing dishes. A shower stool can be obtained from a medical supply store. Personal care activities should be spaced throughout the day.
- Support bars, also obtained from a medical supply store, can be strategically placed in the shower area, on

the walls along hallways, and in a passageway to the restroom. This can help the patient ambulate when fatigued and also help prevent falls.
- If the COPD patient is tempted to adjust his or her own oxygen flow rate, equipment suppliers can put on a locking flowmeter. Increasing flow rate can reduce hypoxic drive and cause hypoventilation.
- Nebulizer parts should be cleaned at least three times a week, using warm water and a common home disinfectant solution for 30 minutes.
- COPD patients often have a difficult time eating. Not only do these patients have intolerance to activities but they also experience changes in their taste due to secretions and medications. Instruct the patient to rinse out his or her mouth prior to eating to help improve taste. Softer foods are often more palatable and require less energy to eat.
- When in the home it is important to not only assess your patient but also the primary caregiver. Many times he or she is experiencing caregiver role strain. Discuss options available and consider having a social worker consulted to assist with counseling and community resources. Contact the physician to discuss your concerns and ideas.

ETHICAL CONSIDERATIONS DISCUSSION

This is a difficult situation. Some elderly patients may not believe that they have a right to question a physician or be fully informed and will simply agree to whatever is suggested. Most families will express their needs, but there are some geographical areas where traditional physician-patient relationships follow a very paternalistic model. This situation provides an opportunity to examine autonomy, paternalism, and veracity. You can see that most of these principles have been placed on the "back burner" if not dismissed altogether in this situation.

Consider the principle of autonomy. You can see that respect for autonomy has been ignored in this situation. The patient was not given the opportunity to participate in his diagnosis and treatment plan so he is no longer a participant in his own care. By disrespecting the patient's right to participate in his care, the physician has placed the patient in a precarious position. The patient is indicating that he would like to know his diagnosis. Most patients at this point need time to resolve life issues and prepare for death. This is a natural function, and by denying the patient this opportunity, not only is the team causing harm, they are not maximizing benefit.

So, what about telling partial truths? One possible response is that before partial truths are told to a patient, the health care professional should consider very carefully the impact of any information and the possible consequences of partial truths. If there is not full disclosure, there is danger for misinterpretation of facts.

To act as a patient advocate and pursue having the patient and family hear the full truth is potentially risky. In some areas, the perceived omnipotence of physicians is still upheld and to act in a way that directly goes against physician orders will likely have consequences. However, as a nurse you must uphold your professional code of ethics. First approach the physician with your concerns. If he or she fails to understand the need for disclosure, then discuss the situation with your supervisor or Ethics Committee.

Bad news is never welcome; however, in the case of terminal illness it provides the patient and family time to prepare for what is coming.

REVIEW QUESTIONS

1. A patient asks the nurse why he doesn't feel sick even though his TB test is positive. The nurse knows the patient has been diagnosed with LTBI. Which explanation is best to provide the patient?
   a. "TB often does not make people feel sick, but it is contagious nevertheless."
   b. "You have latent disease, which just stays in your system but won't ever make you sick."
   c. "You have TB infection, but not active disease. As long as your immune system stays strong, it can keep the infection from making you sick."
   d. "Even though you do not feel sick, the positive test shows that you have the disease and must be treated."

2. Which of the following assessment findings does the nurse expect in the patient with emphysema?
   a. Purulent sputum
   b. Diminished breath sounds
   c. Generalized edema
   d. Dull chest pain

3. A patient with shortness of breath is being tested for lung cancer. Which diagnostic test will be most conclusive?
   a. Chest x-ray
   b. MRI
   c. Sputum culture
   d. Biopsy

4. A patient with recurrent pneumothorax is scheduled to have pleurodesis done in one hour. Which nursing intervention should take priority at this time?
   a. Encourage fluids.
   b. Encourage coughing and deep breathing.
   c. Administer a prn analgesic as ordered.
   d. Administer a prn bronchodilator as ordered.

5. Which of the following assessment findings in the patient with pneumonia most indicates a need to remind the patient to cough and deep breathe?
   a. The patient complains of chest pain.
   b. The patient has removed her oxygen.
   c. The patient develops wheezes and crackles.
   d. The patient has a fever of 101°F (38.3°C).

6. A patient is admitted to the hospital with shortness of breath. The nurse notes increasing confusion and combativeness over the past hour. Which of the following actions is appropriate first?
   a. Assess the patient; check to see if the oxygen is flowing correctly.
   b. Page the physician stat.
   c. Put up the patient's side rails and apply soft restraints.
   d. Administer an intramuscular sedative.

7. Which of the following interventions is most appropriate for the patient with an ineffective breathing pattern?
   a. Encourage the patient to cough and deep breathe.
   b. Teach the patient controlled diaphragmatic breathing.
   c. Encourage oral fluids.
   d. Allow the patient to rest between activities.

8. A patient with end-stage COPD has a nursing diagnosis of impaired gas exchange. Which assessment finding shows that interventions have been effective?
   a. The patient's SaO_2 is 97% on 2 liters of oxygen.
   b. The patient appears comfortable.
   c. The patient is coughing up copious white sputum.
   d. The patient is able to move in bed without difficulty.

References

1. World Health Organization: Tuberculosis Home Page. http://w3.whosea.org/tb/faqs.htm, accessed January 10, 2006.
2. National Heart, Lung, and Blood Institute: Chronic Obstructive Pulmonary Disease Data Fact Sheet. NIH Publication No. 03–5229, March 2003.
3. Global Initiative for Chronic Obstructive Lung Disease. Pocket Guide to COPD Diagnosis, Management, and Prevention, July, 2004. :www.GOLDCOPD.org
4. American Lung Association. Epidemiology & Statistics Unit, Research and Program Services. Trends in Asthma Morbidity and Mortality, May 2005.

Unit Six Bibliography

1. Carroll, P: Exploring chest drain options. RN 63:10, 2000.
2. Dunn, N: Keeping COPD patients out of the ED. RN 64:2, 2001.
3. Global Initiative for Chronic Lung Disease. www.GOLD-COPD.org, accessed January 10, 2006.
4. Hayes, DD: Stemming the tide of pleural effusions. Nursing 2001 31:5, 2001.
5. Lazzara, D: Respiratory distress: Loosening the grip. Nursing 2001 31:6, 2001.
6. Lindgren, VA, and Ames, NJ: Caring for patients on mechanical ventilation. AJN 105:5, 2005.
7. Marion, BS: A turn for the better: Prone positioning of patients with ARDS. Am J Nurs 101:5, 2001.
8. Martinez, FJ, de Oca, MM, White, RI, et al: Lung-volume reduction improves dyspnea, dynamic hyperinflation, and respiratory muscle function. Am J Respir Crit Care Med 6:155, 1997.

5. Yeaw, E: How position affects oxygenation: Good lung down? Am J Nurs 92:26, 1992.
6. Centers for Disease Control/Lung Cancer Statistics. Accessed at http://www.cdc.gov/cancer/lung/statistics.htm, January 10, 2006.
7. American Heart Association: Cigarette Smoking Statistics. www.americanheart.org, accessed July 30, 2005.
8. American Lung Association: Adolescent Smoking Statistics. www.lungusa.org, accessed July 30, 2005.
9. Cardenas, VM, Thun, MJ, Austin H, et al: Environmental tobacco smoke and lung cancer mortality in the American Cancer Society's Cancer Prevention Study II. Cancer Causes Control 8:57, 1997.
9. National Heart, Lung, and Blood Institute: Chronic Obstructive Pulmonary Disease Data Fact Sheet. NIH Publication No. 03–5229, March 2003.
10. Perkins, LA, and Shortall, SP: Ventilation without intubation. RN 63:1, 2000.
11. Petty, TL: COPD: Interventions for smoking cessation and improved ventilatory function. Geriatrics 55:12, 2000.
12. Petty, TL: Smoking Cessation Strategies. National Lung Health Education Program. Accessed January 11, 2006 at http://www.nlhep.org/smoking.html.
13. Sandhu, AK, and Mossad, SB: Influenza in the older adult: Indications for the use of vaccine and antiviral therapy. Geriatrics 56:43–51, 2001.
14. Yeaw, E: How position affects oxygenation: Good lung down? Am J Nurs 92:26, 1992.

SUGGESTED ANSWERS TO

CRITICAL THINKING

■ *Mr. Smith*

1. A complete respiratory history is taken as described in Chapter 29. An open-ended question such as "What happened to bring you to the hospital?" elicits information about the incident. In addition, questions to determine mental status and ability to make decisions and function safely on his own are appropriate. If any concerns arise, a social service consultation will be helpful for discharge planning.

2. Mr. Smith should be instructed to always read label warnings before using any cleaning products in the future and to never mix bleach and ammonia!

■ *Mr. Woo*

Document exactly what you see: "No redness or induration at either the PPD or *Candida* test sites." Date and time your entry, and sign. What does this mean? Everyone has been exposed to, and should react to *Candida* with some degree of redness and induration. The fact that Mr. Woo has no reaction at all may mean that his immune system is not working well, or he is "anergic." Therefore, the fact that his PPD test shows no redness and swelling could just be because of his anergy even though he may be infected with TB. So, this is an unreliable test for him. Mr. Woo will need a chest x-ray and a sputum culture to be sure he is not infected. At this time it is not known whether the QuantiFERON–TB Gold test is accurate in immune-compromised patients.

■ Jim

1. Ask questions based on the WHAT'S UP? format:

   Where (not applicable)

   How does it feel? Does the coughing cause chest pain? Are you short of breath?

   Aggravating and alleviating factors. What makes the cough worse? What seems to help? Do you use any techniques at home that are helpful?

   Timing. How often do you cough during a day? Is it interfering with sleep and rest?

   Severity. How bad is it on a scale of 0 to 10? How much sputum are you coughing up? Is it usually this color?

   Useful other data. Are you experiencing any other symptoms with your cough (such as shortness of breath, nausea, loss of appetite)?

   Patient's perception. Is it better or worse than usual today? How can I help? (The patient with long-standing disease often knows what will help but is hesitant to ask.)

2. The most appropriate nursing diagnosis is ineffective airway clearance related to excessive secretions and ineffective cough.

3. Provide hydration with oral liquids and a room humidifier to liquefy secretions. Administer expectorants as ordered. Instruct the patient in coughing and deep breathing exercises to increase the effectiveness of his cough. Provide good oral care following expectoration of sputum to freshen the patient's mouth. Obtain an order for chest physiotherapy to help loosen and drain secretions.

4.

$$\frac{300 \text{ mg}\ \ |\ \ 5 \text{ mL}}{|\ \ 200 \text{ mg}} = 7.5 \text{ mL}$$

5. "Patient coughed up 200 mL of bright yellow, foul-smelling sputum. Lungs have scattered crackles and wheezes throughout after coughing episode. Expectorant given; fluids encouraged. Mouth care provided."

■ Mr. Franklin

1. You need to do several things at once. You will begin by speaking in a calm voice and trying to help Mr. Franklin to calm himself by doing pursed lip breathing. Assure him that you will help him and won't leave. At the same time, check his oxygen to make sure it is on the ordered number of liters and that his tubing is not kinked or disconnected. Grab the bedside table for him to lean on. Call for someone to page a respiratory therapist to do an NMT if ordered. Have someone bring a pulse oximeter to check his oxygen saturation. Also call for the registered nurse (RN) to administer IV morphine if ordered. All this should take about 1 minute! Once Mr. Franklin is a bit calmer, you can find out what happened. Did the exertion of moving to the bedside commode cause his dyspnea? Check his vital signs and lung sounds, and work with the RN to determine if this represents a change in Mr. Franklin's condition that should be reported to the physician.

2. Teach Mr. Franklin that he should probably stay on bedrest until his acute exacerbation is resolved. Once he is able to start moving around, he should call for help to get up. Review his controlled breathing exercises, which he can use during movement, and encourage rest between activities.

3. "3:00: Patient up on BSC, RR 36 and labored, color gray, appeared very apprehensive. O_2 on at 2 L per min per NC, assisted to lean on overbed table. Encouraged pursed lip breathing. VS 146/64, 102, 36, Sao2 82%. RT paged; administered PRN NMT. LS diminished, no cough. At 3:15, patient appears much calmer, RR 24 and less labored, Sao_2 90%."

unit EIGHT

UNDERSTANDING THE GASTROINTESTINAL, HEPATIC, AND PANCREATIC SYSTEMS

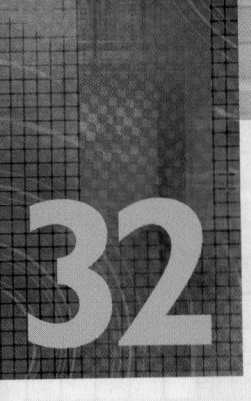

32

Gastrointestinal, Hepatic, and Pancreatic Systems Function, Assessment, and Therapeutic Measures

LAZETTE V. NOWICKI,
LINDA S. WILLIAMS, AND
JANICE L. BRADFORD

KEY TERMS

basal cell secretion test (BAY-zuhl SELL see-KREE-shun TEST)

bowel sounds (BOW'L SOWNDS)

caput medusae (KAP-ut mi-DOO-see)

carcinoembryonic antigen (KAR-sin-oh-EM-bree-ah-nik AN-ti-jen)

colonoscopy (KOH-lun-AHS-kuh-pee)

endoscopy (EN-dohs-kuh-pee)

esophagogastroduodenoscopy (ee-SOFF-ah-go-GAS-troh-doo-AH-den-AHS-kuh-pee)

esophagoscopy (ee-soff-ah-GAHS-kuh-pee)

fluoroscope (FLOOR-o-skohp)

gastric acid stimulation test (GAS-trik ASS-id STIM-yoo-LAY-shun TEST)

gastric analysis (GAS-trik ah-NAL-i-sis)

gastroscopy (gas-TRAHS-kuh-pee)

gastrostomy (gas-TRAHS-toh-mee)

gavage (gah-VAZH)

icterus (ICK-ter-us)

impaction (im-PAK-shun)

jaundice (JAWN-diss)

lavage (lah-VAZH)

lower gastrointestinal series (LOH-er GAS-troh-in-TES-ti-nuhl SEER-ees)

occult blood test (ah-KULT BLUHD TEST)

peripheral parenteral nutrition (puh-RIFF-uh-ruhl par-EN-te-ruhl new-TRISH-un)

peristalsis (pear-is-TALL-sis)

proctosigmoidoscopy (PROK-toh-SIG-moy-DAHS-kuh-pee)

retrograde cholangiopancreatography (RET-roh-grayd koh-LAN-jee-oh-PAN-kree-ah-TOG-rah-fee)

spider angioma (SPY-der AN-jee-OH-mah)

steatorrhea (STEE-ah-toh-REE-ah)

striae (STRIGH-ee)

upper gastrointestinal series (UH-per GAS-troh-in-TES-ti-nuhl SEER-ees)

QUESTIONS TO GUIDE YOUR READING

1. What are the structures of the gastrointestinal tract and of the accessory glands: liver, gallbladder, and pancreas?

2. What are the functions of each organ of the gastrointestinal tract and of the accessory glands: liver, gallbladder, and pancreas?

3. How does age affect the gastrointestinal tract and accessory glands?

4. Which data should you collect when caring for a patient with a disorder of the gastrointestinal system, liver, gallbladder, or pancreas? Differentiate normal and abnormal findings.

5. What are the techniques used in a physical examination of the abdomen conducted for a patient with possible gastrointestinal system, liver, gallbladder, or pancreas disease?

6. How would you prepare, teach, and provide follow-up care for patients having various diagnostic tests of the gastrointestinal tract?

7. What are types and uses of nasogatric and intestinal tubes?

8. What is nursing care for insertion and maintenance of nasogastric tubes?

9. What are therapeutic interventions for patients with gastrointestinal disease?

REVIEW OF NORMAL GASTROINTESTINAL, LIVER, GALLBLADDER, AND PANCREAS ANATOMY AND PHYSIOLOGY

The gastrointestinal (GI) tract (or alimentary tube) is part of the digestive system (Fig. 32.1). It extends from the mouth to the anus and consists of the oral cavity, pharynx, esophagus, stomach, small intestine, and large intestine (or colon). Digestion begins in the oral cavity and continues in the stomach and small intestine. Most absorption of nutrients takes place in the small intestine. The large intestine is where the majority of water is reabsorbed from digested food. Indigestible material, mainly cellulose, is then eliminated from the large intestine.

Oral Cavity and Pharynx

The boundaries of the oral cavity are the hard and soft palates superiorly, the cheeks laterally, and the floor of the mouth inferiorly. Within the oral cavity are the teeth and tongue and the openings of the ducts of the salivary glands.

The teeth begin mechanical digestion, the physical breakup of food into smaller pieces to create more surface area for the chemical digestion brought about by enzymes. The roots of the teeth are in sockets in the jawbones (the mandible and maxillae). The gums, or gingiva, cover the jawbones and surround the bases of the crowns (tops) of the teeth. The tooth sockets are lined with a periodontal membrane (ligament) of dense fibrous connective tissue which cements the roots of the teeth.

The tongue is made of skeletal muscle innervated by the hypoglossal nerve (twelfth cranial nerve). The papillae on the upper surface of the tongue contain taste buds, innervated by the facial and glossopharyngeal nerves (seventh and ninth cranial). The tongue is important for chewing because it keeps food between the teeth. Elevation of the tongue is the first step in swallowing.

The three pairs of salivary glands are the parotid, submandibular, and sublingual glands. Their ducts carry saliva to the oral cavity. The presence of anything in the mouth increases the rate of secretion; this is a parasympathetic response mediated by the facial and glossopharyngeal nerves. Saliva is mostly water, which is used to dissolve food for tasting and moisten the food for swallowing. The only digestive enzyme in saliva that functions in the mouth is amylase, which digests starch to maltose. Usually, however, food does not remain in the mouth long enough for amylase to have any significant effect. There is also lingual lipase, however being activated by acidic pH, it begins its action in the stomach.

The pharynx is a muscular tube that is a passageway for food exiting the oral cavity and entering the esophagus. When a mass of food is pushed backward by the tongue, the constrictor muscles of the pharynx contract as part of the swallowing reflex. This reflex is regulated by the medulla and pons. The uvula closes off the nasopharynx while the epiglottis closes the opening to the larynx.

Esophagus

The esophagus is about 10 inches long and carries food from the pharynx to the stomach. No digestion takes place in the esophagus. **Peristalsis** (rhythmic contraction of muscles) of the muscle layer in the wall of the esophagus is one way; food reaches the stomach even if the body is upside down. At the junction with the stomach, the lumen of the esophagus is surrounded by the lower esophageal sphincter (LES; gastroesophageal sphincter, or cardiac sphincter), a circular smooth muscle. The LES relaxes to permit food to enter the stomach and then contracts to prevent the back-up of stomach contents. Incomplete closure of the LES may allow gastric juice to splash up into the esophagus.

Stomach

The stomach is in the upper left abdominal quadrant, to the left of the liver and in front of the spleen. It is a J-shaped, saclike organ that extends from the esophagus to the duodenum of the small intestine. Some digestion takes place in the stomach, and it also serves as a reservoir for food so that digestion may take place gradually.

The parts of the stomach are shown in Figure 32.2. The LES provides the opening from the esophagus to the stom-

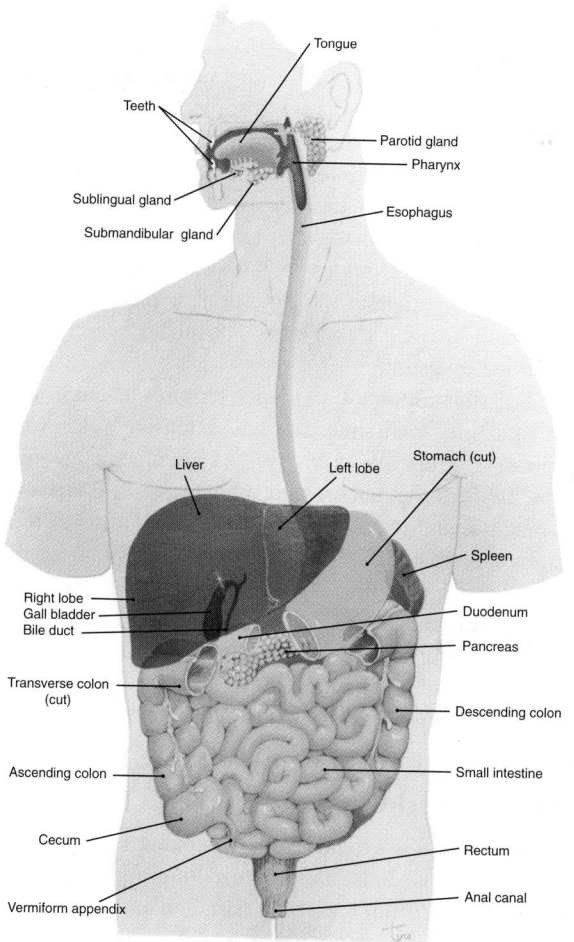

FIGURE 32.1 Anterior view of the digestive system. *(From Scanlon, VC, and Sanders, T: Essentials of Anatomy and Physiology, ed 4. F.A. Davis, Philadelphia, 2003, p 351, with permission.)*

Labels in figure: Tongue, Teeth, Parotid gland, Pharynx, Sublingual gland, Submandibular gland, Esophagus, Liver, Left lobe, Stomach (cut), Spleen, Right lobe, Gall bladder, Bile duct, Duodenum, Pancreas, Transverse colon (cut), Descending colon, Ascending colon, Small intestine, Cecum, Rectum, Vermiform appendix, Anal canal

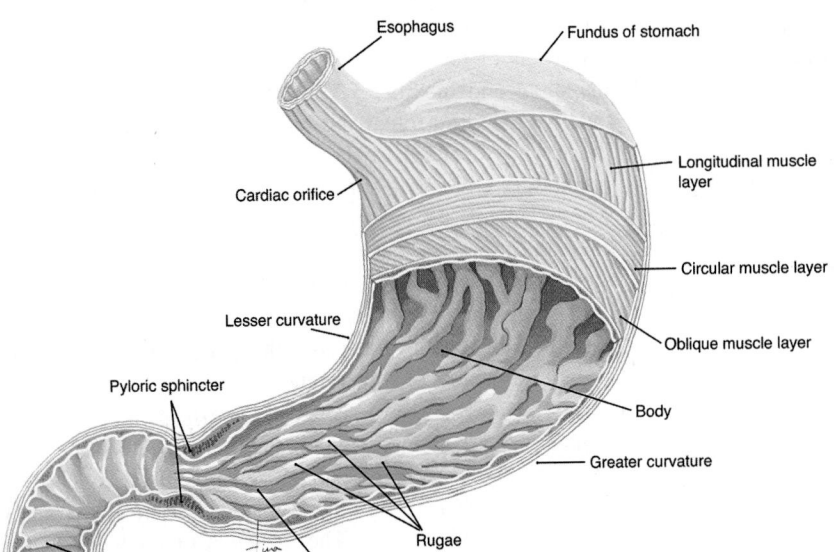

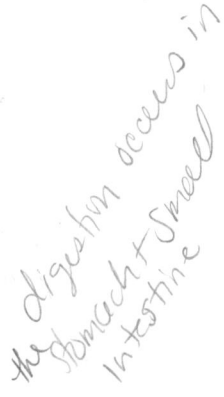

digestion occurs in the Stomach + Small Intestine

FIGURE 32.2 Stomach: anterior view and partial section. *(From Scanlon, VC, and Sanders, T: Essentials of Anatomy and Physiology, ed 4. F.A. Davis, Philadelphia, 2003, p 357, with permission.)*

Important

ach. The fundus forms the upper curve of the stomach. The body of the stomach is the large, central portion, bounded laterally by the greater curvature and medially by the lesser curvature. The pylorus is adjacent to the duodenum, and the pyloric sphincter surrounds the junction of the two organs.

When the stomach is empty, the mucosa has folds called rugae. The rugae flatten out as the stomach fills and permit expansion of the lining. The mucosa contains gastric pits, the glands of the stomach that produce gastric juice. Gastric juice is mostly water and contains mucus, pepsinogen, hydrochloric acid, gastric lipase, and intrinsic factor. Mucus helps form a bolus and protects the mucosal lining. Pepsinogen is an inactive enzyme that is changed to active pepsin by hydrochloric acid; pepsin begins the digestion of proteins to polypeptides. Hydrochloric acid creates the pH of 1 to 2 that is necessary for pepsin to function and to kill most microorganisms that enter the stomach; it also denatures proteins. Gastric lipase helps digest triglycerides. Intrinsic factor aids in the absorption of vitamin B_{12}.

Gastric juice is secreted at the sight or smell of food; this is a parasympathetic response. The presence of food in the stomach stimulates the secretion of the hormone gastrin by the gastric mucosa. Gastrin increases the secretion of gastric juice.

The stomach wall has three layers of smooth muscle: circular, longitudinal, and oblique. These provide for very efficient mechanical digestion to change food to a thick liquid called chyme. The pyloric sphincter contracts when the stomach is churning food and relaxes at intervals to allow small amounts of chyme to pass into the duodenum, then contracts again to prevent the back-up of intestinal contents into the stomach. Carbohydrates are most readily digested by the stomach, followed by proteins and fats.

Small Intestine

The small intestine is about 1 inch in diameter and approximately 20 feet long. Within the abdominal cavity, the coils

of the small intestine are encircled by the colon. The small intestine extends from the stomach to the cecum of the colon. The duodenum is the first 10 inches and contains the hepatopancreatic ampulla (ampulla of Vater), the entrance of the common bile duct and the pancreatic duct. The jejunum is about 8 feet long, and the ileum is about 11 feet in length.

Digestion is completed in the small intestine, and the end products of digestion are absorbed into the blood and lymph. Bile from the liver and enzymes from the pancreas function in the small intestine (Table 32.1). When chyme enters the duodenum, the intestinal mucosa produces the enzymes sucrase, maltase, and lactase, which complete the digestion of disaccharides to monosaccharides; the peptidases, which complete the digestion of proteins to amino acids; and nucleosidases and phosphatases, completing nucleotide digestion.

The absorption of nutrients requires a large surface area, and the small intestine has extensive folds for this purpose. The circular folds (plicae circulares) are macroscopic folds of the mucosa and submucosa. Villi are folds of the mucosa, and microvilli are microscopic folds of the cell membranes on the free surface of the intestinal epithelial cells. Within each villus is a capillary network and a lymph capillary called a lacteal. Water-soluble nutrients (monosaccharides, amino acids, minerals, water-soluble vitamins) are absorbed into the blood in the capillary networks. Fat-soluble vitamins and fatty acids and glycerol are absorbed into the lymph in the lacteals.

Large Intestine

The large intestine extends from the ileum of the small intestine to the anus. It is about 5 feet long and 2.5 inches in diameter. The cecum is the first part, and at its junction with the ileum is the ileocecal valve, which prevents back-up of colon contents into the small intestine. Attached to the cecum is the small, dead-end appendix.

TABLE 32.1   DIGESTIVE SECRETIONS

Organ	Enzyme or Other Secretion	Function	Site of Action
Salivary Glands	Amylase	Converts starch to maltose	Oral cavity
Stomach	Pepsin	Converts proteins to polypeptides	Stomach
	Hydrochloric acid	Changes pepsinogen to pepsin; maintains pH 1–2; destroys pathogens	Stomach
Liver	Bile salts	Emulsifies fats	Small intestine
Pancreas	Amylase	Converts starch to maltose	Small intestine
	Lipase	Converts emulsified fats to fatty acids and glycerol	Small intestine
	Trypsin	Converts polypeptides to peptides	Small intestine
Small Intestine	Peptidases	Converts peptides to amino acids	Small intestine
	Sucrase, maltase, lactase	Converts disaccharides to monosaccharides	Small intestine

The other parts of the colon are the ascending, transverse, and descending colon, which encircle the small intestine; the sigmoid colon, which turns medially and downward; the rectum, which is about 6 inches long; and the anal canal, the last inch that surrounds the anus (clinically, the terminal end of the colon is usually referred to as the rectum).

Although no digestion takes place in the colon, its functions are important. The colon temporarily stores and then eliminates undigestible material. The mucosa absorbs significant amounts of water and minerals, as well as the vitamins produced by the normal bacterial flora.

Elimination of feces is accomplished by the defecation reflex, a spinal cord reflex over which voluntary control may be exerted. When peristalsis propels feces into the rectum, receptors in the smooth muscle layer detect the stretching and generate impulses to the spinal cord. The returning motor impulses cause contraction of the smooth muscle of the rectum and relaxation of the internal anal sphincter, which surrounds the anus. Surrounding the internal sphincter is the external anal sphincter, which is made of skeletal muscle and may be voluntarily contracted to prevent defecation.

The liver, gallbladder, and pancreas are called accessory organs of digestion because they produce or store digestive secretions but are not sites of the digestive process. Mechanical and chemical digestion of ingested foods take place throughout parts of the GI tract.

Liver

The liver fills the right and center of the upper abdominal cavity just below the diaphragm. It has a larger right lobe and a smaller left lobe.

The blood supply of the liver differs from that of other organs. The liver receives oxygenated blood by way of the hepatic artery. By way of the portal vein, blood from the abdominal digestive organs and the spleen is brought to the liver before being returned to the heart. This special pathway is called hepatic portal circulation and permits the liver to regulate blood levels of nutrients or to remove potentially toxic substances such as alcohol from the blood before the blood circulates to the rest of the body.

The only digestive function of the liver is the production of bile by the hepatocytes (liver cells). Bile flows through small bile ducts, converges into larger ones, and leaves the liver by way of the common hepatic duct (Fig. 32.3). The common hepatic duct joins the cystic duct of the gallbladder to form the common bile duct, which carries bile to the duodenum.

Bile is mostly water and bile salts. Its excretory function is to carry bilirubin and excess cholesterol to the intestines for elimination in feces. The digestive function of bile is accomplished via bile salts, which emulsify fats in the small intestine. Emulsification is a type of mechanical digestion in which large fat globules are broken into smaller globules but are not chemically changed. Production of bile is stimulated by the hormone secretin, which is produced by the duodenum when acidic chyme enters the small intestine.

Functions of the Liver

The liver is involved in a great variety of metabolic functions, most of which involve the synthesis of specific enzymes. For the sake of simplicity, these functions may be grouped into categories.

CARBOHYDRATE METABOLISM. The liver regulates the blood glucose level by storing excess glucose as glycogen and changing glycogen back to glucose when the blood glucose level is low. The liver also changes other monosaccharides such as fructose and galactose to glucose, which is more readily used by cells for energy production.

AMINO ACID METABOLISM. The liver regulates the blood levels of amino acids based on tissue needs for protein synthesis. Of the 20 amino acids needed for the production of human proteins, the liver is able to synthesize 12, called the nonessential amino acids, by the process of transamination. The other eight amino acids, which the liver cannot synthesize, are called the essential amino acids. Essential amino acids are required in the diet.

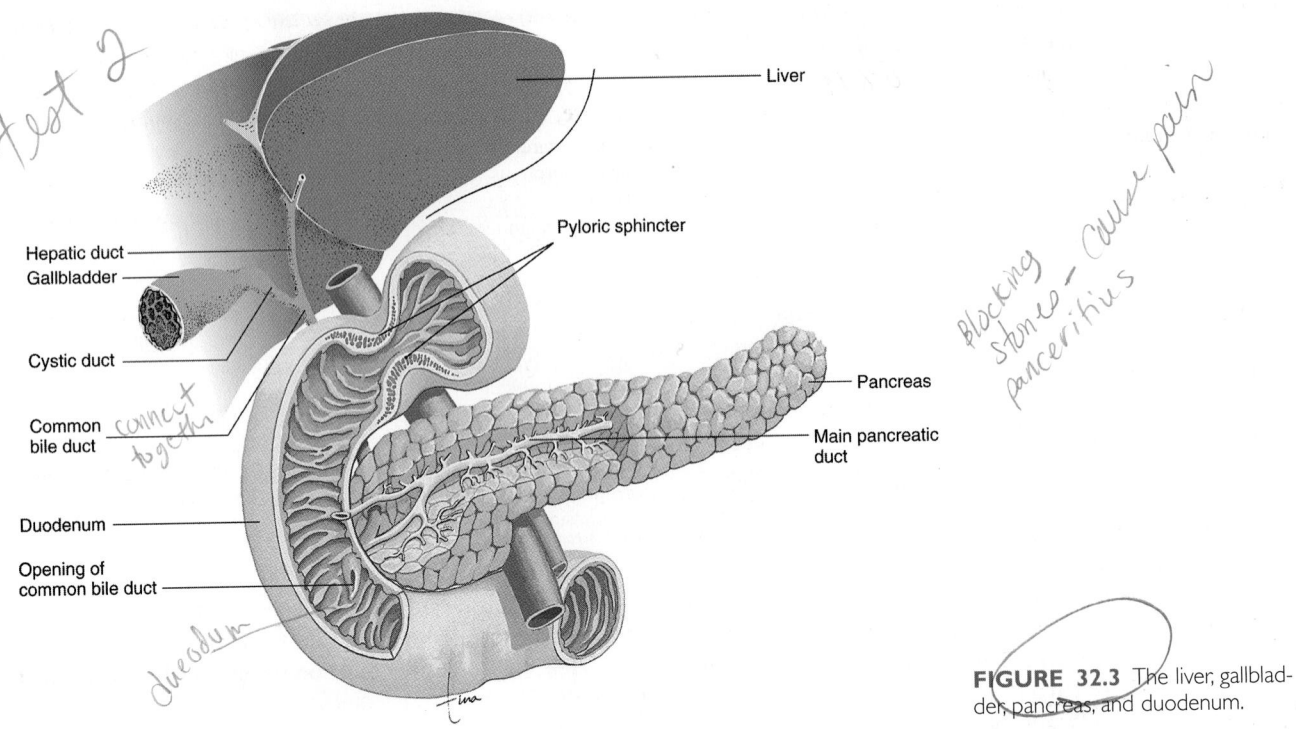

Liver

Hepatic duct
Gallbladder

Cystic duct

Common bile duct

Duodenum

Opening of common bile duct

Pyloric sphincter

Pancreas

Main pancreatic duct

FIGURE 32.3 The liver, gallbladder, pancreas, and duodenum.

Excess amino acids (those not needed for protein synthesis) undergo the process of deamination in the liver; the amino group is removed and the remaining carbon chain is converted to a simple carbohydrate that is used for energy production or converted to fat for energy storage. The amino groups are converted to urea, a nitrogenous waste product that is removed from the blood by the kidneys and excreted in urine.

LIPID METABOLISM. The liver forms lipoproteins for the transport of lipids in the blood to other tissues. The liver also synthesizes cholesterol and excretes excess cholesterol into bile to be eliminated in feces.

The liver is also the main site of the process called beta oxidation, in which fatty acid molecules are split into two-carbon acetyl groups. These acetyl groups may be used by the liver to produce energy, or they may be combined to form ketones to be transported to other cells for energy production.

SYNTHESIS OF PLASMA PROTEINS. The liver synthesizes albumin, clotting factors, and globulins. Albumin, the most abundant plasma protein, helps maintain blood volume by pulling tissue fluid into capillaries. Clotting factors produced by the liver include prothrombin and fibrinogen, which circulate in the blood until needed for chemical clotting. The globulins synthesized by the liver become part of lipoproteins or act as carriers for other molecules in the blood.

PHAGOCYTOSIS BY KUPFFER CELLS. The fixed macrophages of the liver are called Kupffer cells (or stellate reticuloendothelial cells). They phagocytize worn blood cells and pathogens that circulate through the liver. Many of the bacteria that enter the liver come from the colon, after

being absorbed along with water. Portal circulation brings this blood to the liver before entering circulation throughout the remainder of the body. These bacteria are normal flora of the colon but would be harmful elsewhere.

FORMATION OF BILIRUBIN. The fixed macrophages of the liver phagocytize worn red blood cells (RBCs) and form bilirubin from the heme portion of their hemoglobin. The liver also removes from the blood the bilirubin formed in the spleen and red bone marrow and excretes it into bile to be eliminated in feces.

STORAGE. The liver stores the minerals iron and copper; the fat-soluble vitamins A, D, E, and K; and the water-soluble vitamin B_{12}.

DETOXIFICATION. The liver synthesizes enzymes that alter harmful substances to less harmful ones. Alcohol and medications are examples of potentially toxic chemicals. The liver also converts ammonia from the colon bacteria to urea, a less toxic substance.

ACTIVATION OF VITAMIN D. The skin, kidneys, and liver each perform a different role in providing the body with activated vitamin D.

Gallbladder

The gallbladder is a muscular sac about 3 to 4 inches long located on the undersurface of the left lobe of the liver. Bile in the common hepatic duct from the liver flows through the cystic duct (see Fig. 32.3) into the gallbladder, which stores bile until it is needed in the small intestine. The gallbladder also concentrates bile by absorbing water.

When fatty foods or partially digested proteins enter the duodenum, the duodenal mucosa secretes the hormone cholecystokinin. One function of cholecystokinin is to stimulate contraction of the smooth muscle of the wall of the gallbladder. Contraction of the gallbladder forces bile into the cystic duct, then into the common bile duct, which empties into the duodenum.

Pancreas

The pancreas is about 6 inches long, and is located posterior to the greater curvature of the stomach. (See Fig. 32.3.) The digestive secretions of the pancreas are produced by exocrine glands called acini. The small ducts of these glands unite to form larger ducts and finally converge into the pancreatic duct, which joins the common bile duct to enter the duodenum at the hepatopancreatic ampulla. The accessory duct has a direct line from the pancreas into the duodenum.

The pancreatic digestive enzymes are involved in the digestion of all four of the organic molecule categories. The enzyme pancreatic amylase digests starch to maltose. Pancreatic lipase converts emulsified fats to fatty acids and monoglycerides. Trypsinogen is an inactive enzyme that is changed to active trypsin in the duodenum. Trypsin digests

polypeptides to shorter chains of amino acids. Pancreatic juice also contains proteolytic enzymes: chymotrypsin, carboxypeptidase, and elastase. Ribonuclease and deoxyribonuclease, for the digestion of RNA and DNA, respectively, are contributed by the pancreas as well.

The pancreas also produces a bicarbonate juice, which is alkaline because of its high sodium bicarbonate content. The function of bicarbonate juice is to neutralize the hydrochloric acid in gastric juice as it enters the duodenum from the stomach. The pH of duodenal chyme is raised to about 7.5, which prevents corrosive damage to the mucosa and creates the optimal pH for intestinal enzyme action.

Secretion of pancreatic juice is stimulated by the hormones of the duodenal mucosa. Secretin stimulates the production of bicarbonate pancreatic juice, and cholecystokinin stimulates secretion of the pancreatic enzyme juice.

Aging and the Gastrointestinal System, Liver, Gallbladder, and Pancreas

Many changes occur in the aging gastrointestinal (GI) system (Fig. 32.4). The sense of taste becomes less acute, and

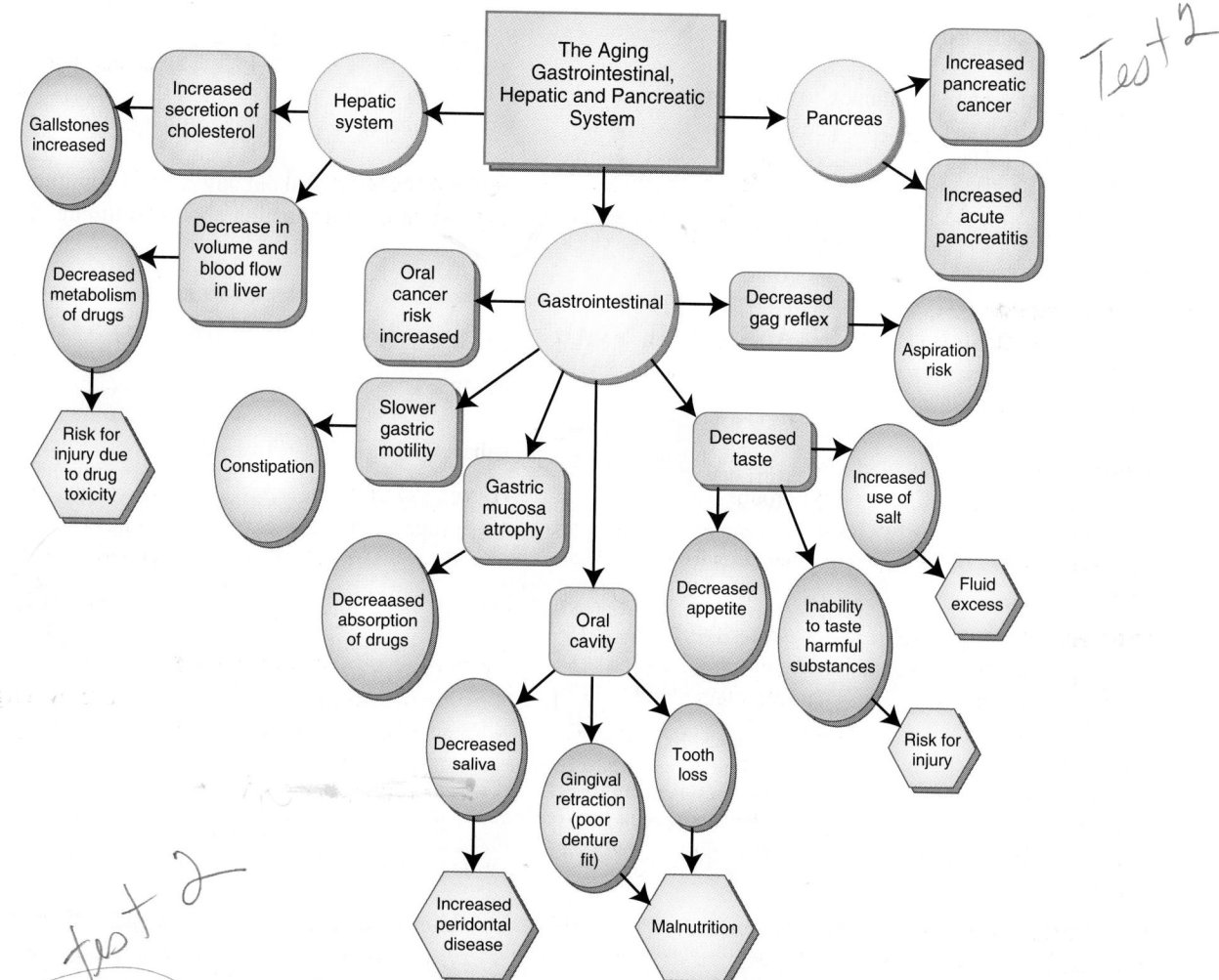

FIGURE 32.4 Aging and its effects on the gastrointestinal, hepatic, and pancreatic systems is shown on this concept map.

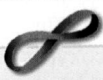

Box 32.1

Gerontological Issues

With increasing age, the liver decreases in volume, mass, and blood flow. These changes are significant because the liver acts to metabolize many drugs. If a patient has impaired liver function, there may be toxic levels of a drug present in the blood. It is important to assess liver function tests and perform a medication review to determine those that are metabolized by the liver. Older adults may require reduced doses of many drugs.

there is greater likelihood of periodontal disease and oral cancer. There may be difficulties with chewing if teeth have been lost. Secretions throughout the GI tract are reduced, and the effectiveness of peristalsis diminishes because of loss of muscle elasticity and slowed motility. Indigestion may become more common, especially if the LES loses its tone, and there is greater chance of peptic ulcer. In the colon, diverticula may form. Constipation may be a problem, as may hemorrhoids. The risk of colon cancer also increases with age.

The liver usually continues to function well into old age, unless damaged by pathogens such as the hepatitis viruses or by toxins such as alcohol (Box 32.1 Gerontological Issues). There is a greater tendency for gallstones to form, sometimes necessitating removal of the gallbladder.

In the absence of specific pathological conditions, the pancreas usually functions well, although acute pancreatitis of unknown cause is somewhat more common in the elderly.

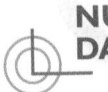

NURSING ASSESSMENT/ DATA COLLECTION

Nursing assessment and data collection of the GI system, liver, gallbladder, and pancreas includes a patient history and physical examination (Tables 32.2, 32.3, and 32.4).

Subjective Data

Health History

Demographic data is obtained, including travel history, which may help in diagnosing the cause of GI symptoms such as diarrhea. Assessment of current signs and symptoms includes asking the WHAT'S UP? questions: where it is, how it feels, aggravating and alleviating factors, timing, severity, useful data for associated symptoms, and perception by the patient of the problem. Also documented are the patient's normal bowel pattern; changes in bowel patterns or habits; a history of any gastrointestinal diseases, such as ulcers, cancer, Crohn's disease, or colitis; or an unexplained weight loss or gain. Information about previous GI surgeries is obtained. Signs or symptoms of disease, such as bloody or tarry stools, rectal bleeding, stomach pain, or abdominal pain, are also noted.

Ask the patient about any nausea, vomiting, or abdominal distention. Information about the timing or other com-

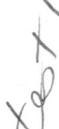

TABLE 32.2 SUBJECTIVE ASSESSMENT OF THE GASTROINTESTINAL SYSTEM

Category	Questions to Ask During History Assessment	Rationale/Significance
Health History	• Assess current symptoms using the WHAT'S UP format. • What are your bowel patterns? How often do you usually have a bowel movement? What is the color? What is the consistency? Any diarrhea or constipation? • Have you had any blood in your stool or on the toilet tissue?	• This will help you adequately assess the patient's current problem. • Changes in bowel habits could indicate new disease process. • Blood in stool could indicate hemorrhoids, early sign of cancer, inflammatory diseases such as ulcerative colitis.
	• Have you had any change in appetite? Nausea and/or vomiting? • Bloating? Excess gas? • Do you have any history or gastrointestinal illnesses or surgeries?	• Appetite changes can be common with gastrointestinal disorders. • Can be associated with GI disorders. • Patient may have a recurring problem.
Medications	• What medications are you currently taking? How do the drugs relate to the GI system? Are they working? How do you know? • Have you recently taken any NSAIDs, aspirin, anticoagulants or steroids? • Do you routinely take laxatives? Fiber?	• Provides baseline information about patient. • These medications can cause gastric upset and/or bleeding. • Patient may have dependency on laxatives.

Category	Questions to Ask During History Assessment	Rationale/Significance
Nutrition **Nutritional Assessment**	• Are taking or have you recently taken antibiotics? • Describe your usual diet. Tell me what you ate yesterday for the entire day.	• Diarrhea due to *C. difficile* can be caused by recent antibiotic use. • Provides information about your patient's nutritional status. Older adults may be on a fixed income and unable to afford adequate nutrition.
	• Do you have any food allergies? • Do you have indigestion, dysphagia, heartburn, nausea, vomiting, diarrhea, constipation, flatulence, or bowel incontinence? • Have you had a change in appetite? • Have you had a change in weight—gain or loss? • Are there any foods that you cannot eat?	• These may interfere with proper nutrition. If patient has any of these symptoms, use the WHAT'S UP format to gather more specific information.
Family History **Cultural Influences**	• Do you have a family history of any gastrointestinal disorders such as cancer? • Are there any cultural considerations I should be aware of regarding your food intake or care?	• Some diseases are thought to be hereditary. • Many societies use herbs, vitamins, or home remedies to care for disorders.

mon triggers of episodes of nausea or vomiting may help the practitioner identify their cause. Such information may also help determine appropriate treatment for any future nausea or vomiting. Abdominal distention in the presence of nausea and vomiting may indicate intestinal obstruction. Patients with liver, gallbladder, or pancreatic disease may also complain of feeling bloated, of having gas or belching frequently, or of right upper quadrant (RUQ) tenderness.

Question the patient about any observed changes in bowel elimination. Diarrhea may be caused by irritation of

TABLE 32.3 SUBJECTIVE ASSESSMENT OF THE LIVER, GALLBLADDER, AND PANCREAS

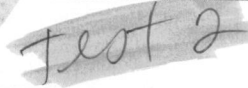

Category	Questions to Ask During History Assessment	Rationale/Significance
Health History	• Do you have abdominal pain? (Use WHAT's UP? to further assess.) Do any foods cause pain? • What do your stools look like?	• Pain can be associated with disease of the liver, gallbladder, or pancreas. Fatty foods can cause pain related to gallbladder disease. • Clay-colored stools indicate liver or gallbladder disease. Black stools may indicate bleeding, which can be related to liver disease. Fatty stools occur with pancreatic disease.
	• Does your abdomen feel distended or full? • How much alcohol do you drink each day? • Do you bruise or bleed easily? • Have you had any recent blood transfusions or blood products, dental procedures, body piercing or tattooing, or intravenous injection with a potentially contaminated needle?	• Fluid in the abdomen, or ascites, occurs with liver disease. • Excess alcohol intake is associated with liver disease and pancreatitis. • Bleeding is associated with liver disease, because clotting factors are made in the liver. • Breaks in skin may be the route of entry for hepatitis (type B or C) or other pathogens.
Nutrition	• Have you experienced nausea and vomiting? • Has your appetite or weight changed?	• These are generalized symptoms that may be associated with disease of the liver, gallbladder, or pancreas. • Anorexia and weight loss accompany many liver, gallbladder, and pancreatic disorders.
Family History	• Does anyone in your family have liver, gallbladder, or pancreatic disease or alcoholism?	• These disorders tend to run in families.
Medications	• Do you use any over-the-counter drugs or herbal remedies?	• Many drugs and herbs are toxic to the liver.

TABLE 32.4 OBJECTIVE ASSESSMENT OF THE GASTROINTESTINAL SYSTEM, LIVER, GALLBLADDER, AND PANCREAS

Category	Physical Assessment Findings	Possible Abnormal Findings/Causes
Height, Weight, and Body Mass Index (BMI)	• Normal height, weight and normal body mass index	• Decreases in height, weight, and BMI could indicate inadequate nutrition or malabsorption problems. • Current weight loss could indicate new onset of a disease such as cancer.
Oral Cavity	• Moist, pink oral mucosa, without lesions, inflammation, tenderness, or discolorations. • Pink, rough tongue. • Teeth should be intact. Dentures should fit properly.	• Foul odor may indicate infection or poor oral hygiene. • Dry tongue with cracked furrows could indicate dehydration possibly due to vomiting or diarrhea. • Broken teeth or ill-fitting dentures can contribute to inadequate nutrition.
Abdomen Inspection	• Abdomen contour should be flat, rounded, or convex. Shape should be symmetrical. • Skin color should be consistent with overall skin tone. No visible scars or discolorations.	• Irregularities in contour such as bulging or masses may be due to distention, tumors, hernia, or previous surgeries. Any scars, dressings, appliances such as an ostomy should be noted. Indicate what the stoma looks like. • Scars may be present if the patient has had previous surgeries or injuries. Striae are present if the skin has been stretched, i.e., with pregnancy or weight gain. Bruising could be related to injury or altered liver function. Note any caput medusae and spider angiomas. Jaundice color may indicate liver or gallbladder disease.
Auscultation	• Soft bowel sounds should be heard in all quadrants every 5-15 seconds. • Circulatory sounds should be absent.	• Hyperactive sounds are heard with increased motility such as diarrhea. Hypoactive sounds are associated with decreased motility such as abdominal surgery, paralytic ileus, or bowel obstruction. • A humming sound may be heard over the liver in patients with chronic liver failure.
Percussion	• Completed by experienced practitioner such as physician or nurse practitioner.	
Palpation	• No pain, muscle tension, rigidity, or masses should be felt on light palpation. The abdomen should feel soft. • Abdominal girth should be appropriate for patient without increasing. • Deep palpation is done by the advanced practitioner.	• Muscle tension, rigidity, or pain may be experienced by many abdominal disorders. • Patients with ascites due to liver disease may have an increased girth that increases as the disease worsens.

the bowel. Constipation may indicate decreased water intake or excessive water loss. Observe the patient's stool for evidence of bacteria (a foul smell), fat (stool floats on the water surface and appears greasy), pus, blood, or mucus. Patients with liver or gallbladder disease may have pale or clay-colored stools.

Ask about the patient's usual work activities and work setting. Document exposure to chemicals such as paint fumes, industrial dyes, acids, farm pesticides, or other liver-toxic substances.

Determine if the patient has had any recent blood transfusions or blood products, dental procedures, body piercing or tattooing, or intravenous injection with a potentially contaminated needle. These procedures cause a break in the skin which can allow an entry point for hepatitis virus (type B or C) as well as other pathogens.

Investigate the patient's activities other than work. Document reports of fatigue along with information about when the fatigue occurs. Ask the patient about stressors such as financial concerns, problems dealing with the health-care environment, and any family or personal problems. Attempt to determine what coping mechanisms the patient usually employs to deal with stressors.

Medications

The patient is asked about medication use such as nonsteroidal anti-inflammatory drugs (NSAIDs), aspirin, vitamins, laxatives, enemas, or antacids. Heavy use of medications that can cause irritation and bleeding in the GI tract, such as NSAIDs or aspirin, should be carefully noted. Elderly patients with arthritis often use these types of medications for pain control. The patient's knowledge of the side effects of these medications should be assessed to identify teaching needs. Elderly patients may use laxatives regularly and develop a dependence on them. Teaching may be needed on normal bowel patterns and laxative use. Also ask the patient what medications are being taken with or without a physician's prescription. Many people do not consider over-the-counter preparations and herbal or natural products that they purchase without a prescription important enough to report and must be asked specifically to do so.

CLOSTRIDIUM DIFFICILE. Question the patient about recent hospitalizations or antibiotic use. Hospitalization or recent antibiotic use is a risk factor for *C. difficile*. With antibiotic use, a decrease in normal flora can result, allowing an overgrowth of *C.. difficile*. The toxins produced by *C. difficile* can cause diarrhea, colitits, toxic megacolon, dehydration, colonic perforation, and sometimes death. Nurses should monitor patients closely for signs of *C. difficle* infection such as diarrhea, nausea, anorexia, and abdominal tenderness or pain. These symptoms should be reported to the physician as this infection can be fatal.

LEARNING TIP

Consider *C. difficle* infection if the patient has diarrhea associated with recent antibiotic use or hospitalization. Educate patients to report its occurrence. Protect your patients with excellent hand hygiene and by following isolation procedures. *C. difficle* can be carried on your hands, nails, rings, or shoes.

CRITICAL THINKING

Mrs. Todd

■ Mrs. Todd, age 74, has arthritis and takes eight aspirin daily for pain control. She is scheduled for an **esophagogastroduodenoscopy** (EGD) for suspected GI bleeding caused by unexplained anemia.
1. What is a likely cause of the GI bleeding?
2. What could you do to help prevent future bleeding episodes for Mrs. Todd?

Suggested answers at end of chapter.

Nutritional Assessment

A diet history should include usual foods and fluids, allergies, appetite patterns, swallowing difficulty, and use of nutritional and herbal supplements. A patient food diary can be used to provide more detailed information. Elderly patients may be on fixed incomes, which may limit their food budget and result in meal skipping or purchasing of inexpensive foods. The elderly patient's daily food intake

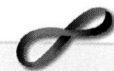

Box 32.2

Gerontological Issues

A complete bowel history should be obtained for older adults before beginning a bowel program. A bowel history includes the following:
   Normal bowel evacuation pattern
   Characteristics of stool
   Presence of any bleeding or mucus with the stool
   Use of products and medications to stimulate or slow bowel function
   Report of usual diet
   Amount of fluids—number and size of beverages, glasses per day (beverages containing caffeine, such as coffee, tea, and sodas, do not count as fluids because of the diuretic effect of caffeine)
   Exercise and physical activity
   Rituals and practices related to bowel function

should be explored, especially if malnutrition, financial limitations, or living alone is noted.

Also explored during a nutritional assessment are patterns of gastric acid reflux, indigestion, heartburn, nausea, vomiting, diarrhea, constipation, flatulence, and bowel incontinence, all of which may interfere with proper nutrition (Box 32.2 Gerontological Issues). Acid reflux can be assessed by asking patients if they experience reflux with a bile taste or awaken with an unpleasant taste in their mouth.

Patients with disease of the liver, pancreas, or gallbladder commonly have changes in appetite such as anorexia or alterations in eating preferences. Ask the patient about any abnormal weight loss or unexpected weight gain and changes in food tolerance, including the type or amount of offending foods. For example, patients with gallbladder disease may report that they feel nauseated or bloated after eating fried or greasy foods. Determine whether the patient ingests alcohol or uses other recreational drugs. If the patient does acknowledge using alcohol or other drugs, record the type, frequency, and amount used.

Family History

Family history of close relatives with conditions that may influence the patient's GI status is assessed. Some GI problems such as colon cancer are thought to be hereditary. The patient's history should note whether there is a family history of liver, pancreas, or gallbladder diseases, such as diabetes mellitus, alcoholism, cancer, heart disease, or bleeding tendencies. These diseases have a high incidence within families.

Cultural Influences

Many cultures have special dietary practices and restrictions (Box 32.3 Cultural Considerations). See Box 32.4 for assessment questions. Understanding these cultural influ-

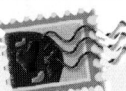

Box 32.3

Cultural Considerations

Most societies of the world use various foods and herbs for maintaining health. With increased attention to herbal therapies in the United States, the U.S. National Institutes of Health is studying 40 foods that are thought to fight disease. Among them are garlic, carrots, soy, cranberry juice, licorice, and green tea. Green tea has been used in Japan and China for centuries as a means of maintaining health and preventing disease.

African Americans

Obesity is seen as positive among many African Americans. They often view individuals who are thin as "not having enough meat on their bones." One needs to have adequate meat on his or her bones so that when an illness occurs, one can afford to lose weight. Many African American diets are high in animal fat and fried foods and low in fiber, fruits, and vegetables.

Appalachians

The diet of some Appalachians is deficient in vitamin A, iron, and calcium. The nurse working with this population needs to do a dietary assessment and teach patients food selections that include adequate vitamin A, iron, and calcium.

Arabs

Many Arabs eat food only with their right hand because it is regarded as the clean hand. The left hand, commonly used for toileting, is considered unclean. Thus, the nurse should feed the Arab patient with the right hand regardless of the nurse's dominant handedness. Additionally, some may not drink beverages with their meals because some individuals consider it unhealthy to eat and drink at the same meal. Likewise, mixing hot and cold foods may be seen as unhealthy.

Muslim Arabs may refuse to eat meat that is not *halal* (slaughtered and prepared in a ritual manner). Because Muslim Arabs are prohibited from ingesting alcohol or eating pork, they may refuse medication that includes alcohol, such as mouthwashes, toothpaste, alcohol-based syrups and elixirs, and products derived from pigs, such as insulin, gelatin-coated capsules, and skin grafts. However, if no substitute is available, Muslims are permitted to use these preparations.

The condition of the alimentary tract has priority over all other body parts in the Arab's perception of health. Gastrointestinal complaints are the most common reason Arab Americans seek care.

Asian Indians

Among Asian Indians, nutritional deficiencies are patterned from their region of emigration. For example,

beriberi (thiamine deficiency) is found in people emigrating from rice-growing areas. Pellagra (niacin deficiency), causing skin and mental disorders and diarrhea, is found in people emigrating from maize-millet areas. Thiamine deficiency is common among people mostly dependent on rice. Thorough milling of rice, washing rice before cooking, and allowing the cooked rice to remain overnight before consumption the following day result in the loss of thiamine.

Asian Indians use chili, which may make it difficult for them to eat food that is tasteless or the use of chili may cause problems with UGI conditions.

Commitment to the sacred cow concept has an impact on Hindus by encouraging dairy and milk use. However, lactose intolerance affects more than 10% of adults. The adequacy or inadequacy to digest lactose may be due to genetic differences among Asian Indians.

Goiter is prevalent among some Asian Indian immigrants resulting from an iodine deficiency in food and water from their homeland. Fluorosis occurs in other parts of India resulting from drinking water high in fluoride. Osteomalacia is prevalent where diets are deficient in calcium and vitamin D. Endemic dropsy is prevalent among Asian Indians emigrating from West Bengal, resulting from using mustard oil for cooking. The nurse needs to be aware of these conditions and their causes when working with Hindus and Asian Indians and teach patients prevention.

Brazilians

There is an increase in gastrointestinal distress among Brazilians when they first come to the United States, partially because many have a lactose intolerance and partially because of different methods of milk pasteurization. The nurse can assist the patient in identifying alternative food sources for Brazilian patients to obtain needed calcium in their diet.

Jewish

Among Jews, the laws regarding food are commonly referred to as the laws of Kashrut, or the laws of what foods are permissible in accordance with the religious law. The term *kosher* means fit for eating; it is not a brand or form of cooking.

Foods are divided into those that are permitted (clean) and forbidden (unclean). The kosher slaughter of animals prevents undue cruelty to the animal and ensures the animal's health for its consumer. Care must be taken that all blood is drained from the animal before eating it.

Among the more conservative and Orthodox Jews, dairy products and meat may not be mixed together, whether in cooking, serving, or eating. This involves separating the utensils used to prepare foods and the plates used to serve them. To avoid mixing foods, religious Jews have two sets of dishes, pots, and utensils: one set for dairy products and one for meat.

Cheeseburgers, meat lasagna, and grated cheese on meatballs and spaghetti are not acceptable. Milk cannot be used in coffee if served with a meat meal. Nondairy creamers can be used as long as they do not contain sodium caseinate, which is derived from milk.

Fish, eggs, vegetables, and fruits are considered neutral and may be used with either dairy or meat dishes. A "U" with a circle around it or a "K" is used on food products to indicate kosher.

When working in a Jewish person's home, the nurse should not bring food into the house without knowing whether the patient is kosher. If the patient is kosher, do not use any cooking items, dishes, or silverware without knowing which are used for meat and which are used for dairy. It is important for the nurse to understand the dietary laws so as not to offend the patient. The nurse should advocate for kosher meals if they are requested and plan medication times accordingly.

Although liberal Jews decide for themselves which dietary laws, if any, they follow, many still avoid pork and pork products out of a sense of tradition and symbolism. It would be insensitive to serve pork products to Jewish patients unless they specifically request it.

Kosher meals are available in hospitals and long-term care facilities. Even though the organization may not have a kosher kitchen, frozen kosher meals can be obtained from several organizations, most of which are located in large cities with large Jewish populations. The kosher kitchen closest to your organization can be obtained by calling the Jewish synagogue nearest the organization to obtain the address and telephone number.

Kosher meals arrive on paper plates with plastic utensils sealed in plastic. The nurse should not unwrap the utensils if the patient is able to do so or change the foodstuffs to another serving dish. Determining a patient's dietary preferences and practices regarding dietary laws should be done during the admission assessment.

Mexican Americans

Good health to Mexican Americans, which is largely a part of "God's will," can be maintained by dietary practices that keep the body in balance. To provide culturally competent care, the nurse must be aware of the hot-and-cold theory of disease when offering health teaching. Many diseases are thought to be caused by a disruption in the hot-and-cold balance theory of the body. Thus, by eating foods of the opposite variety, one may either cure or prevent specific hot-and-cold illnesses and conditions.

Examples of hot disease conditions include infection, diarrhea, sore throats, stomach ulcers, liver conditions, kidney problems, gastrointestinal upsets, and febrile conditions. Foods that are considered "cold" are therefore viewed as remedies for hot illness conditions. Cold foods include fresh fruits and vegetables, dairy products, barley water, fish, chicken, goat meat, and dried fruits. However, there are significant differences in what are considered hot and cold foods and illnesses among Mexican American families depending on their native region in Mexico.

Examples of cold illness conditions include cancer, malaria, earaches, arthritis and related conditions, pneumonia and other pulmonary conditions, headaches, menstrual cramping, and musculoskeletal conditions. Hot substances used to treat these conditions typically include cheeses, liquor, beef, pork, spicy foods, eggs, grains other than barley, vitamins, tobacco, and onions.

ences, respecting them, and assisting the patient to maintain desired cultural practices are important for nutritional maintenance.

Objective Data

Height, Weight, and Body Mass Index

When the GI system is assessed, the patient's height and weight are obtained for planning care. The patient's ideal body weight according to height is obtained using current reference charts. Body mass index (BMI) is calculated to measure body fat and used with waist circumference measurements to determine patient's health risk factors (Table 32.5). Excess waist circumferences (for women, more than 35 inches; for men, more than 40 inches) place people at greater risk for diabetes and cardiovascular disease.

Oral Cavity

Gastrointestinal assessment begins with the oral cavity. The lips are examined for lesions, abnormal color, and symmetry. With a penlight and tongue blade, the oral cavity is inspected

for inflammation, tenderness, ulcers, swelling, bleeding, and discolorations. Any odor of the patient's breath is noted. A foul odor may indicate infection or poor oral care. The tongue should be pink with a rough texture and assessed for signs of dehydration such as dryness, cracks, or furrows. The patient's gums should be pink without swelling, redness, or irregularities. The teeth or dentures are examined for loose, broken, or absent teeth and the fit of the dentures or dental work. Ill-fitting dentures can affect the patient's nutritional intake and obstruct the airway. Loose teeth can become dislodged and aspirated into the airway. Broken teeth can be a source of pain and contribute to poor nutritional intake. The patient's knowledge of dental and oral care is assessed. The ability of the patient to perform oral care is noted and included in the plan of care if there are deficits.

Abdomen

Be prepared to assist with a thorough physical assessment of the patient. Instead of following the usual inspect-palpate-percuss-auscultate (IPPA) format, assess the abdomen start-

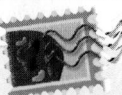

Box 32.4

Cultural Considerations

Questions to ask when performing a cultural nutritional assessment:

1. What types of your cultural foods are available in your community?
2. What are your preferred foods over foods available and eaten?
3. Which foods do you most commonly consume?
4. How and where are your foods chosen and purchased?
5. Who prepares the food in your household?
6. Who purchases the food in your household?
7. How is your food stored for future use?
8. How is your food prepared before eaten?
9. How is any uneaten food discarded?
10. What foods do you eat to maintain your health?
11. What foods do you avoid to maintain your health?
12. What foods do you eat when you are ill?
13. What foods do you avoid when you are ill?

ing with inspection, then auscultation, percussion, and palpation. This is to prevent palpation from changing other assessment findings.

INSPECTION. To inspect the abdomen, patients are placed in a supine position with their arms at their sides. The abdomen is visually inspected to note the condition of the skin and the contour. The contour may be rounded, flat, concave, or distended, depending on the patient's body type. Abdominal pulsatile masses are noted, they may be visible in thin persons or they may indicate an abdominal aortic aneurysm. Irregularities in contour may be due to distention, tumors, hernia, or previous surgeries. Also note

TABLE 32.5 CALCULATING BODY MASS INDEX AND WAIST MEASUREMENT

To calculate body mass index:	Step 1. Multiply body weight (in pounds) by 703. Step 2. Multiply height (in inches) by height. Step 3. Divide answer in step 1 by answer in step 2.
To obtain waist measurement:	Step 1. Place measuring tape at the level of the top of the iliac crest. Step 2. Pull snugly around the waist. Step 3. Read measurement at end expiration.
Findings	Below 18.5 Underweight 18.5–24.9 Normal 25–29.9 Overweight 30 and over Obese

any wounds, tubes, and ostomy device including type and location.

Inspect the patient's skin for scars, **striae** (commonly called stretch marks; light silver-colored or thin red lines on the abdomen), bruising, **caput medusae** (bluish purple swollen vein pattern extending out from the navel), and **spider angiomas** (thin reddish purple vein lines close to the skin surface). Note any petechiae. The patient's abdomen is observed for any visible masses, visible movement or peristalsis, or **jaundice** (also called **icterus,** a yellowing of the skin and the sclerae of the eyes).

Jaundice is a cardinal symptom of liver or gallbladder disease and red blood cell disorders. Old red blood cells are cleared from the circulatory system by phagocytes in the spleen, liver, lymph nodes, and bone marrow. In the process, the compound heme (part of hemoglobin) is split into iron and another substance that is metabolized to bilirubin. The liver is then responsible for converting bilirubin to a water-soluble compound that can be excreted in bile. If the liver is unable to convert or conjugate bilirubin to a water-soluble compound, or if bile drainage is obstructed, serum bilirubin is elevated and pigments are deposited in body tissues.

When serum bilirubin levels elevate, the patient's skin color changes to yellow. The yellow color varies from pale yellow to a striking golden orange. The color intensity is directly related to the amount of elevation of the serum bilirubin. Jaundice can be seen in nearly every body tissue and fluid where there is any amount of albumin. Pigment may occasionally be seen in cerebrospinal fluid or joint fluid. Pigment is not seen in saliva or tears. Urine becomes dark, and if bile flow to the bowel is obstructed, stools will be a light clay color (Box 32.5 Cultural Considerations). Describe any abnormal finding completely in the patient's record, and report your findings promptly.

AUSCULTATION. When auscultating the patient's abdomen, the upper right quadrant is auscultated first (Fig. 32.5). Then a clockwise direction is followed to listen to the other quadrants. The stethoscope is pressed lightly on the abdomen to listen for bowel sounds, which are soft clicks and gurgles that may be heard every 5 to 15 seconds, occurring irregularly 5 to 30 times per minute. **Bowel sounds** at this rate are considered normal. Bowel sounds are produced when peristalsis moves air and fluid through the GI tract and are categorized as normal, hyperactive,

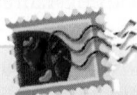

Box 32.5

Cultural Considerations

The nurse should be aware of the variations of assessing for jaundice among people of color. To assess for jaundice in a patient with dark skin, look at the sclerae, conjunctivae, palms of hands, soles of feet, and in the buccal mucosal for patches of bilirubin pigment.

hypoactive, or absent. Hyperactive bowel sounds are usually rapid, high pitched, and loud and may occur with hunger or gastroenteritis. Hypoactive bowel sounds are bowel sounds that are infrequent and can occur in patients with a paralytic ileus or following abdominal surgery. Bowel sounds are considered absent if no sounds are auscultated after listening to all four quadrants for 2 to 5 minutes in each quadrant. However, this timing is an area for further research as in practice auscultation for this amount of time is rarely done. With a bowel obstruction, a high-pitched tinkling sound that is proximal to the obstruction and absent distal to the obstruction may be heard. Abnormal or absent bowel sounds are important findings and should be documented and reported to the physician.

Note the presence of any vascular sounds or bruits (swooshing sounds) that are heard with the stethoscope over the aorta, which are normally not present. Patients with chronic liver failure may have a humming sound over their liver. This finding usually indicates overloaded venous circulation in the liver.

LEARNING TIP

In a complete bowel obstruction, air and fluid are propelled forward by peristalsis proximal to the obstruction. This produces proximal high-pitched bowel sounds when the air and fluid create turbulence as they hit the obstruction and are unable to pass. Absent bowel sounds are heard distal to the obstruction. If a patient has an nasgastric (NG) tube for suction, turn off the suction before listening for bowel sounds.

PERCUSSION. Percussion produces a sound that identifies the density of the organs beneath and is performed by the physician or advanced nurse practitioner. Percussion is used to detect fluid, air, and masses in the abdomen and to identify size and location of abdominal organs (especially the liver and spleen). Tympanic high-pitched sounds indicate the location of air, and dull thuds indicate fluid or solid organs.

PALPATION. Light palpation of the abdomen concludes the physical assessment. If the patient is having pain that area should be palpated last. Using the same quadrant approach as previously mentioned, lightly depress the abdomen not more than 0.5 to 1.0 inch during the palpation (see Fig. 32.5). Note any muscle tension, rigidity, masses, or expressions of pain. Deep palpation of the abdomen is done only by physicians and highly skilled nurses such as nurse practitioners.

Abdominal girth is measured by placing a tape measure around the patient's abdomen at the iliac crest. A mark can be made at the measurement site so that measurements

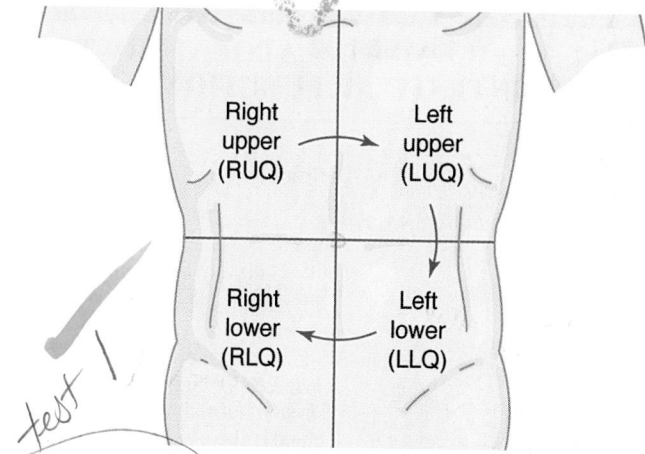

FIGURE 32.5 Abdominal quadrants are auscultated from the right upper quadrant in a clockwise manner.

obtained by others are made at the same location for comparison. Abdominal girth is increased in patients with distention or conditions such as ascites (accumulation of fluid in the peritoneal cavity). Daily measurements should be obtained and recorded to monitor changes when abdominal girth is abnormal.

The advanced nurse practitioner or physician performs all other types of palpation. The liver is not normally palpable, but if enlarged, it may be felt below the right lower rib cage. Rebound tenderness is determined by pressing down on the abdomen a few inches and quickly releasing the pressure. If the patient feels a sharp pain during this procedure, appendicitis may be indicated.

Diagnostic Studies

Use standard precautions when obtaining specimens of body fluids, substances, or blood. Hand hygiene before and after the procedure, wearing gloves, and using goggles if splashing may occur are important.

Laboratory Tests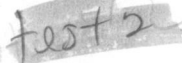

The complete blood cell count (CBC) reveals if anemia or infection is present (Tables 32.6 and 32.7). Anemia may occur with GI bleeding or cancer. Electrolyte imbalances often occur with GI illness as a result of vomiting, diarrhea, malabsorption, or use of GI suction. **Carcinoembryonic antigen** (CEA) and carbohydrate antigen 19-9 are markers used to monitor GI cancer treatment effectiveness and detect recurrence. These markers are also found in patients with cirrhosis, hepatic disease, and alcoholic pancreatitis and in heavy smokers.

Bilirubin is an excellent measure of liver and gallbladder functioning. In addition, certain enzymes such as alanine aminotransferase (ALT; formerly called serum glutamic pyruvic transaminase [SGPT]), aspartate aminotransferase (AST; formerly called serum glutamic oxaloacetic transaminase [SGOT]), and lactic dehydrogenase (LDH) are

TABLE 32.6 COMMON LABORATORY TESTS USED TO ASSESS GASTROINTESTINAL FUNCTION

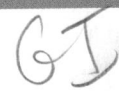

Test	Definition	Normal	Significance of Abnormal Findings
Carcinoembryonic Antigen			
	Blood test to detect protein that is usually found in fetal gut tissue.	Less than 5 ng/mL (nonsmokers)	Increased values indicate possible colorectal cancer, other cancers and inflammatory bowel disease
Complete Blood Cell Count			
Red Blood Cell Count	Blood test to determine size, shape, color and intracellular structure of red blood cells.	4.2–5.2 million/mm³ (women) 4.5–6.2 million/mm³ (men)	Decreased values indicate possible anemia or hemorrhage
Hemoglobin	Blood test to determine the amount of hemoglobin in circulation. Hemoglobin reflects the oxygen-carrying capcity of the blood.	12–16 g/dL (women) 14–18 g/dL (men)	Increased values indicate possible hemoconcentration, caused by dehydration. Decrreased levels can indicate anemia, hemorrhage, or hemo-dilution such as with cirrhosis.
Hematocrit	Measures the percentage of the total blood volume that is made up of RBCs.	38%–46% (women) 42%–54% (men)	Same as hemoglobin.
Electrolytes			
Calcium	Blood test used to determine serum calcium levels.	8.0–10.5 mg/dL	Decreased values indicate possible malabsorption.
Chloride	Blood test used to determine serum chloride levels.	98–107 mEq/L	Decreased values indicate possible malabsorption.
Potassium	Blood test used to determine serum potassium levels.	3.5–5.0 mEq/L	Decreased values indicate possible GI suction, diarrhea, vomiting, intestinal fistulas.
Sodium	Blood test used to determine serum sodium levels	135–145 mEq/L	Decreased values indicate possible malabsorption and diarrhea.
Fecal Analysis			
Stool for Occult Blood	Normally minimal quantities of blood are passed into the GI tract. Stool sample is taken to determine if blood is present in the stool.	Negative	Presence indicates possible peptic ulcer, cancer of the colon, ulcerative colitis.
Stool for Ova and Parasites	Stool sample to determine if pathogenic bacteria, or para-sites are present in the stool.	Negative	Presence indicates infection.
Stool Cultures	Same as above.	No unusual growth	Presence of pathogens may indi-cate *Shigella, Salmonella, Staphylococcus aureus,* or *Bacillus cereus* infections.
Stool for Llipids (Fecal Fat)	Test that measures the fat con-tent in the stool. Used to confirm diagnosis of steatorrhea.	2–5 g per 24 hours (normal diet)	Increased values indicate possible malabsorption syndrome or Crohn's disease, increased in pancreatic disease.

released by damaged liver cells. Elevations in these blood values in the absence of known trauma or heart muscle damage such as a heart attack are excellent indicators of liver damage.

Stool Tests

Stool samples can be tested for **occult blood** (blood not seen by the naked eye). A series of three tests are usually done to increase the chances of detecting blood. False-positive occult blood results can occur with bleeding gums following a dental procedure; ingestion of red meat within 3 days before testing; ingestion of fish, turnips, or horseradish; and use of drugs, including anticoagulants, aspirin, colchicine, iron preparations in large doses, NSAIDs, and steroids.

Stool for ova (eggs) and parasites is collected to detect intestinal infections caused by parasites and their ova. The test usually requires a series of three stool specimens collected every second or third day. The stool specimen is col-

TABLE 32.7 COMMON LABORATORY TESTS FOR LIVER, GALLBLADDER, AND PANCREAS DISORDERS

Test	Definition	Normal Range	Significance
Blood			
Alanine aminotransferase (ALT)	Blood test to determine serum ALT levels. ALT is found mainly in the liver. With injury or disease of the liver, ALT is released into the bloodstream.	5–35 IU/dL	↑ in chronic liver failure and hepatitis
Albumin	Blood test which measures serum protein levels.	3.1–4.3 g/dL	↓ in liver disease
Amylase	Blood test to determine serum levels to detect and monitor pancreatitis.	53–123 U/L	↑ in pancreatitis, gallstones
Ammonia	Blood test to determine serum levels. Ammonia is a by-product of protein catabolism.	12–55 mol/L	↑ in chronic liver failure, hepatitis
Aspartate aminotransferase (AST)	Enzyme found in highly metabolic tissues such as the liver. AST is released into blood stream when cells lyse.	8–20 units/L	↑ in chronic liver failure, viral hepatitis, acute pancreatitis
Bilirubin	Serum blood test used to evaluate liver function.		
Total serum	Sum of the conjugated and unconjugated bilirubin.	0.1–1.0 mg/dL	↑ in liver and gallbladder disease with red blood cell destruction
Conjugated (direct)	Bilirubin which is conjugated in the liver (joined with glucuronide).	0.0–0.4 mg/dL	↑ with gallstones, gallbladder obstruction, extensive liver metastasis
Unconjugated (indirect)	Bilirubin in the blood stream which has not yet passed through the liver.	0.1–1.0 mg/dL	↑ with red blood cell destruction or liver disease such as hepatitis or cirrhosis
Calcium	Blood test to determine serum levels.	9–10.5 mg/dL	↓ with acute pancreatitis, liver disease, or malabsorption
Cholesterol	Blood test to determine serum levels.	150–200 mg/dL	↑ in pancreatitis, gallbladder disease; ↓ may indicate severe liver disease. Patient should fast 12-14 hours prior to test.
Lactic dehydrogenase (LDH)	Blood test to determine levels of this intracellular enzyme which is released with injury or disease.	110–250 IU/L	↑ in liver disease
Potassium	Blood test to determine serum levels. Major cation within the cell.	3.5–5.0 mEq/L	↓ with diarrhea, intestinal fistulas, vomiting, suctioning
Prothrombin time	Blood test used to determine adequacy of clotting mechanism. Used to monitor anticoagulation therapy with warfarin (Coumadin).	11–12.5 s	↑ in liver disease, vitamin K deficiency
Urine			
Urine amylase	Urinalysis examination used to assist in making the diagnosis of pancreatitis.	Depends on test	↑ in acute pancreatitis
Urine bilirubin	Urinalysis exam used to measure predominantly conjugated bilirubin.	Negative	↑ in chronic liver failure, hepatitis, biliary obstruction. Used primarily for screening purposes.
Urobilinogen	Included in a routine urinalysis to support the diagnosis of hemolysis.	0.3–1.0 Ehrlich unit in 2 hr	↑ with destruction of red blood cells, hepatitis, chronic liver failure, obstructive jaundice

lected using a tongue blade, placed in a container with a preservative, and sent immediately to the laboratory. The stool must be examined within 30 minutes of collection. False-negative results can occur as a result of urine in the specimen or if the specimen is not fresh.

Stool cultures (sterile collection technique) are done to determine the presence of pathogenic organisms in the GI tract. Stool can also be examined for lipids (fat). Excessive secretion of fecal fats (**steatorrhea**) may occur in various digestive and absorptive disorders. The stools are collected for 72 hours and stored on ice if necessary before being sent to the laboratory.

(Text continued on page 650)

TABLE 32.8 DIAGNOSTIC PROCEDURES FOR GASTROINTESTINAL SYSTEM

Procedure	Definition/Normal Finding	Significance of Abnormal Findings	Nursing Management
		Noninvasive	
Radiologic Flat Plate of Abdomen	X-ray of the abdomen showing an anterior to posterior view.	Stool or gas may be detected as with constipation or bowel obstruction.	No preparation is necessary.
Upper GI Series	X-ray examination of the esophagus, stomach, duodenum, and jejunum using an oral liquid radiopaque contrast medium. A fluoroscope outlines the contours of the organs. Normal finding should show normal anatomic structures.	Used to detect such things as strictures, ulcers, tumors, polyps, hiatal hernias, and motility problems.	Clear liquid diet night before procedure. NPO for 6–8 hours prior to test. No smoking morning of procedure. Provide increased fluids and laxative after procedure.
Lower GI Series (Barium Enema)	Colon is filled with barium and x-rays are performed to visualize the position, movements, and filling of the colon. Normal finding would be no polyps, inflammation, diverticula, stenosis, or tumors.	Tumors, diverticula, stenosis, obstructions, inflammation, ulcerative colitis, and polyps can be detected.	Patient is placed on a low-residue or clear liquid diet for 2 days before the test. Laxatives, bowel cleansing solutions (such as GoLYTELY), and enemas may be administered the evening before the test. The bowel needs to be adequately cleaned out for adequate visualization during the test. Encourage fluids and possibly laxatives to clear barium from colon.
Computed tomography (CT)	Uses a beam of radiation to allow three-dimensional visualization of abdominal structures. Diluted oral barium or other contrast media may be used to distinguish normal bowel from abnormal masses. Normal finding is no masses.	May show abnormal masses.	Clear liquid diet the morning of the test. If a contrast medium is to be used note allergies to contrast media. Consent form is signed. NPO for 2 to 4 hours before the procedure.
Ultrasonography	High-frequency sound waves are passed through the abdomen to view soft-tissue structures.	Abnormal soft tissue structures.	NPO after midnight.
		Invasive	
Nuclear Scanning (cholescintigraphy, 99mTc Di-isopropyl Iminodiacetic Acid Scintigraphy [DISIDA], Hepatobiliary Imidodiacetic Acid [HIDA] scan, or imidodiacetic Acid [IDA])	Involves injecting a patient with a small amount of intravenous radioactive isotope. Serial images of the gallbladder, bile duct and duodenum are recorded. Normal finding is no evidence of biliary disease, obstruction or ejection problems.	Confirms any biliary disease, ejection problem or obstruction.	Fasts for 2–6 hours prior to procedure. May be given cholecystokinin.
Angiography	A contrast medium is injected and identifies abnormalities of vascular structure and function, observes masses, and notes bleeding sites. A normal finding is no evidence of abnormal vasculature or masses.	Neoplasms of liver, gallbladder or pancreas. May indicate abnormal vasculature.	Ask if allergies to contrast media or iodine. NPO for 2–8 hours prior to test. Stop medications that interfere with clotting about 1 week prior to exam. Assess for bleeding and hematoma formation after the exam.
Endoscopy	Uses a tube and a fiberoptic system (endoscope) for observing the inside of a hollow organ or cavity. The physician can also remove polyps, take biopsy specimens, or coagulate bleeding sites that are identified.	Strictures, polyps, tumors, bleeding.	Consent form is signed for any endoscopic procedure.

Procedure	Definition/Normal Finding	Significance of Abnormal Findings Invasive	Nursing Management
Esophagogastroduo-denoscopy (EGD)	Endoscopy which visualizes the esophagus, the stomach, and the duodenum. Biopsy or cytology specimens can be obtained. Normal findings would indicate all normal structures without inflammation, bleeding or cancer.	Abnormalities such as inflammation, cancer, bleeding, injury, and infection can be detected.	See endoscopy. May use a preoperative checklist. NPO for 8–12 hours. May need to premedicate to relax patient. Monitor vital signs and prevent aspiration after procedure. Monitor for pain, bleeding, fever and dysphagia after the procedure.
Endoscopic retrograde cholangiopancreatography (ERCP)	Endoscopy which permits the physician to visualize the liver, gallbladder, and pancreas. May use contrast medium. An endoscope is passed through the esophagus to the duodenum, where dye is injected that outlines the pancreatic and bile ducts. Normal findings would indicate all normal structures without inflammation, bleeding, or cancer.	Liver, gallbladder, or pancreas disease.	See endoscopy and EGD. NPO after 8 PM the night before exam. Check prothrombin time prior to procedure. Monitor for pain, fever, chills which could indictate infection. Monitor for onset of pancreatitis.
Proctosigmoidoscopy	Examination of the distal sigmoid colon, the rectum, and the anal canal using a rigid or flexible endoscope (sigmoidoscope). Normal finding would be no ulcerations, punctures, laceration, tumors, hemorrhoids, polyps, fissures or fistulas.	Ulcerations, punctures, lacerations, tumors, hemorrhoids, polyps, fissures, fistulas, early malignancies and abscesses can be detected.	Clear liquid diet for 24 hours prior to exam. Laxative the night before exam. Enemas the morning of the exam.
Colonoscopy	Visualization of the lining of the large intestine to identify abnormalities through a flexible endoscope, which is inserted rectally. A biopsy specimen may be obtained or polyps be removed during the colonoscopy. A normal finding would show a normal colon without signs of inflammation, ulcers, polyps, or cancer.	Colon cancer, polyps, inflammation.	Clear liquid diet for 24 hours prior to exam. Bowel preparation (GoLYTELY) the night before exam. Possibly enemas the evening prior to examination and the morning of the examination. Patient will receive conscious sedation during examination. Monitor for complicaitons such as hemorrhage and severe pain. Instruct patient that cramping will last for several hours after test, and blood may be present in stool if specimen was taken.
Gastric Analysis Basal cell secretion test Gastric acid stimulation test	Gastric analysis measures the secretions in the stomach. For the basal cell secretion test, a nasogastric (NG) tube is inserted and the contents of the stomach are suctioned out through the tube using a syringe. Stomach contents are collected at intervals. The gastric acid stimulation test measures the amount of gastric acid for 1 hour after subcutaneous injection of a histamine drug.	Diagnosis of duodenal ulcer, gastric carcinoma, pyloric or duodenal obstruction, and pernicious anemia are made.	Before the basal cell secretion test, the patient should avoid taking any drugs that could interfere with gastric acid secretion, such as cholinergics and antacids. The patient is NPO after midnight the night before the test.
Endoscopic ultrasonography	Endoscopic ultrasonography is performed through the endoscope using sound waves.	Tumors in various GI structures and organs.	Similar to endoscopy.
Percutaneous liver biopsy	The physician generally inserts a needle through the skin and into the liver to withdraw a small sample for examination. Normal finding would be negative for cancer, cirrhosis, hepatitis or other liver diseases.	May identify cancer, cirrhosis, hepatitis, or other causes of liver disease.	Signed consent. Ensure laboratory tests such as CBC, coagulation studies have been ordered and reviewed. NPO for 6–8 hours prior to procedure. Rest several hours after procedure; restricted activity 1 day. Monitor biopsy site pressure dressing for bleeding. Monitor vital signs after procedure. Coughing and straining avoided after the procedure. Medicate for pain.

Handwritten annotations:
test 1 — ulcers — priorty GAG reflex
test 1 — usually afts age 50
test 2 — through the skin, long needle — High risk for Bleeding — Lay on the side to stop Bleeding to Avoid Bleeding

Radiographic Tests

Flat Plate of the Abdomen

A flat plate of the abdomen is an x-ray examination giving an anterior-to-posterior view (see Table 32.8). Radiographs visualize abdominal organs and can detect such abnormalities as tumors, obstructions, and strictures. For an x-ray examination, the patient should be dressed in a hospital gown without any metal such as zippers, belts, or jewelry. Pregnant patients or those thought to be pregnant should avoid x-ray examinations.

Upper Gastrointestinal Series (Barium Swallow)

test 1 ✓

An **upper gastrointestinal series** (UGI series) is an x-ray examination of the esophagus, stomach, duodenum, and jejunum using an oral liquid radiopaque contrast medium (barium) and a **fluoroscope** to outline the contours of the organs. An upper gastrointestinal (UGI) series is used to detect such things as strictures, ulcers, tumors, polyps, hiatal hernias, and motility problems.

The patient receives nothing by mouth (*non per os* in Latin, abbreviated NPO) for 6 to 8 hours before the procedure. Usually the patient has a clear liquid supper the night before the procedure and is then NPO until the procedure is done. Because smoking can stimulate gastric motility, the patient is discouraged from smoking the morning of the procedure. Patient teaching includes information about the patient's diet before and after the procedure, the barium ingestion, and the appearance of stools afterward.

During the procedure, the patient drinks the thick, chalky barium while standing in front of a fluoroscopic tube. X-ray films are taken in various positions and at specific intervals to visualize the outline of the organs and to note the passage of the barium through the GI tract. The patient should understand that the procedure may take several hours depending on the rate at which the barium moves through the patient's gastrointestinal tract.

A laxative is usually ordered after the procedure to expel the barium and prevent constipation or a barium **impaction.** The patient is instructed to drink 12 8-oz glasses of water per day for several days to prevent dehydration, which can lead to constipation. The abdomen is assessed for distention and bowel sounds. The stool is monitored to determine whether the barium has been completely eliminated. Initially, the barium causes the patient's stool to be white, but it should return to its normal color within 3 days. Constipation with distention indicates a barium impaction.

Lower Gastrointestinal Series

test 1

The **lower GI series** (barium enema) is performed to visualize the position, movements, and filling of the colon. Tumors, diverticula, stenosis, obstructions, inflammation, ulcerative colitis, and polyps can be detected. The patient is placed on a low-residue or clear liquid diet for 2 days before the test to empty the bowel. Laxatives, bowel-cleansing solutions (such as GoLYTELY), and enemas may be administered the evening before the test. GoLYTELY is chilled and drunk full strength with no ice, 8 oz every 10 minutes for a total of 4 L. Inform the patient that a watery diarrhea will begin in about 1 hour and continue up to 5 hours as the bowel is cleared. This is necessary for adequate visualization during the procedure. Inadequate bowel preparation may result in poor test results or test cancellation (Fig. 32.6). The patient either receives a clear liquid diet the morning of the test or is NPO after midnight the night before. The area around the rectum should be clean before the patient is sent for the procedure. If the patient has active inflammatory disease of the colon or suspected perforation or obstruction, a barium enema is contraindicated. Active GI bleeding may also prohibit the use of laxatives and enemas.

During the procedure, barium is instilled rectally and x-ray films are taken with or without fluoroscopy. The patient may experience some abdominal cramping and an urge to have a bowel movement during the procedure. The patient is

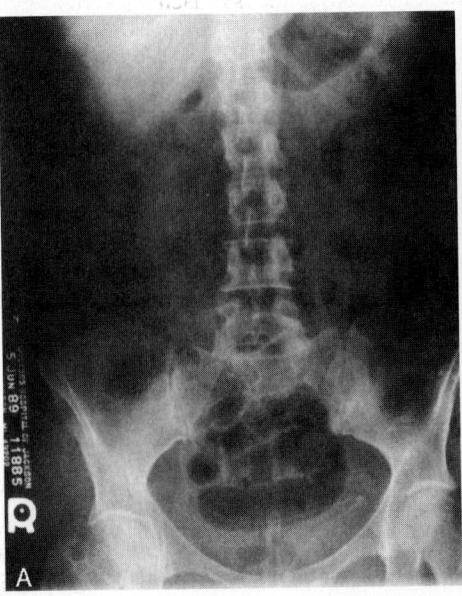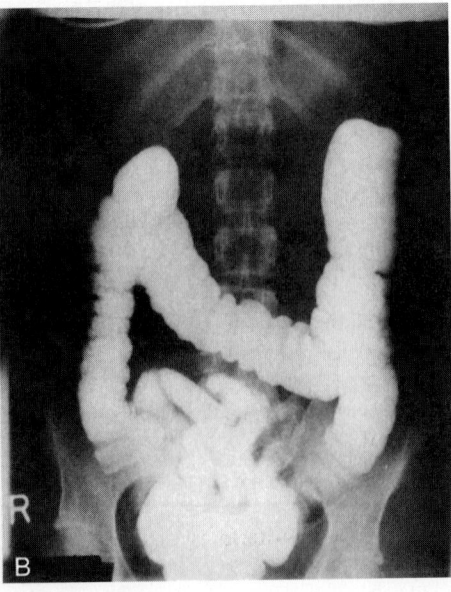

FIGURE 32.6 *(A)* An image of a patient who was poorly prepared for a barium enema. *(B)* An image of a patient who was adequately prepared for a barium enema. *(Courtesy Dr. Russell Tobe.)*

told to take slow, deep breaths and to tighten the anal sphincter. The rate of flow of the barium is slowed until the cramping diminishes. The procedure takes about 15 minutes, and the patient is allowed to use the bathroom immediately after the procedure.

The patient's stools are monitored after the procedure to note if all the barium is passed, as with the UGI series. Constipation development is monitored. The patient is encouraged to drink at least one 8-oz glass of liquid per hour for the next 24 waking hours to help remove the barium. Laxatives may be ordered to help clear the barium from the colon. The patient is told to report any abdominal pain, bloating, or absence of stool, all of which could indicate constipation or bowel obstruction, as well as any rectal bleeding.

CRITICAL THINKING

Mrs. Pearl

■ Mrs. Pearl is a 95-year-old woman undergoing a lower GI series for complaints of abdominal pain. As her nurse, what concerns might you have for Mrs. Pearl as she undergoes this test? How can you address them?

Suggested answers at end of chapter.

Computed Tomography

Computed tomography (CT) uses a beam of radiation to allow three-dimensional visualization of abdominal structures. Diluted oral barium or other contrast media may be used to distinguish normal bowel from abnormal masses. The patient may have a clear liquid diet the morning of the test. If a contrast medium is to be used, any allergies to iodine or contrast media are noted, a consent form is signed, and the patient is NPO for 2 to 4 hours before the procedure.

Nuclear Scanning

Nuclear scanning involves injecting a patient with a small amount of radioactive isotope. The scan may be called a cholescintigraphic, DISIDA, HIDA, or IDA scan, depending on the radioactive isotope and exact procedure that is used. Prior to the procedure, the patient fasts and does not chew gum for at least 2 to 6 hours. After the injection, the isotope is secreted into the bile and goes anywhere the bile goes. Visualization of these areas occurs about 60 minutes after the IV injection. The scanning camera (like a Geiger counter) traces the path of the isotope as it travels through the bile ducts, gallbladder, and intestines. Serial images are recorded. A patient may be given a fatty meal or cholecystokinin to stimulate emptying of the gallbladder. Any biliary disease, ejection problem, or obstruction can be confirmed with this examination. The test takes about 2 hours.

Angiography

Angiography may be ordered for patients with symptoms of arterial occlusive disease of the hepatic, biliary, and pancreatic arterial vessels. It is used to evaluate suspected neoplasms in these organs. Medications that might cause bleeding, such as aspirin, NSAIDs, or anticoagulants, are stopped about 1 week prior to the procedure. A contrast medium is injected and identifies abnormalities of vascular structure and function, masses, and show bleeding sites. Prior to the procedure, the patient usually is NPO for 2 to 8 hours. The injection of contrast medium is done about 1 hour before the examination. Radiographs are taken about every 20 minutes for 1 hour or until the structures are readily viewed. The radiopaque material is iodine based, so ask the patient about any allergies to iodine. Following the procedure, observe for bleeding at the puncture site. Patients with liver disease may have clotting disorders and should be assessed for bleeding or hematomas at the site. Monitor pulses distal to the insertion site.

Liver Scan

A liver scan involves injecting a slightly radioactive medium that is taken up by the liver. An instrument is passed over the liver that records the amount of material taken up by the liver and forms a composite "picture" of the liver. The physician may be able to determine tumors, masses, and abnormal size and patterns of blood vessel. The procedure takes a short time.

Endoscopy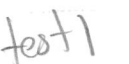

Endoscopy uses a tube and a fiberoptic system (endoscope) for observing the inside of a hollow organ or cavity. In addition to viewing the structures, the physician can also remove polyps, take biopsy specimens, or coagulate bleeding sites that are identified.

A consent form must be signed for any endoscopic procedure.

Esophagogastroduodenoscopy

Esophagogastroduodenoscopy (EGD) visualizes the esophagus (**esophagoscopy**), the stomach (**gastroscopy**), and the duodenum. Abnormalities such as inflammation, cancer, bleeding, injury, and infection can be seen.

The procedure is explained to the patient. Because this is an invasive procedure, patients may be asked to sign an operative consent form, and a preoperative checklist may be necessary, depending on institution policy. To prevent aspiration of stomach contents into the lungs if vomiting occurs, the patient is NPO for 8 to 12 hours before the procedure. Sedatives such as diazepam (Valium) or midazolam (Versed) may be given before the procedure to help relax the patient. The patient may be given atropine sulfate to dry secretions in the mouth. A local anesthetic in spray or gargle form is administered just before the scope is inserted to inhibit the gag reflex.

The patient is placed on the left side, and the flexible fiberoptic endoscope tube is passed orally down the GI tract (Fig. 32.7). Photographs or videotapes of the procedure can be made. Biopsy or cytology specimens can be obtained.

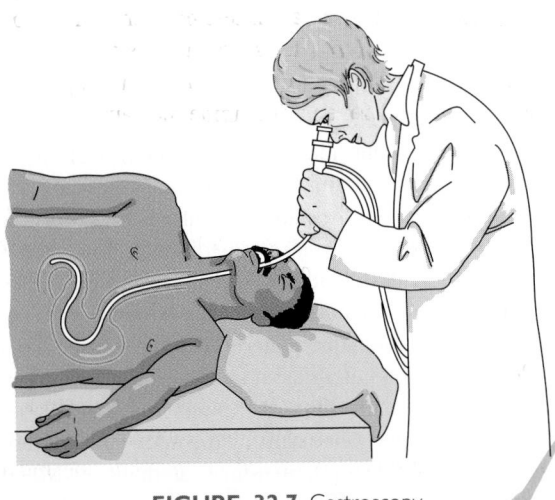

FIGURE 32.7 Gastroscopy.

After the procedure, vital signs are checked as ordered. Patients are placed on one side to prevent aspiration while sedation and the local anesthetic wear off. Patients are NPO until the gag reflex returns (usually within 4 hours). Patients are assessed for signs of perforation, which include bleeding, fever, and dysphagia. Midesophageal perforation can cause referred substernal or epigastric pain. Blood loss secondary to perforation can lead to hematoma formation, which in turn can result in cyanosis and referred back pain. Distal esophageal perforation may result in shoulder pain, dyspnea, or symptoms similar to those of a perforated ulcer. The patient may have a sore throat for a few days.

Endoscopic Retrograde Cholangiopancreatography

Endoscopic **retrograde cholangiopancreatography** (ERCP) permits the physician to visualize the liver, gallbladder, and pancreas (Fig. 32.8). The procedure allows both direct viewing and use of contrast medium. An endoscope is passed through the esophagus to the duodenum, where dye is injected that outlines the pancreatic and bile ducts.

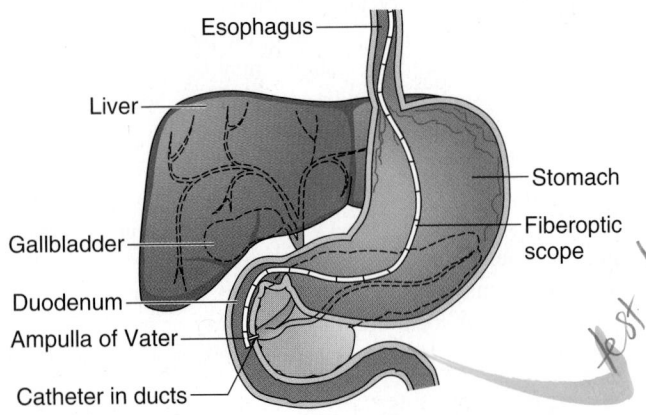

FIGURE 32.8 Endoscopic retrograde cholangiopancreatography. *(Modified from Watson, J, and Jaffe, S: Nurse's Manual of Laboratory and Diagnostic Tests, ed 2. F.A. Davis, Philadelphia, 1995, p 525, with permission.)*

The patient is prepared for an ERCP in the same manner as for an EGD, with nothing by mouth after 8 p.m. the night before the examination. In addition, the patient is asked about allergies to iodine. Ensure that any ordered laboratory studies, such as a prothrombin time, have been done before the procedure and that the patient has removed dentures. Follow-up care is similar to an EGD. In addition, the nurse is alert to patient complaints such as increased right upper quadrant pain, fever, or chills, which may indicate infection. Hypotension, tachycardia or rapid heart rate, increasing RUQ pain, nausea, or vomiting may indicate perforation or the onset of pancreatitis. Report such findings immediately.

Lower Gastrointestinal Endoscopy

PROCTOSIGMOIDOSCOPY. Proctosigmoidoscopy is the examination of the distal sigmoid colon, the rectum, and the anal canal using a rigid or flexible endoscope (sigmoidoscope). Ulcerations, punctures, lacerations, tumors, hemorrhoids, polyps, fissures, fistulas, and abscesses can be detected. Malignancies at an early stage can be detected, so an annual examination for patients 40 years old and older is recommended.

Proctosigmoidoscopy requires the lower bowel to be cleaned out. The patient usually receives a clear liquid diet 24 hours before the test and a laxative the night before the test. The morning of the procedure a warm tap-water enema or sodium biphosphate (Fleet) enema is given. Bowel preparation may not be ordered for patients with bleeding or severe diarrhea.

The patient is positioned in a left lateral knee-to-chest position, which allows the sigmoid colon to straighten by gravity. A rigid proctoscope is used to visualize the rectum. A flexible scope is then used to permit visualization above the rectosigmoid junction. Patients are told they may feel pressure as though they are going to have a bowel movement. During the procedure, one or more small pieces of intestinal tissue may be removed (biopsy specimens). Rectal or sigmoid polyps are removed with a snare. An electrocoagulating current is used to cauterize sites to prevent or stop bleeding. Specimens are labeled and sent to the pathology laboratory immediately for examination.

After the procedure, the patient is allowed to rest for a few minutes in the supine position to avoid orthostatic hypotension when standing. Pain and flatus may occur from instilled air. The patient is observed for signs of perforation such as bleeding, pain, and fever.

COLONOSCOPY. Colonoscopy provides visualization of the lining of the large intestine to identify abnormalities through a flexible endoscope, which is inserted rectally. A biopsy specimen may be obtained or polyps be removed during the colonoscopy.

The patient receives a liquid diet 24 hours before the test and is NPO after midnight before the procedure. A bowel preparation solution such as GoLYTELY is given the night before the procedure. Drinking this solution can be

> **SAFETY TIP**
>
> Older patients may experience fatigue and weakness during bowel preparation and may be unable to complete it. Monitor the patient for distress. Consult the physician if you note any patient distress during bowel preparation. Observe the patient often because defecation urgency, especially in unfamilar surroundings, may create a fall risk.

unpleasant for the patient. In addition, a laxative, suppository (bisacodyl [Dulcolax]), or enema may be needed.

Conscious sedation , for example, midazolam (Versed) is used to relax and ease pain during the procedure. The patient is positioned on the left side with the knees bent. A small amount of air is instilled into the colon to help the physician visualize the bowel. The air causes pressure and may be uncomfortable for the patient. The patient is encouraged to relax and take slow deep breaths through the nose and out the mouth. Vital signs are monitored throughout the procedure to watch for a vasovagal response, which can lead to hypotension and bradycardia.

After the procedure, the patient is monitored until stable. Complications such as hemorrhage or severe pain are reported. When giving the patient discharge instructions, explain that flatus and cramping will occur for several hours after the test, that blood may be present in the stool if a biopsy specimen was taken, and to report problems to the physician.

Gastric Analysis

Gastric analysis measures the secretions in the stomach. Diagnoses of duodenal ulcer, gastric carcinoma, pyloric or duodenal obstruction, and pernicious anemia are made. A diagnosis of pernicious anemia is ruled out by the finding of acid. A diagnosis of gastric carcinoma may be made by the presence of cancer cells in the gastric secretions. There are two tests performed in gastric analysis: the **basal cell secretion test** and the **gastric acid stimulation test.**

Before the basal cell secretion test, the patient should avoid taking any drugs that could interfere with gastric acid secretion, such as cholinergics and antacids. The patient is NPO after midnight the night before the test. For the procedure, a nasogastric (NG) tube is inserted and the contents of the stomach are suctioned out through the tube using a syringe. The NG tube is connected to wall suction, and stomach contents are collected every 15 minutes for 1 hour. The specimens are labeled according to the time they were collected and the order in which they were obtained. The gastric acid is tested for pH using indicator paper or a pH meter. The amount of gastric acid is also measured. Too much hydrochloric acid may indicate a peptic ulcer; too little could be a sign of cancer or pernicious anemia.

The gastric acid stimulation test measures the amount of gastric acid for 1 hour after subcutaneous injection of a histamine drug. If abnormal results occur, radiographic tests or endoscopy can be done to determine the cause.

Ultrasonography

The use of high-frequency sound waves through the abdomen allows the physician to view soft-tissue structures. The sound waves reflect varying images based on the density of the soft tissues in the abdomen. The patient is asked not to take anything by mouth after midnight on the day of the examination. A clear gel is applied to the abdomen and to the transducer on the sonograph. The gel improves the conduction of sound waves and thus improves the images obtained. The transducer is placed on the skin and moved over the abdomen while the technician views the sonograph screen and takes periodic pictures. The procedure takes about half an hour and requires no follow-up care.

Endoscopic Ultrasonography

Endoscopic ultrasonography is performed through the endoscope using sound waves. Tumors can be detected in various GI structures and organs. Preprocedure and postprocedure care are similar to those for endoscopic care. During the test the patient must lie still while a transducer with gel is moved back and forth over the abdomen to produce images.

Percutaneous Liver Biopsy   test 2

If less invasive tests do not aid in diagnosis of liver disease, a liver biopsy may be done. This may be done to identify cancer, cirrhosis, hepatitis, or other causes of liver disease. The physician generally inserts a needle through the skin and into the liver to withdraw a small sample for examination. This procedure places the patient at risk for bleeding because the liver is highly vascular and because many patients with liver disease have reduced clotting ability.

Before the biopsy, ensure that the patient understands the procedure and that a consent has been signed if required by institution policy. You should also ensure that laboratory tests, such as a complete blood cell count and coagulation studies, have been completed and reviewed as ordered. The patient may be ordered nothing by mouth for 6 to 8 hours before the procedure. Baseline vital signs are taken, and a sedative is given if ordered.

During the procedure the nurse assists the physician to position the patient on his or her back or left side and assists the patient to hold very still while the needle is being introduced. The physician may also ask the patient to exhale and hold his or her breath during the needle insertion.

After the biopsy, the patient should remain on bedrest for 24 hours. The patient lies on the right side for the first 2 hours with a small pillow or rolled towel under the biopsy site to provide pressure and prevent bleeding. Vital signs and the site are monitored for signs of bleeding. The patient is advised to avoid coughing or straining. Analgesics are offered for comfort if ordered.

CRITICAL THINKING

Mr. Wozynski

■ Mr. Wozynski is admitted with chronic liver failure and jaundice. What specific laboratory value can you expect to be elevated related to his jaundice? Mr. Wozynski's physician orders a liver biopsy. Why is it important for you to check Mr. Wozynski's laboratory reports before the procedure?

Suggested answers at end of chapter.

THERAPEUTIC INTERVENTIONS

Gastrointestinal Intubation

Gastrointestinal intubation is the placement of a tube within the GI tract for therapeutic or diagnostic purposes (Fig. 32.9). When the GI tube is inserted orally into the stomach it is an orogastric tube. When it is from the nares into the stomach, it is referred to as a nasogastric tube. A nasointestinal tube is a tube inserted from the nares into the intestines. A variety of tubes are available, each designed for

specific purposes (Table 32.9). Orogastric tubes reduce sinus infection risk as they do not block normal drainage of the sinuses as nasal tubes may. Nasogastric and nasointestinal tubes are inserted for a variety of reasons, but the main purposes for their use include the following:

- To remove gas and fluids from the stomach or intestines (decompression)
- To diagnose GI motility and to obtain gastric secretions for analysis
- To relieve and treat obstructions or bleeding within the GI tract
- To provide a means for nutrition (**gavage** feeding), hydration, and medication when the oral route is not possible or is contraindicated
- To promote healing after esophageal, gastric, or intestinal surgery by preventing distention of the GI tract and strain on the suture lines
- To remove toxic substances (**lavage**) that have been ingested either accidentally or intentionally and to provide for irrigation

Feeding tubes include esophagostomy, **gastrostomy,** or jejunostomy tubes (see Fig. 32.9) Nasogastric tubes are usually temporary and short term. Esophagostomy, gastrostomy, or jejunostomy tubes are generally used for longer term nutrition delivery.

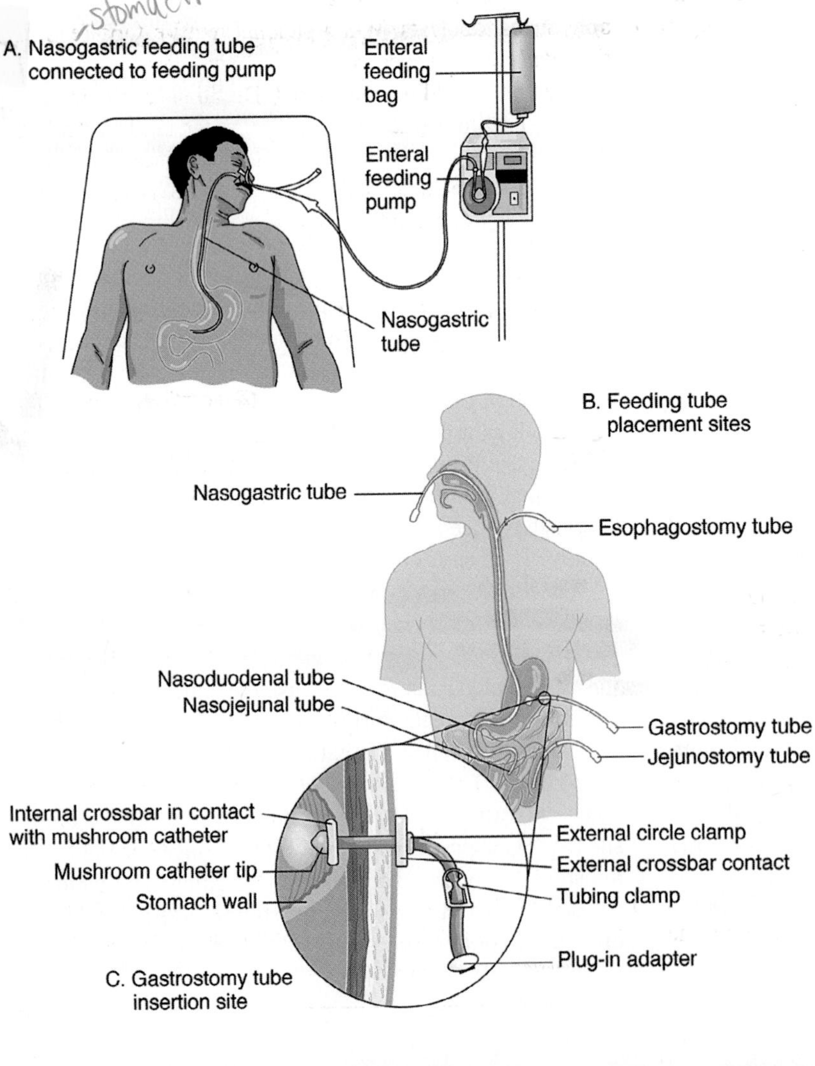

A. Nasogastric feeding tube connected to feeding pump

Enteral feeding bag

Enteral feeding pump

Nasogastric tube

B. Feeding tube placement sites

Nasogastric tube

Esophagostomy tube

Nasoduodenal tube
Nasojejunal tube

Gastrostomy tube
Jejunostomy tube

Internal crossbar in contact with mushroom catheter

External circle clamp

Mushroom catheter tip

External crossbar contact

Stomach wall

Tubing clamp

Plug-in adapter

C. Gastrostomy tube insertion site

FIGURE 32.9 Feeding tubes. *(A)* Nasogastric tube connected to tube feeding pump. *(B)* Feeding tube placement sites (esophagostomy, nasointestinal, gastrostomy, and jejunostomy). *(C)* Gastrostomy tube insertion site.

test 1

TABLE 32.9　GASTROINTESTINAL TUBES

Tube	Uses and Description	Nursing Considerations
	Gastric	
Levin Tube	Single lumen, may be used for gastric decompression, irrigations, lavages, and feedings.	Tube is not vented; avoid use with suction to prevent injury to stomach lining.
Salem Sump Tube	Double lumen, "pigtail" acts as an air vent and prevents excess suction, which could damage stomach lining. Air vent must not be plugged off. Used for decompression, irrigations, and lavage.	May be used with continuous suction because of air vent.
Weighted, Flexible Feeding Tubes with Stylets (Nutriflex, Keofeed)	Small-bore tubes for tubes for tube feedings only; less injury, remains in place for extended periods.	Suction collapses tube. Use a 10-mL syringe or greater, because smaller syringe creates too much pressure and possible rupture of tube.
	Intestinal	
Miller-Abbott Tube	Double-lumen tube used to drain and decompress the small intestine in cases of partial or complete obstruction; one lumen for aspiration, the other to inflate the balloon with mercury so that the tube is weighted and moves by gravity and peristalsis into the small intestine.	Rarely used, this tube is inserted by the physician or a specially trained nurse. Tube is not secured with tape, but passed through gauze taped to patient's forehead to allow tube to advance into intestines. Usually the tube advances 1–2 inches every 2 hours until it reaches small intestine; turning and ambulating the patient, if possible, facilitates tube's advancement.
Cantor Tube, Harris Tube	Single-lumen tubes with distal mercury-filled balloons and proximal drainage ports.	Precautions with mercury disposal.

Handwritten annotations: stomach; Intermittent; Need doctors order; Dobhoff; intestinal tube; make sure pills are powder-crushed; moves the tube down; walking + turning; Need x-ray to make sure its in the right spot leave Sy liss

See Box 32.6 Nursing Care for Insertion and Maintenance of Nasogastric Tubes. Provide emotional support and explanation to the patient and significant others to facilitate the process of tube insertion and maintenance. Assessing tube placement is essential to prevent complications or death from incorrect tube placement. Nasogastric tube placement must be assessed after insertion and then intermittently to ensure that it is in the correct position and not in the lungs (most common), esophagus, pleural space, or brain.

Gastrostomy or jejunostomy tube placement is verified by comparing current length with documented insertion length. The tube may not be in the desired position if the current and insertion tube lengths are different, so the physician should be consulted before using the tube.

Tube Feedings

A tube feeding supplies patients with nutrition when oral intake is not possible. Feedings can be given to the patient as a supplement or to provide the patient's total nutritional needs. If the esophagus and stomach need to be bypassed, tube feedings are delivered directly into the duodenum or proximal jejunum. Reasons for administering tube feedings include inability to swallow, severe burns or trauma to the face or jaw, debilitation, mental retardation, and oropharyngeal or esophageal paralysis. Complications associated with tube feedings are presented in Table 32.10.

Tube Feeding Formulas

Tube feeding formulas are chosen by the physician based on the patient's nutritional needs, the consistency of the formula, the size and location of the tube, the method of delivery, and the convenience for the patient at home. Com-

mercially prepared formulas are composed of protein, carbohydrates, and fats. When patients receive tube feedings, their daily water needs in addition to any water supplied by the feeding should be considered. Dietitians can help calculate the patient's water needs. The water used to flush the tube or administer medications can be considered as satisfying part of the patient's daily total water needs. Dehydration can occur if the patient's water needs are not met.

Method of Feeding Delivery

Feedings are administered either by gravity or by a controlled pump that delivers continuous volume through the

(Text continued on page 658)

CRITICAL THINKING

Mrs. Wood

■ Mrs. Wood is receiving a tube feeding because of dysphagia, the cause of which is being investigated. Mrs. Wood is not receiving any medications. You note that Mrs. Wood's tongue is bright red with deep furrows. She states her mouth is very dry. Her skin remains tented when skin turgor is checked.

1. What do Mrs. Wood's assessment findings indicate?
2. How would you document your assessment findings?
3. Why might Mrs. Wood be exhibiting this condition?
4. What actions could you take for this condition?
5. How would you record the total of Mrs. Wood's 8-hour intake which is tube feeding at 50 mL per hour?

Suggested answers at end of chapter.

Box 32.6

Nursing Care for Insertion and Maintenance of Nasogastric Tubes

1. Explain the procedure and reason for the tube to the patient. Inform the patient how he or she can help by swallowing when instructed to do so if able.
2. Assist patient into high Fowler's position (right side lying as an alternative) as able.
3. Measure tube for correct insertion length: Hold insertion end of tube from nose tip to earlobe to xyphoid process and mark tube with tape at this point.
4. Select naris that is straightest and from which patient breaths the easiest, because tube is inserted more easily in a straight naris.
5. Lubricate tube with water-soluble lubricant before insertion.
6. Insert tube as follows:
   - As tube is inserted, aim it along the floor of the naris and laterally. Rotate the tube gently if resistance is met.
   - Encourage patient to swallow to advance the tube. Drinking water with a straw or ice chips facilitates the swallowing process if patient is able.
   - If patient is unconscious, flex patient's head to bring chin toward chest to help prevent tube from passing into the trachea.
   - Observe for coiling of the tube in patient's mouth.
   - To assist in assessing correct placement, insert tube to level of carina tracheae and listen for air at end of tube. If air is present, remove tube. If no air is heard, advance tube to stomach.
   - If at any time the patient begins to cough uncontrollably, becomes cyanotic, or begins to experience any respiratory distress, remove the tube, allow rest time, and then reattempt insertion.
7. After tube is inserted to premeasured length, confirm gastric placement per institutional policy using the following methods[1]:
   - Flexible feeding tubes should have x-ray confirmation.
   - Aspirate for gastric contents with a 30- or 60-mL catheter-tipped syringe:
   - Gastric fluid—green with sediment; colorless and clear with off-white or tan mucus; brown if digested blood is present.
   - Esophageal contents—scant fluid, aspirate is unreliable for confirmation.
   - Intestinal fluid—light to dark golden yellow to brownish green.
   - Respiratory secretions—off-white or tan mucus.

- Pleural fluid (with stylet perforation)—watery, straw colored, may be blood-tinged from perforation.
- Measure pH of secretions obtained to rule out respiratory placement:
  - Gastric pH range is acidic (1–5).
  - Respiratory and intestinal secretions are alkaline with pH >6.
- If any doubts about gastric placement exist, notify physician for x-ray order to confirm tube placement.
8. Secure tube in place with tape so that pressure is not put on the naris. Provide daily skin care to taped area to prevent skin breakdown. Slipknot a rubber band around tube and pin rubber band to patient's gown.
9. If suction is ordered, low intermittent suction is used with nonvented tubes (Levin); vented tubes (Salem) may have continuous low suction.
10. If patient is NPO, provide frequent care to keep oral mucous membranes moist. When suction is used, prevent excessive intake of ice chips, if ordered, because electrolyte imbalances may result when the water is suctioned out along with electrolytes. Normal saline instead of water can be made into ice chips to help prevent imbalances.
11. Gastric placement is periodically confirmed, especially before instilling anything into the tube[1]:
    - Review any recent chest or abdominal x-ray report with tube status.
    - Verify tube position marking is in original position. If not, reposition as necessary.
    - Bolus feedings/medications: 4 hours after last feeding, aspirate fluid for pH and appearance.
    - Continuous feedings: Note tolerance. If normal along with correct tube marking and any confirming x-ray reports, continue feeding.
    - For patients at high risk of dislodgement (e.g., those who are vomiting or have severe coughing) with tube movement, consider x-ray examination.
12. The tube is flushed at intervals, every 2–4 hours, to maintain patency. When tube feedings are administered, residual feeding amounts are checked at specified intervals (hourly when begun, every 4 hours thereafter) to ensure the feeding is being absorbed.
13. After tube placement, record accurate intake and output, including drainage, vomitus, and irrigation solution instilled (use only normal saline to prevent electrolyte imbalance).

TABLE 32.10 COMMON MECHANICAL, GASTROINTESTINAL AND METABOLIC COMPLICATIONS OF TUBE-FED PATIENTS AND PREVENTION STRATEGIES

Complication	Prevention Strategies
Mechanical	
Tube Irritation	Consider oral tubes and avoid nasal tubes due to sinus infection risk. Oral tubes also help prevent ventilator associated pneumonia.
	Consider using a smaller or softer tube.
	Lubricate the tube before insertion.
	Ensure tube is secured in place.
Tube Obstruction	Flush tube after use.
	Do not mix medications with the tube feeding formula.
	Use liquid medications if available.
	Crush other medications thoroughly (if not contraindicated to crush).
	Use an infusion pump to maintain a constant flow (see Fig. 32.9)
Aspiration and Regurgitation	Feeding should not be started until tube placement is radiographically confirmed.
	Avoid use of blue dye to detect aspiration as it has not been demonstrated to be predictive and the dye can be absorbed in critically ill patients, who then turn blue and can die.
	Elevate head of the patient's bed more than or equal to 30 degrees at all times.
	Discontinue feedings at least 30–60 minutes before treatments requiring head to be lowered (e.g., chest percussion).
	If the patient has an endotracheal tube in place, keep the cuff inflated during feedings.
	Test pH of aspirate with pH paper or meter.
	a. pH of tracheobronchial secretions is alkaline, >7.4.
	b. pH of gastric secretions is acidic, <5.0.
	c. As the tube moves from the acid stomach to the alkaline duodenum, pH will change from acid to alkaline.
	Place a black mark at the point where the tube, when properly placed, exits the nostril.
Tube Displacement	Replace tube and obtain physician's order to confirm with x-ray imaging.
Gastrointestinal	
*Cramping, distention, bloating, gas pains, nausea, vomiting, diarrhea**	Practice good personal hygiene when handling any feeding product.
	Bring formula to room temperature before feeding.
	Initiate and increase amount of formula gradually.
	Change to a lactose-free formula.
	Decrease fat content of formula.
	Adminster drug therapy as ordered (e.g., Lactinex, kaolin-pectin, Lomotil).
	Change to formula with a lower osmolality.
	Change to formula with a different fiber content.
	Evaluate diarrhea-causing medications the patient may be receiving (e.g., antibiotics, digitalis preparations).
Metabolic	
Dehydration	Note the patient's fluid requirements before treatment.
	Monitor hydration status.
	Provide adequate daily water.
Overhydration	Note the patient's fluid requirements before treatment.
	Monitor hydration status.
Hyperglycemia	Initiate feedings at a low rate.
	Monitor blood glucose.
	Use hyperglycemic medication if necessary.
	Select a low-carbohydrate formula.
Hypernatremia	Note the patient's fluid and electrolyte status before treatment.
	Provide adequate fluids.
Hyponatremia	Note the patient's fluid and electrolyte status before treatment.
	Restrict fluids.
	Supplement feeding with rehydration solution and saline.
	Diuretic therapy may be beneficial.
Hypophosphatemia	Monitor serum levels.
	Replenish phosphorus levels before refeeding.
Hypercapnia	Select a low-carbohydrate, high-fat formula.
Hypokalemia	Monitor potassium levels.
	Supplement feeding with potassium if necessary.
Hyperkalemia	Reduce potassium intake.
	Monitor potassium levels.

* The most commonly cited complication of tube feeding is diarrhea.

Modified from Lutz, CA, and Przytulski, KR: Nutritional and Diet Therapy, ed 4. F.A. Davis, Philadelphia, 2006. Reprinted with permission.

[Handwritten margin notes at top: "Important to check Accu: for sugar / 24-Hr. Bag", "temporarily", "test 1 / white solution"]

feeding tube. Gravity feedings are placed above the level of the stomach and dripped in by gravity slowly or given as a bolus feeding over a few minutes. Intermittent feedings are defined as either being delivered by a pump that runs continuously throughout the day and is discontinued each night or as a 4- to 6-hour volume of feeding given over 20 to 30 minutes. Intermittent feedings via a pump allow the stomach to rest at night and more closely simulate normal eating and nutrient absorption patterns. A continuous feeding administered 24 hours a day through a pump allows for small amounts to be given over a long period. Pumps are set at the specified rate to control the speed of the feeding being delivered to the patient.

When feedings are administered, patients must be positioned in a sitting or high-Fowler's position to reduce the risk of aspiration. Monitor the rate carefully to avoid administering feedings too rapidly, and watch for signs that the feeding is not being absorbed. Abdominal distention, patient report of a feeling of fullness, and nausea or vomiting are indicators that the feeding is not being absorbed and should be stopped to prevent aspiration. A residual check to see how much feeding, if any, has not been absorbed is done hourly when the feeding is initiated, then every 4 hours or before giving any medications or adding more feeding for infusion. If there is more than 100 mL or the amount specified by the agency or physician, the feeding should be stopped to prevent vomiting or aspiration and the physician notified. Continuous or intermittent feedings reduce the risk of aspiration, distention, nausea, vomiting, and diarrhea.

If medications are administered during tube feedings, understand possible drug-nutrient interactions. Some medications cannot be given with certain substances. Other medications, such as enteric-coated or sustained-release medications, should not be crushed. Liquid medications should be used when possible to reduce clogging of the tube. Pharmacists and dietitians should be consulted for special considerations.

Gastrointestinal Decompression

Gastrointestinal decompression may be necessary when the stomach or small intestine becomes filled with air or fluid. Swallowed air and GI secretions enter the stomach and intestines and collect there if they are not propelled through the GI tract by peristalsis. Accumulating air or fluid causes distention, a feeling of fullness, and possibly pain in the abdomen. Gastric distention may occur after major abdominal surgery. Ambulating or turning the patient frequently can help prevent this. However, when GI decompression is necessary, a nasogastric tube or occasionally a nasointestinal tube may be inserted and suction applied. Nasointestinal tubes are more difficult and slower to place and may be uncomfortable, so they are not used often. The tube remains in place until full peristaltic activity (active bowel sounds and passage of flatus) has returned. The diet is then progressed as ordered and tolerated by the patient.

Total Parenteral Nutrition

Total parenteral nutrition (TPN; also known as intravenous hyperalimentation) is a method of supplying nutrients to the patient by an intravenous (IV) route. TPN solutions usually contain dextrose (sugar), amino acids (protein), vitamins, minerals, and fat (intralipid) emulsions. TPN solutions are designed to improve the patient's nutritional status, achieve weight gain, and enhance the healing process. The patient with conditions such as burns, trauma, cancer, acquired immunodeficiency syndrome (AIDS), malnutrition, anorexia nervosa, or fever and those undergoing major surgery may need TPN. *[handwritten: all based on Labs]*

Usually, registered nurses are responsible for administering TPN. A filter must be used with TPN solutions but not with lipid solutions, which are given as a separate infusion along with TPN therapy. TPN is started slowly to give the pancreas time to adjust to increasing insulin production for the high amounts of glucose in the TPN. The TPN rate is increased until the ordered rate, as tolerated by the patient, is reached. When TPN is discontinued, the patient must be gradually weaned to allow the pancreas to adjust to decreasing glucose levels. The patient, as ordered, is fed before the TPN is stopped to help prevent hypoglycemia. Signs of hypoglycemia include weakness, shakiness, sweating, and confusion.

It is important to monitor glucose levels as ordered and to look for signs of hyperglycemia in the patient receiving TPN. Refer to agency policy for obtaining glucose levels when a hyperglycemic reaction is suspected in the patient receiving TPN.

During TPN administration, the following laboratory values, as ordered, are usually monitored:

- Complete blood cell count (CBC)
- Albumin
- Glucose
- Electrolytes
- Platelet count
- Prothrombin time (PT)

TPN can be irritating to the peripheral veins because it is five or six times more concentrated than blood. Therefore, TPN dextrose more than 12% is administered through a central venous catheter into a large vein such as the subclavian or internal jugular (see Fig. 6.8). The volume in the large vein dilutes the TPN solution, so it is less irritating. *[handwritten: You must be weaned off TPN / slow the rate down]*

Peripheral Parenteral Nutrition

Peripheral parenteral nutrition (PPN) is a method of supplying nutrients to the patient by an IV route that is not a central vein. PPN is used for less than 10 days when the patient does not need more than 2000 calories daily. PPN solutions can contain a mixture of dextrose (of less than 12%), amino acids, and lipids, in addition to electrolytes or water, which can be found in routine IV solutions. The all-in-one PPN system mixes dextrose, amino acids, and lipids all in one container, which causes less irritation of veins.

NURSING CARE TIP

Patients with any of the following may need to be considered for TPN or PPN:

- Any significant weight loss (10% or more of healthy weight)
- A decrease of oral food intake for more than 3 days
- Any significant sign of protein loss: serum albumin levels below 3.2 g/dL
- Muscle wasting
- Decreased tissue healing
- Persistent vomiting and diarrhea

LEARNING TIP

- Patients may respond to TPN with an elevated serum glucose level, even though they do not have diabetes. This is due to the high concentration of glucose used in TPN. These elevated serum glucose levels do not usually indicate that the patient who does not have diabetes has acquired the disease. After the TPN is discontinued, the serum glucose levels should return to baseline or normal levels.
- Regular insulin is given, as ordered, to control hyperglycemia during TPN therapy. The insulin is ordered on a sliding scale (regular insulin given based on blood glucose levels measured at ordered intervals over 24 hours) or as an additive to the TPN solution, or both.
- Administration of insulin according to a sliding scale requires a current blood glucose level. Based on the obtained glucose level, if it is elevated, specified regular insulin units may be ordered. Usually blood glucose is measured before meals, but for a patient who is not eating, as with most patients receiving TPN, there is no meal time. Instead, specified time intervals are ordered (typically every 6 hours).
- Insulin given on a sliding scale is always regular insulin. Can you figure out why? Regular insulin is rapid acting, which is what is needed to treat the current blood glucose level that was obtained to determine what insulin coverage was needed, if any.

Home Health Hints

- Be familiar with community nutritional support services: Women, Infant's, and Children (WIC) program, elderly nutrition sites, Meals on Wheels, school food programs, and government surplus food programs.
- Observe patient's food preparation facilities to ensure the patient's nutritional needs can be met. Some older patients may have outdated or spoiled food in their refrigerators or cupboards because they are unable to see dates or mold growing on foods.
- Ensure that patients are able to use appliances to heat food safely. Patients with limited vision may not see gas flames and can ignite their clothing. Confused patients might try to heat foods in the cardboard containers. If the patient is able to obtain and learn to use a microwave, it may be a safer cooking appliance.
- A feeding tube can be prevented from kinking by slipping a split straw lengthwise around the area that tends to kink and lightly taping over the split in the straw.
- Wire coat hangers make good hooks for enteral feeding solutions bags. They can be bent and hung over doorways or closet bars.
- If a 60-mL feeding syringe is not available for a bolus tube feeding or tube flushing, a measuring cup and funnel can be used.

REVIEW QUESTIONS

1. The nurse is collecting data on a patient with a ruptured appendix that is painful. Where would the nurse expect the patient's pain to be located?
   a. Right upper quadrant
   b. Right lower quadrant
   c. Left upper quadrant
   d. Left lower quadrant

2. Which of the following is a function of the liver?
   a. Synthesis of plasma proteins
   b. Elimination of carbohydrates
   c. Concentration of bile
   d. Secretion of cholecystokinin

3. The nurse is planning care for a 78-year-old patient's elimination needs. Which of the following interventions should the nurse plan to reduce complications from the aging change of slowed motility?
   a. Decrease ambulation.
   b. Increase dietary fiber.
   c. Increase dairy products.
   d. Decrease fluid intake.

4. The nurse is assessing a patient's bowel sounds. The nurse understands that bowel sounds heard at an irregular rate every 5 to 15 seconds should be documented as which of the following?
   a. Abnormal
   b. Hyperactive
   c. Hypoactive
   d. Normal

5. Which of the following best describes the technique of palpation?
   a. Firmly place the hands on the abdomen, depressing the tissues 1-2 inches.
   b. Lightly depress the abdomen 1/2 to 1 inch.
   c. Randomly feel the patient's abdomen with fingertips.
   d. Light palpation should be completed only by an experienced practitioner.

6. Which of the following nursing measures is most important after an upper or lower GI series?
   a. Offer a laxative as ordered.
   b. Encourage fluids.
   c. Check for return of a gag reflex.
   d. Keep the patient in semi-Fowler's position.

Multiple response item. Select all that apply.
7. A patient is admitted with an order for a Sump tube (Salem sump). The nurse knows this tube is used for :
   a. Supplemental feeding
   b. Decompression
   c. Irrigation
   d. Lavage
   e. Gavage

8. A patient has had a flexible feeding tube inserted. Which of the following should be done to confirm placement?
   a. Aspirate gastric contents for green colored fluid.
   b. Measure the pH of secretions from tube.
   c. Obtain x-ray to check placement.
   d. Look in the back of the mouth to ensure tube has not coiled in the throat.

9. The nurse is caring for a patient who is receiving a TPN infusion. Blood glucose monitoring every 6 hours is ordered to detect which of the following complications?
   a. Hyponatremia
   b. Hyperglycemia
   c. Hypocalcemia
   d. Hyperkalemia

SUGGESTED ANSWERS TO

CRITICAL THINKING

■ Mrs. Todd

1. Daily aspirin use is the most likely cause of her bleeding.
2. Medication teaching including side effects can help Mrs. Todd prevent future bleeding episodes. Assessment of pain relief needs and consultation with the physician will also help.

■ Mrs. Pearl

Mrs. Pearl is at risk for dehydration and electrolyte loss as a result of the laxative and enema preparation and NPO status. This risk is increased because of her age. Her fluid and electrolyte status should be monitored closely.

Mrs. Pearl will likely have a concern about "making it" to the bathroom during the preparation and should have a bedside commode placed within easy reach. Her call light should be answered promptly. If enemas are ordered "until clear," Mrs. Pearl will be at greater risk for fluid and electrolyte loss. If more than two or three enemas are required, the physician should be notified.

Elderly patients can become very fatigued during testing and test preparation. Mrs. Pearl should be allowed plenty of rest before and after the test. She may also have a concern about being able to hold the barium in her bowel during the test without having an "accident." She should be assured that the barium is held in with a balloon on the end of the enema catheter and that bathrooms are nearby.

■ Mr. Wozynski

You can expect to find that Mr. Wozynski's serum bilirubin is elevated because his liver is unable to convert or conjugate bilirubin into a water-soluble compound that can be eliminated in feces. Mr. Wozynski is at risk for bleeding because the liver is highly vascular and prone to bleed when a biopsy specimen is taken. In addition, he may not be manufacturing the necessary amount of prothrombin needed for blood clotting and is less likely to stop bleeding once the biopsy has been performed. It will be especially important to check his coagulation studies and report any elevations to the physician before the biopsy.

■ *Mrs. Wood*

1. Assessment of Mrs. Wood indicates dehydration.
2. Document as follows: "1/20/06 0800 'Mouth very dry.' Tongue bright red with deep furrows, tented turgor. Tube feeding infusing (include solution and rate). Physician notified. K. Ohno LVN."
3. Mrs. Wood's daily water needs are not being met. She is not receiving medications that would incidentally provide water during their administration.
4. Consult a dietitian and/or physician to review Mrs. Wood's daily water needs. Divide the water needs over 24 hours and ensure that water is administered. Ensure tubing is flushed per agency policy, and calculate water used toward daily water needs. Monitor intake and output. Continue assessing Mrs. Wood's signs and symptoms, and report abnormal findings.
5. 50 mL × 8 hours = 400 mL

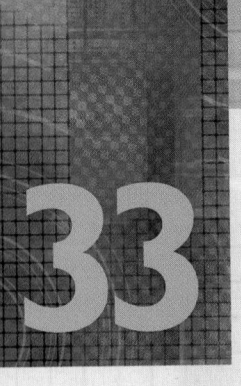

Nursing Care of Patients with Upper Gastrointestinal Disorders

LAZETTE V. NOWICKI

KEY TERMS

anorexia (AN-oh-REK-see-ah)
anorexia nervosa (AN-oh-REK-see-ah ner-VOH-sah)
aphthous stomatitis (AF-thus STOH-mah-TIGH-tis)
bariatric (BAR-ry-AT-rick)
bulimia nervosa (byoo-LEE-mee-ah ner-VOH-sah)
gastrectomy (gas-TREK-tuh-mee)
gastritis (gas-TRY-tis)
gastroduodenostomy (GAS-troh-DOO-oh-den-AHS-toh-mee)
gastrojejunostomy (GAS-troh-JAY-joo-NAHS-toh-mee)
gastroplasty (GAS-troh-PLAS-tee)
Helicobacter pylori (HEH-lick-co-back-tur PIE-lori)
hiatal hernia (high-AY-tuhl HER-nee-ah)
obesity (oh-BEE-si-tee)
peptic ulcer disease (PEP-tick UL-sir di-ZEEZ)
roux-en-Y (roo-ehn-WHY)
steatorrhea (STEE-ah-toh-REE-ah)
stomatitis (STOH-mah-TIGH-tis)

QUESTIONS TO GUIDE YOUR READING

1. What are anorexia, anorexia nervosa, and bulimia nervosa and their therapeutic interventions and nursing care?

2. What is obesity, and what medical, surgical, and nursing management is used to treat it?

3. What nursing care would you give to a patient with stomatitis?

4. How would you care for patients with acute or chronic gastritis?

5. How would you explain the pathophysiology, signs and symptoms, and diagnostic testing for hiatal hernia, peptic ulcer disease, gastric bleeding, and gastric cancer?

6. Describe current pharmacological treatments for peptic ulcer disease?

7. What nursing care would you provide for patients with hiatal hernia, peptic ulcer disease, gastric bleeding, and gastric cancer?

NAUSEA AND VOMITING

Nausea is the subjective feeling of the urge to vomit. Vomiting is the act of expelling stomach contents from the body through the esophagus and mouth. Nausea and vomiting are common occurrences that most people experience at some time. Vomiting is a protective function to rid the body of harmful substances from the gastrointestinal (GI) tract. This reflex is controlled by the vomiting center of the brain. It is a complex process. Many stimuli and conditions that are directly related to the GI tract or independent of it can trigger nausea and vomiting. Viral GI infection and other infections, motion sickness, stress, pregnancy, medications (narcotics), myocardial infarction, uremia, and other conditions may cause nausea and vomiting.

Therapeutic Interventions

Nausea and vomiting may be self-limited and require no intervention. If it is prolonged, however, dehydration and electrolyte imbalances may occur. The loss of hydrochloric acid from the stomach can result in metabolic alkalosis. "Coffee grounds"–appearing emesis (dark brown) occurs from bleeding in the stomach.

Protection of the airway during vomiting is a priority to prevent aspiration. Those at risk of aspiration are persons who are unconscious, older, and experiencing gag reflex impairments. Place these types of persons on their side when they begin to vomit. This allows the gastric contents to be expelled from the mouth rather than pooling at the back of the throat and being aspirated.

If the cause of vomiting is known, it is treated. Various medications can be given to control the nausea and vomiting (e.g., diphenhydramine [Benadryl], hydroxyzine [Vistaril], metoclopramide [Reglan], promethazine [Phenergan], prochlorperazine [Compazine], ondansetron [Zofran], scopolamine [TransdermScop], thiethylperazine [Torecan], trimethobenzamide [Tigan]). For severe or prolonged vomiting, IV fluids and possibly nutrition need to be provided. A nasogastric (NG) tube with suction may be ordered to decompress the stomach. After the vomiting is resolved, clear liquids are started, with water being preferred. If liquids are tolerated, crackers or dry toast may be tolerated as well.

Nursing Process for the Patient with Nausea and Vomiting

Assessment/Data Collection

The nurse identifies characteristics of the episodes of the nausea and vomiting. Medical conditions, medications, and treatments are documented to aid in diagnosing the cause. Signs of early fluid deficit, such as weakness, headache, muscle cramps, restlessness, inability to concentrate, and postural hypotension, are noted and reported for treatment. Late signs include confusion, oliguria, cold clammy skin, and chest or abdominal pain.

Nursing Diagnoses, Planning, and Implementation

Nausea related to various causes

EXPECTED OUTCOME: *Patient will report no nausea.*

- Provide quiet, odor-free, visually clean environment *to avoid triggering stimuli.*
- Give antiemetics as ordered.
- Provide frequent oral care *to remove emesis taste and enhance patient comfort.*
- Explain to patient to avoid triggering fluids or foods to prevent nausea and vomiting.

Risk for aspiration related to decreased gag reflex or unconsciousness

EXPECTED OUTCOME: *Patient's airway and lung sounds will remain clear.*

- Identify patients who are nauseated and are at risk of aspiration *to plan preventive care.*
- Place patient on side if nauseated and vomiting *to protect airway.*

Deficient fluid volume

EXPECTED OUTCOME: *Patient's vital signs will remain within normal limits.*

- Monitor for early signs of hypovolemia in patient with vomiting *to allow treatment and prevent complications.*
- Obtain daily weight on same scale, at same time of day, with same type of clothing *to detect fluid losses. A 1 lb weight loss reflects a fluid loss of 500 mL.*
- Monitor intake and output and vital signs including orthostatic blood pressure per shift or daily or more frequently as patient's condition indicates *to report changes for prompt treatment.*
- Provide fluids as ordered *to hydrate patient. IV fluids may to be used to allow the GI tract to rest. Slightly chilled oral replacement solutions may be used such as sports replacement drinks or ginger ale given in small frequent amounts.*
- Monitor older adults for excess fluid volume during treatment of deficient fluid volume *to prevent and detect fluid overload, which may occur quickly in the older adult.*

Evaluation

The patient's goals are met if nausea is not present, lung sounds remain clear, and vital signs remain within normal limits.

EATING DISORDERS

Anorexia

Anorexia, which is a lack of appetite, is a common symptom of many diseases and can be caused by noxious food odors, certain drugs (as an intended or side effect), emotional stress, fear, psychological problems, and infections. Prolonged anorexia with an inadequate nutritional intake can lead to serious electrolyte imbalances, which in turn can lead to cardiac dysrhythmias. Although eating is the preferred method of weight gain, other measures such as tube feedings and intravenous infusion can be used. Ask patients what causes them to lose their appetite and what improves it to plan care. Nursing actions for the patient with anorexia include documenting accurate intake and output; monitoring vital signs, electrolytes, and electrocardiograms; and monitoring the rate of the intravenous infusion and tube feeding.

Anorexia Nervosa

Anorexia nervosa is an eating disorder that is recognized by the American Psychiatric Association (Box 33.1 Diagnostic Criteria for Anorexia Nervosa). This disease most commonly occurs in females between the ages of 12 and 18 who are from the middle and upper classes of Western culture. Males account for less than 10% of the population with anorexia nervosa. Young women with low self-esteem seem to be at highest risk. Anorexia nervosa is thought to be psychological in origin. Patients may have a phobia of weight gain, are afraid of a loss of control, and are mistrusting.

Signs and Symptoms

Early signs and symptoms of anorexia nervosa include severe weight loss, low self-esteem, compulsive dieting, and an altered body image (patients imagine themselves as fat, although they are within or below normal weight range). As the disease progresses, additional symptoms appear, including amenorrhea in females, electrolyte imbalance, cardiac dysrhythmias, constipation, dry skin, lanugo (downy hair covering body), bradycardia, hypothermia, hypotension, muscle wasting, and facial puffiness. Often patients with anorexia nervosa deny the existence of any problem. They may develop bizarre food rituals and sometimes weigh themselves several times a day. Anorexia nervosa sometimes overlaps with **bulimia nervosa** (compulsive eating with self-induced vomiting).

Box 33.1

Diagnostic Criteria for Anorexia Nervosa

1. Refusal to maintain body weight over a minimum normal weight for age and height
2. Intense fear of gaining weight or becoming fat, even though underweight
3. Disturbance in the way in which one's body weight, shape, or size is experienced
4. In females, the absence of at least three consecutive menstrual cycles when otherwise expected to occur

Therapeutic Interventions

Treating this disorder is complex and requires a multidisciplinary approach. Patients often do not see the need for medical intervention. They do not usually seek help on their own and are often resistant to treatment. When treatment is sought, often through a concerned person's urgings, a medical and psychological workup is necessary. Nutritional status is also evaluated to determine the urgency of intervention. Establishing a trusting relationship, which can be difficult, is a key element in initiating treatment. Early treatment results in a better prognosis.

Often the most important initial intervention for anorexia nervosa is the restoration of nutritional health; up to 18% of anorexia patients eventually die as a result of starvation and complications from it. For those who are underweight with severe weight loss, life-threatening electrolyte imbalances and dysrhythmias or other symptoms, nutrition is supplied by intravenous infusions containing electrolytes. Oral food supplements may also need to be given. Restoring normal weight is a long, slow process. Gains may be small with setbacks along the way. Praise and rewards for small achievements in weight gains (not food intake) are positive reinforcements that aid recovery. Programs that treat eating disorders are often set up on a reward system, with privileges being increased as progress occurs.

The patient's damaged self-image and self-esteem are underlying causes of the disorder that must be addressed in conjunction with the nutritional aspect (Box 33.2 Nutrition Notes). Psychotherapy and behavior modification that includes participation of the patient's significant others are included in treatment of anorexia nervosa. The altered body image is the main focus of therapy. Educating the patient on normal body weight can be helpful. Individual or group therapy is used. Family counseling may be used since childhood events often create the negative self-image. During treatment, a support system is vital to success.

Complications

Chronic poor nutritional health takes its toll on the body. Complications from starvation occur as the body tries to conserve energy. Pulse and blood pressure fall. Heart and kidney failure are a risk. Osteoporosis and muscle loss occur. Vitamin and electrolyte imbalances result. Diabetes may develop with a high morbidity.

Bulimia Nervosa

Bulimia nervosa is compulsive eating with self-induced vomiting, which is commonly known as binge-purge. A high percentage of patients with bulimia are young women.

The bulimic patient typically eats massive amounts of food at one sitting and then purges the food by intentionally inducing vomiting so weight is not gained. Laxatives are also sometimes used by the bulimic patient to purge the body of food to avoid weight gain. Excessive exercise may also be used to control weight.

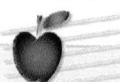

Box 33.2

Nutrition Notes

Supplying Nutrition in Upper Gastrointestinal Conditions

Anorexia Nervosa and Bulimia Nervosa

These eating disorders, which produce severe weight loss, require multidisciplinary treatment. Although correcting the nutritional consequences of these conditions is of major importance, to achieve a cure it is essential to treat the underlying psychological causes.

Obesity

Candidates for gastric banding or gastric bypass surgery should be carefully selected. The procedure should be viewed as one tool to assist with weight control, along with behavioral changes. It is not done to permit overeating because in time the constructed pouch can be stretched, thus negating the surgery. Guidelines include eating three to six small balanced meals daily, chewing thoroughly and eating slowly, drinking most fluids between meals, exercising regularly, and taking a multivitamin-multimineral supplement. Potential complications of these surgeries include nausea, vomiting, bloating, heartburn, staple disruption, obstruction, dumping syndrome, and osteoporosis.

Gastroesophageal Reflux and Hiatal Hernia

Patients with gastroesophageal reflux and hiatal hernia may find symptoms alleviated by protein foods that tighten the cardiac sphincter so normal amounts of dietary protein are suggested. Substances that may be better avoided because they relax the sphincter include fat, caffeine, peppermint, spearmint, chocolate, alcohol, and nicotine. Pepper and decaffeinated coffee may be problematic because they stimulate gastric secretions. Acidic juices may be irritating as well.

Postprandial Hypotension

This refers to a drop in systolic blood pressure of 20 mm Hg or more within 75 to 120 minutes after the beginning of a meal, most often resulting in dizziness and fatigue but also weakness, light-headedness, disturbed speech, and vision changes. Normally the body compensates for the increased blood flow to the digestive tract following meals, but in the elderly, the mechanisms maintaining adequate circulation to the rest of the body become less effective. Most at risk are people with neurological, cardiovascular, or renal diseases. Complications include higher incidence of coronary events, stroke, and total mortality. To prevent postprandial hypotension, a person should limit carbohydrate intake and take frequent small meals. Special additives to delay gastric emptying are sometimes prescribed. Lying in a semirecumbent position for 90 minutes after eating and avoiding excessive exercise for 2 hours after meals can help to manage the condition. Scheduling of antihypertensive medications between rather than just before meals also can be helpful.

Dumping Syndrome

The recommended meal pattern for patients with dumping syndrome includes six small meals per day, high in protein and low in simple sugars; fluids between rather than with meals; and reclining for half an hour after meals. Supplementation with the vitamins B_{12} and D, folic acid, and the minerals calcium and iron may be necessary to prevent deficiencies.

Gastric Cancer

If a patient has a poor prognosis following a total gastrectomy for cancer, dietary interventions should focus on symptoms the patient wishes to control. An overly restricted diet causing the patient discomfort or distress is inappropriate.

Source: Malozemoff, W, and Gentlemen, B: When dinner's done—postprandial hypotension in older adults. Nurs Spect Midwest 5:18, 2004.

Signs and Symptoms

Patients with bulimia nervosa exhibit many of the same signs and symptoms as patients with anorexia nervosa, with a few exceptions. Bulimic patients often have enamel erosion of the front teeth and staining caused by the acid content of the emesis. They also spend a great deal of time locked in the bathroom vomiting, especially after meals. Electrolyte imbalances occur from dehydration. The loss of potassium and sodium may result in dysrhythmias, heart failure, and death. As the electrolyte imbalance worsens, metabolic alkalosis develops as a result of the loss of gastric acid in the stomach contents. Signs and symptoms of metabolic alkalosis include hypokalemia and hypocalcemia. Laxative use results in irregular bowel movements.

Therapeutic Interventions

The treatment for bulimia nervosa is essentially the same as for the patient with anorexia nervosa.

Nursing Process for the Patient with an Eating Disorder

Caring for patients with eating disorders is challenging. Gaining the patient's genuine cooperation by using therapeutic communication and setting realistic, mutual goals is important in establishing trust and preventing relapse. To work with patients with an eating disorder, a therapeutic relationship must be developed to facilitate effective interactions. Empathy, acceptance of the patient, trust, warmth, and being nonjudgmental are important.

Assessment/Data Collection

Collect data related to inadequate nutrition. Note changes in weight (15% or more below expected weight), poor skin turgor, poor muscle tone, lanugo, amenorrhea, electrolyte imbalances, and hypothermia. Data collection findings may also include a normal weight, enamel erosion of front teeth, and metabolic alkalosis for the patient with bulimia. Note abnormal diagnostic studies such as anemia, electrolyte imbalances, altered endocrine studies, and electrocardiographic (ECG) changes.

Nursing Diagnosis, Planning, and Implementation

Imbalanced nutrition: less than body requirements related to inadequate food intake, self-induced vomiting, and/or chronic/excessive laxative use

EXPECTED OUTCOME: *Establish dietary pattern and weight gain toward desired individual weight range.*

- Monitor patient's weight *to determine baseline and monitor patient's progress toward goal.*
- Monitor vital signs and laboratory studies *to detect changes in cardiac function related to electrolyte imbalances.*
- Promote consistent approach *to enhance acceptance of patient and to build trust.*
- Promote pleasant eating environment and record intake *to enhance patient intake.*
- Provide six smaller meals and snacks *to prevent gastric dilation.*

Body image, disturbed related to psychosocial or cognitive/perceptual changes

EXPECTED OUTCOME: *The patient verbalizes satisfaction with body appearance.*

- Assess and document patient's verbal and nonverbal responses to own body *to provide baseline understanding of patient's perceptions of body image.*
- Listen to patient and acknowledge reality of concerns regarding treatment and progress *to establish therapeutic relationship.*
- Monitor frequency of negative statements about self *to determine if interventions are helping patient.*
- Assist with referrals to social services or counseling *to help patient overcome psychosocial issues.*
- Provide care in a nonjudgmental manner *to maintain the patient's dignity.*
- Use positive praise when patient verbalizes positive comments about own body.
- Encourage patient to verbalize consequences of eating disorder that have influenced self-concept *to help patient realize the negative impact of the eating disorder.*

Evaluation

The patient's goals are met if the patient gains weight toward expected weight goal and the patient verbalizes satisfaction with body appearance and increases the number of positive statements about own appearance.

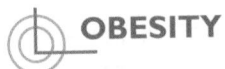 OBESITY

Several methods can be used to diagnose a patient as overweight or obese, although there is no one definitive measure of either. Factors such as age, body frame size, and gender can influence these measurements:

- Height-weight chart: Weight 10% to 20% above ideal body weight is overweight; 20% or more above ideal body weight is **obesity.**
- Waist-to-hip ratio: Waist-to-hip ratio is waist measurement divided by hip measurement. If the result is more than 1.0 in men or 0.8 in women, it indicates that the patient is overweight.
- Body mass index (BMI): BMI is one of the best methods for defining obesity. BMI increases with age. Generally, a BMI of 25 to 29.9 kg/m^2 is defined as being overweight, with more than 30 kg/m^2 being obese (Fig. 33.1). BMI can be calculated using height-to-weight ratios:

$$BMI = Weight\ (kg)/Height\ (m^2)$$
Example: BMI = 68 kg/1.67 m^2 = 68 kg/2.7889 m^2 = 24.38 kg\m^2

Obesity is caused by a caloric intake that exceeds energy expenditure. Only a small percentage of obesity is associated with a metabolic or endocrine abnormality within the body. Heath risks can result from being overweight. Diseases that are associated with obesity are called comorbidites. Comorbidites include, but are not limited to, atherosclerosis, heart disease, diabetes mellitus, hypertension, sleep apnea, osteoarthritis, decreased mobility, lack of self-esteem, and depression. Obesity that interferes with activities of daily living, such as breathing or walking, is known as morbid obesity. Morbid obesity refers to people whose BMI is above 40, which is about 100 lb overweight for men and about 80 lb overweight for women. Surgery can be an option for people whose BMI is above 40 or for people whose BMI is between 35 and 40 and who have life-threatening obesity-related diseases such as severe sleep apnea or heart disease. For more information, go to the National Heart, Lung, and Blood Institute website at www.nhlbisupport.com/bmi, The American Obesity Association at www.obesity.org, or The North American Association for the Study of Obesity at www.naaso.org. For information about surgery, finding a surgeon, chat rooms, and more, visit www.obesityhelp.com.

Persons who are overweight are at risk for developing other diseases. These can include hypertension, type 2 diabetes, heart disease, degenerative joint disease, sleep apnea, and gallbladder disease. When combined with a high-fat diet, there is also an increased risk of breast, colon, rectum,

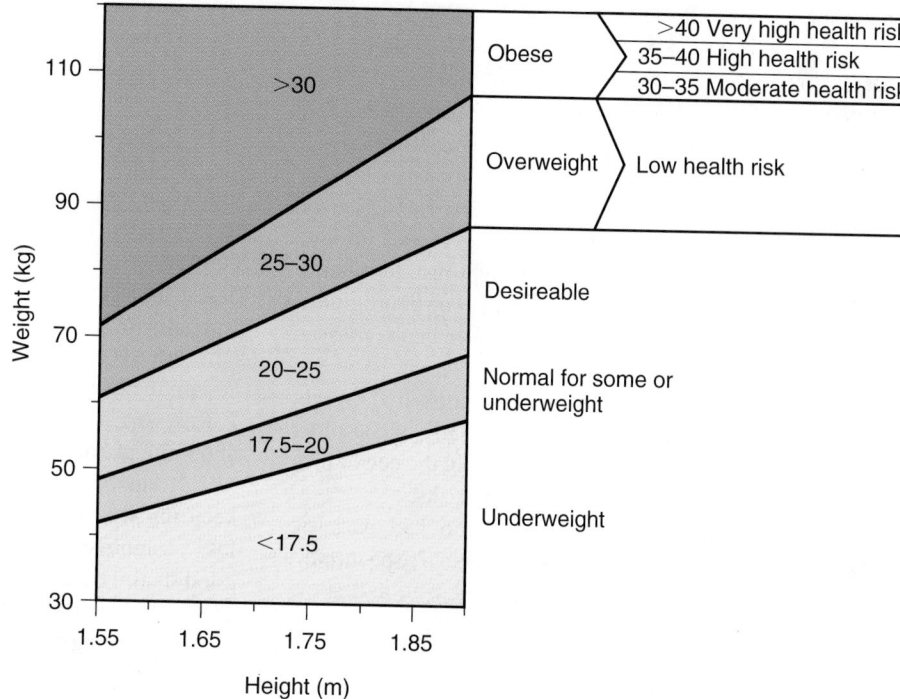

FIGURE 33.1 Body mass index ranges and associated level of health risk with obesity.

and prostate cancer. For more information, visit the Centers for Disease Control and Prevention at www.cdc.gov/nccdphp/dnpa/obesity/defining.htm.

Therapeutic Interventions

Initial treatment for obesity is weight loss through exercise and calorie restriction. For weight loss to occur, it is essential that the patient cooperates and has sustained motivation. Support groups such as Take Off Pounds Sensibly (TOPS) and Weight Watchers can help patients be successful. Behavior modification methods that provide rewards for successful weight loss are often included in a weight loss plan. Short-term use of medications that suppress appetite or block fat absorption may also be used. The patient should receive education regarding a healthy and balanced diet.

Surgical Management

Patients who do not respond to medical methods of weight loss or whose BMI is 40 or above may have surgery to reduce their weight if they meet established criteria for the surgery (Box 33.3 Patient Perspective). Established criteria for surgery may include gross obesity for 5 years, failure to reduce weight with other forms of therapy, body weight 100% above ideal weight, absence of other medical conditions, psychiatric and social stability, and presence of a high-risk condition that weight loss would relieve. Surgical techniques produce weight loss by restriction (limiting how much the stomach can hold), or malabsorption (decreased calorie and nutrient absorption) (see Box 33.2 Nutrition Notes). The field of obesity surgery is called bariatric surgery and is designed to treat severe obesity. The word *bariatric* comes from the Greek word *baros,* which means "weight." Various procedures have been used over the years,

but complications have arisen with some, such as malabsorption, so they are no longer used. For a list of surgical obesity centers and surgical procedures, visit The American Society for Bariatric Surgeons at www.asbs.org.

Gastric Bypass

The **Roux-en-Y** bypass is a common gastric bypass surgery (Fig. 33.2). In the first part of this two-step surgery, a small stomach pouch the size of a thumb is created with staples. This small pouch causes a quick satisfactory feeling of fullness during a meal, which is the key to the success of this procedure. Next, a Y-shaped section of the small intestine is attached to the pouch to allow food to bypass the lower stomach and duodenum. Digestive juice flow is maintained, and food enters the jejunum within 10 minutes of eating. There is little malabsorption of food. This procedure has also been performed laparoscopically.

Vertical Banded Gastroplasty

Vertical banded **gastroplasty** (VBG) is the most commonly used restrictive surgery for weight reduction and control today (see Fig. 33.2). There is little malabsorption of food with this procedure and it is technically easier to perform than gastric bypass surgery. If a reversal procedure is needed, it is easier to reverse the VBG than the gastric bypass. About 30% of patients who have had VBG achieve normal weight. Other methods of gastric banding are currently under study.

Complications of Gastric Restrictive Surgeries

A common side effect of restrictive surgery is vomiting caused by overeating or by not chewing food well. Severe side effects of VBG include erosion of the gastric tissue surrounding the band, breakdown of the staple line, and leaking

---

gastroplasty: gastro—stomach + plasty—repair

Box 33.3

Patient Perspective

Curtis

I am 47, with 8 children. For many years, I experienced weight control problems. By the time I was in high school, I weighed 250 lb, and the weight just kept building from there. I had tried many weight control programs, including some medications that now have been removed from the market.

When I was about 38, I began to look into weight loss surgeries such as the Roux-en-Y. Many of the older techniques were dangerous and risky. Even the newer procedures are major procedure with many risks.

I had spoken to many people who had bariatric surgery. Many pointed out the psychological aspect, talking about how differently people treated you, and some even ending with a divorce. This was a very scary aspect to me.

However, after much research and after reaching a weight of about 380 lb, I arranged to have the surgery done. I had my surgery at a facility that did only bariatric surgery. I felt very comfortable through the whole process. This included all the presurgical testing, including psychological evaluation and counseling.

One of the nice features was that the facility itself was patient friendly, with large chairs, etc. When I had the surgery I had a rough first 24 hours spent in CCU (critical care unit). The nursing staff was very professional and understanding. The care was very personal and responsive to my needs. The staff was very courteous and made me comfortable.

I think that understanding the medical field you are working in is very important to this feeling of patient comfort. Several of my nurses had gone through the procedure themselves. This really helped them to know what I was experiencing. Nurses should be well-informed about the procedures.

It has been 6+ years now and I have continued to keep my weight down around 230 to 250 lb, which is a loss of approximately 120 lb. My health has improved a good deal. I would do it again, even though at about day 21 I would have said "never again."

As nursing professionals, it is very important to treat everyone as a human being and with much respect regardless of the socioeconomic status or medical needs. If patients are treated with respect and caring, it is a step for them in the right direction. I believe it is not only kind but helps in the healing and recovery processes as well. I was treated with a great deal of kindness and respect during my procedure and I greatly appreciated this. Thanks to all the professional nurses out there who do a great job.

---

of the stomach secretions into the abdomen. Leaking of the stomach secretions can lead to peritonitis, a very serious infection of the peritoneum and requires emergency surgery. Infection or death from any of these complications can occur.

Postoperative Care

Postoperative bariatric patients require care similar to that for most types of gastric surgeries. (See section Nursing Management After Gastric Surgery later in this chapter.) The bariatric diet, however, is very different. Patients are started on a clear liquid diet because of the small stomach pouch that has been created. Then the diet progresses to full liquids, pureed foods, and finally, at about 6 weeks after surgery, regular foods as tolerated.

Nursing Process for the Patient Who Is Obese

Assessment/Data Collection

Assessment for the patient with obesity should include measurements of height, weight, and BMI. Information about eating patterns and exercise patterns should be obtained. The nurse should determine if any problems exist for the patient related to excess weight such as physical limitations, social interaction issues, and personal issues (e.g., changes in sexuality or financial status). The nurse should complete a complete physical assessment noting any abnormalities. Assessment should include any areas in which the patient has expressed concerns or problems. Persons who are overweight have an increased risk for other diseases. The nurse should assess for signs and symptoms of these diseases.

Nursing Diagnosis, Planning, and Implementation

Imbalanced nutrition: more than body requirements related to caloric intake greater than metabolic needs and/or decreased activity level

EXPECTED OUTCOMES: The patient will achieve and maintain weight loss to specified weight.

- Establish desired weight goal and monitor weight.
- Modify eating habits and patterns.
- Establish and maintain increased activity pattern.
- In collaboration with a dietician, implement eating plan for patient *to safely reduce weight and maintain adequate protein intake.*
- Discuss realistic weight loss goals of 1 to 2 lb/week *to achieve lasting weight loss effects.*
- Discuss emotions, events, and patterns of eating *to help patient identify when she or he is eating*

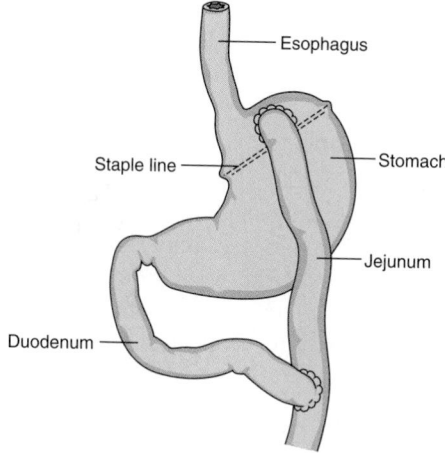

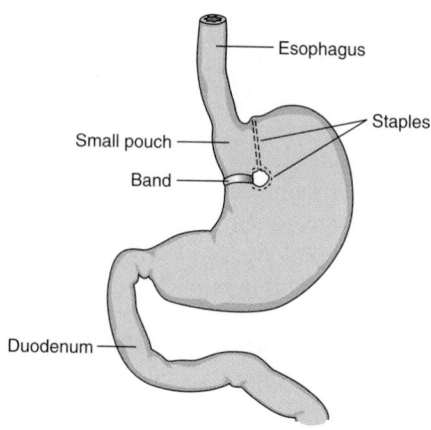

FIGURE 33.2 *(A)* Roux-en-Y gastric bypass. A staple line creates a small pouch at the top of the stomach, which is then attached to the jejunum. Food bypasses most of the stomach and the duodenum and goes into the jejunum. *(B)* Vertical banded gastroplasty for gastric bypass. A small stomach pouch is made with a staple line and a mesh band. A circular window made with staples allows the band to be placed around the pouch. The band restricts and slows food flow from the stomach pouch. As the small pouch fills, there is a feeling of fullness even with small meals.

to satisfy an emotional need versus a physiological hunger.
- In collaboration with physician, establish increased activity pattern *to promote weight loss.*
- Provide preoperative instructions if surgical interventions are planned, *for understanding.*

Evaluation
The patient's goals are met if the patient maintains progressive weight loss to specified weight goal and safely progresses through the perioperative period if a surgical intervention is completed.

ORAL HEALTH AND DENTAL CARE

Good oral health care is important to overall health. Nutritional needs can be a problem if oral problems interfere with

NURSING CARE TIP
For the patient who is obese, it is often necessary to have on hand special equipment for patient care. Some items you may need include:
- Larger hospital bed, wheelchair, or walker
- Patient lifting devices
- Extra pillows to ease breathing
- Larger hospital gowns
- Larger blood pressure cuff

eating and drinking. Respiratory illness and cardiac disease is associated with pathogens in the mouth. Regular oral hygiene and dental care are important in preventing infections (Box 33.4 Common Concerns in Oral Health and Dental Care). Providing oral hygiene using oral chlorhexidine gluconate washes has been shown to be effective in preventing pneumonia in long-term care residents as well as reducing ventilator-associated pneumonia in cardiac surgery patients. This is an easy and inexpensive way to promote patient health.

Aging changes as well as disease and treatment can result in oral inflammation and infection. Those who are immunosuppressed (AIDS) or undergoing chemotherapy or who have vitamin deficiencies are more at risk. Candidiasis is a common oral infection that is often treated with nystatin oral swish and swallow. During data collection, especially in these higher risk patients, the nurse should note any oral signs of inflammation or infection for prompt treatment. This is important to preserve oral comfort and nutrition.

ORAL INFLAMMATORY DISORDERS

Stomatitis

Stomatitis is the general term for inflammation of the oral cavity. There are many causes of stomatitis, such as an infection or a systemic disease. The most common types of stomatitis are **aphthous stomatitis** (canker sores) and herpes simplex virus type I infection (also known as cold sores or fever blisters).

Aphthous Stomatitis (Canker Sores)
Aphthous stomatitis appears as small, white, painful ulcers on the inner cheeks, lips, tongue, gums, palate, or pharynx and typically lasts for several days to 2 weeks. Self-induced trauma such as biting the lips and cheeks can cause these ulcers to develop, as well as stress or exposure to irritating foods. Application of topical tetracycline several times a day usually shortens the healing time. A topical anesthetic such

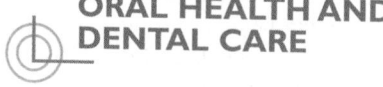

stomatitis: stoma—mouth + itis—inflammation

Box 33.4

Common Concerns in Oral Health and Dental Care

Oral care is important throughout life and has been found to have a link to cardiac health. The importance of daily and ongoing oral care should be considered for all patients, especially older adults.

Patients undergoing dental procedure who have artificial joints or some heart conditions need to take prophylactic antibiotics prior to some dental procedures to prevent bacteria entry and bacterial endocarditis. The dentist should be informed of the patient's history so that appropriate antibiotics can be prescribed.

Xerostomia (Dry Mouth)

As people age, it is not unusual for them to experience a condition known as xerostomia (dry mouth). Also, some medications and radiation treatment of the head and neck areas can cause it. Xerostomia can lead to rampant tooth decay in older adults, putting their dentition at risk.

Prior to any radiation therapy of the head or neck area, a thorough oral examination and any needed restorative dental procedures should be completed.

Although water is used as a common substitute for saliva, it does not contain the necessary compounds such as lubricants to protect the teeth, therefore an artificial saliva substitute should be considered such as Oralbalance gel, Salivart solution, or Salix lozenges.

Dentures

It is helpful to have a person's name implanted into their dentures to avoid lost or mixed up dentures, especially when the person lives in an extended care facility. It can be requested when the dentures are made and the dentist will place a small identity tag in the acrylic of the denture with the person's name on it.

Those with complete dentures still need to be routinely screened by a dentist or dental hygienist for proper denture fit, sore areas, oral cancer detection, and oral fungal infections.

Gingival Recession

As people age, it is not unusual for their gingival (gums) to recede or shrink, exposing the root surfaces of the teeth. This can lead to root sensitivity and/or tooth decay.

In order to protect the teeth from rampant tooth decay due to dry mouth or gingival recession, a fluoride gel or rinse is strongly recommended such as over-the-counter products as Act rinse or Gel-Kam.

Gingivitis

As people get older, the gingivae have a greater tendency to bleed, a condition known as gingivitis. If the supporting tissues in the sockets of the teeth become inflamed, bone loss occurs, resulting in a condition known as periodontitus (pyorrhea). Periodontitus can lead to tooth mobility or loss.

Good oral hygiene habits cannot be overemphasized in the prevention of gum disease. Flossing every day is very important. If the patient is unable to floss due to arthritis or other conditions, an electric toothbrush or a water pic device is helpful in providing oral hygiene.

Candida Albicans Infection (Yeast Infection)

Older adults are susceptible to oral yeast infections (caused by Candida albicans) due to certain medications, systemic conditions, or chemotherapy. Nystatin (Mycostatin, Nadostine) as an oral rinse treats this infection.

Angular Cheilosis

A condition known as angular cheilosis (red, raw corners of the mouth) may develop in people, especially older adults. This can be due to infection, riboflavin (vitamin B_2) deficiency, or loss of facial profile due to worn dentures or not wearing dentures. The cause is treated by, for example, anti-infective medications, vitamins, and dentures.

Source: Contributed by Dr. Ralph Kluk and Dr. Cheryl Kluk.

as benzocaine or lidocaine provides pain relief and makes it possible to eat with minimal pain.

Herpes Simplex Virus Type I Infection

Herpes simplex virus type I (HSV-I) infection may appear as painful cold sores or fever blisters on the face, lips, perioral area, cheeks, nose, or conjunctivae. These lesions recur over time but last only for a few days each time. The onset can be provoked by fever or stress, among other things. Acyclovir ointment can be used to ease the pain, but it does not cure the lesions. Oral acyclovir may reduce recurrences. These lesions are infectious, and standard precautions should be used when ointment is applied or oral care is given.

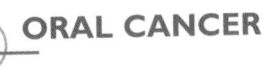

ORAL CANCER

Pathophysiology and Etiology

Oral cancer can occur anywhere in the mouth or throat. If detected early enough, it is curable. Oral cancer is found most commonly in patients who use alcohol or any form of tobacco. The highest incidence of oral cancer is found in the pharynx (throat), with the lowest incidence being on the lips.

Signs and Symptoms

Any oral sore that does not heal in 2 weeks should be assessed by the patient's physician. Cancerous ulcers are often painless but may become tender as the cancer progresses. In the later stages, the patient may complain of difficulty in chewing, swallowing, or speaking or may have swollen cervical lymph glands.

Diagnosis

Biopsy specimens are taken to determine the presence of cancer.

Therapeutic Interventions

Oral cancer treatment varies depending on the individualized diagnosis. Radiation, chemotherapy, and surgery are used alone or in combination to treat oral cancer. Radical or modified neck dissection is performed if the cancer has metastasized to cervical lymph nodes (Fig. 33.3). The tumor is removed along with lymph nodes, muscles, blood vessels, glands, and part of the thyroid, depending on the extent of the cancer. Drains are inserted into the incision to prevent fluid accumulation. A tracheostomy is usually performed to protect the airway and prevent obstruction.

Nursing Management

For the patient undergoing surgery, preoperative and postoperative nursing care is discussed in Chapter 11. Preoperatively, issues that are addressed in planning care include the use of alcohol or tobacco. Referrals to cessation programs and support groups are included in the plan of care. Preoperative teaching would also include how the patient will communicate if a tracheostomy is placed. Postoperatively, major concerns are airway patency, commu-

nication, and nutritional needs. Nursing care for the patient with a tracheostomy is discussed in Chapter 29. The airway must be monitored and secretions controlled to prevent aspiration. Determining that the methods the patient is using for communication are satisfactory is evaluated. Tube feedings are usually given to meet the patient's nutritional needs because swallowing is difficult (discussed in Chapter 32).

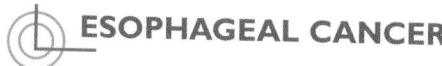 ESOPHAGEAL CANCER

Pathophysiology and Etiology

As with oral cancer, esophageal cancer is associated with the use of tobacco or alcohol. Esophageal cancer is usually detected late because of its location near many lymph nodes that allow it to metastasize. As the cancer progresses, obstruction of the esophagus can occur, with possible perforation or fistula development that may cause aspiration. The appearance of signs and symptoms usually means that the cancer is in the late stages.

Signs and Symptoms

Signs and symptoms may include difficulty swallowing, a feeling of fullness, pain in the chest area after eating, foul breath, or regurgitation of foods if there is obstruction.

Diagnosis

Diagnosis of esophageal cancer is usually made by esophagogastroduodenoscopy (EGD) and biopsy. Mediastinoscopy (endoscopic examination of mediastinum) is used to determine whether the cancer has spread to the lymph nodes and surrounding structures.

Therapeutic Interventions

Treatment for esophageal cancer includes radiation, chemotherapy, and surgery alone or in combination. Surgical procedures include esophageal resection (esophagogastrostomy), Dacron esophageal replacement, or use of a section of colon to replace the esophagus (esophagoenterostomy). If the tumor is inoperable, esophageal dilation or stent placement can be done to relieve dysphagia and allow food to pass through the esophagus.

Nursing Process for the Patient with Esophageal Cancer

The patient with esophageal cancer may undergo various forms of treatment: chemotherapy, radiation, or surgery. Nursing care is provided based on the effects of the therapies which are discussed in Chapters 10 and 11.

Assessment/Data Collection
Patient data are collected for risk factors of esophageal cancer, pain, dysphagia, and nutritional status.

Nursing Diagnosis, Planning, and Implementation
Pain related to tumor and pressure exerted on surrounding tissues

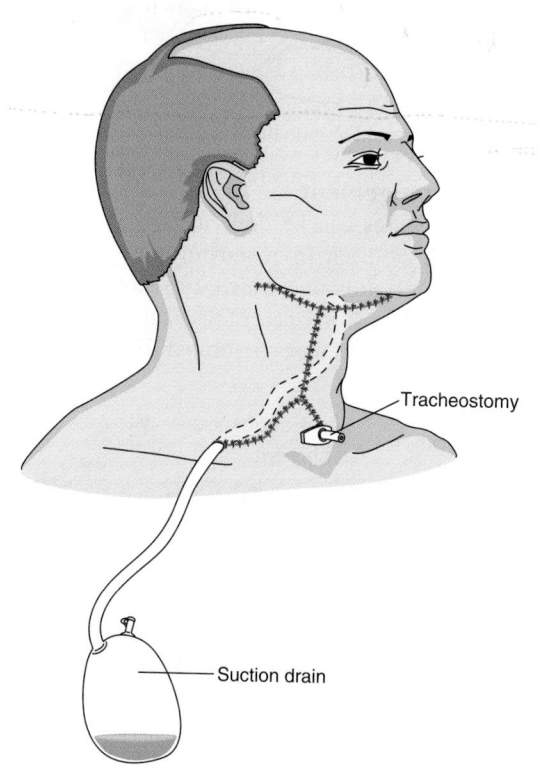

FIGURE 33.3 Radical neck dissection with tracheostomy tube and drains inserted.

EXPECTED OUTCOME: Patient will state a reduction of pain to acceptable level or total relief of pain.

- Assess pain level using pain rating scale *to identify pain level*.
- If surgery is performed, provide pain medications as ordered *to provide pain relief*.

Risk for deficient fluid volume related to decreased intake

EXPECTED OUTCOME: Vital signs remain within normal limits and balanced intake and output over 24 hours.

- Assess fluid intake and swallowing ability with fluids *to plan care*.
- Obtain daily weights *to detect changes in fluid volume*.
- Provide fluids as able to swallow *to ensure adequate intake*.
- Monitor intravenous infusion as ordered *to prevent hypovolemia*.
- Monitor vital signs and report abnormal findings *for prompt treatment*.

Imbalanced nutrition: less than body requirements related to dysphagia

EXPECTED OUTCOME: Patient will maintain weight within normal limits for body frame and laboratory values such as albumin, electrolytes, and lymphocytes will be within normal limits.

- Obtain patient height and weight, and weigh weekly *to monitor changes during care*.
- Identify patient's ability to swallow and eat food *to determine plan of care*.
- Provide oral care frequently *to refresh mouth and encourage desire to eat*.
- Provide nutrition as ordered in form patient is able to tolerate: liquid supplements, tube feedings, total perenteral nutrition (TPN) *to maintain adequate nutrition*.

Evaluation

The goals are met if the patient reports pain is relieved and fluid volume and nutritional needs are met.

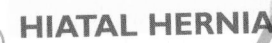

HIATAL HERNIA

Pathophysiology

The esophagus passes through an opening in the diaphragm called the hiatus. A **hiatal hernia** is a condition in which the lower part of the esophagus and stomach slides up through the hiatus of the diaphragm into the thorax (Fig. 33.4). A sliding hiatal hernia is the most common type in which the stomach slides up into the thoracic cavity when a patient is supine and then usually goes back into the abdominal cavity when the patient stands upright. Hiatal hernia occurs most commonly in women and those who are older than age 60, obese, or pregnant. People with hiatal hernia often have gastroesophageal reflux disease (GERD) as well (discussed later).

Signs and Symptoms

A small hernia may not produce any discomfort or require treatment. However, a large hernia can cause pain, heartburn, a feeling of fullness, or reflux, which can injure the esophagus with possible ulceration and bleeding.

Diagnosis

Hiatal hernias are diagnosed by x-ray studies and fluoroscopy.

Therapeutic Interventions

Medical treatment for symptomatic hiatal hernia includes antacids; eating small meals that pass easily through the esophagus; not reclining for 1 hour after eating; elevating the head of the bed 6 to 12 inches to prevent reflux; and avoiding bedtime snacks, spicy foods, alcohol, caffeine, and smoking (see Box 33.2 Nutrition Notes).

Surgical Management

Surgical procedures can be done to prevent the herniated portion of the stomach from moving upward through the hiatus. Fundoplication, in which the stomach fundus is wrapped around the lower part of the esophagus, is the most common surgical procedure performed (Fig. 33.5).

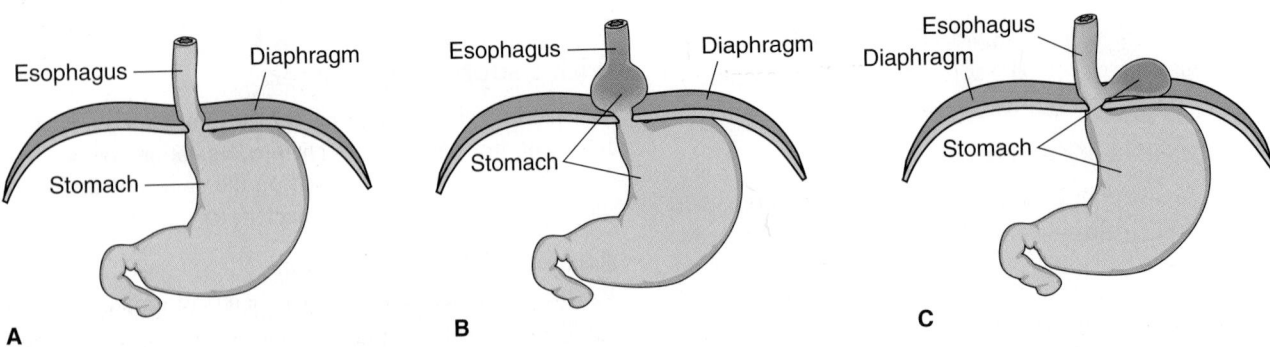

FIGURE 33.4 Hiatal hernia. (A) Normal esophagus and stomach. (B) Sliding hiatal hernia. (C) Rolling hiatal hernia.

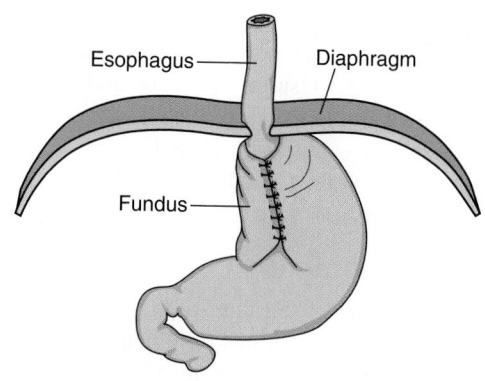

FIGURE 33.5 Hiatal hernia repair. Nissen fundoplication wraps the stomach fundus around the esophagus and then sutures it onto itself to hold it in place.

Nursing Management

Teaching the patient interventions to reduce symptoms of hiatal hernia is included in the plan of care (see section Therapeutic Interventions above). If the patient undergoes surgery, general postoperative nursing care is provided. In addition, following fundoplication, patients are assessed for dysphagia during their first postoperative meal. If dysphagia occurs, the physician should be notified because the repair may be too tight, causing obstruction of the passage of food.

GASTROESOPHAGEAL REFLUX DISEASE

Pathophysiology

Gastroesophageal reflux disease (GERD) is a condition in which gastric secretions reflux into the esophagus. The esophagus can be damaged by acidic gastric secretions and exposure to digestive enzymes. GERD is caused primarily by conditions that affect the ability of the lower esophageal sphincter to close tightly, such as hiatal hernia.

Signs and Symptoms

Signs and symptoms of GERD include heartburn, regurgitation, dysphagia, and bleeding (Table 33.1). Aspiration is a concern. Scar tissue can develop from the inflammation.

Diagnosis

Diagnostic tests include a barium swallow, esophagoscopy, or pH monitoring of the normally alkaline esophagus. GERD often occurs in older people.

Therapeutic Interventions

Interventions for GERD aim to decrease the reflux of gastric secretions into the esophagus. Lifestyle changes are recommended along with medications. Obese patients are encouraged to lose weight. A low-fat, high-protein diet is recommended because fat causes decreased functioning of the lower esophageal sphincter. Caffeine, milk products, and spicy foods should be avoided.

TABLE 33.1 GERD SUMMARY

Signs and Symptoms	Heartburn
	Regurgitation
	Dysphagia
	Bleeding
Diagnostic Tests	X-ray studies, endoscopy, and fluoroscopy
Therapeutic Interventions	Medications to decrease acid, improve gastric emptying, and lower espophageal functioning: antacids, histamine (H₂) receptor antagonists, cytoprotective agents (sucralfate), and cholinergic drugs
	Control of symptoms
	Low-fat, high-protein diet
	Avoid triggers
Complications	Esophagitis
	Barrett's syndrome
	Respiratroy symptoms
Possible Nursing Diagnoses	Acute pain
	Deficient knowledge

[handwritten annotations: "reduce Acid" pointing to cytoprotective agents line; "Tagamin Pepsid Zantat" in right margin]

Medications may include nonprescription antacids for mild symptoms (Mylanta, Tums, Gaviscon). Histamine (H_2) receptor antagonists (acid reducers) that are available in nonprescription and prescription strengths are used for mild to moderate symptoms (cimetidine [Tagamet], famotidine [Pepcid], ranitidine HCl [Zantac], nizatidine [Axid]). Proton pump inhibitors (PPI) reduce acid in the stomach and are used for frequent, severe symptoms and Barrett's esophagus (esomeprazole [Nexium], lansoprazole [Prevacid], omeprazole [Prilosec], pantoprazole [Protonix], rabeprazole [Aciphex]). Prokinetic agents, which are not used as a first choice because of side effects, (metoclopramide [Reglan, Maxolon]) improve gastric emptying and function of the lower esophageal sphincter (see Table 33.4). If surgery is necessary to alleviate symptoms, a fundoplication can be done.

Complications

Complications of GERD can result in esophagitis (inflammation of the esophagus) due to acid reflux. Over time this can lead to changes in the epithelium of the esophagus and lead to Barrett's esophagus. This is a precancerous lesion that puts the patient at risk of developing esophageal cancer. The patient with Barrett's esophagus should have regular endoscopic examinations. Respiratory complications such as bronchospasm, laryngospasm, and aspiration pneumonia can also occur owing to aspiration of gastric contents.

Nursing Process for the Patient with GERD

Assessment/Data Collection

Assessment of the patient with GERD should include evaluation of complaints of heartburn. Note the onset, duration, and characteristics of the pain. Note any precipitating factors as well as anything that relieves the pain.

Nursing Diagnosis, Planning, and Implementation
Acute pain related to inflammation of esophageal tissues

EXPECTED OUTCOME: Patient will state a reduction of pain to acceptable level or total relief of pain.

- Monitor pain level using pain rating scale *to identify pain level.*
- Identify factors that increase pain *to develop teaching plan.*
- Instruct patient regarding factors that aggravate pain *to enhance management of condition.*
- Instruct patient to sleep with head of bed elevated 4 to 6 inches, eat small meals, and avoid lying down for 2 hours after eating *to prevent reflux of gastric contents into esophagus.*
- Instruct patient to avoid smoking and alcohol *as they decrease functioning of the lower esophageal sphincter.*
- Instruct patient to avoid foods that cause discomfort *to avoid pain.*
- Review medication schedule and teach patient to take medications even if symptoms are relieved *since the underlying pathology still exists.*
- If surgery is completed, provide pain medications on routine schedule *to provide optimum pain relief and control.*

Evaluation
The goals are met if the patient is able to manage the medications, pain is controlled, and symptoms are relieved.

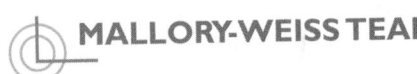 MALLORY-WEISS TEAR

Pathophysiology

A Mallory-Weiss tear (MWT) is a longitudinal tear in the mucous membrane of the esophagus at the stomach junction (gastric cardia). These tears occur from a sudden powerful or prolonged force due to coughing, vomiting, seizures, prolapse of the stomach into the esophagus, or cardiopulmonary resuscitation (CPR). Hiatal hernia is present in most patients with MWTs .

Signs and Symptoms

Bleeding may result from the tear. Up to 15% of GI bleeding occurs from MWTs. Symptoms include bright red bloody emesis or bloody or tarry stools.

Diagnosis

The tear can be diagnosed with an esophagogastroduodenoscopy (EGD). Hemoglobin and hematocrit are checked to determine amount of bleeding.

Therapeutic Interventions

The tears usually self heal without intervention in several days and bleeding stops within a few hours. It is rare to have it happen again. Medications such as a PPI and an antieme-

tic may be given. Alcohol use should be avoided. Up to 75% of those with MWT use alcohol excessively. Rarely, excessive bleeding may occur resulting in shock and or the need for a blood transfusion. Bleeding is treated with epinephrine injection, and during endoscopy, hemaclips can be placed. The prognosis for MWTs is good. The condition is seen in men more often than in women.

Nursing Management

Monitoring the patient for the signs of bleeding and reporting them to prevent complications from hemorrhage are the focus of nursing care. If excessive bleeding occurs, shock symptoms may occur and require prompt intervention. Teaching about medications and the avoidance of alcohol use is also done. See section Gastric Bleeding later in this chapter for more information.

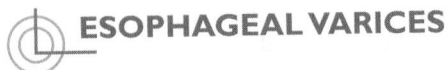 ESOPHAGEAL VARICES

Esophageal varices are dilated blood vessels in the esophagus. If they rupture, it can be a life-threatening event. Varices develop from portal hypertension. This occurs when pressure rises in the portal vein from blocked blood flow in the liver. This is often due to cirrhosis of the liver. Esophageal varices are discussed in Chapter 35.

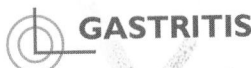 GASTRITIS

Pathophysiology

Gastritis is inflammation of the stomach mucosa and can be acute or chronic. Causes are listed in Box 33.5. Gastritis results when the protective mucosal barrier is broken down and allows autodigestion from hydrochloric acid and pepsin to occur. This results in edema of the tissue and possible hemorrhage. With severe gastritis, the gastric mucosa can become gangrenous and perforate, which can lead to peritonitis (infection of the peritoneum). Scarring may also occur, resulting in pyloric obstruction.

Signs and Symptoms

The major symptom of gastritis is abdominal pain, which is often accompanied by nausea and anorexia. The patient may also experience abdominal tenderness, feeling of fullness, reflux, belching, and hematemesis. If the cause of the gastritis is contaminated food, symptoms including diarrhea usually start within 5 to 6 hours.

Therapeutic Interventions

Treatment of gastritis is removal of the irritating substance and provision of a bland diet of liquids and soft foods along with antacids. Medication therapy may include phenothiazines to control vomiting and antacids and/or histamine

---

gastritis: gastr—stomach + itis—inflammation

test 1 (handwritten)

Box 33.5

Causes of Gastritis

Diet
- Alcohol
- Spicy foods

Microorganisms
- *Helicobacter pylori*
- *Salmonella*

Medications
- Aspirin
- Nonsteroidal anti-inflammatory drugs
- Corticosteroids
- Digitalis
- Chemotherapeutic drugs

Stress
- Physiological
- Psychological

Trauma

Other Factors
- Reflux of bile
- Smoking
- Radiation
- Nasogastric suctioning

Endoscopic procedures

---

receptor antagonists to control pain. With a bland diet, the patient usually recovers in a short period of time.

Chronic Gastritis

Chronic gastritis occurs over time and is classified as type A or type B.

Type A

Chronic gastritis type A is often referred to as autoimmune gastritis and occurs in the fundus (body of stomach). Chronic gastritis type A is diagnosed by endoscopy, upper gastrointestinal (GI) x-ray examination, and gastric aspirate analysis (see Chapter 32). Type A gastritis is often asymptomatic. Patients with type A gastritis usually do not secrete enough intrinsic factor from their stomach cells and as a result have difficulty absorbing vitamin B_{12}, which leads to pernicious anemia (discussed later).

Type B

Type B chronic gastritis affects the antrum and pylorus (lower end of the stomach near the duodenum) and is associated with *Helicobacter pylori* bacterial infection. Type B is the most common type of chronic gastritis. Signs and symptoms include poor appetite, heartburn after eating, belching, a sour taste in the mouth, and nausea and vomiting. Type B gastritis can also be diagnosed by endoscopy, upper gastrointestinal x-ray examination, and gastric aspirate analysis. *H. pylori* infection is treated with antibiotics.

 ## PEPTIC ULCER DISEASE

PUD (handwritten) · *Stomach* · *Duodenum* (handwritten) · *Acid has eroded* (handwritten)

Etiology

Until 1982 the cause of peptic ulcer was poorly understood and thought to be related to stress, diet, and alcohol or caffeine ingestion. However, research results found that **peptic ulcer disease** (PUD) is primarily caused by infection with the gram-negative bacterium *Helicobacter pylori* (*H. pylori*). This bacterium is responsible for 80% of gastric ulcers and more than 90% of duodenal ulcers. Two-thirds of all people are infected with *H. pylori,* and it is most common in those who are elderly, Hispanic, African American, or in lower socioeconomic groups in the United States. The discovery of *H. pylori* has led to changes in treating and curing peptic ulcers. It is not known how *H. pylori* is transmitted, although the oral-oral or fecal-oral route is likely. Contaminated water may also play a role. Vaccines to prevent peptic ulcers are being developed.

Risk factors that contribute to PUD include smoking, chewing tobacco, stress, caffeine, or medications such as steroids, aspirin, and nonsteriodal anti-inflammatory drugs (NSAIDs). Peptic ulcer development is also influenced by smoking, which increases the harmful effects of *H. pylori,* alters protective mechanisms, and decreases gastric blood flow. For more information on *H. pylori,* visit www.cdc.gov or call 1-888-MY-ULCER (1-888-698-5237).

Tagment (handwritten, margin)

LEARNING TIP

Most peptic ulcers are caused by an infection (*H. pylori*) that can be cured with antibiotics.

Pathophysiology

PUD is a condition in which the lining of the stomach, pylorus, duodenum, or the esophagus is eroded, usually from infection with *H. pylori*. The erosion may extend into the muscular layers or the peritoneum. Peptic ulcers occur in the portions of the gastrointestinal tract that are exposed to hydrochloric acid and pepsin. The erosion is due to an increase in the concentration or activity of hydrochloric acid and pepsin. The damaged mucosa is unable to secrete enough mucus to act as a barrier against the hydrochloric acid. Some individuals have more rapid gastric emptying, which, combined with hypersecretion of acid, creates a large amount of acid moving into the duodenum. As a result, peptic ulcers occur more often in the duodenum. Ulcers are named by their location: esophageal, gastric, or duodenal. Duodenal ulcers are more common than gastric ulcers.

Signs and Symptoms

Symptoms vary with the location of the ulcer (Table 33.2). Symptoms, including pain, may not be experienced with gastric or duodenal ulcers until complications such as hemorrhage, obstruction, or perforation develop. If pain does

TABLE 33.2 PEPTIC ULCER DISEASE SUMMARY

Signs and Symptoms	*Gastric:* Intermittent high left epigastric or upper abdominal burning or gnawing pain, increased 1–2 hours after meals or with food. Variable pain pattern may be made worse by food, antacids ineffective. Can lead to gastric cancer. Patient may be malnourished. Hematemesis is more common than melena.
	Duodenal: Intermittent midepigastric or upper abdominal burning or cramping pain, increased 2–4 hours after meals or in the middle of the night; relieved with food or antacids. Patient generally well nourished. Melena is more common than hematemesis.
	Anorexia
	Nausea/vomiting
	Bleeding (stomach secretions or stool positive for occult blood)
Diagnostic Tests	Urea breath test
H. pylori	IgG antibody detection test for *H. pylori*
	Biopsy
	Culture
Peptic Ulcer	Upper GI series (barium swallow)
	Esophagogastroduodenoscopy
Medical Treatment	Antibiotics
	Proton pump inhibitors
	H₂ antagonists
	Bismuth subsalicylate
	Sucralfate (Carafate)
	Antacids
	Bland diet
	Avoiding irritants, such as smoking, caffeine, alcohol
Complications	Bleeding
	Perforation
	Obstruction
Nursing Diagnoses	Acute pain related to disruption of GI mucosa
	Risk for injury related to complications of peptic ulcer activity such as hemorrhage or perforation
	Deficient knowledge related to lack of exposure to peptic ulcer disease and its treatment

fecal occult blood may be found, depending on where the ulcers are located.

Diagnosis

H. pylori can be diagnosed with several tests. The urea breath test is performed by having the patient drink carbon-labeled urea. The urea is metabolized rapidly if *H. pylori* is present, allowing the carbon to be absorbed and measured in exhaled carbon dioxide. An IgG antibody detection test for *H. pylori* identifies whether the patient is infected with *H. pylori*. These are both noninvasive detection tests. Biopsy specimens for the *Campylobacter*-like organism (CLO) biopsy urease test and a histological examination can be obtained during esophagogastroduodenoscopy (EGD). Biopsy is the most conclusive test for *H. pylori*. Cultures of the biopsy specimen may also be done to determine antimicrobial susceptibility.

Peptic ulcers are diagnosed on the basis of symptoms, upper GI series (barium swallow), endoscopy, and EGD.

Therapeutic Interventions

Several treatment options are used to cure *H. pylori* without recurrence (Table 33.3). The first antibiotic treatment for ulcer disease caused by *H. pylori* was approved by the Food and Drug Administration (FDA) in 1996. For better effectiveness, triple therapy with two antibiotics to decrease resistance of the bacteria and a proton pump inhibitor or H₂ antagonist is used. Treatment lasting 14 days has better eradication rates than 10-day treatments. Bismuth subsalicylate (Pepto-Bismol) may also be used for its antibacterial effects. Proton pump inhibitors are powerful agents that stop the final step of gastric acid secretion to reduce mucosa erosion and aid in healing ulcers (Table 33.4). H₂ antagonists block H₂ receptors to decrease acid secretion, although not as powerfully as gastric acid pump inhibitors. A bland diet may

TABLE 33.3 MEDICATION REGIMEN OPTIONS FOR *H. PYLORI* INFECTION

Type of Therapy	Examples of Therapy Options
*Triple Therapy**	• Amoxicillin (Amoxil) + clarithromycin (Biaxin) + omeprazole (Prilosec)
Two antibiotics + proton pump inhibitor	• Amoxicillin (Amoxil) + clarithromycin (Biaxin) + lansoprazole (Prevacid) (available as Prevpac, combined for convenience)
Dual Therapy	• Clarithromycin (Biaxin) + omeprazole (Prilosec)
Antibiotic + proton pump inhibitor or Antibiotic + H₂ antagonist	• Amoxicillin (Amoxil) + lansoprazole (Prevacid)
	• Clarithromycin (Biaxin) + ranitidine bismuth citrate (Tritec)
Other Therapy	
Two antibiotics + bismuth subsalicylate + H₂ antagonist	• Metronidazole (Flagyl) + tetracycline + bismuth subsalicylate (Pepto-Bismol) + H₂ antagonist

*Triple therapy has a better eradication rate.

occur, patients with gastric ulcers commonly experience a burning and gnawing pain in the high left epigastric region. There may be more pain with food ingestion or 1 to 2 hours after a meal. Duodenal ulcers produce cramping or burning pain in the midepigastric or upper abdominal area. The pain occurs 2 to 4 hours after meals or in the middle of the night. This intermittent pain may be relieved by the ingestion of food or antacids. Anorexia and nausea and vomiting may also occur with either ulcer location. Bleeding may occur with massive hemorrhaging or slow oozing. Patients often have low hematocrit and hemoglobin levels, and gastric or

TABLE 33.4 MEDICATIONS USED TO PROMOTE HEALING OF PEPTIC ULCERS

Drug Class/Action	Examples	Route	Side Effects	Nursing Implications
Hyposecretory Agents **H_2 Receptor Blocking Agents** Inhibits gastric acid secretion by blocking H_2 receptors on gastric parietal cells.	Cimetidine (Tagamet)	PO, IM, IV	Fever, rash, headaches, dizziness, somnolence, confusion (especially in elderly), hypotension, diarrhea, neutropenia, gynecomastia, and impotence	Monitor mental status of elderly; do not take antacids within 1 hour of Tagamet; take with meals and at bedtime; interacts with theophylline, phenytoin, warfarin, and beta blockers; continue treatment for at least 8 weeks to ensure healing.
	Ranitidine (Zantac)	PO, IM, IV	All side effects rare, including nausea, constipation, bradycardia, increased liver enzymes, and headache	Give antacids at least 1 hour before or 2 hours after Zantac; can be given in single bedtime dose; use cautiously in patients with liver or renal disease; absorption not affected by food; interacts minimally with other drugs.
	Famotidine (Pepcid)	PO, IV	Headache, diarrhea, constipation, nausea, flatulence, increased blood urea nitrogen and creatinine, and rash	Should not be taken longer than 8 weeks without physician's order; may be given with antacids; can be given in single bedtime dose; has no significant drug interactions.
	Nizatidine (Axid)	PO	Diarrhea, rash, bronchospasms, somnolence, joint pain, and sweating	Give as single bedtime dose or, if given twice a day, one dose at bedtime; assess for excessive drowsiness; monitor and record stools; do not give antacids within 1 hour of Axid; must be taken 4 to 8 weeks for ulcer healing; notify physician if somnolence or rash develops.
Proton Pump Binds to enzyme on gastric parietal cells to prevent final transport of hydrogen to block gastric acid secretion.	Omeprazole (Prilosec)	PO	Abdominal pain, diarrhea, rash, chest pain, and weakness	Give before meal in morning; swallow capsule whole; assess for abdominal pain and bleeding; monitor complete blood cell count and liver enzymes; may be given with antacids; must be taken 4 to 8 weeks for ulcer healing; notify physician if bleeding, diarrhea, headache, or abdominal pain develops.
Binds to an enzyme in the presence of acidic gastric pH, preventing the final transport of hydrogenions into the gastric lumen.	Lansoprazole (Prevacid)	PO	Dizziness, headache, diarrhea, abdominal pain, nausea, rash	Note epigastric or abdominal pain and blood in stool, emesis, or gastric aspirate. Give before meals. Capsules may be opened and sprinkled on applesauce and taken immediately for patients with difficulty swallowing. Do not crush capsule. Tell patient not to chew capsule.
Same as for lansoprazole	Rabeprazole (Aciphex)	PO	Headache	Tell patient to swallow tablets whole.
Antacids Increases gastric pH to reduce pepsin activity; strengthens gastric mucosal barrier and esophageal sphincter tone.	Aluminum-magnesium combinations (Riopan, Maalox, Mylanta, Gelusil)	PO	Mild constipation or diarrhea	Do not give to patients with renal disease; monitor bowel movements and signs of hypermagnesemia; Riopan low in sodium; do not give within 1 to 2 hours of H_2 receptor antagonists, tetracycline, or enteric-coated tablets.
	Calcium carbonate (Tums, Titralac)	PO	Constipation, gastric distention, rebound hyperacidity, hypercalcemia, and hypophosphatemia	Do not give with milk; monitor for symptoms of hypercalcemia and constipation; do not give within 1 to 2 hours of H_2 receptor antagonists, tetracycline, or enteric-coated tablets.
Mucosal Barrier Fortifiers In presence of mild acid condition, forms viscid and sticky gel and adheres to ulcer surface, forming a protective barrier.	Sucralfate (Carafate)	PO	Dizziness, constipation, sleepiness, nausea, and gastric discomfort	Take on an empty stomach, 1 hour before meals and at bedtime; monitor for constipation.

Handwritten annotations: "Blocks (to fix)", "can cause pill dissolved", "Coating them", "Bandaid", "test 1"

also be recommended, and foods known to cause discomfort to the patient, such as spicy foods, carbonated drinks, and caffeine, should be avoided until the ulcer heals. Alcohol should also be avoided during the healing period.

Complications

Major complications can result from PUD. These include bleeding, perforation, and obstruction. Bleeding can occur in varying degrees from occult blood in stool and emesis to massive bright red bleeding. Hemorrhage tends to occur more often with gastric ulcers in older adults. The patient may experience signs and symptoms of shock. Treatment includes stopping the bleeding, replacing fluid and electrolytes, and possibly administering vasopressin to stop the bleeding.

A perforated ulcer is a medical emergency and usually requires surgical intervention. Gastroduodenal contents escape through the perforation into the peritoneal cavity. This can result in peritonitis, septicemia, and hypovolemic shock. Perforation most often occurs with duodenal ulcers and presents with an acute onset of sharp, severe pain. Surgical treatment includes cleaning the peritoneal cavity, closing the perforation, and possibly a vagotomy and hemigastrectomy or pyloroplasty.

Obstruction may be due to scar tissue because of repeated ulcerations and healing in a patient with long-standing PUD. Obstruction frequently occurs at the pylorus causing pain at night and vomiting. A pyloroplasty is completed to correct the problem.

CRITICAL THINKING

Mr. Smith

■ Mr. Smith is a patient on your medical/surgical unit who has a duodenal ulcer. His wife runs to the nursing station and says that you need to help her husband, he is in terrible pain. As you enter the room, you see Mr. Smith curled up in a knee-chest position on the bed. He is crying and is complaining of excruciating abdominal pain.
1. What additional data would you like to gather?
2. What nursing actions would you complete?
3. What emotional support would you offer to Mrs. Smith?
4. What complication do you suspect Mr. Smith is experiencing?

Suggested answers at the end of chapter

Nursing Process for the Patient with Peptic Ulcer Disease

Assessment/Data Collection

The primary focus of nursing care for peptic ulcer disease is educating patients regarding the importance of this diagnosis because ulcers may be caused by an infection that can be cured with antibiotics. Patients may still believe that all ulcers are caused by stress, lifestyle, or diet. Assessing the patient's knowledge aids in providing accurate information to assist the patient in managing peptic ulcer disease. Data are also collected about the patient's disease history. Identifying factors that trigger or relieve symptoms is important.

The nurse should assess and monitor for complications of bleeding, such as occult blood in stool or emesis, perforation, including acute onset of severe pain, obstruction, changes in vital signs, and signs of shock

Nursing Diagnosis, Planning, Implementation, and Evaluation

See Box 33.6 Nursing Care Plan for the Patient with Peptic Ulcer Disease. The care plan should focus on the patient's understanding of the importance of taking all medication as directed, even if symptoms are gone. Patient noncompliance with treatment is a major cause of ulcer recurrence.

STRESS ULCERS
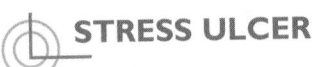

A small number of patients who are critically ill may develop gastric or small intestinal stress ulcers from ischemia. The stress response to the illness causes reduced blood flow to the stomach and small intestine, resulting in ischemia and damage to the mucosa. The damaged mucous barrier allows acid secretions to create ulcers. Preventive treatment has dramatically reduced stress ulcers, which have a high mortality rate because of the multiple bleeding ulcer sites. This treatment includes trauma care that quickly restores oxygen to the stomach, as well as early feeding within 24 hours of the trauma. Placement of a nasogastric (NG) tube allows testing of the gastric pH to ensure that it is higher than 5, as well as providing a means for enteral feeding. In addition, medications are given such as antacids and histamine blockers.

GASTRIC BLEEDING
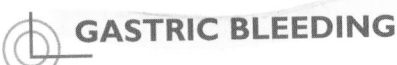

Gastric bleeding may be caused by ulcer perforation, tumors, gastric surgery, or other conditions. Bleeding peptic ulcers are the most common cause of blood loss into the stomach or intestine. Blood loss can be hidden (occult) blood in the stool, observable vomited blood (hematemesis), or black tarry stools (melena). When blood mixes with hydrochloric acid and enzymes in the stomach, a dark, granular material resembling coffee grounds is produced. This material can be vomited or passed through the GI system and mixed with stools. Melena occurs from slow bleeding in an upper GI area.

Signs and Symptoms

With mild bleeding, the patient may experience only slight weakness or diaphoresis (Table 33.5). Severe blood loss (more than 1 L in 24 hours) may result in hypovolemic shock, with signs and symptoms such as hypotension; a weak, thready pulse; chills; palpitations; and diaphoresis.

Box 33.6   NURSING CARE PLAN for the Patient with Peptic Ulcer Disease

Nursing Diagnosis: Acute pain related to gastric mucosal erosion

Expected Outcomes Patient's pain is relieved as evidenced by no report of pain and absence of nonverbal pain cues.

Evaluation of Outcomes Is pain relieved to patient's satisfaction?

Interventions	Rationale	Evaluation
Ask patient to rate pain level on scale of 0 to 10 every 3 hours and as needed. Note location, onset, intensity, characteristics of pain, and nonverbal pain cues.	Prompt assessment can lead to timely intervention and relief of pain.	Does patient rate pain using scale and describe pain?
Ask about for factors precipitating and relieving pain.	Peptic ulcer pain may be relieved by food, antacids, or other interventions.	Is patient able to state precipitating and relieving pain factors?
Ask patient to help identify techniques for pain relief.	Gaining the patient's cooperation increases compliance.	Is patient willing to participate in planning how to relieve pain?
Administer antiulcer medications as ordered.	H_2 receptor antagonists reduce amount of gastric acid produced, and antacids neutralize gastric acid to help relieve pain.	Do medications reduce patient's symptoms?
Provide small, frequent meals four to six times a day.	Small, frequent meals dilute and neutralize gastric acid.	Does patient report relief of gastric pain between meals?
Encourage nonacidic fluids between meals.	Nonacidic fluids decrease irritation to gastric mucosal.	Does patient identify and drink nonacidic fluids?

Nursing Diagnosis: Risk for injury related to complications of peptic ulcer activity such as hemorrhage and perforation

Expected Outcomes Patient's vital signs will be maintained within normal limits and bleeding or hemorrhage will be promptly detected.

Evaluation of Outcomes Are patient's vital signs within normal limits?

Interventions	Rationale	Evaluation
Monitor for signs and symptoms of hemorrhage such as hematemesis (vomiting blood) and melena (blood in the stool).	Rapid assessment can lead to prompt intervention.	Does patient have any bleeding?
Monitor vital signs: blood pressure, pulse, respirations, and temperature.	Severe blood loss of more than 1 L per 24 hours may cause manifestations of shock such as hypotension; weak, thready pulse; chills; palpitations; and diaphoresis.	Are vital signs normal?
Maintain intravenous infusion as ordered.	Normal fluid balance prevents hypovolemia and shock due to hemorrhage.	Are intake and output balanced?
Monitor hematocrit and hemoglobin levels as ordered.	Decreased hematocrit and hemoglobin levels indicate a decrease in circulating blood volume and reduced oxygen-carrying capacity to the tissues.	Are hematocrit and hemoglobin levels normal?

TABLE 33.5 GASTRIC BLEEDING SUMMARY

Signs and Symptoms	Occult blood in stool Hematemesis Melena Hypovolemic shock
Diagnostic Tests	Endoscopy Low hemoglobin and hematocrit
Therapeutic Interventions	Treat hypovolmic shock: NPO, IV fluids, oxygen therapy, NG tube Removal or ligation of bleeding area Medications to decrease gastric acid
Complications	Hypovolemic shock
Possible Nursing Diagnoses	Deficient fluid volume Risk for deficient fluid volume

Therapeutic Interventions

The goal of treatment for a massive GI bleed is to prevent or treat hypovolemic shock and prevent dehydration, electrolyte imbalance, and further bleeding. The patient is kept on nothing by mouth (NPO) status. An intravenous (IV) line is started to replace lost fluids and administer blood if necessary. A complete blood cell count is obtained to determine the amount of blood lost. A urinary catheter is inserted to monitor output. An NG tube is inserted to assess the rate of bleeding, decompress the stomach, monitor the pH of gastric secretions, and administer saline lavage if ordered. Oxygen therapy may be required if the patient has lost a large amount of blood. To prevent aspiration with vomiting, the head of the bed is elevated. The physician may perform endoscopy to help control the bleeding. Drugs may also be instilled into the GI tract by use of an endoscope. For severe cases, surgery may be needed to remove the bleeding area or ligate bleeding vessels. Drugs such as ranitidine (Zantac) are given to decrease the secretion of gastric acid.

Nursing Process for the Patient with Gastric Bleeding

Assessment/Data Collection

The nurse should assess patients at risk for bleeding for signs and symptoms of bleeding. Assess any emesis and stool for occult or obvious bleeding. Assess for signs of hypovolemic shock such as hypotension, tachycardia, tachypnea, chills, palpitations, and diaphoresis. The nurse should also assess for changes in level of consciousness, confusion, dry mucous membranes, reports of thirst, and fatigue which could indicate a decrease in circulating blood volume.

Nursing Diagnosis, Planning, and Implementation
Deficient fluid volume or risk for deficient fluid volume related to vomiting and diarrhea

EXPECTED OUTCOME: Vital signs remain within normal limits and balanced intake and output over 24 hours.
- Monitor color, amount, and frequency of fluid loss *to determine fluid balance changes.*
- Monitor vital signs and report abnormal findings *for prompt treatment.*
- Monitor level of consciousness, mucous membranes, and skin turgor *to assess for changes in fluid volume.*
- Obtain daily weights *to detect changes in fluid volume.*
- Offer oral fluids *to ensure adequate intake.*
- Monitor intravenous infusion as ordered *to prevent hypovolemia.*
- Monitor hematocrit and hemoglobin levels as ordered *to detect a decrease in circulating blood volume.*

Evaluation
If interventions have been effective, vital signs are within the normal range and the patient has a balanced intake and output over 24 hours.

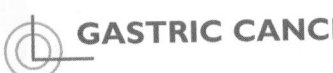

GASTRIC CANCER

Gastric cancer refers to malignant lesions found in the stomach. It is more common in men than in women. *H. pylori* infection plays a role in gastric cancer development. Studies are being done to see whether preventing *H. pylori* infection reduces the development of gastric cancer. Other factors that may be associated with gastric cancer development include pernicious anemia; exposure to occupational substances such as lead dust, grain dust, glycol ethers, or leaded gasoline; and a diet high in smoked fish or meats. A poor prognosis is often associated with gastric cancer because most patients have metastasis at the time of diagnosis (see Box 33.2 Nutrition Notes).

Signs and Symptoms

Gastric cancer is rarely diagnosed in its early stages because symptoms do not appear until late in the disease (Table 33.6). In the early stages, there may not be any symptoms at all, and metastasis to another organ, such as the liver, may have already occurred. The symptoms of gastric cancer are often mistaken for peptic ulcer disease: indigestion, anorexia, pain relieved by antacids, weight loss, and nausea and vomiting. Anemia from blood loss commonly occurs, and occult blood in the stool may be present.

Diagnosis

Diagnosis of gastric cancer is made by upper gastrointestinal x-ray examination, gastroscopy, gastric fluid analysis, and measurement of serum gastrin levels.

Therapeutic Interventions

There is little effective medical treatment available for gastric cancer. Surgical removal of the cancer is the most effective treatment for gastric cancer. Most often the cancer has already metastasized, and surgery is performed only to relieve the symptoms. Chemotherapy and radiation are sometimes used in conjunction with surgery, although they

TABLE 33.6 GASTRIC CANCER SUMMARY

Signs and Symptoms	Rarely detected during early stages Symptoms often mistaken for PUD: indigestion, anorexia, pain, weight loss, nausea, vomiting, anemia Late symptoms include involvement of other organs such as the liver
Diagnostic Tests	X-ray studies Gastroscopy Gastric fluid analysis Serum gastrin levels
Therapeutic Interventions	Medical treatment is not very effective Surgical treatment subtotal or total gastrectomy
Complications	Related to disease and surgery: hemorrhage, acute gastric distention, nutritional problems
Possible Nursing Diagnoses	Acute pain related to gastric erosion and postoperative pain Fear related to body image changes, treatment and life-threatening illness

are not very effective against the cancer. Biological therapies, new cytotoxic agents, and new delivery methods are being studied for use with gastric cancer. Total parenteral nutrition is a method for providing nutrition to the patient who has had a total gastrectomy.

GASTRIC SURGERIES

Subtotal Gastrectomy

Two types of surgical interventions are used to treat upper gastrointestinal diseases. The first type is the subtotal **gastrectomy,** which is used to treat cancer in the lower two-thirds of the stomach. *Subtotal gastrectomy* is a general term used to describe any surgery that involves partial removal of the stomach. There are two types of subtotal gastrectomies: the Billroth I procedure and the Billroth II procedure.

Billroth I Procedure (Gastroduodenostomy) *—subtotal*

In the Billroth I procedure, also known as a **gastroduodenostomy,** the surgeon removes the distal portion (75%) of the stomach (Fig. 33.6). The remainder of the stomach is anastomosed (surgically attached) to the duodenum. This procedure is used to treat gastric problems.

Billroth II Procedure

The Billroth II procedure, **gastrojejunostomy,** involves removal of the distal 50% of the stomach and reanastomosis

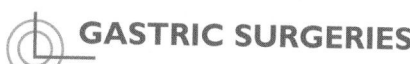

gastrectomy: gastr—stomach + ectomy—to remove
gastroduodenostomy: gastro—stomach + duoden—duodenum + ostomy—mouth or opening
gastrojejunostomy: gastro—stomach + jejeun—jejunum + ostomy—mouth or opening

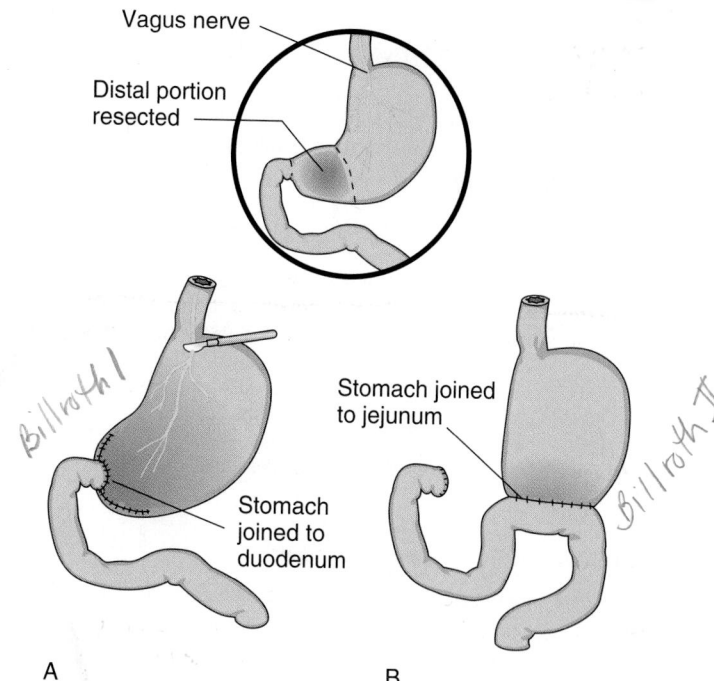

FIGURE 33.6 Subtotal gastrectomy involves removing the distal portion of the stomach. The remaining portion of the stomach is then sutured *(A)* to the duodenum (Billroth I procedure) or *(B)* to the proximal jejunum (Billroth II procedure). Vagotomy may also be performed.

need low carb diet

of the proximal remnant of the stomach to the proximal jejunum (see Fig. 33.6). Because it results in bypassing of the duodenum, the Billroth II procedure is used to treat duodenal ulcers. Pancreatic secretions and bile are necessary for digestion and continue to be secreted into the duodenum from the common bile duct even after the partial gastrectomy.

Total Gastrectomy

Total gastrectomy, the total removal of the stomach, is the treatment for extensive gastric cancer. This surgery involves removal of the stomach, with anastomosis of the esophagus to the jejunum (Fig. 33.7).

Vagotomy

A vagotomy, in which a section of the vagus nerve is cut, may be performed with gastric surgery. Vagotomy eliminates the vagal stimulation for hydrochloric acid and gastrin hormone secretion and slows gastric motility.

Nursing Process for the Patient Having Gastric Surgery

Assessment/Data Collection

The patient's vital signs are monitored postoperatively as ordered. Respiratory status is carefully monitored because the high location of the surgical incision may cause pain, which interferes with deep breathing and coughing. Atelectasis or pneumonia can develop as a result of guarding and shallow breathing. The patient's pain is assessed and relieved, which also helps the patient's ability to deep breathe or cough without pain. The patient's IV site and

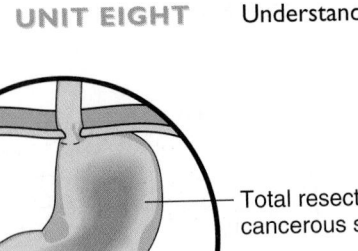

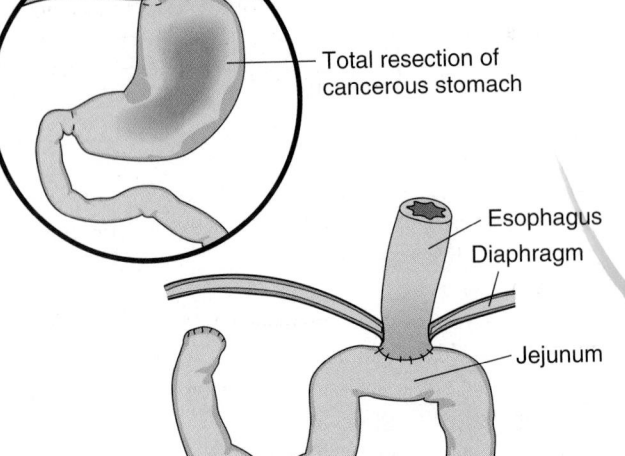

FIGURE 33.7 Total gastrectomy.

infusion are monitored, and intake and output are recorded. The incisional site and dressings are observed for drainage and bleeding.

Bowel sounds are assessed. Patients may have an NG tube inserted during surgery. The drainage from the NG tube is monitored for color and amount. If bleeding or excessive amounts of drainage are noted, they are reported to the physician. Assess the patient for abdominal distention.

Assess patient's reports of fear about the surgery and outcome of the surgery. The patient may report feeling of fear related to the uncertainty of the disease and surgery.

It is important to assess the patient's knowledge about postoperative care and discharge instructions. It is important to teach patients how to assist in their recovery. This includes incisional care, activity or dietary restrictions, and information about prescribed medications. Patients are encouraged to ambulate early to promote a quicker recovery by improving respiratory and gastrointestinal function.

Nursing Diagnosis, Planning, and Implementation
Acute pain related to postoperative pain

EXPECTED OUTCOME: Pain will be controlled or reduced to a tolerable level of 2 to 3 on a pain scale of 0 to 10.

- Evaluate pain regularly, noting characteristics, location, and intensity on pain scale of 0 to 10 *to provide information regarding patient's pain level and effectiveness of interventions.*
- Take vital signs (note if tachycardia, hypertension, or tachypnea is present), *which may indicate acute pain is present.*
- Provide comfort measures such as positioning every 2 hours and backrub *to improve circulation and reduce tension associated with pain.*

- Use relaxation techniques such as deep breathing, guided imagery, music, and distraction therapy *to enhance relaxation and improve pain relief.*
- Medicate as ordered on routine schedule for 24 to 48 hours *to control postoperative pain and prevent pain from becoming unbearable for patient.*
- Ensure functioning of NG tube (usually low-intermittent suction) *to prevent distention and increased pain.*
- Monitor incision noting any drainage, redness, swelling, or increased pain *to assess for postoperative infection, which can increase pain level.*
- Assess religion, culture, beliefs, and circumstances *to determine impact on patient's pain and response to interventions.*
- Instruct patient to inform nurse if adequate pain control is not achieved *to allow for revision of care plan.*
- Notify physician if pain control measures are unsuccessful.
- If NG tube is present, do not irrigate or reposition *to prevent damaging the suture line.*
- Encourage ambulation *to enhance respiratory and gastrointestinal function.*

Evaluation
If interventions have been effective, patient will report a reduction of pain to a tolerable level or total absence of pain.

Fear related to body image changes, treatment, and life-threatening illness

EXPECTED OUTCOME: Patient will understand and discuss disease process and treatment options and possible outcomes of treatment.

- Explain disease process and treatment options, reinforce as needed *to decrease patient's fear of the unknown.*
- Explain all postoperative procedures and interventions (such as medications, NG tube, drains) *to help decrease the patient's fear.*
- Use open communication and convey acceptance of patient's fears *to help patient cope with fears.*

Evaluation
If interventions are effective, the patient will verbalize understanding of the disease process, treatment options, and possible outcomes of treatment.

Complications of Gastric Surgery

Complications that can occur after gastric surgery include hemorrhage, acute gastric distention, nutritional problems, **steatorrhea** (fat in stools), pyloric obstruction, and dumping syndrome.

---

steatorrhea: steatos—fat + rrhea—profuse flow

Hemorrhage

The incidence of hemorrhage after gastric surgery is very low and is most often caused by a dislodged clot at the surgical site or slippage of a suture. The patient experiencing hemorrhage exhibits restlessness, cold skin, increased pulse and respirations, and decreased temperature and blood pressure. The patient may have a change in level of consciousness and become confused. In addition, the patient may vomit bright red blood. To prevent aspiration during vomiting, the patient is turned to one side and the head of the bed is elevated.

Following gastric surgery, patients usually have an NG tube that has been inserted in the operating room. The drainage from the tube should be assessed for color and amount. A small amount of pink or light red drainage may be expected for the first 12 hours, but moderate or excessive bleeding should be immediately reported to the physician. The abdominal dressing should also be assessed for any drainage or bleeding.

Gastric Distention

In the immediate postoperative period, distention of the stomach can occur if an inserted NG tube is clogged or if an NG tube has not been inserted. Symptoms of gastric distention include an enlarged abdomen, epigastric pain, tachycardia, and hypotension. The patient may complain of feeling full and may hiccup or gag repeatedly. These symptoms must be reported to the physician.

The physician usually inserts the NG tube during surgery so that the suture line is not damaged. If suction is desired, a physician's order is required. Irrigating or repositioning the NG tube is not performed by the nurse to prevent harm to the suture line. Any problems with distention or an improperly functioning NG tube are reported to the physician. The physician may need to reposition the NG tube to correct the problem. The patient's vital signs should be monitored until the patient's distention is relieved and the patient is stable.

CRITICAL THINKING

Mr. Wong

■ You are working the evening shift on a surgical unit. A patient, Mr. Wong, has had gastric surgery earlier that morning. He has an intravenous infusion of 1000 mL dextrose 5% 0.45 normal saline over 8 hours and a nasogastric tube to low intermittent wall suction. Mr. Wong is restless and complaining of pain. His bowel sounds are absent, and his abdomen is distended. The suction canister contains no gastric output.

1. What nursing interventions in order of priority are needed to help Mr. Wong?

2. What equipment do you need to care for Mr. Wong?

3. As you monitor the IV, you know it is set for how many drops per minute with a 10-drop factor IV set?

Suggested answers at end of chapter.

Nutritional Problems

Nutritional problems that commonly occur after removal of part or all of the stomach include B_{12} and folic acid deficiency and reduced absorption of calcium and vitamin D. Also, rapid entry of food into the bowel often results in inadequate absorption of food.

Following gastric surgery, patients are NPO until bowel sounds return (usually 24 to 48 hours) or the physician orders a diet. Intravenous fluid provides hydration. However, if patients are to be NPO for a longer time, they may need additional nutritional intake provided by total parenteral nutrition (TPN) through a central line. TPN is an intravenous solution given to meet caloric needs and provide fluids lost in drainage or emesis. Many patients with gastric cancer are malnourished and may require several days of TPN therapy.

After removal of the nasogastric tube, clear fluids may be ordered with progression to full liquids, then soft foods as the patient tolerates. Foods and fluids should be introduced into the diet gradually following gastric surgery. If the patient eats too much or too fast, regurgitation may result.

PERNICIOUS ANEMIA. Vitamin B_{12} deficiency can occur after some or all of the stomach is removed because intrinsic factor secretion is reduced or gone. Normally vitamin B_{12} combines with intrinsic factor to prevent its digestion in the stomach and promote its absorption in the intestines. The parenteral route has traditionally been used. However, vitamin B_{12} is also now available in oral tablets or as a nasal gel. Vitamin B_{12} injections are given daily initially, then weekly, and then monthly for life. Lifelong administration of vitamin B_{12} is required to prevent the development of pernicious anemia, and patients must be taught the importance of complying with this treatment. Symptoms of pernicious anemia include anemia, weakness, sore tongue, numbness and tingling, and gastrointestinal upset.

Steatorrhea

Steatorrhea is the presence of excessive fat in the stools and is the result of rapid gastric emptying, which prevents adequate mixing of fat with pancreatic and biliary secretions. In most cases, steatorrhea can be controlled by reducing the intake of fat in the diet.

Pyloric Obstruction

Pyloric obstruction can occur after gastric surgery as a result of scarring, edema, or inflammation or a combination of these. The signs and symptoms are vomiting, a feeling of fullness, gastric distention, nausea after eating, loss of appetite, and weight loss. As the obstruction increases, it gradually becomes more difficult for the stomach to empty, and symptoms worsen. Conservative methods are used first, such as replacing fluids and electrolytes through intravenous fluids and decompressing the distended stomach using a nasogastric tube. Surgery may be necessary if conservative measures do not relieve the signs and symptoms. Pyloroplasty widens the exit of the pylorus to improve emptying of the stomach.

Dumping Syndrome

Dumping syndrome occurs with the rapid entry of food into the jejunum without proper mixing of the food with digestive juices. On entering the jejunum, the food draws extracellular fluid into the bowel from the circulating blood volume to dilute the high concentration of electrolytes and sugars. This rapid shift of fluids decreases the circulating blood volume and produces symptoms. The symptoms occur 5 to 30 minutes after eating and include dizziness, tachycardia, fainting, sweating, nausea, diarrhea, a feeling of fullness, and abdominal cramping. Additionally, the blood sugar rises, and excessive insulin is excreted in response. This release of insulin causes the patient to have symptoms of hypoglycemia about 2 hours later. Symptoms include weakness, sweating, anxiety, shakiness, confusion, and tachycardia. The patient should immediately eat some candy or drink juice containing sugar to relieve the symptoms.

The treatment for dumping syndrome includes teaching the patient to eat small, frequent meals that are high in protein and fat and low in carbohydrates, especially refined sugars (see Box 33.2 Nutrition Notes). The patient is also taught to avoid fluids 1 hour before meals, with meals, or for 2 hours after meals to prevent rapid gastric emptying. It is best for the patient to lie down after meals to delay gastric emptying. The patient is told that these symptoms may last for up to 6 months after gastric surgery but usually slowly subside over time.

CRITICAL THINKING

Mrs. Lindsay

■ Mrs. Lindsay has had gastric surgery. You have taught her about dumping syndrome, and she is concerned about what she will eat. Create a 1-day meal plan for Mrs. Lindsay.

Suggested answers at end of chapter.

REVIEW QUESTIONS

1. The nurse is planning care for a patient with an eating disorder. The patient is 40 kg, and 68 inches tall. Serum laboratory data: potassium 2.6 mEq/dL, sodium 126 mEq/dL, chloride 95 mEq/dL, calcium 10.8 mg/dL. The nurse understands that which of the following is the most important intervention for this patient?
   a. Weigh the patient daily at the same time.
   b. Maintain IV of dextrose and electrolytes.
   c. Praise intake of any type of food.
   d. Document intake and output.

2. In planning care for patients, the nurse understands that which of the following patients are considered obese?
   a. A 25-year-old woman with body weight 5% above ideal body weight
   b. A 45-year-old man with waist to-hip ratio measurement of 0.5
   c. A 50-year-old man with body mass index of 31 kg/m^2
   d. A 16-year-old girl with anorexia nervosa weighing 45 kg.

3. A patient is diagnosed with aphthous stomatitis (canker sore). Which of the following actions would be appropriate?
   a. Tell patient to avoid brushing teeth until the sore has healed.
   b. Encourage patient to use a mouthwash four times a day.
   c. Apply acyclovir ointment to ease the pain of the lesion.
   d. Teach patient to apply topical tetracycline several times a day to sore.

4. The nurse is caring for a patient with gastritis. Which of the following interventions would be appropriate for a patient with gastritis?
   a. Administer phenothiazine to control vomiting.
   b. Instruct patient that medications such as aspirin rarely cause gastritis.
   c. Monitor patient for bloody diarrhea.
   d. Encourage a regular diet during the acute phase of gastritits.

5. The nurse is planning a teaching session for a patient with a peptic ulcer. Which of the following would the nurse include in the teaching plan as the primary cause of peptic ulcers?
   a. Eating spicy foods
   b. A stressful life
   c. A bacterial infection
   d. Excessive caffeine intake

6. After a teaching session for a patient with a peptic ulcer, the nurse would evaluate the patient as understanding the teaching if the patient stated the purpose of H$_2$ antagonists is which of the following?
   a. Neutralize gastric acid
   b. Form a protective paste
   c. Determine gastric pH levels
   d. Inhibit secretion of gastric acid

7. A patient who has just returned from surgery after a total gastrectomy begins to vomit bright red blood. Which of the following is a priority action for the nurse to take?

a. Increase the IV rate.
b. Take blood pressure.
c. Place patient on side.
d. Administer oxygen.

8. For the patient with dumping syndrome, which of these foods would the nurse instruct the patient to avoid?
   a. Spinach and avocado salad
   b. Coffee and glazed doughnut

c. Sausage and liver
d. Creamed chipped beef

Fill in the blank (calculation)

9. To deliver 1000 mL of 5% dextrose in 0.45 normal saline (at 150 ml per hour using 10 drop tubings), the nurse would monitor the IV infusion at how many drops per minute?

   _____ 25 _____ drops per minute

$$\frac{150mL}{60min} \times \frac{10\ gtts}{mL}$$

$$2.5 \cdot 10 = 25$$

References

1. Calvet, X, Ducons, J, Bujanda, L, et al: Seven versus ten days of rabeprazole triple therapy for *Helicobacter pylori* eradication: a multicenter randomized trial. Am J Gastroenterol 100:1696–1701, 2005.
2. Gene, EL, Calvet, X, Azagra, R, et al: Triple vs. quadruple therapy for treating *H. pylori* infection: a meta analysis. Aliment Pharmacol Therapeut 17:1137–1143, 2003.
3. Marzio, L, Cellini, L., and Anglucci, D: Triple therapy for 7 days vs. triple therapy for 7 days plus omeprazole for 21 days in treatment of active duodenal ulcer with *H. pylori* infection: a double blind placebo controlled study. Digest Liver Dis 35:20–23, 2003.
4. Ulmer, J, Beckerling, A, and Gatz, G: Recent use of proton pump inhibitor-based triple therapies for the eradication of *H. pylori*: A broad data review. Helicobacter 8:95–104, 2003.

SUGGESTED ANSWERS TO

CRITICAL THINKING

■ Mr. Smith

1. Additional data would include: vital signs: looking for signs of shock; assessment of Mr. Smith's abdomen: looking for location of pain, tenderness, rigidity; assess for any vomiting and characteristics of emesis including any blood; and assess for IV site access.

2. Assist Mr. Smith to a comfortable position and stay with him. Call for help. Inform the RN so the physician can be notified immediately and provide data regarding Mr. Smith's change in condition. Administer oxygen, monitor IV fluids, and continue to monitor vital signs. Medicate for pain as ordered.

3. Explain that you will stay with Mr. Smith as you gather data and take vital signs. State that you have informed the RN who will assess Mr. Smith and report findings to the physician now. Explain that the treatments as ordered by the physician will be started: oxygen, IV fluids, pain medication. State that explanations will be provided related to Mr. Smith's care. Invite questions and have nursing assistant provide Mrs. Smith with comfort needs: beverage, tissues, chair.

4. You suspect a perforated duodenal ulcer, which is a medical/surgical emergency.

■ Mr. Wong

1. Prioritize your interventions:
   a. Take Mr. Wong's vital signs to determine whether he is stable. Pain can sometimes increase the blood pressure and pulse rate. However, gastric distention can cause pain, and once the distention is relieved, the pain caused by distention subsides.
   b. Listen to Mr. Wong's bowel sounds. Manipulation of internal organs during abdominal surgery can produce a loss of normal peristalsis for 24 to 48 hours. Expect to hear absent or hypoactive bowel sounds for the first 1 or 2 days.
   c. Next, check placement of Mr. Wong's nasogastric tube by aspirating gastric contents and verifying pH of the contents as ordered. It is important to check for abdominal placement of Mr. Wong's nasogastric tube to make sure it is not misplaced in the lungs. After abdominal placement is determined, if there is a physician's order, the nasogastric tube can be connected to suction equipment, usually set on low intermittent suction.
   d. Next check the suction equipment for ordered settings and to ensure that it is turned on. The suction setting normally is ordered to be on low. A whistling sound is heard when the tube is disconnected from the suction setup. The seals should be tight on the suction canister. When the tubing is hooked to suction, gastric contents should be moving into the suction canister. It is important to make sure equipment is functioning properly to ensure patient safety.
   e. Check the nasogastric tube for clogs only if the physician orders aspiration or irrigation to be done. The tube is gently aspirated with a 60-mL catheter-tipped syringe. If the tube remains clogged, it is gently flushed as ordered with 10 to 20 mL of sterile normal saline.

f. After the gastric distention has been relieved, Mr. Wong's pain level is reassessed to determine if he needs pain medication. Considering that he is less than 1 day postoperative, he probably needs it.

2. Necessary equipment includes stethoscope, 60-mL catheter-tipped syringe, gloves, goggles, and normal saline for irrigation.

3.

$$\frac{1000 \text{ mL} \times 10 \text{ drops/mL}}{(60 \times 8) = 480 \text{ min}}$$

$$= \frac{10{,}000 \text{ drops}}{480 \text{ min}} = 21 \text{ drops/min}$$

■ *Mrs. Lindsay*

Although there are many variations, the following is an example of a 1-day meal plan for Mrs. Lindsay:

Breakfast: one egg, any style; 1/2 orange; one glass milk

Snack: one slice toast with apple butter, jelly, or jam

Lunch: 2 oz ham, 1/2 cup cottage cheese, four asparagus spears

Snack: 1/2 serving chicken salad on bed of lettuce

Dinner: 2 oz broiled fish, 1/2 serving corn, 1/2 serving broccoli

Snack: 1/2 cup yogurt or sherbet

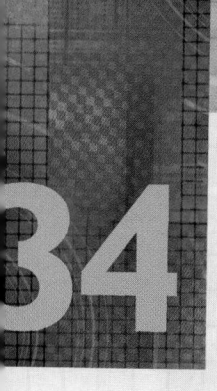

34

Nursing Care of Patients with Lower Gastrointestinal Disorders

LINDA S. WILLIAMS, VIRGINIA BIRNIE, AND RUTH REMINGTON

KEY TERMS

appendicitis (uh-PEN-di-SIGH-tis)
colectomy (koh-LEK-tuh-me)
colitis (koh-LYE-tis)
colostomy (koh-LAH-stuh-me)
constipation (KON-sti-PAY-shun)
diarrhea (DYE-uh-REE-ah)
diverticulitis (DYE-ver-tik-yoo-LYE-tis)
diverticulosis (DYE-ver-tik-yoo-LOH-sis)
enteritis (en-ter-EYE-tis)
fissures (FISH-ers)
fistulas (FIST-yoo-lahs)
hematochezia (HEM-uh-toh-KEE-zee-uh)
hemorrhoids (HEM-uh-royds)
hernia (HER-nee-uh)
ileostomy (ILL-ee-AH-stuh-me)
impaction (im-PAK-shun)
intussusception (IN-tuh-suh-SEP-shun)
megacolon (MEG-ah-KOH-lun)
melena (muh-LEE-nah)
obstipation (OB-sti-PAY-shun)
peristomal (PER-i-STOH-muhl)
peritonitis (per-i-toh-NIGH-tis)
stoma (STOH-mah)
volvulus (VOL-view-lus)

QUESTIONS TO GUIDE YOUR READING

1. What are the causes, signs, and symptoms of constipation and diarrhea?

2. What nursing care and teaching do patients with constipation or diarrhea require?

3. What medical treatment, nursing care, and teaching are appropriate for patients with inflammatory and infectious disorders of the lower gastrointestinal tract?

4. How would you describe Crohn's disease, ulcerative colitis, irritable bowel syndrome, and the nursing care for these conditions?

5. What is nursing care for abdominal hernias?

6. What nursing care and teaching do patients with absorption disorders require?

7. What are the causes, signs and symptoms, therapeutic interventions and nursing care of intestinal obstruction?

8. What are therapeutic interventions and nursing care for lower gastrointestinal bleeding?

9. What are the causes, signs and symptoms, therapeutic interventions, and nursing care of colon cancer?

10. What nursing care and teaching does a patient with an ostomy require?

The lower gastrointestinal (GI) system includes the small and large intestines, rectum, and anus.

 PROBLEMS OF ELIMINATION

Constipation

Pathophysiology

Constipation occurs when the fecal mass is held in the rectal cavity for a period that is not usual for the patient. While the feces are held for a prolonged time in the rectum, more water is absorbed, making the feces drier, harder, more difficult to pass, and sometimes painful to pass.

If a patient repeatedly ignores the urge to have a bowel movement (laxation), the musculature and rectal mucous membrane become insensitive to the presence of feces. Eventually a stronger stimulus is needed to produce the peristaltic rush required for defecation. Prolonged constipation is called **obstipation.**

Etiology

There are many causes of constipation. Medications such as narcotics, tranquilizers, and antacids with aluminum decrease motility of the large intestine and may contribute to constipation. Rectal or anal conditions such as **hemorrhoids** or **fissures** may lead to a delay in defecation because of the associated pain. Metabolic or neurological conditions such as diabetes mellitus, multiple sclerosis, lupus erythematosus, or scleroderma may interfere with normal bowel innervation and function. Colon cancer may cause an obstruction that prevents normal bowel function and leads to constipation. Low intake of dietary fiber and fluids decreases the bulk of the feces and causes constipation. Decreased mobility, weakness, and fatigue, especially in the elderly, reduce the strength of the muscles used for defecation, increasing the likelihood of constipation. Chronic laxative use can also contribute to constipation because the laxative overrides the bowel's ability to recognize the urge to defecate.

Prevention

Regular exercise and a diet high in fiber and fluids are the best preventive measures for constipation. Laxatives should be used only occasionally to prevent dependence and complications.

Signs and Symptoms

Abdominal pain and distention, indigestion, rectal pressure, a sensation of incomplete emptying, and intestinal rumbling are indications of constipation (Table 34.1). The patient may also complain of headache, fatigue, decreased appetite, straining at stool, and elimination of hard, dry stool.

Complications

A variety of problems can result from constipation. Fecal **impaction** may result when the fecal mass is so dry it cannot be passed. Pressure on the colon mucosa from a mass of stool may cause ulcers to develop. Often, small amounts of liquid stool ooze around the fecal mass and cause inconti-

TABLE 34.1   CONSTIPATION SUMMARY

Signs and Symptoms	Abdominal distention
	Indigestion
	Rectal pressure
	Feeling of incomplete emptying
	Straining at stool
	Hard, dry stool
	Intestinal rumbling
Diagnostic Tests	History
	Physical examination
Therapeutic Interventions	High-fiber diet
	2–3 L fluid daily
	Strengthening of abdominal muscles
	Exercise
	Bulk-forming agents
	Stool softeners
Nursing Diagnosis	Constipaton
	Deficient knowledge

nence of liquid stools. The incontinence may be treated with an antidiarrheal medication, which will worsen the constipation if a thorough assessment is not performed to rule out impaction. Straining to have a bowel movement (Valsalva's maneuver) can result in cardiac, neurological, and respiratory complications. If the patient has a history of heart failure, hypertension, or recent myocardial infarction, straining can lead to cardiac rupture and death. Grossly dilated loops of the colon, known as **megacolon,** can occur proximal to the dry fecal mass and obstruct the colon. Abdominal distention occurs, and in severe cases, loops of bowel can be palpated through the abdominal wall.

Chronic laxative abuse can lead to colonic mucosal atrophy, muscle thickening, and fibrosis. These conditions can result in perforation of the colon and necessitate an emergency **colectomy.**

Diagnostic Tests

Constipation is usually self-diagnosed or diagnosed by history and physical examination. If complications are suspected, a radiographic examination, sigmoidoscopy, and stool testing for occult blood may be necessary.

Therapeutic Interventions

Treatment of constipation depends on the cause. Fiber should be added to the diet, and exercises to strengthen abdominal muscles should be done. Behavior changes, such as setting a daily defecation time, appropriately responding to the urge to defecate, and drinking 8 oz of warm water every morning and 2 to 3 L of water every day, if it is not contraindicated for other reasons, can help establish a more normal bowel pattern. Chronic laxative use should be discontinued. Bulk-forming agents such as psyllium (Metamucil) or stool softeners such as docusate sodium (Colace) should be used

---

megacolon: mega—large + colon—colon
colectomy: col—pertaining to colon + ectomy—surgical excision

instead of laxatives. Enemas and rectal suppositories are used only in extreme cases and are discontinued when an acute episode is resolved. A new medication, methylnaltrexone (MNTX), is under study and may be available in the future for use with palliative care patients to treat constipation from opioid use.

Nursing Process for the Patient with Constipation

ASSESSMENT/DATA COLLECTION. The patient may feel self-conscious or embarrassed when interviewed about bowel habits and history. Consideration should be given to the patient's feelings by postponing the discussion until rapport has been established. The nursing history should include the onset and duration of constipation, past elimination pattern, current elimination pattern, occupation, lifestyle (stress, exercise, nutrition), history of laxative or enema use, medical-surgical history, and current medications being taken. The color, consistency, and odor of the stool, as well as any intestinal symptoms, are also important.

After the interview, the patient's abdomen is inspected and palpated for distention and symmetry. Inspection of the perianal area may reveal fissures, external hemorrhoids, or irritation.

NURSING DIAGNOSIS, PLANNING, AND IMPLEMENTATION. Constipation related to irregular defecation habits

EXPECTED OUTCOME: The patient will maintain passage of soft, formed stool every 1 to 3 days without straining.

- Assess normal pattern of defecation, diet and fluid intake, medications, surgeries, and use of laxatives *to help identify factors contributing to constipation.*
- Setting a specific time for defecation, such as after a meal *to facilitate the urge reflex.*
- Place feet on a footstool *to promote flexion of the hips to aid defecation.*
- For constipation caused by decreased motility and muscle tone or a low-fiber diet, a high-fiber, high-residue diet including fresh fruits, vegetables, and whole grains with 2 g of bran added to cereal daily can be eaten *to significantly increase bowel movements and decrease the number of laxatives, enemas, or stool softeners required* (Box 34.1 Nutrition Notes).
- Increase activity through a daily walking program and abdominal exercises designed to improve the muscle tone *to improve peristalsis and promote more spontaneous defecation.*
- Determine patient's access to the bathroom and ability to use the toilet *to ensure barriers to safe toileting, such as unsafe obstructing furniture arrangement or clutter are removed.*
- Increase exercise, fluid if not contraindicated to 2 to 3 L per day, and fiber in the diet *to aid in ability to discontinue laxative use.*

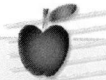

Box 34.1

Nutrition Notes

Treating Constipation with Food Formula

Constipation may be successfully treated with 1 to 2 oz of the following mixture taken with the evening meal: 1 cup applesauce, 1 cup All-Bran cereal, and $\frac{1}{2}$ cup 100% prune juice. Mixture may be stored in the refrigerator for 5 days and then should be discarded. In all cases of constipation, especially when increased fiber is given, adequate fluid intake is essential.

Deficient knowledge related to practices to prevent constipation

EXPECTED OUTCOME: The patient will state understanding and ability to carry out preventive measures for constipation.

- Teach factors leading to constipation and preventive interventions such as increasing fluid intake. *Prevention of constipation may be as simple as correcting the contributing factors.*
- Explain the physiology of defecation and the reason for obeying the urge to defecate when it occurs. *Patient and caregiver education is one of the most important aspects of treatment of constipation.*
- Assure the patient that having a daily bowel movement is not always necessary. *The patient who believes that a daily bowel movement is absolutely necessary needs information and reassurance.*
- Explain that regular laxative use may increase motility and pressure in the bowel and cause further complications *to promote understanding and use of other preventive measures.*

EVALUATION. The plan has been effective if the patient has established a regular bowel function pattern (Table 34.2), and verbalizes understanding of self-care measures and expresses satisfaction with the outcomes.

CRITICAL THINKING

Mrs. Burns

■ Mrs. Burns is a 93-year-old nursing home resident. You see on her chart that she has not had a bowel movement in 5 days. What action would you take?

Suggested answers at end of chapter.

Diarrhea

Diarrhea occurs when fecal matter passes through the intestine rapidly, resulting in decreased absorption of water, elec-

---

diarrhea: dia—through + rhea—to flow

TABLE 34.2 CRITERIA FOR REGULAR BOWEL FUNCTION

1. A regular time for defecation is routine.
2. A regular exercise program is followed.
3. Laxative use is avoided.
4. Water consumption is 2–3 L per day.
5. High-fiber and high-residue foods are added to the diet.
6. Consistency of stools reported are soft and formed.
7. Frequency of stools is every 1 to 3 days.

trolytes, and nutrients and causing frequent, watery stools. Classification and severity of diarrhea are based on the number of unformed stools in 24 hours. Large-volume diarrhea occurs when the volume of feces is increased. Small-volume diarrhea is caused by an increase in peristalsis, without an increase in fecal volume.

Pathophysiology and Etiology

The most common cause of acute diarrhea is a bacterial or viral infection. Bacteria (normal flora) are normally found in the intestines. If these bacteria grow out of control or if bacteria or viruses are ingested in contaminated food or water, infection results. Some bacteria release toxins that irritate the intestinal mucosa, causing an inflammatory response and an increase in mucus production. Hyperperistalsis occurs, which lasts until the irritants have been excreted. The most common infectious agents are *Escherichia coli*, *Campylobacter jejuni*, *Shigella* spp., *Clostridium difficile*, *Giardia* spp., and *Salmonella* spp.

Poor tolerance or allergies to certain foods may cause diarrhea. Foods that most commonly cause diarrhea are additives (such as nutmeg or sorbitol), caffeine, milk products, meats, wheat, and potatoes. Acute diarrhea usually resolves in 7 to 14 days.

Chronic diarrhea may result from inflammatory disease, osmotic agents, excessive secretion of electrolytes, or increased intestinal motility. Inflammatory diseases such as Crohn's disease or ulcerative **colitis** (discussed later) may impair absorption, resulting in frequent, watery stools. Osmotic diarrhea results from ingestion of laxatives or other agents that prevent absorption of water or nutrients in the intestine. Additional causes of malabsorption include surgical resection or disease of certain areas of the intestinal tract, such as the terminal ileum or pylorus. Radiation therapy for cancer also may induce a malabsorption syndrome. Enteral tube feedings commonly result in diarrhea, especially when malnutrition has caused edema in the gut wall, which decreases absorption.

Increased secretion of water and electrolytes by the intestinal mucosa associated with certain hormonal disorders results in high-volume fecal output. An irritable bowel or a neurological disorder may cause increased motility problems. Also, as described earlier, diarrhea can indicate fecal impaction.

---

colitis: col—pertaining to colon + itis—inflammation

Prevention

Proper handling, storage, and refrigeration of all fresh foods minimize contact with infectious agents. Milk and milk products must be kept refrigerated and protected. Hand washing and cleaning of the kitchen and food preparation or serving items are extremely important.

It is best to start enteral feedings slowly with full-strength formula and gradually increase the rate rather than dilute the formula, thus reducing the risk of contaminating the formula by adding to it.

Signs and Symptoms

Initial diarrheal stools are foul smelling and may have undigested food particles and mucus. The stools may also contain blood or pus. Diarrhea resulting from food poisoning usually has an explosive onset and may be accompanied by nausea and vomiting. Abdominal cramping, distention, anorexia, intestinal rumbling, and thirst are common. Fever indicates infection. Weakness and dehydration from fluid loss may occur (Box 34.2 Gerontological Issues).

Diagnostic Tests

The diagnosis of diarrhea is determined by the onset and progression of the disease, absence or presence of fever, laboratory examinations, and visual inspection of the stool. Evidence of bacteria, pus, and blood is checked. Diarrhea mixed with red blood cells and mucus is associated with cholera, typhoid, typhus, large-bowel cancer, or amebiasis. Diarrhea mixed with white blood cells and mucus is associated with shigellosis, intestinal tuberculosis, salmonellosis, regional enteritis, or ulcerative colitis. Bulky, frothy stool is seen in sprue and celiac disease. Pasty stools

---

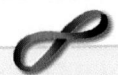

Box 34.2

Gerontological Issues

Diarrhea can cause older people to quickly become dehydrated and hypokalemic because both fluid and potassium are lost in stools. The signs and symptoms of hypokalemia include muscle weakness, hypotension, anorexia, paresthesia, and drowsiness. It can also cause cardiac dysrhythmias, such as atrial and ventricular tachycardia, premature ventricular contraction, and ventricular fibrillation, which can be fatal.

If the older person has decreased mobility, quick access to the bathroom is important. Because of poor muscle control, older patients may be incontinent. This might embarrass patients or cause them to hurry, which increases chances of patients falling and causing other problems such as fracture, dislocation, or hematoma. Also, because older patients' skin is more sensitive resulting from poor turgor and a reduction in subcutaneous fat layers, perirectal skin excoriation can occur secondary to the acidity and digestive enzyme content of diarrheal stools.

usually have a high fat content and may be associated with common bile duct obstruction, sprue, and celiac disease. A "butter stool" appearance is seen in patients with cystic fibrosis.

Therapeutic Interventions

Replacing fluids and electrolytes is the first priority. This is done by increasing oral fluid intake, using solutions with glucose and electrolytes if ordered by the physician. Intravenous fluid replacement may be necessary for rapid hydration, especially in the very young or very old. An elimination diet can be tried to identify foods that may contribute to diarrhea. Foods known to cause diarrhea are eliminated to see if a change in bowel function occurs. Each food item is then added back into the diet, one at a time, to see which ones cause diarrhea. The patient is also encouraged to increase fiber and bulk in the diet.

If the patient has three or more watery stools per day, motility of the intestines can be decreased with the use of drugs, such as diphenoxylate (Lomotil), difenoxin HCl (Motofen), and loperamide (Imodium). If diarrhea is thought to be caused by antibiotics that change the normal flora of the bowel, a *Lactobacillus* granules dietary supplement (Lactinex) may be used to restore the normal flora. Antimicrobial agents are prescribed if infectious agents have been documented.

Nursing Process for the Patient with Diarrhea

ASSESSMENT/DATA COLLECTION. Observation of the patient's behavior and symptoms assists in identifying the cause of diarrhea. Ask the patient to describe any symptoms, when they started, and how long they have been present. Questions should include "Is there any abdominal pain, urgency, or cramping?" and "What time of the day does it happen?" Stool consistency, color, odor, and frequency are documented.

The abdomen is inspected for distention. The patient's usual dietary habits and any changes or recent exposure to contaminated food or water is assessed. Find out if any medications contributed to the diarrhea. If the patient has traveled recently, discover the geographical location and whether exposure to an infected person or someone with similar symptoms occurred.

Assess for symptoms of dehydration, such as tachycardia, hypotension, decreased skin turgor, weakness, thready pulse, dry mucous membranes, and oliguria. Abnormal laboratory studies that may indicate dehydration include increased serum osmolality, increased specific gravity of urine, and increased hematocrit. Decreased serum potassium may result from intestinal loss of potassium.

Data are collected on the patient's coping mechanisms for use if the patient needs to express concerns or anxiety regarding incontinence of liquid stools and embarrassment.

NURSING DIAGNOSIS, PLANNING, AND IMPLEMENTATION. Diarrhea related to infection or possible ingestion of irritating foods

EXPECTED OUTCOME: The patient will maintain formed, soft stool every 1 to 3 days.

- Obtain history including medications regarding diarrhea episode *to help identify cause.*
- Monitor and record stool characteristics, amount, and frequency *to plan care.*
- During acute diarrhea nothing is taken by mouth (NPO) *to promote bowel rest.*
- Give antidiarrheal medications as ordered. *Controlling diarrhea controls comfort and fluid balance.*
- Provide clear liquids, such as water, juices, bouillon, and gelatin, with progression to a low-residue diet when acute diarrhea phase is over (Box 34.3 Nutrition Notes).
- Limit caffeine intake *as it stimulates intestinal motility.*
- Keep skin clean, dry, and protected with a moisture barrier, such as petrolatum or medicated ointment,

---

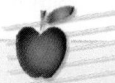

Box 34.3

Nutrition Notes

Deciding When to Refer an Adult with Diarrhea for Medical Care

Most instances of diarrhea in healthy adults are self-limiting and resolve without treatment. Indications for medical consultation include the following:

- Large volumes of stool
- Severe abdominal pain
- Bloody stools
- Protracted duration
- Systemic symptoms such as fever or prostration
- Medical conditions for which fasting, dehydration, or infectious disease are hazardous

Healthy adults at minimal risk of electrolyte imbalance may institute self-treatment as follows:

- For the first 12 hours: Water or oral rehydration solutions at room temperature. Easily absorbed fluids maintain hydration. Hot or cold liquids are more likely to stimulate peristalsis.
- For the second 12 hours: Clear liquids, no caffeine or extremes of temperature. If more than 5% of body weight is lost, seek medical attention.
- For the third 12 hours: Full liquids. Experiment with milk in case temporary lactose intolerance has developed as a result of intestinal inflammation.
- For the fourth 12 hours: Soft diet. Include applesauce or banana for pectin and also rice, pasta, and bread without fat (digested by enzymes usually unaffected in gastroenteritis).
- By the 48th hour: Regular diet. If diarrhea has not resolved and regular diet is not tolerated, seek medical treatment.

after each bowel movement *to protect perianal skin from contact with liquid stools and their enzymes.*
- Consider private patient room *to prevent infection transmission.*
- Identify potentially infected persons or contaminated foods *to prevent the spread of infection.*
- Ensure hand washing by patient, family, and healthcare staff *to prevent the spread of infection.*

Risk for deficient fluid volume related to frequent passage of stools and insufficient fluid intake

EXPECTED OUTCOME: The patient will maintain vital signs and urine output within normal limits.
- Intake and output (including diarrheal stools) are recorded *to determine fluid balance.*
- Weight patient daily *to determine fluid loss.*
- If output is greater than intake, intravenous fluid replacement may be ordered *to maintain fluid*
- balance.
- Encourage fluids when acute diarrhea subsides *to maintain fluid balance.*
- Teach patient signs and symptoms of dehydration to report *to allow prompt treatment.*

EVALUATION. Goals have been met if frequency of diarrheal stools is decreased and fluid and electrolyte balance is achieved.

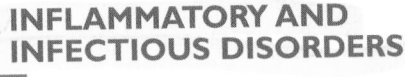

INFLAMMATORY AND INFECTIOUS DISORDERS

Many diseases of the lower GI tract are a result of inflammation in the bowel. Sometimes the inflamed areas become infected, resulting in a worsening of symptoms and necessitating antimicrobial therapy.

Appendicitis

Pathophysiology
Appendicitis is the inflammation of the appendix, the small, fingerlike appendage attached to the cecum of the large intestine. Because of the small size of the appendix, obstruction may occur, making it susceptible to infection. The resulting inflammatory process causes an increase in intraluminal pressure of the appendix.

Signs and Symptoms
Signs and symptoms of appendicitis include fever, increased white blood cells, and generalized pain in the upper abdomen. Within hours of onset the pain usually becomes localized to the right lower quadrant at McBurney's point, midway between the umbilicus and the right iliac crest (Fig.

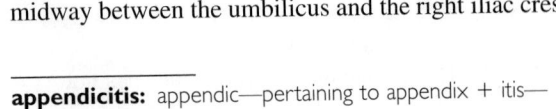
appendicitis: appendic—pertaining to appendix + itis—inflammation

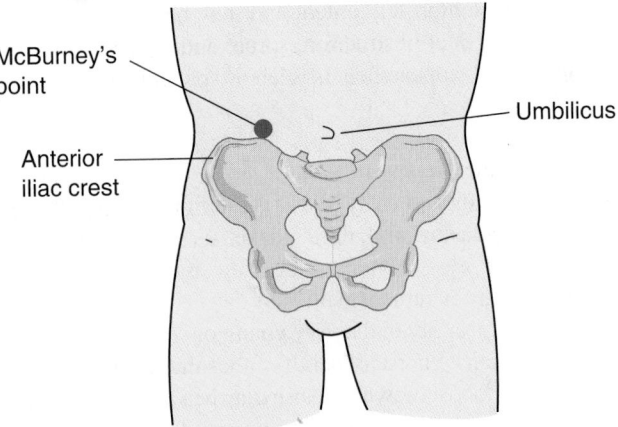

FIGURE 34.1 Pain at McBurney's point is a symptom of appendicitis.

34.1). This is one of the classic symptoms of appendicitis. Nausea, vomiting, and anorexia are also usually present.

Physical examination reveals slight abdominal muscular rigidity (guarding), normal bowel sounds, and local rebound tenderness (intensification of pain when pressure is released after palpation) in the right lower quadrant of the abdomen. Sometimes there is pain in the right lower quadrant when the left lower quadrant is palpated (Rovsing's sign). The patient may keep the right leg flexed for comfort and experience increased pain if the leg is straightened.

Diagnostic Tests
A complete blood cell count (CBC) reveals elevated leukocyte and neutrophil counts. Ultrasound or computed tomographic (CT) scan reveals an enlargement in the area of the cecum.

Therapeutic Interventions
The patient is kept NPO and surgery is done immediately unless there is evidence of perforation or peritonitis. Ice to the site of pain and maintaining semi-Fowler's position may help reduce pain while the diagnosis is being made. The patient is often readied for an appendectomy by emergency department staff.

If the appendix has ruptured, intravenous fluids and antibiotic therapy are started and surgery may be delayed for 8 hours or more. Laxatives and enemas are avoided because they may trigger or complicate a rupture. The use of a heating pad on the abdomen is avoided because the warmth may increase inflammation and risk of rupture.

After surgery, the patient is usually NPO until GI functioning returns, and if the appendix has ruptured, the patient may have an orogastric or nasogastric tube placed to decompress the stomach. When bowel function returns, the diet initially consists of clear fluids and is advanced as tolerated by the patient. Vital signs and abdominal data are collected to monitor for signs and symptoms of peritonitis. Pain control to promote early ambulation, coughing, deep breathing, and turning help prevent respiratory complications.

Complications

Perforation, abscess of the appendix, and peritonitis are major complications of appendicitis. With perforation, the pain is severe and the temperature is elevated to at least 37.7°C (100°F). An abscess is a localized collection of pus separated from the peritoneal cavity by the omentum or small bowel. This is usually treated with parenteral antibiotics and surgical drainage. An appendectomy is done about 6 weeks later.

Peritonitis

Peritonitis is inflammation of the peritoneum that occurs from a variety of causes. It is a serious condition that can be life threatening.

Pathophysiology and Etiology

Trauma, ischemia, or tumor perforation in any abdominal organ causes leakage of the organ's contents into the peritoneal cavity. The most common cause of peritonitis is a ruptured appendix, but it may also occur after perforation of a peptic ulcer, gangrenous gallbladder, intestinal diverticula, incarcerated **hernia,** or gangrenous small bowel. It may also be a complication of peritoneal dialysis. Peritonitis results from the inflammation or infection that is caused by the leakage. The tissues become edematous and begin leaking fluid containing increasing amounts of blood, protein, cellular debris, and white blood cells. Initially, the intestinal tract responds with hypermotility, but this is soon followed by paralysis (paralytic ileus). *no bowel sounds*

Signs and Symptoms

Generalized abdominal pain evolves into localized pain at the site of the perforation or leakage. The area of the abdomen that is affected is extremely tender and aggravated by movement. Rebound tenderness and abdominal rigidity are present. Decreased peristalsis results in nausea and vomiting. Infection causes fever, increased white blood cells, and an elevated pulse. *(hard rigided Board Like -abdoman)*

Therapeutic Interventions

The patient is NPO because of the impaired peristalsis. Fluid and electrolyte replacement is crucial to correct hypovolemia. Abdominal distention is relieved through insertion of an orogastric (or nasogastric) tube with low intermittent suction. Antibiotics are used to treat or prevent sepsis. Depending on the cause of the peritonitis, surgery may be performed to excise, drain, or repair the cause. An ostomy may be formed to divert feces, allowing resolution of the infection. After surgery, the patient usually has a wound drain, a nasogastric (NG) tube, and a urinary catheter. Pain control is essential to overall recovery. Severely compromised patients may receive total parenteral nutrition (TPN) to meet nutritional needs for increased immune function and healing.

Complications

Complications of peritonitis are intestinal obstruction (discussed later), hypovolemia caused by the shift of fluid into the abdomen, and septicemia from bacteria entering the bloodstream. Shock and ultimately death may result. Wound dehiscence or evisceration can occur if the patient has had abdominal surgery.

Diverticulosis and Diverticulitis

Pathophysiology

A diverticulum is a herniation or outpouching of the bowel mucous membrane caused by increased pressure within the colon and weakness in the bowel wall. **Diverticulosis** is a condition in which multiple diverticula are present without evidence of inflammation (Fig. 34.2). Many people have diverticulosis without knowing it because it develops gradually. When food and bacteria are trapped in a diverticulum, inflammation and infection develop. This is called **diverticulitis.**

Etiology

Chronic constipation usually precedes the development of diverticulosis by many years. When the patient is chroni-

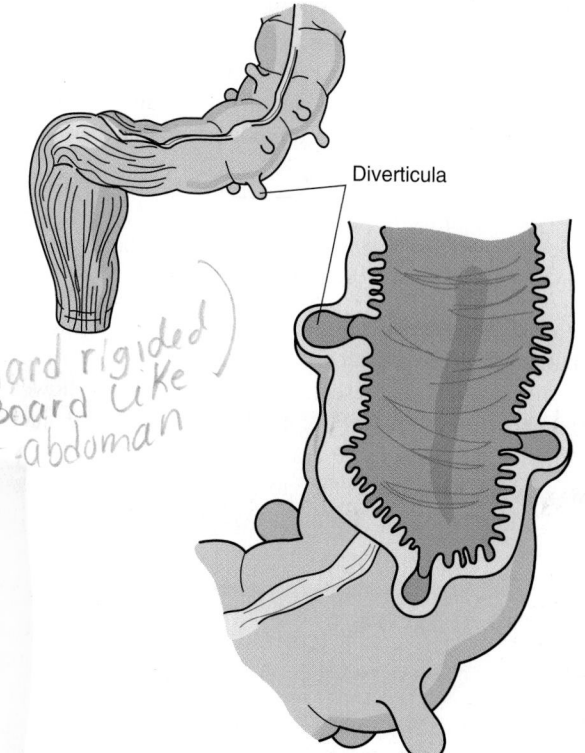

Diverticula

FIGURE 34.2 A diverticulum is a herniation or outpouching of the bowel mucous membrane. Multiple diverticula are called diverticulosis. If they become inflamed or infected, the condition is called diverticulitis.

---

peritonitis: periton—pertaining to peritoneum + itis— inflammation

diverticulosis: diverticul—blind pouch + osis—condition
diverticulitis: diverticul—blind pouch + itis—inflammation

TABLE 34.3 SYMPTOMS ASSOCIATED WITH DIVERTICULITIS

W—Where is the pain?	Usually in the left lower quadrant
H—How does it feel? (Describe quality)	Tender, crampy
A—Aggravating and alleviating factors	Constipation and low-fiber diet may aggravate; treatment of constipation may alleviate
T—Timing (onset, duration, frequency)	Gradual onset, intermittent, gradual increase in frequency of pain events
S—Severity (0–10)	Usually 5–7
U—Useful other data/ associated symptoms	Intermittent rectal bleeding; straining at stool; constipation alternating with diarrhea; elevated white blood cells and sedimentation rate; elevated temperature and pulse rate; and pus, mucus, and blood in stool
P—Patient's perception	Fear diagnosis of cancer

cally constipated, pressure within the bowel is increased, leading to development of diverticula. A major cause of the disease is a decreased intake of dietary fiber. Diverticulosis is most common in the sigmoid colon. A small percentage of patients with diverticulosis develop diverticulitis. People older than age 60 are the most common group to experience diverticulitis.

Prevention

Diverticulitis can be prevented by increasing dietary fiber to prevent constipation and onset of diverticulosis.

Signs and Symptoms

The patient with diverticulosis is generally asymptomatic. When diverticulitis is present, the patient exhibits bowel changes, possibly alternating between constipation and diarrhea (Table 34.3). Steady or crampy pain in the left lower quadrant of the abdomen is the most common symptom. As the condition worsens, bleeding may occur, along with

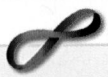

Box 34.4

Gerontological Issues

With age-related weakness in the intestinal wall, approximately 40% of adults older than age 80 have diverticular disease. Clinical manifestation of this condition may include abdominal pain, rectal bleeding, nausea, and vomiting. Patients may not notice the abdominal pain until infection is present. Many times the symptoms are not reported early because patients fear it may be cancer. Blood in the stool, which can be an indication of diverticulitis, may not be seen by the older adult due to impaired vision.

weakness, fever, fatigue, and anemia. Guarding and rebound tenderness may be present. If an abscess develops, the diverticulum may rupture, leading to peritonitis (Box 34.4 Gerontological Issues).

Diagnostic Tests

Diverticulosis is confirmed with sigmoidoscopy, colonoscopy, or barium enema. The diverticula and specific areas of inflammation can be seen during a colonoscopy or sigmoidoscopy. If an abscess is suspected, a CT scan may be done. Barium enema may show irregular narrowing of the colon and thickened muscle walls. A stool specimen may show occult blood. An abdominal x-ray examination may be done to identify a perforated diverticulum.

Therapeutic Interventions

Diverticulosis is managed by preventing constipation. With acute diverticulitis, the patient may be hospitalized for administration of intravenous antibiotics and pain control. A nasogastric tube, intravenous fluids, and NPO status may be ordered until pain, nausea or vomiting, fever, and inflammation decrease. When the acute period is over, a progressive diet is started. Whether or not perforation occurs, surgical resection with anastomosis or a temporary **colostomy** (discussed later) may be done to allow the inflammation to subside and the diseased portion of the colon to rest.

Dietary considerations for a patient with diverticulosis (without evidence of inflammation) include foods that are soft but high in fiber, such as prunes, raisins, and peas. Unprocessed bran can be added to soups, cereals, and salads to give added bulk to the diet. Fiber should be increased in the diet slowly to prevent excess gas and cramping. Some health-care providers recommend avoiding nuts or foods with small seeds that can get caught in diverticula, such as tomatoes and raspberries, but this has not been shown to prevent diverticulitis.

Nursing Process for the Patient with an Inflammatory or Infectious Disorder

Assessment/Data Collection

Assessment of pain is essential for patients with inflammation or infection. Monitor the patient closely and notify the physician immediately if pain increases, especially if associated with abdominal rigidity. Increased pain may indicate that the bowel has ruptured and peritonitis is developing. Abdominal distention is monitored and recorded. With diverticulitis, a firm mass may be palpated in the sigmoid area.

Vital signs are monitored for fever or signs of septic shock. Intake and output are monitored and recorded accurately so that appropriate fluid replacement therapy is ordered. Monitoring for reduced urinary output, dropping blood pressure, and rising pulse rate can show fluid volume deficit. If a fever is noted, the patient may be developing sepsis. All symptoms are reported to the physician promptly.

---

colostomy: colo—pertaining to colon + stoma—mouth or opening

Nursing Diagnosis, Planning, and Implementation

Acute pain related to inflammatory process

EXPECTED OUTCOME: The patient will report pain is at an acceptable level.

- Have patient rate pain on objective scale such as 0 to 10 *to determine pain level.*
- Give analgesics or antispasmodic drugs as ordered *to relieve pain.*
- Use position changes, diversion, and relaxation exercises *to help relieve pain. Semi-Fowler's position may reduce tension on the abdomen.*
- Provide frequent mouth care if an NG tube is in place *to increase comfort.*

Risk for deficient fluid volume related to diarrhea or fluid shifting from the circulation to the peritoneal cavity

EXPECTED OUTCOME: The patient will maintain vital signs and urine output within normal limits.

- Intake and output are recorded *to determine fluid balance.*
- Weight patient daily *to determine fluid loss.*
- Monitor vital signs and urine output and report changes *to detect changes from within normal limits.*
- If output is greater than intake, intravenous fluid replacement may be ordered *to maintain fluid balance.*

For constipation related to low-fiber diet, see section on constipation above.

Evaluation

The goals are met if the patient reports that pain is controlled, vital signs and urinary output are stable, and patient has regular, comfortable bowel elimination.

INFLAMMATORY BOWEL DISEASE

Crohn's Disease (Regional Enteritis)

Pathophysiology

affects, small + Large Bowls

Crohn's disease, also known as regional **enteritis** or granulomatous enteritis, is an inflammatory bowel disease (IBD) that can involve any part of the intestine but most commonly affects the terminal portion of ileum. The inflammation extends through the intestinal mucosa, which leads to the formation of abscesses, **fistulas,** and fissures. As the disease progresses, obstruction occurs because the intestinal lumen narrows with inflamed mucosa and scar tissue.

Etiology

Although the exact cause of Crohn's disease has not been identified, there is a familial tendency. Other possible influences are autoimmune processes and infectious agents. Crohn's disease is most often diagnosed between the ages of

---

enteritis: entero—intestine + itis—inflammation

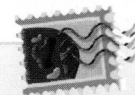

Box 34.5

Cultural Considerations

Ulcerative colitis and Crohn's disease are more common in Caucasians, persons of Jewish descent, and upper middle class urban populations. The incidence of Crohn's disease is increasing rapidly in western Europe and North America. These findings support possible hereditary or environmental risk factors for inflammatory bowel disease.

15 and 30 and occurs more often in women. There are periods of remissions and exacerbations. Physical or psychological stress may trigger exacerbations (Box 34.5 Cultural Considerations). *comes and goes*

Signs and Symptoms

Crampy abdominal pains (unrelieved by defecation), weight loss, and diarrhea occur. Because the crampy pains occur after eating, the patient often does not eat in order to avoid the pain. A lack of eating and poor absorption of nutrients results in weight loss and malnutrition. Chronic diarrhea contributes to fluid deficit and electrolyte imbalance. The inflamed intestine may perforate, leading to the formation of intra-abdominal or anal fissures, abscesses, or fistulas. Some nongastrointestinal symptoms may also occur, including arthritis, skin lesions, inflammatory disorders of the eyes, and abnormalities of liver function.

Complications

In addition to malnutrition, the development of fissures, abscesses, or fistulas is the most common complication of Crohn's disease. Fistulas may include enterovaginal (small bowel to vagina), enterovesical (small bowel to bladder), enterocutaneous (small bowel to skin), enteroentero (small bowel to small bowel), or enterocolonic (small bowel to colon) (Fig. 34.3). Fistulas communicating with organs that then drain externally can cause tremendous skin irritation, as well as increased risk of developing infections. Fistulas are corrected surgically.

Diagnostic Tests

Endoscopy (colonoscopy and sigmoidoscopy), with multiple biopsies of the diseased colon and terminal ileum, is used to diagnose Crohn's disease. Endoscopy identifies areas of normal to severely inflamed mucosa. Crohn's disease is confirmed by granulomas in the biopsy specimen. A barium enema shows a classic "cobblestoning" effect and, as the disease progresses, areas of narrowing in the intestine. A newer test, optical coherence tomography, allows the layers of the bowel to be examined for microscopic inflammation to differentiate this disease from ulcerative colitis.

An elevated sedimentation rate and leukocytosis are present, and serum albumin levels may be low because of malnutrition or poor absorption of protein. A stool examination may reveal fat content and occult blood. Newer diag-

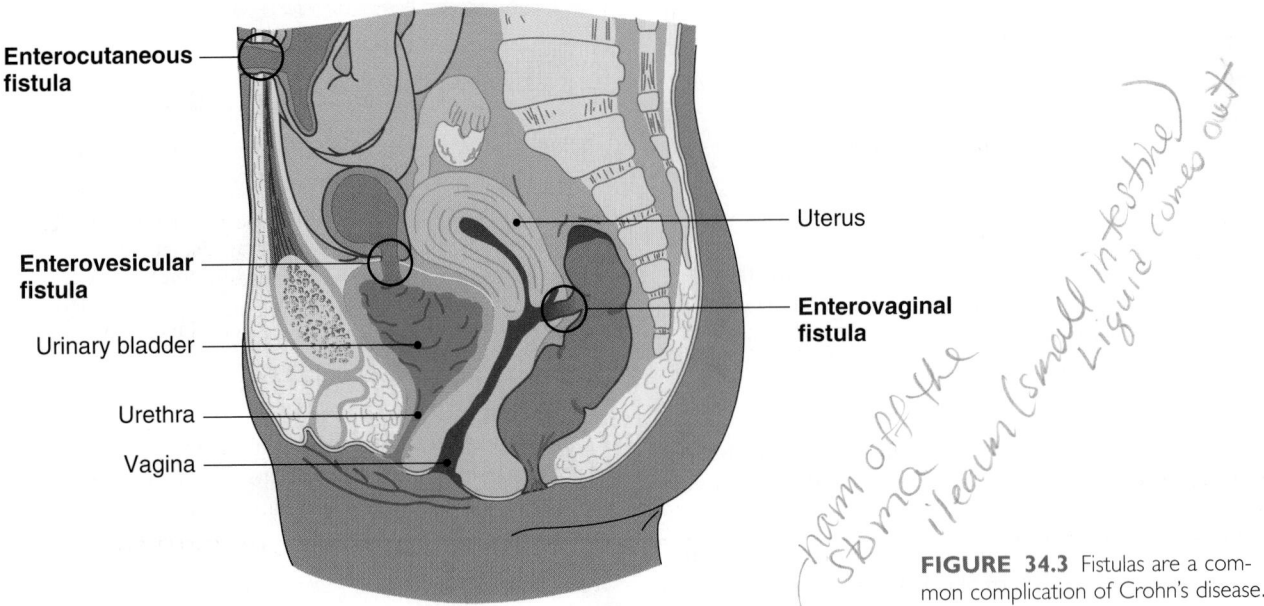

Enterocutaneous fistula

Enterovesicular fistula

Urinary bladder

Urethra

Vagina

Uterus

Enterovaginal fistula

ham off the stoma ileaum (small intestine) Liquid comes out

FIGURE 34.3 Fistulas are a common complication of Crohn's disease.

nostic antibody tests may be useful for IBD. They include: antineutrophil cytoplasmic antibody with perinuclear staining (pANCA), anti–*Saccharomyces cerevisiae* antibody (ASCA), outer membrane porin C (Omp C), and I2 antibody (novel homologue of the bacterial transcription factor families).

Therapeutic Interventions

Management of Crohn's disease is aimed at achieving remission and maintaining it as there is no cure. Symptoms are controlled by reducing the intestinal inflammation that is the underlying cause of the symptoms. More medications are available today offering better control of the disease. The classes of medications used to achieve these goals are aminosalicylates, corticosteroids, immunomodulators, biologics, and antibiotics (see Table 34.4). Treatment is individualized. Aminosalicylates reduce inflammation and have various formulations to be delivered to specific sites in the intestines. Corticosteroids are used during an acute inflammation, then tapered and discontinued. They do not prevent acute episodes. A newer class of steroids, which includes budesonide (Entocort EC), are nonsystemic steroids that act locally rather than affect the whole body. Immunomodulators modify the immune system to decrease inflammation. They may be used with steroids to treat acute episodes as they have a longer onset of action. Biologics selectively target agents in the inflammatory process to block their action and effects. Antibiotics are helpful in Crohn's disease as long-term therapy and when fistulas are present. Antidiarrheal medications such as diphenoxylate with atropine (Lomotil) or loperamide (Imodium) are used. Bulk-forming laxatives may help reduce loose stools and subsequently skin irritation.

Medication is used first for treatment but surgery may eventually be indicated for obstruction, stricture, fistula, abscess, excessive bleeding, perforation, toxic megacolon (loss of muscle tone and dilation in colon), or symptoms that do not respond to treatment. Surgery does not cure Crohn's disease as it can recur elsewhere in the intestines. Surgical procedures include strictureplasty to widen areas of stricture, resection of the affected area with anastomosis, colectomy with ileorectal anastomosis, or proctocolectomy (rectum and colon) with **ileostomy**. See details regarding intestinal ostomies later in this chapter. Symptoms may be relieved for several years with surgery but may recur in the surgical site area. A Kock pouch is not recommended for those with Crohn's disease as the disease may affect the pouch.

A healthy diet is important in overall health but there is no special diet for Crohn's disease. Malnutrition is a concern if the small intestine is affected and nutrients are not absorbed properly. Folic acid and vitamin B_{12} supplements may be needed. Calcium intake may be decreased and osteoporosis a concern. Calcium 1500 mg daily and vitamin D supplements are considered. Foods that increase symptoms should be avoided. Enteral feedings may be required and can be done at night through a gastrostomy tube (G tube) or feeding tube. For acute flare-ups, total parenteral nutrition (TPN) may be used to rest the GI tract. Adequate fluid intake is essential to prevent dehydration if diarrhea is present.

New nutritional therapy is looking at helping the GI tract to heal itself. The therapy may include fish or flaxseed oils to reduce inflammation, psyllium that stimulates bacteria to heal the colon, and probiotics that maintain normal intestinal flora. Research is ongoing in this area.

Nursing Process

Because of the similarities between Crohn's disease and ulcerative colitis, the nursing processes for both are discussed together. See section Nursing Process for the Patient with Inflammatory Bowel Disease below.

---

ileostomy: ileo—pertaining to ileum + stoma—mouth or opening

TABLE 34.4 MEDICATIONS FOR CROHN'S DISEASE AND/OR ULCERATIVE COLITIS

Medication/Action	Examples	Route	Side Effects	Nursing Implications
Aminosalicylates Decrease intestinal inflammation.	Sulfasalazine (Azulfidine)	PO, Rectal	Headache, nausea, anorexia, rash, fever	Contraindicated in sulfa allergy. Some patients do not tolerate sufasalazine but can tolerate others drugs in this class.
	Mesalamine (Asacol, Canasa, Pentasa, Rowasa)	PO, Rectal based on drug	Abdominal pain, diarrhea, nausea, hair loss, headache, dizziness	Monitor for signs of reduced kidney function.
	Olsalazine (Dipentum)	PO	Diarrhea, headache, rash, fatigue	Take with food.
	Balsalazide (Colazal)	PO	Headaches, abdominal pain	Continue drugs even if feeling better to maintain remission.
Corticosteroids Decrease inflammation and suppress immune system. May be used with aminos-alicylates.	Prednisone (Deltasone)	PO	Hypertension, moon face, infection, mood swings, weight gain, osteoporosis	Teach patient not to stop taking medication abruptly.
	Methylprednisolone (Medrol, Solu-Medrol)	PO, IV		
	Hydrocortisone (Cortenema)	Enema		Patient should lie on left side for 30 minutes and retain enema for 1 hour if not all night.
Nonsystemic steroids Reduce inflammation locally for Crohn's disease.	Budesonide (Entocort EC)	PO	Fewer steroid side effects (e.g., moon face and acne)	Grapefruit juice should be avoided. Take in morning. Swallow whole.
Immunomodulators Immunosuppression to reduce inflammation	Azathioprine (Imuran, Azasan)		Headache, N/V, diarrhea, malaise	Report symptoms of infection when taking any immunomodulators.
	6-Mercaptopurine (6-MP, Purinethol)		Headache, N/V, diarrhea, malaise	Monitor for infection.
	Cyclosporine A (Sandimmune, Neoral)	PO	Infections, headache, hypertension	Blood pressure and renal function is monitored.
	Tacrolimus (Prograf)	PO, topi-cally	Infections, headache, hypertension	Blood pressure and renal function is monitored.
	Methotrexate (MTX, Mexate, Rheumatrex)	IM	Bone marrow depression, infections, rash, nausea, diarrhea, stomatitis	Monitor for infections.
Antibiotics In Crohn's disease, reduces intestinal bacteria.	Metronidazole (Flagyl)	PO, IV	Headache, N/V, diarrhea, anorexia, metallic taste, dark urine, tingling of hands, feet	Teach to avoid alcohol. Avoid sun. Interfere with oral contraceptives, warfarin.
	Ciprofloxacin (Cipro)	PO, IV	Headache, N/V, diarrhea, rash, abdominal pain	Do not give with antacids, calcium, iron, zinc. Avoid sun. Interfere with oral contraceptives, warfarin.
Biologics Selectively target inflammatory agents to interfere with inflammatory response.	Infliximab (Remicade)	IV	Headache, chills, fever, hypotension, dyspnea, hives, nausea, rash, sore throat, lymphoma	TB test should be done before therapy begins. Monitor for infections, bone marrow suppression, CNS disorder.

CNS = central nervous system; N/V = nausea and vomiting; TB = tuberculosis.

Ulcerative Colitis *Large intestine*

Pathophysiology

Ulcerative colitis is similar to Crohn's disease. Crohn's disease, however, can occur anywhere in the gastrointestinal system, whereas ulcerative colitis occurs in the large colon and rectum. Multiple ulcerations and diffuse inflammation occur in the superficial mucosa and submucosa of the colon. The lesions spread throughout the large intestine and usually involve the rectum. The patient with ulcerative colitis has increased risk of developing colorectal cancer.

Etiology

Several theories exist to explain the cause of ulcerative colitis. These include infection, allergy, and autoimmune response. Environmental agents such as pesticides, tobacco, radiation, and food additives may precipitate an exacerbation. At one time, a psychological component was suggested in the etiology of ulcerative colitis. However, anyone who experiences chronic intestinal cramps and frequent, sometimes painful bowel movements is going to be discouraged, anxious, and depressed. These behaviors may be a result of the disease, not the cause. Psychological stress may trigger or worsen an attack of symptoms. Ulcerative colitis usually begins between ages 15 and 40.

Signs and Symptoms

Abdominal pain, diarrhea, rectal bleeding, and fecal urgency are common symptoms of ulcerative colitis (Table 34.5). Anorexia, weight loss, cramping, vomiting, fever, and dehydration associated with passing 5 to 20 liquid stools a day may also occur. Along with the potential for fluid and electrolyte imbalance, there is a loss of calcium. Anemia often develops as a result of rectal bleeding. Serum albumin may be low because of malabsorption. Like Crohn's disease, arthritis, skin lesions, inflammatory disorders of the eyes, and abnormalities of liver function may also occur. Symptoms are usually intermittent, with remissions lasting from months to years.

Complications

Malnutrition and its associated problems are complications of ulcerative colitis. Other complications include the potential for hemorrhage during an acute phase, bowel obstruction, perforation, and peritonitis. The risk for colon cancer is also increased in patients with ulcerative colitis. Symptoms outside the GI tract, such as arthritis, skin lesions, and inflammatory disorders of the eyes, may also occur.

Diagnostic Tests

Examination of stool specimens is done to rule out the presence of any bacterial or amebic organisms. The stool is positive for blood. Anemia is often present because of blood loss. Leukocyte levels and erythrocyte sedimentation rate are elevated because of the chronic inflammation. Electrolytes are depleted from chronic diarrhea. There is a protein loss because of liver dysfunction and malabsorption. Endoscopy and barium enema help differentiate ulcerative colitis from other diseases of the colon with similar symptoms. Biopsy specimens taken during sigmoidoscopy and colonoscopy typically show abnormal cells. Optical coherence tomography is used to differentiate this disease from Crohn's disease.

Therapeutic Interventions *Could have TPN*

Medications are used first as treatment. Foods that cause gas or diarrhea should be avoided. Because the offending foods may be different for each patient, foods are tried in small amounts if they are thought to cause symptoms. In general, high-fiber foods, caffeine, spicy foods, and milk products are avoided. Total parenteral nutrition may be needed to meet nutritional needs during acute exacerbations. Diarrhea may increase the need for fluids to prevent dehydration.

Many of the same medication classes as with Crohn's disease are used (see Table 34.4).

Surgery is considered for excessive bleeding, severe symptoms, perforation, or toxic megacolon. Because ulcerative colitis usually involves the entire large intestine, the surgery of choice is total proctocolectomy with restorative proctocolectomy or ileostomy (discussed later in this chapter). Surgery cures ulcerative colitis if the colon is removed.

A restorative proctocolectomy does not require an ostomy bag to be worn, and is the more common surgery performed. Since the anus and sphincter are saved, stool still passes through the anus. The rectum and colon are removed and the ileum, which is made into a pouch, is attached to the anus. A temporary ileostomy is created to allow the pouch to heal. After about 12 weeks, the ileostomy is closed. Several bowel movements per day occur. The stool is of soft consistency. Surgical complications can include an inflammation of the pouch (pouchitis) which is treated with antibiotics or a bowel obstruction.

TABLE 34.5 INFLAMMATORY BOWEL DISEASE SUMMARY

Signs and Symptoms	Abdominal pain or cramping
	Weight loss
	Diarrhea
	Fluid and electrolyte imbalance
	Fissures, fistulas, abscesses
	Arthritis and skin lesions
	Inflammatory eye disorders
	Abnormal liver function
Diagnostic Tests	Endoscopy with biopsy
	Barium enema
	Laboratory examination
	Stool examination
	Absent bowel sounds
Therapeutic Interventions	Medications: anti-inflammatories, antidiarrheal, antibiotics, immuno-suppressants, corticosteroids
	Surgery if necessary
	Avoidance of offending foods
	Elemental formula or TPN if required
Possible Nursing Diagnoses	Constipation
	Diarrhea
	Deficient knowledge

Nursing Process for the Patient with Inflammatory Bowel Disease

Assessment/Data Collection

A history obtained from the patient should include identification of symptoms, including the onset, duration, frequency, and severity. Ask if there has been any correlation between exacerbations of symptoms related to dietary changes or stress. Determine the presence of any food allergies or intolerances that may increase diarrhea. Also, note the daily and weekly intake of caffeine, nicotine, and alcohol because all these stimulate the bowel and can cause cramping and diarrhea.

Assess the patient for nutritional status and signs of dehydration. Ten to 20 lb can be lost in a 2-month period. Perianal skin should be assessed for irritation and excoriation.

Assessment of emotional status, coping skills, and verbal and nonverbal behaviors is essential. The patient may withdraw from family and friends because of frequent bowel movements. Anxiety, sleep disturbances, depression, and denial can be problems. If surgery involving an ileostomy is planned, the patient is at risk for body image problems.

Nursing Diagnosis, Planning, and Implementation

Acute pain related to increased peristalsis and cramping

EXPECTED OUTCOME: The patient will state pain is relieved or at an acceptable level.

- Document the character of the pain (dull, cramping, burning) and if the pain is associated with meals or activity *to plan care.*
- Give analgesics and medications *to relieve cramping, as prescribed.*

Diarrhea related to inflammatory process

EXPECTED OUTCOME: The patient will maintain formed, soft stool every 1 to 3 days.

- Document characteristics of stools, including color, consistency, amount, frequency, and odor *to plan care.*
- Ensure patient has quick access to the bathroom, or provide a bedside commode *to prevent incontinence.*
- Administer antidiarrheal medication as prescribed. *Controlling diarrhea controls comfort and fluid balance.*
- Encourage bedrest *to decrease peristalsis.*
- Keep the environment clean and odor free *to help alleviate anxiety.*
- Teach the patient to avoid high-fiber foods such as whole grains and raw fruits and vegetables, as well as caffeine, alcohol, and nicotine *because they stimulate intestinal motility.*

Risk for deficient fluid volume related to diarrhea and insufficient fluid intake

EXPECTED OUTCOME: The patient will maintain vital signs and urine output within normal limits.

- Record intake and output (including diarrhea stools) *to determine fluid balance.*
- Weight patient daily *to determine fluid loss.*
- Signs of deficient fluid volume are documented and reported to the physician *to allow treatment.*
- Maintain IV fluids as ordered *to maintain fluid balance.*
- Encourage fluids when acute diarrhea subsides *to maintain fluid balance.*
- Teach patient signs and symptoms of dehydration to report *to allow prompt treatment.*

Anxiety related to symptoms and frequency of stools and treatment

EXPECTED OUTCOME: The patient will report anxiety is reduced.

- Answer questions, talk in a calm, confident manner, and actively listen to the patient *to reduce anxiety, which aggravates symptoms of inflammatory bowel disease.*

Impaired skin integrity related to frequent loose stools

EXPECTED OUTCOME: The patient's skin remains intact.

- Keep perianal skin clean, dry, and protected with a moisture barrier, such as petrolatum or medicated ointment, after each bowel movement *to protect perianal skin from contact with liquid stools and their enzymes.*
- Sitz baths may be comforting and helpful in keeping skin clean *to prevent excoriation.*

Ineffective nutrition, less than body requirements, related to malabsorption

EXPECTED OUTCOME: The patient will maintain weight within normal range for height and age.

- Give special liquid (elemental) formula that is absorbed in the upper bowel as ordered *to allow the colon to rest.* milky BAG
- Maintain TPN as ordered to provide nourishment if the patient is unable *to tolerate oral intake.*
- Weight weekly *to detect weight loss.*

CRITICAL THINKING

Judy Moore

■ Judy Moore is an 18-year-old college student who has just been diagnosed with Crohn's disease.

1. What questions can you ask Judy to identify her symptoms?
2. What nursing diagnoses would be relevant for Judy's condition?
3. What can you do to help her adapt to this disease?
4. If Judy's condition were to worsen what manifestations would be exhibited?

Suggested answers at end of chapter.

See Box 34.6 Nursing Care Plan for the Patient with Inflammatory Bowel Disease.

Evaluation

Goals have been met if pain is relieved, frequency of diarrhea stools is decreased, fluid and electrolyte balance is achieved, anxiety is reduced, skin is intact, and weight is within normal range for height and age.

IRRITABLE BOWEL SYNDROME

peristolics is a fixable

Pathophysiology *Little slow*

Irritable bowel syndrome (IBS) is a disorder of altered intestinal motility in which the colon does not contract in a normal pattern. Instead it contracts in a disorderly way that can be violent and last for long times or there can be times when it does not contract at all. The abnormal contractions lead to pattern changes alternating between diarrhea and constipation. Additionally, there is increased abdominal discomfort or pain. Localized prolonged contractions may cause stool to be retained for a long time, causing it to become hardened as water is absorbed from it. Bloating may also occur as air

Stablize the diet, high Brand, avoid

is unable to be expelled. Mucus may be seen in the stool, although this is not abnormal and does not typically cause a problem. The bowel mucosa is normal. IBS is not a disease but rather a functional problem.

Symptoms may be exacerbated by psychological stress or food intolerances. The nerves in the bowel are overly sensitive in persons with IBS. At times of stress in daily living, abnormal contractions may result.

Etiology

There is a hereditary tendency for IBS. IBS is more common in women and in those who are young to middle aged. Flare-ups can be caused by other illnesses, infections, or the menstrual cycle.

Signs and Symptoms

IBS is characterized by complaints of gas, bloating, constipation, diarrhea, or alternating constipation and diarrhea. The patient also has feelings of abdominal bloating, with or without visible abdominal distention. Other symptoms include the rectal passage of mucus, a feeling of incomplete evacuation, abdominal pain, depression, anxiety, and palpitations.

Box 34.6   NURSING CARE PLAN for the Patient with Inflammatory Bowel Disease

Ineffective coping related to inflammatory bowel disease

Patient Outcomes Patient will identify strategies that will promote effective coping.

Evaluation of Outcomes Is the patient able to state strategies for effective coping?

Interventions	Rationale	Evaluation
Ask knowledge of Crohn's disease or ulcerative colitis	Many people have little knowledge of a disease unless they know someone who has it. Inaccurate information must be corrected.	Does the patient verbalize information about ulcerative colitis and its effects on the body?
Encourage the patient to express feelings about the disease and how it may affect his or her life.	Expressing feelings about the disease and its perceived effect enables the patient to identify and talk about concerns. Once identified, these concerns can then be addressed by the health care team.	Does the patient talk about feelings regarding the potential impact of the disease on his or her life?
Determine whether the patient would like to speak with a person of similar age from the Crohn's and Colitis Foundation of America.	Speaking with someone close in age with the same disease lets the patient know that he or she is not the only person having to cope with this disorder. It can also help him or her learn some strategies for effectively coping with the disease.	Does the patient show an interest in speaking with someone with the same disease?
Identify strategies for effective coping that are acceptable to the patient.	Talking about concerns and possible solutions is a positive step. Coping strategies identified with the patient are more likely to be implemented.	Is the patient able to identify strategies for effective coping that he or she believes will work?

Diagnostic Tests

Diagnosis of IBS is made based on history and physical examination. Stool examination, barium enema, upper GI series, and sigmoidoscopy may be done to rule out other disorders. Avoiding milk products for a time may be advised to rule out lactose intolerance.

Therapeutic Interventions

IBS is a chronic condition, but symptoms can generally be controlled. A high-fiber and high-bran diet (psyllium [Metamucil] or methylcellulose [Citrucel]) may help to form softer, larger stools but may increase other symptoms in some people. Foods that cause distress or gas formation are avoided such as fresh fruits or vegetables, spices, milk, coffee, carbonated drinks, and alcohol. Eating smaller, frequent meals can be helpful in reducing bowel contractions. Stress management, behavioral therapy (biofeedback, hypnosis, psychotherapy), and exercise are helpful in relaxing the bowel as well as contributing to overall health.

Various medications are used depending on the type of IBS. Antidepressants are given to block the brain's perception of abdominal pain. For IBS with constipation, citadep (Celexa) or paroxetine HCl (Paxil) are examples of selective serotonin reuptake inhibitors (SSRIs) that are prescribed. Tricyclic antidepressants (such as amitriptyline HCl [Elavil]) are used for IBS with diarrhea as they tend to cause constipation. Antispasmodics such as hyoscyamine (Levbid) or dicyclomine (Bentyl) are used in IBS with diarrhea. For women under age 65 with IBS with constipation, tegaserod maleate (Zelnorm) is prescribed short term to help normalize bowel function by coordinating muscle function. Zelnorm is not effective for all women or men with IBS with constipation.

Nursing Process for the Patient with IBS

Assessment/Data Collection

Height and weight are obtained. Data are collected on the symptoms including pain that the patient experiences. Timing of the symptoms, food and fluid intake, elimination patterns, effects on self-esteem, socialization, and personal and family roles are explored since IBS is a significant cause of missed work and school and also causes social withdrawal and embarrassment for people with it. Knowledge of the syndrome and its treatment are determined. Readiness for managing the syndrome is determined to plan care.

Nursing Diagnosis, Planning, and Implementation

Constipation related to irregular motility of GI tract

EXPECTED OUTCOME: The patient will maintain passage of soft, formed stool every 1 to 3 days without straining.

- Assess normal pattern of defecation, diet and fluid intake, and medications *to help identify factors contributing to constipation for planning care.*
- Ensure fluid intake, if not contraindicated, of 2 to 3 L per day *to prevent hard stools.*

- Explain to increase fiber and bran in diet *to promote soft, larger stools that are easier to pass.*
- Give medication as ordered to control symptoms.

Diarrhea related to irregular motility of GI tract

EXPECTED OUTCOME: The patient will maintain formed, soft stool every 1 to 3 days.

- Obtain history including medications regarding diarrhea episodes *to help identify cause.*
- Monitor and record stool characteristics, amount, and frequency *to plan care.*
- Give antidiarrheal medications as ordered. *Controlling diarrhea controls comfort and fluid balance.*
- Limit caffeine intake *as it stimulates intestinal motility.*
- Keep skin clean, dry, and protected with a moisture barrier, such as petrolatum or medicated ointment, after each bowel movement *to protect perianal skin from contact with liquid stools and their enzymes.*

Readiness for enhanced therapeutic regimen management related to desire to manage symptoms of IBS

EXPECTED OUTCOME: The patient will state understanding and ability to carry out preventive measures to control symptoms.

- Explain IBS including symptoms, aggravating factors, and treatments *to promote understanding for ability to follow therapeutic regimen.*
- Encourage use of food dairy documenting foods eaten and timing of symptom occurrence *to identify food triggers for symptoms including lactose intolerance.* A food diary is available at http://www.healthywomen.org/presskit/aw/fooddiary.pdf.
- Consult registered dietitian and share food diary *to allow identification of food connection with symptoms and meal planning to prevent symptoms.*
- If lactose intolerant, avoid dairy products and substitute yogurt *to reduce symptoms.*

Evaluation

The plan has been effective if the patient has regular bowel function pattern, and verbalizes understanding of self-care measures and expresses satisfaction with the outcomes.

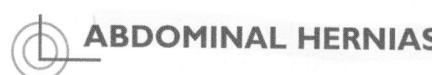

ABDOMINAL HERNIAS

Pathophysiology and Etiology

A hernia is an abnormal protrusion of an organ or structure through a weakness or tear in the wall of the cavity normally containing it, which in this case is the abdominal wall. Hernias are caused by a weakness in the abdominal wall along with increased intra-abdominal pressure, such as the pressure from coughing, straining, and heavy lifting. Obesity, pregnancy, and poor wound healing are also risk factors. The hernial sac is formed by the peritoneum protruding through the weakened muscle wall. Contents of the

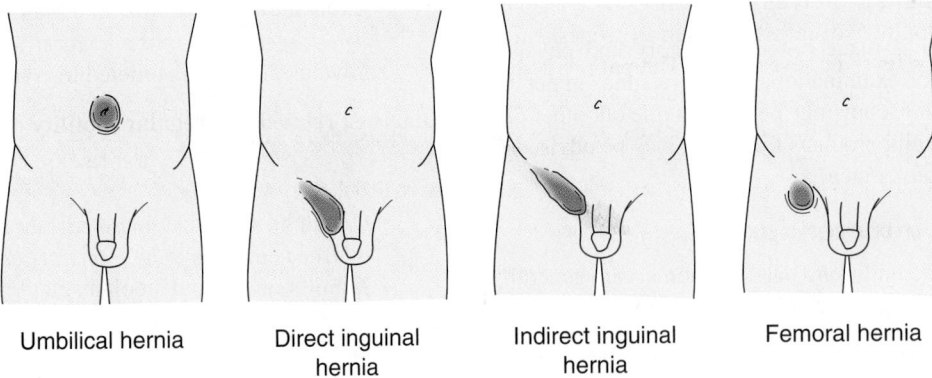

Umbilical hernia   Direct inguinal   Indirect inguinal   Femoral hernia
                              hernia   hernia

FIGURE 34.4 Types of hernias.

hernia can be small or large intestine, or the omentum. Indirect hernias are caused by a defect of structural closure. Direct hernias are acquired and arise from a weakness in the abdominal wall, usually at old incisional sites.

There are many types of hernias (Fig. 34.4). Inguinal hernias are located in the groin where the spermatic cord in males or the round ligament in females emerges from the abdominal wall. This common hernia is an example of an indirect hernia and is usually seen in males.

Umbilical hernias are seen most often in obese women and in children. They are caused by a failure of the umbilical orifice to close. Ventral (incisional) hernias usually result from a weakness in the abdominal wall following abdominal surgery, especially in the obese patient, if a drainage system was used, the patient experienced poor wound healing, or the patient received inadequate nutrition.

Prevention

Congenital defects cannot be prevented. However, reducing strain on abdominal muscles is helpful. Those who do heavy lifting, tugging, or pushing should wear a support binder or avoid the lifting. A healthy lifestyle of maintaining normal weight, not smoking, and eating high-fiber foods is recommended.

Signs and Symptoms

Unless complications occur, there are very few symptoms associated with hernias. An abnormal bulging can be seen in the affected area of the abdomen, especially when straining or coughing. It may disappear when the patient lies down. If the intestinal mass easily returns to the abdominal cavity or can be manually placed back in the abdominal cavity, it is called a reducible hernia. When adhesions or edema occur between the sac and its contents, the hernia becomes irreducible or incarcerated. The trapped loop of bowel becomes strangulated with the blood supply cut off.

Complications

An incarcerated hernia may become strangulated if the blood and intestinal flow are completely cut off. Strangulated hernias do not develop in adults very often. Incarceration leads to an intestinal obstruction and possibly gangrene and bowel perforation. Symptoms are pain at the site of the strangulation, nausea and vomiting, and colicky abdominal pain. Treatment is emergency surgery.

Therapeutic Interventions

Hernias are diagnosed by physical examination. Treatment options include no treatment, observing the hernia, and using short-term support devices or surgery to cure the hernia. A supportive truss or brief applies pressure to keep the reduced hernia in place. Surgery is recommended for inguinal hernias and is indicated if there is strangulation or the threat of bowel obstruction. For symptomatic hernias, surgical procedures include open hernia repair (herniorrhaphy) or hernioplasty (open or laparoscopically). Herniorrhaphy involves making an incision in the abdominal wall, replacing the contents of the hernial sac, sewing the weakened tissue, and closing the opening. Hernioplasty involves replacing the hernia into the abdomen and reinforcing the weakened muscle wall with wire, fascia, or mesh. Bowel resection or a temporary colostomy may be necessary if the hernia is strangulated.

Nursing Management

The patient is instructed to avoid activities that increase intra-abdominal pressure, such as lifting heavy objects. The patient is taught to recognize signs of incarceration or strangulation and the importance of notifying the physician immediately. If a support truss or brief has been ordered, the patient is taught to apply it before arising from bed each morning while the hernia is not protruding. Special attention should be paid to maintenance of skin integrity beneath the truss.

Postoperative Care

Care following inguinal hernia repair is similar to any postoperative care. Patients can perform deep breathing to keep lungs clear postoperatively but should avoid coughing. Coughing increases abdominal pressure and could affect the hernia repair. The male patient may experience swelling of the scrotum. Ice packs and elevation of the scrotum may be ordered to reduce the swelling. Because most patients are discharged the same day as surgery, they are taught to change the dressing and report difficulty urinating, bleeding, and signs and symptoms of infection, such as redness, incisional drainage, or fever or severe pain. The patient is also instructed to avoid lifting, driving, or sexual activities for 2 to 6 weeks as specified by the physician. Most patients can return to nonstrenuous work within 2 weeks.

ABSORPTION DISORDERS

The process of digestion reduces nutrients to a liquid form that can be absorbed through intestinal mucosa into the portal bloodstream. More than 8000 mL of liquid with nutrients and electrolytes is absorbed, mostly proximal to the ileocecal valve.

Pathophysiology and Etiology

Malabsorption occurs when the GI system is unable to absorb one or more of the major nutrients (carbohydrates, fats, or proteins). Some causes of malabsorption are ileal dysfunction, jejunal diverticula, parasitic disease, celiac disease, enzyme deficiency, and inflammatory bowel diseases such as Crohn's disease and ulcerative colitis. The primary malabsorption disorders are tropical sprue, adult celiac disease (nontropical sprue), and lactose intolerance.

The cause of tropical sprue has not been specifically identified but is thought to be related to bacterial infection of the intestine. In adult celiac disease (sometimes called nontropical sprue), a sensitivity to gluten is thought to cause malabsorption of protein. Gluten is a protein found in wheat, barley, oats, and rye (Box 34.7 Nutrition Notes).

A deficiency in lactase, an enzyme that breaks down lactose (milk sugar), causes lactose intolerance. When lactose is not digested, a high concentration of it occurs in the intestines, causing an osmotic retention of water in the colon and watery stools (Box 34.8 Nutrition Notes).

Signs and Symptoms

Weight loss, weakness, and general malaise resulting in malnutrition are associated with malabsorption disorders. Signs

---

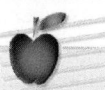

Box 34.7

Nutrition Notes

Treating Celiac Disease

Celiac disease, or gluten-sensitive enteropathy, requires permanent elimination of wheat, rye, oats, and barley from the diet. Careful selection of prepared foods is mandatory because of the widespread use of these grains as thickeners. If a patient with celiac disease ingests gluten, damage to the intestine continues even in the absence of symptoms. Instruction from and followup by a dietitian are indicated to ensure adequate nutritional intake despite the many dietary limitations.

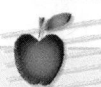

Box 34.8

Nutrition Notes

Managing Lactose Intolerance

Patients with lactose intolerance control their conditions through trial and error because the degree of lactose intolerance varies greatly among patients. Moderate amounts of many lactose-containing foods can be digested when taken with a mixed meal. A dietitian's services may be advised to begin dietary management after diagnosis. Ingredients to avoid include milk, milk solids, lactose, and whey. Low-lactose foods (up to 2 g per serving) include sherbet, cheese aged longer than 90 days, processed cheese, and milk treated with lactate enzyme. In cheese making, the whey containing most of the lactose is removed, so that hard, ripened cheeses such as blue, Brie, Cheddar, Colby, Gouda, Parmesan, and Swiss are classified as low lactose. Some brands of yogurt, a high-lactose food, may be tolerated because they contain bacterial lactate.

---

and symptoms of sprue include frequent loose, bulky, foul stools that are gray in color and have an increased fat content. (Increased fat in stool is called steatorrhea.) Lactose intolerance causes abdominal cramping, excessive gas, and loose stools after eating milk products.

Complications

Vitamin K deficiency and resulting hypoprothrombinemia can increase the risk of bleeding. Calcium deficiency can be severe enough to cause bone pain and neuromuscular hyperirritability, including tetany. Folic acid, vitamin B_{12}, and iron deficiencies can result in glossitis, stomatitis, anemia, and dry, rough skin.

Diagnostic Tests

See Table 34.6 for the diagnostic studies used to identify malabsorption diseases.

Therapeutic Interventions

Folic acid, broad-spectrum antibiotics, and a high-calorie, high-protein, low-fat diet are ordered for patients with tropical sprue. Adults with celiac disease are ordered a high-calorie, high-protein, gluten-free diet to relieve the symptoms and improve nutritional status. However, because gluten is used as a filler or binder in many products, even those labeled "wheat free," diligence in identifying potentially offending foods is essential.

Lactose intolerance is treated by removing foods from the diet that contain lactose, such as milk and milk products. Some fermented milk products, such as cheese and yogurt, may be lower in lactose and better tolerated. Lactaid is an over-the-counter lactase substitute that can be taken when milk products cannot be avoided. It can be added to milk in

TABLE 34.6 DIAGNOSTIC TESTS FOR DISORDERS OF MALABSORPTION

Diagnostic Test	Test Result and Associated Malabsorption Syndrome
Hemoglobin and hematocrit	Decreased if anemia is present.
Mean corpuscular volume	Decreased values are found with malabsorption of vitamin B_{12}.
Upper GI series	Thickening of the intestinal mucosa, narrowed mucosa of the terminal ileum, or a change in fecal transit time are indicative of malabsorption syndrome.
D-Xylose absorption test	Decreased excretion of xylose after 5 hours is indicative of malabsorption.
Sudan stain for fecal fat	Malabsorption can be distinguished from maldigestion if this test shows abnormally large numbers of fat droplets.
72-hour stool collection for fat	Stool fat greater than 5 g per 24 hours after ingestion of 80 g of fat in 2 days implies a fat digestion disorder.

TABLE 34.7 BOWEL OBSTRUCTION SUMMARY

Signs and Symptoms	Abdominal pain Blood and mucus per rectum Feces and flatus cease Visible peristaltic waves in thin person Possible fecal vomiting Bowel sounds high-pitched, tinkling or absent Abdominal distention Fluid and electrolyte imbalance
Diagnostic Tests	Abdominal x-ray examination CT scan CBC and electrolytes
Therapeutic Interventions	NPO status Frequent mouth care Nasogastric tube Fluid and electrolyte replacement Medications: antibiotics, antiemetics, analgesics Surgery
Possible Nursing Diagnoses	Pain Constipation Deficient fluid volume

liquid form or taken as a tablet before eating foods containing lactose. Lactaid digests about 70% of the lactose in foods, making them more tolerable.

Nursing Management

Nursing care involves monitoring fluid and electrolyte balance, nutritional status, and skin integrity. Daily weight and intake and output help determine if fluid loss is occurring. Intake of electrolyte-rich fluids is encouraged to replace losses. Antidiarrheal agents are given if ordered. Electrolyte levels, especially potassium, are monitored as ordered. The patient is instructed in dietary limitations. Nutritional supplements may be ordered if necessary. Perianal skin is kept clean and dry, and barrier ointments are used as needed to protect the skin from excoriation.

INTESTINAL OBSTRUCTION

Intestinal obstructions occur when the flow of intestinal contents is blocked. There are two types of intestinal obstruction, mechanical and paralytic, both of which can be either partial or complete.

Mechanical obstruction occurs when a blockage occurs within the intestine from conditions causing pressure on the intestinal walls such as adhesions, twisting of the bowel, or strangulated hernia. Paralytic obstruction occurs when peristalsis is impaired and the intestinal contents cannot be propelled through the bowel. Paralytic obstruction is seen following abdominal surgeries, trauma, mesenteric ischemia, or infection. The severity of the obstruction depends on the area of bowel affected, the amount of occlusion within the lumen, and the amount of disturbance in the blood flow to the bowel (Table 34.7).

Small-Bowel Obstruction

Pathophysiology

When obstruction occurs in the small bowel, a collection of intestinal contents, gas, and fluid occurs proximal to the obstruction. The distention that results stimulates gastric secretion but decreases the absorption of fluids. As distention worsens, the intraluminal pressure causes a decrease in venous and arterial capillary pressure, resulting in edema, necrosis, and eventually perforation of the intestinal wall.

Etiology

Following abdominal surgery, loops of intestine may adhere to areas in the abdomen that are not healed. This may cause a kink in the bowel that occludes the intestinal flow. These adhesions, or bands of scar tissue, are the most common cause of small bowel obstruction and are usually acquired from previous abdominal surgery or inflammation. Hernias and neoplasms are the next most common causes, followed by inflammatory bowel disease, foreign bodies, strictures, **volvulus,** and **intussusception.** A volvulus occurs when the bowel twists, occluding the lumen of the intestine. Intussusception occurs when peristalsis causes the intestine to telescope into itself (Fig. 34.5). These conditions are mechanical obstructions. Paralytic, or adynamic, ileus is a nonmechanical obstruction that occurs when the intestinal peristalsis decreases or stops because of a vascular or neuromuscular pathological condition. Box 34.9 lists causes of nonmechanical obstructions.

Signs and Symptoms

The patient initially complains of wavelike abdominal pain and vomiting. Initially, flatus and feces that are low in the bowel and blood and mucus may be passed, but this stops as

---

intussusception intus—within + suscept—to receive

Before surgery

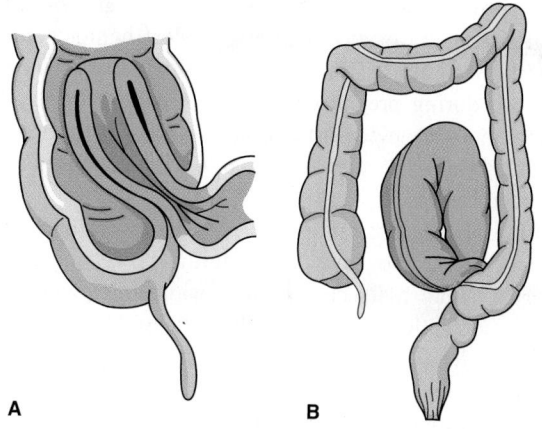

FIGURE 34.5 Mechanical bowel obstructions. (A) Intussusception. (B) Volvulus.

the obstruction becomes worse. The symptoms progress as the obstruction worsens or becomes complete. As the obstruction becomes more extreme, peristaltic waves reverse, propelling the intestinal contents toward the mouth, eventually leading to fecal vomiting. Peristaltic waves may be visible in a thin person. Pain that is sharp and sustained may indicate perforation. In mechanical obstructions, high-pitched, tinkling bowel sounds are heard proximal to the obstruction and are absent distal to it. If the obstruction is nonmechanical, there is an absence of bowel sounds.

Loss of fluid and electrolytes leads to dehydration, with its associated symptoms of extreme thirst, drowsiness, aching, and general malaise. The lower in the gastrointestinal tract the obstruction is, the greater the abdominal distention. An uncorrected obstruction can lead to shock and possibly death.

Diagnostic Tests
Dilated loops of bowel are evident in radiographic studies and CT scans. If strangulation or perforation occurs, leukocytosis is evident. Hemoglobin and hematocrit levels are elevated if the patient is dehydrated, and serum electrolyte levels are decreased.

Therapeutic Interventions
In most cases, the patient is kept NPO and the bowel is decompressed using a nasogastric (or rarely an intestinal) tube, which relieves symptoms and may resolve the obstruc-

tion. An IV solution with electrolytes is initiated to correct the fluid and electrolyte imbalance. Sometimes IV antibiotics are begun. Complete mechanical obstruction requires surgical intervention, such as removal of tumors, release of adhesions, or bowel resection with anastomosis.

Large-Bowel Obstruction *-constipation*
Pathophysiology
Obstruction in the large bowel is less common and not usually as dramatic as small-bowel obstruction. Dehydration occurs more slowly because of the colon's ability to absorb fluid and distend well beyond its normal full capacity. If the blood supply to the colon is cut off, the patient's life is in jeopardy because of bowel strangulation and necrosis.

Etiology
Most large-bowel obstructions occur in the sigmoid colon and are caused by carcinoma, inflammatory bowel disease, diverticulitis, or benign tumors. Impaction of stool may also cause obstruction.

Signs and Symptoms
Symptoms of large-bowel obstruction develop slowly and depend on the location of the obstruction. If the obstruction is in the rectum or sigmoid, the only symptom may be constipation. As the loops of bowel distend, the patient may complain of crampy lower abdominal pain and abdominal distention. Vomiting, if it occurs, is a late sign and may be fecal. High-pitched tinkling bowel sounds may be heard. A localized tender area and mass may be felt on palpation. Large-bowel obstructions, if not diagnosed and treated, can lead to gangrene, perforation, and peritonitis (discussed earlier).

Therapeutic Interventions
Radiological examination reveals a distended colon. If impaction is present, enemas and manual disimpaction may be effective. Other mechanical blockages may require surgical intervention.

Surgical resection of the obstructed colon may be necessary. A temporary colostomy may be indicated to allow the bowel to rest and heal. Sometimes an ileoanal anastomosis is done. A patient who is a poor surgical risk may have a cecostomy (an opening from the cecum to the abdominal wall) to allow diversion of stool.

Nursing Process for the Patient with a Bowel Obstruction
ASSESSMENT/DATA COLLECTION. Each quadrant of the abdomen is auscultated for bowel sounds. The abdomen is palpated for distention, firmness, and tenderness. The amount and character of stool, if any, is documented. Pain is assessed using the institution's pain scale and described according to location and character, such as crampy or wavelike. Daily weight and intake and output are monitored. Skin turgor is assessed for fluid deficit. If a nasogastric tube is in place, the amount, color, and character of drainage is documented. Vital signs are monitored for signs of infection or shock.

Box 34.9

Causes of Nonmechanical Obstruction

- Abdominal surgery and trauma
- Pneumonia
- Spinal injuries
- Hypokalemia
- Myocardial infarction
- Peritonitis
- Vascular insufficiency

NURSING DIAGNOSIS, PLANNING, AND IMPLEMENTATION. Acute pain related to abdominal distention

EXPECTED OUTCOME: Patient will state pain is relieved or at acceptable level.

- Assess pain level using rating scale *to consistently communicate patient level.*
- Give medication for pain as ordered. *Opioids are given cautiously because they may mask symptoms of perforation and decrease intestinal motility.*
- Position patient in semi-Fowler's position *to reduce tension on the abdomen.*
- Maintain oral/nasogastric tube on low intermittent suction as ordered *to relieve discomfort from distention.*
- Maintain NPO status *to rest the bowel and promote comfort.*

Provide frequent mouth care *to promote comfort.*

Deficient fluid volume related to vomiting

EXPECTED OUTCOME: The patient will maintain vital signs and urine output within normal limits.

- Accurately monitor intake and output *to identify fluid deficit.*
- Maintain fluid replacement as ordered *to prevent dehydration.*
- Give ice chips sparingly if ordered by the physician. *When melted ice mixed with electrolytes and hydrochloric acid is removed from the stomach by suction, electrolyte imbalance and metabolic alkalosis occur.*

EVALUATION. Goals are met if the patient states that pain is controlled and fluid is balanced and electrolytes are within normal limits.

CRITICAL THINKING

Mrs. Loos

■ Mrs. Loos is admitted for abdominal pain. She has a history of diabetes mellitus. You find her abdomen large, firm, and tender to touch. She states that she feels nauseated.

1. What do you do?
2. What do you think is happening?
3. How do you document your findings?

Suggested answers at end of chapter.

 ANORECTAL PROBLEMS

Hemorrhoids

Hemorrhoids are varicose veins in the anal canal. They are caused by an increase in pressure in the veins, often from increased intra-abdominal pressure. Internal hemorrhoids occur above the internal sphincter, and external hemorrhoids occur below the external sphincter. Most hemorrhoids are caused by straining during bowel movements. They are common during pregnancy. Prolonged sitting or standing, obesity, and chronic constipation also contribute to hemorrhoids. Portal hypertension related to liver disease may also be a factor.

Internal hemorrhoids are usually not painful unless they prolapse. They may bleed during bowel movements. External hemorrhoids cause itching and pain when inflamed and filled with blood (thrombosed). Inflammation and edema occur with thrombosis, causing severe pain and possibly infarction of the skin and mucosa over the hemorrhoid.

Preventing constipation, avoiding straining during defecation, and good personal hygiene relieve hemorrhoid symptoms and discomfort. Astringents, such as witch hazel, can be used for symptom relief. Sitz baths increase circulation to the area and aid in comfort and healing. Stool softeners can be used to reduce the need for straining. Other anti-inflammatory medications may be tried, such as steroid creams or suppositories. Alternating ice and heat helps relieve edema and pain with thrombosed hemorrhoids.

If hemorrhoids are prolapsed and are no longer reduced by palliative measures, more aggressive measures may be used. Sclerotherapy involves the injection of a sclerosing agent into the tissues around the hemorrhoids, causing them to shrink. Rubber band ligation uses rubber bands placed around the hemorrhoids until the tissue dies and sloughs off. Cryosurgery uses cold to freeze the hemorrhoid tissue. Surgical hemorrhoidectomy involves surgical removal of hemorrhoids, and is used in severe cases.

The patient should be instructed to consume a high-fiber diet and 2 to 3 L of fluid a day to promote regular bowel movements. The effects and side effects, proper dosage, and frequency of local or topical treatments should be explained. If the patient has surgery, analgesics should be given as needed because the many nerve endings in the anal canal can cause severe pain. Comfort measures such as a side-lying position and fresh ice packs should also be used to relieve pain. After the first postoperative day, sitz baths may be ordered. Unfortunately, a side effect of opioid analgesics is constipation, which needs to be avoided, especially in the immediate postoperative period. Because the first bowel movement can be painful and anxiety provoking, stool softeners are given and analgesics administered before the first bowel movement.

Anal Fissures

Anal fissures are cracks or ulcers in the lining of the anal canal. They are most commonly associated with constipation and stretching of the anus with passage of hard stool, although Crohn's disease or other factors may also play a role. The patient may experience bright red bleeding. Pain may be so severe that the patient delays defecation, leading to further constipation and worsening symptoms. Treatment of anal fissures involves measures to ensure soft stools, allowing fissures time to heal. Sitz baths may be used to promote circulation to the area to aid in healing. Anesthetic suppositories and nonopioid analgesics may be ordered for comfort. If conservative measures are not helpful, surgical excision may be necessary.

Anorectal Abscess

An anorectal abscess is a collection of pus in the rectal area. Common causative organisms include *Escherichia coli, Proteus* spp., staphylococci, or streptococci. Symptoms include pain, redness and swelling, fever, and sometimes drainage. Abscesses are treated with antibiotics and surgical incision and drainage of pus. The area may be left open to drain, with packing placed to assist with drainage and healing.

Nursing Management

Nursing care includes dressing or packing changes as ordered. Sitz baths are used to keep the area clean and promote healing, especially after bowel movements. The patient is instructed in the importance of keeping the area clean and dry. Other postoperative care is similar to care following hemorrhoidectomy.

LOWER GASTROINTESTINAL BLEEDING

Etiology

Major causes of lower gastrointestinal bleeding are diverticulitis, polyps (growths in the colon), anal fissures, hemorrhoids, inflammatory bowel disease, and cancer.

Signs and Symptoms

Bleeding from the GI tract is evident in the stools. When blood has been in the GI tract for more than 8 hours and has come in contact with hydrochloric acid, it causes **melena,** or black and tarry stools. The presence of melena indicates bleeding above or in the small bowel. Bleeding from the colon or rectum is usually bright red (**hematochezia**).

Significant blood loss causes hypotension, lightheadedness, nausea, and diaphoresis. The patient may be pale and have cool skin. The onset of tachycardia and worsening hypotension indicate hypovolemic shock and should be reported to the physician immediately.

Diagnostic Tests

A thorough history is necessary to determine underlying disorders that may be causing the bleeding. Decreased hemoglobin and hematocrit levels result from blood loss. Blood urea nitrogen (BUN) may be elevated as a result of breakdown of proteins in the blood by the GI tract. Stool can be tested for occult blood if it is not evident on inspection. Digital examination, colonoscopy, or sigmoidoscopy may be done by the physician.

hematochezia: hemat—blood + chezia—in stool

Therapeutic Interventions

Treatment involves correction of the cause of the bleeding: surgery to correct diverticulosis, to correct inflammatory bowel disease, or to resect cancer may be considered.

Nursing Management

Stools are checked for the presence and amount of blood. Vital signs are monitored for signs of shock. Declining blood pressure and rising heart rate are reported to the physician immediately. The patient is prepared for diagnostic tests and nursing care for the underlying disorder is provided.

COLON CANCER

Colon cancer is one of the most common types of internal cancer in the United States. People with a family history of colon cancer or ulcerative colitis are at higher risk of developing it themselves.

Pathophysiology and Etiology

Colon cancer originates in the epithelial lining of the colon or rectum and can occur anywhere in the large intestine. People with a personal or family history of ulcerative colitis, colon cancer, or polyps of the rectum or large intestine are at higher risk for developing cancer. Colon cancer has also been linked with previous gallbladder removal and dietary carcinogens. A major causative factor is lack of fiber in the diet, which prolongs fecal transit time and in turn prolongs exposure to possible carcinogens. Also, bacterial flora is believed to be altered by excess fat, which converts steroids into compounds having carcinogenic properties.

Signs and Symptoms

Manifestations of colon cancer vary according to the type of tumor and the location (Fig. 34.6). A change in bowel habits is the most common symptom (Table 34.8). Blood or mucus in stools may occur. Although all tumors cause varying degrees of obstruction, those in the descending colon and rectum generally do not cause anemia, weight loss, nausea, or vomiting.

Diagnostic Tests

Home screening for blood in the stool can be done with a home colon cancer test kit. ColonCare is a newer immunological test that looks for small amounts of blood. If blood is found, a physician should be contacted for follow-up. Most colorectal cancers are identified by biopsy done at the time of endoscopy (proctosigmoidoscopy, sigmoidoscopy, or colonoscopy). A CT scan can perform a virtual colonoscopy to view the inside of the colon. In addition to abdominal and rectal examination, other tests include fecal occult blood testing and barium enema. Carcinoembryonic antigen (CEA), a blood test, is used to assess response to treatment of GI cancer. CEA is present when epithelial cells rapidly divide and provides an early warning that the cancer has returned.

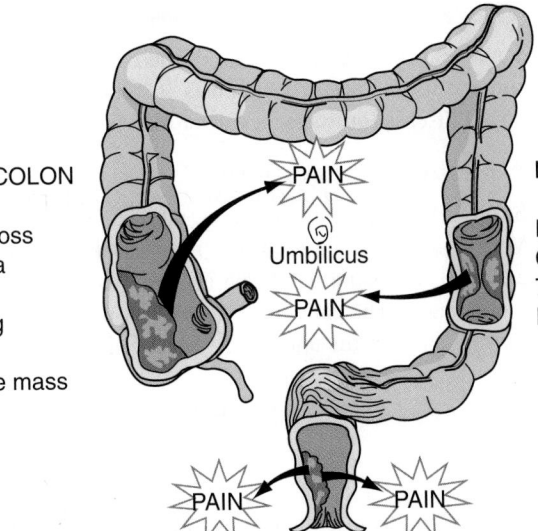

RIGHT COLON

Weight loss
Anorexia
Nausea
Vomiting
Anemia
Palpable mass

LEFT COLON AND RECTUM

Rectal bleeding
Changed bowel habits
Tenesmus
Intestinal obstruction

FIGURE 34.6 Symptoms of carcinoma of the colon. Pain usually radiates toward the umbilicus or perianal area. *(Modified from Black, JM, and Matassarin-Jacobs, E: Medical-Surgical Nursing, ed. 5. Saunders, Philadelphia, 1997, p 1810, with permission.)*

Therapeutic Interventions

Small localized tumors may be excised and treated during endoscopy or laparoscopy. These procedures can also be used as palliative care for patients with advanced tumors who cannot tolerate major surgery.

Surgery is performed to either resect larger tumors and anastomose the remaining bowel or create a fecal diversion by forming an ostomy. A variety of surgical procedures can be done depending on the location and extent of the cancer (Table 34.9). In rectal cancer, an abdominoperineal (A&P) resection is done with the formation of a permanent end colostomy (Fig. 34.7). With an A + P resection, the anus, rectum, and part of the sigmoid colon are removed. There is a perineal wound, often with a drain inserted short-term, where the anus was that will heal. Medical management includes radiation therapy and chemotherapy. When both are used, along with surgery, increased survival rates have been demonstrated.

Complications

Complications include bleeding, complete obstruction of the colon, perforation, anastomosis leaking leading to peritonitis, and extension of the tumor to adjacent organs. Colorectal cancer can metastasize to the lymphatic system and liver.

If the patient has an anastomotic leak, the location of the leak determines the effects that are seen. The patient may need to be NPO for up to 4 weeks to rest the GI tract and prevent more leakage and receive high-dose antibiotic therapy such as ciprofloxacin (Cipro) or metronidazole (Flagyl). Ongoing monitoring includes WBCs, sedimentation rate, and fever. The patient will likely go home with special home care needs. A peripherally inserted central catheter (PICC line) is placed to continue the antibiotic therapy.

Nursing Process for the Patient with Colon or Rectal Cancer

Assessment/Data Collection

Risk factors for colon or rectal cancer are identified by asking questions about the patient's personal and family history: Is there a history of inflammatory bowel disease? What were the patient's dietary habits? What foods were usually eaten, and how much fluid was usually consumed? Prior to diagnosis, did the patient experience constipation or diarrhea? Has there been a change in bowel habits? Has mucus or blood been noted in the stools? What social habits does the patient have? Did the patient smoke, drink alcoholic beverages, exercise? Has there has been a recent weight loss? How much and in what time frame? Does the patient admit to unusual fatigue or insomnia? Stool should be checked for mucus or blood.

If the patient has surgery, postoperative assessment includes monitoring vital signs and the return of flatus and bowel movements. Lung sounds are monitored for response to coughing and deep breathing and early ambulation. Dressings are observed for drainage. Large amounts of drainage or bleeding are reported. If a drain is inserted, often

TABLE 34.8 COLON CANCER SUMMARY

Sings and Symptoms	Change in bowel habits
	Blood or mucus in stools
	Abdominal or rectal pain
	Weight loss
	Anemia
	Obstruction
Diagnostic Tests	Colonoscopy with biopsy
	Sigmoidoscopy with biopsy
	Proctosigmoidoscopy
	Barium enema
	Abdominal and rectal examination
	Fecal occult blood
Therapeutic Interventions	Surgery, possibly colostomy
	Radiation
	Chemotherapy and/or radiation
	Medications: analgesics
	TPN as necessary
	Support and education

TABLE 34.9 INTESTINAL SURGERIES

Types of Intestinal Surgery	Definition	Effect on Stool Elimination
Partial colectomy	Part of colon removed	Anastomosed ends; stool is passed via rectum and anus.
Right colectomy	Right side of colon removed	Anastomosed ends; stool is passed via rectum and anus.
Ileocolectomy	Right side of colon and diseased portion of ileum removed	Anastomosed ends; stool is passed via rectum and anus.
Abdominoperineal resection	Sigmoid colon, rectum, anus removed	End colostomy
Proctosigmoidectomy	Sigmoid colon and rectum removed	Colorectal anastomosis
Total abdominal colectomy	Entire colon removed; rectum and anus remain	Ileorectal anastomosis; ileal pouch
Total proctocolectomy	Entire colon, rectum, and maybe anus removed	Ileostomy; if anus left, ileal pouch

in the perineal wound, moderate amounts of serosan-guineous (light pink) drainage are expected. If the patient has an ostomy, it is monitored (see ostomy section below).

Nursing Diagnosis, Planning, and Implementation
Acute pain related to tissue compression from the tumor

EXPECTED OUTCOME: The patient will report pain relieved or at an acceptable level.

* Have patient identify pain using a rating scale *to identify pain level consistently.*
* Postoperatively, administer analgesics as prescribed *to relive pain.*

Anxiety related to diagnosis of cancer

EXPECTED OUTCOME: The patient will report anxiety relieved.

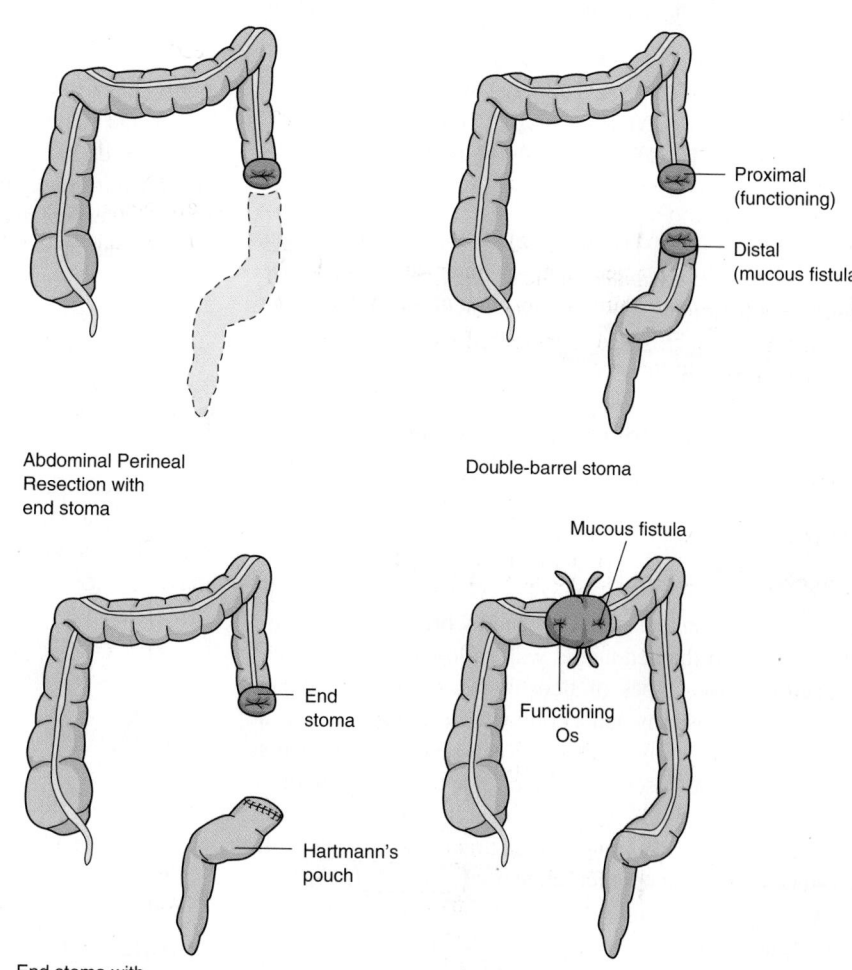

Abdominal Perineal Resection with end stoma

Double-barrel stoma

Proximal (functioning)

Distal (mucous fistula)

Mucous fistula

End stoma

Functioning Os

Hartmann's pouch

End stoma with Hartmann's pouch

Loop stoma (transverse)

FIGURE 34.7 Types of stomas.

- Set aside time to allow the patient who so desires to talk, cry, or ask questions about the diagnosis and planned surgery.
- Provide a quiet, relaxing atmosphere *to help alleviate anxiety*.
- Answer questions accurately *to provide a trusting relationship*.

Imbalanced nutrition: less than body requirements related to nausea and anorexia

EXPECTED OUTCOME: *The patient will maintain weight normal for height and age.*

- Give antiemetics as ordered *to relieve nausea*.
- Identify foods patients like and provide them *to stimulate appetite*.
- Give total parenteral nutrition as ordered *to provide depleted vitamins, minerals, and nutrients if the patient has been anorexic for any length of time or has had a significant weight loss*.
- Provide the patient with a high-protein, high-calorie diet, as ordered, that is low in residue *to decrease excessive peristalsis and minimize cramping*.

Evaluation

Expected outcomes are that the patient verbalizes control of pain and less anxiety, and attains an optimum level of nutrition.

OSTOMY AND CONTINENT OSTOMY MANAGEMENT

An ostomy is a surgically (traditionally abdominal incision or laprascopically) created opening that diverts stool or urine to the outside of the body through an opening on the abdomen called a **stoma.** A stoma is the portion of bowel that is sutured onto the abdomen. A continent ostomy uses an internal reservoir to collect stool. The types of abdominal ostomies include ileostomy, colostomy, and urostomy. (Urinary ostomies are discussed in Chapter 37.) The stomas can be end, loop, or double barrel. See Figure 34.7 for types of ostomies.

Ileostomy   —small bowel of ileum

An ileostomy is an end stoma formed by bringing the terminal ileum out to the abdominal wall following a total proctocolectomy. Two types of ileostomies can be formed: a conventional ileostomy and a continent ileostomy, such as a Kock pouch (sometimes called a Koch pouch) or Barnett's continent internal reservoir which is a modification of a Kock pouch (Fig. 34.8). A conventional ileostomy is a small stoma in the right lower quadrant that requires a pouch at all times because of the continuous flow of liquid effluent.

Continent ileostomies are formed by taking a portion of the terminal ileum to construct an internal reservoir with a nipple valve. A stoma is created and the patient is taught to insert a catheter into the stoma three or four times a day to

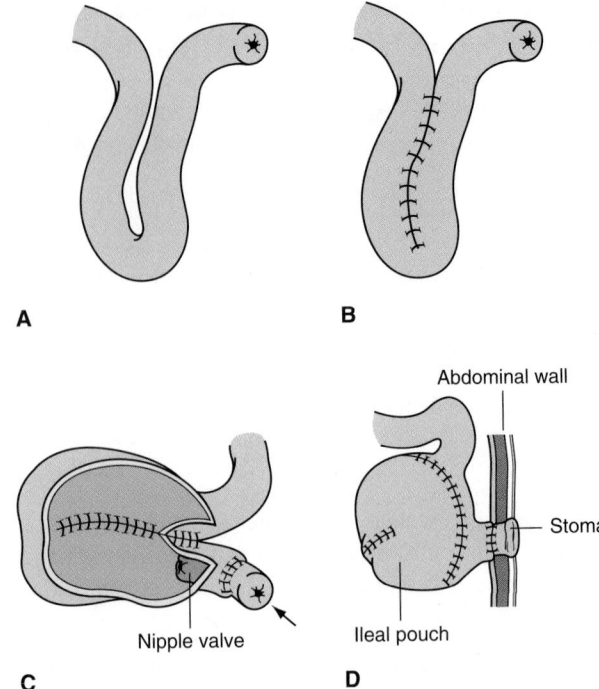

FIGURE 34.8 Surgical formation of continent ileostomy (Kock pouch). (*A*) Loop of terminal ileum. (*B*) Both limbs of ileum are brought together and sutured into a U shape. (*C*) Pouch created with nipple valve. (*D*) Pouch sutured to abdominal wall.

empty the reservoir. A continent ileostomy surgery takes longer and requires additional instruction for the patient to be able to do self-care. It is important that the patient empty the pouch routinely to prevent pouch rupture. Complications can occur, especially for the Kock pouch, such as valve slippage or leaking, pouch rupture, or pouchitis. Corrective surgery may be required.

An ileoanal anastomosis connects the ileum to the anus and avoids the need for a stoma (Fig. 34.9). This is usually a two-step procedure. During the first surgery, the diseased bowel is removed. A reservoir (named by its shape: J [most

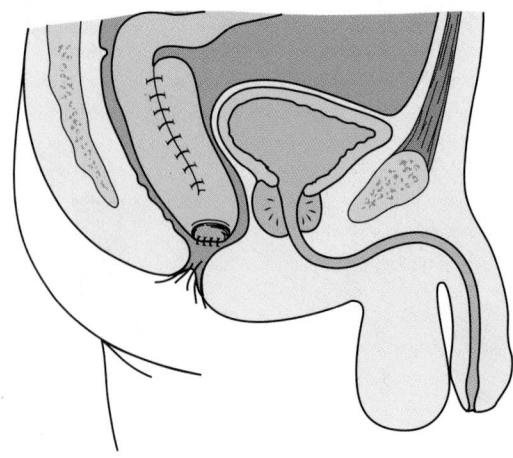

FIGURE 34.9 Ileal J pouch–anal anastomosis. The two-loop ileal pouch is simple to construct, provides adequate storage capacity, and is evacuated spontaneously and fully.

common], S, W, or H pouch) is then formed from part of the ileum and connected to the anus. A temporary ileostomy is also formed to divert stool while the reservoir heals. After about 3 months, the temporary ileostomy is reversed and the patient can have bowel movements from the anus. Problems with perianal skin irritation resulting from frequent liquid stools may occur. An ileorectal anastomosis can also be performed, but this may not be a curative procedure for a patient with ulcerative colitis because the rectum may still be diseased.

Colostomy

A colostomy is named according to where in the bowel it is formed: It may be an ascending, transverse, descending, or sigmoid colostomy. The type of effluent is dependent on the location of the bowel used (Table 34.10).

LEARNING TIP

As stool travels through the colon, water is absorbed and the stool becomes firmer. Therefore, an ileostomy produces the most liquid effluent, followed by an ascending colostomy. A descending or sigmoid colostomy produces the firmest stool. Those with an ileostomy are at increased risk for dehydration due to greater water loss.

End Stoma

An end stoma is formed when the proximal end of the bowel is brought to the outside abdominal wall. If an abdominal perineal resection is done (usually for low rectal cancer), the rectum is removed and the proximal sigmoid or descending colon is brought out as a stoma. Another procedure that may be done involves removing the segment of diseased or injured bowel and using the proximal portion to form the stoma. The remaining limb of bowel is sutured closed and left in the peritoneal cavity so that the rectum is intact. This is called a Hartmann's pouch, or mucous fistula, and may be permanent or temporary depending on the diagnosis. Because the rectum is intact, the patient may feel the urge to defecate. This is normal because the colon continues to produce mucus. As the rectal stump fills with mucus, the

sphincter is triggered and alerts the patient as if it were stool.

Loop Stoma

To create a loop stoma, a loop of bowel, usually the transverse colon, is pulled to the outside abdominal wall and a bridge is slipped under the loop to hold it in place. An incisional slit is made in the top of the exposed colon to allow stool to exit. The entire loop of bowel is not cut through.

Double-Barrel Stoma

With a double-barrel stoma, the bowel is completely dissected and both ends of the colon are brought to the outside abdominal wall to form two separate stomas. The proximal stoma is the functioning stoma that expels stool. The distal stoma is called a mucous fistula because mucus produced by the bowel passes from it. A double-barrel stoma is often temporary, allowing the bowel to rest during healing after trauma or surgery.

Preoperative Care

A wound ostomy continence nurse (WOCN) should be consulted before surgery. The WOCN can help prepare the patient both emotionally and physically for the surgery. In addition, the WOCN has expertise in selecting the stoma site for the surgeon to ensure that it is easy to sit with it, care for it, and wear clothing over it. This involves observing the abdomen as the patient assumes different positions and noting how clothing is worn, such as where the belt rides. The site for the stoma can then be chosen so it is visible to the patient for self-care, avoids skin or fat folds, and is where clothing will not interfere with the appliance. Properly planned stoma placement can prevent agony over discomfort when sitting, inability to perform self-care, and uncomfortable, leaking, or poorly fitting appliances postoperatively.

Routine preoperative instruction, including the importance of coughing and deep breathing, splinting, and early ambulation, is provided. Orders for cleansing of the bowel are performed to reduce the risk for infection following surgery. Unless the patient has chronic diarrhea related to IBD, an oral agent to cleanse the bowel (such as Osmoprep, Go-LYTELY) is given. Oral and intravenous antibiotics are given as ordered.

Nursing Process for the Patient with an Ostomy or Continent Ostomy

Assessment/Data Collection

The patient with a new ostomy has many nursing care needs. In addition to routine postoperative assessment, a stoma should be inspected at least every 8 hours. The stoma should be pink to red, moist (similar to the inside of the mouth), and well attached to the surrounding skin (Fig. 34.10). A bluish stoma indicates inadequate blood supply; a black stoma indicates necrosis. Either complication should be reported to the physician immediately for treatment, which may require that the patient return to surgery. Note edema of stoma. The stoma size gradually decreases over the first few weeks following surgery.

TABLE 34.10 LOCATION OF STOMA AND TYPE OF EFFLUENT

Location of Stoma	Type of Effluent
Ileostomy	Liquid to mushy
Cecostomy, ascending colostomy	Liquid to mushy, foul odor
Right transverse colostomy	Mushy to semiformed
Left transverse colostomy	Semiformed, soft
Descending or sigmoid colostomy	Soft to hard formed

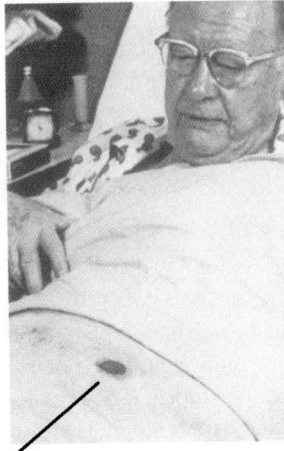

Man above has a descending or "dry" colostomy.

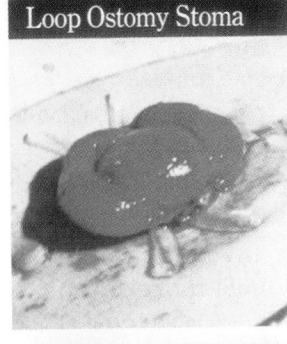

Loop Ostomy Stoma

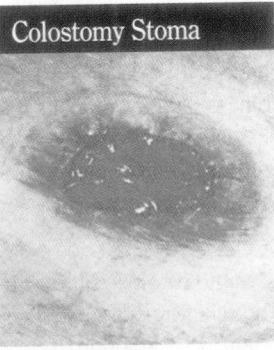

Colostomy Stoma

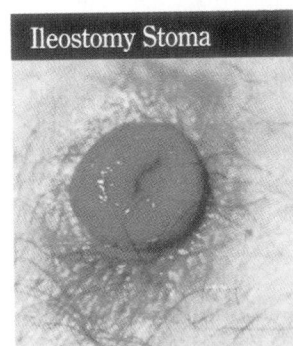

Ileostomy Stoma

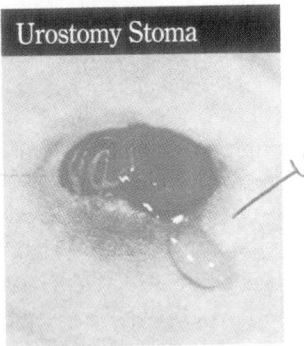

Urostomy Stoma

FIGURE 34.10 Types of stomas. Note moist, pink to red appearance of healthy stoma. *(Reproduced with permission of Hollister Inc., Libertyville, Illinois)*

Skin is assessed for irritation around the pouch and under the pouch each time it is changed. Ostomy discharge (effluent) is monitored and documented. Unexpected changes, such as liquid stool from a descending ostomy, are reported.

For the patient with a continent ostomy pouch, assessing that regular emptying of the pouch is done is important to prevent rupture and leakage. The characteristics of the stool are noted for any type of continent ostomy so that problems can be reported.

Nursing Diagnosis, Planning, and Implementation
See Box 34.10 Nursing Care Plan for the Patient with an Intestinal Ostomy and Table 34.11.

Deficient knowledge related to new ostomy

EXPECTED OUTCOME: Patient will demonstrate how to care for ostomy.

- Determine patient readiness and ability to learn and perform self-care. *The patient experiencing pain,*

nausea, or vomiting is not likely to be ready to look at the ostomy or learn about ostomy care.
- Patients with special needs: blindness, deafness, language barrier, severe arthritis or other physical conditions that limit ability to perform self-care require special instructions or specific type of ostomy appliance *to be able to perform self-care.*
- If the patient is not ready or able to learn, it is important that a family member or caregiver be included in the teaching. *With short hospital stays, teaching time frames are limited and must begin soon after surgery.*
- Ensure referral to home care nurse is made *to continue teaching in the patient's home.*
- Consult a WOCN or equipment supplier if needed for suggestions for appliances *to identify appliances suited to individual patient's needs.* Figure 34.11 shows types of appliances.
- Explain how to change appliance (Fig. 34.12):
  - Depending on the type of appliance used, the appliance will need to be changed as often as every 3 days or rarely every 10 to 14 days.
  - If leakage occurs, the appliance should be changed as soon as possible to avoid **peristomal** skin irritation.
  - The skin barrier that is placed over the stoma on the skin should fit within one-sixteenth to one-eighth inch of the base of the stoma *to prevent skin contact with stool.*
  - The stoma should be measured initially with each appliance change *as the stoma will be edematous until it shrinks over time.*
  - Trace a stoma pattern to teach the patient proper size and shape *because most stomas are not round.*
  - An open-ended or drainable pouch should be used for all colostomies or ileostomies, especially during the first 8 weeks after surgery *to facilitate emptying and comfort.*
- Explain to the patient who has a left-sided (descending or sigmoid) colostomy that the bowel can be regulated either by diet or regular irrigation of the stoma. *Once bowel regulation has been achieved, the patient may use a closed-end pouch or a stoma cap.*
- Explain daily care and hygiene:
  - Empty pouch when it is one-third to one-half full. *The amount of effluent and the frequency of emptying depends on the location of the stoma in the bowel. If the pouch is allowed to get more than half full of stool, the weight of the effluent will pull on the pouch and weaken the seal of the skin barrier.*
  - Once the pouch is emptied, the inside of the tail of the pouch must be cleaned and dried before the clamp is replaced *to help control odor. If a two-*

---

peristomal: peri—surrounding + stoma—mouth or opening

Box 34.10   NURSING CARE PLAN for the Patient with an Intestinal Ostomy

Disturbed body image related to new ostomy

Patient Outcomes Patient will verbalize acceptance of intestinal ostomy before discharge.

Evaluation of Outcomes Is the patient able to verbalize acceptance of the ostomy?

Interventions	Rationale	Evaluation
Ask about knowledge of self-care of ostomies.	Many people have misconceptions regarding ostomies. Identification of misconceptions and "hearsay" knowledge is important to clarify or correct.	Does the patient verbalize appropriate knowledge of ostomy care?
Encourage patient to verbalize feelings about the stoma.	Allowing the patient to express his or her feelings provides opportunity to identify and verbalize concerns, which then can be addressed by health-care providers.	Does the patient discuss his or her feelings regarding the stoma to the nurse or significant other?
Explain the normal characteristics of the stoma before the patient's first look.	Helping the patient understand what to expect will help relieve anxiety. Being available to answer questions immediately also relieves anxiety.	Does the patient look at the stoma without hesitation?
Demonstrate ostomy appliance change and daily care and encourage patient participation.	When the patient observes and participates in self-care, his or her self-concept improves.	Is the patient participating in self-care? Has the patient performed return demonstration of appliance change and emptying of pouch?

piece system is used, the pouch can be taken off, washed out, and replaced.
- Spray deodorants or chlorophyll tablets can be placed in the pouch *to control odor. Chlorophyll is more effective if taken by mouth.*
- Bathe or shower with the appliance in place

but check seal and retape or change it if it is loosening.
- Explain dietary considerations:
  - Identify foods that contribute to odor and gas. *If foods that are known to cause odor or gas are eaten, the patient should know to empty the pouch*

TABLE 34.11   SUMMARY OF RECOVERY FROM INTESTINAL SURGERY

Intestinal Surgery	Elimination Needs	Discharge Teaching needs	Possible Psychological Needs
Partial colectomy	Normal, no appliance needed.	Monitor for constipation.	Fear of cancer
Right colectomy or ileocolectomy	Normal, no appliance needed.	Avoid stress to abdomen: heavy lifting, situps. Soft diet until first doctor visit. Monitor for constipation and report.	Fear of cancer; chronic sorrow related to IBD
Abdominoperineal resection	Pouch	Ostomy care	Fear of cancer Body image changes
Proctosigmoidectomy	Normal, no appliance needed	Soft diet until first doctor visit. Monitor for constipation and report.	Fear of cancer
Total abdominal colectomy	Normal or continent anal passage	Continent ostomy care. Soft diet until first doctor visit. Monitor for constipation and report.	Chronic sorrow related to IBD
Total proctocolectomy	Continent anal passage or pouch	Continent ostomy care. Soft diet until first doctor visit. Monitor for constipation and report.	Chronic sorrow related to IBD

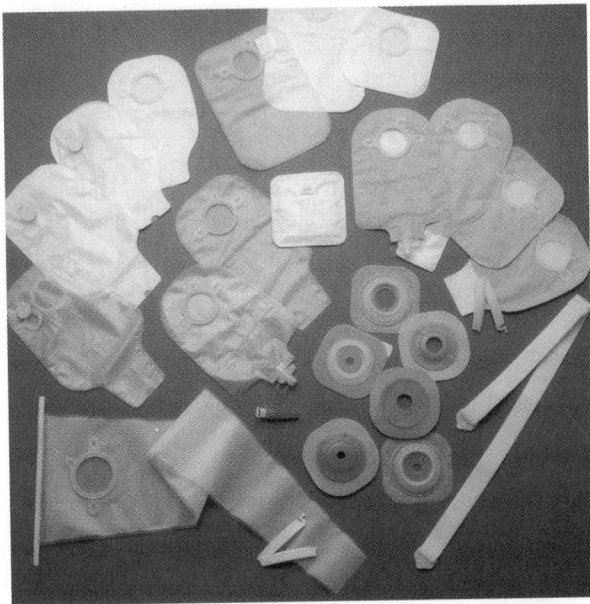

FIGURE 34.11 Appliances used for ostomies. The long sleeve at the lower left of the photograph is used to drain the bowel following irrigation. *(Reproduced with permission of Hollister Inc., Libertyville, Illinois)*

  of flatus more often and to be aware that more odor is probable.
- Identify foods that contribute to and control diarrhea and what to do for constipation. *A list of foods that may contribute to ileostomy blockage must be given to the ileostomy patient* (Table 34.12; Box 34.11 Nutrition Notes).
- Explain colostomy irrigation:
  - Tell that colostomy irrigation is done *to regulate bowel movements at a regular time.* Candidates for irrigation are those with more formed stool (descending or sigmoid portion of colon).
  - Show how to perform irrigation (similar to an enema), with special equipment used to instill fluid into the bowel via the stoma. *Since a stoma does not have a sphincter, specially designed tubing with a cone at the end is used to irrigate the ostomy. The cone blocks the fluid that is being instilled from flowing back out of the stoma.*

Ineffective Therapeutic Regimen Management related to difficulty carrying out self-care measures
- Identify financial ability to obtain supplies. *The cost and availability of ostomy supplies is problematic for many patients. Most insurers, including Medicare, pay for ostomy supplies, although some limit the type of appliance and number allowed per month. Each state-funded Medicaid system is different. The type of appliance needed to eliminate leakage may not always be covered, requiring the patient to either pay the difference or wear what the insurance company will provide. If the patient has no insurance, costs can be high. Some patients find*

Preparation of the Stomahesive Wafer with Sur-Fit Flange

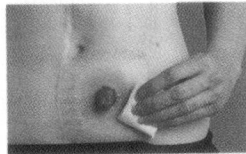

1. Cleanse the peristomal area with water and pat thoroughly dry. Measure your stoma size with the measuring guide provided and trace the proper opening on the white paper backing of the Stomahesive® disc.

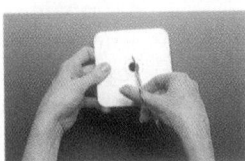

2. Leaving the white paper backing of the wafer in place, cut a hole in the wafer to the same shape and size as the base of the stoma. The best result is usually obtained by cutting from the reverse side of the wafer, using curved, short-bladed scissors.

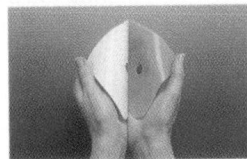

3. Peel the white paper backing from the wafer just prior to application.

4. Gaps between the wafer and the base of the stoma may be further protected by applying Stomahesive® Paste to the wafer.

Application of the Stomahesive Wafer with Sur-Fit Flange

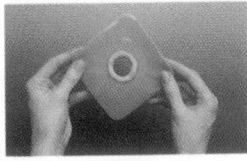

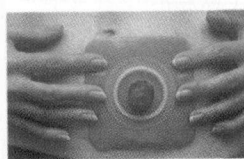

5. Center the enlarged hole over the stoma, place on abdomen, and apply light pressure.

FIGURE 34.12 Preparation to apply an ostomy appliance. *(Courtesy ConvaTec, a Bristol-Myers Squibb Company, Princeton, NJ, with permission.)*

they have to choose whether to purchase ostomy appliances or prescriptions with their limited funds. Fortunately, the pouches in most two-piece systems can be washed out and reused to save money (see Home Health Hints).

Sexual dysfunction related to body image change or erectile dysfunction

EXPECTED OUTCOME: Patient will discuss satisfying acceptable sexual practices for self and partner.

TABLE 34.12 FOODS THAT CAN CAUSE ILEOSTOMY BLOCKAGE

Green leafy vegetables	Mushrooms
Spinach	Nuts
Collards	Dried fruits
Mustards	Raisins
Cole slaw	Figs
Celery	Apricots
Corn, popcorn	Chinese vegetables
Foods with nondigestible	Meats with casings
peels	Sausage
Apples	Hot dogs
Grapes	Bologna
Potatoes	
Coconut	

- Identify if male patient who had an abdominoperineal resection for cancer of the rectum has erectile dysfunction. *This impotence may be transient, depending on the severity of nerve damage or edema associated with the surgery.*
- Ensure consultation with urologist is made if erectile dysfunction is present.
- Encourage patients to discuss any concerns regarding sexuality with his or her sexual partner. *This may help them work through any fears or embarrassment.*

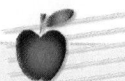

Box 34.11

Nutrition Notes

Anticipating Dietary Management of Ostomies

Ostomy patients receive a soft diet initially, progressing to a general diet as the surgeon prescribes. Stringy, high-fiber foods are avoided initially. These include celery, coconut, corn, cabbage, coleslaw, membranes on citrus fruits, peas, popcorn, spinach, dried fruit, nuts, sauerkraut, pineapple, seeds, and skins of fruits and vegetables. Some patients avoid fish, eggs, beer, and carbonated beverages because they produce excessive odor. Dietary restrictions are usually based on individual tolerance.

Patients with ostomies should be encouraged to do the following:

- Eat at regular intervals.
- Chew food well to avoid blockage at the stoma site.
- Drink adequate amounts of fluid.
- Avoid foods that produce excessive gas, loose stools, offensive odors, and undesirable bulk.
- Avoid excessive weight gain.

- Attractive pouch covers can be purchased and worn *to help disguise the pouch and its contents.*
- Refer to sexual counselor who can suggest alternative sexual positions that may be satisfying to the partners.

Risk for injury related to skin and stomal complications

- Consult WOCN for complications associated with the care of the ostomy. *A WOCN has had specialized instruction in caring for the stoma and peristomal skin and has a wealth of information to offer.*
- Identify allergies. *Allergic dermatitis from sensitivity to the adhesive may develop.*
- Use a skin barrier such as stomahesive *to prevent peristomal skin irritation. The skin around the stoma may become irritated if the opening in the skin barrier around the stoma is cut too large and exposes skin to the GI effluent. Prolonged contact with effluent can lead to a reaction similar to a chemical burn.*
- Ensure tape and adhesive removal is done only when necessary. *If done frequently, it can lead to skin shearing.*
- Leave pouches on for several days or until leakage occurs *to prevent skin shearing from frequent removal.*
- Monitor for peristomal hernia. *Hernias may develop around the stoma as a result of weakened abdominal muscles and cause leakage by the change in body contours associated with the hernia.*
- Use a more flexible ostomy appliance if perisomal hernia present *to fit body contours better.*
- *Monitor for and report stomal prolapse, especially in the older adult patient.* Weakened abdominal muscles contribute to the falling down (or out) of the intestinal mucosa which can make pouching difficult.
- Monitor stoma color and report immediately dusky or blue color *which occurs when there is circulatory compromise. This may arise as a result of vascular collapse, blockage in the mesentery of the intestines, or edema in the intestine from obstruction proximal to the stoma. Usually, necrotic tissue occurs only at the very end of the stoma and will eventually slough off, revealing viable mucosa.*
- Explain signs and symptoms of an ileostomy blockage and how to manage it. Signs of a blockage are absent stool, abdominal cramping, edematous stoma, and stoma color that is pale or dusky.
- If blockage occurs, have patient consider what was eaten in the past 24 hours *because certain foods are considered to cause stomal blockage.* (See Table 34.12.)

- For an ileostomy blockage, have the patient get into a tub of warm water (not too hot or cold), get into a knee-to-chest position, and sip on warm liquid, such as coffee, tea, bouillon, broth, or hot chocolate. *If the blockage is partial, relief will occur fairly soon after these measures are taken.*
- Explain to patient that if no relief is obtained, medical treatment should be sought. *For a complete blockage, an ileostomy lavage must be performed by a physician or WOCN.*

Evaluation

The plan of care has been effective if the patient is able to accept the change in body image, competently care for the ostomy (or caregiver will), carry out self-care, is satisfied with sexual practices, and describes self-care measures to prevent or treat complications.

Rehabilitative Needs

Ensuring that the patient is becoming comfortable with self-care, is able to perform the ostomy appliance change, and is able to return to work or civic activities as before are the goals of care. The patient can generally perform any activity he or she was able to do before the ostomy. Several support resources are available (Table 34.13).

TABLE 34.13 RESOURCES AND SUPPORT GROUPS

United Ostomy Association, Inc. (UOAA)
www.uoaa.org
info[at]uoaa.org
(800) 826-0826 (toll free)

Celiac Sprue Association
PO Box 34700
Omaha, NE 68134
(402) 558-0600
www.csaceliacs.org

Crohn and Colitis Foundation of America, Inc.
386 Park Ave. South
17th Floor
New York, NY 10016-8804
(212) 685-3440 (voice)
(212) 779-4098 (fax)
(800) 932-2423 (toll free)
www.ccfa.org

American Cancer Society (ACS)
(800) ACS-2345
www.cancer.org

National Institute of Diabetes and Digestive and Kidney Diseases, NIH
http://digestive.niddk.nih.gov/ddiseases/pubs/ibs.

Home Health Hints

- Patients with ostomies may be able to have some of their supplies covered by insurance. The home health nurse can work with the medical supply store to assist the patient in receiving the necessary equipment. Most companies will deliver the supplies to the patient's home.
- Foods such as broccoli, cauliflower, Brussels sprouts, and cabbage can cause increased malodorous gas production. Encourage the patient with a colostomy to eat these in moderation. Offer alternative choices such as: green leafy vegetables, carrots, and cucumbers.

- If the patient requires a stool for occult blood test, deliver a collection hat before you visit to assist with obtaining the specimen. Plan to deliver the specimen to the laboratory that day.
- Dietary instruction is important for home health patients with lower GI disorders. Give instructions both verbally and in written format. Written format allows the patient to have the information available for review and to assist with creating a shopping list.

REVIEW QUESTIONS

1. The nurse is collecting data on a patient admitted with a history of severe diarrhea. Findings include cool, pale skin, red tongue with furrows, blood pressure 102/74, pulse 106, respirations 20, temperature 99.9° F (37.7°C). Which of the following actions should the nurse take now?
   a. Report findings to registered nurse
   b. Give acetaminophen (Tylenol) as ordered
   c. Obtain bedside commode
   d. Apply warm blankets

2. The nurse is planning a teaching session for a patient who has a history of constipation and laxative use. Which of the following statements about laxative use would the nurse include in the teaching plan to promote patient understanding?
   a. Laxatives may be used as needed.
   b. Regular laxative use can be harmful.
   c. Daily use of laxatives prevents constipation.
   d. Laxative use has no complications.

Multiple response item. Select all that apply.

3. Which of the following interventions should the nurse include in the plan of care for a patient after an appendectomy to prevent respiratory complications?
   a. Pain control
   b. Early ambulation
   c. Bedrest
   d. Coughing, deep breathing
   e. Turning in bed
   f. Incentive spirometer

4. Which of the following foods would the nurse teach the patient with ulcerative colitis to avoid?
   a. Fresh fruits
   b. White bread
   c. Sweet desert
   d. Meat

5. Following a teaching session, which of the following statements would indicate to the nurse that the patient understood the teaching for postoperative care to prevent respiratory complications after a hernia repair?
   a. "I will cough every hour while awake to keep my lungs clear."
   b. "I will deep breathe four times daily."
   c. " I will cough and deep breathe every hour."
   d. "I will deep breathe every hour while awake."

6. The nurse would evaluate the patient as understanding adult celiac disease teaching if the patient selected which of the following foods to eat?
   a. Pancakes with hash brown potatoes
   b. Tomato juice and waffles
   c. Hard boiled egg, bacon, and blueberries
   d. Banana, cream of wheat cereal, and coffee

Multiple response item. Select all that apply.

7. The nurse is caring for a patient with a small bowel obstruction. The patient is NPO with an orogastric tube to low intermittent suction. Which of the following ongoing data would be a priority for the nurse to monitor and collect?
   a. Intake and output
   b. Pain level
   c. Bowel sounds
   d. Pulse rate
   e. Temperature
   f. Edema

8. The nurse is caring for a patient who has a sudden onset of diarrhea. Which of the following terms should the nurse use to document the patient's black, tarry stool?
   a. Melena
   b. Hematochezia
   c. Hematemesis
   d. Steatorrhea

9. The nurse is developing a teaching plan for a patient who is interested in lifestyle changes to help prevent colon cancer. Which of the following of the patient's dietary habits does the nurse understand may increase the risk for development of colon cancer?
   a. High-fat, low-fiber intake
   b. High intake of milk and milk products
   c. Low-meat and protein intake
   d. Low-fat, high-carbohydrate intake

10. The nurse is caring for a 1-day postoperative patient who has a new end colostomy. Which of the following findings regarding the stoma would be a priority for the nurse to report?
    a. Dusky color
    b. Mucus drainage
    c. Slight bleeding with touch
    d. Round shape

11. A patient with Crohn's disease is to receive sulfasalazine (Azulfidine), 500 mg oral suspension qid.
    The oral suspension is available as 250 mg/5 mL. How many milliliters should the nurse give for the 0800 dose?
    a. 5 mL
    b. 10 mL
    c. 20 mL
    d. 50 mL

SUGGESTED ANSWERS TO

CRITICAL THINKING

■ Mrs. Burns

You need to assess the situation before intervening. First, ask Mrs. Burns or her caregivers if she had a bowel movement that was inadvertently not charted. Next, ask Mrs. Burns if she feels constipated or if she has abdominal discomfort. Assess Mrs. Burns's abdomen for distention and presence or absence of bowel sounds. A digital examination may be necessary to determine if a fecal impaction is present. If simple constipation appears to be the problem, the medical record should be checked for as-needed laxative or enema orders. Once Mrs. Burns has had a bowel movement, laxatives should be discontinued and preventive measures such as regular fluids, fiber, and exercise should be instituted.

■ *Judy Morrow*

1. Characteristics of pain: location, quality, intensity, precipitating factors, relieving factors.

   Characteristics of bowel elimination: frequency, characteristic of stool, amount, color, consistency.

   Nutritional status: Weight loss, appetite, daily food intake, food likes/dislikes, irritating foods, fluid intake.

   Anxiety and coping skills: Support systems, usual coping methods.

2. Acute pain related to increased peristalsis and cramping

   Diarrhea related to inflammatory process

   Risk for deficient fluid volume related to diarrhea and insufficient fluid intake

   Anxiety related to symptoms and frequency of stools and treatment.

   Impaired skin integrity related to frequent loose stools

   Ineffective nutrition, less than body requirements, related to malabsorption

   Ineffective coping related to frequency of stools

3. You need to further assess how Judy perceives that Crohn's disease will affect her lifestyle. What does she know about Crohn's disease? What is she concerned about? How has Crohn's disease affected her ability to sleep, what she eats, her participation in sports, and her relationships with other people?

   Convey a caring manner to Judy by being accepting of her, listening actively to her concerns, and helping her to find acceptable ways of resolving them. Provide her with information that she needs about Crohn's disease. Arrange to have a well-adapted person of approximately the same age from the Crohn's and Colitis Foundation of America meet with her to share coping strategies with her.

4. Increased frequency of stools leading to fluid volume deficit and possibly shock symptoms. Bleeding leading to anemia and hypovolemia and possibly shock symptoms.

■ *Mrs. Loos*

1. You need to further assess Mrs. Loos before deciding what to do. Begin by asking the WHAT'S UP? questions, including exactly where the pain is occurring, how it feels, if there is anything that aggravates or alleviates the pain, when it started, how bad it is on a scale of 0 to 10, whether there are associated symptoms, and if Mrs. Loos has some insight regarding the cause of her problem. Listen for bowel sounds for 5 minutes in each quadrant. Find out when her last bowel movement was.

2. Because of her history of diabetes, you suspect that neuropathy may be causing a nonmechanical bowel obstruction. If assessment findings confirm this possibility, the physician should be contacted. Because of the nausea and the potential obstruction, withhold food and fluids until the physician can be contacted.

3. When documenting, answer the questions what, why, when, where, who, how (either explicitly or implicitly by professional knowledge, in narrative or flow sheet format) for completeness.

   What = Patient is experiencing large, firm, tender to touch abdomen with nausea (additional assessment data should be included).

   Why = Unknown, physician notified

   When = Current date and time

   Where = Abdomen

   How = Unknown

   Who = J. Morgan, LPN

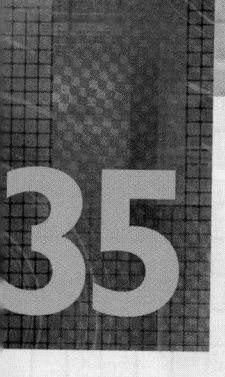

35

Nursing Care of Patients with Liver, Gallbladder, and Pancreatic Disorders

JEAN JEFFRIES

KEY TERMS

ascites (a-SIGH-teez)
asterixis (AS-ter-IK-sis)
cholecystitis (KOH-lee-sis-TIGH-tis)
choledochoscopy (koh-LED-oh-KOS-koh-pee)
choledocholithiasis (koh-LED-oh-koh-li-THIGH-ah-sis)
cholelithiasis (KOH-lee-li-THIGH-ah-sis)
cirrhosis (si-ROH-sis)
colic (KAH-lik)
encephalopathy (en-SEF-uh-LAHP-ah-thee)
extracorporeal shock-wave lithotripsy (EKS-trah-kor-POR-ee-uhl SHAHK-wayv LITH-oh-TRIP-see)
fetor hepaticus (FEE-tor he-PAT-i-kus)
hepatitis (HEP-uh-TIGH-tis)
hepatorenal syndrome (he-PAT-oh-REE-nuhl SIN-drohm)
laparoscopy (LAP-uh-ROS-Koh-pee)
pancreatectomy (partial, total) (PAN-kree-uh-TEK-tuh-mee)
portal hypertension (POR-tuhl HIGH-per-TEN-shun)
T-tube (TEE-toob)
transjugular intrahepatic portosystemic shunt (TRANZ-jug-u-lar in-tra-he-PAT-ik por-to-sis-TEM-ik SHUNT)
varices (VAR-i-seez)

QUESTIONS TO GUIDE YOUR READING

1. How would you explain the causes, risk factors, and pathophysiology of the various types of liver disease?

2. What are current therapeutic interventions for patients with liver disease?

3. What nursing care should you provide for the patient experiencing a liver disorder?

4. What are the causes, risk factors, and pathophysiology of the various pancreatic disorders?

5. What are current therapeutic interventions for pancreatic disorders?

6. What nursing care would you provide for a patient with a pancreatic disorder?

7. What are the causes, risk factors, and pathophysiology of gallbladder disorders?

8. What are current therapeutic interventions for gallbladder disorders?

9. What nursing care would you provide for a patient with a gallbladder disorder?

DISORDERS OF THE LIVER

Hepatitis

Hepatitis is an inflammation of the cells of the liver, resulting from infection by viral agents or exposure to drugs toxic to the liver or occasionally from bacterial infection. Symptoms of hepatitis range from nearly no symptoms to life-threatening symptoms due to death of liver tissue.

Pathophysiology and Etiology

Hepatitis is usually caused by one of six viruses:

- Hepatitis A virus (HAV), sometimes called infectious hepatitis
- Hepatitis B virus (HBV), sometimes called serum hepatitis

---

hepatitis: hepat—liver + itis—inflammation

- Hepatitis C virus (HCV), sometimes called non-A, non-B (NANB) hepatitis
- Hepatitis D virus (HDV)
- Hepatitis E virus (HEV)
- Hepatitis G virus (HGV)

The viral agents vary by mode of infection, incubation period, symptoms, diagnostic tests, and preventive vaccines (Table 35.1). The infecting organism causes inflammation of the liver, with resulting damage to liver cells and loss of liver function. If damage involves the bile canaliculi, obstructive jaundice will occur. If complications do not occur, cells regenerate and normal liver function eventually resumes.

There are an estimated 164,000 new hepatitis A, B, and C infections in the United States each year.[1] The incidence of HAV increased nearly 27% in the mid 1980s and is the most common cause of hepatitis. HAV has a low mortality rate. However, HBV is more common among some groups, including health-care workers and intravenous drug users; it

TABLE 35.1 COMPARISON OF TYPES OF VIRAL HEPATITIS

	Hepatitis A Virus	Hepatitis B Virus	Hepatitis C Virus	Hepatitis D Virus	Hepatitis E Virus
Mode of transmission	Oral-fecal contamination of water, shellfish, eating utensils, or equipment	Blood or body fluids such as saliva, semen, and breast milk; equipment contaminated by blood	Blood transfusions, IV drug use, unprotected sex	Blood or body fluids as with HBV; strongly linked as a confection with HBV	Usually, contaminated water
Incubation period *Symptoms*	3–7 weeks Early (prodromal): fatigue, anorexia, malaise, nausea, or vomiting	2–5 months Early (prodromal): 1–2 months of fatigue, malaise, anorexia, low-grade fever, nausea, headache, abdominal pain, muscle aches May have no early symptoms	1 week to months Same as HBV, usually less severe	Same as HBV Similar to HAV and to HBV but more severe	2–9 weeks Similar to HAV
	Icteric: jaundice, pale stools, amber or dark urine, RUQ pain	Icteric: jaundice, rashes			
Diagnostic tests	Elevated serum liver enzymes (ALT, AST), elevated serum bilirubin, HAV antigen	Elevated serum liver enzymes (ALT, AST), elevated serum bilirubin, HBV antigen	Elevated serum liver enzymes (ALT, AST), elevated serum bilirubin, HCV antigen	Elevated serum liver enzymes (ALT, AST), elevated serum bilirubin, HDV antigen	Elevated serum liver enzymes (ALT, AST), elevated serum bilirubin
Preventive vaccine	Immune globulin	Immune globulin or HBIG	None	HBIG	None
Groups at risk	Individuals in military or day care	IV drug abusers, homosexuals, health-care workers, transplant and hemodialysis patients	Same as HBV	Same as HBV	Travelers to endemic areas

ALT = alanine aminotransferase; AST = aspartate aminotransferase; HBIG = hepatitis B immune globulin;
IV = intravenous; RUQ = right upper quadrant.

has a mortality rate of about 5%. Hepatitis G virus is a recently discovered virus that is transmitted by blood transfusions and IV drug abuse. It may cause hepatitis, but not a lot is known about it yet.

Prevention

The hepatitis viruses are very resistant to a wide range of anti-infective measures, such as drying, heat, ultraviolet light exposure, freezing, and bleach and other disinfectants. At least 30 minutes in boiling water is required to destroy them. The best methods for preventing the transmission of the hepatitis viruses are careful attention to cleanliness and the use of vaccines such as immune serum globulin (ISG) or vaccines to HBV and HAV. Health-care workers must use standard precautions at all times. Infection control precautions should reflect the usual mode of transmission of the particular hepatitis virus.

Immune serum globulin provides temporary, passive, nonspecific immunity to hepatitis. Permanent, active immunity is acquired from the body's own antibodies in response to actual viral infection. The active immunity is to the specific virus to which the body has developed antibodies. Vaccines to HBV are available and provide permanent, active immunity to HBV. Health-care workers are strongly encouraged (and frequently required by employers as a condition of employment) to be vaccinated for HBV. A vaccine for HAV has also been developed.

Public health measures such as health education programs, licensing and supervision of public facilities, screening of blood donors, and careful screening of food handlers are general measures to prevent the transmission of hepatitis viruses.

SAFETY TIP

Protect yourself! Reduce the risk of health-care–associated infections. Comply with current Centers for Disease Control and Prevention (CDC) (www.CDC.gov) hand hygiene guidelines (2006 National Patient Safety Goals from www.JCAHO.org).

Signs and Symptoms

Hepatitis usually shows a typical pattern of loss of liver function. There are generally three stages:

1. The prodromal, or preicteric (prejaundice), stage lasts about 1 week. The patient complains of flu-like symptoms of malaise, headache, anorexia, low-grade fever, possibly dull right upper quadrant (RUQ) pain, nausea, vomiting, and diarrhea or constipation
2. The icteric stage peaks at 2 weeks and lasts 2 to 6 weeks. The patient continues to have fatigue, anorexia, nausea, vomiting, and malaise. The patient is also likely to have jaundice or noticeable

yellowing of the skin, sclerae of the eyes and other mucous membranes; dark amber urine; and clay-colored stools (see Chapter 32). The liver is usually enlarged and tender on examination.
3. The posticteric, or convalescent, stage lasts from 2 to 6 weeks with complete recovery in 6 months if relapse does not occur. The patient usually feels well during this time, but full recovery as measured by the return to normal of all liver function tests may take as long as 1 year.

Hepatitis is considered a reversible process if the patient complies with a medical regimen of adequate rest, good nutrition, and abstinence from alcohol or other liver-toxic agents for at least 1 year after liver function laboratory values return to normal. See Chapter 32 for a more complete discussion of jaundice.

Complications

Hepatitis may lead to fulminant or acute liver failure (see the following). About 5% of hepatitis patients progress to chronic liver failure. Some patients become asymptomatic carriers of the virus; HBV-infected carrier patients have a greater risk of developing cancer of the liver.

Diagnostic Tests   35.1

Serum liver enzymes are elevated. Serum bilirubin and urobilinogen may be elevated. The erythrocyte sedimentation rate is usually elevated from the inflammatory process. In patients with severe hepatitis, prothrombin time may be elevated (Table 35.2). Serological tests may be ordered to determine the specific virus causing the hepatitis. Each virus has specific antigen markers that serological study can reveal. The antigen markers can be further used to determine the degree of healing from the hepatitis. Abdominal x-ray examination may show an enlarged liver.

Therapeutic Interventions   Rest

Treatment is aimed at providing rest and adequate nutrition for healing. There are no specific drugs or other medical therapies for hepatitis. Interferon therapy and antiviral medication may be used for hepatitis B or C, but they may not be effective. A new medication is currently being researched that inhibits replication of the hepatitis C virus. Currently the best treatment is proper rest and nutrition.

Very important

Patients are restricted from any alcohol or drugs that are known to be toxic to the liver (Box 35.1 Common Hepatotoxic Substances). In addition, patients are generally placed on limited activity with bathroom privileges. Because the patient usually experiences malaise, fatigue, and anorexia, rest is advised. As the patient improves, activity may be increased as tolerated as long as the patient does not become fatigued.

Nursing Process for the Patient with Hepatitis

ASSESSMENT/DATA COLLECTION. Assess the patient for subjective complaints such as malaise, fatigue, pruritus (itching), nausea, anorexia, and RUQ abdominal pain. Objective data, such as baseline weight, vomiting, pale

TABLE 35.2 LABORATORY TESTS FOR HEPATITIS

Test	Normal Range	Significance
Alanine aminotransferase	5–35 IU/mL	Found in high concentrations in liver cells; released with death of liver cells
Aspartate aminotransferase	8–20 U/L	Found in high concentrations in liver cells; released with death of liver cells
Erythrocyte sedimentation rate	Adult: Women, 1–20 mm/hr Men, 1–13 mm/hr	Increased with inflammation and tissue damage
Prothrombin time	8.8–11.6 seconds	Liver can no longer make prothrombin
Serological tests		
Anti-HAV	Negative titer	Indicates exposure and probable infection with virus
Anti-HBV	Negative titer	Indicates exposure and probable infection with virus
Anti-HCV	Negative titer	Indicates exposure and probable infection with virus

stools, amber- or dark-colored (tea-colored) urine, and jaundice, are recorded. The patient's vital signs are taken, and a low-grade fever or any abnormal bruising or bleeding is reported immediately. Assess the patient for knowledge of disease process and how to prevent spread of the disease.

NURSING DIAGNOSIS, PLANNING, AND IMPLEMENTATION. Imbalanced nutrition, less than body requirements related to anorexia, nausea, or vomiting

EXPECTED OUTCOME: The patient's weight will be stable and appropriate for height.

- Monitor weight and nutritional intake. *Patient assessment should guide intervention.*
- Provide a high-calorie, high-protein, high-carbohydrate, low-fat diet. *There are no restrictions on what the patient may eat, but the focus is to provide a well-rounded, nutritious diet.*
- Administer antiemetic drugs as ordered *to reduce nausea and increase appetite.*
- Provide frequent, smaller meals. *These may be tolerated better then larger meals.*
- Provide larger meals earlier in the day *because nausea tends to increase during the day.*
- Place the patient in an upright or sitting position for meals *to decrease abdominal discomfort.*
- Serve meals in a quiet environment without unpleasant noise or odors *to increase intake by making eating as pleasant as possible.*
- Teach patient to avoid alcohol and vitamin supplements unless specifically prescribed by the physician. *Alcohol and some vitamins are metabolized by the liver.*

Box 35.1 *toxic to Liver*

Common Hepatotoxic Substances

Ethyl alcohol
Acetaminophen (Tylenol)
Acetylsalicylic acid (aspirin)
Anesthetic agents
   Halothane (Fluothane)
Diazepam (Valium)
Erythromycin estolate (Ilosone)
Isoniazid (INH)
Methyldopa (Aldomet)
Oral contraceptives
Phenobarbital (Luminal)
Phenytoin (Dilantin)
Tranquilizers
   Chlorpromazine (Thorazine)
Industrial chemicals
   Carbon tetrachloride
   Trichloroethylene
   Toluene

Risk for impaired skin integrity related to itching secondary to bilirubin pigment deposits in skin

EXPECTED OUTCOME: The patient's skin will remain intact and free from secondary infection.

- Administer antihistamines as ordered *to decrease the itching*
- Encourage the patient not to scratch, but to press firmly on the itching area. *Scratching can damage skin and increase risk for infection.*
- Encourage the patient to keep fingernails trimmed short *so that vigorous scratching does not tear the skin.*
- Maintain room temperature at a comfortable level to decrease perspiration, *which may increase itching.*

Pain related to inflammation and enlargement of the liver

EXPECTED OUTCOME: Patient will state that pain level is acceptable.

- Monitor pain level on 10-point scale, including "What's Up? questions. *A good assessment should guide treatment.*

- Give analgesics as ordered *to control pain. Lower doses may be necessary for the patient with liver dysfunction. Acetaminophen is generally avoided due to risk of liver toxicity.*
- Encourage nonpharmacological pain relief activities, such as distraction, imagery, and relaxation. *These can supplement and may decrease the need for analgesics.*

Risk for ineffective management of therapeutic regimen related to lack of knowledge of hepatitis and its treatment

EXPECTED OUTCOME: Patient will state how to self-manage the treatment regimen for viral hepatitis, and how to prevent spread of the disease.

- Assess the patient's knowledge of hepatitis. *A good assessment should guide teaching.*
- Teach the patient the necessity of proper home cleanliness, including hand washing after toileting and using soap and hot water to clean eating utensils, cookware, and food preparation surfaces *to reduce spread of hepatitis to others.* (See Home Health Hints.)
- Teach patients how hepatitis affects the body and the importance of adequate rest and proper nutrition. *The patient is more likely to follow a treatment regimen if he or she understands the rationale.*
- Teach the importance of avoiding alcohol and other liver-toxic drugs. *These can further damage an already compromised liver.*
- Teach patient how to prevent spread of the disease to others. Provide guidelines specific to the type of hepatitis the patient has. *Hepatitis is contagious.*

EVALUATION. Management of the patient with hepatitis has been successful if the patient demonstrates the following:

- Maintenance of body weight to within 2 lb of preillness weight
- No breaks, cuts, or tears in skin, and no secondary infections.
- Abdominal pain or other discomfort reported as not greater than 2 to 3 on a 10-point scale
- The effects of hepatitis, how hepatitis is spread, and the necessity of adequate rest, proper nutrition, and necessary sanitation measures can be stated.

For more information, visit Hepatitis Foundation International at www.hepfi.org, www.cdc.gov, or the American Liver Foundation at www.liverfoundation.org.

Acute (Fulminant) Liver Failure

Acute (fulminant) liver failure is an uncommon but gravely serious complication of liver disease and has a mortality rate as high as 50%.

Pathophysiology and Etiology

Acute liver failure results from the sudden massive loss of liver tissue, or necrosis. The cause of liver damage is usually

---

CRITICAL THINKING

Carl

■ Carl is a 23-year-old man admitted to your medical-surgical nursing unit. During the admission process, Carl talks about his trip to an African country as a missionary. He returned to this country 4 weeks ago. During his trip he sustained a serious laceration that required many sutures. Carl also mentions his fondness for seafood and that he has had several "feasts" that have included raw oysters. Carl states that since his return he has lost nearly 8 lb, is nauseated, has frequent headaches, and tires easily. Carl also tells you that he is very irritable, which is different from his usual easygoing manner.

1. What information might lead you to suspect hepatitis A? Hepatitis B?
2. What precautions should be instituted for Carl until a diagnosis is made?
3. What nursing actions might you implement to help Carl improve his nutrition?
4. What medications should Carl avoid?
5. What information should be included in a discharge teaching plan for Carl?

Suggested answers at end of chapter.

---

drug toxicity or HBV in the presence of HDV. The outcome of the disease may be decided within 48 to 72 hours of diagnosis. Possible outcomes are reversal, need for transplantation, or death.

Prevention

Acute liver failure may be avoided by eliminating exposure to hepatitis B or hepatotoxic, liver-damaging substances. Hepatitis B can be transmitted through body fluids, such as blood or semen from unprotected sex; intravenous drug use; blood transfusions; and dialysis. See Box 35.1 for a list of hepatotoxic substances.

Signs and Symptoms

Signs and symptoms of the disorder include hepatic **encephalopathy,** or central nervous system dysfunction (discussed in detail in the section on chronic liver failure). The patient may suddenly lapse into extremely serious illness, starting with confusion and progressing to coma. In a matter of hours the liver shows a rapid reduction in size; a typical sign of onset of acute liver failure. In addition, there is a sudden elevation of liver enzymes and bilirubin. Prothrombin time is elevated. Marked elevation in the prothrombin time is an ominous sign.

Diagnostic Tests

Early diagnosis of acute liver failure is essential so that the process of organ procurement may begin. An otherwise

---

encephalopathy: encephalo—brain + pathy—disease

healthy patient may be a priority organ recipient depending on age and whether or not the patient is alcohol dependent.

Laboratory tests include the serum liver enzymes alanine aminotransferase (ALT) and aspartate aminotransferase (AST). Levels of ALT and AST may rise from 1000 mU/mL to as high as 4000 mU/mL. The serum bilirubin level is more than 2.5 mg/dL. Urobilinogen levels may be elevated. Serum potassium levels drop below 3.5 mEq/L. Blood glucose drops below 70 mg/dL. The prothrombin time is elevated above 25 seconds.

An abdominal x-ray examination may document the change in size of the liver.

Therapeutic Interventions

Medical treatment is directed toward stopping and reversing the damage to the liver. An attempt is made to put the liver completely at rest. The patient is put on complete bedrest. All drugs are discontinued, since they are metabolized by the liver. Dialysis may be ordered if the liver damage is a result of an overdose of a hepatotoxic substance. The patient is ordered a high-calorie, low-sodium, low-protein diet. Lactulose, neomycin, magnesium citrate, or sorbitol may be given to decrease ammonia levels, but they are not always effective. (For information on how these drugs work, see the section on medical treatment for chronic liver failure.) The patient needs intensive amounts of supportive care. It may be possible to support the patient long enough to stabilize him or her for transplantation.

Complications

The patient with acute liver failure experiences metabolic alkalosis, hypokalemia, hypoglycemia, disruption of blood clotting, and possibly sepsis. Metabolic alkalosis is related to disruption of the urea production cycle and the resulting accumulation of bicarbonate. Patients with acute liver failure also experience electrolyte imbalances. The patient's kidneys excrete potassium rather than hydrogen ions in an attempt to correct the alkalosis. The patient usually has hypoglycemia from loss of glycogen stores in the damaged liver, impaired gluconeogenesis (the manufacture of glucose from other nutrients), and an elevated insulin level caused by the stress response. Further, blood clotting disorders that can lead to disseminated intravascular coagulation (DIC) develop when prothrombin time is elevated.

Finally, the patient is at risk for sepsis because of poor white blood cell migration and other responses to infection. Sepsis, abscess formation, endocarditis, and meningitis account for nearly a quarter of the deaths from acute liver failure. Renal failure accounts for about 30% of deaths. Respiratory problems and hypotension also contribute to the deaths from acute liver failure. The patient progresses through encephalopathy to coma and death.

Nursing Process for the Patient with Acute Liver Failure

Nursing care of the patient with acute liver failure is essentially the same as for the patient with terminal chronic liver failure, which is discussed next.

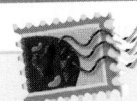

Box 35.2

Cultural Considerations

The incidence of liver disease is more common among Mexican Americans. Risk factors include working in occupations such as mining, factories using chemicals, and farming using pesticides. Additionally, the use of alcohol is increased in men, and cigarette smoking is common.

Egyptian Americans may suffer from schistosomiasis, known as bilharziasis in Egypt. Schistosomiasis can lead to cirrhosis, liver failure, portal hypertension, esophageal varices, bladder cancer, and renal failure. Thus, the nurse may need to screen newer Egyptian American immigrants for this disease.

Alcohol use and abuse is common among African American communities. For many it is a socially accepted behavior and carries little or no stigma. The mortality rate from cirrhosis of the liver among African Americans is nearly twice that of European Americans. The nurse needs to provide counseling, teaching the detrimental effects of alcohol, and work with African American churches and community leaders to help prevent the detrimental effects of alcohol abuse.

Chronic Liver Failure

Chronic liver failure is also called Laënnec's **cirrhosis,** or portal, nutritional, fatty, or alcoholic liver disease. Chronic liver failure is the tenth leading cause of death among the total population and is more common among men than women (Box 35.2 Cultural Considerations).

Etiology

A variety of problems can result in chronic liver failure:
- Laënnec's cirrhosis is caused by chronic excessive alcohol ingestion, especially when excess alcohol is combined with a lack of dietary protein.
- Postnecrotic liver failure may result from massive exposure to hepatotoxins, viral hepatitis, or infection.
- Biliary liver failure is caused by chronic inflammation and obstruction of the gallbladder and bile ducts.
- Cardiac liver failure is caused by chronic severe congestion of the liver from heart failure. The liver congestion causes death of liver cells from lack of nutrients and oxygen.

Pathophysiology

Chronic liver failure is a progressive disease. Healthy liver cells respond to toxins such as alcohol by becoming

---

cirrohsis: cirrh—orange yellow + osis—condition

inflamed. The liver cells are infiltrated with fat and white blood cells and are then replaced by fibrotic tissue. As the disease progresses, more and more liver cells are replaced by fatty and scar tissue. The lobes of the liver are disrupted and the liver becomes hardened and lumpy. Early in the disease, the liver is enlarged, firm, and hard from the inflammatory process. Later, the liver shrinks and is covered with gray connective tissue.

Prevention

Chronic liver failure may be prevented by abstinence from alcohol, eating a balanced diet with adequate amounts of protein, and avoiding exposure to infections or hepatotoxic chemicals. Patients are advised that total abstinence from alcohol should be a lifelong goal.

Signs and Symptoms

Signs and symptoms of impaired liver function include malaise, anorexia, indigestion, nausea, weight loss, diarrhea or constipation, and dull, aching RUQ pain. The liver may be enlarged, firm, and tender. Bruising of the skin, bleeding gums, anemia, and jaundice, also known as icterus, may be present. Jaundice is a common finding with hepatitis. The patient's skin may be dry or contain abnormal pigmentation. The patient may complain of severe pruritus (itching). Laboratory values reflect progressive loss of liver function. As chronic liver failure progresses, signs and symptoms of increasing loss of liver function and complications related to the increasing loss of function develop.

Complications

Complications of chronic liver failure include **hepatorenal syndrome,** blood clotting defects, **ascites, portal hypertension,** and hepatic encephalopathy.

HEPATORENAL SYNDROME. Hepatorenal syndrome is a secondary kidney failure that occurs in about one-third of liver failure patients. Symptoms of hepatorenal syndrome include oliguria without detectable kidney damage, reduced glomerular filtration rate (GFR) with essentially no urine output or less than 200 mL per day, and nearly total sodium retention. Hepatorenal syndrome is considered an ominous sign.

CLOTTING DEFECTS. Blood clotting defects may develop because of impaired prothrombin and fibrinogen production in the liver. Further, the absence of bile salts prevents the absorption of fat-soluble vitamin K, which is essential for some blood clotting factors. Patients with chronic liver failure have a tendency to bruise easily and may progress to disseminated intravascular coagulation (DIC) or hemorrhage.

ASCITES. Ascites is an accumulation of serous fluid in the abdominal cavity. The fluid accumulates primarily because of low production of albumin by the failing liver. An insufficient amount of protein in the capillaries causes plasma to seep into the abdominal cavity. The accumulated fluid causes a markedly enlarged abdomen. The fluid may cause severe respiratory distress as a result of elevation of the diaphragm.

PORTAL HYPERTENSION. Portal hypertension is a persistent blood pressure elevation in the portal circulation of the abdomen. Liver damage causes a blockage of blood flow in the portal vein. Increased resistance from delayed drainage causes enlargement of the visible abdominal veins around the umbilicus (called caput medusae), rectal hemorrhoids, enlarged spleen, and esophageal **varices** (dilated veins) (Fig. 35.1). The most serious result of portal hypertension is bleeding esophageal varices. The walls of the esophageal veins are thin and tear easily. Varices usually develop from the fundus of the stomach upward and may extend into the upper esophagus. The blood-filled, thin-walled varices may tear easily from sudden excessive pressure, such as the intra-abdominal pressure that results from coughing, lifting, or straining, causing severe bleeding.

HEPATIC ENCEPHALOPATHY. Hepatic encephalopathy is caused by the accumulation of noxious substances in the circulation. The failing liver is unable to make the toxic substances water soluble for excretion in the urine. Ammonia, a by-product of protein metabolism, is most commonly the substance causing symptoms. Signs and symptoms of hepatic encephalopathy include progressive confusion; **asterixis,** or flapping tremors in the hands caused by toxins at peripheral nerves; and **fetor hepaticus,** or foul

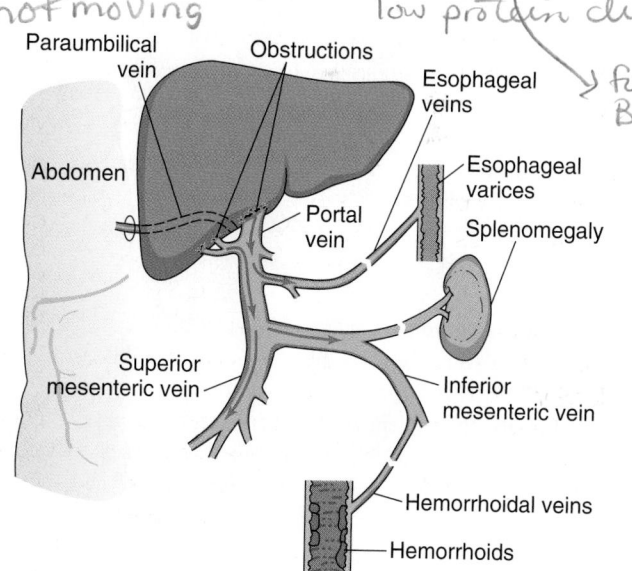

FIGURE 35.1 Portal hypertension. Obstruction of normal blood flow through the liver causes blood to back up into the venous system, leading to esophageal varices, splenomegaly, hemorrhoids, and caput medusae.

---

hepatorenal syndrome: hepato—liver + renal—kidneys + syndrome—group of symptoms

asterixis: a—not + sterixis—fixed postition

fetor hepaticus: fetor—offensive odor + hepat—liver + icas—related to

breath caused by metabolic endproducts related to sulfur. Stages of hepatic encephalopathy are *early, stuporous and confused,* and *comatose.* Signs and symptoms of the stages are as follows:

- Early: The patient exhibits subtle changes in personality, fatigue, drowsiness, and changes in handwriting (the best assessment for the early stage).
- Stuporous and confused: The patient is often belligerent and irritable and develops asterixis, muscle twitching, hyperventilation, and marked confusion.
- Comatose: The patient gradually loses consciousness and becomes comatose.

If levels of toxic substances can be decreased and managed, the patient gradually regains consciousness. Hepatic encephalopathy represents end-stage liver failure and has a mortality rate as high as 90% once coma begins. Figure 35.2 shows signs and symptoms of chronic liver failure.

Diagnostic Tests

Liver serum enzymes, serum bilirubin, urobilinogen, serum ammonia, and prothrombin times are all elevated in chronic

LEARNING TIP

For complications of chronic liver failure, remember the pneumonic CHEAP:
C: Clotting disorders
H: Hepatorenal syndrome
E: Encephalopathy
A: Ascites
P: Portal hypertension

liver failure (Table 35.3). Abdominal radiographs of patients with chronic liver failure may show ascites and enlargement of the liver. An upper gastrointestinal (UGI) series may reveal esophageal varices or evidence of gastric inflammation or ulcers. If the patient is bleeding, other arterial radiological examinations may be done to locate the specific source of bleeding.

A liver scan may be done to show abnormal liver masses or thickening. The physician may order an esopha-

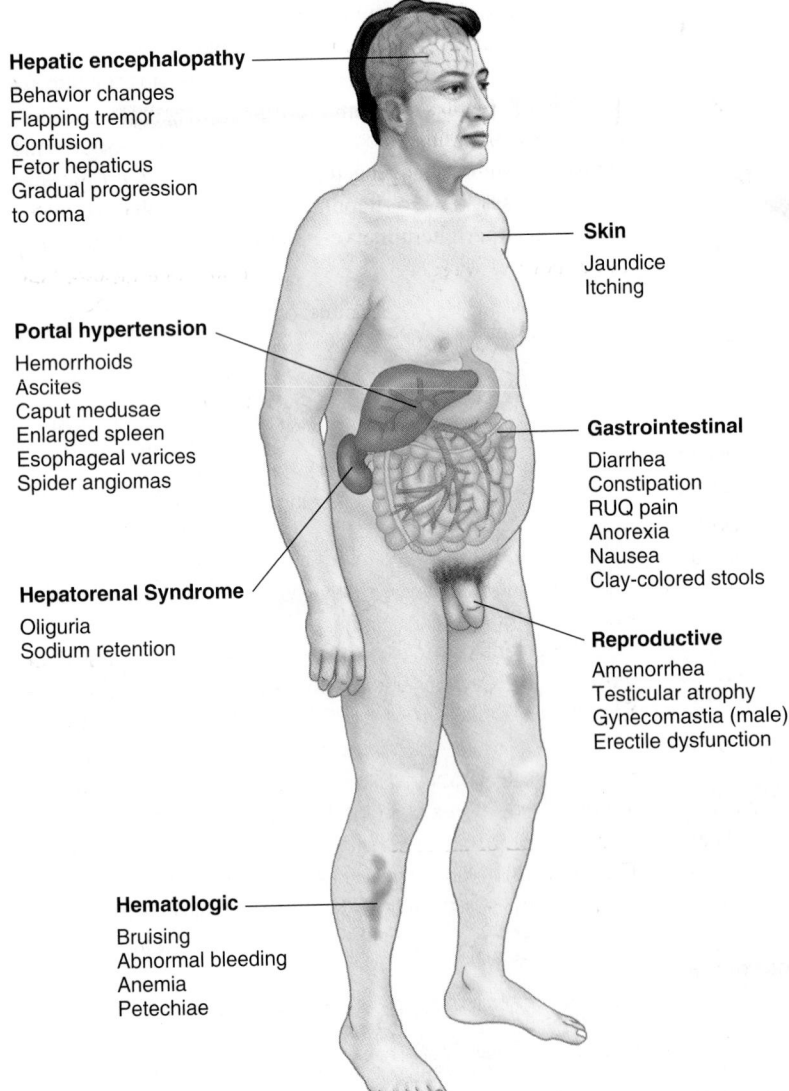

Hepatic encephalopathy

Behavior changes
Flapping tremor
Confusion
Fetor hepaticus
Gradual progression
to coma

Skin

Jaundice
Itching

Portal hypertension

Hemorrhoids
Ascites
Caput medusae
Enlarged spleen
Esophageal varices
Spider angiomas

Gastrointestinal

Diarrhea
Constipation
RUQ pain
Anorexia
Nausea
Clay-colored stools

Hepatorenal Syndrome

Oliguria
Sodium retention

Reproductive

Amenorrhea
Testicular atrophy
Gynecomastia (male)
Erectile dysfunction

Hematologic

Bruising
Abnormal bleeding
Anemia
Petechiae

FIGURE 35.2 Signs and symptoms of chronic liver failure.

TABLE 35.3 LABORATORY TESTS FOR CHRONIC LIVER FAILURE

Test	Normal Value	Significance of Abnormal Findings
Blood		
Alanine amino-transferase (ALT)	5–35 IU/mL	Found in high concentra-tions in liver cells; released with death of liver cells
Albumin	3.5–5.5 g/dL	Decreased because of impaired protein synthe-sis; edema and ascites may result
Ammonia	15–19 µg/dL	Increased because liver cannot metabolize pro-tein end product; con-tributes to hepatic encephalopathy
Bilirubin	0.3–3.0 mg/dL	Increased because the liver is unable to use it to produce bile
Aspartate aminotrans-ferase (AST)	8–20 U/L	Found in high concentra-tions in liver cells; released with death of liver cells
Prothrombin time (PT)	8.8–11.6 sec	Prolonged. Liver can no longer make prothrom-bin; patient bleeds easily
Urine		
Urobilinogen	<4 mg/24 hr	Increase in urine because of filtration of excessive bilinogen in blood

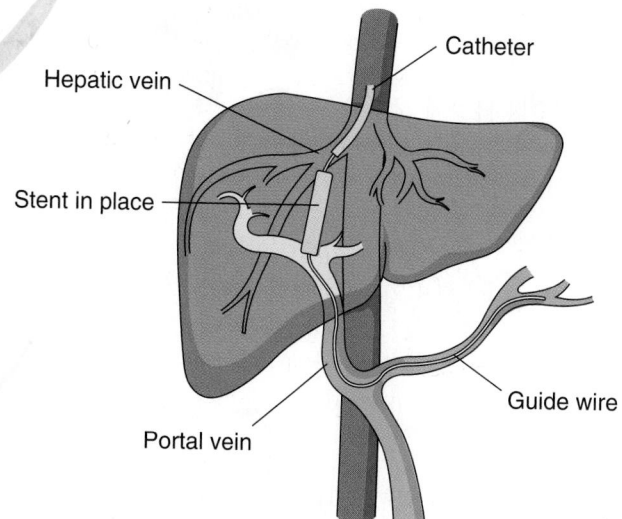

FIGURE 35.3 Transjugular intrahepatic portosystemic shunt. A stent is placed to shunt blood from the portal vein to the sys-temic circulation to divert blood flow around the diseased liver.

gogastroduodenoscopy (EGD) to detect any bleeding and to directly observe the esophagus, stomach, and duodenum. Small surface vessels that are bleeding can be treated by injection sclerotherapy during the EGD. The procedure uses sclerosing agents, which are chemical substances that cause the veins to inflame and scar shut.

The physician may do a liver biopsy to determine the extent and nature of the liver damage. Patients with chronic liver failure undergoing a liver biopsy need careful observa-tion for bleeding after the procedure. (See Chapter 32.)

Therapeutic Interventions

Interventions for chronic hepatic failure seek to remove or to treat the underlying causes of the disease. In addition, med-ical treatment seeks to support liver regeneration and to treat the complications of liver failure. check (K)

Ascites is treated with diuretics, albumin infusions, and fluid and sodium restrictions. Paracentesis is sometimes considered as an emergency measure to remove accumu-lated abdominal fluid, especially when the fluid compro-mises the patient's breathing, causes abdominal discomfort, or poses a threat of ruptured umbilical hernia. Paracentesis is not commonly done because it removes serous fluid, which contains a large amount of albumin that the liver can-not easily replace. Ascites may be treated by the nonsurgical placement of a shunt between the portal and systemic

venous systems, which is called a **transjugular intrahep-atic portosystemic shunt** (TIPS) (Fig. 35.3).

The purpose of the shunt is to sidetrack venous blood around the liver to the vena cava. Shunts are used for patients with severe respiratory compromise and are not as success-ful as originally hoped. Surgical shunts, sometimes called portacaval shunts, may be used to relieve portal hyperten-sion. When shunts are used, less venous blood circulates through the liver and fewer protein endproducts are metabo-lized. For this reason, patients are put on a low-protein diet.

The medical goals for managing bleeding from esophageal varices are as follows:

* Stop the bleeding.
* Treat the fluid volume deficit caused by the bleed-ing.
* Prevent further fluid loss.
* Maintain fluid and electrolyte balance.

Bleeding varices are treated with vasoconstrictors such as vasopressin, with tamponade (direct pressure on the bleeding veins), or with emergency sclerotherapy to close the veins. (pressure)

Tamponade is usually a temporary measure and is done with a multilumen esophagogastric tube such as the Sengstaken-Blakemore tube (Fig. 35.4). Other multilumen tubes such as the Minnesota tube may be used. The Sengstaken-Blakemore tube is inserted through the nose or mouth to the stomach. First the gastric balloon is inflated with 200 mL of air to secure the tube in its proper location. The esophageal tube is then inflated with 50 mL of air to produce tamponade. One to 2 lb of traction may be applied to the tube. Occasionally the patient may wear a football hel-

transjugular intrahepatic portosystemic shunt: trans— across + jugular—jugular vein + intra—within + hepatic—liver + porto—portal (liver circulation) systemic—systemic (circula-tion) + shunt—to divert

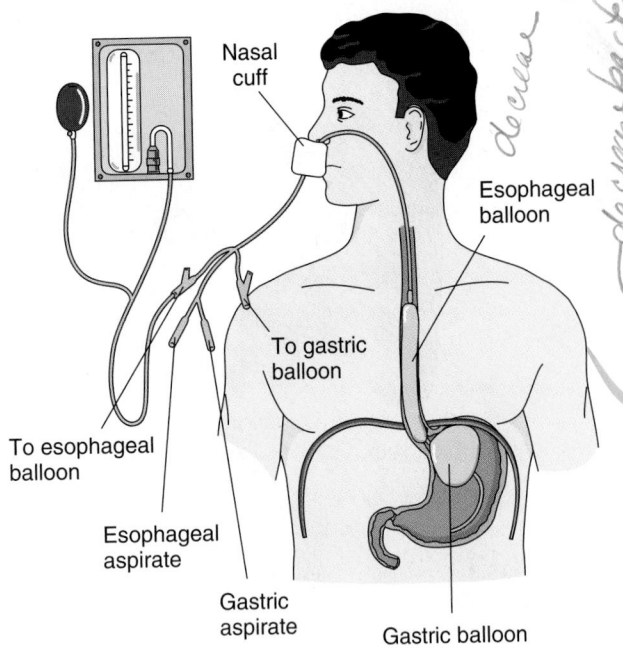

FIGURE 35.4 Balloon tamponade for bleeding esophageal varices. An esophageal balloon compresses bleeding vessels.

met so that the tube can be secured to the face guard rather than putting pressure on the patient's nose. The Sengstaken-Blakemore tube is then connected to nasogastric suction.

Complications that may occur from the use of esophagogastric tamponade include (1) aspiration, (2) erosion of esophageal gastric mucosa, and (3) suffocation. With the balloons inflated, the patient cannot swallow saliva. Oral suction with a Yankauer catheter should be available. Sometimes a Salem sump tube is placed in the upper esophagus before the esophageal balloon is inflated to drain secretions.

Inflation pressure of the esophageal balloon should be maintained between 20 and 25 mm Hg. Agency procedures should clearly state how long the tube may remain in place and how often (and for how long) the esophageal balloon should be deflated. The gastric balloon remains inflated at all times until the procedure is stopped.

If the gastric tube dislodges into the esophagus, the patient can be suffocated. Keep a pair of scissors at the bedside when esophagogastric tamponade is in progress. If the gastric balloon dislodges, cut the inflation ports of the gastric and esophageal balloons to allow quick release of air.

Unfortunately, recurrence of bleeding occurs in about 20% to 60% of patients after successful tamponade. With each new bleeding episode, the risk of mortality increases. Sclerotherapy may be undertaken to prevent recurrence of bleeding. Sclerotherapy can be done without general anesthesia, which is an advantage for the patient with a severely damaged liver. The procedure is usually done as part of an EGD while the patient is sedated with diazepam (Valium) or midazolam hydrochloride (Versed). A topical anesthetic is used. The varices are injected with a sclerosing agent that causes thickening and closing of the dilated vessels. The procedure usually takes about an hour. After the procedure

the patient may complain of chest pain for up to 72 hours. Give the prescribed analgesics and monitor the patient for pain relief. Report severe pain unrelieved by the prescribed analgesic immediately because the patient may be experiencing an esophageal perforation or ulceration, which is a complication of sclerotherapy.

Hepatic encephalopathy is treated by trying to remove the toxic waste material. Saline or magnesium sulfate (MgSO$_4$) enemas may remove some of the toxic waste. The enemas may be given to cleanse the bowel of the noxious substances. Neomycin, an intestinal antibiotic, may be given by mouth, nasogastric tube, or enema. The antibiotic inhibits ammonia formation by reducing colonic bacteria that change ammonium to ammonia. Lactulose may be given by mouth to reduce the pH of the intestine and to "trap" ammonia, allowing it to be excreted in the stool. Hepatic encephalopathy is also treated by restricting or eliminating dietary protein. In severe cases, dialysis may be considered to remove ammonia (Box 35.3 Nutrition Notes). See Box 35.4 Chronic Liver Failure Summary.

Nursing Process for the Patient with Acute and Chronic Liver Failure

ASSESSMENT/DATA COLLECTION. A complete history and physical assessment are done. Be alert to subjective symptoms of liver dysfunction such as malaise, anorexia, indigestion, nausea, severe itching, and dull, aching RUQ pain. Assess the patient for objective evidence of liver problems, such as weight loss, diarrhea or constipation, and an enlarged, firm, and tender liver. Observe the patient for dryness and bruising of the skin, bleeding gums, anemia, jaundice, and any evidence of alterations in thought processes, such as confusion, disorientation, or inability to make decisions.

NURSING DIAGNOSIS, PLANNING, AND IMPLEMENTATION. Common nursing diagnoses for chronic liver failure include the following:

Excess fluid volume related to portal hypertension (ascites)

EXPECTED OUTCOME: Fluid volume will be controlled as evidenced by stable weight, and abdominal girth within normal limits for patient.

- Weigh the patient on admission and daily. *Daily weights are a good measure of fluid retention.*
- Measure and record the patient's abdominal girth (circumference) daily. Mark the place where you measured so the same site will always be measured during subsequent assessments. *This monitors the amount of ascites.*
- Report any weight gain or increase in girth promptly *so treatment can be ordered and complications minimized.*
- Check the patient's vital signs every 4 hours; report changes and any evidence of difficulty breathing or changes in mental status promptly. *These are signs of fluid overload.*

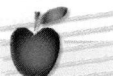

Box 35.3

Nutrition Notes

Supplying Nutrients to Patients with Liver Disease

A registered dietitian may modify the diet daily for patients with liver disease. Usually these patients suffer from severe anorexia, often displaying their best appetites for breakfast. For early or mild disease, protein is encouraged to support healing; later in liver disease, protein may be restricted. For esophageal varices, foods are soft, in addition to other restrictions. For liver failure, the following dietary considerations are necessary:

• Protein is restricted according to the individual's ability to metabolize it.
• Complete protein foods are selected to the provide all the essential amino acids.
• Homogenized milk and eggs are offered because the fat is already emulsified, requiring less bile for digestion.
• Adequate carbohydrates are given to prevent the use of tissue protein for energy.
• Fluid and sodium are likely to be restricted if ascites is present.

   Hepatic encephalopathy is associated with increased serum levels of ammonia and aromatic amino acids. Foods producing high ammonia levels may be restricted (e.g., chicken, salami, ground beef, ham, bacon, gelatin, peanut butter, potatoes, onions, lima beans, egg yolk, buttermilk, blue and cheddar cheeses). Vegetable proteins and special enteral feeding formulas (e.g., Hepatic-Aid II and Travasorb-Hepatic) containing branched-chain amino acids may be given in place of foods containing aromatic amino acids that interfere with formation of dopamine and norepinephrine.

Box 35.4

Chronic Liver Failure Summary

Signs and Symptoms	Malaise, anorexia, nausea Dull RUQ pain Easy bruising Jaundice Ascites
Diagnostic Tests	Elevated ALT, AST, ammonia, bilirubin, PT
Therapeutic Interventions	Treat or remove underlying cause, especially alcohol
Complications	CHEAP (see Learning Tip)
Priority Nursing Diagnoses	Fluid volume excess or deficit Imbalanced nutrition Pain

mineral levels. *These may be better indicators of nutrition if accurate weights are complicated by fluid overload.*
• Assess the patient's bowel sounds, abdominal distention, and evidence of bleeding at least once every 8 hours. *These can signal complications that can further compromise ability to eat.*
• Monitor the patient's diet to ensure that any ordered protein restriction is carried out. *Protein metabolism can contribute to high ammonia levels.*
• Offer the patient frequent, small, high-calorie meals *to reduce feeling of fullness that can occur with larger meals.*
• Make sure that odors and other unpleasant stimuli are eliminated *to prevent further worsening of appetite.*
• Offer frequent mouth care *to increase comfort and make food more palatable.*
• Administer vitamins or supplements as ordered *to correct deficiencies.*

Pain related to abdominal pressure

EXPECTED OUTCOME: Patient will state pain level is acceptable.
• Monitor pain level using a 10-point scale and "What's Up?" questions. *A good assessment should guide treatment.*
• Give analgesics as ordered *to control pain. Lower doses may be necessary for the patient with liver dysfunction. Acetaminophen is generally avoided due to risk of liver toxicity.*
• Encourage nonpharmacological pain relief activities, such as distraction, imagery, and relaxation. *These can supplement and may decrease the need for analgesics.*

• Maintain a low-sodium diet and order fluid restrictions *to reduce fluid retention.*
• If intravenous fluids or albumin have been ordered, assist in careful monitoring of the rate of infusion. *Rapid fluid administration can increase risk of overload.*
• Administer ordered diuretics as scheduled *to reduce fluid volume.*

Imbalanced nutrition: less than body requirements related to anorexia and impaired metabolism of needed nutrients

EXPECTED OUTCOME: Patient's (dry) weight will be within normal limits for height.
• Monitor weight; report unexpected (nonfluid) weight loss *so timely intervention can be implemented.*
• Monitor serum albumin, total protein, vitamin, and

Risk for disturbed thought processes related to elevated ammonia levels

EXPECTED OUTCOME: Patient will remain alert and oriented to person, place, and time.

- Assess the patient's level of consciousness and orientation frequently. *Early recognition of changes allows prompt treatment.*
- Assess neuromuscular function. Neuromuscular function can be assessed by asking the patient to hold his or her arms out straight in front and steady. *If asterixis, or liver flap, is present, the patient's hands will unwillingly dip and return to the horizontal position in a flapping motion.*
- Look for changes in the patient's handwriting. *Changes can indicate altered neuromuscular function.*
- Give lactulose, neomycin, magnesium citrate, or sorbitol as scheduled *to decrease serum ammonia levels.*
- Be aware that lactulose causes loose stools, and do not withhold the medication when the patient develops diarrhea. *Loose stools are a sign that the medication is working, and not a reason to withhold the medication.*
- Question giving medications such as sedatives, narcotics, and tranquilizers. *These may increase the serum ammonia levels and depress level of consciousness (LOC).*
- Reorient the patient to time and place frequently *to reinforce reality.*
- Give simple, clear explanations of care and give the patient time to understand the explanation. *Short, simple explanations are easier to process.*
- Provide a safe environment for the confused or unsteady patient *to prevent injury.*

Risk for ineffective breathing pattern related to excess fluid in the abdomen

EXPECTED OUTCOME: Respirations will be even and unlabored, 16 to 20 per minute.

- Assess the patient's respiratory rate, rhythm, chest movement, skin color, and oxygen saturation frequently *to determine if breathing pattern is effective.*
- Assist the patient to use an incentive spirometer and to cough gently every 2 to 4 hours *to encourage deep breathing and keep airways clear.*
- Elevate the head of the patient's bed *so that the patient's lungs have maximum room for expansion.*
- Reposition the patient at least every 2 hours *to ventilate all areas of the lungs.*
- Assist with treatments to decrease ascites as ordered *to increase room for lung expansion.*
- Administer analgesics as ordered if pain is causing shallow respirations. *Reducing pain with breathing allows for a more effective breathing pattern.*

Risk for deficient fluid volume related to bleeding esophageal varices or gastrointestinal bleeding secondary to clotting dysfunction

EXPECTED OUTCOME: Fluid volume will remain within normal limits without bleeding as evidenced by no signs and symptoms of bleeding, and vital signs within normal limits.

- Monitor gastric secretions, stool, and urine at least every 8 hours, and report any signs of bleeding. *Early identification of bleeding is essential to prompt treatment.*
- Monitor blood clotting laboratory studies such as the prothrombin time and report any abnormal values. *Prolonged values increase the risk for bleeding.*
- Caution the patient to use a soft-bristle toothbrush and an electric rather than straight razor *to avoid injury.*
- Avoid suctioning the patient if possible. *Suctioning can cause varices to bleed.*
- Use a small-gauge needle for injections and apply direct pressure to all puncture sites *to avoid bleeding.*
- Teach the patient to avoid hot, spicy, or irritating foods. *These may irritate the esophageal mucosa and increase risk of bleeding.*
- Instruct the patient to avoid forceful coughing or nose blowing, straining, vomiting, or gagging if at all possible. Administer medications as ordered to prevent their occurrence. *These can increase pressure and risk of bleeding varices.*

Risk for infection related to impaired immune function

EXPECTED OUTCOME: The patient will be free from infection as evidenced by white blood cell count (WBC) within normal limit, afebrile.

- Monitor for signs of infection and report promptly *so treatment can be initiated.*
- Carefully evaluate laboratory studies such as the white blood cell count. *The white blood cell count may not elevate or may elevate slowly because the white cell activity is impaired.*
- Be aware that the earliest warning signs of infection may be subtle changes in the patient's behavior, such as sudden restlessness, an increase in confusion, or irritability. *Early recognition is essential to prompt treatment.*
- Teach the patient careful hand washing and avoidance of people who are ill *to prevent exposure to infection.*

EVALUATION. Nursing care has been effective if the patient demonstrates the following:
- No signs of fluid retention
- Weight stable and appropriate for height
- Abdominal pain or other discomfort reported as not greater than 2 on a 10-point scale
- Alert and oriented demeanor

- Respiratory rate between 16 and 20 respirations per minute with no cyanosis or changes in level of consciousness
- No bleeding, infection, or injuries
- Accurate knowledge of chronic liver failure and proper disease management requirements

PATIENT EDUCATION. Teach patients how chronic liver failure is affecting their bodies. In particular, patients need to know about portal system hypertension and hepatic encephalopathy. In addition, teach:

- How to observe for and report any confusion, tremors, or personality changes
- The importance of adequate rest and avoidance of strenuous activity
- A diet high in calories, low in sodium, and high in protein if hepatic encephalopathy has not developed
- To avoid narcotics, sedatives, and tranquilizers
- To promptly report any bleeding; any sign of low potassium, such as muscle cramps, nausea, or vomiting caused by diuretics; changes in mental status, such as confusion or personality changes; changes in weight; and any increase in current symptoms
- The importance of avoiding alcohol
- The importance of frequent follow-up care and laboratory studies

---

CRITICAL THINKING

Mary

■ Mary, a 76-year-old retired businesswoman, has lived alone for the past 20 years, since the death of her husband. She has a long history of poor nutritional habits but does not use alcohol. She is admitted to your unit with chronic liver failure.

1. What risk factors does Mary have for chronic liver failure?
2. What symptoms would you expect Mary to exhibit with early chronic liver failure?
3. What values do you expect to see for serum albumin? Prothrombin time?
4. What are the two greatest concerns with portal hypertension?
5. What is the usual treatment for ascites?
6. What complication of esophageal tamponade requires that a pair of scissors be at the bedside at all times while tamponade is in progress?

Suggested answers at end of chapter.

Transplantation

Patients with liver disease who do not respond well to medical or surgical treatment may be candidates for a liver transplant. Patients who have chronic liver failure from hepatitis or biliary disease, metabolic disorders, or hepatic vein obstruction may be evaluated for a liver transplant. In gen-

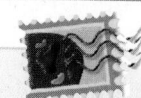

Box 35.5

Cultural Considerations

Jewish law addresses organ transplantation from the perspectives of the recipient, the living donor, the cadaver donor, and the dying donor. If a recipient's life can be prolonged without considerable risk, transplant is ordained. For a living donor to be approved, the risk to the life of the donor must be considered. One is not obligated to donate a part of himself or herself unless the risk is small. This includes kidney and bone marrow donations. The use of a cadaver for transplant is usually approved if it is saving a life. The use of skin for burns is acceptable, although there is no agreement on the use of cadaver corneas. The nurse may need to help the Jewish patient contact a rabbi when making a decision regarding organ donation or transplantation.

---

eral, patients who have cancer are not considered for liver transplantation; the drugs used to suppress tissue rejection by the immune system can cause the cancer cells to grow at an increased rate.

The patient with end-stage liver failure who does not have hypertension, bleeding esophageal varices, infection, or severe cardiac disease is placed on a national list as a potential liver recipient. The patient will be evaluated for emotional and physical stability and must realize that he or she will be on daily medications for life (Box 35.5 Cultural Considerations).

After the surgical implantation of a donor liver, the patient must be closely observed for evidence of donor organ rejection. The patient will be in an intensive care unit (ICU) setting until stable enough to be transferred to a medical unit. The patient will be on drugs such as cyclosporine (cyclosporin A), azathioprine (Imuran), and prednisone (Deltasone) to suppress the immune system responses to foreign protein or tissue rejection. Observe the patient for the following signs of impending rejection:

- Pulse greater than 100 beats per minute
- Temperature greater than 101°F (38°C)
- Complaints of RUQ pain
- Increased jaundice
- Decrease in bile from the **T-tube** or change in bile color

In addition, laboratory studies may show increased serum transaminases (ALT and AST), serum bilirubin, alkaline phosphatase, and prothrombin time. Symptoms of acute tissue rejection usually develop between the fourth and tenth postoperative days.

Monitor urine output and lab studies daily. Bowel sounds and passage of flatus must be documented. The patient who has received an organ transplant needs extended medical follow-up. Teach the patient to promptly report to the physician any symptoms of infection, bleeding episodes, or RUQ pain (Box 35.6 Ethical Considerations).

Box 35.6

Ethical Considerations

Organ Transplantation

Despite widespread public and medical acceptance of organ transplantation as a highly *beneficial* procedure, ethical questions remain. Whenever a human organ is transplanted, a large number of people are involved, including the donor, the donor's family, nursing and medical personnel, as well as the recipient and the recipient's family. Society in general could also be added to this mix because of the high cost of organ transplantation that usually comes from tax dollars or indirectly in the form of increased insurance premiums. Each one of these persons or groups has *rights* that may conflict with another's rights.

Most institutions that perform transplants and organizations that are involved in obtaining organs have developed elaborate, detailed, and involved procedures to help deal with the ethical and legal issues involved in transplantation. Despite these efforts, there are still some ethical issues that should be considered whenever the issue of organ transplantation is raised.

Despite the best efforts of the medical and legal communities to establish criteria for death, there are still some ethical questions about when a person is really dead. Does brain death, the most widely accepted criterion for death, really indicate that a person no longer exists as a human being? Alternatively, are there other criteria that should be examined? Such organs as hearts, lungs, and liver must come from a donor with a beating heart. Might there not be the tendency to declare brain death before it actually occurs?

One of the most difficult ethical issues involved in organ transplantation is the selection of recipients; this can be considered under the principles of *justice or fairness*. There are many fewer organs available than there are people who need them. Many potential ethical dilemmas arise from this fact. Should someone receive an organ because he or she is rich or famous or knows the right people? The national organ recipient list attempts to list and rank all persons who need organs in a nondiscriminatory manner. Some of the important criteria include need, length of time on the list, potential for survival, prior organ transplantation, value to the community, and tissue compatibility.

Nurses can be and often are involved in some aspect of the organ donation process. Many states have passed laws that require health-care workers to ask family members of potential organ donors if they have ever thought about organ donation for their dead or dying loved one. Many nurses, particularly nurses in critical care units, provide care for patients who are potential organ donors. Nurses in operating rooms may help in the surgical procedures that remove organs from a cadaver and that transplant them into a recipient's body. Many nurses provide postoperative care for patients who have received a transplanted organ. Home health care nurses provide follow-up care for these patients at home.

Nurses working with organ transplantation need to be sensitive to the potential for manipulation. Most people who are seeking organ transplantations are desperately ill or near death. They, and their families, can be very easily manipulated or can be very manipulating. On the other side, the families of potential organ donors are usually emotionally distraught because of the sudden and traumatic loss of a loved one. They too are very vulnerable. As a rule, neither the donor nor the donor's family should play any part in the selection of a recipient. Nurses must avoid making statements or giving nonverbal indications of approval or disapproval of potential recipients.

Cancer of the Liver

Cancer of the liver is usually the result of metastasis from a primary cancer at a distant location. The liver is a likely area of involvement if cancer originated in the esophagus, lungs, breast, stomach, colon, pancreas, kidney, bladder, or skin. For some patients, liver cancer is the primary tumor site. Patients with a history of chronic hepatitis B, hepatitis C, nutritional deficiencies, or exposure to hepatotoxins have an increased risk for cancer of the liver.

Symptoms of cancer of the liver include encephalopathy, abnormal bleeding, jaundice, and ascites. Laboratory tests show an elevated serum alkaline phosphatase. Radiological examinations may include abdominal radiographs or radioisotope scans, which show tumor growth. Liver cancer is definitively diagnosed with a positive needle biopsy combined with an ultrasonogram of the liver. Most patients with liver cancer die within 6 months of diagnosis.

Rarely, a patient with liver cancer may be a candidate for surgical removal of the affected portion of the liver. Care of the postsurgical patient is similar to other abdominal surgery patients. If surgery is not an option, the patient may receive chemotherapeutic drugs by injection directly into the affected lobe of the liver or into the hepatic artery. Intra-arterial injection of chemotherapeutic drugs has the advantage of being less toxic to the rest of the body. (See Chapter 10 for care of patients with cancer.)

 DISORDERS OF THE PANCREAS

Pancreatitis

Pancreatitis is an inflammation of the pancreas. It may be either acute or chronic. The two forms of pancreatitis have different courses and are considered two different disorders.

Acute Pancreatitis

Pathophysiology

Inflammation of the pancreas appears to be caused by a process called autodigestion. Recall that the pancreas normally secretes digestive enzymes. For reasons not fully understood, pancreatic enzymes can be activated while they are still within the pancreas and begin to digest the pancreas. In addition, large amounts of the enzymes are released by inflamed cells. As the pancreas digests itself, chemical cascades occur. Trypsin destroys pancreatic tissue and causes vasodilation. As capillary permeability increases, fluid is lost to the retroperitoneal space, causing shock. In addition, trypsin appears to set off another chain of events that causes the conversion of prothrombin to thrombin, so that clots form. The patient may develop DIC. (See Chapter 28.)

Etiology

Pancreatitis is most commonly associated with excessive alcohol consumption. Alcohol appears to act directly on the acinar cells of the pancreas and the pancreatic ducts to irritate and inflame the structures. Biliary disease such as **cholelithiasis** (gallstones) or cholangitis (inflammation of the bile ducts) may also trigger pancreatitis. Gallstones may plug the pancreatic duct and cause inflammation from excessive fluid pressure on sensitive ducts. The irritant effect of bile itself may cause inflammation. Blunt trauma to the abdomen or infection may trigger the process by causing ischemia, inflammation, and activation of the pancreatic enzymes. Drugs such as thiazide diuretics (HydroDiuril), estrogen, opioids, corticosteroids, and excessive serum calcium from hyperparathyroidism are less common causes of pancreatitis.

Elderly patients and patients with a first diagnosis of pancreatitis have a higher mortality rate. In addition, patients who have pancreatitis associated with biliary disease have a higher mortality rate than patients with alcohol-related pancreatitis.

Prevention

Caution patients who drink alcohol to stop. Patients with biliary disease need to seek medical treatment for these conditions so that pancreatitis does not develop as a complication. Monitor patients, especially the elderly, for any abdominal complaints when they are placed on medications that are associated with pancreatitis (Box 35.7 Cultural Considerations).

Signs and Symptoms   *NPO*

Patients with acute pancreatitis are very ill, with dull abdominal pain, guarding, a rigid abdomen, hypotension or shock, and respiratory distress from accumulation of fluid in the retroperitoneal space. The abdominal pain is generally located in the midline just below the sternum, with radiation to the spine, back, and flank. The location and degree of pain indicate the area of the pancreas involved and to some extent the amount of involvement. Respirations are likely to be

---

cholelithiasis: chole—bile + lith—stone + iasis—condition

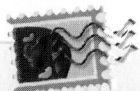

Box 35.7

Cultural Considerations

Pancreatic disease is more common among Mexican Americans and Chinese Americans. Risk factors include working in occupations such as mining, factories using chemicals, and farming using pesticides. The high use of alcohol and cigarette smoking add to the risk of pancreatic disease.

Labs   ALT   AST

shallow as the patient attempts to splint painful areas. Eating makes the pain worse.

The patient may have a low-grade fever, dry mucous membranes, and tachycardia. If the primary cause is biliary, the patient may complain of nausea and vomiting, and jaundice may be evident. The islets of Langerhans in the terminal one-third of the pancreas are usually not impaired.

Complications   *can cause hypovolemia*

It may be useful to think of pancreatitis as a chemical burn to the organ. As with other severe burns, death is likely to occur from secondary causes. From the onset of symptoms, cardiovascular, pulmonary (including acute respiratory distress syndrome), and renal failure are the most likely causes of death. Hemorrhage, peripheral vascular collapse, and infection are also major concerns for patients with pancreatitis. A purplish discoloration of the flanks (Turner's sign) or a purplish discoloration around the umbilicus (Cullen's sign) may occur with extensive hemorrhagic destruction of the pancreas.   *Bleeding occurs*

Diagnostic Tests

Serum amylase (normal: 80 to 180 U/dL) and serum lipase (normal: 0 to 160 U/L) may be elevated 5 to 40 times normal. The levels usually begin to drop within 72 hours. Urine amylase elevates and stays elevated for a longer period of time. Glucose, bilirubin, alkaline phosphatase, lactic dehydrogenase, ALT, AST, cholesterol, and potassium are all elevated. Decreases are measured in serum albumin, calcium, sodium, and magnesium.

X-ray examination may show pleural effusion from local inflammatory reaction to pancreatic enzymes, pulmonary infiltrates, or a change in the size of the pancreas. Computed tomography and ultrasonography can provide more complete information about the pancreas and surrounding tissues.

Therapeutic Interventions

Treatment of acute pancreatitis depends on the intensity of the symptoms. Treatment is concerned with the maintenance of life support until the inflammation resolves, along with preventing or treating complications. Intravenous fluids are administered, such as crystalloid, electrolyte, or colloid (such as albumin) solutions, if the patient experiences hypovolemic shock. Blood or blood products may also be ordered if the patient has significant blood loss from hemorrhage.

The patient may be given antianxiety agents to decrease oxygen demand. The patient may require supplemental oxygen if abdominal pressure, pleural effusion, or acidosis cause an impaired gas exchange or ineffective breathing pattern.

The physician usually orders meperidine hydrochloride (Demerol) for pain because some experts believe morphine can cause spasm of the sphincter of Oddi and increase pain. Pain and anxiety increase pancreatic secretion by stimulating the autonomic nervous system. Phenergan may be ordered to potentiate the Demerol; it may also help reduce nausea.

The patient is usually ordered to have nothing by mouth (NPO) to rest the gastrointestinal tract, although recent research indicates that patients may experience fewer complications if enteral feeding is maintained. The patient may have a nasogastric tube inserted into the stomach and attached to low suction to empty gastric contents and gas. IV odansetron (Zofran) for nausea and a histamine (H₂) antagonist such as famotidine (Pepcid) may help decrease acid stimulation of pancreatic secretion. See Table 35.4 for a summary of medications. If NPO therapy is prolonged or if the patient is malnourished, the patient will need TPN (Box 35.8 Nutrition Notes). A Foley catheter may be inserted to provide accurate output measurements and to assess need for fluid replacement. Strict intake and output must be documented.

Additional typical drug orders include sodium bicarbonate to reverse the acidosis caused by shock, electrolytes such as calcium and magnesium to replace losses, short-acting insulin to combat hyperglycemia, and antibiotics to treat sepsis. See Box 35.9 Pancreatitis Summary.

Nursing Process for the Patient with Pancreatitis

See Box 35.10 Nursing Care Plan for the Patient with Acute and Chronic Pancreatitis

Chronic Pancreatitis

Chronic pancreatitis is continuing pancreatic cellular damage and decreased pancreatic enzyme functioning usually following repeated occasions of acute pancreatitis.

PATHOPHYSIOLOGY. Chronic pancreatitis is a continuous, progressive disease that replaces functioning pancreatic tissue with fibrotic tissue as a result of inflammation. Pancreatic ducts become obstructed, dilated, and finally atrophied. The acinar, or enzyme-producing, cells of the pancreas ulcerate in response to inflammation. The ulceration causes further tissue damage and tissue death, and it may cause cystic sacs filled with pancreatic enzymes to form on the surface of the pancreas. The pancreas becomes smaller and hardened, and progressively smaller amounts of pancreatic enzymes are produced.

ETIOLOGY AND INCIDENCE. The major cause of chronic pancreatitis in men is excessive alcohol ingestion that causes repeated attacks of acute pancreatitis. The major cause in women is chronic obstructive biliary disease that leads to persistent inflammation of the pancreatic ducts.

TABLE 35.4 MEDICATIONS USED FOR LIVER, GALLBLADDER, AND PANCREATIC DISORDERS

Medication Class/Action	Examples	Route	Side Effects	Nursing Implications
Antiemetics Reduce nausea	Metoclopramide (Reglan)	IV, PO, IM	Dry mouth, constipation, drowsiness, extrapyramidal (parkinsonian) symptoms	Monitor for extrapyramidal symptoms. Administer 30 minutes before meals.
	Odansetron (Zofran)	PO, IM, IV	Headache, constipation, diarrhea, extrapyramidal symptoms	Monitor for hypersensitivity, extrapyramidal symptoms.
	Promethazine (Phenergan)	PO, PR, IM, IV	Dizziness, drowsiness, constipation, urinary retention	May be additive when used with opioids; monitor for sedation. Monitor I&O, urinary retention.
Antihistamines Reduce itching	Diphenhydramine (Benadryl)	PO, IM, IV, topical	Drowsiness, dry mouth, confusion in elderly	If using topical preparation, do not apply to open skin.
Anticholinergics Decrease GI secretions	Propantheline bromide (Pro-Banthine) Dicyclomine hydrochloride (Bentyl)	PO PO, IM	Constipation, dry mouth, urinary retention, tachycardia	Contraindicated if patient has glaucoma or prostatic hypertrophy.
Gastric acid-pump inhibitors	Pantroprazole (Protonix)	PO, IV	Headache, diarrhea, abdominal pain	Monitor bowel sounds, liver function (AST, ALT)
Histamine (H₂) antagonists Inhibit gastric acid secretion	Famotidine (Pepcid) Ranitidine (Zantac)	PO, IV PO, IV, IM	Confusion, drowsiness, dizziness	If ordered once a day, give at bedtime. Smoking may interfere with action.

CRITICAL THINKING

Mrs. Samuels

■ Mrs. Samuels, an 85-year-old retired librarian, is admitted to the nursing unit from the emergency department with severe midepigastric pain that radiates to her back. On admission, she is noted to have guarding of the abdomen, and her abdomen is full and tense. Her medical record documents that she had an endoscopic retrograde cholangiopancreatograph (ERCP) 2 days ago for recurrent episodes of RUQ abdominal pain. She has no history of excessive alcohol intake.

1. What is the most common cause of acute pancreatitis? Does Mrs. Samuels fit the description?
2. Why do patients such as Mrs. Samuels have difficulty breathing?
3. Why is Mrs. Samuels at risk for hemorrhage?
4. What laboratory test is most likely to be abnormal in early acute pancreatitis?
5. Why are opioids commonly ordered for acute pancreatitis?
6. Why does the physician usually order a histamine antagonist?

Suggested answers at end of chapter.

Box 35.9

Pancreatitis Summary

Signs and Symptoms	Midline abdominal pain Low-grade fever Nausea and vomiting
Diagnostic Tests	Elevated serum amylase and lipase
Therapeutic Interventions	NPO, NG suction IV fluids and/or nutrition Pain control
Complications	Hemorrhage, shock, infection
Priority Nursing Diagnoses	Pain Imbalanced nutrition Risk for ineffective breathing pattern

---

pancreatitis is made. Death is often not related to pancreatic failure.

PREVENTION. Advise patients with acute pancreatitis from excessive alcohol ingestion that abstinence could prevent recurrence of the pancreatitis and prevent the possibility of chronic pancreatitis. Advise all patients with obstructive biliary disease to seek medical treatment for their condition to prevent the progression from acute to chronic pancreatitis. Carefully monitor patients who are unable to feed themselves for nutritionally adequate diets. Monitor routine laboratory values. Report any trend toward reduced functioning of the pancreas.

SIGNS AND SYMPTOMS. The signs and symptoms of chronic pancreatitis are less severe than acute pancreatitis but more long term. The patient's history will show a pattern of remissions and exacerbations over a period of years. The patient will complain of epigastric or LUQ pain, weight loss, and anorexia. Malabsorption and fat intolerance occur late in the disease. Usually the islets of Langerhans function until late stages of the disease; diabetes mellitus is a late-occurring symptom.

COMPLICATIONS. A variety of complications can result from chronic pancreatitis. Abscesses and fistulas may develop when cysts filled with pancreatic enzymes burst into the abdominal cavity, causing severe inflammation and tissue necrosis. Pleural effusion may develop from inflammation just under the diaphragm. Pancreatic enzymes are essential for normal absorption of nutrients from the intestines. Malabsorption syndrome with fatty stools and diarrhea may develop in response to the limited amount of pancreatic enzymes produced. In addition, biliary obstruction may further complicate fat absorption. As the terminal third of the pancreas becomes involved and the islets of Langerhans

---

Other conditions known to cause chronic pancreatitis are prolonged malnutrition, cancer of the pancreas or duodenum, and prolonged use of enteral feedings, which can cause atrophy of the pancreas. The usual age for chronic pancreatitis to develop is between ages 45 and 60. The patient's mean life span is 25 years after the diagnosis of chronic

---

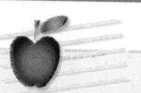

Box 35.8

Nutrition Notes

Nourishing the Patient with Pancreatitis

For acute pancreatitis, the patient may be given ice chips made with electrolyte solutions to minimize gastric secretions and subsequent loss through a nasogastric tube. Nourishment is provided intravenously via TPN. If enteral feedings are started, an elemental formula that has been "predigested" may be selected.

In chronic pancreatitis, the meal pattern is six small meals per day, beginning with clear liquids and progressing to a high-carbohydrate, low-fat diet. Medium-chain triglyceride (MCT) oil may be added to foods because it is absorbed without pancreatic lipase or bile. Pharmaceutical preparations of pancreatic enzymes may be prescribed. Vitamin supplements, including parenteral B_{12}, are commonly administered. When monitoring progress, an increase in serum amylase levels may necessitate the return to a more restricted diet.

(Text continued on page 738)

Box 35.10   NURSING CARE PLAN   for the Patient with Acute and Chronic Pancreatitis

Nursing Diagnosis: Pain related to edema and inflammation

Expected Outcome Patient will state pain level is less than 3 on a scale of 0 to 10.

Evaluation of Outcome Does patient state pain level is less than 3 on a pain scale of 0 to 10?

Interventions	Rationale	Evaluation
Assess the patient every 2 hours for pain by • Asking the patient to rate pain on a scale of 0 to 10. • Observing the patient for pain behaviors such as grimacing, irritability, reluctance to move, or inability to lie quietly.	Intense pain is likely to occur with acute pancreatitis. A pain scale allows for a consistent and individual evaluation of pain. Observation of pain behaviors, such as reluctance to move, shallow respirations, grimacing, or irritability, may be a reliable indicator of pain. However, the patient in pain may have no observable pain behaviors.	Does patient state that pain is less than 3 on a pain scale of 0 to 10, where 0 = no pain and 10 = worst possible pain? Does patient exhibit pain behaviors that differ from his or her report of pain?
Administer analgesics as ordered, before pain becomes severe.	Analgesics are most effective if given before pain becomes too great.	Are analgesics effective?
Assist the patient to a position of comfort, usually high Fowler's or leaning forward slightly.	An upright position keeps abdominal organs from pressing against the inflamed pancreas.	Does positioning promote comfort?
Keep the environment free from excessive stimuli.	Quiet, restful, anxiety-free atmosphere permits the patient to relax and may decrease pain perception.	Does patient state atmosphere is relaxing?
Teach the patient alternative pain control strategies such as guided imagery and relaxation techniques.	Successful use of pain control strategies may decrease the amount of analgesics needed and give the patient a greater sense of control.	Are alternative strategies effective?

Nursing Diagnosis: Imbalanced nutrition: less than body requirements related to pain, medical restrictions (NPO), and treatment (suction)

Expected Outcome Patient will experience improved nutrition as evidenced by stable weight, serum albumin greater than 3.5 g/L.

Evaluation of Outcome Is weight stable? Is serum albumin level greater than 3.5 g/L?

Interventions	Rationale	Evaluation
Assess the patient's nutritional status by		Has patient lost less than 5% of total baseline body weight? Is patient's albumin above 3.5 g/dL?
• Weighing the patient every other day.	A loss of 1 lb of body weight occurs when the body uses 3500 calories more than is taken in.	Does patient have sufficient energy and strength to carry out activities of daily living?
• Monitoring serum albumin levels as ordered.	Serum albumin of 3.5–5.5 g/L indicates normal protein metabolism in the absence of liver or renal disease.	
• Auscultating for bowel sounds.	Bowel sounds must be present before oral nutrition can be provided.	
• Observing for nausea or vomiting.	Nausea, vomiting, and pain are risk factors for inadequate intake.	

Interventions	Rationale	Evaluation
• Monitoring blood sugar at least every 6 hours if the patient is on TPN.	Patients on TPN are more likely to have high blood glucose.	
• Observing for diarrhea, bloating, or steatorrhea (fatty stools). Report steatorrhea immediately.	Diarrhea, bloating, or fatty stools may indicate malabsorption syndrome. Steatorrhea (fatty stools) may indicate that the enzyme replacement doses are not meeting the patient's needs.	
Administer nutritional supplements, including pancreatic enzymes, as ordered.	Provides adequate nutrition.	Does patient take any supplements?
Teach the patient to avoid alcohol.	Alcohol may trigger another episode of pancreatitis.	Does patient verbalize understanding of importance of avoiding alcohol? Is follow-up support for alcohol avoidance provided?
Teach the patient and family the signs and symptoms of diabetes mellitus.	Patients with pancreatitis are at great risk for developing diabetes mellitus.	Does patient verbalize signs and symptoms of diabetes to report?
Teach the patient and family to self-monitor for symptoms of malabsorption syndrome, such as fatty stools, weight loss, dry skin, or bleeding.	Absence of pancreatic enzymes causes problems with digestion of fats, carbohydrates, and proteins.	Does patient verbalize understanding of symptoms of malabsorption to report?

Nursing Diagnosis: Risk for ineffective breathing pattern related to abdominal pressure and pain

Expected Outcome Patient has an effective breathing pattern as evidenced by unlabored respirations, 16–20 per minute, $Sao_2 \geq 95\%$.

Evaluation of Outcome Are respirations unlabored, 16–20 per minute, $Sao_2 \geq 95\%$?

Interventions	Rationale	Evaluation
Assess the patient's breathing patterns: • Observe respirations for depth, regularity, and rate. • Observe respiratory effort. • Observe for evidence of respiratory distress, such as use of accessory muscles, use of intercostal muscles, $Sao_2 < 95\%$, and rapid or difficult breathing.	Abdominal pressure from inflammation and tissue damage under the diaphragm may cause the patient to take shallow, rapid respirations, which can tire the patient.	Are patient's respirations 16–20 per minute, unlabored, and regular? Is patient alert and oriented? Has there been a change in the level of patient's arousal? Does patient exhibit signs of distress?
Administer oxygen as ordered.	Oxygen can decrease the amount of effort the patient must expend to breathe.	Does oxygen help patient breathe easier?
Place the patient in an upright or slightly forward-leaning position.	Relieves pressure on the diaphragm.	Is positioning effective?
Prepare the patient's food by opening cartons and lids. Cut food into bite-size portions.	Decreases the demand for oxygen.	Does patient accept assistance with food preparation?
Teach the patient to move slowly and to take frequent rests.	Helps decrease the demand for oxygen.	Does patient tolerate activity?

(Continued on following page)

Box 35.10 NURSING CARE PLAN **for the Patient with Acute and Chronic Pancreatitis** *(Continued)*

Nursing Diagnosis: Risk for injury related to hemorrhage, or fluid and electrolyte imbalances

Expected Outcome Patient experiences no injury.

Evaluation of Outcome Is there evidence of injury? Are signs and symptoms of impending injury recognized and reported early?

Interventions	Rationale	Evaluation
Monitor sodium, potassium, calcium, and magnesium levels daily.	Electrolyte levels can become imbalanced in pancreatitis.	Do laboratory studies show that patient's electrolytes are within acceptable ranges?
Evaluate neuromuscular status by checking Chvostek's/Trousseau's signs.	These are signs of calcium depletion (see Chapter 5).	Are signs of calcium depletion present?
Monitor the patient's hematocrit, hemoglobin, and blood clotting times frequently.	Destruction of the pancreas can result in hemorrhage.	Does patient have any abnormal bruising, bleeding gums, or pink urine?
Observe abdomen and flanks for Cullen's and Turner's signs.	These are signs of hemorrhage.	
Weigh the patient daily.	To monitor fluid balance.	Is weight stable?
Measure and record intake and output every shift.	To monitor fluid balance.	Is urinary output greater than 30 mL/h?
Observe for nausea and vomiting.	Vomiting can contribute to fluid loss.	Does nausea need to be treated to prevent vomiting?
Report any drop in blood pressure greater than 5% of the patient's baseline.	May indicate severe fluid loss.	Are vital signs stable? Is patient's blood pressure within 5% of baseline?
Monitor TPN and report any difficulties.	TPN must not be stopped abruptly. Patient's blood glucose may drop sharply.	Are blood glucose levels stable?
Teach the patient to report any weakness or muscle twitching.	May indicate electrolyte imbalance.	Does patient verbalize understanding of signs and symptoms of electrolyte imbalance to report?

are destroyed, the patient exhibits symptoms of insulin-dependent diabetes mellitus (discussed in Chapter 40).

DIAGNOSTIC TESTS. Serum amylase and serum lipase levels are only elevated in acute disease. In chronic pancreatitis, enzymes will be normal or below normal. Fecal fat analysis shows higher than normal amounts of fat.

Both computed tomography and ultrasonography show characteristic pancreatic structural changes such as masses, calcification of ducts, cysts, and change in pancreatic size. Endoscopic retrograde cholangiopancreatography (ERCP) can locate specific obstructions and detect ductal leaks.

THERAPEUTIC INTERVENTIONS. Treatment is aimed at promoting comfort and maintaining adequate nutrition. Pain is managed with analgesics. Nutrition is maintained

with the careful replacement of pancreatic enzymes and specially prepared nutritional supplements.

Surgery may be necessary to repair fistulas, drain cysts, or repair other damage. In some cases, ducts or sphincters may be surgically repaired. In other instances, part or all of the pancreas may be removed.

NURSING PROCESS FOR THE PATIENT WITH PANCREATITIS. See Box 35.10, Nursing Care Plan for the Patient with Acute and Chronic Pancreatitis.

Cancer of the Pancreas

Cancer of the pancreas is the fourth leading cause of cancer death in men in the United States, and the fifth leading cause in women, killing more than 30,000 people each year. Nearly 32,000 new cases of cancer of the pancreas are diagnosed yearly[2]; it most often affects people between ages 65 and 79. About 70% of cancers of the pancreas occur in the head of the pancreas. About 30% of cancers are located in the body and tail of the pancreas.

Pathophysiology

Most primary tumors of the pancreas are ductal adenocarcinomas and occur in the exocrine parts of the pancreas. The tumors in the head and body of the pancreas tend to be large. Cancer of the pancreas spreads rapidly by direct extension to the stomach, gallbladder, and duodenum. Cancer located in the body of the pancreas usually spreads further and more rapidly than do masses in the head. Cancer of the pancreas may spread by the lymphatic and vascular systems to distant organs and lymph nodes.

Etiology

The cause of cancer of the pancreas is not known. Cancer of the pancreas has been associated with chemical carcinogens such as high-fat diets and cigarette smoking, diabetes mellitus, excessive alcohol intake, exposure to chemicals such as coke and benzidine, and chronic pancreatitis. It may also occur as a result of metastasis from a primary cancer of the lung, breast, kidney, or thyroid gland or malignant melanomas of the skin.

Signs and Symptoms

The patient with cancer of the pancreas usually experiences vague symptoms early in the disease process. Weight loss, pain, anorexia, nausea, vomiting, and weakness are among the early symptoms. Detection is often difficult because of the nonspecific complaints offered by the patient. The patient may complain of abdominal pain that is worse at night. The pain is described as gnawing or boring, and it radiates to the back. The pain may be lessened by a side-lying position with the knees drawn up to the chest or by bending over when walking. The pain becomes increasingly severe and unrelenting as the cancer grows.

The patient may complain of a bloated feeling or fullness after eating. If the cancer obstructs the bile duct, the patient may have jaundice, dark urine, pruritus, and light-colored stools. The patient often complains of fatigue and depression. The patient's health history may include a recent diagnosis of diabetes mellitus.

Complications

Complications may occur before or after surgical treatment. Preoperative complications include malnutrition, spread of the cancer, and gastric or duodenal obstruction. Postoperative complications include infection, breakdown of the surgical site, fistula formation, diabetes mellitus, and malabsorption syndrome. If the patient has chemotherapy or radiation therapy, complications specific to those therapies may also occur.

Thrombophlebitis is a common complication of cancer of the pancreas. As the tumor grows, by-products of the tumor growth appear to increase the levels of thromboplastic (clotting) factors in the blood, making clotting easier. The potential for thrombophlebitis increases if the patient is confined to bed or has surgery.

Diagnostic Tests

Serum alkaline phosphatase, glucose, and bilirubin levels may be elevated. Amylase and lipase are elevated if the cancer has caused a secondary pancreatitis. Blood coagulation tests, such as clotting time, may be done. Carcinoembryonic antigen (CEA) may be ordered to confirm the presence of cancer (normal: less than 5 ng/mL).

Abdominal radiographs may be ordered to determine the size of the pancreas and the presence of masses. Computed tomography and ultrasonography may be done to more precisely locate any masses in the pancreas. ERCP can be used to visualize the common ducts and to take tissue samples for microscopic analysis. Pancreatic biopsy is necessary for definitive diagnosis of pancreatic cancer. A tissue sample may be obtained by needle aspiration during ultrasonography. This procedure may cause seeding of the tumor along the needle pathway.

Therapeutic Interventions

Medical treatment depends on the staging of the cancer. If diagnosed early, treatment may be aimed at cure. If the patient's cancer has progressed to distant involvement of other organ structures and lymph nodes, treatment is directed at easing symptoms and making the patient more comfortable.

Surgery may include a total or partial **pancreatectomy** or removal of all or part of the pancreas. This is only possible when the tumor is located at the head of the pancreas; tumors in the body and tail of the pancreas have usually spread to other areas and are not resectable. Whipple's procedure is done to remove the head of the pancreas, parts of the stomach nearby, the lower portion of the common bile duct, and the duodenum (Fig. 35.5). Sometimes the gallbladder is also removed. Potential postoperative problems after Whipple's procedure include failure of the suture lines to hold, causing leakage of pancreatic enzymes and bile into the abdomen; pneumonia or atelectasis from shallow breathing because the incision line is directly under the diaphragm; paralytic ileus; gastric retention or ulceration; wound infection; fistula formation; unstable diabetes mellitus; and renal failure.

Other surgical procedures may remove the entire pancreas, stomach, gallbladder, duodenum, and regional lymph nodes, or merely the distal portion of the pancreas and the spleen for smaller, more localized tumors. Even with surgical resection, 5-year survival rates are poor. Postoperative complications similar to those that occur after Whipple's procedure may develop.

Relief of biliary obstruction can sometimes be accomplished by implanting a stent or plastic tube in the common bile duct during an endoscopic procedure. Pain can be reduced by surgical removal of a portion of the greater splanchnic nerve.

Surgery may be followed by chemotherapy and radiation therapy. In some instances, either radiation therapy

---

pancreatectomy: pancreat—pancreas + ectomy—exicsion

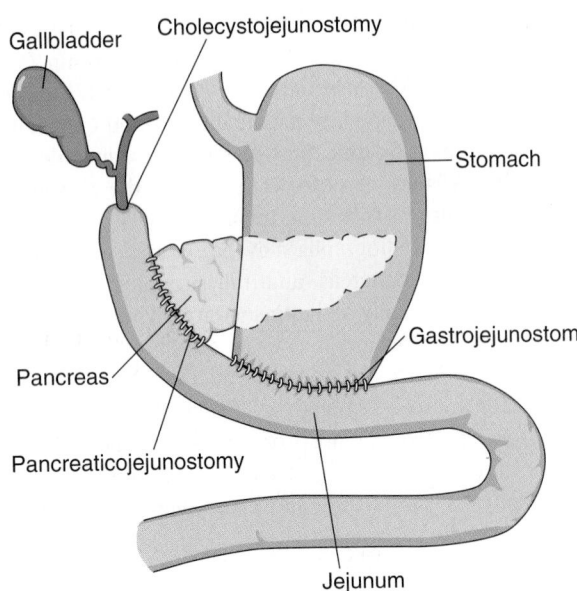

FIGURE 35.5 Pancreatoduodenectomy (Whipple's procedure) for cancer of the head of the pancreas.

or chemotherapy may be used for relief of symptoms if the cancer has become too widespread for surgery. (See Chapter 10 for care of the patient undergoing radiation or chemotherapy.)

Nursing Process for the Patient with Pancreatic Cancer

ASSESSMENT/DATA COLLECTION. Observe the patient with cancer of the pancreas for evidence of malnutrition and fluid imbalance, including weight loss, inelastic skin turgor, vomiting, fatty stools, and complaints of anorexia or nausea. Review laboratory tests, especially blood glucose, liver function studies, and clotting studies. Evaluate the patient every 2 to 4 hours for pain. Observe the skin for bruising, scaling, and yellowing, and question the patient about itching. Evaluate the patient's mental status for evidence of depression.

NURSING DIAGNOSIS, PLANNING, AND IMPLEMENTATION. The patient with cancer of the pancreas will have numerous problems. Interventions for imbalanced nutrition: less than body requirements related to inability to digest food, anorexia, nausea, and vomiting, and pain related to pancreatic tumor or surgical incision are the same as for patients with pancreatitis and are found in Box 35.10 Nursing Care Plan for the Patient with Acute and Chronic Pancreatitis. Other care is listed below. Additional interventions for patients with cancer, including psychosocial interventions, can be found in Chapter 10.

Risk for deficient fluid volume

EXPECTED OUTCOME: The patient will have adequate fluid volume as evidenced by stable vital signs, elastic skin turgor, and moist mucous membranes.

- Monitor the patient's intake and output carefully. *Low intake increases risk of deficient fluid volume; low output is a sign of deficient fluid.*
- Monitor vital signs. *Tachycardia, tachypnea, and low blood pressure may indicate excessive fluid loss.*
- Monitor laboratory values, especially serum sodium, potassium, calcium, and chloride levels. Report abnormal values. *If electrolyte values are low, the physician may order intravenous replacement solutions.*
- Report low serum albumin level (normal is between 3.4–4.8 g/dL) and assist with monitoring intravenous albumin therapy if ordered. *Low albumin places the patient at risk for fluid imbalances.*
- Carefully observe the patient for signs of blood loss *that may indicate abnormal bleeding:*
  - Bruising, bleeding gums, or pink-tinged urine
  - Cullen's sign (bluish discolorations around the umbilicus)
  - Turner's sign (bluish discolorations on the flanks)
  - Bleeding at incision and drain sites and in drainage tubing
- Teach the patient to use a soft-bristle toothbrush. Encourage use of an electric razor rather than a straight razor. *These reduce risk of injury and bleeding.*
- Administer vitamin K as ordered *to replace deficiency and reduce risk for bleeding.*

High risk for impaired tissue integrity related to itching, and leaking around drainage tubes

EXPECTED OUTCOME: The patient's skin will remain intact.

- Assess the patient for any complaints of itching. *Itching leads to scratching, which can cause a break in the skin.*
- Help the patient keep fingernails short *to reduce damage to skin with scratching.*
- Provide frequent skin care with products free of soap or alcohol *to keep the skin clean; soap and alcohol can dry the skin and increase itching and risk for breakdown.*
- Protect skin around drains with skin-protective barrier products and ostomy bags. *Drainage may contain pancreatic enzymes which can be very damaging to skin.*
- Apply products such as calamine lotion as ordered *to decrease itching.*
- Exercise special care of any drains *to prevent unnecessary tension that may cause sutures to give way.*
- Keep all drains patent, and keep drainage tubing and bags free from kinks. *A kinked drain can cause fluid leakage onto the skin.*
- Place the patient in semi-Fowler's position *to help with gravity drainage and reduce risk of fluid leakage.*

PATIENT EDUCATION. Teach the patient and family self-care measures such as blood glucose monitoring, insulin administration, signs and symptoms of hyperglycemia and hypoglycemia (see Chapter 40), and the regimen for pancreatic enzyme replacement. Instruct the patient on how to manage dressing changes if he or she is to be discharged with tubes or drains. The patient and family should know the signs and symptoms of hemorrhage, gastric ulceration, infection, and fistula formation. The patient being cared for at home should have a referral for hospice care or home nursing care.

EVALUATION. The plan of care for the patient with pancreatic cancer is successful if the patient exhibits the following:

- Maintains body weight within 5% of normal body weight and experiences no nausea or vomiting.
- States that pain remains at 3 or less on a pain scale of 0 to 10.
- Has urinary output greater than 40 mL/hr, elastic skin turgor, moist mucous membranes, and pulse and blood pressure within 10% of patient's baseline.
- Has no complaints of sudden, excessive abdominal pain or rigidity; incisions heal at the expected rate.
- Can demonstrate the appropriate self-care procedures for tubes, drains, dressings, and medication administration and states the signs and symptoms of complications that are to be reported immediately.

For more information, visit the National Pancreas Foundation at www.pancreasfoundation.org.

DISORDERS OF THE GALLBLADDER

Cholecystitis, Cholelithiasis, and Choledocholithiasis

Gallstones and inflammations of the gallbladder and common bile duct are the most common disorders of the biliary system. These disorders are also common health problems for people in the United States: Nearly 25 million people have gallstones, and about 500,000 people have their gallbladders removed each year.

Pathophysiology

Cholecystitis is an acute or chronic inflammation of the gallbladder. It is most often a response to obstruction of the common bile duct resulting in edema and inflammation. Often bacteria invade the bile and add to the inflammation and irritation of the gallbladder. Chronic cholecystitis may be the result of repeated attacks of acute cholecystitis or chronic irritation from gallstones. The gallbladder becomes fibrotic and thickened and does not empty easily or completely.

Cholelithiasis is characterized by the formation of gallstones in the gallbladder that are usually composed primarily of cholesterol. **Choledocholithiasis** refers to gallstones in the common bile duct. Although the exact cause of gallstones is unknown, one theory suggests that cholesterol may supersaturate the bile in the gallbladder. After a time, the supersaturated bile crystallizes and begins to form stones. Another type of gallstone is a pigment stone. Pigment stones appear to be composed of calcium bilirubinate, which occurs when free bilirubin combines with calcium.

Etiology and Incidence

Pooling, or stasis, of bile within the gallbladder appears to contribute to the formation of stones. Stasis may be caused by a decreased gallbladder emptying rate or a partial obstruction in the common duct. Excessive cholesterol intake combined with a sedentary lifestyle is linked with an increased incidence of cholelithiasis.

Some low-fat diets have been linked to cholelithiasis because the diet appears to free cholesterol from body tissues; the cholesterol then crystallizes in the gallbladder before it is excreted. Fasting can contribute to cholelithiasis because the gallbladder is less active, and bile becomes concentrated. Further, a family history of cholelithiasis, obesity, diabetes mellitus, pregnancy, some hemolytic blood disorders, and bowel disorders such as Crohn's disease have also been linked to a higher incidence of cholelithiasis.

Cholelithiasis is responsible for about 90% of the cases of cholecystitis, or inflammation of the gallbladder. Women between ages 20 and 50 are about three times more likely to have gallstones than men; especially women with multiple pregnancies, women who are pregnant, or women who are using birth control pills. After age 50, the rate of gallstones is about the same for men and women (Box 35.11 Cultural Considerations). Cholelithiasis is responsible for nearly 800,000 hospital admissions at a cost of more than $2 billion every year. The incidence of gallstones increases with age.

Signs and Symptoms

Signs and symptoms of cholecystitis and cholelithiasis are similar. Objective symptoms include evidence of inflammation, such as an elevated temperature, pulse, and respirations; vomiting; and jaundice. Subjective symptoms include patient complaints of epigastric pain, RUQ tenderness, nausea, and indigestion, especially after eating foods high in fat. The patient may have a positive Murphy's sign, which is the inability to take a deep breath when an examiner's fingers are pressed below the liver margin.

The epigastric pain caused by cholelithiasis may also be called biliary **colic.** The pain is a steady, aching, severe pain in the epigastrium and RUQ that may radiate back to behind the right scapula or to the right shoulder. The pain usually begins suddenly after a fatty meal and lasts for 1 to 3 hours. If the pain is caused by a stone in the common bile

---

cholecystitis: chole—bile + cyst—bladder + itis—inflammation

choledocholithiasis: chole—bile + docho—duct + lith—stone + iasis—condition

colic: colic—spasm

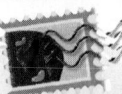

Box 35.11

Cultural Considerations

Gallbladder disease is more common among Mexican Americans. Risk factors include working in occupations such as mining, factories using chemicals, and farming using pesticides. The disease has a lower incidence in blacks in Africa and in blacks living in the Western world. Native Americans have an increased incidence of pancreatic and gallbladder disease. It is unknown how much increased dietary risk factors may contribute to gallbladder disease. The nurse can positively affect the nutritional status of at-risk patients by teaching food preparation practices that use less fat.

duct (choledocholithiasis), the pain may last until the stone has passed into the duodenum. Jaundice is more commonly present with acute choledocholithiasis because the common bile duct is blocked or inflamed.

The biliary colic caused by cholecystitis typically lasts 4 to 6 hours. The pain is made worse with movement such as breathing. The patient usually has nausea, vomiting, and a low-grade fever with the pain.

Patient complaints of heartburn, indigestion, and flatulence are more common with chronic cholecystitis. Patients often report a medical history that suggests repeated attacks of acute cholecystitis (Table 35.5).

Family history of either cholecystitis or cholelithiasis, dietary habits such as high fat intake or a recent low-fat diet, and complaints of flatulence (gas), eructation (belching), nausea, vomiting, or abdominal discomfort after a high-fat meal are common evidence of a gallbladder disorder.

Complications

Complications of cholecystitis include inflammation of the bile ducts (cholangitis), necrosis or perforation of the gallbladder, empyema (a collection of purulent drainage in the gallbladder), fistulas, and adenocarcinoma of the gallbladder. A major complication of choledocholithiasis is acute pancreatitis if the pancreatic duct is obstructed.

Diagnostic Tests

The patient may have an elevated white blood cell count (normal: 5000 to 10,000 cells per mm^3). Serum amylase level may be elevated (normal: 59 to 190 IU/L) if the pancreas is involved or if there is a stone in the common duct.

An abdominal x-ray examination may be done to determine whether the gallstone is primarily calcium. Calcium-based stones are less responsive to medical treatments. Cholesterol stones are highly responsive to medical therapy.

Further examination may include a nuclear scan. For this procedure, the patient will be given an IV injection of a radioactive isotope that is metabolized by the liver and excreted in the bile. The scanning camera then traces the path of the isotope as it travels through the bile ducts, gallbladder, and intestines. This test may be called a PIPIDA scan, DISIDA scan, or HIDA scan, depending on the isotope used.

Sonograms can detect stones and may be able to determine whether the walls of the gallbladder have thickened. An ERCP can be done to directly visualize the pancreatic ducts and bile ducts to determine the presence of stones in the common duct and occasionally to remove stones from the common duct.

Therapeutic Interventions

Treatment of an acute episode of cholecystitis centers on pain control, prevention of infection, and maintenance of fluid and electrolyte balance. Pain control is achieved by using opioid analgesics. The analgesic agent most often ordered is meperidine hydrochloride (Demerol) because morphine sulfate is believed to cause spasms of the gallbladder, biliary ducts, and the sphincter of Oddi. Antispasmodics or anticholinergic drugs such as propantheline bromide (Pro-Banthine) and dicyclomine hydrochloride (Bentyl) may be ordered to decrease the biliary colic. If the patient has nausea and vomiting, an antiemetic such as

TABLE 35.5 SYMPTOMS OF GALLBLADDER DISORDERS

	Acute Cholecystitis	Chronic Cholecystitis	Cholelithiasis and Choledocholithiasis
Biliary colic	Lasts 4–6 hours Worse with movement	Only during acute attack	Sudden onset
Jaundice	Present (if common bile duct is inflamed or blocked)	Present	Lasts 1–3 hours
			Radiates to right scapula or shoulder
Low-grade fever	Present	Present	Present
Nausea, vomiting	Present	Only during acute attack	Present
Repeated attacks		Present	
Heartburn, indigestion, and flatulence		Present	
Complications	Cholangitis Necrosis or perforation Fistulas	Empyema Fistulas Adenocarcinoma	Acute pancreatitis

ondansetron (Zofran) or promethazine (Phenergan) may be ordered (see Table 35.4). Patients are placed on high-protein, low-fat diets after the nausea and vomiting subside (Box 35.12 Nutrition Notes).

Treatment for cholelithiasis usually involves surgical removal of the gallbladder. The surgical procedure may be cholecystectomy via **laparoscopy** or a traditional cholecystectomy. A laparoscopic cholecystectomy is done with a laparoscope through four small puncture wounds in the abdomen.

A traditional cholecystectomy is done through a long, transverse, right subcostal incision. The patient may have a T-tube inserted into the common duct for several days postoperatively to ensure that bile drainage is not obstructed (Fig. 35.6). A Jackson Pratt or Penrose drain may also be inserted at the time of surgery. The drain is removed when drainage is minimal. The patient with a traditional cholecystectomy has incisional pain that creates difficulty with coughing and deep breathing postoperatively because deep breathing causes the diaphragm to press on the operative site. Patients are hospitalized for 2 to 3 days with a traditional cholecystectomy and 24 hours or less with a laparoscopic cholecystectomy.

Some patients are poor surgical risks and have stones in the gallbladder or biliary duct that cannot be removed easily by other methods. Such patients may have a cholecystostomy, which is an incision directly into the gallbladder to remove a stone. If the stone is in the biliary ducts, a choledocholithotomy may be done. The patient usually has a T-tube in place for several days to help remove bile from swollen structures.

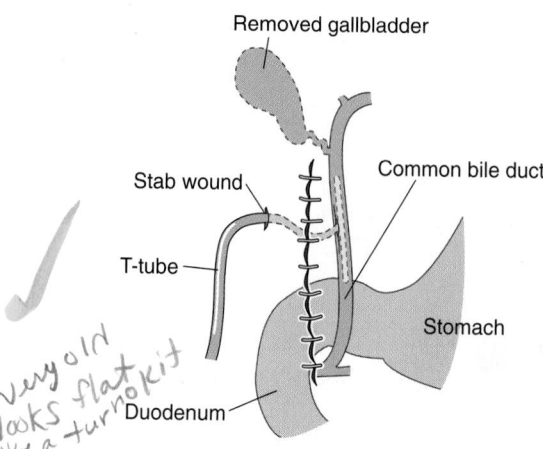

very old looks flat no kit like a turn

FIGURE 35.6 T-tube. A T-tube is used to drain bile after a cholecystectomy until swelling of the duct subsides.

Other methods of treatment include **choledochoscopy, extracorporeal shock-wave lithotripsy** (ESWL), oral drugs to dissolve stones, and direct-contact dissolving drugs. The procedure for a choledochoscopy involves the use of an endoscope to explore the common bile duct and in some instances to snare and remove any stones found.

Extracorporeal shock-wave lithotripsy uses shock waves as a noninvasive method to destroy stones in the gallbladder or biliary ducts. Patients who are considered poor surgical risks and who have few cholesterol stones that are not calcified are the most likely candidates for ESWL. The patient lies face down on a water bag over a lithotriptor (Fig. 35.7). A conductive gel is placed between the patient and the water bag. Ultrasound is used to locate the stone or stones and to monitor the destruction of the stones. The patient requires sedation and strong analgesics during the procedure to reduce the pain and discomfort of the shock waves. After ESWL, the patient is usually put on a course of oral dissolution drugs to ensure complete removal of all stones and stone fragments.

Dissolution of stones with drugs may be attempted with chenodiol (Chenix) or ursodiol (Actigall). Patients who are poor surgical risks because of advanced age or severe health problems and who have cholesterol stones may be given oral dissolution drugs. The major disadvantages to the use of these drugs are that abnormal liver function studies and diarrhea are common side effects. Patients may also have an increase in serum cholesterol while taking the drugs. Treatment with the dissolution drugs may take from 4 months to 2 years. Patients may need to take cholesterol-lowering drugs in addition to the dissolution drugs to lower serum cholesterol and to decrease the probability of stones reforming.

Direct-contact dissolution drugs are administered directly into the gallbladder through a percutaneous transhep-

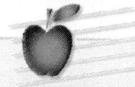

Box 35.12

Nutrition Notes

Modifying the Diet for Patients with Gallbladder Disease

During an acute attack of cholecystitis, a full liquid diet with minimal fat is usually allowed. For treatment of chronic cholecystitis, the patient is instructed to do the following:

- Correct obesity.
- Avoid troublesome and gas-forming foods.
- Decrease dietary fat each day by (1) selecting skim-milk dairy products, (2) limiting fats or oils to 3 tsp, and (3) consuming no more than 6 oz of very lean meat.

Cholelithiasis has been associated with a long overnight fast that permits concentrated bile to remain in the gallbladder for an extended period. Eating a light bedtime snack or drinking two glasses of water on arising if breakfast is delayed alter this risk factor.

---

choledochoscopy: chole—bile + docho—duct + scopy—to examine

extracorporeal shock-wave lithotripsy: extra—outside + tripsy—rub or crush

---

laparoscopy: aparo—pertaining to flank + scopy—to examine

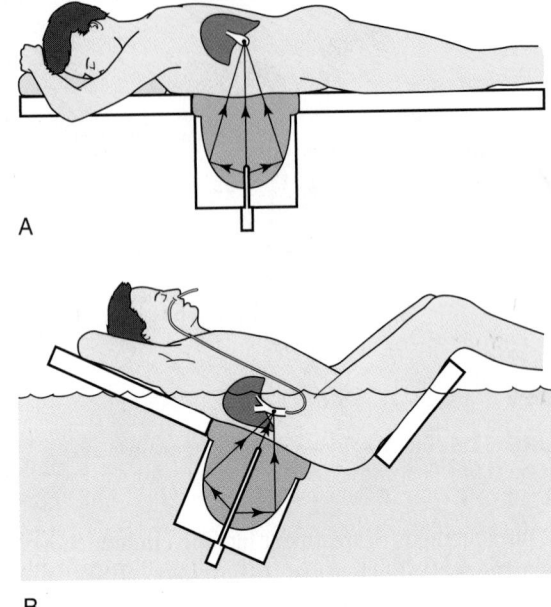

FIGURE 35.7 Extracorporeal shock-wave lithotripsy. Shock waves are transmitted through water to break up gallstones. (A) Position for stones in gallbladder. Patient is lying on a fluid-filled bag. (B) Position for stones in common bile duct. Patient is in a water bath.

Box 35.13

Cholecystitis Summary

Signs and Symptoms	Epigastric/RUQ pain, especially after a fatty meal Elevated temperature, pulse, respirations Jaundice if common bile duct blocked
Diagnostic Tests	WBC count Abdominal x-rays Nuclear scan (HIDA, PIPIDA, or DISIDA) Ultrasound, ERCP
Therapeutic Interventions	Pain control Laparoscopic or open cholecystectomy Extracorporeal shock-wave lithotripsy Low-fat diet
Priority Nursing Diagnoses	Pain Risk for deficient fluid volume Risk for ineffective breathing pattern Risk for impaired skin integrity

atic catheter. The physician inserts a catheter through the wall of the abdomen into the gallbladder and then injects and aspirates the dissolution agent repeatedly during the treatment. Candidates for this procedure are patients who are poor surgical risks and whose gallbladder can be seen during oral cholecystography. Disadvantages of the procedure include abnormal liver function studies, pain at the catheter site, nausea, and elevations in the white blood cell count. See Box 35.13 Cholecystitis Summary.

Nursing Process of the Patient with a Gallbladder Disorder

ASSESSMENT/DATA COLLECTION. Assess the patient frequently for pain, using the "What's Up?" questions. Take the patient's vital signs, particularly the temperature and pulse, frequently to monitor for signs of infection. Weigh the patient and inspect mucous membranes, skin turgor, and urinary output for signs of dehydration. Measure intake and output, including any emesis or drainage from nasogastric tubes or T-tubes. Observe stools and urine for color and consistency. Obstruction of bile flow may result in stools that are clay colored or have a foul, greasy appearance or urine that is dark amber or tea colored. Report either new finding immediately. Evaluate laboratory studies for elevation in the white blood cell count or abnormalities in electrolytes or serum bilirubin levels.

NURSING DIAGNOSIS, PLANNING, AND IMPLEMENTATION. Common nursing diagnoses for the patient with cholecystitis include pain and risk for deficient fluid volume.

Additional nursing diagnoses for the patient with cholelithiasis who has a surgical procedure include risk for impaired skin integrity related to surgical incision and T-tube drainage, and risk for ineffective breathing pattern related to abdominal incision.

Acute pain related to biliary colic

EXPECTED OUTCOME: Patient rates pain as 3 or less on 10-point scale.

- Assess the patient frequently for pain. *Treatment should be based on assessment.*
- Administer meperidine (Demerol) or other analgesics as ordered *to reduce pain.*
- Administer antispasmodics or anticholinergics as ordered *for biliary colic.*
- Assist patient with positioning. *The patient should assume whatever position provides the most comfort.*

Risk for deficient fluid volume related to anorexia, nausea, vomiting, or excessive tube drainage

EXPECTED OUTCOME: The patient will have adequate fluid volume as evidenced by stable vital signs, elastic skin turgor, and moist mucous membranes.

- Monitor intake and output, daily weights, and skin turgor *to monitor fluid balance.*
- Monitor T-tube drainage. Carefully observe the T-

tube drainage unit to prevent kinking of the tubing. *About 250 to 500 mL of yellowish green bile is common within the first 24 hours after surgery. The amount of bile diminishes over the next several days. Pressure in the biliary drainage system from poor drainage may greatly increase the patient's pain and the risk for infection.*

- After surgery, maintain nasogastric tube placement as ordered *to prevent an ileus from developing.*
- Frequently assess for the return of bowel sounds and passage of flatus. *Once bowel sounds return, the nasogastric tube will be removed, and the patient is slowly reintroduced to a solid diet, usually high protein and low fat.*
- Give antiemetics as needed *to control nausea and vomiting.*
- Assist with administration of intravenous fluids and electrolytes as ordered while the patient is on restricted oral intake *to maintain hydration.*

Risk for impaired skin integrity related to surgical incision and T-tube drainage

EXPECTED OUTCOME: The patient's skin will remain intact.

- Inspect the patient's skin and the sclerae of the eyes frequently for jaundice. Report new onset of jaundice or patient complaints of excessive itching. *Jaundice is associated with itching, which can lead to scratching and impaired skin integrity.*
- Inspect the cholecystectomy incision frequently for excessive drainage or evidence of infection such as redness, edema, or warmth. *Drainage or infection can irritate and break down skin.*
- Change dressings frequently *to protect the skin around the incision site from irritating drainage.*
- Use Montgomery straps to secure dressings *to prevent skin irritation from repeated or prolonged exposure to adhesive bandages.*
- Change the patient's position frequently *to reduce risk of pressure ulcers.*
- Protect the skin with a skin barrier product or bag such as those used with colostomies if bile is leaking around the T-tube site. An enterostomal therapist (if available) can be consulted for the best choice of dressing. *A skin barrier can protect skin from breakdown due to contact with bile.*

Risk for ineffective breathing pattern related to abdominal incision

EXPECTED OUTCOME: Patient will have effective breathing pattern as evidenced by rate 16 to 20, even, unlabored, depth within normal limits.

- Monitor respiratory rate, depth, and effort, and ability to cough effectively. *The high abdominal incision can cause pain with deep breathing and coughing.*
- After surgery, encourage the patient to cough and deep breathe at every encounter. Instruct the patient

in the proper techniques before surgery and give the opportunity to practice. *Deep breathing and coughing after any surgical procedure help prevent respiratory tract infections and atelectasis.*

- If the patient is reluctant to cough because of pain, evaluate the pain medication regimen. *Pain must be controlled so the patient is able to cough and deep breathe.*
- Assist the patient with splinting when coughing *to make coughing less painful.*
- Encourage the patient to walk when permitted *to help mobilize secretions.*

PATIENT EDUCATION. Discharge education focuses on diet. Patients are put on high-protein, low-fat diets. Encourage obese patients to lose weight. After a cholecystectomy, fat should be slowly reintroduced into the diet. Once the duodenum becomes accustomed to a constant infusion of bile, the patient's individual tolerance for fat becomes the only restriction for diet.

EVALUATION. The plan of care for a patient with cholecystitis or cholelithiasis is successful if the patient exhibits the following:

- Reports pain not greater than 3 on a pain scale of 0 to 10, or pain that is tolerable
- No weight loss, urinary output greater than 50 mL/h, moist mucous membranes, elastic skin turgor, and no complaints of excessive thirst
- Intact skin with no warmth, redness, swelling, or purulent drainage at the wound site; no jaundice or complaints of itching
- Clear breath sounds and a normal white blood cell count.

CRITICAL THINKING

Donna

■ Donna, a 23-year-old woman, is diagnosed with possible acute cholecystitis. She is 5 feet, 6 inches tall and weighs 138 pounds. She has recently stopped following an extremely low-fat diet after losing nearly 70 pounds. Her physician wishes to delay surgery until her inflammation has subsided.

1. What risk factors does Donna have for cholecystitis?
2. What diagnostic tests might be ordered to confirm Donna's diagnosis of cholecystitis?
3. What medications can you anticipate that the physician will order for Donna?
4. What type of diet will Donna need to eat after discharge?
5. If the diagnosis of cholecystitis is confirmed, what type of surgical treatment might be ordered?

Suggested answers at end of chapter.

Home Health Hints

- For patients with hepatitis, home health nurses are concerned with proper treatment and patient education to prevent transmission in the community.
- If possible, the patient with hepatitis should have a separate bedroom and bathroom. The person cleaning the bathroom should wear disposable gloves or rubber gloves and then clean the gloves with a 10% bleach solution. The family is advised to use liquid soap instead of bar soap.
- Contaminated linens used by a patient with hepatitis should be washed separately from household laundry and in hot water. One cup of bleach should be added

with the detergent to each load. Rubber gloves should be worn to wash the patient's laundry.
- A patient with abdominal ascites needs a hospital bed at home so the patient can be positioned to aid in breathing. A physician's order must be obtained for insurance coverage.
- Measure abdominal girth of the patient with ascites at each visit and record in the nurse's notes. The patient should weigh on the same scale, first thing in the morning, and record the weight so the nurse can document the findings.

REVIEW QUESTIONS

1. Which of the following conditions most places a patient with chronic liver failure at risk for bleeding?
   a. Encephalopathy
   b. Low vitamin K
   c. Elevated liver enzymes
   d. Hepatorenal syndrome

2. A nurse is administering lactulose to a patient with chronic liver disease. The patient states, "That stuff gives me diarrhea. I don't want it." Which response by the nurse is best?
   a. "This keeps your ammonia level under control, so it is important to your care. How many stools have you had today?"
   b. "Diarrhea can cause dehydration—I'll hold the medication."
   c. "I am placing you in charge of your own care, so I will hold this medication at your request."
   d. "The diarrhea should stop after a few doses; it is important to keep taking the medication."

3. A health care worker is diagnosed with hepatitis C virus. Which question is most important to ask during the admission assessment?
   a. "Have you eaten any raw seafood recently?"
   b. "Have you experienced a needle stick?"
   c. "Have you made beds or handled clothing without gloves?"
   d. "Has anyone coughed into your face when you weren't wearing a mask?"

4. An elevation in which laboratory test indicates chronic pancreatitis?
   a. Serum bilirubin
   b. Serum calcium

c. Serum albumin
d. Serum amylase

5. A patient with acute pancreatitis is hospitalized must remain NPO. His serum enzymes are very high. He has been receiving only IV hydration. Which laboratory result indicates the need to consult the dietitian for nutrition support?
   a. Potassium 4.2 mEq/L
   b. Sodium 130 mEq/L
   c. Fasting glucose 82 mg/dL
   d. Serum albumin 2.9 g/dL

6. In planning care for the newly admitted patient with acute pancreatitis, which patient outcome should receive highest priority?
   a. Patient expresses satisfaction with pain control.
   b. Patient verbalizes understanding of medications for home.
   c. Patient increases activity tolerance.
   d. Patient maintains normal bowel function.

7. A patient develops jaundice and dark, amber-colored urine. Which of the following is most likely the cause?
   a. Encephalopathy
   b. Pancreatitis
   c. Bile duct obstruction
   d. Cholecystitis

8. Which meal is most appropriate for the patient with acute cholecystitis?
   a. Chicken broth, low fat custard, gelatin dessert
   b. Cream of chicken soup, milk, gelatin dessert
   c. Meat loaf, mashed potatoes with small amount of gravy, green beans

d. Turkey and cheese sandwich on whole grain bread, apple, milk

9. Which interventions will help a patient who had an open cholecystectomy 24 hours ago to maintain an effective breathing pattern? Select all that apply.
   a. Place in a supine position.
   b. Provide analgesics for pain relief.

c. Encourage coughing and deep breathing.
d. Monitor bowel sounds.
e. Assist with splinting during coughing.
f. Maintain bedrest for 48 hours after surgery.

10. The nurse is to administer promethazine 12.5 mg IM and has 50 mg/mL on hand. How many mL should be drawn up? _____

References

1. Centers for Disease Control: Disease Burden from Hepatitis A, B, and C in the United States. Accessed http://www.cdc.gov/ncidod/diseases/hepatitis/resource/dz_burden02.htm, September 18, 2005.

2. American Cancer Society: Leading Sites of New Cancer Cases and Deaths—2004 Estimates. Accessed http://www.cancer.org/docroot/MED/content/downloads/MED_1_1x_CFF2004_page 10.asp, September 18, 2005.

Unit Eight Bibliography

1. Acambis. Emerging strain of common bacteria *Clostridium difficile,* is highly toxic. April 11, 2005. Accessed November 7, 2005: ttp://www.acambis.com/documents/sites/1/News_releases/SHEA_release.pdf

2. Buckhold, KM: Who's afraid of hepatitis C? Am J Nurs 100:26–31, 2000.

3. Canadian Press: Quebec C. difficile strain has high toxin levels. April 11, 2005. Accessed November 1, 2005: http://www.ctv.ca/servlet/ArticleNews/story/CTVnews/1113222804128_6/?hub-Health

4. Coleman, P, and Watson, NM: Oral care provided by certified nursing assistants in nursing homes. J Am Geriatr Soc 2006 54:138–143.

5. Dharmarajan, TS, and Unnikrishnan, D: Tube feeding in the elderly: The technique, complications, and outcome. Postgrad Med 115:51–61, 2004. http://www.postgradmed.com/issues/2004/02_04/dharmarajan.htm. Accessed November 1, 2005.

6. Dickerson, RN, Tidwell, AC, and Brown, RO: Adverse effects from inappropriate medication administration via a jejunostomy feeding tube. Nutr Clin Pract 18:402–405, 2003.

7. Larson, D, Dozois, E, Sandborn, W, and Cima R: Total laparoscopic proctocolectomy with Brooke ileostomy: a novel incisionless surgical treatment for patients with ulcerative colitis. Surg Endosc 19:1284–1287, 2005.

8. Longstreth, GF, and Yao, JF: Irritable bowel syndrome and surgery: a multivariable analysis. Gastroenterology 126: 1665–1673, 2004.

9. Lutz, CA, and Przytulski, KR: Nutrition and Diet Therapy, ed. 4. F.A. Davis, Philadelphia, 2005.

10. Madsen, D, Sebolt T, Cullen L, et al: Listening to bowel sounds: an evidenced based project. Am J Nurs 105:40–50, 2005.

11. Maloney, J, Ryan, TA, Brasel, KJ, et al: Food dye use in enteral feedings: a review and a call for a moratorium. Nutr Clin Pract 17:169–181, 2002.

12. Marik, P, and Zaloga, G: Meta-analysis of parenteral nutrition versus enteral nutrition in patients with acute pancreatitis. BMJ 328:1407–1410, 2004.

13. McCormick, ME: Endoscopic retrograde cholangiopancreatography. Am J Nurs 99:24HH–JJ, 1999.

14. Medline Plus: Acute cholecystitis. Accessed at http://www.nlm.nih.gov/medlineplus/ency/article/000264.htm January 20, 2006.

15. Metheny NA, Dahms TE, Stewart BJ, et al: Efficacy of dye-stained formula in detecting pulmonary aspiration. Chest 122:276–281, 2002.

16. Molle, E: Getting down to the lower GI tract. Nursing 35:20–21, 2005.

17. National Center for Infectious Diseases: Viral hepatitis. Accessed at http://www.cdc.gov/ncidod/diseases/hepatitis/ January 20, 2006.

18. Parker, M: Acute pancreatitis. Emergency Nurse 11:28–35, 2004.

19. Perceived barriers and benefits were factors in decision making about colorectal screening. John Oliffe (commentator). Evid Based Nurs 2006; 9:31, 2006. doi:10.1136/ebn.9.1.31

20. Persson E, Wilde L: Quality of care after ostomy surgery: a perspective study of patients. Ostomy Wound Manage 51:40–48, 2005.

21. Review: good evidence supports use of polyethylene glycol and tegaserod for constipation. Jane P Joy (commentator). Evid Based Nurs 8:109, 2005. doi:10.1136/ebn.8.4.109

22. Rosemurgy, AS: What's new in surgery: Gastrointestinal conditions. J Am Coll Surgeons 197: 792–801, 2003.

23. Rutgeerts, P, Sandborn, WJ, Feagan, BG et al: Infliximab for induction and maintenance therapy for ulcerative coiltis. N Engl J Med 353:2462, 2005.

24. Sandborn, WJ: Serologic markers in inflammatory bowel disease: state of the art. Rev Gastroenterol Disord 4:167–174, 2004 [review].

25. Sandborn, W: What's new: innovative concepts in inflammatory bowel disease. Colorectal Dis 1(Suppl):3–9, 2006.

26. Sanko, J: Aspiration assessment and prevention in critically ill enterally fed patients: evidence-based recommendations for practice. Gastroenterol Nurs 27:279–285, 2004

27. Stanley, M, Blair, KA, and Gauntlett-Beare, P: Gerontological Nursing—Promoting Successful Aging with Older Adults, ed. 3. F.A. Davis: Philadelphia, 2005.

28. Starr, S, and Hand, H: Nursing care of chronic and acute liver failure. Nurs Stand 6:47–55, 2002.

29. Yeow, JTW, Yang, VXD, Chahwan, ML et al: Micromachined 2-D scanner for 3-D optical coherence tomography. Sensors and Actuators A 117: 331–340, 2004.

30. Wilson, LA: Understanding bowel problems in older people: part 1. Nurs Older People 17:25–29, 2005.

SUGGESTED ANSWERS TO

CRITICAL THINKING

■ Carl

1. Foreign travel within the past 2 months, fatigue, nausea, and irritability suggest hepatitis A virus. Recent possible exposure to materials contaminated with blood or body fluids, fatigue, headache, and nausea suggest hepatitis B virus.

2. Careful hand washing and standard precautions when handling any body fluids or feces should be instituted.

3. The nurse should plan to give an antiemetic if Carl is nauseated. Larger meals should be given early in the day, with Carl in an upright or sitting position. The nurse should also ensure that the environment is free of noxious stimulants such as unpleasant odors. The diet should be high calorie, high protein, high carbohydrate, and low fat.

4. Any medication that is known to be hepatotoxic, such as acetaminophen, aspirin, and diazepam (Valium), should be avoided.

5. Carl should be reminded that cleanliness, especially with food preparation, is essential. He should also be reminded that frequent hand washing is crucial. Carl needs to know that alcohol and other liver-toxic substances should be avoided.

■ Mary

1. Mary has a history of poor nutrition. Her age also puts her at risk.

2. Mary may report that she has malaise, nausea, weight loss, a change in bowel habits, and dull, aching RUQ pain.

3. Serum albumin is usually less than 3.2 g/dL. Her prothrombin time will probably be greater than 25 seconds.

4. Esophageal varices and ascites are the two greatest concerns for the patient with portal hypertension.

5. The physician will usually order diuretics, intravenous albumin infusions, and a sodium-restricted diet.

6. The possibility of suffocation from having the gastric tube dislodge into the esophagus requires that scissors be kept at the bedside at all times during tamponade.

■ Mrs. Samuels

1. The most common cause of acute pancreatitis is excessive alcohol intake. Mrs. Samuels denies alcohol consumption, but she does have the risk factor of having a recent ERCP, which may have dislodged a gallstone or irritated the pancreatic duct.

2. Respiratory distress may result from excess fluid accumulation in the retroperitoneal space and from shallow respirations that seek to decrease pressure from the diaphragm on the inflamed pancreas and surrounding tissues.

3. Pancreatitis is similar to a chemical burn and may cause erosion of major blood vessels in surrounding tissue.

4. Serum amylase may be elevated as much as 40 times more than normal early in acute pancreatitis.

5. Opioids are ordered because pain is intense, and pain with anxiety stimulates the autonomic nervous system, which may stimulate greater production of pancreatic enzymes.

6. Stomach acid stimulates the production of pancreatic enzymes. Histamine antagonists decrease stomach acidity.

■ Donna

1. Some low-fat diets have been linked to the development of cholesterol gallstones, which then irritate the gallbladder and cause inflammation.

2. Donna's physician might order a white blood cell count, which will be elevated if she has cholecystitis. In addition, the physician may order an x-ray, nuclear scan, or ultrasound to visualize the gallbladder and its contents and the common bile duct.

3. You can anticipate that the physician will order an antibiotic, a narcotic such as meperidine hydrochloride, and possibly an antispasmodic such as Pro-Banthine.

4. Donna will need to eat a low-fat diet after discharge. Eventually she may be able to add more fats to her diet as her body adjusts.

5. If the diagnosis is confirmed, Donna will probably have a laparoscopic cholecystectomy unless her surgeon decides that she needs a traditional cholecystectomy.

unit NINE

UNDERSTANDING THE URINARY SYSTEM

36

Urinary System Function, Assessment, and Therapeutic Measures

MAUREEN McDONALD AND JANICE L. BRADFORD

KEY TERMS

cystoscopy (sis-TAHS-koh-pee)
dysuria (dis-YOO-ree-ah)
hematuria (HEM-uh-TYOOR-ee-ah)
incontinence (inn-con-tin-unce)
nephrotoxic (nef-row-tocks-ick)
nocturia (kock-tur-e-ah)
percutaneous (PER-kyoo-TAY-nee-us)
pyelogram (PIE-loh-GRAM)
uremia (yoo-REE-mee-ah)

QUESTIONS TO GUIDE YOUR READING

1. What are the effects of aging on the urinary system?

2. What data should you collect when caring for a patient with a disorder of the urinary system?

3. How do you collect a midstream, clean-catch urine specimen, and 24-hour creatinine clearance specimen?

4. What is the preparation and postprocedure for diagnostic tests of the urinary system?

5. What nursing care is given for patients with incontinence?

6. Which nursing actions can be taken to decrease the risk of infection in catheterized patients?

REVIEW OF ANATOMY AND PHYSIOLOGY

The urinary system consists of two kidneys, two ureters, the urinary bladder, and the urethra. The kidneys form urine, and the rest of the system eliminates urine. The purpose of urine formation is the removal of potentially toxic waste products from the blood; however, the kidneys have other equally important functions as well:

- Regulation of the blood volume, composition, and pressure by the excretion or conservation of water
- Regulation of the electrolyte balance of the blood by the excretion or conservation of minerals
- Regulation of the acid-base balance of the blood by the excretion or conservation of ions such as hydrogen or bicarbonate
- Regulation of all of the above in tissue fluid
- Production of erythropoietin, which then stimulates erythocyte production in the bone marrow.

The process of urine formation thus helps maintain the normal composition, volume, and pH of blood and tissue fluid.

Kidneys

The two kidneys are located in the upper abdominal cavity behind the peritoneum on each side of the vertebral column. The upper portions of both kidneys rest on the lower surface of the diaphragm and are enclosed and protected by the lower rib cage. The kidneys are cushioned by surrounding adipose tissue, which is in turn covered by a fibrous connective membrane called the renal fascia; both help hold the kidneys in place. On the medial side of each kidney is an indentation called the hilus, where the renal artery enters and the renal vein and ureter emerge. The renal artery is a branch of the abdominal aorta, and the renal vein returns blood to the inferior vena cava. The ureter carries urine from the kidney to the urinary bladder.

Internal Structure of the Kidney

A frontal section of the kidney shows three distinct areas (Fig. 36.1). The outermost area is the renal cortex, which contains the parts of the nephrons called renal corpuscles and convoluted tubules. The middle area is the renal medulla, which contains loops of Henle and collecting tubules. The renal medulla consists of wedge-shaped pieces called renal pyramids; the apex, or papilla, of each pyramid points medially. The third area is a cavity called the renal pelvis; it is formed by the expansion of the ureter within the kidney at the hilus. Funnel-shaped extensions of the renal pelvis, called calyces, enclose the papillae of the renal pyramids. Urine flows from the pyramids into the calyces, then to the renal pelvis, and finally into the ureter.

Nephron

The nephron is the structural and functional unit of the kidney. Urine is formed in the approximately 1 million nephrons in each kidney. The two major parts of a nephron

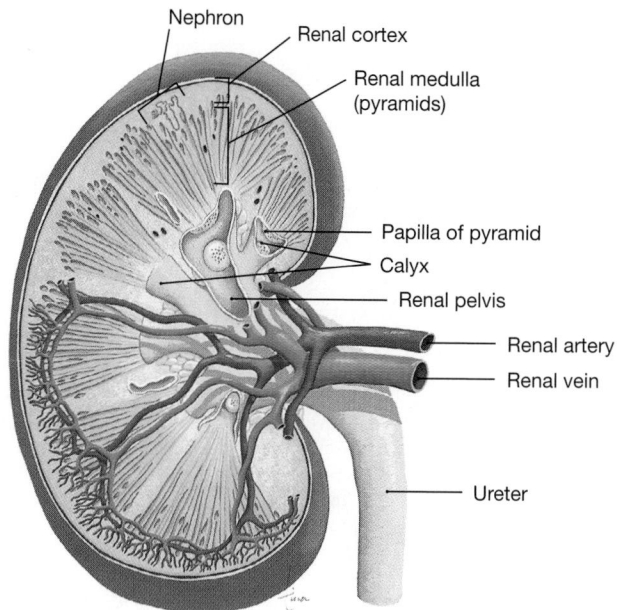

FIGURE 36.1 Frontal section of the left kidney. *(From Scanlon, V, and Sanders, T: Essentials of Anatomy and Physiology, ed. 4. F.A. Davis, Philadelphia, 2003, p 401, with permission.)*

are the renal corpuscle and the renal tubule; these and their subdivisions and blood vessels are shown in Figure 36.2.

A renal corpuscle consists of a glomerulus surrounded by a Bowman's capsule. The glomerulus is a capillary network that arises from an afferent arteriole and empties into an efferent arteriole. The diameter of the efferent arteriole is smaller than that of the afferent arteriole, which helps maintain a fairly high blood pressure in the glomerulus. Bowman's capsule is the expanded end of a renal tubule; it encloses the glomerulus. The inner layer of Bowman's capsule has pores and is highly permeable; the outer layer has no pores and is not permeable. The space between the inner and outer layers contains renal filtrate, the fluid that is formed from the blood in the glomerulus and that will eventually become urine.

The renal tubule continues from Bowman's capsule and consists of the proximal convoluted tubule, the loop of Henle, and the distal convoluted tubule. The distal convoluted tubules from several nephrons empty into a collecting tubule. Several collecting tubules then unite to form a papillary duct that empties urine into a calyx of the renal pelvis. All the parts of the renal tubule are surrounded by the peritubular capillaries, which arise from the efferent arteriole and receive the materials reabsorbed by the renal tubules.

Blood Vessels of the Kidney

The pathway of blood flow through the kidney is an essential part of the process of urine formation. Blood from the abdominal aorta enters the renal artery, which branches extensively within the kidney into smaller arteries. The smallest arteries give rise to afferent arterioles in the renal cortex. From the afferent arterioles, blood flows into the glomeruli (capillaries), to efferent arterioles, to peritubular

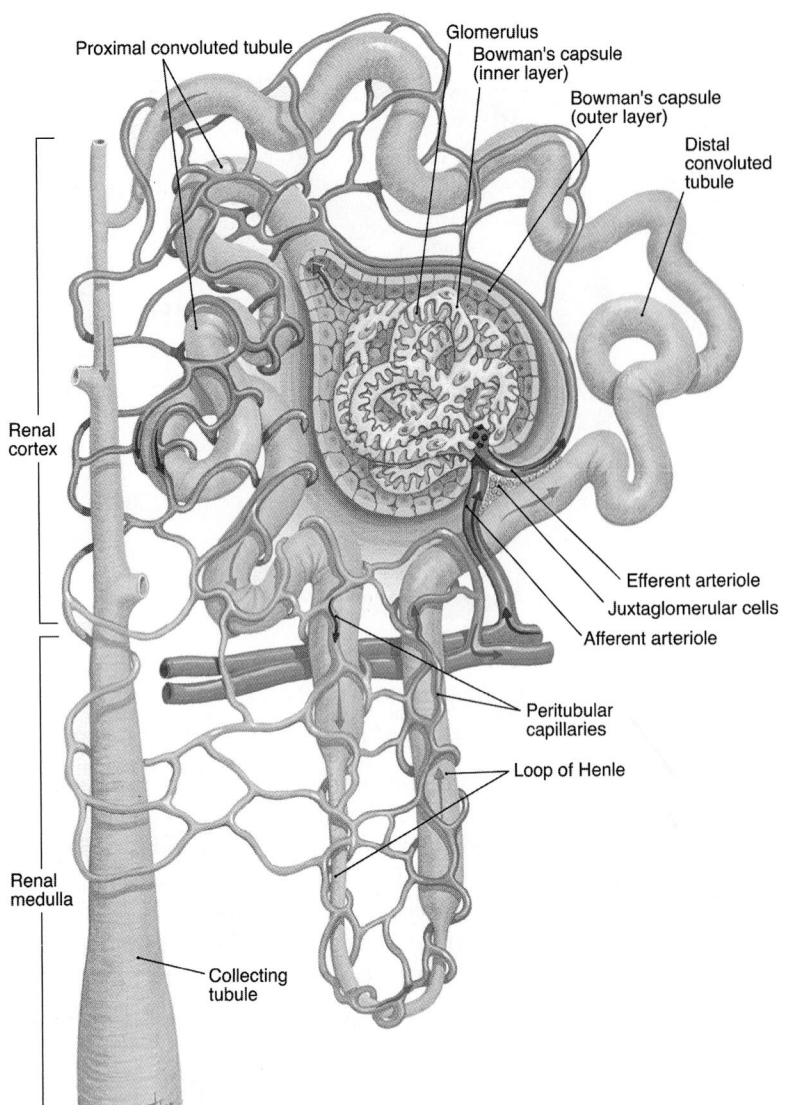

Proximal convoluted tubule

Glomerulus

Bowman's capsule (inner layer)

Bowman's capsule (outer layer)

Distal convoluted tubule

Renal cortex

Efferent arteriole

Juxtaglomerular cells

Afferent arteriole

Peritubular capillaries

Loop of Henle

Renal medulla

Collecting tubule

FIGURE 36.2 A nephron and its associated blood vessels. *(From Scanlon, V, and Sanders, T: Essentials of Anatomy and Physiology, ed. 4. F.A. Davis, Philadelphia, 2003, p 402, with permission.)*

capillaries, to veins in the kidney, to the renal vein, and finally to the inferior vena cava. In this pathway are two sets of capillaries; that is, two sites of exchanges between the blood and the surrounding tissues (in this case, the parts of the nephrons). The exchanges that take place in the capillaries of the kidneys form urine from blood plasma.

Formation of Urine

The formation of urine involves three major processes: glomerular filtration in the renal corpuscles, tubular reabsorption, and tubular secretion.

Glomerular Filtration

Filtering urine

Filtration is the process by which blood pressure forces plasma and dissolved materials out of capillaries. In glomerular filtration, blood pressure forces plasma, dissolved substances, and small proteins out of the glomeruli and into Bowman's capsules. This fluid is then called renal filtrate.

The blood pressure in the glomeruli is relatively high— about 55 mm Hg. The pressure in Bowman's capsule is low,

and its inner layer is permeable, so that approximately 20% to 25% of the blood that enters glomeruli becomes renal filtrate in Bowman's capsules. The larger proteins and blood cells are too large to be forced out of the glomeruli; they remain in the blood. Waste products such as urea and ammonia are dissolved in plasma, so they pass to the renal filtrate, as do dissolved nutrients and minerals. Renal filtrate is similar to blood plasma except that there is far less protein and no blood cells are present.

The glomerular filtration rate (GFR) is the amount of renal filtrate formed by the kidneys in 1 minute; it averages 100 to 125 mL/min. The GFR may change if the rate of blood flow through the kidney changes. If blood flow increases, the GFR increases, more filtrate is formed, and urinary output increases. If blood flow decreases, the GFR decreases, less filtrate is formed, and urinary output decreases.

Tubular Reabsorption

Tubular reabsorption is the recovery of useful materials from the renal filtrate and their return to the blood in the peritubular capillaries. Approximately 99% of the renal filtrate formed is reabsorbed, and normal urinary output is 1000 to 2000 mL per 24 hours. Most reabsorption takes place in the proximal convoluted tubules, whose cells have microvilli that greatly increase their surface area. The distal convoluted tubules and collecting tubules are also important sites for the reabsorption of water. The mechanisms of reabsorption are active transport, osmosis, diffusion, facilitated diffusion, and pinocytosis.

Active transport requires energy in the form of adenosine triphosphate (ATP); the cells of the renal tubule use energy to transport useful materials such as glucose, amino acids, vitamins, and positive ions back to the blood. For many of these substances there is a threshold level of reabsorption—that is, a limit to how much the renal tubules can remove from the filtrate. The level of a substance in the renal filtrate is directly related to its blood level. If the blood level of a substance such as glucose is normal, the filtrate level is normal, the threshold level cannot be exceeded, and no glucose appears in the urine.

Passive transport is the mechanism by which most negative ions are reabsorbed. They are returned to the blood after the reabsorption of positive ions because opposite charges attract.

The reabsorption of water by osmosis follows the reabsorption of minerals, especially sodium. The conservation of water is very important to maintain normal blood volume and blood pressure. The hormones that influence the reabsorption of water or minerals are summarized in Table 36.1.

Small proteins in the filtrate are reabsorbed by pinocytosis; the proteins become attached to the membranes of the tubule cells and are engulfed and digested. Normally, all proteins in the filtrate are reabsorbed and none are found in urine.

TABLE 36.1 EFFECTS OF HORMONES ON THE KIDNEYS

Hormone (Gland)	Function
Aldosterone (Adrenal Cortex)	Promotes reabsorption of sodium ions from the filtrate to the blood and excretion of potassium ions into the filtrate. Water is reabsorbed following the reabsorption of sodium.
Antidiuretic Hormone (Posterior Pituitary)	Promotes reabsorption of water from the filtrate to the blood.
Atrial Natriuretic Hormone (Atria of Heart)	Decreases reabsorption of sodium ions, which remain in the filtrate. More sodium and water are eliminated in the urine.
Parathyroid Hormone (Parathyroid Glands)	Promotes reabsorption of calcium ions from the filtrate to the blood and excretion of phosphate ions into the filtrate.

Source: Scanlon, V, and Sanders, T: Essentials of Anatomy and Physiology, ed. 4. F.A. Davis, Philadelphia, 2003, p 406, with permission.

Tubular Secretion

In tubular secretion, substances are actively secreted from the blood in the peritubular capillaries into the filtrate in the renal tubules. Waste products, such as ammonia and creatinine, excess water-soluble vitamins, and the metabolic products of medications may be secreted into the filtrate to be eliminated in urine. Hydrogen ions may be secreted by the tubule cells to help maintain the normal pH of the blood.

In summary, tubular reabsorption conserves useful materials, tubular secretion may add unwanted substances to the filtrate, and most waste products simply remain in the filtrate and are excreted in urine.

The Kidneys and Acid-Base Balance

Other than exhalation of carbon dioxide by the respiratory system, the kidneys are the organs most responsible for maintaining the normal pH range of blood and tissue fluid. They have the greatest ability to compensate for or correct the pH changes that are part of normal body metabolism or the result of disease.

At its simplest, this function of the kidneys may be described as follows. If body fluids are becoming too acidic, the kidneys secrete more hydrogen ions into the renal filtrate and return more bicarbonate ions back to the blood. This helps raise the pH of the blood back to normal. In the opposite situation, when the body fluids become too alkaline, the kidneys return hydrogen ions to the blood and excrete bicarbonate ions in urine. This helps lower the pH of the blood back to normal.

Other Functions of the Kidneys

Some functions of the kidneys are not related to the formation of urine. These include the secretion of renin, activation of vitamin D, and production of erythropoietin. The production of renin influences urine formation and is considered first.

When blood pressure decreases, the juxtaglomerular cells in the walls of the afferent arterioles secrete the enzyme renin. Renin then initiates the renin-angiotensin-aldosterone mechanism, which results in the formation of angiotensin II. (See Chapter 15.) Angiotensin II stimulates vasoconstriction and increases the secretion of aldosterone, both of which help raise blood pressure.

Vitamin D exists in several structural forms, which are converted to calcitriol, the most active form, by the kidneys. Vitamin D is important for the efficient absorption of calcium and phosphate from food in the small intestine.

Erythropoietin is a hormone secreted by the kidneys during states of hypoxia; it stimulates the red bone marrow to increase the rate of red blood cell (RBC) production. With more RBCs in circulation, the oxygen-carrying capacity of the blood is greater and the hypoxic state may be corrected.

Elimination of Urine

The ureters, urinary bladder, and urethra do not change the composition or volume of urine but are responsible for its elimination.

Ureters

The ureters are behind the peritoneum of the dorsal abdominal cavity. Each ureter extends from the hilus of a kidney to the lower, posterior side of the urinary bladder. The smooth muscle in the wall of the ureter contracts in peristaltic waves to propel urine toward the urinary bladder. As the bladder fills, it expands and compresses the lower ends of the ureters to prevent backflow of urine.

Urinary Bladder

The urinary bladder is a muscular sac below the peritoneum and behind the pubic bones. In women, the bladder is inferior to the uterus; in men, the bladder is superior to the prostate gland. The functions of the bladder are the temporary storage of urine and its elimination.

Urethra

The urethra carries urine from the bladder to the exterior. Within its wall, near the bladder, is an involuntary, internal urethral sphincter. Inferior to that is the external urethral sphincter, which is made of skeletal muscle and is under voluntary control.

In women, the urethra is 1.0 to 1.5 inches long and is anterior to the vagina. In men, the urethra is 7 to 8 inches long and extends through the prostate gland and penis. The male urethra carries semen, as well as urine.

Urination Reflex

Urination (micturition) is a spinal cord reflex over which voluntary control may be exerted. The stimulus is the stretching of the detrusor muscle as urine accumulates in the bladder. Sensory impulses travel to the sacral spinal cord, and motor impulses return along parasympathetic nerves to the detrusor muscle, causing contraction. At the same time, the internal urethral sphincter relaxes. If the external urethral sphincter is voluntarily relaxed, urine flows into the urethra and the bladder is emptied.

Characteristics of Urine

Amount

Normal urinary output is 1000 to 2000 mL per 24 hours. Any changes in fluid intake or other fluid output (such as sweating) change this volume.

Color

The color of urine is often referred to as straw or amber. Dilute urine is a lighter color (straw) than is concentrated urine. Freshly voided urine is clear. Cloudy urine may indicate an infection.

Specific Gravity

The usual range of specific gravity of urine is 1.010 to 1.025; this is a measure of the dissolved materials in urine. (The specific gravity of distilled water is 1.000.) The higher the specific gravity, the more dissolved material is present. Specific gravity of urine is a measure of the concentrating ability of the kidneys; the kidneys must excrete the waste products that are constantly formed in as little water as possible.

pH

The pH range of urine is 4.6 to 8.0, with an average of 6.0. Diet has the greatest influence on urinary pH. A vegetarian diet results in a more alkaline urine; a high-protein diet results in a more acidic urine.

Constituents

Urine is approximately 95% water, which is the solvent for waste products and salts. Nitrogenous wastes include urea, creatinine, and uric acid. Urea is formed by liver cells when excess amino acids are deaminated (metabolized) to be used for energy production. Creatinine comes from the metabolism of creatine phosphate, an energy source in muscles. Uric acid comes from the metabolism of nucleic acids—that is, the breakdown of DNA and RNA. Other solutes are present in small quantities: enzymes and hormones, for example.

Aging and the Urinary System

With age, the number of nephrons in the kidneys decreases, often to half the original number by age 70 or 80 (Fig. 36.3). The GFR also decreases; this is in part a consequence of arteriosclerosis and diminished renal blood flow. The urinary bladder decreases in size, and the tone of the detrusor muscle decreases. This may result in the need to urinate more frequently or in residual urine in the bladder after voiding. Elderly people are also more subject to infections of the urinary tract, and the changes of aging may influence medication therapy for elderly people (Box 36.1 Gerontological Issues).

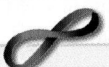

Box 36.1

Gerontological Issues

Age-Related Renal Changes

Certain changes typically occur in the renal system as people age. They include the following:

- The renal mass becomes smaller.
- Renal flow decreases by 50%, with subsequent decreased glomerular filtration rate.
- Tubular function and the exchange of substances decrease.
- Bladder muscles weaken and bladder capacity decreases, leading to increased frequency and nocturia.
- The voiding reflex is delayed.

Also, keep in mind that most drugs are excreted through the kidneys. Consequently, changes in renal function become a serious consideration for older adults who need drug therapy. Decreased renal function could slow the excretion of some drugs, keeping them in the body longer. This can increase the risk of adverse drug reactions, such as toxicity and overdose. It is important to monitor kidney function (such as creatinine and blood urea nitrogen levels) in an older person receiving drug therapy.

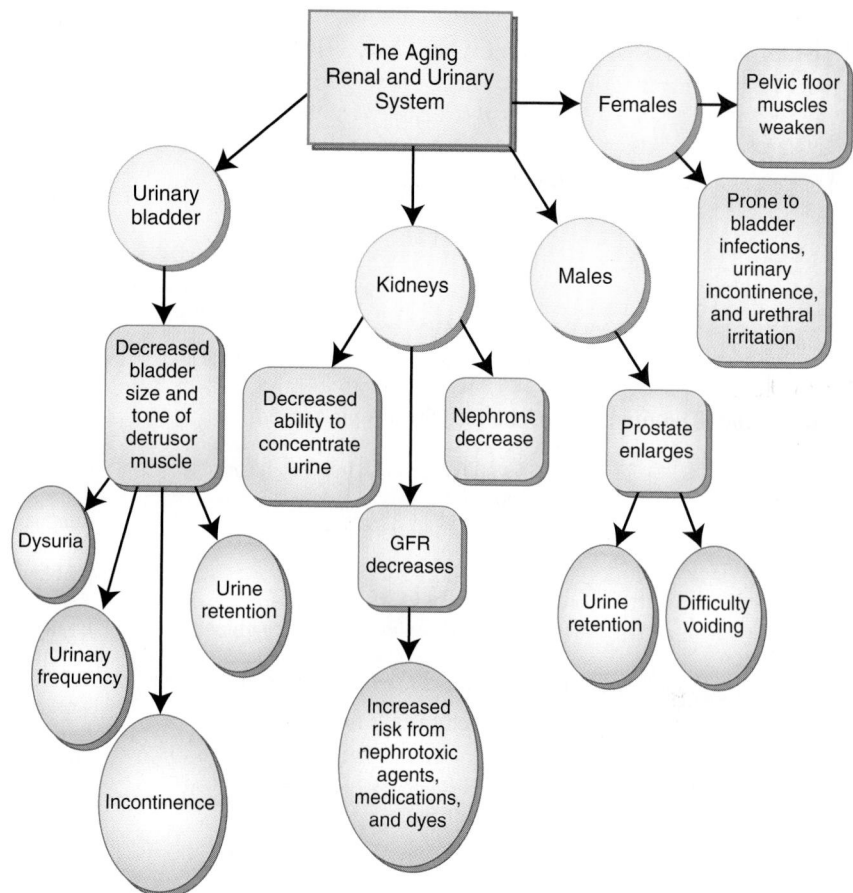

FIGURE 36.3 Aging and the urinary system. This concept map shows the effects the aging process has on the urinary system.

NURSING ASSESSMENT/ DATA COLLECTION OF THE URINARY SYSTEM

Subjective Data: Health History

Table 36.2 describes questions to ask for a health history. Any symptoms should be further assessed using the WHAT'S UP? format found in Chapter 1.

If the patient has impaired kidney function or is in kidney failure, a complete head-to-toe assessment is needed because urinary disease and kidney failure (renal failure) affect every system of the body (see Chapter 37).

Objective Data: Physical Assessment

Objective data to collect is found in Table 36.2. The nurse first inspects the skin for color, texture, edema, or swelling. A patient with chronic renal failure may have a yellow or gray cast to the skin. The presence of crystals on the skin is called uremic frost and is a late sign of waste products building up in the blood (**uremia**). When the wastes are not filtered by the kidneys, they can come out through the skin and look like a coating of frost.

Palpation and percussion of the kidneys is done by physicians and advanced practice nurses. Gentle palpation

and percussion of the bladder may be done by the licensed practical nurse/licensed vocational nurse (LPN/LVN) if urine retention is suspected. If the patient has a feeling of fullness but is unable to urinate, the nurse gently palpates the suprapubic area for a full bladder. Normally, the bladder is not palpable. The bladder may also be percussed. The percussion note sounds dull over a fluid-filled bladder.

Assess for difficulty with cognition, mobility, or manual dexterity. Problems in these areas may be reflected in toileting skill and ability.

Most assessment of the urinary system is done using indirect measures. Assessment of vital signs, lung sounds, edema, daily weights, and intake and output can provide valuable data related to urinary function. The nurse often collects urine specimens for analysis and reports observations about the characteristics of the urine.

Vital Signs

If renal disease is suspected, blood pressure should be assessed and documented while the patient is lying, sitting, and standing. An increase in blood pressure is commonly seen with renal disease. A drop in blood pressure accompanied by a rise in pulse rate as the patient rises to sitting or standing positions is called orthostatic, or postural, hypotension and may indicate fluid deficit (see Chapter 20). A rapid respiratory rate may indicate fluid retention in the lungs.

uremia: ur—urine + emia—blood

(Text continued on page 760)

TABLE 36.2 ASSESSMENT OF THE URINARY SYSTEM

Subjective Assessment		
Category	**Questions to Ask During History Assessment**	**Rationale/Significance**
Age	• How old are you?	• Aging is associated with a gradual loss of nephrons. At about age 80 a person may have 40% fewer functioning nephrons. • Kidneys become less able to concentrate urine • Bladder capacity decreases and may not completely empty with age
Gender	• Male or female	• Women have a high incidence of incontinence. • Men are at risk for prostate problems that can affect voiding patterns.
Race, ethnicity	• What is your ethnic origin? • What is the language you speak at home? • Do you prefer to speak in a language other than English?	• Black males over 40 years of age have a higher incidence of prostate and bladder cancer. Younger men between the ages of 25 and 35 have increased incidence of testicular cancer. • Language barriers may exist for patients who speak another primary language that affect expression of problems and understanding of treatments.
Occupation	• What type of work do you do? • Have you had any exposure to chemicals in your present or past jobs or hobbies? • Has your job affected your heath, if so how?	• Renal cancers may occur with occupational exposure to phenol and ethylene glycol which are nephrotoxic chemicals. • Textile workers, painters, hairdressers, and industrial workers have a higher incidence of bladder tumors. • Stress may predispose hypertension and cardiovascular disease.
Health Habits	• Do you use alcohol, tobacco, recreational drugs, or caffeine?	• Alcohol can irritate the bladder and increase urinary output. • Tobacco use is associated with increased risk of renal cancer.
History of Renal or Urinary Problems	• Do you have any of the following problems with voiding? Pain Increased frequency Blood in urine Bladder or urinary tract infections • Have you noticed any changes in your voiding patterns? Urgency Hesitancy Difficulty starting a stream of urine **Nocturia** Diminished amount of urine Incontinence • Have you had kidney or bladder surgery? • Describe the surgery. • Have you had any changes in the color, odor, clarity or amount of urine? • Have you had any pain in the flank area? • Have you had any pain in the costovertebral angle (the area formed by the rib cage and the vertebral column)? • Have you noticed any swelling of your lower legs in the evening? • Have you noted any swelling of your eyes in the morning?	• Painful voiding may indicate an infection. • Increased urinary urgency with diminished amounts of urine suggests urinary retention. • **Hematuria** may indicate an infection or cancer. • Difficulty obtaining a stream of urine may indicate a prostate obstruction. Nocturia may be noted with nephrotic syndrome, diabetes, and heart failure. • Changes in the amount of urine voiding may indicate renal disease. • Decreased amounts of urine may indicate renal failure. • Increased amounts may indicate diabetes or inability to concentrate urine. • Changes in color, odor, or clarity of urine indicate the possibility of infection. • Flank pain may indicate renal disease. • A renal calculus or stone may produce a dull ache in the kidney area or a colicky pain that periodically radiates to the genital area or the leg on the affected side. • Edema is noted when there is fluid retention with an increase in circulating fluid volume. • Periorbital edema is noted around the eyes in the morning.
Past Medical History	• Have you been diagnosed in the past with any of the following conditions? Urinary tract infections Renal stones Use of indwelling catheters Diabetes Hypertension	• Diabetes is the most common cause of chronic kidney disease worldwide. • Hypertension is another significant risk factor. • Systemic diseases such as gout, lupus, sickle cell disease, coronary artery disease, and atherosclerosis increase the risk of renal disease. • Streptococci infections may precede renal disease.

hematuria: hemat—blood + uria—urine

Category	Questions to Ask During History Assessment	Rationale/Significance
Past Medical History (cont'd)	Heart attacks Angina Gout Lupus erythematosus Sickle-cell disease Beta hemolytic streptococci Systemic infections Cancer Glomerulonephritis Polycystic kidney disease • Do you have any history of falls, motor vehicle accidents, or other trauma? • Do you have any history of renal diagnostic tests? • How many children do you have?	• Delayed diagnosis of renal trauma increases the risk of renal damage secondary to infection, abscess formation, and strictures. • Previous history or renal tests may indicate a previous problem with the renal system. • Increased parity may affect pelvic floor muscles that may lead to stress incontinence.
Family History of Urinary Disorders	• Has anyone in your family had any problems with their kidneys or urinary system? • Has anyone in your family had hypertension, diabetes, or kidney stones?	• The presence of certain renal abnormalities in families increases the likelihood of similar problems occurring in the patient. • Often genetic abnormalities go undetected until later in life with the onset of symptoms. • Positive family history is a risk factor for renal disease. • Polycystic kidney disease is a hereditary disorder where grapelike cysts replace normal kidney tissue.
Current Medications, Over-the-Counter Medications, or Herb Use	• What prescribed medications are you taking? • What over-the-counter medications are you taking? • What herbs or minerals are you taking? • Do you have any allergies to antibiotics, contrast media, or dyes?	• Many drugs may lead to increased risk for renal failure: Gentamicin Amphotericin B NSAIDs ACE inhibitors Rifampin Aminoglycosides • "Chinese herbs" have been reported to cause kidney failure and cancer. These substances contain aristolochic acid, which may be renal toxic. • Contrast media is often used with x-rays to diagnose renal disease.
New Onset of Symptoms	• Have you noticed any new onset of any of the following symptoms? Fatigue Shortness of breath Fever or chills Nausea, vomiting, or anorexia Headaches or blurred vision Lethargy Impaired mentation or confusion Itchy skin Facial swelling around the eyes Metallic taste in your mouth Bone or joint problems	• Fatigue and shortness of breath may be from anemia. Erythropoietin produced in the kidney is necessary to produce red blood cells. • Fever is associated with urinary tract infections. • Uremic toxins may produce itching skin, headache, bone pain, numbness, nausea, and vomiting. • Facial swelling is due to edema. • Metallic taste in the mouth may be due to imbalances of electrolytes. • Bone and joint problems may be due to problems with calcium and vitamin D metabolism.
Diet and Fluid Intake	• Describe your appetite and nutritional status. • Have you noticed any changes in weight over the last year? • How many cups of fluid do you drink daily? • What types of fluid do you drink? • Are you able to shop and cook for yourself?	• Obesity often leads to diabetes, hypertension, and renal disease. • Obese individuals have less body water in relation to weight than a lean person does. This predisposes the obese person to greater risk for renal ischemia from fluid losses and dehydration. • Large intake of protein or dairy products may lead to kidney stone formation. • Anorexia and nausea may be present as renal insufficiency progresses toward renal failure. • Hyperlipidemia is a risk factor for renal disease. • Inability to take care of shopping and cooking can have a direct effect on diet.

(Continued on following page)

TABLE 36.2 ASSESSMENT OF THE URINARY SYSTEM (Continued)

Subjective Assessment (Continued)

Category	Questions to Ask During History Assessment	Rationale/Significance
Pain	• Have you had recent pain in the back, over the bladder, lower abdomen, or perineum? • Have you had any pain or burning with urination? • Have you had any back or leg pain?	• Flank pain or lower abdominal pain may indicate infection, obstruction, or inflammation of the urinary system. • Kidney pain is dull, aching, and steady, and located in the flank area. • Ureteral pain begins in the costovertebral angle and radiates into the lower abdomen and groin. • Bladder pain may be felt over the symphysis pubis. • Back or leg pain may be due to prostrate or metastasis of cancer.

Objective Assessment

Category	Possible Abnormal Findings	Possible Causes
General Survey • Height • Weight • Ethnicity • Posture • Gait • Apparent State of Health	• Hyperlipidemia • Obesity • Ambulation difficulty • Lethargy • Weakness	• Lipids may accumulate in the glomerular cells and promote glomerular fibrosis. • Obesity leads to hypertension and diabetes, both high risks for renal disease. • Weight gain may be secondary to edema • Weight loss may be secondary to renal failure and muscle wasting. • Difficulty ambulating may interfere with voiding patterns and promote incontinence.
Vital Signs • Blood pressure • Pulse • Respiratory rate • Pulse oximetry	• Hypertension • Orthostatic hypotension • Tachycardia • Bradycardia • Irregular heart rates	• Hypertension is related to renal disease and fluid volume overload • Orthostatic hypotension may be due to dehydration. • Hyperkalemia causes arrhythmias.
Cognitive Function and Neurological Status	• Confusion • Lethargy • Insomnia • Diminished deep tendon reflexes • Hyperesthesia • Paresthesias • Peripheral neuropathy • Decreased mentation • Headaches	• Changes in level of consciousness may be due to changes in electrolytes and fluid balance. • Sleep disorders and neuropathies are common and may be a result of altered fluid balance. • Increased levels of urea, creatinine, and parathyroid hormone may interfere with nerve function and contribute to neuropathies. • Headaches occur from fluid volume overload and uremic toxins.
Skin, Hair, and Nail Assessment	• Skin pallor, color, yellow gray cast • Excoriations • Changes in turgor • Bruising • Changes in skin texture • Dry skin • Distal portion of nail beds white • Capillary refill less than 3 seconds • Impetigo—a streptococcal infection of the skin	• Pallor may be due to anemia. • Scratching from pruritus may lead to excoriations. • Dehydration is associated with oliguria. • Edema contributes to nocturia and results from fluid volume overload. • Distal portion of nail beds turn white with renal failure • Increased capillary refill may result from poor blood flow to the extremity or anemia. • Streptococcal infections may precede glomerulonephritis.
Eyes	• Conjunctival pallor • Corneal calcification • Retinal arteriosclerotic changes • Blurred vision	• Anemia • Corneal calcification results from phosphate retention • Retinal changes in blood vessels results from prolonged hypertension or diabetes. • Retinitis pigmentosa may accompany hereditary nephropathies
Ears, Nose, and Throat	• Deafness • Strep throat	• High-frequency deafness may accompany hereditary nephritis • Acute glomerulonephritis may be accompanied with pharyngitis or group A hemolytic streptococcal infections.
Cardiovascular	• Hypertension • Friction rub • Cardiac enlargement of the left ventricle • Dysrhythmias • Angina or chest pain	• Hypertension is the most frequent cause of renal disease. • Hypertension may also be a result of renal disease from alterations of sodium and renal secretion of vasoconstrictors.

Objective Assessment *(Continued)*

Category	Possible Abnormal Findings	Possible Causes
Cardiovascular *(cont'd)*	• Pericardial effusion • Heart failure • Pulmonary edema • Distended neck veins • Edema	• Elevation of blood pressure in glomerular capillary circulation has an adverse effect on the progression of renal disease. • Friction rubs may occur with uremia. • Cardiac enlargement may occur from hypertension or increased fluid volume. • Angina may occur from chronic anemia. • Dysrhythmias may occur as a result of imbalances of K, Mg, and Ca. • Heart disease is the leading cause of death in patients with renal failure. • Edema will occur from decreased albumin in the blood.
Respiratory	• Shortness of breath • Tachypnea • Rales • Acid–base disturbances • Kussmaul's respirations	• Shortness of breath, tachypnea, and rales are often a result of fluid volume overload. • Metabolic acidosis occurs early in renal disease.
Hematological	• Anemia • Bruising • Bleeding tendencies • Infections	• Anemia is a result of decreased erythropoietin production in the kidneys. • Red blood cells have a shortened life span.
Gastrointestinal	• Weight loss • Anorexia • Vomiting • Loss of appetite • Constipation • Diarrhea • Malnutrition • Gastroparesis • Metallic taste in the mouth • Foul urine odor to breath • Ascites • Gastritis • Gastrointestinal bleeding	• Metabolic and hormonal changes in renal disease lead to malnutrition and decreased nutrient intake. • Nausea and changes in taste may lead to diminished appetite. • Urea build-up causes metallic taste in the mouth or foul odor of breath. • Malabsorption of calcium from the intestine.
Genitourinary	• Nocturia • Enuresis • Hematuria • Dysuria • Oliguria • Anuria • Polyuria • Interrupted urine stream • Straining • Hesitancy • Frequency • Dribbling • Urgency • Retention • Bladder distention • Incontinence • Stress incontinence • Cloudy urine • Odor to urine • Fever • Chills • Perineal pain	• Kidneys lose concentrating ability that may result in changes in urine volume. • Obstruction of lower urinary tract, failure to concentrate urine, or urinary tract infection. • Blood in the urine may indicate infection, irritation, obstruction, or cancer in the renal system. • Anticoagulation with medications may produce bloody urine. • Dysuria is a sign of urinary tract infection or interstitial cystitis. • Urine output of 100–400 mL in 24 hours. Oliguria is noted in severe dehydration, shock, transfusion reactions, and end-stage renal disease. Less than 100 mL of urine in 24 hours may be seen in acute renal failure, end-stage renal disease, and bilateral ureteral obstruction. • It is normal to void every 3–4 hours in the day, and once at night. • 1000–1500 mL of urine is excreted daily. Polyuria may be noted with diabetes, diabetes insipidus, and chronic renal failure. • Coffee and alcohol may have a diuretic effect. • Urine flow difficulty may be due to prostate problems. • Acutely inflamed bladder, retention with overflow, and excess fluid intake may increase frequency. • Urinary hesitancy may indicate blockage of the prostrate. • Urinary urgency may indicate cystitis. • Urinary retention can lead to renal failure as fluid causes increased pressure in the kidney. • Incontinence may be a sign of urological disorders or neurological disease. • Cloudy, strong-smelling urine may indicate a urinary tract infection. • Urinary tract infections may cause sepsis in the elderly. • Pain may be due to infection, foreign body in urinary tract, urethritis, pyelonephritis, and renal colic or stone.

(Continued on following page)

TABLE 36.2 ASSESSMENT OF THE URINARY SYSTEM *(Continued)*

Objective Assessment *(Continued)*

Category	Possible Abnormal Findings	Possible Causes
Musculoskeletal	• Osteoporosis • Bone and joint problems • Muscle weakness • Gait disturbances • Fractures	• Vitamin D synthesis decreases with the increase of parathyroid hormone causing changes in the calcium phosphorus ratio and hyperparathyroidism. • Osteodystrophy occurs from low calcium levels, high phosphorus levels, and inability to produce vitamin D. • Physical mobility is necessary to move to a toilet in a timely manner.
Endocrine System	• Hyperlipidemia • Hyperglycemia • Anemia • Hypertension	• Renal disease impairs the kidneys' ability to produce erythropoietin which stimulates red blood cell production in the bone marrow. • Renin produced in the kidney activates angiotensin II which is a potent vasoconstrictor that elevates blood pressure.

Lung Sounds

If the patient retains more fluid than the heart can effectively pump, fluid may be retained in the lungs. This is manifested as crackles, which are popping sounds heard on inspiration and sometimes on expiration when the chest is auscultated. Wheezes may also be present. New-onset crackles and wheezes should be reported to a physician (see Chapter 29 for assessment of the respiratory system).

Edema

Fluid retention may be manifested as edema (excess fluid in tissues). The nurse assesses and documents the degree and location of edema (see Chapter 20). Edema may be generalized in renal failure. The nurse also looks for edema in the area around the eyes (periorbital edema).

Daily Weights

Weight is the single best indicator of fluid balance in the body. Patients with renal disease often have fluid imbalances. The patient should be weighed at the same time each day, in the same or similar clothing, and with the same scale. The nurse is careful not just to document the weight, but also to look at trends in weight gain or loss. If the patient's weight is steadily increasing, fluid retention is suspected and should be reported. A patient undergoing diuresis is expected to have decreasing weights.

Intake and Output

All patients with renal disease should have careful measurement of intake and output with each voiding. The nurse measures and records all liquids taken in, including oral, intravenous, irrigation, tube feeding, and other fluids. Output includes urine, emesis, nasogastric effluent, wound drainage if it is copious, and any other drainage. The nurse should also examine the urine for any abnormalities.

Intake and output totals are analyzed and recorded every 8 or 12 hours or more often for unstable patients. As with daily weights, the nurse notes trends in retention or loss of fluid and reports significant changes to the physician. Accurate documentation is vital because the physician may base medication and intravenous fluid orders on intake and output results.

CRITICAL THINKING

Mr. Nolan

■ It is the end of the shift. As you empty Mr. Nolan's indwelling catheter bag, you find that it has only 50 mL of concentrated urine in it. What do you do?

Suggested answers at end of chapter.

DIAGNOSTIC TESTS OF THE RENAL SYSTEM

Laboratory Tests

Urine Tests

URINALYSIS. A urinalysis (urine analysis) is a commonly performed diagnostic test for the renal system. Urinalysis is an invaluable tool in the diagnosis of kidney disease and other systemic diseases that may affect the kidneys. The results of the urinalysis give information regarding kidney function and various body functions. Table 36.3 lists normal and abnormal findings on a urinalysis.

A routine urinalysis specimen may be collected at any time of day; however, the first morning specimen is best. First morning specimens are usually concentrated and more likely to contain abnormal constituents if they are present. The specimen should be examined within 1 hour of urinating. Urine that cannot be examined promptly should be refrigerated. Urine standing at room temperature longer than 2 hours has more bacteria present, changes in pH, and hemolysis of RBCs. Urine collected for cytology should not be a first morning specimen due to changes in epithelial cells in urine held overnight. Random specimens are done for cytology.

To collect a voided specimen for urinalysis, the nurse has the patient wash the perineum using soap and water or a special towelette from a clean-catch midstream urine collection kit. Women should be directed to wash from the front to the back of the perineum. The patient is instructed to begin

TABLE 36.3 URINALYSIS RESULTS

Test	Normal Results	Abnormal Results and Significance
Color of Urine	Pale yellow to amber	Dark-amber urine suggests dehydration. Yellow-brown to green urine indicates excessive bilirubin. Dark, smoky color suggests hematuria. Orange-red or orange-brown caused by phenazopyridine (Pyridium). Cloudiness of freshly voided urine indicates infection. Nearly colorless urine is seen with a large fluid intake, renal disease, or diabetes insipidus.
Odor of Urine	Aromatic	With infection, urine becomes foul smelling. In diabetic ketoacidosis, the urine has a fruity odor. Urine that has been standing for a while develops a strong ammonia smell.
pH	4.6–8.0	The pH is greatly affected by the food eaten. pH below 4.6 is seen with metabolic and respiratory acidosis. pH above 8.0 is seen when urine has been standing or with infection because bacteria decompose urea to form ammonia.
Specific Gravity	1.010–1.025	Low specific gravity indicates excessive fluid intake or diabetes insipidus. High specific gravity is seen with dehydration. A specific gravity fixed at 1.010 indicates kidney dysfunction. The specific gravity of glomerular filtrate is 1.010.
Protein	0–18 mg/dL 0–150 mg/24 hr	Persistent proteinuria is seen with renal disease from damage to the glomerulus. Intermittent protein in the urine can result from strenuous exercise, dehydration, or fever. As a general rule, protein in the urine is a significant sign of renal problems. Vaginal secretions may contaminate urine and give a positive reading.
Glucose	None	Glucose in the urine indicates diabetes mellitus, excessive glucose intake, or low renal threshold for glucose reabsorption.
Ketones	None	Ketones in the urine indicate diabetes mellitus with ketonuria or starvation from breakdown of body fats into ketones. Can also be seen with carbohydrate-free diets, severe diarrhea, dehydration, and vomiting.
Bilirubin	None	Bilirubin in the urine indicates liver disorders causing jaundice. Bilirubin may appear in the urine before jaundice is visible.
Nitrite	Negative	Nitrites in the urine indicate infection. Bacteria in the urine convert nitrate to nitrite, which gives a positive reading.
Leukocyte Esterase	Negative	A positive leukocyte esterase in the urine indicates infection in the urine. It determines the presence of an enzyme released by WBCs in the urine.
Red Blood Cells	0–4/hpf	Blood in the urine may be caused by kidney stones, infection, cancer, renal disease, or trauma.
White Blood Cells	0–5/hpf	WBCs in the urine indicate infection or inflammation in the urinary tract.
Casts	None to occasional hyaline cast	Casts are formed when abnormal urine contents settle into molds of the renal tubules and may be made of protein, WBCs, RBCs, or bacteria. A few hyaline casts may be found in normal urine. The presence of casts generally indicates renal damage or infection.

hpf = high-power field; RBC = red blood cells; WBC = white blood cells.

to void into the toilet, and then move the collection container under the stream, and then finish voiding into the toilet. This is called a clean-catch midstream specimen. It is used to obtain the cleanest possible specimen. Female patients should be told to separate the labia with one hand and keep them separated while washing and collecting the specimen to decrease the risk of contamination of the specimen. If the female patient is menstruating, this should be specified on the laboratory form. A tampon may be used to prevent contamination of the specimen. The uncircumcised male patient should be directed to retract the foreskin with one hand and keep it retracted while cleansing and voiding. At least 10 mL of urine should be collected.

If a urinalysis is ordered for a patient with a urinary catheter, the nurse obtains the urine specimen. This specimen is considered sterile because it is coming directly from the bladder into the urinary catheter tubing. To obtain the specimen, wear clean gloves and use an alcohol swab to clean the sample port on the catheter tubing. Insert a blunt needle of a syringe (usually 10 mL) into the port and withdraw urine from the tubing into the syringe. Then empty the urine from the syringe into a collection container and safely dispose of the syringe.

Composite urine specimens are collected over a period of time that may range from 2 to 24 hours. These specimens are usually used to examine the urine for specific components such as glucose, electrolytes, protein, 17-ketosteroids, catecholamines, creatinine, and minerals. These specimens may need refrigeration or may have preservatives added to the collection container.

The patient is instructed to void and discard this specimen. The time is noted and is the start time of the test. All subsequent voiding is saved in the container for the designated time period. At the end of the time frame, the patient is asked to void and this is added to the container as the last amount to be added. Reminding the patient to save all of the urine is critical for accurate results. Incomplete collections do not result in accurate results.

Renal Function Tests

A number of blood and urine tests reflect kidney function (Table 36.4). If the kidneys are not functioning adequately, these test results will be elevated. These tests are useful because they provide information about the severity of a patient's kidney disease and also the patient's response to any treatments or medications being used. In this way, clinical progress can be monitored. Renal function tests may still be within the normal range until the glomerular filtration rate is less than 50% of normal. The most accurate way to assess kidney function is to use several tests and analyze the results together.

Diagnostic Procedures

Table 36.5 summarizes diagnostic procedures for the urinary system.

Radiological Studies

With all contrast studies, the patient should be questioned for allergies to iodine and contrast media before the test.

LEARNING TIP

A handy approximation to determine kidney function is to equate the creatinine clearance result to percentage of renal function. For example, a creatinine clearance of 100 mL per minute = 100% renal function, 30 mL per minute = 30% renal function, and 5 mL per minute = 5 % renal function.

Contrast media may be **nephrotoxic** and can worsen renal function. The most severe complication in patients who have allergies is an anaphylactic reaction that causes cardiac and respiratory distress or arrest. When contrast media is used, Metformin hydrochloride (Glucophage) must not be given before and 48 hours after administration of contrast media. Severe lactic acidosis as well as renal failure may occur. MRI and nuclear medicine studies have the advantage of not requiring contrast media to be used.

Endoscopic Procedures

Endoscopic procedures examine the inside of hollow organs with an endoscope. The endoscope is a device consisting of a tube and an optical system. The observations can be done through a natural body opening such as the urethra or a small incision through the skin.

Renal Ultrasound

Ultrasonography is a noninvasive study using sound waves passed into the body through a transducer to detect abnormalities. It is commonly used to examine the anatomy of the urinary tract. Ultrasound requires no contrast media and no preparation. There are also no contraindications to ultrasound.

(Text continued on page 769)

TABLE 36.4 DIAGNOSTIC LABORATORY TESTS FOR URINARY SYSTEM

Test Urine Studies	Definition/Normal Value	Significance of Abnormal Findings
Urinalysis	• Used to establish baseline information, confirm or establish a diagnosis, or determine if further testing needs to be done.	• May be used to monitor the progress of an existing condition or plan a program of care.
Urine Culture	• A urine culture is done to determine the number of bacteria present in the urine and to identify the organism causing infection in the urine. • The urine should be collected before antibiotic treatment is begun to avoid affecting results. The midstream clean-catch system is used to obtain voided specimens. • A physician may order a catheterized specimen if there is a risk of contamination from the vagina, if a female patient is menstruating, or if the patient is incontinent.	• Reference value: <10,000 negative 100,000 positive • A bacterial count of 100,000 or more per milliliter of urine indicates a urinary tract infection. • An amount less than 100,000 may result from contamination during specimen collection. • The urine is cultured to grow and identify the kind of bacteria present. Often a sensitivity test is also ordered to determine what kind of antibiotic will be most effective in eradicating the offending bacteria.

Test Urine Studies	Definition/Normal Value	Significance of Abnormal Findings
Urine Concentration Test or Specific Gravity	• This study evaluates the concentration of urine with specific gravity readings.	• Reference value: 1.05–1.35 • A low specific gravity may be noted in patients with diabetes insipidus, glomerulonephritis, and severe renal damage. • A high specific gravity may occur from diabetes mellitus and high sugar concentrations in the urine, nephrosis, congestive heart failure, and dehydration.
Residual Urine	• This study looks at the amount of urine left in the bladder after voiding. • Increased residual volume may be noted with urethral strictures, sphincter impairment, urethral strictures, or neurogenic bladder.	• Reference value: <50 mL (amount increases with age) • The patient is catheterized immediately after voiding. • If a large amount of urine is present, a urinary catheter may be left in place. • Bladder ultrasound equipment may also be used to determine the amount of urine remaining after voiding.
Quantitative Test for Protein	• A 12- or 24-hour collection is obtained. • Persistent proteinuria is usually seen with glomerular renal disease.	• Reference values: <150 mg/24 in 24 hours <0.15 g in 24 hours
Creatinine Clearance	• The creatinine clearance test measures the amount of creatinine cleared from the blood in a specified period by comparing the amount of creatinine in the blood with the amount of creatinine in the urine.	• Reference value: 85–135 mL/min • The creatinine clearance is computed in the laboratory and is expressed in volume of blood that is cleared of creatinine in 1 minute. • A minimum creatinine clearance of 10 mL per minute is needed to live without dialysis. • To carry out the test, urine is collected for a 24-hour period, and a sample for serum creatinine is collected sometime during the 24 hours. • It is an excellent indicator of renal function. The following procedure should be followed: 1. When the test is begun, the patient is directed to void and discard that urine. 2. Urine is collected for 24 hours, keeping the urine in a large container provided by the laboratory. The container is kept on ice. 3. Twenty-four hours after the test was begun, the patient is instructed to void again. This urine is added to the collection container. 4. The laboratory collects a serum creatinine during this 24-hour period.
Urine Cytology	• Microscopic examination of urine to detect atypical epithelial cells shed from the surface of the urinary tract. • Used as a screening for people with high risk for the development of cancer within the urinary system.	• Atypical cells indicate the need for further testing.
Urine Bladder Cancer Markers (Bladder Tumor Antigen) **BTA** **NMP22**	• Bladder tumor antigen is a protein that is produced by bladder tumor cells. • NMP22 is a protein deposited into the urine during nuclear disruption (apoptosis) of bladder cells.	• Reference value: BTA <14 units/mL NMP22 <10 units/mL • No special preparation necessary. • A single voided specimen collected before noon is taken directly to the laboratory.
Blood Chemistry Studies Kidney Function Tests Serum Creatinine	• Creatinine is a waste product from muscle metabolism and is released into the bloodstream at a steady rate. • Creatinine levels are a very good indicator of kidney function.	• Reference values: 0.6–1.5 mg/dL • A serum creatinine level above 1.5 mg/dL means there is kidney dysfunction. The higher the creatinine level, the more impaired the kidney function.

(Continued on following page)

TABLE 36.4 DIAGNOSTIC LABORATORY TESTS FOR URINARY SYSTEM (*Continued*)

Test Urine Studies	Definition/Normal Value	Significance of Abnormal Findings
Cystatin C (Cys C)	• Cystatin C is a proteinase inhibitor. • It is a small molecule that is produced by all cells with chromosomes and genetic material at their center. • It is produced at a constant rate and filtered out of the blood by the glomerulus and reabsorbed by the tubular epithelial cells. • Cystatin C is a sensitive marker that reflects the glomerular filtration rate independent of body weight and height.	• Reference values: 0.53–0.95 mg/dL <0.70 mg/mL or <0.9 μmol/mL young adults <0.85 mg/mL or 3.5 μmol/mL elderly adults • Cystatin C levels increase with impaired renal function.
Blood Urea Nitrogen (BUN)	• Urea is a waste product of protein metabolism. • The blood urea nitrogen is not as sensitive an indicator of kidney function as the creatinine level. • This is because it is readily affected by increased protein intake, dehydration, and other factors in the body.	• Reference value: 8–20 mg/dL • An elevated BUN level can be caused by the following factors: Kidney dysfunction or failure Decreased kidney blood supply, such as when the patient is in a state of shock or in severe heart failure Dehydration, because the loss of water makes the blood more concentrated (decreased BUN level is seen with overhydration) High-protein diet, because urea formation increases Gastrointestinal bleeding, because blood is absorbed as protein and converted into urea Steroid use, because steroids increase the rate of protein breakdown in the body
Uric Acid	• Uric acid is an end product of purine metabolism and the breakdown of body proteins. • Uric acid is not as diagnostic as creatinine because many factors can cause an elevated uric acid level.	• Reference value: 2–7 mg/dL • An elevated uric acid level can be caused by the following: Kidney disease Gout (patients with gout metabolize uric acid abnormally) Malnutrition Leukemia Use of thiazide diuretics (because of impairing uric acid clearance by the kidney)
BUN-to-Creatinine Ratio	• Evaluates hydration status.	• Reference value: About 10:1 • An elevated ratio is seen with hypovolemia. • A normal ratio with an elevated BUN and creatinine is seen with intrinsic renal disease.
Blood Chemistries Electrolytes Sodium (Na$^+$)	• Sodium is an extracellular electrolyte regulating blood volume.	• Reference value: 135–145 mEq/L • Sodium values usually remain within normal ranges until late stages of renal failure.
Potassium (K$^+$)	• Kidneys are responsible for excreting potassium. • In renal disease K$^+$ is one of the first electrolytes to become abnormal.	• Reference value: 3.5–5.5 mEq/L • Elevated levels of K >6 mEq/L can lead to muscle weakness and cardiac arrhythmias.
Calcium (Ca^{2+})	• Calcium is the main mineral in bone and aids in muscle contraction, neurotransmission, and blood clotting. • In renal disease decreased reabsorption of calcium leads to renal osteodystrophy.	• Reference values: 4.5–5.5 mEq/L and 9–11 mg/dL
Phosphorus	• Phosphorus balance is inversely related to calcium balance. • In renal disease phosphorus levels are elevated.	• Reference values: 2.8–4.5 mg/dL and 0.95–1.45 mmol/L
Bicarbonate (HCO$_3^-$)	• Most patients in renal failure have metabolic acidosis and low serum HCO$_3^-$ levels.	• Reference values: 22–28 mEq/L
Magnesium	• Magnesium is found in the bone and intracellularly. • Most of the serum magnesium is excreted by the kidney. • Chronic renal disease causes magnesium elevations.	• Reference value: 1.3–2.1 mEq/L • Symptoms of elevated magnesium levels include lethargy, nausea and vomiting, and slurred speech.
Serum Albumin	• Low levels may be seen with nephrotic syndrome.	Reference value: 3.5–5.0: g/dL

TABLE 36.5 DIAGNOSTIC PROCEDURES FOR URINARY SYSTEM

Procedure	Definition/Normal Finding	Significance of Abnormal Findings	Nursing Management
		Noninvasive	
Renal Ultrasound or Ultrasonography	• High-frequency sound waves are used to image the kidneys, ureter, and bladder. • Structures of the urinary system can be visualized on a screen. • Ultrasound may also be used for mapping of the kidneys before a biopsy is done.	• A renal ultrasound is used to help diagnose congenital disorders of the kidney, renal abscesses, hydronephrosis, kidney stones, or tumors. • The images identify enlargement of the kidneys, and changes of renal structures with chronic infection.	• A transducer is passed over the skin, which has been covered with a conductive gel. • There is no special preparation or aftercare, and there are no known complications. • Because this study does not expose the patient to radiation frequent studies can be done if necessary.
Bladder Ultrasound	• A portable ultrasound instrument is able to compute bladder volume from 12 cross-sectional readings.	• The bladder is scanned for residual urine volume, bladder wall thickness, bladder calculi, tumors, and diverticula.	• Is used to determine postresidual voiding accurately. • May diminish the number of catheterizations for bladder distention.
Kidney-Ureter-Bladder X-ray Study	• A radiological procedure • This test is also known as a flat plate of the abdomen. • This study examines the size, shape, and position of the kidneys, ureters, and bladder.	• May help to discover renal calculi, kidney size, or masses in the kidney.	• No special care is usually necessary. • If done as preliminary study, bowel prep may be done.
Computed Tomographic (CT) Scan	• A radiological procedure • The computer constructs images of the area scanned from a series of tomograms or cross-sectional slices and displays them on a screen. CT scans are able to distinguish subtle differences in the density of tissues. • A CT scan of the abdomen and pelvis may be done to discover tumors, metastatic cancers, renal cysts, or abscesses. • The scan may also be used for tumor staging or identifying masses.	• The kidneys, ureters, bladder, abdominal and pelvic organs can be evaluated for kidney size, tumors, abscesses, malignant masses, metastases, or lymph node enlargement. • Cysts or abscesses can be identified. • Other uses include identification of nonfunctioning kidneys, renal stones, obstructions, and infections.	• The patient is NPO for 4 hours before the procedure. The patient is asked to hold very still during the procedure. • Contrast media may be given. • If contrast media is given, check for allergies to the dye or iodine. • Push fluids post test to remove dye. • Glucophage should not be given before for 48 hours after contrast is given.
Magnetic Resonance Imaging (MRI)	• A radiological procedure • Computer-generated films produced by the interaction of radio waves and magnetic fields. • Is used to visualize the kidneys, bladder, prostate, testes, and retroperitoneum.	• May be used for staging of cancers of the kidney, bladder, and prostate.	• MRI is contraindicated in any patient with metallic objects in the body, surgical clips, or pacemakers. • Patient preparation includes removal of any metal objects, jewelry, or clothing with metal clips. • Patients with a history of claustrophobia may need to be sedated. • Contrast media may be used.
		Invasive	
Intravenous Pyelogram (IVP)	• A radiological procedure • The intravenous **pyelogram** (IVP) is a common test. • X-ray examination that visualizes the renal tissue, calyces, pelvises, ureters, and the bladder after the intravenous injection of contrast media or dye.	• During the test, a radiopaque dye is injected into a large vein. • The dye is cleared from the blood by the kidneys. • Because the x-rays cannot penetrate the dye, the dye outlines the renal structures.	• Assess patient for allergies to iodine or contrast media prior to the test. • The dye can cause allergic and anaphylactic reactions in people who are allergic to these substances, although this problem is less common since the introduction of a newer radiopaque dye.

(Continued on following page)

pyelogram: pyelo—pelvis of the kidney + gram—radiograph

TABLE 36.5 DIAGNOSTIC PROCEDURES FOR URINARY SYSTEM (Continued)

Procedure	Definition/Normal Finding	Significance of Abnormal Findings	Nursing Management
IVP (cont'd)	• Test provides a rough estimate of renal function.	**Invasive** (Continued) • Radiographs are taken at frequent intervals to see the dye filling the renal pelvis and going down the ureters into the bladder (see Fig. 36.4). • The dye outlines the renal system and identifies: Abnormal size or shape of kidneys Absent kidneys Polycystic kidney disease Tumors Hydronephrosis Renovascular hypertension	• NPO for 8 hours prior to test. • Enemas may be given the evening before the test to empty the colon. • The patient should be warned about a warm, flushing sensation up the arm and sometimes all over the body when the dye is injected. A strange taste may occur as well. • Aftercare for an IVP includes having the patient drink large amounts of fluids to help clear the dye from the kidneys. • On rare occasions, people can develop acute renal failure because the dye is highly concentrated and can obstruct the kidney tubules. • Urine output should be monitored after the test. • IVP is not recommended for patients with renal insufficiency or failure.
Renal Angiography or Arteriogram	• A radiological procedure • Purpose is to visualize renal blood vessels. • The femoral artery is pierced with a needle, and a catheter is threaded up through the femoral and iliac arteries into the aorta and then the renal artery. • A contrast agent is injected to make the renal arterial supply visible on x-ray examination. • The test helps the physician see blood flow to the kidneys to determine the cause and treatment of kidney disease.	Is useful if renal insufficiency is caused by renal vascular disease. The test reveals hypervascular tumors, renal cysts, renal artery stenosis, renal artery aneurysms, pyelonephritis, obstructions, renal infarction, and evaluates renal trauma.	• Angiography is done in the x-ray department with the patient awake during the procedure. • Before the procedure check for allergies to iodine or contrast media. • The patient should be NPO for 4 to 8 hours prior to the test. • An enema or cathartic may be given the evening prior to test. • Patient care following angiography includes bedrest for up to 12 hours to prevent bleeding at the injection site. • Check distal pulses in leg every 30–60 minutes after the procedure. • The patient is instructed not to bend the leg, and the head of the bed is not raised more than 45 degrees. • The nurse monitors vital signs, dressing, and pulses in the affected extremity frequently. • Institution policy should be consulted for specific care guidelines. • Complications of the procedure include: Vessel injury, embolus or clot formation, and allergic reactions.

Procedure	Definition/Normal Finding	Significance of Abnormal Findings	Nursing Management
		Invasive (Continued)	
Nephrotomogram	• A radiological procedure using intravenous contrast media. • A series of x-rays taken from different angles to create a three-dimensional image of the kidney.	• Test is useful in the identification of renal cysts, tumors, areas of nonperfusion, and renal fractures or lacerations following renal trauma.	• Prepare patient as for an IVP. • Check for allergies to contrast media and iodine. • Push fluids post test. • Monitor fluid intake and output before and after the test. • Advantages include the ability to determine kidney function without exposure to contrast agents and the ability to obtain quantitative information that may not be obtainable by other procedures.
Renal Scan	• Nuclear scan • Nuclear scans work on the principle that radioactive substances called radioisotopes injected into the bloodstream can be detected by a special camera called a gamma camera similar to an x-ray machine. • A radioactive isotope that is rapidly excreted by the kidneys is injected intravenously. • Radiation detectors (cameras) placed over the kidney monitor the radioactive material in the kidney. • As the isotope passes through the kidney and into the urine the two kidneys "light up."	• Measures kidney function. • Measures renal blood flow, glomerular filtration rate, tubular function, and excretion of urine. • Outlines kidneys size and shape. • Abscesses, cysts, and tumors may appear as cold spots because of the presence of nonfunctioning kidney tissue. • The main use is for the diagnosis of renovascular hypertension. • May also determine vascular supply to the kidneys in patients with renal trauma, dissecting aneurysm, and other disorders affecting blood flow to the kidneys.	• Assesses the kidneys ability to perfuse blood and secrete urine. • No special preparation is usually necessary. • Determine if any medications the patient is taking will interfere with the test such as nonsteroidal anti-inflammatory drugs or antihypertensive medications. • The patient may be asked to drink two glasses of water prior to the test. • The level of radiation is very low and has no side effects. • Pregnant and nursing mothers are advised to be cautious.
Renal Biopsy	• Renal tissue is obtained for laboratory analysis. • **Percutaneous** renal biopsy is done with a needle through the skin. • Open renal biopsy is done through a surgical incision. • A percutaneous biopsy may be done in the operating room, the radiology department, or the patient's room. • A computed tomographic (CT) scan or ultrasound is done first to locate the kidney for biopsy.	• Renal biopsy is indicated when microscopic examination of kidney tissue is needed to diagnose or treat a renal disorder. • The type of renal disease present or the progress of renal disease is determined. • Biopsy is used to diagnose benign and malignant masses, causes of renal failure, renal transplant tissue, or lupus.	• Before the biopsy, the patient is NPO for 6 to 8 hours. • A mild sedative is given. • The patient should not take anticoagulants before the biopsy because of the risk of bleeding. • A complete blood cell count and coagulation studies are performed prior to the biopsy. • The patient is in a prone position, usually with a sandbag under the abdomen, and the biopsy is taken through the flank area. • For a percutaneous biopsy, a local anesthetic is used. • During the test the patient is instructed to take a breath in and hold it while the needle is being inserted. This prevents the kidney from moving. • Following the biopsy, the patient may be kept in a prone position. • Observe closely for bleeding, because the kidney is highly vascular. • A bandage is applied, and the patient is maintained on bedrest for 24 hours or more. • Urine is inspected for blood with each voiding and compared to the previous voidings for 24 hours.

(Continued on following page)

percutaneous: per—through + cutaneous—skin

TABLE 36.5 DIAGNOSTIC PROCEDURES FOR URINARY SYSTEM (*Continued*)

Procedure	Definition/Normal Finding	Significance of Abnormal Findings	Nursing Management
Renal Biopsy (*cont'd*)		Invasive (*Continued*)	• Vital signs are monitored frequently for 24 hours according to agency policy. • Grossly bloody urine, falling blood pressure, and rising pulse are signs of bleeding and are reported immediately. • Fluids are encouraged if not contraindicated. • Complications include gross hematuria, pain, infection, hypotension, pneumothorax, and hemorrhage. • No heavy lifting for 2 weeks when the patient goes home. • Instruct the patient to notify the physician if flank pain, hematuria, lightheadedness, or fainting occurs.

Cystoscopy	• A **cystoscopy** and pyelogram (C&P) is a minor surgical procedure that involves a rigid or fiberoptic instrument (cystoscope) inserted into the bladder through the urethra.
	• A light at the end of the instrument allows a physician to visualize the interior of the bladder.
	• Commonly a pyelogram is done as well. This involves insertion of a ureteral catheter into the pelvis of the kidney.
	• Radiopaque dye is injected through the catheter and radiographs are taken.
	• A C&P is done for both diagnostic and therapeutic reasons.
		• Cystoscopy allows diagnostic inspection of the urinary tract for urinary calculi, infection, vesicoureteral reflux, prostatic obstruction, bladder tumors and urethral strictures.
		• As part of the diagnosis, a physician can do the following:
		  Inspect the inside of the bladder.
		  Collect a urine specimen from either kidney.
		  Visualize the renal structure with x-rays.
		  Biopsy any suspicious growths in the bladder or ureter.
		• Therapeutic interventions that can be done during a C&P include the following:
		  Removal of small bladder tumors
		  Removal of stones from the bladder
		  Removal of stones from the ureters
		  Dilation of the ureters
		• Abnormal findings include enlarged prostate, urethral strictures, tumors, polyps, and congenital abnormalities.
			• The preparation for a C&P is the same as for any surgery.
			• Care following a C&P includes measuring urine to make sure the patient has not developed urinary retention from swelling of the urinary meatus and encouraging fluid intake.
			• The patient should expect some dysuria for 24 hours following a C&P, and the first one or two voidings may be blood tinged.
			• Complications that can result include urinary tract infection, urinary retention, and perforation of the bladder.

Cystogram or Voiding Cystourethrogram	• A cystogram is an x-ray of the bladder and lower urinary tract. • Contrast media or a radioisotope is instilled into the bladder via a catheter or cystoscope.	• The test is done to evaluate the filling and emptying of the bladder. • The purpose is to visualize the bladder and evaluate vesicoureteral reflux. • Incomplete bladder emptying, distention, or reflux is determined. • Obstruction to urine outflow may be determined.	• No medication, fasting, or special diets are necessary. • The patient is prepared accordingly for either catheter or cystoscope insertion. • After the scan there may be slight dysuria and pink urine for 1–2 days. • Bright red urine, fever, or persistent discomfort should be reported to the physician.

cystoscopy: cysto—bladder + scopy—to examine

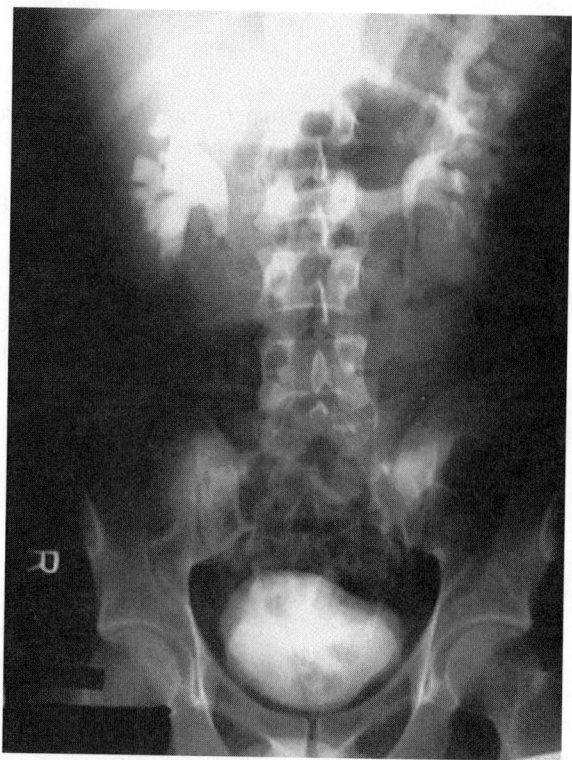

FIGURE 36.4 Intravenous pyelogram x-ray.

Renal Biopsy

A renal biopsy may be done to diagnose or gain more information about kidney disease.

Nursing Process for Diagnostic Tests of the Renal System Assessment

The patient is assessed for baseline understanding of and comfort with testing procedures to plan teaching sessions. Possible contraindications to testing such as renal function and the use of dyes or MRI and metal in the body are assessed and reported.

Nursing Diagnosis, Planning, and Implementation

Anxiety related to unfamiliar environment, procedure, diagnostic test, health status, or severity of disease

EXPECTED OUTCOME: The patient will report increased familiarity or knowledge with the environment, procedure, or diagnostic test prior to the procedure.

- Assess the patient for signs and symptoms of anxiety: verbalization, tenseness, tachycardia, elevated blood pressure, facial pallor, and self-focused behaviors. Anxiety may be manifested by increases in vital signs, pallor, or self-focused behaviors. *A high level of fear may interfere with learning and cooperation.*
- Introduce staff who will be caring for the patient. *Familiarity with staff will decrease anxiety.*
- Orient patient to the environment, equipment, and routines to *decrease anxiety.*
- Include family members or significant others in ori-

entation and teaching sessions *to encourage their support of the patient.*
- Assess the patient's understanding of the procedure *to provide a baseline for teaching.*
- Explain all activities that will take place in the diagnostic area and afterward. *This will reduce fear and promote cooperation during testing.*
- Provide information based on the patient's current needs at the level the patient can understand.
- Reinforce physician's explanations and clarify misconceptions about the diagnostic test or procedure *to help alleviate anxiety.*
- Encourage family members or significant others to provide support to patient without obvious anxiousness. *Anxious family members will convey those feelings to the patient.*
- Identify allergies the patient may have to contrast agents, or drugs prior to diagnostic testing. *This will prevent allergic responses and provide for patient safety.*
- Provide information about injections or invasive procedures that may be done to the patient *to reduce anxiety.*
- Explain any unfamiliar machines or equipment to the patient *to reduce anxiety.*
- Explain that the patient may have to drink increased fluids after the test and that the patient's intake and output will be closely monitored. *Increased fluids help rid the patient of the contrast media after the procedure.*
- Provide information about self-care following the procedure or diagnostic test. *This will facilitate the patient in self-care at home.*

EXPECTED OUTCOME: The patient will experience reduction in anxiety concerning health status or severity of disease.

- Assess the patient for signs and symptoms of anxiety: verbalization, tenseness, tachycardia, elevated blood pressure, facial pallor, and self-focused behaviors. A high level of fear will interfere with teaching and learning as well as diminish cooperation during testing.
- Examine patient's health beliefs. *Health beliefs provide insight to patient behaviors that may affect outcome.*
- Maintain a calm, supportive, and confident manner when interacting with the patient. *This will reduce anxiety.*
- Respond to patient call signals as soon as possible to *reduce anxiety.*
- Acknowledge the patient's anxiety and the perceived threat of the situation to *facilitate communication and trust.*
- Encourage the patient to verbalize feelings or concerns *to provide a baseline of information to develop a teaching plan.*

- Encourage the patient to verbalize specific stressors that may be causing anxiety *to allow individualized care specific to meet patient's needs.*
- Encourage patient to ask questions. *Teaching will be guided by patient-specific needs.*
- Provide the patient with access to timely information regarding the outcome of diagnostic testing *to facilitate trust and promote comfort.*
- Provide consistent reinforcement of information to the patient *to facilitate trust and promote comfort.*
- Reinforce explanations and clarify misconceptions the patient has about diagnostic tests or disease condition *to facilitate trust and promote comfort.*
- Encourage the patient to ask questions concerning self-care and decision making if possible.
- Engage the support of the patient's family throughout diagnostic testing *for patient's coping.*
- Provide a calm environment *to reduce anxiety.*
- Instruct the patient in relaxation techniques and facilitate their use *to reduce anxiety.*

Acute pain related to infection, edema, obstruction, or bleeding along the urinary tract or to invasive diagnostic tests

EXPECTED OUTCOME: Patient will report a decrease in pain and absence of discomfort.

- Assess level of pain, **dysuria**, burning on urination, or abdominal or flank pain *to provide baseline data to evaluate progression of pain and effectiveness of treatment plan.*
- Assess voiding patterns. *Delayed emptying of the bladder or frequent voiding of small amounts or abdominal distention may reflect infection or distention.*
- Evaluate urine for color, odor, consistency, and quantity *to assess for infections or other problems.*
- Encourage fluid intake unless contraindicated *to facilitate dye removal.*
- Provide comfort measures *to relieve pain.*
- Provide analgesics and antispasmodics as prescribed *for pain relief.*
- Report severe pain to the primary care provider. *Severe pain may indicate complications are present or the need for a change in pain control medications.*

Impaired urinary elimination related to complications from diagnostic tests of the urinary system

EXPECTED OUTCOME: The patient will maintain urine output greater than 30 mL per hour in the postprocedure period.

- Encourage fluid intake after renal diagnostic testing *to facilitate dye or contrast removal from the body.*
- Monitor fluid intake and output closely *to ensure adequate renal function.*

- Evaluate urine for color, odor, consistency, and quantity *to assess for complications from diagnostic testing.*
- Observe the patient for hypersensitivity reactions *to contrast media or injectable materials.*
- Assess the patient for pruritus, rashes, breathing difficulties, generalized edema, or urinary retention *to detect possible reaction symptoms.*

Evaluation

If interventions have been effective, the patient will report reduced anxiety, increased understanding of procedure, maintain urine output greater than 30 mL per hour, and decrease in pain.

THERAPEUTIC INTERVENTIONS

Management of Urinary Incontinence

Urinary **incontinence** is defined as the involuntary leakage of urine and is very common. More than 17 million adults have urinary incontinence. The incidence is rising. Incontinence affects approximately 45% of all American women. The highest incidence, 55%, is noted in the 80- to 90-year-old women. An estimated 3.4 million men over the age of 60 are also affected with incontinence. Urinary incontinence is often underdiagnosed because many patients are too embarrassed to talk about the problem.

Most patients do not seek treatment until the problem profoundly affects quality of life. At times, urinary incontinence can be prevented by patient teaching or physician intervention. Incontinence that cannot be prevented is managed by the use of padding and absorptive products worn by the patient. With all kinds of incontinence, it is helpful for the nurse or patient to keep a voiding diary for at least several days to determine when incontinence occurs and to look for any predisposing events. The patient should be referred to a urologist specializing in the area of incontinence for a careful examination to determine the cause and identify potential medical or surgical treatment. Some areas of the country have continence clinics, which can be helpful for patients with this problem. There are several types of incontinence.

Stress Incontinence

Stress incontinence is the involuntary loss of less than 50 mL of urine associated with increasing abdominal pressure during coughing, sneezing, laughing, or other physical activities. Stress incontinence is commonly seen in women following childbirth and after menopause. In men, stress incontinence is associated with prostatectomy and radiation.

Urge Incontinence

Urge incontinence is the involuntary loss of urine associated with an abrupt and strong desire to void. The patient typically complains of being "unable to make it to the bathroom in time." Urge incontinence is the most common type of urinary incontinence in older adults. Patients with stress incon-

---

dysuria: dys—difficult or painful + uria—urination

Box 36.2

Patient Education for Kegel Exercises

The purpose of Kegel exercises is to decrease the incidence of incontinence by strengthening the pubococcygeal muscle, which supports the pelvic organs. By increasing the tone of this muscle, the patient has an increased ability to tighten the muscle that encircles the urinary meatus and stop the flow of urine. This exercise can also help prevent uterine prolapse, enhance sensation during sexual intercourse, and hasten postpartum healing. It may be used by the elderly male patient to control dribbling.

1. Establish awareness of pelvic muscle function by instructing the patient to "pull in" the muscles in the perineum as if to control urination or defecation. The muscles of the buttocks, inner thigh, and abdomen are not used to do Kegel exercises.
2. To help identify the correct muscles to tighten, ask the patient to tighten the muscles that control urination. It can be helpful to use an analogy of an elevator: start squeezing at the bottom floor and then squeeze upward to the top floor.
3. Instruct the patient to tighten the pelvic muscles for 10 seconds, followed by at least 10 seconds of relaxation.
4. Advise the patient to perform these exercises 30 to 80 times per day. Help the patient determine cues to remind the patient to perform the exercises, such as stopping the stream of urine 10 times each time the patient urinates.

Source: Adapted from Urinary Incontinence in Adults: Clinical Practice Guideline. Agency for Health Care Policy and Research, Public Health Service, US Department of Health and Human Services (AHCPR Pub No 92-0038), Rockville, MD, 1992.

tinence or urge incontinence can be taught Kegel exercises to increase perineal muscle tone. Box 36.2 Patient Education for Kegel Exercises explains how to teach patients to perform them.

Functional Incontinence   confusion

Functional incontinence is the inability to reach the toilet because of environmental barriers, physical limitations, loss of memory, or disorientation. People with functional incontinence are often dependent on others and have no other urinary problems. This is a common cause of incontinence in the elderly who are institutionalized.

Overflow Incontinence

Overflow incontinence is the involuntary loss of urine associated with overdistention of the bladder. It occurs with acute or chronic urinary distention with dribbling of urine. The bladder is unable to empty normally despite frequent urine loss. Spinal cord injuries or an enlarged prostate may cause this type of incontinence.

Total Incontinence

Total incontinence is a continuous and unpredictable loss of urine. It usually results from surgery, trauma, or a malformation of the ureter. Bladder training has been tried and proven ineffective. Often the patient with total incontinence is neurologically impaired. In these situations, the nurse's priority is to keep the patient clean and dry using absorptive products. For the male patient, an external condom catheter can be effective in some situations. *Sometimes clamping catheter*

NURSING PROCESS FOR THE PATIENT WITH STRESS OR URGE INCONTINENCE. The medical diagnoses of stress and urge incontinence are also nursing diagnoses. Many nursing interventions can be helpful to decrease these kinds of incontinence. See Box 36.3 Nursing Care Plan for the Patient with Stress Incontinence or Urge Incontinence and Box 36.4 Nursing Care Plan for the Patient with Functional Incontinence.

Management of Urine Retention

Urinary retention is the inability to empty the bladder completely during attempts to void. Urine retention can be caused by many factors. It can be acute, with a sudden onset of retention and no urine output, or chronic, with a slower onset of retention of urine and some urine being expelled. Acute retention often results from surgery and is caused by anesthesia, medications, or local trauma to the urinary structures. Acute retention can be a medical emergency causing extreme pain, a large bladder, and the possibility of bladder rupture or acute renal failure. Chronic urine retention may be related to an enlarged prostate gland, diabetes, pregnancy, a medication effect, strictures, or other causes of obstruction of the urinary tract.

To assess for urinary retention, urine output is determined and the lower abdomen is palpated. Symptoms noted may include urinary frequency and absent or decreased urine output. An enlarged bladder can be palpated, and the dull percussion notes may extend up to and beyond the umbilicus.

A bladder scan assesses the volume of urine in the bladder (Fig 36.5). Sound waves estimate the amount of urine in the bladder. It is painless, noninvasive, and requires no patient preparation. The nurse performs this scan at the bedside. It helps guide the need for catheterization, thereby reducing unnecessary catheterizations and associated risks. The bladder scan may be used instead of catheterization (the gold standard for determining urine retention) after the patient urinates to determine the amount of urine remaining in the bladder. Normally the bladder contains less than 50 mL after urination. A residual volume of 150 to 200 mL of urine indicates the need for treatment for urinary retention. Bladder scanning may also be used as a tool for incontinent patients to plan their care.

Urinary Catheters

Indwelling Catheters

Indwelling urinary catheters (Foley catheters) may be inserted into hospitalized patients for various justifiable

Box 36.3   NURSING CARE PLAN for the Patient with Stress Incontinence or Urge Incontinence

Nursing Diagnosis: Stress incontinence or urge incontinence related to decreased tone of perineal muscles

Expected Outcomes Patient will be continent of urine. Patient will state three actions that can be taken to decrease incidence of stress or urge incontinence.

Evaluation of Outcomes Is the patient continent? Is the patient able to state three actions that can be taken to decrease the incidence of stress or urge incontinence?

Interventions	Rationale	Evaluation
	Stress Incontinence or Urge Incontinence	
Ask about the history of incontinence; have patient keep a voiding journal.	A journal helps identify the severity and timing of incontinence.	Does patient complete the voiding journal?
Instruct patient on how to perform Kegel exercises (see Box 36.2).	Kegel exercises increase perineal muscle tone and help prevent incontinence.	Does patient explain how to perform Kegel exercises?
Work with the patient to incorporate Kegel exercises into normal activities of daily living (e.g., do 10 pelvic muscle contractions during each voiding).	An excellent time to perform Kegel exercises is when voiding because the correct muscles are used.	Does patient perform Kegel exercises when voiding or at other cued times during the day?
Encourage patient to drink at least 2000 mL of fluid per day, preferably 3000 mL per day unless medical reason for fluid restriction.	Concentrated urine is irritating to the urinary tract and can increase the incidence of urge incontinence and dribbling.	Is urine dilute?
Encourage patient to avoid alcohol and caffeine.	Alcohol serves as a diuretic, and caffeine is irritating to the urinary tract.	Does patient explain the need to avoid alcohol and fluids containing caffeine?
Discuss use of and provide small adhesive peripads to wear in underclothing.	Peripads provide protection in case of incontinence.	Does patient have and use peripads if desired?
Refer patient to a continence clinic or to a physician specializing in incontinence.	Specialists in the area of incontinence can use medical or surgical interventions to decrease the incidence of incontinence.	Does patient know resources available to further assist with treatment of incontinence?
Refer patient to supportive and educational groups such as Help for Incontinent People (HIP).	Support groups can help patients deal with the embarrassment of incontinence and learn methods and resources to prevent incontinence.	Does patient know the names and addresses of support groups to help with incontinence?
	Urge Incontinence	
Teach patient to void at frequent intervals (every 2 hours), then gradually increase length of time between voidings.	By emptying the bladder at frequent intervals, the incidence of urge incontinence can be decreased.	Does patient follow a frequent voiding schedule?
Teach urge inhibition techniques (distraction), such as counting back from 100 by sevens and relaxation breathing.	These distraction techniques can help patients reach the bathroom in time to prevent incontinence.	Do distraction techniques help patient prevent incontinence?

Box 36.4   NURSING CARE PLAN for the Patient with Functional Incontinence

Nursing Diagnosis: Functional urinary incontinence related to interference with rapid voiding

Expected Outcomes Patient will be continent of urine. Patient will state three measures to increase continence.

Evaluation of Outcomes Is the patient continent of urine? Is the patient able to state three measures to increase continence?

Interventions	Rationale	Evaluation
Ask about the history of incontinence. Keep a voiding log of when patient is incontinent.	A voiding log helps demonstrate when incontinence is most likely to occur and can help determine the cause of incontinence.	Does the patient cooperate so that a voiding log can be kept?
Determine any acute causes of incontinence, including new onset of urinary tract infection, constipation or impaction, medication effect, or poor fluid intake.	These may be readily treatable causes of incontinence.	Does the patient have any easily treatable causes of incontinence?
Determine if clothing is inhibiting timely voiding. If necessary, Velcro fasteners can be appropriate, or sweat shirts and sweat pants.	Clothing can be difficult to remove for the elderly, resulting in voiding before the clothing can be removed. Clothing can be modified so that it comes off quickly.	Does the patient have easy-to-remove clothing?
Determine if there are any obstacles to reaching appropriate urine receptacle, such as poor lighting, busy bathroom, lack of assistive devices.	Obstacles can make it impossible for the patient to reach the voiding receptacle in time to prevent incontinence.	Does the patient have ready access to a voiding receptacle?
Provide appropriate urinary receptacles, such as a three-in-one commode, female or male urinal, or no-spill urinal.	Assistive devices can be helpful for the patient to increase continence.	Does the patient need and have access to an appropriate assistive device?
Initiate a voiding schedule of every 2 hours, or base schedule on voiding log. Always assist patient to the toilet when patient first awakens and before sleep. Use prompted voiding techniques: check patient regularly, provide positive reinforcement if dry, prompt patient to toilet, praise patient after toileting, return patient to toilet in a specified time.	Frequent scheduled voiding using prompting techniques can increase continence.	Does the patient receive help to do bladder training with prompted voiding?
Teach patient to set up schedule of voiding using environmental cues such as meals, bedtime, and television shows.	Environmental cues help the patient remember when it is time to void.	Can the patient indicate cues throughout the day that prompt voiding?

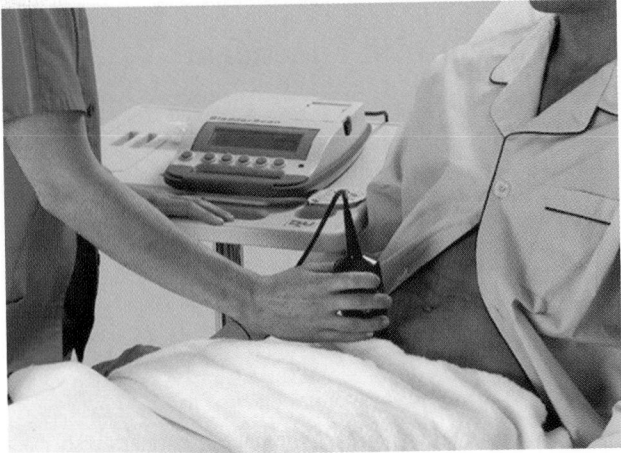

FIGURE 36.5 A bladder scan can be used to determine the volume of urine in a patient's bladder.

reasons, such as shock, heart failure, or urinary tract obstruction. As a general rule, catheters should be avoided if possible because of the high risk of urinary tract infections. Urinary incontinence is not justification for insertion of a catheter. Urinary catheters result in infection of the urinary tract in up to 44% of patients within 72 hours of catheterization, and up to 90% of patients who have indwelling catheters for 17 days develop significant bacterial infection.[1]

Bacteria enter the bladder mainly in one of two ways with an indwelling catheter: (1) through the outlet at the end of the drainage bag contaminating the urine, which is then inadvertently drained back into the bladder; or (2) around the catheter up the urethra and into the bladder. Routine perineal care during the daily bath is sufficient to minimize infection from an indwelling urinary catheter. It has been demonstrated that the incidence of infection is decreased when intermittent straight catheterization is used instead of indwelling urinary catheters. Box 36.5 Guidelines for Care of the Patient with an Indwelling Catheter outlines steps that should be followed to decrease infection in the patient with a catheter (see Home Health Hints).

After an uncircumcised male is catheterized, it is essential that the foreskin is properly positioned over the glans penis and not left retracted to prevent injury. If left retracted, subsequent swelling may make it impossible to pull the foreskin over the glans penis later. This can then cause ischemia of the glans penis, which is an emergency. A physician must be notified immediately and may need to perform an emergency circumcision if the foreskin cannot be properly positioned. Always make sure that the foreskin is positioned properly following catheterization or perineal care.

Intermittent Catheterization

For the patient who is unable to void, the best intervention is intermittent catheterization. A postoperative patient or a patient with a neurological disorder or urine retention may benefit from intermittent catheterization. It reduces the risk of infection as long as the bladder is not allowed to overfill.

Box 36.5

Guidelines for Care of the Patient with an Indwelling Catheter

1. Maintain a closed system. Do not separate the catheter from the tubing of the bag. Instead, collect specimens and irrigate through the sample port in the tubing.
2. Keep the catheter securely taped or fastened to the leg. This decreases traction on the catheter with back-and-forth movement of the catheter that can help bacteria enter the bladder.
3. Encourage fluids to internally irrigate the catheter, if fluids are not contraindicated because of heart or kidney disease.
4. Use good aseptic technique when emptying the drainage bag by hand washing, wearing clean gloves, and using a container designated for that patient only to collect the urine.
5. Wash the perineum with soap and water at least once a day, and again if there is any bowel incontinence.
6. Keep the tubing coiled on the bed and positioned to allow free flow of urine. Keep the catheter bag below the level of the bladder at all times.
7. Do not clamp catheters. Clamping a catheter results in obstruction, which increases infection. Periodic clamping has not been found to be effective in bladder retraining.
8. Remove indwelling catheters as soon as possible.

A full bladder stretches the muscle fibers, which in turn reduces circulation to the bladder and increases the risk of infection.

Intermittent catheterization involves the use of a straight plastic or rubber catheter that is inserted into the urethra every 3 hours or more to empty the bladder. Once the bladder is empty, the catheter is removed. Patients may be taught to do intermittent self-catheterization (ISC) at home. Patients doing ISC may be taught to wash and reuse the same catheter repeatedly when they are in their own environment. In the hospital, however, sterile technique is used.

Suprapubic Catheter

After some surgeries of the urinary tract and in some long-term situations, a suprapubic catheter may be used. This is an indwelling catheter that is inserted through an incision in the lower abdomen directly into the bladder.

Nursing care of a suprapubic catheter involves keeping the area clean and dry, changing the dressing when the site is new, and keeping the catheter taped to prevent tension. A skin barrier such as Stomahesive may help protect the skin from urine leakage. All other care is the same as for any indwelling catheter.

Home Health Hints

- The home health nurse should always have a sterile specimen container. This provides a quick way to get a specimen to the physician's office without the nurse having to obtain the container, saving time and money.
- When catheters plug and irrigation fails, families can be taught to take the catheter out. A syringe for removing water from the balloon should be left in the home for this purpose. The family is instructed to avoid cutting the valve stem. The family should contact the nurse to reinsert the catheter, but in the meantime, the patient's bed or chair can be padded with towels or diapers. Garbage or dry cleaners' bags can be used to line the mattress. The family must be instructed to notify the nurse immediately if the catheter is plugged or has been removed.
- Not all homes have adequate lighting, which is a must

for inserting a catheter. If lighting is inadequate, a caregiver can be asked to hold a flashlight while the nurse inserts the catheter. The nurse should always have a flashlight with him or her. Having two catheters and catheter trays is also wise in case of a defect or contamination.
- Urinary bags can be used safely for up to 4 weeks. Instruct the patient or family to cleanse the bag daily with a 1:10 bleach solution to decrease bacteria.[2]
- To encourage fluid intake, the patient should keep a large container of water (1 to 2 quarts) next to the place the patient sits most of the day. The goal is to drink 2 quarts of water by the end of the day, unless contraindicated by other medical problems. This also simplifies measuring intake. A sports bottle helps to keep water at hand while moving about the home.

Resources

- http://www.kidney.org/
- http://www.niddk.nih.gov/
- http://www.kidneyurology.org/
- http://www.optn.org/
- http://www.nephron.com/virtual.html

REVIEW QUESTIONS

1. A home health nurse visits a patient who is 82 years old, uses a cane, and is not incontinent. Which of the following interventions should be included in the plan of care, based on an understanding of normal age-related changes of the urinary system, to promote patient safety?
   a. Encourage fluids after 6 p.m.
   b. Limit fluids to 1000 mL per day.
   c. Provide a nightlight in the bathroom.
   d. Provide adult briefs to prevent dribbling.

2. Which of the following is the most accurate assessment of fluid balance in the patient with renal failure?
   a. Voiding pattern
   b. Daily weight
   c. Laboratory studies
   d. Skin turgor

3. Which of the following should be included in patient teaching for collecting a midstream urine specimen for culture and sensitivity?
   a. A second voided specimen is preferred.
   b. A 24-hour urine specimen is needed.
   c. As soon as the urine starts to flow, it should be collected in a sterile container.

   d. Women should keep the labia separated while voiding.

Multiple response item. Select all that apply.
4. Which of the following care should the nurse provide following an intravenous pyelogram test?
   a. Maintain NPO
   b. Encourage fluids
   c. Check gag reflex
   d. Measure urine output
   e. Position patient prone
   f. Maintain bedrest for 24 hours

5. A patient is experiencing stress incontinence with frequent involuntary loss of urine. Which of the following directions would be most appropriate when teaching the patient how to perform Kegel exercises?
   a. "Tighten your rectum at frequent intervals throughout the day."
   b. "Keep your abdominal muscles tightened; do this every time you stand up."
   c. "Do at least 20 sit-ups per day."
   d. "When urinating, stop and start the stream of urine by tightening the perineal muscles."

6. Which of the following is the most important nursing action for the nurse to take to prevent urinary tract infection in the catheterized patient?
   a. Force fluids to 4000 mL every 24 hours.
   b. Empty the Foley bag every 4 hours around the clock.
   c. Maintain a closed catheter system.
   d. Wash the perineum every 8 hours.

7. What is the patient's total output for the past 8 hours?
   8 a.m. voided 165 mL
   11:30 a.m. voided 450 mL
   1 p.m. emesis 42 mL
   3 p.m. voided 255 mL
   _____ mL

References

1. Crow, R, Chapman, R, Roe B, et al: Study of Patients with an Indwelling Urinary Catheter and Related Nursing Practice. Nursing Practice Research Unit, University of Surrey, Guildford, UK, 1986.

2. Madigan, E, andNeff, D: (2003) Care of patients with long-term indwelling urinary catheters. Online Journal of Issues in Nursing 8. Retrieved from http://nursingworld.org/ojin/hirsh/topic2/tpc2_1.htm

SUGGESTED ANSWERS TO

CRITICAL THINKING

■ *Mr. Nolan*

You should realize that 50 mL of concentrated urine for 8 to 12 hours is not normal. Further investigation is necessary to determine the cause and seriousness of the problem. Some items to assess follow.

1. Consider Mr. Nolan's diagnosis. Is he in renal failure? Is he severely dehydrated and retaining water?
2. Ask if anyone emptied Mr. Nolan's bag earlier in the shift.
3. Look at the trends in Mr. Nolan's intake and output record. Has his output been decreasing? Is this a change?
4. Has Mr. Nolan been taking in enough fluids?
5. Look at trends in daily weights. Is Mr. Nolan's weight increasing? Is this an expected finding?
6. Listen to Mr. Nolan's lung sounds. Check for edema. Do findings indicate fluid retention?
7. Palpate Mr. Nolan's bladder. Is it distended? Maybe the catheter is blocked.
8. If a problem is identified, the physician should be contacted.

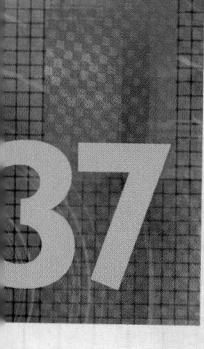

37

Nursing Care of Patients with Disorders of the Urinary System

MAUREEN McDONALD

KEY TERMS

anuria (an-YOO-ree-ah)
azotemia (AY-zoh-TEE-me-ah)
calculi (KAL-kyoo-lye)
cystitis (sis-TIGH-tis)
glomerulonephritis (gloh-MER-yoo-loh-ne-FRY-tis)
hemodialysis (HEE-moh-dye-AL-i-sis)
hydronephrosis (HIGH-droh-ne-FROH-sis)
nephrectomy (ne-FREK-tuh-mee)
nephrolithotomy (NEFF-roh-li-THOT-uh-mee)
nephropathy (ne-FROP-uh-thee)
nephrosclerosis (NEFF-roh-skle-ROH-sis)
nephrostomy (ne-FRAHS-toh-mee)
nephrotoxin (NEFF-roh-TOK-sin)
oliguria (AH-li-GYOO-ree-ah)
peritoneal dialysis (PER-i-toh-NEE-uhl dye-AL-i-sis)
polyuria (PAH-lee-YOOR-ee-ah)
pyelonephritis (PYE-e-loh-ne-FRY-tis)
stent (STENT)
uremia (yoo-REE-mee-ah)
urethritis (YOO-ree-THRIGH-tis)
urethroplasty (yoo-REE-throh-PLAS-tee)
urosepsis (yoo-roh-SEP-sis)

QUESTIONS TO GUIDE YOUR READING

1. What are the predisposing causes, symptoms, laboratory abnormalities, and treatment of urinary tract infections?

2. What are the predisposing causes, symptoms, treatment, and teaching for kidney stones?

3. What are symptoms of cancer of the bladder and cancer of the kidneys?

4. How do you provide care for a patient with an ileal conduit or continent reservoir?

5. How would you explain the pathophysiology associated with diabetic nephropathy, nephrosclerosis, hydronephrosis, and glomerulonephritis?

6. What is the nursing care for patients with diabetic nephropathy, nephrosclerosis, hydronephrosis, and glomerulonephritis?

7. What is the difference between acute renal failure and chronic renal failure?

8. What are common symptoms experienced by the patient in renal failure?

9. What nursing care should be given to patients in renal failure and with a hemodialysis blood access site?

10. How does hemodialysis and peritoneal dialysis work to replace the function of the kidney?

Disorders of the urinary tract include a variety of problems involving the kidneys, ureters, bladder, and urethra. These problems may arise from infection, obstructions, cancer, hereditary disorders, and metabolic, traumatic, or chronic diseases. Some may lead to renal failure if not treated or controlled. Infection may be found in three different anatomical parts of the urinary tract: the urethra, resulting in **urethritis;** the bladder, with a diagnosis of **cystitis;** or the kidneys, with a diagnosis of **pyelonephritis.**

URINARY TRACT INFECTIONS

Urinary tract infection (UTI), a general term, refers to invasion of the urinary tract by bacteria. Normally, the urinary tract is sterile above the urethra. Urinary tract infection is the second most common bacterial disease. More than 100,000 people are hospitalized because of urinary tract infections. In the hospital, urinary tract infections are the most common nosocomial infections. Urinary tract infections are described by their location in the urinary tract. Lower urinary tract infections include urethritis, prostatitis, and cystitis. Upper urinary tract infections include pyelonephritis and ureteritis. Infections may result in chronic renal failure, sepsis, or damage to the kidney.

Predisposing Factors for Urinary Tract Infections

Urinary tract infections are almost always caused by an ascending infection, starting at the external urinary meatus and progressing toward the bladder and kidneys. The majority of UTIs are caused by the bacterium *Escherichia coli,* which is commonly found in stool. Predisposing factors for UTIs include the following:

- Stasis of urine in the bladder can be caused from obstruction such as a clamped catheter or simply from not voiding frequently enough. Urine overdistends the bladder, decreasing the blood supply to the wall of the bladder, which keeps white blood cells (WBCs) from fighting contamination that may have entered the bladder. The standing urine then serves as a culture medium for bacterial growth. Incomplete emptying of the bladder prevents flushing out of the bacteria and allows bacteria to ascend to higher structures.
- Contamination in the perineal and urethral areas can be from fecal soiling, from sexual intercourse in which bacteria are massaged into the urinary meatus, or from infection in the area, such as vaginitis, epididymitis, or prostatitis.
- Instrumentation, or having instruments or tubes inserted into the urinary meatus. The most common

---

urethritis: urethr—urethra (canal that discharges urine from bladder) + itis—inflammation

cystitis: cyst—closed sac containing fluid + itis—inflammation

pyelonephritis: pyelo—pelvis + nephr—kidney + itis—inflammation

cause is urinary catheterization. Bacteria ascend around or within the catheter, causing infection. Within 48 hours of catheter insertion, bacterial colonization begins. Many patients develop a UTI within 2 weeks of placement of an indwelling catheter.

- Reflux of urine from the urethra to the bladder or the bladder to the ureter because of faulty valves to maintain one-way flow. Reflux can be congenital, or it may be acquired as a result of previous infections.
- Previous UTIs are thought to provide a reservoir of persistent bacteria that causes reinfection.
- Women are more susceptible than men due to the short length of the female urethra and close proximity to anus and vagina. Pregnant women may have asymptomatic bacteruria. Untreated, 40% to 50% will develop pyelonephritis. Pregnant women may be prone to infection with group B streptococci. Most commonly, infection occurs in the second and third trimesters.

Older adults have an increased incidence of UTIs due to diminished immune response, diabetes, and neurogenic bladder. Aging increases the risk of lower UTIs and may also mask the symptoms. UTI is the most common cause of acute bacterial sepsis in the patient over 65 years of age. Older men are predisposed to infection because an enlarged prostate causes obstruction of urine flow. In older women, the decline in estrogen can contribute to the risk of UTI.

Signs and Symptoms

UTIs are characterized by common symptoms of dysuria, urgency, frequency, incontinence, nocturia, hematuria, back pain, and cloudy, foul-smelling urine (Box 37.1 Urinary Tract Infections Summary). In the elderly, the most common presenting symptom of UTI is generalized fatigue. The elderly may experience atypical symptoms or present with a change in cognitive functioning, especially noted in patients without dementia. A decline in mental status and fever in any patient with an indwelling catheter meets the diagnostic criteria for a UTI.

Types

Urethritis

Urethritis is inflammation of the urethra that may be due to a chemical irritant, bacterial infection, trauma, or exposure to a sexually transmitted disease. Posttraumatic urethritis can occur with intermittent catheterization or instrumentation of the urethra. Bubble bath and bath salts are common urethral irritants and should not be used by anyone with a history of UTIs. Urethritis can also be caused by spermicidal agents. Gonorrhea and chlamydiosis are sexually transmitted diseases that can cause urethritis in men. It is common to have some degree of urethritis in association with bladder or prostatic infections.

Symptoms of urethritis include urinary frequency, urgency, and dysuria. The male patient may have discharge

Box 37.1

Urinary Tract Infections Summary

Urethritis, Cystitis, Pyelonephritis

Signs and Symptoms	Urinary urgency, frequency, dysuria Flank pain, fever, chills, costovertebral tenderness Cloudy urine with casts, bacteria, and WBCs Urine is positive for nitrites
Diagnostic Tests	Urinalysis culture greater than 100,000 bacteria Elevated WBCs Elevated sedimentation rate Increased neutrophils
Therapeutic Interventions	Antibiotic therapy sensitive to organism cultured from urine
Complications	Pyelonephritis Urosepsis Renal failure
Possible Nursing Diagnosis	Pain Impaired urinary elimination: frequency Ineffective health maintenance

from the penis. A urinalysis or urine culture is done to diagnose urethritis.

The treatment of urethritis is removal of the cause if the cause is a chemical irritant. If urethritis is caused by bacteria, an antibiotic is prescribed based on the results of a culture. Possible organisms include gram-negative rods, gram-positive cocci, and *Chlamydia*. Phenazopyridine (Pyridium), a urinary analgesic, is often used to treat dysuria. The patient should be forewarned that their urine will turn orange while on phenazopyridine. If urethritis is sexually transmitted, it is important that the sexual partner also be treated.

Cystitis

Cystitis is inflammation and infection of the bladder wall. It can be caused by bacteria, viruses, fungi, or parasites. Fungal infections can occur during long-term antibiotic therapy. About 90% of UTIs are caused by *Escherichia coli*. In most cases, the causative organisms first grow in the perineal area and then ascend into the bladder. Catheters are the most common predisposing factor for UTIs in the hospital setting.

Symptoms include dysuria, frequency, urgency, and cloudy urine. Cystitis infection acquired outside the hospital is diagnosed with a routine urinalysis collected as a clean-catch midstream specimen. Changes seen in the urinalysis include cloudy urine and the presence of WBCs, bacteria, and sometimes red blood cells (RBCs) in the specimen.

Nitrites are usually positive. Some laboratories also examine for leukocyte esterase, which is positive if infection is present in the urine. In complicated UTIs, such as one acquired in the hospital or a repeat infection, a urine culture and sensitivity should be done. Hospital-acquired UTIs are often caused by bacteria that are resistant to the usual antibiotics used for UTIs. A sensitivity test can identify which antibiotics will be effective against the offending organism.

The treatment of uncomplicated cystitis is most often a combination of sulfa medication, such as sulfamethoxazole and trimethoprim (Bactrim, Septra). Complicated cystitis is often treated with ciprofloxacin (Cipro). Other antibiotics may be prescribed depending on the results of the urine culture and sensitivity. Estrogen used as an intravaginal cream may prevent recurrent UTIs in postmenopausal women. The patient is told to finish all prescribed medications, force fluids unless contraindicated, and return for a follow-up urinalysis or culture after the antibiotic course is complete to ensure that the infection is gone.

Pyelonephritis

PATHOPHYSIOLOGY. Pyelonephritis is infection of the renal pelvis, tubules, and interstitial tissue of one or both kidneys. Pyelonephritis usually begins with colonization and infection of the lower urinary tract by means of the ascending urethral route. A preexisting condition is usually present such as obstruction, strictures, stones, or vesicoureteral reflux. Risk factors include urological surgery, lymphatic infection, urinary stasis, and decreased immunity. Acute pyelonephritis begins in the renal medulla and spreads to the adjacent cortex. Pathophysiology includes formation of small abscesses throughout the kidney and gross enlargement of the kidney. On occasion, kidney infection is caused by bacteria spreading from a distant site through the bloodstream and entering the kidney through the glomerulus. Urosepsis is a systemic infection arising from a source within the urinary system. Prompt diagnosis and treatment is essential to prevent septic shock and death. Urosepsis can occur in the elderly or persons susceptible to infection.

SIGNS AND SYMPTOMS. Symptoms include fatigue, urgency, frequency, dysuria, flank pain, fever, and chills. Costovertebral tenderness on the right or left side (tenderness posteriorly at angle where rib and vertebrae join when struck gently with heel of examiner's closed fist) is noted which is associated with renal disease. The urine is cloudy with increased WBCs, bacteria, casts, RBCs, and positive nitrites. In contrast to cystitis, the patient with pyelonephritis is much sicker and shows signs of systemic disease. In acutely ill patients, blood cultures may be obtained.

DIAGNOSTIC TESTS. Several tests are helpful to differentiate pyelonephritis from cystitis. With kidney infection, the urinalysis will show casts. Casts are microscopic particles formed in the kidney from abnormal constituents in the urine such as WBCs, RBCs, or pus. The urine specimen will have greater than 100,000 colonies of bacteria per

5,000~10,080

milliliter. The presence of casts always indicates a problem in the kidneys. The complete blood cell count (CBC) will show an elevated WBC count. There will also be an increase in sedimentation rate.   *inflammation*

THERAPEUTIC INTERVENTIONS. Treatment of pyelonephritis includes antibiotics based on the results of the culture and sensitivity (Table 37.1). With severe gram-negative infections, the patient is hospitalized for intravenous (IV) antibiotics. The patient with acute pyelonephritis generally heals completely after treatment and has no lasting

kidney damage. Men who have recurrent UTIs require a 6-week regimen of antibiotic therapy.

COMPLICATIONS. Repeated kidney infections can result in scarring and loss of kidney function, leading to renal failure. Septicemia may occur from bacteria invading the bloodstream. When septicemia results from a urinary cause, it is called **urosepsis.** In the elderly, urosepsis can be the cause of new-onset confusion. The elderly or immuno-

---

urosepsis: uro—urine + sepsis—infection in the blood

TABLE 37.1 MEDICATIONS FOR URINARY TRACT INFECTIONS

Medication/Classification	Action	Route	Side Effects	Nursing Considerations
Cinoxacin (Cinobac) Urinary antiseptic	Antibacterial action in the urine, not systemic. Effective against *E. coli, Klebsiella,* and other gram-negative organisms.	PO	Monitor for photosensitivity, GI upset, and rash	Avoid sunlight, push fluids, may discolor urine.
Methenamine (Mandelamine)* Urinary antiseptic, anti-infective	Effective against gram-negative and gram-positive the organism *E. coli.*	PO	Nausea, vomiting, rash	Do not use with sulfa drugs because it may cause crystalluria.
Trimethoprim-sulfamethoxazole (Bactrim, Septra) Sulfonamides*	Effective against *E. coli* and *Pseudomonas.* Used for uncomplicated UTIs.	PO	Monitor for photosensitivity, GI upset, hemolytic anemia, and rash. Severe hypersensitivity* erythema multiforme or exfoliative dermatitis, sometimes called Stephens-Johnson syndrome.	Requires alkaline urine for best effectiveness. Give with large amounts of water. Contraindicated in severe renal or liver disease.
Sulfisoxazole (Gantrisin) Sulfonamide		PO	Same as above	Requires alkaline urine for best effectiveness. Give with large amounts of water. Contraindicated in severe renal or liver disease.
Ciprofloxacin (Cipro) Fluoroquinolone	Antibacterial action against *Pseudomonas* and other enterobacteria. May be given IV.	PO IV	GI upset, dry mouth, oral and vaginal fungal infections	Avoid aluminum antacids, which may hinder absorption. Avoid in pregnancy. Give with large amounts of water.
Aztreonam (Azactam) Antibiotic	Antibacterial action against *E. coli, Klebsiella, Serratia.*	PO	GI upset	Contraindicated in patients allergic to penicillins and cephalosporins or if creatinine clearance is less than 30 mL/min. Check BUN and creatinine prior to administration.
Phenazopyridine (Pyridium)* Urinary analgesic	Topical analgesic. Relieves pain urgency and frequency associated with UTI.	PO	GI upset, rash, and blue to purple skin discoloration. Nephrotoxic and hepatotoxic.	Urine color changes to red orange.* Avoid in renal insufficiency. Changes urine glucose testing.

drink lots of fluid

compromised patient may develop septic shock from infection in the urinary tract that has invaded the bloodstream, which may result in death.

Nursing Process for the Patient with a Urinary Tract Infection

Assessment/Data Collection

It is important to listen to the patient's concerns about the diagnosis. The patient is asked about pain on urination, flank pain, or general symptoms of infection such as fever, chills, and malaise. The patient's usual pattern of voiding is assessed. Urinary frequency, burning, or pain on urination is noted. Assess the patient for pain in the lower abdomen, flank, or costovertebral angle. The presence of a catheter, recent instrumentation, surgery, or other predisposing factor is determined. The urine is examined for volume, color, concentration, cloudiness, blood, or foul odor. Urinalysis and culture results are examined.

Nursing Diagnosis, Planning, and Implementation

Acute pain related to inflammation of the urethra, bladder, and other urinary structures

EXPECTED OUTCOME: The patient will report relief of pain and discomfort.

- Encourage fluids 2 to 3 L per day *to flush bacteria from urinary tract and* promote renal blood flow.
- Give antimicrobial therapy as ordered *to relieve pain and discomfort from inflammation and infection.*
- Teach patient to finish all prescribed medications *to prevent recurrent infection.*
- Give antispasmodic agents as ordered *to relieve bladder irritability and pain.*
- Administer antipyretics *to relieve fever, pain, and discomfort.*
- Encourage voiding every 3 hours *to empty the bladder and lower bacterial counts, reduce stasis, and prevent reinfection.*
- Teach to avoid cola, coffee, tea, alcohol *as they are urinary irritants.*
- Suggest cranberry juice or vitamin C 500 to 1000 mg per day *to acidify the urine to reduce bacterial growth.*
- Apply heat to suprapubic area *to relieve discomfort.*
- Empty bladder as soon as urge is felt and after sexual intercourse *to flush bacteria out of the body.*
- Avoid substances such as bubble bath and scented toilet paper, which can be irritating.
- Teach to practice good perineal hygiene, and to wipe front to back.
- Teach to wear cotton underwear *to reduce perineal moisture.*

Impaired urinary elimination: frequency, nocturia, dysuria, and incontinence

EXPECTED OUTCOME: Patient will return to previous voiding patterns.

- Monitor urinary elimination including frequency, consistency, volume, and color *to identify signs and symptoms.*
- Administer antimicrobial drugs as ordered *to eliminate symptoms exhibited by microbial growth.*
- Teach patient signs and symptoms of UTI *to monitor effectiveness of treatment and recognize symptoms of recurrence.*
- Encourage adequate fluids *to prevent infection and dehydration.*
- Women should be encouraged to void after sexual intercourse *to flush bacteria out of the urethra.*

Risk for injury related to sepsis, renal failure, kidney injury

EXPECTED OUTCOME: The patient will be free from injury due to sepsis, renal failure, or recurrent infection.

- Administer antimicrobial drugs as prescribed *to prevent recurrent infection or complications from occurring.*
- Teach symptoms of UTI *to monitor symptoms of recurrence or complications.*
- Monitor the patient for signs of bacteriuria and bacteremia such as fever, chills, recurrent pain.
- Explain need for follow-up urine culture and imaging studies *when indicated by recurrent symptoms.*
- Monitor intake and output *to ensure adequate intake and normal output.*
- Teach need for adequate fluid intake *to prevent dehydration and renal impairment.*

Evaluation

The outcomes have been met if the patient verbalizes relief of pain and discomfort, returns to previous voiding patterns, and is free from injury related to sepsis, renal failure, or recurrent infection.

CRITICAL THINKING

Mrs. Milan

■ Mrs. Milan is a 25-year-old woman who recently spent a 3-day weekend getaway with her husband. On Monday she notices that she has symptoms of dysuria, frequency, and urgency. She visits her family practitioner and is diagnosed with a UTI. She is placed on an antibiotic.

1. What do you think could have predisposed Mrs. Milan to developing a UTI?
2. What should Mrs. Milan be taught to prevent further occurrences of a UTI?
3. What urinalysis findings would you expect for Mrs. Milan?
4. What should you include in her teaching plan based on her therapeutic regimen?

Suggested answers at end of chapter.

Patient Education

It is very important that patients be advised to take all of the prescribed antibiotic until it is gone. Commonly, patients take medication for several days until they no longer have symptoms and then stop. Stopping the antibiotic too early allows the infection to continue. It may become chronic and resistant to antibiotics as a result.

Patients who have one UTI commonly develop repeat infections. It is important that they receive health teaching to prevent repeated infections of the urinary tract (Box 37.2 Patient Teaching to Prevent Urinary Tract Infection and Box 37.3 Nutrition Notes).

 UROLOGICAL OBSTRUCTIONS

Obstruction of urine flow in the urinary tract is always a significant problem. Urinary tract obstruction is an interference with the flow of urine at any location along the urinary system. The obstruction of urine flow causes dilation and thinning of the renal tubules with eventual atrophy of renal tissues. When urine does not drain normally from the kidney, local compensation occurs initially. The area decompensates and damage occurs moving the pressure along the continuum of the renal system. The resulting backup of urine and pressure causes dilation and thinning of renal tissue. Renal blood flow is compromised. Eventually renal tissue is destroyed by the compression. The causes of urological obstructions include strictures, stones, and tumors.

Box 37.2

Patient Teaching to Prevent Urinary Tract Infection

1. Void frequently—at least every 3 hours while awake.
2. Drink up to 3000 mL of fluid a day if there are no fluid restrictions from the physician. Preferably drink water.
3. Drink one glass of cranberry juice (10 oz) per day.
4. Take showers; avoid tub baths.
5. Wipe perineum from the front to the back after toileting.
6. Urinate after sexual intercourse.
7. Avoid bubble bath and bath salts, perfumed feminine hygiene products, synthetic underwear, and constricting clothing such as tight jeans.
8. Take prescribed medication for UTIs until it is all gone.
9. If UTI is associated with another source of infection such as vaginitis or prostatitis, ensure that both infections are treated.

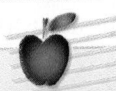 **Box 37.3**

Nutrition Notes

Urinary Tract Infections

An effective intervention for urinary tract infections is increasing fluid intake both for its flushing effect and to excrete urinary drugs. Instructions to increase fluid intake should specify amounts to consume or amount of urine resulting. Patients have developed electrolyte imbalances by overenthusiastically forcing fluids.

Verifying anecdotal evidence of the effect of cranberry juice in preventing urinary tract infections, certain compounds have been identified in cranberries that prevent *E. coli* from adhering to cells in the urinary tract. Cranberry juice has been useful in preventing urinary tract infections and daily intake of 8 to 16 oz of cranberry juice (at least 30% concentration) is recommended for patients with indwelling catheters to prevent UTI.

Urethral Strictures

A urethral stricture is a narrowing of the lumen of the urethra caused by scar tissue. Urethral strictures are becoming more prevalent due to the rising incidence of sexually transmissible diseases. Increasingly in young adults, gonococcal and chlamydial infections may result in urethral strictures. Most strictures are acquired from injury or infection. Strictures from urethral injury tend to be localized to the area where the injury occurred. Some strictures are a result of trauma from insertion of catheters or surgical instruments. Strictures may also be caused by trauma from straddle injuries, a result of direct application of force to the perineal area, as well as untreated gonorrhea and congenital abnormalities.

The patient with a urethral stricture has a diminished urinary stream and is prone to develop UTIs because of obstruction of urine flow. Urethral strictures are often seen in elderly men. The problem becomes more apparent when attempts to insert a urinary catheter are unsuccessful because of the narrowed lumen.

Initially the treatment of a urethral stricture is mechanical dilation by a urologist, who inserts instruments to stretch open the urethra and then inserts a urinary catheter. If the stricture continues to be a problem after dilation, the area can be surgically repaired (**urethroplasty**).

The dilation process is often done at the bedside when the patient is awake. This is a painful experience for the patient, and it is helpful and caring to encourage the urologist to order pain medication before the procedure. The nursing diagnosis of acute pain is very relevant. An indwelling catheter is generally inserted after the dilation, so the nursing diagnosis of risk for infection is also present. Patients need teaching about how to prevent UTIs (see Box 37.2 Patient Teaching to Prevent Urinary Tract Infection).

---

urethroplasty: urethro—urethra + plasty—surgical repair

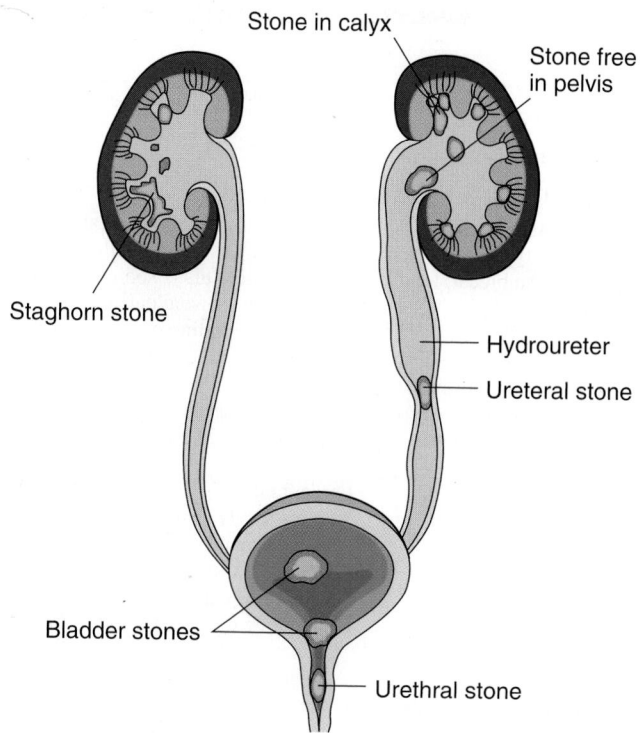

FIGURE 37.1 Location of calculi in the urinary tract.

Renal Calculi

Renal **calculi** (kidney stones; one stone is a calculus) are hard, generally small stones that form somewhere in the renal structures. The stones are masses of crystals and protein that form when the urine becomes supersaturated with a salt capable of forming solid crystals. Symptoms occur when the stones become impacted in the urinary tract. When stones are found in the kidneys, the condition is called nephrolithiasis (Fig. 37.1).

Pathophysiology

Normally, the dissolved substances in urine, including urinary salts, are diluted and readily excreted from the body. Calculi are formed when urinary salts are concentrated enough to settle out; there is often a nucleus around which the salts collect and deposit. Substances that can serve as a nucleus include pus, blood, dead tissue, a catheter, and crystals. Stones usually grow on the papillae or in the renal tubules, calyces, or renal pelvis. Stones may also form in the ureter or bladder. Stones less than 5 mm are readily passed in the urine. The following are common urinary salts that make up renal calculi, which are arranged in order of frequency:

1. Calcium oxalate
2. Calcium phosphate
3. Magnesium ammonia
4. Uric acid
5. Cystine

The majority of renal calculi contain calcium, either in the form of calcium oxalate or calcium phosphate, but it is also possible to have combination stones (Table 37.2).

Etiology

Causes of calculi formation include a family history of stones, chronic dehydration (causing more concentrated urinary salts), and infection, because the latter provides a nucleus for stone formation (Table 37.3). Additional causes of calcium stones include dietary factors (Box 37.4 Nutrition Notes). Excessive amounts of calcium in the water in some geographical areas may also be a factor. Immobility causes stone formation because of the resulting urinary stasis; in addition, calcium leaves the unstressed bones during immobility, so more calcium is in the blood, which is then filtered through the kidneys. Stones are more common in men than women. The risk peaks between the ages of 30 and 50.

Signs and Symptoms

Symptoms of renal calculi include excruciating flank pain and renal colic; when the stone is lodged in the ureter, it is common to have pain radiate down to the genitalia. The pain results when the stone prevents urine from draining. Additional symptoms include hematuria from irritation by the stone, dysuria, frequency, urgency, and enuresis. The patient may also have costovertebral tenderness. Some patients develop nausea, vomiting, and diarrhea because of the proximity of the gastrointestinal structures (Box 37.5 Renal Calculi Summary).

Diagnostic Tests

The diagnosis of renal calculi may be made initially by doing a kidney-ureter-bladder (KUB; flat plate of the abdomen) examination or an intravenous pyelogram. Both of these tests will identify the anatomical location of the stone. Renal ultrasound may be done to identify a stone in the renal pelvis, calyx, or ureter. Urinalysis may indicate gross or microscopic hematuria and could indicate abrasion of the urinary tract. The presence of crystals or urinary pH may indicate calculus type.

Therapeutic Interventions

Renal calculi are treated medically if possible. Most stones are flushed out of the body during urination. Patients can pass stones in the urine if they are 5 mm or smaller; larger stones do not pass. If patients experience severe renal colic, they are admitted to the hospital. Intravenous fluids are administered to hydrate the patient and help flush the stone out of the body. All urine is strained to detect passage of stones, and pain medication such as morphine is given. If the patient is unable to pass the stone and infection, impaired renal function, or severe pain continues, intervention is needed. The solubility of stone-forming substances can be changed by altering the pH of the urine. Calcium stones may be treated with thiazide diuretics and allopurinol (Alloprim, Zyloprim). Surgical removal may be required for large stones, obstructions, or intractable pain.

LITHOTRIPSY. Lithotripsy therapy is the use of sound, laser, or dry shock-wave energies to break the stone into small fragments. The stones can then be removed or urinated out. Forms of lithotripsy include extracorporeal shock-wave lithotripsy (ESWL), electrohydraulic lithotripsy, laser

TABLE 37.2 OVERVIEW OF RENAL CALCULI

Type of Stone	Features	Possible Causes	Interventions
Calcium oxalate, calcium phosphate, or mixture	Accounts for two-thirds of stones Small, rough, and hard Shaped like needles Colors vary from gray to white	Excessive calcium Excessive urea Hyperparathyroidism, Cushing disease, immobility, osteolysis from tumors of the breast, lung	Force fluids Restrict protein and sodium in the diet Administer hydrochlorothiazide Treat hyperparathyroidism (Calcibind) cellulose sodium phosphate may prevent calcium stones by binding calcium from food in the GI system
Struvite—magnesium ammonium phosphate	Second most common type of stone Calculi crumble easily Stones have a yellow color	Infection by urea splitting microbes, usually *Proteus.* May cause abscess formation in the kidney.	Force fluids Decrease urine pH Administer antibiotics
Uric acid stones	Dye enhancement needed for x-ray visualization Small Color varies from yellow to red Hard	Gout High uric acid levels Decreased fluid intake	Force fluids Administer sodium citrate to alkalinize urine Administer allopurinol to reduce urinary uric acid levels Low-purine diet. Avoid shellfish, anchovies, asparagus, organ meats, and mushrooms.
Cystine stones	Small, smooth calculi Smooth, waxy stones	Cystine-containing crystals appear in the urine	Force fluids Low-protein diet, urine is alkalinized Penicillamine given to decrease amount of cystine in urine
Triamterene	Type of stone recently identified	Triamterene ingestion	Withhold triamterene (Dyrenium) from at-risk patients.

lithotripsy, and percutaneous ultrasonic lithotripsy. With ESWL, the patient is immersed in a tub of water and ultrasonic shock waves are used to break up the stone into sand particles (Fig. 37.2), which are then urinated out. The patient is anesthetized for the procedure. Some of the newer lithotripters do not require submersion and use other means of initiating shock waves. After the procedure, the patient is usually discharged home after being told to increase fluid intake to help flush the sand particles out and to notify the urologist if there are any problems. Blood in the urine is common after lithotripsy. The patient is told to strain all urine to identify passage of stone fragments. Occasionally, a stent is put in place to facilitate the passage of the stone fragments.

SURGERY FOR RENAL CALCULI. For some patients, surgery may be necessary. The surgical procedure depends on the location of the stone. With any of these surgical procedures, postprocedure bleeding is a concern. Endoscopic procedures or open surgery can be used. Endoscopic procedures for the bladder include a cystoscopy for small stones and a cystolitholapaxy for larger stones. For cystolitholapaxy, an instrument is inserted through the urethra to the bladder to crush the stone; the stone is then washed out with an irrigating solution. If the stone is lodged in a ureter, the urologist may insert an instrument into the ureter through a cystoscope to crush the stone or use an ultrasonic lithotripsy instrument to break the stone into fragments. Postoperative care following these procedures is similar to care following any cystoscopy (see Chapter 36). The open surgery procedure for stones in the bladder is a cystotomy and for the ureter is a ureterolithotomy.

TABLE 37.3 MEDICATIONS AFFECTING STONE FORMATION

Acetazolamide (Diamox)	Decreases urinary citrates and increases uric acid concentration in urine.
Adrenocorticosteroids	Increases urinary calcium.
Allopurinol	Used to prevent uric acid calculi. May cause the rarer xanthine calculi.
Antacids such as magnesium trisilicate (Gaviscon)	May cause rare silicon based calculi. Phosphate finding nonabsorbable antacids can increase urinary calcium.
Aspirin	Increases urinary uric acid levels in patients with hyperuricemia.
Chemotherapeutic agents and external radiation	May cause cellular breakdown and cause acute hyperuricemia.
Hydrochlorothiazide (used to prevent calcium calculi)	May cause uric acid calculi by increasing urinary uric acid levels.
Furosemide (Lasix)	May cause hyperuricemia.
Vitamin C in large doses	Increases oxalate excretion in urine.
Vitamin D	Increases calcium and oxalate excretion in urine.

Box 37.4

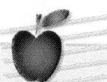

Nutrition Notes

Renal Calculi

Concentrated urine enhances the formation of crystals so sufficient fluid should be consumed to produce 2000 mL of urine per day. About 3000 mL or 13 cups of water per day are necessary to produce this amount of urine.

Approximately 80% of kidney stones are composed of calcium oxalate, which led to early prescriptions for low-calcium diets, but it was later found that a high-calcium intake binds dietary oxalate in the gastrointestinal tract and prevents its absorption, thereby reducing urinary oxalate formation. If a low-oxalate diet is prescribed, foods such as beets, rhubarb, spinach, cocoa, and instant coffee may be restricted.

Uric acid kidney stones can be a complication of gout, which is a disorder of purine metabolism. Purines are endproducts of digestion of certain proteins and are present in some medications. High-purine foods include organ meats, anchovies, herring, sardines in oil, meat extracts, consommé, and gravies. Low-purine foods include fruits, milk, cheese, eggs, refined grains, sugars, coffee, tea, carbonated beverages, tapioca, yeast, and vegetables (except asparagus, beans, cauliflower, mushrooms, peas, and spinach).

For kidney stones, a percutaneous **nephrolithotomy** is performed, in which a scope is inserted through the skin into the kidney to aid in breaking up the stone and to irrigate the renal pelvis. Often a nephrostomy tube is left in place at first to prevent the stone fragments from passing through the urinary system. If the stone is very large, it may be necessary to do a nephrolithotomy, which is a surgical incision into the kidney to remove the stone. A pyelolithotomy is done to remove stones lodged in the renal pelvis.

Prevention of Renal Calculi

The patient may be advised to avoid foods that increase the risk of recurrent calculus development. Box 37.4 (Nutrition Notes) discusses foods that may contribute to calculi (see also Box 37.6 Cultural Considerations). Encourage fluid intake to prevent dehydration. Consult with the physician and dietitian to determine which foods should be avoided, depending on the type of stone found. Encourage the patient to walk, which promotes the excretion of stones and reduces bone calcium resorption (release).

Complications of Renal Calculi

The presence of renal calculi increases the risk for UTIs because of obstruction of the free flow of urine. Untreated obstruction of a stone in a ureter or the urethra can also

Box 37.5

Renal Calculi Summary

Signs and Symptoms	Costrovertebral angle pain Groin pain Renal colic Flank pain radiating to genitalia Hematuria Anuria Restlessness Pallor Temperature Diminished or absent bowel sounds with ileus
Diagnostic Tests	Urinalysis Crystals and urine pH 24-hour renal creatinine clearance BUN Creatinine KUB—reveals most calculi Retrograde pyelography Ultrasound
Therapeutic Interventions	Treat pain to prevent shock Chemolysis—stone dissolution using infusions of chemicals to dissolve stone Surgery—lithotripsy Nephrolithotomy Pyelolithotomy Percutaneous nephrostomy tube
Complications	Shock Sepsis Hydronephrosis Hydroureter Renal failure
Possible Nursing Diagnosis	Acute pain related to calculi Risk for infection related to obstructed urinary flow and instrumentation Deficient knowledge related to lack of knowledge about renal calculi

result in retention of urine and damage to the kidney. This process is called **hydronephrosis** (discussed later).

Nursing Process for the Patient with Renal Calculi

ASSESSMENT/DATA COLLECTION. Patients with stones are often in extreme pain and should be monitored routinely

---

nephrolithotomy: nephro—kidney + lith—stone + otomy—incision

hydronephrosis: hydro—pertaining to water + nephrosis—degenerative change in kidney

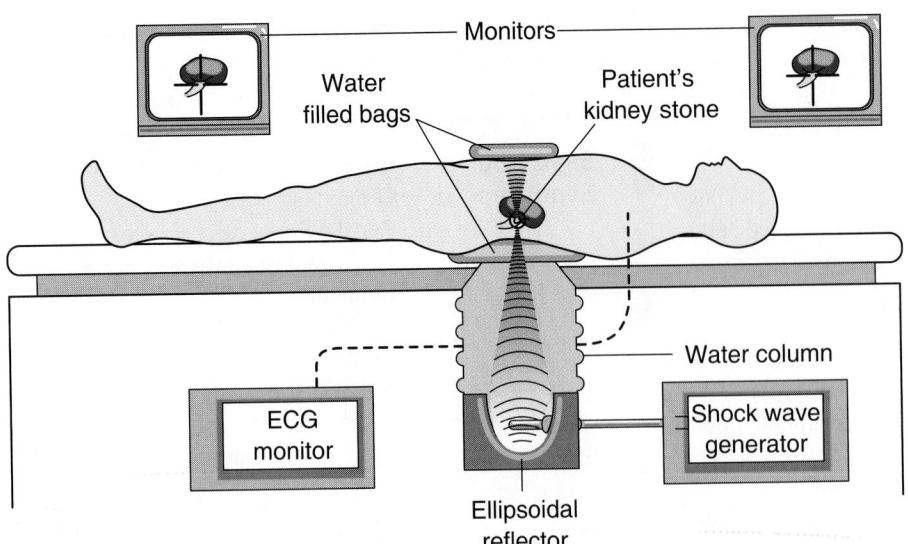

FIGURE 37.2 Extracorpeal shock-wave lithotripsy.

for pain. A health history may identify a family history or patient history of previous stone formation. People who have had stones usually have a recurrence. Also, patients over 60 years of age should be ruled out for abdominal aneurysms. Renal colic usually begins suddenly, progresses rapidly, and peaks over a 30-minute period. Flank pain may radiate to the genitalia. Diminished or absent bowel sounds may progress to an ileus. The patient may also be restless, pale, and lightheaded. Nursing care of a patient with a renal calculus always involves careful measurement of intake and output and observation of the urine for abnormalities such as hematuria, pyuria, or passage of a stone. Obstruction may occur at the bladder neck or urethra. With obstruction, **anuria** or **oliguria** is noted. This is an emergency and must be treated immediately to preserve kidney function. Temperature is monitored for onset of fever, which would indicate infection. Blood pressure may decrease if severe pain causes shock. A special strainer is used to strain all urine for stones. If a stone is found, it is saved for analysis in the laboratory. The patient is also asked about a recent history of infection, dietary or activity changes, or other risk factors for renal

---

anuria: an—without + uria—urine
oliguria: olig—small + uria—urine

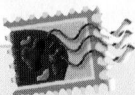

Box 37.6

Cultural Considerations

Recurrent Calculus Development

Filipino immigrants are at high risk for developing renal stones, hyperuricemia, and gout. A shift from a traditional Filipino diet to a U.S. diet increases the occurrence of hyperuricemia, with some older Filipinos developing gout. The nurse may need to assist Filipino patients to identify food choices that will help prevent these conditions.

---

calculi. If the cause can be identified, teaching can be done to help prevent recurrent calculi.

NURSING DIAGNOSIS, PLANNING, AND IMPLEMENTATION. Acute pain related to the presence of, obstruction, or movement of a stone within the urinary system

EXPECTED OUTCOME: *Patient verbalizes the relief of pain or ability to tolerate pain.*

- Ask severity, location, and duration of pain using pain scale. *Pain is typically in the flank or costovertebral angle and may radiate to the pelvic, groin, or abdominal area.*
- Monitor patency of drains, and catheters in preoperative and postoperative patients. *Obstruction of urine flow will increase and intensify pain.*
- Encourage fluid intake unless contraindicated *to promote the passage of stone, dilute the urine, and reduce the risk of further stone formation.*
- Administer pain medication as ordered *to promote comfort.*
- Apply heat to flank area *to reduce pain and promote comfort.*
- Monitor vital signs and blood pressure; observe for bleeding in preoperative and postoperative patients. *Abnormalities may indicate an infection.*
- Strain urine through gauze or strainer *to identify any stones that may have been passed.*
- Monitor urine amount, color, clarity, and odor *to ensure patency of urinary system or tubes. Foul smelling or cloudy urine may indicate an infection.*
- Ambulate if possible *to facilitate the passage of the stone through the urinary system.*

Risk for infection related to the introduction of bacteria from obstructed urinary flow and instrumentation

EXPECTED OUTCOME: *Patient will remain infection free.*
- Monitor urine amount, color, clarity, and odor *to*

ensure patency of urinary system or tubes. Foul smelling or cloudy urine may indicate an infection.

- Assess for elevation in temperature, chills, cloudy, foul-smelling urine *as indicators of infection.*
- Encourage fluids *to flush bacteria and stones, and prevent further stone formation.*

Deficient knowledge related to lack of knowledge about prevention of recurrence, diet, and symptoms of renal calculi

EXPECTED OUTCOME: Patient will verbalize an understanding of the factors related to the recurrence of renal calculi, infection, and treatment options.

- Monitor for recurrence of renal stones. *Recurrence may indicate knowledge deficit.*
- Note family history of renal stones. *Stones have a higher incidence in patients with a positive family history.*
- Determine the relationship between activity and stones. *Sedentary lifestyle or limited mobility may increase risk of stone formation.*
- Ask the patient's understanding of possible courses of therapy to treat renal stones.
- Teach the patient the importance of maintaining a fluid balance of 3000 mL per day. *Low-solute urine prevents stasis and stone formation.*
- Teach patient about medications used to prevent recurrence of renal stones.
  - *Diuretic agents (thiazide type) increase tubular reabsorption of calcium, making it less available for calculi formation in the urinary tract.*
  - *Allopurinol (Zyloprim) reduces uric acid production.*
  - *Antibiotics are used to prevent chronic urinary tract infections which may precede renal calculus formation.*

- As applicable, teach patient about management of stones. *Most stones pass spontaneously. There may be pain, nausea, and vomiting. Management consists of fluids, pain management, and antibiotics. Mechanical interventions with percutaneous catheters and nephroscopic procedures or surgery can be used to eliminate stones.*
- Teach patient to strain all urine. *Stone fragments may continue to pass for weeks after stone crushing or lithotripsy.*
- Teach patient to report signs of infection, pain not relieved by medication, nausea, chills, or the appearance of foul-smelling urine *for treatment.*

EVALUATION. Outcomes have been achieved if the patient remains comfortable, free from infection, and gains understanding about prevention of the reoccurrence of renal stones.

Hydronephrosis *not on test*

Hydronephrosis is a condition that results from untreated obstruction in the urinary tract. The kidney enlarges as urine collects in the pelvis and kidney tissue. It is usually treatable once the condition is detected. The obstruction of urine flow can be from a stricture in a ureter or the urethra, from kidney stones, from a tumor, or from an enlarged prostate. Because of the unrelieved obstruction, urine backs up and distends the ureters and then progresses to the kidney (Fig. 37.3). The capacity of the renal pelvis is normally 5 to 8 mL. Obstruction in the pelvis quickly distends the renal pelvis. Kidney pressure increases as the volume of urine increases. This enlargement of the kidney can be either unilateral or bilateral. The unrelieved pressure on the kidneys from the urine causes the kidneys to become sacs filled with urine instead of functioning kidneys. Sometimes, in a matter of hours, the blood vessels and renal tubules can be damaged extensively.

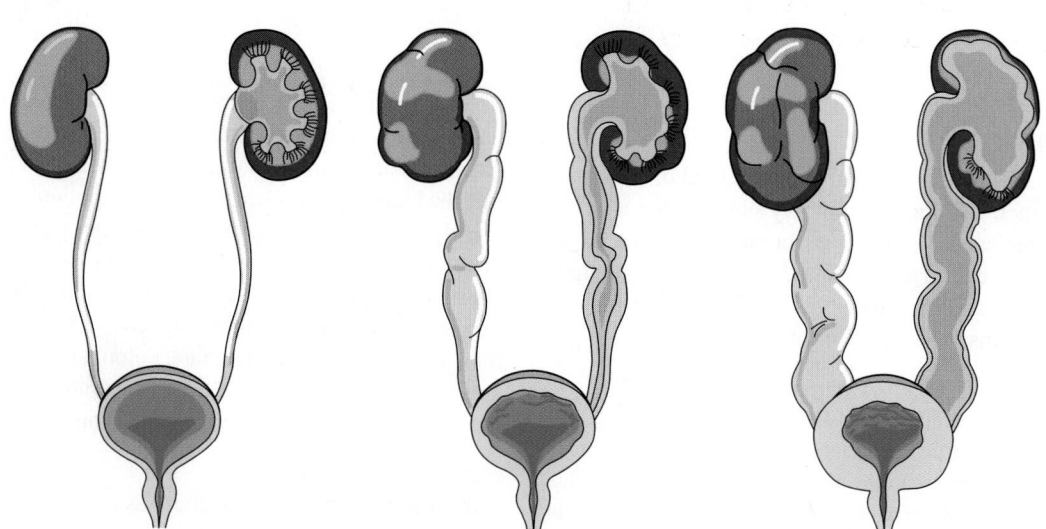

FIGURE 37.3 Hydronephrosis. Progressive thickening of bladder wall and dilation of ureters and kidneys results from obstruction of urine flow.

If the onset of obstruction is gradual, the patient initially may be asymptomatic. Patients often develop UTIs because of the obstruction of urine flow and may have symptoms of frequency, urgency, and dysuria. As the disease progresses, flank and back pain may occur. Eventually the patient develops symptoms of renal failure (discussed later).

The treatment of hydronephrosis always involves relieving the obstruction. Initial removal of the obstruction may be done by insertion of an indwelling urinary catheter. Long-term correction of the obstruction depends on the cause and includes treatments and surgeries to relieve obstruction from strictures, stones, tumor, or an enlarged prostate. At times, the obstruction cannot be relieved because a stone is too large or removal of tumor growth would result in death of the patient. In these situations, **stents**, which are tiny tubes, may be placed inside the ureters during a cystoscopy and pyelogram (C&P) to hold them open or a **nephrostomy** tube may be inserted directly into the kidney pelvis to drain urine. A nephrostomy tube exits through an incision in the flank area and allows urine to drain into a collecting bag, so that function of the kidney can be maintained. Figure 37.4 shows a stent in place in a ureter and a nephrostomy tube.

Complications associated with hydronephrosis include increased incidence of UTIs because of obstruction of urine flow and kidney failure from unrelieved pressure on the kidneys.

Intake and output are carefully measured. Urine retention can worsen the condition and must be recognized and reported promptly. If the patient has a nephrostomy tube, ensure that it is draining adequately and prevent kinking or clamping of the tube. Kinking of the tube results in continuation of the hydronephrosis, and the resulting pressure will destroy kidney function. If both a nephrostomy tube and urinary catheter are present, output from each should be measured and documented separately.

TUMORS OF THE RENAL SYSTEM

Cancer of the Bladder

Cancer of the bladder is the most common kind of cancer of the urinary tract. It is more commonly seen in men ages 50 to 70. Bladder cancer is twice as common in men as in women. Bladder cancer is rare in men and women younger than 40 years of age. It is more common in whites than in African Americans.

Etiology

There is a strong correlation between cigarette smoking and bladder cancer. Specific chemicals that cause bladder cancer have been found in cigarette smoke. The more cigarettes smoked, the greater the risk. The lung absorbs the chemicals

nephrostomy: nephr—pertaining to the kidney + ostomy—surgically formed artificial opening to the outside

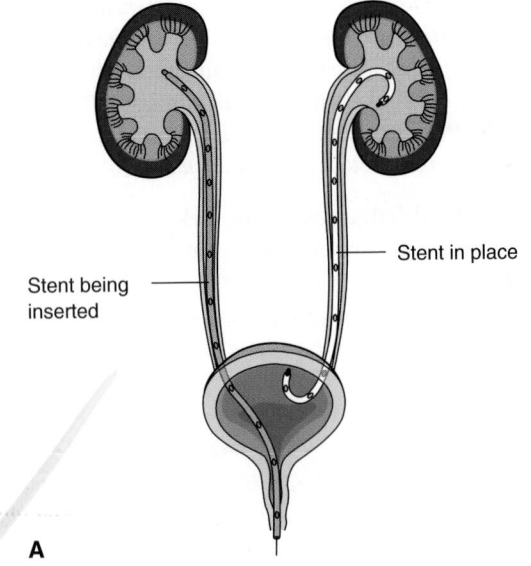

Stent being inserted

Stent in place

A

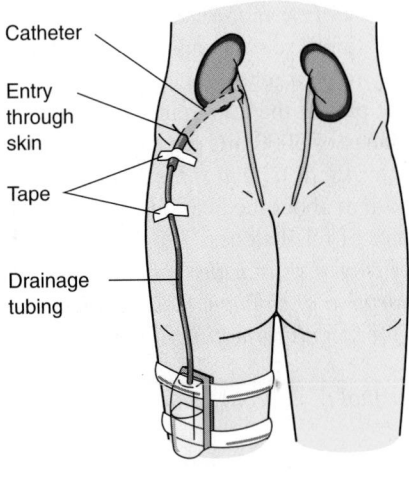

Catheter

Entry through skin

Tape

Drainage tubing

B   **Posterior view**

FIGURE 37.4 (A) Ureteral stents. (B) Nephrostomy tube inserted into renal pelvis; catheter exits through an incision on flank.

from tobacco. These chemicals are then passed via the bloodstream to the kidneys and collected in the urine. These chemicals accumulate in the urine and damage the cells that line the bladder. Exposure to industrial pollution such as aniline dyes, benzidine and naphthylamine, leather finishings, metal machinery, and petroleum processing products also increases the incidence. It can take about 25 years after exposure to chemicals for bladder cancer to develop. Cancer may also arise from the prostate, colon, and rectum in males and the lower reproductive tract in women. Bladder cancer is often diagnosed at a later stage in women.

Pathophysiology

Cancer of the bladder often starts as a benign growth on the bladder wall that undergoes cancerous changes. Most bladder cancers begin in the inner lining of the bladder called the urothelium. The cancers are called transition cell cancers.

They come in a variety of forms and can behave in different ways. Some occur as small wartlike growths on the inside of the bladder. Others form large tumors that grow into the muscle wall of the bladder and require surgical removal. If the bladder cancer affects only the inner lining of the bladder, it is known as a superficial cancer. If the cancer has spread to the muscle wall, it is called an invasive cancer. Common sites for metastasis include the liver, bones, and lungs.

Signs and Symptoms

Cancer of the bladder usually causes painless hematuria. The patient may notice that the urine is darker or more reddish in color than usual. Blood in the urine is one of the seven warning signs of cancer from the American Cancer Society. Initially the bleeding is intermittent, which often causes the patient to delay seeking treatment. As the disease progresses, the patient experiences frank hematuria, bladder irritability, urinary retention from clots obstructing the urethra, and fistula formation (an opening between the bladder and an adjoining structure such as the vagina or bowel). Other common signs and symptoms of bladder cancer include pelvic pain, pain in the lower back, painful urination, changes in bladder habits, and inability to void.

Diagnostic Tests

Routine urinalysis can detect signs of bladder cancer. A urine test for the enzyme telomerase has been found to be 90% accurate in detecting bladder cancer in early and late stages. Urine for cytology can be obtained to determine if cancer cells are present in the urine. Urine culture should also be done. Symtoms of bladder infection may be similar to those that accompany bladder cancer. Diagnosis of cancer of the bladder may also be made with a cystoscopy and transurethral biopsy. An intravenous pyelogram (IVP) may also be done.

Therapeutic Interventions

Treatment depends on the kind of bladder cancer and the severity. For small, confined tumors, chemotherapeutic agents are instilled into the bladder through a urinary catheter, allowed to dwell, and then removed along with the catheter. Systemic chemotherapy is also used and can be helpful to prolong life when other treatments are no longer indicated. The bacille Calmette-Guérin (BCG) vaccine may be instilled into the bladder to prevent recurring tumors.

Photodynamic therapy in which drugs are given that make tumors sensitive to light may be used. When light is applied to the tumor area, cancer cells are killed.

Surgical treatment of cancer of the bladder includes a number of procedures. A cystoscopy and pyelogram with fulguration (destruction of tissue with electrical current) may be done to burn off cancerous tissue. An alternate method is use of a laser to destroy tumor tissue. Advances in surgical techniques involve robotic and laparoscopic techniques. If the bladder requires removal, then robotic laparoscopic radical cystectomy with urinary diversion is an option. In this robotic procedure, surgical robotic equipment, which imitates surgical movements guided by the

surgeon, allows more precision, steadiness, and maneuverability, as well as the use of small openings rather than larger incisions into the abdomen. Recovery time is reduced as a result.

INCONTINENT URINARY DIVERSION. If it has been determined that the patient has a potentially curable disease with significant bladder involvement, complete removal of the bladder and creation of a urinary diversion may be done. A urinary diversion means that urine leaves the body in a different manner. A common incontinent surgery for urinary diversion is called an ileal conduit, an involved surgery in which a 6- to 8-inch section of the ileum or colon is removed and used as a conduit for urine. The remaining portions of the bowel are stitched back together. The surgeon is careful to keep the blood and neurological supply intact to the section of bowel that has been removed. The isolated section of bowel is closed off on one end, the ureters are stitched into it, and the other end is brought out as a stoma on the abdomen that almost continuously drains urine (Fig. 37.5). The urine from an ileal conduit contains mucus because it comes through the ileum, which normally secretes mucus. The patient must wear an ostomy appliance at all times over the stoma to collect urine. Box 37.7 (Application of a Disposable Pouch to an Ileal Conduit) explains how to apply an appliance to an ileal conduit stoma.

CONTINENT URINARY DIVERSION. Continent urinary diversion surgeries are being done for patient convenience. One version is the Kock pouch (continent internal ileal reservoir), which is created from a segment of ileum that has been made into a reservoir for urine (see Fig. 37.5). The ureters are implanted into the side of the reservoir. A special nipple valve is constructed and is the passageway through which the patient inserts a catheter at 4- to 6-hour intervals to drain urine. Another type of this surgery is the Indiana pouch (see Fig. 37.5). A reservoir is created using a portion of the ascending colon and terminal ileum, making a larger pouch than the Kock pouch. Additional versions of this type of surgery use other parts of the bowel and include the Mainz pouch or Florida pouch.

ORTHOTOPIC BLADDER SUBSTITUTION. The newest surgery is formation of an orthotopic bladder using a section of the intestines to make a neobladder (*neo* = new) and implanting both the ureters and the urethra into the neobladder. Various types of orthotopic bladder substitution surgery include the Studer pouch, hemi-Kock pouch, and ileal W-neobladder. After this surgery, the patient can void through the urethra, although incontinence may be a problem and intermittent catheterization may be needed.

Nursing Management

Nursing care of the postoperative patient is similar to care following any major surgical procedure. (See Chapter 11.) Specific postoperative care should be aimed at preventing complications of shock, atelectasis, deep vein thrombosis, and paralytic ileus. It is important to ensure that there is ade-

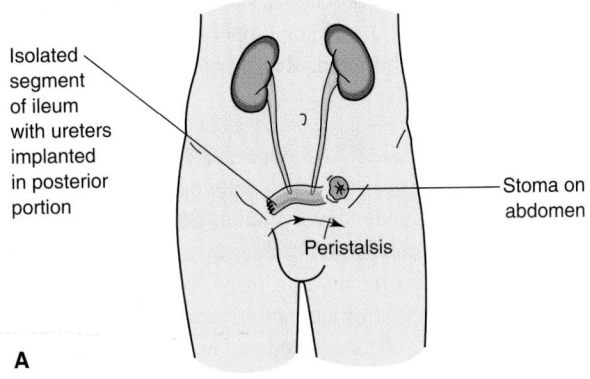

Isolated segment of ileum with ureters implanted in posterior portion

Stoma on abdomen

Peristalsis

A

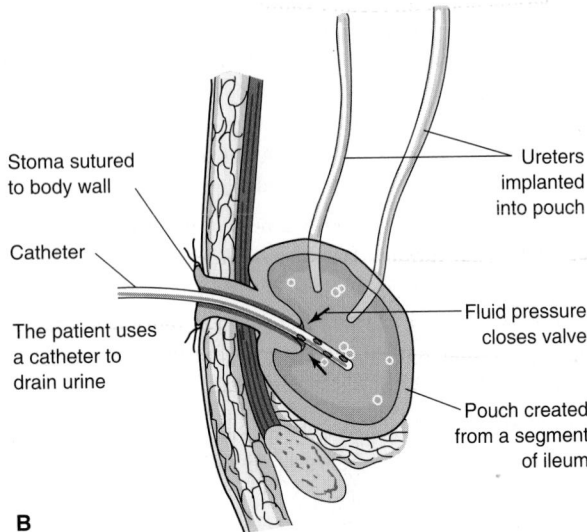

Stoma sutured to body wall

Catheter

The patient uses a catheter to drain urine

Ureters implanted into pouch

Fluid pressure closes valve

Pouch created from a segment of ileum

B

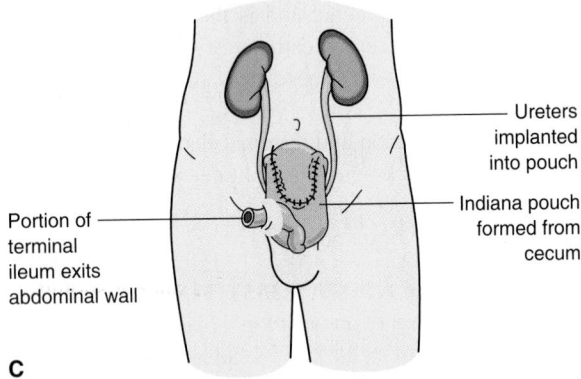

Ureters implanted into pouch

Indiana pouch formed from cecum

Portion of terminal ileum exits abdominal wall

C

FIGURE 37.5 Urinary diversion surgery. (A) Ileal conduit. (B) Kock pouch. (C) Indiana pouch.

quate urinary output and to detect and report any obstruction of urine drainage early to prevent complications. The skin around the stoma will require special care to prevent skin breakdown. The patient needs to be taught how to care for the urinary diversion after surgery, either by frequent draining with a catheter or by wearing an appliance. Be sensitive to the patient's anxiety about caring for the urinary diversion. Body image disturbance may occur because of the change in body function. A consultation with a nurse

---

Box 37.7

Application of a Disposable Pouch to an Ileal Conduit

1. Gather all supplies: a washcloth and towels and water, a pouch to apply with a stomahesive flange, and wicks such as gauze to absorb continually flowing urine. Wear clean gloves.
2. Empty the old pouch.
3. Gently remove soiled pouch by pushing down on skin while lifting up on the flange. Discard soiled pouch and flange.
4. Place a towel around the stoma to catch urine.
5. Cut an opening in the flange that is only 1/16 to 1/8 inch larger than the stoma. Once stomal shrinkage is complete, a presized pouch can be used that fits the stoma.
6. Remove paper backing from the stomahesive and set the flange to one side.
7. Clean the skin around the stoma with water. Pat dry. Immediately wrap the stoma in wicks to absorb urine. Otherwise urine will leak onto the skin, and the flange will not adhere.
8. Center the flange over the stoma, remove the wick, and immediately apply the flange. Then snap the pouch onto the flange. NOTE: The flange and pouch may be snapped together before application to the stoma.
9. Use the heat of your hand to compress the flange to ensure a good seal.
10. Ensure that the bottom of the pouch is closed off, or connect to a urinary catheter bag at night or if patient is in bed most of the time.

---

who specializes in wound, ostomy, and continence care (WOC nurse, or sometimes referred to as an enterostomal therapy nurse, which was the original name for this specialty) or an ostomy support group may be helpful both before and after surgery.

Cancer of the Kidney

Pathophysiology and Etiology

Cancer of the kidney is rare but serious. Kidney cancer accounts for 3% of all adult malignancies. Risk factors include smoking, obesity, hypertension, years of kidney dialysis, radiation exposure, asbestos, and exposure to industrial pollution. Most patients are between 50 and 70 years of age. During the last 30 years there has been an increased incidence in renal cell cancer, with an increase of 43% since 1973. This is probably due to the use of CT scans and ultrasound evaluation of the abdomen. More than 50% of tumors are found incidentally. Males have twice the incidence of females. Often the cancer has metastasized before it is diagnosed because the kidney has such a large volume of circulating blood, which increases the risk for spread of the tumor. In addition, there are few early symptoms of the disease.

Signs and Symptoms

The three classic symptoms of kidney cancer are hematuria, dull pain in the flank area, and a mass in the area. Often symptoms of kidney cancer do not occur until there is invasion of the surrounding tissue by the tumor. Less specific symptoms include fever, weight loss, night sweats, hypertension, anemia, polycythemia, swelling in the legs, fatigue, anorexia, and constipation. Symptoms of metastasis may be the first manifestation of kidney cancer and include weight loss, cough, bone fractures, liver abnormalities, and increasing weakness.

Diagnostic Tests

A number of diagnostic tests will be done, including an IVP, cystoscopy and pyelogram, ultrasound examination of the kidneys, computed tomographic (CT) scans of the abdomen, and magnetic resonance imaging (MRI). A definitive diagnosis is made with a renal biopsy.

Therapeutic Interventions

Surgery is the commonly used treatment for cancer of the kidney. A radical **nephrectomy** removes the entire kidney along with the adrenal gland and other surrounding structures, including fascia, fat, and lymph nodes, in the area. Radiation therapy, immunotherapy, or chemotherapy may be used following the surgery. Newer surgical techniques allow nephron sparing surgery in which only the tumor is removed and the healthy part of the kidney is saved.

Nursing Management

Nursing care of the nephrectomy patient is similar to postoperative care following any major surgery. (See Chapter 11.) Because the kidney is highly vascular, it is essential that the nurse observe for onset of bleeding and any signs of hypovolemic shock. Urine output is monitored. Changes in urine amount or color, bleeding, and signs of infection are reported. The patient should be assessed for shortness of breath or diminished breath sounds on the affected side. Surgically induced or spontaneous pneumothorax may occasionally occur after a nephrectomy.

RENAL SYSTEM TRAUMA

Renal trauma is the most common injury to the urinary system. The kidneys are highly vascular and have a lot of mobility so they are vulnerable to vascular and tissue damage. There are many causes of trauma to the kidney, ureters, and bladder, such as motor vehicle accidents, sports injuries, falls, gunshot wounds, and stabbing. Young males are at greatest risk for renal system trauma. Patient assessment includes a history of the injury, inspection of the abdomen and flank for asymmetry and bruising, or swelling of the

flank area. Flank pain and hematuria may be present. Diagnostic tests include urinalysis, IVP, ultrasound, CT, and MRI. Treatment depends on the extent of the injury and ranges from bedrest to surgical intervention. Nursing care includes measuring intake and output, monitoring vital signs, and providing IV fluids and pain relief.

Bladder trauma may occur with pelvic fractures and multitrauma from a blow to the lower abdomen when the bladder is full. The weakest part of the bladder wall, which is the dome located at the top of the bladder, may rupture. Urine leaks out of the peritoneal cavity and around the bowel. The patient may have symptoms of hematuria, abdominal pain, inability to void, shock, and pelvic hematoma noted on rectal examination. IVP and x-ray of the abdomen may be done. A urinary or suprapubic catheter should be in place until the bladder heals.

POLYCYSTIC KIDNEY DISEASE

Polycystic kidney disease is a hereditary disorder that can result in renal failure. The disease affects men and women equally. Polycystic kidney disease is characterized by formation of multiple cysts in the kidney that can eventually replace normal kidney structures. The cysts are grapelike and contain serous fluid, blood, or urine. The patient generally first shows signs of the disease in adulthood. The initial symptoms include a dull heaviness in the flank or lumbar region and hematuria. Other symptoms include hypertension and urinary tract infections. People with the inherited type of polycystic kidney disease may also experience aneurysms in the brain and diverticulosis in the colon. As the disease progresses, the patient develops symptoms of renal failure (discussed later). The renal cysts are usually diagnosed with ultrasound imaging. Ultrasound uses no dyes or radiation so it is safe for all patients including pregnant women. Often there is a strong family history of polycystic kidney disease.

There is no treatment to stop the progression of polycystic kidney disease. Complications such as urinary tract infections are treated as needed. Headaches that are severe due to hypertension or seem to feel different might be caused by aneurysms in the brain. The patient should see a physician with severe or recurring headache. As the disease progresses, treatment for hypertension and eventual renal failure may be necessary. Because polycystic disease is hereditary, patients should be counseled about the risks of children inheriting it.

CHRONIC RENAL DISEASES

Diabetic Nephropathy

Diabetic **nephropathy** is the most common cause of renal failure. It is a long-term complication of diabetes mellitus in

---

nephrectomy: nephr—kidney + ectomy—excision

nephropathy: nephro—pertaining to the kidney + pathy—disease which the effects of diabetes result in damage to the small blood vessels in the kidneys. Microalbuminuria may be detected within 5 years of the onset of type I diabetes and 10 to 15 years after the onset of type 2 diabetes. Renal damage shows up approximately 15 to 20 years after onset of type 1 diabetes (insulin dependent), but it may also be a complication of type 2 diabetes (non–insulin dependent). Risk factors for the development of diabetic nephropathy include hypertension, genetic predisposition, smoking, and chronic hyperglycemia. Careful control of blood glucose levels reduces the risk of nephropathy in patients with diabetes.

Pathophysiology

Multiple factors contribute to diabetic nephropathy. Diabetic nephropathy begins with increased osmotic pressure due to hyperglycemia, increases diuresis and compensatory cell growth and expansion, and increases the glomerular filtration rate. Widespread atherosclerotic changes occur in the blood vessels of patients with diabetes, decreasing the blood supply to the kidney. Abnormal thickening of glomerular capillaries damages the glomerulus, allowing protein to leak into the urine. Patients with diabetes also commonly develop pyelonephritis and renal scarring. Another complication of diabetes, neurogenic bladder, causes incomplete bladder emptying. This results in retention of urine, which can cause infection or obstruction of urine, further damaging the kidneys.

Initially patients lose only small amounts of protein in their urine (microalbuminuria); this disease can be detected only with careful watching by the physician, utilizing frequent examinations of the urine. As the disease progresses, high-output renal failure (nonoliguria) can develop, in which a large amount of diluted urine is excreted without the usual amounts of waste products dissolved in the urine. The patient can lose large amounts of protein in the urine and may develop nephrotic syndrome, which causes massive edema because of low levels of albumin in the blood. As renal function decreases, the patient needs smaller doses of insulin because the kidney normally degrades insulin. Because the kidney is no longer able to break down insulin and excrete it, small doses of insulin circulate in the body for long periods.

Symptoms

The progression of nephropathy is marked by microalbuminuria advancing to proteinuria. Hypertension accelerates the renal damage. As diabetic nephropathy progresses, urine output decreases, toxic wastes accumulate, and the patient develops chronic renal failure. See Chronic Renal Failure section below for symptoms.

Diagnostic Tests

Diabetic nephropathy is diagnosed by careful watching of the patient with diabetes for onset of protein spillage or microalbuminuria in the urine, which is an early sign of the disease. Serum creatinine levels and 24-hour creatinine clearance tests are then done to confirm the presence and extent of diabetic nephropathy.

Therapeutic Interventions

In the early stages of diabetic nephropathy, strict control of blood glucose levels and blood pressure and a restricted-protein diet can help slow the progress of the disease and reduce symptoms. As the disease progresses to renal failure, the patient needs dialysis to maintain life. Unfortunately, other complications related to diabetes cause patients to tolerate dialysis less well than patients with renal failure from other causes. Kidney or kidney-pancreas transplant, when available, is the treatment of choice for the patient with diabetic nephropathy and often improves the patient's chance for a healthier life.

Complications

Patients with diabetic nephropathy often have a guarded prognosis because they are vulnerable to all the complications of long-term diabetes in addition to kidney disease. The risk of cardiovascular disease is significant with the progression of protein spilling in the urine.

Nephrotic Syndrome

Nephrotic syndrome is the excretion of 3.5 g or more of protein in the urine per day. Nephrotic syndrome may occur as a result of other disease processes. In nephrotic syndrome, large amounts of protein are lost in the urine from increased glomerular membrane permeability. As a result, serum albumin and total serum protein are decreased. Normally, albumin and other serum proteins maintain fluid within the vascular space. When levels of these proteins are low, fluid leaks from the blood vessels into tissues, resulting in edema. With very low levels of protein, ascites and massive widespread edema (anasarca) occur. In response to the low protein levels, the liver produces lipoproteins. As a result, serum cholesterol, low-density lipoproteins, and triglyceride levels are elevated. Urine may appear foamy from lipoproteinemia. Loss of immunoglobulins may lead to increased susceptibility to infection. Elevated blood pressure readings are noted.

Treatment is focused on the cause and symptoms of nephrotic syndrome. To control edema, sodium intake is restricted. A low to moderate protein intake is ordered to prevent build-up of nitrogen wastes (nitrogen wastes result from protein metabolism) from impaired kidney function. Protein intake is based on the severity of urinary protein loss. Diuretics may be used. Lipid-lowering drugs may be tried. Anticoagulants are given for thrombosis. In some cases, corticosteroids may be used.

Complications of nephrotic syndrome include impaired immune function, nutritional imbalances, and most importantly increased blood coagulation. Nursing care focuses on the edema and preventing infection. For edema, daily weights, careful intake and output measurement, and abdominal girth measurement are performed and documented. Edematous tissue must be protected from injury. Preventing malnutrition is challenging but important in maintaining normal body functions.

Nephrosclerosis

Hypertension damages the kidneys by causing sclerotic changes in the small arteries and arterioles, such as arteriosclerosis with thickening and hardening of the renal blood vessels (**nephrosclerosis**). The arteriosclerotic changes in the kidney blood vessels result in a decreased blood supply to the kidney (ischemia of the kidney) and can eventually destroy the kidney. The remaining nephrons try to compensate with vasodilation to increase blood flow to the glomeruli. This results in increased glomerular pressure and filtration, which thickens the blood vessels. The high pressure within the kidneys causes the vessels to weaken and hemorrhage. Large areas of the kidney become damaged. Symptoms of nephrosclerosis include proteinuria, hyaline casts in the urine, and, as it progresses, symptoms of renal failure.

The treatment of nephrosclerosis is to reduce blood pressure and treat the hypertension. The patient is placed on antihypertensive medications or, if already on these, changed to stronger antihypertensive medications. The patient is placed on a low-sodium diet. If the patient develops renal failure, dialysis will be used to maintain life.

The prognosis is often poor because by the time the patient has developed nephrosclerosis, there is widespread arteriosclerosis throughout the body. Arteriosclerosis makes the patient prone to myocardial infarctions or cerebrovascular accidents.

The major nursing diagnosis that is relevant when the patient develops nephrosclerosis is impaired health maintenance. The priority is to help the patient learn as much about the control of hypertension as possible. The patient should also be taught the symptoms of renal failure. Once the patient has lost renal function, the nursing care plan for renal failure is appropriate.

CRITICAL THINKING

Mr. Stevens

■ Mr. Stevens is a 35-year-old African American man admitted to the intensive care unit with uncontrolled hypertension. His blood pressure is controlled by intravenous medication. His laboratory tests show protein and hyaline casts in the urine. He is diagnosed with nephrosclerosis.

1. What data should the nurse collect as part of the morning evaluation of the patient's condition?
2. What other renal function tests are appropriate for the nurse to check?
3. What teaching does Mr. Stevens need when his condition is more stable?

Suggested answers at end of chapter.

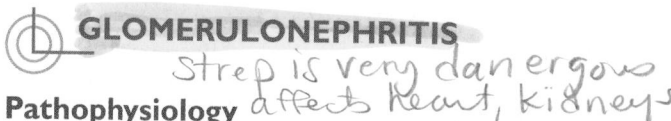

GLOMERULONEPHRITIS

Pathophysiology

[handwritten: Strep is very dangerous affects heart, kidneys]

Glomerulonephritis is an inflammatory disease of the glomerulus. It can be caused by a variety of factors including immunological abnormalities, toxins, vascular disorders, and systemic diseases. Inflammation occurs as a result of the deposition of antigen-antibody complexes in the basement membrane of the glomerulus or from antibodies that specifically attack the basement membrane. The resulting immune reaction in the glomerulus causes inflammation, which in turn causes the glomerulus to be more porous, allowing proteins, white blood cells, and red blood cells to leak into the urine.

Etiology

Acute Poststreptococcal Glomerulonephritis

Glomerulonephritis can be caused by a variety of factors but is most commonly associated with a group A beta-hemolytic streptococcal infection following a streptococcal infection of the throat or skin. This is the most common cause in children and young adults. Antibodies form complexes with the streptococcal antigen and are deposited in the basement membrane of the glomerulus, inducing damage from inflammation. Damaged glomeruli become unable to filter blood correctly and protein leaks into the urine. Edema, oliguria, and hypertension result. Glomerulonephritis generally develops about 6 to 10 days after the preceding infection. The disease has an abrupt onset. Other kinds of bacteria and viruses can also be the offending infectious agent.

Goodpasture's Syndrome

Occasionally glomerulonephritis is caused by an autoimmune response, in which the person for some unknown reason forms antibodies against his or her own glomerular basement membrane. Glomerulonephritis caused by an autoimmune response usually progresses rapidly and often leads to renal failure.

Chronic Glomerulonephritis

Chronic glomerulonephritis occurs over years as a result of glomerular inflammatory disease. There may be no history of renal disease before the diagnosis. Often proteinuria and hematuria may have been noted previously before the diagnosis. Lupus erythematosus and insulin-dependent diabetes mellitus may precede chronic glomerular injury. It is often discovered during an examination for another concern. Ultrasound, CT scan, or renal biopsy is used to diagnose the cause.

Symptoms

The symptoms of glomerulonephritis include fluid overload with oliguria, hypertension, electrolyte imbalances, and

---

nephrosclerosis: nephro—pertaining to the kidney + sclerosis—hardening

glomerulonephritis: glomerulo—glomerulus + nephr—kidney + itis—inflammation

Box 37.8

Glomerulonephritis Summary

Signs and Symptoms	Fluid volume overload Hypertension Electrolyte imbalances Edema Periorbital edema Flank pain
Diagnostic Tests	Urinalysis shows red cells, WBCs, protein, and casts Urine dark or cola colored Foamy urine from protein Creatinine, urea level elevated
Therapeutic Interventions	Treatment is symptomatic Nonsteroidal antiinflammatory drugs Steroids
Complications	Renal failure
Possible Nursing Diagnosis	Fluid volume excess related to compromised renal regulation Decreased tissue perfusion related to anemia, CHF, edema

edema (Box 37.8 Glomerulonephritis Summary). Edema may begin around the eyes (periorbital edema) and face and progress to the abdomen (ascites), lungs (pleural effusion), and extremities. Flank pain may be present. Blood urea nitrogen (BUN) and creatinine levels may be elevated. Urinalysis shows red blood cells, white blood cells, albumin, and casts. The urine is dark or cola colored from old red blood cells and may be foamy because of proteinuria.

Diagnostic Tests

Glomerulonephritis is diagnosed with urinalysis, which shows protein, casts or RBCs, and elevated serum levels of nitrogenous wastes (creatinine, urea). Hypertension may be present. Kidney ultrasound, x-ray, or biopsy may be done to determine abnormal kidney shape, size, blood flow, inflammation, or scarring of the glomeruli. *weight, intake + output*

Therapeutic Interventions

Most cases of acute glomerulonephritis resolve spontaneously in about a week, but some progress to renal failure. Treatment is primarily symptomatic. Sodium and fluid restrictions may be ordered along with diuretics to treat fluid retention. Medications may be given to control hypertension. If associated with a streptococcal infection, antibiotics are given to treat any remaining infection. If fluid overload is severe, dialysis may be done.

Complications

The prognosis is good for acute glomerulonephritis acquired in childhood, and the majority of children recover completely. Adults who develop glomerulonephritis may recover renal function or progress to chronic glomerulonephritis. Some patients develop rapidly progressive glomerulonephritis, which can quickly lead to renal failure. Chronic glomerulonephritis is a slow process characterized by hypertension, gradual loss of renal function, and eventual renal failure.

Nursing Management

Nursing care for a patient with glomerulonephritis focuses on symptom relief. Vital signs are monitored because the patient may be critically ill. During the acute phase, rest is encouraged. Edema is controlled with fluid and sodium intake restrictions. Protein intake may be limited if the kidneys are not filtering protein waste products (as seen by increased serum BUN and creatinine levels). Other care is discussed in the section Chronic Renal Failure. Teaching the patient about preventing glomerulonephritis is important. Antibiotics for diagnosed streptococcal throat infections should be taken for prevention.

RENAL FAILURE

Renal failure, also called kidney failure, is diagnosed when the kidneys are no longer functioning adequately to maintain normal body processes. This results in dysfunction in almost all other parts of the body as a result of imbalances in fluid, electrolytes, and calcium levels, as well as impaired RBC formation and decreased elimination of waste products. Renal failure can be acute, with sudden onset of symptoms, or chronic, occurring gradually over time. For more information on kidneys, visit the American Kidney Fund at http://www.kidneyfund.org/, the National Kidney Foundation at www.kidney.org, and the American Association of Kidney Patients at www.aakp.org.

Acute Renal Failure

Acute renal failure (ARF) is the sudden (hours to days) loss of the kidneys' ability to clear waste products and regulate fluid and electrolyte balance. There is a rapid accumulation of toxic wastes from protein metabolism in the blood (**azotemia**). In azotemia, the serum urea level (measured by BUN) and creatinine levels are elevated. Most types of acute renal failure are reversible if diagnosed and treated early; however, ARF can lead to chronic renal failure. Acute renal failure is often associated with a urine output of less than 30 mL/hr or 400 mL/day. It may be caused by hypotension, vascular obstruction, glomerular disease, acute tubular necrosis (ATN) in which the tubules are damaged after administration of diagnostic contrast media.

---

azotemia: azo—nitrogenous waste products + temia—blood

NURSING CARE TIP

To protect patients' kidneys, be aware of the following:

- The patient's renal function status: Serum BUN and creatinine levels will tell you this.
- Nephrotoxic substances:
  - Diagnostic contrast media (dyes) in presence of dehydration or renal impairment
  - Medications—IV aminoglycosides (gentamicin [Garamycin], tobramycin [Tobrex], amikacin [Amikin], cisplatin [Platinol])
  - Chemicals—arsenic, carbon tetrachloride, lead, mercuric chloride
- Preventive measures:
  - Before administering nephrotoxic dyes or medications, check serum BUN and creatinine levels.
  - With contrast media (dye) tests, encourage fluids before and after to dilute and flush, flush, flush the dye away!

Make sure peak and trough drug levels of nephrotoxic drugs are obtained on an ongoing basis per institutional policy.

Pathophysiology

In acute renal failure, rapid damage to the kidney causes waste products to accumulate in the bloodstream, resulting in the symptoms of renal failure. The patient becomes oliguric, with urine output decreasing to less than 20 mL/h. Treatment is directed toward correcting the cause, supporting the patient with dialysis, and prevention of complications that may lead to permanent damage. Many patients with acute renal failure recover completely. Approximately 50% of patients with intrarenal ARF die as a result of complications of infection, pneumonia, or septicemia.

ARF can progress through four stages, with an intrarenal cause taking a longer recovery time frame since there is actual renal damage. Once an event causes ARF in the initial phase, symptoms occur in hours to days.

OLIGURIC PHASE. In the oliguric phase, less than 400 mL of urine in 24 hours is produced. Fifty percent of those with ARF experience this phase, which occurs from 24 hours to 7 days after the initial phase. This phase can last up to 2 weeks to several months. Prognosis for renal recovery is decreased the longer this phase lasts.

In the oliguric phase, fluid is retained, electrolytes become imbalanced, and waste products are not excreted as urine output decreases. Signs of fluid overload are seen. Serum potassium rises while sodium is lost in the urine, creating a normal or low serum sodium level. The longer this phase lasts, the more effects are seen. These may include metabolic acidosis from reduced hydrogen ion excretion and sodium bicarbonate levels, increased phosphate and decreased calcium levels, abnormal blood cells (RBC, WBC, platelets), neurological effects ranging from confusion, seizures to coma, and finally effects on all body systems as is seen in CRF (discussed later).

DIURETIC PHASE. As the kidneys begin to be able to again excrete waste products, 1 to 3 L/day of urine is produced. The osmotic diuresis occurs from the elevated waste products (urea) which the body is attempting to eliminate. The kidneys are not yet able to concentrate urine and so dehydration and hypotension are a concern. It is important for the nurse to monitor for hypovolemia, hyponatremia, and hypotension in this phase. Serum BUN and creatinine levels are high until the end of this phase, at which time they begin to return to normal. This phase may last from 1 to 3 weeks.

RECOVERY PHASE. In this final phase, recovery begins as the glomerular filtration rate rises. Waste product levels (BUN, creatinine levels) decrease greatly within the first 2 weeks of this phase. However, recovery can take up to 1 year. Those who do recover usually do so without complications. Older adults are more at risk for reduced recovery of renal function. In those who do not recover renal function, chronic renal failure occurs.

Etiology

Acute renal failure is often classified as prerenal, intrarenal, or postrenal. These categories relate to the causes leading to acute renal failure. Each category is associated with the location of the cause in the kidney. Understanding the cause can point to the direction of treatment plans helpful to the patient.

PRERENAL FAILURE. Prerenal (before the kidney) failure is associated with a decrease or interruption of blood supply to the kidneys. This type of renal failure accounts for 55% to 60% of all cases of acute renal failure. The causes may include a decrease in blood pressure as a result of dehydration, blood loss, shock, or trauma to or blockage in the arteries that carry blood to the kidneys. When the nephrons receive an inadequate blood supply, they are unable to make urine and the waste products are not adequately removed. The use of nonsteroidal anti-inflammatory drugs (NSAIDs) and cyclooxygenase-2 (COX) inhibitors can also lead to prerenal failure. These drugs impair the autoregulatory responses of the kidney by blocking prostaglandin, which is necessary for renal perfusion.

Prerenal failure can be diagnosed by evaluating possible causes. If dehydration is the cause, then an IV fluid challenge may be given. With increased IV fluid, more blood flows to the kidneys for filtering, which increases urine output and waste product filtering. An arteriogram of the renal arteries is helpful to determine if the blood supply to the kidneys is decreased or blocked; angioplasty may be used to open the blockage. The serum creatinine increases and cre-

TABLE 37.4 COMMON NEPHROTOXINS

Antibiotics	Analgesics	Other Drugs	Heavy Metals	Contrast Dyes	Organic Solvents
Aminoglycosides	Nonsteroidal anti-	ACE inhibitors	Lead	Contrast media used for	Gasoline
Tetracyclines	inflammatory drugs	Dextran	Mercury	diagnostic testing	Glycols
Cephalosporins	Acetaminophen	Mannitol	Arsenic	such as intravenous	Kerosene
Sulfonamides	Salicylates	Interleukin-2	Copper	pyelograms, cardiac	Turpentine
Vancomycin		Cisplatin	Gold	catheterizations	Tetrachloroethylene
Amphotericin B		Amphetamines	Lithium		
		Heroin			

ACE = angiotensin-converting enzyme.

atinine clearance decreases. Urinalysis may be helpful in determining the cause as well.

INTRARENAL FAILURE. Intrarenal failure (inside the kidney) occurs when there is damage to the nephrons inside the kidney. The most common causes are ischemia, reduced blood flow, and toxins. Other causes are from infectious processes leading to glomerulonephritis, trauma to the kidney, exposure to **nephrotoxins**, allergic reactions to radiographic dyes, and severe muscle injury, which releases substances that are harmful to the kidneys (Table 37.4).

A number of substances can be toxic to the kidneys (nephrotoxic) when they enter the body. Kidney damage is most likely to occur when these substances enter the body in high concentrations or when there is preexisting kidney damage for some other reason. Environmental nephrotoxins, such as insecticides and lead paint, may be ingested by children. Many commonly administered medications can be nephrotoxic. Aminoglycosides are nephrotoxic antibiotics; when they are administered, blood levels of the drugs are carefully monitored to avoid toxic levels.

Contrast media used during tests such as intravenous pyelograms and CT scans can cause kidney damage when the patient is dehydrated or has preexisting renal damage. The medium can precipitate out in the tubules, damaging the kidney. It is important for the patient to be adequately hydrated before and after any diagnostic test using a contrast medium to decrease the incidence of toxicity.

POSTRENAL FAILURE. Postrenal (after the kidney) failure is associated with an obstruction that blocks the flow of urine out of the body. Only 5% of cases of acute renal failure are classified as postrenal. In this case, the blood supply to the kidneys and nephron function initially may be normal, but urine is unable to drain out of the kidney, resulting in back-up of urine and impaired nephron function. Common causes are kidney stones, tumors of the ureters or bladder, and an enlarged prostate that blocks the flow of urine.

Diagnosis of causes of postrenal failure can be done with x-ray examination of the kidneys, ureters, and bladder. Cystoscopy will show presence of tumors, stones, or prostate enlargement. Renal ultrasound can measure the kidney size, detect tumors and blockages, and reveal cystic disease. Surgical intervention may be needed to correct the problem.

Therapeutic Interventions

Acute renal failure is treated by relieving the cause. Prevention of permanent damage is the goal of treatment. Signs and symptoms are managed as they develop and supportive care is given. Treatment may include restoring fluid and electrolyte balance, discontinuing nephrotoxic drugs that may have caused the problem, bypassing urinary tract obstructions with catheters, or short-term continuous renal replacement therapy to filter blood and restore potassium and other electrolytes to normal. Some symptoms such as anemia may not have time to develop in the patient with ARF as they do in CRF. The care of the patient with acute renal failure is similar to care of the patient with chronic renal failure, as explained in the next section.

CONTINUOUS RENAL REPLACEMENT THERAPY (CRRT). CRRT is a therapy to remove fluid and solutes in a controlled, continuous manner in unstable patients with acute renal failure. Unstable patients may not be able to tolerate rapid fluid shifts as occurs in hemodialysis so CRRT provides an alternative therapy that results in less dramatic fluid shifting. CRRT can be used along with **hemodialysis,** which is necessary if severe symptoms of **uremia** (hyperkalemia) are present. CRRT is not as complex as hemodialysis and can be done for more than a month if needed. Temporary vascular access is used with CRRT.

During CRRT, a permeable hemofilter is attached to the vascular access. Blood flows through the hemofilter and excess fluids and solutes move into a collection bag. The remaining blood returns to the patient via the venous access. If desired, replacement fluid and electrolytes can be given through the vascular access. Monitoring intake and output, fluid and electrolytes, daily weights, hourly vital signs, and vascular access is important.

Chronic Renal Failure

Chronic renal failure (CRF) affects approximately 290,000 people in the United States. The incidence is on the rise. It is a progressive, irreversible deterioration in renal function where the body is unable to maintain metabolic, fluid, and electrolyte balance. It occurs with a gradual decrease in the

nephrotoxins: nephro—kidney + toxin—poison

hemodialysis: hemo—blood + dialysis—passage of a solute through a membrane

uremia: ur—urea + emia—in the blood

function of the kidneys over time. The result is nitrogenous waste products in the blood and uremia. Chronic renal disease affects every body system (Box 37.9 Renal Failure Summary).

Etiology

The causes of chronic renal failure are numerous; the most common ones include diabetes mellitus resulting in diabetic nephropathy, chronic high blood pressure causing nephrosclerosis, glomerulonephritis, and autoimmune diseases. Diabetes and hypertension account for close to 70% of all chronic renal disease.

Pathophysiology

When a large proportion of the nephrons are damaged or destroyed because of acute or chronic kidney disease, renal

---

Box 37.9

Renal Failure Summary

Signs and Symptoms	Decreased urine output
	Acute renal failure symptoms appear rapidly
	Fatigue
	Nausea and vomiting
	Shortness of breath
	Platelet dysfunction
Diagnostic Tests	Urinalysis
	Elevated BUN, creatinine
	Urine Na level less than 10 mEq/L
	Acidosis
	Anemia
	Electrolyte abnormalities
	Elevated K, Mg
	Hypertension
	Pericarditis
	Platelet dysfunction
	Dialysis
Therapeutic Interventions	Transplant
	Diet
Complications	Progressive renal failure
	Headache
	Uremic encephalopathy—lethargy, coma, seizures
	Hypertension
	Accelerated atherosclerosis
	Heart failure
	Pulmonary edema
	Uremic pericarditis
	Anorexia, nausea, and vomiting
	Impotence
	Anemia
	Dry itchy skin, ecchymosis, and subcutaneous bruises
	Osteomalacia
	Osteoporosis
Possible Nursing Diagnosis	Fluid volume excess related to edema and failure of renal regulatory mechanism
	Electrolyte abnormalities related to edema and failure of renal regulatory mechanism
	Imbalanced nutrition: less than body requirements due to hypercatabolic state
	Sexual dysfunction related to neuropathy
	Urinary retention related to neuropathy
	Anxiety related to illness
	Infection related to suppression of immune system
	Noncompliance related to apathy or denial
	Ineffective coping related to loss of control

TABLE 37.5 LOSS OF NEPHRONS AND CREATININE LEVEL RELATIONSHIP

Normal Creatinine: 0.5–1.5 mg/dL

Nephron Loss	Creatinine Level
50%	2 × normal
75%	4 × normal
90%	markedly elevated

Contributed by Carol Duell.

failure occurs (Table 37.5). As the nephrons die off, the undamaged ones increase their work capacity and take over the work previously done by the dead ones, so the patient may experience significant kidney damage without showing symptoms of renal failure.

Chronic renal failure is a progressive disease process. In the early, or silent, stage (decreased renal reserve), the patient is usually without symptoms, even though up to 50% of nephron function may have been lost. This stage is often not diagnosed.

The renal insufficiency stage occurs when the patient has lost 75% of nephron function and some signs of mild renal failure are present. Anemia and the inability to concentrate urine may occur. The BUN and creatinine levels are slightly elevated. These patients are at risk for further damage caused by infection, dehydration, drugs, heart failure, and use of diagnostic x-ray dyes. The goal of care is to prevent further damage, if possible, by control of blood sugar levels and blood pressure.

End-stage renal disease (ESRD) occurs when 90% of the nephrons are lost. Patients at this stage experience chronic and persistent abnormal kidney function. The BUN and creatinine levels are always elevated. These patients may make urine but not filter out the waste products, or urine production may cease. Dialysis or a kidney transplant is required to survive.

Uremia (urea in the blood) is present in chronic renal failure. Patients eventually develop problems in all body systems (Table 37.6). If left untreated, the patient with uremia dies, often within weeks.

Symptoms of Renal Failure

Patients in either acute or chronic renal failure have multiple symptoms. Some of the more common symptoms associated with renal failure are explained next (Fig. 37.6).

Disturbance in Water Balance

Patients with renal failure experience disturbances in the removal and regulation of water balance in the body and

TABLE 37.6 EFFECTS OF RENAL FAILURE ON BODY SYSTEMS

Body System	Disease Process
Cardiovascular	Hypertension due to fluid overload and accelerated arteriosclerosis
	Congestive heart failure/pulmonary edema due to fluid overload, increased pulmonary permeability, left ventricular failure
	Angina due to coronary artery disease, anemia
	Dysrhythmias due to electrolyte imbalance, coronary artery disease
	Edema due to fluid overload and a decrease in osmotic pressure
	Pericarditis due to presence of waste products in the pericardial sac
Gastrointestinal	Stomatitis due to fluid restriction, presence of waste products in the mouth, secondary infections
	Anorexia, nausea, vomiting due to uremia
	Gastritis/gastrointestinal bleeding due to urea decomposition in gastrointestinal tract releasing ammonia that irritates and ulcerates the stomach or bowel; patient is also under stress, increasing ulcer formation, and may have platelet dysfunction
	Constipation due to electrolyte imbalances, decrease in fluid intake, decrease in activity, phosphate binders
	Diarrhea, hypermotility due to electrolyte imbalance
Hematopoietic	Anemia due to impaired synthesis of erythropoietin, a substance needed by the bone marrow to stimulate formation of RBCs; also due to decreased life span of RBCs from uremia and interference in folic acid action
	Bleeding tendency due to abnormal platelet function from effects of uremia
	Prone to infection due to a decrease in immune system function from uremia; renal patients can rapidly become septic and die from septic shock
Integumentary	Dry, itchy, inflamed skin due to calcium-phosphate deposits in the skin and urochrome, and a pigment of uremia, causes the skin to be pale gray, yellow bronze; skin will have an odor of urine because skin is an organ of excretion and the body attempts to remove toxins; there is also a decrease in function of oil and sweat glands
Neurological	Confusion due to uremic encephalopathy from an increase in urea and metabolic acids
	Peripheral neuropathy due to effects of waste products on neurological system
	Cerebrovascular accidents due to accelerated atherosclerosis
Pulmonary	Pleurisy/pleural effusion due to waste products in the pleural space causing inflammation with pleurisy pain and collection of fluid resulting in effusion
Reproductive	Loss of libido, impotence, amenorrhea, infertility due to a decrease in hormone production
Skeletal	Bone disease due to renal osteodystrophy from hyperphosphatemia and hypocalcemia

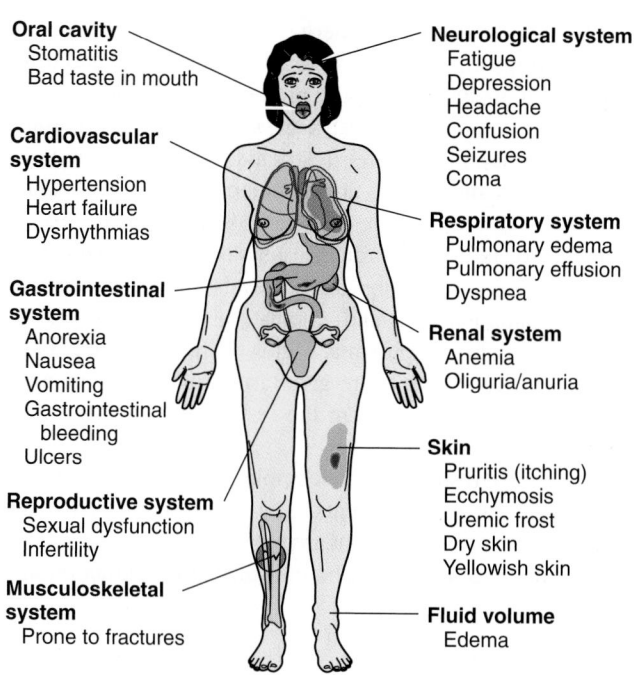

Oral cavity
Stomatitis
Bad taste in mouth

Cardiovascular system
Hypertension
Heart failure
Dysrhythmias

Gastrointestinal system
Anorexia
Nausea
Vomiting
Gastrointestinal bleeding
Ulcers

Reproductive system
Sexual dysfunction
Infertility

Musculoskeletal system
Prone to fractures

Neurological system
Fatigue
Depression
Headache
Confusion
Seizures
Coma

Respiratory system
Pulmonary edema
Pulmonary effusion
Dyspnea

Renal system
Anemia
Oliguria/anuria

Skin
Pruritis (itching)
Ecchymosis
Uremic frost
Dry skin
Yellowish skin

Fluid volume
Edema

FIGURE 37.6 Symptoms of chronic renal failure.

show signs of fluid accumulation. An early symptom is edema (swelling) of the extremities, sacral area, and abdomen. Patients may complain of being short of breath. Crackles and wheezes may be present on auscultation of the lungs, which are signs of fluid accumulation in the lungs. The blood vessels in the neck may be distended, and the patient may be hypertensive. These patients may produce a large amount of dilute urine (**polyuria**), small amounts of urine (oliguria), or no urine (anuria).

Disturbance in Electrolyte Balance

As kidney function decreases, the kidneys lose their ability to absorb and excrete electrolytes. Important electrolytes are sodium, potassium, and magnesium. When the kidneys are unable to maintain normal amounts of electrolytes in the blood, these substances accumulate at high levels and may be life threatening.

When the kidneys are unable to regulate sodium levels adequately, the patient may show signs of hypernatremia, an excessive sodium level in the blood, which causes water retention, edema, and hypertension. Hyponatremia, too little sodium, may occur when too much sodium is lost. This can occur when the patient has experienced prolonged episodes of vomiting or diarrhea or is urinating large amounts of diluted urine. Patients with hyponatremia may show signs of confusion. The sodium may be normal or low in renal failure due to being diluted from excess fluid.

Hyperkalemia (high level of potassium) presents a life-threatening situation. The patient may exhibit signs of dysrhythmia and cardiac arrest if the potassium level is too

polyuria: poly—much + uria—urine

high. Patients complain of muscle weakness, abdominal cramping, and diarrhea. The nurse may identify that the patient is confused or demonstrates disinterest in care. Hyperkalemia exists when the potassium level exceeds 5 mEq/L. These patients should be placed on a cardiac monitor and observed for cardiac dysrhythmias. A potassium level above 7 mEq/L may be life threatening. A high potassium level in the patient with renal failure may be caused by a diet high in potassium-rich foods, injuries, or blood transfusions. Monitoring daily laboratory values, restricting potassium intake, and reporting abnormalities are important. Intravenous insulin, glucose, or calcium gluconate may be used as a temporary measure to drive excess potassium into the cells. Sodium polystyrene sulfonate (Kayexalate) may be given either orally or as a retention enema; it causes the potassium to be eliminated through the stool. The definitive treatment for hyperkalemia is hemodialysis, which removes potassium from the body. Dietary education is extremely important. The patient is instructed to avoid foods that are high in potassium (Box 37.10 Foods High in Potassium).

Calcium levels decrease because the kidneys are unable to produce the hormone that activates vitamin D, the vitamin that is necessary for the absorption of calcium. Hypocalcemia exists when the calcium level falls below 8.5 mg/dL. Also associated with a low calcium level is hyperphosphatemia, a phosphorus level above 5 mg/dL. These imbalances cause the bones to release calcium, causing patients to be prone to fractures. These patients should ambulate regularly to prevent further calcium loss from the bone. Many patients with chronic renal failure who are on dialysis develop hypercalcemia due to hyperparathyroidism (excess release of parathyroid hormone). Cinacalcet (Sensipar) reduces excess levels of parathyroid hormone, which reduces calcium levels.

Phosphates are also found in some foods. Medications to bind phosphate are given to patients with high phosphate levels. Calcium carbonate (Tums, Caltrate), calcium acetate (PhosLo), sevelamer hydrochloride (Renagel), or lanthanum (Fosrenol) are examples of commonly ordered phosphate binders. These must be given to the patient with meals, so that the medicines can bind with the phosphates in the stool and be eliminated. High phosphorus levels may cause severe

Box 37.10

Foods High in Potassium

- Citrus fruits and juices
- Bananas
- Salt substitutes
- Potatoes, sweet and white
- Excessive dairy products
- Excessive meats
- Chocolate

itching, and patients may have open sores from scratching, placing them at risk for infections. Patients may also have muscle cramps and aches.

Disturbance of Removal of Waste Products

With azotemia, the patient may show signs of weakness and fatigue, confusion, seizures, twitching movements of extremities (asterixis), nausea, vomiting, and lack of appetite and may complain of a metallic or bad taste in the mouth. There may be a smell of urine on the patient's breath. The patient may have yellowish pale skin and complain of itching due to urea crystals on the skin. Dialysis to remove the excessive waste products in the blood is the only treatment of the underlying causes of these symptoms.

Disturbance in Maintaining Acid-Base Balance

Renal failure affects hydrogen ion excretion, causing a disturbance in the acid-base balance that results in metabolic acidosis. Patients may complain of a headache, fatigue, weakness, nausea, vomiting, and lack of appetite. As the acidosis progresses, the patient shows signs of lethargy, stupor, and coma. Respirations become fast and deep as the lungs attempt to blow off carbon dioxide to correct the acidosis (Kussmaul's respirations). See Chapter 5 for a more detailed discussion of acid-base balance.

Disturbance in Hematological Function (Primarily Seen in CRF)

Over time, disturbances in blood cells occur from chronic renal failure. Usually with treatment there is not time for this to occur in ARF. Failing kidneys do not produce adequate erythropoietin, the hormone that stimulates red blood cell production. Nutritional deficiencies and blood loss during dialysis also contribute to anemia. Regular injections of epoetin (Epogen, Procrit), a synthetic form of erythropoietin, help restore RBC production and prevent anemia. A common side effect of erythropoietin is the development of hypertension.

Impaired white blood cell and immune functions contribute to an increased risk for infection. The patient should be protected from potential sources of infection.

Impaired platelet function creates a risk for bleeding. The patient should be protected from injury, and signs of bleeding, such as blood in stool or emesis, are reported.

Therapeutic Interventions for Renal Failure

Renal insufficiency and early renal failure are treated based on symptoms with a restricted diet and fluid intake, medications, and careful monitoring for onset of serious problems that warrant initiation of dialysis. In later stages, dialysis is necessary to replace lost kidney function. A kidney transplant, when available, may return the patient to a nearly normal state of health.

Diet

Dietary recommendations are individualized by the dietitian and physician based on the patient's needs. Calories are high to maintain weight and energy needs. Protein is usually restricted to limit nitrogen intake but may be increased for the patient on dialysis because protein is lost during the dialysis process. Sodium is restricted to minimize sodium and fluid retention. Potassium is restricted, especially later in the disease when the kidneys are unable to eliminate it. Calcium is increased or supplemented because of poor absorption related to faulty vitamin D activation. Phosphorus is restricted because of high blood levels related to hypocalcemia. Saturated fat and cholesterol are restricted for patients with hyperlipidemia. Fluids are restricted to prevent overload. Most patients are given iron, folic acid, vitamins, and minerals to supplement the restricted diet (Box 37.11 Nutrition Notes).

Because restrictions are complex, the diet is a source of frustration for many patients. The nurse should assist the patient to identify foods that are palatable yet within the diet plan. The dietitian should be consulted for instruction and assistance.

Medications

Early in the disease, diuretics are given to increase output, and angiotensin-converting enzyme (ACE) inhibitors, calcium channel blockers, or beta-blocking agents may be used to control hypertension. Phosphate binders are given with meals to reduce phosphate levels. Calcium and vitamin D supplements are used to raise calcium levels. Agents to lower potassium levels are used if necessary. All drug therapy is closely monitored because diseased kidneys are unable to effectively remove medications from the body. The patient with diabetes needs less insulin since one of the functions of the kidneys is to break down insulin. Since it is not being broken down, it remains in the body longer, and therefore less is needed as the kidney disease progresses.

Dialysis

Dialysis is started when the patient develops symptoms of severe fluid overload, high potassium levels, acidosis, pericarditis, vomiting, lethargy, fatigue, or symptoms of uremia that are life threatening. Both peritoneal and hemodialysis involve the movement and diffusion of particles from an area of high concentration to an area of low concentration through a semipermeable membrane. The substances move from blood through the semipermeable membrane into the dialysate. Fluid and electrolyte imbalances can be corrected with dialysis. Dialysis can also be used to treat drug overdoses.

HEMODIALYSIS. Hemodialysis involves the use of an artificial kidney to remove waste products and excess water from the patient's blood. During the dialysis procedure, the patient's blood and the dialyzing solution flow in opposite directions through the dialyzer across an enclosed semipermeable membrane. The dialysate contains electrolytes and water in a balanced mix that resembles blood plasma. On the other side is the patient's blood with metabolic waste products, excess water and electrolytes. The waste products from the patient's blood move into the dialysate by diffusion

Box 37.11

Nutrition Notes

Understanding Dietary Changes in Renal Disease

Patients with impaired renal function require careful coordination of diet with current physiological status, which may change frequently, necessitating the services of a dietitian who specializes in renal treatment. Six national meal-planning systems were developed for renal insufficiency with/without diabetes, hemodialysis with/without diabetes, and peritoneal dialysis with/without diabetes. The following principles are offered as general guidelines.

- Maintaining caloric intake is essential to avoid catabolism of tissue for energy.* Simple carbohydrates and monounsaturated and polyunsaturated fats are given freely because their endproducts, carbon dioxide and water, are less likely than protein to tax the kidney. Patients with diabetes and uremia may receive more sugar than usual because treatment of the uremia may take precedence over the diabetes; however, patients with type IV hypertriglyceridemia may have to limit carbohydrates.
- Protein may be restricted when the patient's kidneys are failing but increased when the patient is treated with dialysis to compensate for losses in the dialysate.

Sometimes proteins of high biological value (e.g., eggs, meat, and dairy products) are prescribed because they are more easily converted to body protein than those of low biological value. In other situations, vegetarian diets may be given, with the plant proteins carefully selected to manage potassium and phosphorus serum levels.

- Sodium may be restricted, depending on blood pressure, edema, and laboratory findings.
- Potassium may be restricted for patients with oliguria. Salt substitutes are often potassium compounds that are to be avoided. Potassium content in foods varies with processing and preparation methods so patients should choose from prescribed foods only.
- Fluid restriction may be altered daily according to output. Renal insufficiency patients may receive 500 mL plus the amount of the previous day's output.

In short, renal diets are individualized for the patient's current condition. Nurses should not expect different patients to be served the same meals or even the same patient to require the same restrictions from one day to the next.

*A special oral supplement such as *ReNeph LP/HC* (low protein, high calorie) from Ross Laboratories may be prescribed for patients who are unwilling to eat enough food.

Lutz, CA, and Przytulski, KR: Nutrition and Diet Therapy, ed. 4. F.A. Davis, Philadelphia, 2006.

---

through the membrane because of the difference in their concentrations. The dialysate solution carries the waste products away, and the cleansed blood is returned back into the patient's body through another tube (Fig. 37.7). A hemodialysis treatment takes 3 to 4 hours and is done three or four times a week. Hemodialysis is done at a hemodialysis center (Fig. 37.8) or in the hospital if the patient develops a complication and needs hospitalization.

Hemodialysis provides a rapid and efficient way to remove waste products from the blood. It is also an excellent means to correct excessive fluid-overloaded states such as occur in heart failure.

Hemodialysis is not without side effects. Following a treatment, the patient normally feels weak and fatigued, sometimes even too tired to eat. Sudden drops in blood pressure may cause the patient to become weak, dizzy, and nauseated. Cardiac dysrhythmias and angina may occur. Fluid and electrolyte levels drop rapidly and cause the patient to feel lethargic and have muscle cramps. Patients are given large amounts of heparin, an anticoagulant used to keep the blood from clotting while it is in the artificial kidney; this may cause bleeding from the puncture sites, gastrointestinal tract, nose, or other sites if injury occurs.

See Box 37.12 Nursing Care of the Patient Receiving Hemodialysis.

Vascular Access. Hemodialysis requires a permanent way to access the bloodstream for blood removal and return to the body during dialysis. Typical vascular access options are a vascular access graft or an arteriovenous (AV) fistula. Grafts and fistulas are placed in the arm when possible. It is imperative that IV angiocaths are not placed in a cephalic or basilic vein in patients who may need grafts or fistulas in the future.

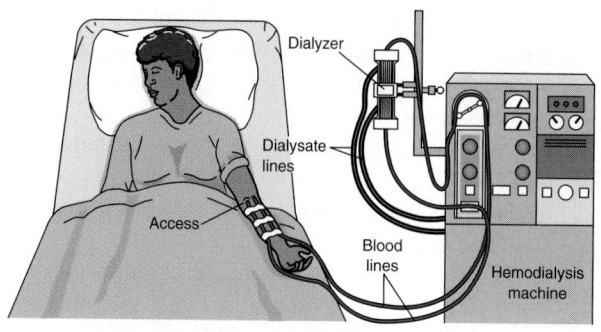

FIGURE 37.7 Hemodialyis.

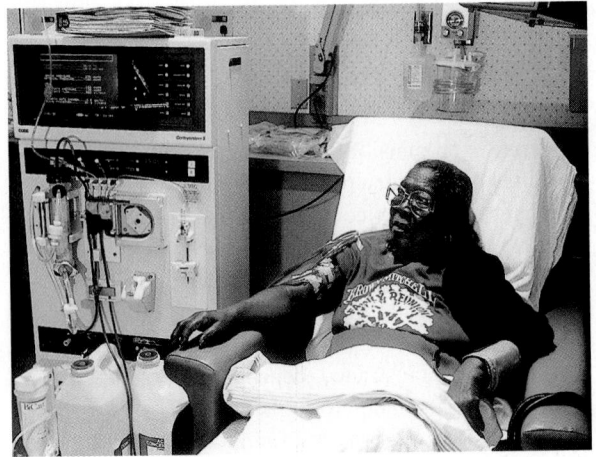

FIGURE 37.8 Patient undergoing hemodialysis at dialysis center.

A temporary access is used for patients requiring hemodialysis before a graft or fistula is placed or is usable. A central venous catheter with two or three ports is placed in the subclavian vein, the jugular vein, or the femoral vein for temporary access. Central catheters cannot be used long term due to the risk of infection. A newer access system is the LifeSite Hemodialysis Access system, which is an implantable port for blood access. Two systems are implanted for hemodialysis. No maturation time is required. This system can be used longer than temporary access catheters.

An arteriovenous graft (AV graft) uses a tube of synthetic material to attach to an artery and a vein. Needles are inserted into the graft to access the patient's blood. Traditional graft material is not self-sealing and requires time for tissue growth to serve as a plug for the hole that the needle makes before it can be used. This may take 1 to 2 weeks. The Vectra vascular access graft is self-sealing and does not require tissue growth so it can be used almost immediately after surgical implantation. This self-sealing property also decreases postdialysis bleeding time and reduces time required for the dialysis session.

An AV fistula is made by sewing a vein and artery together under the skin (Fig. 37.9). AV fistulas may take 2 to 4 months to mature. A temporary access device is usually needed until the fistula matures.

Vascular Access Care. Arteriovenous grafts and fistulas are regularly checked for patency by palpating for a thrill (a tremor) and auscultating for a bruit (swishing sound) at the site of the graft or fistula. Any decrease or cessation of bruit or thrill indicates occlusion. If a thrill or bruit is diminished or not present, the physician is notified immediately by the nurse. Special care of the access site must be taken because this is the patient's only way to eliminate waste products (Box 37.13 Care of Blood Access Graft or Fistula). It is important that the site be carefully monitored per institution policy to detect any clotting or problems at the site. Early detection of clotting allows the surgeon an opportunity to save the access by performing a declotting procedure rather than a total revision.

Box 37.12

Nursing Care of the Patient Receiving Hemodialysis

1. Consult with the physician about medications to hold before hemodialysis. Some medications, such as antihypertensives, can be harmful when they become effective during dialysis and can reduce blood pressure to dangerously low levels. Other medications are water soluble and will be dialyzed out of the body, and thus are not effective.
2. Ensure that the patient is weighed both before dialysis in the morning and after dialysis to document weight loss as a result of fluid removal.
3. If the patient has laboratory tests ordered and blood needs to be drawn, coordinate this process with the dialysis nurse, who can obtain the blood samples and save the patient unnecessary needle sticks.
4. Try to get morning care done early and breakfast given before dialysis. After dialysis, patients are often exhausted and need rest.
5. When the patient returns from dialysis, weigh the patient, assess the access site for bleeding, and make sure the vital signs are stable. Administer medications that were held if not contraindicated and vital signs are stable.
6. Protect the patient's dialysis access as outlined in Box 37.13 Care of Blood Access Graft or Fistula.

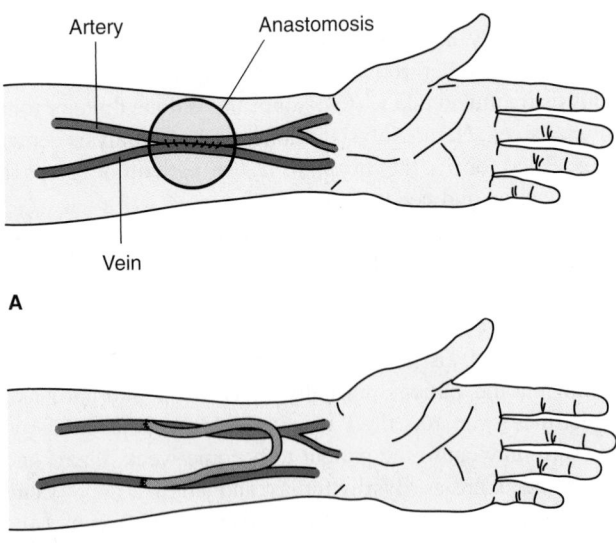

FIGURE 37.9 Hemodialysis access sites. (A) Arteriovenous fistula. (B) Arteriovenous graft.

Box 37.13

Care of Blood Access Graft or Fistula

Dialysis access sites should not be utilized for any purpose other than dialysis.

1. Watch for signs of bleeding or infection at the site.
2. Listen for a bruit at the site by placing the diaphragm of a stethoscope gently on the site. A bruit is a swishing sound made as the blood passes through the access site.
3. Gently palpate the site for a thrill, which is a buzzing or pulsing feeling that indicates good blood flow through the access site.
4. *Do not* take blood pressure, use a tourniquet, draw blood, or start any intravenous lines in the affected arm. Injections should be avoided if possible.
5. Many hospitals have the patient wear a red arm bracelet to signify that the arm should be protected. A sign above the bed may also be used.
6. Teach the patient to keep the site clean and not to bump or cut it.
7. Teach the patient not to lift heavy objects or carry a purse on the access arm.
8. Teach the patient to avoid wearing constrictive clothing or jewelry over the site.
9. Teach the patient to avoid prolonged bending or sleeping on the arm with an access.
10. Notify the physician if signs of bleeding, reduced circulation, or infection occur in the access extremity: coldness, numbness, weakness, redness, fever, drainage, or swelling.

Postoperative Care. Initially, neurovascular checks are performed hourly for vascular surgery. Neurovascular checks include extremity movement and sensation, presence of numbness or tingling, pulses, temperature, color, and capillary refill (less than 3 seconds normally). Peripheral pulses are palpated to feel the thrill and auscultated to hear the bruit. If a pulse is absent or weak or the extremity is cool or dusky, the physician is notified immediately. Dressings or incisions are checked, and any drainage, hematoma, or infection development is documented and reported as needed. Vascular surgery pain is usually mild. Severe pain may indicate an occlusion of the graft. Arteriovenous grafts can cause distal ischemia or "steal syndrome" because too much of the arterial blood is being "stolen" from the distal extremity. This is usually seen postoperatively and may require surgical correction to restore blood flow to the extremity.

Blood pressure readings and IVs should not be done in the extremity in which the access is placed. The extremity with the vascular access should be elevated postoperatively. Range of motion exercises should be encouraged. Patients are taught care of the access (see Box 37.13).

PERITONEAL DIALYSIS. Peritoneal dialysis provides continuous dialysis treatment and is done by the patient or family in the home. The peritoneal membrane is used as a semipermeable membrane across which excess wastes and fluids move from blood in peritoneal vessels into a dialysate solution that has been instilled into the peritoneal cavity. A peritoneal catheter is placed into the patient's peritoneal space between the two layers of the peritoneum below the waistline. This catheter is used to perform an exchange. The exchange process has three steps: filling, dwell time, and draining.

The fill step involves instilling a bag of sterile dialyzing solution (dialysate) into the patient's peritoneal cavity through the catheter. The amount of solution is usually 1500 to 2000 mL. The solution is left to dwell in the abdomen for several hours, allowing time for the waste products from the blood to pass through the peritoneal membrane into the dialysate solution (Fig. 37.10).

The solution is then drained out of the body and discarded. This process is repeated three or four times a day and is continuous for the patient. Several different treatment plans use this exchange process; the treatment plan that best suits the patient's needs is determined by the patient and the dialysis team.

Continuous ambulatory peritoneal dialysis (CAPD) is the most commonly used treatment plan. Usually three exchanges are done during the day and one before bedtime. Other treatment plans allow for the use of a computerized machine called a cycler to regulate the exchanges during sleeping hours. Sometimes medications are added to the dialyzing solutions, such as heparin to prevent clotting of the catheter, insulin for the patient with diabetes, or antibiotics if there is infection.

Patient and family education is extremely important for peritoneal dialysis to be successful. The patient must be taught and be able to demonstrate that he or she is able to do a successful exchange. Sterile technique while performing the exchanges is imperative and the exchanges should be done in a clean environment. A major complication is peritonitis (infection of the peritoneum), which can be life threatening. The major cause of peritonitis is poor technique when connecting the bag of dialyzing solution to the peritoneal catheter. The first sign of peritonitis is usually abdominal pain. Refer to Chapter 34 for additional signs and symptoms of peritonitis. If any symptoms of peritonitis occur, the patient must contact the physician immediately, so that antibiotic treatment can begin. The patient should be taught to care for the exit site (the site where the

---

peritoneal dialysis: peritoneal—peritoneum + dialysis— passage of a solution through a membrane

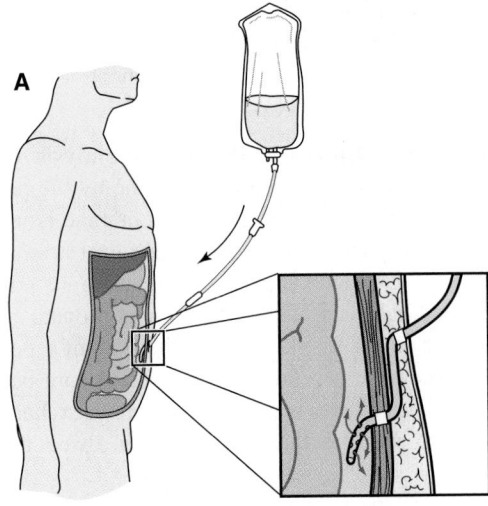

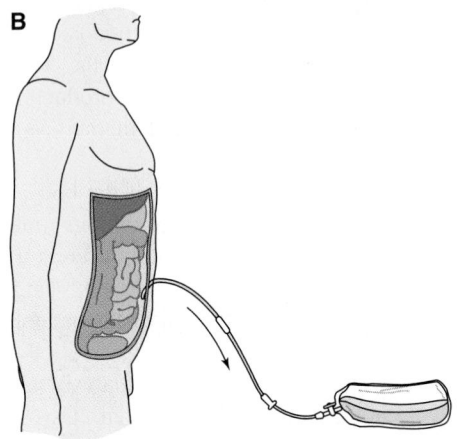

FIGURE 37.10 *(A)* Peritoneal dialysis works inside the body. Dialysis solution flows through a tube into the abdominal cavity, where it collects waste products from the blood. *(B)* Periodically the used dialysis solution is drained from the abdominal cavity, carrying away waste products and excess water from the blood.

LEARNING TIP

Differences between hemodialysis (HD), peritoneal dialysis (PD), and continuous renal replacement therapy (CRRT) include the following:

- *Patient Access:* HD requires vascular access either temporary (acute renal failure) or permanent surgical graft or fistula (chronic renal failure). PD requires insertion of a catheter into the peritoneal cavity. CRRT requires temporary vascular access such as a central line.
- *Equipment:* HD requires a specialized complex dialyzer. PD and CRRT do not require the specialized dialyzer, although machines are available for these therapies.
- *Training:* HD requires a skilled HD nurse. CRRT can be done by a non–HD nurse in a critical care setting. PD can be done by the patient.
- *Timing:* HD is intermittent. PD and CRRT are continuous.
- *Solute removal:* HD and PD use the principles of osmosis and diffusion, which require a dialysate solution. CRRT uses convection, so no dialysate is needed.
- *Cardiovascular effects:* HD may cause hypotension, which is a risk in the unstable patient. PD and CRRT have few cardiovascular effects. CRRT can be used on the unstable patient.

catheter comes out of the abdomen) and the need to inspect both the site and the dialysate solution for any signs of infection.

Dietary education is also important. A dietitian can assist the patient in making appropriate choices for adequate calories, protein, and potassium intake. The peritoneal dialysis patient generally has fewer dietary and fluid restrictions than the patient on hemodialysis because dialysis is continuous and maintains serum waste levels. Proteins are lost through the peritoneal membrane into the dialysate fluid, so increased dietary protein is needed. This loss increases with peritonitis, which further increases permeability.

Kidney Transplantation

Kidney transplantation is another treatment for renal failure. Kidney transplantation is extremely successful. An advantage of transplant compared to dialysis is that it reverses many of the physiological changes noted with renal failure. The patient is also not dependent upon dialysis and dietary restrictions.

A kidney transplant is a procedure in which a donor kidney is placed in the abdomen of a patient with chronic renal failure (Fig. 37.11). This healthy transplanted kidney functions as a normal functioning kidney does. The donated kidney can come from a family member, a living, non-related donor, or a cadaver donor. Tissue and blood types must match so that the body's immune system does not reject the donated kidney. Patients receive special drugs to help prevent rejection; these drugs must be taken for the rest of the patient's life. Sometimes even with these drugs, the body rejects the kidney and the patient needs to go back on dialysis (Box 37.14 Cultural Considerations and Box 37.15

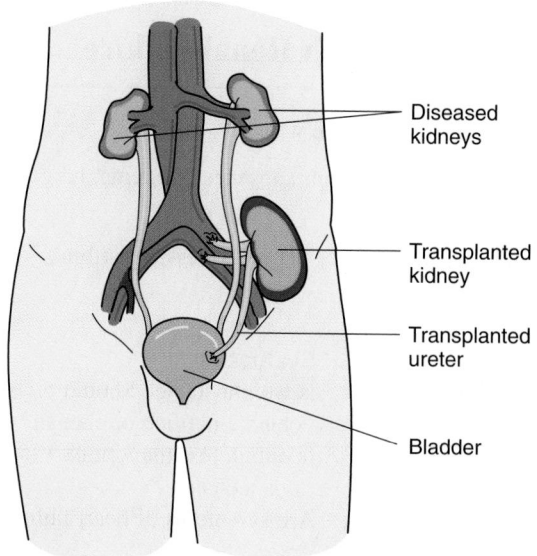

FIGURE 37.11 A transplanted kidney is placed in the abdomen. The patient's kidneys are usually left in place.

Patient Perspective). For more information, visit the Transplant Society at www.a-o-t-a.org.

Nursing Process for the Patient with Renal Failure

Assessment/Data Collection

Renal failure progressively affects all body systems. There may be fewer effects in ARF if it is short term and there is not time for some effects to develop. In chronic renal failure,

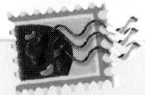

Box 37.14

Cultural Considerations

Renal Function and Assessment

Because many Vietnamese people believe that the body must be kept intact, even after death, they may object to removal of body parts or organ donation.

Jewish law views organ transplantation from the recipient, the living donor, the cadaver donor, and the dying donor differently. If the recipient's life can be prolonged without considerable risk, transplant is ordained. For a living donor to be approved, the risk to the life of the donor must be considered. One is not obligated to donate a part of himself or herself unless the risk is small. The use of a cadaver for transplant is usually approved if it is saving a life. The nurse may need to assist the Jewish patient to contact a rabbi when making a decision regarding organ donation or transplantation.

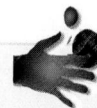

Box 37.15

Patient Perspective

Kidney Transplantation: Pat

My experience with a kidney transplant spans three decades, but my overall renal illness experience also spans several years of illness and dialysis before the transplant. I think the biggest changes I have seen over the years are the involvement of patients in their own care options, as well as increased technical advances that allow transplantation to be much more successful. Some of the feelings experienced before transplantation are fear, uncertainty, and—if awaiting a donor—the guilt of knowing someone must die before you can live.

Thirty years ago there were no support groups and no one to talk to except family and doctors. Today, there are many support mechanisms in place for patients and families both before and after transplantation. As a nurse, you can help patients by knowing these support resources for referral. After a transplant, it is wonderful to feel better, almost immediately. However, as wonderful as transplantation is, the side effects of the antirejection medications may be immediately felt, while other problems take years to develop. Unfortunately, no patients escape the side effects of the medications. I have had breast cancer, osteoarthritis, cataracts, ulcers, skin cancer, anemia, weight gain, and other side effects of prednisone and Imuran (azathioprine). However, I can assure you that this is much better than the alternative of dialysis.

more effects are seen since the disease has time to progress. Data should be collected for signs and symptoms in all body systems. Family history of renal disease and patient history of health problems such as hypertension, diabetes, systemic erythematous lupus, or urinary disorders are noted in the history. Also noted are medications the patient takes as they may be nephrotoxic and require adjustments. Recent changes in weight are documented.

Signs and symptoms vary depending on the severity of renal failure and cause. Common signs are hypertension, abnormal laboratory values (creatinine, BUN), or changes in urine. See signs and symptoms section for other effects of renal failure.

Nursing Diagnosis, Planning, Intervention, and Evaluation

See Box 37.16 Nursing Care Plan for the Patient with Renal Failure for nursing care.

Box 37.16   NURSING CARE PLAN **for the Patient with Renal Failure**

Nursing Diagnosis: Excess fluid volume related to kidney's inability to excrete water

Expected Outcomes Fluid volume will be stable as evidenced by stable weight, absence of edema, lung sounds clear, and blood pressure within patient's normal parameters.

Evaluation of Outcomes Is weight stable? Is edema absent? Are lungs clear? Is blood pressure within patient's normal parameters?

Nursing Interventions	Rationale	Evaluation
Monitor weight daily at same time; report gain of greater than 2 pounds.	Those retaining fluid will have weight gain.	Is weight stable? Should physician be notified of change?
Monitor intake and output.	This monitors degree of fluid retention.	Is output less than intake? Is this a change?
Monitor and report shortness of breath, tachycardia, crackles in lungs, frothy sputum, heart irregularities, hypotension, cold clammy skin.	These are symptoms of heart failure that may accompany fluid overload.	Are symptoms of heart failure present?
Watch for new onset of jugular vein distention with patient's head raised to 30- to 45-degree angle.	Fluid overload causes right-sided heart failure resulting in distended jugular veins.	Are jugular veins distended? Is this a new finding?
Monitor vital signs, including orthostatic blood pressure.	Blood pressure changes reflect fluid volume.	Is blood pressure increased?
Monitor for edema.	Edema is a symptom of fluid overload.	Is edema present? Is this a change?
Monitor activity tolerance.	Reduced activity tolerance may indicate heart failure related to fluid retention.	Is patient's tolerance of activity stable? Worsening?
Monitor serum protein and albumin levels.	Low serum protein and albumin levels contribute to edema.	Are levels within normal limits?
Maintain sodium and fluid restrictions (often 600 mL plus the previous day's urine output) as ordered. Develop a plan with specific allotted amounts of fluid at each meal and for medications. Teach patient importance of each.	For those on dialysis, fluid intake is adjusted so that weight gains are no more than 1–3 kg between dialysis sessions.	Does patient understand and maintain sodium and fluid restriction?

Nursing Diagnosis: Impaired skin integrity related to dryness, excess fluid, crystal deposits

Expected Outcomes Patient will maintain intact skin.

Evaluation of Outcomes Does patient report no itching or dryness? Is patient's skin intact?

Interventions	Rationale	Evaluation
Observe skin for open areas and signs of infection.	Detects early signs of problems.	Is skin intact?
Bathe with tepid water, oils, or oatmeal.	Bathe regularly to reduce crystals with nondrying items to reduce itching and dryness and promote comfort.	Does patient report no itching or skin dryness?
Apply lotion to skin after bathing.	Lotion is used for itching to reduce dry skin.	Is skin dry?

Nursing Diagnosis: Activity intolerance related to anemia secondary to impaired synthesis of erythropoietin by the kidneys

Expected Outcomes Patient will be able to perform activities important to him or her.

Evaluation of Outcomes Does patient state satisfaction with level of activity tolerance?

Interventions	Rationale	Evaluation
Assess for pale mucous membranes and skin color, dyspnea, chest pain.	These are signs and symptoms of anemia.	Does patient exhibit symptoms of anemia?
Monitor hemoglobin (Hgb), hematocrit (Hct).	Low hemoglobin and hematocrit indicate anemia.	Are Hgb and Hct within normal limits?
Watch for signs of bleeding.	Bleeding will worsen anemia.	Are signs of bleeding present?
Administer erythropoietin as ordered. Assist with blood transfusion as necessary.	Erythropoietin stimulates production of red blood cells by bone marrow.	Are Hgb and Hct rising with use of erythropoietin?
Have patient space activities with rest periods.	Rest periods decrease demand for oxygen.	Is patient able to tolerate activities with rest periods?

Nursing Diagnosis: Risk for injury related to bleeding tendency from platelet dysfunction and use of heparin during dialysis, and tendency for gastrointestinal bleeding

Expected Outcomes Patient will not experience bleeding. If bleeding occurs, it will be recognized and stopped quickly.

Evaluation of Outcomes Are signs and symptoms of bleeding absent or recognized and reported quickly?

Interventions	Rationale	Evaluation
Observe for and report blood in stool or emesis, easy bruising, bleeding from mucous membranes or puncture sites and report immediately if present.	Bleeding must be recognized quickly to prevent complications.	Does patient exhibit signs of bleeding?
Monitor Hgb, Hct, clotting studies, and platelets and report results.	Declining Hgb and Hct indicate blood loss.	Are lab results stable?
	Declining platelet count or rising clotting times indicate increased risk for bleeding.	Are vital signs stable?
Monitor vital signs.	Falling blood pressure and rising pulse may indicate volume deficit from bleeding.	Can medications be given by another route?
Avoid giving injections if possible.	Injections can cause bleeding into tissue.	Does pressure stop bleeding?
If bleeding, apply gentle pressure to site if possible.	Pressure promotes hemostasis.	
Teach patient to prevent injury to self and symptoms of bleeding to report.	Injury can cause bleeding. Understanding of symptoms of bleeding encourages early reporting.	Does patient verbalize understanding of instruction?
Protect patient from injury if confusion or seizures occur.	Waste product accumulation or hyponatremia puts patient at risk of altered mental status or seizures.	Does patient require protection such as seizure precautions? Is patient free from injury?

(Continued on following page)

Box 37.16   NURSING CARE PLAN **for the Patient with Renal Failure** *(Cont'd)*

Nursing Diagnosis: Risk for infection related to impaired immune system function

Expected Outcomes Patient will not develop infection as evidenced by WBCs and temperature within normal limits, no signs and symptoms of infection.

Evaluation of Outcomes Are WBCs and temperature within normal limits?

Interventions	Rationale	Evaluation
Monitor for signs and symptoms of infection and report promptly to physician.	Early recognition of infection and prompt treatment help prevent complications.	Does patient exhibit symptoms of infection?
Protect patient from any source of infection, including infected roommates, visitors, or nursing staff.	Exposure to pathogens increases risk for infection.	Does anyone in contact with the patient have an infection?
Maintain skin integrity.	Intact skin protects against infection.	Is skin intact?
Staff and patient practice good handwashing technique.	Handwashing helps control spread of infection.	Is good handwashing being practiced?
Culture any suspected site of infection as ordered by physician.	A culture identifies pathogens and guides treatment.	Is a culture necessary?
Consult with physician about influenza and pneumonia vaccines.	Patients with impaired immune function are at risk for influenza and pneumonia.	Has the patient been vaccinated?
Teach patient and family signs and symptoms of infection to report to physician.	Early reporting of symptoms allows for prompt initiation of treatment.	Do patient and family verbalize understanding of symptoms to report?

Nursing Diagnosis: Imbalanced nutrition, less than body requirements related to restricted diet, anorexia, nausea, and vomiting, and stomatitis secondary to effect of excessive urea on the gastrointestinal system

Expected Outcomes Patient will maintain ideal weight. Serum protein and albumin levels are within normal limits.

Evaluation of Outcomes Are weight and lab values at desired levels?

Interventions	Rationale	Evaluation
Monitor weekly weight and serum protein and albumin levels.	Weight and laboratory results provide information about nutrition status.	Are weight and laboratory values stable?
Consult dietician for low-protein diet planning and teaching.	Low-protein diets decrease formation of waste products (urea, creatinine).	Does patient understand low-protein diet?
Initiate a calorie count—consult dietitian for assistance.	A calorie count can provide information about the adequacy of the patient's diet.	Is patient receiving adequate calories?
Provide frequent oral care.	Oral care enhances appetite and reduces urine taste in mouth.	Does oral care enhance appetite?
Offer frequent small feedings and dietary supplements.	Smaller feedings are better tolerated and reduce risk of nausea.	Does patient tolerate small feedings?
Offer medications ordered for nausea before meals.	Nausea reduces appetite and must be controlled.	Are antiemetics effective?
Ensure bowel movement daily or according to patient's usual pattern.	Constipation can interfere with appetite.	Are patient's bowels functioning normally for him or her?

CRITICAL THINKING

Mrs. Jackson

■ Mrs. Jackson is a single, 56-year-old woman with a 20-year history of type 1 diabetes, hypertension, hyperlipidemia, chronic anemia, and a total knee replacement. She has been diagnosed with chronic renal failure. She was admitted to a medical unit for treatment of shortness of breath and renal failure which will include hemodialysis. She has had increasing shortness of breath, has pitting edema, urine output of about 375 mL/day, and is having premature ventricular contractions (PVCs) as seen on the cardiac monitor. Her admitting laboratory values are: Na 131, K 6, Cl 97, Ca 10, iron (Fe) 64, WBC 4000, RBC 3.12, Hgb 10.1, Hct 32, creatinine 7, BUN 30. Her blood glucose level yesterday was: 7 a.m. 154 mg/dL, noon 122 mg/dL, 5 p.m. 188 mg/dL. She has sliding-scale insulin ordered. She is

having an echocardiogram and chest x-ray done. She is having a two-tailed subclavian catheter placed for blood access. She is withdrawn and quiet.
1. What would be the first thing the nurse would address after getting the report?
2. What do her physical symptoms indicate and the laboratory values reflect?
3. What should the nurse say to Mrs. Jackson related to her withdrawn behavior?
4. What should the nurse identify related to Mrs. Jackson's understanding of self-care?
5. What teaching is needed for the diagnostic tests?
6. What care is required for the blood access?
7. What type of insulin is used for sliding-scale insulin coverage? Why?

Suggested answers at end of chapter.

REVIEW QUESTIONS

Multiple response item. Select all that apply.
1. When teaching a patient about preventing urinary tract infections, which of the following information should the nurse include?
   a. Void frequently.
   b. Drink large amounts of citrus juices.
   c. Eat large amounts of vegetables.
   d. Wash the perineum every 8 hours.
   e. Void after sexual intercourse.

2. A patient is admitted to the hospital with a diagnosis of a kidney stone. Which of the following interventions should be included in the plan of care?
   a. Restrict fluids.
   b. Strain all urine.
   c. Increase calcium intake.
   d. Maintain bedrest.

3. The nurse is taking a history on a patient with a diagnosis of bladder cancer. Which of the following would the nurse expect to find in the patient's history?
   a. Tobacco use
   b. Vegetarian diet
   c. Caffeine use
   d. Alcohol use

4. While changing the pouch at the stoma site of an ileal conduit, the nurse notes the stoma is constantly spilling urine. Which of the following actions should the nurse take?
   a. Notify the physician of the constant spillage.
   b. Continue changing the pouch.

   c. Remove the overflow of urine with a straight catheter.
   d. Irrigate the stoma with a sterile solution of normal saline.

5. The nurse is caring for a patient with glomerulonephritis. Which of the following interventions would the nurse recommend be included in the patient's plan of care?
   a. Increase fluid intake.
   b. Decrease sodium intake.
   c. Increase potassium intake.
   d. Decrease carbohydrate intake.

6. The nurse is planning a teaching session for a patient with diabetic nephropathy. Which of these should the nurse include in the teaching plan to aid in slowing the progress of the disease?
   a. Increase protein in diet.
   b. Restrict protein in diet.
   c. Increase potassium intake.
   d. Decrease potassium intake.

7. The nurse is caring for a postoperative patient who is receiving 0.9% normal saline IV at 125 mL/hour, morphine for pain control, and garamycin IVPB every 8 hours for 24 hours. The patient is allergic to iodine. Morning labs are WBC 8500, Hgb 12.4 g/dL, creatinine 2.2 mg/dL. Which of these findings is a priority for the nurse to report to the RN?
   a. WBC
   b. IV rate of 125 mL/hour

c. Allergies

d. Creatinine level

8. A patient with renal failure who is on hemodialysis asks for a snack in the afternoon. His potassium level remains high. Which of the following foods would be contraindicated?

a. Banana

b. Gelatin dessert

c. Clear carbonated beverage

d. Cranberry juice

9. A patient is returning to the medical unit after a dialysis session. The nurse notes bleeding from the patient's vascular access in the left arm. Which of the following is the nurse's first action?

a. Call the physician.

b. Notify the dialysis nurse.

c. Apply pressure to site.

d. Take patient's blood pressure.

10. The nurse is assessing a patient who has had a new right AV fistula created. How is the patency of the fistula checked?

a. Auscultate the left brachial pulse.

b. Auscultate and palpate the right radial pulse.

c. Measure blood pressure in the right arm.

d. Palpate for thrill and auscultate bruit over the fistula.

11. A patient is to receive 1600 mg of Renagel (sevelamer) orally with meals. Renagel 400-mg tables are available. How many tablets should the nurse give?

_____ tablets

Unit Nine Bibliography

1. Ackley, B, and Ladwig, G: Nursing Diagnosis Handbook: A Guide To Planning Care, ed 5. Mosby, St Louis, 2005.
2. Burrows-Hudson, S: Chronic kidney disease: an overview. AJN 105:40–49, 2005.
3. Cannon, J. Recognizing chronic renal failure…..the sooner the better. Nursing 2004 34:50–53, 2004.
4. Carpenito-Moyet, L: Handbook of Nursing Diagnosis. Lippincott Williams & Wilkins. New York, 2006.
5. Castner, D, and Douglas, C: Now onstage: chronic kidney disease. Nursing 2005 35:58–64, 2005.
6. Chertow, GM, Raggi, P, McCarthy, JT, et al: The effects of sevelamer and calcium acetate on proxies of atherosclerotic and arteriosclerotic vascular disease in hemodialysis patients. Am J Nephrol 23:307–314, 2003.
7. Coburn, S, and Mitchell, S: Acute Renal Failure. AJN 102(Suppl) 2002.
8. Daniel, J, Chantrel, R, Offner, M, et al: Comparison of cystatin C, creatinine, and creatinine clearance vs. GFR for detection of renal failure in renal transplant patients. Renal Failure 26:253–257, 2004.
9. Goldenberg, I, and Matetzky, S: Nephropathy induced contrast media: pathogenesis, risk factors, and preventive strategies. Can Med Assoc J 172:1461–1471, 2005.
10. Goldrick, B: Emerging infections. AJN 105:31–34, 2005.
11. Gray, M: Assessment and management of urinary incontinence. Nurse Practitioner 30:33–43, 2005.
12. Gulanick, M, Klopp, A, Myers, J, and Puzas, M: (2003). Nursing Care Plans Mosby. St. Lewis.
13. Hawkins, C, and Zazworsky, D. Self-management of chronic kidney disease. AJN 105:40–48, 2003.
14. Holcomb, S: Evaluating chronic kidney disease risk. Nurse Practitioner 30:12–25, 2005.
15. Johnson, D: Evidence based guide to slowing the progression of early renal insufficiency. Intern Med J 34:50–57, 2004.
16. Johnson, C, Levey, A, Coresh, J, et al: clinical practice guidelines for chronic kidney disease in adults: Part I. Glomerular filtration rate, proteinuria, and other markers. Am Fam Physician 70:869–876, 2004.
17. Johnson, C, Levey, A, Coresh, J, et al: Clinical practice guidelines for chronic kidney disease in adults: Part II. Glomerular filtration rate, proteinuria, and other markers. Am Fam Physician 70:1091–1097, 2004.
18. Legg, V: Complications of chronic kidney disease. AJN 105: 40–48, 2005.
19. Lewis, S, Heitkemper, M, and Dirksen, S: Medical-Surgical Nursing Assessment and Management of Clinical Problems. Mosby, St Louis, 2004.
20. Lutz, CA, and Przytulski, KR: Nutrition and Diet Therapy, ed. 3. F.A. Davis, Philadelphia, 2005.
21. Lynch, DM: Cranberry for prevention of urinary tract infections. Am Fam Physician 11:2175, 2004.
22. Madigan, E, and Felber, N: Care of Patients with long term indwelling urinary catheters. Online Journal of Issues in Nursing 8:130,2003. Downloaded : 7/11/05 from http:// Weblinks2.Epnet.Com/Delivery/Printsave.Asp?Tb=0&_ Ug=Sid+F2246be-0d4b-4fbb.
23. McCance KL, and Huether, SE: Pathophysiology, ed. 4. The Biologic Basis for Disease in Adults and Children. Mosby, St. Louis, 2001.
24. Motwani, B, and Khayr, W: Staphylococcus saprophyticus urinary tract infection in men. Infect Dis Clin Pract 12:341–342, 2004.
25. Newman, D: Stress urinary incontinence in women. AJN 103:46–55, 2003.
26. Newman, DK, Gaines, T, Snare, E: Innovation in bladder assessment: use of technology in extended care. J Gerontol Nurs 31:33–41, 2005.
27. Neyhart, C: The patient with progressive renal insufficiency and a failing renal transplant: a unique practice challenge. Nephrol Nurs J 29:227–242, 2002.
28. Peterson, A, and Webster, G: Management of urethral stricture disease: developing options for surgical intervention. Indian J Surg 67:971–976, 2004.
29. Ramakrishnan, K, and Scheid DC: Diagnosis and management of acute pyelonephritis in adults.Am J Fam Physician 71:933–942, 2005.
30. Saad, T, and Vesely, T: Venous access for patients with chronic kidney disease. J Vasc Interven Radiol 15: 1041–1045, 2004.
31. Saint, S: How to prevent urinary catheter-related infections in the critically ill: recognizing when indwelling devices must be used and when they should not. J Crit Ill 15:419–423, 2000.
32. Schaeffer, AJ: What do we know about the urinary tract infection-prone individual? J Infect Dis 183(Suppl 1):S66, 2001.
33. Schonder, K: The dangers of over-the-counter medications in kidney disease. Nephrology Incite. Issue 18. Downloaded 8/12/05 from http://Ikidney.Com/Ikidney/Infocenter/ Nephrologyincite/Archive/Otcmedstoavoid.

34. Sheffield, J, and Cunningham, FG: Urinary tract infection in women. Obstet Gynecol 106:1085–1092, 2005.
35. Simerville, J, Maxted,W, and Pahira, J: Urinalysis: a comprehensive review. Am Fam Physician 71:1153–1162, 2005.
36. Simmons Holcomb, S: Keeping kidney function flowing. Nursing Made Incredibly Easy 2:30–41, 2004.
37. Simmons Holcomb, S: Evaluating chronic kidney disease risk. Nurse Practitioner 30:12–25, 2005.
38. Small, K, and McMullen, M: When clear becomes cloudy. AJN 105:72aa–72gg, 2005.
39. Snively, C, and Gutierrez, C: Chronic kidney disease: prevention and treatment of common complications. Am Fam Physician 70:1921–1928, 2004.
40. Specht, J: 9 Myths of incontinence in older adults. AJN 105:58–67, 2005.
41. Stevens, E: Bladder ultrasound: avoiding unnecessary catheterizations. Medsurg Nurs 14:249–253, 2005.
42. Tambyah, PA, and Maki, DG: Catheter-associated urinary tract infection is rarely symptomatic. Arch Intern Med 160:678–682, 2000.
43. Toughill, E: Bladder matters: indwelling urinary catheters. AJN 105:35, 2005.
44. Wallace, M, and Sadovsky, R: What physicians are forgetting about urinalysis. Cortlandt Forum March:27–37, 2005.
45. Ward, K: Kidneys, don't fail me now! Nursing Made Incredibly Easy 3:18–26, 2005.
46. Wells, C: Optimizing nutrition in patients with chronic kidney disease. Nephrol Nurs J 30:637.648, 2003.
47. Wilson, LA: Urinalysis. Nurs Stand 19:51–54, 2005.

SUGGESTED ANSWERS TO

CRITICAL THINKING

■ *Mrs. Milan*

1. Sexual intercourse can be a predisposing factor to UTI, especially if the patient does not urinate after intercourse.
2. Mrs. Milan should be cautioned to always urinate after intercourse. See also Box 37.2 Patient Teaching to Prevent Urinary Tract Infection.
3. The urinalysis will show WBCs, bacteria, RBCs, and positive nitrites.
4. Teaching should include the need to take all of the medication until it is gone even if she feels better. The reason for this is to ensure the infection is completely resolved so it does not return due to some remaining bacteria. She should return for a urine culture after the therapy is complete.

■ *Mr. Stevens*

1. Weight, intake and output, blood pressure, and laboratory tests should be assessed as part of the morning evaluation.
2. BUN, serum creatinine, and potassium levels should also be checked.
3. Mr. Stevens should be taught that he needs to take antihypertensive medications, keep his follow-up visits to his physician, follow a low-sodium diet, and restrict fluids if ordered.

■ *Mrs. Jackson*

1. Collect data related to her breathing and respiratory status first. Then address the cardiovascular system to see how she is tolerating the dysrhythmia. Obtain Mrs. Jackson's weight and intake and output to monitor fluid balance.
2. Shortness of breath and pitting edema related to fluid overload; urine output 375 mL/day is due to renal failure; PVCs are due to elevated K. Na is low due to dilutional effect of excess fluid. K is retained due to renal failure. WBC low due to renal failure. RBC, Hgb, Hct low due to anemia from renal failure. Creatinine and BUN are not excreted and are elevated due to renal failure. Blood glucose is elevated due to diabetes.
3. Therapeutic conversation suggestions: "Mrs. Jackson, would you like to talk about your diagnosis?" "How do you feel about your diagnosis?" "Do you have questions or concerns?" "What are your usual coping methods?" Provide explanations for procedures and interventions.
4. Determine Mrs. Jackson's understanding of what renal failure is, how it is treated, how to follow the renal diet and fluid restrictions, and the action and importance of medications. Identify barriers to self-care and her support systems.
5. Teaching includes that the chest x-ray and echocardiogram require no preparation and are not painful.
6. A two-tail subclavian blood access is dedicated for hemodialysis. It is not used for any other purpose. Monitoring includes observing the site for signs of infection—redness, warmth, swelling, tenderness, drainage, and fever.
7. Regular insulin because it is rapid acting. Sliding-scale insulin is used to treat a current blood glucose. A rapid-acting insulin will affect a current blood glucose so only rapid-acting insulin is used.

unit TEN

UNDERSTANDING THE ENDOCRINE SYSTEM

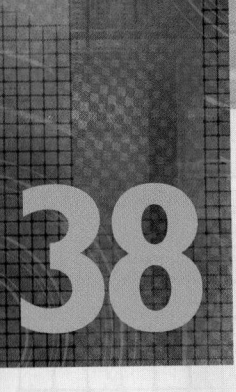

38

Endocrine System Function and Assessment

PAULA D. HOPPER AND
JANICE L. BRADFORD

KEY TERMS

affect (AF-feckt)
exophthalmos (EKS-off-THAL-mus)

QUESTIONS TO GUIDE YOUR READING

1. What are the glands of the endocrine system?

2. What is the function of each of the hormones in the endocrine system?

3. What are the effects of aging on endocrine system function?

4. What data should you collect when caring for a patient with a disorder of the endocrine system?

5. What nursing care should you provide for patients undergoing testing for an endocrine disorder?

NORMAL ANATOMY AND PHYSIOLOGY

The endocrine system consists of the endocrine (ductless) glands, which secrete chemicals called hormones. Unlike other organ systems, the glands of the endocrine system are anatomically separate (Fig. 38.1). Their hormones are involved in the composition and volume of interstitial fluid; all aspects of metabolism, energy balance, and growth/development; contraction of smooth and cardiac muscle; glandular secretion; reproduction; and the establishment of circadian rhythms. Each hormone is secreted in response to a particular and specific stimulus, is circulated by the blood throughout the body, and exerts its effects on certain target tissues that have receptors for that hormone. The effects of the hormone often reverse the stimulus and ultimately lead to decreased secretion of the hormone. This is called a negative feedback system; many hormone secretions are regulated this way. Some hormones are secreted in response to hormones from other endocrine glands.

Pituitary Gland

The pituitary gland, called the hypophysis, is suspended by a short stalk from the hypothalamus in the brain. The two major regions are the posterior pituitary (neurohypophysis) and anterior pituitary (adenohypophysis).

Posterior Pituitary Gland

The posterior pituitary gland stores antidiuretic hormone (ADH; sometimes called vasopressin) and oxytocin, which are actually produced by the hypothalamus. Their release is stimulated by nerve impulses from the hypothalamus.

Antidiuretic hormone increases the amount of water reabsorbed by the kidney tubules, which decreases urinary output. The water is reabsorbed back into the blood, thereby maintaining normal blood volume and normal blood pressure. The stimulus for secretion of ADH is a decrease in the water content of the body—that is, dehydration. When body water is lost and not replaced, specialized cells in the hypothalamus called osmoreceptors detect the elevated blood osmotic pressure (increased concentration) and transmit impulses to the posterior pituitary to secrete ADH to prevent

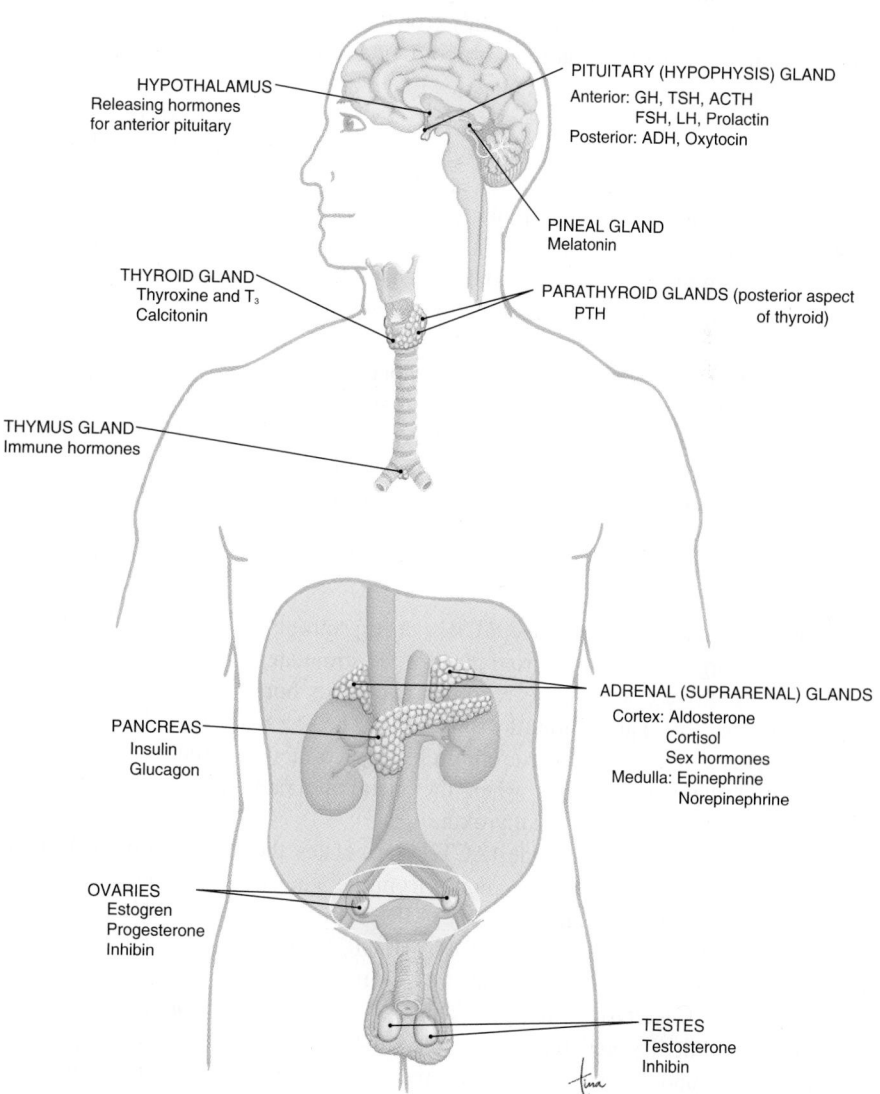

FIGURE 38.1 Glands of the endocrine system. *(From Scanlon, V., and Sanders, T: Essentials of Anatomy and Physiology, ed. 5. F.A. Davis, Philadelphia, 2007, with permission.)*

the further loss of water in urine. In cases of great fluid loss, as in severe hemorrhage, the large amount of ADH secreted is especially important because it causes arteriole vasoconstriction, which increases blood pressure to homeostatic levels.

Oxytocin causes contraction of the smooth muscle in the uterus and mammary glands. At the end of pregnancy, stretching of the cervix generates sensory impulses to the hypothalamus, which then transmits impulses to the posterior pituitary for the release of oxytocin. Oxytocin causes strong contractions of the myometrium to bring about delivery of the baby and the placenta. This is an example of a positive feedback mechanism. During breastfeeding, the sucking of the baby generates sensory impulses from the mother's nipple to the hypothalamus. The subsequent release of oxytocin causes contraction of the smooth muscle cells around the mammary ducts. This release of milk is called milk ejection (or letdown).

Anterior Pituitary Gland

The anterior pituitary gland secretes its hormones in response to releasing hormones from the hypothalamus. The anterior pituitary synthesizes and secretes growth hormone, thyroid-stimulating hormone, adrenocorticotropic hormone, prolactin, follicle-stimulating hormone, and luteinizing hormone.

Growth hormone (GH, or somatotropin) increases cell division in those tissues capable of mitosis, which is one of the ways it is involved in growth. It also increases the transport of amino acids into cells and their use in protein synthesis. Growth hormone also increases the release of fat from adipose tissue and the use of fats for energy production; this is important even after growth in height has ceased. The secretion of GH is regulated by growth hormone–releasing hormone (GHRH) and by growth hormone–inhibiting hormone (GHIH, or somatostatin), both from the hypothalamus. GHRH is produced during hypoglycemia or when there is a high blood level of amino acids (to be turned into protein). GHIH is secreted during hyperglycemia, when carbohydrates are available for energy production and the mobilization of fat is not necessary.

Thyroid-stimulating hormone (TSH, or thyrotropin) has only one target organ: the thyroid gland. TSH stimulates growth of the thyroid and the secretion of two of its hormones, thyroxine (T_4) and triiodothyronine (T_3). The secretion of TSH is stimulated by thyrotropin-releasing hormone (TRH) from the hypothalamus when the metabolic rate decreases and there is a need for thyroxine.

Adrenocorticotropic hormone (ACTH) stimulates the secretion of cortisol and related hormones from the adrenal cortex. Corticotropin-releasing hormone (CRH) from the hypothalamus stimulates the release of ACTH. CRH is produced during any type of physiological stress situation, such as injury, disease, exercise, or hypoglycemia.

Prolactin initiates and maintains milk production by the mammary glands. The hypothalamus produces both prolactin-releasing hormone (PRH) and prolactin-inhibiting hormone (PIH). Prolactin is not secreted in high enough levels to produce milk until pregnancy is over and the levels of estrogen and progesterone (from the placenta) have dropped. The action of a nursing infant reduces PIH, thus the prolactin level rises.

Follicle-stimulating hormone (FSH) is a gonadotropic hormone; that is, its target organs are the ovaries or testes. In women, FSH initiates growth of ova in ovarian follicles and secretion of estrogen by the cells of those follicles. In men, FSH initiates sperm production in the seminiferous tubules of the testes. FSH is secreted in response to gonadotropin-releasing hormone (GnRH) from the hypothalamus. Another hormone called inhibin (from the ovaries or testes) decreases the secretion of FSH.

Luteinizing hormone (LH) is another gonadotropic hormone whose secretion is increased by GnRH from the hypothalamus. In women, LH causes ovulation and stimulates the ruptured ovarian follicle to become the corpus luteum and begin secreting progesterone, as well as estrogen. In men, LH stimulates the secretion of testosterone by the interstitial cells of the testes.

Thyroid Gland

The thyroid gland consists of two lobes connected by a middle piece called the central isthmus; the gland is located on the front and sides of the trachea just below the larynx. Three hormones are produced by the thyroid gland. T_4 and T_3 are produced in the thyroid follicles, require iodine (T_4 has four iodine atoms, T_3 has three iodine atoms), and have the same functions. Calcitonin is the third hormone produced by the thyroid gland; it is produced by parafollicular cells.

T_4 and T_3 increase energy production and protein synthesis. They increase cellular respiration of glucose and fatty acids, which increases the metabolic rate—that is, energy and heat production. These hormones are the most important daily regulators of metabolic rate; their activity is reflected in the functioning of the heart, brain, muscles, and virtually all other organs. They are essential for normal physical growth, mental development, and reproductive maturation.

The direct stimulus for secretion of T_4 and T_3 is TSH from the anterior pituitary. The sequence of events is as follows: A decrease in the metabolic rate (energy production) is detected by the hypothalamus, which secrets TRH. TRH stimulates the anterior pituitary to secrete TSH, which stimulates the thyroid to increase secretion of T_4 and T_3, which increase energy production to raise the metabolic rate. As the metabolic rate rises, negative feedback decreases the secretion of TRH from the hypothalamus until the metabolic rate decreases again.

The third thyroid hormone, calcitonin, targets bone tissue and therefore is especially important during childhood when bone growth is accelerated. Calcitonin inhibits resorption of calcium and phosphate by osteoclasts, thereby lowering the blood levels of these minerals and retaining them in bones. This one function of calcitonin has two important results: the maintenance of normal blood levels of calcium and phosphate and the maintenance of a strong, stable bone matrix.

The stimulus for secretion of calcitonin is hypercalcemia (a high blood calcium level). When the blood calcium level rises, increased calcitonin ensures that no more will be removed from bones until need for blood calcium returns.

LEARNING TIP

An easy way to remember the function of calcitonin is to remember calciTONin TONes down serum calcium.

Parathyroid Glands

There are usually four parathyroid glands, two on the back of each lobe of the thyroid gland. The hormone they produce is called parathyroid hormone (PTH), which is an antagonist to calcitonin; it maintains normal blood levels of calcium and phosphate. Besides bone, the target organs of PTH are the small intestine and kidneys.

PTH increases the resorption of calcium and phosphate from the bones to the blood, which raises their blood levels. Absorption of calcium and phosphate from food in the small intestine is also increased by PTH through its action of activating vitamin D (calcitriol) in the kidneys. PTH also increases the resorption of calcium by the kidneys and the excretion of phosphate (more than is obtained from bones). Therefore, the overall effect of PTH is to raise the blood calcium level and lower the blood phosphate level.

Secretion of PTH is stimulated by hypocalcemia (a low blood calcium level) and is inhibited by hypercalcemia. In adults, PTH is probably the most important regulator of the blood calcium level. Calcium ions in the blood are essential for normal excitability of neurons and muscle cells and for the process of blood clotting.

Adrenal Glands

The two adrenal (also called suprarenal) glands are located one on top of each kidney. Each adrenal gland consists of an inner adrenal medulla and an outer adrenal cortex.

Adrenal Medulla

The cells of the adrenal medulla are called chromaffin cells. They secrete epinephrine and norepinephrine, which are collectively called catecholamines and are sympathomimetic (mimicking the sympathetic nervous system). Secretion of both hormones is stimulated by sympathetic impulses from the hypothalamus in stressful situations. The functions of the catecholamines mimic and prolong those of the sympathetic nervous system, which enable the individual to respond physiologically to stress situations.

Of the two hormones, epinephrine is secreted in larger amounts (approximately four times that of norepinephrine) and has many effects. It increases the heart rate and force of contraction, stimulates vasoconstriction in skin and most

viscera and vasodilation in skeletal muscles, dilates the bronchioles, decreases peristalsis, stimulates the liver to convert glycogen to glucose, increases the use of fats for energy, and increases the rate of cell respiration. The most significant function of norepinephrine is to cause vasoconstriction in the skin and most viscera, thereby raising blood pressure.

Adrenal Cortex

The adrenal cortex secretes three types of steroid hormones: mineralocorticoids, glucocorticoids, and sex hormones. The sex hormones are small amounts of male androgens and even smaller amounts of female estrogens. Their function is not known with certainty, although they may contribute to the growth spurt that often occurs just before puberty and to the libido (sex drive) in adult women.

LEARNING TIP

An easy way to remember the hormones of the adrenal cortex is to remember salt, sugar, and sex. Mineralocorticoids promote salt retention, glucocorticoids affect sugar (carbohydrate) metabolism, and androgens and estrogens are sex hormones.

Aldosterone is the most abundant of the mineralocorticoids, and its target organs are the kidneys. Aldosterone increases the reabsorption of sodium ions and the excretion of potassium ions by the kidney tubules. This means that sodium ions are returned to the blood and potassium ions are eliminated in urine. This function of aldosterone has important consequences. As sodium ions are reabsorbed, hydrogen ions may be excreted in exchange; this is one mechanism to prevent the accumulation of hydrogen ions that would lead to acidosis. Also, as sodium ions are reabsorbed, water and negative ions such as bicarbonate follow and are thus returned to the blood. Although the reabsorption of water is an indirect effect of aldosterone, it is important for the maintenance of normal blood volume and blood pressure.

Secretion of aldosterone may be stimulated in several ways: a low blood sodium level, a high blood potassium level, or loss of blood or dehydration that lowers blood pressure. Low blood pressure activates the renin-angiotensin mechanism of the kidneys, which culminates in the formation of angiotensin II. One function of angiotensin II is to increase secretion of aldosterone. The hormone called atrial natriuretic peptide (ANP), secreted by the atria of the heart when blood pressure or blood volume rises, seems to inhibit secretion of aldosterone (and renin) and thereby promotes elimination of sodium ions and water by the kidneys.

Cortisol is the most abundant of the glucocorticoids and has many target tissues. Cortisol stimulates gluconeogenesis (the conversion of triglycerides, lactic acid, and some amino acids to glucose) in the liver. It also increases lipolysis and protein breakdown to liberate fatty acids and amino acids, respectively, for gluconeogenesis. The goal is to increase capabilities of energy production. By providing these secondary energy sources to most cells, cortisol ensures that whatever glucose is present will be available for the brain (the glucose-sparing effect).

Cortisol also has an anti-inflammatory effect because it blocks the effects of histamine and stabilizes the lysosomes in cells. Normal cortisol secretion seems to limit the inflammation process to what is useful for tissue repair and to prevent excessive tissue destruction. Excess cortisol has damaging effects, however: It raises blood glucose levels, decreases the immune response, and delays healing of damaged tissue.

The direct stimulus for cortisol secretion is ACTH from the anterior pituitary gland. Cortisol is also a "stress" hormone, and any type of physiological stress (injury, disease, malnutrition) stimulates the hypothalamus to secrete CRH. CRH increases the secretion of ACTH by the anterior pituitary, which increases cortisol secretion by the adrenal cortex.

Pancreas

The pancreas extends from the curve of the duodenum to the spleen. The endocrine portions of the pancreas are called islets of Langerhans (pancreatic islets); they contain alpha cells, which produce glucagon, and beta cells, which produce insulin. Delta cells in the islets secrete somatostatin, which inhibits secretion of both insulin and glucagon.

The functions of glucagon are all related to energy production. Glucagon stimulates the liver to catabolize glycogen to glucose (glycogenolysis) and to increase gluconeogenesis to use fats and excess amino acids for energy production. The overall effect, therefore, is to raise the blood glucose level for cellular uptake and respiration.

The secretion of glucagon is stimulated by hypoglycemia, a low blood glucose level. Such a state may occur during physiological stress situations such as exercise or simply being between meals.

Insulin increases the transport of glucose from the blood into cells by increasing the permeability of cell membranes to glucose (brain and liver cells, however, are not dependent on insulin for glucose intake). Inside cells, glucose is broken down in cellular respiration to release energy. The liver and muscles are also stimulated by insulin to change glucose to glycogen (glycogenesis) to be stored for later use. Insulin also enables cells to take in fatty acids and amino acids to use in the synthesis of lipids and proteins (not energy production). Insulin, therefore, decreases the blood glucose level by increasing the use of glucose for energy, promoting the storage of excess glucose, and decreasing energy production from other food sources.

Secretion of insulin is stimulated by hyperglycemia, a high blood glucose level. This state occurs after meals, especially those high in carbohydrates. It should be apparent that insulin and glucagon function as antagonists and that normal secretion of both hormones ensures a blood glucose level that fluctuates within normal limits. Table 38.1 reviews endocrine hormone function.

Aging and the Endocrine System

Most of the endocrine glands decrease their secretions with age, but normal aging usually does not lead to serious hor-

TABLE 38.1 REVIEW OF ENDOCRINE FUNCTION

Hormone	Function(s)	Regulation of Secretion
	Hormones of the Posterior Pituitary Gland	
Oxytocin	Promotes contraction of myometrium of uterus (labor)	Nerve impulses from hypothalamus, the result of stretching of cervix or stimulation of nipple
	Promotes release of milk from mammary glands	Secretion from placenta at the end of gestation—stimulus unknown
Antidiuretic hormone (ADH)	Increases water reabsorption by the kidney tubules (water returns to the blood)	Decreased water content in the body (alcohol inhibits secretion)
	Hormones of the Anterior Pituitary Gland	
Growth hormone (GH)	Increases rate of mitosis	GHRH (hypothalamus) stimulates secretion
	Increases amino acid transport into cells	
	Increases rate of protein synthesis	GHIH—somatostatin (hypothalamus) inhibits secretion
	Increases use of fats for energy	
Thyroid-stimulating hormone (TSH)	Increases secretion of thyroxine and T_3 by thyroid gland	TRH (hypothalamus)
Adrenocorticotropic hormone (ACTH)	Increases secretion of cortisol by the adrenal cortex	CRH (hypothalamus)
Prolactin	Stimulates milk production by the mammary glands	PRH (hypothalamus) stimulates secretion PIH (hypothalamus) inhibits secretion
Follicle-stimulating hormone (FSH)	In women: Initiates growth of ova in ovarian follicles Increases secretion of estrogen by follicle cells	GnRH (hypothalamus) stimulates secretion Inhibin (ovaries or testes) inhibits secretion

Hormone	Function(s)	Regulation of Secretion
	Hormones of the Anterior Pituitary Gland (*Continued*)	
FSH (cont.)	In men:	GnRH (hypothalamus)
	Initiates sperm production in the testes	
Luteinizing hormone (LH)	In women:	
	Causes ovulation	
	Causes the ruptured ovarian follicle to become the corpus luteum	
	Increases secretion of progesterone by the corpus luteum	
	In men:	GnRH (hypothalamus)
	Increases secretion of testosterone by the interstitial cells of the testes	
	Hormones of the Thyroid Gland	
Thyroxine and triiodothyronine (T_4 and T_3)	Increase energy production from all food types	TSH (anterior pituitary)
	Increase rate of protein synthesis	
Calcitonin	Decreases the reabsorption of calcium and phosphate from bones to blood	Hypercalcemia
	Hormones of the Parathyroid Glands	
Parathyroid hormone (PTH)	Increases the reabsorption of calcium and phosphate from bone to blood	Hypocalcemia stimulates secretion. Hypercalcemia inhibits secretion.
	Increases absorption of calcium and phosphate by the small intestine	
	Increases the reabsorption of calcium and the excretion of phosphate by the kidneys; activates vitamin D	
	Hormones of the Pancreas	
Glucagon (alpha cells)	Increases conversion of glycogen to glucose in the liver	Hypoglycemia
	Increases the use of excess amino acids and fats for energy	
Insulin (beta cells)	Increases glucose transport into cells and the use of glucose for energy production	Hyperglycemia
	Increases the conversion of excess glucose to glycogen in the liver and muscles	
	Increases amino acid and fatty acid transport into cells and their use in synthesis reactions	
Somatostatin (delta cells)	Decreases secretion of insulin and glucagon. Slows absorption of nutrients.	Rising levels of insulin and glucagon
	Hormones of the Adrenal Medulla	
Norepinephrine	Causes vasoconstriction in skin, viscera, and skeletal muscles	Sympathetic impulses from the hypothalamus in stress situations
Epinephrine	Increases heart rate and force of contraction	
	Dilates bronchioles	
	Decreases peristalsis	
	Increases conversion of glycogen in glucose in the liver	
	Causes vasodilation in skeletal muscles	
	Causes vasoconstriction in skin and viscera	
	Increases use of fats for energy	
	Increases the rate of cell respiration	
	Hormones of the Adrenal Cortex	
Aldosterone	Increases reabsorption of Na^+ ions by the kidneys to the blood	Low blood Na^+ level
	Increases excretion of K^+ ions by the kidneys in urine	Low blood volume or blood pressure
		High blood K^+ level
Cortisol	Increases use of fats and excess amino acids for energy	ACTH (anterior pituitary) during physiological stress
	Increases gluconeogenesis	
	Increases use of glucose	
	Anti-inflammatory effect: stabilizes lysosomes and blocks the effects of histamine	

Abbreviations: K^+ = potassium; Na^+ = sodium.
  Source: Adapted from Scanlon, VC, and Sanders, T: Essentials of Anatomy and Physiology, ed 4. F.A. Davis, Philadelphia, 2003.

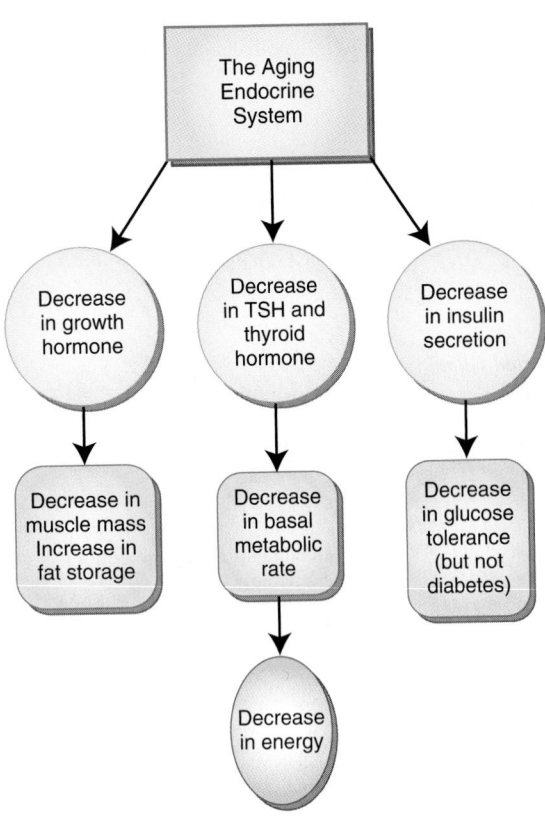

FIGURE 38.2 Effects of aging.

mone deficiencies or illness (Fig. 38.2). Unless specific pathological conditions develop, the endocrine system usually continues to function adequately in old age.

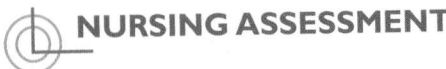

NURSING ASSESSMENT

Health History

When performing a health history, a number of questions can be asked to determine whether an endocrine problem exists. Often, however, you might be aware of a history of an endocrine disorder, such as diabetes or hypothyroidism. When a disorder exists or is suspected, you can do a more focused assessment. Assessment of individual disorders is provided in Chapters 39 and 40. Table 38.2 offers general questions that can help you identify new problem areas. If the assessment reveals abnormalities, they should be reported to a registered nurse or physician.

NURSING CARE TIP

Some patients call diabetes mellitus "sugar." So instead of asking if anyone in their family has diabetes, you may need to ask if anyone has "sugar."

TABLE 38.2 SUBJECTIVE ASSESSMENT OF THE ENDOCRINE SYSTEM

Category	Questions to Ask	Rationale
Neuromuscular	Have you noticed muscle spasms or twitching?	These symptoms may be associated with excessive antidiuretic hormone secretion (SIADH) or calcium depletion resulting from hypoparathyroidism.
	Do you have numbness, tingling, or pain in your feet, legs, or hands?	These may be associated with neuropathy resulting from diabetes mellitus. Numbness and tingling may also indicate hypocalcemia related to hypoparathyroidism.
Nutrition/Fluid Balance	Have you gained or lost weight without trying?	Actual weight gain may be associated with hypothyroidism. Weight gain due to water retention may result from Cushing's syndrome, or SIADH.
		Weight loss may result from uncontrolled diabetes or hyperthyroidism. Weight loss due to dehydration may be related to Addison's disease.
	Have you noticed excessive thirst or urination?	Excessive thirst and urination are classic symptoms of diabetes mellitus and diabetes insipidus.
	Have you noticed a change in your energy level?	Lack of energy may be associated with uncontrolled diabetes, hypothyroidism, hyperthyroidism, Addison's disease, or pituitary disorders.
Metabolic	Do you generally tolerate changes in environmental temperature?	Hypothyroidism can cause cold intolerance. Hyperthyroidism can cause heat intolerance.
Mood/Memory	Have you noticed a change in your mood or memory?	Mental function may be dull with hypothyroidism. Mood swings may occur with Cushing's syndrome. Agitation or confusion may result from hypoglycemia in a person with diabetes.
Family History	Does anyone in your family have a thyroid problem, diabetes, or another endocrine disorder?	Some disorders are hereditary.

SIADH = syndrome of inappropriate antidiuretic hormone.

TABLE 38.3 ENDOCRINE-RELATED CAUSES OF ABNORMAL PHYSICAL ASSESSMENT FINDINGS

Category	Abnormal Assessment Finding	Possible Causes
Mood	Depressed mood or affect	Hypothyroidism
	Nervousness	Hyperthyroidism, pheochromocytoma
	Agitation	Low blood sugar
Nutrition/Fluid Balance	Weight gain	Decreased metabolic rate in hypothyroidism, fluid excess
	Weight loss	Increased metabolic rate in hyperthyroidism; uncontrolled diabetes, dehydration
	Poor skin turgor	Dehydration due to water loss in Addison's disease, diabetes mellitus, diabetes insipidus
Integumentary	Hyperpigmentation of skin	Addison's disease
	Dry, scaly skin	Hypothyroidism
	Dusky lower extremities with weak peripheral pulses	Circulatory changes in diabetes mellitus
Vital Signs	Change in pulse or temperature	Elevated due to increased metabolic rate in hyperthyroidism
		Decreased due to slowed metabolic rate in hypothyroidism
	Elevated blood pressure	Increased catecholamine release in pheochromocytoma or fluid retention in Cushing's syndrome
	Decreased blood pressure	Sodium and water loss in Addison's disease
Neuromuscular	Tremor	Hyperthyroidism, hypoglycemia, or pheochromocytoma
Head and Neck	Exophthalmos (bulging eyes)	Fat deposits and edema behind the eyes in Graves' disease
	Fat pads on neck and shoulders ("buffalo hump"), round "moon" face	Accumulation of fat in Cushing's syndrome
	Enlarged thyroid gland	Excessive stimulation by TSH in hypothyroidism or hyperthyroidism

Physical Assessment of the Patient with an Endocrine Disorder

Physical assessment starts with height, weight, and vital signs. Compare findings with the patient's baseline assessment if available. Table 38.3 includes common endocrine-related causes of physical assessment abnormalities.

Inspection

Observe the patient for mood and **affect** (emotional tone) throughout the physical assessment. Inspect the neck for thyroid enlargement. Look for eyes that bulge (**exophthalmos**). Note posture, body fat, and presence of tremor. Observe skin and hair texture and moisture. Note the presence of a moon-like face or "buffalo hump" on the upper back. Observe the lower extremities for skin and color changes that might indicate circulatory impairment. See Table 38.3 for rationales for these observations.

Palpation

The thyroid gland is the only palpable endocrine gland. The licensed practical nurse/licensed vocational nurse (LPN/ LVN) may assist a physician or nurse practitioner to palpate the thyroid gland. The practitioner stands behind or in front of the seated patient and palpates the gland while the patient swallows a sip of water (Fig. 38.3). You can assist with positioning the patient, providing water, and instructing the

patient to take a sip of water and hold it in his or her mouth until told to swallow. The thyroid gland should never be palpated in a patient with uncontrolled hyperthyroidism because this can stimulate secretion of additional thyroid hormone.

Palpate all peripheral pulses. The posterior tibial and dorsalis pedis pulses may be diminished in patients with circulatory impairment. Palpate skin turgor by gently pinching

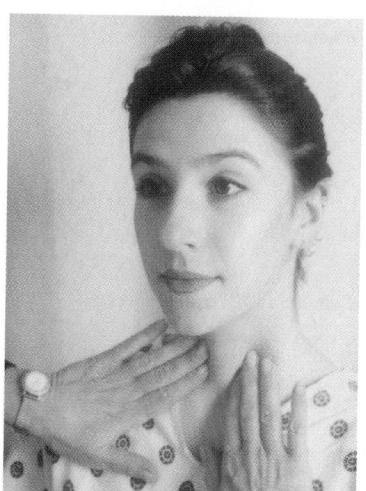

FIGURE 38.3 Thyroid palpation *(From Dillon, P M: Nursing Health Assessment: A Critical Thinking Approach, ed. 2. F. A. Davis, Philadelphia, 2007, with permission.)*

---

exopthalmos: exo—outward + ophthalmos—eye

a small piece of skin. If a "tent" remains, the patient may be dehydrated as a result of water loss, as in ADH deficiency.

Auscultation and Percussion

Auscultation and percussion are not usually part of an endocrine assessment.

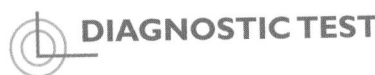 DIAGNOSTIC TESTS

Hormone Tests

Serum Hormone Levels

Many hormones can be measured from a simple blood specimen. This is useful in diagnosing hypofunctioning or hyperfunctioning gland states. See Table 38.4 for some commonly measured hormones.

Stimulation Tests

Stimulation tests may also help determine endocrine gland function. For this type of test, a substance is injected to attempt to stimulate a gland. The hormone secreted by that gland is then measured in the blood to determine how well it responded to the stimulation. For example, in a TRH stimulation test, TRH is injected. If the pituitary gland responds appropriately, TSH is secreted. If the thyroid gland responds appropriately to the TSH, T_3 and T_4 levels rise. Failure of the TRH to stimulate TSH and thyroid hormone indicates a pituitary or thyroid condition. Further studies might be done to determine the cause.

Suppression Tests

Suppression tests are the opposite of stimulating tests. For this type of test, a substance is injected that is expected to suppress a hormone's release. For example, if dexametha-

TABLE 38.4 COMMON ENDOCRINE-RELATED LABORATORY TESTS

Test	Normal Values*	Significance
	Thyroid Tests	
Thyroid-stimulating hormone	0.5–5.0 U/mL	↑ in primary hypothyroidism ↓ in primary hyperthyroidism
Trüodothyronine (T₃)	80–200 ng/100 mL	↓ in hypothyroidism ↑ in hyperthyroidism
Thyroxine (T₄)	4–12 µg/100 mL	↓ in hypothyroidism ↑ in hyperthyroidism
	Parathyroid Tests	
Parathyroid hormone	<25 pg/mL	↑ in primary hyperparathyroidism ↓ in primary hypoparathyroidism, parathyroid trauma during thyroid surgery
Calcium	8.5–10.5 mg/100 mL	↑ in some cancers, hyperparathyroidism ↓ in hypothyroidism
Phosphorus	2.4–4.7 mg/dL	↑ in hypoparathyroidism ↓ in hyperparathyroidism
	Pituitary Tests	
Growth hormone	<5 ng/mL	↑ in acromegaly ↓ in small stature
Antidiuretic hormone	2.3–3.1 pg/mL	↑ in SIADH ↓ in diabetes insipidus
Urine specific gravity	1.010–1.025	↓ in diabetes insipidus
Adrenocorticotropic hormone	<120 pg/mL at 6–8 a.m.	↑ in Addison's disease ↓ in Cushing's syndrome, long-term corticosteroid therapy
	Adrenal Tests	
Cortisol	5–25 µg/100 mL	↑ in Cushing's syndrome, stress ↓ in Addison's disease, steroid withdrawal
Vanillylmandelic acid (VMA; urine test)	0.7–6.8 mg/24 h	↑ in pheochromocytoma
	Pancreas Tests	
Fasting plasma glucose (FPG)	70–100 mg/dL	↑ in stress, Cushing's syndrome FPG 101–125 = pre-diabetes FPG ≥126 = diabetes mellitus ↓ in hypoglycemia, Addison's disease
Oral glucose tolerance test	Blood glucose less than 140 mg/dL at 2 hours	BG 140–199 at 2 hours = pre-diabetes BG ≥200 at 2 hours = diabetes mellitus
Glycosylated hemoglobin	4%–7%	↑ in poor diabetes control

SIADH = syndrome of inappropriate antidiuretic hormone.
*All normal values are for a fasting test.

CRITICAL THINKING

Mrs. Hackworth

■ Mrs. Hackworth is tired all the time, and the nurse practitioner orders a TSH level drawn. The result is higher than normal.
1. She asks, "If my thyroid level is high, then why am I so tired?" How should you respond?
2. After further testing, the NP places Mrs. Hackworth on levothyroxine (Synthroid) 50 μg daily. Her pharmacist supplies Synthroid 0.05 mg. Is her dose correct?

Suggested answers at end of chapter.

CRITICAL THINKING

Mrs. Trombley

■ Mrs. Trombley is having a 24-hour urine test done. You begin the test at 0600, and it progresses well until you learn that the nursing assistant helped her up to void in the toilet at noon, forgetting to save her urine.
1. What do you do?
2. How can you prevent this from happening again?
3. How would you document this incident?

Suggested answers at end of chapter.

sone (a steroid hormone) is injected, cortisol release from the adrenal cortex is expected to be suppressed via a negative feedback mechanism. If the cortisol level is not suppressed, adrenal cortex dysfunction is suspected.

Urine Tests

Sometimes it is helpful to measure the amount of hormone or hormone by-product excreted in the urine during a 24-hour period. Examples are cortisol and vanillylmandelic acid, a product of catecholamine metabolism.

To collect a 24-hour urine specimen, you must obtain a special urine container from the laboratory. It is usually an opaque container that protects the specimen from light; it may have preservative in it. Check with the laboratory to find out whether the specimen needs to be kept on ice during the test and whether the patient needs to be on a special diet before or during the test. To keep a specimen on ice, fill a bath basin with ice and place the container in the basin. The ice must be refilled every few hours to keep the specimen cold. When initiating the test, ask the patient to urinate and discard the urine. The time of this first discarded voiding is considered the start of the test. Any urine collected from this time forward for 24 hours is saved. At the end of the 24-hour period, the patient is again asked to urinate, but this time the urine is saved. The entire collection is then labeled and sent to the laboratory. Instruct the patient how to do the test, place a sign on the toilet with the start and stop time of the test, and remind all staff to save the urine.

If the patient is incontinent or otherwise unable to participate in the test, a catheter may need to be inserted. If the patient already has an indwelling catheter, a new bag and tubing should be attached before the start of the test. The laboratory should be consulted to determine the need for a preservative or ice. Preservative can be added to the catheter bag if necessary. If ice is necessary, the bag should be kept in a basin of ice rather than hanging on the side of the bed.

If the specimen must be protected from light, the bag can be covered with dark plastic or foil.

Other Laboratory Tests

Some laboratory tests may indirectly reflect the function of an endocrine gland. For example, a serum calcium level helps indicate PTH or calcitonin secretion, and a blood glucose level reflects insulin secretion.

Nuclear Scanning

A thyroid scan may be done to determine the presence of tumors or nodules. For this test, a radioactive material is injected or radioactive iodine is taken orally. The material is taken up by the thyroid gland. After a specified time, the thyroid gland is scanned with a scintillation camera. The scan will show "hot spots," which are nodules that are not malignant, or "cold spots" (areas that do not take up the radioactivity), which indicate malignancy. Cold spots can then be biopsied to confirm a diagnosis. Because such a small amount of radioactive material is used, there is no risk to the patient. The patient should be aware that the test takes approximately 30 minutes to complete.

Radiographic Tests

A computed tomographic (CT) scan or magnetic resonance imaging (MRI) may be done to locate a tumor or identify hypertrophy of a gland.

Ultrasound

Ultrasound may be done of the thyroid or parathyroid glands to determine if they are enlarged or to find masses.

Biopsy

Biopsy is done to obtain tissue to examine for possible cancerous cells. The thyroid gland can be biopsied either by needle aspiration under local anesthesia or using a surgical incision.

REVIEW QUESTIONS

1. Which hormones are secreted by the posterior pituitary gland? Choose all that apply.
   a. Antidiuretic hormone
   b. Thyroid-stimulating hormone
   c. Growth hormone
   d. Luteinizing hormone
   e. Oxytocin
   f. Calcitonin

2. What are the functions of T_4 and T_3?
   a. Retention of salt and water
   b. Maintenance of blood sugar
   c. Maintenance of blood pressure
   d. Regulation of energy production

3. Which hormone maintains strong bones?
   a. ADH
   b. Insulin
   c. Calcitonin
   d. TRH

4. The nurse is doing an admission assessment on a new resident to a nursing home. The patient's face and shoulders seem to have a lot of fat, but the patient's arms and legs are thin. Which of the following disorders might these findings relate to?
   a. Cushing's syndrome
   b. Diabetes insipidus
   c. Diabetes mellitus
   d. Pheochromocytoma

5. When explaining a thyroid scan to a patient, which of the following statements is correct?
   a. "You will take a special pill, and then an ultrasound will be taken of your neck."
   b. "You will receive an injection of radioactive material, and then a special camera will take pictures of your thyroid gland."
   c. "You will be placed into a special machine, and x-rays will be taken of your neck. It may be noisy."
   d. "You will be given a special drink, and then magnetic energy is used to visualize the thyroid area."

SUGGESTED ANSWERS TO

CRITICAL THINKING

■ *Mrs. Hackworth*

1. "It's not your thyroid hormone that is high, it's your thyroid-stimulating hormone. That means your pituitary gland has to work extra hard to try to stimulate your thyroid gland."

$$\frac{50 \text{ μg}}{} \Big| \frac{1 \text{ mg}}{1000 \text{ μg}} = 0.05 \text{ mg}$$

■ *Mrs. Trombley*

1. The specimen must include all urine for a 24-hour period. Restart the test from noon.

2. To prevent this from happening again, try placing an incontinence pad or other large item directly over the toilet as a reminder to the patient. Be sure there is a sign posted above the toilet or on the toilet handle, and communicate with the nursing assistants why the urine needs to be saved.

3. "Patient voided in toilet at 1200. 24-hour urine test restarted; importance of saving urine explained to patient and staff. RN notified." Note that it is not appropriate to "blame" the nursing assistant for making a mistake.

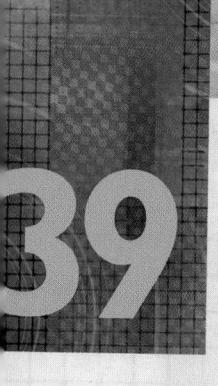

39

Nursing Care of Patients with Endocrine Disorders

PAULA D. HOPPER

KEY TERMS

amenorrhea (ay-MEN-uh-REE-ah)
autoimmune (AW-toh-im-YOON)
dysphagia (dis-FAYJ-ee-ah)
ectopic (ek-TOP-ik)
euthyroid (yoo-THY-royd)
goitrogenic (GOY-troh-JEN-ik)
goitrogens (GOY-troh-jenz)
hyperplasia (HIGH-per-PLAY-zee-ah)
hypophysectomy (HIGH-pah-fi-SEK-tuh-mee)
hypovolemic (HIGH-poh-voh-LEEM-ik)
myxedema (MIK-suh-DEE-mah)
nephrogenic (NEFF-roh-JEN-ik)
nocturia (nok-TYOO-ree-ah)
osmolality (ahs-moh-LAL-i-tee)
pheochromocytoma (FEE-oh-KROH-moh-sigh-TOH-mah)
polydipsia (PAH-lee-DIP-see-ah)
polyuria (PAH-lee-YOO-ree-ah)
psychogenic (SIGH-koh-JEN-ik)
tetany (TET-uh-nee)

QUESTIONS TO GUIDE YOUR READING

1. What are the disorders caused by variations in the hormones of the pituitary, thyroid, parathyroid, and adrenal glands?

2. How would you explain the pathophysiology of each of the endocrine disorders presented?

3. What are the etiologies, signs, and symptoms of each of the disorders?

4. What is current therapeutic treatment of each of the selected endocrine disorders?

5. What data would you collect when caring for patients with each of the endocrine disorders discussed?

6. What nursing care will you provide for patients with each of the disorders?

7. How will you know if your nursing interventions have been effective?

A variety of disorders can be found within the endocrine system. Although the causes vary, the pathophysiology usually involves either too little or too much hormone activity. Insufficient hormone activity may be the result of hypofunction of an endocrine gland or insensitivity of the target tissue to its hormone. Excessive hormone activity may be the result of a hyperactive gland, **ectopic** hormone production, or self-administration of too much replacement hormone (Table 39.1). If you can remember the function of each hormone in the body, understanding the problems involved with an altered amount of each hormone becomes easier.

Most endocrine disorders are either primary or secondary. A primary disorder is a problem within the gland that is out of balance. Secondary disorders are caused by problems outside the gland, such as an imbalance in a tropic hormone, certain drugs, trauma, surgery, or a problem in the feedback mechanism. For example, if the thyroid gland is diseased and causing hypothyroidism, it would be considered a primary problem. Sometimes hypothyroidism is caused by not enough thyroid-stimulating hormone from the pituitary gland, even though the thyroid gland is healthy. This would be considered a secondary problem.

LEARNING TIP

If you can remember what each hormone does in the body, it will be easier to remember what results from imbalances of that hormone. Most symptoms of hormone hyperactivity are the opposite of symptoms of that hormone's hypoactivity.

PITUITARY DISORDERS

Pituitary disorders often involve several hormone imbalances at once, caused by general hypopituitarism or hyperpituitarism. Problems involving all the pituitary hormones at once are rare. For simplicity, imbalances are considered separately here.

TABLE 39.1 CAUSES OF ENDOCRINE PROBLEMS

Insufficient Hormone Activity	Excess Hormone Activity
Gland hypofunction	Gland hyperfunction
Lack of tropic or stimulating hormone	Excess tropic or stimulating hormone
Target tissue insensitivity to hormone	Ectopic hormone production
	Self-administration of too much replacement hormone

ectopic: ec—away from normal + topic—place

TABLE 39.2 ANTIDIURETIC HORMONE DISORDERS SUMMARY

	Insufficient ADH	Excess ADH
Disorder	Diabetes insipidus	SIADH
Signs and Symptoms	Polyuria, polydipsia, hyponatremia, dehydration	Fluid retention, weight gain, hyponatremia
Diagnostic Tests	Urine specific gravity, urine and plasma osmolality	Serum and urine sodium and osmolality
Therapeutic Interventions	Synthetic ADH replacement	Treat cause
Priority Nursing Diagnoses	Risk for deficient fluid volume	Risk for excess fluid volume

Disorders Related to Antidiuretic Hormone Imbalance

Antidiuretic hormone (ADH; also called arginine vasopressin [AVP]) is synthesized in the hypothalamus and stored and secreted by the posterior pituitary gland. A decrease in ADH activity results in diabetes insipidus (DI). An increase in ADH activity is called syndrome of inappropriate antidiuretic hormone (SIADH). Table 39.2 compares DI and SIADH. Note how symptoms of too little ADH (water loss) are opposite from symptoms of too much ADH (water retention).

Diabetes Insipidus

PATHOPHYSIOLOGY. Diabetes insipidus is caused by a deficiency of ADH. Recall that ADH is responsible for reabsorption of water by the distal tubules and collecting ducts in the kidneys. If ADH is lacking, adequate reabsorption of water is prevented, leading to diuresis. In **nephrogenic** diabetes insipidus, there is enough ADH but the kidneys do not respond to it. Patients may urinate from 3 to 15 L per day. This leads to increased serum **osmolality** (concentrated blood) and dehydration. The increased osmolality and decreased blood pressure normally trigger ADH secretion, which causes water retention and dilutes the blood; in patients with DI, this does not occur. Increased osmolality also leads to extreme thirst, which usually causes the patient to drink enough fluids to maintain fluid balance. In an unconscious patient or a patient with a defective thirst mechanism, however, dehydration may quickly occur if the problem is not recognized and corrected. For more information, check out the Nephrogenic Diabetes Insipidus Foundation at www.ndif.org.

ETIOLOGY. The primary causes of diabetes insipidus are tumors or trauma to the pituitary gland. Surgery in the area of the pituitary and certain drugs, such as glucocorticoids or alcohol, may also cause DI. Occasionally, the cause is **psychogenic,** in which the patient drinks large quantities of

nephrogenic: nephro—kidney + genic—to produce
psychogenic: psycho—related to the mind + genic—to produce

water in the absence of true disease. Nephrogenic DI occurs mostly in males and may be inherited or acquired. It is diagnosed when the kidneys do not respond to ADH. It can be triggered by certain drugs or neoplasms or by damage to the kidneys from pyelonephritis, polycystic disease, or other causes.

SIGNS AND SYMPTOMS. The patient with DI urinates frequently (**polyuria**), and nighttime urination (**nocturia**) is present. This results in high serum osmolality and low urine osmolality. Urine specific gravity is decreased, making the urine diluted and light in color.

The patient experiences extreme thirst (**polydipsia**), and consumes large volumes of water. Often patients crave ice-cold water. If urine output exceeds fluid intake, dehydration occurs, with characteristic symptoms of hypotension, poor skin turgor, and weakness. **Hypovolemic** shock occurs if fluid balance is not restored. Dehydration and electrolyte imbalances result in a decrease in level of consciousness and death if the problem is not corrected.

The patient with DI may develop an enlarged bladder and kidney damage from constantly trying to "hold" too much urine.

DIAGNOSTIC TESTS. Diagnosis is based initially on a history of risk factors and reported symptoms. Urine specific gravity is less than 1.005 (normal: 1.010 to 1.025), and can be monitored by laboratory tests or by using reagent strips at the bedside. Plasma and urine osmolality are measured and compared to each other. The actual amount of sodium in the blood may be normal, but it appears elevated in relation to the decreased amount of water. A computed tomographic (CT) scanning or magnetic resonance imaging (MRI) may show a pituitary tumor.

A water-deprivation test may be done. For this test, the patient is deprived of water for up to 6 hours. Body weight and urine osmolality are tested hourly. If the urine continues to be diluted, even though the patient is not drinking and is losing weight as a result of volume depletion, DI is suspected. In the second stage of the test, the patient receives an injection of ADH, with a final urine test done 1 hour later. If the DI is nephrogenic, the kidneys do not respond to the injected ADH.

ADH levels can be measured in plasma or urine following administration of hypertonic saline or fluid restriction. The normal response would be elevated ADH; if it is not elevated, DI is suspected. The urine glucose level may also be checked to rule out diabetes mellitus.

THERAPEUTIC INTERVENTIONS. Hypotonic intravenous (IV) fluids such as 0.45% saline may be ordered to replace intravascular volume without adding excessive sodium. IV fluids are especially important if the patient is unable to take oral fluids.

Medical treatment of DI involves replacement of ADH. In acute cases, vasopressin, a synthetic form of ADH, is given by the intravenous or subcutaneous route, along with intravenous fluid replacement. In patients who require long-term therapy, synthetic ADH (desmopressin, or DDAVP) in the form of a nasal spray is used, usually twice a day. Other drugs, such as chlorpropamide (Diabinese), help the kidneys respond better to ADH. Thiazide diuretics may decrease urine flow in the absence of ADH (even though they usually are used to increase urine output!). If a pituitary tumor is involved, treatment usually involves removal of the pituitary gland (**hypophysectomy**).

NURSING PROCESS FOR THE PATIENT WITH DIABETES INSIPIDUS. Assessment/Data Collection. When doing a nursing assessment of a patient with DI, place special attention on fluid balance. Daily weights are the most reliable method for monitoring the amount of fluid that is being lost. Accurate intake and output measurement is also helpful. Skin turgor will be poor and mucous membranes will be dry and sticky if the patient is becoming dehydrated. Monitor skin integrity because dehydration increases risk of breakdown. Monitor vital signs for signs of shock. Use a reagent strip (dipstick) or urimeter to measure urine specific gravities. Monitor serum electrolytes and osmolality as ordered, and watch for changes in level of consciousness. Assess the patient's understanding of his or her disease and treatment. Once treatment is initiated, continue to monitor fluid balance, being especially alert to signs of fluid overload.

Nursing Diagnosis, Planning, and Implementation. Deficient fluid volume related to failure of regulatory mechanisms

EXPECTED OUTCOME: *Fluid balance will be maintained as evidenced by urine specific gravity between 1.010 and 1.025, skin turgor within normal limits, and stable daily weight.*

- Monitor daily weight, I&O, vital signs, and urine specific gravity. *Decreased weight, output greater than intake, low blood pressure, elevated pulse rate, and high urine specific gravity may all indicate fluid deficit.*
- Provide free access to oral fluids if the DI is not psychogenic. If the patient's thirst mechanism is not intact, give the patient fluids every hour. *Oral fluids are essential to replace the excess lost in diuresis. If the patient is alert with an intact thirst mechanism, the patient can usually manage this independently.*
- Encourage the patient to participate in maintaining intake and output records, monitoring weight, and checking urine specific gravity, if able. *This involves the patient and helps prepare him or her for self-monitoring at home.*
- Report a significant drop in blood pressure and a rising pulse to the registered nurse or physician *because these may be signs of hypovolemic shock.*

---

polyuria: poly—much + uria—urine
nocturia: noct—night + uria—urine
polydipsia: poly—much + dipsia—thirst
hypovolemic: hypo—deficient + vol—volume + emic—blood

hypophysectomy: hypophysis—pituitary + ectomy—surgical removal

Risk for ineffective health maintenance related to deficient knowledge

EXPECTED OUTCOME: *Patient will verbalize and demonstrate understanding of medication administration and self-monitoring of disease.*

- Assess patient's understanding of his or her disease process and treatment. *Teaching should build on baseline knowledge.*
- Teach the patient about DI. *The patient will have to self-medicate and monitor his or her disease at home.* Include:
  - Basic pathophysiology of the disease
  - How to administer medications and monitor their effectiveness
  - How to measure urine specific gravity and the significance of results
  - Signs and symptoms of dehydration and fluid overload
- Stress the importance of monitoring daily weight: losses or gains of greater than 2 pounds in a day should be reported to the physician. *Weight loss or gain can indicate fluid imbalance and need for a change in medication regimen.*
- Advise the patient to wear identification, such as a medical alert bracelet, that identifies the disorder. *Faster treatment can be initiated if emergency personnel are aware of DI diagnosis.*

Evaluation. If treatment has been effective, signs of dehydration will be absent and weight and vital signs will be stable. The patient should be able to explain what is happening in the disease, symptoms to report, and demonstrate how to manage self-care.

Syndrome of Inappropriate Antidiuretic Hormone

PATHOPHYSIOLOGY. Syndrome of inappropriate antidiuretic hormone (SIADH) results from too much ADH in the body. This causes excess water to be reabsorbed by the kidney tubules and collecting ducts, leading to decreased urine output and fluid overload. As fluid builds up in the bloodstream, osmolality decreases and the blood becomes diluted. Normally, a decreased serum osmolality inhibits release of ADH. In SIADH, however, ADH continues to be released, adding to the fluid overload.

ETIOLOGY. Certain lung cancers, pancreatic cancer, or Hodgkin's disease may be ectopic sites of production of an ADH-like substance. Some drugs, such as tricyclic antidepressants and general anesthetics, may increase ADH secretion. Head trauma or surgery or a brain tumor affecting pituitary function may also cause SIADH. It may also be a complication of treatment of diabetes insipidus.

SIGNS AND SYMPTOMS. Symptoms of SIADH include symptoms of fluid overload, such as weight gain (usually without edema) and dilutional hyponatremia (Box 39.1 Manifestations of Dilutional Hyponatremia). The actual amount of sodium in the blood may be normal, but it

---

Box 39.1

Manifestations of Dilutional Hyponatremia

Bounding pulse
Elevated or normal blood pressure
Muscle weakness
Headache
Personality changes
Nausea
Diarrhea
Convulsions
Coma

---

appears low because of the diluting effect of the retained fluid. Serum osmolality is less than 275 mOsm/kg. The urine is concentrated because water is not being excreted. Muscle cramps and weakness may occur because of electrolyte imbalance. Because the osmolality of the blood is low, fluid may leak out of the vessels and cause brain swelling. If untreated, this results in lethargy, confusion, seizures, coma, and death.

DIAGNOSTIC TESTS. Serum and urine sodium levels and osmolality are measured. Serum ADH is high. Additional testing may be done to diagnose and locate an ADH-secreting tumor. Occasionally, a water load test may be done, which involves administering a specific amount of water, then measuring blood and urine sodium and osmolality hourly for 6 hours. The patient with SIADH retains the water instead of excreting it. This test can cause an unsafe fluid overload, so is not done unless necessary for diagnosis.

THERAPEUTIC INTERVENTIONS. Treatment is aimed at eliminating the cause. If a tumor is secreting ADH, surgical removal may be indicated. Symptoms may be alleviated by restricting fluids to 800 to 1000 mL per 24 hours. Hypertonic saline fluids may be administered intravenously, and oral salt may be encouraged to maintain the serum sodium level. If the cause is inoperable cancer, drugs such as furosemide (Lasix) and demeclocycline (Declomycin) may be used to block the action of ADH in the kidney.

LEARNING TIP

Remember "a pint's a pound the world around." So each time the patient gains 1 pound of fluid, it is equal to approximately 1 pint or 480 mL!

NURSING PROCESS FOR THE PATIENT WITH SYNDROME OF INAPPROPRIATE ANTIDIURETIC HORMONE. Assessment/Data Collection. Fluid overload with hyponatremia is the primary concern for the patient with SIADH. To monitor fluid balance, assess vital signs, weight, intake and output, urine specific gravity, skin turgor, and edema. Auscultate lung sounds for crackles, a sign of fluid overload. Determine the patient's ability to maintain a fluid restriction. Assess level of consciousness and neuromuscular function. Monitor laboratory tests, including serum sodium level, as ordered by the physician. Assess the patient's understanding of the disease process and treatment.

Nursing Diagnosis, Planning, and Implementation. Excess fluid volume related to compromised regulatory mechanism

EXPECTED OUTCOME: Fluid balance will be maintained as evidenced by weight and serum sodium within normal limits, lungs clear.

- Monitor daily weight, I&O, vital signs, and urine specific gravity. *Increased weight, intake greater than output, elevated blood pressure, bounding pulse, and low urine specific gravity may all indicate fluid overload.*
- Maintain fluid restriction *to reduce serum dilution and normalize serum sodium.*
  - Fluids high in sodium, such as broth, cola, or tomato juice, may help correct dilutional hyponatremia.
- Promote comfort and choice during fluid restriction. *Fluid restrictions are not pleasant for patients, and measures to increase comfort can help increase compliance.*
  - Offer hard candy
  - Provide ice chips (counted as half the volume of fluid; that is, 100 mL of ice chips equal approximately 50 mL of water).
  - Allow the patient to participate in planning the types and times of fluid intake.
- Provide calibrated cups *to help the patient maintain the restriction independently if able.*
- Report a change in level of consciousness immediately, and monitor the patient for seizures. *These are signs of serious fluid imbalance.*

Risk for ineffective health maintenance related to knowledge deficit

EXPECTED OUTCOME: Patient will verbalize and demonstrate understanding of self-care.

- Assess patient's understanding of his or her disease process and treatment. *Teaching should build on baseline knowledge.*
- Explain the importance of maintaining the fluid restriction to the patient. *The patient must understand the fluid restriction to maintain it and manage it at home if it is to be continued.*
- Instruct the patient to report any weight gain greater than 2 pounds in 1 day, a change in urine output, or acute thirst. *These are signs of fluid overload or risk for overload.*

- Encourage use of medical alert bracelet or other identification *so emergency personnel will have information if needed.*

Evaluation. Weight should stabilize at the preillness level once treatment is begun. Serum sodium level should be within normal limits. Patients should be able to verbalize the cause of their symptoms and demonstrate self-care, including ability to maintain a fluid restriction if necessary.

CRITICAL THINKING

Mrs. Jackson

■ You are caring for Mrs. Jackson, a 78-year-old woman who has just returned to your unit following hip surgery. During the next 2 days, you notice that her weight increases from 118 to 124 pounds and she seems lethargic, but the nurse's report didn't indicate concern about it. You check her ankles and sacrum for edema but find none. In the afternoon, her son rushes out of the room and tells you she is becoming confused, adding that this is not like her at all.

1. What could be happening?
2. What assessment can you do to gather further data to support your suspicions?
3. What will you do?
4. Based on her weight gain, about how much water is she retaining?

Suggested answers at end of chapter.

Disorders Related to Growth Hormone Imbalance

Growth hormone (GH), also called somatotropin, is responsible for normal growth of bones, cartilage, and soft tissue. GH is synthesized and secreted by the anterior pituitary gland. An excess or deficiency of GH may be related to a more generalized problem with the pituitary gland. A deficit of GH results in dwarfism. Excess GH results in gigantism or acromegaly (Fig. 39.1).

Dwarfism

PATHOPHYSIOLOGY. Dwarfism, also called short stature, occurs when growth hormone is deficient in childhood. A deficiency of GH in adults does not affect growth.

ETIOLOGY. Growth hormone may be deficient as a result of a pituitary tumor or failure of the pituitary to develop. It may be the result of infection or other trauma to the pituitary gland. It may also be deficient in some cases of neglect or severe emotional stress, causing psychosocial dwarfism. Malnutrition is the most common cause worldwide. Sometimes the cause is not known (Box 39.2 Cultural Considerations).

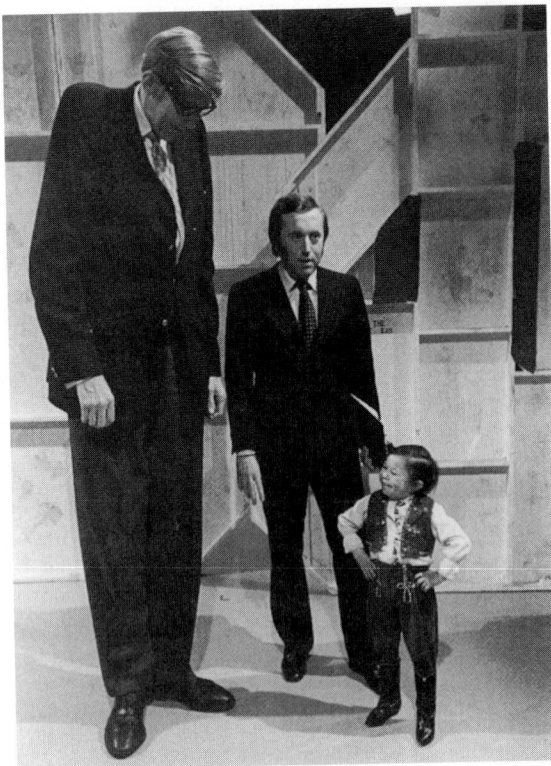

FIGURE 39.1 Gigantism and dwarfism. *(From Tamparo, CD, and Lewis, MA: Diseases of the Human Body, ed. 3. F.A. Davis, Philadelphia, 2000, p. 247, with permission.)*

SIGNS AND SYMPTOMS. Children may grow to only 3 to 4 feet in height but have normal body proportions. Sexual maturation may be slowed, related to involvement of additional pituitary hormones. Dwarfism in children is sometimes accompanied by mental retardation. In adults, symptoms include weakness, hypoglycemia, sexual dysfunction, skin changes, and increased risk for cardiovascular and cerebrovascular disease. Headaches, mental slowness, and visual disturbances may also occur.

DIAGNOSTIC TESTS. Growth hormone levels in the blood are measured by a routine laboratory test. A growth hormone stimulation test may be done by measuring GH response to induced hypoglycemia. An MRI may help determine the presence of a pituitary tumor; radiographic studies may be used to determine bone age.

THERAPEUTIC INTERVENTIONS. Treatment of dwarfism in a child is administration of growth hormone. In the past, GH was derived from human pituitary glands, so treatment was expensive. Now GH can be made in a laboratory using genetic engineering, and it is more readily available to those who need it. It is administered by injection. Surgery may be indicated if a tumor is the cause.

NURSING PROCESS FOR THE PATIENT WITH DWARFISM. Assessment/Data Collection. Assessment of the adult with dwarfism includes mental status, ability to cope with the effects of the disorder, and understanding of the treatment plan. Also assess for signs of cardiovascular disease and other complications of the disorder.

Nursing Diagnosis, Planning, and Implementation. Because the disorder in an adult has likely been present since childhood, most related problems will not be new to the patient. The priority for the nurse, then, is to approach the patient with respect while assessing current problems that may need attention.

Disturbed body image related to short stature

EXPECTED OUTCOME: *Patient will express feelings of acceptance of self.*

- Approach patient with an attitude of acceptance and caring *to help develop trusting nurse-patient relationship.*
- Provide an opportunity for patient to verbalize feelings. *Expressing feelings may help reduce anxiety.*
- Consult occupational therapist if necessary *to provide techniques to assist patients to adapt to an environment that is geared toward people of average height.*
- Provide information about support groups. *A support group can help the patient feel less alone.*

Evaluation. The goal has been achieved if the patient is able to express his or her feelings of acceptance of the disorder, and demonstrate adaptive techniques.

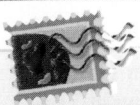

Box 39.2

Cultural Considerations

Dwarfism, mostly related to a limited gene pool, often occurs among Amish communities. Ellis–van Creveld syndrome is prevalent among the Amish of Lancaster County, Pennsylvania. This syndrome is characterized by short stature and an extra digit on each hand, with some individuals having a congenital heart defect and nervous system involvement resulting in a degree of mental handicap.

CRITICAL THINKING

Adoption

■ Three siblings were adopted to a loving home after having been in several foster homes. After a year in their new home, each child suddenly grew 6 to 8 inches. What do you think happened?
Suggested answer at end of chapter.

Acromegaly

Acromegaly is a rare excess of growth hormone that affects adults, usually in their 30s or 40s. If a GH excess occurs in children, the condition results in gigantism.

PATHOPHYSIOLOGY. Acromegaly occurs as a result of oversecretion of GH in an adult. Bones increase in size, leading to enlargement of facial features, hands, and feet. Long bones grow in width but not length because the epiphyseal disks are closed. Subcutaneous connective tissue increases, causing a fleshy appearance. Internal organs and glands enlarge. Impaired tolerance of carbohydrates leads to elevated blood glucose.

ETIOLOGY. Excess secretion of growth hormone can be caused by pituitary **hyperplasia,** a benign pituitary tumor, or excess if GH-releasing hormone due to hypothalamic dysfunction.

SIGNS AND SYMPTOMS. Often the first symptom noticed is a change in ring or shoe size. The nose, jaw, brow, hands, and feet enlarge (Fig. 39.2). The teeth may be displaced, causing difficulty chewing, or dentures may no longer fit. The tongue becomes thick, causing difficulty in speaking and swallowing (**dysphagia**). The patient may develop sleep apnea. Vertebral changes may lead to kyphosis. Visual disturbances may occur because of tumor pressure on the optic nerve. Headaches are a result of tumor pressure on the brain. Diabetes mellitus may develop because GH increases blood glucose and causes an increased workload for the pancreas. (See Chapter 40.) Osteoporosis and arthritis may occur. Erectile dysfunction may occur in men and **amenorrhea** in women. With treatment, soft tissues reduce in size, but bone growth is permanent.

DIAGNOSTIC TESTS. Serum growth hormone levels are measured, and radiographs show abnormal bone growth. Growth hormone may also be measured following a large dose of oral glucose. Normally, glucose suppresses GH release. If it continues to be released even after a glucose load, acromegaly is suspected. MRI is done to locate a pituitary tumor.

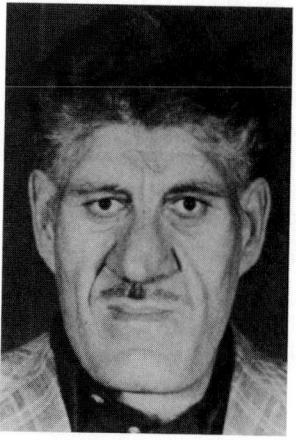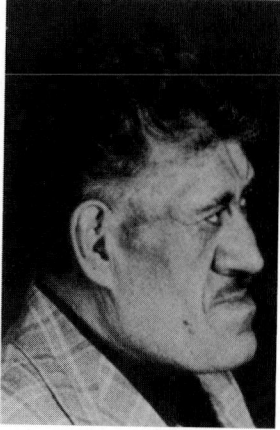

FIGURE 39.2 Patient with acromegaly. *(From Martin, JB, Reichlin, S, and Brown, GM: Clinical Neuroendocrinology. F.A. Davis, Philadelphia, 1977, p. 353, with permission.)*

---

hyperplasia: hyper—excessive + plasia—formation or deviation
dysphagia: dys—bad + phagia—swallowing
amenorrhea: a—not + men—month + orrhea—flow

THERAPEUTIC INTERVENTIONS. Treatment is aimed at the cause. Bromocriptine (Parlodel) or octreotide (Sandostatin) may decrease GH levels. Hypophysectomy or radiation may be indicated if a tumor is the cause. If the pituitary is removed, lifelong replacement of thyroid hormone, corticosteroids, and sex hormones is important to maintain homeostasis.

NURSING PROCESS FOR THE PATIENT WITH ACROMEGALY. Assessment/Data Collection. The nurse caring for the patient with acromegaly is concerned with the patient's response to the disease. Assess safety in relation to impaired eyesight, chewing, swallowing, and sleep apnea. Monitor serum glucose levels for onset of diabetes mellitus. Assess knowledge and acceptance of the disease. If hypophysectomy is planned, assess the patient for anxiety related to the surgery and perform a preoperative baseline neurological assessment.

Nursing Diagnosis, Planning, and Implementation. Disturbed body image related to changes in appearance

EXPECTED OUTCOME: *Patient will express feelings of acceptance of self.*

- Approach patient with an attitude of acceptance and caring *to help develop trusting nurse-patient relationship.*
- Encourage the patient to be accepting of self *because most changes will be permanent and require patient to become accustomed to a changed self-image.*
- Provide information about support groups. *A support group can help the patient feel less alone.*

Risk for injury related to poor eyesight, sleep apnea, dysphagia

EXPECTED OUTCOME: *Patient will not experience injury.*

- Assess for increased risk of injury. *An accurate assessment will guide interventions.*
- Maintain safe, uncluttered environment *to prevent injury from falls related to poor eyesight.*
- Request swallowing evaluation from speech therapy if indicated. *A speech therapist can diagnose swallowing problems and make recommendations.*
- Observe for sleep apnea and discuss with physician if indicated. *Sleep apnea, if present, will require sleep studies and treatment.*

Additional nursing diagnoses are identified if diabetes mellitus or other problems exist.

Patient Education. Teach the patient and significant others about the disease and treatment. If the patient is having a hypophysectomy, be sure he or she understands that some symptoms will be relieved but that bone growth and visual changes may not reverse. Stress the need for lifelong hormone replacement after surgery. See section on care of the patient undergoing hypophysectomy later in this chapter.

Evaluation. The patient who is effectively treated will have some soft tissues return to normal size. The patient will be safe and free from injury. The patient should be able to accurately describe self-care requirements.

Pituitary Tumors

Most tumors of the pituitary gland are benign adenomas. However, even benign tumors in the brain can cause many symptoms, including visual disturbances, symptoms of increased pressure in the brain, and symptoms related to hormone imbalances, as described earlier. Treatment for pituitary tumors is usually hypophysectomy (surgical removal of the pituitary gland). Radiation may also be used, either alone or as an adjunct to surgery.

Care of the Patient Undergoing Hypophysectomy

Removal of the pituitary gland is called hypophysectomy. Figure 39.3 shows the transsphenoidal approach to the gland. Some tumors may necessitate removal via a transfrontal craniotomy (entry through the frontal bone of the skull).

PREOPERATIVE CARE. Ensure that the patient understands the physician's explanation of surgery. Perform and document a baseline neurological assessment. Prepare the patient for what to expect following surgery. Instruct the patient to avoid any actions that increase pressure on the surgical site, such as coughing, sneezing, nose blowing, straining to move bowels, or bending from the waist. Because coughing can raise intracranial pressure and is therefore contraindicated, instruct the patient in deep breathing exercises or use of an incentive spirometer.

POSTOPERATIVE CARE. Perform routine neurological assessments to monitor for neurological damage. Also be sure to check urine for specific gravity because diabetes insipidus may occur following pituitary surgery. If a patient has had transsphenoidal surgery, he will have nasal packing and a "mustache dressing," which is placed under the nose to collect drips. These are left in place and not removed unless ordered by the physician. Monitor the dressing for signs of

cerebrospinal fluid (CSF) leakage. CSF contains glucose, so glucose testing strips can be used to determine if drainage is actually CSF or just nasal discharge. Remind the patient to avoid any actions that increase pressure on the surgical site. Obtain orders for stool softeners and antitussives as needed. Tooth brushing is avoided until the incision line is healed. The patient may use floss and mouth rinses. The patient is placed on hormone replacement therapy following hypophysectomy. Pituitary hormones are difficult to replace, so target hormones are generally given. These may include thyroid hormone, glucocorticoids, intranasal desmopressin, and sex hormones. Instruct the patient about how to administer the hormones, as well as side effects to report.

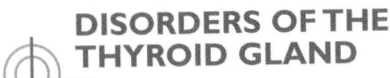 DISORDERS OF THE THYROID GLAND

Triiodothyronine (T_3) and thyroxine (T_4) are thyroid hormones secreted by the thyroid gland. These hormones may be collectively referred to as thyroid hormone (TH). Deficient secretion of TH results in hypothyroidism; excess TH results in hyperthyroidism. For more information on disorders of the thyroid gland, visit the American Thyroid Association at www.thyroid.org.

Hypothyroidism

Hypothyroidism occurs primarily in women 30 to 60 years old. If hypothyroidism occurs in an infant, the result is cretinism. Hypothyroidism that develops in an adult is called **myxedema.**

Pathophysiology

Primary hypothyroidism occurs when the thyroid gland fails to produce enough TH even though there is enough thyroid-stimulating hormone (TSH) being secreted by the pituitary gland. The pituitary responds to the low level of TH by producing more TSH. Secondary hypothyroidism is caused by low levels of TSH, which fail to stimulate release of TH. Tertiary hypothyroidism results from inadequate release of thyrotropin-releasing hormone (TRH), secreted by the hypothalamus. Most cases of hypothyroidism are primary (Table 39.3).

Because thyroid hormones are responsible for metabolism, low levels of these hormones result in a slowed metabolic rate, which causes many of the characteristic

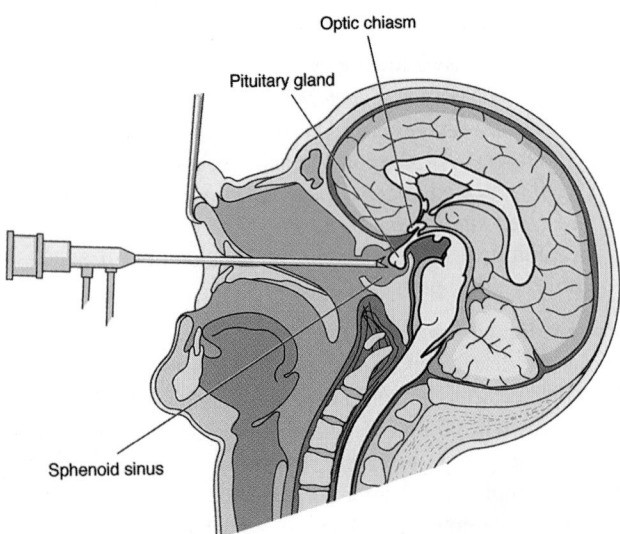

FIGURE 39.3 Transsphenoidal approach to pituitary gland for hypophysectomy.

Optic chiasm

Pituitary gland

Sphenoid sinus

TABLE 39.3 THYROID HORMONE ABNORMALITIES

	Hyperthyroidism	Hypothyroidism
Primary	TH↑ TSH↓	TH↓ TSH↑
Secondary (Pituitary Cause)	TH↑ TSH↑	TH↓ TSH↓

myxedema: myx—mucus + edema—swelling

symptoms of hypothyroidism. Other symptoms are related to myxedema, which refers to a nonpitting type of edema that occurs in connective tissues throughout the body.

Etiology

Primary hypothyroidism may be a result of a congenital defect, inflammation of the thyroid gland, or iodine deficiency. Hashimoto's thyroiditis is an **autoimmune** disorder that eventually destroys thyroid tissue, leading to hypothyroidism. Secondary or tertiary hypothyroidism may be caused by a pituitary or hypothalamic lesion or by postpartum pituitary necrosis, a rare disorder in which the pituitary is destroyed following pregnancy and delivery. Treatment of hyperthyroidism, whether with medication or thyroidectomy, can lead to secondary hypothyroidism. Peripheral resistance to TH may also occur.

Signs and Symptoms

Manifestations primarily are related to the reduced metabolic rate and include fatigue, weight gain, bradycardia, constipation, mental dullness, feeling cold, shortness of breath, decreased sweating, and dry skin and hair (Table 39.4). Heart failure may occur because of decreased pumping strength of the heart. Altered fat metabolism causes hyperlipidemia. Myxedema causes water retention, with puffiness in the face, eye area, and feet. Fluid may also accumulate around the heart, causing altered cardiac function. See Box 39.3 Patient Perspective.

Complications

If the metabolic rate drops so low that it becomes life threatening, the result is myxedema coma. This usually occurs in patients with longstanding, untreated hypothyroidism and can be triggered by stress, such as infection, trauma, or exposure to cold. The patient becomes hypothermic, with a temperature less than 95°F (35°C) and a decreased respiratory rate. Depressed mental function and lethargy may occur. Blood glucose drops. Cardiac output drops, which in turn can reduce perfusion of kidneys. Nonpitting edema of the hands and feet may develop. Death may occur as a result of respiratory failure. If you note changes in mental status or vital signs, the physician should be contacted immediately. Treatment of myxedema coma involves intubation and

---

autoimmune: auto—pertaining to self + immune—exempt

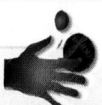

Box 39.3

Patient Perspective

Mary

When I turned 40-something, I began to notice a few changes in my body. I seemed to be easily fatigued, but I attributed that to moving our family across country and all the adjustments that needed to be made. I also noticed weight gain, most notably around my waist. Again, I thought, "well, I **am** 40-something," but it seemed no matter how much I exercised and watched what I ate, I couldn't lose weight. Worse, I was gaining! One day a friend of mine pointed out that I always seemed tired. Each time she called to do something, my reply was always the same, "I'd love to, but not today, I am just so tired."

Things started to get worse; I began losing hair by the handfuls each time I shampooed. It was so bad that every time I went to my hair stylist she had to reassure me that I wasn't going bald. However, my hair just didn't seem as full as it once did. I began to notice dry skin (I thought it was just our hard water) and constipation (I thought I had irritable bowel syndrome). Finally, I went to the doctor for a physical, including laboratory test, which included a TSH and free T_4. The diagnosis came back: I had hypothyroidism and was started on Synthroid. I noticed the effect on my energy almost immediately. Now I am able to exercise effectively. I have lost nearly all the weight I gained and my husband no longer complains about having to clean out the drain in our shower every time I wash my hair. I am thankful for the diagnosis and treatment because I feel like myself again.

mechanical ventilation. The patient is slowly rewarmed with blankets. Intravenous levothyroxine (Synthroid) is given, and any underlying cause is treated.

Diagnostic Tests

T_3 and T_4 levels are low, and TSH may be high or low, depending on the cause. If the pituitary is functioning normally, TSH is elevated in an attempt to stimulate an increase

---

TABLE 39.4 SYMPTOMS OF THYROID DISORDERS

	Hypothyroidism	Hyperthyroidism
Cardiovascular	Bradycardia, decreased cardiac output, cool skin, cold intolerance	Tachycardia, palpitations, increased cardiac output, warm skin, heat intolerance
Neurological	Lethargy, slowed movements, memory loss, confusion	Fatigue, restlessness, tremor, insomnia, emotional instability
Pulmonary	Dyspnea, hypoventilation	Dyspnea
Integumentary	Cool, dry skin; brittle, dry hair	Diaphoresis; warm, moist skin; fine, soft hair
Gastrointestinal	Decreased appetite, weight gain, constipation, increased serum lipid levels	Increased appetite, weight loss, frequent stools, decreased serum lipid levels
Reproductive	Decreased libido, erectile dysfunction	Decreased libido, erectile dysfunction, amenorrhea

in TH. Serum cholesterol and triglycerides are elevated. Antibodies are usually present in autoimmune disease.

Therapeutic Interventions

Primary hypothyroidism is easily treated with oral thyroid replacement hormone. Some patients still use TH from animal thyroids. Most patients now take synthetic thyroid hormone (levothyroxine). Doses are started low and are slowly increased to prevent symptoms of hyperthyroidism or cardiac complications.

Nursing Process for the Patient with Hypothyroidism

See Box 39.4 Nursing Care Plan for the Patient with Hypothyroidism.

Patient Education

Instruct the patient in the importance of consistent use of thyroid replacement medication and regular blood tests to monitor TSH. The patient needs to be aware that too much thyroid hormone will cause symptoms of hyperthyroidism. Such symptoms should be reported to the physician immediately. In addition, if the patient is experiencing mental status changes, discuss the need to avoid driving or operating machinery until symptoms are resolved.

CRITICAL THINKING

Mae

■ Mae is a 59-year-old woman who is tired all the time and has gained 16 pounds during the past year. Her physician does some blood tests and prescribes levothyroxine PO. Laboratory results show low T_3 and T_4 and elevated TSH.

1. Why is Mae's TSH elevated?
2. What will happen to Mae's caloric requirements as she begins treatment? Why?
3. Why should you teach Mae to check her pulse?

Suggested answers at end of chapter.

Hyperthyroidism

Hyperthyroidism is most often diagnosed in young women. Graves' disease, which is one cause of hyperthyroidism, is more common in young women. Multinodular goiter is more common in older women.

Pathophysiology

Hyperthyroidism results in excessive amounts of circulating thyroid hormone (thyrotoxicosis). Primary hyperthyroidism occurs when a problem within the thyroid gland causes excess hormone release. Secondary hyperthyroidism occurs because of excess TSH release from the pituitary, causing overstimulation of the thyroid gland; tertiary hyperthyroidism is caused by excess TRH from the hypothalamus. A high level of thyroid hormone increases the metabolic rate.

It is also believed to increase the number of beta-adrenergic receptor sites in the body, which enhances the activity of norepinephrine. The resulting fight-or-flight response is the cause of many of the symptoms of hyperthyroidism.

Etiology

A variety of disorders can cause hyperthyroidism. Graves' disease is the most common cause; it is thought to be an autoimmune disorder because thyroid-stimulating antibodies are present in the blood of affected patients.

Multinodular goiter, in which thyroid nodules secrete excess TH, is also sometimes associated with hyperthyroidism. A pituitary tumor may secrete excess TSH, which overstimulates the thyroid gland. A thyroid tumor may secrete TH. Patients taking thyroid hormone for hypothyroidism may take too much. Each of these problems can cause excess circulating TH and symptoms of hyperthyroidism.

Radiation exposure may predispose a patient to develop hyperthyroidism. Heredity may also play a role in autoimmune hyperthyroidism.

Signs and Symptoms

Many signs and symptoms are related to the hypermetabolic state, such as heat intolerance, increased appetite with weight loss, and increased frequency of bowel movements. Nervousness, tremor, tachycardia, and palpitations are caused by the increase in sympathetic nervous system activity, and may be more common in younger patients. Heart failure may occur because of tachycardia and the resulting inefficient pumping of the heart. See additional signs and symptoms in Table 39.4. If treatment is not begun, the patient may become manic or psychotic. Additional signs that occur only with Graves' disease include thickening of the skin on the anterior legs and exophthalmos (bulging of the eyes; Fig. 39.4) caused by swelling of the tissues behind

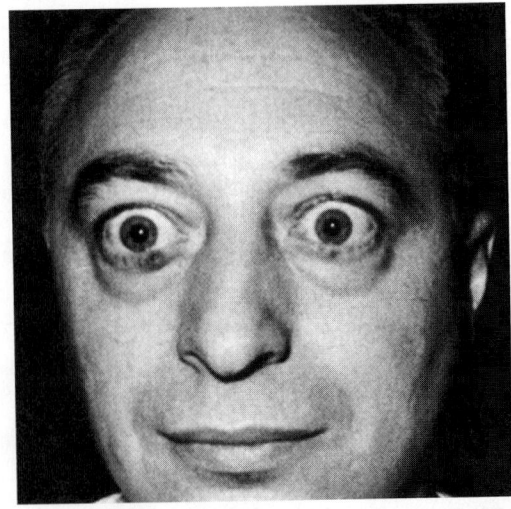

FIGURE 39.4 Exophthalmos caused by Graves' disease. *(From Tamparo, CD, and Lewis, MA: Diseases of the Human Body, ed. 4. F.A. Davis, Philadelphia, 2005, p 339, with permission.)*

Box 39.4 NURSING CARE PLAN for the Patient with Hypothyroidism

Nursing Diagnosis: Activity intolerance related to fatigue

Expected Outcomes (1) Patient reports lessening fatigue after treatment initiated. (2) Patient is able to carry out usual activities of daily living (ADLs).

Evaluation of Outcomes (1) Does patient report lessening fatigue? (2) Is patient able to carry out ADLs?

Interventions	Rationale	Evaluation
Assist patient with self-care activities.	Patients with fatigue may have difficulty carrying out activities independently.	Are patient's self-care needs being met? Is assistance needed?
Allow for rest between activities.	Rest periods will enable patient to conserve energy for activities.	Does patient state rest is adequate?
Slowly increase patient's activities as medication begins to be effective.	As thyroid replacement therapy becomes effective, patient's fatigue will subside.	Does patient tolerate increases in activity?

Geriatric

When getting elderly patients up, watch for orthostatic hypotension.	Orthostatic hypotension is common in elderly and may cause falls.	Does patient's blood pressure drop when changing positions?

Nursing Diagnosis: Constipation related to slowed gastrointestinal motility

Expected Outcomes (1) Soft, formed stool passed at preillness frequency. (2) Patient identifies measures to prevent constipation in future.

Evaluation of Outcomes (1) Are bowels moving according to patient's pre-illness pattern? (2) Does patient verbalize measures to prevent constipation?

Interventions	Rationale	Evaluation
Monitor and record bowel movements.	A record helps determine if a problem exists.	Does record show a problem?
Help patient follow usual pre-illness pattern (e.g., after morning coffee).	A schedule allows bowel movement to occur before stool becomes hard and dry.	Is patient able to identify and implement usual self-care for bowels?
Increase fluids to eight 8-ounce glasses of water daily if cardiovascular status stable.	Adequate fluid intake helps prevent hard, dry stools.	Does patient take adequate fluids?
Add fiber to diet: fresh fruit, vegetables, bran.	Fiber helps increase the number of bowel movements.	Does patient tolerate fiber? Is it effective?
Encourage regular ambulation.	Activity increases peristalsis.	Is patient able to ambulate or engage in other activity?
Use bedside commode or bathroom rather than bedpan.	The sitting position aids in evacuation.	Is sitting position effective?
Obtain physician order for stool softener if needed.	Soft stools are passed more easily.	Is stool softener needed? Effective?
If stool is impacted, break up stool digitally and gently remove.	Breaking up stool eases evacuation.	Is stool impacted? Is digital disimpaction effective?
Avoid use of enemas.	Enemas can cause fluid and electrolyte imbalances and can damage mucosa.	Does patient understand need to avoid enemas?

(Continued on following page)

Box 39.4   NURSING CARE PLAN for the Patient with Hypothyroidism *(Continued)*

Nursing Diagnosis: Impaired skin integrity related to dry skin, inactivity

Expected Outcomes (1) Skin is soft and moist. (2) Skin remains intact.

Evaluation of Outcomes Is skin soft, moist, and intact?

Interventions	Rationale	Evaluation
Assess skin daily for breakdown.	Skin lesions are more effectively treated when identified early.	Is breakdown present?
Avoid use of soap on dry areas. Try bath oil.	Soap is drying to skin.	Does use of bath oil help?
Use nondrying lotion following bath.	Lotion helps trap moisture in skin. Some lotions contain alcohol, however, which is drying.	Does patient state relief with use of lotion?
Encourage/assist with position changes at least every 2 hours.	Changing position enhances circulation to the skin, promoting healing and preventing breakdown.	Does patient change position at least every 2 hours? Are pressure areas prevented?

Nursing Diagnosis: Imbalanced nutrition, more than requirements, related to decreased metabolic rate

Expected Outcomes (1) Patient will return to pre-illness weight. (2) Patient will verbalize understanding of dietary recommendations.

Evaluation of Outcomes (1) Is patient approaching pre-illness weight? (2) Is patient able to explain dietary recommendations and how they will be implemented?

Interventions	Rationale	Evaluation
Weigh weekly and record.	Weekly weights record progress without the frustration of daily fluctuations.	Is patient losing or maintaining weight?
Consult dietitian for therapeutic diet until hypothyroidism is controlled.	The dietitian can provide food choices for gradual weight loss if necessary.	Does patient verbalize understanding of and ability to follow diet?
Encourage regular exercise within limits of fatigue.	Exercise promotes weight control.	Does patient verbalize understanding of and ability to follow exercise plan?
Counsel patient that weight should normalize once hypothyroidism is controlled.	Thyroid replacement hormone increases the metabolic rate, allowing return to normal weight.	Does patient verbalize understanding of instruction?
Geriatric		
Allow patient to help determine acceptable diet modifications.	Older patients may have long-standing dietary habits that are hard to change.	Is patient satisfied with weight loss plan?

the eyes. Other eye changes include photophobia and blurred or double vision.

Elderly patients may not exhibit the typical signs and symptoms of hyperthyroidism so be especially alert for this. These patients may present with heart failure, atrial fibrillation, fatigue, apathy, and depression.

Complications

THYROTOXIC CRISIS. Thyrotoxic crisis (also called thyroid storm) is a severe hyperthyroid state that can occur in hyperthyroid individuals who are untreated or who are experiencing another illness or stressor. It may also occur following thyroid surgery in patients who have been inadequately prepared with antithyroid medication. Thyrotoxic crisis can result in death in as little as 2 hours if untreated. Symptoms include tachycardia, high fever, hypertension (with eventual heart failure and hypotension), dehydration, restlessness, and delirium or coma.

If thyrotoxic crisis occurs, treatment is first directed toward relieving the life-threatening symptoms. Acetaminophen is given for the fever. Aspirin is avoided because it binds with the same serum protein as T_4, freeing additional T_4 into the circulation. Intravenous fluids and a cooling blanket may be ordered to cool the patient. A beta-adrenergic blocker, such as propranolol, is given for tachycardia. Oxygen is administered and the head of the bed is elevated because the high metabolic rate requires more oxygen. Once symptoms are controlled and the patient is safe, the underlying thyroid problem is treated.

HYPOTHYROIDISM. Another complication of hyperthyroidism can be hypothyroidism. This can occur as a result of long-term disease or as a result of treatment. Patients with a history of hyperthyroidism should be monitored for recurrent hyperthyroidism or the onset of hypothyroidism.

Diagnostic Tests

Serum levels of T_3 and T_4 are elevated. TSH is low in primary hyperthyroidism or high if the cause is pituitary. A thyroid scan can be done to locate a tumor. The thyroid gland may be enlarged; palpation of the thyroid in a patient suspected to be hyperthyroid should only be performed by a physician. TSI (thyroid-stimulating immunoglobulin) is present in Graves' disease. Rarely, a TRH stimulation test may be done.

Therapeutic Interventions

Several medications can be used to treat hyperthyroidism. Propylthiouracil (PTU) and methimazole (Tapazole) inhibit the synthesis of TH. Propranolol (Inderal) is a beta-blocking medication that relieves the sympathetic nervous system symptoms. Oral iodine suppresses the release of thyroid hormone.

Radioactive iodine (^{131}I or RAI) may be used to destroy a portion of the thyroid gland. The patient takes one oral dose of RAI. Dietary iodine normally goes to the thyroid gland, where it is used to make thyroid hormone. When RAI is given, the radioactivity destroys some of the cells that make thyroid hormone.

Sometimes medications alone control hyperthyroidism. If this does not occur, surgery is planned. If surgery is the treatment chosen, antithyroid medications are given to calm the thyroid before surgery. They help slow the heart rate and reduce other symptoms, making surgery safer. Iodine also reduces the vascularity of the thyroid gland, decreasing the risk of bleeding during surgery. Adequate preparation of the patient is important because a **euthyroid** state helps prevent a postoperative thyrotoxic crisis. Nursing care of the

patient undergoing a thyroidectomy is discussed later in this chapter.

Nursing Process for the Patient with Hyperthyroidism

ASSESSMENT/DATA COLLECTION. Monitor the patient with hyperthyroidism closely until normal thyroid activity is restored. Monitor vital signs and report any increases in pulse and blood pressure to the registered nurse or physician. Monitor lung sounds because crackles may indicate heart failure. Assess level of anxiety and ability to cope with symptoms. Monitor weight and bowel function. Assess eyes for risk for injury caused by exophthalmos, and note degree of muscle weakness. Never palpate the thyroid gland of a patient with hyperthyroidism because palpation may stimulate release of thyroid hormone and precipitate a thyrotoxic crisis.

NURSING DIAGNOSIS, PLANNING, AND IMPLEMENTATION. **Hyperthermia related to hypermetabolic state**

EXPECTED OUTCOMES: Body temperature will be within normal limits.

* Monitor temperature. *Temperature may be elevated due to hypermetabolic state.*
* Administer acetaminophen as ordered *to reduce temperature.*
* Apply cooling blanket as ordered. *External cooling may be necessary if acetaminophen is not effective.*
* If a cooling blanket is necessary, set to one to two degrees below current temperature, and wrap extremities with towels *to prevent shivering, which can further increase temperature.*

Diarrhea related to increase in peristalsis

EXPECTED OUTCOMES: Patient will maintain fluid and electrolyte balance.

* Provide a low-fiber diet. *Fiber can increase peristalsis and stools.*
* Provide small frequent meals of bland foods (bananas, rice, applesauce) *that are less likely to worsen diarrhea.*
* Monitor electrolytes, especially sodium and potassium. *Diarrhea can cause electrolyte loss.*
* Monitor for dehydration. *Diarrhea causes fluid loss.*
* Keep skin clean and dry; apply barrier cream *to protect skin from injury from stool.*

Imbalanced nutrition, less than requirements, related to increased metabolism

EXPECTED OUTCOMES: The patient will maintain weight in proportion to height.

* Determine healthy weight for height, *so the expected outcome is realistic for the patient.*
* Monitor weight weekly *to make sure interventions are working.*
* Consult dietician for high-calorie diet with six meals *to meet caloric requirements.*

---

euthyroid: eu—normal, healthy + thyroid

Disturbed sleep pattern related to sympathetic stimulation

EXPECTED OUTCOMES: The patient will state feeling rested upon awakening.

- Provide a quiet, restful environment *to assist the patient to fall asleep.*
- Ask the patient if music or earplugs are desired *to mask environmental noise.*
- Administer propranolol or sedative as ordered *to reduce sympathetic stimulation and calm patient.*

Anxiety related to sympathetic stimulation

EXPECTED OUTCOMES: Patient will state anxiety is controlled.

- Provide the patient with accurate information about the disorder and treatment, and that proper treatment will correct symptoms. *Fear of the unknown can produce anxiety.*
- Administer propranolol or antianxiety agent as ordered *to reduce sympathetic stimulation and calm patient.*
- Offer massage, music, or other relaxation techniques preferred by the patient. *These may promote relaxation.*

Risk for injury related to hypermetabolic state and eye involvement

EXPECTED OUTCOMES: Patient will remain safe and without injury.

- Report changes in vital signs to the physician. *Prompt treatment can reduce complications.*
- Administer lubricating saline eyedrops as ordered *to protect eyes from drying.*
- Advise use of dark, tight fitting glasses *to protect eyes from light and injury.*
- Gently tape eyes shut with nonallergic tape for sleeping. *Exophthalmos may prevent the patient from fully closing the eyes.*
- Elevate the head of the bed *to reduce edema behind the eyes.*
- Provide a low-sodium diet. *This may decrease edema behind the eyes.*
- Teach patient to notify physician immediately if eye pain or vision changes occur. *These can be signs of pressure from edema on optic nerve, which can cause permanent damage if not corrected.*

PATIENT EDUCATION. Teach the patient about the disease and symptoms of hyperthyroidism or hypothyroidism to report. Also teach the patient how to take medications and the importance of routine follow-up laboratory testing.

EVALUATION. If the plan of care is effective, the patient will remain free from complications or injury. Eyes will be comfortable and free from injury. Body temperature will be kept within normal limits. Diarrhea will be controlled, and complications of diarrhea such as skin breakdown and

dehydration avoided. The patient's weight should remain stable. The patient should report that he or she is rested on awakening and that anxiety is controlled.

Care of the Patient Receiving Radioactive Iodine

If radioactive iodine is used, it is usually given orally in one dose. If the dose is high, such as for the patient with thyroid cancer, the patient is hospitalized. Patients receiving lower doses may be treated as outpatients. You should limit time spent with the patient and maintain a safe distance when providing direct care (see Chapter 10). Pregnant caregivers should avoid caring for patients receiving radioactive iodine. Urine, vomitus, and other body secretions are contaminated and should be disposed of according to hospital policy. Flush the toilet twice following disposal of contaminated material. The radiation safety officer and hospital policy should be consulted for specific precautions.

At home, the patient is instructed to avoid close contact with family members for about a week and to use careful hand washing after urinating. Oral contact with others should be avoided, and eating utensils should be washed thoroughly with soap and water. Hospital teaching protocols should be used for specific patient teaching. If the treatment is being administered for hyperthyroidism, inform the patient that symptoms will subside in about 6 to 8 weeks.

Side effects are rare, and may include a sore throat or nausea. Sore throat is easily treated with acetaminophen, and nausea can be reduced by taking the dose on an empty stomach. Encourage the patient to drink plenty of fluids to help remove the RAI from the body. In addition, the patient should be aware of symptoms of hypothyroidism to be reported because hypothyroidism may occur up to 15 years after the treatment.

Goiter

Pathophysiology and Etiology

Enlargement of the thyroid gland is called a goiter. The thyroid gland may enlarge in response to increased TSH levels. TSH is elevated in response to low TH, iodine deficiency, pregnancy, or viral, genetic, or other conditions. When a goiter is caused by iodine deficiency or other environmental factors, it is called an endemic goiter.

Some foods and medications are **goitrogens.** These substances interfere with the body's use of iodine and include such foods as turnips, cabbage, broccoli, horseradish, cauliflower, and carrots (Box 39.5 Nutrition Notes). Some **goitrogenic** medications include propylthiouracil, sulfonamides, lithium, and salicylates (aspirin).

A goiter may be associated with a hyperthyroid, hypothyroid, or euthyroid state. Goiter that occurs with hyperthyroidism is sometimes called a toxic goiter. Once the cause of the goiter is removed, the gland usually returns to normal size.

---

goitrogenic: goitro—goiter + genic—producing

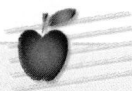

Box 39.5

Nutrition Notes

Relating Nutrition to Thyroid Disorders

Iodine Deficiency

Inland areas of all continents have iodine-poor soils. People in developing countries with only local food sources are still subject to endemic goiter; however, addition of iodine to table salt has significantly reduced the occurrence of endemic goiter in developed countries.

Vegetables in the cabbage family contain goitrogens, substances that block the body's absorption or utilization of iodine, but the risk is small. At higher risk of iodine deficiency are strict vegetarians who consume sea salt, which contains virtually no iodine, rather than iodized salt.

Iodine Excess

Saltwater fish, shellfish, and seaweed are naturally high in iodine so that iodine toxicity from seaweed has occurred in Japan. Excessive iodine can be manifested as either hyperthyroidism or hypothyroidism, sometimes producing "iodine goiter."

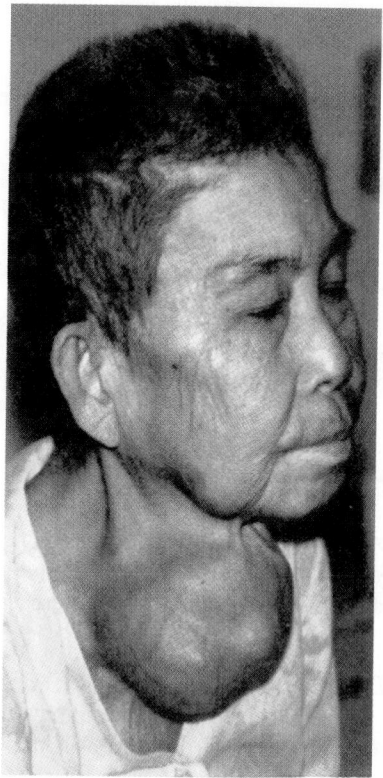

FIGURE 39.5 Patient with goiter.

Signs and Symptoms

The thyroid gland is enlarged, and swelling may be apparent at the base of the neck (Fig. 39.5). Alternatively, it may enlarge posteriorly, which can interfere with swallowing or breathing. The patient may have a full sensation in the neck. Symptoms of hypothyroidism or hyperthyroidism may be present.

Diagnostic Tests

A thyroid scan shows an enlarged thyroid gland. Serum T_3 and T_4 levels are measured to determine thyroid function. Additional diagnostic studies may be done to determine the cause or evaluate the size of the gland.

Therapeutic Interventions

Treatment is aimed at the cause. If goitrogens are suspected, the patient is given a list of foods to be avoided. If iodine deficiency is a problem, it is added to the diet with supplements or iodized salt. Hypothyroidism or hyperthyroidism is treated if indicated. Levothyroxine (Synthroid) may be given to reduce TSH levels via negative feedback. A thyroidectomy may be necessary if the gland is interfering with breathing or swallowing.

Nursing Care

Be careful to assess the effect of the goiter on breathing and swallowing. Stridor, a whistling sound, may be heard if the airway is obstructed. Stridor is an ominous sign and should be reported to the physician immediately. If the patient experiences difficulty swallowing, notify the physician and collaborate with the dietitian to provide soft foods or liquid nutrition. A swallowing study might be ordered, which can assist a speech pathologist or other expert to make specific recommendations for safe swallowing.

Cancer of the Thyroid Gland

Although thyroid cancer is rare, it is the most common cancer of the endocrine system (Box 39.6 Cultural Considerations). Women are affected more often than men. Most tumors of the thyroid gland are not malignant.

Etiology

Thyroid hyperplasia may lead to thyroid cancer. Other causes include exposure to radiation, iodine deficiency, and prolonged exposure to goitrogens. Tendency to develop some forms of thyroid cancer is inherited.

Signs and Symptoms

A hard, painless nodule may be palpable on the thyroid gland. Difficulty breathing or swallowing or changes in the voice may occur if the tumor is near the esophagus and trachea. Most patients with cancer of the thyroid have normal TH levels.

Diagnostic Tests

A thyroid scan shows a "cold" nodule. This is because malignant tumors of the thyroid do not take up the radioactive iodine administered for the scan. A fine-needle aspiration biopsy confirms the diagnosis. A "hot" nodule indicates a benign tumor.

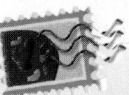

Box 39.6

Cultural Considerations

Because of the Chernobyl nuclear disaster in Russia in 1988, Russian immigrants are at exceptionally high risk for developing pituitary, thyroid, and parathyroid disorders and cancers. The proximity of Estonia, Latvia, Lithuania, Poland, and other Eastern European countries to Russia places immigrants and long-term visitors from these countries at risk also. The nurse needs to be alert for endocrine disorders among these populations and assist patients to arrange genetic counseling for those who desire it.

Therapeutic Interventions

A partial or total thyroidectomy may be done. Chemotherapy, radioactive iodine therapy, or external beam radiation may also be used, alone or following surgery.

Nursing Care

Nursing care is determined by the symptoms the patient is experiencing. See Chapter 10 for care of the patient with cancer.

Nursing Process for the Patient Undergoing Thyroidectomy

Patients may undergo thyroidectomy for cancer of the thyroid, hyperthyroidism, or a goiter that is causing dyspnea or dysphagia. See Chapter 11 for general care of a patient having surgery.

A total thyroidectomy is usually performed if cancer is present. After a total thyroidectomy, lifelong replacement hormone must be taken. A subtotal (partial) thyroidectomy may be done for hyperthyroidism, leaving a portion of the thyroid gland to secrete TH.

Preoperative Care

Before undergoing a thyroidectomy, the patient should be in a euthyroid state. This is accomplished with the use of antithyroid medication. Saturated solution of potassium iodide (SSKI) may also be administered to decrease the size and vascularity of the gland, reducing the risk of bleeding during surgery.

Do a baseline assessment of vital signs and voice quality, so you can compare findings postoperatively. Explain what the patient can expect before, during, and after surgery and clarify misconceptions. Preoperative teaching should include how to perform gentle range-of-motion exercises of the neck, how to support the neck during position changes, and how to use an incentive spirometer after surgery. See Chapter 11 for routine preoperative care.

Postoperative Care

ASSESSMENT/DATA COLLECTION. Monitor vital signs, oxygen saturation, drain (if present), and dressings every 15 minutes initially, progressing to every 4 hours, as ordered.

Decreased blood pressure with increased pulse should alert you to the possibility of shock related to blood loss. Tachycardia and fever, along with mental status changes, may indicate thyrotoxic crisis. Check the back of the neck for pooling of blood. Because of the location of the surgery, observe for signs of respiratory distress, including an increase in respiratory rate, dyspnea, or stridor. Ask the patient to speak to detect hoarseness of the voice, which may indicate trauma to the recurrent laryngeal nerve. Monitor the patient's serum calcium levels and watch for evidence of **tetany** (discussed later in this chapter). Report abnormal findings to the physician immediately.

NURSING DIAGNOSIS, PLANNING, AND IMPLEMENTATION. Risk for ineffective airway clearance due to edema at surgical site

EXPECTED OUTCOMES: Patient will maintain a clear airway.
- Notify physician of respiratory distress immediately; keep a tracheostomy set at the bedside. *Although not common, a tracheostomy may be needed in an emergency if edema obstructs the airway.*
- Maintain patient in semi-Fowler's position *to help reduce edema and promote comfort.*
- Monitor neck dressing. *If the dressing seems to get tighter, it may be a sign that the patient's neck is swelling, which could impair the airway.*
- Use room humidifier or humidified oxygen *to keep airways and secretions moist.*
- Remind the patient to do coughing and deep breathing exercises every hour. *This keeps the airway clear of secretions.*
- Have suction equipment available *in case patient is unable to cough up secretions effectively.*
- Encourage the patient to use the incentive spirometer *to assist with deep breathing.*
- Assess the patient's swallowing and gag reflexes before offering clear liquids *to guard against aspiration.*

Risk for injury (tetany, thyrotoxic crisis) related to surgical procedure

EXPECTED OUTCOMES: Complications will be recognized and treated quickly.
- Monitor for numbness or tingling around the mouth or muscle spasms and report immediately if they occur. *These are symptoms of tetany that must be treated immediately. Tetany is most likely to occur 24 to 72 hours postoperatively.*
- Monitor vital signs frequently and report changes immediately. *Elevated vital signs may be signs of thyrotoxic crisis, which is most likely to occur up to 18 hours postoperatively.*

Pain related to surgical procedure

EXPECTED OUTCOMES: Patient will state that pain level is acceptable.

- Administer acetaminophen or opioids as ordered. Avoid aspirin products. *Aspirin binds to the same protein as thyroid hormone, and can precipitate a thyrotoxic crisis.*
- Use pillows or sandbags to support the patient's head. *Unexpected movement may be painful.*

Risk for ineffective health maintenance related to knowledge deficit

EXPECTED OUTCOMES: *Patient will verbalize understanding of follow-up care. Patient's weight will stabilize at appropriate weight for height.*

- Assist the patient with gentle range-of-motion exercises, avoiding hyperextension of the neck, which can cause strain on the incision line. *Avoidance of neck movement due to pain can result in contracture.*
- Consult dietitian to assist the patient with potential dietary changes needed following surgery. *With correction of metabolic alterations, dietary needs may be significantly altered.*
- Teach the patient the importance of follow-up care *to avoid complications.*
  - How to administer replacement hormone if indicated.
  - How to change the dressing and to report bleeding or signs of infection at the site.
  - Importance of immediately reporting unusual irritability, fever, or palpitations.
  - Importance of follow-up lab work for thyroid function.

EVALUATION. If the plan has been effective, complications caused by surgery will not occur or will be recognized and reported early. Pain will be prevented or controlled, and the patient will demonstrate understanding of dietary modifications and postoperative self-care.

Complications

THYROTOXIC CRISIS. Thyrotoxic crisis may result from manipulation of the thyroid gland during surgery, with the subsequent release of large amounts of thyroid hormone. This is a rare complication because the use of antithyroid drugs before surgery has become routine. For more information on thyrotoxic crisis, see the section on hyperthyroidism earlier in this chapter.

TETANY. Tetany is caused by low calcium levels and is characterized by tingling in the fingers and perioral area (around the mouth), muscle spasms, twitching, and cardiac dysrhythmias. Muscle spasms in the larynx can lead to respiratory obstruction. Watch carefully for symptoms of tetany and report them immediately if they occur because if the problem is not recognized quickly, death can result.

Tetany can occur if the parathyroid glands are accidentally removed during thyroid surgery. Because of the proximity of the parathyroid glands to the thyroid, it is sometimes difficult for the surgeon to avoid them. In the absence of

parathyroid hormone, serum calcium levels drop and tetany results. Intravenous calcium gluconate is given to treat acute tetany.

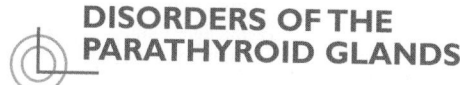 DISORDERS OF THE PARATHYROID GLANDS

Recall that the parathyroid glands secrete parathyroid hormone (PTH) in response to low serum calcium levels. PTH raises serum calcium levels by promoting calcium movement from bones to blood and by increasing absorption of dietary calcium. Decreased PTH activity is called hypoparathyroidism. Increased PTH activity is called hyperparathyroidism.

Hypoparathyroidism

Pathophysiology

A decrease in PTH causes a decrease in bone resorption of calcium, a decrease in calcium absorption by the GI tract, and decreased resorption in the kidneys. This means that calcium stays in bones instead of being moved into the blood, and more calcium is excreted from the body. The result is a decreased serum calcium level, called hypocalcemia. As calcium levels fall, phosphate levels rise.

Etiology

The most common causes of hypoparathyroidism are heredity and the accidental removal of the parathyroid glands during thyroidectomy. Because of the proximity of the glands to the thyroid, it is sometimes difficult to avoid removing them. Hypoparathyroidism also occurs following purposeful removal of the parathyroid glands for hyperparathyroidism or cancer. Another cause is hypomagnesemia, which impairs secretion of PTH. Hypomagnesemia can occur with chronic alcoholism or certain nutritional problems.

Signs and Symptoms

Calcium plays an important role in nerve cell stability. Hypocalcemia causes neuromuscular irritability. In acute cases, tetany may occur (see previous section on tetany), with numbness and tingling of the fingers and perioral area, muscle spasms, and twitching. (See Table 39.5.) Positive Chvostek's and Trousseau's signs are early indications of tetany. To check Chvostek's sign, tap on the patient's facial nerve just in front of the ear. Spasm of the face is a positive result, indicating hypocalcemia. To elicit Trousseau's sign, place a sphygmomanometer on the patient's arm and pump it to above the patient's systolic pressure. Spasm of the thumb and fingers occurs within 3 minutes if the patient has hypocalcemia. See Chapter 5 for pictures of these tests.

 LEARNING TIP

To remember which test is which, remember **CH**vostek's sign is assessed near the **CH**eek.

TABLE 39.5 PARATHYROID DISORDERS SUMMARY

	Insufficient PTH	Excess PTH
Disorder	Hypoparathyroidism	Hyperparathyroidism
Signs and Symptoms	Hypocalcemia, neuromuscular irritability, tetany; positive Chvostek and Trousseau signs	Hypercalcemia, fatigue, pathological fractures
Diagnostic Tests	Serum PTH, calcium, and phosphate	Serum PTH, calcium, and phosphate
Therapeutic Management	Calcium replacement; high-calcium, low-phosphorus diet	Calcitonin, parathyroidectomy
Priority Nursing Diagnoses	Risk for injury related to tetany	Risk for injury related to bone demineralization

In chronic hypoparathyroidism, the patient is lethargic and experiences muscle spasms. Calcifications may occur in the eyes and brain, leading to psychosis. Cataracts can develop. Bone changes are evident on x-ray examination. Convulsions may occur. Death can result from laryngospasm if treatment is not provided.

Diagnostic Tests

Chvostek's and Trousseau's signs are present. Laboratory studies show decreased serum calcium and PTH levels and increased serum phosphate. Radiographs show bone changes.

Therapeutic Interventions

Acute cases of hypoparathyroidism are treated with intravenous calcium gluconate. Long-term treatment includes a high-calcium diet (Box 39.7 Dietary Sources of Calcium), with oral calcium and vitamin D supplements. Thiazide diuretics may also be used because they reduce the amount of calcium excreted in the urine. Magnesium is given if hypomagnesemia is present.

Nursing Process for the Patient with Hypoparathyroidism

ASSESSMENT/DATA COLLECTION. The patient at risk for hypoparathyroidism should be closely monitored for symptoms of tetany. If you suspect tetany, check for Chvostek's and Trousseau's signs. Monitor respirations closely for stridor, a sign of laryngospasm.

NURSING DIAGNOSIS, PLANNING, AND IMPLEMENTATION. Risk for injury related to tetany

Box 39.7

Dietary Sources of Calcium

Milk
Cheeses
Yogurt
Sardines
Oysters
Salmon
Cauliflower
Green leafy vegetables

EXPECTED OUTCOME: The patient will remain free from injury; signs of tetany will be recognized and treated quickly.

- Monitor for signs of tetany and report immediately to RN or physician *so treatment can be instituted quickly.*
- Make sure a tracheostomy set, endotracheal tube, and intravenous calcium are available *for emergency use if laryngospasm occurs.*
- Consult a dietitian for high-calcium diet teaching. *The patient may need a lifelong high-calcium diet.*
- Teach the patient about the importance of diet and medication therapy, and follow-up laboratory testing. *The patient needs to understand self-care for follow-up at home.*

EVALUATION. Injury is prevented through early recognition and reporting of signs and symptoms of tetany. The patient should be able to describe correct treatment and self-care measures for home.

Hyperparathyroidism

Pathophysiology

Overactivity of one or more of the parathyroid glands causes an increase in PTH, with a subsequent increase in the serum calcium level (hypercalcemia). This is achieved through movement of calcium out of the bones and into the blood, absorption in the small intestine, and reabsorption by the kidneys. PTH also promotes phosphate excretion by the kidneys.

Etiology

Hyperparathyroidism is usually the result of hyperplasia or a benign tumor of the parathyroid glands, or it may be hereditary. Some cancers can also make a substance that mimics PTH and causes hypercalcemia. Secondary hyperparathyroidism occurs when the parathyroids secrete excessive PTH in response to low serum calcium levels. Serum calcium may be reduced in kidney disease because of the kidneys' failure to activate vitamin D, which is necessary for absorption of calcium in the small intestine.

Signs and Symptoms

Signs and symptoms of hyperparathyroidism are caused primarily by the increase in serum calcium level, although many patients are asymptomatic. Symptoms include fatigue, depression, confusion, increased urination, anorexia, nausea, vomiting, kidney stones, and cardiac dysrhythmias. The increased serum calcium level also causes gastrin secretion, resulting in abdominal pain and peptic ulcers. Because calcium is being removed from bones, bone and joint pain and pathological fractures may occur. With severe hypercalcemia, the result may be coma and cardiac arrest.

Diagnostic Tests

Laboratory studies include serum calcium, phosphate, and PTH levels. Radiographs may show decreased bone density. Nuclear scanning may be used to help locate the parathyroid glands if surgical removal is planned.

Therapeutic Interventions

The patient is monitored for bone changes and decline in renal function. Hydration with intravenous normal saline lowers the calcium level by dilution. Furosemide (Lasix) is given to increase renal excretion of calcium. Alendronate (Fosamax) or calcitonin may be given to prevent calcium release from bones. Estrogen therapy might be used in women, although side effects must be considered.

If hypercalcemia is severe or if the patient is at risk for bone or kidney complications, surgery to remove the diseased parathyroid glands (parathyroidectomy) is performed. If possible, some parathyroid tissue is left intact to continue to secrete PTH.

Preoperative and postoperative care is similar to that of the patient undergoing thyroid surgery, with special attention paid to calcium and PTH levels. The patient will likely be on calcium and vitamin D supplements following surgery. A new procedure, called minimally invasive radio-guided parathyroidectomy, can be done under local anesthesia through a small incision.

Nursing Process for the Patient with Hyperparathyroidism

ASSESSMENT/DATA COLLECTION. Assess the patient for symptoms related to hypercalcemia, including muscle weakness, lethargy, bone pain, anorexia, nausea, vomiting, behavioral changes, and renal insufficiency. Monitor serum calcium levels as ordered.

NURSING DIAGNOSIS, PLANNING, AND IMPLEMENTATION. Nursing diagnoses depend on assessment findings. Risk for injury usually takes priority.

Risk for injury (fracture, complications of hypercalcemia) related to calcium imbalance

EXPECTED OUTCOME: The patient remains free from injury.
- Monitor for and report signs or symptoms of calcium imbalance promptly. *Prompt treatment can prevent serious complications.*
- Encourage oral fluids *to prevent dehydration and kidney stones and help excrete calcium.*
- Encourage strengthening and weight-bearing exercises *to help keep calcium in the bones.*
- Provide a safe environment for ambulation; assist the patient with ambulation if necessary. *A fall could result in fracture if bones are demineralized.*

- Encourage smoking cessation. *Smoking causes bone loss.*
- Teach patient symptoms to report and use of long-term medications *so patient can manage self-care at home.*

EVALUATION. If the plan is effective, symptoms of hypercalcemia will be recognized and reported quickly, and complications and injury will be prevented.

DISORDERS OF THE ADRENAL GLANDS

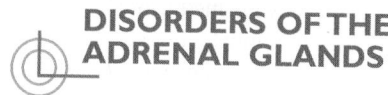

Adrenal disorders may involve the adrenal medulla or the adrenal cortex. A rare tumor of the adrenal medulla, called a **pheochromocytoma**, causes hypersecretion of epinephrine and norepinephrine. Hyposecretion of epinephrine is rare and generally causes no symptoms. Hypersecretion of cortisol from the adrenal cortex results in Cushing's syndrome. Hypofunction of the adrenal cortex results in Addison's disease.

Pheochromocytoma

Pathophysiology

A pheochromocytoma is an uncommon tumor that arises from the chromaffin cells of the adrenal medulla. Occasionally, a pheochromocytoma occurs outside the adrenal gland. The tumor autonomously secretes catecholamines (epinephrine and norepinephrine) in excessive amounts. Ninety percent of pheochromocytomas are benign.

Etiology

The cause of pheochromocytoma is unknown. About 5% of cases are hereditary.

Signs and Symptoms

Because norepinephrine is the fight-or-flight hormone, patients with a pheochromocytoma have exaggerated fight-or-flight symptoms. These might be fairly constant, or occur in "attacks." Manifestations include hypertension, tachycardia (with heart rate greater than 100), palpitations, tremor, diaphoresis, feeling of apprehension, and severe pounding headache. Nausea and vomiting are occasionally present. Blood glucose may increase because catecholamines inhibit insulin release from the pancreas. Constipation may occur because catecholamines relax the bowel. The most prominent characteristic is intermittent unstable hypertension. Diastolic pressure may be greater than 115 mm Hg. If hypertension is uncontrolled, the patient is at risk for stroke, vision changes, and organ damage. It is estimated that about 0.1% of cases of hypertension are caused by a pheochromocytoma.

Diagnostic Tests

Patients with a suspected pheochromocytoma have a 24-hour urine test for metanephrines and vanillylmandelic acid

---

pheochromocytoma: pheo—dark + chromo—color + cyt—cell + oma—tumor

(VMA). These are endproducts of catecholamine metabolism. A blood test for metanephrines may also be done. The patient should avoid caffeine and medications for 2 days before and during the test. Check institution policy for other dietary restrictions. If results are elevated, a CT scan or MRI is done to locate the tumor.

Therapeutic Interventions

Treatment for pheochromocytoma is surgical removal of one or both adrenal glands. However, the patient must be stabilized before surgery. Alpha-blocking medications such as phenoxybenzamine (Dibenzyline) dilate blood vessels to control acute hypertension. Beta-blocking medication may be added to block beta-adrenergic receptors in the heart and lungs, reducing other fight-or-flight symptoms.

Nursing Process for the Patient with Pheochromocytoma

ASSESSMENT/DATA COLLECTION. Monitor vital signs frequently, and report elevations promptly.

NURSING DIAGNOSIS, PLANNING, AND IMPLEMENTATION. Risk for injury related to hypertensive crisis

EXPECTED OUTCOME: Patient will be free from injury related to hypertension.

- Monitor vital signs and report elevated pulse and blood pressure promptly. *Prompt treatment helps prevent complications.*
- Approach the patient calmly and maintain a quiet environment. *Stress may precipitate a hypertensive episode.*
- Administer alpha and beta blockers as ordered *to control symptoms.*
- Teach the patient how the medications will reduce symptoms, and the importance of avoiding foods and beverages containing caffeine, *so the patient can participate in self-care.*
- If patient has surgery, continue careful monitoring *as manipulation of tumor can increase catecholamine release.*

EVALUATION. If interventions have been effective, the patient's vital signs will be within normal limits, and complications will be avoided.

Adrenocortical Insufficiency/ Addison's Disease

Adrenocortical insufficiency (AI) is the insufficient production of the hormones of the adrenal cortex. Primary AI is called Addison's disease.

Pathophysiology

Adrenal insufficiency is associated with reduced levels of cortisol, aldosterone, or both hormones. A deficiency in androgens may exist. In primary disease, ACTH levels from the pituitary may be elevated in an attempt to stimulate the adrenal cortex to synthesize more hormone. In secondary disease, deficient ACTH fails to stimulate adrenal steroid

synthesis. In most cases, the adrenal glands are atrophied, small, and misshapen and are unable to produce adequate amounts of hormone.

Etiology

Addison's disease is thought to be autoimmune; that is, the gland destroys itself in response to conditions such as tuberculosis, fungal infection, infection related to acquired immunodeficiency syndrome (AIDS), or metastatic cancer. It may also be associated with other autoimmune diseases, such as Hashimoto's thyroiditis. Adrenalectomy also results in adrenal insufficiency.

Secondary AI may be caused by dysfunction of the pituitary or hypothalamus. In addition, prolonged use of corticosteroid drugs may depress ACTH and corticotropin-releasing hormone production, which in turn reduces steroid hormone production. A patient receiving long-term corticosteroid therapy is particularly at risk for AI if the drugs are abruptly discontinued. Because the pituitary has been suppressed for a prolonged period, it may take up to a year before ACTH is produced normally again.

NURSING CARE TIP

Always slowly taper corticosteroid therapy to avoid adrenal crisis.

Signs and Symptoms

The most significant sign of Addison's disease is hypotension. This is related to the lack of aldosterone. Remember that aldosterone causes sodium and water retention in the kidney and potassium loss. If aldosterone is deficient, sodium and water are lost and hypotension and tachycardia result. Low cortisol levels cause hypoglycemia, weakness, fatigue, weight loss, confusion, and psychosis. In primary AI, increased ACTH may produce hyperpigmentation of the skin, causing the patient to have a tanned or bronze appearance. Anorexia, nausea, and vomiting may also occur, possibly as the result of electrolyte imbalances. Women may have decreased body hair because of low androgen levels.

Complications

If a patient is exposed to stress, such as infection, trauma, or psychological pressure, the body may be unable to respond normally with secretion of cortisol and an adrenal crisis can occur. Loss of large amounts of sodium and water and the resulting fluid volume deficit cause profound hypotension, dehydration, and tachycardia. Potassium retention can cause cardiac dysrhythmias. Hypoglycemia may be severe. Coma and death result if treatment is not initiated. Treatment of adrenal crisis involves rapidly restoring fluid volume and cortisol levels. Intravenous fluids (containing glucose) and large doses of glucocorticoids are administered. Electrolytes are replaced as needed. The cause of the crisis should be identified and treated.

Diagnostic Tests

Serum and urine cortisol levels are measured. Blood glucose is low. Blood urea nitrogen (BUN) and hematocrit levels may appear to be elevated because of dehydration. An ACTH stimulation test may help determine whether the adrenal glands are functioning. Serum sodium and potassium levels are monitored.

Therapeutic Interventions

Long-term treatment consists of replacement of glucocorticoids (hydrocortisone) and mineralocorticoids (fludrocortisone). Patients will need hormone replacement therapy for the rest of their lives. Hormones are given in divided doses, with two-thirds of the daily dose given in the morning and one-third in the evening to mimic the body's own diurnal rhythm. Remember that steroid hormones are our natural stress hormones and so are naturally elevated during times of stress. Therefore, during times of stress or illness, doses need to be increased to two to three times normal. The patient may also be placed on a high-sodium diet.

Nursing Process for the Patient with Addison's Disease

ASSESSMENT/DATA COLLECTION. The patient with Addison's disease should be assessed for understanding of and compliance with the treatment regimen. Monitor daily weights or intake and output to track fluid status. Monitor serum glucose levels and symptoms of hyperkalemia and hyponatremia. Report changes in mental status. If the patient is in crisis, monitor vital signs closely and report any signs of fluid volume deficit such as orthostatic hypotension or poor skin turgor to the physician immediately.

NURSING DIAGNOSIS, PLANNING, AND IMPLEMENTATION. Risk for deficient fluid volume related to deficient adrenal cortical hormones

EXPECTED OUTCOME: Fluid volume will be stable as evidenced by stable weights and vital signs, and skin turgor within normal limits.

- Monitor fluid status and report changes promptly *so treatment can be initiated.*
- Administer steroid replacements as ordered *to maintain fluid and electrolyte balance.*

Risk for ineffective health maintenance related to deficient knowledge about self-care of Addison's disease

EXPECTED OUTCOME: The patient will verbalize understanding of self-monitoring and self-medication at home.

- Assess patient's understanding of his or her disease process and treatment. *Teaching should build on baseline knowledge.*
- Teach the patient the importance of hormone replacement. Doses are generally taken two-thirds in the morning and one-third in the evening. *The patient who does not secrete endogenous adrenocortical hormones must rely on replacements.*
- Help the patient identify the causes and symptoms of stress, and explain the need to increase medica-

tion dosage by two to three times during times of stress or illness according to the physician's instructions. *Since these hormones are normally increased during times of stress, it is important that the patient understand how to increase the dose during stress to prevent adrenal crisis.*

- Advise patient he or she may need to increase salt intake in hot weather *because of fluid and salt losses.*
- Recommend medical alert identification to the patient. *A patient in adrenal crisis may not be able to provide a medical history to emergency personnel, and identification can prevent delay of treatment.*
- If ordered by the physician, teach the patient and significant other how to use an emergency intramuscular hydrocortisone injection kit. *IM medication may be needed during stress or times when the patient is unable to take oral medications.*

EVALUATION. If nursing care is effective, the patient's fluid status will be stable, and the patient and family will be able to describe proper self-care of Addison's disease.

Cushing's Disease/Syndrome

Cushing's *disease* is characterized by excess cortisol secretion resulting from secretion of too much adrenocorticotropic hormone (ACTH) by the pituitary. Cushing's *syndrome* refers to symptoms of cortisol excess caused by other factors. See Table 39.6 for a comparison of adrenal insufficiency and Cushing's syndrome.

Pathophysiology

Recall that cortisol, aldosterone, and androgens are the three steroid hormones secreted by the adrenal cortex. Cortisol is essential for survival and is normally secreted in a diurnal rhythm, with levels increasing in the early morning. Secretion is increased during times of stress. In Cushing's syndrome, cortisol is hypersecreted without regard to stress or time of day. When levels of cortisol are very high, effects related to excess aldosterone and androgens are also seen.

LEARNING TIP

Remember from Chapter 38, an easy way to remember the hormones of the adrenal cortex is to think salt, sugar, and sex. Aldosterone promotes salt retention, cortisol affects sugar (carbohydrate) metabolism, and androgens are sex hormones.

Etiology

Cushing's disease is caused by the hypersecretion of ACTH by the pituitary. This is most often the result of a pituitary adenoma. Sometimes ACTH is produced by a tumor in the

TABLE 39.6 ADRENAL CORTEX HORMONE SUMMARY

	Hypofunction	Hyperfunction
Disorder	Adrenocortical insufficiency, Addison's disease	Cushing's syndrome
Signs and Symptoms	Sodium and water loss, hypotension, hypoglycemia, fatigue	Weight gain, sodium and water retention, hyperglycemia, buffalo hump, moon face
Diagnostic Tests	Serum and urine cortisol	Serum and urine cortisol
Therapeutic Management	Glucocorticoid and mineralocorticoid replacement	Alter steroid therapy schedule; surgery if tumor
Priority Nursing Diagnoses	Risk for fluid volume deficit	Risks for fluid volume excess, glucose intolerance, infection

lungs or other organs. The high levels of ACTH cause adrenal hyperplasia, which in turn increases production and release of cortisol.

The most common cause of Cushing's syndrome is prolonged use of glucocorticoid medication (e.g., prednisone) for chronic inflammatory disorders such as rheumatoid arthritis, chronic obstructive pulmonary disease, and Crohn's disease.

Signs and Symptoms

Most signs and symptoms of Cushing's syndrome are related to excess cortisol levels. Weight gain, truncal obesity with thin arms and legs, buffalo hump, and moon face result from deposits of adipose tissue at these sites (Fig. 39.6). Cortisol also causes insulin resistance and stimulates gluconeogenesis, which result in glucose intolerance. Some patients develop secondary diabetes mellitus. (See Chapter 40.) Muscle wasting and thin skin with purple striae occur as a result of cortisol's catabolic effect on tissues. Catabolic effects on bone lead to osteoporosis, pathological fractures, and back pain from compression fractures of the vertebrae. Because cortisol has anti-inflammatory and immunosuppressive actions, the patient is at risk for infection. Hyperpigmentation of the skin may occur. Approximately 50% of patients experience mental status changes from irritability to psychosis (sometimes referred to as steroid psychosis). Sodium and water retention are related to the mineralocorticoid effect. As sodium is retained, potassium is lost in the urine, causing hypokalemia. (See Chapter 5 to review these electrolyte imbalances.) Androgen effects include acne, growth of facial hair, and amenorrhea in women.

Diagnostic Tests

Suspicion of Cushing's disease or syndrome may initially be based on a cushingoid appearance. Plasma and urine cortisol and plasma ACTH are measured. A 24-hour urine test for cortisol may be collected. A dexamethasone suppression test may be done. Serum potassium is measured. Additional tests to locate the cause of excess endogenous cortisol may be done.

Therapeutic Interventions

If a pituitary or other ACTH-secreting tumor is present, surgical removal or radiation therapy to the pituitary may be employed. If the adrenals are the primary cause of the problem, radiation or removal of the adrenal gland or glands may

be performed. Drugs such as ketoconazole block production of adrenal steroids.

If the cause of Cushing's syndrome is administration of steroid medication, an every-other-day schedule or once-a-day dosing in the morning may reduce side effects. Usually steroids are prescribed as a last resort for chronic disorders that are unresponsive to other treatment. The patient and physician must weigh the risks and benefits of continuing the medication. The physician may order a high-

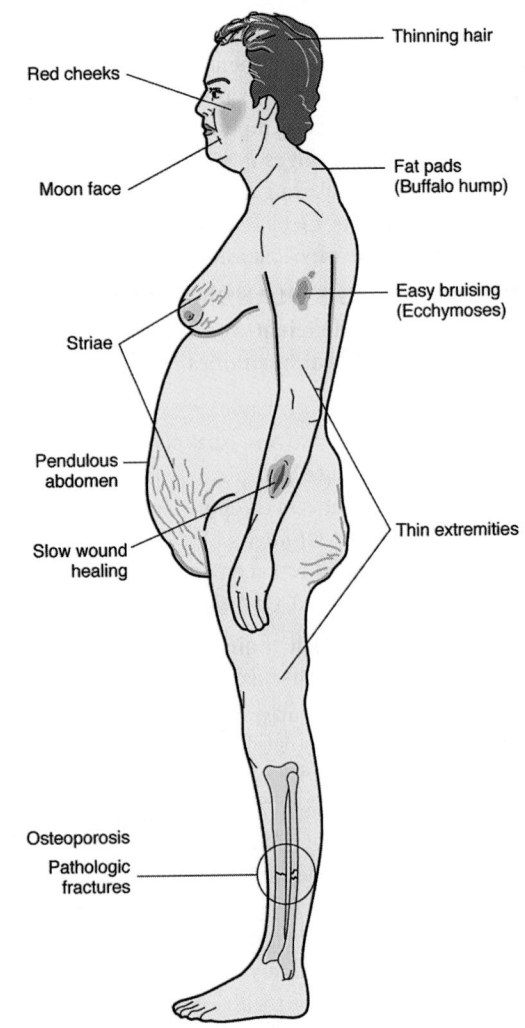

FIGURE 39.6 Physical manifestations seen in Cushing's syndrome.

- Thinning hair
- Red cheeks
- Fat pads (Buffalo hump)
- Moon face
- Easy bruising (Ecchymoses)
- Striae
- Pendulous abdomen
- Thin extremities
- Slow wound healing
- Osteoporosis
- Pathologic fractures

potassium, low-sodium, high-protein diet. Potassium supplements may be ordered. If the patient has high blood sugar, appropriate therapy for diabetes should be instituted. (See Chapter 40.)

Nursing Process for the Patient With Cushing's Disease

ASSESSMENT/DATA COLLECTION. When caring for the patient with Cushing's disease or syndrome, assess the patient's drug history. Monitor vital signs and complications related to fluid and sodium excess. Auscultate the lungs for crackles, and assess extremities for edema. Assess skin integrity, and monitor capillary glucose as ordered by the physician. Watch for signs of infection.

NURSING DIAGNOSIS, PLANNING, AND IMPLEMENTATION. Risk for excess fluid volume related to sodium and water retention

EXPECTED OUTCOME: Fluid volume will be stable as evidenced by stable daily weights.

- Monitor fluid status and report changes promptly *so treatment can be initiated.*

Risk for impaired skin integrity due to thin fragile skin

EXPECTED OUTCOME: The patient's skin will remain intact.

- Assist patient to change positions at least every 2 hours *to prevent pressure ulcers.*
- Observe skin and monitor for breakdown with every position change. *Early recognition and treatment of a problem can prevent further breakdown.*
- Use a lift sheet to move patient in bed *to prevent friction and sheer.*
- Avoid harsh soaps and hot water. *These can dry skin and increase risk for injury.*
- Use moisturizing cream *to keep skin from drying.*
- Secure IVs and dressings without tape whenever possible. *Removal of tape can tear fragile skin.*
- Consider a specialty pressure-reducing mattress if the patient is very thin or unable to move *to reduce risk of pressure ulcer.*
- Consult dietitian if nutritional status is poor. *Poor nutrition further increases risk for skin breakdown and poor healing.*

Risk for infection related to immune suppression

EXPECTED OUTCOME: Patient will be infection-free as evidenced by WBC and temperature within normal limits.

- Use good hand washing technique before and after patient care. *Hand washing is important in reducing exposure to pathogens.*
- Instruct the patient in good hand washing, and in the importance of avoiding others who are ill. *The patient with an impaired immune system is more likely to contract illness from others.*
- Consult dietitian if nutritional status is poor. *Poor nutrition further impairs immune function.*

- Report signs or symptoms of infection promptly *so treatment can be initiated.*
- Encourage flu and pneumonia vaccinations *to help prevent illness in event of exposure.*

Risk for injury related to impaired glucose tolerance

EXPECTED OUTCOME: Blood glucose will remain within normal limits.

- If glucose intolerance occurs, be prepared to administer insulin *because oral hypoglycemics are not usually effective.*
- Refer the patient and family to diabetes education classes *because diabetes is a complex disease that requires knowledge of self-care.*
- See Chapter 40 for care of the patient with diabetes.

Disturbed body image related to cushingoid appearance

EXPECTED OUTCOME: Patient will express feelings of acceptance of self.

- Approach patient with an attitude of acceptance and caring *to help develop trusting nurse-patient relationship.*
- Provide an opportunity for patient to verbalize feelings. *Expressing feelings may help reduce anxiety.*

EVALUATION. If care has been effective, complications of fluid overload will be recognized and treated early. The patient will have intact skin and be free from signs of infection. The patient will demonstrate skill in self-care of diabetes if indicated, and will verbalize acceptance of self in spite of changes in appearance.

Nursing Care of the Patient Undergoing Adrenalectomy

Preoperative Care

Monitor the patient for electrolyte imbalance and hyperglycemia. Abnormalities must be corrected before surgery. To prevent adrenal crisis, glucocorticoids are administered because removal of the adrenals causes a sudden drop in adrenal hormones. Prepare the patient for adrenalectomy or hypophysectomy, depending on which surgery will be performed.

Postoperative Care

See care of the patient undergoing hypophysectomy earlier in this chapter. Following adrenalectomy, the patient receives routine postoperative care. In addition, the patient is closely monitored for changes in fluid and electrolyte balance and adrenal crisis. Patients who undergo bilateral adrenalectomy must take replacement glucocorticoid and mineralocorticoid hormones for the remainder of their life. If only one adrenal gland is removed, the remaining gland should eventually produce enough hormone to enable the patient to discontinue replacement hormone.

See Table 39.7 for a summary of endocrine disorders and Table 39.8 for a summary of medications used for endocrine disorders.

TABLE 39.7 SUMMARY OF ENDOCRINE DISORDERS

Hormone	Hypofunction	Hyperfunction
Antidiuretic hormone	Diabetes insipidus—water loss	SIADH—water retention
Growth hormone	Dwarfism—short stature	Acromegaly, gigantism—bone and tissue overgrowth
Thyroid hormone	Hypothyroidism—slow metabolism	Hyperthyroidism—increased metabolism
Epinephrine	Rare	Pheochromocytoma—hypertension
Parathyroid hormone	Hypoparathyroidism—low serum calcium, osteoporosis, tetany	Hyperparathyroidism—high calcium, weakness
Cortisol	Addison's disease—sodium and water loss	Cushing's syndrome—sodium and water retention, hyperglycemia; see text

TABLE 39.8 MEDICATIONS USED FOR ENDOCRINE DISORDERS

Medication Class	Examples/Action	Route	Side Effects	Nursing Implications
Medications for ADH disorders	Vasopressin (Pitressin): replaces ADH	IM, IV, SC	Water retention	Check daily weights and urine specific gravity.
	Desmopressin (DDAVP): replaces ADH	PS, IV, SC, Intranasal	Water loss, dehydration	
	Demeclocycline (Declomycin): reduces ADH release	PO	Photosensitivity, allergy, water loss	Do not give demeclocycline with dairy products or antacids.
Medications for growth hormone disorders	Bromocriptine (Parlodel): reduces growth hormone release	PO	Dizziness, hypotension, nausea	Monitor blood pressure, serum growth hormone.
	Octreotide (Sandostatin): supresses growth hormone	SC, IM, IV	Uncommon: dizziness, nausea, constipation	Teach patient self-administration.
	Somatropin (Humatrope): replaces growth hormone	SC, IM	Insulin resistance, hypothyroidism	Monitor growth; teach patient self-administration.
Medications for thyroid disorders	Levothyroxine (Synthroid): replaces T3 and T4	PO, IM, IV	Tachycardia, insomnia, nervousness, weight loss	Monitor vital signs and thyroid laboratory results.
	Propylthiouracil (PTU): inhibits synthesis of thyroid hormones	PO	Nausea, vomiting, agranulocytosis	Monitor WBC and differential, thyroid function.
	Methimazole (Tapazole): inhibits synthesis of thyroid hormones	PO	Rash, agranulocytosis	
Medications for parathyroid disorders	Calcium gluconate: replaces calcium	PO, IV	Dysrhythmia, cardiac arrest, constipation	Monitor vital signs and ECG during IV therapy. Do not take PO calcium with other medications.
	Alendronate (Fosamax): inhibits resorption of bone; keeps calcium in bones	PO	Abdominal pain, constipation, diarrhea, nausea	Do not take with calcium supplements or caffeine.
Medications for adrenal disorders	Phenoxybenzamine (Dibenzyline): blocks action of epinephrine at alpha receptors in pheochromocytoma	PO	Orthostatic hypotension	Monitor vital signs.
	Hydrocortisone: replaces cortisol in adrenal insufficiency	PO, IV	Cushing's effects	Teach patient to take with food and not to discontinue abruptly.
	Fludrocortisone (Florinef): replaces aldosterone in adrenal insufficiency	PO	Fluid retention, heart failure, hypokalemia	Monitor daily weights, vital signs, and serum potassium.

CRITICAL THINKING

Mrs. Tercini

■ Mrs. Tercini is a 62-year-old woman admitted to your unit in addisonian crisis. She is lethargic, with a blood pressure of 86/58, pulse 112, and respirations 18. While interviewing her daughter, you learn that Mrs. Tercini has a history of Cushing's syndrome treated with bilateral adrenalectomy 25 years ago. She has been taking 150 μg fludrocortisone (Florinef) and 200 mg hydrocortisone daily ever since. Three days ago she developed the flu.

1. Why is an adrenalectomy done to treat Cushing's syndrome?
2. What is the most effective schedule for Mrs. Tercini's medication?
3. What precipitated this addisonian crisis?
4. Why is Mrs. Tercini's blood pressure low?
5. How could this crisis have been prevented?
6. Fludrocortisone is available as 0.1-mg tablets. How many should you administer?

Suggested answers at end of chapter.

REVIEW QUESTIONS

1. Which disorder results from too much cortisol secretion in the body?
   a. Addison's disease
   b. Hypothyroidism
   c. Cushing's disease
   d. Pheochromocytoma

2. A patient with SIADH asks the nurse why he has gained 10 pounds. Which response is best?
   a. "SIADH causes an increase in appetite. As soon as you are effectively treated, the weight should drop back to normal for you."
   b. "You are retaining a lot of sodium and potassium, and that causes you to gain a lot of water weight."
   c. "You have too much of a hormone in your system that causes you to retain water. The extra 10 pounds is likely water weight."
   d. "Your kidneys are not working correctly, so they can't get rid of extra water from your system."

3. Which assessment finding should the nurse expect to see in the patient with uncontrolled diabetes insipidus? Choose all that apply.
   a. Edema
   b. Polyuria
   c. Heat intolerance
   d. Diarrhea
   e. Polydipsia
   f. Dehydration

4. Which of the following instructions should the nurse provide to the patient who is being discharged after a thyroidectomy?

   a. "You must take your thyroid replacement every day just as the physician prescribes."
   b. "You must weigh yourself daily and report any gain or loss of more than 1 pound."
   c. "You will need to return to the physician's office for a weekly blood pressure check."
   d. "You will need to restrict your sodium and potassium intake."

5. Which of the following nursing assessments is most important in the patient with hyperthyroidism and risk for thyrotoxic crisis?
   a. Intake and output
   b. Breath sounds
   c. Bowel sounds
   d. Vital signs

6. Which action by the nurse is most important following hypophysectomy?
   a. Performing a routine neurological assessment
   b. Encouraging the patient to cough and deep breathe
   c. Monitoring for tracheal edema
   d. Assisting with use of an incentive spirometer

7. Which of the following statements by the patient with hypothyroidism indicates to the nurse that the plan of care has been effective?
   a. "I feel so much better now that my energy is returning."
   b. "I'm really glad the diarrhea has stopped."
   c. "I'm so glad I won't have to take medication for very long."
   d. "My fingers aren't tingling any more."

SUGGESTED ANSWERS TO

CRITICAL THINKING

■ *Mrs. Jackson*

1. Her weight gain is most likely caused by fluid retention, which can be a result of heart failure or SIADH, among other things.
2. Assess edema, lung sounds, and vital signs. Check intake and output during the past 2 days. Monitor mental status and level of consciousness. Check recent lab work to see if her serum sodium is low. You also check a book on the unit and recall that anesthetics and morphine are possible causes of SIADH. Morphine can also cause confusion.
3. Notify the registered nurse of your findings and your suspicions. Be prepared to place Mrs. Jackson on a fluid restriction. Reassure her son that the physician is being notified of the changes he noted.
4.

$$\frac{6 \text{ pounds} \mid 480 \text{ mL}}{\mid 1 \text{ pound}} = 2880 \text{ mL or almost 3 liters}$$

■ *Adoption*

The children's growth hormone secretion was probably suppressed because of psychosocial stress. Once they felt secure in a loving environment, growth hormone levels returned to normal.

■ *Mae*

1. Mae's TSH is elevated because her pituitary gland is working overtime to try to stimulate the underactive thyroid gland.
2. Mae's metabolism has been slow, so she has been burning fewer calories. When she starts on thyroid replacement hormone, her metabolic rate will return to normal and she will need more calories. Intake of calories should be balanced with the possible need for weight loss.
3. If Mae receives too much thyroid hormone, she will have symptoms of hyperthyroidism, including an increased pulse rate. She should know how to check her pulse and to call her physician if it is elevated.

■ *Mrs. Tercini*

1. Cushing's syndrome is caused by too much cortisol. The adrenal cortex is responsible for secreting cortisol.
2. Mrs. Tercini should take two-thirds of her daily dose of hydrocortisone and fludrocortisone in the morning and one-third in the evening. This most closely mimics the body's natural corticosteroid secretion.
3. The flu probably triggered this crisis. Illness is a stressor, and normally the body secretes steroids during stress. Because Mrs. Tercini's body is unable to produce steroids, she experiences symptoms of hypoadrenalism during stressful times.
4. Mrs. Tercini's blood pressure is low because she has insufficient circulating mineralocorticoids. Without aldosterone, sodium and water are lost and blood pressure drops.
5. Mrs. Tercini should have taken extra medication when she became ill.
6.

$$\frac{150 \text{ μg} \mid 1 \text{ mg} \mid 1 \text{ tab}}{\mid 1000 \text{ μg} \mid 0.1 \text{ mg}} = 1.5 \text{ tablets}$$

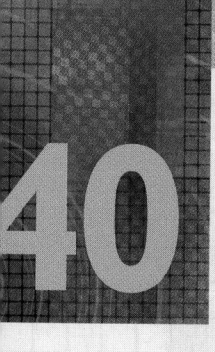

40

Nursing Care of Patients with Disorders of the Endocrine Pancreas

PAULA D. HOPPER

KEY TERMS

diabetes mellitus (DYE-ah-BEE-tis mel-LYE-tus)
endogenous (en-DAH-jen-us)
gastroparesis (GAS-troh-puh-REE-sus)
glycosuria (GLY-kos-YOO-ree-ah)
hyperglycemia (HIGH-per-gligh-SEE-mee-ah)
hypoglycemia (HIGH-poh-gligh-SEE-mee-ah)
ketoacidosis (KEE-toh-ass-i-DOH-sis)
Kussmaul's (KOOS-mahlz)
nephropathy (ne-FROP-uh-thee)
neuropathy (new-RAH-puh-thee)
polyphagia (PAH-lee-FAY-jee-ah)
postprandial (POST-PRAN-dee-uhl)
preprandial (PREE-PRAN-dee-uhl)
retinopathy (RET-i-NAH-puh-thee)

QUESTIONS TO GUIDE YOUR READING

1. What are the pathophysiologies of type 1 and type 2 diabetes mellitus?

2. What are risk factors for type 1 and type 2 diabetes mellitus?

3. What are the signs and symptoms of diabetes mellitus?

4. What are the causes, signs and symptoms, and treatment of high and low blood glucose levels?

5. Why are persons with diabetes prone to complications such as heart disease, blindness, and kidney failure? How can you help your patients prevent these complications?

6. What diagnostic tests are used to diagnose and monitor diabetes mellitus and its complications?

7. What therapeutic interventions help patients with diabetes control their blood glucose levels?

8. How do the different insulins and oral hypoglycemic agents lower blood glucose levels? What should you know when administering these medications?

9. How would you apply the nursing process to the patient with diabetes mellitus?

10. What measures can be taken to increase the safety of the diabetic patient undergoing surgery?

11. What is reactive hypoglycemia? How is it diagnosed and treated?

DIABETES MELLITUS

Diabetes mellitus (be careful not to confuse this with diabetes insipidus) is a group of metabolic diseases in which defects in insulin secretion or action result in high blood sugar level (**hyperglycemia**). According to the latest Centers for Disease Control and Prevention (CDC) data, approximately 20.8 million people in the United States have diabetes mellitus, and 6.2 million of those do not know it. The direct and indirect cost (such as lost work time) of diabetes in the United States is about $132 billion per year. The incidence of diabetes mellitus varies by race and ethnicity. In the United States, Hispanic, black, Native American, Alaska Native, and Asian American populations have a higher rate of diabetes than non-Hispanic white ethnic groups.[1]

Diabetes is a serious disease that can cause complications such as blindness, kidney failure, heart attacks, and strokes. It is a leading cause of lower limb amputations in the United States. With good education and self-care, patients with diabetes can prevent or delay these complications and lead full, productive lives. A major role of the nurse is helping the patient learn to care for herself or himself effectively.

Pathophysiology

Body tissues, and the cells that compose them, use glucose for energy. Glucose is a simple sugar provided by the foods we eat. When carbohydrates are eaten they are digested into sugars, including glucose, which is then absorbed into the bloodstream. Carbohydrates provide most of the glucose used by the body; proteins and fats can indirectly provide smaller amounts of glucose. Glucose is able to enter the cells only with the help of insulin, a hormone produced by the beta cells in the islets of Langerhans of the pancreas (Fig. 40.1). When insulin comes in contact with the cell membrane, it combines with a receptor that allows activation of special glucose transporters in the membrane (Fig. 40.2). By helping glucose enter the body's cells, insulin lowers the glucose level in the blood. Insulin also helps the body store excess glucose in the liver in the form of glycogen.

Another hormone, glucagon, is produced by the alpha cells in the islets of Langerhans. Glucagon raises the blood glucose when needed by releasing the stored glucose from the liver and muscles. Insulin and glucagon work together to keep the blood glucose at a constant level.

Diabetes results from faulty production of insulin by the beta cells in the pancreas, or from inability of the body's cells to use insulin. When glucose is unable to enter body cells, it stays in the bloodstream; hyperglycemia results, and the cells are denied their energy source. Abnormal glucagon secretion may also play a role in type 2 diabetes.

---

diabetes mellitus: diabetes—passing through + mellitus—sweet

hyperglycemia: hyper—excessive + glyc—glucose + emia—in the blood

Types and Causes

Type 1 Diabetes Mellitus

Type 1 diabetes (formerly called juvenile diabetes mellitus, insulin-dependent diabetes mellitus, or IDDM) is caused by destruction of the beta cells in the islets of Langerhans of the pancreas. When the beta cells are destroyed, they are unable to produce insulin. Insulin must then be injected for the body to use food for energy. See Box 40.1 Patient Perspective for Dave's story about having type 1 diabetes. Only 5% to 10% of people with diabetes have type 1 diabetes.

It is believed that the pancreas may attack itself following certain viral infections or administration of certain drugs (this is called an autoimmune response). Almost 90% of patients newly diagnosed with type 1 diabetes have islet cell antibodies in their blood. These antibodies might be present for years before actual symptoms of diabetes develop. About 10% of people with type 1 diabetes cases also have a genetic predisposition to its development. The patient with type 1 diabetes is most often young and thin and is prone to develop **ketoacidosis** when blood glucose is elevated. (See Table 40.1 for a comparison of type 1 and type 2 diabetes.) Diabetic ketoacidosis is discussed later in this chapter. Research studies are ongoing to try to find ways to prevent type 1 diabetes once antibodies have been detected.

LATENT AUTOIMMUNE DIABETES OF ADULTHOOD (LADA). This is a new type of type 1 diabetes that has recently been identified. Some patients who were initially diagnosed with type 2 diabetes were later found to have islet cell and insulin antibodies (which are usually associated with type 1), and their blood glucose levels were not controlled with oral medications. However, beta cell destruction tended to occur more slowly than with type 1 diabetes. This is possibly because of differences in the antibodies or the individual's response to the antibodies. Some experts distinguish patients with LADA as either thin or obese because the disorder has slightly different characteristics depending on the patient's body fat.

Type 2 Diabetes Mellitus

Ninety percent to 95% of people with diabetes have type 2 diabetes mellitus (formerly called adult-onset diabetes mellitus, non–insulin-dependent diabetes mellitus, or NIDDM). In type 2 diabetes mellitus, tissues are resistant to insulin. Insulin is still made by the pancreas, but in inadequate amounts. Sometimes the amount of insulin is normal or even high, but because the tissues are resistant to it, hyperglycemia results. Glucagon levels may be elevated.

Heredity is responsible for up to 90% of cases of type 2 diabetes. Obesity is also a major contributing factor. Often the patient with a new diagnosis of type 2 diabetes is obese, relates a family history of diabetes, and has had a recent life stressor such as the death of a family member, illness, or loss of a job.

---

ketoacidosis: keto—ketones + acid—acidic + osis—condition

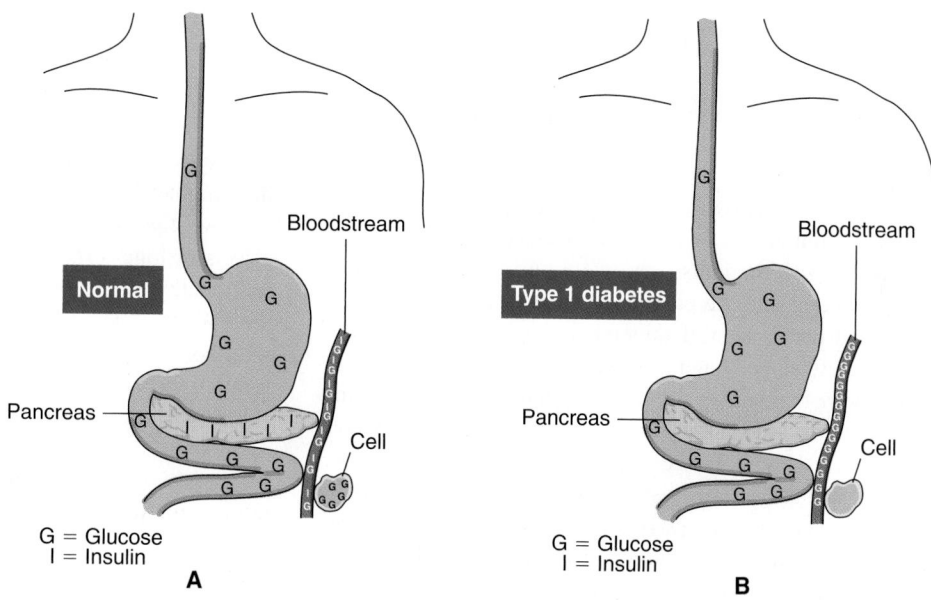

FIGURE 40.1 Maintenance of blood glucose levels. *(A)* Normal physiology: Foods (especially carbohydrates) are broken down into glucose, which is absorbed into the bloodstream for transport to the cells. Insulin, produced by the beta cells of the islets of Langerhans in the pancreas, is needed to "open the door" to the cells, allowing the glucose to enter. *(B)* In type 1 diabetes mellitus, the pancreas does not produce insulin. Because glucose is unable to enter the cells, it builds up in the bloodstream, causing hyperglycemia. *(C)* In type 2 diabetes mellitus, insulin production is reduced and/or cells are resistant to insulin. Less glucose enters the cell, and hyperglycemia results.

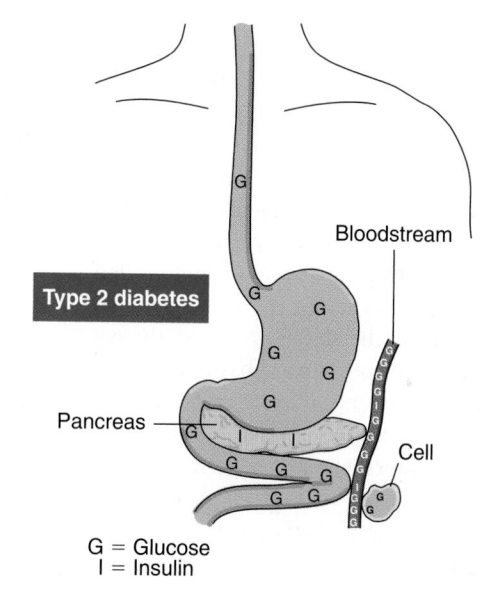

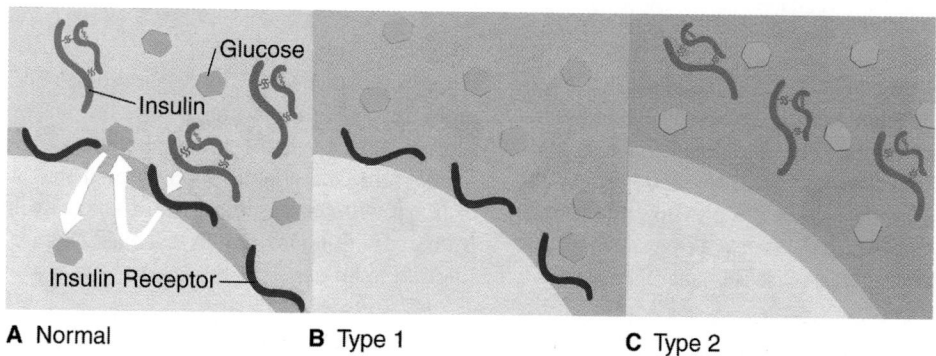

FIGURE 40.2 *(A)* Cell membrane in normal state, with insulin receptors and insulin to regulate glucose intake. *(B)* Cell membrane in type 1 diabetes: insulin not present, glucose remains outside of cell. *(C)* Cell membrane in type 2 diabetes: without insulin receptors, glucose remains outside cell *(From Scanlon VC, Sanders T: Essentials of Anatomy and Physiology, ed 4. F.A. Davis, 2003, Philadelphia, p 225, with permission.)*

Box 40.1

Patient Perspective

Dave

I was diagnosed with type 1 diabetes mellitus at age 3 years. I remember being left in a children's ward of the hospital with the nuns (who were nurses) in their habits and looking into the parking lot as my parents got in the car and drove away. I remember the fear and horror of being left alone. Later, I remember my doctor teaching my mother and me about the diet and monitoring my urine for glucose and ketones. This was all we had in those days (the early 1960s). I was supposed to test my urine before meals and at bedtime, just like we monitor blood glucose today. Every time I saw my doctor he would review and change my treatment based on the results. Insulin then was extracted from pig and cow cadavers.

I remember my life being pretty normal except at holidays. When my brothers and sisters were getting Halloween candy and Christmas candy canes, I felt odd and left out. My mom was really tough and observant and I had to be sneaky to get away with stealing a treat or two left momentarily unobserved by those around me. I was thrilled when sugarless candy became available around age 10 or so and I could have my own candies to hoard for myself.

Hypoglycemic reactions were always a trauma-filled event at our house. They came at unexpected times, and my mom sometimes blamed herself. I can honestly say that my mom deserves more credit than I have ever given her for my good fortune with my diabetes. She did not have glucometers, glycohemoglobin tests, or even diabetes specialists and educators; she just had the desire of a mother who did everything she could to make sure I had and did everything right as far as she knew.

In my late teens I took everything my doctor and my mom had done for me and trashed them. I lived with reckless abandon: I did what I wanted, ate what I wanted, and didn't even think about the disease I lived with until I was about 30. I worked hard those years in construction, and

the physical activity probably delayed the complications that might otherwise have occurred.

At age 35, I began to experience the inevitable effects of long-term hyperglycemia. I developed diabetic retinopathy, the leading cause of adult-onset blindness in the United States. My vision was restored in my left eye with laser surgery. It would take another surgery (vitrectomy) to bring the vision in my right eye back to the 20/60 it is now from the 20/2000 it was before the surgery.

About that time I was referred to an endocrinologist who specialized in diabetes, and my treatment took a remarkable turn for the better. The endocrinologist began to aggressively change my medications, insulin regimen, exercise program, and diagnostic testing, all with the purpose of controlling blood glucose and preventing the onset and advancement of diabetic complications. This aggressive plan of action was taught to me by a registered nurse certified diabetes educator who worked with my doctor. I must also give enormous credit to the office staff nurses who were an integral part of the team, supporting me throughout the whole experience. The doctors and nurses made my education both understandable and pertinent. They basically put the ball in my court, and then it was up to me to take control of my own life. My wife was more than supportive throughout this time period too, and sacrificed much for the new array of medications and doctor's appointments that took a huge chunk out of our family finances.

I have mentioned briefly those involved in my life with diabetes. I take no credit for any of the results though; I believe it was God who made these choices available and miraculously reversed the effects of disease in my body. To the amazement of medical professionals, He continues to bless me with good health. It is because of all I have gone through with diabetes that I have recently completed my nursing degree and hope to become a diabetes educator myself.

TYPE 2 DIABETES IN YOUTH. More and more children and adolescents are developing type 2 diabetes, which in the past only occurred in adults. This is related to increasing obesity and decreasing activity levels in children today. Many experts are concerned about the growing number of obese children in the United States because of their increased risk for diabetes, heart disease, and other obesity-related problems.

Gestational Diabetes

Gestational diabetes mellitus (GDM) may develop during pregnancy, especially in women with risk factors for type 2 diabetes. The extra metabolic demands of pregnancy trigger

the onset of diabetes. Blood glucose usually returns to normal after delivery, but the mother has an increased risk for type 2 diabetes in the future. If the mother with GDM is overweight, she should be counseled that weight loss and exercise will decrease her risk of later developing diabetes. Mothers with GDM require specialized care and should be referred to an expert in this area.

Prediabetes

Prediabetes refers to blood glucose levels that are above normal but do not meet the criteria for diagnosing diabetes. Prediabetes usually occurs prior to the onset of type 2 diabetes. It is diagnosed by evaluating glucose tolerance or fast-

TABLE 40.1 COMPARISON OF TYPE 1 AND TYPE 2 DIABETES

	Type 1 (IDDM)	Type 2 (NIDDM)
Onset	Rapid	Slow
Age at onset	Usually <40	Usually >40
Risk factors	Virus, autoimmune response, heredity	Heredity, obesity
Usual body type	Lean	Obese
High blood glucose complication	Ketoacidosis	Hyperosmolar, Hyperglycemic, Nonketotic syndrome
Treatment	Diet, exercise; must have insulin to survive	Diet, exercise; may need oral hypoglycemics or insulin to control blood glucose level

ing glucose levels (see tests of diabetes below). Individuals with prediabetes may be able to prevent the onset of diabetes with weight loss and exercise.

Other Types of Diabetes

Secondary diabetes may develop as a result of another chronic illness that damages the islet cells, such as pancreatitis or cystic fibrosis. Prolonged use of some drugs, such as steroid hormones, phenytoin (Dilantin), thiazide diuretics, and thyroid hormone, may also impair insulin action and raise blood glucose. Maturity-onset diabetes of the young (MODY) is an inherited defect in insulin secretion that usually occurs in individuals under the age of 25. Less common causes include pancreatic trauma and other endocrine disorders.

Metabolic Syndrome

A newer finding is the link between diabetes and a condition called metabolic syndrome, sometimes called syndrome X. According to the American Heart Association and the National Heart, Lung, and Blood Institute, metabolic syndrome is diagnosed when at least three of the following criteria are met[2]:

- Elevated waist circumference (abdominal obesity)
- Triglyceride level of 150 mg/dL or higher
- High-density lipoprotein (HDL) ("good") cholesterol lower than 40 mg/dL for men and lower than 50 mg/dL for women
- Blood pressure level of 130/85 mm Hg or higher
- Fasting glucose of 100 mg/dL or higher

Other risk factors include physical inactivity, aging, hormonal imbalance, and genetic predisposition. Hispanic Americans are at higher risk than Caucasians. A major factor is the growing obesity epidemic in the United States.

Any patient who fits this profile should be monitored closely for the onset of type 2 diabetes and heart disease. Patients should be counseled on the importance of a diet low in saturated fats and cholesterol, weight loss, physical activity, and control of blood pressure.

Signs and Symptoms of Diabetes

Classic symptoms of diabetes mellitus include **polydipsia** (excessive thirst), **polyuria** (excessive urination), and **polyphagia** (excessive hunger). Because glucose is unable to enter the cells, the cells starve, causing hunger. The large amount of glucose in the blood causes an increase in serum concentration, or osmolality. The renal tubules are unable to reabsorb all the excess glucose that is filtered by the glomeruli, and **glycosuria** results. Large amounts of body water are required to excrete this glucose, causing polyuria, **nocturia,** and dehydration. The increased osmolality and dehydration cause polydipsia. High blood glucose may also cause fatigue, blurred vision, abdominal pain, and headaches. Ketones may build up in the blood and urine of patients with type 1 diabetes (ketoacidosis).

Diagnostic Tests

FASTING PLASMA GLUCOSE. Diagnosis of diabetes mellitus is based on plasma glucose levels measured by a laboratory. According to the American Diabetes Association,[3] a normal plasma glucose level is less than 100 mg/dL, although different laboratories may have slightly different normal values. When the fasting plasma glucose (drawn after at least 8 hours without eating) is ≥126 mg/dL, diabetes is diagnosed. A second test may be required if the first test is not clearly diagnostic. If the fasting plasma glucose is between 100 and 125 mg/dL, the patient has impaired fasting glucose (IFG).

CASUAL PLASMA GLUCOSE. Sometimes it is not feasible to check a fasting plasma glucose. A casual plasma glucose (CPG) is checked without regard to the last meal. Diabetes is diagnosed if the CPG is ≥200 mg/dL, with symptoms of diabetes.

ORAL GLUCOSE TOLERANCE TEST. Another test to diagnose diabetes is the oral glucose tolerance test (OGTT). An OGTT measures blood glucose at intervals after the patient drinks a concentrated carbohydrate drink. Diabetes is

LEARNING TIP

Remember the classic symptoms of diabetes by the **3 Ps:** polydipsia, polyuria, and polyphagia.

polydipsia: poly—many or much + dipsia—thirst
polyuria: poly—many or much + uria—urine
polyphagia: poly—many or much + phagia—to eat
glycosuria: glyc—glucose + uria—urine
nocturia: noc—by night + uria—urine

diagnosed when the blood glucose level is ≥200 mg/dL after 2 hours. A result between 140 and 199 mg/dL at 2 hours diagnoses impaired glucose tolerance (IGT).

GLYCOHEMOGLOBIN. The glycohemoglobin test (also called glycosylated hemoglobin, or HbA_{1c}) is used to gather baseline data and to monitor progress of diabetes control (not to diagnose diabetes). Glucose in the blood attaches to hemoglobin in the red blood cells. Red blood cells live about 3 months in the body. When the glucose that is attached to the hemoglobin is measured, it reflects the average blood glucose level for the previous 2 to 3 months. A normal HbA_{1c} is 4% to 6%. This is a helpful measurement when blood glucose levels fluctuate and a single measurement would be misleading. It also assists in determining the degree of effectiveness of a patient's treatment plan. Newer methods allow this test to be done in a physician's office while the patient waits. Glycohemoglobin testing might be inaccurate in some people, such as those with anemia. These individuals may have a glycated serum protein test, which is a similar test that indicates glucose levels over a period of 1 to 2 weeks instead of 3 months. See Table 40.2.

ADDITIONAL TESTS. Because diabetes affects so many body systems, additional tests recommended for baseline data include a lipid profile, serum creatinine and urine microalbumin levels to monitor kidney function, urinalysis, and electrocardiogram.

CRITICAL THINKING

Mr. McMillan

■ Mr. McMillan is a 50-year-old patient brought into the emergency department with extreme fatigue and dehydration. After the physician sees him, you ask Mr. McMillan some additional questions. Based on the patient's answers, you request that the physician add a glucose level to the laboratory tests ordered. The result is 1400 mg/dL.

1. What questions would you ask Mr. McMillan if you suspected diabetes?
2. Why was Mr. McMillan fatigued?
3. Why was he dehydrated?

Suggested answers at end of chapter.

Prevention

Although there is currently no known way to prevent type 1 diabetes, there are ways to prevent type 2 diabetes. Research studies have shown that patients at risk for diabetes, even those who already have IGT or IFG, can prevent or delay the onset of diabetes with weight loss and regular exercise. Losing as little as a 5% to 7% body weight through a half hour of exercise 5 days a week, and reducing fat and calories can reduce the risk of diabetes by 58%.[4] Patients at risk should have their plasma glucose checked regularly.

TABLE 40.2 CORRELATION BETWEEN HbA_{1c} AND MEAN FASTING PLASMA GLUCOSE (FPG)[2]

HbA_{1c} (%)	FPG (mg/dL)
6	135
7	170
8	205
9	240
10	274
11	310
12	345

Therapeutic Interventions

The only cure for diabetes is a pancreas (or islet cell) transplant. However, diabetes can be controlled. Treatment begins with diet and exercise. Insulin is added in patients with type 1 diabetes and insulin or oral hypoglycemic medication as needed in those with type 2 diabetes. Blood glucose monitoring and education are also important to good diabetes control.

To monitor the effectiveness of treatment, patients should have regular health care follow-up visits. See Box 40.2 Summary of Diabetes Goals and Recommendations proposed by the American Diabetes Association for 2006.

Goals of Treatment

The American Diabetes Association recommends that patients maintain a **preprandial** (premeal) plasma glucose level of 90 to 130 mg/dL, peak **postprandial** glucose <180 mg/dL, and glycohemoglobin level of less than 7% to prevent or delay complications of diabetes. Because of the risk for cardiovascular disease, they also recommend maintaining blood pressure <130/80 mm Hg.[3] The American Association of Clinical Endocrinologists recommends even stricter goals: preprandial plasma glucose of <110 mg/dL, 2-hour postprandial glucose <140 mg/dL, and HbA_{1c} ≤6.5%.[5] All goals may be adjusted in individual circumstances. For example, the patient who does not feel symptoms of **hypoglycemia** might have a higher preprandial glucose goal to prevent undetected hypoglycemic episodes.

Medical Nutrition Therapy

The goal of medical nutrition therapy (MNT) is to achieve and maintain blood glucose and lipid levels as near to normal as possible to prevent long-term complications. For some, especially those with type 2 diabetes, weight loss and blood pressure control may be additional goals of nutrition therapy.

Because the patient with diabetes has a limited amount of insulin, either **endogenous** (from within the body) or

---

preprandial: pre—before + prandial—meal
postprandial: post—after + prandial—meal
hypoglycemia: hypo—deficient + glyc—glucose + emia—in the blood
endogenous: endo—within + genous—to produce

Box 40.2

Summary of Diabetes Goals and Recommendations

Capillary plasma glucose should be measured at least three times a day for patients using multiple insulin injections. Blood pressure should be measured at every office visit. Target levels are:

- HbA$_{1c}$ (every 3–6 months)   <7%
- Preprandial capillary glucose   90 to 130 mg/dL
- Peak postprandial capillary glucose   <180 mg/dL
- Blood pressure   <130/80 mm Hg

Blood lipids should be measured at least yearly. Target levels are:

- LDL   <100 mg/dL
- Triglycerides   <150 mg/dL
- HDL   >40 mg/dL

Urine should be checked for microalbumin yearly. Patient should receive:

- Yearly flu vaccine for all patients ≥6 months of age
- One lifetime pneumococcal vaccine for adults
- Aspirin therapy, 75–162 mg/day, if >21 years of age
- Statin therapy to achieve an LDL reduction of 30% to 40% regardless of baseline LDL levels if >40 years of age
- Smoking cessation counseling
- Yearly comprehensive foot examination
- Dilated comprehensive eye examination within 3 to 5 years of onset of type 1 diabetes, or at diagnosis of type 2 diabetes, and every year thereafter.

Source: Adapted from American Diabetes Association: Clinical Practice Recommendations 2006. Diabetes Care 29(Suppl 1): 2006.

---

injected, it is important to eat an amount of food that will not exceed the insulin's ability to carry it into the cells. The meal plan should include consistent amounts of carbohydrates, proteins, and fats each day (Box 40.3 Nutrition Notes). Because carbohydrates contribute most to the blood glucose level, it is most important that carbohydrates are consistent from one day to the next. If a patient eats a small amount of carbohydrate one day and a large amount the next, the blood glucose will fluctuate, leading to complications. It is possible to relax nutrition restrictions somewhat if the patient is willing to test blood glucose frequently at home and adjust treatment accordingly. This requires in-depth instruction by a diabetes educator.

In the past, the commonly prescribed meal plan was the American Diabetes Association (ADA) diet, which was based on a basic meal plan with lists of amounts of foods that could be exchanged to vary the menu. The ADA no longer recommends a single meal plan, but rather advocates a complete assessment by a specially trained dietitian and individualized nutrition therapy recommendations and teaching.

A variety of meal plans are available, as shown in Table 40.3. Because diabetes increases the risk of high serum cholesterol and triglycerides, all plans limit fat intake. Patients who use fat replacers (in foods such as fat-free baked goods or ice cream) should be aware that they still have food value and calories, so they cannot be considered "free" foods. Most plans also encourage the use of complex carbohydrates such as grains, pastas, vegetables, and fruits. Simple sugars, which may raise blood glucose more than complex carbohydrates (they have a higher *glycemic index*), are used less but are not prohibited as they were in the past. Sodium intake is limited in individuals with hypertension. Protein is limited in patients with any degree of kidney impairment. Any meal plan should be chosen to fit the patient's lifestyle and food preferences. Patient preferences based on ethnic background should also be considered (Box 40.4 Cultural Considerations).

The success of MNT is evaluated by monitoring glucose levels, HbA$_{1c}$, lipids, weight, blood pressure, and kidney function.

Exercise

Exercise is an important factor in controlling blood glucose and lipid levels. Exercise lowers blood glucose, both immediately and for approximately 24 hours after the exercise. Insulin is not needed for glucose to enter exercising muscle cells. Exercise also improves blood lipid levels and circulation, which is important for the person with diabetes, who already has an increased risk of cardiovascular disease. Patients are instructed to exercise on a regular basis, ideally 30 minutes on most days of the week, to keep blood glucose levels stable and promote health.

Some patients with complications of diabetes must be careful in their exercise choices. For example, a patient with **retinopathy** should not do anything that causes straining. (See Long-Term Complications later in this chapter.) A patient with **neuropathy** or foot problems should limit weight-bearing exercise. A physician or exercise physiologist should be consulted for an individualized exercise plan.

Persons with diabetes should always carry a quick source of sugar when exercising in case the blood glucose drops too low. Individuals on intermediate-acting insulin are taught to avoid exercising at the time of day when their blood glucose is at its lowest point (i.e., when insulin or medication is peaking) and to have a carbohydrate snack before exercising if blood glucose is less than 100 mg/dL. Exercising at similar times each day also helps prevent blood glucose fluctuations.

Patients should be cautioned to avoid exercise when their glucose level is higher than 250 mg/dL and ketones are present in the urine or if glucose is more than 300 mg/dL without ketones. This indicates that insufficient insulin is

---

retinopathy: retino—nervous tissue of the eye + pathy—illness
neuropathy: neuro—nervous system + pathy—illness

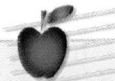

Box 40.3

Nutrition Notes

Individualizing Medical Nutrition Therapy in Diabetes Mellitus

A certified diabetes educator can use many approaches in the nutritional management of diabetes. This permits a meal plan based on the patient's abilities and commitment. Several meal-planning approaches are described in Table 40.3 and commonly used ones are detailed below. The education of the patient with diabetes is a process that may take months, and should not be expected to be accomplished in a single visit or with a paper handout.

Overall goals and strategies differ for the type 1 and type 2 diabetics. In general, a patient with type 1 diabetes needs to prevent wide swings in blood glucose levels through careful timing of meals and snacks in relation to insulin therapy and activity. A patient with type 2 diabetes uses diet modifications to maintain near-normal glucose, blood pressure, and lipid levels and to lose weight as necessary.

Using MyPyramid

A basic educational tool, the MyPyramid, can be adapted for a first-level meal plan for the newly diagnosed person with diabetes. The physician or diabetes educator can select the kilocalorie level appropriate for the patient and common household measures are used as guidelines.

Using ADA Exchange Lists

A food guide called the ADA *Exchange Lists*, published jointly by the American Dietetic Association and the American Diabetes Association, is used by some patients with diabetes. This system is composed of six lists of foods plus a "free food" list. Foods in each list contain similar energy nutrients (carbohydrate, protein, and fat). For example, corn is on the starch list rather than the vegetable list because it is closer in composition to a slice of bread than to green beans. Individual food items within an exchange list are essentially equal to each other in nutrient composition and can thus be exchanged or "swapped" for each other. Exchanges were designed to be approximately equal in nutrients, not in volume; therefore, portion sizes vary widely. For instance, one fruit exchange is equal to $1\frac{1}{4}$ cup of whole strawberries but to only three dates. To correctly use this method of meal planning, patients must choose the prescribed number of items from each appropriate list: starch, fruit, milk, vegetable, meat, and fat.

A specific meal plan should be given to the patient with the exchange lists. A meal plan is a food guide that shows the number of choices or exchanges the patient should eat at each meal and snack. A meal plan based on exchange lists allows patients a variety of food choices yet requires minimal calculation. Even experienced users of the exchange list system should be advised to weigh or measure their portions several times per week to avoid portion inflation.

Using Carbohydrate Counting

Carbohydrate counting is a three-level approach to teaching meal planning that focuses on carbohydrates, but patients are told to eat about the same amount of protein each day and to choose low-fat foods. With this system, the patient keeps track of the units or exchanges of carbohydrates eaten throughout the day to keep carbohydrates and insulin balanced. Carbohydrate counting is based on classifying carbohydrates together, whether from starch, fruit, or milk. For example, one slice of whole wheat bread, one orange, and 8 oz of skim milk are each equivalent to one carbohydrate unit or exchange. This method offers more flexible food choices within a day's meal plan than the exchange list system and may achieve better control of blood glucose. Despite those advantages, however, carbohydrate counting may entail weighing and measuring food, keeping food records, monitoring blood sugar before and after eating, and controlling body weight. Mastery of level III of carbohydrate counting permits adjusting short-acting insulin dosage using insulin-to-carbohydrate ratios and is often a prerequisite for starting insulin pump therapy.

Using the Glycemic Index

All carbohydrates are not metabolized identically. Foods containing equal amounts of carbohydrate impact blood glucose levels differently. The glycemic index is a classification of foods according to the speed and degree of change in blood glucose levels. Compared with a standard of 100 for white bread, glucose has a glycemic index of 138, sucrose (table sugar) 83, and fructose 26. Baked russet potatoes and cornflakes have higher glycemic indices than sucrose, whereas sweet potatoes have a lower one. Because most meals contain a combination of nutrients, the glycemic index should not be a primary strategy but might be an adjunct to another meal planning system for highly motivated patients.

TABLE 40.3 MEAL-PLANNING APPROACHES FOR DIABETES

Approach	Comments	Availability
Food Pyramid	Initial phase of teaching Provides a basic foundation in normal nutrition. Does not emphasize meal consistency.	A colorful version is available from the National Dairy Council, 10255 West Higgins Road, Suite 900, Rosemont, IL 60018-4233 1-708-803-2000
Dietary Guidelines	Initial phase of teaching Provides a basic foundation in normal nutrition, 40 pages in length. Does not emphasize meal consistency.	United States Department of Agriculture Home & Garden Bulletin #232, Local Cooperative Extension Office
The First Step in Diabetes	Initial phase in teaching	The American Dietetic Association, 216 West Jackson Boulevard, Suite 800, Chicago, IL 60606-6995 1-800-366-1655
Meal Planning	Combines Food Pyramid and Dietary Guidelines, and provides information on meal consistency in a simplified format.	
CHO Counting	Progressive teaching tool that leads to maximum control of blood glucose and lipid levels. Decreased emphasis on balance and variety.	The American Dietetic Association, 216 West Jackson Boulevard, Suite 800, Chicago, IL 60606-6995 1-800-366-1655
Month-O-Meals	Each book contains 28 complete and interchangeable menus for breakfast, lunch, dinner, and snacks. Excellent approach for the patient who "just wants to be told what and when to eat."	The American Dietetic Association, 216 West Jackson Boulevard, Suite 800, Chicago, IL 60606-6995 1-800-366-1655
Exchange Lists of the American Dietetic and the American Diabetes Associations	Allows the health-care educator to distribute all of the energy nutrients. More emphasis on the importance of eating a balanced diet than the CHO counting approach. Time consuming to learn and teach	The American Dietetic Association, 216 West Jackson Boulevard, Suite 800, Chicago, IL 60606-6995 1-800-366-1655

Source: Lutz, CA, and Przytulski, KR: Nutrition and Diet Therapy, ed. 4, F.A. Davis, Philadelphia, 2005.

available and glycogen may be released during exercise, further increasing the serum glucose.

Medication

INJECTED INSULIN. The individual with type 1 diabetes has no endogenous insulin and therefore must administer insulin daily. At this time, insulin cannot be taken by mouth because it is a protein and is therefore digested. Insulin is generally given subcutaneously, although fast-acting insulin may be ordered via the intramuscular or intravenous route in urgent situations, or sometimes inhaled. There are several types of insulin and schedules by which it may be given. The type and schedule are determined by the physician, in collaboration with the patient, based on the patient's lifestyle and willingness to spend time on injections. In general, the more frequent the injections, the better the glucose control.

Insulin injections should be given in a different subcutaneous site each time to avoid injury to the tissues. A sample rotation chart is shown in Figure 40.3. Because each area absorbs insulin at a slightly different rate, it is advisable to use one area for a week, then move on to the next area. Within that area, each injection should be spaced at least 1 inch from the previous injection. Most experts recommend using primarily the torso (abdomen and buttocks) to provide more uniform absorption. Aspirating for blood before injection and rubbing the site following injection are not recommended with insulin injections.

Patients who desire tighter control of blood glucose levels and a more flexible lifestyle may choose to use an insulin pump (Fig. 40.4). This is a small device that delivers subcutaneous insulin continuously in small (basal) amounts. The patient can then add a bolus of insulin with the push of a button before meals or snacks. This provides insulin levels that are more normal, like a person without diabetes.

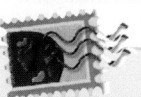

Box 40.4

Cultural Considerations

The diabetic diet for ethnic individuals may need a significant adjustment from the U.S. menu. An exchange list of foods for these patients will not be followed because their food choices are different. The patient may be labeled noncompliant, when in reality the health-care worker has been culturally insensitive.

The nurse can consult the American Diabetes Association in Washington, DC (1-800-342-2383) to obtain meal plans for ethnic individuals such as Asians, Hispanics, African Americans, and Native Americans. Some helpful web sites include www.diabetes.org/espanol and www.eatright.org.

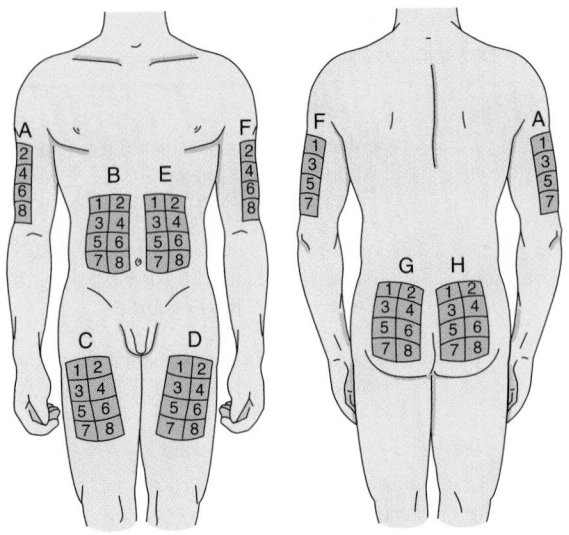

Rotation sites for injection of insulin.

FIGURE 40.3 Sample insulin rotation chart.

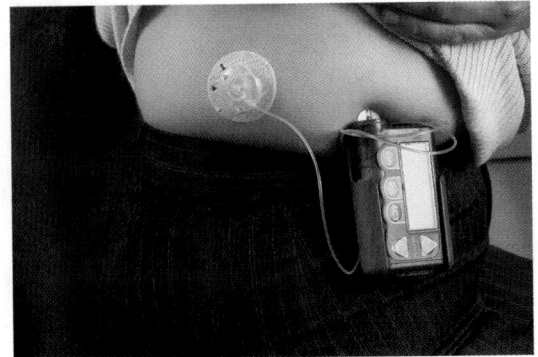

FIGURE 40.4 Patient wearing insulin pump.

Insulin is synthetically produced in a laboratory and is either identical to human insulin, or one or two amino acids different (called insulin analogs). In the past, insulin was derived from cows and pigs; this is no longer available in the United States, but may be available from other countries. Be careful to check the source when preparing insulin for injection (especially if you work in home care, where patients could purchase their insulin online from another country), because insulins from different sources may act slightly differently. Some individuals may be allergic to beef or pork preparations or may refuse them based on cultural practices.

Once insulin is injected, a period elapses before it begins to lower blood glucose. This time is called the *onset* of action. The *peak* action time occurs when the insulin is working at its hardest and the blood glucose is at its lowest point. It is during this peak time that the patient is most at risk for an episode of low blood glucose. *Duration* is the length of time the insulin works before it is used up. Onset, peak, and duration are determined by whether the insulin is short-, intermediate-, or long-acting (Table 40.4). It is important for the individual with diabetes and the nurse to

be aware of the onset, peak, and duration of any insulin given. This assists in making decisions such as when to give insulin, when to exercise, and when to be alert to low blood glucose symptoms.

LEARNING TIP

The Evens-and-Odds Rule: to remember the onset, peak, and duration of intermediate-acting insulin, think *evens*—2, 12, and 24 hours. To remember short-acting insulin, think *odds*—1, 3, and 5 hours. These times are not exact, but they are a great memory booster when you need to think fast.

In the past, most patients with diabetes used an injection of intermediate-acting insulin before breakfast and possibly a second injection before supper. Many patients are now choosing to take more frequent injections of short-acting insulin before meals or a combination of short- and intermediate-acting or long-acting insulins to achieve better, "tighter" control. These patients are often taught to adjust their insulin dose based on blood glucose level and the amount of carbohydrates eaten. Tighter control can mean fewer complications in the long run.

One regimen that is becoming more common because it mimics normal insulin secretion is sometimes called

TABLE 40.4 ONSET, PEAK, AND DURATION OF INSULINS

Insulin Type	Example	Sample Brand Names	Onset	Peak	Duration
Very short acting	Insulin lispro,	Humalog	15–30 min	30–90 min	≤5 hr
	Insulin aspart	NovoLog	10–20 min	1–3 hr	3–5 hr
	Insulin human rDNA origin (for inhalation)	Exubera*			
Short acting	Regular	Humulin R, Novolin R	1/2–1 hr	2–5 hr	5–8 hr
Intermediate acting	NPH	Humulin N, Novolin N	1–2 hr	6–12 hr	18–26 hr
Long acting	Ultralente	Humulin U	4–6 hr	14–24 hr	26–36 hr
	Insulin glargine	Lantus AE	70 min	No peak	24 hr

Note: A variety of premixed formulas are also available.
Note: All insulins listed are injected except Exubera.
*Data for onset, peak, and duration not currently available.

"basal-bolus" insulin. This consists of an injection of a basal insulin once a day, often at bedtime, to provide a constant small amount of insulin in the bloodstream. Then an injection of very short-acting insulin is injected before meals to mimic the extra insulin that is secreted normally with meals.

When two insulins need to be given at the same time, they can often be mixed together to prevent having to give more than one injection. See Box 40.5 How to Mix Insulins in one syringe. Preset mixtures of intermediate- and short-acting insulins are available for patients who have difficulty learning to mix insulins.

LEARNING TIP

When mixing insulins, remember *clear to cloudy*. Always draw up the clear insulin first. This involves injecting air into the cloudy vial first. This is because if the clear is drawn up last, the vial may be contaminated by the cloudy insulin, altering the action of the clear insulin. If cloudy insulin is unknowingly contaminated by clear insulin, the clear will become cloudy and its effect will be diminished. *Note: Lantus insulin cannot be mixed with other insulins.*

Box 40.5

How to Mix Insulins

1. Assemble equipment: insulins, syringe (be sure it is large enough to hold the entire insulin dose), alcohol swab, physician's order.
2. Check physician's order to confirm correct insulin types and doses of regular (clear) and an intermediate-acting (cloudy) insulin.
3. Roll the bottle of cloudy insulin to mix. Do not shake, because this will cause bubbles.
4. Wipe tops of both vials with alcohol swab.
5. Draw up and inject an amount of air equal to the dose of intermediate-acting insulin into the cloudy vial. Remove syringe from vial.
6. Draw up and inject an amount of air equal to the dose of short-acting insulin into the clear vial.
7. Draw up the correct amount of clear insulin. Double-check amount with another nurse if this is the institution's policy.
8. Remove the syringe and insert into the cloudy vial. Carefully draw up the correct amount of insulin. If too much insulin is accidentally drawn into the syringe, the syringe must be discarded and the process repeated. Double-check again with another nurse according to institution policy.
NOTE: Some insulins cannot be mixed. Check a drug reference before mixing.

During times of stress or illness, some patients who usually take the same insulin doses every day are placed on "sliding-scale" insulin. This involves determining each dose of short-acting insulin based on blood glucose results, usually before meals and at bedtime. For example, a sliding-scale order might read, "For blood glucose <200, no insulin; 201 to 250, 2 units regular insulin; 251 to 300, 4 units regular insulin; 301 to 350, 6 units regular insulin; >350 call physician."

INHALED INSULIN. A new short-acting human insulin that can be inhaled, Exubera, was approved by the Food and Drug Administration (FDA) in January 2006. Exubera is a dry powder insulin that can actually enter the circulation via the lungs faster than a subcutaneous injection. It can reduce lung function slightly, so patients must have pulmonary function tests before using it. It cannot be used by patients who smoke or who have quit smoking within the last 6 months. Some are concerned that patients may overuse inhaled insulin because it is easier to administer than injections, which will increase the risk of low blood glucose. It can be used alone or to supplement other treatment in type 2 diabetes, and may be used in conjunction with long-acting injected insulin in type 1 diabetes.

PROBLEMS WITH INSULIN THERAPY. Two problems that can occur with glucose control are the Somogyi effect and the dawn phenomenon. The Somogyi effect may be at fault when the patient's blood glucose seems to be rising in spite of increasing insulin doses. If insulin levels are too high, the blood glucose may drop too low, stimulating release of counterregulatory hormones (epinephrine, glucagon, corticosteroids, growth hormone) that then elevate the blood glucose. The low glucose levels often occur during the night, and the patient may report night sweats or morning headaches. The high morning glucose is then interpreted as hyperglycemia, and the insulin dose may be further increased, compounding the problem.

The dawn phenomenon is thought to occur because of the natural release of growth hormone and cortisol during the early morning hours. This causes hyperglycemia on arising in the morning.

CRITICAL THINKING

Mrs. Evans

■ Mrs. Evans is a 68-year-old woman with type 2 diabetes who resides in an assisted living facility. She is on 42 units of NPH insulin every morning.

1. If Mrs. Evans eats her breakfast at 8:00 every morning, when should she take her insulin?
2. At what time of day should she be alert for symptoms of low blood sugar?
3. What could happen if Mrs. Evans has a busy day and misses her lunch?

Suggested answers at end of chapter.

The patient might be asked to monitor blood sugar between 2 and 4 a.m. in addition to bedtime and morning testing to assess whether the Somogyi effect or the dawn phenomenon is occurring. Correction of the Somogyi effect involves reducing the insulin dose. The dawn phenomenon is treated with careful adjustment of meals and insulin; moving the evening insulin dose to bedtime may cause the insulin to peak when the blood glucose is highest.

ORAL HYPOGLYCEMIC MEDICATION. The patient with type 2 diabetes may be able to control blood glucose levels with medical nutrition therapy and exercise alone. Oral hypoglycemic medication or insulin may also be prescribed. Oral hypoglycemics are not insulin pills. Remember that if insulin is ingested, it is digested, because it is a protein. Because most oral hypoglycemic agents depend on at least a partially functioning pancreas, most are not useful for patients with type 1 diabetes. See Table 40.5 for a list of frequently used oral hypoglycemic agents.

Most insulins and oral hypoglycemics should be administered before meals (check individual drugs for specific timing). Care should be taken to prevent passage of more than 30 minutes between medication administration and the meal because this may result in a hypoglycemic episode.

If blood glucose levels are not controlled with oral hypoglycemic agents, insulin may be necessary for the person with type 2 diabetes. This does not mean the person has type 1 diabetes. Insulin may be necessary to control blood glucose, but it is not necessary to sustain life, as it is for the person with type 1 diabetes.

NEW DEVELOPMENTS IN DIABETES MEDICATION. Researchers are constantly looking for new medications that will help control blood glucose levels. One new medication is exenatide (Byetta), an injectable drug that was first isolated in the saliva of the Gila monster! It is an "incretin mimetic," meaning it mimics natural incretins in the body. Incretins are hormones secreted by the gastrointestinal (GI)

TABLE 40.5 ORAL HYPOGLYCEMIC AGENTS

Medication Class/Action	Examples	Side Effects	Nursing Implications
Insulin Stimulators			
Sulfonylureas Stimulate insulin secretion by pancreas, increase insulin receptor sensitivity	Glipizide (Glucotrol) Glimepiride (Amaryl) Glyburide (Micronase, Diabeta)	Hypoglycemia, weight gain, possible increased risk of cardiovascular disease.	Monitor for hypoglycemia. Teach patient to avoid alcohol.
Meglitinides Stimulate insulin secretion by pancreas	Repaglinide (Prandin), nateglinide (Starlix)	Hypoglycemia, weight gain	Monitor for hypoglycemia. Dosed with meals to improve postprandial hyperglycemia; multiple dosing less convenient. Hold dose if patient skips meal.
Insulin Sensitizers			
Biguanide Decreases glucose production by liver; increases glucose uptake by muscle	Metformin (Glucophage)	Nausea, diarrhea, decreased appetite	Give with meals. May enhance weight loss. Withhold if patient is having tests involving contrast dye. Contraindicated in renal and hepatic disease and CHF. Notify physician of early symptoms of lactic acidosis: hyperventilation, myalgia, malaise.
Combination agents	Metformin/glyburide (Glucovance) Metformin/rosiglitazone (Avandamet)	See individual agents.	See individual agents.
Thiazolidinediones (glitazones) Reduces insulin resistance in muscles. Improves blood lipids; may lower blood pressure and improve cardiovascular risk.	Pioglitazone (Actos), rosiglitazone (Avandia)	Nausea, weight gain, and fluid retention	Give with meal. Works well with obese patients. Avoid with liver disease; monitor liver enzymes. May alter effectiveness of some birth control pills.
Absorption Delayers			
Alpha-glucosidase inhibitors (AGIs) Lower postprandial glucose by reducing rate of carbohydrate digestion and absorption.	Acarbose (Precose), miglitol (Glyset)	Flatulence, bloating	Give at start of each meal. No weight gain or hypoglycemia risk. Multiple dosing less convenient. If used in combination with another drug and hypoglycemia occurs, treat with milk or glucose tablets, not table sugar.

CHF = congestive heart failure.

tract that stimulate insulin release in response to nutrients in the intestine. Byetta works in conjunction with oral hypoglycemic agents, and stimulates insulin secretion, lowers production of glucagon, slows gastric emptying, and promotes weight loss.

Another new drug, pramlintide (Symlin), is an injectable agent that is used with insulin. It is a synthetic analog of amylin, a naturally occurring hormone that reduces glucose levels following meals. It may also promote weight loss in individuals who are overweight. Symlin carries with it an increased risk of hypoglycemia.

Self-Monitoring of Blood Glucose

The ability to test blood glucose levels at home has been a major advance in diabetes care. Blood glucose can be better controlled because of the availability of monitoring at any time, in any place. A variety of blood glucose monitors are on the market at a reasonable price (Fig. 40.5). Most of the cost involved in monitoring is in the test strips that must be used. Health insurance programs sometimes cover this cost.

Self-monitoring of blood glucose (SMBG) is generally done before meals and at bedtime by the individual on insulin who wishes to maintain tight control of blood glucose. Less frequent schedules may be prescribed for patients who are unable or unwilling to test four times a day or for patients not on insulin. Some may test before breakfast and supper, and some may vary testing times from day to day. Patients are also often recommended to periodically test 2 hours after meals. New noninvasive devices are being developed, such as a monitoring device that resembles a wrist watch. It is worn on the arm, and it checks glucose levels by extracting fluid from the arm every 20 minutes. An excellent test for long-term monitoring is the HbA_{1c} blood test, described earlier. It is usually done every 3 to 4 months.

The physician should be consulted for desirable blood glucose ranges because these may differ for each patient.

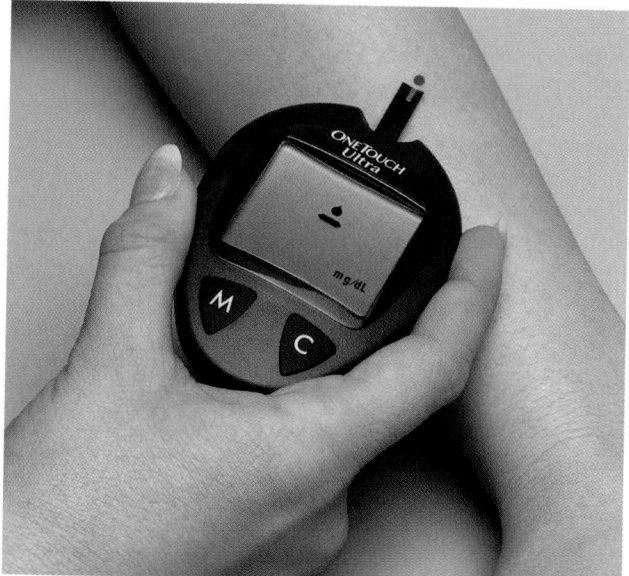

FIGURE 40.5 OneTouch Ultra glucose monitor. *(Courtesy Life Scan.)*

The American Diabetes Association recommends a preprandial goal of 90 to 130 mg/dL for most patients. Patients who are prone to insulin reactions (hypoglycemia) or small children or the elderly may have higher goal ranges, such as 100 to 150 mg/dL. Lower blood glucose levels for these populations could increase the risk of hypoglycemia.

Urine Glucose and Ketone Monitoring

Urine may also be tested for glucose and for ketones. Urine glucose testing was done routinely before the development of SMBG. A variety of dipsticks and tape products are available for urine testing. If glucose appears in the urine, the patient is warned that the blood glucose is elevated, but the actual level is unknown. Most people have glucose in their urine when their blood glucose is more than about 180 mg/dL. It is difficult to base treatment on urine glucose levels, and so routine urine testing for glucose is no longer recommended.

Urine should be tested for ketones during acute illness or stress, when blood glucose levels are consistently above 300 mg/dL, during pregnancy, or when symptoms of ketoacidosis are present. If ketones are present, the patient knows an insulin deficiency is present and should notify the physician. Patients with type 1 diabetes are most at risk for developing ketoacidosis; however, it is wise for the patient with type 2 diabetes to test for ketones if risk factors are present.

An important aspect of blood or urine monitoring is the interpretation of results. Monitoring is useless if the results are not used to improve blood glucose control. The patient should be instructed to keep a diary of blood glucose levels (Fig. 40.6). Some patients have computer software that graphs results. The patient may be taught by a diabetes educator to interpret the trends in the results, or the diary may be taken on a regular basis to the health-care provider for interpretation and adjustment of the treatment plan.

See Box 40.6 Diabetes Summary for diabetes symptoms, diagnosis, and treatment.

Transplant

If the patient is determined to be an appropriate candidate, a pancreas transplant may be considered. This is especially beneficial in the patient with kidney disease, who can receive both a kidney and pancreas transplant at the same time. Another promising treatment is the use of pancreatic islet cell transplant.

Acute Complications of Diabetes

The individual with diabetes is at risk for a variety of complications. Acute complications related to high and low blood glucose levels are treatable and can often be prevented with appropriate care.

Hyperglycemia

When calories eaten exceed insulin available or glucose used, high blood glucose (hyperglycemia) occurs. The most common cause of hyperglycemia is eating more than the meal plan prescribes. Another major cause is stress. Stress causes the release of counterregulatory hormones, including epinephrine, cortisol, growth hormone, and glucagon. These hormones all increase the blood glucose level. In a person

Day		Break-fast	Lunch	Supper	Bedtime	Urine Ketones	Notes
Sunday	Time	7:00	11:30	6:00	11:00		
	Glucose	186	108	116	142		
	Insulin	38N,6R		16N,2R			
Monday	Time	7:30	12:00	6:00	10:45	6:00-neg	Ate cake at Betty's party at 3 pm-oops!
	Glucose	171	97	302	180		
	Insulin	38N,6R		16N,2R			
Tuesday	Time						
	Glucose						
	Insulin						
Wednesday	Time						
	Glucose						
	Insulin						
Thursday	Time						
	Glucose						
	Insulin						
Friday	Time						
	Glucose						
	Insulin						
Saturday	Time						
	Glucose						
	Insulin						

FIGURE 40.6 Sample diary of blood glucose results and insulin use.

without diabetes, this is an adaptive function. However, the patient with diabetes is unable to compensate for the increased blood glucose with increased insulin secretion, and hyperglycemia occurs.

Patients must be able to recognize signs and symptoms of high blood glucose levels and know what to do if they occur (Table 40.6). For many patients, these are similar to the symptoms they experienced when they were first diagnosed with diabetes. Chronic high blood glucose levels can lead to long-term complications (discussed later in this chapter).

Hypoglycemia

Low blood glucose, or hypoglycemia, occurs when there is not enough glucose available in relation to circulating insulin. This is sometimes referred to as an insulin reaction. Hypoglycemia is usually defined as a blood glucose level below 50 mg/dL, although patients may feel symptoms at higher or lower levels. Occasionally, symptoms occur as a result of a rapid drop in blood glucose, even though the actual glucose level is normal or high. Causes of hypoglycemia may include skipping a meal, exercising more than usual, or accidentally administering too much insulin. An occasional hypoglycemic episode, treated promptly, should not lead to chronic complications. Repeated or extremely low blood glucose levels can cause neurological damage because there is not enough glucose for brain function. It is therefore important to teach patients how to prevent and treat low blood sugar (see Table 40.6).

Symptoms of low blood glucose include hunger, sweating, pallor, tremor, palpitations, and headache. These symptoms are caused by activation of the sympathetic nervous system. As hypoglycemia progresses, the brain is deprived

CRITICAL THINKING

Jeff

■ Jeff is a 16-year-old who is having trouble with repeated insulin reactions. He says he has not had this trouble before, and it is interfering with his new job. What questions might you ask as you do your assessment to help him figure out how to prevent future reactions?

Suggested answers at end of chapter.

of glucose and neurological symptoms such as irritability, confusion, seizures, and coma may occur.

If you find someone with symptoms of an altered blood glucose but are unable to identify whether it is high or low, do a blood glucose test. However, if the patient is exhibiting neurological symptoms, treat for low blood glucose immediately. The blood glucose may then be checked and further treatment provided as indicated.

To treat low blood glucose, administer a "fast sugar"— 15 g of carbohydrate that will enter the bloodstream quickly. This may be 4 oz of orange juice, commercially available glucose tablets, or another quickly available source of sugar (Box 40.7 Fast Sugars). If the patient is not alert or is unable to safely swallow, subcutaneous glucagon can be given. If the patient is hospitalized, intravenous (IV) glucose can be administered by the RN. Recheck glucose in 15 minutes. If the blood glucose does not return to normal, repeat the procedure every 15 minutes until relief occurs. Do not overtreat hypoglycemia with too much sugar because this may cause

Box 40.6

Diabetes Summary

Signs and Symptoms	Polyuria Polydipsia Polyphagia Fatigue Blurred vision Headache Abdominal pain
Diagnostic Tests	Fasting plasma glucose HbA$_{1c}$ (glycosylated hemoglobin) Oral glucose tolerance test Additional testing for complications
Therapeutic Interventions	Diet Exercise Insulin Oral hypoglycemic medication Self-monitoring of blood glucose levels Education
Complications	Hypoglycemia, Hyperglycemia DKA, HHNKS
Priority Nursing Diagnoses	Risk for ineffective health maintenance, risk for imbalanced nutrition Risk for injury: complications

Box 40.7

Fast Sugars

4 oz orange juice
6 oz regular (not diet) soda
Miniature box of raisins
Commercial glucose tablets
6–8 Life Savers

hyperglycemia and rebound hypoglycemia. Many nurses added sugar to orange juice in the past; this is no longer recommended.

If the next meal is more than 1 hour away, follow the treatment with a protein and complex carbohydrate snack, such as crackers with cheese or peanut butter, or half of a sandwich. If symptoms worsen, call 911, or contact the physician for the hospitalized patient. Check hospital or agency policy for specific protocol for treating hypoglycemic episodes.

Some elderly patients with poor autonomic nervous system function or patients taking beta-adrenergic–blocking medication such as propranolol or atenolol (that block the sympathetic response) may not feel the symptoms of hypoglycemia. These patients should check glucose levels more frequently and keep the levels in a safe range to prevent hypoglycemic episodes.

Individuals with diabetes should be instructed to keep a fast sugar in their purse or pocket at all times. Fast sugars may also be stored in bedside tables, cars, and desks at work.

TABLE 40.6 COMPARISON OF HIGH AND LOW BLOOD GLUCOSE LEVELS

	Hyperglycemia	Hypoglycemia
Causes	Overeating Stress Illness Too little insulin or medication	Undereating, skipping a meal Too much insulin or medication Exercise
Symptoms	Polyuria Polydipsia Polyphagia Blurred vision Headache Lethargy Abdominal pain Ketonuria (if type I) Coma	Hunger Sweating Tremor Blurred vision Headache Irritability Confusion Seizures Coma
Treatment	Confirm hyperglycemia with glucose meter; if greater than 300 mg/dL, check urine for ketones and increase fluid intake. Assess cause of hyperglycemia, teach prevention. Return to prescribed treatment plan if applicable. Call physician for medication adjustment if indicated or if blood glucose is >200 mg/dL for 2 days. Call physician if patient is ill or vomiting.	Confirm hypoglycemia with glucose meter (if patient is not acutely ill). Administer 15 g fast-acting carbohydrate. Recheck glucose in 15 minutes; if still low, readminister carbohydrate. Continue cycle of checking glucose and administering fast sugar until hypoglycemia subsides; if symptoms worsen, call physician or emergency help. Glucagon subcutaneously or dextrose 50% IV may be administered if ordered. Assess cause of hypoglycemia, teach prevention.

Diabetic Ketoacidosis

PATHOPHYSIOLOGY. Diabetic ketoacidosis (DKA) occurs when blood glucose levels become very high and insulin is deficient. This most commonly occurs in individuals with type 1 diabetes. DKA is often the reason a person with undiagnosed type 1 diabetes first seeks help. It may also be the result of stress or illness in a person with previously diagnosed type 1 (or rarely, type 2) diabetes. When there is insufficient insulin to allow glucose into cells, the cells starve. The body then breaks down fat to be used for energy. The fat breakdown releases an acid substance called ketones. As ketones build up in the blood, ketoacidosis occurs.

The body attempts to compensate for acidosis by deepening respirations, thereby blowing off excess carbon dioxide. (See the section on metabolic acidosis in Chapter 5.) The deep, sighing respiratory pattern is called **Kussmaul's** respirations. The expired air has a fruity odor caused by the ketones and may be mistaken for alcohol. Some nurses have likened the odor to Juicy Fruit chewing gum.

With such high blood glucose and the accompanying polyuria, the body becomes dehydrated very quickly. Tachycardia, hypotension, and shock can result. Acidosis also causes potassium to leave the cells and accumulate in the blood (hyperkalemia). Potassium is then lost in large amounts in the urine. The combination of dehydration, potassium imbalance, and acidosis causes the patient to develop flulike symptoms, including abdominal pain and vomiting. The patient loses consciousness and death occurs if DKA is not treated. The mortality rate for DKA is about 5%.

THERAPEUTIC INTERVENTION. Treatment includes IV fluids, IV insulin, and blood glucose monitoring, often initially in an intensive care unit (ICU) setting. You can assist with monitoring hourly blood glucose levels and notify the RN or physician when the desired level is reached. Glucose should be added to the IV when the blood glucose drops to about 180 mg/dL to avoid hypoglycemia. Potassium should also be monitored closely, since it is essential to have normal levels for cardiac function. Arterial blood gases help monitor acidosis. The cause of the DKA should be identified and treated.

Prevention of ketoacidosis involves careful monitoring of blood glucose levels at home. If the blood glucose rises above 300 mg/dL, the patient should use a urine dipstick made to detect ketones. If ketones are present, the patient should drink water and recheck with the next urination. If ketones are still present, the physician should be notified. Patients should be instructed to never stop their insulin without a physician's supervision.

Hyperosmolar, Hyperglycemic, Nonketotic Syndrome

PATHOPHYSIOLOGY. Hyperosmolar, hyperglycemic, nonketotic (HHNK) syndrome occurs primarily in type 2 diabetes, when blood glucose levels are high as a result of stress or illness. Because the person with type 2 diabetes has some insulin production, cells do not starve and DKA usually does not occur. HHNK occurs more often in the elderly.

As the blood glucose rises (hyperglycemic), polyuria causes profound dehydration, producing the hyperosmolar (concentrated) state. Blood glucose may rise as high as 1500 mg/dL, and electrolyte imbalances occur. Because ketoacidosis is not present, the patient may not feel as physically ill as the patient with DKA and may delay seeking treatment. Symptoms of HHNK develop slowly and include extreme thirst, lethargy, and mental confusion. Shock, coma, and death occur if HHNK is left untreated. The mortality rate for HHNK is between 10% and 20%.

THERAPEUTIC INTERVENTION. Treatment includes IV fluids and insulin, and glucose monitoring. Electrolytes are closely monitored. The cause of HHNK should be identified and treated. HHNK syndrome can be prevented with careful monitoring of glucose levels at home. Patients should be instructed to drink plenty of fluids if blood glucose levels are beginning to rise, especially in times of stress and illness. They should also know when to call their physician with high blood glucose results.

Long-Term Complications

Over time, chronic hyperglycemia causes a variety of serious complications in persons with diabetes. These involve the circulatory system, eyes, kidneys, skin, and nerves. Most of the complications involve either the large blood vessels in the body (macrovascular complications) or the tiny blood vessels, such as those in the eyes or kidneys (microvascular complications). The Diabetes Control and Complications Trial (DCCT), a large research study completed in 1993, showed that individuals with type 1 diabetes who maintain tight control of blood glucose experience fewer long-term complications than individuals who take traditional care of their diabetes.[6] Similarly, the United Kingdom Prospective Diabetes Study (UKPDS), completed in 1998, showed that individuals with type 2 diabetes who maintain an HbA_{1c} below 7% can significantly reduce complications. In fact, for every percentage of decrease in HbA_{1c}, there were 25% fewer deaths from diabetes-related complications.[7] Unfortunately, even tight control does not guarantee the prevention of all complications.

Macrovascular Complications

CIRCULATORY SYSTEM. Individuals with diabetes develop atherosclerosis and arteriosclerosis faster than the general population. They are more likely to have hypertension and elevated low-density lipoprotein (LDL) cholesterol and triglyceride levels. High blood glucose may also affect platelet function, leading to increased clotting. These problems lead to a higher incidence of strokes, heart attacks, and poor circulation in the feet and legs. The risk of cardiovascular disease and strokes is two to four times more common in persons with diabetes than in the general population.

Blood glucose and blood pressure control is vital to help prevent these deadly complications. Patients should also avoid smoking, and maintain normal weight. Aspirin therapy to reduce platelet aggregation is recommended for patients older than 21 years of age with diabetes.

Microvascular Complications

EYES. Small blood vessels can become diseased, eventually leading to retinopathy in most patients with diabetes. Retinopathy involves damage to the tiny blood vessels that supply the eye. Small hemorrhages occur, which can cause blindness if not corrected. Twenty-three percent of all adults with diabetes report some vision impairment.[8] Newer laser surgery techniques may help improve vision after hemorrhages occur. Diabetes is also associated with a high incidence of cataracts. Patients with diabetes should have a yearly dilated eye examination.

KIDNEYS. Nephropathy is caused by damage to the tiny blood vessels within the kidneys. Up to 40% of patients with diabetes develop some degree of nephropathy. Native Americans, Hispanics, and African Americans have the highest risk. A primary risk factor for diabetic nephropathy is poor control of blood glucose. If nephropathy occurs, the kidneys are unable to remove waste products and excess fluid from the blood. Diabetes is the leading cause of end-stage renal (kidney) disease (ESRD) in the United States. When the kidneys have lost most of their function, patients may have their blood cleansed artificially by either hemodialysis or peritoneal dialysis. (See Chapter 37.) The only cure for ESRD is a kidney transplant.

Patients should be taught the importance of blood glucose control to prevent or delay kidney disease. Angiotensin-converting enzyme inhibitor (ACEI) and angiotensin receptor blocker (ARB) medications have also been shown to slow the development of kidney problems in patients with diabetes. Patients who have both diabetes and hypertension should be placed on an ACEI or ARB. Routine urine tests are done to check for microalbuminuria (tiny amounts of protein in the urine) or microalbumin-to-creatine ratios. If microalbuminuria occurs, a low-protein diet may help delay further development of nephropathy. A trained renal dietitian should work with the patient and physician in determining the best diet for the patient.

Nerves

Another complication of diabetes is neuropathy, which is damage to nerves as a result of chronic hyperglycemia. Neuropathy can cause numbness and pain in the extremities, erectile dysfunction (impotence) in males, sexual dysfunction in women, **gastroparesis** (delayed stomach emptying), and other problems. Unfortunately, pain caused by neuropathy is difficult to treat with traditional analgesics. Some antidepressant and anticonvulsant drugs may be helpful, and in some cases local injections of anesthetics may be used. A new drug, pregabalin (Lyrica), that reduces painful nerve impulses was recently approved by the FDA specifically for

nerve pain. Improved control of blood glucose levels may also help.

Infection

Persons with diabetes are prone to infection for several reasons. If injuries occur, healing may be slow because of impaired circulation. There may not be enough blood supply to heal the wound or fight an infection. For the same reason, it may be difficult for IV antibiotics to reach an infected site, and topical antibiotics may be preferable. In the presence of hyperglycemia, white blood cells become sluggish and ineffective, further reducing the body's ability to fight infection.

The incidence of periodontal (gum) disease, caused by bacteria in plaque, is also increased in individuals with diabetes. Patients must be taught to maintain good oral hygiene and make regular visits to the dentist.

Foot Complications

The combination of vascular disease, neuropathy, and risk for infection makes patients with diabetes prone to foot problems. Consider the patient who has no feeling in his or her feet because of neuropathy. If the patient steps on a tack, it may not be felt right away. Vascular disease will prevent a good blood supply from preventing infection and promoting healing. If infection sets in, it is slow to resolve and may progress to necrosis and gangrene. Pressure points on the feet may also break down (Fig. 40.7). One woman had a Bic pen in her shoe all day and did not realize it! Neuropathy can also lead to deformities of the feet, further increasing the risk for injuries.

For these reasons, diabetes is the leading cause of amputation of the lower extremities. Patients should be taught to protect their feet at all times by wearing well-fitting shoes and by washing, drying, and inspecting their feet daily (Box 40.8 Foot Care Tips). If any sores are noted, the patient should not delay in seeking treatment. During routine visits to the physician, the patient should be sure to remove shoes and socks so the feet can be thoroughly examined. The physician or diabetes specialist can test sensation in the feet with tiny filaments. Loss of protective sensation

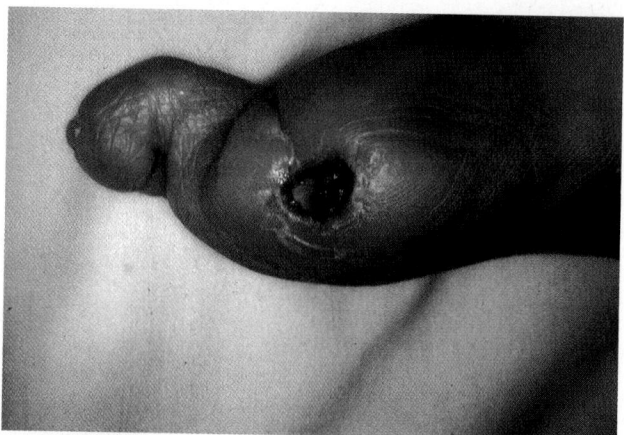

FIGURE 40.7 Diabetic foot ulcer at site of amputated toe. *(From Goldsmith, LA, Lazarus, GS, and Tharp, MD: Adult and Pediatric Dermatology. F.A. Davis, Philadelphia, 1997, p 438, with permission.)*

---

nephropathy: nephro—of the kidney + pathy—illness
gastroparesis: gastro—stomach + paresis—partial paralysis

is an early risk factor for amputation, so any reduction in sensation is a warning sign that extra care must be taken. A podiatrist (foot doctor) can be consulted if problems occur. Specialized wound treatment centers have new healing techniques that have prevented many amputations (Box 40.9 Ethical Considerations).

CRITICAL THINKING

Mr. Jones

■ Mr. Jones is a 54-year-old banker with type 2 diabetes admitted to your unit with a tiny red area on his right heel. His admitting blood glucose is 360 mg/dL. The lesion is so small you wonder what the fuss is about. While doing his assessment, you find that he wore a new pair of shoes to work all day about a month ago and has been avoiding seeing his physician about the resulting red area. He is placed on IV antibiotics, and within 3 days the red area has broken open and has yellow drainage. He is sent home with topical antibiotics and crutches, to be followed by a visiting nurse. The wound takes 6 months to fully heal.

1. List three risk factors for foot problems.
2. Why did the sore take so long to heal?
3. Why do you think crutches are necessary?
4. Why might topical antibiotics work better than IV antibiotics?
5. The nurse documents the following description of Mr. Jones' wound: "Small red open area on heel, with yellow drainage on dressing." What is wrong with this charting? How can you improve it?

Suggested answers at end of chapter.

Box 40.8

Foot Care Tips

Wash and dry feet every day. Use warm (not hot) water to avoid burns.

Apply lotion that does not contain alcohol, avoiding areas between toes.

Inspect feet for sores or red areas daily (have a family member help if necessary).

Report any abnormalities immediately.

Wear leather shoes and cotton socks.

Never go barefoot.

Avoid garters and tight socks.

Avoid crossing legs.

Cut toenails to natural shape of nail—not into corners.

See a podiatrist for calluses or problem toenails (avoid "bathroom surgery").

Have feet checked at least once a year, preferably three to four times a year, for loss of sensation.

Box 40.9

Ethical Considerations

Refusal of treatment

Mr. Mann is 55 years old and has had diabetes for more than 20 years. He has not managed his diabetes well and has subsequently suffered many complications. Mr. Mann does not regularly test his blood sugar, so he does not always get the appropriate amount of insulin. In addition, he does not eat properly. He picks up fast food during his lunch break and he binges on various snack foods before he eats his dinner, or sometimes instead of eating his dinner.

Mr. Mann is not aware of the importance of taking care of himself to prevent long-term complications of diabetes. He is now seeking health care because of a neglected leg ulcer. He tried to treat it at home with over-the-counter remedies, but it did not improve, and it is now infected. Part of his foot is gangrenous and an amputation is recommended. The first time the surgery is mentioned, Mr. Mann becomes outraged and refuses to discuss it. He says he is "not going to leave this earth without all his parts." After further discussions with Mr. Mann, it is clear that he understands the consequences of his condition. He is more annoyed by the drainage from the ulcer than worried about the progressive gangrene. This is a complex case. Questions that should be asked may include:

• Does Mr. Mann *really* understand his current situation and likely consequences?
• Can Mr. Mann be treated without his permission?
• Should action be taken to have someone else named as Mr. Mann's guardian, despite his apparent competence?
• What would a "non compos mentis" (unconscious or incompetent) diagnosis mean for Mr. Mann's future care planning?
• Does disagreement with the medical establishment in itself denote incompetence?
• Does the level of risk if treatment is refused make any difference in the health professional's response?
• What if Mr. Mann's refusal is based on religious or cultural beliefs?
• Should his wishes be supported at all costs?
• What are the nurse's responsibilities?
• How does the application of ethical theory help to sort out the critical elements of this case?

Special Considerations for the Patient Undergoing Surgery

Surgery is a stressor. The counterregulatory hormones released during stress cause the blood glucose to rise, even if the patient has been fasting. High blood glucose levels interfere with immune function and healing, and can promote an environment conducive to infection. Tight blood glucose control during hospitalization and surgery has been shown to significantly reduce complications. Check with the physician for changes in insulin orders. Often patients are placed on intravenous infusions of glucose and insulin during and immediately after surgery, in place of longer acting insulins. FPG levels should be maintained at less than 110 mg/dL at all times, and postprandial glucose should be less than 180 mg/dL.[9] Monitor blood glucose levels every 2 to 4 hours or as ordered, and monitor carefully for signs and symptoms of hypoglycemia or hyperglycemia. If a patient uses a pump at home, check with a diabetes resource nurse and try to see that the patient can continue to use it during hospitalization.

Patients who were not previously on insulin may be placed on insulin during surgery and postoperatively. They can generally return to their presurgical treatment plan after the stress of surgery is past.

Nursing Process for the Patient with Diabetes Mellitus

Assessment/Data Collection
A complete history and physical assessment should be carried out because diabetes affects every body system. Some areas on which to focus are shown in Table 40.7. It is especially important to assess each patient's knowledge of diabetes and its care so that appropriate teaching can be done.

Nursing Diagnosis, Planning, and Implementation
Because diabetes affects so many different areas, nearly any nursing diagnosis may be appropriate. It is important to assess each patient as an individual and choose diagnoses based on assessment findings. A sample care plan is shown for a diagnosis of risk for ineffective health maintenance because patients with diabetes must learn to care for themselves to maintain their health (Box 40.10 Nursing Care Plan for the Patient with Diabetes Mellitus). The actual pres-

ence of the defining characteristics should be confirmed with the patient before choosing any nursing diagnosis. Once diagnoses have been identified, planning takes place. This should be done with the patient and family. Diabetes affects not only the person with the disease, but the entire family as well. The desired outcome for the plan of care is that the patient is knowledgeable about and able to care for his or her disease. Consult the dietitian, social worker, certified diabetes educator (CDE), home care nurse, outpatient education programs, and other resources as needed. (See Home Health Hints.)

Evaluation
The best indicator of the success of a care plan for diabetes is controlled blood glucose and glycohemoglobin levels. The patient should also be without symptoms of hypoglycemia or hyperglycemia and be able to state what to do if they do occur. Long-term complications should be minimized. Another important indicator is the patient's statement of satisfaction and comfort with the plan and his or her ability to carry it out on a daily basis.

Diabetes Self-Management Education

The individual with diabetes must receive diabetes self-management education (DSME) if at all possible. No amount of care from a physician or nurse can replace the self-care required of the person with diabetes. The involvement of family or significant others is also important for the success and well-being of the person with diabetes.

If the patient is hospitalized at diagnosis, the initial instruction is done in the hospital. However, with hospital stays becoming shorter, you must not waste any time. Begin assessing baseline knowledge and teaching as soon as the patient is feeling physically well enough to learn. Depending on your state nurse practice act, this is usually the responsibility of the primary or registered staff nurse, although aspects of the instruction may be delegated to the LPN/LVN. Some hospitals have a Certified Diabetes

TABLE 40.7 ASSESSMENT OF THE PATIENT WITH DIABETES MELLITUS

Acutely Ill Patient with Newly Diagnosed Diabetes		Patient with Previously Diagnosed Diabetes	
Subjective Data	**Objective Data**	**Subjective Data**	**Objective Data**
• History of current problem	• Vital signs	• History of diabetes: type, onset, duration, degree of blood glucose control	• Labs: blood glucose level, HbA$_{1c}$, BUN, creatinine, ketones, cholesterol, triglycerides
• History of stress, illness, virus	• Lab values—electrolytes, blood glucose, ketones	• Knowledge of self-care and degree of compliance	• Condition of legs and feet; pulses, presence of circulatory or sensation impairment
• Family history of diabetes • Current medications • Other medical or surgical conditions	• Signs of dehydration • Fruity breath • Presence of complications if suspect diabetes was undiagnosed for period of time	• Support systems • History of complications	
• Knowledge of diabetes self-care			

Box 40.10   NURSING CARE PLAN for the Patient with Diabetes Mellitus

Nursing Diagnosis: Risk for ineffective health maintenance related to knowledge deficit in the patient with newly diagnosed diabetes mellitus

Expected Outcomes Blood glucose levels within parameters negotiated with health care provider. Patient states satisfaction with understanding of diabetes self-care.

Evaluation of Outcomes Are blood glucose levels within parameters negotiated? Does patient state satisfaction with understanding of diabetes self-care?

Interventions	Rationale	Evaluation
Assess knowledge of diabetes self-care.	Teaching should be initiated only if a knowledge deficit exists.	Does patient exhibit knowledge of diabetes self-care?
Assist patient to collaborate with health care provider to determine appropriate blood glucose levels and action to be taken if glucose levels are too high or too low.	Appropriate blood glucose levels may be different for each patient. The patient should know what blood glucose levels require notification of the health care provider.	Are blood glucose levels within parameters negotiated with health care provider? Does patient state appropriate blood glucose levels and action to take if glucose is high or low?
Teach patient to assess glucose levels before meals and at bedtime or as ordered by health care provider. Ensure that patient knows how to obtain glucose monitor and instruction for home use.	Good blood glucose control depends on knowledge of glucose levels and trends.	Does patient demonstrate correct use of glucose monitor or state how monitor and instruction will be obtained?
Teach patient how to administer insulin or oral hypoglycemic agent. Ensure that meals are timed appropriately with medications. Replace any uneaten foods to prevent hypoglycemia.	If most medications are taken without food to supply calories, hypoglycemia can occur. Check individual medication for specific instructions.	Does patient state correct meal and medication schedule?
Teach technique for administering insulin if indicated.	The patient and family should be familiar with the injection procedure.	Does patient demonstrate correct injection technique?
Observe for symptoms of hypoglycemia and hyperglycemia and treat as necessary. Teach causes, prevention, recognition, and treatment of hypoglycemia and hyperglycemia.	If the patient has a good understanding of hypoglycemia and hyperglycemia, most episodes can be prevented. If hypoglycemia or hyperglycemia does occur, prompt treatment is essential to prevent complications.	Does patient state causes, prevention, symptoms, and treatment of hypoglycemia? Does patient carry fast sugar at all times?
Consult with dietician for nutrition therapy instruction.	The dietitian is trained to provide in-depth meal plan instruction.	Is patient able to state plan for obtaining appropriate meals?
Consult with social worker or case manager as needed.	Some patients may not have the resources or support to carry out effective self-care.	Does patient state availability of adequate resources for self-care at home?

Interventions	Rationale	Evaluation
Provide patient with information regarding comprehensive diabetes education. Remind patient that only survival skills have been taught during initial instruction.	Instruction provided in the hospital usually is not comprehensive. Outpatient diabetes classes can provide additional self-care and health promotion information.	Does patient state plan for obtaining further diabetes education after discharge?
Assist patient to obtain medical alert card or tag that identifies diabetes.	If the patient is ever unresponsive for any reason, the health care provider would need to be aware of diabetes.	Does patient state plan to carry or wear identification at all times?
Geriatric		
Assess ability to see and manipulate syringe, glucose monitor, and other equipment. Obtain assistive devices as needed.	The elderly patient may have poor eyesight or other sensory deficits.	Is patient able to manipulate equipment to safely care for self?

Educator (CDE) who provides classroom or bedside instruction. The dietitian should be contacted to provide nutrition instruction.

Most hospitals have policies or management plans describing the instruction to be provided by the nurse. Generally this encompasses "survival skills," which include the basic information the patient needs initially to survive at home. Survival skills include medication administration, glucose monitoring, meal plan basics, and what to do if high or low blood glucose levels occur. A variety of helpful aids, such as pamphlets and videos, are available. Diabetes equipment suppliers provide kits that are full of samples and information. These are a significant help when you are teaching a patient. Also advise the patient to purchase a medical alert bracelet or necklace.

It is difficult to know how to operate and teach glucose monitoring with the variety of glucose monitors available. Many drugstores and medical supply stores not only sell the monitors but also provide training for the patient and family. You can obtain this information by calling local medical suppliers or by contacting the diabetes educator.

After discharge, the patient should be referred to outpatient diabetes classes for further instruction. If classes are unavailable or if the patient is unable to leave home, a referral to a visiting nurse should be given. It is usually advisable to have a nurse present for the patient's first insulin injection at home. The ADA recommends that DSME include information about the following:

- Disease process and treatment options
- Nutrition therapy
- Importance of physical activity
- Medications
- SMBG (and urine ketone monitoring when appropriate)
- Preventing, detecting, and treating acute complications
- Preventing, detecting, and treating chronic complications
- Goal setting and problem solving
- Psychosocial adjustment to daily life
- Preconception, pregnancy, and gestational diabetes management[10]

Two websites that might be helpful to both you and your patients are www.diabetes.org and www.lifeclinic.com/focus/diabetes/resources.asp.

Because many people with diabetes are elderly, it is important to be aware of their special needs (Box 40.11 Gerontological Issues).

REACTIVE HYPOGLYCEMIA

Reactive hypoglycemia occurs when the blood glucose drops below a normal level, usually below 50 mg/dL. Hypoglycemia is most often a complication of diabetes treatment, but at times it may occur without the presence of diabetes. It may be a warning sign of impending diabetes.

Box 40.11

Gerontological Issues

Diabetes care can be a challenge for many older adults. Syringe magnifiers and talking glucose meters are available for those with impaired vision. Family members may be taught to draw up a week's supply of insulin for the patient to store in the refrigerator. Home meal programs may help ensure an adequate diet. Older adults should also have an emergency call system in their home and regular contact with family members or other support people.

Pathophysiology

Low blood glucose may occur as an overreaction of the pancreas to eating. The pancreas senses a rising blood glucose and produces more insulin than is necessary for the use of that glucose. As a result, the blood glucose drops to below normal. Some experts believe that this is a rare condition and that many "hypoglycemic" episodes are due to activation of the sympathetic nervous system for other reasons, without true hypoglycemia.

Signs and Symptoms

Low blood glucose causes release of epinephrine, which in turn causes the blood glucose to rise. Epinephrine release causes a fight-or-flight reaction, which may produce shaking, sweating, and palpitations. Headache, chills, and confusion may also occur. Symptoms are the same as those described earlier related to hypoglycemia in diabetes.

Diagnosis

Diagnosis is often based on a 5-hour glucose tolerance test, with below-normal readings between 2 and 5 hours. However, with the availability of home glucose monitors, it is now preferable for patients to monitor blood glucose levels at home. Readings should be taken in the morning on arising, 2 hours after each meal, at bedtime, and during symptoms of hypoglycemia. These results may then be taken to the physician for interpretation.

Therapeutic Intervention

Treatment includes frequent small meals and avoidance of fasting. Simple sugars are avoided because they may aggravate symptoms. A high-protein, low-carbohydrate diet is stressed. See Table 40.8 for a sample diet.

TABLE 40.8 SAMPLE MEAL PLAN FOR HYPOGLYCEMIC DIET

Exchange Group	Sample Menu
Morning	
1 fruit	$^1/_2$ cup unsweetened orange juice
1 starch	$^3/_4$ cup whole-grain cereal
1 meat	1 oz low-fat cheese or meat
$^1/_2$ skim milk	$^1/_2$ cup skim milk
Free	Decaffeinated coffee
Mid-morning	
1 meat	1 tbsp peanut butter
1 starch	4 whole-grain crackers
Noon	
Chef salad:	
2–4 meat	2–4 oz lean meat
1 vegetable	Lettuce, tomatoes
1 fat	Dressing
1 fruit	1 small piece fresh fruit
1 skim milk	1 cup skim milk
1 starch	2 breadsticks ($4 \times {}^1/_2$ in)
Mid-afternoon	
1 meat	1 oz low-fat cheese
1 starch	4 whole-grain crackers
Evening	
2–4 meat	2–4 oz lean meat
1 starch	$^1/_2$ cup potato or pasta
1 vegetable	$^1/_2$ cup vegetable
1 fat	Lettuce salad with dressing
1 fruit	1 piece fresh fruit
Free	Decaffeinated coffee or tea
Bedtime	
1 starch and 1 meat	$^1/_2$ sandwich (1 slice whole-grain bread and 1 oz lean meat)
1 vegetable	Fresh vegetables
Free	Decaffeinated beverage

ETHICAL CONSIDERATIONS DISCUSSION

The principles of autonomy, nonmaleficence, and beneficence come into play in this case. Preservation of the patient's autonomy regardless of personal feelings or even mounting evidence is paramount. The only exception is when the patient is not making decisions based on sound and accurate information (does he *really* know what to expect should he refuse treatment?), and secondly when the patient can be considered not of sound mind (non compos mentis). We all make decisions that may appear to others to be unwise, but it is a basic human right to make such decisions.

The principle of "do no harm" has significant application in this case. If the patient's wishes are upheld, the respect for autonomy and choice means that the patient's integrity and humanity are intact, therefore no harm has been done. Conversely, should the patients' wishes be overridden and he is forcibly subjected to treatment "for his own good," then the patient was harmed at a fundamental level because there has been infringement of basic human rights. The role of the patient as an active participant in treatment planning must be protected.

Doing good, like doing no harm, can also be applied. Should the patient's choice be upheld, then the nurse is supporting the principle of beneficence. However, if the patient is forced to have the treatment against his will, the outcome for the patient's foot may be good but his basic rights have been violated.

Home Health Hints

- Patients with newly diagnosed diabetes may be anxious and overwhelmed. Instruction may need to be repeated several times before they understand. Don't get discouraged; as patients adapt to new routines, they will become more involved and develop a better understanding of the education. Offer praise and positive reinforcement for all accomplishments.
- Some home glucose monitoring devices have a memory that the nurse can access on the visit. It gives the date, time, and blood glucose result. This is a good indication of compliance with self-monitoring performed by patient or caregiver.
- Assist your patients in obtaining the necessary supplies to manage their diabetes. Many medical supply companies can deliver these supplies to the home. Work with your agency to identify companies that are reliable in your area.
- Remember to call the patient the day before performing a venipuncture for a fasting blood sugar and remind him or her not to eat after midnight.
- Older patients tend to skip meals. Assist them to identify easy but nutritious meals, such as frozen dinners that are low in sodium, such as Healthy Choice products. Meals-on-Wheels is another option since they are able to deliver meals that are tailored to special diets.
- Prefilled syringes should be stored in the refrigerator flat or with needles pointing up. This prevents crystals from settling and clogging the needles.
- Patients can discard used syringes and needles in a hard plastic container such as a Clorox bottle with a screw top.
- If the patient has a visual or dexterity problem, suggest getting a syringe magnifier. A pharmacist or occupational therapist may be able to assist with obtaining one.

- Help the patient learn to use a mirror to look at the bottom of the feet or have a family member examine the patient's feet. The patient should remove shoes and socks at each physician visit for a thorough foot inspection. Catching a "red spot" early is the goal.
- Instruct the patient on the importance of wearing comfortable shoes. The patient should avoid sandals, high heels, flip flops, or ill-fitting shoes. If necessary, the physician can request a podiatry consult. The podiatrist can arrange for the patient to be measured and fitted with special shoes that properly fit his or her feet. Special shoes may be covered by Medicare.
- The patient should keep a pair of nonskid slippers at the bedside. If the patient needs to get up in the night to use the restroom, putting on secure slippers can help prevent the possibility of stepping on something and causing a foot injury.
- Due to decreased skin sensation in some persons with diabetes, hot water heaters should be set below 120°F (48.8°C).
- Even if patients have had diabetes for many years, observe them preparing and injecting their insulin. This provides an opportunity to praise good technique or correct bad habits.
- Diabetic patients with vision problems can become isolated and depressed. Assist your patient with obtaining vision aids that can help improve social outlets. Many communities have stores that specialize in low-vision products, such as a magnifier that attaches to a computer. This can help them gain some independence and facilitate communication with family and friends via email, or to join an online support group to share experiences and discuss feelings with others who have similar physical ailments.

REVIEW QUESTIONS

1. Which of the following is the best definition of diabetes mellitus?
   a. It is a group of metabolic diseases in which high blood glucose results from defective insulin secretion or action.
   b. It is a disease that causes polyuria and polydipsia.
   c. It is a disease characterized by macrovascular and microvascular complications.
   d. It is a complex disease of protein and fat metabolism.

2. Which of the following is a risk factor for type 2 diabetes mellitus?

   a. Cardiovascular disease
   b. Obesity
   c. Age younger than 40 years
   d. Virus exposure

3. Diabetes is diagnosed when the fasting blood glucose is greater than _____.

4. Which of the following symptoms is most commonly associated with hyperglycemia?
   a. Tremor
   b. Flank pain
   c. Sweating
   d. Polyuria

5. Protein in the urine is a sign of which long-term complication of diabetes?
   a. Nephropathy
   b. Neuropathy
   c. Retinopathy
   d. Gastroparesis

6. What is the best way for patients to avoid long-term complications of diabetes?
   a. See the doctor for a complete check-up every 6 months.
   b. Check feet daily.
   c. Maintain blood sugar levels under 130 mg/dL.
   d. Follow a strict 1500-calorie diet.

7. Which breakfast menu is most appropriate for a patient with diabetes?
   a. Two eggs, two strips bacon, orange juice, coffee
   b. Oatmeal with artificial sweetener, whole grain toast, tea
   c. One half grapefruit, cranberry juice, bagel with sugar-free jelly
   d. One slice whole grain toast with peanut butter, skim milk, orange juice

8. Place the steps for mixing insulin in correct sequential order.
   a. Draw up cloudy insulin
   b. Draw up clear insulin
   c. Roll cloudy vial
   d. Inject air into cloudy insulin
   e. Inject air into clear insulin
   f. Clean vial tops with alcohol

9. For which of the following blood glucose results would the nurse administer a fast sugar?
   a. 48
   b. 80
   c. 126
   d. 223

10. A patient who is preparing for surgery asks the nurse why his physician took him off his oral hypoglycemic and placed him on sliding scale insulin. Which response by the nurse is best?
    a. "It helps us maintain better control of your blood sugar during surgery. You will most likely be back on your pills before you go home."
    b. "The stress of surgery often exacerbates diabetes. We will teach you how to give insulin before you go home."
    c. "Oral hypoglycemics are ineffective during times of stress. Insulin is the only way to keep your blood sugar under control."
    d. "The oral agents must not be controlling your blood sugar any longer. I will check and see which insulin you will be going home with."

11. Which meal plan is best for the patient with reactive hypoglycemia?
    a. High-carbohydrate meals
    b. Small, frequent meals
    c. Avoidance of fats and proteins
    d. Three medium to large meals daily

References

1. Centers for Disease Control: National Diabetes Fact Sheet. Accessed January 19, 2006 at http://www.cdc.gov/diabetes/pubs/pdf/ndfs_2005.pdf.
2. American Heart Association/National Heart, Lung, and Blood Institute scientific statement: Metabolic syndrome: new guidance for prevention and treatment. Accessed January 17, 2006, at http://www.americanheart.org/presenter.jhtml?identifier=3033454.
3. American Diabetes Association: Clinical Practice Recommendations 2006. Diabetes Care 29(Suppl 1):S47, 2006.
4. Tuomilehto, J, Lindstrom, J, Eriksson, JG, et al: Prevention of type 2 diabetes mellitus by changes in lifestyle among subjects with impaired glucose tolerance. N Engl J Med 344:1343–1350, 2001.
5. American College of Endocrinologists: Outpatient diabetes mellitus consensus conference recommendations. Revised July 8, 2005. Accessed at http://www.aace.com/pub/odimplementation/PositionStatement.pdf.

6. The Diabetes Control and Complications Trial Research Group: The effect of intensive treatment of diabetes on the development and progression of long-term complications in insulin-dependent diabetes mellitus. N Engl J Med 329:14, 1993.
7. U.K. Prospective Diabetes Study Group: Intensive blood-glucose control with sulphonylureas or insulin compared with conventional treatment and risk of complications in patients with type 2 diabetes. Lancet 352:837, 1998.
8. Centers for Disease Control and Prevention: Data and Trends. Diabetes Public Health Resources. Accessed 8/25/2005 at http://www.cdc.gov.
9. Levetan, C: Blood glucose in the hospital. Diabetes Forecast, September 2005.
10. American Diabetes Association. National Standards for Diabetes Self-Management Education. In Clinical Practice Recommendations 2006. Diabetes Care 29(Suppl 1): S78–S85, 2006.

Unit Ten Bibliography

1. American Diabetes Association: Clinical Practice Recommendations 2006. Diabetes Care 29(Suppl 1): 2006.
2. Bacoka, J: Action stat: Thyroid storm. Nursing 31:88, 2001.
3. Diabetes Control and Complications Trial Research Group: The effect of intensive treatment of diabetes on the development and progression of long-term complications in insulin-dependent diabetes mellitus. N Engl J Med 329: 14, 1993.
4. Daub, KF: Pheochromocytoma, up close and personal. Nursing 32:hn1–hn3, 2002.
5. Isomaa, B, Almgren, P, and Tuomi, T: Cardiovascular morbidity and mortality associated with the metabolic syndrome. Diabetes Care 24:4, 2001.

6. Jankowski, CB: Irradiating the thyroid: How to protect yourself and others. Am J Nurs 96:51, 1996.

7. Kumrow, D, and Dahlen, R: Thydroidectomy: Understanding the potential for complications. Medsurg Nursing 11:S228–S235, 2002.

8. Lutz, CA, and Przytulski, KR: Nutrition and Diet Therapy, ed. 4. F.A. Davis, Philadelphia, 2005.

9. Nabhan, F, Emanuele, MA, and Emanuele, N: Latent autoimmune diabetes of adulthood. PostGrad Med 117:3, 2005.

10. Riddle, MC: Managing type 2 diabetes over time: Lessons from the UKPDS. Diabetes Spectrum 13: 194–196, 2000.

11. Sachse, D: Acromegaly. Am J Nurs 101:69–77, 2001.

12. Sammer, CE: How should you respond to hypoglycemia? Nursing 31:7, 2001.

13. UK Prospective Diabetes Study Group: Intensive blood-glucose control with sulphonylureas or insulin compared with conventional treatment and risk of complications in patients with type 2 diabetes. Lancet 352:837–853, 1998.

14. Watson, R: Assessing endocrine system function in older people. Nursing Older People 12:27–28, 2000.

SUGGESTED ANSWERS TO

CRITICAL THINKING

■ *Mr. McMillan*

1. "Have you been eating or drinking more than usual? Have you been urinating more than usual? Do you get up at night to urinate? Does anyone in your family have diabetes?"

2. Fatigue occurs because the glucose is unable to enter the cells without insulin, so they are starving.

3. Mr. McMillan is dehydrated because he is losing excessive amounts of urine as his kidneys lose excess glucose.

■ *Mrs. Evans*

1. Mrs. Evans should take her insulin no earlier than 7:30 a.m.

2. She should be alert for low blood sugar at midafternoon to just before supper. Although her insulin peaks between 1:30 and 7:30 p.m., her chances of having a hypoglycemic episode are slim once she has eaten her supper.

3. If she misses a meal, her blood sugar will drop further, increasing her risk of a hypoglycemic episode.

■ *Jeff*

What kind of new job is it? What schedule is he working? Is it more physically strenuous than his previous job? Does it interfere with his usual meal schedule? What other changes has he experienced in his life that may have affected his blood glucose?

■ *Mr. Jones*

1. Poor circulation, neuropathy, and slow wound healing place Mr. Jones at risk for problems.

2. Circulation to the foot may be poor, and white blood cells are sluggish if the blood glucose is high.

3. Any pressure on the foot while walking may further impair circulation. He should not bear weight on the affected foot.

4. If circulation to the area is poor, IV antibiotics may not reach the sore.

5. "Small red open area on right posterior heel, 1 cm × 1.5 cm, 2 mm deep, 2-cm area of yellow drainage on dressing." In addition, many agencies are now taking instant photos of wounds to include in the chart. If no camera is available, a drawing of the size and shape is helpful.

unit ELEVEN

UNDERSTANDING THE GENITOURINARY AND REPRODUCTIVE SYSTEM

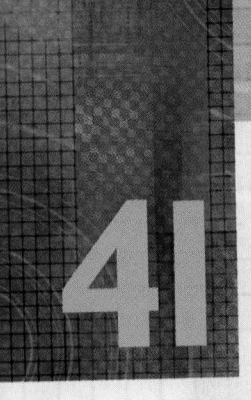

41

Genitourinary and Reproductive System Function and Assessment

DEBRA PERRY-PHILO AND
JANICE L. BRADFORD

KEY TERMS

adnexa (ad-NEK-sah)
bimanual (by-MAN-yoo-uhl)
circumcised (SIR-kum-sized)
colposcopy (kul-POS-koh-pee)
conization (KOH-ni-ZAY-shun)
culdoscopy (kul-DOS-koh-pee)
curet (kyoo-RET)
cystic (SIS-tik)
ejaculation (ee-JAK-yoo-LAY-shun)
epispadias (EP-i-SPAY-dee-ahz)
erection (e-REK-shun)
gravida (GRAV-id-ah)
gynecomastia (JIN-e-koh-MASS-tee-ah)
hydrocele (HIGH-droh-seel)
hypospadias (HIGH-poh-SPAY-dee-ahz)
hysterosalpingogram (HIS-tur-oh-SAL-pinj-oh-gram)
hysteroscopy (HIS-tur-AHS-koh-pee)
insufflation (in-suff-LAY-shun)
libido (li-BEE-doh)
mammography (mah-MOG-rah-fee)
menarche (me-NAR-kee)
menopause (MEN-oh-pawz)
orgasm (OR-gazm)
para (PAR-ah)
salpingoscopy (SAL-ping-AHS-koh-pee)
transillumination (TRANS-i-loo-mi-NAY-shun)
varicocele (VAR-i-koh-seel)

QUESTIONS TO GUIDE YOUR READING

1. What is the normal anatomy of the reproductive system?

2. What are the normal functions of the reproductive system?

3. What data should you collect when caring for a patient with a disorder of the reproductive system?

4. Which diagnostic tests are commonly performed to diagnose disorders of the reproductive system?

5. What nursing care should you provide for patients undergoing each of the diagnostic tests?

6. Which therapeutic measures are commonly used for patients with disorders of the reproductive system?

REVIEW OF NORMAL ANATOMY AND PHYSIOLOGY

The male and female reproductive systems produce gametes (sperm and egg cells [ova]) and facilitate the union of gametes in fertilization following sexual intercourse. Ideally, in women, the uterus provides the site for the developing embryo/fetus until birth.

Female Reproductive System

The female reproductive system consists of paired ovaries and fallopian tubes, a single uterus and vagina, and external genitalia (Fig. 41.1). The mammary glands may be considered accessory organs to the system.

Ovaries

The ovaries are a pair of oval structures, about 5 cm long and 2.5 cm wide, on either side of the uterus in the pelvic cavity (Fig. 41.2). The ovarian ligament extends from the medial side of the ovary to the uterine wall, and the broad ligament of the uterus is a fold of the peritoneum that also attaches to the ovaries. These ligaments help keep the ovaries in place.

The ovaries produce egg cells by the process of meiosis, more specifically called oogenesis, which begins at puberty and ends at **menopause,** usually occurring between the ages of 45 and 55. This process is cyclical in that usually one mature ovum is produced and released every 28 days and is under hormonal control (covered in the section on the

menopause: men—month + pause—stop

menstrual cycle). The follicles of the ovary produce the hormone estrogen and later, as the corpus luteum, secrete progesterone as well.

Fallopian Tubes

Each fallopian, or uterine, tube is about 13 cm long; the lateral end with its fringelike fimbriae approach but do not touch the ovary, and the medial end attaches and opens into the uterus. The fallopian tube is lined with ciliated epithelium; in the wall is smooth muscle. The sweeping of the cilia and the peristaltic contractions of the smooth muscle usually ensure that the ovum (called "zygote" after fertilization), will reach the uterus. Fertilization usually takes place within the fallopian tube, and the zygote is swept into the uterus within 4 to 5 days.

Uterus

The uterus is a muscle which is about 8 cm long and 5 cm wide. It is superior to the urinary bladder and medial to the ovaries in the pelvic cavity. Ligaments help keep the uterus in place, tilted forward over the top of the bladder. During pregnancy the uterus increases greatly in size, and contains the placenta which nourishes the embryo (later called the fetus), and expels the infant near the end of gestation.

The fundus of the uterus is the upper portion above where the fallopian tubes enter laterally. The body is the large central portion. The cervix is the narrow, lower end, which opens into the vagina. The uterus is divided into three muscle layers. The outermost layer of the uterine wall is the perimetrium, a fold of the visceral peritoneum. The myometrium is the middle, smooth muscle layer. During

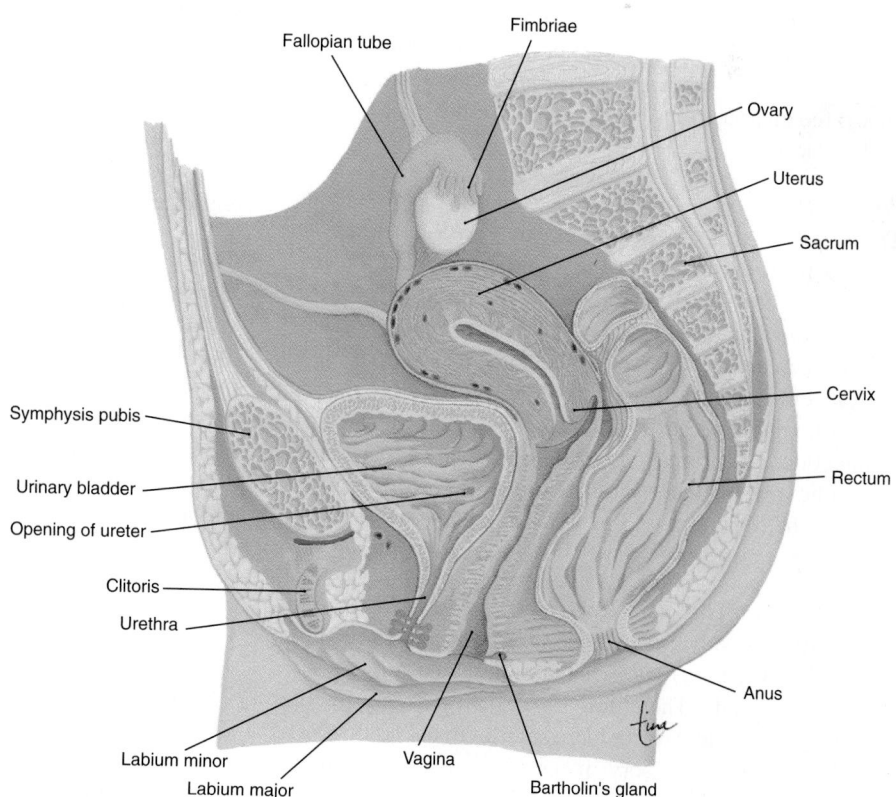

FIGURE 41.1 Female reproductive system in a midsagittal section. *(From Scanlon, VC, and Sanders, T: Essentials of Anatomy and Physiology, ed. 3. F.A. Davis, Philadelphia, 1999, p 446, with permission.)*

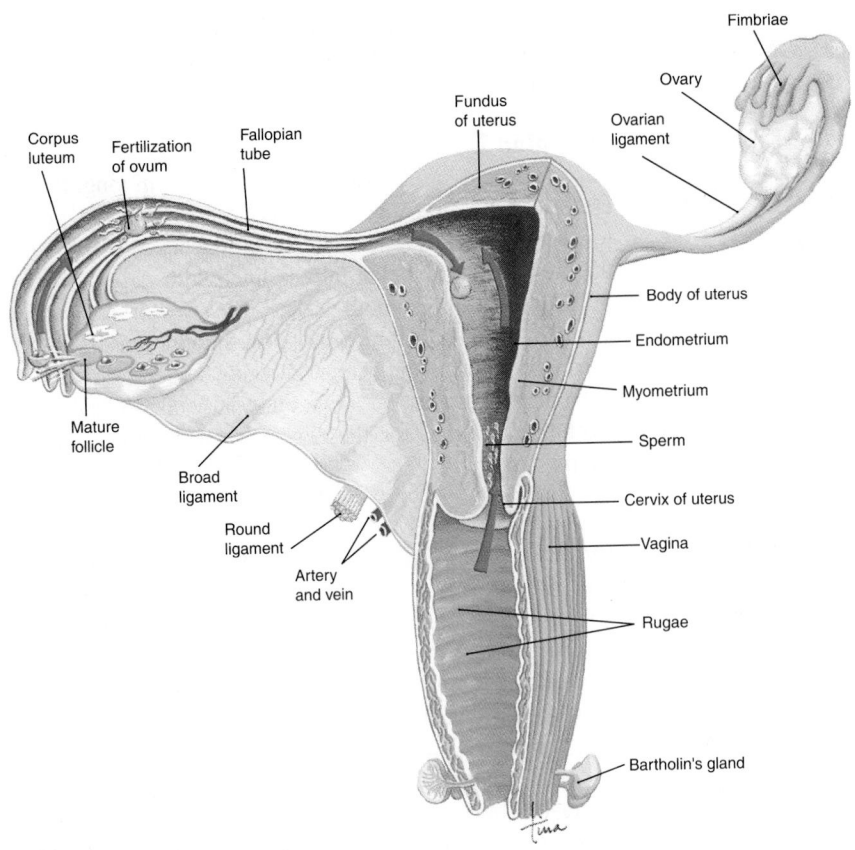

FIGURE 41.2 Female reproductive system in an anterior view and a longitudinal section. (*From Scanlon V., Sanders T.: Essentials of Anatomy and Physiology, ed. 5. F.A. Davis, Philadelphia, 2007, p. 464, with permission.*)

pregnancy these cells increase in size to accommodate the growing fetus, and during labor and delivery, oxytocin causes coordinated contractions of this middle layer to expel the fetus.

The lining of the uterus is called the endometrium, and is a highly vascular mucous membrane, part of which is lost and regenerated with each menstrual cycle. During pregnancy, the endometrium helps in forming the maternal side of the placenta.

Vagina

The vagina is a muscular tube about 7 to 9 cm long that extends from the cervix to the vaginal orifice in the perineum. It is between the urethra and the rectum. The functions of the vagina are to receive sperm from the penis during sexual intercourse, to serve as the exit for menstrual blood flow, and to serve as the birth canal at the end of pregnancy.

After puberty, the vaginal mucosa is relatively resistant to infection. The normal bacterial flora of the vagina creates an acidic pH, which retards microbial growth. Prior to puberty, the hymen, a fold of mucous membrane, provides mechanical protection.

External Genitals

Also called the vulva, the female external genital structures are the clitoris, mons pubis, labia majora and minora, and Bartholin's glands. The clitoris is a small mass of erectile tissue, approximately 6 mm long, anterior to the urethral orifice. Its function is sensory; it responds to sexual stimulation, and its vascular sinuses become filled with blood.

The mons pubis is a pad of fat over the pubic bones, covered with skin and pubic hair. Extending posteriorly from the mons are the lateral labia majora and the medial labia minora; these are paired folds of skin. The area between the labia minora is the vestibule; it contains the openings of the urethra and vagina. The labia cover these openings and prevent drying of their mucous membranes. Bartholin's glands, also called vestibular glands, are within the floor and at the base of the vestibule; their ducts open into the mucosa at the vaginal orifice. Their secretion keeps the mucosa moist and lubricates the vagina during sexual intercourse.

Mammary Glands

Enclosed within the breasts and surrounded by adipose tissue, the mammary glands produce milk after pregnancy. The milk enters the lactiferous ducts, which converge at the nipple. The skin around the nipple is a pigmented area called the areola. The formation of milk occurs secondary to hormonal influence. During pregnancy, high levels of estrogen and progesterone prepare the glands for milk production. Prolactin from the anterior pituitary causes the production of milk after pregnancy. The sucking of the infant on the nipple stimulates the release of oxytocin from the posterior pituitary gland, which in turn stimulates the release of milk as well as contraction of the uterine muscle.

The Menstrual Cycle

The menstrual cycle depends on follicle-stimulating hormone (FSH) and luteinizing hormone (LH) from the anterior pituitary gland and estrogen and progesterone from the ovaries. These hormones bring about changes in the ovaries and uterus. A cycle may be described in terms of three phases: menstrual phase, follicular phase, and luteal phase.

The menstrual phase involves the loss of the endometrium during menstruation, which may last 2 to 8 days, with an average duration of 3 to 6 days. At this time, secretion of FSH is increasing and several ovarian follicles, each with a potential ovum, begin to develop. Table 41.1 includes a summary of these hormones.

During the follicular phase, FSH stimulates growth of ovarian follicles and secretion of estrogen by the follicle cells. The secretion of LH also increases, but more slowly. FSH and estrogen promote the growth and maturation of the ovum, and estrogen stimulates the growth of blood vessels to regenerate the endometrium. This phase ends with ovulation, when a sharp increase in LH causes rupture of a mature ovarian follicle and an egg is released.

During the luteal phase, LH causes the ruptured follicle to become the corpus luteum, which begins to secrete progesterone in addition to estrogen. Progesterone stimulates further growth of blood vessels in the endometrium and promotes the storage of nutrients such as glycogen. As progesterone secretion increases, LH secretion decreases, and if the ovum is not fertilized, the secretion of progesterone also begins to decrease. Without progesterone, the endometrium cannot be maintained and begins to slough off in menstruation. FSH secretion begins to increase (as estrogen and progesterone decrease), and the cycle begins again. Although an average cycle is 28 days, cycles of 23 to 35 days may also be considered normal.

Male Reproductive System

The male reproductive system consists of the testes and a series of ducts and glands. Sperm are produced in the testes and are transported through the reproductive ducts: epididymis, ductus deferens, ejaculatory duct, and urethra (Fig. 41.3). The reproductive glands are the seminal vesicles, prostate gland, and bulbourethral glands, all of which produce secretions that become part of semen.

Testes

The testes are located in the scrotum between the upper thighs, where the temperature is slightly lower than body temperature, which is necessary for the production of viable sperm. Each testis is about 5 cm long and 3 cm wide and contains the seminiferous tubules in which spermatogenesis (meiosis) takes place. In contrast to oogenesis, once started at puberty, spermatogenesis is a constant rather than cyclical process and usually continues throughout life. Also in the testes are specialized cells that produce the hormones testosterone and inhibin. Spermatogenesis is initiated by FSH from the anterior pituitary. LH from the anterior pituitary stimulates the secretion of testosterone, which contributes to the maturation of sperm. The secretion of inhibin is stimulated by testosterone; inhibin decreases the secretion of FSH, which helps keep the rate of spermatogenesis fairly constant. The functions of these hormones are summarized in Table 41.2.

The head of the sperm cell contains the 23 chromosomes, and has an acrosome on the tip that contains enzymes to digest the membrane of the egg cell during fertilization. Attached to the head is a midpiece with high numbers of mitochondria, and attached to the midpiece is a flagellum, which provides motility. Sperm from all the seminiferous tubules of a testis pass through tubules leading to the epididymis.

Epididymis, Ductus Deferens, and Ejaculatory Ducts

The epididymis is a tube about 4 to 6 meters long that is coiled on the posterior side of a testis. Smooth muscle within its wall propels sperm from the testes into the ductus deferens.

Also called the ductus deferens, the vas deferens extends from the epididymis in the scrotum to the ejaculatory

TABLE 41.1 HORMONES OF FEMALE REPRODUCTION

Hormone	Secreted By	Functions
Follicle-stimulating hormone	Anterior pituitary	Initiates development of ovarian follicles Stimulates secretion of estrogen by follicle cells
Luteinizing hormone	Anterior pituitary	Causes ovulation Converts ruptured ovarian follicle into corpus luteum Stimulates secretion of progesterone by corpus luteum
Estrogen	Ovary (follicle) Placenta	Promotes maturation of ovarian follicles Promotes growth of blood vessels in endometrium Initiates development of secondary sex characteristics Promotes growth of duct system of mammary glands
Progesterone	Ovary (corpus luteum) Placenta	Promotes further growth of blood vessels in endometrium Inhibits contractions of the myometrium during pregnancy Promotes growth of secretory cells of mammary glands
Inhibin	Ovary (corpus luteum)	Decreases secretion of FSH toward end of cycle
Prolactin	Anterior pituitary	Promotes production of milk after birth
Oxytocin	Posterior pituitary	Promotes release of milk

Source: Scanlon, VC, and Sanders, T: Essentials of Anatomy and Physiology, ed. 4. F.A. Davis, Philadelphia, 2003, p 448, with permission.

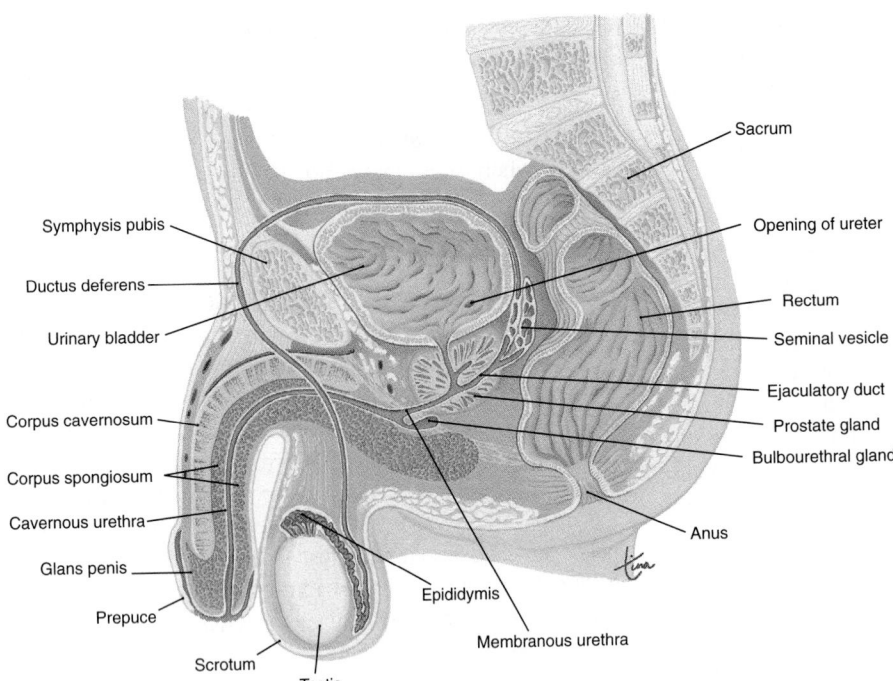

Sacrum

Opening of ureter

Rectum

Seminal vesicle

Ejaculatory duct

Prostate gland

Bulbourethral gland

Anus

Symphysis pubis

Ductus deferens

Urinary bladder

Corpus cavernosum

Corpus spongiosum

Cavernous urethra

Glans penis

Prepuce

Scrotum

Testis

Epididymis

Membranous urethra

FIGURE 41.3 Male reproductive system in a midsagittal section. *(From Scanlon, VC, and Sanders, T: Essentials of Anatomy and Physiology, ed. 4. F. A. Davis, Philadelphia, 2003, with permission.)*

duct within the pelvic cavity. Exterior to the body, the vas deferens is contained within the spermatic cord, a connective tissue sheath. Testicular blood vessels and nerves share the spermatic cord; and the cord opens into the abdominopelvic wall at the inguinal canal. Within the pelvic cavity, the vas deferens loops over the ureter and extends down the posterior side of the urinary bladder to join the ejaculatory duct.

Each of the two ejaculatory ducts receives sperm from the ductus deferens and the secretion of the seminal vesicle on its own side. Both ejaculatory ducts empty into the urethra.

Seminal Vesicles, Prostate Gland, and Bulbourethral Glands

The paired seminal vesicles are posterior to the urinary bladder. Their secretion is alkaline and contains fructose, prostaglandins, and clotting proteins. The alkalinity neutralizes the urethra and the acidic environment of the female reproductive tract. The fructose is used for adenosine triphosphate (ATP) production, the prostaglandins enhance motility, and the clotting proteins coagulate the semen after

ejaculation. The duct of a seminal vesicle joins the ductus deferens on its side to form the ejaculatory duct.

The prostate is a muscular gland that surrounds the first 2 to 3 cm of the urethra as it emerges from the urinary bladder. The secretion of the prostate is alkaline and contributes to sperm motility. The smooth muscle of the prostate contracts during **ejaculation,** causing the expulsion of semen from the urethra.

The bulbourethral glands are located below the prostate gland and empty into the urethra. Their alkaline secretion coats the interior of the urethra just before ejaculation, which neutralizes any acidic urine that might be present.

The alkaline secretions of the male reproductive glands work to ensure that many sperm remain viable in the acidic environment of the vagina. The normal bacterial flora of the vagina create an acidic pH in the vaginal environment, but the pH of semen is about 7.4 and permits sperm to remain motile.

Urethra and Penis

The urethra is the last of the male reproductive ducts, and its longest portion is within the penis. The penis is an external

TABLE 41.2 HORMONES OF MALE REPRODUCTION

Hormone	Secreted By	Functions
Follicle-stimulating hormone	Anterior pituitary	Initiates production of sperm in the testes
Luteinizing hormone	Anterior pituitary	Stimulates secretion of testosterone by the testes
Testosterone	Testes	Promotes maturation of sperm
		Initiates development of male secondary sex characteristics
Inhibin	Testes	Decreases secretion of FSH to maintain a constant rate of spermatogenesis

Source: Scanlon, VC, and Sanders, T: Essentials of Anatomy and Physiology, ed. 4. F.A. Davis, Philadelphia, 2003, p 440, with permission.

genital organ; its distal end is called the glans penis and when uncircumcised is covered with a fold of skin called the prepuce, or foreskin. Within the penis are three layers of erectile or cavernous tissue. Each consists of a framework of smooth muscle and connective tissue that contains blood sinuses, which are large, irregular vascular channels.

When blood flow through these sinuses is minimal, the penis is flaccid (soft). Sexual stimulation causes the arteries to the penis to dilate; the sinuses fill with blood, and the penis becomes erect and firm. This is brought about by parasympathetic impulses. The culmination of sexual stimulation is ejaculation, which is brought about by peristalsis of the reproductive ducts and contraction of the prostate gland.

Aging and the Reproductive System

For women, there is a definite end to reproductive capability; this is called menopause and is defined as having occurred when menses have ceased for 12 months. Menopause usually occurs between the ages of 45 and 55. Estrogen secretion decreases, and ovulation and menstrual cycles become irregular and finally cease. The decrease in estrogen has other effects as well. See Figure 41.4 for a mindmap on the effects of aging.

For most men, testosterone secretion continues throughout life, as does sperm production, although both diminish with advancing age. Perhaps the most common reproductive problem for older men is enlargement of the prostate gland, called benign prostatic hyperplasia (see Figure 41.4).

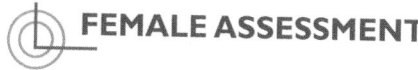

FEMALE ASSESSMENT

Assessment of women's reproductive health can seem challenging because of the complex relationship of physical and psychosocial factors. Hormones not only affect a multitude of body functions, they also can influence moods and mental functioning. Reproduction involves not only physical processes, but also relationships, role identifications, and self-esteem issues.

Normal Function Baselines

Knowing about expected functioning of the reproductive system is the nurse's best preparation for nursing assessment. Regular, relatively pain-free shedding of an appropriate amount of the endometrial lining of the uterus is expected from puberty through midlife or later. Intercourse is normally expected to be free of pain and infection, to occur when desired by both partners, to be satisfying, and generally to result in pregnancy within a few months (unless precautions are taken). A pregnancy is expected to last approximately 40 weeks and to produce a healthy child. Physical and psychological sexual characteristics and function including **libido** are expected to be adequately maintained by hormones. Sexual functioning, desire, and fertility are expected to change throughout the process of aging. Although individuals may vary somewhat from these expected descriptions, these serve as a baseline for assessment of possible disorders. Chapter 42 further defines specific female reproductive system disorders.

Much of what happens in female reproductive system disorders occurs inside the body and may not show external signs. Skill in asking appropriate questions, documenting patient statements, and describing observations is essential. Descriptions of symptoms should be thorough and follow the WHAT'S UP? format described in Chapter 1. Short quotes of the patient's own words to describe change that you have noticed may add valuable information, but be careful to use critical thinking skills when interviewing and documenting rather than just quoting indiscriminately. Because many signs and symptoms of reproductive system disorders occur in a cyclic fashion, the patient may be asked to keep an accurate written record of occurrences, noting times and dates to identify patterns.

History

Subjective assessment of the female reproductive system includes general personal information as well as menstrual, obstetrical, gynecological, sexual, family, and psychosocial histories. See Table 41.3 for specific questions to ask.

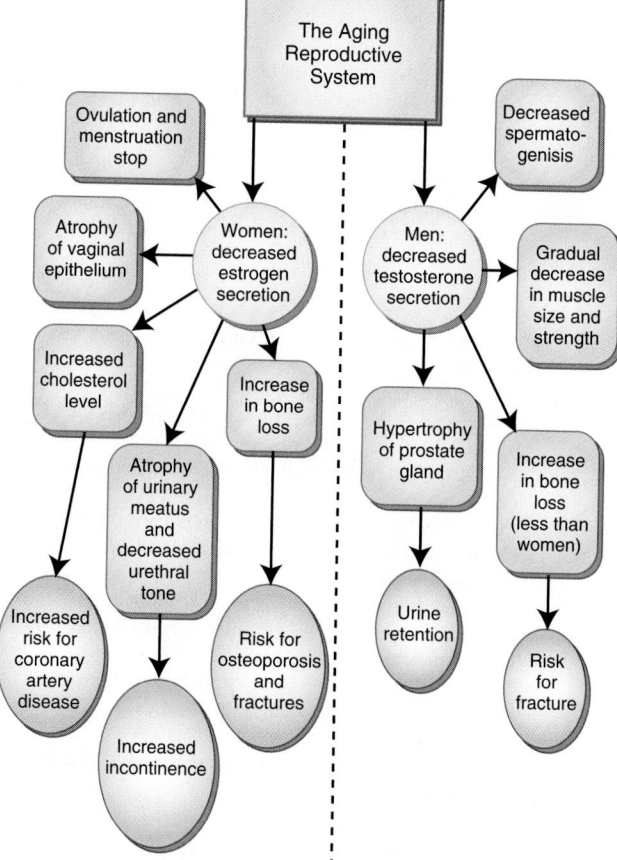

FIGURE 41.4 Aging and the reproductive system. This concept map shows the effects the aging process has on the reproductive system.

---

libido: sexual desire

TABLE 41.3 SUBJECTIVE ASSESSMENT OF THE FEMALE REPRODUCTIVE SYSTEM

Category	Questions to Ask During History Assessment	Rationale/Significance
Personal History	• Have you ever been diagnosed or treated for any health problems?	• Data may reveal general state of health, knowledge/practice of health promotion behaviors, meaning of health, expectations related to care.
	• Have you had any recent weight changes? What type of change (if any)?	• Weight changes may reflect physical or psychological pathology.
	• Are you experiencing pain? (Quality/quantity/character if patient reports pain).	• Subjective indication of pain may indicate a variety of disorders.
	• Do you have any allergies? (Agent/type of reaction)	• Allergy status should always be assessed to guide possible intervention should treatment be needed.
	• Are you using any medications? (Include prescription, over-the-counter and herbal remedies.) How much/how often do you take the medication?	• May lead to health issues not yet revealed. Medication use reflects meaning of health and pattern of health behaviors in many patients. Use of alternative treatments should be identified, and may guide possible interventions should treatment be needed.
	• Do you smoke, use caffeine, drink alcohol, or use recreational drugs? How much/how often?	• Recreational behaviors may indicate risk of health disorders. Smoking increases risk of coagulation disorders with use of contraceptives containing estrogen.
	• Do you exercise? What type of exercise do you do? How often?	• Exercise is recognized as an activity that improves health status, in general, and for many disorders.
	• How many hours of sleep do you get in a 24-hour period of time? Do you feel you get enough rest?	• May indicate state of health or lead to discussion of social issues that lead to stress and, ultimately, physical disorders.
	• Do you feel under stress? How do you deal with stress?	• May indicate social issues that may lead to physical disorders.
	• Have you been hit, kicked, slapped, or made to do anything sexually against your will since your last visit?	• Abuse screening should be considered during all primary care visits; may indicate need for intervention or guide care.
Menstrual History	• At what age did you begin menstruating (**menarche**)? How often do you menstruate and how long do your periods last? How heavy is your flow?	• May reveal abnormalities of cycle and lead to a diagnosis of benign/malignant tumors, endometriosis, pregnancy, anemia, endocrine disorders.
	• At what age did you enter menopause (if applicable)?	
Obstetric/ Gynecological History	• How many pregnancies and deliveries have you had? Were your deliveries vaginal or cesarean section? Did you have any complications following your deliveries?	• May indicate health of reproductive system, knowledge/meaning of health maintenance practice, and risk for disease.
	• Have you had previous treatment/surgery on your reproductive organs?	• May indicate past health issues related to the reproductive organs and need for current evaluation related to issues.
	• Have you had any itching of your perineum or have you noted any vaginal discharge (describe)?	• Subjective report of itching or discharge may indicate disorder of inflammation or lead to diagnosis of sexually transmitted disease.
	• When was your last Pap/pelvic exam? What were the results?	• May reflect meaning of health and guide current care.
	• Do you do BSE? How often? Have you noticed any breast changes?	• If changes have been noted by the patient, they should be evaluated by the primary care provider for the possible pathology.
	• Did you breastfeed? How long?	• Breastfeeding may offer some protection against breast cancer. If patient currently breastfeeding, may help guide care and diagnosis.
Sexual History	• Are you sexually active? How many partners do you have? Of what gender? Is your sexual activity satisfying?	• May indicate risk of sexually transmitted diseases, risk of unintended pregnancy, and indicate state of sexual satisfaction/intimacy.
	• When did you become sexually active?	• Early onset of sexual activity increases risk of cervical cancer.
	• What contraceptive method(s) do you use (if sexually active with a male)? How do you use them?	• May reflect meaning of health, high-risk health behaviors, and risk for unintended pregnancy or sexually transmitted disease.

menarche: men—month + arche—beginning

Category	Questions to Ask During History Assessment	Rationale/Significance
Sexual History (Cont'd)	• Have you ever been diagnosed with a sexually transmitted disease? When, what type, and how was it treated? That you are aware, was treatment successful?	• May indicate high-risk sexual behavior patterns or potential for active disease and, therefore, indicate need for diagnostic testing and treatment.
Family History	• Do you have a family history of cardiovascular problems, cancer, osteoporosis, thyroid abnormalities?	• May indicate underlying cause of or risk for sexual/physical abnormalities of the reproductive system.
Psychosocial History	• Are you married or in a significant relationship? Is the relationship satisfying?	• Relevant to determine financial, social, and emotional support.
	• Are you employed? Where?	

NURSING CARE TIP

It is helpful to have women retain a monthly calendar of their menstrual cycle, and bring it to any appointment during which discussion of the cycle may take place.

An obstetrical history includes number of pregnancies, pregnancy outcomes, and complications. These are generally documented using abbreviations of Latin words: G = number of pregnancies (from the Latin word **gravida**); P = births, whether alive or stillborn (regardless of number of fetuses) after 20 weeks' gestation (from the Latin word **para**); A = abortions, whether spontaneous or therapeutic (from the Latin word *abortus;* a spontaneous abortion is sometimes called a miscarriage). Roman numerals follow the letter to specify the number of each. For example, three pregnancies—twins, one single birth, and one spontaneous abortion—are recorded as GIII, PII, AI. This may also be written as $G_3P_2A_1$. Note, however, that some hospitals use different notation, further delineating history, such as number of premature or full-term births, number of living children, and number of therapeutic abortions. If you are uncertain of how to document, check your institutional history forms.

LEARNING TIP

Remember the word gravida by thinking of gravity and that a woman is generally heavier when pregnant.

You will also want to ask about any tests, surgeries, or treatments done on the reproductive organs and excretory system. Medications the patient is taking (for whatever reasons), height to weight ratio, and marked changes in weight may also provide significant data for diagnostic and care planning purposes concerning reproductive system disorders.

gravida: number of pregnancies
para: number of deliveries after 20 weeks' gestation

LEARNING TIP

There are many things to remember when asking health history questions. Making up an index card for your pocket or purchasing a prepared one from a medical bookstore can provide a handy reference.

Many nurses feel awkward asking reproductive history questions, and patients may also feel some uneasiness with this line of questioning. A matter-of-fact attitude, an assurance of confidentiality, and an adequate explanation about why the information is needed tend to encourage patient comfort and cooperation.

Breast Assessment

Palpation

Palpation is the most important assessment technique for breast examination because it can be used to identify alterations from normal consistency, to confirm the presence of lumps, and to locate areas of tenderness. Even mammograms are not sensitive enough to detect a small percentage of masses that can be felt by the patient or health-care provider.

Breast Self-Examination

Self-palpation during breast self-examination (BSE), if done regularly and thoroughly, may be even more sensitive than physician or nurse palpation because the patient becomes so familiar with her own breasts that she is more likely to notice subtle changes that an infrequently visited health practitioner might overlook. BSE is one of the most important health protection skills that nurses can teach to women. The few moments spent monthly on this activity may mean the difference between life and death or comfort and extreme suffering for women.

See Table 41.4 for additional objective assessments.

Patient Teaching

The examination procedure is simple. BSE should be done regularly once per month. A good time to perform BSE is 1 week following menses, when hormonal influence, which may result in edema and swelling of normal breast tissue

TABLE 41.4 OBJECTIVE ASSESSMENT OF THE FEMALE REPRODUCTIVE SYSTEM

Category	Physical Assessment Findings	Possible Abnormal Findings/Causes
Clinical Breast Examination	• Observe and palpate for presence of swelling, lumps, skin changes, nipple exudate.	• Changes may indicate breast cancer, fibrocystic breast disease.
External Genitalia: Mons Pubis, Clitoris, Labia Majora/Minora, Bartholin's Glands	• Observe for color, symmetry, hair distribution, lesions, swelling or exudate.	• Changes may indicate vulvular cancer, developmental abnormalities, infection, or injury.
Vagina	• Observe for shape, bulges, color changes, lesions, exudate.	• Changes may indicate infection, structural abnormalities, or injury.
Internal Genitalia: Uterus/cervix, fallopian tubes, ovaries (by trained personnel)	• Palpate for tenderness, size, shape, mobility. Observe for color, lesions, exudate, bleeding.	• Changes may indicate infection, structural abnormalities, cervical cancer, polyps, endometriosis, fibroid/malignant tumors, pregnancy, or injury.
Perineum	• Observe for lesions, shape.	• Abnormalities may indicate infection, structural abnormalities, or injury.
Anus	• Observe for shape, color changes, lesions.	• Abnormalities can indicate hemorrhoids, or injury.
Inguinal Nodes	• Palpate for swelling, tenderness.	• May indicate infectious process or regional malignancy.

structures, is at a minimum. For women who no longer have a regular menstrual period, any regular monthly schedule is fine. Although most women's breasts are not exactly the same size, marked differences between the breasts or a change in the size of one breast should be checked with a health-care provider. Puckering or dimpling of skin, asymmetrical movement, and different pointing position of the nipples should also be reported to a health-care provider. Whether the breasts are examined in parallel lines, a spiral formation, or a wedge pattern is probably insignificant. It is important, however, to encourage that the examination be methodical and cover all areas of the breast, the tail of Spence, and the axilla (Fig. 41.5).

PATIENT CARE TIP

Some women do BSE the day their telephone bill arrives each month because it is a dependable monthly reminder.

CRITICAL THINKING

Breast Health Education

■ Holly, age 24, states, "Why should I do breast exams at my age? I probably won't get breast cancer until I'm older, if I get it at all."

1. What should your response to Holly include?
2. Why would this be a good time to provide education about health maintenance?

Suggested answers at end of chapter.

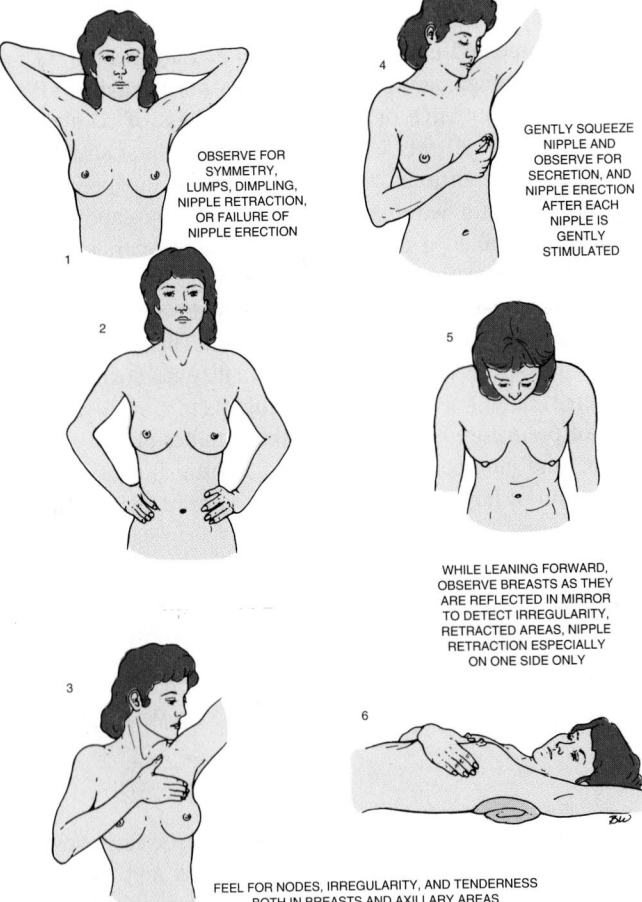

FEEL FOR NODES, IRREGULARITY, AND TENDERNESS BOTH IN BREASTS AND AXILLARY AREAS

BREAST SELF EXAMINATION

FIGURE 41.5 Breast self-examination. *(From Venes, DJ (ed): Taber's Cyclopedic Medical Dictionary, ed. 19. F.A. Davis, Philadelphia, 2001, with permission.)*

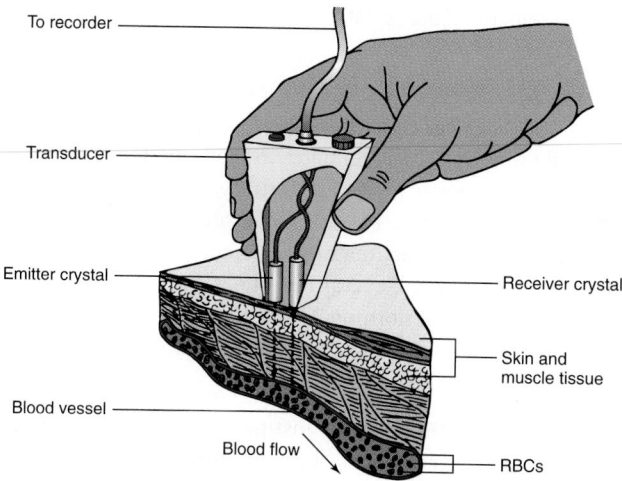

FIGURE 41.6 Diagnostic testing by ultrasound. *(Modified from Cavanaugh, BM: Nurse's Manual of Laboratory and Diagnostic Tests, ed. 3. F.A. Davis, Philadelphia, 1999, p 687, with permission.)*

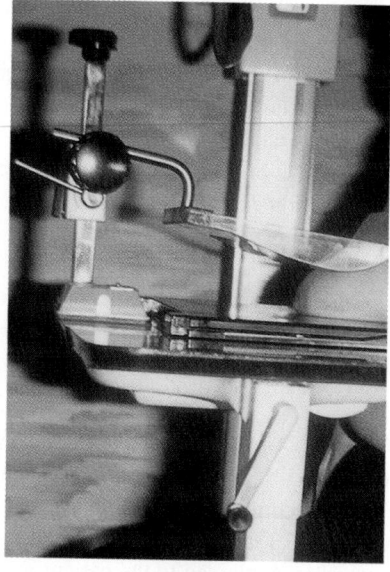

FIGURE 41.7 Mammogram procedure. *(Photo courtesy of Dinesh Patel, MD. Medical Oncology, Internal Medicine, Zanesville, OH.)*

Diagnostic Tests of the Breasts

Ultrasound and Mammography

Further assessment of the breast may be done by other methods. Ultrasound examination is done by bouncing high-frequency sound waves off the tissues within the breast to determine the density of the tissues and to map the breast structures (Fig. 41.6). This is mainly useful for distinguishing fluid-filled (**cystic**) lumps from solid tumors but may also be used to guide a needle for fine-needle aspiration of cystic fluid or core needle biopsies.

Mammography is a radiographic (x-ray) examination of the breast. A special machine is used that spreads and flattens the breast tissue to a thin layer to more effectively show benign and malignant growths, which might be hidden by breast structures on typical chest examination (Fig. 41.7). Generally, at least two radiographs are taken of each breast, with the machine compressing the breast top to bottom and side to side to give comparison views of any lumps from more than one angle. If suspicious or unclear spots are seen, additional views may be taken. The American Cancer Society recommends from age 20 throughout life that women do monthly BSE, from ages 20 to 39 that they add a breast examination by a health professional every 3 years, and from age 40 that they have a yearly mammogram and breast examination by a health professional. Those who experience breast symptoms or have a strong family history of breast cancer may be advised to have more frequent examinations.

PATIENT TEACHING. Patients preparing for mammography should be advised to bathe and not to apply deodorant, powder, or any other substance to the upper body because these may cause false shadows on the test. They should be instructed that if a shadow is seen on a mammogram, further testing will be done to determine the reason for the shadow.

Thermography, Tomography, and Magnetic Resonance Imaging

There are several other less commonly used methods for diagnosis of breast disorders. Thermography is a method of mapping the breast using photographic paper, which records temperature variations throughout the tissue in different colors. Tomography takes very precise x-ray pictures of the breast, layer by layer, as it would look if it were in thin slices, and then stores these pictures in a computer. This allows for precise measurement of the position of tumors without the displacement caused by flattening the breast for a mammogram. Tomography, however, is much more expensive than mammography, so it is not a practical method to use for general screening of all women to detect possible breast cancers. Magnetic resonance imaging (MRI) uses radiofrequency radiation and magnetic fields to map the breast tissue. The equipment needed for this method is expensive, and it is unavailable in some areas.

PATIENT TEACHING. Ask patients preparing for MRI whether they have any metal inside their bodies, such as orthopedic wires, metal sutures, or artificial joint replacements, because heat is generated by the MRI and the procedure may be contraindicated.

Biopsy

If suspicious lesions are found in the breast by any of these assessment methods, the lesion may be again assessed using one of the other methods and then a biopsy performed to confirm the diagnosis. This procedure involves removing a small portion of tissue, fluid, or cells from the breast or

---

cystic: baglike

mammography: mammo—breast + graphy—recording

lymph nodes for microscopic examination. This may be done by surgically removing a portion of tissue or by aspirating fluid or cells through a needle that is placed into the lump or lesion. Needle biopsies are often done with local anesthetic and may take place in a clinic or physician's office. More extensive biopsies may require a general anesthetic. A frozen section examination may be done in the laboratory by moistening and rapidly freezing a section of tissue, slicing it very thinly, and immediately examining it by microscope. This allows for diagnosis to be made during the course of an operation, so that the patient is spared an additional later operation for removal of cancerous tissue.

NURSING CARE. As with any surgical intervention, be prepared to set out the sterile equipment and supplies needed for the procedure and ensure that a signed consent has been obtained after the risks and benefits of the procedure have been explained to the patient by the primary care provider. Following the biopsy, assess the patient for excessive bleeding and instruct about signs of impairment of healing processes. It is important that biopsy samples be clearly labeled, packaged appropriately for transport to laboratory facilities, and delivered promptly. Consult the laboratory for information about the transport container and whether a cell fixative is required in the container.

Assessment of the patient's psychological condition during breast diagnosis procedures is essential. Most women know someone who has had breast cancer. Although breast cancer screening procedures can seem routine to health-care workers, they may be a cause of much anxiety for patients and their families. An understanding and calm nurse who can explain the procedures can help the assessment phase to be less traumatic.

SAFETY TIP

Use at least two patient identifiers (neither to be the patient's location) whenever collecting laboratory samples or administering medications or blood products, and use two identifiers to label sample collection containers in the presence of the patient. 2006 National Patient Safety Goals from www.JCAHO.org.

Additional Diagnostic Tests of the Female Reproductive System

There are many tests to assess reproductive system function; this is presently an area of rapid change. The names of the individual procedures may also vary among institutions or according to particular methods used (e.g., a **salpingoscopy** is also called a falloposcopy, and a laparoscopy is the same as a peritoneoscopy). For this reason, this chapter is limited to general descriptions of categories of medical and surgical assessment procedures rather than attempting to name all tests.

Hormonal Tests

Hormonal tests are commonly used to assess functioning of the endocrine system as it relates to reproduction. They may be used to measure potential fertility, to find reasons for abnormal menses, to assess hormone-producing tumors, and to determine whether treatments to adjust hormone levels have been effective. Several hormones may be assessed at any one time. Some hormonal tests are time specific, and the samples can be useless if not gathered within a certain time range.

NURSING CARE. Consult institution policy for specific instructions for each test. Explain the procedure to the patient and provide support. Women who are undergoing hormonal tests may feel embarrassed, worried about their femininity and potential fertility, and depressed because of repeated tests, often with little positive result. Some may fear loss of their spouse's love (and perhaps relationship) if they are diagnosed with alterations in hormonal levels or functioning leading to infertility.

Pelvic Examination

The pelvic examination allows visual inspection of the vagina and cervix, as well as sampling of mucus, discharge, cells, and exudates. Palpation of portions of the reproductive system and some treatments may also be done as part of the procedure (Fig. 41.8).

NURSING CARE. Be prepared to assist the health-care provider with the examination. Explain the procedure as you set out the supplies. Vaginal specula range from tiny virginal sizes to extra large. The appropriate size is related to the size and shape of the woman's (or child's) pelvis and whether she has had children or not. For a small child, a nasal speculum may be used. A clean basin of warm tap water to warm the speculum and a small amount of surgical lubricant should be placed near but not on the speculum (because some tests may be affected by water or lubricant). If reusable equipment is being used, be sure it has been sterilized between patients. Two clean gloves for the examiner should be placed nearby, and a light should be adjusted to illuminate the area. Other equipment may be set out according to the tests or treatments that will be carried out during the pelvic examination.

Instruct the patient to empty her bladder before the examination, change into a gown, and remove her underclothing. Instruct the patient to lie either on her back with her arms resting down at her sides (to aid relaxation of abdominal muscles) or in a side-lying position, according to the health-care provider's preference. Provide a sheet large enough so that there is plenty of room for her legs to spread while the sheet still covers the patient on both sides.

Bimanual Palpation

Because much of the reproductive system is not visible even with a speculum, **bimanual** palpation is often done during a

---

salpingoscopy: salpingo—tube + scopy—looking

bimanual: bi—two + manual—hands

A   B

C   D

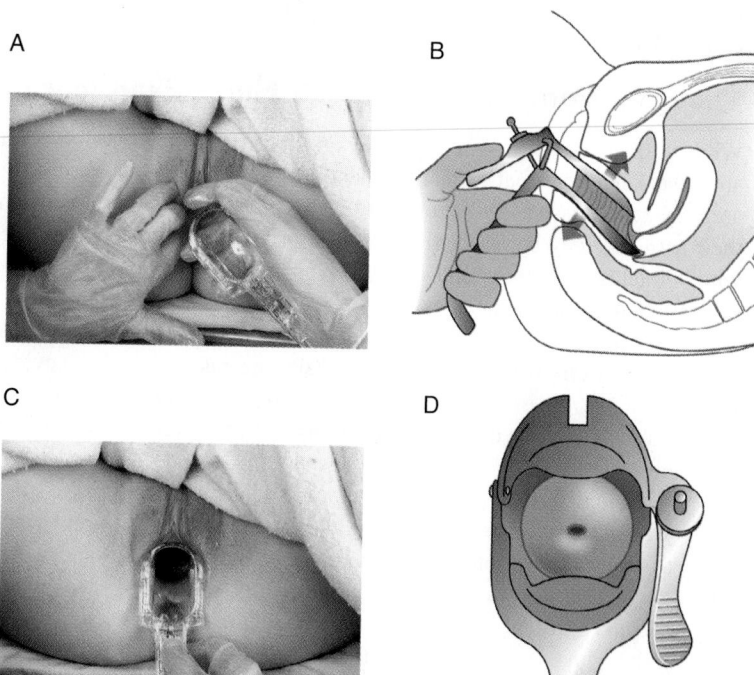

FIGURE 41.8 Pelvic exam with pap smear
(From Dillon, PM: Nursing Health Assessment: A Critical Thinking Case Studies Approach, ed. 2. F.A. Davis, Philadelphia, 2007, with permission)

pelvic examination. One hand is placed on the abdomen and the other gloved hand is inserted deeply into the vagina. The uterus and **adnexa** are moved about between the two hands to feel the size, shape, and consistency of the uterus and adnexa and to check for any abnormal growths.

NURSING CARE. Explain the procedure and support the patient. Some women may be fearful, embarrassed, or tense and may find the procedure uncomfortable. Active relaxation strategies may decrease discomfort. See Box 41.1 Thoughts from a Sexual Assault Nurse Examiner for the experiences of a sexual assault nurse examiner.

Cytology
Cytology is the study of cells taken as tissue samples. There are several ways that cells from the reproductive system may be removed for microscopic examination. During a Pap smear, one or more small samples of cells are gently scraped away from the surface of the cervical canal using a small wooden spatula, tiny cylindrical brush, and/or long cotton-tipped applicator. They are then smeared or rolled onto microscopic slides and sprayed with a fixative to preserve them for viewing, or placed into a fixative solution for later preparation and viewing in a laboratory. Cells may also be collected by **conization,** which involves removing a small cone-shaped sample from the cervical canal, or by punch biopsy, which removes a small core of cells. Endometrial biopsy specimens are samples of cells taken from the lining of the uterus by scraping with a small spoon-shaped tool called a **curet,** which is inserted through the cervix. Small

---

adnexa: ad—together + nexa—to tie (usually refers to ovaries and tubes)

conization: coniz—cone-forming + ation—process

curet: scoop

CRITICAL THINKING

Reproductive Assessment

■ How might the age of the patient change your approach, plans, and teaching for patients who have disorders of the reproductive system? Consider your approach, plans, and teaching for each of the following scenarios.

1. A 2-year-old child is brought into the clinic by her mother because she has a foul-smelling discharge coming from her perineal area and a slight yellowish discharge from her vagina.

2. A 19-year-old woman comes to the doctor's office where you work for renewal of her yearly birth control pill prescription. Your employer enforces regular checks for cervical changes by renewing the prescription only after a Papanicolaou (Pap) smear is done. As you start setting out the Pap smear materials, your patient expresses some reluctance to have a Pap smear today because she is so sore already.

3. Your 56-year-old patient comes in to "get things checked out" because she hurts every time that she and her husband have intercourse.

Suggested answers at end of chapter.

biopsy specimens may also be taken by cutting or removing a suspicious lesion. Cells may be observed for changes indicative of hormonal secretion, cellular maturation, or abnormalities such as are seen with viral growths and cancerous or precancerous conditions.

NURSING CARE. Add appropriate sample collection materials and fixatives to the pelvic examination supplies

Box 41.1

Thoughts from a Sexual Assault Nurse Examiner (SANE)

When patients come in to see me they are in crisis. They are unsure how or what to feel and whom to trust. They are very apprehensive. As patients gives me the history of their assaults, they begin to trust me. They see someone who is interested in them and who believes them. By the time I actually start the head-to-toe physical examination, they know they are safe. Often when I am performing the physical examination, I start small talk and take an interest in their lives that has nothing to do with the assault. When they are discharged from my care, they are more animated, talkative, and sometimes smiling.

The patient I remember the most was a child who's father was molesting her when her mother went to work. She was about 6 years old. When she came to the hospital, she wasn't talking to anybody, let alone a nurse in a scary hospital at midnight. I spent 4 hours with this child. We colored, played, and talked about her brothers. By the end of the night, she allowed me to do an examination on her. And she trusted me enough to let the physician come in and look at her. Unfortunately, in her young life, she had a reason to be scared. Her life became much worse before it got better. Her father tried to kill her mother and himself as a result of this.

So many of us have grown up with pop culture television and we think of forensic examiners as professionals working with dead people. In fact, forensic nursing is caring for patients as it applies to the law. As a sexual assault nurse examiner, I care for those people who have experienced interpersonal violence. And in caring for this special population of patients, I care for them through the nursing process. I not only care for their physical trauma but also care for their spiritual needs; lastly, I collect evidence for the prosecution of a crime. I advocate for their safety needs, and help provide for their physical needs. I provide a bridge to the legal and mental health systems.

I began forensic nursing 8 years ago when the concept was still new. We were navigating uncharted waters and were unsure what the end result would bring. What we quickly learned is when you deliver good nursing care to patients, the end result can be a positive change in their lives, and that is the reward of the job: making a positive difference in patients' lives, giving them some tools to help in their recovery process. Having the patient and family look at you and say "thank you for helping me" is what we all went into nursing for.

Becoming a sexual assault nurse examiner has made me become a more empathic person, a more compassionate nurse, and a better citizen within my community.

according to the type of cytological examination being done. For a Pap smear, this may include one or two clear glass slides, fixative spray, cytobrush and/or wooden cervical spatula, and transport box for the slides. In some settings, or for larger cell samples in most settings, a sterile collection container which includes a preservative solution may be used. Consult the procedure manual or health-care provider concerning specific types of instruments to put out for biopsies and Pap smears. Cells die and degrade rapidly once removed from the patient, so they must be packaged securely for transport to laboratory facilities. Always label specimens carefully.

Prepare the patient by explaining the procedure and providing support. The woman may be fearful of cancer or other abnormality. Removal of the sample may cause pain, bleeding, swelling, or, later, inflammation, so the patient is monitored after the procedure and alerted to watch for and report these complications if they occur. Document the woman's status after the procedure on the chart and record that the sample was sent to the laboratory.

Swabs and Smears

Swabs and smears are done to determine which microorganisms are causing infection, and consequently which antibiotics should be used.

NURSING CARE. Add sample collection materials, including swabs, slides, and sterile saline in site-specific receptacles, and a gonorrhea/*Chlamydia* collection kit, to pelvic examination equipment if symptoms of vaginal infection are present. It is important to place samples of discharge or exudate into culture media that support growth. Clear media are required for some and charcoal media for others, so both types should be set out. Viral swabs require a special collection kit. *Chlamydia* samples are especially difficult to transport to laboratories, and special kits are available for this pathogen. Some microorganisms, such as yeasts and *Trichomonas,* can be identified well from smears on slides. Wet mounts are smears of discharge spread onto a slide. These must be taken to the microscope immediately after they are obtained. Sodium chloride and potassium hydroxide are dropped onto individual wet mount slides before they dry to aid in identification of some microorganisms. Support the patient, who may be anxious about possible sexually transmitted diseases and effects on relationships.

Sonography

Ultrasound assessment (also called sonography) may be done to determine size, shape, development, and density of structures associated with the female reproductive system, as well as fetal measurements and some types of prenatal diagnoses. This procedure is especially useful for differentiating cysts from solid tumors, as well as locating ectopic pregnancies and intrauterine devices. Ultrasound may also be used to guide needles for obtaining samples of fluid or cells. Either external or vaginal transducers may be used to send and receive the signals for this procedure. Vaginal transducers are placed in a plastic sheath before insertion into the vagina. A full bladder may be required for some ultrasound tests.

NURSING CARE. Explain the procedure and support the patient. The pressure of the transducer on the skin or in the vagina may be painful if the adjacent structures are inflamed or swollen, or if the bladder is very full.

Radiographic Procedures

Several radiographic procedures may be used for diagnosis of reproductive system problems. Computed tomographic (CT) scanning and MRI are used to locate tumors of the reproductive system. Structures of the female reproductive system may also be outlined by taking x-ray pictures of cavities that have been filled with a radiopaque substance. During a **hysterosalpingogram,** dye is injected into the uterus until it comes out the ends of the fallopian tubes. This test is useful for identifying congenital abnormalities in the shape or structure of the uterus and blockages of the fallopian tubes.

NURSING CARE. Prepare the patient for this test according to the x-ray department policy and the physician's orders (they may include a laxative, suppository, or enema). Ensure that the patient understands the procedure and that appropriate consents are signed as required. Ask about allergies to iodine or shellfish because contrast media may contain iodine. Notify the charge nurse immediately if the patient reports an allergy. After the procedure, assess for nausea, light-headedness, and signs of allergic reaction and promote comfort, as some cramping may occur. Discharge teaching should include signs of infection and advice that the x-ray dye may stain clothing. Provide a perineal pad following the procedure and advise the patient to wear a perineal pad until any vaginal drainage stops.

Endoscopic Examinations

Several types of endoscopic examinations are done to visually inspect internal areas to diagnose (and sometimes treat) reproductive system disorders. The names of the tests vary according to the area inspected, but all these generally make use of a fiberoptic light and lens system, which is inserted through a tube called a cannula into a small incision. A laparoscopy is done to view the abdominal cavity and is useful for identifying problems such as endometriosis (Fig. 41.9). A salpingoscopy is performed to see the inside of the fallopian tubes and a **hysteroscopy** to see the inside of the uterus. A binocular microscope is used with an endoscope that is introduced into the vagina to closely study lesions of the cervix during a **colposcopy.** During **culdoscopy,** an endoscope is introduced into the vagina and through a small incision in the vagina into the cul-de-sac of Douglas, a cavity behind the uterus, in order to observe for abnormalities in this region (Fig. 41.10).

NURSING CARE. Preoperatively the patient is prepared for an endoscopic examination according to institutional protocol. This generally involves asking the patient whether she has fasted as instructed, assessing vital signs, recording the time of last voiding, helping the patient into the operating room gown, and obtaining a signature on the consent form. General anesthesia may be given for some endoscopic procedures. Explain what to expect and provide

---

hysterosalpingogram: hystero—womb + salpingo—tube + gram—record

hysteroscopy: hystero—womb + scopy—looking
colposcopy: colpo—vagina + scopy—looking
culdoscopy: culdo—cul de sac + scopy—looking

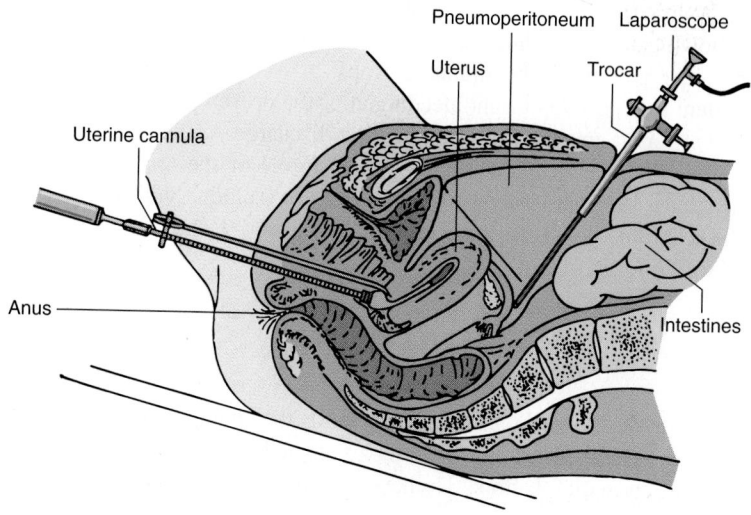

FIGURE 41.9 Laparoscopy. *(Modified from Cavanaugh, BM: Nurse's Manual of Laboratory and Diagnostic Tests, ed. 3. F.A. Davis, Philadelphia, 1999, p 571, with permission.)*

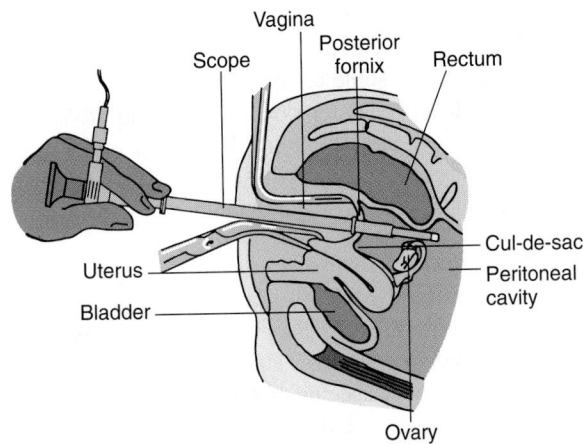

FIGURE 41.10 Culdoscopy. *(Modified from Cavanaugh, BM: Nurse's Manual of Laboratory and Diagnostic Tests, ed. 3. F.A. Davis, Philadelphia, 1999, p 566, with permission.)*

support for the woman. The patient may be anxious about possible disorders.

Postoperatively, provide comfort measures. These procedures produce almost no blood loss. The woman may experience pain in the neck, shoulders, and upper back if carbon dioxide (CO_2) gas was pumped into the body compartment being examined. Called **insufflation,** this is done to increase the distance between structures, so that it is easier for the physician to see and diagnose possible disorders. The CO_2 remaining after completion of the examination travels to the highest level of the body before being absorbed, so lying flat for a few hours after the examination may decrease discomfort. If incisions were made through the abdominal wall for insertion of the endoscope and for insufflation, these are tiny and a Band-Aid or small dressing is applied.

PATIENT TEACHING. Advise the patient to observe the sites for redness, bleeding, or any drainage, seeking evaluation by the physician promptly if these should occur or otherwise approximately 1 week later for suture removal (according to physician preference). If the endoscopic procedure was done transvaginally, provide a perineal pad following the procedure and advise the patient to wear a perineal pad until the drainage stops. Also instruct the patient to report any bright bleeding after the operative day, and to report any fever or foul-smelling discharge.

Further detail about some specific forms of the tests that have been described in this chapter are included with the disorders to which they apply in Chapters 42 and 43. Also see Table 41.5.

⚕ MALE ASSESSMENT

As with the female reproductive system, the male reproductive system is a complex interaction of both physical and psychosocial factors. Unlike women, however, men

may find it much more difficult in our society to talk about or admit to having problems related to reproductive health. From toilet training through adulthood, men are expected to have behaviors associated with maleness. Unfortunately, by the time some boys reach manhood, their male identity may be defined by the successful functioning of their sex organs.

One of the important first steps in obtaining a male reproductive assessment is to provide a comfortable, nonjudgmental, confidential atmosphere for discussion. This means you must first be knowledgeable and comfortable with sexual issues. Nurses do not hesitate to ask female patients about their menstrual history and should be equally comfortable in asking men about their **erection** or ejaculation history. Be open and straightforward with all questions and answers. It may be necessary at times to use more commonly expressed sexual words instead of medical terminology. You will discover that many men do not know the function of their prostate gland or the difference between ejaculation and **orgasm.** Use the assessment as an opportunity to teach men the facts about their own sexual functioning.

History

There are some basic questions to ask a male patient during a reproductive assessment (Table 41.6). Additional questions related to sexual function include the following:

1. "Are you having any problems getting or keeping an acceptable erection?" Additional questions might be whether the patient can have an erection anytime (with or without a sex partner); if erection problems occur when he is under stress or taking medication; or if he is involved in substance abuse. "Do you have erections first thing in the morning or during sleep?" If the patient is able to get an erection, is it straight and firm enough for penetration? Does the erection last long enough for him to reach orgasm?

2. "Are you able to ejaculate during orgasm? Do you have any painful sensations related to the experience? Does any fluid come out during the ejaculation process, and if so, is it a small, moderate, or large amount, and is it clear, cloudy, or brown in color?" The amount and color may depend on whether the patient has had recent sexual activity or genitourinary surgery or may indicate a congenital anomaly or infection.

3. For patients younger than 40 years old: "Do you practice monthly testicular self-examinations?" Men younger than age 40 should be encouraged to perform monthly testicular examinations as a cancer prevention measure.

4. For patients older than 40 years: "When was the last time you had a prostate examination?" A digital rectal examination (DRE) should be a regular part of a man's routine physical after age 41. Prostate cancer is treatable when detected early.

As mentioned earlier, a professional, matter-of-fact attitude, along with an explanation as to why the questions

---

insufflation: in—in suffl—to blow + ation—process

TABLE 41.5 DIAGNOSTIC PROCEDURES FOR THE FEMALE REPRODUCTIVE SYSTEM

Procedure	Definition/Normal Finding	Significance of Abnormal Findings	Nursing Management
Noninvasive			
Breast Self-Examination (BSE)/Clinical Breast Examination (CBE)	Assessment of breast tissue by patient (BSE) or health-care provider (CBE) through inspection and palpation	Abnormal physical exam may indicate pathology and indicates need for further assessment.	Educate about appropriate technique and witness a return demonstration of BSE. Education about BSE may be demonstrated during CBE.
Ultrasound/Sonography	High-frequency sound waves bounce off tissue to map tissue structure and determine tissue density. Also may be used to guide biopsy procedure.	May help to determine abnormal lesions, abnormalities of tissue structure, or presence of abnormal fluid volume	Follow institutional guidelines for patient preparation and support which may be determined by testing goals.
Mammography X-ray	Radiographic examination of tissue. X-ray may be used with dye contrast injected into body before procedure.	May help to determine abnormal lesions or abnormalities of normal tissue structure	Educate patient not to apply lotions/powders to skin over area to be tested by mammogram. If dye is used, inquire about past allergic reaction to dye and/or watch for allergic response after procedure.
Thermography/Computed Tomography (CT)/ Magnetic Resonance Imaging (MRI)	Precise pictures of tissue using temperature (thermography), x-ray (computed tomography), or radiofrequency (MRI)	May help to determine abnormal lesions or abnormalities of normal tissue structure	Ask patient about presence of metal or wire inside their bodies before MRI as the procedure may then be contraindicated.
Hormonal Tests	Assessment of endocrine function related to reproduction	Abnormal hormone levels may reflect fertility potential, find reasons for abnormal menses, assess for hormone-producing tumors, or evaluate if adjustment of hormone levels have been effective.	Explain procedure to patient and provide support.
Invasive			
Pelvic Examination/ Bimanual Examination	Inspection and palpation of external/internal reproductive organs by health-care provider	Abnormal physical examination may detect pathology or may indicate need for further testing.	Consult institutional policies for specific instructions for each test. Explain procedure to patient and provide support.
Biopsy/Cytology/ Swabs/Smears	Obtainment of body cells/tissue through aspiration or excision, or swabbing/scrapping of tissue/exudate	May diagnose pathology or infection	Consult institutional policies for specific instructions for each test. Explain procedure to patient and provide support.
Endoscopy/Laparoscopy	Use of fiberoptic light and lens system to inspect internal structures	May help to determine abnormal lesions or abnormalities of normal tissue structure. Biopsies may be taken of tissue during procedure.	Explain procedure to patient and provide support. Observe for postprocedure complications.

are necessary, can put both you and the patient at ease during the assessment.

Physical Examination

The physical examination is generally performed by a physician or practitioner trained in physical assessments. The examination begins with the patient's general appearance. He is observed for male patterns of hair growth on the head, face, chest, arms, and legs. Normal male pubic hair pattern is in an upside-down triangular shape, with hair growth up toward the umbilicus. The patient's height and muscle mass are noted. Men are commonly taller than 5 feet, 6 inches tall, weigh more than 135 pounds, and have shoulders that are broader than their hips. The presence of excess breast tissue

may indicate **gynecomastia,** an excess of female hormones. Abnormal findings in either hair patterns or muscle mass often indicate a hormone imbalance.

The penis, scrotum, and testes (testicles) are examined by observation and palpation. On observation, the penis is normally flaccid (soft) and hanging straight down. The size can vary greatly and should not be a concern unless it is unusually small (microphallus) or edematous. The left testis generally hangs slightly lower in the scrotum than the right.

The penis is examined for warts, sores (evidence of sexually transmitted diseases), swelling, curves, or lumps

gynecomastia: gyneco—female + mastia—breast

TABLE 41.6 SUBJECTIVE ASSESSMENT OF THE MALE REPRODUCTIVE SYSTEM AND SEXUAL HEALTH

Category	Questions to Ask During History Assessment	Rationale/Significance
Medication	Are you using any medications? (Include prescription, over-the-counter, and herbal remedies.) How much/how often? (For medications that affect sexual desire, erection, or ejaculation, refer to Chapter 43.)	Loss of sexual desire, erection, ejaculation, orgasm, or fertility can occur as a result of some medication use.
Family History	Do you have a family history of genetically transmitted diseases (e.g., heart problems, hypertension, diabetes)? Did your mother use DES during pregnancy?	These conditions put one at high risk for circulation problems that interfere with erections, congenital anomalies of reproductive organs.
Personal Habits and Health Promotion Behaviors	Do you smoke, use caffeine, drink alcohol, use recreational drugs, or use steroids? How much/how often? Do you use hot tubs, engage in long-distance drives, or ride a bike? How much/how often? Do you use contraceptives? What type of contraceptives do you use? How do you use them? Do you do TSE? Have you noticed any changes in your testicles or other reproductive organs?	These habits may lead to decreased blood flow to penis, loss of erection; decreased testosterone (male hormone) interferes with erection and fertility; excessive heat decreases sperm production. Data will reveal knowledge/practice of health promotive behaviors, meaning of health, as well as history of changes/abnormalities.
Personal Health History	Did you have mumps during adolescence, or have you recently had an infection or fever?	Some infectious processes may lead to decreased sperm production.
Mental Health	Are you experiencing stress? How do you deal with stress? Are you having problems with a sexual partner? Have you ever or are you experiencing performance anxiety or depression?	Decreased sexual desire and ability to have an erection may result from mental and/or emotional issues.
Circulatory/ Respiratory	Have you ever been diagnosed with or treated for heart problems/surgery, high blood pressure, sickle cell disease, lung disease, or sleep apnea?	Decreased circulation can lead to inability to have usable erection; decreased respiratory function can result in activity intolerance, loss of erection, congenital anomalies of reproductive organs.
Gastrointestinal	Have you ever been diagnosed/treated for liver infection/disease or bowel problems?	Liver infections/disease can lead to decreased testosterone and increased estrogen production, loss of erection; gastrointestinal/bowel problems can lead to pain, loss of desire; surgery may result in loss of blood or nerve flow.
Musculoskeletal	Do you have painful joints, pelvic/lower back pain, or nerve damage?	Pain, loss of desire; limited movement/positions, loss of erection, ejaculation, and orgasm may result from musculoskeletal problems.
Neurological	Have you ever experienced a stroke or suffered from multiple sclerosis or Parkinson's disease?	Limited movement/positions, loss of sensations, loss of control can result from neurological problems.
Metabolic/Endocrine	Have you ever suffered from diabetes, obesity, or thyroid problems?	Diabetes mellitus can result in circulation problems, retrograde ejaculation, nerve damage; obesity can result in decreased male hormones, excess female hormones.
Genitourinary	Have you ever been diagnosed with a congenital deformity of the penis/testicles, suffered from prostate problems, or experienced erection/ejaculation problems? Have you ever been diagnosed with a sexually transmitted disease? When, what type, and how was it treated? That you are aware, was treatment successful? Do you have any lesions, pain, discharge, swelling of the reproductive organs? Have you noticed any abnormalities/changes in size, shape, color of your external reproductive organs? (Describe).	Difficulty with penetration, erection problems, retrograde ejaculation, infertility may be associated with genitourinary abnormalities. Lesions, pain, discharge, swelling, or other abnormalities of the external reproductive organs may indicate infection, structural abnormalities such as varicocele, or other disease processes such as cancer.
Sexual Practices	Are you sexually active? How many partners do you have? Of what gender? How often do you have intercourse (including positions, timing with female ovulation cycle if heterosexual)? Is the amount/type of sexual activity satisfying? Do you masturbate, or use lubricants?	Some sexual practices can lead to a decrease in quality and quantity of sperm that reach the female egg.

DES = diethylstilbestrol.

894

along the shaft. The examiner also makes sure the urethral opening is at the tip of the penis and not on the underside of the shaft (**hypospadias**) or on the dorsum of the shaft (**epispadias**). If the man is not **circumcised,** the foreskin should be pulled back carefully and the glans inspected for signs of inflammation or foul-smelling discharge. The practitioner should be sure to replace the foreskin in the forward position after the examination is completed.

The scrotum and testes are carefully examined and palpated. Both testes should be present and a normal size (approximately 2 cm × 4 cm). The testes are egg shaped and should feel smooth and rubbery when lightly palpated between the thumb and fingers. The epididymis can be felt along the top edge and posterior section of each testis. The testes and scrotum are palpated for any lumps, cysts, or tumors. If a fluid-filled mass (**hydrocele**) is found, further evaluation should be done. A simple noninvasive test called **transillumination** is used to determine if the mass is fluid filled or solid. With the room lights out, a flashlight is held behind the scrotum. If the mass is fluid, a red glow appears; if it is solid, it appears opaque. Each spermatic cord (made up of veins, arteries, lymphatics, nerves, and the vas deferens) is palpated and should feel firm and threadlike. If

a condition called a **varicocele** is present, the area feels like a bag of worms. A varicocele, which is swelling of the veins of the spermatic cord, is one of the most common problems associated with male infertility.

The male patient is also examined for inguinal hernias by pressing up through the scrotum into each of the inguinal rings while asking him to cough or bear down. Each side is examined separately while he is in the standing position. A hernia feels like a pulsation against the examining fingertips.

A digital rectal examination may be done by an experienced practitioner. During DRE, the prostate gland is palpated by inserting a gloved, lubricated finger into the rectum while the man is in a knee-to-chest position. The entire posterior lobe of the gland can be felt this way. The gland should feel slightly firm and without any lumps. If the prostate gland feels very hard or soft, enlarged, or contains any lumps, a rectal ultrasound with needle biopsy is often ordered. A swollen, painful prostate generally indicates that an infection is present. Remind all men older than age 40 that unless they have had a complete removal of the prostate gland, they still need a DRE performed every year. Many men are under the impression that any prostate surgery means the gland has been completely removed. When simple surgery is performed, prostate tissue is left in the body and will begin to regrow over time. This prostatic tissue can become cancerous and needs to be monitored with a yearly DRE.

See Table 41.7 for a summary of objective assessments of the male reproductive system.

hypospadias: hypo—under + spadias

epispadias: epi—upon + spadias

circumcised: circum—around + cised—cut

hydrocele: hydro—water + cele—hernia

transillumination: trans—across + illumin—light + ation—process

varicocele

TABLE 41.7 OBJECTIVE ASSESSMENT OF THE MALE REPRODUCTIVE SYSTEM

Category	Physical Assessment Findings	Possible Abnormal Findings/Causes
Clinical Breast Examination	• Observe and palpate for presence of swelling, lumps, skin changes, nipple exudates.	• Changes may indicate breast cancer, though rare in males.
Glans of Penis	• Observe for lesions, exudate, tenderness. Observe for placement of the urethra. If foreskin is present, attempt to reduce to observe for lesions, exudate, inflammation.	• Lesions, exudate, tenderness can indicate presence of infective or disease process, injury. • Epispadias/hypospadias may be noted when observing for placement of the urethra.
Shaft of Penis	• Observe for lesions, tenderness, shape.	• Lesions, exudate, tenderness can indicate presence of infectious or disease process, injury. • Irregularity of shape may indicate structural abnormalities/diseases.
Scrotum	• Visualize and palpate for swelling, pain, lesions.	• Inguinal herniation may be noted. • Swelling may occur with heart or renal failure, local inflammation, injury.
Testes	• Palpate for descent, pain, lesions, size, shape, consistency. Palpate for lesions/swelling of epididymitis.	• Absence of palpated testes may indicate nondescent. • Testicular lesion can indicate testicular cancer. • Swelling, pain can indicate infectious process.
Spermatic Cord	• Palpate for swelling, size, consistency, pain	• Presence of swelling, pain can indicate infection or varicocele.
Inguinal Ring (by trained personnel)	• Palpate for bulge, pain.	• Bulge, pain may indicate inguinal hernia.
Inguinal Lymph Nodes	• Palpate for swelling, pain.	• Swelling, pain may indicate infectious process or regional malignancy.
Digital Rectal Exam: DRE (by trained personnel)	• Observe external rectum for lesions, exudate. Palpate for pain, swelling, penile exudate.	• Pain, swelling, exudate may indicate benign changes, infectious process, cancer, or injury.

Testicular Self-Examination

All men after puberty should do monthly testicular self-examination (TSE) to detect any tumors or other changes in the scrotum. See Box 41.2 Guidelines for Monthly Testicular Self-Examination for instructions that can be used to teach a man how to examine his testicles. Also see Figure 41.11.

CRITICAL THINKING

Testicular Evaluation

■ Tony is a 20-year-old who complains of a "bump" on his right testicle. He comes into the health clinic and asks if he can take any medication for his "disease."
1. What would be the best action?
2. What should your health assessment include?

Suggested answers at end of chapter.

Breast Self-Examination

Although breast cancer in men is rare, it can occur. Men, like women, should perform monthly breast self-examination.

Diagnostic Tests of the Male Reproductive System

Ultrasound

An ultrasound may be done to diagnose or evaluate a variety of male reproductive or genitourinary problems. A transrectal ultrasound may be done to diagnose prostate cancer. For this procedure, a rectal probe transducer is inserted into the rectum and sound waves are used to evaluate the prostate gland. An enema may be ordered before the procedure. No special aftercare is necessary.

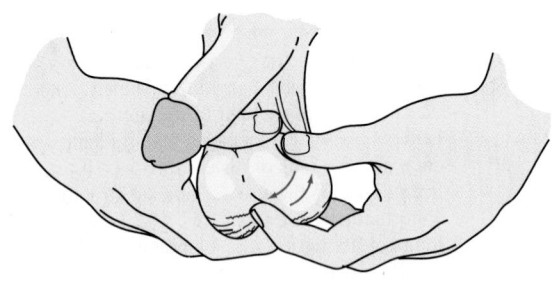

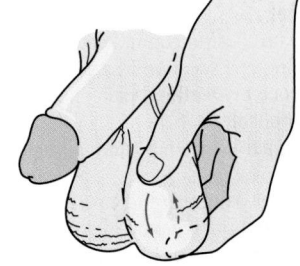

FIGURE 41.11 Testicular self-examination.

Box 41.2

Guidelines for Monthly Testicular Self-Examination

The examination is easiest during or right after a warm shower or bath, when the scrotum is relaxed and the testicles are hanging low. Choose 1 day a month to always do the examination.
1. Raise the penis up out of the way and look for any difference in size or shape of each side of the scrotum (sac). The left side usually hangs a little lower than the right.
2. Using both hands; hold the scrotum in the palms. Begin, one at a time, to gently roll each testicle between the thumb and first three fingers, feeling for any lumps or hard spots.
3. Identify the parts. The testicles should feel round, smooth, and egg shaped. The epididymis along the top and back side should feel soft and a little bit tender. The spermatic cord is a tube that runs from the epididymis and usually feels firm, smooth, and movable.
4. See your doctor immediately if you feel any lumps or unusual changes.

Pelvic or scrotal ultrasound helps evaluate and locate masses. Ultrasound may also be done to guide a needle during a fine-needle biopsy.

Cystourethroscopy

Cystourethroscopy may be done to evaluate the degree of obstruction by an enlarged prostate gland. For this procedure, a Foley catheter is inserted and a dye is injected into the bladder. Radiographs are taken with the dye in the bladder and while voiding after the catheter has been removed.

NURSING CARE. The procedure is explained to the patient, and possible allergic reaction to dyes is assessed and communicated to the physician as necessary. The patient is instructed to void before the procedure. A sedative or analgesic may be ordered to help the patient relax during the procedure.

After the procedure, intake and output are measured for 24 hours and alteration from the patient's normal pattern or absence of urination are reported to the physician. Fluids are encouraged to promote excretion of the dye.

Laboratory Tests

PROSTATE-SPECIFIC ANTIGEN. The normal value of prostate-specific antigen (PSA) is less than 4 ng/L. PSA is a glycoprotein produced by prostate cells. An elevated level indicates prostatic hypertrophy or cancer.

PROSTATIC ACID PHOSPHATASE. Normal value of prostatic acid phosphatase (PAP) is less than 3 ng/mL. PAP is an enzyme that normally affects metabolism of prostate cancer cells. An elevated level indicates prostate cancer.

OTHER TESTS. If prostate cancer is suspected or diagnosed, additional tests may be done. Acid phosphatase may be elevated in metastatic prostate cancer. Alkaline phosphatase and serum calcium levels may be elevated if metastasis to the bone has occurred. See Table 41.8 for a summary of diagnostic procedures.

Tests for Infertility

Various hormone levels may be measured, including FSH, LH, testosterone, and adrenocorticotropic hormone (ACTH) to help determine causes of infertility in male patients.

Semen analysis may be done to provide information about causes of infertility or to evaluate whether a vasec-

tomy has been effective. Semen may be analyzed for sperm count, motility, and shape. Other tests determine whether the semen contains adequate nutrients to support sperm, whether antibodies to the sperm are present, and the ability of the sperm to penetrate an ovum.

NURSING CARE. The patient is instructed to refrain from ejaculation for 3 days before collecting the semen sample to avoid altering findings. Generally, specimens are collected on three separate occasions over a period of 4 to 6 days. Masturbation and ejaculation directly into a sterile container are recommended to avoid loss of semen. Condoms and lubricants should be avoided. The sample should be taken to the laboratory within 1 hour of collection. Additional tests of the male reproductive system are discussed in Chapter 43.

TABLE 41.8 DIAGNOSTIC PROCEDURES FOR THE MALE REPRODUCTIVE SYSTEM

Procedure	Definition/Normal Finding	Significance of Abnormal Findings	Nursing Management
Noninvasive			
Testicular Self-Examination (TSE)	Palpation of testes by patient.	Abnormalities may indicate pathology and require further evaluation.	Instruct patient on appropriate technique and witness a return demonstration.
Ultrasound	High-frequency sound waves bounce off tissue to map tissue structure and determine tissue density. Also may be used to guide biopsy procedure.	May help to determine abnormal lesions, abnormalities of tissue structure, or presence of abnormal fluid volume.	Follow institutional guidelines for patient preparation and support which may be determined by testing goals.
Hormonal Tests/Antigen Level Testing	Blood test to measure hormone or antigen levels.	Abnormal hormone levels may reflect fertility potential. Abnormal antigen levels may indicate pathology.	Consult institutional policies for specific instructions for each test. Explain procedure to patient and provide support.
Invasive			
Digital Rectal Examination	Palpation of internal reproductive organs, especially prostate gland, through rectum.	Abnormal physical exam may indicate pathology and indicates need for further testing.	Educate patient about procedure and provide support.
Cystourethroscopy	Insertion of a Foley catheter and dye into the bladder to evaluate for obstruction (usually an enlarged prostate) by radiography.	Obstruction may cause difficulty with urination.	Educate patient about the procedure and postprocedure care. Instruct patient to void before procedure. Measure intake and output for 24 hours following the procedure. Observe for allergic reaction.

REVIEW QUESTIONS

1. Which male reproductive duct carries sperm into the abdominal cavity?
   a. Urethra
   b. Epididymis
   c. Ductus deferens
   d. Ejaculatory duct

2. Which of the following is the usual site of fertilization?
   a. Ovary

   b. Uterus
   c. Vagina
   d. Fallopian tube

3. Which procedure is most helpful in distinguishing a fluid-filled mass from a solid mass of the breast?
   a. BSE
   b. Mammogram

c. Clinical breast examination

d. Ultrasound

4. Which of the following items should be placed out in preparation for a Pap smear? Choose all responses that are correct.
   a. 50-mL syringe
   b. Vaginal speculum
   c. Lubricant
   d. Clean gloves
   e. Slides and fixative spray
   f. Normal saline

5. When obtaining the history of a 17-year-old male during a sports physical, what important screening practice should be discussed?

a. Yearly DRE

b. Monthly TSE

c. Yearly PSA

d. Bimonthly bimanual examination

6. A patient has just had a laparoscopy to investigate the causes of her infertility. Why should the nurse instruct her to lie flat in the bed for a few hours?
   a. She could rupture her abdominal incision.
   b. Her blood pressure will be extremely low because of blood loss.
   c. The carbon dioxide left over from the test will travel upward and cause pain.
   d. Her uterus needs to be at the same level as her heart to prevent excessive swelling.

SUGGESTED ANSWERS TO

CRITICAL THINKING

■ Breast Health Education

1. The answer should include basic breast health statistics, risks, as well as proper assessment practice and techniques as discussed in this chapter. Technique should be demonstrated and a return demonstration received during the visit. The patient should also verbalize understanding of risks related to breast health and proper BSE technique to verify teaching was effective.

2. Questions about breast health and self-assessment practices provide an opportunity for the nurse to educate a patient about health facts and technique. Patient questions can also be a cue to patient readiness and willingness to learn.

■ Reproductive Assessment

1. Calm fears. Explain simply. Allow the parent to stay with the child if appropriate. Consider whether the child has possibly been abused. (If so, evidence needs to be collected and a report filed with the appropriate child protection authorities.) Place a nasal speculum out for examination. Place a forceps out for removal of a possible foreign body (not uncommon at this age). Teach that this is a normal part of the body that is to be protected and taken care of.

2. Assess knowledge and maturity. Set out supplies for a Pap smear and for swabs and smears. Teach while getting supplies ready. Explain that vaginal soreness generally needs to be treated and that the doctor must know more about the problem to do so effectively. Explain that inflammations can interfere with Pap smear results, so it may have to be repeated later after treatment. Explain culture and sensitivity testing. Teach about risk reduction and inform that oral contraceptives do not offer a barrier.

3. Try to put the woman at ease through general conversation. Set out supplies for a Pap smear (if needed) and for swabs and smears. Teach while getting supplies ready. Discuss aging and the effects of decreased estrogen in general and specifically on vaginal tissues. Inform that there are several ways to deal with the problems resulting from decreased estrogen, such as oral hormonal replacements, water-soluble vaginal lubricants, vaginal creams, estrogen patches, and estrogen receptor modulator medication.

■ Testicular Evaluation

1. Palpable scrotal changes can be present from a variety of reproductive and/or genitourinary abnormalities. Before Tony's question can be answered, a complete history needs to be obtained and a clinical exam of the genitalia performed.

2. The history should explore:
   • If TSEs are regularly performed and if changes have been noted.
   • If Tony is sexually active and has, recently or in the past, been knowingly exposed to a sexually transmitted disease.
   • If there has been pain associated with the "bump" or exudate noted from the penis.

The assessment should include:
   • Visual inspection of the size, shape, symmetry and color of the scrotum and its contents.
   • Palpation to assess for abnormalities and pain.
   • Cultures to rule out sexually transmitted diseases.
   • An inguinal exam to rule out herniation.

Ultimately, based on this complaint, a testicular tumor should be ruled out.

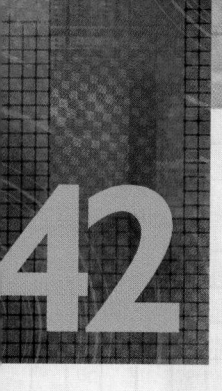

42

Nursing Care of Women with Reproductive System Disorders

DEBRA PERRY-PHILO AND
LINDA HOPPER COOK

KEY TERMS

agenesis (ay-JEN-uh-sis)
amenorrhea (AY-men-oh-REE-ah)
anteflexion (AN-tee-FLECK-shun)
anteversion (AN-tee-VER-zhun)
augmentation (AWG-men-TAY-shun)
balanitis (BAL-uh-NIGH-tis)
cautery (KAW-ter-ee)
colporrhaphy (kohl-POOR-ah-fee)
contraceptive (KON-truh-SEP-tiv)
cryotherapy (KRY-oh-THER-uh-pee)
culdocentesis (KUL-doh-sen-TEE-sis)
culdotomy (kul-DOT-uh-mee)
cystocele (SIS-toh-seel)
cytolytic (SIGH-toh-LIT-ik)
dermoid (DER-moyd)
dilation and curettage (DIL-AY-shun and kyoor-e-TAHZH)
dysmenorrhea (DIS-men-oh-REE-ah)
dyspareunia (DIS-puh-ROO-nee-ah)
dysplasia (dis-PLAY-zee-ah)
ectasia (ek-TAY-zee-ah)
fibrocystic (FIGH-broh-SIS-tik)
hypertrophy (high-PER-truh-fee)
hypoplasia (HIGH-poh-PLAY-zee-ah)
hysterectomy (HISS-tuh-RECK-tuh-mee)
hysterotomy (HISS-tuh-RAH-tuh-mee)
imperforate (im-PER-foh-rate)
in vitro fertilization (in-VEE-troh FER-ti-li-ZAY-shun)
laparotomy (LAP-uh-RAH-tuh-mee)
laser ablation (LAY-zer uh-BLAY-shun)
leiomyoma (LYE-oh-my-OH-mah)
mammoplasty (MAM-oh-PLAS-tee)
marsupialization (mar-SOO-pee-al-i-ZAY-shun)
mastalgia (mass-TAL-jee-ah)
mastectomy (mass-TECK-tuh-mee)
mastitis (mass-TIGH-tis)
mastopexy (MAS-toh-PEKS-ee)
myomectomy (MY-oh-MECK-tuh-mee)
panhysterectomy (PAN-hiss-tuh-RECK-tuh-mee)
pedicle (PED-i-kuhl)
perimenopausal (PER-ee-MEN-oh-PAWS-uhl)
phytoestrogens (FY-toh-ES-troh-jenz)
postcoital (post-KOH-i-tal)
rectocele (RECK-toh-seel)
retroflexion (RET-roh-FLECK-shun)
retrograde (RET-roh-grayd)
retroversion (RET-roh-VER-zhun)
salpingo-oophorectomy (by-LAT-er-uhl sal-PINJ-oh-ah-fuh-RECK-tuh-mee)
teratoma (ter-uh-TOH-muh)
vaginosis (VAJ-i-NOH-sis)

QUESTIONS TO GUIDE YOUR READING

1. How would you explain the pathophysiology of each of the disorders of the female reproductive system?

2. What are the etiologies, signs, and symptoms of each of the disorders?

3. What care would you provide for patients undergoing tests for each of the disorders?

4. What is current therapeutic management for each of the disorders?

5. What data should you collect when caring for patients with disorders of the female reproductive system?

6. What nursing care will you provide for patients with each of the covered disorders?

7. How will you know if your nursing interventions have been effective?

8. How do different forms of contraceptives available vary in effectiveness?

Reproductive system disorders can be frightening, irritating, frustrating, embarrassing, and in some cases fatal. They involve not just body parts but also roles, relationships, and sense of identity and purpose in life. Nurses can play an important role in helping women with these disorders. Women's health is an area where much research is being done. The Nurses' Health Study, conducted at Harvard Medical School, is a large ongoing study on many topics related to women's health. You can learn about it at www.nurseshealthstudy.org.

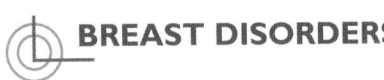

BREAST DISORDERS

Benign Breast Disorders

Much has been done in recent years to educate the general public concerning breast cancer. It is the most commonly diagnosed cancer in women.[1] Heightened awareness of the risks of breast cancer, however, sometimes results in excessive anxiety among women with benign breast conditions. The following section covers benign, or noncancerous, breast disorders.

Cyclic Breast Discomfort
PATHOPHYSIOLOGY, ETIOLOGIES, AND SIGNS AND SYMPTOMS. The most common breast symptoms result from cyclic variations in hormone levels. Swelling, tenderness, and sometimes pain (**mastalgia**) can be related to hormone-mediated changes within the breast tissues that prepare them for their potential role of breastfeeding.

TREATMENT. If persistent or severe, these symptoms may be treated with oral contraceptives that modify hormone levels or nonsteroidal anti-inflammatory drugs (NSAIDs) to control pain. Explaining that cyclic discomfort is temporary and not from a disease process helps to allay fears.

Fibrocystic Breast Disease
Fibrocystic breast disease is common in women between the ages of 30 and 50. Many refer to it as simply "fibrocystic breast changes."

PATHOPHYSIOLOGY, ETIOLOGIES, AND SIGNS AND SYMPTOMS. Overresponsiveness of cells in the breasts to hormonal stimulation (especially estrogen) may cause long-term changes resulting in replacement of normal tissue with fibrous tissue, **ectasia** (overdevelopment) of cells, and blockage of ducts so that cysts form around trapped fluid. This makes the breasts feel somewhat hard and lumpy, and sometimes painful. These changes often occur during the reproductive years, and can respond to hormonal variations during the menstrual cycle. It usually subsides with menopause.

DIAGNOSIS AND TREATMENT. Fibrocystic breast changes can be identified on palpation. A mammogram or ultrasound may be done to assist in diagnosis. Needle or excisional biopsy may be done to rule out malignancy. Treatment for fibrocystic breast changes is based on patient symptoms. Often, no treatment is necessary. Analgesics, primarily NSAIDs, may be needed for discomfort. Herbal remedies, such as evening primrose oil, or supplemental vitamin therapy may offer symptomatic relief, but these therapies remain controversial. Limitation of dietary fat and caffeine and addition of oral contraceptive use may be helpful to control hormonal changes that result in discomfort.

Although **fibrocystic** changes are not cancerous, more frequent mammography or ultrasound may be advised as fibrocystic changes may make it more difficult to feel early cancerous lumps during breast self-examination (BSE). Some types of breast cysts are associated with a higher cancer risk. Needle aspiration may be used to treat cystic lesions.

Mastitis
PATHOPHYSIOLOGY, ETIOLOGIES, AND SIGNS AND SYMPTOMS. Breast infection with inflammation (**mastitis**) occurs as a result of injury and introduction of bacteria into the breast. This condition most commonly occurs while breastfeeding. The breast becomes swollen, hot, red, and painful and may form an abscess.

TREATMENT. Mastitis may be treated either with antibiotics or by incision and drainage (I&D) of the abscessed area. NSAIDs, warm packs, and breast supports are often used to control pain and swelling.

NURSING CARE AND TEACHING. You may assist with an I&D by setting out the equipment: a wrapped sterile sharp-pointed scalpel blade, a blade handle, clean gloves, and dressing materials. A dressing may be applied over the I&D site to absorb drainage.

Patient teaching should include instructions to wash hands carefully to prevent the spread of infection. If the patient is breastfeeding, it is often continued to promote drainage of the breast, mother/infant bonding, and infant nutrition. The infant is often already colonized with the bacteria so further exposure is not thought to be detrimental.

> ### NURSING CARE TIP
> If a mother is breastfeeding, frequent changes in feeding positions as well as exercising good hygiene techniques, such as hand washing when handling the breasts, may help to prevent mastitis.

Malignant Breast Disorders
Etiology
Research has identified factors that increase the risk of development of breast cancer: increasing age, personal or family

---

mastalgia: mast—breast + algia—pain
ectasia: extension

fibrocystic: fibro—fibrous + cystic—saclike
mastitis: mast—breast + itis—inflammation

history of breast cancer, high-fat diet, high alcohol intake, treatment with estrogens (especially when used without progestins), early menarche, late menopause, no pregnancy or late first pregnancy, no breastfeeding, or breastfeeding for a short period of time following delivery.

Prevention

Exercising moderation in fat and alcohol consumption, using nonhormonal methods of birth control, and managing menopausal symptoms can reduce risk of breast cancer. However, there are many factors that cannot be controlled, so the importance of early detection cannot be overemphasized. Recent research has discovered genes (BRCA1 and BRCA2) that are linked with susceptibility to breast cancer. These findings offer the possibility of very early identification of women at the most risk of developing breast cancer (and also ovarian cancer for those with BRCA1). They can then be monitored closely for any changes and receive early treatment if cancer develops.

Diagnostic Tests

Breast self-examination and clinical breast examinations are important parts of identification of cancer. Cancerous growths tend to be harder, less mobile, less painful, more irregularly shaped, and have less clearly defined borders than benign growths. The prognosis is good for women who have breast cancers removed in the early stages but gets worse when treatment begins during the later stages of the disease process. Teaching and encouraging the regular use of BSE and appropriate use of mammography can save lives. Refer to Chapter 41 for more about BSE and for explanations about diagnostic tests used to assist in determining whether tumors of the breast are malignant.

Staging

The spread (metastasis) of cancerous cells from the primary site to other areas of the body by way of the blood or lymph is denoted by staging classifications. (See Chapter 10.) The lower numbers indicate less cancer spread.

Therapeutic Interventions and Complications

There are five main treatment options for breast cancer: radiation therapy, chemotherapy, hormonal therapy, modification of biological response, and surgery. These options may be used separately or in combination depending on the condition of the patient and the stage of the disease.

The possibility of metastases necessitates drastic treatment of the whole body in many cases to prevent secondary cancer growth at other sites. Both radiation and chemotherapy generally combat cancer by destroying rapidly reproducing cells. These treatments are effective against cancer but also tend to destroy normal body cells that reproduce rapidly, such as hair and the cells lining the mouth, vagina, and gastrointestinal tract. Interventions to help preserve these tissues and maintain nutrition can be helpful (see Chapter 10).

Hormonal therapy may be undertaken to deprive cancer cells of hormones that stimulate their growth. Because breast cancer cells are often estrogen sensitive, this may be accomplished by decreasing circulating estrogen levels with drugs or by blocking the use of estrogen by cancer cells as occurs with use of the drug tamoxifen citrate. Interference with estrogen levels, however, may produce menopausal symptoms and increase the risk of osteoporosis and heart disease.

Substances that modify the body's biological responses may be given to intensify positive responses of the body (e.g., stimulate the immune system) or to decrease negative body responses. Some examples of biological response modifiers are interferons, tumor necrosis factor, interleukins, and various experimental immunotherapy formulations. This is an area of much research and is likely to expand greatly during the next few years.

Breast surgeries to remove cancerous tissue can be disfiguring and have profound effects on the patient's self-concept. The amount of tissue removed varies depending on the size, nature, and invasiveness of the cancer. A lumpectomy removes just the tumor and a margin around it. A **mastectomy** may be partial (removing only part of the breast), simple (removing breast tissue of one or both breasts), or radical (removing breast tissue, underlying muscle, and surrounding lymph nodes). Recently, surgical practice has shifted from mainly radical mastectomies to more breast-conserving surgeries with the addition of radiation therapy, and result in similar survival rates being demonstrated.

Nursing Care

See Box 42.1 Nursing Care Plan for Care of the Patient Undergoing a Mastectomy.

Alternative therapies are also available for many cancers. See Chapter 4 for information about helping patients evaluate alternative and complementary therapies. The American Cancer Society and cancer treatment centers also have people who can answer questions about experimental and alternative therapies and discuss research findings. For more information about breast cancer, visit the American Cancer Society at www.cancer.org.

(Text continued on page 904)

CRITICAL THINKING

Julie

■ Julie, age 32, reports pain and grapelike "lumps" in her breasts.

1. What questions would you ask to further assess the complaint?
2. What diagnostic tests would you expect to be suggested (if any)?
3. What treatment options might be used?

Suggested answers at end of chapter.

---

mastectomy: mast—breast + ec—away + tomy—cutting

Box 42.1   Nursing Care Plan for the Patient Undergoing a Mastectomy

Nursing Diagnosis: Risk for anxiety related to uncertainty about diagnosis, prognosis, and treatments

Expected Outcomes Patient will verbalize and demonstrate a decrease in anxiety.

Evaluation of Outcomes (1) Does the patient report a decrease in anxiety following education and explanation of the procedure? (2) Do patient's vital signs, verbal, and nonverbal behavior suggest a decrease in anxiety?

Interventions	Rationale	Evaluation
Assess vital signs and observe verbal and nonverbal behavior.	An increase in blood pressure, pulse and respirations as well as observation of mild to severe agitation may reflect an anxiety state.	Are the patient's vital signs within normal range for the patient? Is verbal and nonverbal behavior consistent with an anxiety state?
Assess patient's current knowledge of the procedure and level of anxiety related to the procedure.	Knowledge dispels unreasonable fears and helps patient to prepare to cope with stressors.	Does patient express satisfaction with amount and type of information?
Teach patient what to expect about the surgical experience based on patient's understanding, concerns, and willingness to learn.		Does patient evidence adequate understanding of the procedure as well as understanding of what to expect afterward?
Support the physician's explanations, answer questions, and refer to knowledgeable sources.		

Nursing Diagnosis: Risk for ineffective breathing pattern related to pain with chest movement

Expected Outcomes Effective breathing pattern with clearance of mucus from air passages

Evaluation of Outcomes (1) Are respirations regular, easy, and unlabored? (2) Is respiratory rate and oxygen saturation within a normal range for the patient? (3) Are lung sounds clear?

Interventions	Rationale	Evaluation
Assess patient's vital signs, oxygen saturation, pain level, and lung sounds.	A change in vital signs, a decrease in oxygen saturation, an unacceptable pain level as defined by the patient, and unclear lung sounds may reflect an ineffective breathing pattern related to pain.	Are the patient's vital signs and oxygen saturation within normal range for the patient? Does patient report pain at an acceptable level? Are lung sounds clear?
Medicate to relieve pain as necessary.	Pain may inhibit deep breathing efforts.	Does patient evidence pain or guarding during chest movement?
Encourage deep breathing and coughing each hour.	This helps to loosen secretions and to prevent atelectasis, pneumonia, and inadequate oxygenation of tissues.	Does chest sound clear? Are skin color and oxygen saturation adequate?
Encourage use of an incentive spirometer each hour when awake.	To encourage deep breathing	Does patient use spirometer correctly?

Nursing Diagnosis: Risk for ineffective tissue perfusion and integrity related to damage to blood and lymph vessels and tension at surgical incision site

Expected Outcomes Incision will heal by primary intention without excessive bleeding or swelling.

Evaluation of Outcomes Are vital signs within normal range for the patient?
Is dressing dry and intact?

Are edges of the incision well approximated, with scant bleeding/serous drainage, and mild edema/erythema? Is range of motion appropriate to post-operative time period?

Interventions	Rationale	Evaluation
Monitor vital signs, oxygen saturation, and peripheral vascular status according to hospital policy and as necessary.	Vital signs, oxygen saturation, and peripheral vascular signs reflect circulatory status.	Are vital signs stable and within normal range? Is dressing dry?
Avoid use of the affected arm for blood pressure, venipunctures, and injections.	Restrictive and invasive procedures might further compromise tissue integrity of the affected arm.	Is arm protected?
Check for bleeding, amount and color of drainage if a drain device is used, and swelling.	Excessive bleeding and swelling may further compromise tissue perfusion.	Does incisional area look swollen, smooth, or shiny? Are drainage amount and color appropriate?
Measure circumference of arms daily and compare.	Swelling causes an increase in circumference.	Is affected arm larger than unaffected arm?
Elevate affected arm if swelling occurs. *Lymphedema (elevate arm)*	Gravity aids fluid return to the heart.	Does elevation prevent swelling?
Place items where patient may easily reach them.	Excessive movement of the arm may exert tension on incision and increase bleeding.	Can patient reach items without abducting the arm over 90 degrees?
Encourage reasonable exercise of the affected arm following post-mastectomy exercises that are approved by the institution.	Reasonable exercise promotes circulation, preserves muscle and joint function, and increases self-care ability. *Prevents contracture*	Is patient moving the arm appropriately and gradually increasing range of motion and self-care ability?
Provide education for the patient related to post-operative self-care and signs and symptoms of ineffective healing.	Early assessment and intervention help prevent the development of serious complications.	Does patient demonstrate and verbalize understanding related to appropriate post-operative self-care?

Nursing Diagnosis: Risk for ineffective coping related to cancer threat and body image disturbance

Expected Outcomes Patient verbalizes ability to cope; seeks help and support appropriately.

Evaluation of Outcomes (1) Does patient take interest in care of condition? (2) Does patient ask appropriate questions related to care and verbalize appropriate concerns?

Interventions	Rationale	Evaluation
Maintain an open and trusting therapeutic relationship.	Effective communication is based on trust.	Is patient talking about concerns?
Allow grieving to take place.	Loss of a breast disturbs many aspects of body image, and cancer threatens one's sense of security and reasonableness of life.	Is patient willing able to talk about loss?
Encourage patient to express feelings and concerns.		
Encourage active problem solving.	Active problem solving promotes self-efficacy and combats depression.	How are family members interacting with patient? How is patient responding to family members and friends?
Help patient remember previous successes in coping and strategies used.	Memory of prior success can encourage hope for future success.	Is patient planning for the future? Is patient taking an active interest in her personal appearance?
Refer to appropriate agencies for further support as needed (e.g., American Cancer Society, Reach for Recovery, local support groups,	Social support can assist individuals to meet their needs while developing effective coping skills and strategies.	Does patient have sufficient coping skills or supports available to promote healthy living?

Breast Modification Surgeries

Mammoplasty is surgical modification of the breast. This may be done to restore a normal shape after removal of cancerous tissues. Many women, however, undergo mammoplasty electively to reduce or increase the size or to improve the shape of their breasts. Because nurses are very aware of the dangers involved with surgery, psychosocial issues may seem to be a trivial reason to voluntarily assume such risks to life and health. However, body image is an important component of quality of life. Patients' informed decisions should be respected if they choose this surgery. It is essential that you present a caring and nonjudgmental attitude.

Breast Reduction and Mastopexy

Generally, in breast reduction operations the nipple is separated from the surrounding tissue except for a small section with the blood vessels and nerves that supply it (Fig. 42.1). A large wedge of tissue is removed from the bottom of the breast, the edges are sewn together, and the nipple is reimplanted in a higher position. This not only decreases the overall size of the breast, which may help with back, neck,

and head pain, it also corrects excessive sagging—a common problem for women with large breasts.

A **mastopexy** involves the removal of some skin and fat with subsequent resuturing so that the breast tissues are held higher on the chest to correct sagging breasts. This procedure usually does not remove as much tissue as a breast reduction.

Augmentation and Reconstruction Mammoplasty

Augmentation is a surgery to increase the size of the breasts. An implant—either a bag containing saline solution or silicone gel or a transplanted portion of the patient's own body tissues from another area—is inserted through an incision and positioned either under or over the pectoral muscles (Fig. 42.2).

For reconstructive mammoplasty, use of the patient's own tissues is generally safer than use of artificial implants because no foreign material is introduced into the body. For situations in which significant amounts of tissue are needed for reconstruction, a portion of tissue may be moved from one area of the body to another as a **pedicle** graft. Pedicle literally means "little foot" because the graft remains attached to a stalk (containing the blood vessels and nerves) somewhat resembling a little leg with a foot (the graft) attached. Figure 42.3 shows two options for mastectomy graft repair—using the latissimus dorsi muscle and overlying tissue on the side of the chest or using the rectus abdominis muscle of the abdomen with its overlying tissue. For both these procedures, a portion of muscle is separated from its usual attachment. Tissues overlying a part of the muscle are excised and left attached to the muscle. This segment of

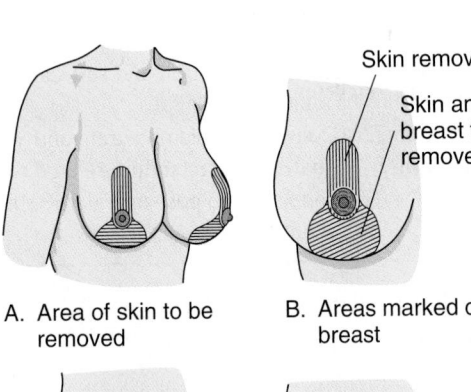

A. Area of skin to be removed

B. Areas marked on breast

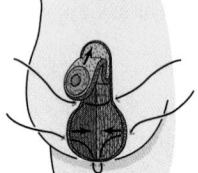

C. Wedge of breast tissue removed, areola pulled up, gap closed

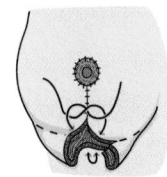

D. Excess tissue removed, skin closed with stitches

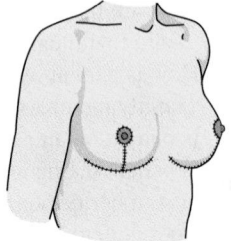

E. Post-operative appearance

FIGURE 42.1 Breast reduction. *(Modified from Love, SM: Dr. Susan Love's Breast Book, ed. 3. Perseus Publishing, Cambridge, MA, 2000; used with permission.)*

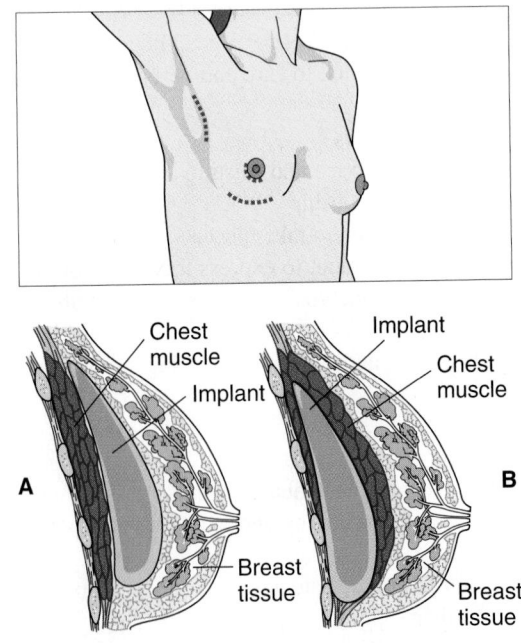

FIGURE 42.2 Breast implants. *(A)* Implant over muscle. *(B)* Implant under muscle. *(Modified from Love, SM: Dr. Susan Love's Breast Book, ed. 3. Perseus Publishing, Cambridge, MA, 2000; used with permission.)*

mammoplasty: mamm(o)—breast + plasty—to mold

pedicle: ped—foot + icle—little

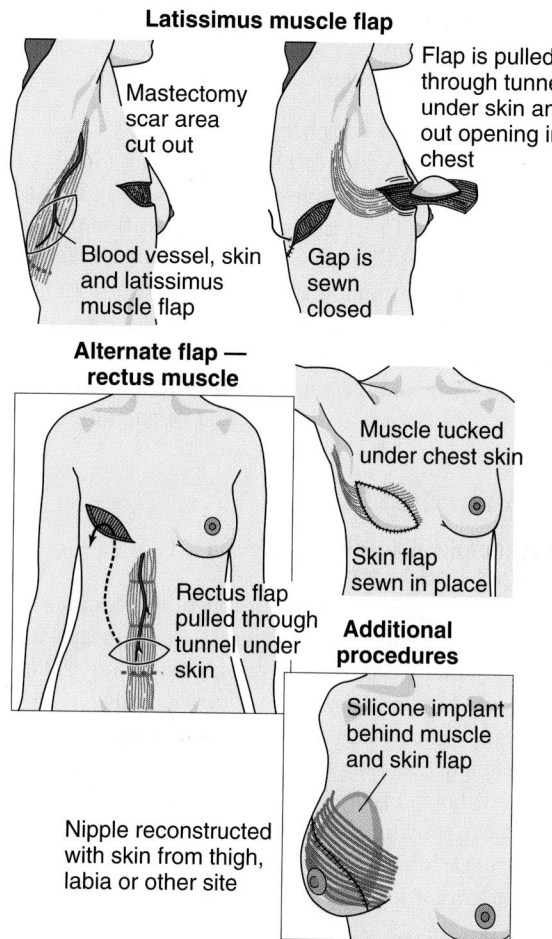

FIGURE 42.3 Mastectomy reconstruction. *(Modified from Love, SM: Dr. Susan Love's Breast Book, ed. 3. Perseus Publishing, Cambridge, MA, 2000; used with permission.)*

tissue is then pulled under the skin and superficial layers to an incision at the mastectomy site. There it is brought to the surface and attached to reconstruct a breast shape. Tissue from the buttock area or the abdomen may also be grafted onto a mastectomy site without a pedicle.

Complications

Any of these surgeries may be complicated by infection or impaired healing. The use of silicone implants has been less than satisfactory for many women. Some women have experienced hardening of breast tissues and others have developed serious autoimmune disease problems after receiving silicone gel implants. Although actual etiologies of all the problems are uncertain, many surgeries have been undertaken recently to remove silicone implants, and saline implants are now used more often.

Nursing Care and Teaching

Carefully assess the healing process when changing dressings and explain to the patient how to assess healing, as not all tissues successfully attach at the new site. Failure of attachment can require surgical revision. Signs of poor attachment include unnatural color of the incision, graft, or surrounding tissues; swelling; drainage; gaping of incision

Box 42.2

Breast Disorders Summary

Signs and Symptoms	Swelling, tenderness, pain, redness Palpable lumps Leakage of fluid/blood from nipple Changes in contour of skin of breast/nipple
Diagnostic Tests and Findings	BSE/CBE Culture and sensitivity Mammography/ultrasound Excisional/fine-needle biopsy
Therapeutic Interventions	NSAIDs Caffeine avoidance Hormone therapy Anti-infectives if infection present Incision and drainage if abscessed area Lumpectomy/mastectomy/breast reconstruction Chemotherapy/radiation Biological response modifiers
Complications	Hormone therapy may cause menopausal symptoms. Breast surgery may have profound negative effect on patient's self-concept.
Priority Nursing Diagnoses	Acute pain r/t distention of the breast Fear r/t diagnosis of breast lesion and possible cancer Deficient knowledge r/t health status and treatment

BSE = breast self-examination; CBE = clinical breast examination; NSAIDs = nonsteroidal anti-inflammatory drugs; r/t = related to.

lines; and sloughing of the graft or edges of the site. See Box 42.2 for a Breast Disorders Summary.

MENSTRUAL DISORDERS

Flow and Cycle Disorders

Pathophysiology, Etiologies, and Signs and Symptoms

There are many types of menstrual abnormalities (Table 42.1). Causes can include stress, pregnancy, hormonal imbalances, metabolic imbalances (such as obesity, anorexia nervosa, and loss of too much body fat through excessive exercise), tumors (both benign and malignant), infections, organ diseases (such as liver, kidney, or thyroid disease), blood or bone marrow abnormalities, and the presence of foreign bodies in the uterus (such as intrauterine devices).

TABLE 42.1 MENSTRUAL FLOW DISORDERS

Disorder	Description
Amenorrhea	Menses absent for more than 6 months or three of previous cycles
	Called primary amenorrhea when menarche has not occurred by age 17
	Called secondary amenorrhea when menses are absent after menarche
Oligomenorrhea	Menstrual cycles of more than 35 days
Hypomenorrhea	Less than the expected amount of menstrual bleeding
Menorrhagia	Passing more than 80 mL of blood per menses
Hypermenorrhea	Menses lasting longer than 7 days
Polymenorrhea (also called Metrorrhagia)	Menses more frequently than 21-day intervals
Menometrorrhagia (also called Metromenorrhagia)	Overly long, heavy, and irregular menses

Menstrual abnormalities can be distressing and can result in anemia, persistent fatigue, and sexual dysfunction. Establishment of a comfortable and open professional relationship is essential for communication about such concerns.

Diagnostic Tests

Appropriate testing to determine the cause of menstrual abnormalities can involve a thorough medical history and physical examination. Papanicolaou (Pap) smear, cervical and vaginal cultures, laparoscopy, ultrasound, pregnancy testing, urine testing, and extensive blood testing may be done to screen for any of the disorders that may influence the menstrual cycle and flow. Generally, health-care providers initially test to rule out the most likely causes and then begin to test for more obscure disorders until the cause of the disorder is identified. For example, reproductive hormone levels are likely to be tested before kidney or liver function, unless the latter disorders are evident in the initial history and physical examination.

Therapeutic Interventions

Medical treatment of menstrual disorders generally involves manipulation of hormone levels. Surgical treatment of menstrual disorders can involve **dilation and curettage (D&C)**, **laser ablation** of endometrial tissue, and **hysterectomy.** During D&C the cervix is first dilated (opened wider) and then a curet—a sharp, spoonlike instrument—is inserted through the cervix and used to scoop out the inner lining of the uterus. Laser ablation involves targeted burning of

endometrial tissue so that scar tissue that does not bleed forms. Hysterectomy (removal of the uterus), a last-resort treatment, is described later in this chapter.

Nursing Care and Teaching

Estimation of the amount of blood lost during menses may be difficult because pad counts can vary widely depending on the frequency of pad changes and the portion of the pad that contains blood. The only accurate way to estimate menstrual flow is by weighing the pads (sealed in a biohazard bag) and then subtracting the weight of the original pads. A 1-g increase in pad weight equals approximately 1 mL of blood loss. You can document what the patient says for blood loss, but be sure to quote it and in parentheses place "patient estimate" after the quote.

Dysmenorrhea

Pathophysiology, Etiologies, and Signs and Symptoms

Painful menstruation, or **dysmenorrhea,** is a common problem in women, although few find it to be incapacitating. Primary dysmenorrhea is not pathological and is thought to be caused mainly by the action of endogenous prostaglandins, which stimulate uterine contractions producing cramping pain. Secondary dysmenorrhea occurs after normal menses, without discomfort, and may be caused by some pathological condition such as endometriosis, pelvic infection, **retroversion** of the uterus, fibroid tumors, or reproductive disorders caused by other body system pathology.

Diagnostic Tests

Hormonal tests such as estrogen and progesterone levels may be required for primary dysmenorrhea, but laparoscopic examination, biopsies, cultures, and various other reproductive function tests (explained later in the chapter) may be required for investigation of secondary dysmenorrhea.

Therapeutic Interventions

Primary dysmenorrhea may be treated with drugs that inhibit prostaglandin synthesis, such as aspirin and nonsteroidal anti-inflammatory drugs (NSAIDs). Correction of secondary causes of dysmenorrhea may include such measures as hormonal adjustment, usually with oral contraceptives or hormone replacement therapy (HRT), dilation and curettage, or other surgical or medical intervention based on the primary cause.

Nursing Care and Teaching

Several nonprescription preparations are available for treatment of dysmenorrhea, but patients should be advised to read the labels carefully because aspirin and NSAIDs (the main component of many of the drugs) may be bought less expensively. Other added drugs in these compounds, such as diuretics, may not be necessary. If dysmenorrhea is related to uterine retroversion, assuming a knee-to-chest position may relieve the discomfort. Sudden development of dys-

---

dilation and curettage: dilat(e)—to widen + ation—the process of + curet—scoop + tage—doing

laser ablation: laser—light amplification by stimulated emission of radiation + ab—away + lat—to carry + ion—the process

hysterectomy: hyster—womb + ec—away + tomy—cutting

dysmenorrhea: dys—painful + men(o)—month + rrhea—flow

retroversion: retro—back + version—turning

menorrhea in a woman with no previous menstrual discomfort should always be investigated.

Premenstrual Syndrome

Pathophysiology, Etiologies, and Signs and Symptoms

Premenstrual syndrome (PMS) is a recurrent problem for many women and may involve water retention; headaches; discomfort of joints, muscles, and breasts; changes in affect, concentration, and coordination; and sensory changes. Few women find PMS serious enough to interfere with work or relationships. The impact of ovarian hormones, aldosterone, and neurotransmitters such as monoamine oxidase and serotonin on PMS is not well understood, and further research is needed.

Therapeutic Interventions

A variety of drugs have been given to combat PMS with varying degrees of success. Some commonly used PMS medications include drugs that affect prostaglandin production, hormonal balance, and neurotransmitter production and reuptake, as well as diuretics and supplements of calcium, magnesium, vitamin E, and vitamin B_6. Patients should be warned, however, that dosages of vitamins should not be increased without professional advice because vitamins are medications (as well as nutrients) and high doses of some vitamins can lead to physiological damage.

Nursing Care and Teaching

Being understanding and nonjudgmental is especially important. Some women who suffer from severe PMS may have been treated as if they are psychologically unbalanced because of the interaction of hormones and neurotransmitters and because of outdated ideas concerning PMS. You can help by providing educational materials on lifestyle measures, such as restriction of alcohol, caffeine, nicotine, salt, and simple sugars; participation in regular exercise; and development of stress management skills that can help women who have a tendency to experience PMS.

Endometriosis Final EXAm

Pathophysiology, Etiologies, and Signs and Symptoms

Endometriosis is a condition in which functioning endometrial tissue is located outside the uterus (Fig. 42.4). Several theories have been proposed to explain development of endometriosis, including faulty developmental differentiation of cells, transport of endometrial cells via blood and lymph to other parts of the body, and **retrograde** menstruation—a backward leakage of blood and tissue out through the fallopian tubes during the menstrual period.

Endometriotic cells grow in areas of sufficient blood supply, extending into other tissues such as intestinal walls, ovaries, and other abdominal structures. On a cyclic basis, mediated by ovarian hormones, these cells build up and slough just as they would in the uterus, but the sloughing

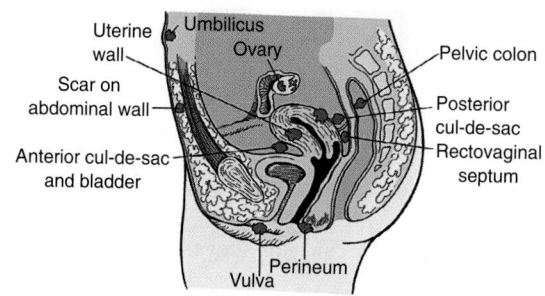

FIGURE 42.4 Possible sites of endometriosis.

and bleeding occur in the enclosed abdominal cavity or into the tissues that they have invaded. The build-up of the blood and cells can result in pain, swelling, damage to abdominal organs and structures, scar tissue development, and infertility.

Therapeutic Interventions

Surgical intervention may be required, especially if scar tissue develops into tight bands, which can cause strangulation of sections of bowel or ureters. Reduction of estrogen and prevention of ovulation either with medications or by surgical removal of the ovaries can be very effective but result in infertility and menopausal symptoms. Analgesics may be required.

Nursing Care and Teaching

The severity and persistence of the pain of endometriosis may lead to overuse of pain medication, so it is important to teach patients alternative pain relief strategies such as relaxation exercises and application of heat to the abdomen or back.

Menopause

Pathophysiology and Signs and Symptoms

Menopause is the permanent cessation of menstrual cycles resulting from decreased hormone production. This is a natural part of aging, but it is placed within this section because several related uncomfortable symptoms and conditions can occur. The climacteric (perimenopause) is the period of gradual decline in hormone production before the permanent end of menses and may last from months to several years. **Perimenopausal** physical symptoms vary widely and may include erratic menses, atrophy of urogenital tissues with a marked decrease in the amount of natural lubrication, a pH shift toward alkalinity (encouraging yeast overgrowth), and vasomotor instability (resulting in hot flashes and night sweats).

Estrogen protects women against several disease processes; the risk of heart disease and osteoporosis increases with declining estrogen production. Mental changes may also occur because of the complex interplay of reproductive hormones and neurotransmitters. It is important to acknowledge mental symptoms such as irritability,

---

retrograde: retro—backward + grade—step

perimenopausal: peri—around + men(o)—month + pausal—stopping

Lola

■ Lola, age 53, has been experiencing menopausal "hot flashes" during the afternoons as she works in her office.

1. What treatments can you suggest to help with her symptoms?
2. If she considers HRT, what information do you need to share with her?

Suggested answers at end of chapter.

anxiety, insomnia, memory problems, and mild depression as a normal, temporary result of hormonal changes, so that perimenopausal women do not doubt their sanity.

Therapeutic Interventions

Hormone replacement therapy (HRT) is a controversial treatment for perimenopausal symptoms. Medications such as conjugated estrogens (Premarin), estradiol, and medroxyprogesterone acetate (Provera) may be prescribed. The National Heart, Lung, and Blood Institute (NHLBI) of the National Institutes of Health conducted a major research project to study the risks and benefits of combined estrogen and progestin therapy for healthy women. However, the project was halted in July 2002, 3 years early, because of very worrisome results. Positive findings with HRT included a one-third reduction in hip fractures, a 24% reduction in total fractures, and a 37% decrease in colorectal cancer. Disturbing findings included a 26% increase in breast cancer, a 41% increase in strokes, a 29% increase in heart attacks, doubling of venous thromboembolism rates, and an overall 22% increase in cardiovascular disease. It is uncertain what to make of these data because there was no differ-ence in total mortality when comparing women treated with HRT and those given a placebo. Long-term results will continue to be examined, but for now, the risks of HRT have been deemed too great to continue the study.[2] The NHLBI continues to research these issues. Stay updated on the latest findings at http://www.nhlbi.nih.gov/whi/whi_faq.htm.

Dietary changes with the inclusion of **phytoestrogens,** which are present in foods/herbs such as soy, tofu, flax seeds, black cohosh, and dong quai, may provide the benefits of estrogen replacement without necessitating the inclusion of HRT. Women should discuss food and herb supplements with their primary care providers before using them.

Prevention of osteoporosis begins in early adulthood. Fair-skinned, Caucasian women are at greatest risk for bone loss. Throughout life, adequate intake of calcium and vitamin D (preferably from foods) and regular weight-bearing exercise help to maximize bone mass. At menopause, some women may receive HRT or intensive treatment with bone-building medications to retard bone loss. See Table 42.2 for a summary of medications used for hormonal problems.

Complications

It is important to note that resumption of vaginal bleeding after menstruation has finally ceased can be a sign of endometrial cell disorder caused by either benign changes, such as polyps, or malignant changes of internal reproductive organs. Bleeding that occurs following previous cessation should always be investigated.

Nursing Care and Teaching

Patients who are perimenopausal often ask nurses about how to cope effectively with symptoms. Planning ahead for hot flashes by dressing in clothing that may be removed or applied in layers makes adjustment easier. Not allowing hot flashes to interrupt activities is an important strategy, as is

---

phytoestrogens: phyto—plant + estrogens—hormones

TABLE 42.2 MEDICATIONS FOR DISORDERS RELATED TO HORMONAL ALTERATIONS (BREAST DISORDERS, MENSTRUAL DISORDERS, MENOPAUSE)

Medication Class/Action	Examples	Route	Side Effects	Nursing Implications
Oral Contraceptives/ HRT Interfere with gonadotropin-releasing hormone, luteinizing hormone (LH), and follicle-stimulating hormone (FSH) release; maintain stable hormonal levels, relax uterus, limit endometrial proliferation, promote vasomotor stability, prevent bone loss	**Combination:** **Progesterone and Estrogen** Norethindrone/levonorgestral/medroxyprogesterone and ethinyl estradiol/conjugated estrogens (Ortho-Novum, Alesse, Prempro)	PO	Hypertension, breakthrough bleeding, amenorrhea, headache, increased risk of gallbladder/liver disease and thromboembolitic disorders secondary to hypercoagulation, glucose intolerance, decreased breast milk production, depression	Educate patient regarding use and side effects. Include education about the "ACHES" side effects presented later in this chapter, as they may indicate presence of serious, detrimental body system involvement.

Medication Class/Action	Examples	Route	Side Effects	Nursing Implications
	Estrogen Only	PO		
	Conjugated estrogens (Premarin)			
	Progesterone Only	PO		
	Norethindrone/ medroxyprogesterone (Micronor, Provera)			
NSAIDs Inhibit prostaglandin synthesis, therefore interrupt pain receptors and produce anti-inflammatory effect	Ibuprofen (Motrin, Nuprin, Advil)	PO	Peptic ulcer or GI perforations, GI bleeding, bleeding tendency, rash, pruritus, liver/renal dysfunction	Avoid with aspirin allergy; administer with milk or food, caution about side effects, use during pregnancy, or using when on anticoagulant therapy.
	Naproxen (Aleve)	PO		
	Ketoprofen (Orudis)	PO		
Antineoplastic Medications Acts as estrogen antagonist to inhibit growth of estrogen-dependent tumors	Tamoxifen citrate (Novo-Tamoxifen)	PO	Vasomotor changes, menstrual changes, increased vaginal discharge, endometrial hyperplasia/polyps, rash, bone pain, retinopathy (with high doses)	Report vaginal bleeding, leg cramps, shortness of breath, weakness. Promote use of non-hormonal contraceptives when using medication.

engaging in satisfying and calming activities that contribute to a sense of serenity. Treatment of vaginal symptoms with a water-soluble moisture restorer or lubricant or with an estrogen cream (following prescription directions) can help. Eating a healthy diet that is light in caffeine, sugar, and alcohol can help women better control their bodies and minds. Looking forward to new challenges rather than toward the past may help to counteract depressive tendencies occurring with hormonal changes. It is important to remind perimenopausal women that they may still be fertile after several months of **amenorrhea.** To prevent conception, they need to continue to practice birth control until they receive confirmation from their primary care provider that menopause is complete.

See Box 42.3 for a summary of menstrual disorders.

IRRITATIONS AND INFLAMMATIONS OF THE VAGINA AND VULVA

Several causative agents can irritate the vulva and the vagina. Signs and symptoms are often similar, but there are some differences in the discharge produced in response to the disorders. See Table 42.3 for common vaginal irritations and inflammations that are not generally sexually transmitted. See Chapter 44 for information on sexually transmitted diseases.

Pathophysiology, Etiologies, and Signs and Symptoms

The normal vaginal environment is a balanced ecosystem with a pH of less than 4.2 as a result of lactic acid and hydrogen peroxide production by cells in the vagina. This acidic pH protects against the growth of many pathogenic microorganisms. A variety of normal resident microorganisms coexist relatively harmoniously unless the ecological balance is destroyed. Candidiasis, bacterial **vaginosis,** and **cytolytic** vaginitis are all instances of overgrowth of normally present, nonpathogenic microorganisms. Trichomoniasis also is included here because it can be transmitted nonsexually (on fomites, such as toilet seats), as well as sexually, and it grows well when the vaginal environment is disturbed.

Several conditions can predispose patients to an overgrowth of resident microbes: poor nutrition (especially diets high in simple sugars), inconsistent control of blood glucose levels in patients with diabetes, stress, pregnancy, marked hormonal fluctuations, pH changes, prolonged overheating of the genital area with little aeration (as happens with sitting still for long periods in overly restrictive clothing), and changes in the balance of vaginal flora types because of antibiotic treatment or douching. Patients who have a compromised immune system may experience frequent overgrowth of resident microbes, and, conversely, vaginal infections can make women more susceptible to

---

amenorrhea: a—without + men(o)—month + rrhea—flow

vaginosis: vagin—vagina + osis—condition

Box 42.3

Menstrual Disorders Summary

Signs and Symptoms	Increase/decrease in menstrual flow Increased pain with menses or generalized abdominal pain Structural change of the internal reproductive organs Fluid retention Headaches Breast pain/lesions/swelling Mood changes
Diagnostic Tests and Findings	Hormone levels Pregnancy test Pap smear Cervical/vaginal cultures Urine testing Ultrasound Laparoscopy Biopsy
Therapeutic Interventions	Medication to stabilize hormone levels NSAIDs D&C, laser ablation, hysterectomy Treatment of underlying causes Vitamin/mineral supplements Diuretics/SSRIs/dietary changes (PMS)
Priority Nursing Diagnoses	Deficient fluid volume r/t increased bleeding Pain r/t cramping Sexual dysfunction r/t menstrual disorders

D&C = dilation and curettage; NSAIDs = nonsteroidal anti-inflammatory drugs; r/t = related to; SSRIs = serotonin reuptake inhibitors.

infection with sexually transmitted diseases, such as gonorrhea and human immunodeficiency virus (HIV). Frequent and persistent yeast infections may be one sign of HIV. Vaginosis (overgrowth) and vaginitis (inflammation) can sometimes produce irritation and inflammation in the male sexual partner as well and may lead to urethritis, **balanitis,** excoriation, and sores on the penis. A variety of anti-infective medications are used for these disorders (Table 42.4). If the male partner is not also treated, he may reactivate the problem for the woman. Therefore, several types of medication come in "partner packs" for both partners to use.

balanitis: balan—acorn (shape of glans penis) + itis—inflammation

Nursing Care and Teaching of the Patient Undergoing Diagnostic Testing

The patient may feel embarrassed to speak about what is bothering her. A safe question to begin with for most patients is, "Hello. What can I write on your chart as the reason for your visit today?" If embarrassment is evident, a comment that you need to know a bit about what materials to put out for examination purposes often defuses an uncomfortable situation. As you set up materials for a pelvic examination, swabs, and cultures, you can explain that some information is needed to determine how to treat the problem. (See Chapter 41.) Often this is a good time to ask about the discharge and other signs and symptoms using the WHAT'S UP? format. (See Chapter 1.) Allow the patient privacy while she changes into a gown. Return to the room if requested as a chaperone, assistant, and support for the woman. NOTE: If any wet mount slides are made, these must be taken to the laboratory immediately while still wet. Use standard precautions to transport samples. Although swabs may be taken for culture, the health-care provider may prescribe medication before the results of the swabs return because such irritations are so uncomfortable.

SAFETY TIP

Use at least two patient identifiers (neither to be the patient's location) whenever collecting laboratory samples or administering medications or blood products, and use two identifiers to label sample collection containers in the presence of the patient (2006 National Patient Safety Goals from www.JCAHO.org).

Nursing Care and Teaching of the Patient Undergoing Treatment

Vaginal inflammations and infections may require oral medication or local application of medication either in cream, suppository, or medicated douche form. Depending on the practice standards in the area, the nurse may apply this for patients who are unable to do this for themselves or may teach patients to self-administer. Anatomically, the vagina slopes back toward the sacrum for approximately the length of an adult finger (although it can stretch longer). Application is easiest when the patient is lying down ready to sleep because vaginal medications tend to run out when the patient stands or sits. Medicated douches may be administered with the patient sitting on a bedpan with the bed in semi-Fowler's position or, if self-administered, while sitting on a toilet. Most vaginal medications come with an applicator that either injects a dose of creamy medication or pushes a firmer, shaped dose of medication off the end of the tube when the plunger is depressed. Consult instructions supplied with the medication. Patients should be instructed to use all the medication as prescribed and to wear an absorbent pad to prevent possible staining of clothing.

TABLE 42.3 COMMON VAGINAL IRRITATIONS AND INFLAMMATIONS

Disorder and Etiology	Signs and Symptoms	Discharge/ Examination	Diagnostic Tests	Usual Treatment
Candidiasis: *Candida albicans, glabrata,* or *tropicalis* overgrowth	Burning, itching, redness of vulva; burning on urination	White, cottage cheese appearance	Wet mount slides (yeasts look like tiny, budding tree branches); may be cultured	Antifungals (drugs mostly ending in *-azole*)
Bacterial vaginosis: *Gardnerella vaginalis, Mycoplasma,* or anaerobe overgrowth	None or vulvar or vaginal irritation	White or gray, homogeneous, foul-smelling discharge; pH higher than 4.5	Wet mount slides show "clue cells" or release fishy odor when potassium hydroxide is applied	Drugs such as metronidazole or clindamycin
Trichomoniasis: *Trichomonas vaginalis* (may be transmitted by inanimate objects or sexually)	Itching, irritation, foul odor, redness, dysuria	Discharge may be frothy; pH higher than 4.5; "strawberry cervix" resulting from petechiae	Wet mount slides treated with normal saline show motile cells with flagella (like tiny whips); may also be cultured	Metronidazole, 2-g single dose
Cytolytic vaginosis: Lactobacilli overgrowth, stress, some medications	Burning, irritation, pain with intercourse	Nonodorous, thick, white, pasty, or dry and flaking	Lower than normal pH as tested with pH indicator tape (or litmus strip); may be cultured	Depends on cause; alkaline douches may be prescribed
Contact vulvo vaginitis: contact with allergens or irritating chemicals such as contraceptive creams or bubble baths	Itching, burning, redness	Generally no change from normal discharge, though may be increased	History and physical information, recent contact with chemicals	Avoidance of the offending substance; warm sitz baths or application of hydrocortisone cream
Atrophic vaginitis: estrogen levels too low to support estrogen-sensitive vaginal tissues	Vulvovaginal irritation, less lubrication, dyspareunia, increased tendency for resident microbe overgrowth	May have little or increased discharge; discharge may be watery, yellow, or green; may be blood-tinged	Maturation index may be determined during Pap test to identify atrophic cellular changes, but diagnosis is usually by history and physical information only	HRT (oral, patch, or vulvovaginal cream) or water-soluble lubricant replacing vaginal lubricants

TABLE 42.4 MEDICATIONS FOR IRRITATIONS AND INFLAMMATIONS OF THE VAGINA AND VULVA

Medication Class/Action	Examples	Route	Side Effects	Nursing Implications
Antibiotics				
Inhibit bacterial protein synthesis	Clindamycin (Cleocin)	Intravaginal	Candidiasis, pruritus, rash, hypersensitivity, abdominal pain Overgrowth of other infectious organisms	Education on correct use; use as directed even if symptoms cease. Report change in symptoms.
Antifungals				
Believed to bind to sterol in fungal cell membrane, thereby altering cell permeability	Fluconazole (Diflucan) Miconazole (Monistat) Terconazole (Terazol) Clotrimazole (Gyne-Lotrimin)	PO Topical to external genitalia; intravaginal	Pruritus, rash, hypersensitivity, abdominal pain	Education on correct use; use as directed even if symptoms cease. Report side effects.
Antiprotozoal				
Enters cells of microorganisms that contain nitroreductase, interferes with DNA synthesis and causes cell death	Metronidazole (Flagyl)	PO	Dizziness, weakness, insomnia, abdominal cramping, anorexia, nausea/diarrhea/emesis, vaginal dryness, overgrowth of other infectious organisms	Teach patient to avoid alcohol use while on medication and for 48 hours after completion. Use medication as directed, even if symptoms cease. Take with meals. Treat partner.

TOXIC SHOCK SYNDROME

Pathophysiology, Etiologies, and Signs and Symptoms

Toxic shock syndrome (TSS), first identified in 1978, is primarily associated with superabsorbent tampon use during menstruation but can also occur with use of nasal packings, or in other individuals with no specific risk factors. It is a severe systemic infection with strains of *Staphylococcus aureus,* which produce an epidermal toxin. The effect of the toxin on the liver, kidneys, and circulatory system makes this a life-threatening condition. A streptococcal infection can cause a similar syndrome.

Individuals with TSS may experience a sudden high fever with sore throat, headache, dizziness, confusion, redness of the palms and soles of the feet, skin rashes, blisters, and petechiae followed by peeling of the skin. Muscle weakness, muscle pain, and gastrointestinal upset also have been reported. Signs and symptoms such as these should be reported to the health-care provider immediately.

Prevention

Tampon makers have removed the highly absorbent fibers that were most often associated with the syndrome from their product lines, and TSS is now rare. Women can also reduce their risk of developing TSS by substituting sanitary pads for tampons at least part of the time (nighttime use may work well); changing tampons every 4 hours; washing hands carefully before inserting anything into the vagina; not leaving female barrier contraceptives in place for longer than needed; and not using tampons or female barrier contraceptives in the first 12 weeks after giving birth.

Nursing Care and Teaching

All menstruating women should be taught measures to prevent TSS. They should also be taught to recognize symptoms of TSS because early identification and treatment can save lives.

DISORDERS RELATED TO THE DEVELOPMENT OF THE GENITAL ORGANS

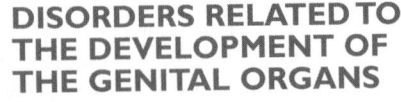

Pathophysiology, Etiologies, and Signs and Symptoms

Several types of congenital malformations of the reproductive organs may affect the health of female patients. Genetic or environmental factors during pregnancy may cause these, and they may require medical or surgical treatment at some point in life. **Agenesis** of structures means that they never

developed. **Hypoplasia** of reproductive tract portions means that they are underdeveloped. **Imperforate** means that expected openings do not exist. Blind pouches exist where cavities should meet but do not. The uterus can form in several different configurations, including a double uterus.

Many malformations are discovered during childhood or early adolescence, but some are identified when patients seek medical help because of dysmenorrhea, **dyspareunia** (pain with intercourse), infertility, repeated spontaneous abortions (miscarriages), or preterm labor when pregnant.

Diagnostic Tests

Procedures such as ultrasonography, hysterosalpingography, computed tomography (CT), magnetic resonance imaging (MRI), and endoscopic examinations may be used to determine the type and extent of developmental defects.

Therapeutic Interventions

Some defects can be repaired surgically, but others cannot. Depending on the type and location of the defect, surgeries may be done by endoscopy or by surgical incision. Absence of hormone-producing tissue may be overcome by hormone supplements.

Nursing Care and Teaching

Patients who have these problems may struggle with self-esteem issues, such as feeling that they are somehow incomplete or have been cheated of something they desire. You can show that you are willing to listen if and when the patient wishes to talk while allowing her as much privacy as she desires.

Displacement Disorders

Pathophysiology, Etiologies, and Signs and Symptoms

The pelvic organs are suspended within the pelvis by ligaments and supported by muscles and fascia. The pubococcygeal muscle runs from the pubis to the coccyx and supplies support from below. Pregnancies (especially those producing large babies) and rapid or traumatic deliveries may result in stretching and injury of the supporting structures, which can cause displacement of the uterus, vagina, bladder, or bowel from its normal position. The observation that some children have defective muscular support of the pelvic organs and that prolapse is more prevalent in some families seems to suggest that congenital defects and genetic inheritance may also influence displacement disorders even without pregnancy. Scarring from sexually transmitted diseases also may cause some displacement of the pelvic organs. Aging generally increases the problem because the effects of gravity over time contribute to stretching, and lower estrogen levels weaken estrogen-dependent supportive tissues. Chronic

---

hypoplasia: hypo—little + plasia—shape (or form)
imperforate: im—not + perforate—pierced
dyspareunia: dys—painful or abnormal + pareunia—mating

---

agenesis: a—without + genesis—production

constipation, obesity, and lack of exercise also worsen these problems.

Therapeutic Interventions

A pessary is a supportive (usually ring-shaped) device that is placed in the proximal end of the vagina to help support the pelvic organs. These are usually removed daily at bedtime for cleaning, but some types are designed to remain in the vagina for months at a time. When pessary use is begun, it is important that the woman return to the physician for a recheck after an initial period of use to determine whether the pessary is causing pressure damage to tissues. Because the pessary is a foreign object in the vagina, increased vaginal discharge may be expected. Discharge should not be pink, bloody, or purulent.

Nursing Care and Teaching

Teach patients to eat a healthy diet to avoid obesity and constipation and how to do Kegel exercises to keep the pubococcygeal muscle strong to support the organs in the pelvic cavity. There are several variations of such exercises. The important idea is that the appropriate muscles are exercised adequately to strengthen and build up the ability to control muscle contractions.

1. To find the pubococcygeal muscle, tighten while urinating so that the flow of urine stops.
2. Squeeze the muscle that stopped urinary flow tightly, holding for 10 seconds, and totally relaxing the muscle afterward. Repeat 15 times per day.
3. Practice controlling the muscle by contracting and relaxing it to move the pelvic floor upward and downward very slowly. Thinking of an elevator helps some women. Repeat this 15 times per day.

NURSING CARE TIP

Teach patients to do Kegel exercises while waiting in lines to use otherwise wasted time to promote their health. Another suggestion is to plan specific times of day or activities that would include Kegel exercises, such as while in a car or working at a computer.

These exercises can be done anywhere and are not apparent to anyone watching.

Cystocele

Pathophysiology, Etiologies, and Signs and Symptoms

Cystocele occurs when the bladder sags into the vaginal space because of inadequate support (Fig. 42.5). A feeling of pelvic pressure and stress incontinence are common with this condition.

Therapeutic Interventions

Kegel exercises or the use of a pessary may help. If these measures are ineffective, anterior **colporrhaphy**, which is a surgical repair of the anterior portion of the vagina, may be necessary to correct this problem. Another possible surgical treatment involves resuspending the bladder.

---

cystocele: cysto—bag (bladder) + cele—hernia
colporrhaphy: colpo—vagina + rrhaphy—suture

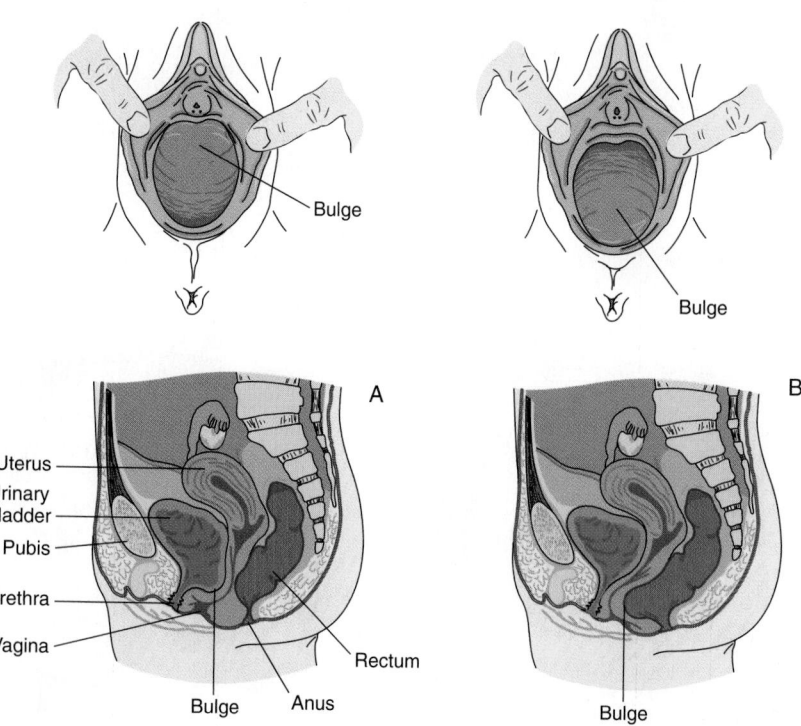

FIGURE 42.5 *(A)* Cystocele. *(B)* Rectocele.

Rectocele

Pathophysiology, Etiologies, and Signs and Symptoms

Rectocele occurs when a portion of the rectum sags into the vagina because of inadequate support (see Fig. 42.5). A feeling of pelvic pressure, as well as fecal incontinence, constipation, and hemorrhoids, may result.

Therapeutic Interventions

Kegel exercises may help strengthen the supporting muscles. The patient should maintain bowel regularity with a high-fiber diet to avoid further discomfort and sagging from bowel overdistention. Posterior colporrhaphy may be necessary to correct this problem.

Uterine Position Disorders

Pathophysiology, Etiologies, and Signs and Symptoms

The most common variations in position of the uterus are **anteversion, anteflexion,** retroversion, and **retroflexion** (Fig. 42.6). In anteversion, the uterus lies too far forward, and in retroversion, it lies too far backward. In anteflexion,

---

rectocele: recto—rectum + cele—hernia
anteversion: ante—front + version—turning
anteflexion: ante—front + flexion—bending
retroflexion: retro—back + flexion—bending

---

the upper portion of the uterus bends forward, and in retroflexion, it bends backward.

Symptoms that may result from these uterine displacements include painful menstruation and intercourse, infertility, and repeated spontaneous abortion.

Therapeutic Interventions

A pessary may correct some positional problems. If infertility or recurrent spontaneous abortion is involved or the condition is very painful, surgery to correct the condition may be undertaken.

Uterine Prolapse

Pathophysiology, Etiologies, and Signs and Symptoms

Uterine prolapse occurs when the uterus sags into the vagina (Fig. 42.7). The amount of sagging can vary and may increase over time as a result of the effects of gravity, poor pelvic support, and excessive lifting or straining. In first-degree prolapse, less than half the uterus sags into the vagina. In second-degree prolapse, the entire uterus sags into the vagina. In third-degree prolapse, the uterus sags outside the body.

Uterine prolapse can be very uncomfortable, resulting in back pain, pelvic pain, pain with intercourse (or inability to have intercourse), urinary incontinence, constipation, and the development of hemorrhoids. The pressure on the uterus also may compromise circulation, resulting in tissue necrosis. Vaginal vault prolapse may also occur in

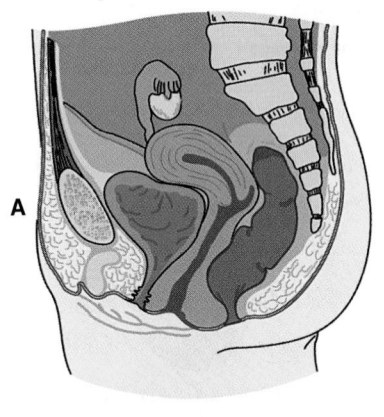
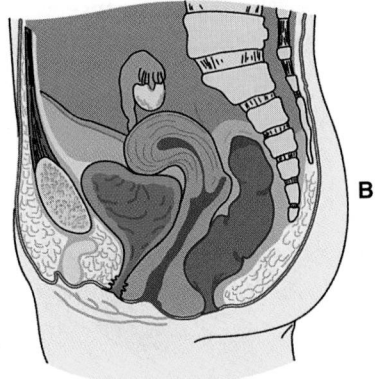
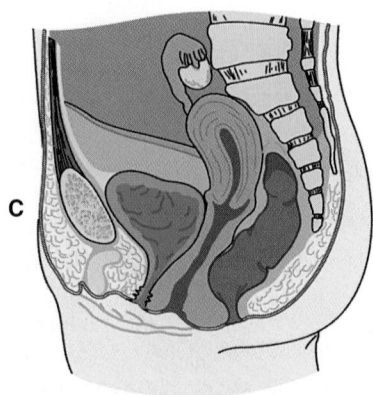
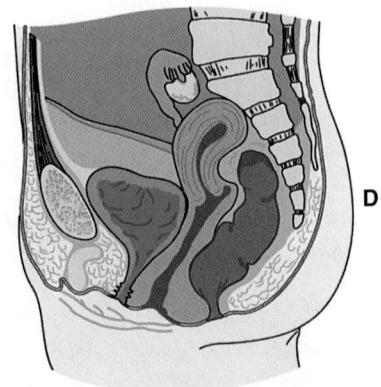

FIGURE 42.6 Uterine positions. (A) Anteversion. (B) Anteflection. (C) Retroversion. (D) Retroflexion.

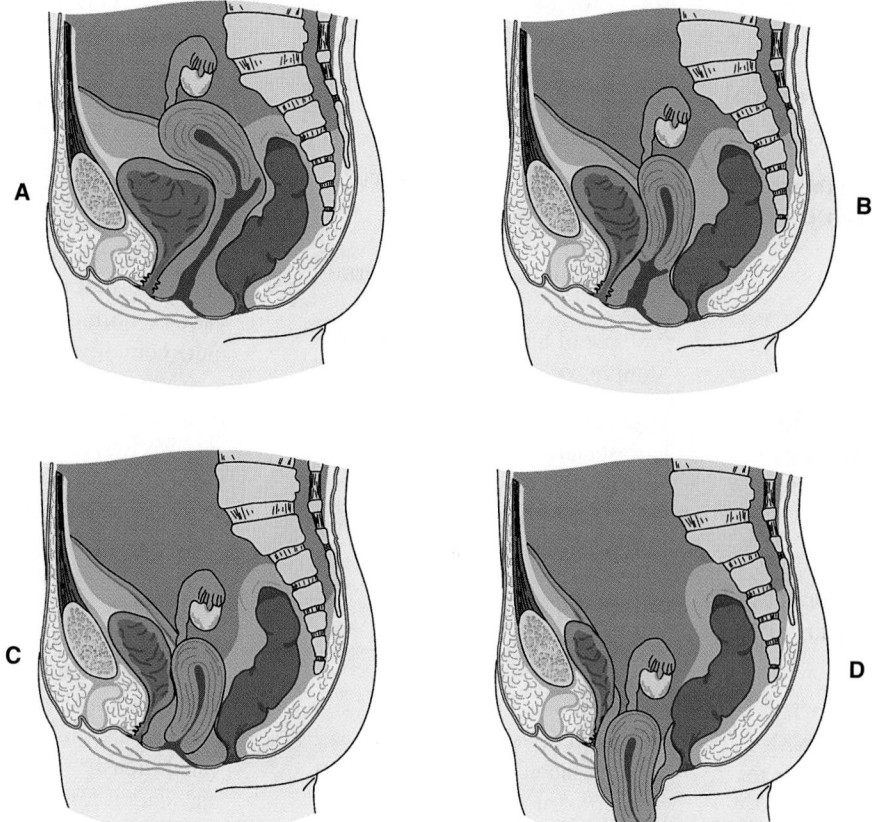

FIGURE 42.7 Uterine prolapse. (A) Normal uterus. (B) First-degree prolapse: Descent within the vagina. (C) Second-degree prolapse. (D) Third-degree prolapse: The vagina is completely everted.

women who have had a hysterectomy, so that the vagina turns inside out and sags downward with similar signs and symptoms. This condition generally requires surgical resuspension.

Therapeutic Interventions

Some of the more minor uterine displacements may be treated with use of a pessary. Kegel exercises may be more effective in prevention of uterine prolapse than in treatment because, once the tissues become stretched sufficiently for the uterus to sag into the vagina, the continued weight of the uterus prevents adequate contraction of the muscles. Surgery may be done to correct this problem. Although the uterus may be resuspended by shortening the muscles and fascia, hysterectomy is the more common treatment unless further childbearing is desired.

See Box 42.4 for a summary of structural disorders.

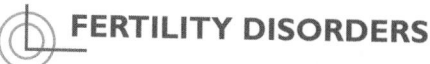 **FERTILITY DISORDERS**

Infertility is a complicated problem that must be considered according to the causative factors. Some couples with infertility may have multiple reproductive problems. Both male and female partners should be examined. (See Chapter 43 for greater detail on male reproductive system disorders.) Often the woman sees the health-care provider first and may be given a specimen container and advised to give the container to her partner for provision of a semen sample for

analysis. See Table 42.5 for a summary of fertility disorders and diagnostic tests.

Nursing Care and Teaching of the Patient Undergoing Fertility Testing

An understanding attitude is very important because infertility can be a cause of low self-esteem, as well as relationship problems. Patients who have been undergoing diagnostic testing or treatment for infertility can become very discouraged with the process and the expense, especially if it has been ineffective. Having to plan your sexual activity around a health-care provider's directions can compromise feelings of spontaneity, enjoyment, and privacy. Extensive questioning by nurses can aggravate the situation, but avoiding conversation may convey a lack of caring. A friendly, "Which test shall I help you get ready for today?" may well be enough to get the needed information. Many women undergoing infertility testing are very well informed about the test they will be having and can tell you so that you know which equipment to set out.

On the first infertility investigation visit, the nurse may teach or give a handout to the patient about keeping a precise record of her oral temperatures with a basal thermometer each morning on awakening, before any other activity. The first day of her menses is day 1 on the temperature chart. Changing levels of hormones result in slight temperature changes, which can be used to identify when ovulation seems to be occurring and when particular hormone levels

---

Box 42.4

Structural Disorders of the Genital Organs Summary

Signs and Symptoms	Pain with menses or sexual intercourse Infertility Spontaneous abortion or preterm labor Prolapse of uterus, bladder, or rectum into vagina or outside of body
Diagnostic Tests and Findings	Physical examination Ultrasound Hysterosalpingography CT or MRI scan Endoscopy
Therapeutic Interventions	Kegel exercises Surgery Hormone supplements
Priority Nursing Diagnoses	Acute/chronic pain r/t structural abnormality/surgery Urinary incontinence or constipation r/t structural abnormalities Sexual dysfunction r/t disturbance in self-concept Grief r/t absence/loss of reproductive status

CT = computed tomography; MRI = magnetic resonance imaging.

---

should be tested. Because many factors may influence temperature and cycles, explain that it may take a few months of recording to clearly identify her own pattern.

You may assist with office procedures such as endometrial biopsy, which may be done during a pelvic examination 2 or 3 days before menses is expected. A pregnancy test should be done before this procedure to avoid interfering with a pregnancy. Consult your procedure manual, laboratory manual, or health-care provider for what materials to set up. The woman may receive pain medication and paracervical block anesthesia for the procedure. Assess pulse and blood pressure. A vasovagal reaction treatment kit containing epinephrine (or atropine, according to the health-care provider's choice), a tourniquet, and a syringe should be kept handy for injection if a vasovagal reflex occurs during the procedure. Vasovagal reflex is a reflex stimulation of the vagal nerve that can happen when the cervix, larynx, or trachea is manipulated and results in slowing of the heart rate and decreased cardiac output, so that the blood pressure drops markedly.

Therapeutic Interventions

Treatment of infertility is designed to ensure that an adequate amount of sperm and an ovum can be in close proximity in the most conducive environment for fertilization.

Removal of barriers such as scar tissue may require surgery. Depending on the results of blood tests and the **postcoital** test (described in Table 42.5), adjustments of environmental factors may involve such actions as sperm washing to avoid destructive antigen-antibody responses, changing the pH of the seminal fluid to encourage sperm motility, treating the female partner to prevent substances in her genital tract fluids from disabling the sperm, or adjusting her hormone levels. The number of sperm or ova available may be increased through use of such fertility drugs as clomiphene citrate or various hormone preparations. Infertility treatments are quite complicated and expensive and change periodically as a result of ongoing research. In-depth coverage of these treatments is beyond the scope of this book.

Various methods may be used to bring the gametes into close proximity. If the problem involves inability to get the sperm close enough to the ovum (as may happen with ejaculatory problems), the physician may place a semen sample from the male partner closer to the ovum via a small catheter. **In vitro fertilization** (IVF) involves bringing ova and sperm together outside the bodies of the participants. Ova may be harvested using a long needle or an endoscope after hormonal preparation of the woman. Sperm may be obtained through masturbation; intercourse with a nonlubricated, nonspermicidal condom; or electrical stimulation of ejaculation for patients with spinal cord injuries.

For those whose sperm is unable to successfully penetrate the ovum, procedures involving gamete micromanipulation may be done. Under a microscope, an ovum from the female partner is partially opened by removing a portion of the outer covering to facilitate sperm penetration, or sperm may be injected into the ovum. This fertilized ovum is then reinserted into the woman's body.

When measures to improve the chances of conception using the partners' own gametes are unsuccessful, gametes from donors may be utilized. Artificial insemination by injecting another man's sperm into the genital tract of the female patient is the simplest of the donor procedures. Ova also may be harvested from a donor woman and used for in vitro fertilization using the male partner's sperm if possible. Both these procedures allow for genetic inheritance from one member of the couple. If genetic inheritance is not possible or desirable (as with familial disease carriers), both donor sperm and ova may be used for in vitro fertilization to be transferred into the female patient. Surrogacy is a situation in which an embryo from one couple is placed into a "host" mother for growth of a baby for the couple, and is a topic of much ethical debate.

Nursing Care and Teaching of the Patient Undergoing Treatment

Patients who are undergoing infertility treatment may experience many upsetting and distressing feelings. Feelings of inadequacy, frustration, depression, and anger are common.

---

postcoital: post—after + coital—pertaining to intercourse
in vitro fertilization: in—inside + vitro—glass + fertiliz—fruitful + ation—process

TABLE 42.5 FERTILITY DISORDERS

Disorder	Pathophysiology/Etiology	Diagnostic Tests
Male	Possible anatomic abnormalities, hormonal factors, genetic defects, inflammatory conditions, immune system disorders, difficulties with sexual function or technique, psychological factors, or exogenous influences such as drug use, radiation or chemical exposure, trauma, and excessive testicular temperatures (as may occur with prolonged hot tub use or too-tight clothing)	Semen analysis of number, condition, and movement of the sperm and composition of seminal fluid using various tests
Female: Ovulation	Possible anatomic and physiological abnormalities of ovaries; hormonal balance problems related to hypothalamus, thyroid, or adrenal glands; or polycystic ovary syndrome	Basal body temperature charting, midluteal serum progesterone blood levels, luteinizing hormone levels, blood or urine testing, ultrasound monitoring of a follicle for evidence of release of ovum, endometrial biopsy, observation of male hair distribution, and other hormone testing as indicated
Tubal	Possible obstruction of the fallopian tubes resulting from anatomic variations, scarring, or adhesions; prior surgeries; and inflammatory processes involving other abdominal tissues	Hysterosalpingography (described in Chapter 41), laparoscopy
Uterine	Possible abnormalities in shape or blockages within the uterus (rare cause of infertility but a potential cause of pregnancy loss before maturity), menstrual disorders involving the endometrium	Hysteroscopy (described in Chapter 41), removal of tissue samples using curet or endoscope
Other Sources of Infertility	Possible reproductive environmental factors such as destructive antigen-antibody responses, inappropriate pH of seminal fluid for maximal sperm motility, or substances in female partner's genital tract fluids that disable sperm	Postcoital test: couple is advised to have intercourse when luteinizing hormone and estrogen levels are high, then a specimen of cervical mucus is taken from the woman 2–12 hours later for analysis of reproductive environment

If the infertility was caused by something the patient perceives as avoidable, such as sexually transmitted disease, guilt feelings may add to the psychological discomfort. Any or all of the previously described tests may be completed and some repeated many times without success in identification of underlying etiology for infertility, and may result in repeated disappointments. Some patients cling to the hope that new tests and treatments are being developed that may help them, whereas others feel that they are being used as a "guinea pig" for development of new strategies. The beginning of menses may signal a time of mourning for these couples. Depression may result after failed IVF attempts. Strained relationships may develop between marriage partners, especially if there is disagreement about the value of testing or the importance of having children.

Usually more than the desired number of embryos is implanted because it is expected that not all will survive and because this is more cost effective with less physical risk for the mother. However, this requires heart-wrenching decisions of whether to "reduce" (abort) extra pregnancies or to risk having more than the desired number of children at once as a result of the fertility treatments.

Offer a listening ear while being careful not to give advice about treatment modalities. There are many ongoing debates among researchers and practitioners as to the value of particular procedures; consequently, strategies may vary widely from one health-care provider to another. Encourage open communication among the patient, the health-care provider, and the patient's significant other, and encourage decision making that is informed and based on the patient's values.

Many varieties of assistive reproductive technology are available, and the number is increasing with research. Most of the procedures are called by acronyms (names developed by using first letters of each descriptor). For example, *GIFT* means "gamete intrafallopian transfer" (gametes are placed together in the fallopian tube with the hope that fertilization will occur). *ZIFT* means "zygote intrafallopian transfer" (fertilization of gametes occurs outside of the body; the conceptus is then placed into a woman's fallopian tube to make the journey to the uterus). Acronyms can be a useful shortcut but can be confusing. Most nurses probably do not need to know all acronyms of infertility treatments unless they work in a gynecologist's office or infertility clinic. Knowing that words in all capital letters are generally acronyms helps understanding of many procedures.

REPRODUCTIVE LIFE PLANNING

Reproductive life planning is a more comprehensive term than *contraception* and implies reasoned decisions related to pregnancy timing and whether or not to have children. Nurses can contribute to the overall health and quality of life for women and families by assisting them to find the information they need to make wise choices.

There are many different types of birth control available and several additional types are in developmental and testing stages. General categories of agents are discussed in this chapter. General knowledge of how the different types of contraceptives work can assist the nurse in answering patients' questions or helping patients find additional information. This section is not intended to be a substitute for discussion with the health-care provider or for information supplied with individual products.

No numerical statements of effectiveness are included here because several different sets of statistics are currently in use. It seems likely that as products improve, hormone dosages are changed, or more data come in from users, the numbers will be adjusted. Methods are introduced in the order of general effectiveness from most to least effective (with the exception that experimental methods are discussed at the end regardless of their efficacy). Consult your clinic or health-care provider for an approved, current comparison list of methods for distribution.

For some patients, the distinction of whether the birth control method actually prevents conception or only interferes with implantation or maintenance of a pregnancy is an important factor in their decision. If a patient believes life begins at conception, any action other than prevention of conception would be considered equivalent to abortion.

Oral Contraceptives

Oral **contraceptive** medications are among the most widely used forms of birth control in North America. Most contain an estrogen and a progestin in combination, although some (minipills) contain only a progestin. Some work to prevent conception by inhibiting ovulation or changing the environment of the reproductive tract so that activity of the sperm is inhibited. Others do not prevent conception but make implantation less likely and hasten the breakdown of the corpus luteum so that pregnancy-sustaining hormones are not produced. Many of the adverse effects that occurred in the past have been overcome by adjustment of dosage levels.

Oral contraceptives may also be used in some instances to regulate irregular menses to decrease dysmenorrhea, or to decrease the symptoms associated with endometriosis or cyclic breast changes. There is much debate about whether hormonal contraceptive agents may offer some protection against some sexually transmitted diseases (STDs) based on lower statistical rates of STDs among oral contraceptive users. However, cellular changes of the cervix seen with hormonal contraceptive use actually tend to be associated with higher rates of some sexually transmitted diseases.[3] Unless some specific mechanism of prevention is demonstrated by research, it seems irresponsible to suggest that oral contraceptives alone offer protection against anything other than pregnancy. Therefore, women should still be advised about the risks of contracting sexually transmitted diseases while taking an oral contraceptive.

Advantages, Disadvantages, Side Effects, and Risks

Oral contraceptives are very effective. Improvement of dysmenorrhea, endometriosis, increased regularity of menses, and decrease in menstrual flow may occur; however, some women experience menstrual changes such as amenorrhea, irregular or prolonged menses, and intermenstrual spotting. They require a great deal of commitment because irregular use decreases effectiveness. To encourage regular use, oral contraceptives are generally dispensed in containers labeled with the days of the week, and some companies include unmedicated pills in the package to be taken during the time of hormone cessation for menses, so that the woman only has to remember to take a daily pill, not specific to her cycle.

Some women experience side effects such as acne, fluid retention, headaches, breast swelling and discomfort, mid cycle bleeding, and sometimes depression. Use of an oral contraceptive also has some risks. Higher rates of blood clot formation, strokes, high blood pressure, heart attacks, and worsening of diabetes are rare occurrences with some hormonal contraceptives and are generally related to preexistent disease entities. Women who smoke or have diabetes, high blood pressure, heart disease, or a history of thrombophlebitis should receive counseling about the risks of oral contraceptives and education about alternative methods of contraception.

Oral contraceptives decrease the risk of endometrial and ovarian cancer, but there is debate about risk of breast cancer, and cervical **dysplasia** (cell changes that may become cancerous) sometimes occurs among oral contraceptive users. Women should definitely be advised to have regular annual (or more frequent if abnormalities develop) Pap smears while taking oral contraceptives.

Many medications can alter the effectiveness of oral contraceptives, and women should be warned always to alert health-care providers and pharmacists that they are on an oral contraceptive whenever a new medication is to be started or a regular medication is discontinued. Use of hormonal contraceptives increases the risk of vitamin B deficiencies, so a healthy diet with good sources of B vitamins is advisable.

LEARNING TIP

Side effects of oral contraceptives can be serious. Teach your patient to watch for "ACHES," and to contact her primary care provider immediately if they occur. ACHES stands for:
Abdominal pain
Chest pain
Headache
Eye pain
Severe leg pain

---

contraceptive: contra—against + ceptive—taking in (conceiving)

dysplasia: dys—painful or abnormal + plasia—shape or form

Contraceptive Implants

Contraceptive implants are small permeable tubes surgically implanted through a small incision under the skin; they slowly release medication for long-term contraception. Implants have been used with varying success. Currently, none is being used due to the unreliability of effectiveness and complications related to use. However, the use of a single tube is being considered. An implant containing nomegestrol acetate (Uniplant) implanted under the skin of the upper arm or in the gluteal region has been tested in clinical trials and has been found to be effective for 1 year. It will likely be available in the near future.

Depot Medications

Medroxyprogesterone acetate (Depo-Provera) is a contraceptive agent available in a slow-release (depot) form that can be injected intramuscularly. Medication is continuously released for 3 months.

Advantages, Disadvantages, Side Effects, and Risks

The main advantage of depot medications is that the woman does not have to remember to take medication daily. Disadvantages are that the medication is not immediately effective, so another method is necessary for the first 2 weeks after the initial injection, and that fertility may not return for several months to 1 year after cessation of injections.

Alterations in menstrual flow, especially amenorrhea, are the most commonly noted side effects. Weight gain of 5 to 10 pounds is also common, which can lead to discontinuation of use. Other side effects and risks are similar to those encountered with oral contraceptives that contain progesterone only.

Estrogen-Progestogen Contraceptive Ring

A newer method is an estrogen-progestogen contraceptive ring (NuvaRing). It works in much the same manner as other hormonal contraceptives by slowly releasing hormones. The user inserts the ring into the vagina around the cervix, similar to a diaphragm. The ring is left in place for 3 weeks and then removed for 1 week in order for menses to occur.

Advantages, Disadvantages, Side Effects, and Risks

Not having to remember daily medication can be an advantage to the contraceptive ring, but failing to remove it at the right time may disrupt the regularity of the menstrual cycles. With consistent use, it is very effective in preventing pregnancy. Since it does not provide a barrier over the cervix, there is less risk of infection than with a diaphragm or cervical cap. A common side effect is an increase in normal vaginal discharge. Other side effects and risks are similar to other low-dose hormonal contraceptives.

Transdermal Contraceptive Patch

A transdermal patch is now available that contains norelgestromin and ethinyl estradiol (Ortho Evra). This patch is placed on the abdomen, upper arm, or buttock following a menstrual period and left in place for 1 week. A new patch is placed on the body each week for 3 weeks. After 3 weeks, the patch is removed and not replaced for 1 week in order for menses to occur.

Advantages, Disadvantages, Side Effects, and Risks

The contraceptive patch has been found to be similar to oral contraceptives in effectiveness, side effects, and risks, without having to remember to take a pill each day. Bathing, swimming, and other activities can continue as the patch will remain where placed.

Barrier Methods

Barrier methods of birth control are less effective in preventing pregnancy than most of the previously mentioned methods when used alone. Barriers are intended to prevent sperm from reaching the ovum. There are several forms of barrier contraceptives. Used in combination, effectiveness of barrier methods and spermicidal preparations come close to that of oral contraceptives. Spermicidal preparations may be purchased without a prescription.

Condoms

Condoms are to be used once and then discarded into an appropriate waste receptacle. They should be stored in a cool, dry place before use and should not be stored tightly pressed because heat and continued pressure can weaken them. Storage in a wallet or glove compartment is not advisable. Petroleum-based substances, such as Vaseline, can also weaken condoms, so use of water-soluble lubricants (preferably spermicides) should be advised.

ADVANTAGES, DISADVANTAGES, SIDE EFFECTS, AND RISKS OF MALE CONDOMS. Male condoms have long been used for contraception because they are a relatively inexpensive, totally reversible method that men can control at the time of intercourse. They provide some barrier protection against transmission of sexually transmitted disease organisms as well. An electron microscopic study of a sample of nonlubricated latex condoms, however, found that the majority of those viewed had surface abnormalities, including cracking and melted areas. Patients should be informed that barrier methods can reduce risk but do not absolutely prevent transmission of STDs, especially in areas of contact not covered by the barrier. The main disadvantages of condom use are interruption of foreplay for application, decreased sensation, and the possibility of slippage or breakage during intercourse. These disadvantages may be overcome by incorporating application of the condom by the female partner as a part of foreplay; using thinner, lubricated, or textured condoms to increase sensation; using the correct size condom with a reservoir or applied with approximately half an inch at the tip of the condom loose enough to serve as a reservoir for the semen (Fig. 42.8); and removal from the vagina before relaxation of the erection.

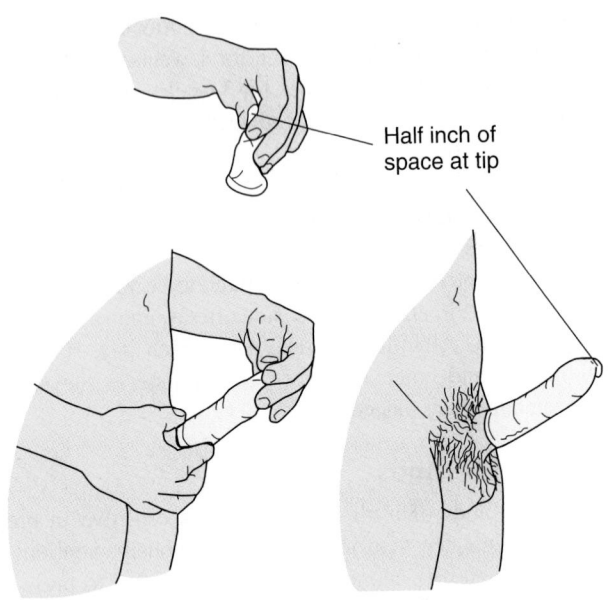

FIGURE 42.8 Correct application of a condom.

ADVANTAGES, DISADVANTAGES, SIDE EFFECTS, AND RISKS OF FEMALE CONDOMS.

Female condoms are a more recent innovation that allows female initiation of contraception, as well as some barrier protection against infection with sexually transmitted diseases. Coverage of the labia by the condom may provide more of a barrier than male condoms (Fig. 42.9). Disadvantages are greater expense than male condoms, decreased sensation, the necessity to apply before intercourse, and the possibility of flaws in the condom material.

Diaphragms and Cervical Caps

Diaphragms and cervical caps work in the same manner by blocking the entry of sperm through the cervix (Fig. 42.10). The barrier effect is enhanced by simultaneous use of a spermicide. Application of a spermicide to the edges of each device, and placement of a small amount in their cups before use, increases effectiveness.

ADVANTAGES, DISADVANTAGES, SIDE EFFECTS, AND RISKS.

These methods are relatively inexpensive, are female initiated, and work without systemic medication. Diaphragms and cervical caps require initial fitting and a prescription to buy them, may need to be refitted after childbirth and the loss or gain of weight, and can last for years. These devices should be replaced periodically as the manufacturer recommends or whenever there is any evidence of hardening, cracking, or thin spots. They need to be washed with soap and water, dried, and stored in a case away from heat and sunlight between uses.

Women and their partners may experience irritation or allergic reaction to the spermicide or the contraceptive device material, which would require changing birth control methods. All these methods require that the device be inserted before intercourse and left in place for several hours after intercourse. (See package insert for recommendations.)

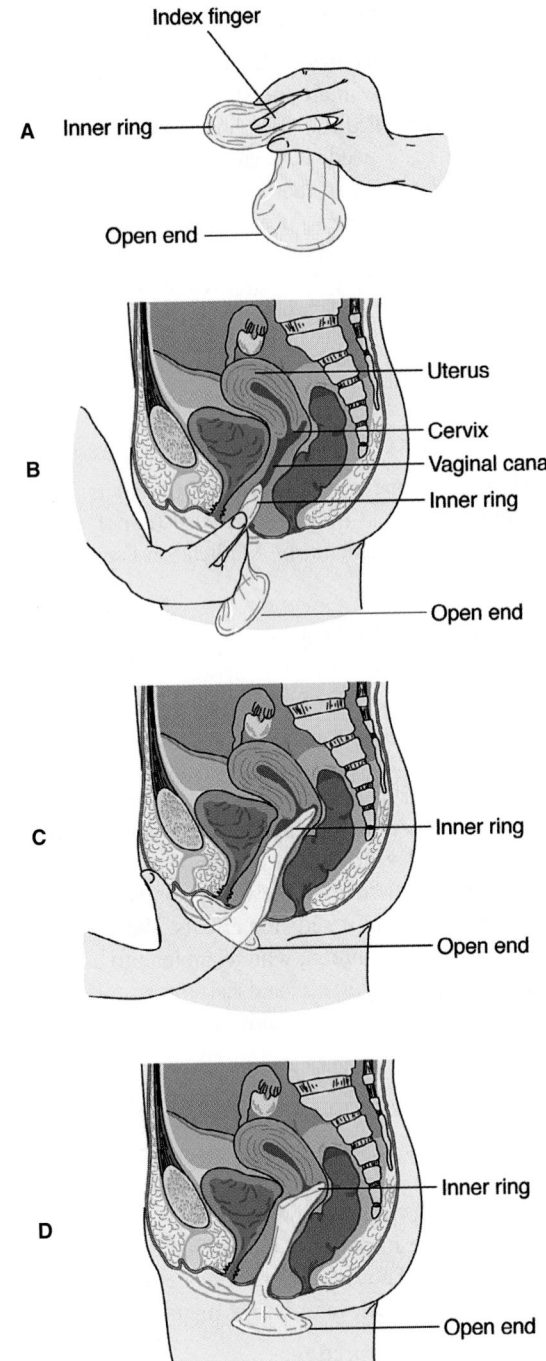

FIGURE 42.9 Female condom application. (A) Inner ring is squeezed for insertion. (B) Sheath is inserted similar to a tampon. (C) Inner ring is pushed up as far as it can go with index finger. (D) Condom in place.

An increase in incidence of urinary tract infection has been reported with use of the diaphragm, and risk of toxic shock syndrome increases with prolonged uninterrupted use of cervical barriers. Adequate fluid intake, voiding shortly after intercourse, and removal of the device when 8 hours have passed since intercourse all help to prevent these potential problems. If urinary tract infections are recurrent using the diaphragm, changing to a cervical cap may decrease the

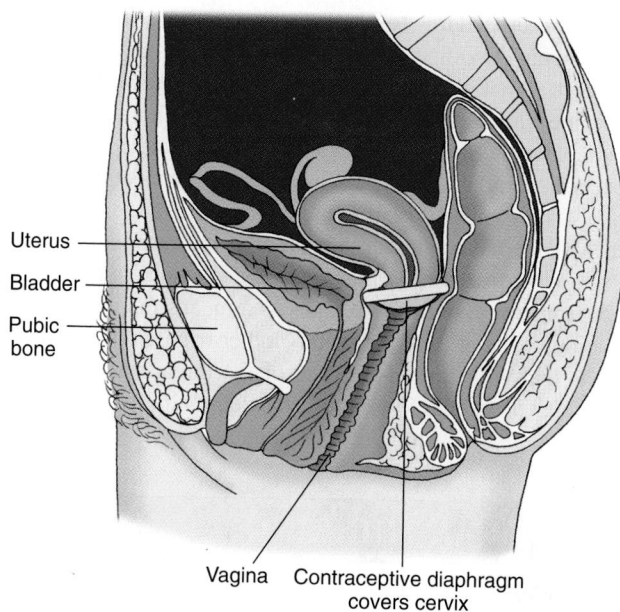

Uterus

Bladder

Pubic
bone

Vagina   Contraceptive diaphragm
covers cervix

FIGURE 42.10 Contraceptive diaphragm.

occurrence because there is less pressure against the bladder through the anterior vagina.

Spermicides

Spermicidal agents may be used alone, although use in combination with a barrier method is much more effective. They come in a variety of forms, such as creams, gels, foams, and suppositories, which kill or disable sperm so that fertilization does not occur.

Advantages, Disadvantages, Side Effects, and Risks

Spermicidal preparations are relatively inexpensive and can be male or female initiated. They do not produce systemic effects, and no hormones are involved. They are less effective alone than with the previously described methods. Spermicides require application before each act of intercourse and are considered by some patients to be somewhat messy. Many contain the same ingredient—nonoxynol 9. If genital irritation or a rash occurs with a spermicide, the patient should read labels carefully to avoid future contact with the same ingredient.

Intrauterine Devices

The presence of a foreign object in the uterus is thought to alter the environment, so that implantation is less likely to occur. Intrauterine devices (IUDs) are generally made from a form of plastic and may contain copper wire or a supply of a progestin that is slowly released into the system to further alter the uterine environment, so that fertilization or implantation is hindered.

Advantages, Disadvantages, Side Effects, and Risks

The main advantage of an IUD is continued contraception without the necessity of remembering to take medication and without the side effects associated with medications. The

disadvantages are changes in menstrual bleeding (especially increases in bleeding), cramping, and increased risk of pelvic inflammatory disease (PID). Rarely, an IUD has caused a uterine perforation. IUDs are contraindicated for women who have never been pregnant, those with uterine abnormalities, those with PID, and those who have a history of anemia or heavy menstrual flow. Expulsion or displacement of the IUD can occur, so women should be taught to feel for the presence of the external string before intercourse.

Insertion Procedure

Insertion of an IUD is generally done as a physician's office procedure with a nurse assisting. Usually this is done during the first 7 days of the menstrual cycle because the cervix is generally slightly dilated at this time. If you are assisting with this procedure, you will need to put out a vasovagal reaction treatment kit, an IUD insertion kit containing one or more uterine "sounds," a tenaculum (a special long forceps) for grasping the cervix, and the IUD package. The IUD is generally inserted into the vagina through a tube that comes packaged with the IUD, which temporarily holds the IUD flat or folded so that it requires less room for insertion. When the IUD is pushed out the end of the tube, it springs into a shape that helps to keep it inside the uterus. One potential danger associated with IUD insertion is vasovagal reflex stimulation (previously described in association with endometrial biopsy). Periodically assess pulse or blood pressure during the procedure and notify the health-care provider of slowing of the heart rate or a decrease in blood pressure.

Natural Family Planning

Periodic abstinence, or natural family planning, is less effective than the previously described methods. It is a method by which couples control their fertility by restricting intercourse to "safe periods" in which risk of conception is low. Many signs may be assessed to determine "safe" days, including temperature changes, cervical consistency and mucus changes, calendar timing, and awareness of symptoms of fertility.

Slight body temperature changes can indicate ovulation. During the first half of the menstrual cycle, the temperature remains low, with a marked drop just before ovulation occurs. With ovulation the temperature rises and stays higher for the last half of the cycle. Women who use this assessment method should use a basal body temperature thermometer when they awaken, before doing anything else, and record it on a chart.

Cervical consistency and mucus changes may also help pinpoint ovulation. As hormone levels change, the consistency of cervical mucus changes. As ovulation approaches, there is an increase in the amount of mucus and the mucus becomes more clear, thin, slippery, and stretchable than at other times of the month. Around the time of ovulation the cervix becomes softer to touch and more open than at other times of the cycle.

Following the calendar can work fairly well if a woman's menstrual periods are regular, but becoming aware of her pattern may take time. Symptoms such as breast tenderness and mid cycle discomfort (mittelschmerz) may also help identify ovulation. Users of this method should be advised to abstain for approximately 3 days before ovulation and 3 to 4 days after because the sperm and ovum can survive for a long period in the female genital tract.

Advantages and Disadvantages

The advantages of this method are that it requires no expense or medication, and it is the only birth control method presently approved by the Catholic Church. The disadvantages are that it requires the cooperation of both partners and may interfere with spontaneity of sexual expression. It is generally not very effective as a means of birth control. It may be difficult to be accurate about ovulation times because infectious and inflammatory processes may affect temperature readings, infections and feminine hygiene products may affect cervical mucus, and irregularity of flow and symptoms may make prediction difficult.

Less Effective Methods

Coitus Interruptus

Coitus interruptus involves removal of the penis from the vagina before ejaculation occurs.

ADVANTAGES, DISADVANTAGES, AND RISKS. Although this method requires no expense or preparation, it is not very effective. Excellent control of ejaculation is required, and even the small amount of sperm that may be present in preejaculatory fluid may result in pregnancy.

Postcoital Douching

The intended purpose of postcoital douching is to wash sperm out of the reproductive tract or to kill or immobilize sperm that the douche solution contacts.

ADVANTAGES, DISADVANTAGES, AND RISKS. This is relatively inexpensive and female initiated, but it is not very effective. Sperm move very rapidly once deposited, and douching may actually push the sperm upward.

Breastfeeding

Breastfeeding is sometimes used as a method of birth control because the high blood levels of prolactin that occur with breastfeeding may suppress ovulation.

ADVANTAGES, DISADVANTAGES, AND RISKS. This method costs nothing but is not very effective. Prolactin levels can vary widely, and ovulation may resume at any time without any noticeable signs, resulting in pregnancy before even experiencing a menstrual period after the previous birth.

Ongoing Research: Future Possibilities for Contraceptive Choices

Many researchers have tried to develop effective and reversible male contraceptives. A plant called *Tripterygium*, used in Chinese herbal medicine, when taken orally yields substances that can limit numbers and mobility of sperm, but it also has active ingredients that suppress immunity somewhat, so further investigation is necessary. Reversible injection procedures to block the seminal vas deferens are also being investigated, as are reversible injection procedures to block the fallopian tubes. Reversible birth control vaccines are also being investigated for both men and women with the goal of causing an immune response to occur at some vital point in the process of conception.

Some questions related to contraceptive vaccines include the unknown long-term repercussions of stimulating the body to respond with immunity to itself and whether governments could use vaccines as a means to control populations without their consent. Another frightening possibility is that with further removal of the threat of pregnancy, even fewer people would use barrier methods and STDs would increase even more dramatically.

CRITICAL THINKING

Jessica

■ You have just observed a patient who looks to be about 13 years old announce loudly at the clinic reception desk that she is "ready to be a responsible adult" and would like some birth control.
1. What information needs to be gathered from her?
2. What do you think she needs to know?
3. How can contraceptive teaching capitalize on her desire to be a responsible adult?

Suggested answers at end of chapter.

Sterilization

Actions

Permanent sterilization can be accomplished by either interrupting the fallopian tubes or vas deferens (vasectomy) (Fig. 42.11) or by removing the uterus and suturing the proximal end of the vagina closed. Tubal interruption may be done by tying a suture or placing a ring or clip around each fallopian tube, by coagulating a section of the tubes, or by surgically removing a portion of the tube and suturing the ends. These procedures are usually done by laparoscope in an outpatient setting, as an additional procedure performed during a cesarean section, or within a few days following a vaginal delivery. A new nonsurgical procedure (Essure) uses an endoscope to implant a tiny insert into each fallopian tube to block patency.

Advantages, Disadvantages, Side Effects, and Risks

Although this method is not absolutely certain to be permanent, the failure rate is low and has been decreasing recently with newer surgical methods. Reversal is sometimes requested at a later time to reestablish fertility. This requires microsurgery with anesthesia and has a poor success rate.

Patient Teaching

Patients should be advised by their surgeon about the complications of the surgery and of reversal before they

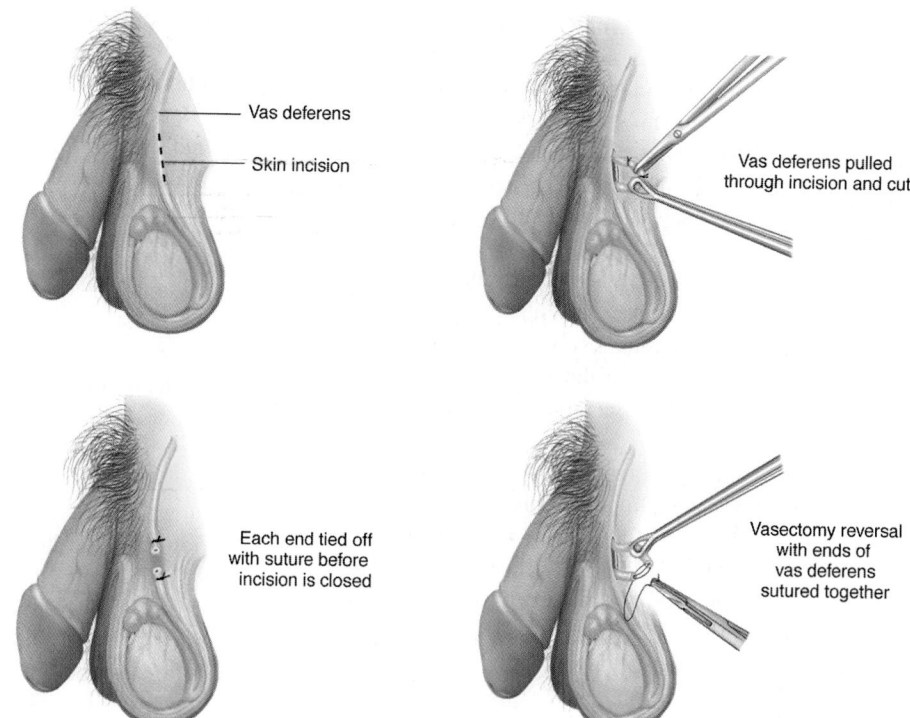

Vas deferens

Skin incision

Vas deferens pulled through incision and cut

Each end tied off with suture before incision is closed

Vasectomy reversal with ends of vas deferens sutured together

FIGURE 42.11 Vasectomy and reversal.

sign a consent form for sterilization. If any uncertainty about the surgery is evident, the physician should be notified promptly.

PREGNANCY TERMINATION

Termination of pregnancy (abortion) is a difficult topic. Discussions about it are often highly charged with emotion. Both pro-life and pro-choice advocates argue on the basis of human rights—the former based on supposed rights of the fetus and the latter on supposed rights of the mother—because of the humanity of each party. There are very few people on either side of the philosophical argument, however, who would describe abortion as a healthy medical intervention. Most agree that abortion is a problematic solution to a difficult situation. There are instances in which carrying a pregnancy to term threatens the life of the mother. There are also many more instances in which a pregnancy is inconvenient or undesired.

Therapeutic Abortion for Ectopic Pregnancy

An ectopic pregnancy is the implantation of a fertilized ovum in an area other than the uterus. It may occur because of an abnormally shaped uterus or fallopian tubes that are obstructed as a result of abnormal development, scarring from STDs or other inflammatory processes, or for unknown reasons. This is a life-threatening situation for the mother, and currently abortion is the only treatment.

Therapeutic Abortion for Prenatal Abnormalities

Development of a variety of prenatal testing methods has introduced the possibility of knowing many things about a baby before birth. Prenatal testing may be done using ultra-

sound, samples of fluid taken from the amniotic sac or the placental villi, or blood samples from the mother. From these tests, several genetic diseases and congenital deformities can be identified. After anomalies are diagnosed, some patients choose to abort the baby. This is a very difficult decision to consider even in instances in which the baby has a fatal defect that will not allow it to live outside the uterus. It is important to provide information about alternatives to abortion and possible treatments for their child when a patient has a serious prenatal diagnosis. No one should feel pressured to make the decision quickly to abort, but legal requirements and increasing risk for the mother may limit the time to decide. Abortion because of fetal abnormality may result in much grieving and guilt for the patient and her family.

Methods of Abortion

Several methods are available. The method is determined primarily by the length of the gestation and the goal of inflicting as little trauma to the mother's reproductive system as possible while still inducing pregnancy loss. Periods for the different abortion methods and the allowable reasons for legal abortion vary according to the laws of the state, province, or country.

Chemical Agents

The "morning after pill," or emergency contraceptive treatment, consists of postcoital administration of sufficient estrogen or an estrogen/progestin combination to cause sudden sloughing of the endometrial lining of the uterus, preventing implantation of a possibly fertilized ovum. For this to be effective, the initial dose is generally given within 72 hours of intercourse. This treatment is used in case of unexpected unprotected sexual intercourse (as with sexual assault) or unexpected risk of conception (as with condom failure). Nausea and cramping may accompany the shedding of the uterine lining, and an antiemetic may be taken to manage nausea. No advance planning before intercourse is required, so this can be abused as a casual form of birth control. These patients may need education about appropriate birth control methods.

Another example of postcoital contraception is the drug RU-486, which is a progestin antagonist. It prevents the binding of progestins at their receptors, resulting in a chemically induced abortion up to the 10th week of pregnancy. Nausea and cramping may accompany expulsion of uterine contents. There is much debate about whether RU-486 should be used at all or only within specific guidelines. The United States Food and Drug Administration approved RU-486 in 2000 in an accelerated drug-approval process, but legislative bills have been introduced and reintroduced to stipulate regulations for health-care providers prescribing RU-486. Undoubtedly RU-486, as well as methotrexate (a cancer medication) and misoprostol (a medication to prevent stomach ulcers), all of which can stimulate abortion, will continue to be the subject of much debate.

Abortion Methods for Early Pregnancy

Early in a pregnancy (during approximately the first 13 weeks) there are three primary means of pregnancy termination—menstrual extraction, vacuum aspiration, and D&C. Menstrual extraction is removal of the endometrial lining by manual suction and can be done during the first 7 weeks following the last menstrual period (LMP). This can be done without anesthesia and without cervical dilation by inserting a small cannula into the cervix and aspirating with a large syringe. Vacuum aspiration is a similar process that is used from confirmation of pregnancy through the first 13 weeks. It requires cervical dilation and is generally done with local anesthesia. The patient returns home 1 to 4 hours after the procedure. D&C may also be used during the first 13 weeks. In this procedure, the cervix is dilated and the uterine contents are scooped away with a curet rather than being removed by suction.

Abortion Methods for Later Pregnancy

During the second trimester, the fetus is much larger, so more dilation is required. A dilation and evacuation (D&E) may be performed in much the same manner as a D&C. Generally, dried laminaria (a type of seaweed) or some other absorbent substance is placed inside the cervical canal. This absorbs fluid and swells, thus gradually dilating the cervix. Prostaglandin may be administered either by suppository into the vagina or by injection into the amniotic sac; this usually induces uterine contractions and results in delivery a few hours later. Unfortunately, a live fetus too premature to survive may be born by this method and continue to breathe for a time until death.

An induction with either a saline or urea injection may be used for pregnancies beyond 16 weeks. A portion of amniotic fluid is removed and replaced with concentrated saline or urea solution, which kills the fetus and stimulates contractions. Sometimes saline and prostaglandins are used in combination to terminate a pregnancy.

Hysterotomy involves removal of the uterine contents through an abdominal incision in the same manner as a cesarean section. This procedure is rarely done for pregnancy termination.

Risks and Complications

Abortion involves risks. Some are the same risks inherent in childbirth, such as possible hemorrhage or introduction of infection, but there are additional risks related to interruption of natural processes and the aggressiveness with which the products of conception are removed during abortion. During an uncomplicated childbirth, the uterine lining is not scraped or forcefully emptied by suction. Natural hormonal preparation for term childbirth contributes to uterine contraction after the birth, which decreases blood loss, but no such preparation occurs for abortion. Artificial dilation of the cervix may cause injury, as may introduction of the instruments used for abortion. Injured tissues are more likely to become sites for growth of microorganisms than are intact tissues. Finally, the possibility of infertility as a result of complications related to abortion, although relatively uncommon, is a risk.

Some possible physical complications following therapeutic abortion are injuries to the uterus or cervix, excessive bleeding, infection, retention of some products of conception, and possible failure of abortion. Rarely, second-trimester abortions can be complicated by amniotic fluid embolism, in which amniotic fluid is absorbed into the uterine circulation because of disruption of placental attachments with instruments. Amniotic fluid in the mother's circulatory system can result in circulatory collapse and disseminated intravascular coagulation (DIC). DIC is a serious derangement of the body's blood clotting controls and, although rare, can be fatal. Clotting mechanisms are overstimulated, so that the blood begins to form clots in vessels all over the body. In response to this hypercoagulation, fibrinolytic mechanisms are overstimulated and the patient may suffer severe and widespread bleeding. Treatment of this disorder is difficult because the normal mechanisms for both sides of this clotting/clot dissolving equation are hypersensitive.

Nursing Care and Teaching

Aftercare is very important. Abortion patients rarely stay overnight, and complications may occur after they are discharged. They should be carefully assessed after the procedure for signs of bleeding. Instruct that bleeding should not exceed that of a heavy period, that the passage of clots larger than a quarter may be a sign of complications, and that the discharge should not become foul smelling. Patients should be given a phone number (available 24 hours per day, 7 days per week) to call if fever, chills, excessive bleeding, or foul-smelling discharge occur. The patient should be advised to abstain from sexual intercourse for the time specified by

---

hysterotomy: hystero—womb + tomy—cutting

the health-care provider (usually about 3 weeks). A grief response may occur after a pregnancy termination, even if the baby was definitely unwanted and the patient does not have strong beliefs against abortion. There is much debate about frequency of postabortion syndrome or whether such a condition exists. However, loss and trauma have occurred in any case, and reorganization of the self takes time. Availability of psychological counseling for women after abortion is very important. Women should be given a number to call if they experience psychological discomforts. The need for birth control should be assessed.

Ethical Issues

Ethically an individual nurse should not be required to assist in any treatment that demands that he or she act in a way that contradicts personal moral beliefs. This would violate the nurse's rights. However, there is also an ethical duty to provide care to patients for whom the nurse is responsible. Therefore, it is wise for nurses who have moral objections to abortion to carefully choose their work setting. For example, choosing to work in day surgery in a hospital that performs

abortions and refusing to care for abortion patients is not a legitimate option. One way that nurses can positively influence the abortion situation is by teaching about family planning, which may lower the number of requests for abortions. Another way might be to become involved with agencies that help pregnant women to have viable alternatives to abortion. See Box 42.5 Ethical Considerations.

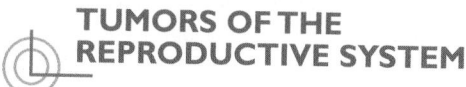

TUMORS OF THE REPRODUCTIVE SYSTEM

Benign Growths

Fibroid Tumors

PATHOPHYSIOLOGY, ETIOLOGIES, AND SIGNS AND SYMPTOMS. Fibroid tumors, or **leiomyomas** (plural form is leiomyomata), are benign tumors made up of endometrial cells that have implanted on or within the walls of the uterus. These can grow very large and may cause pain or menstrual

---

leiomyoma: leio—smooth + myom(a)—fibroid

Box 42.5

Ethical Considerations

Abortion

The famous case of *Roe vs Wade* (1973) changed the legal status of therapeutic abortion in the United States but added a great deal of confusion to its ethical and moral status. A careful reading of the *Roe vs Wade* decision reveals that the court made no decision about the ethics or morality of elective (therapeutic) abortion. Rather, the court said that according to the U.S. Constitution, all people, including women, have a right to determine what they can do with their bodies *(right to self-determination)* and a right to privacy. Therefore, during the first trimester a woman and her physician may decide to terminate a pregnancy without interference from the state. During the second trimester, the state may regulate the circumstances under which an abortion may occur to protect the woman's health. Once the fetus is viable, the state may also prohibit abortion. Although a woman may have a right to obtain an abortion, there is not a right to require the death of the fetus should a viable fetus be identified after the abortion procedure. Pro-choice groups put the right to self-determination and privacy central to their concerns. Pro-life groups generally believe that abortion is fundamentally killing and therefore wrong.

One of the central issues in the debate is the status of the fetus. Is the fetus considered a person with individual rights separate from those of the woman who is pregnant? Another central question is when does human life begin? Is abortion at any stage of pregnancy morally acceptable? Each fertilized egg contains the essential genetic material

for the development of a unique individual. However, many fertilized eggs never successfully implant in the uterus in the natural process of conception. Does such a factor make the timing of the procedure a critical element? Related to this problem is the status of frozen embryos created through in vitro fertilization. They too contain the essential, unique genetic material for the development of a human person. If every embryo should be respected as potential human life, what moral obligation do we have toward those embryos? What about those embryos left in freezers unclaimed? Should we implant them into childless women? Should we use cells that are otherwise scheduled to be destroyed in order to treat disease or further the understanding of genetic disorders?

The issues around abortion are huge, and there are no easy suggested answers. There are many resources that can provide information and guidance to the public about the variables. However, health-care workers are not only members of the public, they are the people on the front line interacting and serving women who are having these procedures. Anyone who decides to work in an establishment like an abortion clinic or a unit where terminations occur is expected to be fully prepared to participate in treatments and procedures. The fundamental question of if this procedure is right or wrong, for whatever reason, has no bearing in such a facility. The staff must be comfortable in their belief that the service they are providing is congruent with their internal and professional value set.

disorders, exert pressure on the bladder or bowel, cause necrosis because of pressure on the blood supply to tissues, and interfere with fertility.

THERAPEUTIC INTERVENTIONS. Because fibroids are estrogen sensitive, medical treatment may involve hormone suppression. Surgical treatment may involve **myomectomy** or hysterectomy. Myomectomy is removal of only the fibroid tumor and may be chosen to preserve fertility. Myomectomy may be done surgically through an abdominal or vaginal incision or with a laser introduced through a laparoscope. Hysterectomy may be necessary for very large fibroids or those that cause severe bleeding or discomfort.

Polyps

PATHOPHYSIOLOGY, ETIOLOGIES, AND SIGNS AND SYMPTOMS. Polyps are generally benign growths that grow inside the uterus or on the cervix and may bleed after intercourse or between menstrual cycles. These are generally teardrop shaped and are attached by a stalk. Polyps develop most often after the age of 42.

THERAPEUTIC INTERVENTIONS. Polyps are generally removed vaginally or transcervically by separating the stalk from the uterus and then stopping the bleeding by use of chemical, electrical, or laser **cautery.** Removal of polyps in the vagina may be done without anesthetic in a physician's office. Removal of polyps transcervically requires cervical dilation and is more likely to be done in a hospital with anesthesia.

Reproductive System Cysts

PATHOPHYSIOLOGY, ETIOLOGIES, AND SIGNS AND SYMPTOMS. Several types of cysts may affect women's health. Cysts of the ovaries may develop associated with incomplete ovulation, **hypertrophy** of the corpus luteum after ovulation, or inflammation of the ovary. Most ovarian cysts eventually will shrink spontaneously and merely cause discomfort for a time. Chocolate cysts are formed when endometrial cells bleed into an enclosed space, as occurs with endometriosis. These are called chocolate cysts because they are filled with old blood that has become chocolate colored. Cystoadenomas are benign growths that can sometimes undergo cellular transformation and become cancerous. Any pelvic mass in a postmenopausal woman has a high potential for malignancy and should be investigated.

THERAPEUTIC INTERVENTIONS. Most cysts are not surgically removed, but excessive size, interference with fertility, and high cancer potential may make needle drainage, biopsy, laparoscopic surgery, or **laparotomy** advisable. If cysts are painful, application of heat to the abdomen or back may help promote comfort.

Polycystic Ovary Syndrome

PATHOPHYSIOLOGY AND ETIOLOGY. Polycystic ovary syndrome (PCOS) is a complex abnormality of endocrine balance of unknown etiology. Multiple cysts on the ovaries are a sign that was discovered early and for which the disease was named, but they are not present in all cases. There seem to be strong genetic links with such family history as too much or too little hair (especially for women), severe acne, diabetes, irregular menses, and infertility. Many of the symptoms of PCOS are a result of excessive levels of insulin in the blood because of insulin resistance. Excess insulin in turn stimulates secretion of androgens.

SIGNS AND SYMPTOMS. Women with PCOS often present with infertility, obesity, and menstrual disturbances. They may also exhibit masculinization because of the excess androgen secretion. They have a higher risk for diabetes mellitus, elevated blood pressure, coronary artery disease, and endometrial cancer.

DIAGNOSTIC TESTS. Diagnostic tests may include blood tests to rule out other causes of endocrine abnormality, tests to determine whether ovulation is occurring (such as mid luteal progesterone levels and basal body temperature graphing), endometrial biopsies to determine the level of proliferation and to check for endometrial cancer, and blood tests to determine lipid levels and glucose tolerance.

THERAPEUTIC INTERVENTIONS. Medical treatments may involve blood pressure medications, lipid control medications, and oral hypoglycemics. Diet and exercise may be recommended for weight reduction, control of lipid levels, and cardiac health. Oral contraceptives may be used to normalize hormone levels and protect the endometrium for those not desiring to conceive. Ovulation-inducing medication may be used for those women who desire to conceive. If masculinization is a problem, antiandrogen medications may be prescribed. In severe cases, gonadotropin-releasing hormone (GnRH) agonists may be used to produce medical suppression of the ovaries, with results similar to removal of the ovaries. This is followed 6 months later with an estrogen/progestin combination to protect the bones from development of osteoporosis.

Bartholin's Cysts

PATHOPHYSIOLOGY, ETIOLOGIES, AND SIGNS AND SYMPTOMS. Bartholin's cysts are actually infected or obstructed Bartholin's glands at either side of the vaginal opening. Excessive swelling of Bartholin's glands results in pain with sitting and with intercourse.

THERAPEUTIC INTERVENTIONS. Incision and drainage may alleviate the discomfort. If Bartholin's cyst formation occurs often, **marsupialization**—the surgical formation of a

---

myomectomy: myom(a)—fibroid + ec—away + tomy—cutting
cautery: branding iron
hypertrophy: hyper—too much + trophy—nourishment (growth)
laparotomy: laparo(o)—abdominal wall + tomy—cutting

marsupialization: marsupial—pouch + ization—process of making pouch around an opening made into a gland to facilitate drainage—may be necessary. Sitz baths may be ordered to cleanse the area and to promote comfort and healing.

Dermoid Cysts

PATHOPHYSIOLOGY, ETIOLOGIES, SIGNS AND SYMPTOMS. Rarely, for unknown reasons, a **dermoid** cyst (also called a cystic **teratoma**) may develop from a germinal cell of an ovary. This cell divides and differentiates into various tissue types such as skin, teeth, bones, hair, and even extremities in a disordered arrangement. This type of cyst may grow quite large and may occur on both ovaries at the same time.

THERAPEUTIC INTERVENTIONS. Dermoid cysts are removed by laparoscopy or laparotomy. If the cyst contains glandular tissue that is secreting hormones, adjustment of hormone levels to normal may take some time. Although most teratomas are benign, some are malignant, especially in postmenopausal women, so a biopsy is generally done on the tissue.

NURSING CARE AND TEACHING. Growth of a dermoid can be a frightening experience for a woman. Reassurance that this is merely a disordered group of cells identical to the other cells in her body, rather than a monster or deformed baby, is important.

Malignant Disorders

It is sometimes difficult to distinguish benign growths from malignant growths without biopsy results, and some benign growths can become cancerous. Malignancies can occur in all parts of the reproductive system and can occur at all ages. Although reproductive system cancers are more common in older age groups, ovarian tumors can occur even in young children. Both male and female children of women who were given diethylstilbestrol (DES) in the past to prevent premature delivery in high-risk pregnancies have experienced a high incidence of developmental defects and cancers of the reproductive organs.

Many different types of genital cancer are possible, and discussion of every type in detail is beyond the focus of this book. This section presents a general overview of the most common cancers. Cancerous changes often can be observed or noticed, and if investigated and treated early enough, cure is often complete.

LEARNING TIP

Three C changes that may indicate cancer are changes in color, contour, and consistency of a tissue.

Vulvar Cancer

PATHOPHYSIOLOGY, ETIOLOGIES, AND SIGNS AND SYMPTOMS. Although vulvar cancer is not common, alertness to changes in visible parts of the reproductive system such as the vulva can result in early diagnosis, requirement of less drastic treatment, and end with more positive results. Persistent itching of the vulva or appearance of white or red patches, rough areas, skin ulcers, or wartlike growths on the vulva should not be ignored; these can be signs of precancerous or cancerous changes. Risk factors for development of vulvar cancer are an STD of any type, precancerous or cancerous changes of the anus or any of the genitalia, immune system depression, and smoking.

DIAGNOSTIC TESTS. Regular Pap smears and physical examinations can identify lesions. Biopsy of suspicious lesions is necessary to diagnose vulvar cancer.

THERAPEUTIC INTERVENTIONS. If discovered early, vulvar cancer may be treated with removal or destruction of cancerous cells. If not diagnosed early, it may require surgical removal of the entire vulva and associated lymph nodes (a radical vulvectomy) with subsequent skin grafting from other areas of the body for repair.

Cervical Cancer

PATHOPHYSIOLOGY, ETIOLOGIES, AND SIGNS AND SYMPTOMS. Changes in the cells of the cervix (called cervical intraepithelial neoplasia [CIN]) can progress to cervical cancer. Dysplastic cells (those with dysplasia) are generally less differentiated or less ordered than expected for their cell type.

Some identified risk factors for development of cervical cancer include starting sexual activity at an early age, having multiple sexual partners, having several pregnancies, smoking, and being infected with human papillomavirus or herpes simplex virus type II (HSV-II). Use of oral contraceptives for several years may also increase a woman's risk of developing cervical cancer, although part of the difference in incidence may be because women using oral contraceptives may not be using barrier protection against STDs. Although some women experience slight spotting or a serosanguineous discharge with cervical cancer, many are asymptomatic until the cancer is widespread.

DIAGNOSTIC TESTS. Pap smears are the best method of screening for cervical cancer presently available, but some work is being done on self-tests that women can collect. A Pap smear determines the degree of cellular change, or dysplasia. Ranking systems vary, but Pap smear results are usually presented in categories that range from no atypical cells seen to invasive cancer evident (0 to IV). This procedure has significantly reduced the incidence of invasive cervical cancer over the years since its introduction because cellular changes can be identified early enough for treatment before the cells become cancerous. Schiller's test may be done if a patient has an abnormal Pap smear. This involves painting the cervix with iodine. Dysplastic cells stain differently than normal ones. Biopsy is done to confirm

dermoid: derm—skin + oid—form
teratoma: terat—monster + oma—growth

a cancer diagnosis. Recommendations for frequency of screening vary, but most recommend that Pap smears begin at either age 21 or with the start of sexual activity and be done yearly unless abnormalities develop. After a period of normal Pap smears, some health-care providers advocate longer intervals for low-risk people.

THERAPEUTIC INTERVENTIONS. Treatments for pre-invasive neoplasia include **cryotherapy** (freezing), laser therapy (burning), and surgical removal of the involved area with a loop excision instrument or by conization (Fig. 42.12). All these procedures are done through the vagina, so there are no external incisions. After any of these treatments the patient is advised not to douche, use tampons, or have intercourse for approximately 2 weeks to allow for healing to take place. She should be advised to report immediately if fever, bloody vaginal discharge, or foul-smelling vaginal discharge occurs. For invasive cancers, hysterectomy, radiation implant, or chemotherapy may be done.

Endometrial Cancer
PATHOPHYSIOLOGY, ETIOLOGIES, AND SIGNS AND SYMPTOMS. Endometrial cancer is the most common type of uterine cancer. Most develop in response to relative estrogen excess. Abrupt changes in bleeding patterns, especially bleeding in a menopausal woman, may indicate endometrial cancer development. Estrogen excess can develop for many reasons. Estrogen levels fluctuate widely in the perimenopausal period. Obesity results in increased estrogen production that is not balanced by progestins. Estrogen replacement therapy for menopausal symptoms without the addition of progestins also has been associated with an increase in endometrial cancer, but addition of a progestin may decrease the risk of endometrial cancer to

less than that of untreated women. Whether alcohol consumption increases the risk of endometrial cancer by interfering with estrogen metabolism is still a matter of debate. Some endometrial cancer, however, is unexplained by any presently known risk factors.

DIAGNOSTIC TESTS. Diagnosis is generally done by endometrial biopsy, but MRI may be used to evaluate invasiveness and involvement of lymph nodes.

THERAPEUTIC INTERVENTIONS. Depending on the stage of endometrial cancer and metastasis, treatment with hysterectomy, radiation, or chemotherapy may be used.

Ovarian Cancer
PATHOPHYSIOLOGY, ETIOLOGIES, AND SIGNS AND SYMPTOMS. Ovarian cancer is an especially insidious killer because cellular changes in the ovaries often are asymptomatic until the cancer is quite advanced. Little is known about what prompts these cells to undergo malignant changes. Risk factors are not definitely identified, but some proposed factors include low fertility and number of children, late menopause, a family history of reproductive or colon cancers, and a diet rich in animal fats. Use of hormonal contraception may help prevent this because it results in less ovulation during the woman's lifetime.

DIAGNOSTIC TESTS. Identification of abnormal growths on the ovaries may begin with bimanual examination, so it is important for women, especially in the older age groups, to continue to have regular pelvic examinations even if they are not sexually active and even if they have had a hysterectomy. Various blood tests measuring tumor marker substances, ultrasonography, CT scanning, and MRI may also be used to assist in diagnosis.

THERAPEUTIC INTERVENTIONS. Treatment may involve surgical removal of the ovaries by laparoscopy or

---

cryotherapy: cryo—cold + therapy—treatment

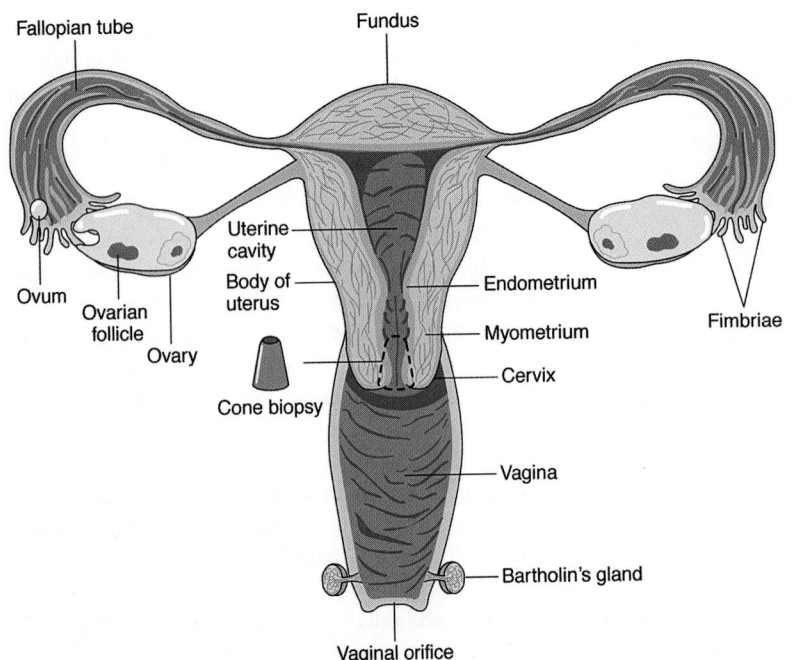

FIGURE 42.12 Conization

laparotomy. Sometimes the ovaries are removed to prevent the disease in women who have a high familial risk. Radiation and combination chemotherapy may also be used.

Nursing Care and Teaching of Patients with Malignant Disorders

Radiation therapy for cancers of the reproductive system may involve the placement of radioactive implants into the patient's body for 24 to 72 hours. Avoid prolonged contact with the patient and perform care with as much of the patient's body between you and the implant as possible (e.g., for cervical implants, stand at the head of the bed rather than at the foot). Prevent inappropriate radiation of the patient's other body parts by such actions as maintaining patency of a urinary catheter to avoid unnecessary exposure of the bladder. Follow institutional guidelines for radiation precautions. Do not give care to patients with radioactive implants if you are pregnant. A foul-smelling vaginal discharge is expected after radiation by implant because of tissue destruction caused by the radiation; document the amount and character of the discharge. Chemotherapy treatments often cause severe nausea, as well as anorexia and sores of the mouth, vagina, and anus. See Chapter 10 for care of patients receiving chemotherapy.

See Box 42.6 for a summary of tumors of the reproductive system.

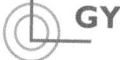 **GYNECOLOGICAL SURGERY**

Endoscopic Surgeries

Many of the surgeries performed on the reproductive system may be done using an endoscope. The scopes used contain not only magnifying lenses and a light source but may also include tiny tools for performing surgery, for removal of small areas of diseased tissue and samples, for suction, and for cauterization of bleeding vessels. Because endoscopic surgeries require tiny incisions (usually less than 1 inch long), there is less tissue disruption and very little bleeding when compared with traditional surgical techniques. Smaller incisions also present less risk of infection than traditional methods, and recuperation is generally more rapid with fewer complications. Overall the danger to the patient is generally low for endoscopic surgeries; however, not all surgical situations may be satisfactorily handled in this way. The size of the cannula restricts the size of tissues that can be removed, unless they can be divided into smaller sections and then pulled out through the cannula. If affected areas are widespread, the scope may not be able to reach all sites. Traditional surgery still may have to be done when endoscopic surgery has been ineffective, and this can be frustrating to patients. However, information gained through the prior endoscopic surgery may decrease the time required for the traditional surgery.

Laparoscopies are the most common type of endoscopic surgical procedure employed for women's reproductive system surgeries. This method can be used for access to the abdominal cavity and the anterior portions of the repro-

---

Box 42.6

Tumors of the Reproductive System Summary

Signs and Symptoms	Menstrual pain/dysfunction
	Infertility
	Incontinence
	Constipation
	Vaginal bleeding
	Abdominal/perineal pain/swelling
	Androgen characteristics
	Obesity
	Diabetes
	Coronary artery disease
Diagnostic Tests and Findings	Physical examination
	Laparoscopy
	Ultrasound
	CT or MRI scan
	Biopsy
	Alteration in hormone levels
Therapeutic Interventions	Surgery
	Chemical/electrical/laser cautery
	Oral contraceptives and medications
	Incision/drainage/marsupialization
Priority Nursing Diagnoses	Acute/chronic pain r/t lesion/ surgery.
	Urinary incontinence or constipation r/t lesion/surgery.
	Impaired body image r/t body structure abnormality.
	Sexual dysfunction r/t disturbance in self-concept.
	Grief r/t absence/loss of reproductive status.

CT = computed tomography; MRI = magnetic resonance imaging; r/t = related to.

---

ductive organs. Tubal ligations, tubal repairs, removal of ectopic pregnancy implantations, removal of small tumors, removal of endometriotic sections of tissue, and aspiration of fluid-filled cysts can all be done by this method.

Culdoscopies may be done to access the area at the back of the uterus. A **culdotomy,** which is an incision into the upper posterior portion of the vagina, is necessary to insert the cannula. A **culdocentesis,** which is the removal of fluid from the cul-de-sac of Douglas, may be done during a culdoscopy. Aftercare is much the same as for laparoscopy, although the patient should be informed that a small amount of vaginal spotting may be expected from the incision but heavy, purulent, or foul-smelling discharge could indicate infection. (See Chapter 41.)

---

culdotomy: culdo—cul-de-sac + tomy—cutting
culdocentesis: culdo—cul-de-sac + centesis—puncturing

Colposcopies are generally used to screen, diagnose, or treat problems of the cervix. The binocular microscope attached to the scope cannula, which is introduced into the vagina, allows the physician to examine dysplastic cells while they are still in their normal place and to treat cervical dysplasia as previously described. Hysteroscopy may be used to treat problems within the uterus. Removal of polyps and other growths, modification of congenital malformations such as septa (walls of tissue where there should be none), and laser ablation of endometrial tissue may all be done during hysteroscopy. The endoscope may be inserted further into the fallopian tubes to perform a salpingoscopy, allowing surgical or laser opening of blocked tubes.

Nursing Care and Teaching

Postoperative care involves careful assessment for signs of possible excessive internal bleeding, including checks of vital signs, skin color and temperature, and pain. Measures to reduce the discomfort produced by residual carbon dioxide from insufflation may include instruction to lie flat for a few hours, massaging of the back and shoulders, and administration of pain medication. Instruction about possible danger signs, any medications, and when and where to go for suture removal complete the discharge teaching.

Hysterectomy

Removal of the uterus (hysterectomy) may be done for a variety of reasons, including abnormally heavy or painful menstruation, large fibroids or other benign tumors, severe uterine prolapse, and cancer of the uterus. It should not be done merely as a sterilization procedure because the risks involved in hysterectomy surgery are much greater than risks associated with tubal ligation. The surgery is usually performed through an abdominal incision, but it may be done vaginally in some cases. The vagina is left intact except for suturing of the proximal end, which had been attached to the uterus, forming a blind pouch. Although less vaginal lubrication is present after hysterectomy, nerve routes are maintained and satisfactory sexual intercourse is expected to continue.

The uterus alone may be removed, and in some cases the tubes and ovaries may also be removed—a procedure called total abdominal hysterectomy with **bilateral salpingo-oophorectomy** (TAH-BSO), or **panhysterectomy**. If the ovaries are removed, the woman undergoes immediate menopause and may suffer from symptoms associated with menopause, including the increased risks of cardiovascular disease and osteoporosis. Because removal of the ovaries is usually done because of the presence of estrogen-dependent cancer, estrogen replacement is not usually feasible in these cases, and extra care, comfort, and explanation from nurses are necessary. See Box 42.7 Nursing Care Plan for the Patient Undergoing Hysterectomy. In addition to the nursing diagnoses covered, also assess for anxiety related to surgery and resulting body image changes and for ineffective coping.

---

bilateral salpingo-oophorectomy: salpingo—tubal + oophor—ovary + ec—from + tomy—cutting

panhysterectomy: pan—all + hyster—uterus + ec—from + tomy—cutting

---

BOX 42.7   NURSING CARE PLAN **for the Patient Undergoing Hysterectomy**

Nursing Diagnosis: Risk for ineffective tissue perfusion related to surgical incision and removal of the uterus (and possibly the ovaries)

Expected Outcomes Incision(s) will heal by primary intention without excessive bleeding.

Evaluation of Outcomes (1) Are vital signs within normal range for patient? (2) Is dressing dry and intact and/or does perineal pad show <3cm stain every hour? (3) Are edges of the incision well approximated, with scant bleeding/serous drainage, and mild edema/erythema (if applicable)?

Interventions	Rationale	Evaluation
Monitor vital signs and oxygen saturation according to hospital policy and as necessary.	Vital signs and oxygen saturation reflect tissue perfusion status.	Are vital signs stable and within normal range?
Check for bleeding or other discharge on perineal pad and on abdominal dressing (if applicable).	Excessive bleeding may compromise tissue perfusion and slow healing. Vaginal discharge gives clues to healing of incision at the proximal end of the vagina.	Is pad or dressing dry? Is discharge foul smelling?
Assess wound healing (if applicable) twice a day (bid) and report any evidence of infection or inadequate healing promptly.	Early treatment of inadequate wound healing decreases postoperative complications.	Is incisional area swollen, reddened, or draining purulent material?

Nursing Diagnosis: Risk for impaired urinary elimination related to manipulation of the bladder and ureters during surgery, anticholinergic drugs, fluid intake changes, and fear of pain

Expected Outcomes Patient will have urinary output 30 mL/hr or more without difficulty.

Evaluation of Outcomes (1) Is patient able to void and effectively empty bladder when voiding? (2) Is patient voiding at least 30 mL per hour?

Interventions	Rationale	Evaluation
Assess urinary output after surgery. Report if less than 30 mL/hr or unable to void.	Inadequate urinary output can be an evidence of dehydration, low glomerular perfusion, kidney dysfunction, damage to ureter, or urinary retention.	Is output adequate? Is patient able to void without discomfort?
Assess bladder fullness using Doppler monitoring or scratch test (listening with a stethoscope, lightly scratch abdomen as you move downward from xiphoid until you hear change in sound indicating top of the bladder).	Urinary retention can cause damage to kidneys, ureters, and bladder. Scratch test and Doppler monitoring cause less discomfort and pressure to an abdominal incision area.	Does patient feel she is emptying fully when voiding? Does Doppler indicate residual urine after voiding? Where is level of sound change with scratch test?
Medicate for pain on a fixed schedule for operative day and first postoperative day (unless patient declines pain medication).	Maintenance of a consistent blood level of medication in the immediate postoperative period provides relief of pain and promotes voiding without fear of discomfort.	Does patient state that she is comfortable?

Nursing Diagnosis: Risk for constipation and gas related to manipulation of the bowel during surgery, opioid analgesics and anticholinergic drugs, diet changes, less exercise than usual, and fear of pain when passing stool

Expected Outcomes Patient will pass soft formed stool without excessive gas discomfort by third postoperative day.

Evaluation of Outcomes (1) Are bowel sounds active in all four quadrants? (2) Is patient passing gas without difficulty? (3) Is patient able to have a formed bowel movement within 3 days of surgery?

Interventions	Rationale	Evaluation
Assess for active bowel sounds in all four abdominal quadrants before giving anything orally.	Manipulation of the bowel during surgery or anesthetics and other medications may interfere with bowel function.	Are bowel sounds sluggish, active, or hyperactive?
Encourage high fluid intake, and graduate diet toward a high-fiber, regular diet as soon as patient is able to tolerate it (or doctor's orders prescribe).	Adequate fluid and fiber in the diet softens the stool for easy passage.	Are bowel sounds present in all four quadrants? Is patient drinking well? Is patient ready for more normal foods, as well as liquids?
Encourage adequate exercise.	Reasonable exercise promotes peristalsis and relives gas discomfort.	Has patient dangled at bedside the day of surgery and then walked increasing amounts each day following?
Assess quantity and quality of pain. Control pain with analgesics, especially before administering suppository or enema.	The presence of pain may inhibit defecation.	Is patient passing intestinal gas without difficulty? Does patient express satisfaction with pain control and report pain at an acceptable level?
Give stool softeners, laxatives, suppositories, or enemas as ordered (check bowel protocol or standing orders).	Soft stool is easier to pass.	Has patient passed soft formed stool by the third day after surgery?

REVIEW QUESTIONS

1. A breastfeeding patient says "My doctor said I have mastalgia. What does that mean?" Which response by the nurse is best?
   a. "That means you may have an infection in your breasts."
   b. "Mastalgia is just the normal discomfort that is associated with breastfeeding."
   c. "The word mastalgia just means breast pain; it can occur with monthly cycles of hormone levels."
   d. "Mastalgia is the medical term for fibrocystic breast disease. It is important to have it treated promptly."

2. Which response by the nurse is most appropriate when a 60-year-old woman who has been menopausal for several years relates that she has begun having vaginal bleeding again?
   a. "Ignore it—it is perfectly normal."
   b. "Try taking some ibuprofen. That may reduce the bleeding."
   c. "You should see a doctor to have that checked as soon as possible."
   d. "Give it time—bleeding after menopause usually goes away within a month."

3. During an endometrial biopsy, for which of the following signs and symptoms of vasovagal response should the nurse observe?
   a. Pain in the chest and abdomen
   b. Cramping and diaphoresis
   c. High blood pressure and tachycardia
   d. Bradycardia and falling blood pressure

4. Which of the following medications can be used to treat vasovagal response during gynecologic procedures?
   a. Atropine
   b. Morphine
   c. Epinephrine
   d. Norepinephrine

5. The nurse is discharging a patient with endometriosis from an office visit. She says her medication helps but does not relieve all her discomfort. What other measures can the nurse recommend?
   a. "Check with the health food store. There are several herbal remedies that can be very effective."
   b. "Try using the relaxation exercises you learned in your childbirth classes. A warm compress to your abdomen might also help."
   c. "You can double up on your pain medication on occasion, but you shouldn't do it on a regular basis."
   d. "If the medications aren't effective, then it is time to talk to the doctor about a hysterectomy."

6. The nurse enters the room of a patient who is 1 day post left-sided mastectomy and notes a phlebotomist taking blood from her left antecubital space. What should the nurse do first?
   a. Nothing; the nurse is not the phlebotomist's supervisor.
   b. Nothing; blood pressures should be avoided in the affected arm, but blood draws are safe.
   c. Stop the phlebotomist and point out that needlesticks must be avoided in the affected arm.
   d. Notify the physician.

7. Following a panhysterectomy, what should the nurse teach the patient to expect?
   a. Heavy bleeding for a week
   b. Symptoms of menopause
   c. Painful intercourse for approximately 6 months
   d. Monthly cramping but no menstrual flow

8. A patient who has just returned from an abdominal panhysterectomy is at risk for impaired urinary elimination. At least how many mL should be in her catheter bag 8 hours post operatively? _____

9. Which of the following is the least effective form of contraception?
   a. Douching
   b. Condom with spermicide
   c. Diaphragm with spermicide
   d. Oral contraceptive medication

SUGGESTED ANSWERS TO

CRITICAL THINKING

■ *Julie*

1. Questions to further assess Julie's complaint should include: Do you do BSEs? Has there been a change in the characteristics of the "bumps"? Are the pain and lumps related to your menstrual cycle? Are the lumps mobile or fixed? Have you noticed any skin or nipple changes of your breasts? Have you noticed any leakage of fluid or blood from your breasts? Are you breastfeeding or have you recently delivered an infant? Have you had a fever?

2. A possible screening mammogram may be considered, realizing that breast tissue is dense at this age and a mammogram is not as accurate as it will be after about age 40. Diagnostic tests may include breast ultrasound and needle/excisional biopsy.

3. Treatment options will be based on the etiology. Treatment for fibrocystic breast changes may include oral contraceptives and dietary changes, including limiting fat and caffeine. Treatment for mastitis (unlikely, but a possible diagnosis based on complaint) may include antibiotics, warm compresses, breast supports, or excision. Treatment for breast cancer may include lumpectomy, mastectomy, chemotherapy, radiation, as well as reconstruction at some point.

■ *Lola*

1. Interventions that may help control Lola's discomfort related to hot flashes include possible inclusion of HRT therapy, inclusion of phytoestrogens into her diet, limiting caffeinated foods or beverages, dressing in layers so that some may be removed as needed, and lowering the thermostat as needed.

2. Information that should be shared with Lola concerning HRT therapy should include the risks as well as benefits according to most recent studies. Risks include increased risk of stroke, cardiovascular disease, breast cancer, and thomboembolism. Benefits include symptomatic relief and decreased risk of complications from osteoporosis.

■ *Jessica*

1. Some important information from Jessica would include her true age (laws vary concerning birth control for minors), her intentions, her family situation, whether she is already sexually active, and what information she wants.

2. She needs to know that being sexually active involves more risks than just pregnancy. Discussion of STDs is vital. Discussion of violence, potential for abuse, long-term effects, and psychological suffering, which may accompany early sexual activity, may also be important. The choices of birth control should be explained, including the risks, effectiveness, disadvantages, and advantages of each method.

3. Although focusing on her desire to be a responsible adult is an admirable attitude, potential scenarios can be presented for her "responsible" consideration, such as the following: What would she do if contraceptive failure resulted in a pregnancy? How would she feel if she contracted an incurable or permanently damaging sexually transmitted disease that she might pass on to someone else? How would she react now to being "dumped" by someone she cares for who is less responsible and mature? Asking about her goals and plans in life may be significant. Counseling that evidences concern for the individual at this stage may do a lot to postpone sexual activity until the patient is more mature. It is important for her to realize that choosing to delay sexual activity at this time may be the most responsible and health-promoting life decision she can make.

References

1. Centers for Disease Control and Prevention: Health, United States, 2005. http://www.cdc.gov/nchs/data/hus/hus05.pdf#summary. Accessed January 22, 2006.
2. National Institutes of Health. National Heart, Lung, and Blood Institute: NHLBI stops trial of estrogen plus progestin due to increased breast cancer risk, lack of overall benefit. NIH News release, July 9, 2002. http://www.nhlbi.nih.gov/new/press/02-07-09.htm.
3. Cates, W, Padian, NS: The interrelationship of reproductive health and sexually transmitted diseases. In Goldman, MB, and Hatch, MC (eds): Women and Health. Academic Press, San Diego, 2000, p 381.

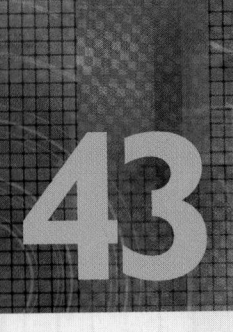

43

Nursing Care of Male Patients with Genitourinary Disorders

DEBRA PERRY-PHILO

KEY TERMS

cryptorchidism (kript-OR-ki-dizm)
epididymitis (EP-i-DID-i-MY-tis)
erectile dysfunction (e-RECK-tile dis-FUNK-shun)
hydrocele (HIGH-droh-seel)
orchiectomy (or-ki-EK-toh-mee)
orchitis (or-KIGH-tis)
paraphimosis (PAR-uh-fih-MOH-sis)
phimosis (fih-MOH-sis)
priapism (PRY-uh-pizm)
prostatectomy (PRAHS-tah-TEK-tuh-mee)
prostatitis (PRAHS-tuh-TIGH-tis)
retrograde (RET-roh-GRAYD)
suprapubic (SOO-pruh-PEW-bik)
tamponade (TAM-pon-AYD)
urodynamic (YOO-roh-dye-NAM-ik)
vasectomy (va-SEK-tuh-mee)

QUESTIONS TO GUIDE YOUR READING

1. How would you explain the pathophysiologies associated with male genitourinary and reproductive disorders?

2. What are the etiologies, signs and symptoms, and treatments of prostate disorders?

3. What nursing care will you provide for patients with male genitourinary or reproductive disorders?

4. What are disorders of the testes and penis, and how do they impact sexual function?

5. What are some physical and emotional causes of erectile dysfunction?

6. What is the nurse's role in helping men cope with the loss of sexual function?

7. Which disorders of the male reproductive system interfere with fertility?

8. What are the treatment options for male infertility?

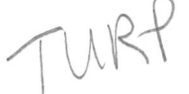
Problems affecting the male genitals and urinary system are generally difficult areas for both the patient and the nurse to deal with because of the sexual nature of the male anatomy. It is important to realize that sexuality is a natural part of each of us as human beings and should not be avoided when we provide care to patients. Very often the nurse is in an ideal position to provide important sexual health-care teaching to patients. If the patient is approached in a confident, confidential manner, it can be a positive learning experience for both the patient and the nurse.

PROSTATE DISORDERS

The prostate gland sits at the base of the bladder and wraps around the upper part of the male urethra like a doughnut. The primary purpose of the prostate is to provide alkaline secretions to semen and to aid in ejaculation. The prostate does not contain any hormones; however, many men fear that prostate problems and treatment will cause problems with their erections or their "nature" (sexual activities).

Prostatitis

Pathophysiology

Prostatitis, or inflammation of the prostate gland, can occur any time after puberty. The problem may be chronic or a single, acute episode. The inflammation causes the prostate gland to swell, resulting in pain, especially when standing. It eventually may lead to difficulty in passing urine as a result of an inward squeezing of the urethra that causes a mild obstruction.

Etiology

There are three basic types of prostatitis: acute bacterial, chronic bacterial, and nonbacterial. Bacterial prostatitis is most common in older men. It results in edema and inflammation of all or part of the prostate gland.

The bacteria primarily responsible for the infection are gram-negative organisms such as *Escherichia coli;* however, gram-positive and gonococcal bacteria may also play a part. The prostate gland may become infected by the following:

- Bacteria ascending the urethra
- Infected urine refluxing from the bladder into the prostatic ducts
- Bacteria in the blood or lymph supply to the gland
- Surgical instrumentation or other forms of urethral trauma.

Prevention

Ways to avert prostatitis are regular and complete emptying of the bladder to prevent urinary tract infection (UTI), avoiding excess alcohol (more than 2 to 3 oz per day—alcohol is a bladder irritant), and avoiding certain high-risk sexual practices. Avoiding contamination of the urinary tract and factors that produce congestion of the prostate gland are the best preventive measures.

Signs and Symptoms

The most common symptoms are the same ones that occur with any UTI: complaints of urgency, frequency, hesitancy, and dysuria. Because of the location and role of the prostate gland, the patient may complain of low back, perineal, and postejaculation pain; he may also have a fever and chills.

Complications

One complication of acute bacterial prostatitis is urinary retention. If the prostate is extremely swollen, it prevents complete bladder emptying. For most men, the most troublesome complication may be a temporary problem with erections. Ascending infections, prostatic abscess, **epididymitis,** and prostatic calculi (stones) are some of the more serious and rare complications of prostatitis.

Diagnostic Tests   PSA-Blood test

The first test performed is a careful, gentle, digital rectal examination (DRE) of the prostate. The prostate gland is examined by the health-care provider by insertion of a gloved finger into the rectum. The examiner may find a warm, irregular, swollen, painful prostate gland. A urine culture generally is positive for bacteria. The examiner may also gently massage the prostate gland and order an expressed prostate secretion (EPS) test that reveals bacteria and a large number of white blood cells.

Therapeutic Interventions

Acute bacterial prostatitis is usually treated medically with antibiotic therapy. The preferred treatment is trimethoprim and sulfamethoxazole (Bactrim) for 30 days. Other antibiotics, including the fluoroquinolones (ciprofloxacin, ofloxacin), may be used for chronic prostatitis (Table 43.1).

Other forms of treatment may include anti-inflammatory agents, stool softeners, warm sitz baths, prostatic massage, and diet changes such as decreasing spicy foods and alcohol. Patients should also avoid alpha-adrenergic agonist medications, which can cause urinary retention. In some cases, prostate surgery is necessary to remove the obstruction.

Nursing Process for the Patient with Prostatitis

ASSESSMENT/DATA COLLECTION. Begin the assessment by asking the patient to describe signs and symptoms that indicate evidence of a UTI, such as sudden fever, chills, and complaints of urgency, frequency, hesitancy, dysuria, and nocturia. In addition, the patient may have complaints of pain in the lower back, in the perineum, or after ejaculating. Ask the patient if he has ever had a UTI or prostate infection in the past. Care must be taken to assess urinary retention resulting from obstruction. Obtain a urine culture and assist with collection of the EPS specimen, if requested, as part of the patient assessment.

NURSING DIAGNOSIS, PLANNING, AND IMPLEMENTATION. The nursing diagnoses and interventions for patients with prostatitis may include:

(Text continued on page 938)

---

prostatitis: prostat—prostate gland + itis—inflammation

epididymitis: epi—upon + didym—testis + itis—inflammation

TABLE 43.1 MEDICATIONS USED FOR DISORDERS OF THE MALE REPRODUCTIVE ORGANS

Medication Class	Medication/Action	Route	Side Effects	Nursing Implications
Medications Used for Infections *Antibiotics*	Sulfonamides: Trimethoprim/ sulfamethoxazole (Bactrim; Septra) *Block bacterial synthesis of essential nucleic acids*	PO or IV	GI upset Anorexia Rash Urticaria Photosensitivity CNS disturbance Crystals in urine	Instruct patient to maintain hydration; take medication on empty stomach with 8 oz water. Avoid unnecessary sunlight.
	Fluoroquinolones: Ofloxacin (Floxin) Levofloxacin (Levaquin) *Inhibit cell wall synthesis*	PO or IV	GI upset Dizziness Headache CNS disturbances Flatulence Rash Photosensitivity Rare but serious: Tendon rupture	Do not administer with antacids. Caution with other medication use; renal, hepatic or CNS disorders.
Medications Used for Cancer of the Male Reproductive System: *Testosterone-Suppressing/Blocking Agents*	Leuprolide (Lupron) *Initially stimulates then inhibits follicle-stimulating and follicle-luteinizing hormones (FSH and LH) to suppress testosterone*	SQ or IM	GI upset Insomnia Sexual dysfunction Tremor Bone pain Constipation Gynecomastia CNS disturbance Photosensitivity Serious: Elevated liver enzymes Arrythmias MI	Store drug at room temperature and protect from light. Instruct patient that signs and symptoms may increase initially. Monitor for side effects.
	Goserelin (Zoladex) *Analogue to luteinizing-releasing hormone; works on pituitary to decrease follicle-stimulating hormone to decrease sex hormones*	Implanted	GI upset CNS disturbance Bone pain Sexual dysfunction Skin disorders Gynecomastia Serious: Arrythmias Hypertension Urinary obstruction Spinal cord compression	Inject into upper abdominal wall. Do not aspirate syringe. Educate patient medication may increase testosterone initially, thus increase incidence of signs and symptoms.
	Flutamide (Eulexin) *Inhibits androgen uptake and/or binding in tissues*	PO	GI upset Fatigue Sexual dysfunction Incontinence Constipation Rash Photosensitivity Gynecomastia Serious: Hypertension Hepatotoxicity Blood dyscrasias	Instruct patient that urine color changes to amber/yellow-green; avoid excess exposure to sun; promptly report side effects. Monitor hepatic function tests.
	Diethylstilbestrol (DES) (estrogen preparation) *Decreases FSH and LH to decrease testosterone*	PO or IV	GI upset CNS disturbance Visual disturbance Serious: Seizures Hypertension Thromboembolism*	Give with or after meals. Use cautiously with other disease processes or with conditions that lead to prolonged immobilization.

because of testosterone

minipres-relaxes smooth muscle. Also can be used for B/P

enlarged prostate

Medication Class	Medication/Action	Route	Side Effects	Nursing Implications
Medications Commonly Used for BPH *Alpha-Adrenergic Antagonists and Alpha-Reductase Inhibitors*	Tamsulosin (Flomax) Terazosin (Hytrin) Alfuzosin (Uroxatral) Doxazosin (Cardura) Alpha-adrenergic antagonists *Relax smooth muscle; produce vasodilatation*	PO	GI upset Dry mouth CNS disturbance Visual disturbance Palpitations Urinary urgency Sexual dysfunction Serious: Profound hypotension	Warn patient dizziness may occur with onset of use; report side effects. Monitor blood pressure/pulse. Do not crush or chew tablets. Caution with driving or use of heavy machinery.
	Finasteride (Proscar) Dutasteride (Avodart) *Alpha-reductase inhibitors. Inhibit enzyme responsible for formation of potent androgen from testosterone*	PO	Sexual dysfunction Gynecomastia Decreased volume of ejaculation	Do not chew or crush tablets. Baseline PSA and DRE before use. Instruct patient on side effects. Caution with liver dysfunction.
Medications Commonly Used for Erectile Dysfunction *Vasodilators, Smooth Muscle Relaxers, Hormone Replacement*	Sildenafil (Viagra) Tadalafil (Cialis) Vardenafil (Levitra) *Relax smooth muscle; produce vasodilation*	PO	GI upset Dizziness Headache Visual disturbance Flushing Rash Rare but serious: Prolonged erection Arrhythmias MI Stroke	Take about 1 hr before sexual activity (may be taken 0.5–4 hr before). Assess cardiovascular status before use; may be contraindicated. Avoid use when taking nitroglycerin preparations.
	Alprostadil (Caverject injection or Muse suppository) Prostaglandin E1 *Relax smooth muscle; produce vasodilation*	Intracavernosal injection or intraurethral suppository	Flulike symptoms Diarrhea Penile pain/fibrosis Urethral burning/bleeding Prolonged erection CNS disturbance Flushing Serious: Hypotension Seizures Heart rate disturbance	Monitor vital signs. Inform patient erection should occur in 2–5 min and not last for >4 hr. Instruct patient to report side effects immediately.
	Yohimbine *Herbal vasodilator*	PO	GI upset Tremors CNS disturbance Insomnia Tachycardia Serious: Hypertension OR severe hypotension Arrhythmias Cardiac failure	Assess for other medical conditions before use. Monitor blood pressure, renal and hepatic function.
	Testosterone transdermal (Testoderm, Androderm) Testosterone cypionate (Depotestosterone injection) *Testosterone replacements; produce androgen effects*	Transdermal patch IM	Gynecomastia Acne Nausea Insomnia Edema Male pattern baldness Itching Erythema Skin irritation Bladder irritability	Rule out cancer before use. Monitor hepatic function. Instruct patient to report side effects, prolonged erection, difficulty urinating.

CNS = central nervous system; DRE = digital rectal examination; GI = gastrointestinal; MI = myocardial infarction; PSA = prostate-specific antigen.
*NOTE: This medication promotes profound defects of the reproductive organs in offspring when taken by pregnant women. Even though this discussion is related to male disorders, it is prudent to acknowledge this fact at this time.

Impaired urinary elimination related to obstruction

EXPECTED OUTCOME: Patient will be able to void with urinary residual <25% of bladder capacity.

- If suspicion of urinary retention is present, determine urinary residual volume by catheterizing patient or obtaining a bladder ultrasound immediately after voiding. *Incomplete emptying of the bladder may lead to increased discomfort or ascending infection.*
- Have the patient complete a bladder log including patterns of elimination and urine loss, as well as volume/type of fluid consumed for 3 to 7 days. *This will provide for an objective verification of intake and output volumes and aid in determination of urinary retention.*
- Educate patient about avoidance of risk factors for urinary retention (e.g., alpha-adrenergic agonists, overfilling of the bladder). *These are modifiable variables that may limit retention of urine.*

Ineffective health maintenance: knowledge deficit related to cause, treatment, and prevention of prostatitis

EXPECTED OUTCOME: Patient will verbalize understanding of disorder and meet goals for health plan.

- Determine patient's current knowledge and understanding about cause and treatment of prostatitis. *This will allow for additional and/or correct information to be provided about the disorder for appropriate understanding.*
- Provide patient with additional and/or correct information about the cause and treatment of prostatitis. *This will allow the patient to have a full understanding of the etiology and care related to the disorder and increase likelihood of patient compliance.*
- Include patient's partner in care. *Some treatment options may also include treatment of the partner (e.g., sexually transmitted diseases such as gonorrhea, chlamydiosis, or trichomoniasis; see Chapter 44).*
- Encourage use of antibiotics as directed, and advise to take medication until finished *in order to best treat infection and prevent development of antibiotic-resistant bacteria.*

Impaired comfort related to swelling and irritation of the prostate gland

EXPECTED OUTCOME: Patient will state that comfort is at an acceptable level.

- Use a culturally appropriate pain scale to help patient identify comfort level. *This will aid in understanding comfort level as defined by the patient and aid in guiding appropriate interventions.*
- Encourage appropriate use of anti-inflammatory medication as ordered. *This will decrease inflammation and promote comfort.*
- Encourage use of comfort measures such as warm sitz baths or prostatic massage, as needed, *to decrease swelling and promote comfort.*
- Consult physician about need for stool softeners. *Firm stool will further irritate the prostate during defecation and increase discomfort.*

Anxiety related to sexual concerns

EXPECTED OUTCOME: Patient will identify presence of anxiety and verbalize concerns about sexuality.

- Identify source of concern related to sexual activity and meaning assigned to disorder as described by the patient. *This will help in guiding interventions that are appropriate for the patient related to etiology of concern.*
- Explore coping skills previously used by the patient to relieve anxiety, reinforce these skills, and explore other outlets for stress. *Coping mechanisms that have been helpful in the past may aid patient in dealing with current stressors that result in anxiety.*
- Encourage the patient to discuss possible complications and questions about sexual practices with his health-care provider. *In some cases, sexual intercourse is encouraged as a means of relieving prostatic congestion; in other situations, it may be contraindicated.*

EVALUATION. A clean urine culture with complete disappearance of signs and symptoms of prostatitis is the desired outcome. Maintaining an acceptable comfort level, understanding the cause and treatment plan, and verbalizing concerns related to the disorder are also desired throughout the care process. Prevention of chronic prostatitis can generally be achieved with patient education.

PATIENT EDUCATION. Teach the patient the causes, prevention, and treatment of prostatitis. Include risk factors such as the use of indwelling urinary catheters, poor hygiene or risky sexual practices, excessive intake of bladder irritants such as alcohol, ignoring signs and symptoms of UTIs, and poor compliance with the antibiotic treatment plan.

Encourage the patient to wash his hands and sitz bath equipment before and after each treatment. Fluids such as water and cranberry juice should be encouraged up to 2500 to 3000 mL per day unless contraindicated by heart failure or other chronic illness. Bladder irritants in the form of caffeine products (e.g., coffee, tea, cola, and chocolate), citrus juices, and alcohol should be taken in very limited amounts. Encourage the patient to empty his bladder every 2 to 3 hours even if he does not feel the urge to urinate.

Benign Prostatic Hyperplasia

Enlargement of the prostate gland is a normal process in older men. It begins at about age 50 and happens in 75% of men older than age 70. Benign prostatic hyperplasia (BPH) is a nonmalignant growth of the prostate that gradually causes urinary obstruction. According to current studies,

BPH does not increase a man's risk of developing cancer of the prostate.

Pathophysiology

There is a slow increase in the number of cells in the prostate gland, generally the results of aging and the male hormone dihydrotestosterone. As the size of the prostate gland increases, it begins to compress or squeeze the urethra shut. The narrowing of the urethra means the bladder must work harder to expel the urine. More effort and a longer time is required to empty the bladder. Eventually the narrowing causes an obstruction and may lead to urinary retention or eventually distention of the kidney with urine (hydronephrosis).

It is the location of the enlargement, not the amount, that causes the problem. A small growth in the prostate gland closest to the urethra may cause more problems with urination than a growth the size of an orange in the outer portion of the gland.

Etiology

There is no known cause of BPH other than normal aging. Some men think they may have caused the problem by certain sexual practices; however, there is no scientific proof at this time. Some factors that are being investigated in research studies are high-fat diet, ethnic background, and lifestyle issues.

Prevention

Because there is no known cause, there is no proven method to prevent enlargement of the prostate gland. There are many new treatments that are aimed at slowing down the enlargement process. One such treatment that is being researched is the herbal supplement saw palmetto.

Signs and Symptoms

Symptoms of BPH are usually identified in two ways; they are either problems related to obstruction or problems related to irritation. Symptoms related to obstruction include decrease in the size or force of the urinary stream, difficulty in starting a stream, dribbling after urination is thought to be completed, urinary retention, and a feeling that the bladder is not empty. The patient may also experience overflow incontinence or an interrupted stream, where the urine stops mid stream and then starts again.

Symptoms related to irritation include nocturia, dysuria, and urgency. A prostatic symptom index score sheet has been developed, and health-care providers are asking their older patients the questions as a way of assessing the seriousness of their symptoms and determining treatment options.

Complications

When BPH is untreated and obstruction is prolonged, serious complications may occur. Urine that sits in the bladder for too long can back up into the kidneys and cause hydronephrosis, renal insufficiency, or **urosepsis;** it can also damage the bladder walls, leading to bladder dysfunction, recurrent UTIs, or calculi (stones).

Diagnostic Tests

The first step is a medical history, including specific questions about the patient's symptoms. A DRE of the prostate is then conducted by the health-care provider to assess for enlargement and whether the gland is hard, lumpy, or "boggy." Primary tests include urinalysis and blood work. BUN (blood urea nitrogen), serum creatinine, and prostate-specific antigen (PSA) levels may be elevated. Secondary tests include **urodynamic** flow studies which may show a decreased urine flow rate. Transrectal ultrasound of the prostate and cystoscopy may reflect structural abnormalities.

Therapeutic Interventions

If the patient has no symptoms or only mild ones, the most current medical approach is "watchful waiting." The health-care provider watches for any increase in symptoms or signs that the urethra is becoming obstructed. Treatment of symptoms may include use of a catheter (indwelling or intermittent), encouraging oral fluids, and antibiotics for UTI.

Conservative medical treatment includes the use of medication to either relax the smooth muscles of the prostate and bladder neck or block the male hormone to prevent or shrink tissue growth. Alpha-adrenergic antagonists are medications that relax the smooth muscles, such as tamsulosin (Flomax), terazosin (Hytrin), and doxazosin (Cardura). These medications are also used to treat high blood pressure, so patients need to work closely with their health-care providers to avoid overdose or the negative side effects of postural hypotension (see Table 43.1).

The most commonly used medications to block the action of the male hormone in the prostate gland are finasteride (Proscar) and dutasteride (Avodart). All these medications must be taken on a long-term, continuous basis to achieve results. Conservative measures are used initially unless there are recurring infections, repeated gross hematuria, bladder or kidney damage, evidence of cancer, or unsatisfactory lifestyle changes.

Nonsurgical invasive treatments, some of which are experimental, are available in some areas of the country in addition to surgical options. These include the transurethral microwave antenna (TUMA), which involves heat applied directly to the gland, and may inhibit growth, and the prostatic balloon, which dilates the urethra by stretching or compressing urethral tissue. Prostatic stents may be used to open the passageway for urine to flow more freely.

Surgical Treatment

TRANSURETHRAL RESECTION OF THE PROSTATE. During the past 50 years, transurethral resection of the prostate (TURP) has been the surgical treatment used most often to relieve obstruction caused by an enlarged prostate (Fig. 43.1). Several other transurethral options also exist. Transurethral incision of the prostate (TUIP) uses surgical

---

urosepsis: uro—urine + sepsis—systemic infection

urodynamic: uro—urine + dynamic—force

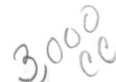

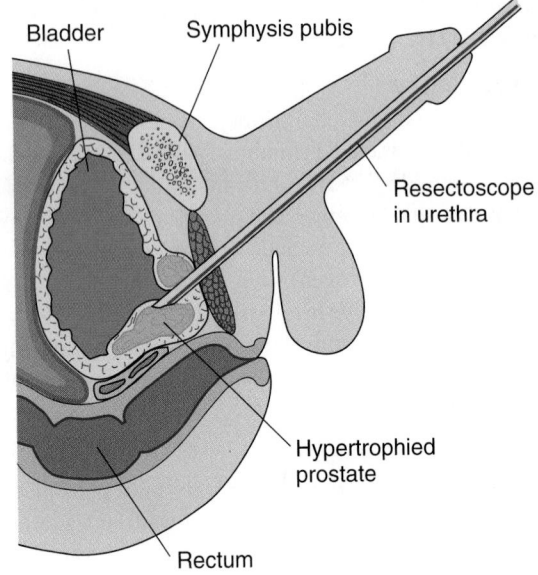

FIGURE 43.1 Transurethral resection of the prostate.

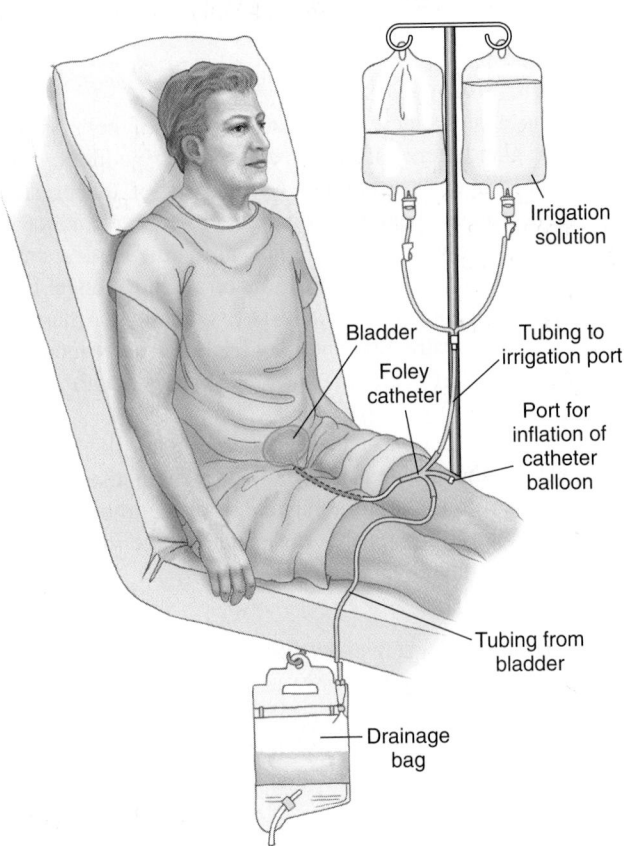

FIGURE 43.2 Bladder irrigation.

incisions into the gland to relieve obstruction. Transurethral ultrasound-guided laser-induced prostatectomy (TULIP) uses laser to relieve obstruction.

For TURP, the patient is anesthetized and the surgery is performed using an instrument called a resectoscope. The resectoscope is inserted into the urethra and the prostate gland is "chipped" away a piece at a time. Special surgical instruments are now being used that "vaporize" or "microwave" the pieces and cut down on the amount of bleeding during surgery. During routine TURP, the "chips" are flushed out using an irrigating solution and are sent to the laboratory to be analyzed for possible evidence of cancer. The prostate gland is not completely removed but peeled away like the rind of an orange. The prostatic tissue that is left eventually grows back and can cause obstruction again at a later time. Patients need to be reminded to continue having yearly prostate examinations.

As the tissue is removed during TURP, bleeding occurs. A Foley catheter is left in place with 30 to 60 mL of sterile water inflating the balloon. The balloon is overfilled and may be secured tightly to the leg or abdomen to **tamponade** (compress) the prostate area and stop the bleeding. Irrigation solution generally flows continuously (Fig. 43.2); manual irrigation may be done for the first 24 hours to help maintain catheter patency by removing clots and chips. The health-care provider will remove the Foley catheter after the danger of hemorrhage has passed.

You may need to save "serial urines" after the Foley catheter has been removed. To do this, each time the patient urinates, save some of the urine in a transparent cup, and make sure to line up the cups in order (usually on a shelf in the bathroom). This way you or the physician can see whether the urine is becoming progressively less bloody and clearer with each void.

Complications associated with prostate surgery depend on the type and extent of the procedure performed. The main

medical complications include clot formation, bladder spasms, and infection. Less common complications may be urinary incontinence, hemorrhage, and erectile dysfunction (Box 43.1 Nursing Care Plan for the Postsurgical Patient Having Transurethral Resection of the Prostate for Benign Prostatic Hyperplasia).

Retrograde ejaculation is a common side effect of prostate surgery. When any of the prostate gland is removed, there is a decrease in the amount of semen produced and a part of the ejaculatory ducts may be removed. The result is that less semen is pushed outside the body, and instead it "falls back" into the bladder. This causes no harm; the semen is simply passed during the next urination.

It is important to understand that erection, ejaculation, and orgasm are all separate actions. Erection means the penis becomes hard, ejaculation is the release of semen, and orgasm is felt as pulsations along the urethra. Unless additional problems are present, the patient continues to have erections and orgasmic sensations but decreased or no ejaculation.

RADICAL PROSTATECTOMY. When the prostate gland is very large, is causing obstruction, or is cancerous, a radical **prostatectomy** is performed to remove the entire prostate gland.

---

retrograde: retro—backward + grade—step
prostatectomy: prostat—prostate gland + ectomy—excision

Open Prostatectomy. Several approaches may be taken during traditional radical surgery (Fig. 43.3). In the **suprapubic** approach, an incision is made through the lower abdomen into the bladder. The gland is removed, and the urethra is reattached to the bladder. The retropubic approach is similar except there is no incision into the bladder. A perineal prostectomy involves making an incision between the scrotum and anus and removing the gland. This procedure is rarely done because of the increased risk of contamination of the incision (close to the rectum), and risk of urinary incontinence, erectile dysfunction, or injury to the rectum.

An open prostatectomy means a longer hospital stay compared with other BPH surgeries. A suprapubic catheter and care for an abdominal incision increase the length of stay and the risk for complications. Follow-up home care for

wound dressing changes and catheter care is an important aspect of nursing interventions for these patients.

Minimally Invasive Prostatectomy. Newer techniques use laparoscopy and even tiny robot arms to perform radical prostatectomy through five small "porthole" incisions in the abdomen. The surgeon makes all the decisions about the surgery while guiding the robotic arms. The robotic arms allow more precision and maneuverability, especially in small areas. Because robotic surgery is so much less invasive, studies are showing better results with less post-operative bleeding and incontinence and shorter hospital stays.

Nursing Process for the Patient with BPH and TURP

ASSESSMENT/DATA COLLECTION. Begin by asking the patient if he has ever had treatment or surgery for

---

suprapubic: supra—above + pubic—pubic bone

(Text continued on page 944)

Box 43.1   NURSING CARE PLAN for the Postsurgical Patient Having Transurethral Resection of the Prostate for Benign Prostatic Hyperplasia

Nursing Diagnosis: Risk for injury (bleeding) related to surgical intervention

Expected Outcomes Urine will become progressively more clear, with no abnormally heavy bleeding.

Evaluation of Outcomes (1) Is urine clearing? (2) Is bleeding reported promptly?

Interventions	Rationale	Evaluation
Closely monitor urinary output in terms of amount, color, and presence of clots at least every hour for the first 24 to 48 hr postoperatively. Monitor serial urines.	Careful monitoring and reporting of changes can help prevent major complications.	Is urine becoming progressively less bloody and more clear with each void?
Explain to patient that some bloody urine is normal after a TURP, as long as it does not suddenly get much worse. Also explain that a little blood mixed with irrigating fluid in a Foley bag may look worse than it actually is.	Seeing the catheter bag filled with bloody drainage may be upsetting to a patient or his family.	Is patient aware of what to expect in Foley bag?
Encourage patient to drink up to 2500 mL per day (unless contraindicated by other medical conditions) of water, noncitrus juices, and other noncaffeinated, nonalcoholic beverages.	Increasing urine flow can help flush blood from bladder.	Is patient drinking adequate amounts?
Teach patient to avoid constipation (stool softener, fluids, prune juice) and heavy lifting.	These can increase pressure in the abdomen and cause bleeding.	Does patient verbalize understanding of instructions?
Advise patient to lie down if urine becomes bright red or has large clots.	Activity can increase bleeding.	Does patient reduce activity if bleeding increases?
Teach patient to avoid aspirin and NSAIDs until risk of bleeding is over.	Aspirin and NSAIDs reduce platelet function and increase risk of bleeding.	Does patient verbalize understanding?

(Continued on following page)

Box 43.1 NURSING CARE PLAN for the Postsurgical Patient Having Transurethral Resection of the Prostate for Benign Prostatic Hyperplasia *(Continued)*

Nursing Diagnosis: Acute pain related to bladder spasms, obstruction, or surgical process

Expected Outcomes (1) Patient states pain has decreased to acceptable level. (2) Patient identifies at least two comfort measures.

Evaluation of Outcomes (1) Does patient state that pain is decreased to acceptable level? (2) Is patient able to identify at least two measures that will help relieve pain?

Interventions	Rationale	Evaluation
Monitor pain every 2 to 4 hr for first 48 hr and within 30 min of any intervention using a culturally specific scale.	A pain scale is a more accurate measure of pain.	Does patient verbalize pain as increasing or decreasing on the scale?
Monitor for signs of pain related to bladder spasms, obstruction, or surgical process, such as facial grimaces, irrigation solution that does not flow into bladder, urinating around catheter, multiple clots.	Relief of mechanical cause of pain promotes comfort, rest, and healing.	Is patient free from signs of pain related to bladder spasms, obstruction, or surgical process?
Give prescribed medication (analgesics, antispasmodics such as B&O suppository) and monitor response.	Medications relieve symptoms.	Does patient state relief when medications are given?
Irrigate catheter as ordered.	Removal of clots reduces spasms and pain.	Does irrigating solution go in and out easily? Are clots being removed?
Educate regarding and support use of nonpharmacologic methods to control pain such as relaxation and deep breathing techniques.	Relaxation calms spasms and relieves pain. Nonpharmacologic measures should be used with, not in place of, medication.	Is patient able to relax?

Nursing Diagnosis: Urge urinary incontinence related to poor sphincter control

Expected Outcomes (1) Patient identifies at least two methods to achieve dryness. (2) Patient verbalizes satisfactory control of dribbling.

Evaluation of Outcomes (1) Does patient identify ways to prevent incontinence? Do they help? (2) Does patient verbalize satisfaction with outcome?

Interventions	Rationale	Evaluation
Teach Kegel (pelvic floor) exercises (see Chapter 42)—to be practiced every time patient urinates and throughout the day.	Strengthens muscle tone to hold urine after catheter is removed.	Is patient able to start and stop urine stream?
Discuss use of condom catheter or penile pads.	Specific urine control devices are available for men.	Does patient indicate an informed choice of incontinence products?
Instruct patient to continue drinking 2000 to 4000 mL of noncaffeinated, nonalcoholic beverages each day.	Adequate nonirritating fluid intake is important for healing and preventing UTI.	Does patient drink adequate fluids even though he dribbles?
Encourage patient to discuss long-term (>6 months) incontinence problems with physician. National incontinence support groups are available.	Patient may need to learn self-catheterization or try medication.	Does patient verbalize understanding of what to do if incontinence continues?

Nursing Diagnosis: Ineffective therapeutic regimen management related to lack of knowledge of postoperative restrictions and care

Expected Outcomes (1) Patient avoids activities that increase intra-abdominal pressure resulting in excessive bleeding. (2) Patient verbalizes understanding of how to prevent postoperative infection.

Evaluation of Outcomes (1) Does patient verbalize understanding of how to prevent bleeding? (2) Is infection prevented?

Interventions	Rationale	Evaluation
Teach patient to avoid lifting heavy objects (>10 lb), stair climbing, driving, strenuous exercise, constipation, straining during bowel movements, and sexual activities until approved by physician (about 6 weeks).	Heavy lifting or straining can disrupt the healing process and result in tissue damage or excess bleeding.	Does patient verbalize understanding of reasons for limitation of heavy lifting and straining?
Instruct patient on proper catheter care using verbal, written, and demonstration techniques (some patients are sent home before catheter is removed). Include the following information: • Keep catheter bag secured to abdomen or thigh and below bladder. • Wash catheter/meatal junction with soap and water once daily. • Use clean technique to change from leg bag to night drainage bag. • Report signs and symptoms of UTI to physician immediately. • Encourage oral fluids.	Urinary tract infections are extremely dangerous and can cause death following genitourinary surgery in an elderly patient.	Can patient give a return demonstration of proper catheter care? Is patient free from signs and symptoms of infection?
Teach all patients to report bleeding that is not stopped with resting, fever, swelling, or difficulty urinating to physician promptly.	These are signs of complications that may require prompt intervention.	Does patient verbalize understanding of signs and symptoms to report?

Nursing Diagnosis: Anxiety related to concerns over loss of sexual functioning following prostate surgery

Expected Outcomes (1) Patient verbalizes normal sexual changes that happen after prostate surgery. (2) Patient identifies support systems if needed.

Evaluation of Outcomes Is patient able to verbalize understanding of expected body function following prostate surgery?

Interventions	Rationale	Evaluation
Explain to patient that he will probably have retrograde ejaculation into bladder after surgery. It is not harmful and semen will come out when he urinates.	Removal of the prostate gland often results in retrograde ejaculation.	Does patient understand what will happen when he ejaculates?
Instruct patient to talk with urologist if erection problems occur.	Urologists who specialize in treatment of erectile dysfunction can be helpful.	Is patient aware of local support services?

B&O = belladonna and opium; NSAIDs = nonsteroidal anti-inflammatory drugs; TURP = transurethral resection of the prostate; UTI = urinary tract infection.

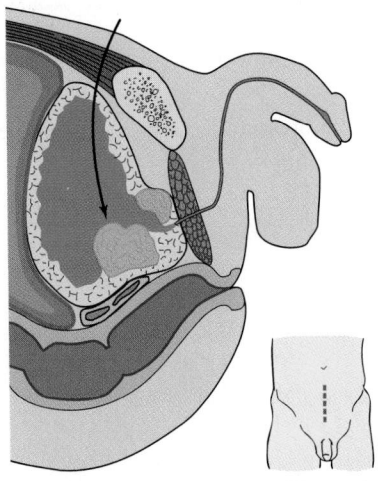

A. Suprapubic prostatectomy

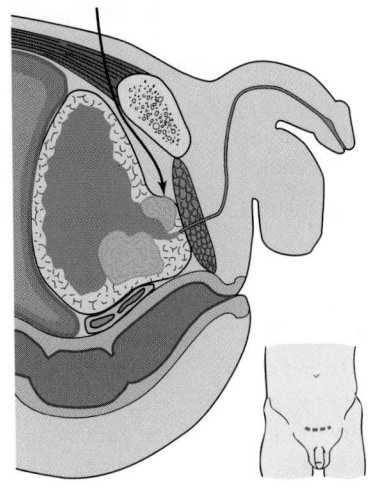

B. Retropubic prostatectomy

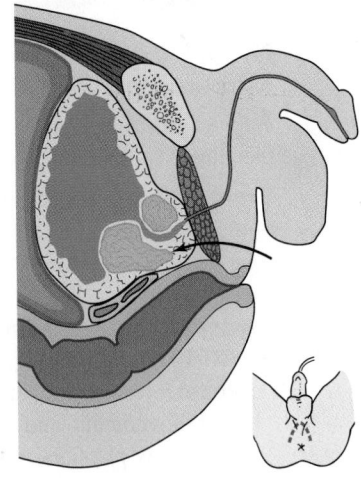

C. Perineal prostatectomy

FIGURE 43.3 *(A)* Suprapubic prostatectomy. *(B)* Retropubic prostatectomy. *(C)* Perineal prostatectomy.

prostate trouble. Assess amount and type of fluid intake per day and whether the patient has noticed any of the symptoms of BPH. Monitor output, and, if he is not catheterized, assure that urine retention is being managed appropriately.

NURSING DIAGNOSES, PLANNING, AND INTERVENTIONS. Nursing diagnoses for patients with mild or no symptoms are directed at knowledge deficits related to prevention of UTIs, knowing when to report an increase in symptoms to the health-care provider, and taking medication exactly as the health-care provider orders. Instruct patients to report changes in urinary output or difficulty voiding. Advise the patient to keep a log book of intake and output and difficulty voiding. Assure that patients scheduled for prostate surgery understand what to expect after surgery.

For nursing care of the patient following TURP see Box 43.1 Nursing Care Plan for the Postsurgical Patient Having Transurethral Resection of the Prostate for Benign Prostatic Hyperplasia. In addition, each patient experiences individual responses and needs. Care plans must be individualized, keeping in mind that the majority of these patients are elderly and have secondary medical problems such as cardiovascular disease.

EVALUATION. A patient should be discharged home with a minimum of bladder discomfort, light pink to clear urine, no evidence of UTI, and knowledge related to self-care at home. Home care nursing may be required if the patient lives alone or does not have the capacity to provide for meals, toileting, or transportation for the follow-up visit. See Box 43.2 Benign Prostatic Hyperplasia Summary.

Cancer of the Prostate

Cancer of the prostate is the second most common cause of cancer death in American men older than 60 years of age. The incidence of prostate cancer has been on the rise for many years, and just recently has begun to drop slightly. The

---

CRITICAL THINKING

Mr. Atkinson

■ Mr. Atkinson is a 68-year-old African American farmer with an enlarged prostate. He lives on a 75-acre farm with his wife and one son. He is scheduled for a TURP in 6 weeks.

1. Mr. Atkinson is currently taking terazosin (Hytrin), and his physician wants him to increase his dose from 2 mg to 5 mg q hr until surgery. He has a bottle at home of 2-mg tablets. How should you instruct him to take his medication? What side effect should he be advised to watch for?
2. What postoperative instructions should he be given in light of his occupation?
3. What should you tell him if he asks about how the surgery will affect his "nature" (sexual activities)?

Suggested answers at end of chapter.

---

cause for this is unknown. Most prostate cancers are very slow growing and often do not cause a major threat to health or life.

Pathophysiology

Prostate cancer depends on testosterone to grow. The cancer cells are usually slow growing and begin in the posterior (back) or lateral (side) part of the gland. The cancer spreads by one of three routes. If it spreads by local invasion, it will move into the bladder, seminal vesicles, or peritoneum. The cancer may also spread through the lymph system to the pelvic nodes and may travel as far as the supraclavicular nodes. The third route is through the vascular system to bone, lung, and liver. Prostate cancer is staged or graded based on the growth or spread.

Box 43.2

Benign Prostatic Hyperplasia (BPH) Summary

Signs and Symptoms	• **Related to Obstruction:** Decrease in size/force of stream, difficulty in starting stream, dribbling, interrupted stream, urinary retention, overflow incontinence • **Related to Irritation:** Nocturia, dysuria, urgency
Diagnostic Tests	• **Primary:** Urinalysis, BUN, serum creatinine, prostate-specific antigen (PSA) • **Secondary:** Urodynamic flow studies, transrectal ultrasound, cystoscopy
Therapeutic Interventions	• **Conservative:** Alpha-blockers, testosterone blockers • **Nonsurgical:** Transurethral microwave antenna (TUMA), prostatic balloon, prostatic stents • **Transurethral:** Transurethral incision of the prostate (TUIP), transurethral ultrasound-guided laser-induced prostatectomy (TULIP), transurethral resection of the prostate (TURP) • **Radical Prostatectomy:** Suprapubic, retropubic, perineal, laparoscopic, or robotic resection
Complications	• Ascending or localized infection • Injury to surrounding tissues during surgery • Impaired sexual function related to tissue injury
Priority Nursing Diagnoses	• Impaired urinary elimination related to obstruction • Ineffective health maintenance: knowledge deficit related to causes, treatment, and prevention of BPH • Pain (acute or chronic) related to urine retention, bladder spasms, surgery

Etiology

Age is the primary risk factor. Prostate cancer is found most often in men older than age 65 and is rare in men younger than age 40. Other risk factors are higher levels of testosterone, high-fat diet, and immediate family history.

Prostate cancer rates are highest in African American men and lowest in American Indian and Native Alaskan men.[1] Occupational exposure to cadmium (e.g., welding, electroplating, alkaline battery manufacturing) has been identified as an added risk factor.

Signs and Symptoms

Symptoms are rare in the early stage of prostate cancer. Later stages include symptoms of urinary obstruction, hematuria, and urinary retention. In the advanced (metastatic) stage, symptoms may be bone pain in the back or hip, anemia, weakness, weight loss, and overall tiredness.

Complications

Early complications of prostate cancer are related to bladder problems, such as difficulty in urinating, and bladder or kidney infection. As the cancer metastasizes, the patient may develop problems such as pain, bone fractures, weight loss, and depression; eventually death may occur if treatment is not successful.

Diagnostic Tests

A routine DRE of the prostate is the first test; often the examiner finds a hard lump or hardened lobe. Blood tests looking for high levels of prostate-specific antigen (PSA) or prostatic acid phosphatase (PAP) are done. When there is a palpable tumor, the health-care provider may order a transrectal ultrasound and biopsy to help confirm the diagnosis. Bone scans and other tests may be ordered to determine if the cancer has spread outside the prostate gland.

Therapeutic Interventions

Prostate cancer in the early stages may be treated with testosterone-suppressing medications, such as leuprolide (Lupron) or goserelin (Zoladex); surgery, such as TURP or radical prostatectomy; or a combination of medication and radiation therapy. In later stages, the treatment is usually a radical prostatectomy, radiation therapy, or implantation of radioactive "seeds" into the prostate (brachytherapy). Metastatic prostate cancer treatment involves relief of symptoms or blocking testosterone by bilateral **orchiectomy,** estrogen therapy (diethylstilbestrol [DES]), administration of antiandrogen (flutamide [Eulexin]), or use of agents such as leuprolide and goserelin. Sometimes chemotherapy is used to help relieve symptoms from the cancer spread.

Brachytherapy, external-beam radiation therapy, and radical prostatectomy combinations are showing favorable results in the treatment of advanced cancer. Gene therapy, vaccine, and immune-based interventions are the latest medical treatment options under investigation in the war against

---

orchiectomy: orchi—testes + ectomy—excision

prostate cancer. Nontraditional prostate cancer prevention using vitamin E and selenium continue to be investigated.

RADICAL PROSTATECTOMY. The radical prostatectomy procedure is generally reserved for patients with cancer of the prostate or when the gland is too large to resect using the TURP method.

The patient returns from surgery with a large indwelling catheter in the urethra and may also have a suprapubic catheter. Often there is a Penrose or sump drain in place to remove fluids from the abdominal cavity and allow the wound to heal from the inside outward. Special care must be taken to keep the incision and drain sites clean and dry. Dressings should be changed according to institution policy using sterile technique.

There are more complications associated with radical prostatectomy than any other treatment option. The major complications are hemorrhage, infection, loss of urinary control, and erectile dysfunction.

Patient Education

All men older than age 40 should be encouraged to have a yearly DRE of the prostate. Prevention and early detection are the best ways to fight prostate cancer.

PENILE DISORDERS

Problems of the penis, aside from sexually transmitted diseases, are fairly rare but may cause great concern and worry for the patient. Most men have difficulty seeking help for a "private" problem. It is important to be sensitive when assessing or providing care for these patients.

Peyronie's Disease

Peyronie's disease often gives the penis a curved or crooked look when it is erect. Fibrous bands or plaques form mainly on the dorsal (top) part of the layer of tissue that surrounds one of the corpora cavernosa of the penis. The plaque may be caused by injury or inflammation of the penile tissue, or it may come and go spontaneously. If the plaque is thick enough, it can cause curvature, painful erection, difficulty in vaginal penetration, and erectile dysfunction. When conservative treatments such as vitamin E, steroids, or ultrasound do not work, surgery may be needed to remove the plaque. Patients need to be reassured that the problem is not life threatening and can be treated.

Priapism

Priapism is a painful erection that lasts too long. Anytime an erection lasts for longer than 4 to 6 hours it can become a medical emergency. The small veins in the corpora cavernosa spasm, so the blood cannot drain back out of the penis as it should. When the blood cannot drain, the tissue of the

penis does not get oxygen and there can be permanent tissue damage. There may be a complete loss of erection ability after the priapism episode. Prolonged priapism can also prevent the patient from passing urine, which can lead to painful bladder and kidney problems. Some causes of priapism are prolonged sexual activity, sickle cell anemia, leukemia, widespread cancer, spinal cord injury or tumors, and use of medication or recreational drugs such as crack cocaine. Treatment in the emergency department may include ice packs, sedatives, analgesics, injection of medications directly into the penis to relax the vein spasms, needle aspiration, and irrigation of the corpora. If all else fails, surgery is done to drain the blood out of the penis.

Phimosis and Paraphimosis

Phimosis is the term used to describe a condition in which the foreskin of an uncircumcised male becomes so tight it is difficult or impossible to pull back away from the head of the penis. It may make it impossible to clean the area underneath. Smegma, a cottage cheese–like secretion made by the glands of the foreskin, becomes trapped under the foreskin and is an excellent place for the growth of bacterial and yeast infections. Treatment usually begins with antibiotics and warm soaks to the area. The physician may then cut a small slit in the foreskin to relieve the pressure and treat the infection. A full circumcision may be recommended if the problem continues or if a condom catheter is necessary for urine drainage. Phimosis is generally prevented by teaching uncircumcised males to pull the foreskin back carefully, wash with mild soap and water daily, and replace the foreskin to its normal position.

Paraphimosis occurs when the uncircumcised foreskin is pulled back, during intercourse or bathing, and not immediately replaced in a forward position. This causes constriction of the dorsal veins, which leads to edema and pain. Moderate to severe paraphimosis is a medical emergency and requires immediate care by a physician. The longer the problem continues, the greater the risk of circulation problems and possible gangrene. Again, prevention through daily cleaning and replacing the foreskin in its normal place is important.

Cancer of the Penis

Cancer of the penis has been found in men who were not circumcised as babies or have acquired the human papillomavirus (HPV). The tumor looks like a small, round, raised wart. It is one form of cancer that may be spread to the sex partner. Several research studies have found a link between cancer of the penis and cancer of the uterine cervix. Cancer of the penis may be treated with minor surgery such as a circumcision or laser removal of the growth. If the cancer has spread, the treatment may mean cutting away part or all of

---

priapism: priap—phallus + ism—condition of

phimosis: phimo—muzzling + osis—condition
paraphimosis: para—abnormal + phimo—muzzling + osis—condition

the penis, radiation, or chemotherapy. Finding and treating any wartlike tumor in its earliest stages is an important part of patient education.

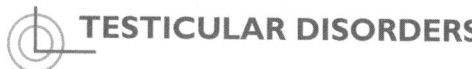 TESTICULAR DISORDERS

Cryptorchidism

Cryptorchidism (undescended testes) is a congenital condition in which a baby boy is born with one or both of his testes not in the scrotum. The testes normally drop down (descend) into the scrotum in the last 1 to 2 months before the boy is born. Many times the testes descend into the scrotum on their own by 2 years of age. If they do not descend by the age of 2, surgery should be done to correct the problem. Testes that are not brought down into the scrotum decrease a man's chances of producing a child, usually because excessive body heat damages sperm production in the testes. Studies have shown that the chances of testicular cancer are also higher if the condition is not corrected before the child reaches his teen years. If normal male sex characteristics do not develop during puberty because the testosterone level is too low, extra testosterone medication may be given. Testosterone can be administered in the form of a daily pill, by long-term injection, or by patch.

Hydrocele

A **hydrocele** is a collection of fluid in the scrotal sac. Hydroceles are not dangerous and generally do not cause any pain. The cause is not known, and it can happen at any point during the lifetime. No treatment is necessary unless the hydrocele is so large that it causes discomfort or embarrassment or is a threat to the blood supply to the testes. If treatment is needed, the health-care provider aspirates, or surgically drains, the fluid.

Varicocele

A varicocele is a condition sometimes called varicose veins of the scrotum. The main blood supply to the testes travels along the spermatic cord. The veins become dilated, and when the man is standing, the area in the scrotum begins to feel like a "bag of worms." The patient may complain of a pulling sensation, a dull ache, or scrotal pain. The sensations are most often felt when standing up. Most varicoceles occur on the left side because of the way the scrotal vein enters at a sharp angle from the left renal vein.

A varicocele is often not discovered until a couple tries to have a baby and is unable to conceive. It is believed that the varicose veins may increase the temperature of the testes and cause damage to the sperm. The most successful treatment is surgical repair of the varicose veins.

---

cryptorchidism: crypt—hidden + orchid—testis + ism—condition

hydrocele: hydro—water + cele—swelling

Epididymitis

The epididymis is a small tube along the back of the testes where sperm is matured for its last 10 to 12 days before it is ready to be ejaculated. Epididymitis is inflammation or infection of the epididymis that may be caused by bacteria, viruses, parasites, chemicals, or trauma. Epididymitis may be facilitated by sexual or nonsexual contact, a complication of some urological procedures, or reflux (backflow) of urine. The problem may also be associated with prostate infections and is usually painful, with the scrotal skin being tender, red, and warm to the touch.

Epididymitis is treated with antibiotics; the partner is also treated if it was sexually transmitted. Depending on the severity of the pain, the patient may be placed on bedrest with the scrotum elevated, possibly on ice packs, and also given analgesics. The pain and tenderness usually go away in about a week, although the swelling may last for several weeks. Complications may include chronic epididymitis, abscess formation, and sterility.

Orchitis

Orchitis is a rare inflammation or infection of the testes. The problem may be caused by trauma or surgical procedures, chemical substance, infection from epididymitis, UTI, or systemic diseases such as influenza, infectious mononucleosis, tuberculosis, gout, pneumonia, or mumps (after puberty). The patient has swollen, extremely tender testes, red scrotal skin, and a fever. Interventions are basically the same as for epididymitis and include bedrest, scrotal support, antibiotics, and medication to relieve pain and fever. Complications such as sterility from mumps orchitis can be prevented by giving boys the mumps vaccine at an early age.

Cancer of the Testes

Pathophysiology and Etiology

Cancer of the testes is the most common solid tumor in men 15 to 40 years of age and peaks between 20 and 34 years of age. The etiology of testicular cancer is unknown. Some of the known risk factors are cryptorchidism, family history, mother's use of DES (an estrogen preparation once used to prevent spontaneous abortion) while pregnant, white race, and high socioeconomic status. The tumors are mostly a germ cell type of cancer formed during normal embryo development.

Prevention

The best prevention is monthly testicular self-examination (TSE). The procedure is simple and easy to learn and should be taught to males between ages 15 and 40. See Chapter 41 for instructions on TSE.

Signs and Symptoms

Early warning signs of cancer may include a small, painless lump on the side or front of the testes. The patient may also notice that the scrotum is swollen and feels heavy. Late

---

orchitis: orch—testis + itis—inflammation

symptoms of back pain, shortness of breath, difficulty swallowing, breast enlargement, and changes in vision or mental status indicate metastasis of the cancer.

Complications

Emotional complications can range from fear of cancer and death to feelings of loss of masculine body image and sexual function. Physical complications may involve dealing with pain and the effects of metastasis to areas such as the lungs, abdomen, or lymph nodes. Other less common areas of cancer spread are the liver, brain, and bone. Treatments such as surgery, chemotherapy, and radiation therapy can all have negative side effects on the patient and require special care.

Diagnostic Tests

When a tumor is found, several laboratory and radiographic tests are done. An ultrasound of the testes is done first. If the test shows cancer, a chest x-ray examination is done to look for spread to the lungs. A scan of the lymph nodes, liver, brain, and bones may also be ordered. Blood is drawn to look for what are called tumor markers. An example of a tumor marker for testicular cancer is beta human chorionic gonadotropin (bHCG). An exploration, biopsy, and removal of the testes are done to decide the stage of the tumor.

Testicular tumors may be staged or classified in several ways. The simplest way to stage a testicular tumor is as follows:

- Stage I—tumor only in the testes
- Stage II—tumor spread to groin lymph nodes
- Stage III—tumor spread past lymph nodes, usually to the lungs

Therapeutic Interventions

Intervention depends on the stage of the cancer. All treatment begins with complete removal of the cancerous testes, spermatic cord, and local lymph nodes. Stage I tumor treatment then includes radiation to the groin area lymph nodes. Treatment for stage II involves chemotherapy. Stage III or metastatic cancer is treated with both radiation and chemotherapy. If the cancer is found in the beginning stages, the chances for complete recovery are about 75%. All patients should have regular follow-up testing.

Nursing Care

Nursing care is directed first at prevention, by teaching young men to practice monthly testicular self-examination and to see their health-care provider if they notice any changes. If a diagnosis of cancer has been made, provide emotional support for the patient. If the patient wants to have children, he should be encouraged to make deposits in a sperm bank before any surgery or treatment is started. The patient and his partner may have many questions about sexual activities as they go through treatment. Encourage them to talk with their health-care provider or a sex therapist about ways to express love and tenderness toward one another. Helping patients deal with pain and the side effects of chemotherapy or radiation therapy are also important nursing interventions for these men. See Chapter 10 for care of the patient with cancer.

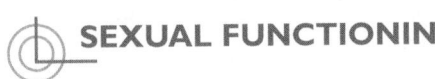

CRITICAL THINKING

Mr. Cunningham

■ Mr. Cunningham is a 23-year-old college student engaged to be married next spring. While taking a shower one day he discovers a lump on his left testis.
1. What should he do?
2. What are the treatment options if Mr. Cunningham has cancer of the testes?
3. How can you help Mr. Cunningham cope with the diagnosis?

Suggested answers at end of chapter.

SEXUAL FUNCTIONING

Vasectomy

A **vasectomy** is the surgical cutting and sealing off of the vas deferens to prevent sperm from reaching the outside of the body. This 15- to 30-minute surgery is performed most often as a permanent birth control method but may also be performed on some men during prostate gland removal. The male patient should carefully discuss the surgery with his physician, so there is a clear understanding of the results following the procedure.

The testes continue to produce the male hormone testosterone and sperm. The prostate gland, along with the seminal vesicles, still ejaculate semen, but the semen does not contain sperm. There should be no major change in the way the ejaculate looks or feels following the procedure. The patient should be encouraged to continue using another birth control method for about 6 weeks after surgery to be sure there are no sperm left in the tract above the surgical site. A semen sample should be sent to be evaluated for the absence of sperm before the procedure is considered successful. The sperm continue to be produced in the testes but are absorbed by the body.

There are times when the man may decide he wants to have more children and asks to have the vasectomy "undone." The surgical procedure to reverse a vasectomy is called a vasovasotomy. Using microscopic instruments, the surgeon reconnects the two pieces of the vas deferens. During the surgery the physician generally tries to determine whether the testes are still producing good sperm. If the vasectomy was done less than 10 years before, the fertility success rate is higher. A vasovasotomy is generally not an option if the vasectomy procedure is more than 10 years old.

Erectile Dysfunction

Problems with getting or keeping an erection can happen at any age and have been a concern of men and their partners for centuries. It is a unique problem because it affects not

---

vasectomy: vas—vas deferens+ ectomy—excision

Injection Method. After careful evaluation, a patient or his partner may be taught how to inject a medication into the penis using a 26- or 27-gauge needle on a tuberculin syringe or a prefilled autoinjector. The injections are nearly painless and produce a natural erection in 10 to 15 minutes. The erection may last 1 to 2 hours, and patients are generally limited to a maximum of three injections per week. The dosage is regulated on an individual basis. The most serious side effect is priapism, which requires immediate reversal in a physician's office or emergency room. When the patient is taught and monitored carefully, the risk of complications is minimal.

Transurethral Suppository. In order to facilitate medication dispersion and absorption, a patient may choose to use a suppository. The patient is instructed to urinate before use of the suppository. A tiny pellet (microsuppository) is inserted into the urethra using a specialized single-dose applicator. The medication usually begins to work in 5 to 10 minutes, and the effects last for approximately 30 to 60 minutes. Side effects can occur with high medication doses.

OTHER NONSURGICAL TREATMENTS. Sexual Devices And Techniques. There are a variety of sexual aids, such as vibrators and dildos (hollow penises), that may be alternatives for patients who do not want or cannot afford expensive medical treatment. They should be encouraged to talk with a health-care provider or qualified sex therapist before trying these alternatives.

Suction devices are another nonsurgical treatment option. This is an external cylinder vacuum device that fits over the penis and draws the blood up into the corporeal bodies, causing an erection. A penile ring is then slipped onto the base of the penis. Once the cylinder is removed, sexual intercourse can begin. Special care must be taken to remove the penile ring within 15 to 20 minutes to prevent tissue damage. The suction device may be used alone or with intracorporeal injection therapy for patients who have difficulty keeping an erection. The companies that manufacture the suction devices provide free videotapes and written patient instruction booklets.

SURGICAL TREATMENTS. Penile Implants (Prostheses). Penile implants are a pair of solid or fluid-filled chambers that are surgically placed into the corporeal bodies in the penis to produce an erection. This treatment option has been used successfully for more than 25 years. There are two basic types of implants—noninflatable and inflatable (Fig. 43.4). The noninflatable type is economical, can be surgically implanted in less than an hour, and provides firmness for penetration. The inflatable device contains a sterile saline solution that fills the cylinders using a manual pumping action. When activated, the inflatable implant provides both firmness and an increase in diameter of the penis. Although the inflatable device is more expensive and has a greater risk of mechanical failure, it provides a more natural-appearing and natural-functioning erection than the noninflatable implant.

Penile implants are considered secondary treatment options because they have a risk of complications such as mechanical failure, infection, and erosion. Patients at greatest risk for complications are those with uncontrolled diabetes and those with severe circulation problems. Patients should be taught that an implant will not restore ejaculation or orgasm if these functions have been lost before the surgery. Surgery recovery time varies from 4 to 6 weeks; the patient must receive approval from the health-care provider before having sexual intercourse.

Vascular Surgery. If a younger man (younger than age 35) has an erection problem caused by poor blood flow into the penis or from blood leaking out of the penis, rapidly causing the loss of the erection, corrective surgery may be performed. A bypass graft may be done to increase the blood flow into the penis or to go around a blockage (e.g.,

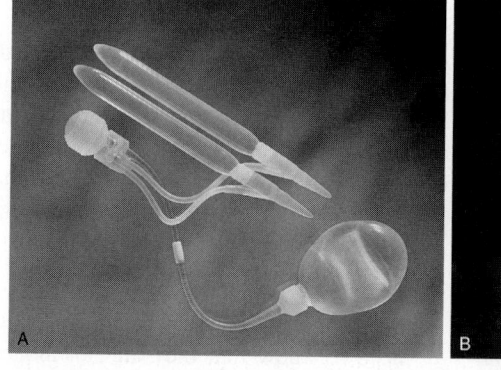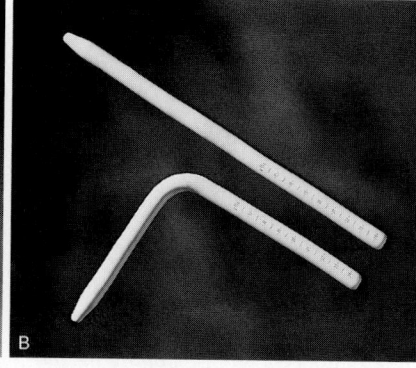

FIGURE 43.4 Penile implants. *(A)* Inflatable penile implant. Inflatable cylinders are implanted in the penis, the small hydraulic pump in the scrotum, and the fluid-filled reservoir in the lower abdomen. Sterile radiopaque saline from the reservoir fills the cylinders to provide an erection. *(B)* Malleable penile implant. Malleable rods are implanted into the penis. The penis is always firm, but the rods can be bent close to the body when erection is not desired. *(Alpha-1 implant [A] and Acu-Form implant [B] photographs courtesy Mentor Urology, Santa Barbara, CA.)*

Peyronie's disease). If the blood leaves the corporeal bodies too fast, a procedure to ligate (tie off) the leaking veins may be successful. Neither surgery works well in older men because the bypass graft rapidly becomes obstructed and the natural tendency of the older body is to form collateral circulation around the veins that are tied off.

Nursing Process for the Patient with Erectile Dysfunction

ASSESSMENT/DATA COLLECTION. Before the assessment begins, it is important to provide privacy and ensure confidentiality. A complete sexual history, often conducted by a nurse, is taken, with special focus on factors related to the circulatory, nervous, and endocrine systems. The questions cover the following:

- Medical problems
- Surgical treatments that might interfere with blood flow or nerve supply to the groin or spine
- Genitourinary problems
- A complete list of medications used, including over-the-counter drugs and any evidence of substance abuse
- General lifestyle patterns, including stress factors, depression, and excessive use of alcohol, caffeine, or nicotine
- Sexual patterns and practices

A physical examination is performed by the physician or health practitioner to assess for any evidence of congenital deformities, hormonal imbalance, decreased circulation, or nerve damage. Throughout the assessment process, it is important to observe for any signs of psychological or emotional distress.

NURSING DIAGNOSES, PLANNING, AND IMPLEMENTATION. Nursing diagnoses and interventions related to sexual dysfunction may include:

Anxiety related to effect of pathology on sexual performance

EXPECTED OUTCOME: Patient will identify presence of anxiety and verbalize concerns about sexual dysfunction.

- Identify source of concern related to sexual activity and meaning assigned to disorder as described by the patient. *This will help in guiding interventions that are appropriate for the patient related to the etiology of concern.*
- Explore coping skills previously used by the patient to relieve anxiety. Reinforce these skills, and explore other outlets for stress. *Coping mechanisms that have been helpful in the past may aid patient in dealing with current stressors that result in anxiety. This will also allow the patient to sort through issues related to sexual dysfunction and be an active participant in working toward resolution.*

Ineffective health maintenance related to knowledge deficit of cause and treatment of sexual dysfunction

EXPECTED OUTCOME: Patient will verbalize understanding of the cause and treatment options for erectile dysfunction.

- Determine patient and partner's current knowledge and understanding about cause and treatment of the disorder. *This will allow for additional and/or correct information to be provided about sexual dysfunction for appropriate understanding.*
- Provide patient and partner with additional and/or correct information about cause and treatment of disorder. *This will allow the patient to have a full understanding of the etiology and care related to the disorder, and increase likelihood of patient compliance and success of treatment.*
- Refer patient and partner (as appropriate) for medical treatment, psychological treatment, or counseling. *An individualized treatment plan (determined by the etiology) is needed to move toward restoration of sexual functioning.*

Self-esteem disturbance related to inability to practice usual/expected sexual activity

EXPECTED OUTCOME: Patient will verbalize effect of sexual dysfunction on feelings of self-esteem.

- Provide privacy and be verbally and nonverbally nonjudgmental when allowing patient and his partner to express concerns about sexual dysfunction. *Treatment success rates are generally higher when a rapport is established with the caregiver and the partner is included in the decision-making process.*
- Validate the patient's feelings and let the patient know he is normal. *A sensitive nurse who has an understanding of sexual health can best direct those who need intervention.*
- Support realistic expectations about treatment and outcomes *as unrealistic, unmet expectations will lead to further self-esteem impairment.*

EVALUATION. The best indicator of a positive outcome is restoration of erectile function with a verbal account of understanding the disorder and satisfaction with the treatment process. Sometimes the physical problem is easier to correct than the emotional scars that the problem has created. It is important to evaluate both the physiological and emotional outcomes of treatment.

PATIENT EDUCATION. The nurse plays an important role in public education related to erectile dysfunction. Men need to know that they are not alone with their problem. More than 20 million men in the United States experience ongoing problems with erections. The majority of the causes are physical, and help is available through health-care providers who specialize in treating erectile dysfunction.

Conservative treatment options are tried first, with surgical interventions reserved as a last resort. Treatment may be as simple as a change in lifestyle or in medication. Men need to be encouraged to seek help from appropriate health-care providers and recognize that erectile dysfunction is a treatable condition with positive outcomes.

See Box 43.3 Male Sexual Dysfunction Summary.

CRITICAL THINKING

Mr. Kittle

■ Mr. Kittle presents to the clinic with a complaint of not being able to sustain an erection long enough for sexual intercourse that is satisfactory for himself and his partner.

1. You have never had a patient tell you his sexual problems, and you feel a little uncomfortable. How should you respond?
2. What will your assessment include?
3. What treatment options might be offered?

Suggested answers at end of chapter.

Infertility

A growing number of couples in the United States are having difficulty conceiving children. Several factors can interfere with a man's ability to father a child.

Physiology

Eight fundamental male physiological factors are necessary for normal conception to occur:

- Proper endocrine function between the hypothalamus, pituitary gland, and testes
- At least one testis that produces quality sperm
- An epididymis, or storage place, to mature the sperm
- A duct system to transport sperm from the testes to the outside of the body
- Glands that secrete the right type and amount of seminal fluid to nurture and transport the sperm
- An intact nervous system that helps provide an erection and ejaculation
- Semen that meets the following criteria: volume 1.5 to 5 mL, a concentration of more than 20 million sperm per milliliter, 50% to 60% of the sperm classified as grade 2 mobility, 60% to 80% of sperm with a normal shape, pH between 7.2 and 7.8, a small amount of fructose (sugar, a food supply), and sperm (semen) that first coagulates and then liquefies
- A basic knowledge of sexual practices, along with a willing partner

Etiology

The factors related to infertility are divided into three general categories: pretesticular, testicular, and posttesticular.

Box 43.3

Male Sexual Dysfunction Summary

Signs and Symptoms
- Report of problems with obtaining and keeping an erection
- Reported dissatisfaction with sexual performance

Diagnostic Tests
- Primary: History and physical
- Secondary: Vascular flow evaluation, apnea studies

Therapeutic Interventions
- Counseling
- Medication to increase blood flow to the penis
- Surgical implants or repair of structural disorders

Complications
- Infection
- Injury to surrounding tissue during surgical treatment

Priority Nursing Diagnoses
- Anxiety related to effect of pathology on sexual performance
- Ineffective health maintenance: knowledge deficit related to cause and treatment of sexual dysfunction
- Self-esteem disturbance related to inability to practice usual/expected sexual activity

PRETESTICULAR (ENDOCRINE) FACTORS. The first factor involves the proper functioning of the hypothalamus, the pituitary gland, and the testes. These endocrine functions are complex and are a rare cause of infertility. Examples of endocrine causes might be pituitary or adrenal tumors, thyroid problems, or uncontrolled diabetes.

TESTICULAR FACTORS. The two most common causes of male infertility are a varicocele (40% to 50%) and idiopathic causes (40%). It is believed that a varicocele lowers the sperm count by raising the blood flow and temperature in the testes. Sperm cannot live if the temperature is too high or too low.

Congenital anomalies such as Klinefelter's syndrome (a chromosomal defect) or cryptorchidism result in absent or damaged testes. Failure of a part of the male reproductive system to develop as a result of the mother's use of DES or other drugs during pregnancy may also result in fertility problems.

Certain disease or inflammatory processes may cause damage to the storage area (epididymitis) or to the testes themselves (mumps orchitis). Any high fever or viral infection can interfere with the production of sperm for up to 3 months.

Medications, radiation, substance abuse, environmental hazards, and lifestyle practices have all been identified as possible factors that can interfere with spermatogenesis (sperm production). Medications such as cimetidine (Tagamet), sulfasalazine (Azulfidine), anabolic steroids (testosterone), anticancer drugs (cyclophosphamide [Cytoxan], methotrexate), recreational drugs (cocaine, marijuana), and antihypertensives (methyldopa) have all been identified as possible causes of infertility. Radiation damage, whether as treatment for cancer or job related, tends to depend on the dosage received. A small amount of radiation causes temporary loss of sperm. Permanent sterility occurs with large doses or prolonged treatment. The relation between use of drugs such as cocaine and marijuana and infertility has been documented in several studies, but there is no clear indication of the amount or length of time it takes for these substances to cause infertility problems. Environmental hazards such as pesticides, Agent Orange, and lead poisoning have been listed as possible causes of infertility and are still under investigation. Excessive use of hot tubs and saunas, wearing tight jeans, and long-haul truck driving have all been identified as raising the temperature level in the scrotum to the extent that the sperm production is decreased.

POSTTESTICULAR FACTORS. The most common factor in post–testicular surgery infertility is the result of surgery or injury along the pathway from the testes to the outside of the man's body. Examples of surgical causes are vasectomy, bladder neck reconstruction, pelvic lymph node removal, or any surgery that causes retrograde ejaculation. Congenital anomalies and various types of infections may also cause infertility problems.

Prevention

Prevention involves possible lifestyle changes to avoid excessive heat to the scrotum, substance abuse, exposure to toxins, and environmental hazards. Problems related to medication or infections should be discussed with the healthcare provider.

Signs and Symptoms

A couple is considered infertile if they have been unsuccessful at becoming pregnant after at least 1 year of unprotected intercourse. If pregnancy has occurred during the year but there was no delivery, the problem is generally considered a female rather than a male factor.

Diagnostic Tests

Diagnosis begins with a detailed history and physical examination that looks for known male causes of infertility.

History

SEXUAL PRACTICES. Assessment includes frequency of intercourse, positions, timing (according to ovulation cycle), use of contraceptives, problems with premature ejaculation, and erection problems.

LIFESTYLE PRACTICES. Weight lifting or use of steroids, hot tubs, or saunas; tight jeans; use of nicotine, caffeine, alcohol, or marijuana; and the strength of desire for children on the part of the man are all assessed.

OCCUPATION. High stress, long periods of sitting, and exposure to environmental toxins are determined.

MEDICAL-SURGICAL HISTORY. Assessment includes any sexually transmitted viruses or diseases, endocrine problems, congenital urinary problems, serious illnesses or groin injuries, cancer, and treatment with chemotherapy or radiation.

Physical Examination

The examiner (generally a primary care practitioner) will observe for normal hair pattern and growth, muscle development, size of testes, and any evidence of a varicocele or hydrocele.

Diagnostic Tests

A semen analysis is done after collecting several specimens following a special collection technique. It is analyzed to see if it contains the right amount and type of healthy sperm needed for a pregnancy. Infection should be ruled out. There are several other tests that may be done, depending on the level of desire and the financial resources of the couple. Many insurance companies do not pay for the tests or treatment options for infertility.

Therapeutic Interventions

Treatment may be as simple as making a change in sexual or lifestyle practices. If the couple is able to handle the emotional and financial strain, they may try male surgery to correct a varicocele or a variety of in vitro fertilization procedures. The success rates for in vitro fertilization range from 8% to 60% and generally cost several thousand dollars each time an attempt is made. Another possible option that should be presented to the couple is adoption.

You can play an important role in the emotional support a couple needs during infertility studies. It is important that the couple feel comfortable in communicating their feelings and frustrations with one another and their healthcare provider. You may need to be the communication link, explaining various tests and cost factors and discussing how long the couple may want to continue trying the various treatment options. It may also help them to talk with other couples or attend a support group designed for couples experiencing infertility. For more information, visit http://www.nlm.nih.gov/medlineplus/infertility.html.

REVIEW QUESTIONS

1. A patient with benign prostatic hyperplasia expresses concern that he has cancer. Which response by the nurse is best?
   a. "Don't worry; prostatic hyperplasia is not the same thing as cancer."
   b. "Since it is called benign, you don't have to worry about it. No treatment should be necessary; you will just need to have it watched."
   c. "Hyperplasia means your prostate is growing too many cells. They are not cancerous, but they could interfere with your ability to urinate, so it is important to have it treated."
   d. "You are correct, it is a form of cancer, but it is very slow growing and very treatable. Your doctor will recommend treatments for you."

2. Which of the following is the most commonly used surgical treatment for BPH?
   a. TUIP
   b. TUMA
   c. TURP
   d. TULIP

3. A patient who is 1 day post–transurethral resection of the prostate says he is having pain in his bladder, and the nurse notices urine leakage around his catheter. Which of the following responses by the nurse is best?
   a. "Bladder spasms are common after your surgery. Take some deep breaths while I get a B&O suppository."
   b. "You should not be experiencing spasms. I will notify the RN right away."
   c. "Spasms can be very painful. Would you like an injection of Demerol?"
   d. "Your catheter is leaking; we will need to replace it right away."

4. A nurse working in a nursing home notes that it is difficult but not impossible to retract the foreskin for washing on an elderly gentleman. Which action is correct?
   a. Avoid retracting the foreskin for cleaning to prevent paraphimosis. The penis secretes an anti-bacterial substance that is self-cleaning.
   b. Gently retract the foreskin for cleaning, then replace it and notify the physician.
   c. Retract the foreskin for cleaning, and leave it retracted to prevent infection.
   d. Retract the foreskin and leave it retracted until the physician can evaluate it.

5. Which of the following is the most common cause of erectile dysfunction?
   a. Endocrine problems
   b. Circulatory problems
   c. Nervous system problems
   d. Excessive alcohol use

6. A patient is admitted to a medical unit for complications of diabetes. The nurse asks if he is satisfied with his level of sexual functioning, and he becomes tearful. Which initial response by the nurse is best?
   a. "You seem upset with my question. Are you having a problem you would like to talk about?"
   b. "Impotence is common with diabetes. Don't let it worry you."
   c. "What kind of sexual dysfunction are you experiencing?"
   d. "I am sorry you are having problems with your sexual functioning. Would you like a referral to a sex therapist?"

Multiple response item. Select all that are correct.
7. What are common complications of varicocele?
   a. Infertility
   b. Infection
   c. Erectile dysfunction
   d. Pain
   e. Priapism
   f. Cancer

8. Which of the following might be included in the treatment plan for male infertility?
   a. Penile implants
   b. Prostatectomy
   c. TURP
   d. Decrease in nicotine and alcohol use

Reference

1. American Cancer Society: Incidence and Mortality Rates by Site, Race, and Ethnicity, US, 1997–2001. Accessed www.cancer.org, August 8, 2005.

SUGGESTED ANSWERS TO

CRITICAL THINKING

■ *Mr. Atkinson*

1. $$\frac{5 \text{ mg} \quad | \quad 1 \text{ tablet}}{2 \text{ mg}} = 2.5 \text{ tablets}$$

   Mr. Atkinson should be alert for signs of hypotension, such as dizziness or lightheadedness on arising. He should not drive until effects/side effects of the medication are known.

2. Mr. Atkinson should be instructed not to lift anything heavier than 10 lb for the first 6 weeks, and he will not be able to plow or drive for the first 6 weeks. It is important that his son understand his father's limitations and how important it is for him or someone else to help out with the farm chores.

3. Mr. Atkinson will notice a change in his ejaculation (either very little ejaculate or none at all). If he could get an erection before surgery, the chances are very good that he will continue to be able to have intercourse; however, he will not ejaculate.

■ *Mr. Cunningham*

1. Mr. Cunningham should be encouraged to see his health-care provider immediately for an evaluation to rule out cancer of the testes.

2. Depending on the stage of the cancer, he will have the cancerous testis, cord, and lymph nodes removed. He may need chemotherapy or radiation treatments as well.

3. Mr. Cunningham should be encouraged to make deposits at a certified sperm bank before any treatments. It is also important to include his future wife and his family in the decision-making process and encourage them to share their feelings and concerns with one another. Cancer support groups may also be helpful to Mr. Cunningham.

■ *Mr. Kittle*

1. It is okay to "pretend" here! Act like you are perfectly comfortable, and that you hear this sort of thing every day. (Of course, you would never pretend to know something you don't—it is always okay to say you don't know.) Have a matter-of-fact communication style. If you get nervous and forget what questions you should ask, start with something general like, "Can you tell me more about your symptoms?"

2. Subjective and objective assessment related to Mr. Kittle's erectile dysfunction should include assessing for medical and surgical factors that might affect his ability to obtain and sustain an erection. This history should primarily focus on the cardiovascular, respiratory, neurological, and reproductive systems. A psychosocial assessment to identify presence of stress, fear, depression, fatigue or problems with interpersonal relationships should also be performed. A medication review may lead to identification of substances that influence erectile ability.

3. Treatment options will depend on the cause. Options may include: Psychotherapy/support group therapy, oral/absorbable/injectable medications, surgical implants or vascular surgery, and nonsurgical devices/techniques which include vibrators and dildos.

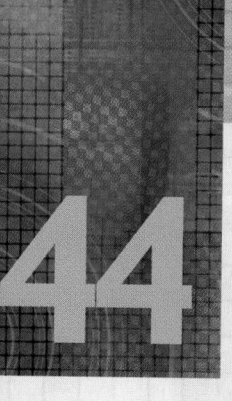

44

Nursing Care of Patients with Sexually Transmitted Diseases

DEBRA PERRY-PHILO AND
LINDA HOPPER COOK

KEY TERMS

cervicitis (SIR-vi-SIGH-tis)
chancre (SHANK-er)
condylomata acuminata (KON-di-LOH-ma-tah ah-KYOOM-in-AH-tah)
condylomatous (KON-di-LOH-ma-tus)
conjunctivitis (kon-JUNK-ti-VIGH-tis)
cytotoxic (SIGH-toh-TOCK-sick)
electrocautery (ee-LECK-troh-CAW-tur-ee)
electrocoagulated (ee-LECK-troh-coh-AG-yoo-LAY-ted)
endometritis (EN-doh-me-TRY-tis)
epidemiological (EP-i-DEE-me-ah-LAHJ-i-kuhl)
gummas (GUM-ahs)
hepatosplenomegaly (he-PAT-oh-SPLE-noh-MEG-ah-lee)
herpetic (her-PET-ik)
lymphadenopathy (lim-FAD-e-NAH-puh-thee)
mucopurulent cervicitis (MYOO-koh-PYOOR-uh-lent SIR-vi-SIGH-tis)
ophthalmia neonatorum (ahf-THAL-mee-ah NEE-oh-nuh-TOR-uhm)
proctitis (prock-TIGH-tis)
puerperal (pyoo-ER-per-uhl)
sacral radiculopathy (SAY-krul ra-DIK-yoo-LAH-puh-thee)
salpingitis (SAL-pin-JIGH-tis)
serological (SEAR-uh-LAJ-ik-uhl)
urethritis (YOO-ree-THRIGH-tis)
verrucous (ve-ROO-kus)
vesicular (ve-SIK-yoo-ler)
vulvovaginitis (VUL-voh-VAJ-i-NIGH-tis)

QUESTIONS TO GUIDE YOUR READING

1. What pathogens are involved with each of the common sexually transmitted diseases (STDs)?

2. What are the signs and symptoms of each of the common STDs?

3. What teaching would you provide to promote prevention of STDs?

4. What are current treatment options for the common STDs?

5. What nursing care will you provide for patients with STDs?

6. How will you know if your nursing interventions have been effective?

Sexually transmitted diseases (STDs) are infections that may be transmitted through intimate contact with the genitals, mouth, or rectum of another individual. Some STDs may also be spread by other routes such as blood or body fluids. A nurse's best protection against catching diseases from blood and body fluids of infected patients is the strict practice of standard precautions and maintaining his or her own healthy, intact skin.

Physically, STDs may cause tremendous suffering through pain, scarring of genitourinary structures, damage to other body organs, infertility, birth defects, nervous system damage, development of cancer, and even death of infected patients and sometimes their children. Psychologically and socially, these diseases also have profound effects on individuals, families, and relationships. Guilt about passing on an incurable disease to a loved one or feelings of betrayal because of being infected as a result of someone else's choices is only part of the emotional consequences of STDs.

Changing social values have been associated with increasing incidence of almost all types of sexually transmitted diseases, including some previously rare diseases related to anal intercourse. Coexistence of more than one STD in an individual is also occurring more often. There are more than 50 diseases and syndromes associated with sexually transmitted diseases; the more common ones are discussed here. Human immunodeficiency virus (HIV) and acquired immunodeficiency syndrome (AIDS) are discussed separately in Chapter 19.

Symptoms, diagnostic techniques, and treatment regimens vary for different geographical areas, depending on availability of equipment for diagnosis and health-care provider preferences. As an introduction for practical/vocational nurses, general overviews are presented in this chapter.

One of the most important ways you can help those who experience STDs is by being kind, polite, nonjudgmental, and sensitive to the patient's communication. Maintaining an open posture and eye contact that is appropriate for the patient's culture relays a sense of openness and willingness to talk and preserves the possibility of continuing health promotion with these individuals in the future.

DISORDERS AND SYNDROMES RELATED TO SEXUALLY TRANSMITTED DISEASES

Vulvovaginitis

Vulvovaginitis is an inflammation of the vulva and vagina and can be asymptomatic or involve redness, itching, burning, excoriation, pain, swelling of the vagina and labia, and discharge. A variety of sexually transmitted and nonsexually

---

vulvovaginitis: vulvo—vulva + vagin—vagina + itis—inflammation

SAFETY TIP

Observe standard precautions and careful hand washing to avoid contact with infectious organisms. Go to www.cdc.gov and type in "hand hygiene" for complete guidelines.

---

transmitted infectious agents can cause vulvovaginitis. The odor, consistency, and color of the discharge varies with the different microbes involved. Nonsexually transmitted vaginitis, vulvovaginitis, and vaginosis are described in Chapter 42. Some microorganisms may be acquired either by sexual or nonsexual routes, so they are also mentioned in this chapter. Bartholin's glands may develop abscesses as a result of infection with nonsexually transmitted microbes or STDs such as gonorrhea and chlamydia.

Urethritis

Both STDs and nonsexually transmitted microorganisms can cause **urethritis** in men and women. In men, inflammation of the urethra, prostate, and epididymis can result in difficult, painful, and frequent urination and a urethral discharge, which may be clear, cloudy, or yellow. Female partners of men with urethritis may also suffer from urethritis, but they may also develop **mucopurulent cervicitis** (MPC) and a variety of other symptoms of the particular infection. Some causative agents for urethritis include *Neisseria gonorrhoeae, Chlamydia trachomatis, Ureaplasma urealyticum, Trichomonas vaginalis, Candida albicans,* and herpes simplex. Often this disease category is divided into gonococcal urethritis caused by *N. gonorrhoeae* (GU) and nongonococcal urethritis (NGU).

Mucopurulent Cervicitis

Mucopurulent cervicitis (MPC) is an inflammation of the cervix that can produce a mucopurulent yellow exudate on the cervix or may have no noticeable symptoms. MPC during pregnancy can result in **conjunctivitis** and pneumonia in newborn infants, as well as **puerperal** infection of the mother. MPC can be caused by such organisms as *Chlamydia trachomatis, N. gonorrhoeae, T. vaginalis, Candida albicans,* and herpes simplex. MPC may spread to become pelvic inflammatory disease (PID).

Proctitis and Enteritis

Proctitis is inflammation of the rectum and anus that may be due to either nonsexually transmitted microbes or to STDs.

---

urethritis: ureth—urethra + itis—inflammation
mucopurulent cervicitis: muco—involving mucus + purulent—involving pus + cervic—cervix + itis—inflammation
conjunctivitis: conjunctiv(a)—lining of the eyelids and sclera of the eye + itis—inflammation
puerperal: childbirth
proctitis: proc—anus + itis—inflammation

This is especially prevalent among those who practice both heterosexual and homosexual anal intercourse. Enteritis, which is inflammation of the lining of the intestine, may occur as a result of contamination during anal intercourse. Infection with *Campylobacter* spp, *Shigella* spp, and *Giardia lamblia* can be a problem for homosexual men. Care of patients who have gastrointestinal disorders is discussed in Unit 8.

Genital Ulcers

Genital ulcers are formed when papules or macules erode and leave often painful raw, pitted, or excoriated areas on or around the genitals. Not all genital ulcers are caused by STDs—injury, some non-STD viruses, some types of drug reactions, radiation, and some forms of cancer can also produce genital ulcers. STDs that can produce genital ulcers include syphilis, herpes, and HIV. Genital ulcers from one type of disease may increase the risk of infection with other STDs during sexual activity because the open areas present an easy portal of entry for the infecting organism.

Cellular Changes

Cellular changes can also be caused by STDs, including **condylomatous** (wartlike) growths and dysplasia or neoplasia, which may result in precancerous or cancerous conditions. Herpes viruses, HIV, and human papillomavirus (HPV) have all been linked to the development of cancer.

Pelvic Inflammatory Disease

Pathophysiology, Etiologies, and Signs and Symptoms

Pelvic inflammatory disease (PID) is an infection of the upper genital tract that may cause chronic pelvic pain due to inflammation. The primary sources of infection include *Chlamydia trachomatis* and *N. gonorrhoeae,* but it may result from any organism that is associated with a sexually transmitted infection. These organisms can invade the endocervical canal, resulting in **cervicitis**, and move upward resulting in infection of the endometrium (**endometritis**), fallopian tubes (**salpingitis**), and pelvic cavity. The chronic inflammation results in extensive scarring and adhesions, which can cause infertility and increase the risk of ectopic pregnancy. Increased risk for PID occurs with a history of multiple sexual partners, sexually transmitted diseases (STDs), substance abuse, frequent vaginal douching, and IUD (intrauterine device) contraceptive use.

Some women with PID are asymptomatic or have minimal symptoms. Other women present with lower abdominal pain and tenderness, purulent vaginal discharge or vaginal bleeding, pain with sexual intercourse, fever, nausea and

vomiting, and pain with urination. Findings during physical examination include adnexal tenderness upon palpation, and pain of the uterus and cervix when moved during a bimanual examination. Laboratory tests may reveal positive culture of causative organism(s) and leukocytosis. Urinary tract infection may need to be ruled out.

Therapeutic Interventions

With serious infection, hospitalization and intravenous antibiotics may be indicated. Intravenous therapy can be changed to oral therapy after 48 hours if status improves. Laparoscopic surgery may be done to release adhesions and reduce complications. Testing and treatment for other sexually transmitted diseases should be considered for both the patient and her partner. Education on the cause of the infection and prevention of future episodes are essential.

SEXUALLY TRANSMITTED INFECTIONS

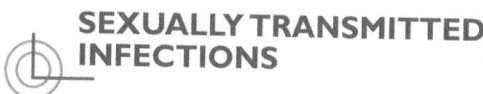

Chlamydia

Etiology and Signs and Symptoms

Chlamydia is the most commonly diagnosed STD in the United States. It can be transmitted sexually and by blood and body fluid contact. There are several different strains of the bacteria *Chlamydia trachomatis*. Chlamydia is often asymptomatic in women (a "silent" STD), but it can cause urethritis, MPC, and conjunctivitis. Fitz-Hugh–Curtis syndrome, a surface inflammation of the liver, can also be caused by *C. trachomatis*. This inflammation may cause nausea, vomiting, and sharp pain at the base of the ribs that sometimes refers to the right shoulder and arm. Chlamydia is a frequent cause of pelvic inflammatory disease (PID) and infertility, and it increases the risk of ectopic pregnancy. The infection can be passed from mother to baby during birth, resulting in neonatal pneumonia and conjunctivitis. It also increases the risk of HIV infection.

Lymphogranuloma venereum (LGV) is also caused by some strains of *C. trachomatis* but is more commonly seen in tropical climates or among people who emigrated from these areas. This disease also causes urethritis and proctitis, and it inflames lymph nodes that drain the pelvic area, resulting in draining sores and fistula development. Scarring from this disease can complicate vaginal deliveries.

Diagnostic Tests

There are several tests for chlamydia. Samples are gathered in a special collection tube to send to a laboratory for culture. Culturing is difficult and expensive and generally requires 2 to 6 days for results. A newer type of testing, called nucleic acid amplification testing (NAT or NAAT) identifies the presence of chlamydial DNA or RNA in urine, cervical, or urethral specimens. Because this disease is so common, it is wise to set out an unopened *Chlamydia* collection kit within easy reach of the health-care provider for each pelvic examination.

---

condylomatous: condyl—rounded projection + oma(t)—growth + ous—like

cervicitis: cervic—cervix + itis—inflammation

endometritis: endo—inside + metr—womb + itis—inflammation

salpingitis: salping—tube + itis—inflammation

Therapeutic Interventions

Antibiotics are generally given to treat chlamydia in adults. These antibiotics include erythromycin, azithromycin, doxycycline, ofloxacin, and levofloxacin (Table 44.1). Erythromycin or azithromycin is used during pregnancy, as other antibiotics may pose an increased risk to the fetus. Use of an ophthalmic ointment or solution containing silver nitrate, erythromycin, or tetracycline is recommended as treatment of the neonate shortly after birth for the prevention of conjunctivitis. This is done regardless of whether or not the mother is diagnosed with chlamydia, as asymptomatic or undiagnosed chlamydia is common, and this simple treatment can prevent serious complications later. Institutional policies and state regulations determine the type of eye preparation to be used and whether administration of the medications requires specific consent of the parents.

See Box 44.1 Common STDs Summary.

Gonorrhea

Etiology and Signs and Symptoms

According to the Centers for Disease Control and Prevention (CDC), 361,705 new cases of gonorrhea were reported to the CDC in 2001 (the most recently available complete statistics), but it is estimated that only half of all cases actually get reported. The cost of care and treatment of gonorrhea in the United States is approximately $56 million each year.[1] It is caused by the bacterium *N. gonorrhoeae*, and may be transmitted vaginally, rectally, orally, or via contact with other mucous membranes, or through contact with blood and body fluids. It can produce a variety of signs and symptoms. Men may be asymptomatic or may have urethritis with a yellow urethral discharge. Women who have gonorrhea may have either no noticeable symptoms or have a sore throat, MPC, urethritis, or abnormal menstrual symptoms such as bleeding between periods. Many cases of PID are caused by gonorrhea. Intercourse with an infected partner during menstruation may be especially risky for development of PID because removal of the cervical mucous barrier can promote the growth of the gonococcus in the higher reproductive tract. Gonorrhea can also cause Fitz-Hugh–Curtis syndrome. Fever, nausea, vomiting, and lower abdominal pain may be present. Gonorrhea may also infect the throat and the rectum and may cause disseminated gonococcal infection, resulting in inflammation of the joints, skin, meninges, and lining of the heart.

Newborns born to mothers who have gonorrhea can develop **ophthalmia neonatorum,** which involves inflammation of the conjunctivae and deeper parts of the eye and can, ultimately, result in blindness. The newborn may also experience a gonorrheal infection at other sites following birth. Abscesses may develop where fetal scalp monitors were attached during labor, and infection of the nose, lungs, and rectum may occur.

Diagnostic Tests

Diagnosis is done by microscopic examination of smears and cultures of the discharge or identification of bacterial DNA (nucleic acid testing) in the urine. More than one test may be done to verify the diagnosis.

Therapeutic Interventions

Development of antibiotic resistance by *N. gonorrhoeae* and coinfection with other microorganisms, such as *Chlamydia trachomatis,* is making treatment more complicated. Cefixime, ceftriaxone, ciprofloxacin, or ofloxacin is recommended for the treatment of gonorrhea (see Table 44.1). It is also recommended that the patient be treated for chlamydia as coinfection is common. Ophthalmia neonatorum may be prevented by use of antibiotic eye preparations which contain silver nitrate, erythromycin, or tetracycline. It is recommended, as with prophylactic treatment of chlamydial conjunctivitis, that all infants be treated shortly after birth regardless of diagnostic status of the mother. The treatment is simple, and may prevent a devastating outcome for the newborn. Institutional policies and state regulations determine the type of eye drops to be used and whether administration of the drops requires specific consent of the parents.

CRITICAL THINKING

Mrs. Miller

■ Mrs. Miller delivered an infant boy 1 hour ago. The nurse is currently applying erythromycin ointment to the infant's eyes bilaterally. Mrs. Miller asks if the medication is necessary.

1. How will you respond?
2. Should *all infants* receive prophylactic eye treatment at birth?

Suggested answers at end of chapter.

Syphilis

Etiology and Signs and Symptoms

Syphilis is an ancient disease that has not disappeared, although it is overshadowed by more commonly occurring diseases such as chlamydia. The primary stage of syphilis begins with the entry of the *Treponema pallidum* spirochete through the skin or mucous membranes. Between 3 and 90 days later, a papule develops at the site of entry, then sloughs off, leaving a painless, red, ulcerated area called a **chancre** (Fig. 44.1). Chancres may also develop in other areas of the body at this time. Chancre formation is generally the only symptom of this stage of syphilis. The chancre eventually heals, but the spirochete remains active in the infected individual and can be passed on to others. Secondary syphilis begins 2 to 8 weeks later and affects the body more generally, causing such problems as flulike symptoms, joint pain,

---

ophthalmia neonatorum: ophthalmia—eye disease + neonatorum—of the newborn

chancre: hard ulceration

TABLE 44.1 MEDICATIONS USED TO TREAT STDs

STD Medication Drug Classification	Medication/Mode of Action	Route	Side Effects	Nursing Implications
Chlamydia Antibiotics	Macrolides: Erythromycin Azithromycin Inhibit bacterial protein synthesis	PO or IV	Abdominal pain Cramping GI upset Rash. Overgrowth of nonsusceptible bacteria.	Administer on empty stomach. Do not administer with antacids. Caution with hepatic disorders.
	Tetracyclines: Doxycycline *Inhibit protein synthesis by binding to ribosomes*	PO or IV	GI upset Anorexia Dysphagia Photosensitivity Rash Urticaria Increased pigmentation May increase anticoagulation	Do not administer during pregnancy due to bone/teeth effects. Do not take with antacids or dairy products. Administer on empty stomach. Avoid unnecessary exposure to sunlight.
	Fluoroquinolones: Ofloxacin Levofloxacin *Inhibit cell wall synthesis*	PO or IV	GI upset Dizziness Headache CNS disturbances Flatulence Rash Photosensitivity Rare but serious: Tendon rupture	Safety under age 18 not established. Do not administer with antacids. Caution with other medication use; renal, hepatic, or CNS disorders.
Gonorrhea Antibiotics	Cephalosporins: Ceftriaxone Cefixime *Inhibit cell wall synthesis*	PO, IM, or IV	GI upset CNS disturbance Rash Pruritus Elevated liver enzymes Pain at injection site	Caution with penicillin allergies; renal, or hepatic dysfunction. Avoid excess sun exposure.
	Fluoroquinolones: Ciprofloxacin Ofloxacin *(see information above)*			
Syphilis Antibiotics	Penicillin: *White milky not in IV* Penicillin G *Inhibits cell wall synthesis* Tetracyclines: Tetracycline Doxycycline *(see information above)*	PO, IM, or IV	GI upset CNS disturbance Rash Itching Fever Chills Pain at injection site Allergy	Administer deep IM or slow IV. Apply ice packs to injection site prn. Administer PO on empty stomach. Instruct patient to report fever/rash.
Trichomoniasis Amebicides/ Antiprotozoals	Metronidazole *Bind to DNA to inhibit synthesis and cause cell death*	PO or IV	GI upset Anorexia Headache Metallic taste or dry mouth Dysuria Rare but serious: Seizures and peripheral neuropathy ECG changes	Administer with food. Caution use with alcohol; abstain for a minimum of 48 hr following treatment to prevent severe flulike reaction.
Herpes Antivirals	Acyclovir Valacyclovir Famciclovir *Inhibit DNA synthesis*	PO, IV, or topical	GI upset CNS disturbance Rash Urticaria Elevated liver enzymes/BUN levels	Use systemic preparations cautiously with CNS, hepatic, or renal disorders. Infuse IV slowly. Maintain hydration. Caution patient that viral transmission can still occur during treatment.
Genital Warts Antimitotics and Acidic Agents	Podophyllin/ trichloroacetic acid (TCA)/bichloroacetic acid (BCA)	Topical application to wart(s)	Local reactions (e.g., pain, burning, inflammation, erosion, itching)	Instruct patient to return for repeated applications as necessary. Avoid medication contact with eyes or tissue surrounding lesion.

CNS = central nervous system; GI = gastrointestinal.

Box 44.1

Common STDs Summary

	Chlamydia	Gonorrhea	Syphilis	Trichomoniasis	Herpes Simplex	Condylomata (HPV)
Signs and Symptoms	Conjunctivitis; in men, urethritis, epididymitis, prostatitis; in women, MPC, urethritis	In men, urethritis, penile discharge, epididymitis, prostatitis; in women, MPC, urethritis, abnormal menses	Primary syphilis, chancre; secondary syphilis, flulike symptoms, rashes, condylomatous growths	Genital redness, swelling, itching, burning, foul discharge; in men, urethritis, prostatitis; in women, "strawberry cervix"	Vesicles/ulcerations in mouth, genitals; flulike symptoms, lymphadenopathy, urethritis, cystitis, MPC	Fleshy tumors, primarily on genitalia
Diagnostic Tests	NAT Culture	NAT Culture	VDRL, ELISA, RPR, FTA-ABS	Microscopic examination	Culture, Western blot	Colposcope examination biopsy, visualization of lesions
Therapeutic Interventions	Antibiotics (see Table 44.1)	Antibiotics (see Table 44.1)	Penicillin	Metronidazole	Antiviral medication (Table 44.1)	Wart removal, interferon therapy
Complications	Fitz-Hugh-Curtis syndrome, increased susceptibility to HIV infection; PID, infertility, transmission to baby at birth; coinfection with gonorrhea	PID, disseminated gonococcal infection, Fitz-Hugh-Curtis syndrome, transmission to baby at birth, coinfection with chlamydia	Tertiary syphilis, gummas damage heart, circulatory system, nervous system; transmission to fetus during pregnancy	Preterm delivery, infertility, increased risk of HIV transmission	Lifelong infection, disseminated infection, nervous system invasion, increased risk of cervical cancer, transmission to baby at birth	Cancers of the reproductive organs and anus, including cervical cancer, transmission to fetus during pregnancy
Priority Nursing Diagnoses	Pain related to inflammation, skin lesions; Fear related to unknown outcome of disease; Risk of transmission to others					

ELISA = enzyme-linked immunosorbent assay; FTA-ABS = fluorescent treponemal antibody absorption; HPV = human papillomavirus; MPC = mucopurulent cervicitis; PID = pelvic inflammatory disease; RPR = rapid plasmin reagin; VDRL = Venereal Disease Research Laboratory.

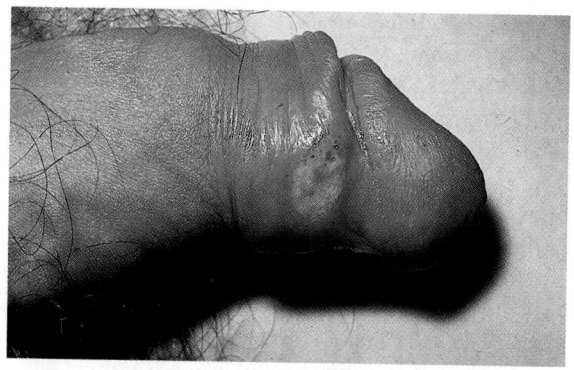

FIGURE 44.1 Syphilis chancre. *(From Reeves, JRT, and Maibach, H: Clinical Dermatology Illustrated: A Regional Approach. F.A. Davis, Philadelphia, 1991, p 88)*

hair loss, skin rashes (primarily on the soles of the hands and feet), mouth sores, and condylomatous growths in moist areas of the body.

Serious damage can occur if syphilis is untreated in the early stages. The disease may not progress to the tertiary (or late) stage for 3 to 15 years. At this stage, it can involve any organ system of the body. In the tertiary stage, the spirochete may form **gummas,** which are tumors of a rubbery consistency that can break down and ulcerate, leaving holes in body tissues. The gummas can damage the heart, circulatory system, and nervous system (neurosyphilis). Ulceration of gummas can destroy areas of vital tissue and lead to mental and physical disability or early death.

Syphilis can be passed on to the unborn children of women who carry the spirochete, resulting in **hepatosplenomegaly,** increase in bilirubin, destruction of red blood cells, birth defects (especially of the face), **lymphadenopathy,** and a baby who can transmit the spirochete through nasal drainage. If left untreated, syphilis during pregnancy may cause lesions in various organs of the unborn baby and result in higher rates of spontaneous abortion, stillbirth, and premature birth.

Diagnostic Tests

Several tests for syphilis exist, and a combination may be used for accurate diagnosis. Cultures may be done but are difficult to grow. **Serological** (blood) tests include the Venereal Disease Research Laboratory (VDRL) test, the rapid plasma reagin (RPR) test, and the automated reagin test (ART). These tests indirectly check for syphilis by detecting the presence of antibodies that the body forms in response to treponema and, unfortunately, in response to some other disorders, so false-positive results can occur. Diagnosis of neurosyphilis is even more difficult because some testing of cerebrospinal fluid may result in false-

negative results. Treponemal enzyme-linked immunosorbent assay (ELISA), fluorescent treponemal antibody absorption (FTA-ABS), and polymerase chain reaction (PCR) tests for treponemal DNA are some newer methods that reduce the risk of false results.

Therapeutic Interventions

Penicillin G is the treatment of choice for patients diagnosed with syphilis (see Table 44.1). For those who are allergic to penicillin, doxycycline and tetracycline are recognized as treatment options. When HIV and syphilis are seen in the same individual, symptoms of neurosyphilis are more likely to occur.

Trichomoniasis

Etiology and Signs and Symptoms

Trichomoniasis is generally a sexually transmitted disease, but it may be transmitted through nonsexual contact with infected articles because it can survive for quite a long time outside the body. Carriers of *Trichomonas vaginalis* may be asymptomatic for several years until changes in vaginal or urethral conditions encourage an outbreak of the disease. A decrease in resident bacteria, injuries to the vaginal tissues, and development of lesions from other STDs or from some forms of cancer may activate the organism. Symptoms include redness, swelling, itching, and burning of the genital area; pain with intercourse and voiding; and a frothy, foul-smelling discharge. Men with trichomonal infection can develop prostatitis and infertility, and men who are also infected with HIV are more likely to transmit it to others. Women who are pregnant risk preterm delivery and low birth weight babies.

Diagnostic Tests

Visualization of the cervix during pelvic examination shows a characteristic "strawberry cervix." When wet-mount slides of the discharge are viewed under a microscope, the organisms can be identified by their motility and whiplike flagella. Trichomoniasis may produce abnormal Papanicolaou (Pap) smear readings, which require that more frequent Pap smears be done to provide adequate surveillance of cellular changes.

Therapeutic Interventions

The drug treatment of choice is metronidazole (see Table 44.1). Some strains of *Trichomonas* may exhibit resistance to this medication, but generally succumb to much higher doses of the drug. Because some people carry the organism without symptoms, sexual partners should also be treated regardless of symptoms.

Herpes

Etiology and Signs and Symptoms

Herpes infection is caused by the herpes simplex virus types I and II (HSV-I and HSV-II). Herpes viruses have an affinity for tissues of the skin and nervous system and can lie dormant in nervous system tissues and then reactivate periodically when the body undergoes stress, fever, or immune system compromise. Both HSV-I and HSV-II can cause "fever blisters" of the mouth (Fig. 44.2), as well as genital

---

gummas: from the word meaning "rubber"—rubber tumors
hepatosplenomegaly: hepato—liver + spleno—spleen + megaly—enlargement
lymphadenopathy: lymph—lymph nodes + adeno—node + pathy—disorder
serological: sero—blood + logical—science

CRITICAL THINKING

Kerri

■ Kerri presents to the health clinic with a complaint of generalized redness, swelling, itching, and burning of her external genitalia. Following history, physical, and microscopic examination, trichomoniasis is diagnosed. Kerri is upset, stating she has been in a monogamous relationship for 2 years.

1. What should your response to Kerri include?
2. Kerri is placed on metronidazole (Flagyl), but you are not comfortable with the dose prescribed, so you look it up. You find that she should receive 7.5 mg/kg every 6 hours. Kerri weighs 140 pounds. What should her dose be every 6 hours?
3. What teaching should you provide for Kerri?

Suggested answers at end of chapter.

lesions. However, HSV-I is more frequently associated with oral lesions and HSV-II with genital lesions.

Genital HSV-II outbreaks are more severe than genital HSV-I outbreaks. After infection, vesicles develop, spontaneously rupture, and produce painful ulceration of the underlying skin tissues. Asymptomatic latent periods are generally interspersed between the **vesicular** outbreaks. Although not as common, the virus may still be transmitted even during latent periods.

An initial outbreak following infection with the herpes virus occurs 2 days to 2 weeks after exposure and may produce a flulike condition. Urethritis, cystitis, and MPC with vaginal discharge may also be evident. Infection of the spinal nerve roots by HSV may result in **sacral radiculopathy,** causing retention of urine and feces. Although rare, dis-

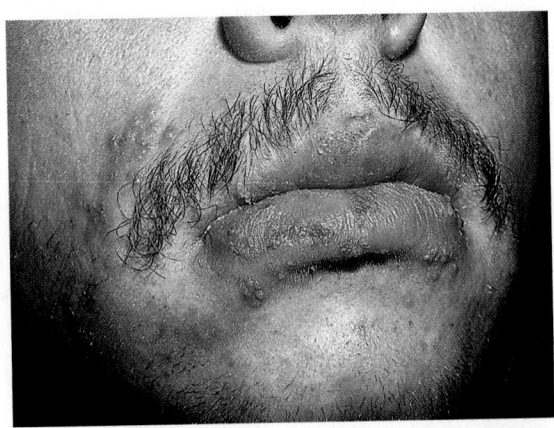

FIGURE 44.2 Herpes simplex. *(From Reeves, JRT, and Maibach, H: Clinical Dermatology Illustrated: A Regional Approach. F.A. Davis, Philadelphia, 1991, p 64)*

vesicular: vesicul—blister + ar—type
sacral radiculopathy: sacral—sacrum + radiculo—root + pathy—disorder or disease

seminated herpes infection can result in inflammation of the spinal cord, meninges, nerve pathways, and lymph nodes. Urethral strictures and increased risk for development of cervical cancer in women are also consequences of herpes.

It is estimated that one in five of all pregnant women carry herpes, although most of their babies do not develop **herpetic** disease. If infected, the baby's skin, eyes, mucous membranes, and nervous system may be involved and death from disseminated herpes infection may occur. The greatest risk of herpes transmission from mother to child during pregnancy occurs if there is an active genital lesion at the time of delivery. If an active genital lesion is present when a woman is close to the time of delivery, a cesarean section is likely to be performed. However, an active lesion at any time during pregnancy poses a risk for transmission.

Diagnostic Tests

Testing for HSV requires special viral collection kits for swabbed or scraped specimens from lesions. Follow the directions on the viral collection kit as well as institutional policies. Blood tests are improving; the Western blot assay can determine whether the person has HSV-I or HSV-II antibodies.

Therapeutic Interventions

There is presently no known cure for herpes infection, although antiviral medications such as acyclovir, valacyclovir, and famciclovir may be given to decrease the severity of symptoms (see Table 44.1). Only acyclovir, a treatment that may reduce the risk of transmission of the herpes virus to the fetus, may be given during pregnancy. See also Box 44.2 Nursing Care Plan for the Patient with Genital Herpes.

Genital Warts

Signs and Symptoms

Condylomata acuminata (genital warts) is a common sexually transmitted viral disease, and its incidence is increasing rapidly. Infection with human papillomavirus (HPV) produces the condylomata—soft, raised, **verrucous** fleshy tumors, which may also have fingerlike projections and resemble cauliflower (Fig. 44.3). Lesions most commonly develop on the external genitalia and perineum, as well as on the internal vaginal wall and cervix in women. However, lesions can also develop on other areas of the body after contact with the virus. Some people remain asymptomatic, but can still transmit the infection. More than 100 types of HPV have been identified, and several have been closely linked to the development of cancers of the reproductive organs and anus in both males and females. There may be a long latent period of as much as 3 years' duration from the time of exposure to development of the warts.

herpetic: herpet—herpes + ic—pertaining to
condylomata acuminata: condyl—rounded projection + oma—growth + ta—pluralizes the word (singular form is condyloma) + acuminata—genital growths
verrucous: verruc—wart + ous—like

Box 44.2 NURSING CARE PLAN for the Patient with Genital Herpes

Nursing Diagnosis: Pain related to inflammation, skin lesions

Expected Outcome The patient will express pain relief at an acceptable level and will rest and move well.

Evaluation of Outcome Does patient state relief of pain level is acceptable?

Interventions	Rationale	Evaluation
Assess pain using the WHAT'S UP? format.	Assessment of the characteristic of the pain assists the nurse in providing appropriate relief measures.	Can patient describe the pain characteristics?
Recommend pain relief measures appropriate to the type and location of the pain (both alternative measures, such as heat, ice, and change of position, and medication may be offered).	Not all types of pain respond well to the same treatment.	Does patient express satisfactory relief of pain? Does patient move and rest without evidence of pain?
Document results of pain relief measures.	Documentation alerts other caregivers about what works and does not work, thus providing more consistent, effective pain relief.	Have you gained sufficient information from patient to document results?
Instruct patient about self-care for pain and STD treatment at home.	Most STDs are treated at home.	Does patient verbalize understanding of self-care measures?

Nursing Diagnosis: Risk for transmission of infection to others related to lack of knowledge about transmission, symptoms, and treatment

Expected Outcome Patient will verbalize understanding of measures to prevent transmission to others.

Evaluation of Outcome Does patient verbalize understanding of transmission prevention? Does patient practice preventive behaviors?

Interventions	Rationale	Evaluation
Assess patient's understanding of transmission, symptoms, complications, and treatment of STDs.	New instruction should be based on patient's previous knowledge.	Is patient's current understanding accurate? What teaching is necessary?
Assess whether patient is engaging in high-risk behaviors.	If patient is continuing to engage in high-risk behaviors, the risk for infection of others is high.	Is patient protecting self and others appropriately?
Use universal precautions and strict aseptic technique for *all* procedures involving blood and body fluids.	The health team, in addition to other patient contacts, must be protected.	Are universal precautions observed?
Instruct patient in appropriate strategies to reduce risk of infecting others: • Abstinence • Monogamy (if no active infection) • Use of barrier methods and spermicides • Adherence to treatment regimen	These measures may help prevent transmission of infection to others.	Does patient verbalize understanding of methods to prevent transmission and intent to practice them?
Teach patient signs and symptoms of STDs to report immediately.	Prompt treatment of patient and partners further reduces risk of transmission of infection.	Does patient verbalize understanding of signs and symptoms to report?

(Continued on following page)

Box 44.2   NURSING CARE PLAN for the Patient with Genital Herpes *(Continued)*

Nursing Diagnosis: Fear related to diagnosis of an incurable illness and effects on sexual relationships and reproduction

Expected Outcome Patient will verbalize realistic and accurate information about disease process and relate control of excessive fear.

Evaluation of Outcome Does patient relate accurate knowledge? Is fear manageable?

Interventions	Rationale	Evaluation
Assess patient's fears.	Fear is a normal response and may be appropriate.	What does patient fear?
If fear is based on misconceptions, provide factual information.	When fear is based on misconceptions, they should be corrected.	Are fears based on factual information?
Allow patient to verbalize feelings. Be empathetic, but do not offer false hope.	Sharing fears may help patient gain insight into dealing with them.	Is patient able to verbalize feelings?
Explain all procedures and treatments.	Unfamiliar procedures or treatments may contribute to fear.	Does patient understand procedures and treatments?
Help patient identify support systems and coping strategies that have worked in the past.	Methods that have worked for patient before are likely to be helpful again.	Does patient have effective coping skills and support systems?

HPV can be passed on from a pregnant woman to her fetus, resulting in the growth of genital warts on the baby, HPV infection of the baby's respiratory tract, and a possible future increased risk of cancer development. HPV infection during pregnancy can cause particularly difficult problems. Genital warts tend to grow more rapidly in pregnant women and to bleed more easily with injury than in nonpregnant women.

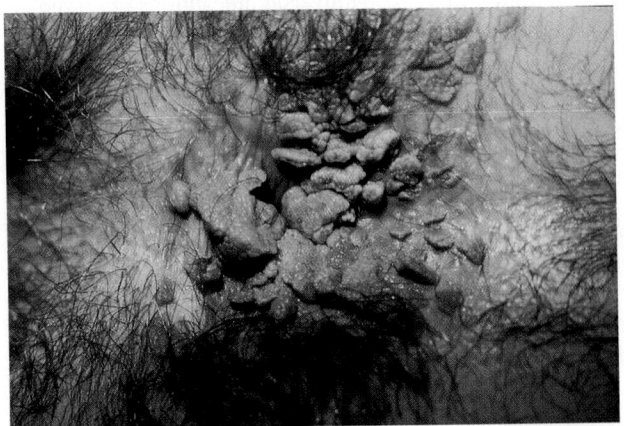

FIGURE 44.3 Condylomata, commonly known as genital warts. *(From Lemone, P, and Burke, KM: Medical-Surgical Nursing: Critical Thinking in Client Care. Addison-Wesley, Menlo Park, CA 1996, p 2079, with permission.)*

Diagnostic Tests

Diagnosis may be made by applying dilute acetic acid (vinegar) to the skin of the external genital area, vagina, cervix, and anus and then closely examining with a colposcope the areas that turn a lighter color. Biopsy specimens of the suspicious areas can be sent for further study of the cells. Other tests to diagnose HPV include an antigen test and the Southern and dot blot tests, which use radioactive probes. Cancerous changes stimulated by this virus may be identified on Pap smears.

Therapeutic Interventions

There is presently no known cure for papillomavirus infection. The warts may be treated by freezing, burning, or chemically destroying them or by manipulating the patient's immune system to attack the virus. Cryotherapy (freezing) of the warts may be done by touching each wart with a cryoprobe or a liquid nitrogen–soaked swab. Warts may also be burned or **electrocoagulated** with an **electrocautery** or a laser. Heat causes the proteins to coagulate, resulting in death of the wart tissue. Podophyllin, trichloroacetic acid (TCA), and bichloroacetic acid (BCA) are some of the chemical agents that may be applied topically to treat the

electrocoagulated: electro—electrical + coagul—curdled or hardened + ated—process completed
electrocautery: electro—electrical + cautery—branding iron

warts (see Table 44.1). Some options are not appropriate for use during pregnancy because of their **cytotoxic** effects, which might damage the fetus, but cryosurgery and laser destruction of the wart tissue may be done during pregnancy. All treatments may require multiple applications and generally result in a great deal of discomfort as the warts degenerate, ulcerate, and slough over a long period. Wart removal does not cure the infection, and new wart growth can occur after treatment.

Various types of immunotherapy have been used against HPV. Interferons are proteins produced by the body that can inhibit viral growth. Several types of interferons have been used to combat HPV. These substances may be applied topically, injected into the condyloma, or administered systemically. Interferons can produce side effects of flulike symptoms, a drop in the number of white blood cells, and changes in liver function. Systemic interferon treatment, however, may offer the advantage of being able to attack warts all over the body at the same time, rather than individually as with topical treatments, thus speeding the process of treatment. Research to develop vaccines against HPV strains is ongoing, but the multitude of varieties makes this difficult.

Home Care

Patients who have genital warts (condylomata acuminatam) burned off need to recuperate at home. If the burns (there may be multiple areas treated) are near the urethra or rectum, the patient may need a Foley catheter inserted to avoid contamination and irritation of the lesions after treatment. Also, the patient is instructed to increase dietary roughage and fluids to prevent constipation. Consult the health-care provider for orders on care of the burns. Use sterile technique for dressing changes, and premedicate the patient for pain control as needed for dressing changes.

Hepatitis B

Etiology and Signs and Symptoms

There are several main hepatitis viruses, but this section deals only with hepatitis B virus (HBV), which is generally considered within the STD category because it can be transmitted through sexual contact with blood and body fluids. (See Chapter 35 for a full discussion on hepatitis.) Early signs of hepatitis are loss of appetite, rashes, malaise, muscle and joint pain, headaches, nausea, and vomiting. As the virus affects the liver, the urine may darken and the stool color lighten (as a result of changes in bile excretion), liver enzymes may rise, and jaundice may appear. Enlargement of the spleen, enlargement and tenderness of the liver, necrosis of liver cells, cirrhosis, coma, and death may follow if the disease is severe. Chronic asymptomatic carrier status may follow hepatitis virus infection, with an increased risk of liver cancer.

During pregnancy, hepatitis B virus may be transmitted to the unborn baby, which can result in acute hepatitis and the possibility of becoming a chronic carrier of HBV.

Diagnostic Tests

Diagnosis of hepatitis is generally made using a variety of blood tests based on antigen and antibody responses.

Therapeutic Interventions

Supportive medical care with avoidance of drugs that require liver metabolism may help the patient through the active stage of the disease. Treatment of the disease may involve injection of serum immune globulins to confer passive immunity. It is recommended that all babies of HBV-positive mothers receive HBV immune globulin less than 12 hours after birth and then be immunized with HBV vaccine 1 week, 1 month, and 6 months after birth. See Chapter 35 for more information. Interferon alpha is also available for patients with chronic hepatitis B.

Prevention

Prevention is better than treatment and may be accomplished by using HBV vaccine. This is especially recommended for health-care workers who come in contact with blood and body fluids. Standard precautions should be used when contact with any body fluids is expected.

Genital Parasites

Etiology and Signs and Symptoms

Genital parasites are not a true STD, but they may be transmitted during close body contact. The two most commonly seen parasites are pubic lice (*Phthirus pubis,* commonly called "crabs" because of the shape of the lice) and scabies (*Sarcoptes scabiei*). These parasites cause itching, redness, and, for scabies, tracks under the skin where the females burrow to lay their eggs.

Diagnostic Tests

History, physical assessment, and direct visual or magnified view of the parasites aids in diagnosis.

Therapeutic Interventions

Parasites are treated with topical insecticides. Advise the patient to refer to package inserts for application instructions and precautions to avoid reinfection.

REPORTING OF SEXUALLY TRANSMITTED DISEASES

The nurse may be required to facilitate the reporting and public health follow-up of STDs by filling in patient information on the STD reporting form and placing the form in the patient's chart for completion by the health-care provider. The requirements for reporting STDs may vary for different states, provinces, and countries. In some areas, laboratories are also required to submit a report form for positive reportable STD tests. Laboratory reports that are not followed by a health-care provider's report may result in investigation of the situation by an STD investigator. Generally, the report form has spaces for listing of sexual contacts who should be notified of possible STD exposure. Depending on the laws of the state, province, or country,

---

cytotoxic: cyto—cell + toxic—poison

health-care providers may notify identified sexual contacts or patients may do so themselves. Contacts may also be notified by a public health authority that they have been listed as a sexual contact by an anonymous person who has tested positive for a particular STD.

NURSING PROCESS FOR SEXUALLY TRANSMITTED DISEASES

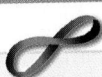

Assessment/Data Collection

STDs are usually assessed, diagnosed, and treated in health-care providers' offices and in clinics. It is important to evaluate the patient's reason for seeking health care with every outpatient visit. Sometimes patients visit clinics or health-care providers' offices for stated reasons other than STDs, yet their real concern is an STD.

The nurse should inquire about whether the patient is presently experiencing any irritation, pain, lesions, or discharge of the genital region when an individual presents with complaints that could lead to an STD diagnosis. Explaining to the patient the need to know what examination supplies to prepare for an appropriate assessment may allow him or her to share concerns and true reasons for the visit. Establishing a rapport and conveying acceptance may also facilitate communication. Often the nurse is present during the examination to assist the health-care provider and to serve as a chaperone or patient support person.

STDs may also be discovered in hospitalized patients. Nurses are often the ones who bathe and give perineal care to patients. It is important to be aware of signs and symptoms in older adults as well as younger people (Box 44.3 Gerontological Issues). Unusual discharges, redness, blisters, swollen areas, ulcers, and evidence of parasites in the genital area may be observed during patient care. STD awareness can sensitize you to the possible significance of patient complaints such as persistent pelvic pain, dysuria, discharges, and rectal soreness. Such problems should be accurately documented and reported, so that further investigation and possible treatment can take place.

Box 44.3

Gerontological Issues

Older adults retain interest and are capable of engaging in sex. Do not assume that because an older adult is single or widowed he or she is not sexually active.

Older adults who have enjoyed active and fulfilling sex lives with a spouse or partner may seek that in new relationships. Older adults who engage in high-risk sexual behaviors (multiple partners, genital-anal sex, no use of barriers during sexual intercourse) are also at risk for sexually transmitted diseases.

NURSING CARE TIP

Neighbors, friends, or family members may seek information from you because they know nurses are educated about health issues. Such questions may be stated in indirect terms, such as, "I have a friend who is having a problem. . . ." You can provide accurate information and stress the importance of diagnosis and treatment to prevent the serious consequences of untreated STDs, without asking probing or embarrassing questions.

Nursing Diagnoses, Planning, and Implementation

Nursing diagnoses and interventions for patients with an STD may include:

Pain related to inflammation or skin lesions

EXPECTED OUTCOME: The patient will express pain relief at an acceptable level.

- Assess pain using a culturally appropriate scale. *This will aid in providing appropriate relief measures.*
- Recommend pain relief measures appropriate to the type and location of the pain (see Chapter 9). *Not all pain will respond to the same treatment.*
- Document results of pain relief measures. *This will communicate to others effective pain interventions.*
- Instruct patient about self-care for pain and STD treatment *to promote resolution of infectious process and related symptoms.*

Risk for transmission of infection to others

EXPECTED OUTCOME: Patient will verbalize understanding of measures to prevent transmission to others.

- Assess whether patient is engaging in high-risk behaviors *to determine risk of transmission to others.*
- Assess patient's understanding of symptoms, complications, treatment, and transmission of STDs. *This will allow for additional, appropriate information to be given.*
- Use universal precautions and strict aseptic technique for *all* procedures involving blood and body fluids *to limit risk of transmission of infectious organism to health-care members.*
- Instruct patient in appropriate strategies to reduce risk of infecting others, such as abstinence, monogamy, use of barrier and spermicidal contraceptives, and adherence to the treatment regimen *in order to reduce the risk of disease transmission.*
- Explain importance of follow-up evaluation *in order to affirm treatment was successful.*

Ineffective sexuality pattern related to illness and risk for transmission of infectious organism

EXPECTED OUTCOME: Patient will describe acceptable, alternative sexual practices and safer sex practices.

- Provide privacy and be verbally and nonverbally nonjudgmental when allowing patient and patient's partner to express concerns about sexual practice. *Treatment success rates are generally higher when a rapport is established with the health-care provider and the partner is included in the decision-making process.*
- When teaching patients, the terms *safe sex* and *STD prevention* are misnomers. You should more accurately refer to information about barrier methods as *safer sex* practices, which may decrease the risk of (but not absolutely prevent) transmission of STDs (Table 44.2).
- Discuss alternative sexual expression, as appropriate, *as this may allow for intimacy when desired sexual expression is not recommended.*
- Support realistic expectations about treatment and outcomes. *Unrealistic expectations may lead to additional undesired issues related to sexuality pattern.*

Fear related to diagnosis of possible incurable illness

EXPECTED OUTCOME: Patient will verbalize realistic and accurate information about the disease process and relate that fear is at an acceptable level.

- Assess patient's fears as *understanding basis of fear will aid in implementation of coping strategies.*
- If fear is based on misconceptions, provide factual information. *Knowledge may decrease fear.*
- Allow patient to verbalize feelings, while being empathetic. *Sharing fears may help patient gain insight into dealing with issues of concern.*
- Explain all procedures and treatments. *Unfamiliar practices may increase fear.*
- Help patient identify support systems and coping strategies that have worked in the past. *These may be helpful in dealing with current fears.*

Health-seeking behaviors related to lack of knowledge about STDs

EXPECTED OUTCOME: Patient will verbalize correct understanding related to STD prevention and testing.

- Assess the patient's health beliefs and correct misconceptions. *Many myths about sexual activity are sincerely believed by some patients (Table 44.3).*

TABLE 44.2 BARRIER METHODS FOR SAFER SEX

Barrier	Related Information
Male condoms	Latex condoms are less likely to break during intercourse than other types.
	Lubrication decreases the chances of breakage during use, but only water-soluble lubricants should be used, because substances such as petroleum jelly (Vaseline) may weaken the condom.
	Condoms should never be inflated to test them, because this can weaken them.
	Condoms should be applied only when the penis is erect.
	Either condoms with a reservoir tip or regular condoms that have been applied while holding approximately 1/2 inch of the closed end flat between the fingertips allow room for expansion by the ejaculate without creating excessive pressure, which might break the condom.
	The penis should be withdrawn after ejaculation before the erection begins to subside while holding the top of the condom securely around the penis to avoid spillage.
	Condoms should never be reused and should be discarded properly after use so that others will not come in contact with the contents.
Female condoms	Female condoms should be applied before any penetration occurs (even preejaculation fluid can contain microorganisms).
	Lubrication decreases the chances of breakage during use, but only water-soluble lubricants should be used, because substances such as petroleum jelly may weaken the condom.
	Female condoms should never be reused and should be discarded properly after use so that others will not come in contact with the contents.
Cervical caps or diaphragms	These may provide some protection for the cervix only. They are not effective barriers against STD infection.
Rubber gloves, rubber dental dams, split (opened) male condoms	These may provide some barrier protection for manual and oral sexual activity. Although some groups suggest that male condoms may be split down one side and opened or rubber dental dam material may be taped over areas that have lesions to avoid direct contact with blood and body fluid, especially during sadomasochistic sexual activity, this *very-high-risk behavior* is not recommended.
Double condoms	Anal intercourse is a *very-high-risk activity* for transmission of many types of STDs, as well as many intestinal organisms, and is not recommended. Homosexual networks advise wearing double condoms and using water-soluble lubricants, preferably containing nonoxynol-9, to decrease risk somewhat if engaging in this type of sexual activity.

TABLE 44.3 COMMON MYTHS ABOUT SEXUALLY TRANSMITTED DISEASES

Myth	Factual Data
People who have STDs are easily identifiable.	Inspection of the potential partner's genitals before sexual activity may decrease the risk (if one does not participate in sexual activity with a person who has visible lesions), *but* • Not all people who are infected have visible symptoms. • There is no standard personality or physical profile for people who can be infected with STDs—*anyone* can be infected.
Avoiding persons who have a history of casual sex, intravenous drug use, homosexual activity, bisexual activity or a previous sexual relationship with persons who engage in these high-risk practices effectively protects one from infection with STDs.	Avoiding people with these types of history may decrease risk, *but* • Not everyone is honest when responding to questions about sexual history. • Not everyone is aware of their previous partners' histories or the histories of others with whom their previous partners have had sexual relationships. • Asking these kinds of questions is difficult and may be postponed at times until emotional factors complicate such communication.
STDs never happen the first time. Intact genital skin is impervious to the germs (and gentle sexual activity does no harm).	Only one contact with one microorganism is necessary for infection. Intact skin is the body's first line of defense, *but* • Some microorganisms can be transmitted without a noticeable tissue injury. • Minor injuries can occur during many types of sexual activity, including vaginal intercourse.
Condoms prevent the spread of all STDs.	Condoms can greatly decrease the risk of STDs, *but* • Condoms can have tiny channels in the rubber (or other elastic material), which can allow microorganisms to pass through. • Condoms can break, slip off, or be applied improperly. • Petroleum-based lubricants may weaken latex condoms. • Condoms do not provide a barrier for any area other than the penis and most of the vagina (or anus). Some STDs may still be transmitted by contact of surrounding uncovered tissues.
The female condom prevents all transmissions of STDs.	It does cover more surface area, but it may have problems similar to male condoms (see previous).
Manual, oral, and anal stimulation cannot transmit STDs.	Contact of hands to genitals can allow for transmission of microorganisms through breaks in the skin. Oral sex can transmit some STD-causing microorganisms. Anal intercourse is a very high-risk activity for transmission of STDs because anal tissues are easily injured and the gastrointestinal tract can be a reservoir for many microorganisms.
Nonoxynol-9 spermicide kills all STD germs.	Nonoxynol-9 can reduce the risk of transmission of STDs, *but* • Nonoxynol-9 is *not* guaranteed to kill all microorganisms.
People get AIDS only by homosexual sexual activity or by blood transfusion. A woman cannot transmit HIV to a man. A man cannot transmit HIV to a woman.	Homosexual activity may result in a higher incidence of transmission of human immunodeficiency virus, *but* • HIV can be transmitted during heterosexual activity. • The gender of the individual does not protect him or her from being infected with HIV.
Sexual activity during menstruation is less likely to result in STDs.	Sexual activity during menstruation is more likely to result in transmission of some microorganisms that cause STDs because of the vulnerability of the lining of the uterus caused by sloughing of the outer layers of cells and because blood and cellular debris may serve as a nutritious medium for growth of microorganisms.
Lesbian sexual activity cannot transmit STDs.	Transmission of microorganisms can occur by contract with mouth, anal, or genital tissues or fomites (inanimate objects, such as vibrators and other sex paraphernalia) that have been contaminated with microorganisms from an infected individual—regardless of the original source of the infection.
Individuals who have not been infected after sexual activity with several people are naturally immune to STDs.	There is no known natural immunity to STDs. The individual may not yet have had contact with someone with an active STD.
Those who have had an STD and have been cured of it by taking medicine are now immune to that disease.	Infection that has been eradicated by medication does not confer immunity.
People can be certified free of all STDs by having a blood test and taking a simple medication if an infection is present.	Testing of those who suspect they may have contracted an STD and treatment (if possible) may decrease the spread of STDs, *but*

Myth	Factual Data
	• No one test identifies all STDs. Some are identified by examination, and not all infected people show symptoms.
	• Some STDs do not show positive test results for long periods yet may be transmitted by the individual while the tests are still negative.
	• People may be infected with more than one causative agent at a time and each must be treated (if possible). One STD may obscure the symptoms of other concurrent STDs, so that one or more types may go unnoticed and untreated or may not be evident until other STDs have been treated.
	• There are no known cures for some STDs.
Oral contraceptive (OC) pills give protection against STDs.	OC preparations are *not* antibiotics—they provide only some protection against conception.
	Use of a barrier method with spermicide along with the OC can decrease risk of STDs, as well as pregnancy.

• Explain the importance of patients knowing the sexual and lifestyle history of any potential partner before sexual activity has occurred. *Having a sexual relationship with someone is the* **epidemiological** *equivalent of engaging in sexual activity with all of that person's previous partners.*

• Provide pamphlets or other reading materials *to reinforce teaching.*

• Explain that abstinence or lifelong monogamy of both sexual partners in a relationship is the only sure prevention against sexually transmitted diseases. *These practices eliminate risk of exposure.*

• Educate the patient that consumption of alcohol or other psychoactive drugs can reduce inhibitions and may result in unintended sexual encounters, which can transmit STDs. *Avoiding or limiting alcohol and other drug consumption when with potential partners may help prevent STD infection from occurring.*

Evaluation

Goals have been met if the patient is able to state that pain is controlled at an acceptable level; verbalizes understanding

of transmission prevention and practices preventive behaviors; describes acceptable, alternative sexual practices and safer sexual practices; and relates accurate information and reduction in fear.

For more information on STDs, visit http://www.cdc.gov/std/healthcomm/fact_sheets.htm and http://www.ashastd.org/.

---

epidemiological: epi—on + demio—people + logical—pertaining to

---

CRITICAL THINKING

Stephanie

■ As you seat a young woman in an examining room of the clinic where you work, she comments, "I am new to this area and I've heard that there are three guys in this town who have syphilis and are spreading it around. Is that true?"

1. What are some concerns this question might reflect?

2. You find out that Stephanie knows very little about syphilis. List in outline form a teaching plan that includes the information that is important for Stephanie to know about syphilis.

Suggested answers at end of chapter.

REVIEW QUESTIONS

1. Which of the following pathogens causes syphilis?
   a. *Treponema pallidum*
   b. *Chlamydia trachomatis*
   c. Human papillomavirus
   d. Human immunodeficiency virus

2. What signs and symptoms of STDs should nurses assess for in all patients? Choose all that are correct.
   a. Itching
   b. Discharge
   c. Dysuria

   d. Genital ulcers
   e. Genital warts
   f. Rectal pain

3. A young woman is seen at a walk-in clinic and is diagnosed with an STD. She says, "How could I have an STD? I only have sex with my boyfriend. I don't sleep around!" Which of the following responses is best?
   a. "You are right, that should have kept you safe. There just are no guarantees."

b. "If your boyfriend is not infected, then obviously you have had sex with someone else."

c. "You or your boyfriend could be infected from past sexual encounters. He should also be tested at this time for STDs."

d. "Even lifelong monogamy cannot prevent many STDs."

4. A home care nurse is preparing to change a dressing on a patient who had genital warts removed the previous day. Which intervention should be completed first?
   a. Clean the wounds.
   b. Remove the old dressing.
   c. Assess for drainage.
   d. Administer an analgesic.

5. An older man is admitted to the hospital with mental status changes. As the nurse begins the shift assessment, the patient begins to cry and says his doctor thinks his problems stem from an untreated syphilis infection when he was in the military as a young man. Which response by the nurse is best?
   a. "Why didn't you have it treated when it occurred?"
   b. "What's done is done; it's unfortunate that treatment is too late now."
   c. "That must be upsetting for you. Do you want to talk about it?"
   d. "Don't cry; I am sure there is treatment that can help now."

6. A nurse has completed instruction related to risk reduction with a 17-year-old woman. Which statement by the patient indicates that teaching has been effective?
   a. "I should avoid drinking alcohol when I will be in situations with potential sex partners."
   b. "If I make sure my partners wear condoms, I will be protected from STDs."
   c. "Use of a barrier method of birth control will prevent infection with an STD."
   d. "As long as I know my partner well, I am safe."

Reference

1. Centers for Disease Control: Antimicrobial Resistance and Neisseria Gonorrhoeae Factsheet. Accessed http://www.cdc.gov/std/gisp/revisedARfactsheet.pdf August 10, 2005.

Unit Eleven Bibliography

1. Adas, J, and Santoro, N: Endocrine mechanisms and management for abnormal bleeding due to perimenopausal changes (management of abnormal uterine bleeding). Clin Obstet Gynecol 48:295–311, 2005.
2. American Cancer Society: Cancer Facts and Figures. Retrieved 5/26/05 from http://www.cancer.org/docroot/STT/stt_0.asp.
3. Cookson, M: Prostate cancer: screening and early detection. Cancer Control 8:133–140, 2001.
4. Elmore, J, Armstrong, K, Lehman, C, and Fletcher, S: Screening for breast cancer. JAMA 293:1245–1256, 2005.
5. Epperly, TD, and Moore, KE: Health issues in men: Part I. Common genitourinary disorders. Am Fam Physician 61:3657, 2000.
6. Fact sheet: Chlamydia. US Department of Health and Human Services, Bethesda, MD. Retrieved January 25, 2006, from http://www.niaid.nih.gov/factsheets/stdclam.htm.
7. Furo, S: Sexually Transmitted Diseases in Women. Lippincott, Williams & Wilkins, Philadelphia, 2003.
8. Healthy Pregnancy: Fertility Awareness and Infertility. The National Women's Health Information Center (NWHIC). Retrieved 5/26/05 from http://www.4woman.gov/Pregnancy/infertility.htm.
9. Jarvis, C: Physical Examination & Health Assessment, ed. 4. Saunders, St Louis, 2004.
10. Kaunitz, A: Beyond the pill: new data and options in hormonal and intrauterine contraception. Am J Obstet Gynecol 192:998–1004, 2005.
11. Kerlikowske, K, Smith-Bindman, R, Ljung, B, and Grady, D: Evaluation of abnormal mammography results and palpable breast abnormalities. Ann Intern Med 139:274–84, 2003.
12. Lewis, JH, Rosen, R, and Goldstein, I: Erectile dysfunction: A panel's recommendations for management. Am J Nurs 103:48–56, 2003.
13. Lewis, RW: Epidemiology of erectile dysfunction. Urol Clin North Am 28:209–216, 2001.
14. Meredith, CE: Erectile dysfunction. In Meredith, CE, and Karlowicz, KA (eds). Urologic Nursing: A Study Guide. Society of Urologic Nurses and Associates, Pitman, NJ, 1995, pp 137–141.
15. Meredith, CE: Male infertility. In Karlowicz, KA (ed.). Urologic Nursing: Principles and Practice (pp. 360–372). Saunders, Philadelphia, 1995, pp 360–372.
16. Morbidity and Mortality Weekly Report: Sexually Transmitted Diseases Treatment Guidelines 2002. (May 10, 2002). Centers for Disease Control: 51(RR-6).
17. Nurse's prescribing reference: Summer 2005. 12(2). New York: Prescribing Reference, Inc.
18. Pap Smear Screening Recommendation Changes. UNMC Department of Obstetrics and Gynecology: Olson Center for Women's Health, 2004. Retrieved 6/21/05 from http://www.unmc.edu/olson/education/papguidelines.htm.
19. Roehrborn, CG: Benign prostatic hyperplasia: Highlighting the latest data, 2003. Accessed medscape.com/viewarticle/437088.
20. Slowey, MJ: Polycystic ovary syndrome: new perspective on an old problem. South Med J 94:190, 2001.
21. Weinstock, M, and Neides D: (2004). The Resident's Guide to Ambulatory Care, ed. 5. Anadem, Columbus, OH, 2004.

SUGGESTED ANSWERS TO

CRITICAL THINKING

■ Mrs. Miller

1. You can educate Mrs. Miller about the possibility of neonatal infections from *C. trachomatis* or *N. gonorrhoeae*, especially of the eyes. Institutional and governmental policies related to treatment should be explained. Care should be taken to explain to Mrs. Miller that treatment is widely used, so as not to make her feel she has a condition she has not been told about.

2. Because the benefits for prophylactic eye treatment of the neonate for *C. trachomatis* and *N. gonorrhoeae* exposure are generally seen as greater than the risks, it is recommended by governmental agencies and supported by most institutional policies to treat all newborns, regardless of known exposure, shortly after birth.

■ Kerri

1. Explain to Kerri the fact that trichomoniasis is generally considered to be an STD, but that the organism that causes the disorder can be transmitted through infected articles (during nonsexual contact), can survive a long time outside the body, and that one can be asymptomatic for many years following exposure to the organism before an outbreak occurs.

2.

$$\frac{7.5 \text{ mg}}{\text{kg}} \left| \frac{1 \text{ kg}}{2.2\#} \right| \frac{140\#}{} = 477 \text{ mg}$$

Her dose will probably be rounded to 500 mg every 6 hours.

3. Teach Kerri that it is possible that her partner could have an undiagnosed infection, and that the possibility of being infected during a monogamous relationship is real. Treatment should be provided to Kerri's partner regardless of symptoms. Also, reinfection may occur if both partners are not treated. Also, be sure to tell her that she should abstain from alcohol for at least 48 hours following completion of the metronidazole. Patients who drink alcohol while taking it are VERY likely to vomit.

■ Stephanie

1. Concerns might include (a) a wish to speak with a health-care worker; (b) uncertainty about whether patient information will be kept confidential (give assurance that if you knew about anyone with syphilis, it would be your professional responsibility to keep it confidential); (c) fear that she might have become infected through heterosexual contact; (d) a desire to protect herself by avoiding those who have syphilis; and (e) a desire for information about syphilis and its transmission routes.

2. The teaching plan might include information about (a) the spirochete that causes syphilis; (b) signs and symptoms; (c) diagnostic tests; (d) means of transmission; (e) strategies for risk reduction; (f) treatment; (g) research; and (h) rights and responsibilities of those who have the disease.

unit TWELVE

UNDERSTANDING THE MUSCULOSKELETAL SYSTEM

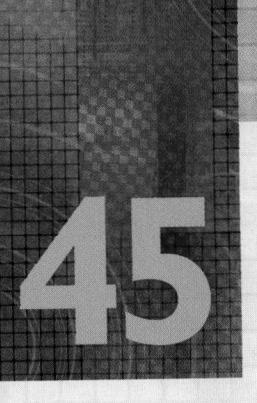

45

Musculoskeletal Function and Assessment

RODNEY B. KEBICZ AND
JANICE L. BRADFORD

KEY TERMS

arthroscopy (ar-THROSS-scop-ee)
arthrocentesis (AR-throw-sen-tee-sis)
articular (ar-TIK-yoo-lar)
bone (BOWN)
bursae (BURR-sah)
crepitation (crep-i-TAY-shun)
hemarthrosis (heem-ar-THROW-sis)
joint (JOYNT)
muscle (MUSS-uhl)
synovitis (sin-oh-VIGH-tis)
vertebrae (VER-te-bray)

QUESTIONS TO GUIDE YOUR READING

1. What is the normal structure and function of the musculoskeletal system?

2. What areas are included in a nursing assessment of the musculoskeletal system?

3. What areas are reviewed when performing a neurovascular assessment?

4. How would you describe diagnostic tests for musculoskeletal problems?

5. What nursing care would you provide for each musculoskeletal diagnostic test?

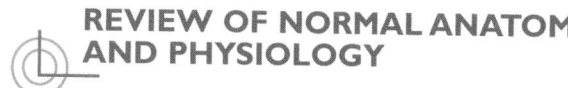

REVIEW OF NORMAL ANATOMY AND PHYSIOLOGY

The skeletal and muscular systems may be considered one system because they work together to enable the body to move. The skeleton is the framework that supports the body and to which the voluntary **muscles** are attached. The skeletal framework includes the **joints,** or articulations, between **bones.** Contraction of a muscle pulls a bone and changes the angle of a joint. It is important to remember that movement would not be possible without the proper functioning of the nervous, cardiovascular, and respiratory systems. Voluntary muscles require nerve impulses to contract, a continuous supply of blood provided by the circulatory system, and oxygen provided by the respiratory system.

SKELETAL SYSTEM TISSUES AND THEIR FUNCTIONS

The tissues that make up the skeletal system are bone tissue; cartilage, which covers most joint surfaces; and fibrous connective tissue, which forms the ligaments that connect one bone to another and also form part of the structure of joints. The tissues of the muscular system are skeletal (also called striated or voluntary) muscle; fibrous connective tissue, which forms the tendons that connect muscle to bone; and the fasciae, the strong membranes that enclose individual muscles. Smooth muscle (also called involuntary or nonstriated) has the same function as skeletal muscle (i.e., contraction) but is not considered part of the skeletal system tissues as it is not involved with articulation or skeletal movement.

Besides its role in movement, the skeleton has other functions. It protects organs and tissues from mechanical injury. For example, the brain is protected by the skull and the heart and lungs are protected by the rib cage. Flat and irregular bones contain and protect the red bone marrow, the hematopoietic (blood-forming) tissue. The bones are also a storage site for excess calcium, which may be removed from bones to maintain a normal blood calcium level. Calcium in the blood is necessary for blood clotting and for the proper functioning of nerves and muscles.

Although the primary function of the muscular system is to move or stabilize the skeleton, the voluntary muscles collectively contribute significantly to heat production, which maintains normal body temperature. Heat is one of the energy products of cellular respiration, the process that produces adenosine triphosphate (ATP), the direct energy source for muscle contraction. Another important function of the muscular system is that it aids in returning blood from the legs through muscular compression on the leg veins.

Bone Tissue and Growth of Bone

Bone tissue is composed of bone cells, called osteocytes, within a strong nonliving matrix made of calcium salts and the protein collagen. In compact bone, the osteocytes and matrix are in precise arrangements called osteons (or haver-

sian systems). Compact bone is very dense and to the unaided eye appears solid. In spongy bone, the arrangement of cells and matrix is less precise, giving the bone a spongy appearance. Compact bone forms the diaphyses (shafts) of the long bones of the extremities and covers the spongy bone that forms the bulk of short, flat, and irregular bones.

A living bone is covered by a fibrous connective tissue membrane called the periosteum, which is the anchor for tendons and ligaments because the collagen fibers of all these structures merge to form connections of great strength. This membrane also contains the blood vessels that enter the bone itself (most of the bone has a very good blood supply) and bone-producing cells called osteoblasts that are activated to initiate repair when bone is damaged.

The growth of bone from fetal life until a person attains final adult height depends on many factors. Proper nutrition (particularly vitamins and minerals) provides the raw material to produce bone matrix: comprised of calcium, phosphorous, and protein. Vitamin D is essential for the efficient absorption of calcium and phosphorus from food in the small intestine. Vitamins A and C do not become part of bone but are needed for the production of bone matrix (a process called calcification or ossification). Hormones directly necessary for growth include growth hormone (GH) from the anterior pituitary gland, thyroxine from the thyroid gland, and insulin from the pancreas. Growth hormone increases mitosis and protein synthesis in growing bones; thyroxine stimulates osteoblasts, as well as increasing energy production from food. Insulin is essential for the efficient use of glucose to provide energy. If a child is lacking any of these hormones, growth is much slower and the child does not reach his or her genetic potential for height.

Bone is not a fixed tissue, even when growth in height has ceased. There is a constant removal and replacement of calcium and phosphate (usually the rates are equal) to maintain normal blood levels of these minerals. Parathyroid hormone secreted by the parathyroid glands increases the removal of calcium and phosphate from bones; the hormone calcitonin from the thyroid gland promotes the retention of calcium in bones, although its greatest effects may be during childhood.

Osteoblasts produce bone matrix during normal growth to replace matrix lost during normal turnover and to repair fractures. Other cells called osteoclasts reabsorb bone matrix when more calcium is needed in the blood and during normal growth and fracture repair when excess bone must be removed as bones change shape.

The sex hormones, estrogen from the ovaries or testosterone from the testes, are important for the retention of calcium in adult bones. For women after menopause, more calcium may be removed from bones than is replaced, leading to a thinning of bone tissue and the possibility of spontaneous fractures.

Structure of the Skeleton

The 206 bones of the human skeleton are in two divisions: the axial skeleton and the appendicular skeleton. The axial skeleton consists of the skull, hyoid, vertebral column, and rib cage; all are flat or irregular bones and contain red bone marrow (hematopoietic tissue). The appendicular skeleton consists of the bones of the arms and legs and the shoulder and pelvic girdles, by which the extremities attach to the axial skeleton (Fig. 45.1).

The long bones of the limbs are those of the arm, forearm, hand, and fingers and those of the thigh, leg, foot, and toes. All long bones have the same general structure: a central diaphysis, or shaft, with two ends called epiphyses. The diaphyses of long bones contain yellow bone marrow, which is mostly adipose—that is, stored energy. The bones of the wrist and ankle are short bones (except for the calcaneus, which is an irregular bone). The scapula is considered a flat

bone, and the pelvic girdle is made of irregular bones. These bones contain red bone marrow.

Skull

The skull consists of 8 cranial bones and 14 facial bones and also contains the 3 auditory bones found in each middle ear cavity. The cranial bones that enclose and protect the brain are frontal, two parietal, two temporal, occipital, sphenoid, and ethmoid (Fig. 45.2). All the joints between cranial bones and those between most of the facial bones are immovable joints called sutures (comprised of dense collagenous connective tissue). The mandible is the only movable facial bone. It articulates with the temporal bone of the skull forming a combined hinge and planar joint called the temporo-

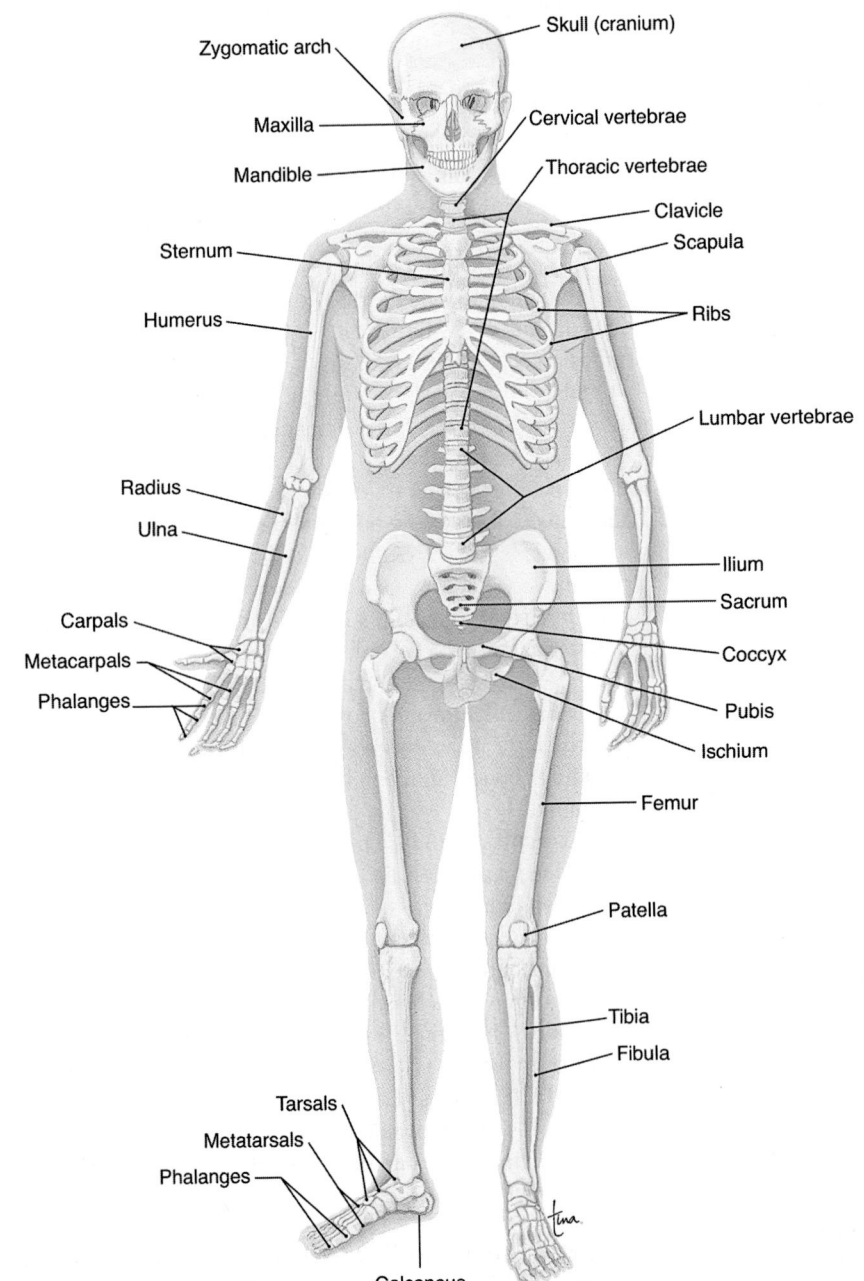

FIGURE 45.1 The full skeleton in anterior view. *(Modified from Scanlon, VC, and Sanders, T: Anatomy and Physiology, ed. 5. F.A. Davis, Philadelphia, 2007, with permission.)*

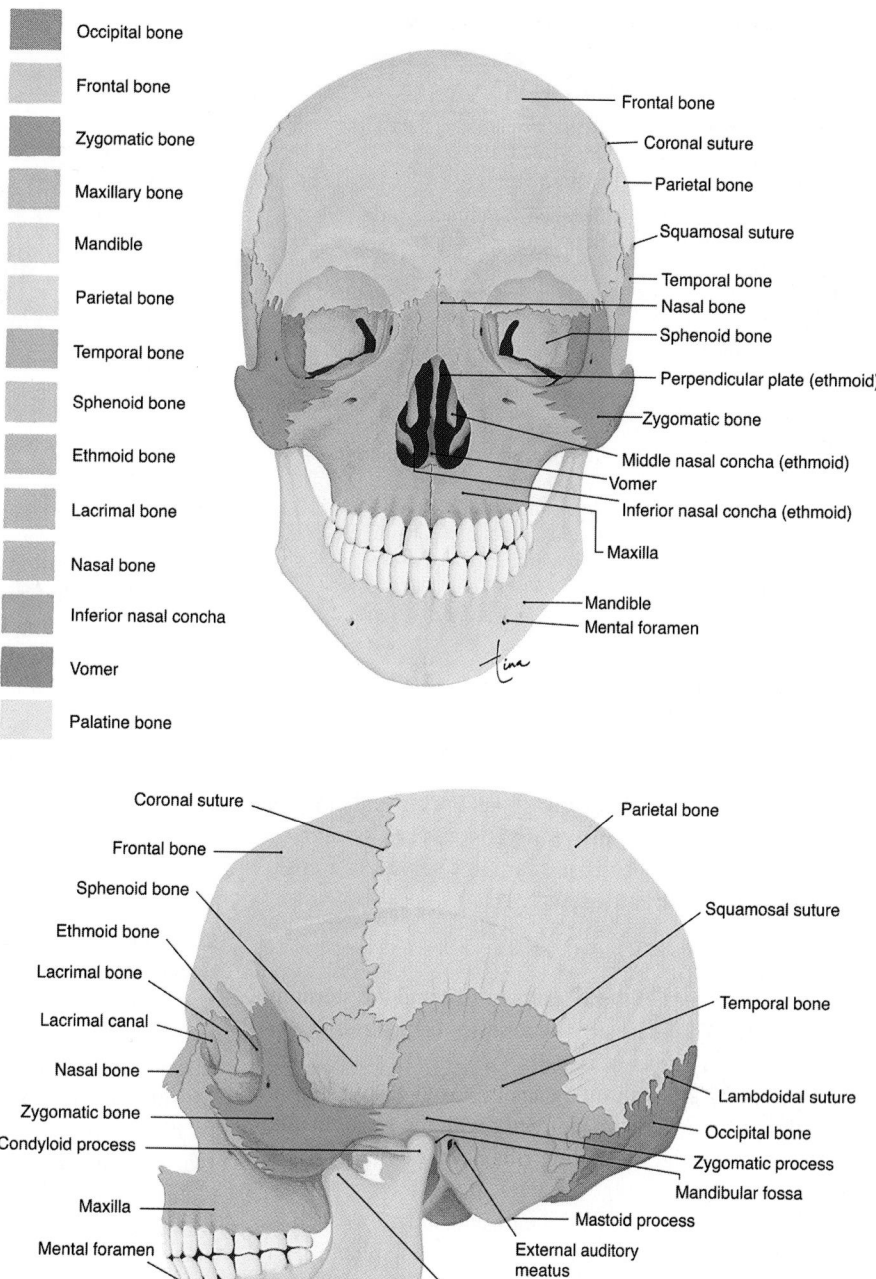

Occipital bone
Frontal bone
Zygomatic bone
Maxillary bone
Mandible
Parietal bone
Temporal bone
Sphenoid bone
Ethmoid bone
Lacrimal bone
Nasal bone
Inferior nasal concha
Vomer
Palatine bone

Frontal bone
Coronal suture
Parietal bone
Squamosal suture
Temporal bone
Nasal bone
Sphenoid bone
Perpendicular plate (ethmoid)
Zygomatic bone
Middle nasal concha (ethmoid)
Vomer
Inferior nasal concha (ethmoid)
Maxilla
Mandible
Mental foramen

Coronal suture
Frontal bone
Sphenoid bone
Ethmoid bone
Lacrimal bone
Lacrimal canal
Nasal bone
Zygomatic bone
Condyloid process
Maxilla
Mental foramen
Mandible
Body

Parietal bone
Squamosal suture
Temporal bone
Lambdoidal suture
Occipital bone
Zygomatic process
Mandibular fossa
Mastoid process
External auditory meatus
Coronoid process

FIGURE 45.2 Anterior *(upper)* and lateral *(lower)* views of the skull. *(Modified from Scanlon, VC, and Sanders, T: Anatomy and Physiology, ed. 5. F.A. Davis, Philadelphia, 2007, with permission.)*

mandibular joint (Table 45.1). The maxillae are the upper jaw bones, which also form the front of the hard palate (part of the roof of the mouth). The rest of the facial bones are shown in Figure 45.2.

Vertebral Column

The vertebral column (or spinal column) is made of individual bones called **vertebrae** (see Fig. 45.1). From top to bottom there are 7 cervical, 12 thoracic, 5 lumbar, 5 sacral fused into 1 sacrum, and 4 or 5 coccygeal vertebrae fused into 1 coccyx.

The first cervical vertebra, the atlas, articulates with the occipital bone of the skull and forms a pivot joint with the axis, the second cervical vertebra. The thoracic vertebrae articulate with the posterior ends of the ribs. The lumbar vertebrae are the largest and strongest. The sacrum permits the articulation of the two hip bones, at the sacroiliac joints. The coccyx serves as an attachment point for some muscles of the perineum.

The vertebrae as a unit form a flexible backbone that supports the trunk and head and contains and protects the spinal cord. Openings, or intervertebral foramina, between

TABLE 45.1 JOINTS OF THE APPENDICULAR SKELETON

Type of Joint and Description	Examples
Symphysis—disk of fibrous cartilage between bones	Between vertebrae Between pubic bones
Ball and socket—movement in all planes	Scapula and humerus (shoulder) Pelvic bone and femur (hip)
Hinge—movement in one plane	Humerus and ulna (elbow) Femur and tibia (knee) Between phalanges (fingers and toes)
Combined hinge and planar	Temporal bone and mandible (lower jaw)
Pivot—rotation	Atlas and axis (neck) Radius and ulna (distal to elbow)
Gliding—side-to-side movement	Between carpals (wrist)
Saddle—movement in several planes	Carpometacarpal of thumb

Modified from Scanlon, VC, Sanders, T: Essentials of Anatomy and Physiology, ed. 5. F.A. Davis, Philadelphia, 2007, p. 120, with permission.

the vertebrae allow for the exit of spinal nerves and entry of blood vessels. The joints between vertebrae are symphysis joints in which a disk of fibrous cartilage serves as a cushion and permits slight movement.

Rib Cage

The rib cage consists of the 12 pairs of ribs and the sternum, or breast bone. All the ribs connect posteriorly with the thoracic vertebrae. The seven pairs of true ribs articulate directly with the sternum by means of costal cartilages; the three pairs of false ribs join indirectly with the sternum, and the inferior two pairs of floating ribs do not connect to the sternum at all.

The rib cage protects the heart and lungs, as well as upper abdominal organs such as the liver and spleen, from mechanical injury. During breathing, the flexible rib cage is pulled upward and outward by the external intercostal muscles to expand the chest cavity and bring about inhalation.

Appendicular Skeleton

The bones of the appendicular skeleton are shown in Figure 45.1. The important joints of the appendicular skeleton are summarized in Table 45.1.

Structure of Synovial Joints

All freely movable joints (this excludes amphiarthroses and synarthroses) are synovial joints in that they share similarities of structure (Fig. 45.3). On the joint surface of each bone is the **articular** cartilage, which provides a smooth surface. The joint capsule is similar to a sleeve. It is made of fibrous connective tissue and forms a strong sheath that encloses the joint. Lining the joint capsule is the synovial membrane, which secretes synovial fluid into the joint cav-

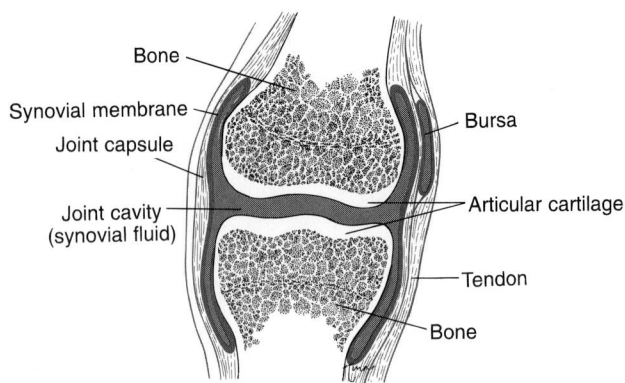

FIGURE 45.3 Longitudinal section through a typical synovial joint. *(Modified from Scanlon, VT, and Sanders, T: Workbook for Essentials of Anatomy and Physiology, ed. 5. F.A. Davis, Philadelphia, 2007, with permission.)*

ity. Synovial fluid is a mixture of hyaluronic acid, proteins, fat, and cells that provides a slippery consistency that prevents friction as the bones move.

Many synovial joints also have **bursae,** which are small sacs of synovial fluid between the joint and the tendons that cross over the joint. Bursae permit the tendons to slide easily as the joint moves.

MUSCLE STRUCTURE AND ARRANGEMENTS

One muscle is made of thousands of muscle cells (fibers), which are specialized for contraction. When a muscle contracts, it shortens and pulls on a bone. Each muscle fiber receives its own motor nerve ending, and the numbers of fibers that contract depend on the job the muscle has to do. Muscles are anchored to bones by tendons, which are made of fibrous connective tissue. A muscle usually has at least two tendons, each attached to a different bone. The more stationary muscle attachment is called its origin; the more movable attachment is the insertion. The muscle itself crosses the joint formed by the two bones to which it is attached, and when the muscle contracts, it pulls on the insertion and moves the bone in a specific direction. The muscle causing this particular action is termed the agonist.

The approximately 700 muscles in the body are arranged to bring about a variety of movements (Fig. 45.4). The general types of arrangements are the agonist with opposing antagonists and the cooperative synergists.

Antagonistic muscles have opposite functions; such arrangements are necessary because muscles can only pull, not push. If the biceps brachii, for example, flexes the forearm, an antagonist, the triceps brachii, is needed to extend the forearm. Other examples of antagonists are the quadriceps femoris and hamstring groups, the pectoralis major and the latissimus dorsi, and the tibialis anterior and gastrocnemius.

Synergistic muscles have similar functions or work together to perform a particular function. The brachioradialis is a synergist to the biceps brachii for flexion of the forearm; the sartorius is a synergist to the quadriceps group for

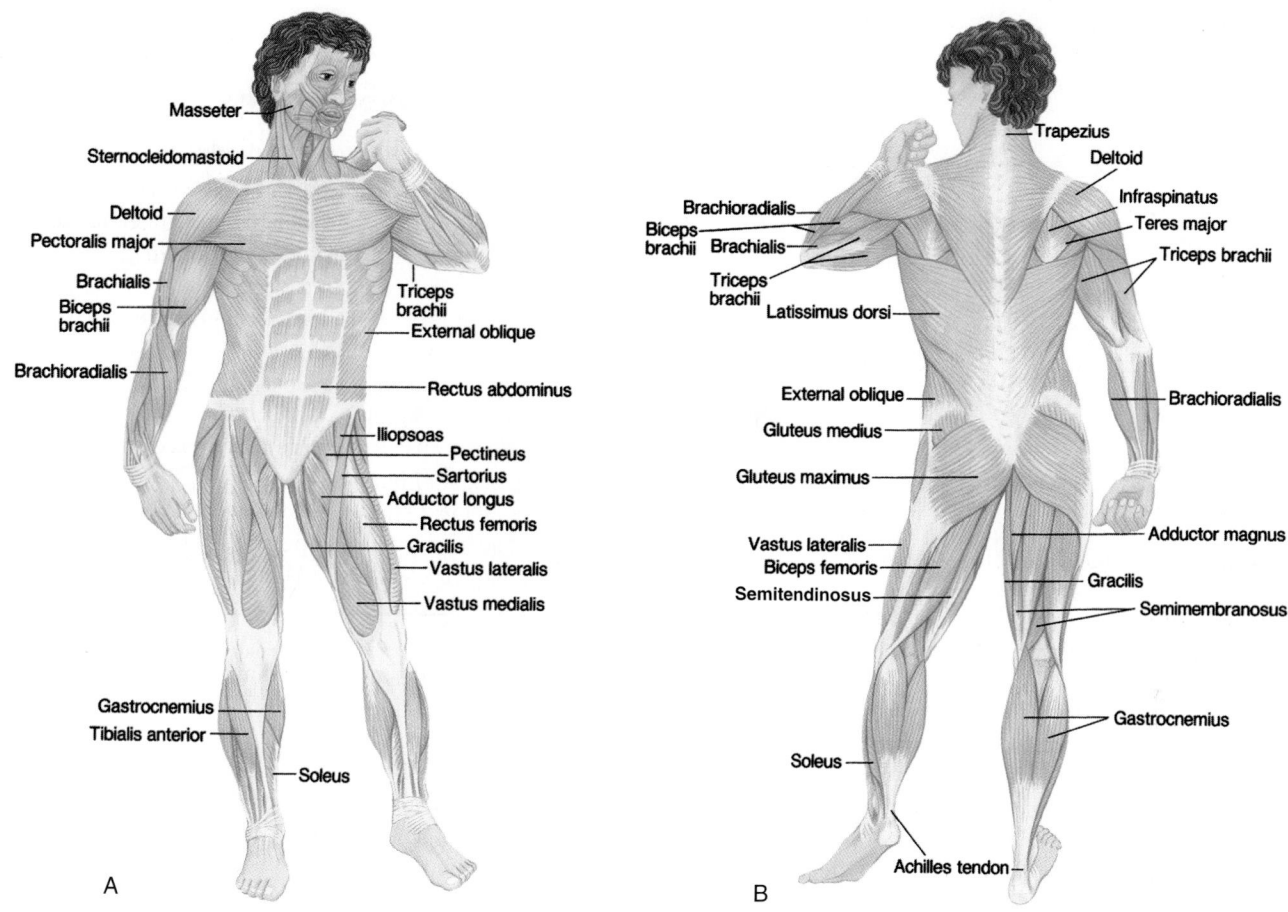

FIGURE 45.4 Major muscles. *(A)* Anterior view. *(B)* Posterior view. *(Modified from Scanlon, VC, and Sanders, T: Essentials of Anatomy and Physiology, ed. 5. F.A. Davis, Philadelphia, 2007, with permission.)*

flexion of the thigh. Synergists are necessary to provide slight differences in angles when joints are moved. Without synergism we would be unable to maintain our balance or have the fine motor control needed to do such movements as writing or talking.

ROLE OF THE NERVOUS SYSTEM

Skeletal muscles are voluntary muscles in that consciously controlled nerve impulses cause contraction. Such nerve impulses originate in the motor areas of the frontal lobes of the cerebral cortex. The coordination of voluntary movement is a function of the cerebellum. Neurons in the CNS (central nervous system) regulate muscle tone, the state of slight contraction usually present in muscles. Good muscle tone is important for posture and for good coordination.

Neuromuscular Junction

Each of the thousands of fibers in a muscle has its own motor nerve ending; the neuromuscular junction is the termination of the motor neuron at the muscle fiber (see Fig. 50.2). The axon terminal is the enlarged distal tip of the motor neuron. It contains vesicles of the neurotransmitter acetylcholine. The membrane of the muscle fiber, called the sarcolemma, contains receptor sites for acetylcholine. The

synaptic cleft is the minute space between the axon terminal and the sarcolemma. The inactivating enzyme acetylcholinesterase is available in the synaptic cleft.

When a nerve impulse arrives at the axon terminal, it causes the release of acetylcholine, which diffuses across the synaptic cleft and bonds to the acetylcholine receptors on the sarcolemma. This makes the sarcolemma permeable to sodium ions, which rush into the cell and generate an electrical impulse (an action potential) along the entire sarcolemma. This electrical change triggers a series of reactions in the internal units of contraction called sarcomeres. Put simply, filaments of the protein actin slide over filaments of another protein called myosin, and the sarcomere shortens. All the thousands of sarcomeres in a muscle fiber shorten, and the entire cell contracts. If a muscle has little work to do, few of its many muscle fibers contract, but if the muscle has more work to do, more of its muscle fibers contract.

AGING AND THE MUSCULOSKELETAL SYSTEM

The amount of calcium in bones depends on several factors (Fig. 45.5). Good nutrition is certainly one factor, but age is another, especially for women. One function of estrogen or

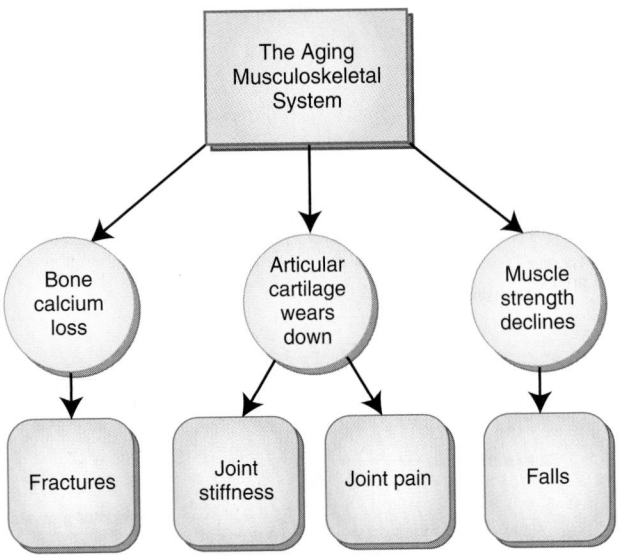

FIGURE 45.5 Aging and the musculoskeletal system. This concept map shows the effects the aging process has on the musculoskeletal system.

testosterone is the maintenance of a strong bone matrix. For women after menopause, bone matrix loses more calcium than is replaced. Calcium loss can lead to weakened bones that may result in bone fractures. Weight-bearing joints are also subject to damage after many years. Often the articular cartilage wears down and becomes rough, leading to pain and stiffness.

Muscle strength declines with age as the process of protein synthesis decreases. Such loss of strength need not be exaggerated because aging muscles benefit from regular exercise, which has been shown to increase strength and reduce falls and accidents (Box 45.1 Gerontological Issues).

NURSING ASSESSMENT OF THE MUSCULOSKELETAL SYSTEM

The initial assessment begins with a history that includes the effects the condition is having on the patient's life. It then proceeds to a physical and psychosocial assessment (Table 45.2). Frequent neurovascular assessments may be needed if there is a risk of circulation impairment, such as if the patient has a fracture or musculoskeletal surgery (Table 45.3).

Subjective Data

History
The patient's history should include the following:
- If there was an injury, how it happened and when it happened
- Occupation and activities, including sports and other physical activities
- Risk factors for musculoskeletal problems and family history of musculoskeletal problems (to detect hereditary problems)

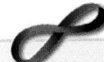

Box 45.1

Gerontological Issues

Age-Related Changes in the Older Adult
Age-related changes can lead to impaired mobility, an increased risk for falls, and pain. Common age-related musculoskeletal changes include the following:
- Muscle mass and strength decline.
- Number of muscle cells decrease and are replaced by fibrous connective tissue.
- Elasticity of ligaments, tendons, and cartilage decrease, resulting in weaker bones.
- Intervertebral spaces decrease from loss of water, causing a loss of height.
- Posture and gait change. (Men develop a wider stance and take smaller steps; women have a narrow stance and walk with a waddling gait.)

- Current health status, including ongoing or chronic medical conditions (such as heart disease, diabetes, lung conditions)
- Diet history (including whether calcium and vitamin D intake are adequate to ensure proper bone and muscle maintenance and repair)
- Information specific to the patient's musculoskeletal problems

Patients with musculoskeletal problems frequently report pain or related stiffness and tenderness as a major concern. The pain may be acute or chronic and may limit the patient in everyday life. Assessment includes previous diagnoses, pain severity, medications, treatments, and procedures the patient uses to alleviate the pain. The WHAT'S UP? model can be used to assess the patient's pain (see Chapter 1.)

Objective Data

Physical Assessment
Three areas of musculoskeletal assessment are important: inspection, palpation, and range of motion (ROM). If the patient is able to walk, inspect the patient's posture and gait, noting poor posture or alterations in movement, such as limping. Note the use of mobility aids, such as a cane or walker. Document other gross deformities, such as unequal limbs, malalignment, or contractures. Spinal deformities are especially significant because they can compromise breathing and balance. Inspect the joints and muscles of the arms, hands, legs, and feet for deformity, redness, swelling, increased temperature, or **crepitation** (grating sound as joint or bone moves). Also note the patient's general nutritional status (e.g., normal, obese, emaciated).

After inspection, gently palpate for warmth, swelling, and tenderness in the areas of swelling, redness, and areas where the patient reported pain (being careful to minimize the pain this may cause). For example, reddened joints

TABLE 45.2 ASSESSMENT OF THE MUSCULOSKELETAL SYSTEM

Category	Questions to Ask During History Assessment	Rationale/Significance
	Subjective Assessment	
Demographic	• Age, gender, socioeconomic status • Occupation	• Increased age, being female, and lower socioeconomic status increases risk of musculoskeletal injury/problems. • Enables you to begin planning for discharge teaching if the patient has to alter his or her employment.
Previous Health History	• Activities patient participates in • Risk factors for musculoskeletal problems • Family history • Diet history	• Provides information regarding the level of activity the patient had before the concern. • Smoking and a sedentary lifestyle are risk factors for musculoskeletal problems. • Some musculoskeletal conditions have genetic and familial tendencies. • Dietary intake such as calcium and vitamin D influence some musculoskeletal disorders.
History of Injury or Present Concern	• Allergies • History of the injury (if there was one) • Pain (Use Pain Assessment Scale [PAS])	• Prevents exposure to medication or compounds used in diagnostic tests, treatments, and therapies. • Provides information that helps in the diagnosis of the problem, as well as making you aware of possible complications of the injury. • Provides information about severity of the condition and effectiveness of the treatment and therapy.
Psychosocial Assessment	• Determine if deformities, changes in body image, self-concept, socialization, or employment are present • Determine coping skills	• The patient may need assistance with strategies to cope with the stress of a possible chronic musculoskeletal condition. • Some musculoskeletal conditions require lifestyle alterations that can cause increased stress and difficulties in coping.
	Objective Assessment	
Physical Assessment	• Inspect, palpate, and observe range of motion [ROM] of affected areas • Assess color, warmth, circulation, and movement (CWCM) of affected areas • Palpate all pulses below involved area	• Altered gait, tone, size, shape, posture, contractures, deformities, ROM, pain, and effects on activities of daily living (ADLs) can be determined. • Nerve function, sensation, movement, weakness, and the potential development of compartment syndrome can be determined. • Alterations may indicate altered vascular integrity (and therefore tissue integrity) of affected area or demonstrate developing compartment syndrome.

should be palpated for **synovitis** (swollen synovial tissue within the joint) or the presence of bony nodes. In some cases, joints and muscles may seem healthy but are tender when palpated.

Next, assess joint mobility. Stabilize the body area proximal to the joint being moved. Observe the patient's ROM for performing independent activities of daily living. Pay particular attention to the hands and observe movement in finger joints. For a quick and easy assessment of range of motion in the hands, ask the patient to touch each finger, one by one, to the thumb (known as opposition) and then to make a fist.

Also assess the size, shape, strength, and tone of muscles. Evaluate bilateral muscle strength by asking the patient to grip your hands. This enables you to feel the strength and equality. Pushing an extremity against your hand provides a general indication of muscle strength. More specific evalua-

tion is performed by a physical therapist (PT) or an occupational therapist (OT). Using a scale of 0 to 5 (0 = paralysis and 5 = moving a muscle against resistance), the PT or OT measures the strength of each muscle group and rates it as a

TABLE 45.3 NEUROVASCULAR ASSESSMENT

Assess for	Note and Report
Color	Pallor, cyanosis, redness, or discoloration
Temperature	Unusual coolness or warmth
Pain	Pain that is worse on passive motion, pain that no longer responds to analgesics
Movement	Alterations in movement
Sensation	Alterations in feeling, tingling or paresthesias
Pulses	Diminished or absent distal pulses
Capillary refill	Nailbed that does not blanch in 3–5 seconds

synovitis: synovia—joint + itis—inflammation

fraction. For example, 5/5 means that the patient reached a 5 out of 5 possible on the muscle strength scale.

Psychosocial Assessment

Deformities resulting from arthritis or other musculoskeletal disorders can affect a patient's body image and self-concept (see Chapter 46.) Chronic pain may keep the patient from socializing or from working. Many work days are lost as a result of both acute and chronic musculoskeletal problems. Patients often avoid social events and tend to withdraw from people. Data collection should include questions related to the psychological effects of the musculoskeletal disorder.

Patients may experience a tremendous amount of psychological stress resulting from the pain, loss of income, and withdrawal from friends and family. The nurse assesses the patient's ability to cope, asking what coping strategies have been used in the past for other life stressors. Support systems for the patient need to be identified, especially spiritual and social systems. As needed, consult the appropriate member of the health-care team (social work, clergy, support groups) to ensure that the patient's psychosocial needs are being met.

CRITICAL THINKING

Mr. Smith

■ Mr. Smith, age 80, is brought to the emergency department with a fractured left hip. He is positioned for comfort while you collect data.

1. What information should you obtain in Mr. Smith's history?
2. What should be assessed in Mr. Smith's physical examination?

Suggested answers at end of chapter.

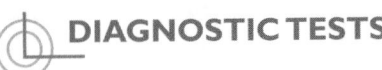

DIAGNOSTIC TESTS

Diagnosis of musculoskeletal problems is assisted by laboratory tests and diagnostic imaging (including x-ray examinations and nonradiological tests). Specific tests for patients with connective tissue diseases are described in Chapter 46.

Laboratory Tests

Serum Calcium and Phosphorus

Bone disorders commonly cause changes in calcium and phosphorus (or phosphate) levels. When a person is healthy, calcium and phosphorus have an inverse relationship. This means that when serum calcium increases, serum phosphorus decreases, and vice versa. Some disorders, however, cause an increase in both values or a decrease in both values. Calcium and phosphorus levels are regulated by calcitonin from the thyroid gland and parathyroid hormone from the parathyroid glands. When these glands are not functioning properly, alterations in calcium and phosphorus levels can occur (Table 45.4)

Serum calcium tends to decrease in patients with osteoporosis or in people who consume inadequate amounts of calcium in their diets. Serum calcium levels increase in patients with bone cancer, particularly those with metastatic disease.

Alkaline Phosphatase

Alkaline phosphatase (ALP) is an enzyme that increases when bone or liver tissue is damaged. In metabolic bone diseases and bone cancer, ALP increases to reflect osteoblast (bone-forming cell) activity.

Myoglobin

Myoglobin is a protein found in striated (skeletal or cardiac) muscle. It is what causes the red color of muscle. When skeletal or cardiac muscle is damaged myoglobin levels rise in the blood.

TABLE 45.4 DIAGNOSTIC LABORATORY TESTS FOR MUSCULOSKELETAL SYSTEM

Test	Normal Value	Significance of Abnormal Findings
Serum Calcium	8.5–10. 5 mg/dL	Hypercalcemia—may be related to metastatic bone disease or extended immobilization. Hypocalcemia—may be due to poor dietary intake. Can ultimately lead to rickets in a child or osteomalacia (bone softening) or osteoporosis in the elderly.
Serum Phosphorus	2.6–4.5 mg/dL	Usually evaluated with serum calcium. A number of disorders can be associated with high or low serum phosphorus.
Alkaline Phosphatase (ALP)	45–115 U/L (male) 30–100 U/L (female)	ALP increases may indicate bone abnormality (examples: Paget's disease, metastatic bone cancer). ALP is increased when new bone is formed.
Creatine Kinase (CK)	60–400 U/L (male) 40–150 U/L (female)	IM injections can cause a rise in CK.
Isoenzyme CK3 (MM)	95%–100%	High levels indicate need for further testing for muscle disease. Can be used as a screening test for malignant hyperthermia. Will be increased in rhabdomyolysis.
Myoglobin	50–120 µg/mL	Increased myoglobin can indicate MI or skeletal muscle destruction.

Serum Muscle Enzymes

When muscle tissue is damaged, a number of serum enzymes are released into the bloodstream, including skeletal muscle creatine kinase (CK-MM [CK3]), aldolase (ALD), aspartate aminotransferase (AST), and lactate dehydrogenase (LDH). These enzymes increase in certain muscle diseases such as muscular dystrophy, polymyositis, and dermatomyositis.

LEARNING TIP

Rhabdomyolysis is a very serious and potentially fatal condition associated with muscle destruction due to such things as injury (especially crushing), high fever, convulsions, or prolonged muscle compression (such as from lying in a coma) can have CK levels greater than five times normal. If the patient suffered muscle destruction, look at the patient's CK, myoglobin, and serum potassium levels to assess for rhabdomyolysis. The three laboratory values will be elevated.

Radiographic Tests

SAFETY TIP

For any radiographic test requiring injection or instillation of a medication or contrast solution, it is important for the nurse to assess for allergies or untoward responses resulting from previous examinations or exposures. Many of the contrast mediums used have alternate substances available in case of allergies. If the patient is unable to do so, then it is the nurse's responsibility to inform the technologist of the allergies or previous adverse responses experienced by the patient.

Standard X-Rays

An x-ray examination can determine bone density, texture, changes in alignment and bone relationship, erosion, swelling, and intactness. In addition, x-ray examinations can be useful in identifying certain soft tissue damage (e.g., ligaments and tendons) because of alterations in bone position and spacing.

Although there is no special nursing care associated with x-ray examinations, you should inform patients that they will have to lie still during the examination and that the x-ray table will be cold and hard (Table 45.5).

Computed Tomography

Tomograms are radiographs that focus on a particular slice of bone or soft tissue, such as ligaments and tendons. Com-

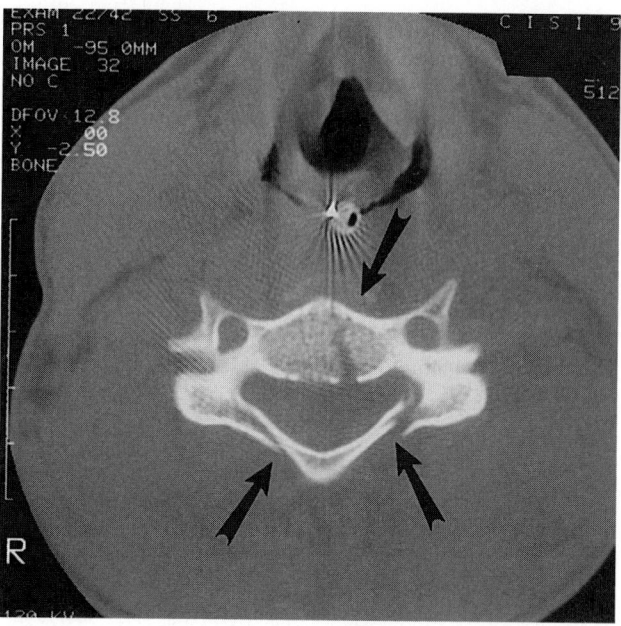

FIGURE 45.6 Computed tomography scan of fifth cervical vertebra showing a burst fracture of the vertebral body *(top arrow)* and both laminae *(bottom arrows)*. *(From McKinnis, LN: Fundamentals of Musculoskeletal Imaging, ed. 2. F.A. Davis, Philadelphia, 2005, p 164, with permission.)*

puted tomography (CT) is especially helpful for diagnosing problems of the joints or vertebral column (Fig. 45.6). It may be used with or without a contrast medium (similar to a dye), which is given orally or intravenously.

Inform patients that they must lie completely still during the test and that they will be surrounded by the scanner during the test. Headphones are worn for communication with the technician and to listen to soothing music of the patient's choice. Reports of claustrophobia and annoying clicking sounds made by the scanner while it is rotating are common. (See Table 45.5.)

Arthrography

An x-ray examination of any synovial joint can be performed for patients with suspected joint trauma. The most common joints tested are the knee and shoulder (see Table 45.5).

Myelogram

During a myelogram, a contrast medium is injected into the subarachnoid space so that the spine and spinal cord can be visualized. Inform patients that they may be positioned head down for a short period to allow the contrast medium to flow up to the level of the neck. This test is not performed as frequently as it used to be. It is usually reserved for those patients unable to have a CT or MRI or for complicated spinal surgery revisions (see Table 45.5).

Other Diagnostic Tests

Magnetic Resonance Imaging

Magnetic resonance imaging (MRI), with or without contrast media, is a commonly performed test to diagnose mus-

TABLE 45.5 DIAGNOSTIC PROCEDURES FOR MUSCULOSKELETAL SYSTEM

Procedure	Definition/Normal Finding (if applicable)	Significance of Abnormal Findings	Nursing Management (if applicable)
		Noninvasive	
Standard X-Rays	Visualization of skeletal abnormality or deformity. Can also be used to visualize dense or inflamed tissues and joints.	Aids in treatment plan and provides additional information for care. Example: broken ribs will necessitate increased attention to respiratory system.	Inform patient of what to expect during ordered procedures.
Computed Tomography	Radiographic "slices" of bone or soft tissue. Provides a better image.		Check for allergies to contrast medium (or if allergic to contrast media or iodine). NPO for 4 hours before test.
Magnetic Resonance Imaging (MRI)	Electromagnets provide a three-dimensional visualization of the area. Produces the best image available.		
Ultrasonography	Visualization of bone or soft tissue using sound waves.		Inform the patient that the jellylike conducting substance will feel cold when applied.
Nerve Conduction Studies	Electromyography (EMG)—the electrical testing of nerves and muscles.	Alterations usually indicate a problem with the nerves or the muscles.	Inform the patient that there may be some discomfort during the nerve and muscle stimulation as well as when the needles are inserted (if needed).
		Invasive	
Arthrography	Injection of air or a contrast medium into a synovial joint which is then x-rayed.	Aids in the diagnosis of joint abnormalities.	Inform patient that the test is uncomfortable during injection. Joint swelling is common after the procedure. Apply ice and elevate limb. Avoid physical activity for 12–24 hours.
Myelogram	Visualization of the spine and spinal cord after injection of a contrast medium.		Assess for headache and nausea post test. Maximum head raise is 45 degrees for at least 3 hours post procedure (or as ordered by physician).
Nuclear Medicine Scans	Injection of a radioisotope to help visualize bone and other soft tissue abnormalities.	Finding a "hot spot" usually indicates metastases or bone infection.	Inform the patient that the test is not dangerous. Inform patient that the test may take up to 90 minutes.
Gallium/Thallium Scans	Injection of radioactive element which migrates to bone, brain, breast, and inflammatory tissue.		Check if the facility you work in recommends that children and pregnant women stay a few feet away from the patient for the first 48 hours.
Arthroscopy	Direct visualization of the joint and its capsule using an instrument inserted into the joint space.		Assess CWCM frequently. Monitor for complications. Apply ice and keep limb elevated to minimize swelling (if ordered by physician).
Arthrocentesis	Withdrawal of synovial fluid from a joint space. Used for analysis of the synovial fluid or for reduction of excess fluid pressure.		Monitor for infection, inflammation or hemarthrosis.
Bone or Muscle Biopsy	Needle aspiration (closed) or surgical extraction (open) of bone or muscle tissue.		Monitor site of biopsy for bleeding. Provide normal wound care for open biopsy. Perform neurovascular assessments prn.

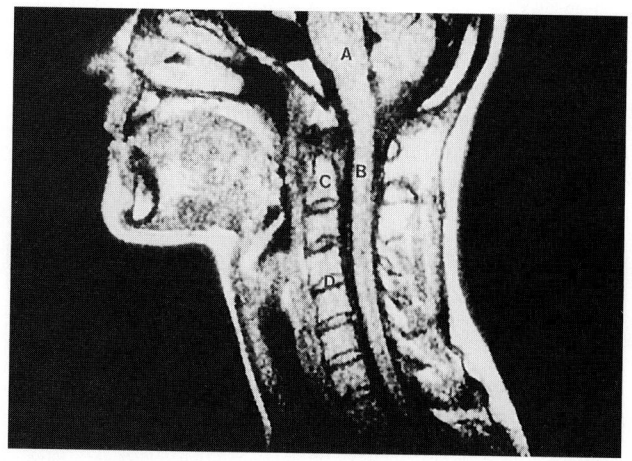

FIGURE 45.7 Magnetic resonance image of a normal cervical spine. *(A)* Cerebellum. *(B)* Spinal cord. *(C)* Marrow of C2 vertebral body. *(D)* C4-5 intervertebral disk. *(From McKinnis, LN: Fundamentals of Orthopedic Radiology. F.A. Davis, Philadelphia, 1997, p 26, with permission.)*

culoskeletal problems, especially those involving soft tissue (see Table 45.5) (Fig. 45.7). MRI is more accurate than CT for diagnosing many problems of the vertebral column. If the patient has had previous spinal surgery, a contrast medium is used.

The image is produced by interaction of magnetic fields and radio waves. For very large patients or those who are claustrophobic, the open MRI offers a comfortable alternative to the traditional machine (Box 45.2 Patient Perspective).

The use of an electromagnet in the machine necessitates the removal of anything metal or with metal components from the patient's body. Pacemakers, surgical clips, and any other internally implanted metal device or apparatus are contraindications for MRI.

 SAFETY TIP

Check with the facility where the MRI will take place for all contraindications for metal implants within a person's body to prevent injury to the patient.

Nuclear Medicine Scans

Several tests are performed using radioactive material to help visualize bone and other tissues. A bone scan allows visualization of the entire skeleton. The patient is injected with a radioisotope 2 to 3 hours before the scan. The radioisotope is attracted to bone and therefore travels to bone tissue.

For an accurate test, the patient must be able to lie still for up to 90 minutes during scanning. Patients who are elderly, restless, agitated, or in pain may therefore find this test uncomfortable. Sedatives or analgesics may have to be administered before or during the procedure. The physician looks for "hot spots," which indicate areas where the radioactive substance is concentrated. These hot spots indicate abnormal bone metabolism, a sign of bone disease (see Table 45.5).

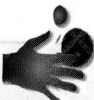 **Box 45.2**

Patient Perspective

Emily: Undergoing an MRI

I was told that the MRI scanner was small and could cause feelings of claustrophobia. When asked if I was claustrophobic, I said no and so was not offered an antianxiety medication before the procedure. I really am not claustrophobic, but I decided to keep my eyes closed during the test to be sure to prevent these feelings. As the table I was lying on moved into the scanner, my heart began beating fast. I shut my eyes and imagined myself walking on the beach, which is a favorite place for me. The cool air that was blowing in the machine I imagined to be the wind blowing. That air really is essential in keeping you cool and the claustrophobic feeling away. I had on headphones through which the music I had brought with me was playing. I focused on the music and sang along to myself as I "walked on the beach." I felt calmer as I did this. Through the headphones the technician kept me informed of how much longer the test would be and when the loud pounding noise would start. This really helped and I did not mind the noise. I knew that I had to be very still for the test, so I gave myself pep talks. "Okay, only 10 more minutes. Just lie still and this will be over soon."

Then, halfway through the MRI, I accidentally opened my eyes for an instant. "Uh, oh." I quickly shut them again with my heart racing and a feeling of panic rising. The wall of the MRI machine was only inches from my face. I quickly focused on the music again, told myself I could get through this, and focused on calming myself down by "going back to the beach." Before I knew it, the test was over and I was told that because I held so still it was a great test that went more quickly than usual. I sure was glad to hear that! My personal coping techniques really helped me through the MRI. Without them I would have panicked and been unable to complete the test. The information the nurse gave me helped me know what to expect during the procedure so I could prepare myself to cope with the test. Providing information to your patients on what to expect during the test, as well as coping methods to use, can help them successfully complete an MRI.

LEARNING TIP

Hot spots are created because increased circulation occurs in abnormal bone areas, resulting in increased amounts of the radioactive substance being transported to the abnormal area.

Gallium/Thallium Scans

A gallium or thallium scan is similar to a bone scan but is more specific and sensitive as a diagnostic test. Gallium not only migrates to bone but also to brain and breast tissues and is therefore used to diagnose problems in these tissues as well.

Traditionally used for heart problems, thallium is now used for evaluation of bone cancers. Thallium is best for detecting osteosarcoma. Like the bone scan, these scans are not harmful to the patient.

Arthroscopy

An arthroscope allows the surgeon to directly visualize a joint (see Table 45.5). The knee and shoulder are the joints most often evaluated. Because **arthroscopy** is an invasive procedure performed under local or light general anesthesia, the patient is treated as a surgical candidate.

Arthroscopy is done in same-day surgery settings. The surgeon makes several small incisions and distends the joint with injected saline. The scope is inserted and the joint is visualized from different angles. The joint is moved through range of motion, so tears, defects, or other soft tissue damage can be assessed and or repaired through the scope using special instrumentation. Depending on the extent of the procedure, a bulky or small dressing wrapped with an elastic bandage may be applied.

The nurse in the postanesthesia care unit (PACU) assesses the neurovascular status of the surgical limb frequently (see Table 45.3). If the patient had a diagnostic arthroscopy and no surgical repair, the PACU nurse encourages the patient to exercise the leg, including straight-leg raises. A mild analgesic usually relieves pain, and the patient returns to regular activities in 24 to 48 hours. If a surgical repair was performed, the patient may have activity restriction and need a stronger analgesic, such as oxycodone with acetaminophen (Tylox, Percocet).

Although complications are not common, monitor and teach the patient to watch for and report to the physician the following:

- Thrombophlebitis (blood clot and vein inflammation)
- Infection (fever or warmth, pain, redness, swelling at surgical site)
- Increased joint pain

---

arthroscopy: arthro—joint + scopy—to examine

If a repair was done during the surgery, the patient is seen by the physician in 1 week to check for complications and progress. The patient may need crutches for the first week to limit weight bearing, depending on the surgical procedure performed. Physical or occupational therapy may be ordered (see Home Health Hints).

CRITICAL THINKING

Mrs. Jones

■ Mrs. Jones was walking down the street when, without warning, she suddenly fell to the ground with extreme pain in her left leg. She was taken to the hospital, where it was determined that the greater trochanter of her left femur was fractured.

1. What information should you obtain from Mrs. Jones?
2. What possible condition may be the cause of her fracture?
3. What tests may be performed to identify the condition creating her problem?

Suggested answers at end of chapter.

Bone or Muscle Biopsy

Bone or muscle tissue can be surgically extracted for microscopic examination to confirm cancer, infection (bone biopsy), inflammation, or damage (muscle biopsy). Muscle can also be biopsied to diagnose malignant hyperthermia, a genetic disorder (see Chapter 11). Two techniques are used to retrieve muscle tissue: a needle (closed) biopsy or an incisional (open) biopsy.

A closed biopsy can be performed in the patient's room or special procedures area. After local or general anesthesia, the physician inserts a long needle into the tissue for extraction of a sample.

The open biopsy is performed in the operating suite under general anesthesia. A small incision is made and a section of bone or muscle is removed. A sterile pressure dressing is applied because bone is highly vascular.

The nurse inspects the biopsy site for bleeding, swelling, and hematoma formation. Increased pain that is unresponsive to analgesic medication may indicate bleeding in the soft tissue. The area is not moved for 8 to 12 hours to prevent bleeding. Vital signs and neurovascular assessments are monitored (see Table 45.3).

Ultrasonography

Sound waves are used to detect osteomyelitis (bone infection), soft tissue disorders, traumatic joint injuries, and surgical hardware placement. The technologist applies a jellylike conducting substance over the area to be tested. A transducer is moved over the area while the ultrasound machine records the images (see Table 45.5).

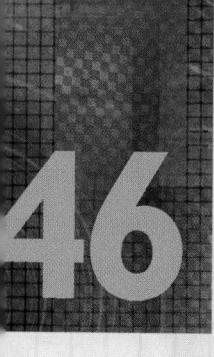

46

Nursing Care of Patients with Musculoskeletal and Connective Tissue Disorders

RODNEY B. KEBICZ

KEY TERMS

arthritis (ar-THRYE-tis)
arthroplasty (AR-throw-PLAS-te)
avascular necrosis (a-VAS-kue-lar ne-KROW-sis)
fasciotomy (fash-e-OTT-oh-me)
hemipelvectomy (hem-e-pell-VEC-toe-me)
hyperuricemia (HIGH-per-yoor-a-SEE-me-ah)
osteogenesis imperfecta (AHS-TEE-oh-gen-i-sis
   im-per-FEC-ta)
osteomyelitis (AHS-tee-oh-my-LIGHT-tis)
osteosarcoma (AHS-tee-oh-sar-KOH-mah)
polymyositis (PAH-lee-my-oh-SIGH-tis)
replantation (re-plan-TAY-shun)
scleroderma (SKLER-ah-DER-ma)
synovitis (sin-oh-VIE–tis)
vasculitis (VAS-kue-LIGH-tis)

QUESTIONS TO GUIDE YOUR READING

1. What are the signs and symptoms and complications of fractures?

2. Which nursing interventions are appropriate when caring for a patient in a cast or traction?

3. What are causes, prevention, and nursing care for osteomyelitis?

4. What are the risk factors for the development of osteoporosis?

5. What signs and symptoms may be seen in patients with Paget's disease?

6. What is the pathophysiology, treatment, and nursing care for gout?

7. Which nursing interventions are appropriate when caring for patients with systemic lupus erythematosus, scleroderma, and polymyositis?

8. How would you differentiate between the care for osteoarthritis and rheumatoid arthritis?

9. What would you include when preparing a plan of care for the patient with a fractured hip or undergoing a total joint replacement?

10. What patient education would be included for a patient with a lower extremity amputation and prosthesis?

BONE AND SOFT TISSUE DISORDERS

The musculoskeletal system is the second largest system in the body. A variety of injuries and diseases can affect bone, soft tissue, or both. Common problems are discussed in this section.

Strains

A strain is a soft tissue injury that occurs when a muscle or tendon is excessively stretched. Causes of strains include falls, excessive exercise, and lifting heavy items without using proper body mechanics. Back and ankle injuries are common. Strains can be mild, moderate, or severe. A mild strain causes minimal inflammation; swelling and tenderness are present. A moderate strain involves partial tearing of the muscle or tendon fibers. Pain and inability to move the affected body part result. The most severe strain occurs when a muscle or tendon is ruptured, with separation of muscle from muscle, tendon from muscle, or tendon from bone. Severe pain and disability result from this injury.

RICE is an acronym for rest, ice, compression, and elevation. These four components are the basis of therapy for strain injuries. Immediately after a strain, ice should be applied to decrease pain, swelling, and inflammation. Applying an elastic bandage (compression) and elevating the affected area (if appropriate) provide support and minimize swelling. Once inflammation subsides, heat application (15 to 30 minutes four times a day) brings increased blood flow to the injured area for healing. Activity is limited (depending on the severity of the injury, casting may even be required for immobilization) until the soft tissue heals, and anti-inflammatory drugs are prescribed. Muscle relaxants may also be used. Exercise may begin as early as 2 to 5 days after the injury (depending on the severity of the injury), but it may take 1 to 3 weeks of immobility before exercise can begin. For more severe strains, surgery to repair the tear or rupture may be needed. These procedures are done on an ambulatory, same-day-surgery basis.

Sprains

A sprain is excessive stretching of one or more ligaments that usually results from twisting movements during a sports activity, exercise, or fall. Like strains, sprains also vary in severity. A mild sprain involves tearing of just a few ligament fibers and causes tenderness. In a moderate sprain, more fibers are torn but the stability of the joint is not affected. A moderate sprain is uncomfortable, especially with activity. A severe sprain causes instability of the joint and usually requires surgical intervention for tissue repair or grafting. Pain and inflammation prevent mobility.

For mild sprains, RICE is used for several days until swelling and pain diminish. Anti-inflammatory drugs are also used to decrease inflammation and control pain. Moderate sprains may need immobilization with a brace or cast until healing occurs.

Dislocations

Dislocations are a common injury in which the ends of the bones are forced from their normal position. They are usually caused by trauma as in falls or contact sports or a disease such as rheumatoid arthritis. Any joint large or small may become dislocated. Severe pain along with lost range of motion of the joint and joint deformity occurs. Immediate medical treatment is required to preserve function. Splint the extremity as it is found, apply ice, and seek help. Do not move the extremity as blood vessels, mucles, and nerves could be damaged.

NURSING CARE TIP

It is important for those with disease processes that could result in dislocation or fractures to use lift sheets when moving the patient rather than pulling on their arms. Always follow institutional policy for moving patients or you could be found liable for a patient's injury.

Bursitis

Bursae (fluid-filled sacs) cushion tendons during movement to prevent friction between the bone and tendon. Several joints have bursae (shoulder, elbow, hip, knee, ankle, heel). Inflammation of a bursa occurs from repetitive movement, sleeping on the side and compressing the bursa, arthritis, or gout. Prevention is key as it may become harder to cure over time. Muscle stretching and strengthening, move often, avoid repetitive movements for long periods, use cushion seats, and do not lean on your elbows to protect the bursae and prevent compression.

Symptoms of bursitis include achy pain, stiffness, or burning pain over the joint area which worsens with activity. Usually pain decreases in about a week. The condition can become chronic if it lasts more than 6 months. Treatment includes resting the joint, application of ice 20 minutes several times per day until joint warmth is gone, then switching to heat, elevating the joint, ultrasound, massage, foam mattress toppers, nonsteroidal anti-inflammatory drugs (NSAIDs), or physical therapy.

Rotator Cuff Injury

Short tendons that are connected to muscles around the shoulder form the rotator cuff. The cuff covers the top, front, and back of the shoulder. Muscle contraction causes these tendons to tighten and move or rotate the shoulder. Various injuries can occur. The top tendon of the cuff (supraspinatus tendon) and bursa may become impinged in the narrow space under the acromion bone. This causes inflammation when the arm is repeatedly moved forward and pain results. This is known as chronic impingement syndrome. Over time the tendon may finally tear from the bone.

Symptoms of rotator cuff injury include shoulder aching, increased pain with lifting the arm, pain that is greater at night, weakness, and sometimes limited range of motion. A magnetic resonance image (MRI) can help diagnosis rotator cuff injury. For minor injury, resting the shoulder, NSAIDs, ice, and physical therapy are recommended. For a more severe injury, arthroscopic and or small incision surgery may be needed to relieve the impingement or repair the tear. A sling or special brace is worn after surgery. Physical therapy for rehabilitation after surgery is used.

Carpal Tunnel Syndrome

Pathophysiology

Carpal tunnel syndrome results in the compression of the median nerve within the carpal tunnel when swelling in the tunnel occurs. This swelling can result from edema, trauma, rheumatoid arthritis, or repetitive hand movements (repetitive motion injury) as used in some occupations such as typing or cash register operation.

Signs and Symptoms

Carpal tunnel syndrome usually results in slow-onset finger, hand, and arm pain and numbness. Painful tingling and paresthesias may also be present. Eventually, fine motor deficits and then muscle weakness may develop.

Diagnosis

Diagnosis is based on signs and symptoms, along with the patient's history. A positive Phalen's test (numbness with wrist flexion) is indicative of carpal tunnel syndrome. Electromyography (EMG) can also be used to detect nerve abnormalities.

Therapeutic Interventions

Medical treatment focuses on relieving the inflammation and resting the wrist. A splint is often ordered for the patient to wear. Medications to reduce pain and inflammation are ordered, such as aspirin and NSAIDs. Cortisone may be injected into the carpal tunnel to decrease pain and inflammation.

For some patients, surgery may be necessary. The surgeon may use an open incision or may perform an endoscopy. The median nerve is released from compression during the surgery, thus correcting the problem of the nerve and the surrounding area becoming inflamed. Physiotherapy helps in the recovery of function.

Nursing Management

Educate the patient on methods to prevent carpal tunnel syndrome, such as frequent short breaks during the work day, interspersing ongoing tasks with repetitive movements throughout the day, and using ergonomically appropriate devices to minimize the pressure placed in the area of the wrist.

Provide pain relief as ordered, and if surgery is performed, provide routine preoperative and postoperative care. Postoperatively elevate the patient's hand and use a splint as ordered for up to 2 weeks. Lifting is restricted for several weeks. The patient is taught to report signs and symptoms of neurovascular compromise, such as numbness and tingling, coolness, lack of pulse, pale skin or nailbeds, or limited movement. The patient may need family assistance with activities of daily living (ADLs).

Fractures

A fracture is a break in a bone and can occur at any age and in any bone. Some fractures are minor and are treated on an ambulatory basis; others are more complex and require surgical intervention with hospitalization and rehabilitation.

Pathophysiology

Bone is a dynamic, changing tissue. When it is broken, the body immediately begins to repair the injury (Fig. 46.1). For an adult, within 48 to 72 hours after the injury a hematoma (blood clot) forms at the fracture site because bone has a rich blood supply. Various cells that begin the healing process are attracted to the damaged bone. In about a week or so, a nonbony union called a callus develops and can be seen on x-ray examination. As healing continues, osteoclasts (bone-destroying cells) resorb any necrotic bone and osteoblasts (bone-building cells) make new bone as a replacement. This process is sometimes referred to as bone remodeling. Young, healthy adult bone completely heals in about 6 weeks; however, it can take up to a year before the whole process of remodeling is complete. An older person takes longer to heal, and children tend to heal more quickly.

Causes and Types

The major reason for a fracture is trauma from either a fall or accident (usually motor vehicle) or some type of crushing injury. Bone disease, such as osteoporosis and metastatic bone cancer, malnutrition, and regular drinking of soda pop (phosphoric acid added to pop may interfere with calcium absorption), can lead to fractures as can various drugs (e.g., certain drugs used to treat human immunodeficiency [HIV] and certain drugs used to treat endometriosis) that as a side effect cause a decrease in bone density. Fractures resulting from any of these diseases are referred to as pathological fractures. One of the most common types of fracture is the hip fracture, which occurs most frequently in middle-aged and older adult women who have osteoporosis (irreversible bone loss).

Fractures can be classified in several ways: by the extent of the fracture, the extent of the associated soft tissue damage, or the configuration of the bone after it breaks. A fracture that is complete, breaking the bone into two separate pieces, is called a displaced fracture. An incomplete fracture does not divide the bone into two pieces; it may also be referred to as a nondisplaced fracture. Complete fractures have the potential to be life threatening because sharp bone fragments can sever blood vessels and nerves.

A fracture may also be classified as open or closed. In an open (or compound) fracture, the bone breaks the skin. A closed fracture does not disrupt the skin. Open fractures are more likely to become infected than closed fractures.

Another way to describe a fracture is by the way that the bone breaks, such as in a spiral or oblique fashion (Fig. 46.2). These fractures may be open or closed, complete or incomplete. Table 46.1 describes the types of fractures.

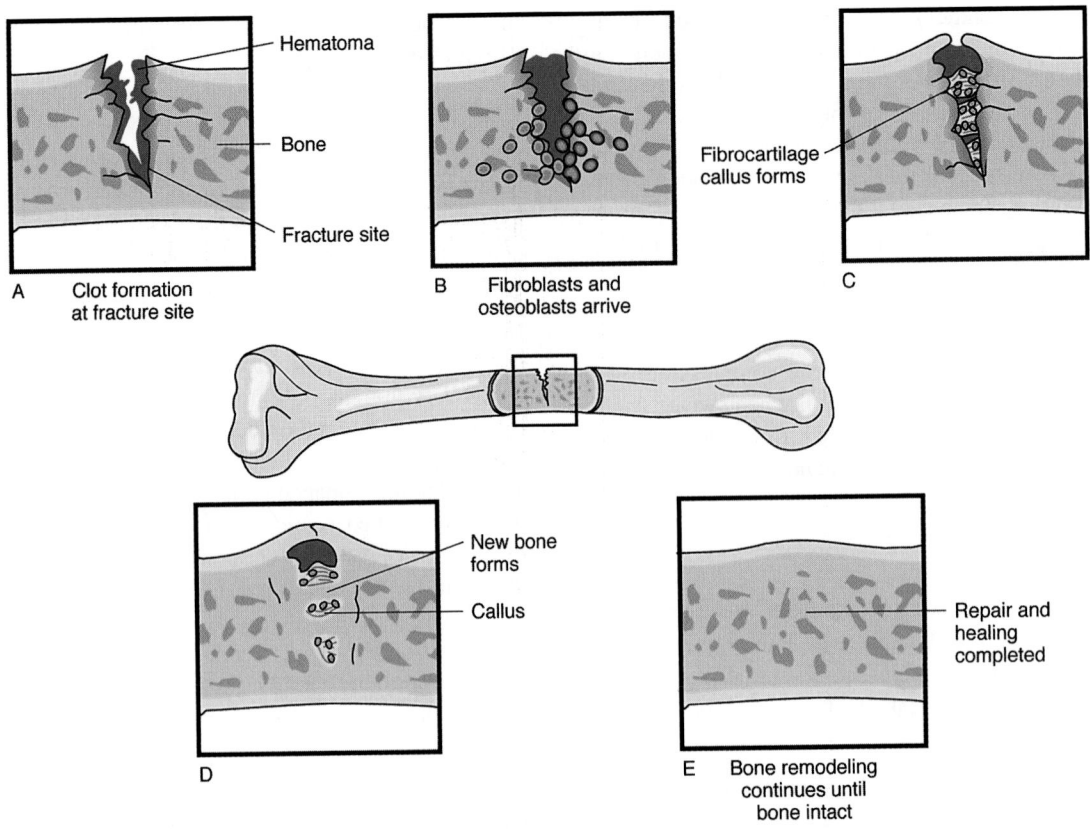

FIGURE 46.1 Fracture healing phases.

Signs and Symptoms

This section focuses on fractures of upper and lower extremities. If the patient sustains a hairline (microscopic) fracture, the signs and symptoms are not readily observable. The patient may complain of tenderness over the site of the injury or more severe pain when moving the affected part of the body. The patient with a hip fracture usually complains of pain either in the groin area (the hip is a deep joint) or at the back of the knee (referred pain). If the fracture is displaced, the limb is often shortened because of contraction of the muscles pulling on the bone sections.

In addition to pain, patients with more complex fractures experience limb rotation or deformity and shortening of the limb (if a limb bone is broken). Range of motion is decreased. If the affected part is moved, a continuous grating sound (crepitation) caused by bone fragments rubbing on each other may be heard. The extremity should not be moved (to try and reposition the bone alignment) if crepitation is present.

Inspect the skin for intactness. A patient with a closed fracture may have ecchymosis (bruising) over the fractured bone from bleeding into the soft underlying tissue. Ecchy-

TABLE 46.1 TYPES OF FRACTURES

Fracture Type	Description
Avulsion	Piece of bone is torn away from the main bone while still attached to a ligament or tendon.
Comminuted	Bone splintered or shattered into numerous fragments. Often occurs in crushing injuries.
Impacted	Bone is forcibly pushed together, resulting in bone being pushed into bone.
Greenstick	Bone is bent and fractures on the outer arc of the bend. Often seen in children.
Interarticular	Fracture involves bones within a joint.
Displaced	Bone pieces are out of normal alignment. One or both pieces may be out of alignment.
Pathological (also called neoplastic)	Caused by bone's being weakened either by pressure from a tumor or an actual tumor within the bone.
Spiral	Fracture curves around the shaft of the bone.
Longitudinal	Fracture occurs along the length of the bone.
Oblique	Fracture occurs diagonally or at an oblique angle across the bone.
Stress	Results in the bone being fractured across one cortex. This is an incomplete fracture.
Transverse	Bone fractured horizontally.
Depressed	Bone pushed inward. Often seen with skull and facial fractures.

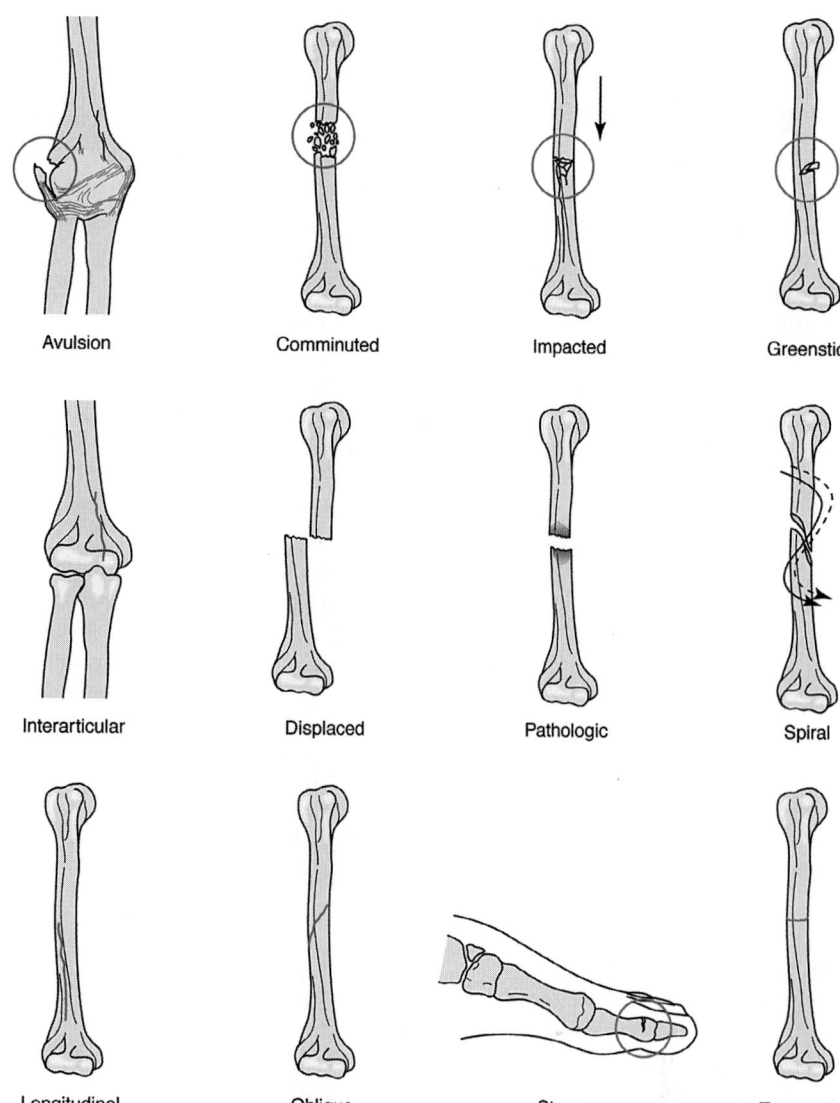

FIGURE 46.2 Types of fractures.

Avulsion, Comminuted, Impacted, Greenstick, Interarticular, Displaced, Pathologic, Spiral, Longitudinal, Oblique, Stress, Transverse

mosis may not develop for several days after the injury. Swelling may also be present and can impair blood flow, causing marked neurovascular compromise. In an open fracture, one or more bone ends pierce the skin, causing a wound, thus increasing the possibility of infection.

Diagnostic Tests

An x-ray examination usually visualizes bone fractures, showing bone malalignment or disruption. Computed tomography may be needed to help detect fractures of complex areas, such as the hip and pelvis. Magnetic resonance imaging is useful in determining the extent of associated soft tissue damage.

For patients experiencing moderate to severe bleeding, a hemoglobin and hematocrit level is obtained. If extensive soft tissue damage is present, the erythrocyte sedimentation rate (ESR) is usually elevated, indicating the expected inflammatory response. The physician may order a serum calcium level to determine baseline values because bone repair requires a sufficient amount of calcium and other minerals.

Emergency Treatment

A patient with a suspected fracture often has injuries elsewhere in the body. Assess the patient for respiratory distress, bleeding, and head or spine injury. If any of these problems occurs, emergency treatment is provided before concern is given to extremity or other fractures.

The treatment of fractures depends on the type and extent of the injury. Emergency treatment is essential to prevent possible life-threatening complications. Box 46.1 Urgent Management of Fractures describes the emergency interventions for the patient with an extremity fracture.

LEARNING TIP

For emergency care of a suspected fracture, do not try to reposition the limb. Remember: Splint it as it lies. Also, ensure that the limb is secured above and below the break to minimize movement and bone grating.

Box 46.1

Urgent Management of Fractures

1. Immediately immobilize affected limb. If movement is required before splinting, support limb above and below fracture.
2. Unless there is bleeding apply splints and padding (above and below fracture site) directly over the clothing. If bleeding is present visualization may be necessary before pressure can be applied where bleeding is originating. Keep patient covered to preserve body heat.
3. If the fractured extremity is a leg bone, the unaffected extremity can be used as a splint by bandaging both legs together. An arm can be bandaged to the chest or put into a sling to minimize further tissue damage.
4. Assess color, warmth, circulation, and movement (CWCM) of the limb distal to the fracture.
5. Open fractures require the protruding bone be covered with a clean (sterile preferred) dressing.
6. Do not attempt to "straighten" or realign the fractured extremity. Move the affected limb as little as necessary.
7. Transport to an emergency department as soon as possible.

Fracture Management

The goals of fracture management are reduction, or realignment, of bone ends; immobilization of the fractured bone (with bandages, casts, traction, or a fixation device); prevention of deformity or further injury; preservation or restoration of function; promotion of early healing; and pain relief.

CLOSED REDUCTION. Closed reduction is the most common treatment for simple fractures. While manually pulling on the bone (limb), the physician manipulates the bone ends into realignment. Analgesia and/or conscious sedation is typically used before the procedure. An x-ray examination is done to confirm that the bone ends are aligned before the area is immobilized.

BANDAGES AND SPLINTS. For some areas of the body, such as the clavicle or wrist, an elastic or muslin bandage or a splint may be used to immobilize the bone during the healing phase. Splints can be used when the fracture has some associated soft tissue damage that needs care or if there is an expectation of swelling. It is important that the splint be well padded, thereby preventing skin breakdown or unnecessary pressure. Perform neurovascular assessments to ensure adequate blood flow to the area (see Chapter 45).

CASTS. Casts provide a strong support for fractured bones, thereby aiding in early mobility and decreased pain. They are also used to correct deformities and to support weak joints while restricting movement. The type of cast used depends on the reason the cast is applied. For more extensive fractures or for weight-bearing areas, a more rigid and durable cast is used for immobilization. Once the need for the cast is resolved (e.g., when bone healing is complete), the cast is removed.

Several types of materials are used for casts, including the traditional plaster of Paris (anhydrous calcium sulfate) and a variety of synthetic products such as fiberglass. Plaster is used for large casts and for weight-bearing areas. Because of a chemical reaction that occurs when the plaster is wet, the cast feels hot when applied for about 30 minutes and then feels cool, taking anywhere from 24 to 72 hours to completely dry. The cast is dry when it feels hard and firm, is odorless, and is shiny white. Keep the wet cast open to air and turn the patient about every 2 hours to expose all sides of the cast to the air to aid in drying and prevent mold growth. A wet cast should be handled with the palms of the hand ("palming the cast") to prevent indentations or a change in the shape of the cast (Fig. 46.3). This prevents the possibility of pressure points forming inside the cast. Unlike plaster of Paris, synthetic material casts such as fiberglass harden quickly and dry in less than 2 hours.

A casted limb is elevated for 24 to 48 hours, and ice can be applied over the injury to reduce swelling. Assess the cast for dryness, tightness, drainage, and odor. A serious complication of a cast being too tight is compartment syndrome (discussed later). If the cast becomes too tight, the physician orders it to be cut (bivalved) with a cast cutter to relieve pressure and prevent pressure necrosis of the underlying skin (Fig. 46.4). If a wound is present or an odor is detected, a window opening into the cast is created to treat the underlying skin problem, often an infected area. The cast window should always be taped in place when wound care is not being provided to prevent the skin from "popping up" through the window and developing pressure points and ischemia. See Box 46.2 Nursing Interventions for a Patient with a Cast.

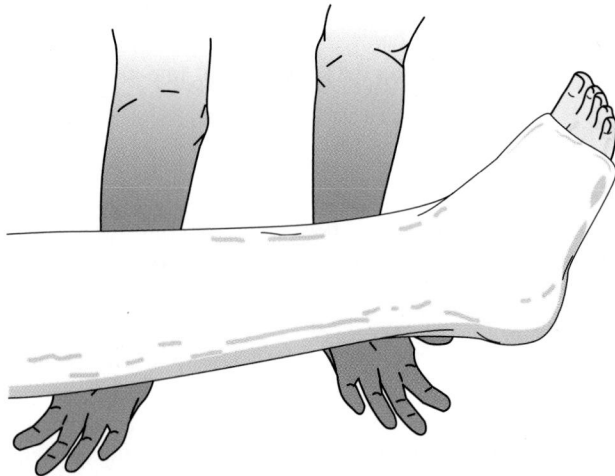

FIGURE 46.3 A wet plaster cast is moved with the palms of the hand to prevent making indentations in the plaster that could become pressure points.

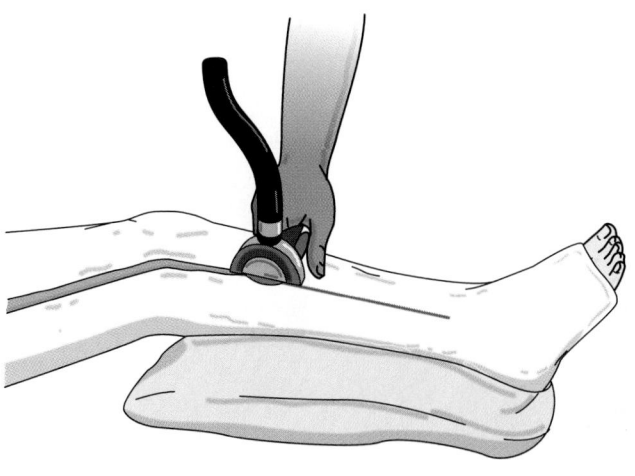

FIGURE 46.4 Bivalving a cast with a cast saw.

TRACTION. Casts can be worn in or out of a hospital setting, but traction for fracture treatment often requires that the patient be hospitalized. As a general definition, traction is the application of a pulling force to a part of the body to provide fracture reduction (positioning bone fragments in correct alignment), reduce movement, or pain relief. Although still used in certain situations, improvements in surgical techniques and orthopedic devices have greatly decreased the use of traction.

Traction is classified as either continuous or intermittent. Continuous traction is required for fracture management; intermittent traction, although not commonly used, may be applied for patients experiencing muscle spasm. Traction can also be performed manually for short periods of time (e.g., to maintain traction on a leg when removing Buck's traction for skin assessment or skin care). The most common types of traction are either skin or skeletal. Skin traction typically involves the use of a Velcro boot (Buck's traction), sling (Russell's traction or knee sling), belt (pelvic), or halter, which is secured around a part of the body (Fig. 46.5). This type of traction does not promote bone alignment or healing but is used instead for relief of painful muscle spasms that often accompany fractures. Buck's traction is indicated for patients with hip fractures and is frequently applied to prevent further trauma while the patient is waiting for surgery. Occasionally, the patient's physical condition or inflammation surrounding the fracture prohibits early surgical intervention, thus necessitating the application of skin (Buck's) traction. When traction is being applied to the skin, there is a restriction as to the amount of weight that can be applied. The weight applied is usually between 5 and 10 lb (2.2 to 4.5 kg). Skeletal traction, also called balanced suspension, involves the use of pins (Steinmann), screws, wires (Kirschner), or tongs (Gardner-Wells, Crutchfield), which are surgically inserted into the

---

Box 46.2

Nursing Interventions for a Patient with a Cast

1. Assess color, warmth, circulation, movement (CWCM) every 1 to 2 hours for 24 hours and then qid and prn.
   a. Assess cast for tightness (ask patient) and for rough or frayed edges of the cast (can interfere with skin integrity).
   b. Ensure patient can move (wiggle) all digits distal to the cast.
2. With newly applied casts (wet)
   a. Never grasp a wet cast to hold or move it (and do not place on any surface that can cause an indentation)—only use the palms of the hands (finger pressure on a wet cast can cause pressure points on the inside surface)
   b. Ensure patient is turned every 1 to 2 hours to prevent "flattening" of cast surface during drying.
   c. With hip spicas or any cast with an abductor bar, do not use bar to move limb or to help with turns.
   d. Inform patient that plaster casts give off heat when drying. Ensure cast air dries (may require 24 to 72 hours for complete drying). Do not cover cast or use drying aids such as blow dryers. Place cast on absorbent surfaces not plasticized pillows.
   e. Protect skin integrity by ensuring rough edges of cast are properly covered.
   f. Ensure patient knows to keep cast dry during bathing. (Cover with plastic and prevent water seeping into cast ends.)
   g. Synthetic casts (e.g., fiberglass) can be exposed to water (e.g., for hydrotherapy) as needed but require complete drying afterward.
3. Tissue integrity within the cast.
   a. When assessing CWCM assess visible skin for signs of impaired integrity.
   b. Cast edges can be smoothed and covered with stockinettes or gauze and tape (ensure there are no tape allergies) to prevent rubbing of cast.
   c. Monitor for signs and symptoms of infections such as foul odor, heat, redness, and pain.
   d. Skin products should not be used on affected limb.
   e. Visible blood on the surface of the cast has to be monitored. (Outline area with a pen to observe for increasing size of area.) Shadowing of blood not quite reaching the surface of the cast is fairly common but also has to be circled and monitored.
   f. Never place any object inside the cast. Teach patient potential for skin damage if this is done.

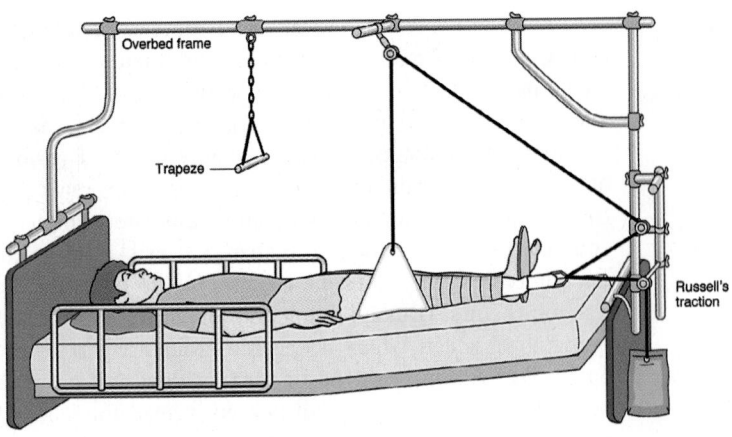

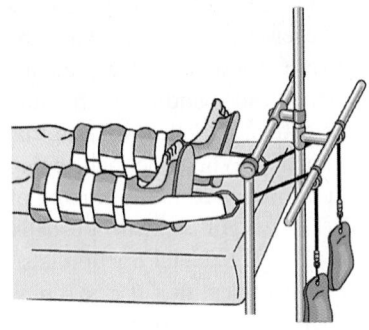

FIGURE 46.5 Types of skin traction. *(A)* Russell's traction. *(B)* Buck's (boot) traction.

bone for the purpose of alignment while the fracture heals (Fig. 46.6). From 20 to 40 lb (9 to 18 kg) of weight is usually applied for skeletal traction, as ordered.

Balanced suspension maintains the traction while allowing the patient some mobility in bed. A Thomas (or T) splint with Pearson's attachment can be used to provide balanced suspension for the lower extremity. The patient's leg rests on a suspended sheepskin-covered splint (see Fig 46.6). Balanced traction methods require countertraction to ensure the patient does not move toward the pull and therefore minimize the effectiveness of the traction. Usually the patients' weight as well as elevating the foot of the bed provides the countertraction necessary.

Caring for the patient in traction includes frequently monitoring neurovascular status for impaired blood flow,

> **LEARNING TIP**
>
> When applying manual traction, usually done by the physician, it is important to maintain a firm, smooth, continuous "pull" on the extremity and not a jerking or yanking motion. The limb is kept in anatomical position and correct alignment is maintained while providing manual traction.

checking the equipment to ensure proper functioning, and monitoring skin condition for pressure points or irritation from equipment. Traction must be maintained at all times for fractures. All knots, ropes, weights, and pulleys are inspected

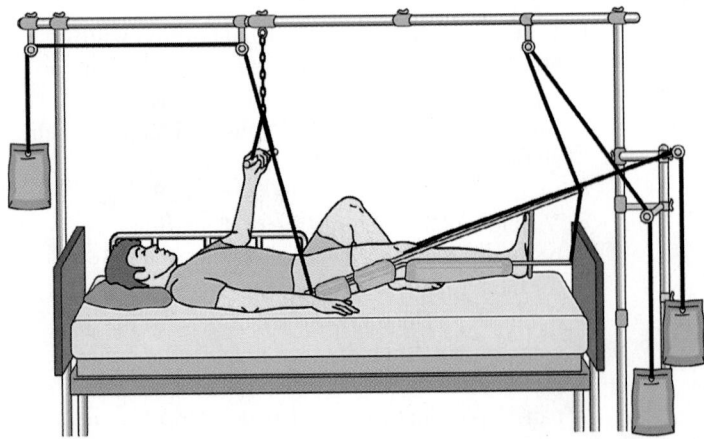

FIGURE 46.6 Balanced suspension and skeletal traction for femur fracture.

every 8 to 12 hours for any loosening and intactness. Weights are to hang unobstructed and should never touch the floor or be removed or lifted. The patient's feet should not rest against the end of the bed. It is important that the traction not be inhibited by any form of friction or impedance. Assistance should be obtained to reposition the patient in bed to prevent lifting injuries, especially with heavy weights in use.

For patients in skeletal traction, pin sites are observed for redness, drainage, odor, swelling, and excessive warmth. Clear, odorless drainage is expected. Some agencies or physicians advocate special solutions or ointments for the skin around the pins (pin care). Others recommend no cleaning to maintain skin integrity. Follow agency policy or physician's order for pin care. Depending on the type of pin used, the pin ends may be covered to protect the patient (and health-care workers) from being injured.

Patients who have traction may be immobilized for an extended period and often experience problems associated with immobility. For example, pressure ulcers on heels are common among older adult patients in traction. Unfortunately, loss of bone density is also a complication of immobility, which may create an additional impairment for normal healing. Another common concern is the person's psychosocial health. Ensure that the patient does not become socially isolated because of the need for extended bedrest.

OPEN REDUCTION WITH INTERNAL FIXATION. An open reduction with internal fixation (ORIF) is a treatment reserved for patients who cannot be managed by casts or traction. One of the most common indications for this surgical procedure is fractured hips. Fractures of the hip involve the proximal femur and affect the older adult more than any other age group. ORIF of the hip allows early mobilization while the bone is healing.

As the name implies, the bone ends are realigned (reduced) by direct visualization through a surgical incision (open reduction [OR]). The bone ends are held in place by internal fixation (IF) devices such as metal plates and screws or by a prosthesis with a femoral component similar to that for total joint replacement (Fig. 46.7). For hip surgery, the IF device is not removed after the fracture heals. For ankle or long bone surgery, the hardware may be removed after healing because of loosening or pain (Box 46.3 Nursing Care Plan for the Patient After Open Reduction with Internal Fixation [ORIF] of the Hip).

EXTERNAL FIXATION. An alternative treatment for some fractures is external fixation. External fixation is used when there has been severe bone damage, such as in crushed or splintered fractures, or if there have been numerous fractures along the bone. After the fracture is reduced, the physician surgically inserts pins into the bone; the pins are held in place by an external metal frame to prevent bone movement (Fig. 46.8). External fixation is ideal for the patient who has an open fracture with soft tissue damage that needs to be treated at the same time. Like skeletal traction, the patient with this device is at risk for complications of skeletal pins,

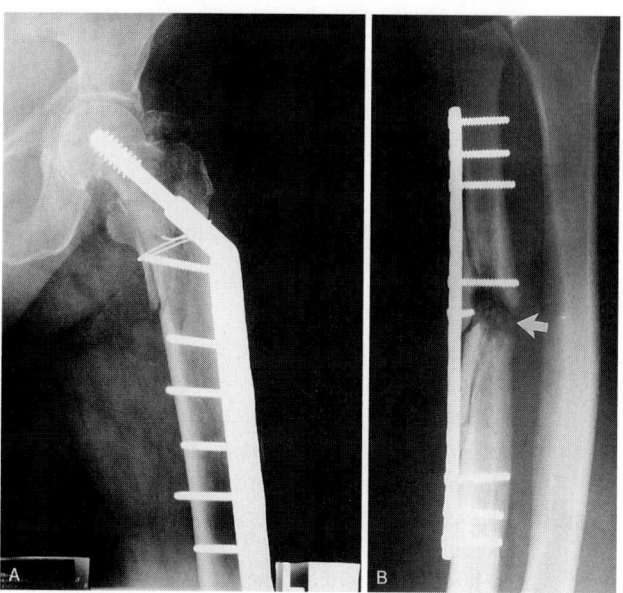

FIGURE 46.7 Internal fixation. *(A)* Intertrochanteric fracture of the hip with fracture fixation via a side plate and screw combination device. *(B)* Side plate and screw fixation of radial fracture. *(From McKinnis, LN: Fundamentals of Orthopedic Radiology. F.A. Davis, Philadelphia, 1997, with permission.)*

CRITICAL THINKING

Mrs. Brown

■ Mrs. Brown, a long-time resident of Happy Hills Care Center, was found lying in the dayroom on her left side, moaning and holding her left leg at 10 a.m. (1/4/07). She cried out with any movement and said she fell and broke her leg. The supervisor notified the paramedics and Dr. Jones. Her vital signs are blood pressure 150/84, pulse 100, respirations 20. Her left leg is noticeably shorter than her right leg. The licensed practical nurse (LPN) remained with Mrs. Brown and instructed her not to move until help arrived. The LPN got blankets and a pillow for her head. The paramedics arrived quickly and took Mrs. Brown to nearby Grace Hospital by ambulance, where she was diagnosed as having a nondisplaced femoral neck (hip) fracture. Dr. Jones ordered 5 lb of Buck's traction. Mrs. Brown is restless and picking at her bedcovers when you assess her at the beginning of your shift.

1. How should the LPN/LVN document the incident of Mrs. Brown's fall at the care center?
2. What is the purpose of Buck's traction for Mrs. Brown?
3. What are your nursing responsibilities while caring for Mrs. Brown?
4. What might explain Mrs. Brown's restlessness?

Suggested answers at end of chapter.

Box 46.3   NURSING CARE PLAN for the Patient After Open Reduction with Internal Fixation (ORIF) of the Hip

Pain related to surgical wound

Patient Outcome Patient states that pain relief is satisfactory.

Evaluation of Outcome Does patient state that pain is absent or at tolerable level (pain rated 0 to 2 on pain assessment scale)?

Intervention	Rationale	Evaluation
Give pain medication as needed; anticipate need for pain medication.	Pain medication relieves pain, especially if given before pain is severe.	Does patient state pain is relieved?
Give pain medication before activity (e.g., session with physical therapist).	Increased activity can cause pain.	Is patient restless or agitated during activity?
Use nondrug pain relief measures, such as distraction, guided imagery, other relaxation techniques.	Analgesic therapy is enhanced with complementary pain relief measures.	Does patient report pain relief is enhanced with music or relaxation?
Use fracture bedpan.	Fracture bedpans are more comfortable and easier to position for patients.	Is patient able to use fracture pan with comfort?

Impaired physical mobility related to hip precautions and surgical pain

Patient Outcome Patient will maintain desired level of activity.

Evaluation of Outcome Does patient maintain activity desired?

Intervention	Rationale	Evaluation
Reinforce transfer and ambulation techniques.	Activity is restricted due to hip precautions and weight-bearing limitations.	Does patient transfer and ambulate as instructed by physical therapist?
Place overhead frame and trapeze on bed; teach patient how to use it.	Patient mobility is increased and pain decreased with use of trapeze for movement.	Does patient use overhead frame and trapeze for movement in bed with less pain?
Monitor patient for and take measures to prevent complications of immobility: turn patient every 2 hours and check skin; keep heels off bed; teach patient to deep breathe and cough q2hr; teach use of incentive spirometer.	Immobility complications can occur if preventive measures are not used.	Does patient experience complications of immobility?
Apply thigh-high elastic stockings or sequential compression device to unaffected limb as ordered.	Helps prevent blood clots.	Is patient free from blood clots?
Give anticoagulants as ordered.		
Get patient out of bed as soon as ordered.		
Ambulate patient as early as possible.		
Remind patient to practice leg exercises.		

CRITICAL THINKING

Tommy Martin

■ Tommy, age 18, was in a motor vehicle accident that resulted in a fractured pelvis and femur. He is to be in skeletal traction for several weeks.

1. Identify three nursing diagnoses related to Tommy's physical or emotional well-being.
2. What are some nursing interventions for these diagnoses?

Suggested answers at end of chapter.

which includes pin reaction, compromised circulation, and infection. Pin sites are observed frequently for signs and symptoms of infection. Pin site care varies from facility to facility. The overriding principle is to ensure that strict aseptic technique is always maintained as the pin is a

NURSING CARE TIP

If you have to move an extremity that has an external fixation device, grasp the device and lift, raise, or move the limb as needed. By grasping the device, there is less movement of the healing bone and therefore less trauma to the site of healing and less pain with movement. Care must be taken not to loosen any fasteners holding the pins in place.

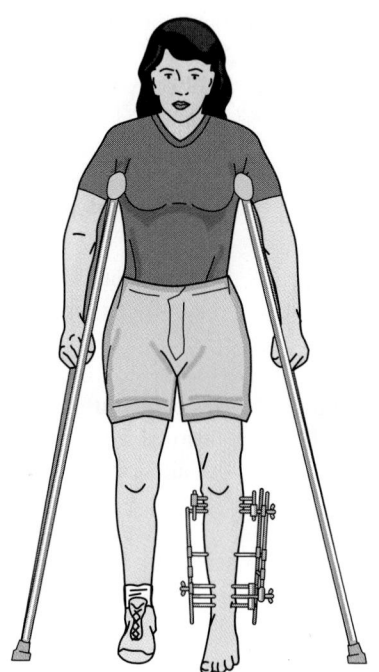

FIGURE 46.8 External fixation for complex fractures and wound care.

pathway for microorganisms to directly enter bone tissue and cause osteomyelitis. See Box 46.4 Nursing Care Plan for the Patient with External Fixation of the Lower Extremity.

NONUNION MODALITIES. Although most bones heal properly with the correct treatment, some patients experience malunion (malalignment of healed bone) or nonunion (delayed or no healing). A number of variables influence how a bone heals, including age, nutritional status, and the presence of other diseases that alter the healing process, such as diabetes mellitus.

Several methods for treating nonunion are available, including electrical bone stimulation and bone grafting. For selected patients, bone stimulation may be effective in promoting healing; the exact mechanism of action is not known. Bone grafting involves adding packed bone to the fracture site in an attempt to facilitate healing. Bone-stimulating compounds such as Osteoset, Pro Osteon, or Allomatrix are being used to promote bone growth in patients. These compounds are used during surgical procedures as glue, cement, or filler.

Another fracture healing method is low-intensity pulsed ultrasound (also called Exogen therapy). Ultrasound treatment has provided excellent results for slow-healing fractures, as well as for new fractures. The patient applies the treatment for about 20 minutes each day.

Complications of Fractures

Monitor for possible complications and implement interventions to prevent them. The most common complications include impaired neurovascular status, hemorrhage, infection, and thromboembolitic complications. Although they do not occur often, acute compartment syndrome and fat embolism syndrome (more common with fractures of long bones) can be life-threatening complications of fractures.

NEUROVASCULAR. Neurovascular checks are done to detect abnormalities. Decreased or absent pulses, cool skin temperature, and dusky color indicate circulation alterations. Numbness and tingling, decreased sensation, and mobility indicate neurological alterations. These findings should be reported to the physician promptly.

HEMORRHAGE. Bone is highly vascular, and damage to or surgery on bone (particularly the large long bones of the extremities) can cause bleeding. Assess for bleeding and monitor vital signs carefully. Hypovolemic shock may result from severe hemorrhage (see Chapter 8).

INFECTION. Trauma predisposes the body to infection, especially when the skin, the body's first line of defense, is disrupted. Wound infections, pin site infections, drainage tube infections, and osteomyelitis (bone infection) are common. Hospital-acquired infections, such as pneumonia or urinary tract infection, can occur in patients who are immobilized for extensive periods while their fractures heal.

THROMBOEMBOLITIC COMPLICATIONS. Deep vein thrombosis or pulmonary embolus (PE) (see Chapter 31)

Box 46.4   NURSING CARE PLAN for the Patient with External Fixation of the Lower Extremity

Risk for infection related to skin integrity impairment

Patient Outcomes Patient does not develop an infection.

Evaluation of Outcome Does patient remain free from infection?

Interventions	Rationale	Evaluation
Inspect dressings, wounds, pin sites for signs and symptoms of infection.	Signs and symptoms of infection could include warmth, redness, heat, swelling, drainage, pain.	Are any wounds infected?
Monitor color of and measure wound drainage.	Wound drainage color and amount can indicate severity of infection.	Does wound have large amount of purulent drainage?
Change dressings or provide wound and pin care per facility policy using aseptic technique.	Use of aseptic technique minimizes chance of infection. Pin wound sites should be free of crusting, which promotes infections because of decreased skin integrity.	Are pin sites clean with no crusting?
Monitor vital signs frequently.	Alterations in vital signs can indicate infection.	Are vital signs within baseline findings?

Impaired physical mobility related to the external fixation (EF) device

Patient Outcomes Patient will maintain desired level of mobility/activity.

Evaluation of Outcome Has patient maintained desired level of mobility and activity?

Interventions	Rationale	Evaluation
Reinforce transfer and ambulation techniques.	Depending on severity of fracture and size of EF device, there may be special needs to transfer and ambulate.	Does patient transfer and ambulate as instructed?
Place overhead frame and trapeze on bed; teach patient how to use them.	Patient mobility is increased and pain decreased with use of trapeze for movement.	Does patient use overhead frame and trapeze for movement with less pain?
Teach patient how to move limb using EF device.	Providing patient with instruction on moving the extremity promotes independence and minimizes pain.	Does patient move the extremity using EF device?
Assess patient for and take measures to prevent complications of immobility. Promote early ambulation to minimize complications.	Immobility complications can occur if preventative measures are not used.	Does patient have any complications of immobility?
Include other disciplines such as the physiotherapist in promoting and teaching about ambulation.	EF devices allow for earlier ambulation. Physiotherapy can provide initial or reinforce the education needed to promote ambulation (e.g., with crutch walking).	Has patient used information learned from other disciplines to aid ambulation?

Disturbed body image related to external fixation device

Patient Outcomes Patient will not experience disturbed body image while EF device is in place.

Evaluation of Outcome Does patient experience disturbed body image resulting from EF device?

Interventions	Rationale	Evaluation
If possible, explain to patient pre-operatively what EF device will look like.	Preparing patient for what to expect postoperatively increases likelihood of acceptance and minimizes the unknown.	Was patient able to verbalize why device is to be used and what device will look like?
Reinforce the idea that EF device will decrease discomfort and allow for earlier ambulation.	Promoting early ambulation and increased comfort enhance acceptance.	Did patient understand benefit of EF device allowing for early ambulation and increased comfort?
Provide psychological support and an environment of acceptance.	Accepting your patient and allowing for discussion of concerns promotes a sense of well-being and acceptance of EF device.	Did patient feel comfortable in expressing concerns related to body image?

can develop in patients who are immobile because of trauma or surgery. Thromboembolitic complications are the most common problems of lower extremity surgery or trauma and the most fatal complication of musculoskeletal surgery, particularly in the older adult. Leg exercises, early ambulation, and anticoagulant therapy, usually using low molecular weight heparin, such as dalteparin (Fragmin) or enoxaparin (Lovenox), help prevent these problems.

ACUTE COMPARTMENT SYNDROME. Compartments are sheaths of fibrous tissue that support and partition nerves, muscles, and blood vessels, primarily in the extremities (Fig. 46.9). There are several compartments within each extremity. Acute compartment syndrome (ACS) is a serious problem in which the pressure within one or more extremity compartments increases, causing massive circulation impairment to the area. An external device such as a cast or bulky dressing can increase pressure when there is tissue swelling or compression in the area. The early symptom of ACS is the patient's report of severe, increasing pain that is not relieved with narcotics and occurs more on active movement than passive movement. Decreased sensation follows before ischemia becomes severe. In severe ACS, the patient has the six Ps:

- Pain (severe, unrelenting, and increased with passive stretching)
- Paresthesia (painful tingling or burning)
- Paralysis (late symptom)

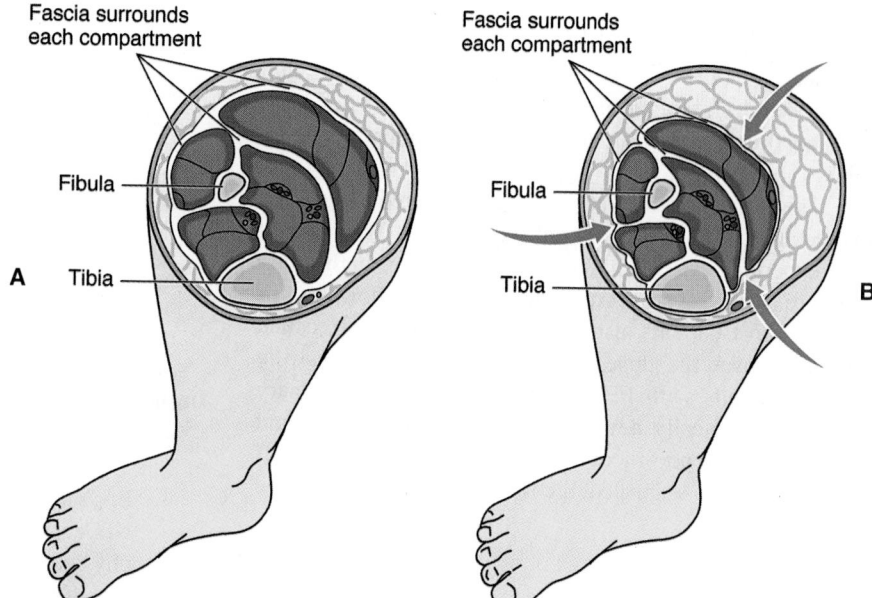

FIGURE 46.9 (A) Lower leg compartments. Each compartment contains muscles, an artery, a vein, and a nerve. (B) Compartment syndrome. Increased pressure in a compartment compresses structures within the compartment.

- Pallor (but there may be warmth or redness over the area)
- Pulselessness (late and ominous sign)
- Poikilothermia (temperature matches environment; i.e., the extremity is cool to touch)

Relief of pressure is the goal. It may be accomplished by removing the source of pressure, such as bivalving a cast, or by performing a **fasciotomy,** which is an incision into the fascia that encloses the compartment. This incision allows the compartment tissue room to expand and relieves the pressure. If more than one compartment has increased pressure, multiple fasciotomies are required. These surgical wounds remain open until the pressure decreases. Then they are closed and may require skin grafting. If this condition continues without pressure relief, tissue necrosis, infection, extremity contracture, or renal failure may result. Renal failure is a potentially fatal complication of ACS.

CRITICAL THINKING

Mr. Andrews

■ Mr. Andrews has suffered a nondisplaced fracture of his right femur. He has a cast on from his groin to the middle of his foot. An hour ago he received 10 mg of morphine intravenously (IV), and he is complaining of continuing and increasing pain.

1. What nursing assessment should now be performed?
2. What might be happening with Mr. Andrews?
3. What interventions may be necessary?

Suggested answers at end of chapter.

FAT EMBOLISM SYNDROME. Fat embolism syndrome (FES) is another serious complication in which small fat globules are released from yellow bone marrow into the bloodstream. The globules then travel to the lung fields, causing respiratory distress. This process most often occurs when long bones (especially the femoral shaft) are fractured or when the patient has multiple fractures. The older adult patient with a fractured hip is also at a high risk for FES. This condition can occur up to 72 hours after the initial injury or procedure.

The earliest manifestation of FES is altered mental status resulting from a low arterial oxygen level. The patient then experiences tachycardia, tachypnea, fever, high blood pressure, and severe respiratory distress (shortness of breath). Most patients also have a measleslike rash, called petechiae, over the upper body. Even when aggressively treated, patients with FES often die from the pulmonary edema that typically develops. Note early FES signs and symptoms and report them to the physician immediately. If a fat embolism is suspected, the following actions should be taken:

- Promote oxygenation by administering oxygen at 2 L per minute via nasal cannula.
- Place patient in high-Fowler's position or raise head of bed as tolerated by patient.
- Maintain bedrest and keep movement of extremity to a minimum.
- Prepare patient for a chest x-ray examination or lung scan.
- Prepare patient for arterial blood gas (ABG) determination.
- Administer intravenous fluids as ordered.
- Administer corticosteroids as ordered.
- Provide emotional support and calm environment.

Nursing Process for the Patient with a Fracture

Caring for the patient with a fracture requires coordinated care with other health team members.

ASSESSMENT/DATA COLLECTION. The most important aspect of monitoring the patient with a fracture is frequent checking of neurovascular status (circulation, sensation, mobility) distal to the fracture site (Chapter 45). As mentioned earlier, acute compartment syndrome is a potentially limb- or life-threatening complication that results when blood flow is impaired.

Pain is managed by both medications and complementary therapies. Bone pain can be excruciating and must be treated aggressively. For the patient who cannot report pain, such as a cognitively impaired or comatose patient, ensure that pain relief is maintained by regularly scheduled analgesic administration.

NURSING DIAGNOSIS, PLANNING, AND IMPLEMENTATION. Determination of the appropriate nursing diagnosis depends on the type of fracture. See Box 46.3 Nursing Care Plan for the Patient After Open Reduction with Internal Fixation [ORIF] of the Hip.

Acute pain related to fractured bone

EXPECTED OUTCOME: Patient will report relief from pain using pain assessment scale.

- Provide analgesics and anti-inflammatories as ordered *to relieve pain and swelling.*
- Ensure proper positioning and alignment *to minimize discomfort and promote pain relief.*
- Assess for compartment syndrome if patient has a cast in place *to prevent neurovascular complications.*
- Apply ice as ordered *to decrease swelling and pain.*
- Teach alternative measure of pain relief *to maximize means to relieve pain.*

Impaired physical mobility related to bone fracture

EXPECTED OUTCOME: Patient will demonstrate increased mobility.

- Encourage independence *to promote mobility.*
- Utilize other disciplines such as occupational and physiotherapy *to encourage and promote patient mobility.*

---

fasciotomy: fascia—fibrous tissue + otomy—opening into

- Provide equipment and resources such as crutches and wheelchairs *to improve mobility.*

Risk for peripheral neurovascular dysfunction related to increased tissue volume or restrictive envelope

EXPECTED OUTCOME: *Patient will maintain peripheral pulses, warm skin, sensation, and ability to move extremity.*

- Assess and monitor frequently for compartment syndrome.
- Assess for swelling of affected limb (especially if patient has a cast or tight dressing).
- Keep limb elevated above heart *to minimize edema.*
- Administer anti-inflammatory agents as ordered.
- Monitor for increasing pain even after analgesic administration.

NURSING CARE TIP

A confused or comatose patient may not be able to report pain, the most reliable indicator of pain. Nonverbal indicators (e.g., grimacing, restlessness, elevated blood pressure and heart rate) are not reliable for pain assessment and should not be used to determine pain absence. You need to prevent the patient's pain by anticipating it and treating it in advance. You can do this by recognizing causes of pain and understanding that the effects of mild but repetitive pain (as in turning several times a day) can adversely affect the patient (such as by leading to exhaustion). Causes of pain include conditions or diseases (such as fractures, surgery, trauma, or cancer), procedures (such as turning or wound care), and biomedical devices (such as orthopedic fixation devices, wound drains, urinary catheters, nasogastric tubes, and chest tubes).

With few patients being medicated before painful procedures, some of which may be done several times a day (turning), confused or comatose patients are at greater risk for lack of pain relief. Provide analgesics as ordered before painful procedures and on a regular basis when pain is assumed to be present to keep your patients comfortable. For anticipated pain, the acronym APP (assume pain present) can be used.

Use pain assessment tools designed for those who are cognitively impaired to ensure that their pain is adequately relieved. The **P**ain **A**ssessment **IN A**dvanced **D**ementia (PAINAD) is a tool that was developed for this purpose. Search the web to view it or visit http://www.amda.com/caring/may2004/painad.htm. Share pain research findings with administrators in your institution to establish policies that support proactive pain management for all patients.

EVALUATION. The outcome is met if the patient reports or demonstrates pain is within tolerable levels on a pain assessment scale, demonstrates increased physical mobility, and maintains peripheral pulses, warm skin, sensation, and ability to move extremity.

PATIENT EDUCATION. If the patient has a cast, review the appropriate instructions for cast care (see Box 46.2 Nursing Interventions for a Patient with a Cast). Health teaching is also important for care of the extremity after cast removal (Box 46.5 Extremity Care Following Cast Removal). If the patient has a wound, teach the patient and caregiver how to assess and dress the wound (and provide pin care if needed), and when to report changes such as signs and symptoms of infection.

Teach the importance of adequate protein, calories, vitamins, and minerals for healing to occur. Unless otherwise contraindicated, milkshakes and instant breakfast preparations are good sources of additional protein and calories, as well as a source of calcium.

Osteomyelitis

Osteomyelitis is an infection of bone that can be either acute or chronic. A bone infection lasting less than 4 weeks is considered acute; one that lasts more than 4 weeks is chronic.

Pathophysiology

Regardless of the type of osteomyelitis, the infection results from invasion of bacteria into bone and surrounding soft tissues. Inflammation occurs, followed by ischemia (decreased blood flow) (Fig. 46.10). Bone tissue then becomes necrotic (dies), which retards healing and causes more infection, often as a bone abscess.

Pathogens enter bone in several ways. Direct inoculation means that an injury to the body allows the offending microbes direct access to bone tissue. An open fracture is an example of that process. Contiguous spread occurs when surrounding soft tissue becomes infected. An example is the patient with cellulitis whose infection then spreads to underlying bone. In hematogenous spread, an infection beginning in another part of the body migrates to bone. For instance, a

---

Box 46.5

Extremity Care Following Cast Removal

- Ensure skin properly cleansed. Soak rather than rub skin to remove dry scales.
- The extremity likely will be weak with decreased ROM—move it gently and provide analgesics prn.
- When extremity is not in use, provide support with pillows or orthotic device until strength and movement return.
- Ensure active and passive ROMs are performed as per PT and patient tolerance will allow.
- Lower extremity swelling can be prevented with elastic support stockings.

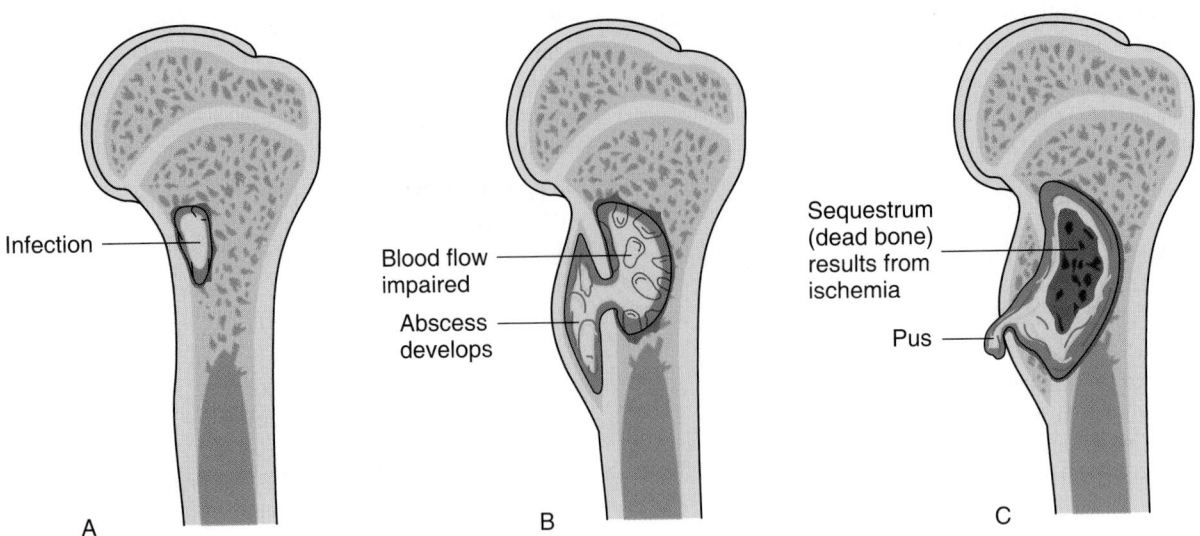

FIGURE 46.10 Sequence of osteomyelitis development. *(A)* Infection begins. *(B)* Blood flow is blocked in the area of infection. An abscess with pus forms. *(C)* Bone dies within the infection site, and pus formation continues.

patient with a total hip replacement may acquire osteomyelitis from a urinary tract infection.

Causes and Types

Penetrating trauma leads to acute osteomyelitis by direct inoculation. The most common pathogens causing osteomyelitis are *Pseudomonas aeruginosa, Staphylococcus aureus,* and *Proteus.* The leading cause of contiguous spread is a slow-healing foot ulcer in the patient who has diabetes mellitus or peripheral vascular disease. Multiple organisms may be present in the wound and subsequently the bone. Hematogenous spread results from bacteremia (infection of the blood), underlying disease, or nonpenetrating trauma. Long-term intravenous catheters are primary sources of infection.

Signs and Symptoms

The patient with acute osteomyelitis has fever, as well as local signs of inflammation, such as tenderness, redness, heat, pain, and swelling. Pain (particularly over the area of infection), may be the only apparent complaint. Ulceration, drainage, and localized pain are typical signs and symptoms of chronic osteomyelitis.

Diagnostic Tests

The patient with osteomyelitis typically has an elevated leukocyte (white blood cell) count, an elevated erythrocyte sedimentation rate, and positive bone biopsy for infection. Some patients also have a positive blood culture. MRIs, x-ray examinations, and CT scans can show areas of infection.

Therapeutic Interventions

Long-term antibiotic therapy is the treatment of choice for patients with bone infection. Infection in bone tissue is difficult to resolve and may require weeks to months of medication. Antibiotic therapy alone may not resolve the infection. Patients with chronic osteomyelitis may require surgery to remove necrotic bone tissue or replace it with healthy bone tissue. Amputations are reserved for patients who have massive infections that have not responded to one or more of the conventional treatments.

Nursing Management

Patients often administer their intravenous antibiotics at home rather than have a costly stay in a hospital. Teach the patient and caregiver about the side effects, toxicity, interactions, and precautions for antibiotic therapy. A home care nurse may be needed to assist the patient.

If a soft tissue wound is present, ensure that sterile technique is used for dressing changes. The home health nurse may teach the patient and family how to perform dressing changes, the importance of hand washing prior to dressing changes, and how to avoid the spread of pathogens.

Osteoporosis

Osteoporosis is a common metabolic disorder in which the bone loses its density, resulting in fragile bones and possibly fractures. The wrist, hip, and vertebral column are most commonly involved. Over 10 million people have osteoporosis, and 18 million more have low bone mass according to the National Osteoporosis Foundation. Both women and men develop osteoporosis, although it is often thought that only women are affected. Women are at greatest risk because their bones are smaller than men's bones. To protect against osteoporosis, good health habits through age 30 are important. They include adequate calcium and vitamin D intake (ages 11 to 25: 1200 to 1500 mg/day), weight-bearing exercise, avoiding alcohol, and not smoking.

Pathophysiology

Bone is living tissue that is resorbing (breaking down) old tissue (osteoclast cells) and constantly building new tissue (osteoblast cells). Bone density (mass) peaks between 30 and 35 years of age. After these peak years, the rate of bone breakdown exceeds the rate of bone building as we age.

Trabecular (cancellous) bone is lost first, followed by a loss of cortical (compact) bone. The result is irreversible bone loss that makes the inside of bones porous and weaker. As a result, over 1,000,000 fractures occur annually, and 700,000 of these are vertebral fractures. Hip fractures are the second most common, accounting for more than 300,000 per year. The mortality rate for hip fractures is about 50% during the first year after the fracture. For postmenopausal women, decreased estrogen appears to slow down the absorption of calcium, resulting in an increased bone loss.

Cause and Types

Osteoporosis is either primary or secondary. Primary osteoporosis is the most common and is not associated with another disease or health problem. Risk factors for primary osteoporosis include the following:

- Caucasian or Asian heritage, postmenopausal, female (less estrogen available to protect bone)
- Sedentary lifestyle
- Decreased calcium intake
- Lack of vitamin D (to absorb calcium)
- Excessive alcohol consumption
- Cigarette smoking
- Excessive caffeine intake
- Small boned, petite body build

Secondary osteoporosis results from an associated medical condition, such as hyperparathyroidism; having renal dialysis; drug therapy, such as steroids and certain antiseizure drugs, sleeping medications, hormones for endometriosis, or cancer drugs; and prolonged immobility, such as that seen with patients who have a spinal cord injury.

Signs and Symptoms

Most women do not realize they have osteoporosis until they fracture a bone. During the late middle years, the classic "dowager's hump," or kyphosis of the spine, is usually present. The patient's height decreases and back pain may be present. The patient may be embarrassed by the change in body image and may have curtailed social activities. Some patients have difficulty finding clothes that fit comfortably.

Diagnostic Tests

X-ray examination of the bone is not helpful in diagnosing bone loss in its early stages. Computed tomography and quantitative CT scans detect early spinal changes and measure bone density. Ultrasound can also be used to screen bone mass. Dual-energy x-ray absorptiometry (DXA) is used as a screening tool to measure bone mineral content. This test is noninvasive and is currently the most widely used technique to measure bone density.

Serum calcium and vitamin D levels may be decreased, and serum phosphorus may be increased. With severe bone loss, alkaline phosphatase levels may be elevated, confirming bone damage.

Therapeutic Interventions

The cornerstone of treatment for osteoporosis is medication and avoidance of modifiable risk factors to prevent bone loss.

MEDICATION. Medication may be used for prevention or treatment purposes. The current drugs of choice are calcium supplements, vitamin D, and bisphosphonates, such as alendronate (Fosamax) and risedronate (Actonel).

Calcium is also important to prevent bone loss. If serum calcium falls below normal levels, the parathyroid glands stimulate the bone to release calcium into the bloodstream. The result is demineralized bone. Therefore, calcium supplements are an important aspect of treatment. Teach the patient to drink plenty of fluids to prevent calcium-based urinary stones. Vitamin D supplementation, to aid calcium absorption, may also be necessary for patients who have inadequate sunlight exposure (institutionalized people) or who cannot metabolize vitamin D.

Alendronate and risedronate are used to prevent or slow the progress of osteoporosis. They suppress osteoclast activity to prevent the breakdown of bone. Although side effects are not common, serious cases of esophagitis and esophageal ulcers have been reported. Therefore, teach the patient to take the drug early in the morning and follow it with a full glass of water. The patient should not lie down for at least 1 hour after taking the drug.

A newer drug class for osteoporosis is the selective estrogen receptor modulator (SERM). Raloxifene (Evista) increases bone mass 2% to 3% each year. SERM drugs are designed to mimic estrogen in some parts of the body while blocking its effects elsewhere. Recently approved for use is the newest drug class for osteoporosis, recombinant human parathyroid hormone. Teriparatide (Forteo) is used for men and women at a great risk for fracture. Teriparatide increases bone mass by increasing the action and number of osteoblasts. It is considered a bone formation agent.

Other drugs that may be used include testosterone (the male hormone that helps build bone), calcitonin (nasal spray, injection), and sodium fluoride. All these medications have major disadvantages and are consequently not commonly given. Any drug used to prevent or control osteoporosis must be administered under the supervision of a physician, including supplements.

DIET. Increasing calcium and fluids are the main dietary considerations for women. Calcium intake should be 1000 mg/day for those age 25 to 65 and 1500 mg for those over age 65. Teach patients what foods are high in calcium, such as dairy products and dark green, leafy vegetables. If the patient consumes excessive caffeine or alcohol, teach about the need to avoid these substances. For more information, visit the National Osteoporosis Foundation at www.nof.org.

Exercise

Weight-bearing exercise, especially walking, stimulates bone building. The patient should wear well-supporting, nonskid shoes at all times and avoid uneven surfaces that could contribute to falls. Resistance exercise such as weight training or the use of some of the equipment available at fitness centers is also beneficial.

FALL PREVENTION. Osteoporotic bone may cause a pathological fracture in which the hip breaks before the fall.

For other patients, a fall can cause a hip or other fracture. Therefore, fall prevention programs in hospitals and nursing homes are important.

In collaboration with the physical or occupational therapist, case manager, or discharge planner, assess the patient's home environment. The patient and family are taught how to create a hazard-free environment, such as avoiding scatter rugs and slippery floors. Walking paths in the home must be kept free of clutter to prevent falls. If needed, a walker or cane provides additional support.

Paget's Disease

Paget's disease, also called osteitis deformans, is a metabolic bone disease in which increased bone loss results in large, disorganized bone deposits throughout the body. It is primarily a disease of the older adult.

Pathophysiology

Three phases of the disorder have been described: active, mixed, and inactive. A prolific increase in osteoclasts (cells that break down bone) causes massive bone deformity and destruction. Osteoblasts (bone-building cells) then react to form new bone. However, the result is disorganized in structure. Finally, when osteoblastic activity exceeds the osteoclastic activity, the inactive phase occurs. The newly formed bone becomes sclerotic with increased vascularity.

Paget's disease can affect one or multiple bones. The most common areas involved are the femur, skull, vertebrae, and pelvis.

Causes and Types

The exact cause of this disease is not known, but it tends to run in families. Paget's disease may be the result of a latent viral infection contracted in young adulthood. It is more common in Europe than in the United States.

Signs and Symptoms

Most patients with Paget's disease have no obvious symptoms, particularly when the disorder is confined to one bone. Pain is a major symptom in many. For patients with more severe disease, signs and symptoms are varied and potentially fatal.

Diagnostic Tests

Diagnosis may be made solely on x-ray findings. Radiographs of pagetic bone show punched-out areas indicating increased bone resorption. The overall mass of bone may be enlarged, depending on the phase of the disorder. Deformities, fractures, and arthritic changes are not uncommon. Bone scans can also be used to help in the diagnosis.

The primary laboratory findings are an increased alkaline phosphatase (ALP) and an increase in urinary hydroxyproline. Pyrilinks and Osteomark are urine tests that can be used in place of the urinary hydroxyproline test. ALP reflects bone damage. Urinary hydroxyproline indicates an increase in bone turnover. The higher the level, the more severe the disease. Calcium levels in both blood and urine are elevated as damaged bone releases calcium into the bloodstream.

Therapeutic Interventions and Nursing Management

Nonsurgical management is employed to relieve pain and promote a reasonable quality of life for the patient. For mild disease, nonsteroidal anti-inflammatory drugs (NSAIDs) are given.

MEDICATION. The purpose of drug therapy for the patient with Paget's disease is to relieve pain and decrease bone loss. Calcitonin (Calcimar) is a thyroid hormone that is often effective in initiating a remission of the disease. It appears to decrease bone loss while also decreasing pain. If effective, the ALP level decreases. The usual duration of therapy is 6 months, followed by 6 months of etidronate disodium (Didronel) or another bisphosphonate drug. Its action is similar to that of calcitonin, and it must be taken on an empty stomach. Alendronate is a bone resorption inhibitor and calcium regulator. Intravenous dosing for 5 days may initiate a disease remission.

Plicamycin (Mithramycin, Mithracin) is a potent anticancer drug and antibiotic that is reserved for patients with severe hypercalcemia or severe disease with neurological involvement. This drug suppresses both osteoclastic and osteoblastic activity within days, but it has serious adverse effects. As with all drugs, observe for toxic effects such as liver and kidney failure. The platelet count is monitored because the drug can decrease platelet production. When liver enzymes become too high, the drug is temporarily discontinued until they return to baseline.

Nursing management for Paget's disease focuses on pain relief and support for symptoms. Teaching about the disease, medications, and other therapies is done.

Bone Cancer

Bone tumors may be benign or malignant. Malignant tumors may be either primary (originating in the bone) or metastatic, originating from another location and migrating to bone. Primary bone tumors tend to develop in people under 30 years of age and account for only a small percentage of bone cancers. Metastatic lesions are much more common and most often affect the older adult. The pathophysiology depends on the type of bone cancer. The cause of bone cancer is not known.

Primary Malignant Tumors

Osteosarcoma, or osteogenic sarcoma, is the most common primary malignant bone tumor as well as being the most fatal bone tumor. It is a fairly large tumor that typically metastasizes to the lung within 2 years of diagnosis and treatment. Osteosarcoma most frequently affects the arms and legs (particularly around the knees), but can be found in other bones. This type of cancer usually affects young people between the ages of 10 and 25, and boys are twice as likely to develop the disease. Long bones of the legs and arms are most often the sites of origin. More than 50% of osteosarcomas occur in the distal femur in young men.

---

osteosarcoma: osteo—bone + sarc—flesh + oma—tumor

The disease itself is relatively rare, with an occurrence rate of approximately two per million people. Pain and swelling in an arm or leg that worsens with exercise or at night are some of the manifestations of osteosarcoma. A lump in the area or an unexplained limp may also be cause for further investigation. X-rays, bone biopsy, CT scan, bone scan, and MRI are some of the diagnostic tests that can be performed to help in the diagnosis of the malignancy. Older patients with Paget's disease may also develop these lesions. Chemotherapy and surgical excision of the affected bone with bone grafting or amputation of the affected limb are the treatments most commonly used for osteosarcomas.

Ewing's sarcoma is the most malignant bone tumor. In addition to local pain and swelling, systemic signs and symptoms, including low-grade fever, leukocytosis, and anemia, are common. The pelvis and lower extremity are most often affected in children and young men.

Patients with a *chondrosarcoma* (cancer of cartilaginous cells) have a better prognosis than those with the previously described types of bone cancer. This type of cancer occurs in middle-aged and older people.

METASTATIC BONE DISEASE. Primary malignant tumors that occur in the prostate, breast, lung, and thyroid gland are called bone-seeking cancers because they migrate to bone more than any other primary cancer. Once cancer has metastasized, multiple bone sites are typically seen. Pathological fractures and severe pain are major concerns in managing metastatic disease. See Chapter 10 regarding caring for patients with cancer.

Signs and Symptoms

Primary tumors cause local swelling and pain at the site. A tender, palpable mass is often present. Metastatic disease is not as visible, but the patient complains of diffuse severe pain, eventually leading to marked disability.

Diagnostic Tests

Diagnosis of bone cancer is made by x-ray examination, computed tomography, bone scan, bone biopsy, or MRI. Chapter 45 discusses these tests in detail.

The patient with metastatic disease has an elevated ALP level and possibly an elevated erythrocyte sedimentation rate, indicating secondary tissue inflammation.

Therapeutic Interventions

Management of bone cancer depends on the type and extent of the tumor. The treatment of primary bone tumors is usually surgery, often combined with chemotherapy or radiation. The surgeon attempts to salvage the limb and performs a resection of the tumor. For patients with Ewing's sarcoma or early osteosarcoma, external radiation may be the treatment of choice to reduce tumor size and pain.

Care of the postoperative patient is similar to that for any patient undergoing musculoskeletal surgery. Monitoring neurovascular status of the operative limb to be operated on is a vital nursing intervention (see Chapter 45). Other general postoperative care is discussed in Chapter 11.

For metastatic bone disease, surgery is not appropriate. External radiation is given primarily for palliation. The radiation is directed toward the most painful sites in an attempt to shrink them and provide more comfort for the patient.

Nursing Management

Nursing care for the patient with bone cancer is not unlike that for patients with any other type of cancer. Help the patient adjust to the diagnosis and refer the patient to resources such as the American Cancer Society and its various support groups. Chapter 10 describes the nursing care associated with chemotherapy and radiation therapy. For more information, visit the American Cancer Society at www.cancer.org.

CONNECTIVE TISSUE DISORDERS

Connective tissue disorders comprise a group of more than 100 diseases in which the major signs and symptoms result from joint involvement. Some connective tissue diseases affect only one part of the body; others affect many body organs and systems. Several disorders are discussed here, including gout, systemic lupus erythematosus, progressive systemic sclerosis, **osteogenesis imperfecta**, **polymyositis**, osteoarthritis, and rheumatoid **arthritis.**

Gout

Gout is an easily treated systemic connective tissue disorder. Men, especially those middle aged and older, are affected more than women. Patients with gout are seldom hospitalized for their disease.

Pathophysiology

Uric acid is a waste product resulting from the breakdown of proteins (purines) in the body. Urate crystals, formed because of excessive uric acid (**hyperuricemia**) build up and are deposited in joints and other connective tissues, causing severe inflammation. When an "attack" of gout occurs, the patient has severe pain and inflammation in one or more small joints, usually the great toe. The inflammation may resolve in several days with or without treatment. Months or years may pass between attacks, and the patient may have no signs or symptoms of joint inflammation between episodes. Urate deposits may appear under the skin (tophi) (Fig. 46.11) or in the kidneys or urinary system, causing stone (calculi) formation (see Chapter 37).

Causes and Types

The causes and types of gout are well known. Primary gout is the most common and is caused by an inherited problem with purine metabolism. Uric acid production is greater than the kidneys' ability to excrete it. Therefore, the amount of

---

polymyositis: poly—many + myo—muscle + itis—inflammation
arthritis: arthr(on)—joint + itis—inflammation
hyperuricemia: hyper—excessive + uric—uric acid + emia—in blood

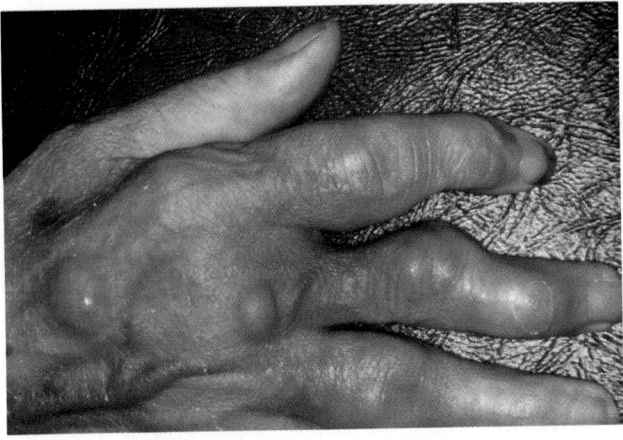

FIGURE 46.11 Gout: subcutaneous nontender lesions near joints. *(From Goldsmith, LA, Lazarus, GS, Tharp MD, et al: Adult and Pediatric Dermatology. F. A. Davis, Philadelphia, 1997, p 405, with permission.)*

uric acid in the blood increases. About 25% of patients have a family history of primary gout. Acute attacks of gout may be triggered by stress, alcohol, illness, trauma, dieting, or certain medications.

Patients with secondary gout also experience hyperuricemia, but the increase is the result of another health problem, such as renal insufficiency, or medications, such as diuretic therapy and certain chemotherapeutic agents.

Signs and Symptoms

ACUTE GOUT. Patients with acute gout have one or more severely inflamed joints due to the uric acid crystals, usually small joints, often in the joint of the great toe. The joint is swollen, red, hot, and usually too painful to be touched.

CHRONIC GOUT. Patients with chronic gout may not have obvious signs and symptoms. Tophi are not commonly seen today because management of patients with gout has improved. If they are present, they tend to appear most often in the outer ear. Renal stones develop in about 20% of patients with gout. Various diagnostic tests may be needed to determine stone formation.

Diagnostic Tests

Diagnosis of gout is based on an elevated serum uric acid level. Joint fluid aspiration analysis can identify uric acid crystals in the synovial fluid, further confirming the diagnosis of gout.

Therapeutic Interventions

MEDICATION. The treatment of secondary gout is management or removal of the underlying cause. Drug therapy is the first-line treatment for primary gout. When the patient has an acute gout episode, the physician usually prescribes either colchicine or an NSAID to reduce the inflammatory response to urate crystals. The patient usually takes these medications until joint inflammation subsides.

Uricosuric agents (medications used to decrease uric acid) are the drug of choice when trying to decrease serum levels. Allopurinol (Zyloprim) is the preferred drug for chronic gout. Allopurinol decreases uric acid production,

necessitating several weeks of therapy before the medication becomes effective. The patient must take it every day to keep the uric acid level within the normal range. Probenecid (Benemid) may also be used temporarily to increase renal excretion of uric acid. The patient's serum uric acid level is monitored periodically.

DIET. For patients with gout, certain foods should be avoided or consumed in moderation (Box 46.6 Health Promotion for Patients with Gout). The patient should avoid all forms of aspirin and diuretics because they can trigger an attack. Increasing daily fluid intake is also important to help prevent kidney stones. The patient should also avoid alcohol (especially beer) as this too can provoke an attack.

Systemic Lupus Erythematosus

The word *lupus* comes from the Latin word for wolf, and was originally associated with leg ulcers. However, it became associated with facial ulcers, and the butterfly facial rash that patients with lupus may develop is one of the most defining characteristics of lupus. The rash is red, and thus the word *erythematosus,* meaning reddened, was added to describe the disease.

Most patients with lupus have the systemic type, but a small percentage have the type that affects only the skin, a condition called discoid lupus erythematosus. Discoid lupus is not life threatening; systemic lupus erythematosus (SLE) can be life threatening because it is a progressive, systemic inflammatory disease that can cause major body organ and system failure. Although this definition seems similar to the definition of rheumatoid arthritis (RA), one distinct difference exists. Patients with SLE typically have more body organ involvement earlier in their disease than patients with RA.

Pathophysiology

SLE is an autoimmune disease characterized by spontaneous remissions and exacerbations. The body's immune system normally produces antibodies to fight invaders such as bacteria, viruses, and other materials foreign to the body. In SLE, the body does not recognize itself and begins to produce antibodies directed at the foreign "self." These anti-

---

Box 46.6

Health Promotion for Patients with Gout

- Avoid high-purine (protein) foods, such as organ meats, shellfish, and oily fish (e.g., sardines).
- Avoid alcohol.
- Drink plenty of fluids, especially water.
- Avoid all forms of aspirin and drugs containing aspirin.
- Avoid diuretics.
- Avoid excessive physical or emotional stress.

bodies attack the self antigens and form immune complexes. Production of abnormal antibodies (antinuclear antibodies [ANAs]), immune complex formation, and complement system activation results in autoimmune effects on the patient's healthy connective tissue. Many of the manifestations result from recurring injuries to the patient's vascular system. The immune complexes that result lodge in the blood and organs, leading to inflammation, damage, and possibly death.

The cause of SLE is unknown, but the disorder tends to occur in families. Identified chromosomal markers indicate a genetic link. There is evidence that environmental factors also play a critical role in the development of SLE. Infections, high stress levels, various hormones and drugs (especially antibiotics such as sulfa and penicillin), and ultraviolet (UV) light have all been linked to triggering SLE. Exacerbation of symptoms often occurs prior to the start of menstruation and during pregnancy, demonstrating the link hormones have in triggering SLE.

African Americans, Hispanics, Native Americans, and Asians are two to three times more likely to develop SLE than others. Lupus most often affects women between ages 15 and 40 and at a rate 10 to 15 times more often than for men. Women represent 90% of all cases of SLE.

With improved therapy, the mortality rate for patients with the disease has improved greatly over the past 30 years. The leading causes of death are kidney failure, heart failure, and central nervous system involvement.

Signs and Symptoms

Unfortunately, there is no classic description of patients with SLE. Some patients have a very mild form of the disease in which only the skin and joints are affected. Others have devastating effects when the disease affects multiple body systems at the same time.

The classic feature of lupus is the characteristic raised, reddened butterfly rash found over the bridge of the nose that extends to both cheeks, although only half of patients develop it (Fig. 46.12). The rash is usually dry and may itch. It commonly is photosensitive, tends to worsen during an exacerbation, and can be triggered by exposure to ultraviolet light or by physical stressors, such as pregnancy or infection. Instead of the butterfly rash, some patients have discoid (coinlike) skin lesions on other parts of the body. During flare-ups, a fever develops which can rise to more than 100° F (38° C). Fatigue, arthralgia or arthritis, myalgia, malaise, weight loss, mucosal ulcers, and alopecia are other possible signs and symptoms of SLE. Table 46.2 lists other possible signs and symptoms of SLE.

Diagnostic Tests

Skin lesions can be biopsied and examined microscopically for signs of inflammation. Patients with suspected SLE are evaluated using the same immunologically based laboratory tests that are used to assess patients with rheumatoid arthritis. These tests include ESR (to detect systemic inflammation) and ANA titers (to detect the presence of abnormal antibodies). There are also two subtypes of ANA: anti-DNA and anti-sm antibodies, which are only found in patients

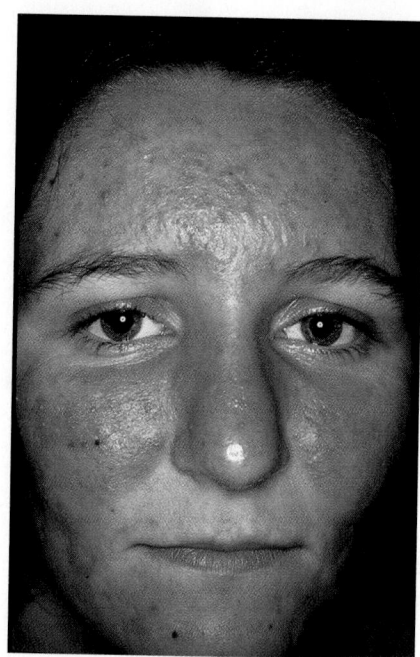

FIGURE 46.12 Lupus erythematosus: red papules and plaques in butterfly pattern on face. *(From Goldsmith, LA, Lazarus, GS, Tharp, MD, et al: Adult and Pediatric Dermatology. F.A. Davis, Philadelphia, 1997, p 230, with permission.)*

with SLE and can be useful when the physician is attempting to confirm a diagnosis of SLE. A new blood test has been developed that aids in the diagnosis of SLE. Systemic lupus erythematosus patients make antibodies against serine/arginine–rich (SR) proteins (which are important in cell division). Seventy percent of SLE patients react positively to the SR proteins. This new diagnostic tool should help in identifying those SLE patients who do not produce some of the other antibodies looked for in the diagnosis of SLE. Although no laboratory test confirms a diagnosis of lupus, the results of the immunological tests may support the diagnosis.

Therapeutic Interventions

Treatment of SLE focuses on decreasing inflammation and preventing life-threatening organ damage. At present, the therapy of choice includes medications to treat the symptoms or the body systems affected. Research is ongoing regarding the possible cause of SLE. Researchers have found the general location of a gene that is believed to predispose a person to lupus. Identifying the genetic cause of lupus will enable researchers to develop new methods of therapy, including gene therapy. Prevention of exacerbations (flares) is important, and therefore taking preventative measures is suggested. Minimizing exposure to the sun and wearing sunscreens helps those patients who are photosensitive. Regular exercise and keeping immunizations up to date are also helpful.

MEDICATION. Medications are prescribed according to the patient's needs. NSAIDs, acetaminophen, corticosteroids, antimalarials (chloroquine [Aralen], hydroxychloroquine

TABLE 46.2 CHARACTERISTICS OF SYSTEMIC LUPUS ERYTHEMATOSUS (SLE)

Manifestations

Central Nervous System
- Headache, epilepsy, psychoses
- Peripheral or sensory neuropathies
- Personality changes, mild alterations in cognition

Cardiovascular
- Inflammation of pericardium (pericarditis)
- Alteration in circulation, particularly to digits (Raynaud's phenomenon)

Pulmonary
- Pleural effusions

Renal
- Inflammation of Kidney Glomerulonephritis

Gastrointestinal
- Peritonitis

Musculoskeletal
- Arthralgias (due to inflammation), especially of the hands, wrists, and knees
- Myalgias

Skin
- Butterfly rash across bridge of nose
- Rash is reddened and raised

Constitutional Signs and Symptoms
- Increased temperature
- Malaise, tiredness
- Weight loss

[Plaquenil]), immunomodulating drugs, and anticoagulants may all be part of the medication regimen. Topical cortisone preparations may help reduce skin inflammation and promote fading of skin lesions.

Patients who experience joint inflammation are usually placed on an NSAID. Patients with organ or major body system involvement are given more potent drugs that suppress the immune process, including oral steroids such as prednisone or immunomodulating agents such as azathioprine (Imuran) or cyclophosphamide (Cytoxan). These drugs have serious side effects, and patients receiving them are monitored very carefully. In addition to monitoring for a variety of side effects, patients must be taught to avoid people with infections because they are immunocompromised while taking any of these medications.

Nursing Process for the Patient with Systemic Lupus Erythematosus

ASSESSMENT/DATA COLLECTION. Determine the extent and severity of signs and symptoms, such as pain, fatigue, skin lesions, and fever. Individualize the plan of care as every patient with SLE is unique.

NURSING DIAGNOSIS, PLANNING, AND IMPLEMENTATION. See nursing process sections on osteoarthritis and rheumatoid arthritis for:

Acute pain related to joint swelling
Chronic sorrow related to loss of health, role changes, and having a chronic disease

Fatigue related to chronic disease process
Disturbed body image related to alterations in skin integrity
Self-care deficits

Ineffective coping related to chronic disease condition and alteration in body integrity

EXPECTED OUTCOME: *Patient will make appropriate decisions related to personal life and condition.*
- Assess patient's coping pattern and ability to have a baseline.
- Provide support and reassurance to patient to let patient know someone is there for them.
- Assist in problem solving without taking over to help when needed but improving self-confidence.
- Encourage inclusion of support systems and resources to utilize all avenues available to help.
- Include input from other disciplines such as social work and clergy to ensure all alternatives are considered.

Risk for impaired skin integrity related to disease condition and increased susceptibility to UV light

EXPECTED OUTCOME: *Patient will maintain skin integrity.*
- Teach importance of protecting self from UV light (decrease sun exposure, wear sunscreen and appropriate clothing) *to minimize flare-ups.*
- Ensure good hygiene *to help minimize infections and promote skin integrity.*
- Apply topical creams and ointments as ordered *to help with inflammation and discomfort.*

EVALUATION. The outcome is met if patient makes appropriate decisions related to personal life and condition and skin integrity is maintained.

CRITICAL THINKING

Mr. Wolf

■ Mr. Wolf is experiencing a relapse of SLE and requires administration of prednisone. The doctor's order states: prednisone 55 mg PO in two equal doses. Prednisone is available as 1-mg, 2.5-mg, and 5-mg tablets. Which of the following combinations of drug would be most appropriate to administer for each dose?

1. Administer four 5-mg tablets in the morning and five 5-mg tablets in the evening.
2. Administer five 5-mg tablets in the morning and four 5-mg tablets in the evening.
3. Administer two and one half 1-mg tablets and five 5-mg tablets in the morning and evening.
4. Administer one 2.5-mg tablet and five 5-mg tablets in the morning and evening.

Suggested answers at end of chapter.

PATIENT EDUCATION. Teach the patient about skin care and ways to prevent disease exacerbations. Skin care includes use of a mild soap, patting the skin dry, using lotion, avoiding drying agents, protecting from sunlight with sun block of SPF 30, cover with clothing and hats, and avoid tanning beds. Exercise can prevent muscle weakness and fatigue. The patient should be encouraged to be immunized against specific infections. Methods of stress reduction should be identified and utilized.

The Arthritis Foundation and the Lupus Foundation are national organizations that can provide information, assistance, and community support groups for patients diagnosed with lupus. For more information, visit the Lupus Foundation of America at www.lupus.org.

Scleroderma

The term **scleroderma** is Greek in origin meaning "hard skin." It is similar to SLE in that it can affect multiple organs and other connective tissues. Scleroderma is not as common as SLE but has a higher mortality rate. There are two types of scleroderma: localized and systemic. As the name implies, systemic scleroderma can affect any part of the body. Among other names for systemic scleroderma are diffuse and progressive systemic scleroderma; however, since scleroderma is not necessarily progressive, this term is not encouraged. What is more frequently seen is the term *systemic sclerosis* (SSc).

Pathophysiology

Scleroderma is characterized by inflammation that ultimately develops into fibrosis (scarring) and then sclerosis (hardening) of tissues. The disease is an autoimmune response to the body's normal tissues. Like some of the other systemic connective tissue diseases, abnormal antibodies damage healthy tissue, resulting in inflammation, which then triggers overproduction of collagen, which is deposited in the skin. The collagen produced is insoluble and when deposited in the skin causes inflammation. Edema in the skin ultimately results in loss of elasticity and tissue function. The same process can occur internally, affecting blood vessels and organs.

SSc is relatively rare in that it affects approximately 300,000 Americans. It affects women three to four times more often than men. It can occur at any age but usually develops between ages 25 and 55. The disease tends to progress rapidly and does not respond well to treatment. Spontaneous remissions and exacerbations can occur. There is a relationship between scleroderma and Raynaud's syndrome; approximately 95% of patients with scleroderma have Raynaud's phenomenon.

Signs and Symptoms

Although arthritis and fatigue are commonly seen, the most obvious sign of SSc is manifested at first by pitting edema, starting in the upper extremities. The skin is taut, shiny, and without wrinkles. The swelling is replaced by tightening, hardening, and thickening of skin tissue. The skin then loses its elasticity, range of motion is decreased, and skin ulcers may appear. As the disease progresses, the patient loses range of motion and the affected area becomes contracted.

The same pathophysiological process affects certain body systems, especially the kidneys, lungs, heart, and gastrointestinal tract. If any of these systems are affected, the corresponding signs and symptoms are present. For example, gastrointestinal tract involvement usually manifests as esophagitis, dysphagia (difficulty swallowing), and decreased intestinal peristalsis caused by decreased smooth muscle elasticity.

The prognosis is thought to be worse when the patient has CREST syndrome, a group of signs and symptoms occurring at the same time:

Calcinosis (calcium deposits)
Raynaud's phenomenon (severe vasospasms of the small vessels in the hands and feet)
Esophageal dysmotility (decreased activity)
Sclerodactyly (scleroderma of the finger digits)
Telangiectasia (spiderlike skin lesions)

Diagnosis

The patient's clinical history and physical manifestations (particularly the sclerotic changes that occur in the skin) aid in the diagnosis of scleroderma. Biopsies of the skin, laboratory tests (ANA, and most recently anti–Scl-70 antibodies and anticentromere antibodies [ACA]), pulmonary function tests, and electrocardiographic (ECG) or x-ray examinations (including esophageal studies) are used to determine the severity of organ involvement or if other diagnostic testing is not helpful in diagnosing this condition.

Therapeutic Interventions

The goal of medical management is to slow the progression of the disease. Systemic steroids, such as prednisone, and immunosuppressant drugs are used in large doses and in combination during a flare-up of SSc.

Other care approaches are directed toward symptom management. Skin-protective measures can help minimize the chance of ulcerations or irritation. For example, teach the patient to use mild soaps and lotions to moisturize the skin.

If the patient has esophageal involvement, small, frequent, bland meals are better tolerated than large, spicy ones. Difficulty swallowing may necessitate cutting the food into smaller, more manageable portions or by providing food that is pureed (thicker liquids are easier to swallow than thin liquids). Medications to treat esophageal reflux, such as antacids and histamine blockers, may be prescribed.

Patients who have Raynaud's phenomenon or other types of **vasculitis** usually experience severe pain when small blood vessels constrict. Joints may also be painful. Pain management is a priority in the care of patients with SSc. A bed cradle or footboard keeps bed covers away from skin. Socks and gloves may keep the fingers and toes warm, thus diminishing pain. Minimizing exposure to cold and

---

scleroderma: sclero—hardening + derma—skin

vasculitis: vascul—blood vessel + itis—inflammation

avoiding stressful situations, stopping smoking, and taking certain medications, such as calcium channel blockers, anti-adrenergic agents, and angiotensin-converting enzyme (ACE) inhibitors, can all help promote circulation or minimize the likelihood of an attack. Research has suggested that antioxidant therapy may provide another approach to treating SSc.

Rehabilitative therapy may be needed to help the patient be as independent as possible with activities of daily living and mobility. Collaborate with other members of the interdisciplinary team to individualize care.

Osteogenesis Imperfecta

Osteogenesis imperfecta (OI) is a rare inheritable disease that is also called fragilitas ossium or brittle bones disease. It is a congenital abnormality characterized by skeletal bone fragility. The fragility predisposes the person to pathological fractures and bone deformities. In addition, there is connective tissue involvement which can cause changes or abnormalities in the eyes, ears, joints, skin, and teeth.

Pathophysiology

In OI, osteoblasts and fibroblasts synthesize collagen abnormally, resulting in fragile bones, multiple fractures (especially of the long bones), bone deformities (resulting from improper healing and weak callus formation along with thinner, smaller, and shorter bones), fragile and discolored teeth, loose joints, and thin, easily damaged skin. There are four types of OI classified according to severity and characteristics, with type 1 being the most common and least severe form of the condition.

Signs and Symptoms

There is much variation in the signs and symptoms for a person with OI. Some of the symptoms common to all types of OI include:

* Fragile bones (easily broken or bent)
* Triangular-shaped face
* Potential hearing loss
* Scoliosis (spine curvature) which may create respiratory problems
* Loose joints
* Alterations in muscle tone or development
* Blue, purple, or gray tint to sclerae
* Brittle or discolored teeth
* Smooth, thin skin

OI types II, III, and IV symptoms also include:

* Decreased height (may only grow to 3 feet tall)
* Barrel-shaped rib cage

Diagnosis

The diagnosis of OI may be based on clinical features of the patient. Most frequently, the diagnosis is made because of the frequency of fractures the patient (usually an infant or child) experiences without an apparent cause. Most OI patients can have 40 to 100 fractures by the time they reach puberty depending on the type of OI they have. It is also not uncommon for type II OI babies to be born with fractures and to either be born dead or die shortly after birth. The only test currently available is a biopsy of the skin assessing the collagen fibers. The test can take weeks to get results and is not definitive.

Therapeutic Interventions and Nursing Care

There is no treatment for OI. Therapy consists of treating the fractures and trying to minimize the bone deformities that result from the disease. Splints, casts, and braces are utilized to aid in healing the fractures and maintaining structure and function. Medications such as pamidronate (Aredia), a bone resorption inhibitor, are being trialed to see if bone density can be increased with the hope of decreasing fractures and improving mobility while decreasing the associated pain. Gene therapy is also being suggested as a means to treat OI; however, this form of therapy will not be soon available. Nursing care requires careful handling of the patients with the understanding that no matter how careful you may be, fractures will still occur. It is important to teach the family and for the nurse to understand that it is not necessarily something that they did that causes the fractures, rather it is the pathological process causing the breaks. The Osteogensis Imperfecta Foundation (www.oif.org) is an excellent resource for patients, family, and the health-care team.

Polymyositis

Polymyositis is a disease with an unknown cause that results in diffuse inflammation of skeletal muscle, leading to weakness, atrophy, and degeneration. When a rash is present with muscle inflammation, the disease is called dermatomyositis. The disease is progressive; however, remissions and exacerbations are common. Women are affected more than men, especially in their middle-aged years.

The shoulder and pelvic girdle muscles (proximal muscles) are most commonly affected. The patient may have associated conditions such as arthritis, fatigue, and possibly Raynaud's phenomenon (spasms and constriction of small vessels in the hands and feet). Patients with dermatomyositis also have the classic heliotrope (lilac) rash and periorbital (around the eyes) swelling. Malignant tumors occur in patients with these diseases more often than in the rest of the population.

Patients are treated symptomatically, using an interdisciplinary approach, to maintain optimum function. The drug of choice is high doses of prednisone. Side effects, such as immunosuppression, can occur with prednisone.

Muscular Dystrophy

Muscular dystrophy (MD) is a group of nine disorders resulting in loss of muscle tissue and progressive muscle weakness. A number of the disorders are diagnosed in childhood (e.g., Duchenne's MD is most common in children); however, other forms of MD, such as myotonic MD, are most common in adults. In addition, individuals with MD are now living longer into adulthood as a result of advances in treatment.

Pathophysiology and Etiology

Muscular dystrophy has a genetic origin. However, the exact cause is unknown. Skeletal (voluntary) muscle fibers degenerate and atrophy. This loss of muscle tissue results in muscle weakness and wasting. Muscle tissue is replaced by connective tissue. These changes in muscle tissue result in increasing disability and deformity. Life expectancy after diagnosis depends on the type of MD as well as the speed and severity of progression. Involvement of the heart and lungs also influences the life expectancy. In some forms of MD, young adulthood (mid to late 20s) is the average life expectancy.

Signs and Symptoms

Signs and symptoms usually become apparent in childhood. Difficulty walking and muscle weakness in the arms, legs, and trunk are indicators of MD. Individuals with MD may have difficulty raising their arms above their heads or climbing stairs. Other signs and symptoms include frequent falls, developmental delays involving muscle skills, drooping eyelids (ptosis), drooling, intellectual retardation (only in some types of MD), contractures, and skeletal deformities.

Diagnosis

An increase in serum creatinine phosphokinase (CPK) caused by muscle atrophy is present in MD. Electromyography (EMG) and muscle biopsy can be used for diagnosis. Lactic dehydrogenase (LDH) and the isoenzymes, myoglobin (urine or serum), creatinine (urine or serum), CPK isoenzymes, and aspartate aminotransferase (AST) levels may also be altered in patients with MD. There are also tests looking for gene mutations for some of the various types of MD.

Therapeutic Interventions

Goals include supportive care and prevention of complications. Treatment regimens focus on controlling symptoms and maximizing quality of life. Keeping the patient as active as possible is a priority in the planning of care. Exercise programs (e.g., range of motion, physical therapy) help prevent muscle tightness, contractures, and atrophy. Splints and braces provide support during ADL. Surgery may be done to correct deformities. The potential benefit of gene therapy is currently being investigated. Some of the current research indicates that gene therapy could prove effective with some types of MD.

Nursing Process for the Patient with Muscular Dystrophy

ASSESSMENT/DATA COLLECTION. Assess for muscle weakness, noting what areas of the body are affected and the severity of the weakness. Asking the patient and family what activities can be done with and without assistance helps determine the plan of care.

NURSING DIAGNOSIS, PLANNING, AND IMPLEMENTATION. Impaired physical mobility related to muscle weakness

EXPECTED OUTCOME: Patient's mobility will increase or be maintained for as long as possible.
- Provide assistive devices (e.g., braces, splints, wheelchair) *to assist with mobility.*
- Provide active and passive range-of-motion exercises and other physical therapy *to prevent contractures and improve muscle strength.*
- Encourage the patient to do as much as possible *to increase independence and help maintain muscle function.*
- Include disciplines such as physiotherapy and occupational therapy *to provide equipment and devices that will help with independence and mobility.*

Ineffective breathing pattern related to muscle weakness

EXPECTED OUTCOME: Patient will demonstrate normal respiratory function and normal oxygen saturation.
- Monitor respiratory function (rate and effort) every 4 hours.
- Monitor oxygen saturation and keep above 90%.
- Administer oxygen at 2 L/minute or as ordered if oxygen saturation drops below 90%.
- Position patient to increase respiratory efficiency.
- Teach and prepare patient about lung function studies to evaluate lungs
- Teach patient to minimize chances of infection (e.g., stay away from crowds) and to ensure early attention to respiratory alterations

EVALUATION. The outcome is met if the patient improves or maintains physical mobility and the patient's oxygen saturation is normal.

PATIENT EDUCATION. The patient and family need to understand the importance of physical therapy in maintaining function and preventing complications. National organizations and support groups provide information, resources, and emotional support. Family members need to encourage the patient to have activity and rest periods. As with any neuromuscular condition, the patient needs to avoid exposure to the cold and persons with infections. For more information on muscular dystrophy, visit www.mdausa.org or www.mdac.ca.

Osteoarthritis

Osteoarthritis (OA) is the most common type of connective tissue disorder, affecting more than 20 million people in the United States. The term *arthritis* means inflammation of the joint, but OA is not a primary inflammatory process. Therefore, some health-care providers may refer to this disorder as *degenerative joint disease.* This term better reflects its pathophysiology.

TABLE 46.3 OSTEOARTHRITIS AND RHEUMATOID ARTHRITIS SUMMARY

	Osteoarthritis	Rheumatoid Arthritis
Pathophysiology	Articular cartilage and bone ends deteriorate Joint is inflamed	Inflammatory cells cause synovitis Synovium becomes thick and fluid accumulates, causing swelling and pain Joint becomes deformed
Etiology	Primary (idiopathic): • Cause unknown • Risk factors include age, obesity, activities causing joint stress Secondary: • Causes include trauma, sepsis, congenital abnormalities, metabolic disorders (Paget's disease), rheumatoid arthritis	Autoimmune disease Can occur at any age (including juvenile rheumatoid arthritis) Cause unknown Familial history possible
Signs and Symptoms	Joint pain and stiffness Pain increases with activity and decreases with rest Nodes on joints of fingers (Heberden's nodes, Bouchard's nodes)	Symptoms vary according to disease process Early symptoms: • Bilateral and symmetrical joint inflammation • Redness, warmth, swelling, stiffness, pain • Stiffness after resting (morning stiffness) • Activity decreases pain and stiffness • Low-grade fever, weakness, fatigue, anorexia (mild weight loss) • Organ system involvement Late symptoms: • Joint deformity • Secondary osteoporosis
Therapeutic Interventions	Medication: • NSAIDs • Acetaminophen • Muscle relaxants • Cox-2 inhibitors Balanced rest and exercise Splinting of joint to promote rest Heat and cold Diet for weight loss Complementary therapies Surgery for total joint replacement	Medication: • Salicylates • NSAIDs • Gold treatment • Methotrexate • Prednisone Heat and cold Balanced rest and activity Surgery for total joint replacement
Possible Nursing Diagnoses	Chronic pain Impaired physical mobility Body image disturbance	Chronic pain Self-care deficits Ineffective health maintenance

ADLs = activities of daily living; NSAIDs = nonsteroidal anti-inflammatory drugs.

Pathophysiology

Osteoarthritis occurs when the articular cartilage and bone ends of joints slowly deteriorate (Table 46.3). The joint space narrows, bone spurs develop, and the joint may become somewhat inflamed. The repair process is not able to overcome the rapid loss of cartilage and bone, eventually resulting in joint deformities, pain, and immobility, leading to the patient's functional decline. Weight-bearing joints (hips and knees), hands, and the vertebral column are most often affected (Fig. 46.13).

Causes and Types

The most common type of OA is primary (idiopathic) osteoarthritis. The cause of OA is unknown, but several risk factors have been identified. Aging, obesity, and physical activities that create mechanical stress on joints are major risks. Each of these factors cause prolonged or excessive "wear and tear" on synovial joints. The majority of people older than 60 years of age have some degree of symptomatic joint degeneration. Native Americans are affected more often than other groups, but the reason for this is unknown.

Patients with secondary osteoarthritis develop joint degeneration as a result of trauma, sepsis, congenital anomalies, certain metabolic diseases (such as Paget's disease), or systemic inflammatory connective tissue disorders such as rheumatoid arthritis.

Signs and Symptoms

The patient usually seeks medical attention when joint pain and stiffness become severe or the patient has problems with everyday activities. One or more joints may be affected, most commonly in the hands, hips, knees, spine, and feet. Joint pain intensifies after physical activity but lessens following rest. If the vertebral column is involved, the patient

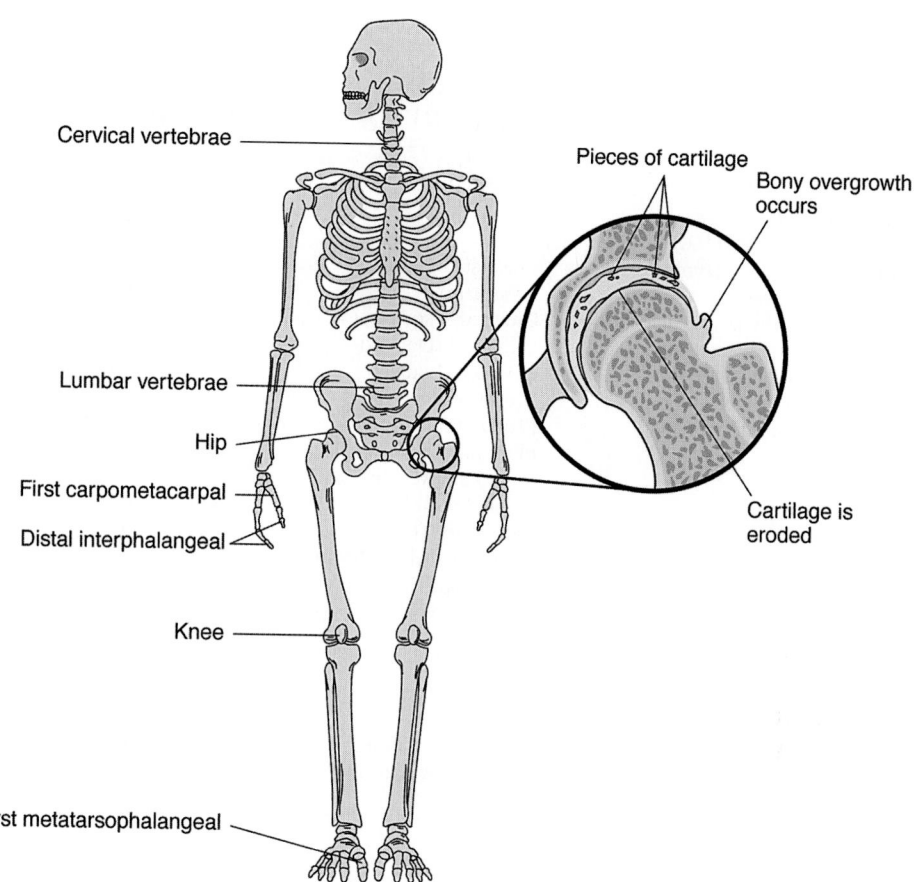

Cervical vertebrae

Pieces of cartilage

Bony overgrowth occurs

Lumbar vertebrae

Hip

First carpometacarpal

Distal interphalangeal

Knee

Cartilage is eroded

FIGURE 46.13 Common joints affected by osteoarthritis and the changes that result in the joint.

First metatarsophalangeal

complains of radiating pain and muscle spasms in the extremity innervated by the area affected.

About half of patients with OA have bony nodes on the joints of their fingers, called Heberden's and Bouchard's nodes. Women tend to have them more often than men, and they may or may not be painful. The nodes have a familial tendency and are often a cosmetic concern to female patients.

Diagnostic Tests

X-ray examinations are useful in outlining joint structure and detecting bone changes. A computed tomographic (CT) scan or magnetic resonance imaging (MRI) may be used to diagnose various joint involvement. Analysis of synovial fluid can aid in the diagnosis of OA while ruling out other pathological conditions of the joint.

Therapeutic Interventions

There is no curative therapy currently available for OA. Management of patients with OA centers on pain control, which is accomplished by drug therapy, other pain relief measures, or ultimately surgery. An interdisciplinary approach is needed to prevent decreased mobility and preserve joint function.

Synvisc is injected directly into osteoarthritic knees and acts like healthy, cushioning synovial fluid. Pain is relieved and flexibility restored when the knee joint is again lubricated and cushioned. For more information about this therapy, visit www.synvisc.com.

CRITICAL THINKING

Mr. Dennis

■ Mr. Dennis is a 59-year-old overweight carpenter who visits his physician with complaints of knee and wrist pain. He has noticed that it is becoming increasingly difficult to climb a ladder or use a hammer. The physician suspects osteoarthritis.

1. What data collection questions should be included in a patient history?
2. What risk factors does he have?
3. What other signs and symptoms might he have?

Suggested answers at end of chapter.

MEDICATION. Drug therapy, often used in combination with other therapies to reduce pain, is commonly used for patients with OA. The most typically used drugs are nonsteroidal anti-inflammatory drugs (NSAIDs) (Table 46.4). These drugs have analgesic and anti-inflammatory effects but may cause side effects if not carefully monitored. Common side effects include gastrointestinal (GI) distress; bleeding tendencies, which can be severe; and sodium and fluid retention. Older adult patients receiving NSAIDs on a routine basis should be carefully monitored for congestive heart failure or high blood pressure as a result of fluid reten-

TABLE 46.4 COMMON DRUGS USED TO TREAT CONNECTIVE TISSUE DISEASES: OSTEOARTHRITIS, RHEUMATOID ARTHRITIS, AND OTHERS

Medication Class/Action	Examples	Route	Side Effects	Nursing Implications
Nonsteroidal anti-inflammatory drugs (NSAIDs) Block activity of enzyme cyclooxygenase (COX-1, COX-2), which makes prostaglandins that produce inflammation, fever, pain; support platelets, and protect stomach lining (COX-1 only)	Acetylsalicylic acid (aspirin) Diclofenac sodium (Voltaren) Diflunisal (Dolobid) Etodolac (Lodine; osteoarthritis only) Fenoprofen (Nalfon) Flurbiprofen (Ansaid) Ibuprofen (Motrin) Indomethacin (Indocin) Ketoprofen (Orudis) Naproxen (Aleve, Naprosyn) Oxaprozin (Daypro) Piroxicam (Feldene) Nabumetone (Relafen) Sulindac (Clinoril) Tolmetin (Tolectin)	PO PO PO PO PO PO PO PO PO PO PO PO PO PO PO	Vary with drug: Nausea, vomiting, diarrhea, constipation, anorexia, rash, dizziness, headache, drowsiness, edema, ulcers, bleeding	Teach risk of GI bleeding greatest with COX-1 inhibitors Those with asthma higher risk for allergic reaction. Avoid use in children/teens with chickenpox or influeneza to prevent Reye's syndrome
Corticosteroids Reduce inflammation and swelling	Prednisone (Cortan, Deltasone, Orasone)	PO	Weight gain, fat deposits, edema, hypertension, infection, fractures, poor wound healing, GI bleeding, depression, mood swings	Daily weight Monitor I&O. Assess for infection. Give with food/milk Medic Alert ID Not used for osteoarthritis
Disease-modifying antirheumatic drugs (DMARDs) For rheumatoid arthritis, ankylosing spondylitis, lupus. Reduce symptoms, prevent joint damage, and preserve joint function by suppressing immune or inflammatory systems.			Vary with drug: Infection, alopecia, bone marrow suppression, kidney/liver damage.	Slow-acting drugs may take months for effect. Other drugs used to control symptoms until effective. Effect stops when drug stops
Gold Preparations	Auranofin (Ridaura) Aurothioglucose (Solganal)	PO IM		
Immunosuppressives	Azathioprine (Imuran) Cyclophosphamide (Cytoxan) Cyclosporine (Sandimmune, Neoral) Methotrexate (Mexate) Leflunomide (Arava; rheumatoid arthritis only) d-Penicillamine (Cuprimine, Depen). Sulfasalaine (Azaline, Azulfidine, Sulfzine) Etanercept (Enbrel)	PO IV, PO PO IM also PO PO PO		
Antitumor Necrosing Factor *Antimalarials*	Chloroquine (Aralen) Hydroxychloroquine (Plaquenil)	PO, IM PO		

tion. Topical creams such as capsaicin (ArthriCare) may also be ordered and applied to the joints. COX-1 and COX-2 inhibitors previously were frequently ordered for OA but ongoing concerns related to adverse cardiac events have resulted in a voluntary recall by the manufacturers, and therefore they are typically not being prescribed for patients with OA.

REST AND EXERCISE. Joint pain from OA tends to decrease with rest; therefore, pain is less severe in the morning. Activities should be scheduled at this time. A severely inflamed joint may be splinted by the occupational or physical therapist to promote rest to a selected joint. However, rest must be balanced with exercise to prevent muscle atrophy from disuse. Exercise has been identified as a means to maintain general health and weight, range of motion, and muscle strength, while decreasing anxiety and depression. To minimize muscle atrophy and to stabilize and protect arthritic joints, patients should be encouraged to perform exercises to strengthen their quadriceps if they have OA of the knee.

Joints should always be placed in their functional position—that is, a position that does not lead to contractures. For example, only a small pillow should be placed under the head when sleeping to prevent excessive neck flexion.

HEAT AND COLD. The patient with OA usually prefers heat therapy unless the joint is acutely inflamed. Hot packs, warm compresses, warm showers, moist heating pads, and paraffin dips provide sources of heat for the patient. Cold therapy minimizes inflammation while altering cutaneous pain receptors, thereby decreasing pain. Cold packs should be applied for no longer than 20 minutes at a time.

Diet

The obese or overweight patient benefits from losing weight to decrease joint stress on weight-bearing joints, thereby reducing pain. If the patient is on medications that can alter fluid volumes (corticosteroids), a diet low in sodium may be appropriate.

COMPLEMENTARY THERAPIES. The popularity of complementary therapies to reduce pain and stress has grown tremendously. Imagery, music therapy, acupressure, acupuncture, and other holistic modalities that foster the mind-body-spirit connection work well for many people. Homeopathic therapies such as glucosamine and chondroitin have been suggested to improve OA. Recent studies have demonstrated that these two therapies are effective in OA therapy; however, further research must be conducted before they become an accepted and recommended therapy for OA.

SURGERY. If the patient's pain is not successfully managed, a total joint replacement (TJR) may be indicated. A TJR is the most common type of **arthroplasty** (see section on musculoskeletal surgery).

---

arthroplasty: arthro—joint + plasty—creation of

Nursing Process for the Patient with Osteoarthritis

ASSESSMENT/DATA COLLECTION. The patient's complaint of pain is assessed and the joints observed for signs of inflammation or deformity. Also assessed are function, alterations in activities of daily living (ADLs), and mobility (see Chapter 45).

NURSING DIAGNOSIS, PLANNING, IMPLEMENTATION, AND EVALUATION. Chronic pain related to chronic inflammatory disease

EXPECTED OUTCOME: Patient will state pain is within tolerable levels (pain assessment scale 0 to 10).

- Ensure patient is aware that his or her pain is acknowledged by the nurse so that he or she knows the pain is accepted.
- Provide analgesics as ordered *to help alleviate painful sensations.*
- Collaborate with interdisciplinary team such as pain clinic to explore alternative pain relief measures such as surgery.
- Consider alternative methods of therapy such as guided imagery, distraction, acupuncture, and biofeedback to use all possible methods of pain control.

Activity intolerance related to pain

EXPECTED OUTCOME: Patient will participate in ADLs as tolerated.

- Promote as much independence as possible *to promote activity.*
- Assist with ADLs as necessary *to ensure patient does not become exhausted.*
- Provide pain relief measures prior to activity, which will help them increase their activity level.
- Ensure nursing interventions are performed in "groups" *to minimize patient exertion.*
- Collaborate with interdisciplinary team (e.g., occupational therapy, home care physiotherapy) *to utilize their resources and knowledge.*

Chronic sorrow related to altered body image, altered role, pain, and ongoing losses

EXPECTED OUTCOME: Patient will verbalize improvement in feelings of sorrow

- Allow for time to discuss feelings and anticipate trigger events *to ensure the patient is aware of what may increase his or her feelings of sorrow.*
- Encourage use of interdisciplinary team such as social worker, psychologist, clergy, or spiritual advisor *to provide alternate methods of dealing with sorrow.*
- Encourage use of support groups to enable the patient to discuss his or her concern with others experiencing the same problems.

Disturbed body image related to changes in joint function and structure

EXPECTED OUTCOME: *Patient will demonstrate acceptance of changes in body image.*

- Encourage patient to discuss feelings and concerns *so patient knows nurse understands what patient is experiencing.*
- Provide information and clarify misconceptions *to ensure that the patient is aware of the expected problems and concerns.*
- Encourage socialization *to improve on the person's perceptions of how he or she "looks" to others.*
- Encourage sharing with support groups so that the patient discusses his or her concerns with others experiencing the same problems.

Impaired physical mobility related to altered joint function and pain

EXPECTED OUTCOME: *Patient will demonstrate improved physical mobility.*

- Administer analgesics and anti-inflammatory agents as ordered *to improve joint function and decrease pain.*
- Encourage active ROM exercises *to prevent or minimize further alteration in joint function*
- Ensure proper positioning and alignment *to promote joint function and decrease pain.*
- Use interdisciplinary team such as physiotherapy and occupational therapy *to utilize resources and knowledge from other sources.*

Self-care deficit related to chronic degenerative joint disease

EXPECTED OUTCOME: *Patient will be able to provide own self-care.*

- Encourage independence to decrease feelings of despair about being unable to care for self.
- Assist when necessary to minimize frustration when patient unable to perform self-care function.
- Teach patient about assistive devices *to help with ADLs to promote self-care.*
- Collaborate with interdisciplinary team such as home care, occupational therapy, or physiotherapy *to acquire assistive devices and use alternate resources.*

EVALUATION. The outcome is met if patient reports pain is within tolerable levels on pain assessment scale of 0 to 10, verbalizes improvement in feelings of sorrow, demonstrates acceptance of changes in body image, demonstrates improved physical mobility, and is able to provide own self-care.

PATIENT EDUCATION. A vital function of each member of the health-care team is health teaching. The patient with OA is seldom admitted to the hospital for treatment of OA unless surgery is scheduled. However, many patients with OA are admitted for other reasons, and their arthritis needs must also be considered in the comprehensive plan of care.

Most patients residing in nursing homes also have OA, which can affect their participation in recreational activities, as well as their ADLs.

In any setting, including the home, patients can be taught ways to protect their joints and conserve energy. Nurses need to teach patients and their families how to promote health. For information on educational materials and self-help courses, visit the Arthritis Foundation at www.arthritis.org.

Rheumatoid Arthritis

Rheumatoid arthritis (RA) is a chronic, progressive, systemic inflammatory disease that destroys synovial joints and other connective tissues, including major organs. It affects women three times more often than men and Native Americans more often than other ethnic groups. Rheumatoid arthritis can occur at any age; when it occurs in children it is called juvenile RA (JRA). The peak onset of RA is 30 to 60 years of age, and it affects 1% to 3% of the population in the United States. The etiology of RA is still unknown; however, there are indications that genetic predisposition and the environment play a role in triggering its development.

Pathophysiology

Inflammatory cells and chemicals cause **synovitis,** an inflammation of the synovium (the lining of the joint capsule). As the inflammation progresses, the synovium becomes thick and fluid accumulation causes joint swelling and pain. A destructive pannus (new synovial tissue growth infiltrated with inflammatory cells) erodes the joint cartilage and eventually destroys the bone within the joint (Fig. 46.14). Ultimately the pannus is converted to bony tissue, resulting in loss of mobility. Joint deformity and bone loss are common in late RA (see Table 46.3).

Synovial joints are not the only connective tissues involved in RA. Any connective tissue may be affected, including blood vessels, nerves, kidneys, pericardium, lungs, and subcutaneous tissue. The result of body system involvement is malfunction or failure of the organ or system. Death can occur if the disease does not respond to treatment.

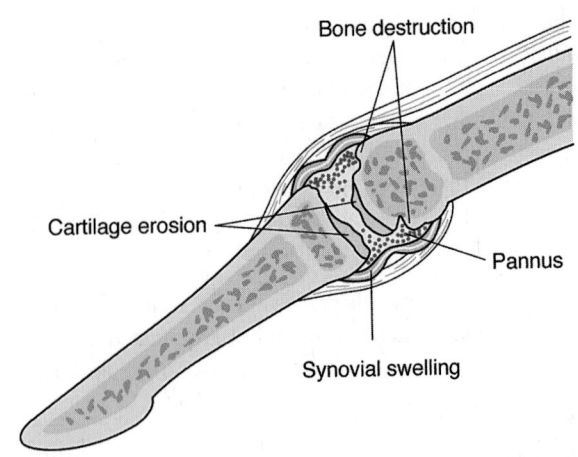

FIGURE 46.14 Rheumatoid arthritis.

Many patients experience spontaneous remissions and exacerbations (flare-ups) of RA. The symptoms of the disease may disappear without treatment for months or years. Then the disease may exacerbate just as unpredictably. Exacerbations usually occur when the patient experiences physical or emotional stress, such as surgery or infection.

Etiology

The exact cause of RA is unknown. An autoimmune response occurs that affects the synovial membrane of the joints; it is unknown what triggers the initial response. Antibodies (called rheumatoid factor) are often found in patients with RA. It is suggested that these antibodies join with other antibodies and form antibody complexes. These complexes lodge in synovium and other connective tissues, causing local and systemic inflammation, and may be responsible for the destructive changes of RA in body tissues.

The origin of the rheumatoid factor is not clear, but a genetic predisposition is likely. RA affects people with a family history of the disease two to three times more often than the rest of the population.

Signs and Symptoms

Signs and symptoms vary as the disease progresses differently in patterns and rates from person to person. In general, the signs and symptoms can be divided into early and late manifestations.

The typical pattern of joint inflammation is bilateral and symmetrical. The disease usually begins in the upper extremities and progresses to other joints over many years (Fig. 46.15). Affected joints are slightly reddened, warm, swollen, stiff, and painful. The patient with RA often has morning stiffness lasting for up to an hour, and those with severe disease may complain of stiffness all day. Generally, activity decreases pain and stiffness.

Because of the systemic nature of RA, the patient may have a low-grade fever, malaise, depression, lymphadenopathy, weakness, fatigue, anorexia, and weight loss. As the disease worsens, major organs or body systems are affected. Joint deformities occur as a late symptom, and secondary osteoporosis (bone loss) can lead to fractures.

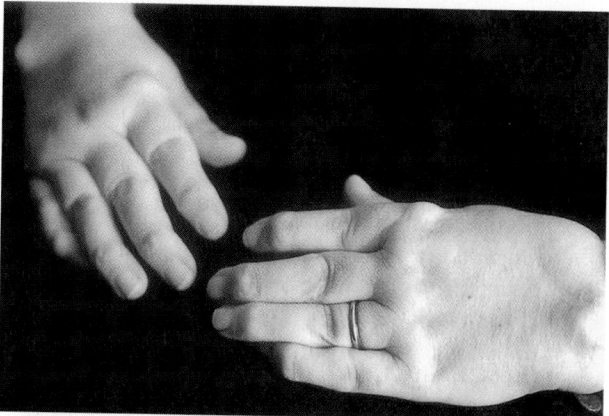

FIGURE 46.15 Joint abnormalities in hands of patient with rheumatoid arthritis.

Several associated syndromes are seen in some patients with rheumatoid arthritis. For example, Sjögren's syndrome is an inflammation of tear ducts (causing dry eyes) and salivary glands (causing dry mouth). Felty's syndrome is less common and is characterized by an enlarged liver and spleen and leukopenia (decreased white blood cell count).

Diagnosis

No specific diagnostic test confirms RA, but several laboratory tests help support the diagnosis. An increase in white blood cells and platelets is typical, unless the patient has Felty's syndrome. A group of immunologic tests are usually performed, and typical findings for patients with RA include the following:

- Presence of rheumatoid factor (RF) in serum
- Decreased red blood cell (RBC) count
- Decreased C4 complement
- Increased erythrocyte sedimentation rate (ESR)
- Positive antinuclear antibody (ANA) test
- Positive C-reactive protein (CRP) test

RF can indicate the aggressiveness of the disease. However, it is not specific to RA and can also be found in systemic lupus erythematosus, connective tissue disease, and myositis. The ESR is also obtained to evaluate the effectiveness of treatment. If the disease responds to treatment, the ESR decreases. The higher the ESR, the more active the disease process.

LEARNING TIP

ESR is a general screening test for inflammation. It measures the amount of time it takes for RBCs to settle to the bottom of a test tube. In the presence of inflammation, RBCs settle faster in the tube. Therefore, the ESR increases with the presence of inflammation.

X-ray examination and MRI detect joint damage and bone loss, especially in the vertebral column. A bone or joint scan assesses the extent of joint involvement throughout the body. For some patients, an **arthrocentesis** may be performed; the synovial fluid is cloudy, milky, or dark yellow with inflammatory cells present.

Therapeutic Interventions

Like patients with osteoarthritis, patients with RA experience chronic joint pain. Pain can interfere with mobility or the ability to perform ADLs. Drug therapy is often needed to relieve or reduce pain as well as to slow the progression of the disease.

MEDICATION. Treatment for RA includes disease-modifying antirheumatic drugs (DMARDs), which can prevent joint destruction, deformity, and disability with early single or combination drug use; NSAIDs; and corticosteroids. (See Table 46.4.) Newer DMARDs such as leflunomide (Arava) and etanercept (Enbrel) are used to slow the progression of RA. Leflunomide taken orally has anti-proliferative and anti-inflammatory properties. Etanercept inhibits tumor necrosis factor, which is involved in the inflammatory process, and is given subcutaneously twice a week. Low-dose methotrexate (MTX) or gold therapy is given to induce disease remission. NSAIDs such as aspirin and ibuprofen are prescribed for pain and stiffness, although they do not slow the disease process. Prednisone is a corticosteroid used to induce disease remission. Many of these medications have potentially serious side effects that must be monitored carefully.

Complementary therapies that may help decrease inflammation or pain include capsaicin cream, fish oil, magnetic therapy, and antioxidants such as vitamin C, vitamin E, and beta carotene (see Chapter 4).

HEAT AND COLD. Heat applications or hot showers help decrease joint stiffness and make exercise easier for the patient. For acutely inflamed, or "hot," joints, cold applications are preferred. As for patients with osteoarthritis, a program that balances rest and exercise later in the day is most beneficial for the patient.

SURGERY. If nonsurgical approaches are not effective in relieving arthritic pain, the patient may have a total joint replacement (discussed later). In general, patients with RA who have surgery are not as successful when compared with patients with osteoarthritis. The presence of a systemic disease predisposes patients with RA to more postoperative complications.

Nursing Process for the Patient with Rheumatoid Arthritis

ASSESSMENT/DATA COLLECTION. A thorough history and physical assessment are needed for the patient with RA because the disease can involve every system of the body. In addition to assessing physical signs and symptoms, assess the patient for psychosocial, functional, and vocational needs.

After having the disease for approximately 15 years, fewer than half of RA patients are totally independent in their ADLs. These limitations may place a burden on family members, who must be included in the care of the patient with RA. Many patients with the disease are young or middle aged. RA can impair their ability to work, depending on the type of job they have. The health-care team assesses the patient's work skills to determine the need for changes in the workplace or a need to train for a new type of work.

NURSING DIAGNOSIS, PLANNING, AND IMPLEMENTATION. Acute pain related to chronic disease process

EXPECTED OUTCOME: Patient will report relief from pain.
- Provide analgesics as ordered *to relieve pain.*
- Ensure proper positioning and alignment *to minimize discomfort and promote pain relief.*
- Teach alternative measure of pain relief to maximize means *to relieve pain.*
- Encourge maintenance of normal weight *to prevent excess wear and tear of joints.*

Disturbed body image related to changes resulting from disease process

EXPECTED OUTCOME: Patient will come to accept alterations in body.
- Encourage patient to discuss feelings and concerns *to provide the nurse with an understanding of what the patient is experiencing.*
- Provide information and clarify misconceptions *to ensure that the patient is aware of the expected problems and concerns.*
- Encourage socialization *to improve on the person's perceptions of how they "look" to others.*
- Encourage sharing with support groups *so that the patient discusses their concerns with others experiencing the same problems.*

Fatigue related to chronic pain and suffering and difficulty with mobilization

EXPECTED OUTCOME: Patient will have decreased episodes of fatigue.
- Ensure regular rest periods throughout the day *to not overexert the patient.*
- Assist as required *to minimize the amount of energy the patient needs to use.*
- Teach patient the need to delegate *to ensure they do not overexert.*
- Teach energy conservation techniques *to reduce workload.*

Self-care deficit related to chronic degenerative disease process

EXPECTED OUTCOME: Patient will be able to provide own self-care.
- Encourage independence *to decrease feelings of despair about being unable to care for self.*
- Assist when necessary *to minimize frustration when patient unable to perform self-care function.*
- Teach patient about assistive devices to help with ADL *to promote self-care.*
- Collaborate with interdisciplinary team such as home care, occupational or physiotherapy *to acquire assistive devices and use alternate resources.*

Impaired physical mobility related to chronic inflammation of joints

EXPECTED OUTCOME: Patient will have improved physical mobility.
- Administer analgesics and anti-inflammatory agents *to reduce pain and increase mobility*
- Administer heat and cold therapy *to aid in joint function and movement.*
- Encourage continued mobilization *to minimize complications of immobility.*
- Collaborate with other disciplines *to help with maintaining mobility.*

EVALUATION. The outcome is met if patient reports pain is within acceptable levels on pain assessment scale of

0 to 10, demonstrates acceptance of changes in body image, has decreased episodes of fatigue, is able to provide own self-care, and demonstrates improved physical mobility.

CRITICAL THINKING

Mrs. Summers

■ Mrs. Summers is a 48-year-old nurse who has had upper extremity joint pain and swelling for about 4 years. She was recently diagnosed with rheumatoid arthritis (RA) but has no systemic involvement other than extreme fatigue at this time. She is concerned that she will have to give up providing direct patient care on a busy medical unit in the local hospital.

1. What questions might you ask her at this time about her illness?
2. What should you teach her about pain management?

Suggested answers at end of chapter.

Patient Education

The patient with RA needs extensive patient education regarding the disease process, medication management, and the comprehensive plan of care. Many fads and myths published in popular tabloids are available, and some publicized "cures" can actually be harmful to the patient.

In collaboration with health team members, help the patient plan a daily schedule that balances rest and exercise. Child care responsibilities and other day-to-day activities need to be scheduled. A vocational counselor may be necessary for job training if the patient needs to pursue a different occupation. Patients who are unable to work may be able to qualify for disability benefits through the Social Security program.

Inform the patient about community resources. For example, the local chapter of the Arthritis Foundation provides support groups, information, and other resources for patients with RA and other types of connective tissue disorders. (See Web link in section on osteoarthritis.)

MUSCULOSKELETAL SURGERY

Some health problems cannot be managed conservatively and require surgery. Other disorders are initially treated medically but may need surgery if treatment is unsuccessful. The most common surgeries are discussed here.

Total Joint Replacement

Total joint replacement (TJR) is most often performed for patients who have some type of connective tissue disease in which their joints become severely deteriorated. TJR may also be done for patients on long-term steroid therapy, such as patients with SLE or asthma. Long-term use of steroids, trauma, and complications of joint replacement can cause

avascular necrosis (AVN), a condition in which bone tissue dies (usually the femoral head) as a result of impaired blood supply. Advanced AVN is very painful and usually does not respond to conservative pain relief measures. The primary goal of TJR is to relieve severe chronic pain and improve ability to carry out ADLs when no other treatment is successful.

The most common surgeries are the total hip replacement (THR) and total knee replacement (TKR), although any synovial joint can be replaced. Another term used for joint replacement is *arthroplasty*. The replacement devices, sometimes referred to as prostheses, are made of metal, ceramic, plastic, or a combination of these materials. Some prostheses are held in place by cement. Others are secured by the patient's bone as it grafts and connects to the prosthesis. Bone substitutes, also called biologics, are being used more often when the amount of available bone is insufficient to provide a good base of support for the replacement devices. Bone glues and fillers such as Osteoset or Pro Osteon and bone stimulants such as Allomatrix help in providing better support for the prosthetics used.

Total Hip Replacement

A THR uses a two-piece device consisting of an acetabular cup that is inserted into the pelvic acetabulum and a femoral component that is inserted into the femur to replace the femoral head and neck (Fig. 46.16). The average life span of a cemented THR is about 10 years. Noncemented prostheses used in younger patients may last longer.

PREOPERATIVE CARE. Total joint surgery is an elective procedure and scheduled far enough in advance to allow ample time for preoperative teaching and screening. A case

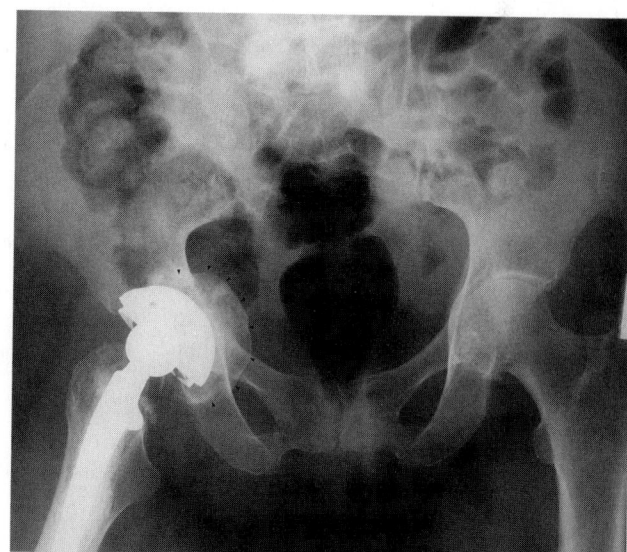

FIGURE 46.16 Total hip arthroplasty of arthritic right hip. *(From McKinnis, LN: Fundamentals of Orthopedic Radiology. F.A. Davis, Philadelphia, 1997, with permission.)*

---

avascular necrosis: a—without + vascular—blood + necrosis—death

manager (registered nurse or social worker) may be assigned to assess the patient's needs and the support systems that are available postoperatively. It is important for the patient to have a caregiver who can assist the patient after surgery.

In addition to the normal preparations for preoperative care (see Chapter 11), the orthopedic patient requires some preoperative baseline assessments. The nurse assesses the neurovascular status (circulation, sensation, mobility) of the extremity to be operated on as well as the patient's level of pain preoperatively. Preoperative mobility can also be assessed to help determine the effectiveness of the surgery postoperatively. The patient may require an IV to be started as the surgeon frequently orders a prophylactic antibiotic preoperatively to minimize the chance of an infection (especially osteomyelitis) developing. The patient is taught about the surgery and what to expect postoperatively. Some patients are scheduled to meet with the physical therapist to learn postoperative exercises and how to ambulate with a walker or crutches. Some institutions have total joint education programs, which are a series of educational sessions designed to make the recovery process smoother and more effective for the patient.

Depending on the amount of blood loss during surgery, some patients receive postoperative blood transfusions. Because total joint surgery is an elective procedure, the physician may order autologous blood donation by the patient. The patient donates blood before surgery per guidelines (e.g., time frames specified, hemoglobin levels normal), which is then available for reinfusion postoperatively as needed. This predeposited blood donation is cost effective and reassures patients who are concerned about receiving blood from other donors.

Patients are often admitted to the hospital the morning of surgery. The patient's length of stay is about 3 to 5 days, depending on the patient's age and progress. Some hospitals have joint camp programs where a group of patients undergoing joint replacements are admitted on the same day, undergo their surgery, and then recover together during activities such as physical therapy with each other for support. Patients have been known to recover more easily in this type of supportive environment and are typically discharged in about 3 days.

POSTOPERATIVE CARE. In addition to providing the general postoperative care that all patients undergoing general or epidural anesthesia require, plan and implement interventions to help prevent the following common complications of THR (see Chapter 11).

Hip Dislocation. The most common postoperative complication for the patient having a THR is subluxation (partial dislocation) or total dislocation. Dislocation occurs when the femoral component becomes dislodged from the acetabular cup. Frequently, if a dislocation occurs, there is an audible "pop" followed by immediate pain in the affected hip. In addition to the pain, the patient experiences shortening of the surgical leg, and possibly rotation of the surgical leg. If any of these signs and symptoms occur, notify the surgeon immediately and keep the patient in bed. Additional analgesics may be ordered until the patient can be taken to the operating room. Under anesthesia, the surgeon manipulates the hip back into alignment and immobilizes the leg until healing occurs.

Prevention of dislocation is a major nursing responsibility. Correct positioning of the surgical leg is critical. The primary goals are to prevent hip adduction (across the body's midline) and hyperflexion (bending forward more than 90 degrees). To accomplish these goals, place the patient returning from the postanesthetic care unit (PACU) in a supine position with the head slightly elevated. A trapezoid-shaped abduction pillow (sometimes called a triangular pillow), splint, wedge, or regular bed pillows may be used between the legs to prevent adduction (Fig. 46.17). The patient can be turned to either side (even the operative side if the patient is comfortable enough) or to the side specified by the physician, with hip adduction avoided. The patient is turned with the abductor pillow or three regular pillows (one proximal and two distal) in place between the legs. When turning, it is important to turn the hip and legs simultaneously to minimize the chance of dislocation. Support for the leg and abductor pillow is also required when the patient is turned on his or her side to decrease the chance of dislocation.

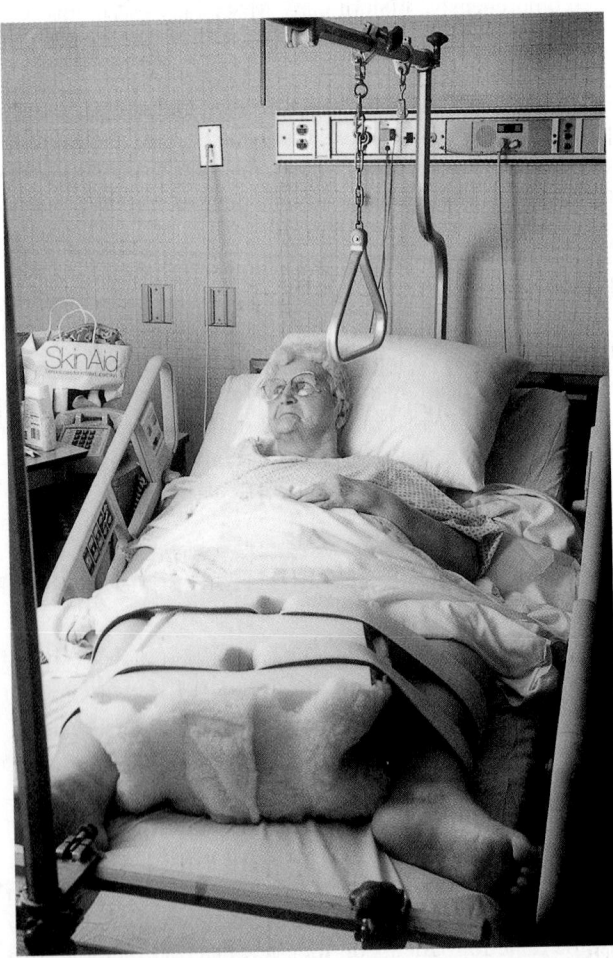

FIGURE 46.17 Abductor pillow is used to prevent adduction and hip dislocation.

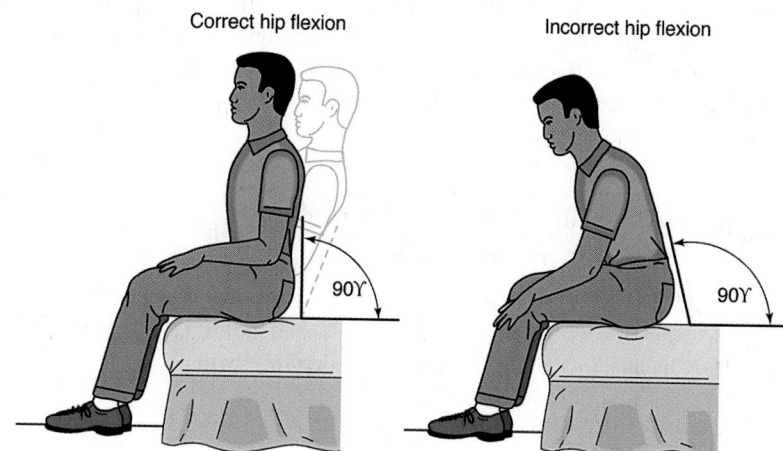

Correct hip flexion

Incorrect hip flexion

90Υ

90Υ

FIGURE 46.18 Hip flexion after total hip replacement should be 90 degrees or less to prevent dislocation.

To prevent hyperflexion, some surgeons initially allow the patient to sit at no more than a 60-degree angle in a reclining chair. The patient's position is progressed to 90 degrees, the maximum allowed to prevent hyperflexion (Fig. 46.18). While the patient is on bedrest, the use of a fracture (also called a slipper) pan when toileting the patient is recommended to minimize discomfort and to prevent the possibility of dislocation.

Skin Breakdown. Because most patients having total joint replacements are older, skin breakdown is a major concern as part of postoperative care. Turning the patient at least every 2 hours (more often if high risk) and keeping the heels off the bed are the key nursing interventions to prevent pressure ulcers. Heels, elbows, and the sacrum are vulnerable and can break down in 24 hours. A reddened area that does not blanch is a stage 1 pressure ulcer and must be treated aggressively to prevent progression to other stages. Prophylactic application of DuoDerm dressings, as well as heel protectors help to decrease the chance of skin breakdown of the heels.

Patients who are incontinent must be kept clean and dry. Toileting the patient every 2 hours and using a protective barrier cream also help prevent skin problems related to incontinence. Adequate diet and hydration are also important to prevent skin breakdown. Box 46.7 (Nursing Interventions Following Total Hip Replacement) describes additional nursing interventions that meet the needs of postoperative patients recovering from THR.

Infection. Orthopedic surgery patients are at an increased risk for infection because of the nature of the surgery and because the patients are often older adults with an already increased risk for postoperative complications. In addition to the preoperative prophylactic intravenous antibiotic, the surgeon can administer antibiotics intraoperatively, and may continue antibiotics for 24 hours postoperatively.

Depending on the institution's policies, the surgeon may or may not remove the initial dressing. Regardless of who removes the dressing, meticulous aseptic care of the surgical wound is important to minimize the chance of infection. Care of the incision, as well as exit sites for drains,

needs to be performed aseptically. When doing dressing changes, observe the incision routinely for signs and symptoms of infection (redness, swelling, warmth, odor, pain, drainage [yellow, green, or brown tinged]). Monitor temperature carefully. An older patient may not experience a fever but may appear confused instead.

Infection may not occur during the patient's hospital stay but can occur 1 or more years later. If this late infection

Box 46.7

Nursing Interventions Following Total Hip Replacement

- Ensure hip that the hip is not allowed to become adducted. Use triangular (abductor) pillow or pillows.
- Turning patient requires abductor pillow to remain in place. Turn patient as a whole, not allowing hip or legs to fall forward or backward. Use pillows to support raised limb.
- Monitor for skin integrity of opposite heel (often used to help mobilize in bed so is prone to friction and pressure sores. Apply protective devices for heels.
- Ensure limb remains in abduction when moving patient out of bed.
- Prevent postoperative pneumonia by encouraging deep breathing and coughing and use of incentive spirometer.
- Pain control is of the utmost importance. Provide regularly scheduled analgesics and ensure breakthrough analgesia is provided prn. Decreased pain allows for earlier mobilization and less complications of immobility.
- Monitor level of consciousness and orientation. Many older patients have alterations in their mental status after surgery due to anaesthetics, analgesics, blood loss, and environmental changes.

does not respond to antibiotics, the prosthesis may be removed and replaced. To prevent infection, antibiotics are often instilled directly into the wound during surgery as beads, as part of the cement mixture, or as an irrigating solution.

CRITICAL THINKING

Mrs. Jacobs

■ Mrs. Jacob's is 78 years old and has had a left THR 3 days ago. When changing her dressing you notice a purulent discharge. Cefaclor (Ceclor) 500 mg PO q8hr is ordered. It is available as a 375-mg/5-mL suspension. How many milliliters should Mrs. Jacobs be given?

Suggested answers at end of chapter.

Bleeding. Like any surgical wound, some bleeding is expected. In joint replacement surgery, up to two-thirds of the blood loss can occur postoperatively. The patient often has at least one surgical drain (e.g., Hemovac or Jackson-Pratt) that is emptied every 8 to 12 hours or as required for the first day or two. Monitor the dressing for signs of bleeding and reinforce the dressing if needed. On the second or third postoperative day, the patient's hemoglobin and hematocrit may decrease to the point that blood transfusion is needed. The patient may receive the preoperatively donated autologous blood or may receive salvaged operative or postoperative blood. Using a cell saver (sometimes called an orthopat, which stands for orthopedic patient auto-transfusion) during surgery, about 50% of blood that is lost can be recovered and saved for reinfusion into the same patient. Postoperatively, blood can be replaced by collecting shed blood via suction into a reservoir, then filtering and reinfusing it within 6 hours of collection. Monitoring for blood loss and signs of shock is an important nursing consideration.

Neurovascular Compromise. For any musculoskeletal surgery or injury, frequent neurovascular checks for circulation (color, warmth, pulses), sensation, and movement are performed distal to the surgical procedure or injury (and compared to the unaffected side) when vital signs are checked. The procedure and significance of these assessments are described in Chapter 45.

Pain. Because patients undergoing THR are in chronic pain preoperatively, some patients report that they have less pain postoperatively than they had before surgery. Initially pain is typically managed by epidural analgesia, patient-controlled analgesia (PCA), or injections with analgesics. After the first postoperative day, the patient usually progresses to oral opioid analgesia with a drug (such as Percocet or Tylenol with codeine). Proper positioning also helps minimize surgical discomfort.

Ambulation. Care for the patient having a THR is interdisciplinary. The patient usually gets out of bed and into a chair the night of surgery or early the next day. Ensure that the patient does not adduct or hyperflex the surgical hip during transfer to the chair. The chair should have a straight back and be high enough to prevent excessive flexion. The toilet seat should also be raised for the same purpose. Permitted amounts of weight bearing depend on the type of prosthesis that is used. In general, weight bearing as tolerated or full weight bearing is used for cemented prostheses. If an uncemented device is used, the patient may be restricted to toe-touch, or partial weight bearing, or featherweight bearing.

Early ambulation helps prevent postoperative complications such as atelectasis and deep vein thrombosis (DVT). The physical therapist works with the patient for ambulation with a walker or crutches. Crutches are reserved for young patients. After 4 to 6 weeks, the patient is progressed to a cane. The patient does not need an ambulatory device if there is no limping.

Thromboembolitic Complications. Patients having hip surgery are at greatest risk for DVT or pulmonary embolus (PE). Older adult patients are especially at risk because of compromised circulation. Obese patients and those with a history of thromboembolitic (TE) problems are also at an exceptionally high risk for potentially fatal problems.

Thigh-high elastic stockings and sequential compression devices (SCDs) may be used while the patient is hospitalized (see Chapter 11). The surgeon orders an anticoagulant medication to help prevent clot formation, including subcutaneous low molecular weight heparin (such as enoxaparin [Lovenox], dalteparin [Fragmin]) or oral warfarin (Coumadin). Occasionally, heparin is still used, and if so, it is important to monitor for heparin-induced thrombocytopenia, which can occur as early as 3 days after the start of heparin therapy. The ordered daily dosage of these drugs is determined by coagulation studies. Partial thromboplastin times are monitored for patients on heparin. International normalized ratio (INR) reported with prothrombin time is monitored when giving warfarin.

NURSING CARE TIP

When giving enoxaparin or dalteparin, follow manufacturer's instructions for administration. The air bubble should not be removed from the pre-filled syringe before administration to ensure the whole dose is given.

Because most DVTs occur in the lower extremities, leg exercises are started in the immediate postoperative period and continued until the patient is fully ambulatory. The physical therapist teaches the patient how to perform foot and ankle exercises such as heel pumping, foot circles, and straight-leg raises (SLRs). The patient also performs quadriceps-setting exercises (quad sets) by straightening the legs and pushing the back of the knees toward the bed. Remind the patient to do several sets of these exercises each day to improve muscle tone and to help prevent blood clots in the leg.

Self-Care. Because of restrictions in hip flexion, patients are instructed not to bend forward to tie shoes or put on pants. The occupational therapist provides adaptive or assistive devices, such as dressing sticks and long-handled shoe horns, to assist the patient in being independent in activities of daily living.

If the patient is medically stable, he or she is discharged home for rehabilitation or to a subacute care unit, rehabilitation unit, or nursing home for short-term rehabilitation, lasting a week or less. The rehabilitation program that began in the hospital continues after discharge until the patient is independent in ambulation and self-care.

Before hospital discharge, the interdisciplinary team provides patient education for home care, including hip precautions that need to be used until the surgeon reevaluates the patient at the 6- to 8-week follow-up visit (Box 46.8 Educating the Patient After Total Hip Replacement and Home Health Hints).

Total Knee Replacement

The knee is the second most commonly replaced joint. It requires three components for replacement: a femoral component, a tibial component, and a patellar button (Fig. 46.19).

Care for the patient with a TKR is similar to that required for a patient with a hip replacement except dislocation and, therefore, preventive positioning are not a concern. Postoperatively, there is usually a bulky dressing along with the normal surgical drain in place. Once again, it is impor-

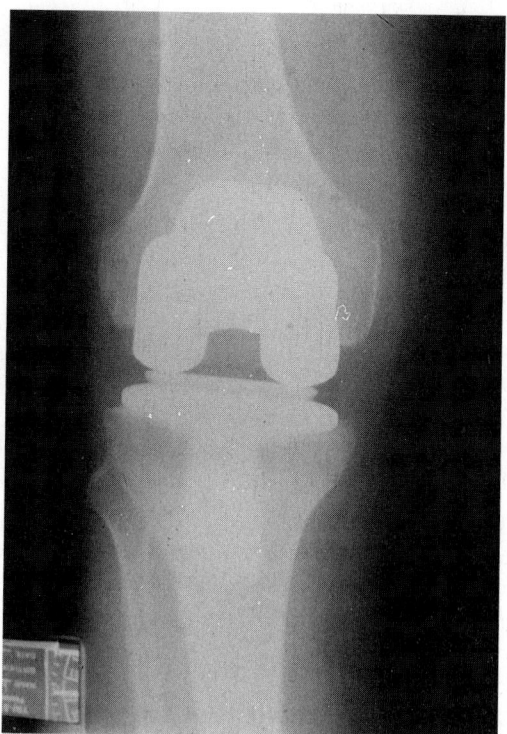

FIGURE 46.19 Knee joint replacement. *(From Richardson, JK, and Iglarsh, ZA: Clinical Orthopaedic Physical Therapy. Saunders, Philadelphia, 1994, p 651, with permission.)*

tant to monitor for bleeding along with the normal postoperative interventions. Although precautions to prevent dislocation are not applicable for the patient with a knee replacement, other medical complications described for THR, such as deep vein thrombosis, may be seen in the patient undergoing knee replacement (see Box 46.7 Nursing Interventions Following Total Hip Replacement).

Postoperatively, a continuous passive motion machine (CPM) may be used for the operative leg. This motorized machine has a flexible extremity rest (for either the leg or arm) that glides back and forth on a track (Fig. 46.20). The CPM is set at the degree of flexion and speed ordered by the physician and is usually begun in the PACU. The CPM can be applied by a nurse, physical therapist, or technician and is used either intermittently up to 8 to 12 hours a day or continuously while the patient is in bed. The purpose of CPM is to keep the knee joint mobile. Nursing care associated with the use of the machine is summarized in Box 46.9 Application of a Continuous Passive Motion (CPM) Machine. A postoperative knee splint may be worn until straight leg raises (indicating leg strength has returned) can be done by the patient.

Amputation

Simply defined, an amputation is the removal of a body part, which can be as limited as removing part of a finger or as devastating as removing nearly half the body. Amputations may be surgical as a result of disease or traumatic as a result of an accident. Surgical amputations are the most common type and are most often scheduled as elective surgery.

Box 46.8

Educating the Patient After Total Hip Replacement

Safety Measures to Prevent Hip Dislocation

- Keep legs abducted (away from center of body) with pillows.
- Bending at the waist (hip) cannot be greater than 90 degrees.
- Getting up from a sitting position requires pushing straight up off of the chair or bed without leaning forward.
- Walkers can be used to assist walking.
- Physiotherapy and occupational therapy can provide equipment that aids in putting on socks and shoes.
- Sleep with pillows between legs until physician states otherwise.
- Sexual activity can be started when tolerated provided hip safety measures followed.

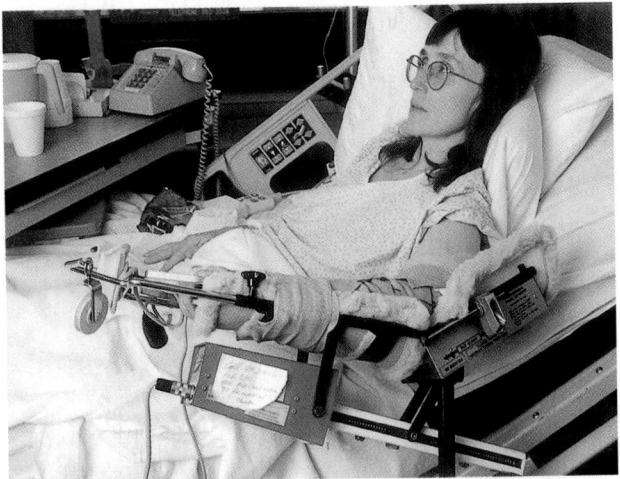

FIGURE 46.20 A continuous passive motion machine can be used following knee or elbow (as shown here) joint replacement to increase joint mobility and enhance recovery. The CPM machine slowly moves along the track at the set degree of flexion and speed.

SURGICAL AMPUTATIONS. The main indication for surgical amputations is ischemia from peripheral vascular disease in the older adult. The rate of lower extremity amputation is much greater in the diabetic patient than in the nondiabetic patient (see discussion of diabetes in Chapter 40). Surgical amputations may also be done for bone tumors, thermal injuries (frostbite, electric shock), crushing injuries, congenital problems, or infections.

TRAUMATIC AMPUTATIONS. Traumatic amputations occur from accidents, often in young and middle-aged adults.

Box 46.9

Application of a Continuous Passive Motion (CPM) Machine

- Position joint (knee) over flexion point of machine.
- Padding (e.g., sheepskin) is particularly important at proximal end near gluteal fold.
- Ensure speed and angle settings are correct and monitored according to facility policy. A minimum of every shift is required.
- The patient is provided the controls to stop the machine prn unless he or she is mentally incompetent to do so. If unable to self monitor, ensure patient is checked frequently.
- Assess how well patient tolerates the speed and angle of movement.
- Speed and angle adjustments are determined by agency policy, physiotherapist, or the physician.
- Ideal utilization is three times a day for at least 1 hour per session.

Industrial machinery, motor vehicles, lawn mowers, chain saws, and snow blowers are common causes of accidental amputation.

Because in these patients the amputated part is usually healthy, attempts at **replantation** may occur. One of the most common replantations is one or more fingers. The current recommendation for prehospital care of the severed body part is to wrap it in a cool, slightly moist cloth and place it in a sealed plastic bag. The bag may be submerged in cold water until the body part is transported to the hospital.

The surgical procedure is performed by specialists who operate using a microscope. Nerves, vessels, and muscle must be reattached. These procedures are generally performed at large tertiary care centers that have specialty practitioners and equipment for replantation.

LEVELS OF AMPUTATION. The most common surgical amputation is part of the lower extremity. The loss of any or all of the small toes presents little problem. However, the loss of the great toe is more important because balance and gait are affected. Midfoot amputations are preferred over below-the-knee amputations (BKAs) for peripheral vascular disease. For the Syme amputation, the surgeon removes most of the foot but leaves the ankle intact for ambulation and weight bearing.

If the lower leg is amputated, a BKA is preferred over an above-the-knee amputation (AKA) to preserve joint function. The higher the level of amputation, the more energy is required for ambulation. Hip disarticulation (removal through the hip joint) and **hemipelvectomy** (removal through part of the pelvis) are reserved for young patients who have cancer or severe trauma. Rarely, a hemicorporectomy (hemipelvectomy plus a translumbar amputation) is performed as a last resort for young patients with cancer. This radical surgery removes nearly half of the body and requires both bowel and urinary diversion surgeries (ostomies) as well.

Upper extremity amputations are usually more significant than lower extremity amputations and more often result from trauma. The arms and hands are necessary for performing activities of daily living. Early replacement with a prosthesis is crucial for the patient with an upper extremity amputation.

PREOPERATIVE CARE. Patients who are scheduled for elective amputations have the advantage of time for preoperative teaching, prosthesis fitting, and adjustment to the loss of part of their bodies. Preoperative teaching is started in the surgeon's office. Postoperative and rehabilitative care is reviewed with the patient and family or significant other. Those patients experiencing a traumatic amputation have no opportunity to prepare for the significant changes that will result from the accident. Preoperative care will not only involve physical needs being met but also significant psy-

---

replantation: re—again + plant—to plant + ation—process
hemipelvectomy: hemi—half + pelv—pelvis + ectomy—removal of

chological and emotional concerns will have to be addressed (this will also have to continue postoperatively).

Preoperatively, the patient should be referred to a certified prosthetist-orthotist (CPO) to begin plans for replacing the removed body part with a prosthesis.

Disturbed body image is a common nursing diagnosis for the patient having an amputation. If possible, it is helpful for the preoperative patient to meet with a rehabilitated amputee. Assess the patient's reaction to having an amputation with the expectation that the patient will experience many of the stages of loss and grieving. Support systems and coping mechanisms are identified that can help the patient through the surgery and postoperative period. Ensure that appropriate support is provided by other disciplines such as social work and clergy.

POSTOPERATIVE CARE. In addition to the general postoperative care, plan and implement interventions to help prevent postoperative complications (see Chapter 11).

Hemorrhage. When a patient loses part of the body, either by surgery or trauma, blood vessels are severed or damaged. The patient returns from surgery with a large pressure dressing that is secured with an elastic wrap. Assess the closest proximal pulse between the heart and the amputated body part for strength and compare findings with the nonsurgical extremity. Assess the bulky dressing for bloody drainage. If blood is on the dressing when the patient is admitted to the PACU or the surgical unit, circle, date, and time the area of drainage and closely monitor for enlargement. If bleeding continues, the surgeon is notified immediately. A tourniquet should be readily available in the event that severe hemorrhage occurs.

After the dressing is removed, observe for adequate perfusion to the skin flap at the end of the residual limb, referred to as the stump. The skin should be pink in a light-skinned patient and not discolored (lighter or darker than other skin pigmentation) in a dark-skinned patient. The residual limb should be warm but not hot.

Infection. Infection of the wound can be problematic, especially if the infection enters the bone (**osteomyelitis**). Inspect the wound for intense redness or drainage. Localized infections usually do not cause an increase in body temperature. If temperature is elevated, it could indicate a serious wound infection, a systemic infection, or some other type of infection. Traumatic amputations are at risk for developing infection due to the nature of the injury and the likelihood of exposure to environmental pathogens from the source of the amputation.

Pain. In addition to the usual incisional pain that is expected following a surgical procedure, phantom limb pain occurs in as many as 80% of all amputees (surgical or traumatic). The patient complains of severe pain where the removed body part was located. The pain may be described as either intense burning, a crushing sensation, or cramping.

Phantom limb pain can be triggered by touching the residual limb, feeling fatigued, or experiencing emotional stress. It is reported that phantom limb pain can also be triggered by pressure or changes in the weather. Although it occurs most often in the immediate postoperative period, phantom limb pain may occur at any time during the first postoperative year or sometimes even years after the amputation. The pain may be mild to severe. The cause is not clear.

Never doubt that the patient is experiencing phantom limb pain. Treat the pain aggressively with medications and complementary therapies. The surgeon prescribes medication based on the type of pain sensation the patient experiences. For example, anticonvulsants, such as phenytoin (Dilantin), are used for knifelike pain. Beta-blocking agents, such as propranolol (Inderal), are appropriate for burning sensations, and gabapentin (Neurontin) or amitriptyline (Elavil) can be used for nerve pain. To complement traditional therapy, a number of therapies may be useful, including biofeedback, massage, imagery, hypnosis, acupuncture, acupressure, and distraction.

Mobility and Ambulation. To reduce surgical swelling, cold application may be ordered. Alternately, the residual limb may be elevated on a pillow for 24 hours or less. Continued use of a pillow for elevation can lead to flexion contractures, especially for patients with a BKA or an AKA. If the hip becomes contracted, using a prosthesis will not be possible because the patient will not be able to walk. Check the limb periodically to ensure that it lies completely flat on the bed. The patient should avoid positions of flexion such as sitting for long periods. If the patient is able, lying prone (on stomach) for 30 minutes four times daily helps prevent contracture.

Postoperative care of the patient experiencing an amputation is interdisciplinary, often requiring an extensive rehabilitation program in a subacute unit, nursing home, or on an ambulatory basis. The physical therapist teaches the patient muscle-strengthening exercises that help with ambulation and transfers and prevent flexion contractures. A trapeze and overhead bed frame aid in strengthening the upper extremities and help the patient move around in the bed.

Prosthesis. The residual limb must be prepared for wearing the prosthesis. A temporary prosthesis may be worn until the swelling subsides.

The residual limb is wrapped at least every 8 hours using an elastic wrap (such as an Ace wrap) in a figure-of-eight fashion (Fig. 46.21). It is important to perform neurovascular checks and assess the residual limb for infection and alterations in tissue integrity at each rewrapping. Begin with the most distal portion and proceed proximally until the bandage is secured to the most proximal joint. The bandage should be tighter at the distal end.

The prosthesis requires special care which the patient should be taught:

---

osteomyelitis: osteo—bone + myel—bone marrow + itis— inflammation

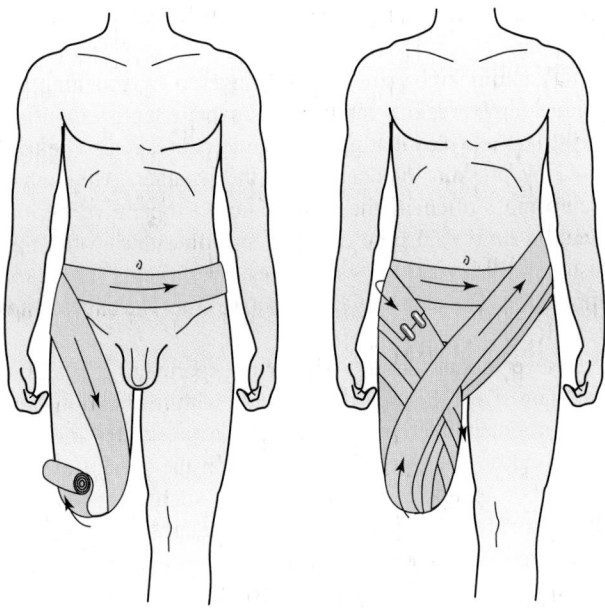

FIGURE 46.21 Application of elastic wraps on an above-the-knee amputation helps mold the stump for a prosthesis.

- The prosthesis socket is cleaned with mild soap/water and dried.
- Clean inserts and liners regularly.
- Use garters to keep socks in place.
- Grease parts as instructed.

- Shoes are replaced when worn out with same height and type.

Lifestyle Adaptation. The patient may feel that life will be markedly changed as a result of the amputation. With the technological advances in prostheses, most patients who worked before surgery are able to return to their jobs after surgery. If the discharge planner or case manager thinks it is needed, a job analysis may be conducted by a vocational analyst or specialized case manager. Many patients with amputations are able to bowl, ski, hike, and experience all the recreational hobbies that they were able to do before surgery.

A supportive family or significant other is vital to help the patient adjust to body image change. Consider the need for a sexual counselor or psychologist if indicated. For any patient with an amputation, help the patient set realistic expectations.

For the patient who is not a candidate for a prosthesis, home adaptations for a wheelchair may be needed. The patient must have access to toileting facilities and areas necessary for self-care. Structural changes in the living environment may be necessary before the patient can be discharged from rehabilitation.

A small percentage of amputees return to their nursing home environment without prostheses. These patients need rehabilitation to ensure that they can be as independent as possible.

Home Health Hints

- Instruct the patient with rheumatoid arthritis to rest during acute inflammations and to stop activity if pain develops.
- If equipment or modifications to the home are needed following hospitalization for an orthopedic problem, it is best if they can be arranged or obtained before discharge. Equipment can include raised toilet seats, hand-held reachers, walkers, canes, wheelchairs, and hand rails.
- Physical and occupational therapy are usually ordered for the orthopedic patient discharged from the hospital. They can work with them to help with ambulation, activities of daily living, teaching them how to use assistive devices, and also obtaining the above listed assistive devices.
- Physical and/or occupational therapy can also be ordered to assist the patient regain strength following surgery. The home health nurse can work with the therapist to educate the patient on the prescribed exercises.
- Peak incidents of DVT after hip or knee surgery is highest by the fifth postoperative day and that risk persists for up to 12 weeks. Be alert for signs of DVT: warmth, redness, edema, Homans' sign, and protective behavior of the affected leg.

- Many times the patient is discharged home still requiring Lovenox injections to prevent DVT formation. The nurse needs to educate the patient on how to administer the injection in the abdomen. If the patient cannot do this and no one is available to teach him or her, the home health nurse can make visits in order to administer the injection.
- Home health nurses frequently remove staples and sutures. Always carry several of each type of removal device in your car. Remember staples, scissors, or other items that are "sharp" need to be disposed of in a biohazard container.
- Research has shown that pain or fear of falling may prevent a patient from moving and functioning to maximum potential. Encourage patients to wear flat, sturdy, rubber-soled shoes to prevent slipping, tripping, or turning an ankle.
- Encourage the patient to dispose of all throw rugs, unnecessary furniture, or other possible fall hazards in the home.
- Patients who use walkers can get pressure ulcers on their palms. One way to relieve the pressure is to wear padded cycling gloves that leave the fingers free.

- A patient on crutches can use the crutch to prop a casted leg or foot.
- Patients who are having a difficult time putting on antiembolism stockings can be instructed on an easy way of slipping them on. Using a plastic grocery bag,

instruct the patient to tie a knot on the closed end. Slip the bag over the foot, and then put the stocking on over the bag. Once the stocking is on over the heel, the patient or caregiver can pull the bag out using the knot that was tied.

REVIEW QUESTIONS

1. The nurse is caring for a patient who just had a plaster cast applied. Which action should the nurse take to facilitate cast drying?
   a. Cover the cast with blankets to provide extra warmth.
   b. Turn the patient every 2 hours.
   c. Increase the room temperature.
   d. Apply a heating pad.

2. A patient with multiple fractures of the femur returns from surgery for surgical repair with an external fixation device in place. Which of the following nursing interventions would be appropriate to properly care for the pins inserted into the patient's leg?
   a. Do not touch the pins.
   b. Follow agency protocol for pin care.
   c. Cleanse with hydrogen peroxide qid.
   d. Loosen the screws holding the pins when cleaning.

Multiple response item. Select all that apply.

3. Which of the following actions can the nurse take to help prevent osteomyelitis for a patient with an open fracture?
   a. Wash hands prior to dressing changes.
   b. Wear a protective gown.
   c. Wear a mask.
   d. Wear goggles.
   e. Wear sterile gloves to apply new dressing.

4. A patient is postmenopausal, has osteoporosis, has lost 2 inches of height, is thin, and has never exercised regularly. Which of these interventions should be included in the plan of care to prevent further bone loss?
   a. Decrease participation in ADLs.
   b. Decrease weight-bearing activities.
   c. Encourage regular exercise.
   d. Encourage weight gain.

5. A priority nursing diagnosis for the patient with Paget's disease includes which of the following?
   a. Pain
   b. Deficient knowledge
   c. Excess fluid volume
   d. Deficient fluid volume

6. Which of the following lab values would the nurse expect to be elevated in the patient with gout?

   a. WBC
   b. RBC
   c. Uric acid
   d. Ammonia

7. A butterfly rash is a classic symptom of which of the following disorders?
   a. Lupus
   b. Paget's disease
   c. Rheumatoid arthritis
   d. Osteosarcoma

8. A patient with osteoarthritis who had a right total knee replacement tells the nurse that her other knee is becoming painful. Which of these is the most appropriate instruction to help the patient preserve function of her left knee?
   a. Reduce dietary purines.
   b. Maintain ideal body weight.
   c. Maintain normal uric acid levels.
   d. Begin a jogging program.

9. A patient is scheduled for a right total hip replacement. The nurse should include which of the following postoperative leg positions in the preoperative teaching plan?
   a. Maintain legs in adduction.
   b. Maintain legs in abduction.
   c. Maintain internal leg rotation.
   d. Maintain more than 90-degree hip flexion.

10. Following amputation, which of these assessments should the nurse consider a priority to monitor for potential postoperative amputation complications?
    a. Sacral edema
    b. Level of consciousness
    c. Stump dressings
    d. Blood sugars

11. Which of the following findings would indicate a complication of a left fibula fracture?
    a. The patient has an increased red blood cell count.
    b. The patient has a decreased pulse, respiration and BP.
    c. The patient has a decreased CD4 lymphocyte count.
    d. The patient has an absent left pedal pulse.

12. A patient has a 36-hour-old fractured femur. He had morphine 5 mg intramuscularly 1 hour ago and is reporting severe unrelieved pain. Which nursing action is most appropriate?
   a. Give pain medication.
   b. Adjust the traction.
   c. Bivalve the cast.
   d. Notify the physician.

13. A patient who had a total knee replacement is to receive Toradol 15 mg intramuscularly every 6 hours as needed for pain. The Toradol comes as 30 mg/mL. How many milliliters should the nurse give?

_____ mL

SUGGESTED ANSWERS TO

CRITICAL THINKING

■ Mrs. Brown

1. When documenting, answer (either explicitly or implicitly by professional knowledge, in narrative or flow sheet format) what, why, when, where, who, and how for completeness.

   What? Patient found on the floor lying on her left side, moaning and holding her leg, crying out with any movement.

   Why = Fell

   When = 10 a.m. on Date

   Where = Dayroom

   Who = Mrs. Brown (patient)

   DATE 1000 Found on floor in dayroom lying on left side, moaning and holding left leg, crying out with any movement. Stated, "I fell. I think my leg is broken." Supervisor immediately notified, and paramedics and Dr. Jones called. Vital signs BP 150/84, P 100, R 20. Left leg shorter than right. Remained with patient and instructed not to move until paramedics arrive. Blankets applied and pillow placed under head for comfort. 1030 taken by ambulance to Grace Hospital. I. Smith, LPN

2. The purpose of the traction is to reduce the muscle spasms that often accompany fractures and to increase comfort.

3. Nursing responsibilities include the following:
   a. Check neurovascular status frequently.
   b. Check equipment, including rope, pulleys, knots, and weights at least every shift.
   c. Do not allow the weights to rest on the floor.
   d. Do not allow the traction to be impeded in any way.
   e. Monitor the patient's skin often for areas of potential breakdown.
   f. Remove and rewrap the elastic bandages, maintaining the traction, at least every shift. Provide skin care during this time.
   g. Monitor area of the fracture for bruising and increased diameter of the limb.
   h. Monitor for pain (using pain assessment scale) frequently.
   i. Turn and position regularly.

4. Her restlessness is most likely the result of pain. She may be unable to state that she is in pain. Evaluate behaviors such as restlessness and other nonverbal cues to evaluate pain management needs. She may also be experiencing shock as a result of blood loss from the fracture. Monitor vital signs, and check the area of the fracture for increased signs of bruising or swelling.

■ Tommy Martin

1. Possible nursing diagnoses may include:
   a. Pain related to injury and immobility
   b. Potential for social isolation related to extended need for immobilization
   c. Potential complications of inactivity: Constipation, impaired skin integrity related to extended need for traction
   d. Deficient diversional activity related to extended need for bedrest

2. Nursing interventions may include:
   a. Monitor pain level, provide analgesics as ordered, assess pain relief. Assess position for comfort. Provide backrubs prn.
   b. To address social isolation, encourage Tommy's friends to come visit; have an occupational therapist assess Tommy's needs; and alternate family visitors.
   c. To avoid complications of inactivity, ensure Tommy's diet includes fiber and adequate hydration 1.5 to 2 L/day; give stool softener especially if on opioids as ordered; monitor daily defecation; ensure Tommy does the exercises recommended by occupational and physical therapists; reposition him every 2 to 3 hours; have trapeze set up for Tommy to use; use skin assessment tool to determine risk for skin breakdown; assess for pressure points and signs and symptoms of skin breakdown.
   d. To alleviate boredom, encourage Tommy to listen to music; encourage visitors; and ensure access to hobbies, videos, books, magazines, and comics.

■ *Mr. Andrews*

1. Nursing assessments should include the following:
   a. Perform a neurovascular check.
   b. Perform a further pain assessment.
   c. Ask Mr. Andrews to move his limb and see if the pain worsens.
   d. Take his vital signs.
   e. Assess for the 6 *Ps* (pulselessness, paresthesia, paralysis, pallor, pain, poikilothermia).
2. He might be experiencing compartment syndrome.
3. Interventions may include the following:
   a. Bivalving cast
   b. Possible fasciotomy

■ *Mr. Wolf*

4. Give one 2.5-mg tablet and five 5-mg tablets in the morning and evening. Although response number 3 could have been done, there is an increased chance of administering less than ordered when you have to split a tablet in half (especially if it is not scored). Also there are less pills to administer in response d which also provides a psychological advantage to the patient's thinking. Responses a and b do not follow the doctor's order of giving equal doses.

■ *Mr. Dennis*

1. "What is your typical day on the job like?"
   a. "Do certain activities increase joint pain?"
   b. "When is your pain worse—after activity or after rest?"
   c. "How long have you experienced joint pain?"
   d. "What relieves the joint pain?"
2. Risk factors include that he is overweight, is in late middle age, and has a physically demanding job.
3. Other signs and symptoms may include bony nodules on his fingers (such as Heberden's nodes) and secondary inflammation causing joint swelling.

■ *Mrs. Summers*

1. Ask:
   a. The nature of her pain
   b. If it is worse after activity or rest
   c. If she experiences joint stiffness and, if so, when
   Follow the WHAT'S UP? method of pain assessment.
2. Teach her to do the following:
   a. Balance rest with exercise.
   b. Use ice for very hot, swollen joints.
   c. Use heat to decrease stiffness.

■ *Mrs. Jacobs*

Unit Analysis Method:

$$\frac{500 \text{ mg}}{} \left| \frac{5 \text{ mL}}{375 \text{ mg}} \right. = 6.7 \text{ mL}$$

Unit Twelve Bibliography

1. American Association of Orthopedic Surgeons. (November 2004). Osteogenesis Imperfecta. http://orthoinfo.aaos.org/fact/thr_report.cfm?Thread_ID=308&topcategory=About%20Orthopaedics&all=all.
2. Bajnoczy, S: Artificial disc replacement—evolutionary treatment for degenerative disc disease. AORN J 82:192–206, 2005.
3. Bailey, J: Getting a fix on orthopedic care. Nursing 33:58, 2003.
4. Campbell, S (commentator): Review: wearing graduated compression stockings during air travel reduces the risk of deep venous thromboembolism. Evid Based Nurs 9:18. doi:10.1136/ebn.9.1.18, 2006.
5. Curry, L, and Hogstel, M: Osteoporosis. Am J Nurs 102:26, 2002.
6. Forster, F (commentator): Relaxing hip precautions increased patient satisfaction and promoted quicker return to normal activities after total hip arthroplasty. Evid Based Nurs 8:115. doi:10.1136/ebn.8.4.115, 2005
7. Forster, F (commentator): Older African-Americans with osteoarthritis of the knee preferred to avoid total knee replacement surgery. Evid Based Nurs 8: 32, 2005.
8. Freeman, TR: Teriparatide: A novel agent that builds new bone. J Am Pharmaceut Assoc 43:535–537, 2003.
9. Griffiths, P (commentator): Review: evidence from individually randomised trials shows that hip protectors do not reduce hip fractures in elderly people. Evid Based Nurs 8:24, 2005.
10. Ho, KT, and Reveille, JD: The clinical relevance of autoantibodies in scleroderma. Arthritis Res Ther 5:80–93, 2003.
11. McDonald, H (commentator): Patients who wore standard magnetic bracelets reported reduced pain from osteoarthritis of the hip or knee compared with patients wearing placebo bracelets. Evid Based Nurs 8:89. doi:10.1136/ebn.8.3.89, 2005.
12. Miller, R: KidsHealth. Childhood Cancer: Osteosarcoma. http://kidshealth.org/parent/medical/cancer/cancer_osteosarcoma_p3.html.
13. Morrison, RS, Magaziner, J, McLaughlin, MA, et al: The impact of post-operative pain on outcomes following hip fracture. Pain 103(3):303-11, 2003.
14. Olofsson, B, Lundstrom, M, Borssen, B, et al: Delirium is associated with poor rehabilitation outcome in elderly patients treated for femoral neck fractures. Scand J Caring Sci 19:119–127, 2005.
15. Pasero, C, and McCaffery, M: Pain in the critically ill. Am J Nurs 102:59, 2002.
16. Schuurmans, MJ. Duursma, SA, Shortridge-Baggett, LM, et al: Elderly patients with a hip fracture: The risk for delirium. Appl Nurs Res 16:75–84, 2003.
17. van Schoor, N, Smit JH, Twisk JW, et al: Prevention of hip fractures by external hip protectors. JAMA 289: 1957–1962, 2003.
18. Warden, V, Hurley, AC, and Volicer, L: Development and psycometric evaluation of the pain assessment in advanced dementia (painad) scale. J Am Med Dir Assoc 4:9–15, 2003.

unit THIRTEEN

UNDERSTANDING THE NEUROLOGICAL SYSTEM

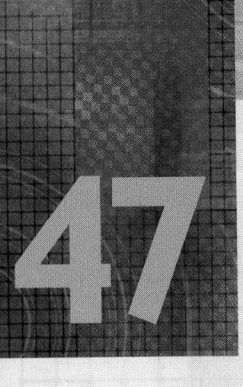

47

Neurological Function, Assessment, and Therapeutic Measures

JENNIFER WHITLEY AND
JANICE L. BRADFORD

KEY TERMS

anisocoria (an-i-soh-KOH-ree-ah)
aphasia (ah-FAY-zee-ah)
cerebrovascular (SER-ee-broh-VAS-kyoo-lur)
contractures (kon-TRAK-churs)
decerebrate (dee-SER-e-brayt)
decorticate (dee-KOR-ti-kayt)
dysarthria (dis-AR-three-ah)
dysphagia (dis-FAYJ-ee-ah)
electroencephalogram (ee-LEK-troh-en-SEFF-uh-
  loh-gram)
myelogram (MY-e-loh-gram)
nystagmus (nis-TAG-muss)
paresis (puh-REE-sis)
paresthesia (PAR-es-THEE-zee-ah)
subarachnoid (SUB-uh-RAK-noyd)

QUESTIONS TO GUIDE YOUR READING

1. What is the normal anatomy of the nervous system?

2. What is the normal function of the nervous system?

3. What data should you collect when caring for a patient with a disorder of the nervous system?

4. What are the effects of aging on the nervous system?

5. What diagnostic tests are commonly performed to diagnose disorders of the nervous system?

6. What nursing care should you provide for patients undergoing each of the diagnostic tests for disorders of the nervous system?

7. What are common therapeutic measures used for patients with disorders of the nervous system?

REVIEW OF NORMAL ANATOMY AND PHYSIOLOGY

The nervous system is one of the body's control systems; by means of electrochemical impulses, we are able to detect changes and feel sensations, initiate appropriate responses to changes, and organize and store information for future use. Some of this is conscious activity, but much of it is reflexive in nature and happens without our awareness.

The nervous system has two divisions. The central nervous system (CNS) consists of the brain and spinal cord. The peripheral nervous system (PNS) consists of cranial nerves and spinal nerves, which include the nerves of the autonomic nervous system (ANS).

Nerve Tissue

Nerve tissue consists of neurons and specialized supporting cells called neuroglia. There are many kinds of neurons (nerve cells or nerve fibers), but they all have the same gen-

eral structure (Fig. 47.1). The cell body contains the nucleus and is essential for the continued life of the neuron. All neuron cell bodies are found in the brain, spinal cord, or within the trunk of the body; in these locations, most are protected by bone. A neuron may have one or many dendrites, which are extensions that carry impulses toward the cell body. A neuron has one axon that transmits impulses away from the cell body. It is the cell membrane of the dendrites, cell body, and axon that carries the electrical nerve impulse.

In the peripheral nervous system, axons and dendrites are wrapped in specialized neuroglial cells called Schwann cells. The concentric layers of cell membrane of a Schwann cell's plasma membrane form the myelin sheath. Myelin is a phospholipid that electrically insulates neurons from one another. The spaces between adjacent Schwann cells along an axon are called nodes of Ranvier (neurofibril nodes). Only the nodes of the neuron cell membrane depolarize when an electrical impulse is transmitted, which makes impulse conduction rapid. The nuclei and cytoplasm of Schwann cells are outside the myelin sheath and form the neurolemma. If a

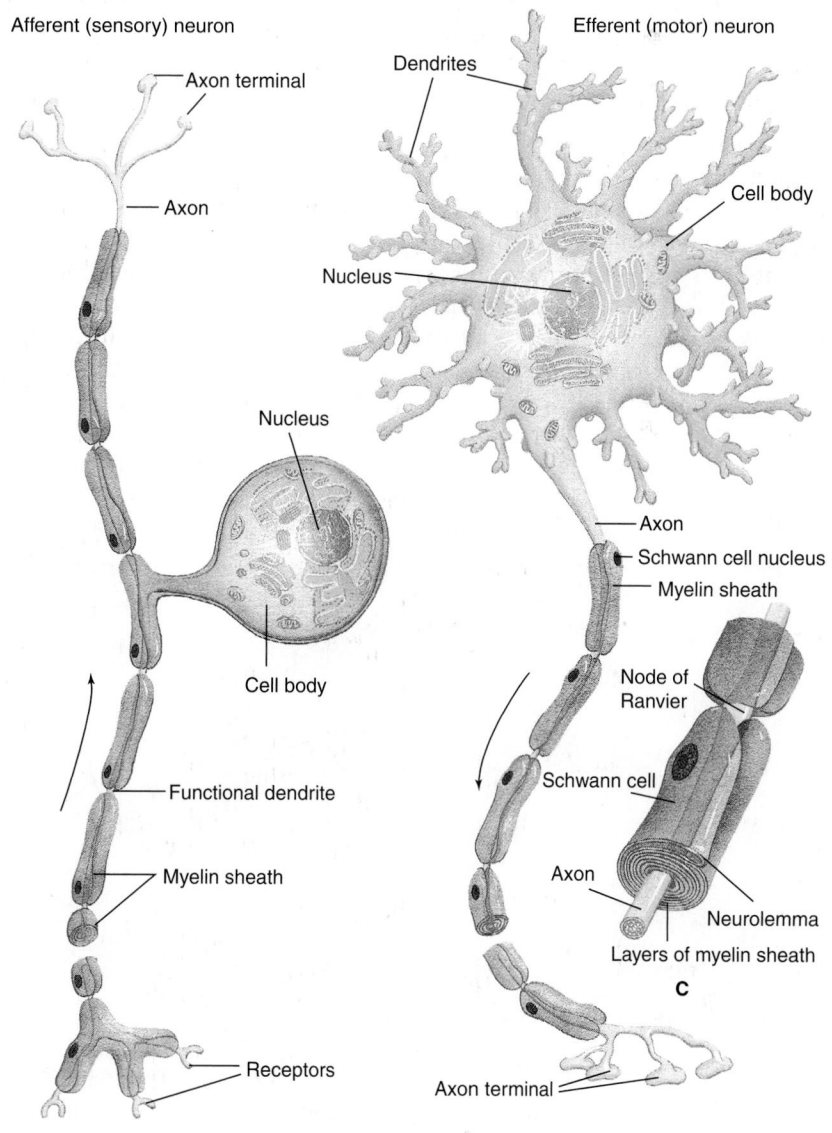

FIGURE 47.1 Structure of sensory and motor neurons. *(From Scanlon, VC, and Sanders, T: Essentials of Anatomy and Physiology, ed. 4. F.A. Davis, Philadelphia, 2003, p 157, with permission.)*

TABLE 47.1 NEUROGLIA

Name	Function
Oligodendrocytes	Produce the myelin sheath to electrically insulate neurons of the CNS
Microglia	Capable of movement and phagocytosis of pathogens and damaged tissue
Astrocytes	Contribute to the blood-brain barrier, which prevents potentially toxic waste products in the blood from diffusing out into brain tissue; disadvantage: some useful medications cannot cross it, which becomes important during brain infection, inflammation, or other disease
Ependyma	Line the ventricles of the brain; many of the cells are ciliated; involved in the circulation of cerebrospinal fluid

peripheral nerve is severed and reattached, the individual axons may regrow through the tunnels provided by the neurolemma. In the central nervous system, the myelin sheaths (but not a neurolemma) are formed by oligodendrocytes, another type of neuroglial cell. See Table 47.1 for the names and functions of the other neuroglial cells.

Synapses

When the axon of a neuron must transmit an impulse to the dendrite or cell body of another neuron, the impulse must cross a small gap called a synapse. An electrical impulse is incapable of crossing this microscopic space, so at synapses impulse transmission becomes chemical. The end of the axon (the presynaptic neuron) is called the synaptic end bulb and contains a chemical neurotransmitter that is released into the synapse by the arrival of the electrical impulse. The neurotransmitter diffuses across the synapse and combines with specific receptor sites on the postsynaptic membrane

(Fig. 47.2). At excitatory synapses, the neurotransmitter makes the postsynaptic membrane more permeable to sodium ions, which rush into the cell, initiating an electrical impulse on the membrane of the postsynaptic neuron. The neurotransmitter is then inactivated to prevent continuous impulses. For example, the neurotransmitter acetylcholine is inactivated by the chemical called acetylcholinesterase; each transmitter has its own specific inactivator.

Some synapses are inhibitory synapses in that the neurotransmitter makes the postsynaptic membrane more permeable to potassium ions, which leave the cell and make the membrane resistant to the electrical charge required for an impulse. Thus, the electrical impulse is stopped. Inhibitory synapses are important for things such as slowing the heart rate or balancing the excitatory impulses transmitted to skeletal muscles, which prevents excessive contraction and is important for coordination.

At chemical synapses, impulse transmission is one-way only because the neurotransmitter is released only by the presynaptic neuron; the impulse cannot go backward. This is important for the normal activity of the functional types of neurons. The relative complexity of synapses also makes them a potential target for the actions of medications.

Types of Neurons

A useful classification of neurons according to their function: a neuron is either a sensory neuron, a motor neuron, or an interneuron. Sensory (afferent) neurons transmit impulses from receptors to the central nervous system. Receptors are specialized to detect external or internal changes and then generate electrical impulses. Sensory neurons from receptors in the skin, skeletal muscles, and joints are called somatic; those from receptors in internal organs are called visceral sensory neurons.

Motor (efferent) neurons transmit impulses from the central nervous system to effectors—that is, muscles and

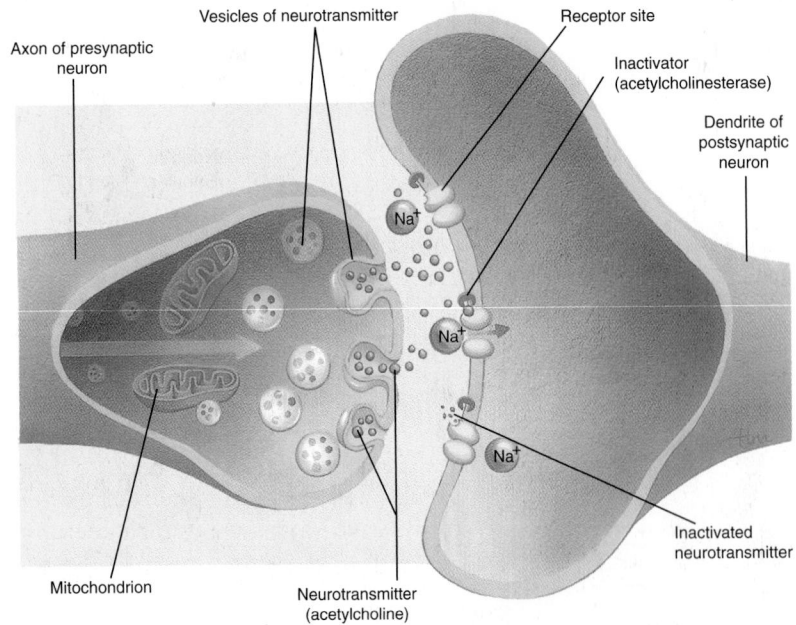

FIGURE 47.2 Structure of a synapse, and the effect of a neurotransmitter such as acetylcholine. *(From Scanlon, VC, and Sanders, T: Essentials of Anatomy and Physiology, ed. 5. F.A. Davis, Philadelphia, 2007, with permission.)*

glands. Motor neurons to skeletal muscle are called somatic; those to smooth muscle, cardiac muscle, and glands are called visceral. Sensory and motor neurons make up the peripheral nervous system. Visceral motor neurons form the autonomic nervous system, a specialized part of the PNS.

Interneurons are found entirely within the central nervous system. Each is specialized to transmit sensory or motor impulses or to integrate these functions. Such integration is involved in thinking and learning.

LEARNING TIP

To remember the difference between afferent and efferent, try these clues:
- Afferent: A is for affect or sense.
- Efferent: E is for effect (action).
- Or, think of the alphabet—A before E: You have to feel or sense (afferent) a stimulus before you can take action (efferent).

Nerves and Nerve Tracts

A nerve is a group of peripheral axons, dendrites, or both, with blood vessels and connective tissue. Most peripheral nerves are mixed; that is, they contain both sensory and motor neurons. An example of a purely sensory nerve is the optic nerve for vision; the autonomic nerves are purely motor nerves.

A nerve tract is a group of thickly myelinated neurons within the central nervous system; such tracts are often called white matter because the myelin sheaths of the individual neurons are white. A nerve tract within the spinal cord carries either sensory or motor impulses; those within the brain may have sensory, motor, or integrative functions.

Nerve Impulse

A nerve impulse, which may also be called an action potential, is an electrical change brought about by the movement of ions across the neuron cell membrane. When a neuron is not carrying an impulse, it is in a state of polarization with a positive charge outside the membrane and a relatively negative charge inside the membrane. Sodium ions are more abundant outside the cell, and potassium and negative ions are more abundant inside the cell. A stimulus makes the membrane very permeable to sodium ions, which rush into the cell, making the inside positive and the outside relatively negative. This reversal of charges is called depolarization and spreads from the point of the stimulus along the entire neuron membrane.

Immediately following depolarization, the membrane becomes very permeable to potassium ions, which rush out of the cell. This is called repolarization and restores the positive charge outside and the negative charge inside. The sodium and potassium pumps return the sodium ions back outside and the potassium ions inside, and the neuron is polarized again and ready to respond to another stimulus.

A neuron is capable of transmitting hundreds of impulses per second, and at speeds of many meters per second.

Spinal Cord

The spinal cord transmits impulses to and from the brain and is the integrating center for the spinal cord reflexes. The spinal cord is within the vertebral canal formed by the vertebrae and extends from the foramen magnum of the occipital bone to the intervertebral disk between the first and second lumbar vertebrae. The spinal nerves emerge from the intervertebral foramina.

In cross section, the spinal cord is oval shaped; internally it has an H-shaped mass of gray matter surrounded by white matter (Fig. 47.3). The gray matter is where the cell bodies of motor neurons and interneurons are located. The white matter is the myelinated axons. These nerve fibers are arranged in tracts based on their functions; ascending tracts transmit sensory impulses to the brain, and descending tracts transmit motor impulses from the brain to motor neurons. The central canal of the spinal cord is a small tunnel that is continuous with the ventricles of the brain; it contains cerebrospinal fluid (CSF).

Spinal Nerves

There are 31 pairs of spinal nerves, named according to their respective vertebrae: 8 cervical pairs, 12 thoracic pairs, 5 lumbar pairs, 5 sacral pairs, and 1 very small coccygeal pair. These nerves are often referred to by letter and number: the second cervical nerve is C2, the tenth thoracic is T10, and so on.

In general, the cervical nerves supply the back of the head; the neck, shoulders, and arms; and the diaphragm (the phrenic nerves). The first and second thoracic nerves also contribute to peripheral nerves in the arms. The remaining thoracic nerves supply the trunk of the body. The lumbar and sacral nerves supply the hips, pelvic cavity, and legs. The small coccygeal pair (Co1) supplies the area around the coccyx.

Each spinal nerve has two roots, which are neurons entering or leaving the spinal cord. The dorsal root is made of sensory neurons that carry impulses into the spinal cord. The dorsal root ganglion is an enlargement of this root that contains the cell bodies of these sensory neurons. The ventral root is the motor root; it is made of motor neurons that carry impulses from the spinal cord to muscles or glands (their cell bodies are in the gray matter of the spinal cord). When the two roots merge, the nerve thus formed is a mixed nerve.

Spinal Cord Reflexes

A reflex is an involuntary, predictable response to a stimulus, an automatic reaction triggered by a specific change. Spinal cord reflexes are those that do not depend directly on the brain, although the brain may inhibit or enhance them.

REFLEX ARC. A reflex arc is the pathway nerve impulses travel when a reflex is elicited. There are five parts:

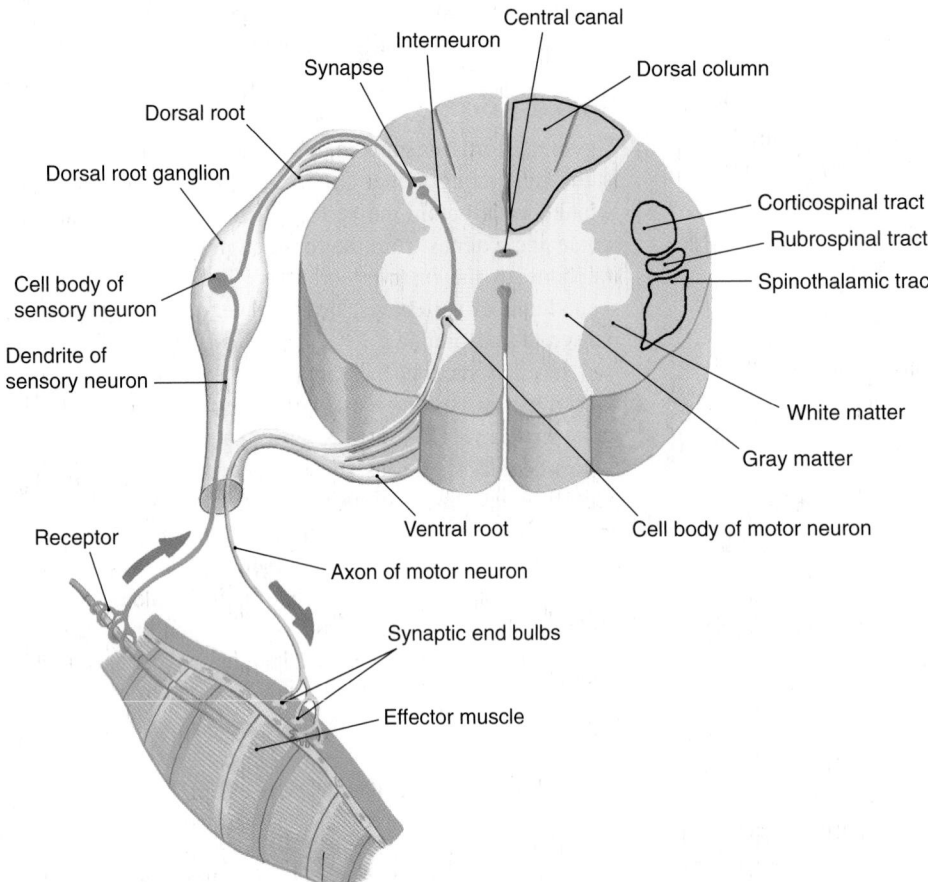

Central canal

Interneuron

Synapse

Dorsal column

Dorsal root

Dorsal root ganglion

Corticospinal tract

Rubrospinal tract

Spinothalamic tract

Cell body of
sensory neuron

Dendrite of
sensory neuron

White matter

Gray matter

Receptor

Ventral root

Cell body of motor neuron

Axon of motor neuron

Synaptic end bulbs

Effector muscle

FIGURE 47.3 Spinal cord in cross section, with nerve roots and meninges. *(From Scanlon, VC, and Sanders, T: Essentials of Anatomy and Physiology, ed. 4. F.A. Davis, Philadelphia, 2003, p 160, with permission.)*

1. Receptors detect a change (the stimulus) and generate impulses.
2. Sensory neurons transmit impulses from receptors to the central nervous system (CNS).
3. The CNS contains one or more synapses and the interneurons that may be part of the pathway.
4. Motor neurons transmit impulses from the CNS to an effector.
5. The effector performs its characteristic action.

The spinal cord reflexes include stretch reflexes and flexor reflexes. In a stretch reflex, a muscle that is stretched automatically contracts; an example is the familiar patellar, or knee-jerk, reflex, but all skeletal muscles have such a reflex. The purpose of these reflexes is to keep us upright (because gravity exerts a constant pull on the body) without our having to think about it. They also avoid possible injury from overstretching a muscle. Flexor reflexes may also be called withdrawal reflexes; the stimulus is something painful and the response is to pull away from it. Again, this occurs without the need for conscious thought; the brain is not directly involved.

The clinical testing of certain spinal cord reflexes provides a way to assess the functioning of their reflex arcs. For example, if the patellar reflex were absent, the problem might be in the quadriceps femoris muscle, the femoral nerve, or the spinal cord itself. If the reflex is present, how-

ever, it indicates that all parts of the reflex arc are functioning normally.

Brain

The brain consists of many parts that function as an integrated whole. The major parts are the medulla, pons, and midbrain (the brainstem); the cerebellum; the hypothalamus and thalamus; and the cerebrum (Fig. 47.4).

Ventricles

The ventricles are four cavities within the brain: two lateral ventricles are located within the cerebral hemispheres, the third ventricle lies midline within the thalamus, and the fourth ventricle is midline between the brainstem and cerebellum. Each ventricle contains a capillary network called a choroid plexus, which forms cerebrospinal fluid from blood plasma.

Medulla

The medulla is just above the spinal cord and extends to the pons. It regulates our most vital functions. Within the medulla are cardiac centers that regulate heart rate, respiratory centers that regulate breathing, and vasomotor centers that regulate the diameter of blood vessels and therefore blood pressure. Also in the medulla are reflex centers for coughing, sneezing, swallowing, and vomiting.

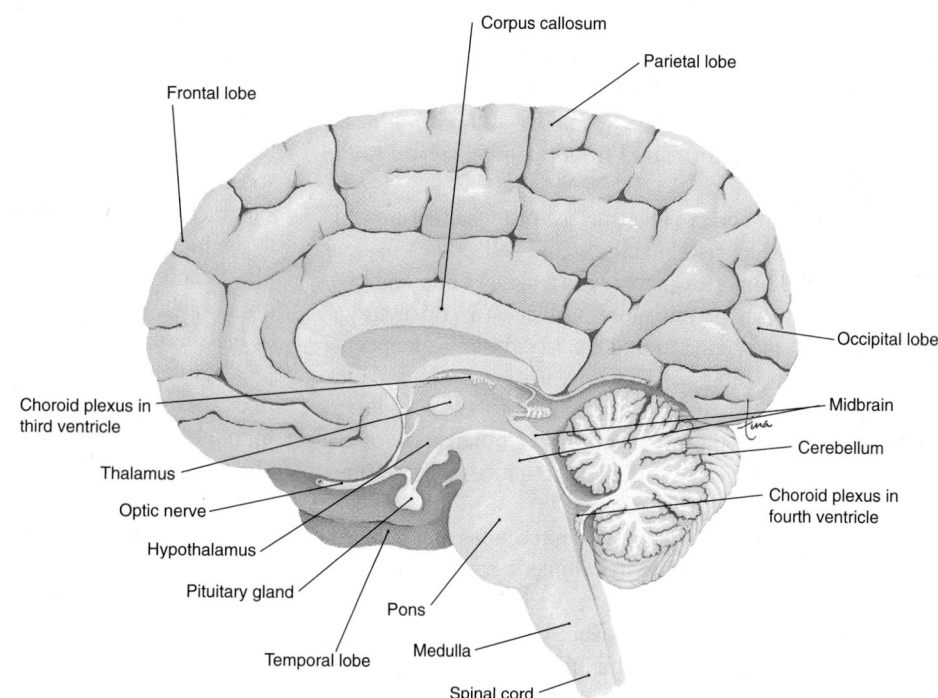

FIGURE 47.4 The brain's mid-sagittal section; medial surface of the right cerebral hemisphere. *(From Scanlon, VC, and Sanders, T: Essentials of Anatomy and Physiology, ed. 4. F.A. Davis, Philadelphia, 2003, p 167, with permission.)*

Pons

The pons is anterior to the cerebellum and superior to the medulla. Within the pons are two respiratory centers that work with those in the medulla to produce a normal breathing rhythm.

Midbrain

The midbrain extends from the pons to the hypothalamus and encloses the cerebral aqueduct, a tunnel that connects the third and fourth ventricles. Primarily a reflex center, the midbrain regulates visual reflexes (coordinated movement of the eyes), auditory reflexes (turning the ear toward a sound), and righting reflexes that keep the head upright and contribute to balance.

Cerebellum

The cerebellum is posterior to the medulla and pons, separated from them by the fourth ventricle; it is overlapped by the occipital lobes of the cerebrum. The functions of the cerebellum are concerned with the involuntary aspects of voluntary movement: coordination, the appropriate direction and endpoint of movements, and the maintenance of posture and balance or equilibrium. For the maintenance of balance, the cerebellum (and midbrain) uses sensory information provided by the receptors in the inner ear that detect movement and changes in position of the head.

Hypothalamus

The hypothalamus is located above the pituitary gland and below the thalamus. It has many diverse functions:

- Production of antidiuretic hormone (ADH) and oxytocin; these hormones are then stored in the posterior pituitary gland. ADH increases the reabsorption of water by the kidneys and thus helps maintain blood volume. Oxytocin causes contractions of the myometrium of the uterus to bring about labor and delivery.
- Production of releasing hormones that stimulate secretion of the hormones of the anterior pituitary gland. An example is growth hormone–releasing hormone (GHRH), which stimulates the anterior pituitary to secrete growth hormone.
- Regulation of body temperature by promoting responses such as shivering in a cold environment or sweating in a warm environment.
- Regulation of food and fluid intake; the hypothalamus is believed to respond to changes in blood nutrient levels or chemicals secreted by adipose tissue and bring about feelings of hunger or fullness.
- Integration of the functioning of the autonomic nervous system (discussed in a later section).
- Stimulation of visceral responses in emotional situations, such as an increased heart rate with anger or fear. The neurological basis of emotions is not well understood, but the hypothalamus brings about physiological changes by way of the autonomic nervous system.

Thalamus

The thalamus is above the hypothalamus and below the cerebrum; its functions are primarily concerned with sensation. Sensory pathways to the brain (except olfaction) to the brain converge in the thalamus, which begins to integrate sensations, permitting more rapid interpretation by the cerebrum. The thalamus is also capable of suppressing minor sensations, which permits the cerebrum to concentrate on more important sensations with less distraction.

Cerebrum

The two cerebral hemispheres form the largest part of the human brain. The right and left hemispheres are connected by the corpus callosum, a band of about 300 million nerve fibers that transfer information from one hemisphere to the other.

The cerebral cortex is the surface of the cerebrum; it is gray matter that consists mainly of the cell bodies of neurons. The cerebral cortex is folded extensively into convolutions (or gyri) that permit more surface area for neurons. The grooves between the folds are called fissures (deeper) or sulci (shallower). Interior to the gray matter is white matter, myelinated axons that connect the parts of the cerebral cortex to one another and the cerebrum to other parts of the brain. The cerebral cortex is divided into lobes, whose functions have been extensively mapped.

The frontal lobes contain the motor areas that generate the impulses that bring about voluntary movement. Each motor area controls movement on the opposite side of the body. Also in the frontal lobe, usually only the left lobe, is Broca's motor speech area, which controls the movements involved in speaking.

The parietal lobes contain the general sensory areas for the cutaneous senses, conscious muscle sense (proprioception), and taste (gustation). This is where these sensations are felt and interpreted.

The temporal lobes contain sensory areas for hearing and olfaction (smell). Also in the temporal and parietal lobes, usually only on the left side, are speech areas involved in the thought that precedes speech.

The occipital lobes contain the visual areas that receive impulses from the retinas of the eyes. Perception and interpretation of sight occurs here.

In all lobes of the cerebral cortex are association areas that enable us to learn, remember, and think; they also help form our individual personalities. These are complex behaviors that require integration of several cerebral and lower brain areas.

Deep within the white matter of the cerebral hemispheres are masses of gray matter called the basal ganglia. Their functions are concerned with certain subconscious aspects of voluntary movement: regulation of muscle tone, inhibiting tremor, and use of accessory movements such as arm swinging when walking.

Meninges and Cerebrospinal Fluid

The meninges are the three layers of connective tissue that cover the central nervous system. The outermost is the dura mater, made of thick, fibrous connective tissue. The middle layer is called the arachnoid mater, which has a weblike appearance; the inner layer is the pia mater, a very thin connective tissue on the surface of the brain and spinal cord. Between the arachnoid mater and the pia mater is the **subarachnoid** space, which contains cerebrospinal fluid.

---

subarachnoid: sub—below + arachnoid—middle layer of the meninges

Each of the four ventricles of the brain contains a choroid plexus, a capillary network that forms cerebrospinal fluid from blood plasma. This is a continuous process, and the cerebrospinal fluid then circulates from the ventricles to the central canal of the spinal cord and to the subarachnoid spaces around the brain and spinal cord. From the cranial subarachnoid space, cerebrospinal fluid is reabsorbed back to the blood through arachnoid villi that project into the cranial venous sinuses between the two layers of the cranial dura mater. The rate of reabsorption usually equals the rate of production.

As the tissue fluid of the CNS, cerebrospinal fluid permits the exchanges of nutrients and wastes between the blood and CNS neurons. It also acts as a cushion or shock absorber for the CNS. The pressure and constituents of cerebrospinal fluid may be determined by means of a lumbar puncture (spinal tap) and may be helpful in the diagnosis of diseases such as meningitis.

Cranial Nerves

The 12 pairs of cranial nerves emerge from the brainstem, with the exception of pair one which originates from the temporal lobe and pair two from the occipital lobe. Some are purely sensory nerves, whereas others are mixed nerves. The impulses for sight, smell, hearing, taste, and equilibrium are all carried by cranial nerves to their respective sensory areas in the brain. Other cranial nerves carry motor impulses to muscles of the face or to glands. Cranial nerves III, VII, IX, and X contain axons of both the somatic and autonomic nervous systems. The functions of all the cranial nerves are summarized in Table 47.2.

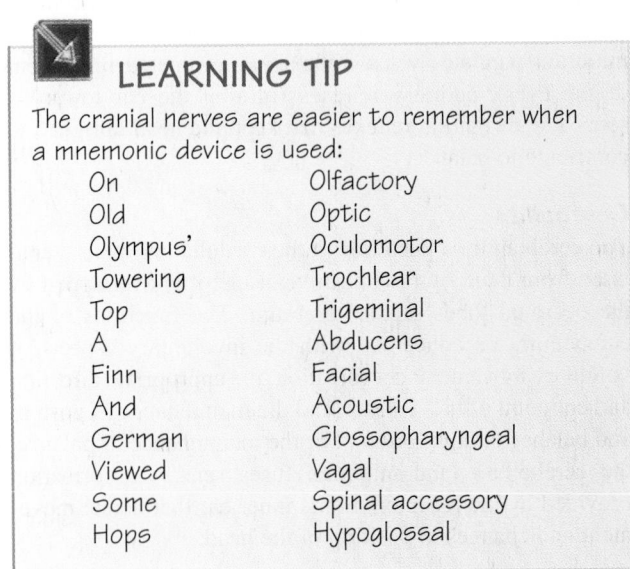

LEARNING TIP

The cranial nerves are easier to remember when a mnemonic device is used:

On	Olfactory
Old	Optic
Olympus'	Oculomotor
Towering	Trochlear
Top	Trigeminal
A	Abducens
Finn	Facial
And	Acoustic
German	Glossopharyngeal
Viewed	Vagal
Some	Spinal accessory
Hops	Hypoglossal

Autonomic Nervous System

The ANS is part of the peripheral nervous system in that it consists of the motor portions of some cranial and spinal nerves. These are the visceral motor neurons to visceral effectors—that is, smooth muscle, cardiac muscle, and glands. The ANS has two divisions, sympathetic and

TABLE 47.2 CRANIAL NERVES

Number	Name	Function
I	Olfactory	Sense of smell
II	Optic	Sense of sight
III	Oculomotor	Movement of eyeball; constriction of pupil for bright light or near vision
IV	Trochlear	Movement of eyeball
V	Trigeminal	Sensation in face, scalp, and teeth; contraction of chewing muscles
VI	Abducens	Movement of eyeball
VII	Facial	Sense of taste; contraction of facial muscles; secretion of saliva
VIII	Vestibulocochlear	Sense of hearing; sense of equilibrium
IX	Glossopharyngeal	Sense of taste; secretion of saliva; sensory for cardiac, respiratory, and blood pressure reflexes; contraction of pharynx
X	Vagus	Sensory in cardiac, respiratory, and blood pressure reflexes; sensory and motor to larynx (speaking); decreases heart rate; contraction of alimentary tube (peristalsis); increases digestive secretions
XI	Accessory	Contraction of neck and shoulder muscles; motor to larynx (speaking)
XII	Hypoglossal	Movement of the tongue

parasympathetic; often they function in opposition to each other, and their activity is integrated by the hypothalamus.

An autonomic nerve pathway from the CNS to a visceral effector consists of two motor neurons that synapse in a ganglion outside the CNS (Fig. 47.5). The first neuron is called the preganglionic neuron, from the CNS to the ganglion. The second neuron is called the postganglionic neuron, from the ganglion to the visceral effector. The ganglia are actually cell body collections of the postganglionic neurons.

Sympathetic Division

The cell bodies of the sympathetic preganglionic neurons are in the thoracic and some of the lumbar segments of the spinal cord. The axons of these neurons extend to the sympathetic ganglia, most of which are in two chains just lateral to the spinal column. Within the ganglia are the synapses between the preganglionic and postganglionic neurons; the axons of the postganglionic neurons then go to the visceral effectors. One preganglionic neuron often synapses with many postganglionic neurons to many effectors; this permits widespread responses in many organs.

The sympathetic division is dominant in stressful situations such as fear, anger, anxiety, and exercise, and the responses it brings about involve preparedness for physical activity, whether or not it is actually needed. (Table 47.3 summarizes both ANS divisions.) The heart rate increases, vasodilation in skeletal muscles supplies them with more oxygen, the bronchioles dilate to take in more air, and the liver changes glycogen to glucose to provide energy. Relatively less important activities such as digestion are slowed, and vasoconstriction in the skin and viscera permits greater blood flow to more vital organs such as the brain, heart, and muscles.

The neurotransmitters of the sympathetic division are acetylcholine and norepinephrine. Acetylcholine is released by sympathetic preganglionic neurons; its inactivator is acetylcholinesterase. Norepinephrine is released by most sympathetic postganglionic neurons at the synapses with the effector cells; its inactivator is catechol-O-methyltransferase.

Parasympathetic Division

The cell bodies of the parasympathetic preganglionic neurons are in the brainstem and the sacral segments of the spinal cord. The axons of these neurons are in cranial nerve pairs III, VII, IX, and X and in some sacral nerves, and they extend to the parasympathetic ganglia. These ganglia are close to or actually in the visceral effector and contain the postganglionic cell bodies, with very short axons to the cells of the visceral effector. One preganglionic neuron synapses with just a few postganglionic neurons to only one effector. This permits localized responses.

The parasympathetic division dominates during relaxed, nonstressful situations to promote normal functioning of several organ systems. Digestion proceeds normally, with increased secretions and peristalsis; defecation and urination may occur, and the heart beats at a normal resting rate (see Table 47.3.)

Acetylcholine is the neurotransmitter at all parasympathetic synapses, both preganglionic and postganglionic; it is inactivated by acetylcholinesterase.

CRITICAL THINKING

Mrs. Stevens

■ Mrs. Stevens receives albuterol treatments for her chronic obstructive pulmonary disease. The medication opens her airways effectively, but after her treatments, she often complains that her heart is racing. What part of the peripheral nervous system do you think this medication affects?

Aging and the Nervous System

With age, the brain loses neurons, but this is only a small percentage of the total and is not the usual cause of mental

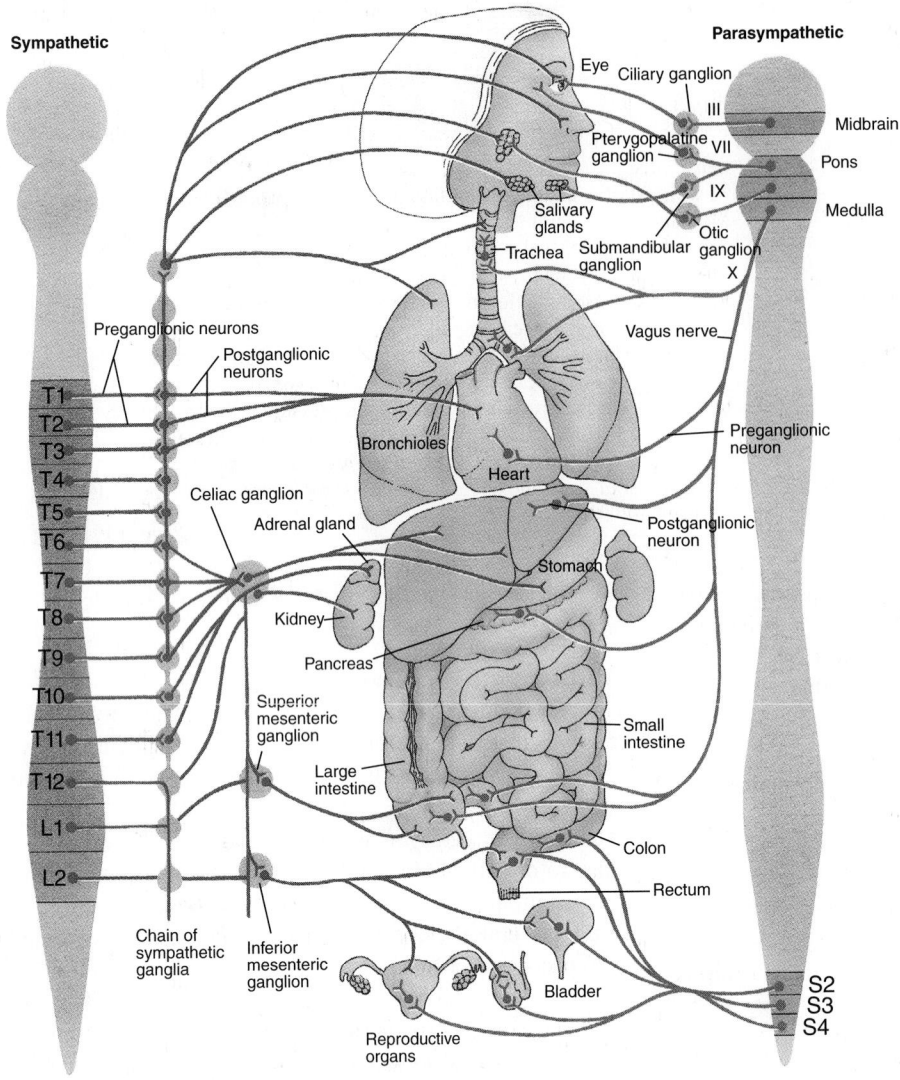

Sympathetic

Parasympathetic

Eye Ciliary ganglion

III

Pterygopalatine
ganglion   VII

Midbrain

Pons

IX

Salivary
glands

Submandibular
ganglion

Otic
ganglion

Medulla

Trachea

X

Preganglionic neurons

Vagus nerve

Postganglionic
neurons

T1
T2
T3
T4
T5
T6
T7
T8
T9
T10
T11
T12
L1
L2

Bronchioles

Heart

Preganglionic
neuron

Celiac ganglion

Adrenal gland

Postganglionic
neuron

Stomach

Kidney

Pancreas

Superior
mesenteric
ganglion

Large
intestine

Small
intestine

Colon

Rectum

S2
S3
S4

Chain of
sympathetic
ganglia

Inferior
mesenteric
ganglion

Bladder

Reproductive
organs

FIGURE 47.5 Autonomic
nervous system *(From Scanlon, VC,
and Sanders, T: Essentials of Anatomy and
Physiology, ed. 4. F.A. Davis, Philadelphia,
2003, p 180, with permission.)*

TABLE 47.3 FUNCTIONS OF THE AUTONOMIC NERVOUS SYSTEM

Organ	Sympathetic Response	Parasympathetic Response
Heart (cardiac muscle)	Increase rate	Decrease rate (to normal)
Bronchioles (smooth muscle)	Dilate	Constrict (to normal)
Iris (smooth muscle)	Pupil dilates	Pupil constricts (to normal)
Salivary glands	Decrease secretion	Increase secretion (to normal)
Stomach and intestines (smooth muscle)	Decrease peristalsis	Increase peristalsis for normal digestion
Stomach and intestines (glands)	Decrease secretion	Increase peristalsis for normal digestion
Internal anal sphincter	Contract to prevent defecation	Relax to permit defection
Urinary bladder (smooth muscle)	Relax to prevent urination	Contract for normal urination
Internal urethral sphincter	Contract to prevent urination	Relax to permit urination
Liver	Change glycogen to glucose	None
Sweat glands	Increase secretion	None
Blood vessels in skin and viscera (smooth muscle)	Constrict	None
Blood vessels in skeletal muscle (smooth muscle)	Dilate	None
Adrenal glands	Increase secretion of epinephrine and norepinephrine	None

From Scanlon, VC, and Sanders, T: Essentials of Anatomy and Physiology. ed. 5. F.A. Davis, Philadelphia,
2007, p. 191, with permission

LEARNING TIP

Sympathetic—S for STRESS RESPONSE: The autonomic nervous system is a primitive response that affects humans automatically and involuntarily, thus increasing the likelihood of survival. It is often referred to as the fight-or-flight response. When you think of the sympathetic nervous system, think about getting away from a man-eating lion: you need dilated pupils to see the path better; copious production of sweat to lose heat through evaporation; increased rate and force of heartbeat to ensure that enough blood gets to the extremities so you can run faster; dilated bronchioles to get more oxygen to your muscles; decreased digestion so you won't get hungry while you are trying to get away from the lion; decreased urine output so you won't have to stop for the restroom; and increased mental alertness so you are always aware of where the lion is.

Parasympathetic—P for PEACEFUL: The parasympathetic nervous system brings the body back to balance and rest. It is sometimes referred to as the rest-and-digest response. Think, "I just got away from a man-eating lion, now my body can go back to normal and start digesting and urinating again!"

This is a great way to remember the responses, rather than an accurate description of the exact physiology involved.

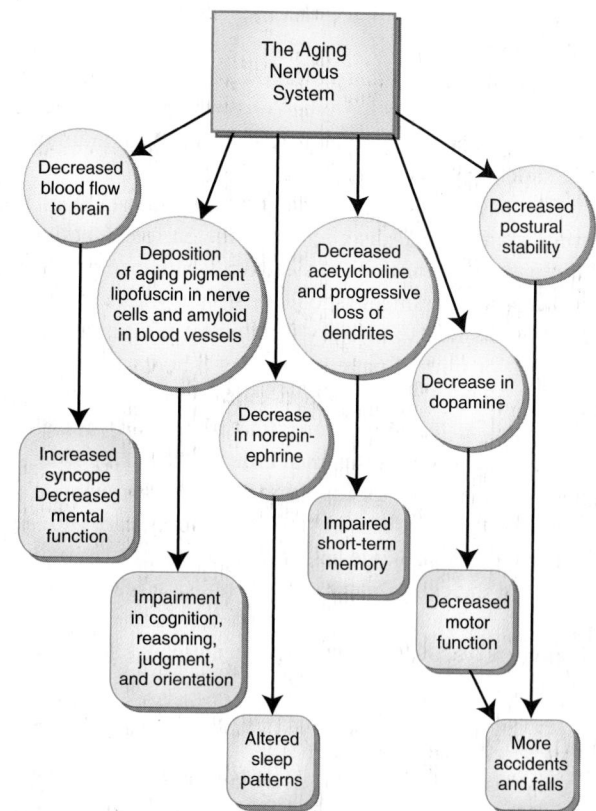

FIGURE 47.6 Aging and the neurological system. This concept map shows the effects the aging process has on the neurological system.

impairment in the elderly; far more common causes of mental changes include depression, malnutrition, hypotension, and the side effects of medications. Some forgetfulness is to be expected, however, as is a decreased ability for problem solving (Fig. 47.6).

NURSING ASSESSMENT/ DATA COLLECTION OF THE NEUROLOGICAL SYSTEM

The focus of the nursing neurological assessment is to establish the present function of the patient's neurological system and to detect changes from previous assessments. A complete neurological assessment, intended to determine the existence of neurological disease, is typically performed by a physician or nurse practitioner. A baseline neurological assessment should be performed on every patient admission (Table 47.4). In addition to giving valuable information about the current functioning of the patient's neurological system, the assessment provides baseline data for comparison purposes. This is especially important if the patient

has chronic neurological deficits on admission. Consider a patient admitted for placement of a prosthetic hip, who has had a previous **cerebrovascular** accident resulting in **paresis** of the right arm. A complete neurological assessment would document that the right arm is weaker than the left. If during the postoperative course you assess that both arms are equal in strength, you would want to notify the physician so the patient could be further assessed for possible causes of weakening of the left arm.

The results of the baseline assessment are invaluable in planning and implementing safe care. For example, patients who give a history of seizure activity need careful monitor-

TABLE 47.4 BASIC NEUROLOGICAL ASSESSMENT

1 Assess level of consciousness (patient's response to verbal or tactile stimulation) and orientation.
2 Obtain vital signs (specifically blood pressure, pulse, and respirations).
3 Check pupillary response to light.
4 Assess strength and equality of hand grip and movement of extremities.
5 Determine ability to sense touch or pain in extremities.

cerebrovascular: cerebro—brain + vascular—vessels
paresis: partial paralysis

ing, and all staff members who interact with such patients should be aware of how to respond to a seizure. Patients with **dysphagia** (difficulty swallowing) may need to have restrictions placed on the types of food or fluids they can have. This information must be consistently communicated to all staff involved in the patient's care.

The patient's admitting diagnosis, the presence of any chronic neurological disorders, and the current functioning of the patient's neurological system all influence how often neurological assessments should be done. Orders for neurological assessments may vary from every 15 minutes for an acutely ill or injured patient, to every 8 hours for a patient who is close to being discharged, to every 24 hours for a resident living in long-term care. It is always appropriate to assess a patient more often than ordered, based on observed changes in the patient's condition, and to communicate the findings of those assessments to the primary care provider. The changes noted while assessing the patient may indicate changes in the central nervous system. Rapid detection and intervention may mean the difference between chronic dysfunction and recovery or even between life and death for the patient.

Subjective Data

To understand the patient's neurological status, ask about past and current symptoms, use of prescribed and over-the-counter medications, use of recreational drugs, past surgeries, treatments, and risk factors such as family history, diet, exercise, sedentary lifestyle, caffeine intake, and recent stressors. Assessment of symptoms, as with other

dysphagia: dys—difficult + phagia—eating

body systems, includes asking the WHAT'S UP? questions (Table 47.5).

Health History

The nurse obtains a history of the patient's general health and then focuses on any neurological symptoms. Symptoms of neurological disorders vary in type, location, and intensity. It is important to remember that some neurological disorders can affect the patient's ability to think, remember, speak, or interpret stimuli. It may be necessary to question significant others about duration and severity of symptoms. Some patients may not be able to recognize their own neurological deficits. In these cases, the significant other usually initiates contact with the health-care system and provides the medical and social history. See Table 47.5 for sample questions to ask if the patient has a neurological problem.

In addition to using these questions, the nurse observes the patient during the health history. Is he or she shifting positions and exhibiting signs of discomfort? Is the patient able to change position and move about easily? Is he or she able to carry on a coherent conversation?

Physical Assessment

The physical assessment of the patient begins when you first meet the patient and make an overall evaluation of the patient's mental and physical status. The neurological system is assessed using inspection, palpation, and percussion (with a reflex hammer). When conducting the mental status and cognitive portions of the assessment, be aware that fatigue, illness, or medications can alter findings. When interpreting findings, consider the patient's age, educational background, and cultural orientation.

TABLE 47.5 SUBJECTIVE ASSESSMENT OF THE NEUROLOGICAL SYSTEM

Category	Questions to Ask During History Assessment	Rationale/Significance
Mental Status	• What is your name? What is the month? Year? Where are you now?	• Disorientation is often an initial sign of a neurological disorder.
Intellectual Function	• Subtract 7 from 100, then 7 from that answer, and so on (serial 7s).	• Most people with intact neurological function can complete serial 7s in about 1\1\2 minutes.
Thought Content	• What would you do if you smelled smoke? • Where would you put milk?	• Assessment of the patient's ability to interpret information and act appropriately is an important safety issue and activity of daily living.
Perception	• Show patient pencil and pen and ask what each is.	• Agnosia (inability to interpret or recognize familiar objects) can occur in cerebral vascular accidents and brain lesions.
Language Ability	• Read the following sentence, _____.	• Different types of aphasia can result from injury to different parts of the brain.
Memory	• Repeat these four or five words_____, and repeat them again in five minutes.	• Impaired memory can be affected by both delirium and dementia. Delirium can cause impaired immediate and short-term memory, whereas dementia not only affects immediate and short-term memory but also the ability to learn new information. Can also be related to stroke.
Pain	• On a scale of 1–10 with 0 as no pain and 10 as the worst you have ever had, what is your pain level?	• Pain perception may be altered or impaired by spinal injury, medications or alcohol, stress, and level of consciousness. Some spinal injuries may be critical but the patient will not complain of pain.

Level of Consciousness

Level of consciousness exists along a continuum from full wakefulness, alertness, and cooperation to unresponsiveness to any form of external stimuli. A fully conscious patient responds to questions spontaneously. As consciousness becomes impaired, a patient may show irritability, a shortened attention span, or an unwillingness to cooperate. The level of consciousness should be the first thing assessed during a neurological examination because the information obtained can be used to modify the remainder of the examination if necessary. Keep in mind that a decrease in the level of consciousness can be caused by problems such as hypoxia, hypoglycemia, and intoxication, not just dysfunction of the neurological system.

Many health-care institutions use the Glasgow Coma Scale (GCS), which is an international scale used to assess level of consciousness (LOC) and document findings (Table 47.6). The GCS is based on simple and clearly defined parameters of patient responses that provide for consistent assessment data. It is used to evaluate patients who have a potential for rapid deterioration in consciousness. The GCS assesses three parameters of consciousness: eye opening, verbal response, and motor response.

In the first section of the GCS, individuals are numerically scored according to their ability to open their eyes. Spontaneously opening their eyes receives a score of 4, opening with verbal stimulation a 3, with a painful stimulus such as pressure on the nailbeds or trapezius muscle a 2, and no response receives a 1. When initiating a painful stimulus use only enough pressure to elicit a response. Consider the patient's physical ability to respond, taking into consideration trauma, medical condition, and medications. For example, a patient who cannot open his or her eyes because of facial trauma may still have an intact neurological system.

The second section of the GCS addresses the patient's orientation to person, place, and time, often referred to as "oriented times 3." A patient who is fully oriented receives a score of 4. Typical questions include "What is your name? Where are you? What day is it?" (Keep in mind that we all forget the date from time to time!) You can also ask if they know what season it is (spring, fall, etc.). A resident of a nursing home may consider the facility his or her home and is not necessarily considered disoriented. Be sure your question is appropriate to the patient's living conditions, lifestyle, and medical condition. If the patient is unable to speak because of a stroke (expressive **aphasia**) or being intubated, do not rule out the possibility that the patient is oriented. Give expressively aphasic patients yes-or-no questions such as "Are you in a grocery store? Are you in a bowling alley? Are you in a hospital?" Patients may be able to answer with a shake of the head, or blinks, or hand squeezes as instructed.

Motor response is scored based on following commands or a response to pain. Ask the patient to move the fingers or toes and the raise arms or legs. You will also want to evaluate the equality of strength bilaterally by having the patient squeeze your fingers and show resistance against your hands by raising the arms. Ask the patient to push against your hands with each foot. Localizing pain indicates that the patient has an adequate level of consciousness to recognize where the pain is coming from and to attempt to push it away. An example is the patient who pushes against your hand when pressure is applied to the nailbed. Abnormal flexion posturing, characterized by flexion of the arms at the elbow and bringing the hands up toward the chest with the legs extended (**decorticate** posturing; Fig. 47.7A), indicates significant impairment of the cerebral functioning. A score of 3 is given to patients who exhibit abnormal flexion posturing. Abnormal extension posturing, or **decerebrate** posturing, indicates damage in the area of the brainstem (Fig. 47.7B). In this case, both the upper and lower extremities are extended and the arms are internally rotated. Abnormal extension posturing is scored as a 2.

The total possible score on the GCS ranges from 3 to 15. A score of less than 7 indicates a comatose patient and a score of 15 indicates the patient is fully alert and oriented. When used to score the effects of a head injury, a score of 13 or 14 indicates mild head injury, 9 to 12 indicates moderate injury, and any score of 8 or below indicates severe head injury. For all the categories of the GCS, the type of painful stimuli required to elicit a response should be documented. Deterioration in the patient's condition (i.e., a lowering of the GCS score) should be reported to the physician promptly.

Mental Status

Mental status can be affected not only by the aging process but also can be due to a variety of neurological disorders and injuries. A traumatic brain injury can result in memory impairment, delayed amnesia, affective disorders, and dementia. To assess for cognitive impairment, the Mini-Mental State Examination (MMSE) or Confusion Assessment Method (CAM) can be used. (Find more about these at

TABLE 47.6 GLASGOW COMA SCALE

Eye Opening	Spontaneous	4
	To verbal stimulus	3
	To painful stimulus	2
	No response	1
Verbal Response	Normal conversation	5
	Confused conversation	4
	Inappropriate words	3
	Incomprehensible sounds	2
	No response	1
Motor Response	Obeys commands	6
	Localizes pain	5
	Withdraws from pain	4
	Abnormal flexion	3
	Abnormal extension	2
	No response	1

aphasia: a—absence + phasia—speech
decorticate: de—down + corticate—cerebral cortex
decerebrate: de—down + cerebrate—cerebrum

A. Decorticate posturing

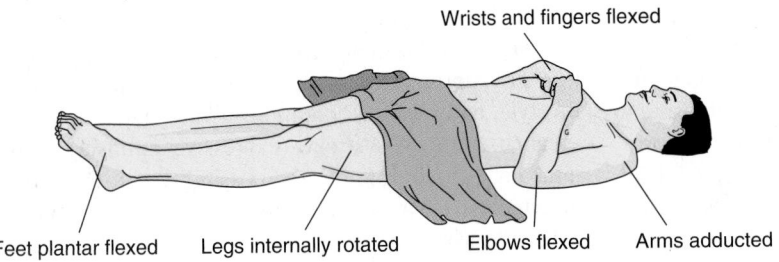

Wrists and fingers flexed

Feet plantar flexed   Legs internally rotated   Elbows flexed   Arms adducted

B. Decerebrate posturing

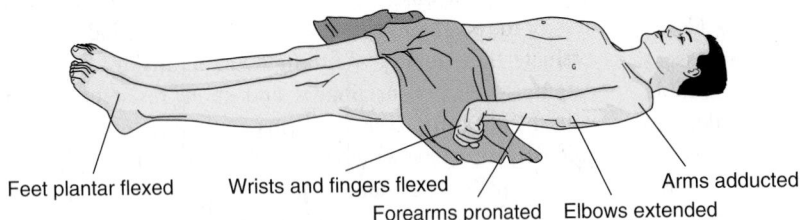

Feet plantar flexed   Wrists and fingers flexed   Arms adducted

Forearms pronated   Elbows extended

FIGURE 47.7 Abnormal posturing. *(A)* Decorticate posturing. *(B)* Decerebrate posturing

www.GeronurseOnline.org, an excellent collaborative website that provides best practice information related to older adults.) A change in mental status should be taken seriously, especially when the patient is on a variety of medicines or has had a recent medicine alteration. A primary cause of delirium and acute states of confusion is adverse effects from medications.

When you assess cognitive function, you are evaluating the patient's thinking capacity. You want to determine their length of attention span, ability to concentrate, judgment, memory, orientation, perception, problem solving ability, and motor function.

You can learn a great deal about a patient's mental capacities and emotional state by simply interacting with the patient. Behavior, mood, hygiene, grooming, and choice of dress reveal pertinent information about mental status. Mental status examinations can be performed to determine patients' cognitive functioning, thought processes, and perceptions by observing the patient's verbal and nonverbal responses to questions and specific requests. Table 47.5 includes some ways to assess these areas.

Assessment of the Eyes

Assessment of pupillary response is an important part of the neurological assessment and cranial nerve evaluation. The size of the pupils at rest is documented. Many institutions use a millimeter gauge for measuring pupils (Figure 47. 8). This allows an objective description of the size. If the patient's pupils are unusually large or small, you should determine if the patient has had any medications that might affect the size of the pupils. If the patient's pupils are unequal in size (**anisocoria**), without a correlating diagnosis or symptoms, ask the patient or his or her significant others if the patient normally has unequal pupils. Development of unequal pupils in a patient who previously had equal pupils is an emergency and should be reported to the physician immediately. Any deviation from the normal round shape of the pupils is documented.

Once the resting size of the pupils has been noted, the next step is to assess their response to light. In a darkened room, a light source (such as a flashlight) is directed at the pupil from the lateral aspect of the eye. This allows the examiner to see the direct and the consensual response to the light. A consensual response means that when one pupil is exposed to direct light, the other pupil also constricts. Absence of a consensual response may indicate a pathological condition in the area of the optic chiasm. Typically, the speed of the reaction to light is described as brisk, sluggish, or absent. Differences in the speed or size of constriction between the two pupils should be reported to the practitioner. Upon completion of the assessment of the pupils, document PERRL (pupils equal, round, and reactive to light) if no abnormalities are found.

Accommodation is the process of visual focusing from far to near. To evaluate for accommodation the patient

---

anisocoria: aniso—unequal + coria—pupil

Pupil gauge (mm)

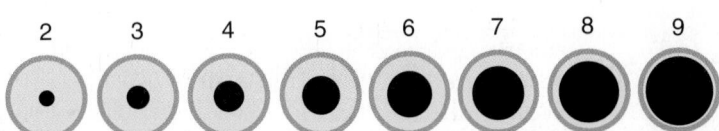

2   3   4   5   6   7   8   9

FIGURE 47.8 Assessment of pupil size.

focuses on an object at a distant point and then refocuses on the object at a near point. Pupils should constrict with the adjustment to the near object and the eyes should converge. PERRLA is used to note that pupils are equal, round, and reactive to light and accommodation.

The eyes are evaluated for range of motion and for smoothness and coordination of movements. Eyes that move in the same direction in a coordinated manner are said to have a conjugate gaze. Conversely, a dysconjugate gaze is movement of the eyes in different directions. Some patients may be unable to move one or both eyes in a specific direction; this is called ophthalmoplegia. It is often documented as "limited extraocular movements." Always document what the limitation is (e.g., "Patient is unable to look laterally with left eye"). This allows colleagues to compare their findings with yours and detect any changes.

Nystagmus is involuntary movement of the eyes. Nystagmus varies in the speed of the movement and the direction. Horizontal nystagmus is the most common. Common causes of nystagmus are phenytoin (Dilantin) toxicity and injury to the brainstem.

Assessment of Muscle Function

Assess muscle groups systematically in the upper extremities and then the lower extremities, comparing right to left. Muscle groups are compared for symmetry of size and strength. The patient's age and general physical condition should be kept in mind when evaluating muscle strength. One does not expect the same amount of strength from a 75-year-old woman as from a 20-year-old man. If the patient has chronic neurological deficits, ask if the results of the assessment are different from his or her usual level of function.

Many health-care providers use a 5-point scale to document muscle strength. A score of 5 indicates a patient who is able to move the extremity against gravity and the resistance of the examiner, displaying normal muscle strength. If the examiner is able to provide more resistance than the patient can overcome with active movement, the score is 4. If the patient is able to move the extremity only against gravity, but not resistance, the score is 3. If gravity must be eliminated by having the examiner support the extremity to allow the patient to move the extremity, the score is 2. A score of 1 is given if there is no active movement of the extremity, but a minimum muscular contraction can be palpated. If the examiner is unable to detect any muscular function, a score of 0 is given.

To test the deltoid muscles, ask the patient to raise his or her arms at the shoulder. Have the patient resist as you push down on the upper arms. The biceps are tested by having the patient flex the arm at the elbow and bring the palm toward the face, then resist as you attempt to straighten the arm by pulling on the forearm. Tell the patient to "make a muscle." With the arm similarly flexed, ask the patient to straighten the arm while you resist the movement.

Hand grasps are tested by having the patient squeeze your fingers. Remember to cross your index and middle fingers to prevent the patient from hurting your fingers. If the patient does not release the grasp when told to, it is a reflex grasp, not a response to command. A reflex palmar grasp may indicate a pathological condition of the frontal lobe.

Assess the patient for arm drift by asking the patient to hold both arms straight in front with the palms upward while keeping the eyes closed. A downward drift of the arm, or rotation so that the palm is down, indicates impairment of the opposite side of the brain. If a pathological condition is present, arm drift may be apparent before differences in muscle strength can be detected.

Assessment of leg muscle strength begins with the iliopsoas muscle. Place your hand on the patient's thigh and ask the patient to raise the leg, flexing at the hip. Hip adductors are tested by having the patient bring his or her legs together against your hands. The hip abductors and gluteus medius and minimus are tested by having the patient move the legs apart against resistance. Hip extension by the gluteus maximus is tested by placing the hand under the thigh and having the patient push down with the leg. The quadriceps femoris extends the knee and is tested by having the patient attempt to straighten the leg at the knee. The hamstrings are responsible for knee flexion and are evaluated by having the patient attempt to keep the heel of the foot against the bed or chair rung. Dorsiflexion is tested by having the patient pull the toes toward the head. Plantar flexion is tested by having the patient push against the examiner's hand with the ball of the foot.

Babinski's reflex is tested by firmly stroking the sole of the foot. Normal response is flexion of the great toe. If the great toe extends and the other toes fan out, neurological dysfunction should be suspected if the patient is more than 6 months old. Deep tendon reflexes are not usually part of a routine nursing assessment. The patient's gait should be assessed to detect any neurological dysfunction and also to assess ability to ambulate safely. Patients who stagger, weave, or bump into objects may need assistance when out of bed.

Romberg's test is performed by having the patient stand with feet together and eyes closed. Be sure to stand close to the patient, especially if he or she is an older adult, to prevent falling. A negative Romberg's test means that the patient experiences minimal swaying for up to 20 seconds. A patient who experiences swaying or who leans to one side is said to have a positive Romberg's test. A positive Romberg's test may be seen in cerebellar dysfunction.

 SAFETY TIP

A positive Romberg's test in an older adult is expected as a result of normal aging changes in the cerebellum. Be sure to protect the patient with a positive result from falls.

Assessment of Cranial Nerves

The cranial nerves are usually not examined in depth during routine bedside neurological assessment. Testing requires a patient who is able to cooperate with the examiner. Table

TABLE 47.7 ASSESSMENT OF CRANIAL NERVES

Nerve	Test
Olfactory nerve	Ask patient to identify common scents such as cinnamon and coffee.
Optic nerve	Ask patient to read something; tell how many fingers you are holding up.
Oculomotor nerve	Check pupils for reaction to light and accommodation.
Oculomotor, trochlear, and abducens nerves	Ask patient to follow your finger while it is moved in front of his or her eyes in the positions of a clock: 1, 3, 5, 7, 9, and 11 o'clock.
Trigeminal nerve	Ask patient to identify touch on different parts of the face with eyes closed.
Facial nerve	Ask patient to frown, smile, wrinkle forehead; check for symmetry.
Vestibulocochlear nerve	Have patient identify whisper close to each ear. Observe gait for balance.
Glossopharyngeal and vagus nerves	Watch for uvula and palate to rise when patient says "ahh." Touch back of throat with cotton tipped applicator to elicit gag reflex.
Spinal accessory nerve	Ask the patient to turn head and shrug the shoulders against resistance.
Hypoglossal nerve	Ask the patient to stick out the tongue and move it from side to side.

47.7 provides basic testing techniques that provide a superficial assessment of cranial nerve function.

Assessment Summary

In all cases, the findings of the neurological examination should be correlated with the remainder of the assessment findings. A decreased level of consciousness, coupled with a decreased oxygen saturation on pulse oximetry, point to hypoxia as a cause. Correlation of vital signs with neurological signs is particularly important. Bradycardia, increasing systolic blood pressure, and widening pulse pressure, commonly referred to as Cushing's response, are late indications of increasing intracranial pressure. These findings, in conjunction with a unilateral dilated pupil, may indicate impending herniation of the brain (discussed further in Chapter 48).

CRITICAL THINKING

Tim Thompson

■ You are caring for Tim, a 78-year-old man admitted with heart problems. As you enter his room with his afternoon medications, you find Tim confused. He thinks he is at home, that the year is 1968, and he does not understand who you are or why you are there. He recognizes his wife, who is at his bedside, and knows his own name.

1. How would you describe and document his mental status?
2. What additional data do you need to decide how to proceed?
3. What may have contributed to his confusion?

Suggested answers at end of chapter.

 DIAGNOSTIC TESTS

Laboratory Tests

Specific diagnostic blood tests do not exist for neurological disorders. However, depending on the history and physical

examination, the practitioner may include laboratory tests to look for underlying causes of symptoms: thyroid hormone levels, vitamin B_{12}, complete blood count, electrolytes, creatine kinase and isoenzymes (CK), VDRL, liver function, and renal function. Measurement of erythrocyte sedimentation rate (ESR) and white blood cell (WBC) count may indicate an infection, such as meningitis. Hormone levels, such as prolactin or cortisol, may indicate dysfunction of the pituitary gland related to a brain tumor. Anticholinesterase testing and antibody titers are useful in diagnosing myasthenia gravis (MG).

Lumbar Puncture

Cerebrospinal fluid may be obtained via lumbar puncture and evaluated for glucose and protein levels, presence of bacteria and white blood cells, levels of immunoglobulin, antibodies, and culture and sensitivity. Cerebrospinal fluid samples should be sent to the laboratory immediately following the procedure.

Typically, the lumbar puncture needle is placed at the level of L3–4 or L4–5 in an adult. Because the spinal cord ends at the L1 level, this placement prevents damage to the cord by the needle. If there is any difficulty inserting the needle, this may be done under fluoroscopy to help guide needle placement.

Nursing Care

Assure that informed consent has been obtained prior to the procedure. Assist the patient into a side-lying position with his or her back as close to the edge of the bed nearest the practitioner as possible. Depending on the patient's condition, you may need to help the patient flex his or her knees up to the chest (Fig. 47.9). This position maximizes the space between the vertebrae, which makes it easier for the practitioner to insert the needle. An alternative position is to have the patient sit with the back perpendicular to the edge of the bed. Leaning over a bedside table may help the patient maintain the position. During the procedure, you may be asked to assist the physician with equipment handling.

After the lumbar puncture is completed, instruct the patient to remain on bedrest with the head of the bed flat for 6 to 8 hours, as ordered by the physician, and to increase

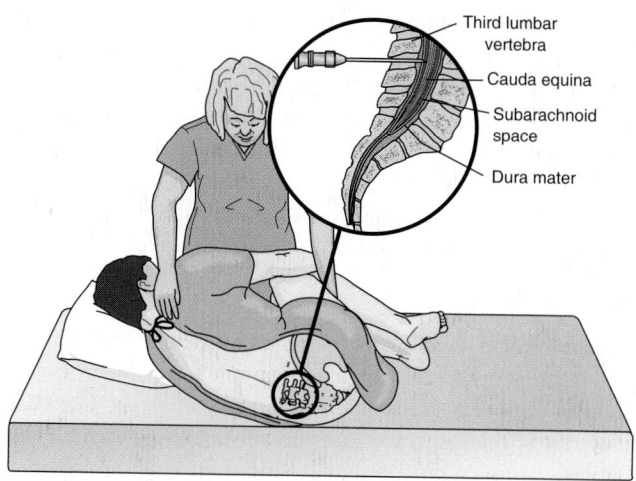

Third lumbar vertebra
Cauda equina
Subarachnoid space
Dura mater

FIGURE 47.9 Position for lumbar puncture.

oral intake of fluids. Keeping the head flat decreases the likelihood of leakage of cerebrospinal fluid from the puncture site, which can result in a severe headache. Increasing fluid intake promotes replacement of the fluid that was removed. Label and send the specimens to the laboratory as ordered. Check the puncture site for swelling or drainage of cerebrospinal fluid and report any leakage to the health-care provider. Assess the movement and sensation to the lower extremities frequently for the first 4 hours after the procedure. Assess the patient for headache and, if necessary, obtain an order for an analgesic.

NURSING CARE TIP

The idea of a needle being introduced into the spinal canal is frightening to many people. Give simple, clear directions to the patient; help the patient maintain his or her position; and provide emotional support throughout the procedure.

X-Ray Examination

Spinal x-ray examinations are done to determine the status of individual vertebrae and their relationship to one another. If the patient experiences pain with certain movements, he or she may be asked to flex and extend the area of the spine being examined while the radiographs are taken. This allows detection of abnormal movement of the vertebrae. If the patient has possibly sustained trauma to the spine, particularly the cervical spine, radiographs are taken before immobilizing devices are removed. Skull radiographs may be taken to detect skull fractures or foreign bodies. No special nursing care is required.

Computed Tomography

A computed tomographic (CT) scan is used for diagnosing neurological disorders of the brain or the spine. Some of the disorders that can be detected by CT are hemorrhage, ventricle size, cerebral atrophy, tumors, skull fractures, and

abscesses. CT is used when MRI is contraindicated because of metal aneurysm clips or other metal implants. The scan may be performed with or without radiopaque contrast material to enhance the clarity of the images that are recorded. If contrast material is used, a series of images is filmed, and then the contrast material is given intravenously and another series of images is filmed. The patient should be questioned about any allergies to contrast material, iodine, or shellfish. The blood urea nitrogen (BUN) and creatinine levels should be checked before administration of contrast material because it is excreted through the kidneys. Patients with elevated BUN and creatinine or known renal disease may be unable to tolerate the contrast material. Contrast material is most commonly used if a tumor is suspected or following surgery in the area to be scanned. CT scans are commonly used in emergency evaluations because they can be done quickly, an important consideration if the patient is ventilated or unstable.

Nursing Care

During the CT scan, the patient must lie still on a moveable table. Noncontrast scans take approximately 10 minutes; contrast scans take between 20 and 30 minutes. Patients who are receiving dye should be warned that they may feel a sensation of warmth following the injection; warmth in the groin area may make them feel as though they have been incontinent of urine. Nausea, diaphoresis, itching, or difficulty breathing may indicate allergy to the dye and should be reported immediately to the physician or nurse practitioner. Sedation may be required for patients who are agitated or disoriented. Patients who are in pain may require pain medication before the examination.

Magnetic Resonance Imaging

Magnetic resonance imaging (MRI) gives a more detailed picture of soft tissue than a CT scan. It is not as useful when looking for bony abnormalities. MRI is used for diagnosis of degenerative diseases such as multiple sclerosis, arteriovenous malformations, small tumors, hemorrhages, and cerebral and spinal cord edema. An MRI of the mediastinal cavity will determine if the thymus gland is enlarged and facilitate the diagnosis of myasthenia gravis. It is a longer procedure and may be difficult for unstable, disoriented, or ventilated patients. As with a CT scan, the MRI can be done with or without contrast material. Some facilities have the capability to perform magnetic resonance angiograms (MRAs). This test allows visualization of blood vessels and assessment of blood flow without being as invasive as a traditional angiogram.

Nursing Care

Because of the magnetic fields being used, there are restrictions placed on patients undergoing an MRI and the health-care personnel who work within the MRI facility. Individuals with pacemakers or any type of metallic prosthesis are not able to undergo MRI or be in the room when one is performed. This is because the magnetic field is so strong that it could dislodge the prosthesis or pacemaker. Patients are asked to remove all metal objects, such as jewelry or hair clips, before the procedure. Individuals who may have accidentally acquired metallic foreign bodies (e.g., metal slivers in the eye or shrapnel that was not removed) may need an x-ray examination to determine the presence or absence of such objects. Even permanent make-up and tattoos can cause problems because of the metallic salts in the dyes. Other contraindications include gross obesity, claustrophobia, agitation and inability to cooperate, and inability to lie flat. It may be difficult for the patient to lie in one position for a prolonged period. The patient's need for pain medication should be assessed before the procedure. Use of pillows for positioning may improve comfort. The narrow, tunnel-like structure of the MRI unit causes claustrophobia in some patients; some patients may require use of sedatives or open MRI units. Warn the patient that the procedure involves a noisy "knocking" sound. Encourage the use of deep breathing, guided imagery, and other relaxation techniques.

SAFETY TIP

Educate patients to consider that they may someday need a life-saving MRI before having tattoos or permanent make-up applied!

Angiogram

An angiogram is an x-ray study of blood vessels that is used when an abnormality of cerebral or spinal blood vessels is suspected or to obtain information about blood supply to a tumor. Following injection of a local anesthetic, a catheter is inserted through the femoral artery and advanced until contrast material can be injected into the appropriate vessels. The dye then shows the vessels on the radiograph and provides information about the structure of specific vessels, as well as overall circulation to the area.

Nursing Care

Before an angiogram, the patient receives a clear liquid diet and has an intravenous needle in place. Informed consent must be obtained. BUN and creatinine levels are evaluated because the contrast material is excreted through the kidneys. Potential for bleeding is assessed by prothrombin time and partial thromboplastin time tests because a puncture is being made in a large artery. Typically, the patient receives some type of sedation before being transported to the angiography suite. During the injection of the contrast material, the patient may complain of severe heat sensations and a metallic taste in the mouth. The patient must lie still while the radiographs are being taken, and so should be told about the sensations he or she may experience. Patients who are disoriented or agitated may require sedation to complete the test.

Following the procedure, pressure is maintained on the catheter insertion site and the patient is kept flat in bed for 6 to 8 hours to prevent bleeding from the insertion site. The patient may turn from side to side but must keep the affected leg straight. In addition to assessing vital signs, evaluate the catheter insertion site and the presence and quality of the popliteal and pedal pulses in the affected leg. Decrease or loss of the pedal pulse may indicate a clot in the femoral artery and should be reported to the physician immediately. Patients should be encouraged to increase oral intake in addition to the intravenous fluids that are administered to aid in the excretion of the contrast material.

Myelogram

A **myelogram** is an x-ray examination of the spinal canal and its contents. Following a lumbar puncture, cerebrospinal fluid is removed and sent for laboratory analysis. Contrast material is then injected into the subarachnoid space. The patient is moved into various positions and radiographs are taken. Compression of nerve roots, herniation of intravertebral disks, and blockage of cerebrospinal fluid circulation may all be detected by myelogram.

Nursing Care

Following the procedure, the patient is kept on bedrest with the head elevated. This lessens the possibility of the contrast material getting into the cerebral cerebrospinal fluid circulation. The contrast material used for myelograms can lower the seizure threshold in some patients. Any patient with a known seizure disorder should have serum levels of anticonvulsants evaluated and be carefully observed for signs of seizures.

Because of their invasive nature, a separate informed consent form may be required for the lumbar puncture and myelogram. The physician performing the test explains the risks, benefits, and possible complications of the examination. Patients who need these diagnostic procedures may have cognitive deficits; therefore, it may be necessary to obtain consent from the legal next of kin.

Electroencephalogram

Evaluation of the electrical activity of the brain is obtained by use of an **electroencephalogram** (EEG). Electrodes are attached to the scalp with an adhesive. Electrical activity is transmitted through the electrodes to a tracing. Analysis of the tracing can identify areas of abnormality, such as a seizure focus or areas of slowed activity.

Nursing Care

Before the test, make sure that the patient's hair is clean and dry. The physician may write orders to withhold sedatives to prevent interference with the EEG, and patients may be weaned from their anticonvulsants if the goal of the test is to identify the seizure focus during a seizure. These patients must be very carefully monitored and protected from harm. Typically, they undergo videotaping while the EEG is performed. Following the procedure, the adhesive must be

---

myelogram: myelo—referring to the spinal cord + gram—picture

electroencephalogram: electro—electrical activity + encephalo—referring to the brain + gram—picture

washed from the hair. Assist the hospitalized patient to do this as soon as possible, before it becomes hardened and difficult to remove.

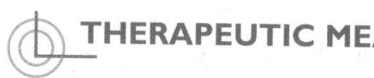

THERAPEUTIC MEASURES

Moving and Positioning

Patients who have pain may need help in changing positions and ambulating. Use of heat, cold, or analgesics may allow the patient to be more independent in mobility. Patients with paresis, paralysis, or **paresthesia** may be partially or completely dependent in moving and positioning. Take care to maintain the body in functional positions when routine position changes are made. If the patient experiences sensory loss, ensure that no part of the body is inadvertently compressed (e.g., a hand caught under a hip or the scrotum compressed between the legs). Pressure ulcers are of primary concern with the patient who is unable to move independently. Collaborate with the physical therapist to determine positioning techniques that maximize the chance of useful recovery.

Contractures and footdrop are complications that are often associated with neurological disorders. Contractures are permanent muscle contractions with fibrosis of connective tissue that occur from lack of use of a muscle or muscle group. They cause permanent deformities and prevent normal functioning of the affected part. Footdrop occurs when the feet are not supported in a functional position and become contracted in a position of plantar flexion (Fig. 47.10). Use footboards, high-top tennis shoes, and splints to help prevent footdrop. Splints are commonly used to prevent contractures of the upper and lower extremities and to keep the affected part in a functional position. If splints are used, the patient must be evaluated for discomfort and skin breakdown at the splint site.

Mobilization should be begun as soon as a patient is medically stable. Initially this may involve the use of a cardiac chair if the patient is unable to bear weight. Transfer of the patient to a bedside chair or use of ambulation aids may require a multidisciplinary approach. Be careful to recognize any physical or cognitive deficits that may affect safety and adjust the environment to protect the patient. This includes communicating any safety concerns to unlicensed personnel who interact with the patient.

Activities of Daily Living

The effects of neurological disorders on activities of daily living (ADLs) may range from an inconvenience to complete dependence. Patients may have trouble bending over to put on their shoes and socks, lifting a full cooking pot, or caring for an infant. A high-level quadriplegic may be completely unable to perform ADLs but can be taught to direct his or her own personal care. Patients should be encouraged to use strategies learned in occupational or physical therapy.

Assessment of a hospitalized patient should include a discussion of the strategies the patient normally uses at home to accomplish ADLs. Every attempt should be made to continue to use these strategies. This is particularly true if the patient is admitted to a long-term care facility. Patients who have normal cognitive function should be included in care planning and encouraged to work collaboratively with caregivers. If the strategies the patient uses during ADLs must be changed (e.g., if the patient's transfer technique is unsafe), the rationale for the changes should be explained to the patient and significant others. If patients have impaired cognitive function, try to maintain a specific routine that is as close to their normal environment as possible. Normalizing routines may help patients adapt to a change in environment and maximize their ability to function.

Communication

The communication problems associated with neurological disorders have a variety of etiologies. Some neurological disorders cause difficulty speaking (**dysarthria**). Dysfunction of the lips, tongue, or jaw makes speech difficult or impossible to understand. When dysarthric individuals know what they want to say but cannot be understood, they can become very frustrated. This frustration is compounded if the patients are treated as if they have cognitive deficits merely because they have difficulty communicating.

Patients who have had a stroke can experience different types of aphasia. Expressive aphasia is difficulty or inability to verbally communicate with others. The patient may be able to speak in sentences but inappropriately substitute words, such as "The sky is dish." Word-finding difficulty is another type of expressive aphasia. These patients may tell you "I want a. . . ." and then be unable to complete the sentence. In severe cases of aphasia, the patient may make sounds that resemble words or may only utter sounds. For individuals with no intelligible speech or with word-finding difficulty, a picture board with commonly used items may

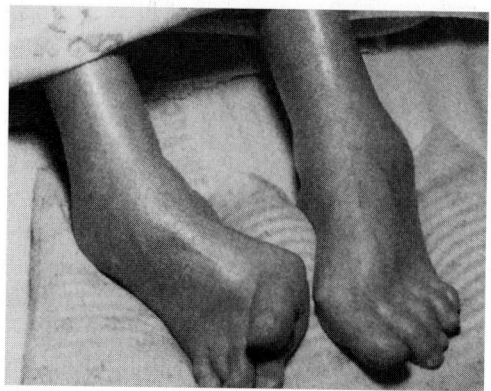

FIGURE 47.10 Contractures, footdrop. *(From Hegner, B: Assisting in Long Term Care, ed. 3. Delmar Publishers, Albany, NY, 1998, with permission.)*

---

paresthesia: para—beside + asthesia—sensations

dysarthria: dys—dysfunctional + arthria—movement of the joints used in speech

facilitate communication. (See an example of a picture board in Chapter 49.) Keep in mind that patients with expressive aphasia may answer yes to all questions rather than just those for which yes is correct. The same is true of answering no. This is one reason why a nurse should never ask a patient, "Are you Mrs. Gonzalez?" An aphasic patient may say yes even if that is not her name. Instead, ask the patient to state her name. If she cannot state her name, check her identification band.

For patients who substitute words, simply correct the substitution and continue the conversation. Patients with expressive aphasia are often very aware of and frustrated by their difficulty communicating. Give them time to try to express themselves. If you cannot understand them, offer possibilities based on the situation. If the patient is sitting in the chair, ask if he or she wants to go back to bed or wants to use the bathroom. If the patient is restless, ask if he or she is in pain.

Some patients use the same word in response to all questions, and for a few patients that word is a profanity. This is very difficult for significant others to deal with, particularly if swearing is not something the patient normally did. Make it clear to the family that you understand that this behavior is part of the patient's illness.

Receptive aphasia affects the patient's ability to understand spoken language. Again, the severity of the aphasia varies. Some patients may understand simple directions such as "sit down" or "squeeze my fingers." In other cases, the nurse may need to pantomime the action the nurse wants the patient to perform, such as showing the patient pills and then mimicking taking the pills and drinking water.

SAFETY TIP

If the patient has receptive aphasia, assume that he or she cannot understand or follow safety instructions, such as "Do not stand up until I get back." Even going around the corner to get water can give a patient enough time to try to stand up and subsequently fall.

Nutrition

Alterations in the ability to maintain an adequate nutritional intake can have many causes. The level of consciousness may be depressed enough that the patient does not recognize that she or he is hungry or thirsty. Decreased level of consciousness or cranial nerve dysfunction may impair the patient's ability to swallow safely. Severe weakness may limit the patient's ability to take in enough food to meet the body's requirements. These conditions are often compounded by the increased metabolic rate that accompanies neurological injury or illness.

If there is any question of the patient's ability to swallow, a swallowing evaluation should be performed by a speech therapist. Some institutions use a radiological examination to evaluate the ability to swallow. A small amount of barium is added to food or fluid, and fluoroscopy is used while the patient swallows. This allows visualization of the path of the food or fluid. Patients with swallowing difficulty (dysphagia) may have better success with foods or thick liquids rather than thin fluids. Liquids may be thickened with special thickening agents to allow easier swallowing. All patients should be positioned as upright as possible while eating or drinking, and patients who have difficulty swallowing should be monitored during eating.

If weakness or fatigue is the cause of decreased nutritional intake, several modifications are possible. Serving small portions of food frequently can increase intake. Using high-protein, high-calorie foods and supplements increases the nutritional content of small amounts of foods.

For patients who are unable to swallow or who cannot swallow enough food, enteral tube feedings may be required. If enteral feedings are anticipated to be for a short duration, a nasogastric tube may be used. The disadvantages of nasogastric tubes include impairment of the integrity of nasal skin and the risk of aspiration. The risk of aspiration in neurologically impaired patients who have cognitive impairments is increased because these patients may pull out the nasogastric tube because they do not understand its purpose. If long-term enteral feedings are anticipated, a gastrostomy tube may be placed directly through the abdominal wall into the stomach. This feeding method has the advantage of reducing the risks of aspiration and eliminating nasal skin breakdown.

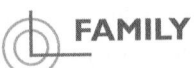

When working with patients who have a neurological deficit, whether acute or chronic, in the hospital, extended care facility, or at home, the family needs to be included in their care and rehabilitation. Depending on the patient's diagnosis and prognosis, the family will need support from staff. It is rewarding to see the patient who has had an accident and recovers with rehabilitation, but it is also rewarding to promote quality of life for the patient with Alzheimer's disease and his or her family. It is important to communicate to the family regarding patient improvements and information about the illness. Include the family in the patient's care, such as bathing, feeding, and grooming. Suggest that the family participate in physical therapy sessions. Education is of vital importance, especially if the patient is going to be discharged home. Direct the patient and family to support groups and case managers for information regarding financial assistance and community resources during rehabilitation.

REVIEW QUESTIONS

1. Which neurons carry impulses from the CNS to effectors?
   a. Mixed
   b. Motor
   c. Afferent
   d. Sensory

2. Which structure in the CNS regulates body temperature?
   a. Hypothalamus
   b. Temporal lobe
   c. Pons
   d. Pituitary

3. Which of the following is a symptom of increasing intracranial pressure that should be reported immediately to the primary care provider?
   a. Constricted pupils
   b. Decreasing level of consciousness
   c. Narrowing pulse pressure
   d. Bradypnea

Multiple response item. Select all that apply.
4. What are the normal effects of aging on the CNS?
   a. Increased postural stability
   b. Reduced blood flow to the brain
   c. Impaired short-term memory
   d. Sleep disturbances
   e. Loss of deep tendon reflexes

5. A patient asks what to expect when she has an angiogram. Which response by the nurse is best?
   a. "A small needle will be inserted into your spinal column to withdraw fluid for examination."
   b. "You will be in a large machine that uses magnetic energy to create images; it has a noisy knocking sound."
   c. "Electrodes will be placed on your head to monitor electrical activity in your brain."
   d. "A catheter will be placed in your femoral artery, and dye will be injected that will make your vessels show up on x-ray."

6. Which of the following activities should be encouraged when a patient returns from a CT scan using a contrast medium?
   a. Ambulation
   b. Drinking fluids
   c. Turning side to side
   d. Coughing and deep breathing

7. Which of the following nursing interventions can help prevent footdrop?
   a. Position the patient in the left lateral position.
   b. Provide daily foot massage.
   c. Apply high-top tennis shoes.
   d. Maintain the patient in an upright position as much as possible.

SUGGESTED ANSWERS TO

CRITICAL THINKING

■ Mrs. Stevens

Albuterol is an adrenergic agonist (sometimes called a sympathomimetic), which is given to stimulate the sympathetic nervous system, resulting in open airways in patients with respiratory disease. However, it can also stimulate the cardiac system and cause a rapid heart rate and increased blood pressure. Be sure to monitor vital signs in patients receiving medications that affect the autonomic nervous system.

■ Tim Thompson
1. He is alert but confused, oriented to person only.
2. The nurse should ask his wife if this has ever happened before; check his medical history for any disorders that may contribute to neurological dysfunction; do a quick neurological assessment to determine if any additional deficits exist; check vital signs and pulse oximetry if available; and notify the physician immediately if the symptoms are a new finding.
3. Some possible explanations to explore include hypoxemia, stroke, worsening heart problems causing inadequate flow of blood to the brain, hypoglycemia, or even confusion (delirium) related to a sudden transition from home to an unfamiliar environment.

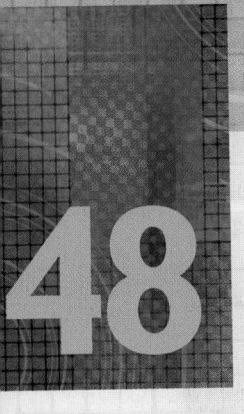

48

Nursing Care of Patients with Central Nervous System Disorders

JENNIFER WHITLEY

KEY TERMS

akinesia (AH-kin-EE-zee-uh)
ataxia (ah-TAK-see-ah)
bradykinesia (BRAY-dee-kin-EE-zee-ah)
contracture (kon-TRAK-chur)
contralateral (KON-truh-LAT-er-uhl)
craniectomy (KRAY-nee-EK-tuh-mee)
cranioplasty (KRAY-nee-oh-plas-tee)
craniotomy (KRAY-nee-AHT-oh-mee)
delirium (de-LEER-ee-um)
dementia (dee-MEN-cha)
dysreflexia (DIS-re-FLEK-see-ah)
encephalitis (en-SEFF-uh-LYE-tis)
encephalopathy (en-SEFF-uh-LAHP-ah-thee)
hemiparesis (hem-ee-puh-REE-sis)
hydrocephalus (HIGH-droh-SEF-uh-luhs)
ipsilateral (IP-si-LAT-er-uhl)
laminectomy (LAM-i-NEK-toh-mee)
meningitis (MEN-in-JIGH-tis)
neurodegenerative (new-roh-de-JEN-er-uh-tiv)
nuchal rigidity (NEW-kuhl re-JID-i-tee)
paraparesis (PAR-ah-puh-REE-sis)
paraplegia (PAR-ah-PLEE-jee-ah)
photophobia (FOH-tuh-FOH-bee-ah)
postictal (pohst-IK-tuhl)
prodromal (proh-DROH-muhl)
quadriparesis (KWA-dri-puh-REE-sis)
quadriplegia (KWA-dri-PLEE-jee-ah)
turbid (TER-bid).

QUESTIONS TO GUIDE YOUR READING

1. What are the causes, risk factors, and pathophysiology of central nervous system infections, including meningitis and encephalitis?
2. What nursing interventions are appropriate for a patient with a central nervous system infection?
3. What are the differences in the varying types of headaches?
4. What education should you provide for the patient experiencing headaches?
5. What are causes and types of seizures?
6. How would you care for someone during a seizure?
7. How would you recognize a patient developing increased intracranial pressure?
8. What nursing interventions can help prevent increased intracranial pressure?
9. What are the causes, risk factors, and pathophysiology of injuries to the brain and spinal cord?
10. What nursing care will you provide for a patient with an injury to the brain or spinal cord?
11. What are the causes, risk factors, and pathophysiology associated with neurodegenerative disorders such as Parkinson's, Huntington's, or Alzheimer's disease?
12. What nursing care will you provide for a patient with a neurodegenerative disorder?
13. What nursing interventions are appropriate for the patient with dementia?

Disorders of the central nervous system (CNS) include problems originating in the brain and spinal cord. Because the CNS is the control center for the entire body, disorders in this system can cause symptoms in any part of the body, ranging from pain to paralysis, confusion, and coma. This chapter presents nursing care of patients with these disorders.

CENTRAL NERVOUS SYSTEM INFECTIONS

Infectious agents can enter the central nervous system via a variety of routes (Table 48.1). Anything that depresses the patient's immune system such as steroid administration, chemotherapy, radiation therapy, or malnutrition can make the patient more vulnerable to infection.

Meningitis

Meningitis is an inflammation of the brain and spinal cord that may be caused by either bacterial or viral infection. Any microorganism that enters the body can result in meningitis. Bacterial meningitis is a serious infection that is spread by direct contact with discharge from the respiratory tract of an infected person. Viral meningitis, also called aseptic meningitis, is more common and rarely serious. It usually presents with flulike symptoms, and patients recover in 1 to 2 weeks.

Pathophysiology and Etiology

The most common bacteria causing meningitis include *Neisseria meningitidis, Streptococcus pneumoniae,* and *Haemophilus influenzae* type b (Hib). With current immunization standards in the United States, the *H. influenzae* type b has decreased in recent years. *N. meningitides,* the cause of meningococcal meningitis, and *S. pneumoniae,* the cause of pneumococcal meningitis, are the major causes of bacterial meningitis. The infection generally begins in another area, such as the upper respiratory tract, enters the blood, and invades the CNS, causing the meninges to become inflamed and intracranial pressure to increase. Vessel occlusion and

TABLE 48.1 ROUTES OF ENTRY FOR CENTRAL NERVOUS SYSTEM INFECTIONS

Route of Entry	Examples
Bloodstream	Insect bite
	Otitis media
Direct extension	Fracture of frontal or facial bones
Cerebrospinal fluid	Dural tear
	Poor sterile technique during procedure
Nose or mouth	Meningococcus meningitis
In utero	Contamination of amniotic fluid
	Rubella
	Vaginal infection

TABLE 48.2 CRANIAL NERVES AFFECTED BY MENINGITIS

Cranial Nerve Affected	Manifestation
III, IV, VI	Ocular palsies
	Unequal and sluggishly reactive pupils
VII	Facial weakness
VIII	Deafness and vertigo

necrosis of areas in the brain may occur. Cranial nerve function may be transiently or permanently affected by meningitis. Some of the effects are listed in Table 48.2.

Prevention

Vaccines are available against Hib and *S. pneumoniae.* Hib vaccinations are begun during the newborn period, but the vaccine against *S. pneumoniae* is not effective under the age of 2 years and is recommended for those individuals over the age of 65 who have a chronic medical condition. In addition to vaccines, current standards for prevention include early diagnosis and prompt treatment of individuals who have come in contact with diagnosed patients.

Signs and Symptoms

The most common symptom of meningitis is headache, caused by tension on blood vessels and irritation of the pain-sensitive dura mater. A high fever and stiff neck are present and the patient may experience **photophobia**. The patient with meningococcal meningitis usually presents with petechiae on the skin and mucous membranes.

Nuchal rigidity (pain and stiffness when the neck is moved) is caused by spasm of the extensor muscles of the neck. Positive Kernig's and Brudzinski's signs are often seen in patients suffering from meningitis. Both signs are caused by inflammation of the meninges and spinal nerve roots. To elicit Kernig's sign, the examiner flexes the patient's hip to 90 degrees and tries to extend the patient's knee. The sign is positive if the patient experiences pain and spasm of the hamstring. Brudzinski's sign is positive when flexion of the patient's neck causes the hips and knees to flex (Fig. 48.1). Nausea and vomiting associated with meningitis are caused by direct irritation of brain tissue and by increased intracranial pressure (ICP).

Encephalopathy refers to the mental status changes seen in patients with meningitis. These are manifested as short attention span, poor memory, disorientation, difficulty following commands, and a tendency to misinterpret environmental stimuli. Late signs of meningitis include lethargy and seizures.

Complications of Meningitis

Resolution of meningitis depends on how quickly and effectively the disease is treated. Some individuals experience no

---

meningitis: mening—membranous covering of the brain + itis—inflammation

photophobia: photo—light + phobia—fear or intolerance
encephalopathy: encephalo—brain + pathy—illness

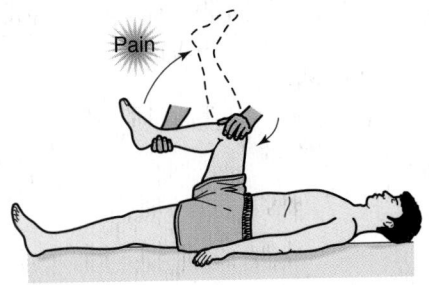
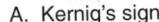
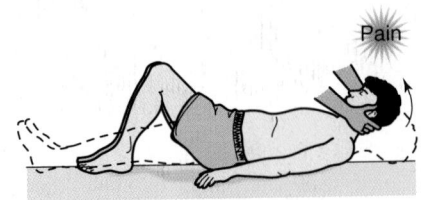

A. Kernig's sign

B. Brudzinski's sign

FIGURE 48.1 *(A)* Kernig's sign. *(B)* Brudzinski's sign.

lasting effects, while other patients have permanent neurological deficits. Cranial nerve damage may leave the patient blind or deaf. Seizures may continue to occur even after the acute phase of the illness has passed. Cognitive deficits ranging from memory impairment to profound learning disabilities may occur.

Diagnostic Tests

A lumbar puncture is the most informative diagnostic test for a patient with suspected meningitis (see Chapter 47). Viral meningitis is characterized by clear cerebrospinal fluid with normal glucose level and normal or slightly increased protein level. No bacteria are seen, but the white blood cell count is usually increased. In contrast, the cerebrospinal fluid of an individual with bacterial meningitis is **turbid,** or cloudy, because of the massive number of white blood cells. Bacteria are identified by Gram stain and culture, and a sensitivity test is done to identify the most effective antibiotic. The bacteria utilize the glucose normally found in cerebrospinal fluid (CSF), thereby lowering the glucose level. The amount of protein in the cerebrospinal fluid is elevated. A magnetic resonance image (MRI) or computed tomographic (CT) scan may be done to evaluate for complications.

Therapeutic Interventions

Meningitis can be fatal if not promptly treated. Antibiotics are administered for bacterial meningitis. Symptom management is the same for viral or bacterial meningitis. Antipyretics such as acetaminophen are used to control the fever; a cooling blanket may also be used. Care should be taken to avoid cooling the patient too much because shivering increases the metabolic demand for oxygen and glucose. A quiet, dark environment lessens the stimulation to a patient who has a headache or photophobia (sensitivity to light) and who may be agitated, disoriented, or at risk for seizures.

Analgesics are given to lessen head and neck pain. Corticosteriods and anti-inflammatory agents are given to decrease swelling. Nausea and vomiting are controlled by administering antiemetic medications. The patient with meningococcal meningitis should be placed in isolation because this disease can be transmitted to others.

Patients may become agitated. An important aspect of nursing care focuses on keeping patients from harming themselves. It is very upsetting to families to see a loved one acting agitated or disoriented. Therefore, it is important to teach the family about symptoms and treatment goals for the patient (Box 48.1 Meningitis Summary).

Encephalitis

Pathophysiology

Encephalitis is an inflammation of brain tissue. Nerve cell damage, edema, and necrosis cause neurological findings localized to the specific areas of the brain affected. Hemorrhage may occur in some types of encephalitis. Increased

---

Box 48.1

Meningitis Summary

Signs and Symptoms	Nuchal rigidity Positive Kernig's and Brudzinski's signs Fever Photophobia Petechial rash on skin and mucous membranes Encephalopathy
Diagnostic Tests	Lumbar puncture with CSF analysis, C&S Complete blood count C&S nose and throat
Therapeutic Interventions	Antimicrobials (if bacterial) Seizure precautions Antipyretics Pain management Reduction of environmental stimuli Education
Complications	Seizures, IICP, hearing loss, vision impairment, cognitive defects
Possible Nursing Diagnoses	Hyperthermia r/t meningitis Risk for injury r/t positive culture in CSF Acute pain r/t nuchal rigidity

CSF = cerebrospinal fluid; C&S = culture and sensitivity; IICP = increased intracranial pressure; r/t = related to.

---

encephalitis: encephalo—brain + itis—inflammation

intracranial pressure (ICP) may lead to herniation of the brain (see section on increased intracranial pressure).

Etiology

Viruses are the most common cause of encephalitis. They may be specifically related to a particular time of year or geographical location. Some viruses, such as West Nile virus, are carried by ticks or mosquitoes. Others are systemic viral infections, such as infectious mononucleosis or mumps, which spread to the brain. Parasites, toxic substances, bacteria, vaccines, and fungi are other potential causes of encephalitis.

Herpes simplex is the most common noninsectborne virus to cause encephalitis. The majority of individuals harbor herpes simplex virus type 1 in a dormant state. This is the virus responsible for sores on the oral mucous membranes, commonly called cold sores. Infectious diseases, fever, and emotional stress are possible reasons for the virus becoming active, but the exact mechanism is not known.

Signs and Symptoms

As with meningitis, headache and fever are common presenting symptoms. The patient may also complain of nausea, vomiting, and general malaise. These symptoms usually develop over a period of several days. Additional symptoms include nuchal rigidity, confusion, decreased level of consciousness, seizures, sensitivity to light, **ataxia,** abnormal sleep patterns, and tremors. The patient may have **hemiparesis.**

The patient with herpes encephalitis develops edema and necrosis (sometimes associated with hemorrhage), most commonly in the temporal lobes. This significant cerebral edema causes increased ICP and can lead to herniation of the brain. If the patient becomes comatose before treatment is begun, the mortality rate may be as high as 70% to 80%. The first 72 hours, when cerebral edema is worst, is the most likely time for death to occur.

Complications of Encephalitis

Patients who have had encephalitis are often left with cognitive disabilities and personality changes. Ongoing seizures, motor deficits, and blindness may also occur. Deterioration in cognition and personality changes are particularly stressful for significant others. The patient's behavioral control is a major factor in determining discharge plans. Assist significant others to realistically assess the patient's functional level and the family's ability to care for the patient. In-home care, outpatient therapy, and adult day care are options to explore. For some severely impaired individuals, custodial care may be the only feasible and safe discharge option.

Diagnostic Tests

CT scan, MRI, lumbar puncture to obtain cerebrospinal fluid, and electroencephalogram (EEG) are used to diagnose encephalitis. Cerebrospinal fluid analysis typically reveals increased white blood cell count and protein level and normal glucose levels. Breakdown of blood after cerebral hemorrhage results in yellow-colored CSF.

Therapeutic Interventions

No specific treatment is currently available for insectborne encephalitis. Careful neurological assessment and treatment of symptoms may help prevent complications and improve survival. Anticonvulsants, antipyretics, and analgesics are administered to reduce seizures, fever, and headache. Corticosteriods are used to decrease the swelling from the inflammation. Sedatives may be given for irritability. Antiviral medications such as acyclovir (Zovirax) may also be used, especially for herpes simplex.

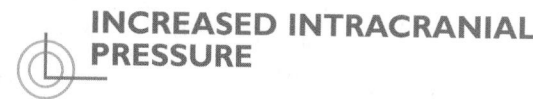

INCREASED INTRACRANIAL PRESSURE

Pathophysiology and Monitoring

Any patient with an intracranial pathological condition is potentially at risk for increased intracranial pressure. ICP is the pressure exerted within the cranial cavity by its components (blood, brain, and cerebrospinal fluid). The normal ICP is 0 to 15 mm Hg. This pressure fluctuates with normal physiological changes, such as arterial pulsations, changes in position, and increases in intrathoracic pressure (e.g., coughing or sneezing). Common causes of increased ICP include brain trauma, intracranial hemorrhage, and brain tumors. Prompt detection of changes in neurological status indicating increased intracranial pressure allows intervention aimed at preventing permanent brain damage.

The skull is a rigid compartment containing three components: brain, blood, and cerebrospinal fluid. If an increase in one component is not accompanied by a decrease in one or both of the other components, the result is increased intracranial pressure (IICP) (Fig. 48.2). The consequences of increased ICP depend on the degree of elevation and the speed with which the ICP increases. Patients with slow-growing tumors may have significantly increased intracranial pressure before they develop symptoms. Conversely, patients with a subarachnoid hemorrhage may sustain a sudden sharp increase in intracranial pressure.

The normally functioning body has several methods of compensating for increased intracranial pressure. Cerebrospinal fluid can be shunted into the spinal subarachnoid space. Hyperventilation may trigger constriction of cerebral blood vessels, decreasing the amount of blood within the cranial vault. These compensatory mechanisms are temporary and not particularly effective if the increase in ICP is sudden and severe.

Signs and Symptoms

Initial symptoms of increased ICP include restlessness, irritability, and decreased level of consciousness because cerebral cortex function is impaired. If not intubated, the patient may hyperventilate, causing vasoconstriction as the body attempts to compensate. As the pressure increases, the ocu-

---

hemiparesis: hemi—one side + paresis—partial paralysis

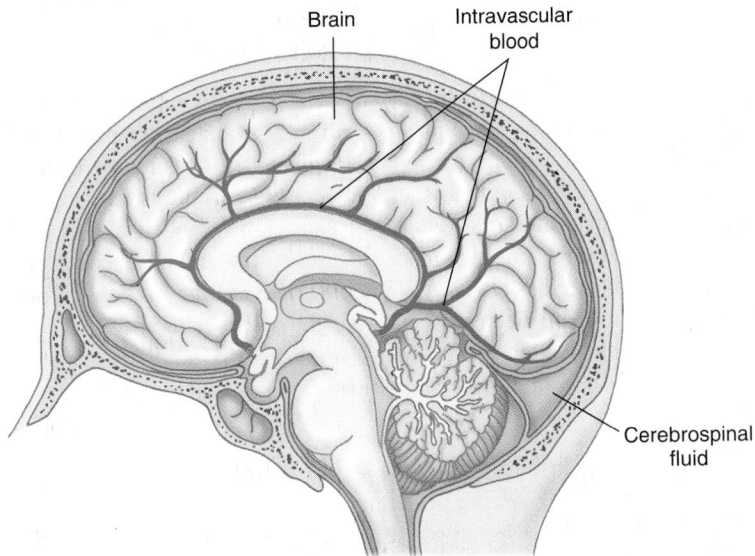

FIGURE 48.2 Any increase in brain tissue, blood, or cerebrospinal tissue can increase intracranial pressure.

lomotor nerve may be compressed on the side of the impairment. Compression of the outermost fibers of the oculomotor nerve results in diminished reactivity and dilation of the pupil. As the fibers become increasingly compressed, the pupil stops reacting to light. If the compression continues and the brain tissue exerts pressure on the opposite side of the brain from the injury, both pupils become fixed and dilated.

Vital sign changes are a late indication of increasing intracranial pressure. Cushing's response is a classic late sign of increased ICP. Cushing's response (or Cushing's triad) is characterized by bradycardia, bradypnea, and arterial hypertension (increasing systolic blood pressure while diastolic blood pressure remains the same), resulting in widening pulse pressure. By the time these symptoms appear, the intracranial pressure is significantly increased and interventions may not be successful.

Monitoring

ICP monitoring allows for early detection of changes in the pressure on the brain, before changes in symptoms can be seen. The most common method of monitoring ICP in adults is by placing a catheter in the ventricle of the brain, in the cerebral parenchyma, or in the subdural or subarachnoid space. This can be done at the bedside or in surgery. Each of these methods requires anesthetizing the scalp and drilling a burr hole into the skull.

Placement of a catheter into one of the lateral ventricles is referred to as external ventricular drainage (Fig. 48.3). This method allows for pressure monitoring as well as drainage of cerebrospinal fluid to reduce intracranial pressure. Disadvantages to this method include difficulty in locating the ventricle for insertion of the catheter and clotting of the catheter by blood in the cerebrospinal fluid.

To allow communication with the subarachnoid space, a subarachnoid bolt can be tightly screwed into the burr hole after the dura has been punctured (Fig. 48.4). The advantage of a subarachnoid bolt is ease of placement. Disadvantages include occlusion of the sensor portion of the bolt with brain tissue and inability to drain CSF. An intraparenchymal monitor is placed directly into brain tissue. Some physicians believe that this most accurately reflects the actual situation within the skull. These monitors cannot be used to drain CSF and may become occluded by brain tissue.

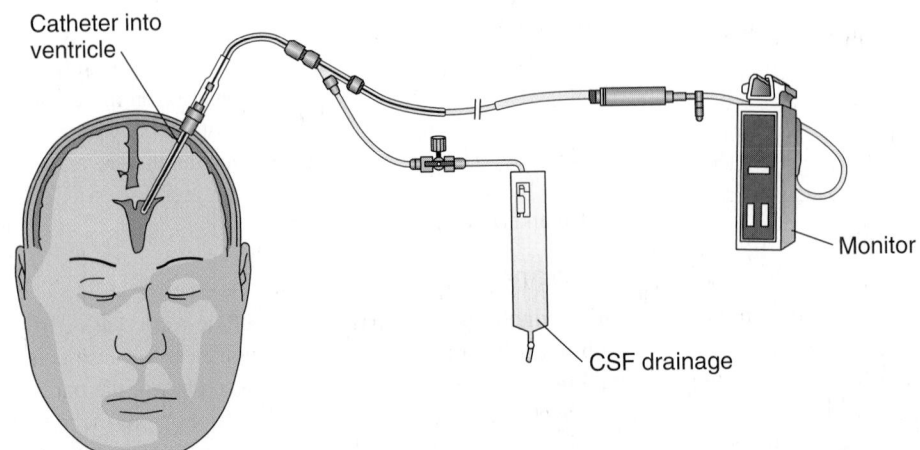

FIGURE 48.3 Ventricular drain. A catheter into the ventricle allows ICP monitoring and CSF drainage.

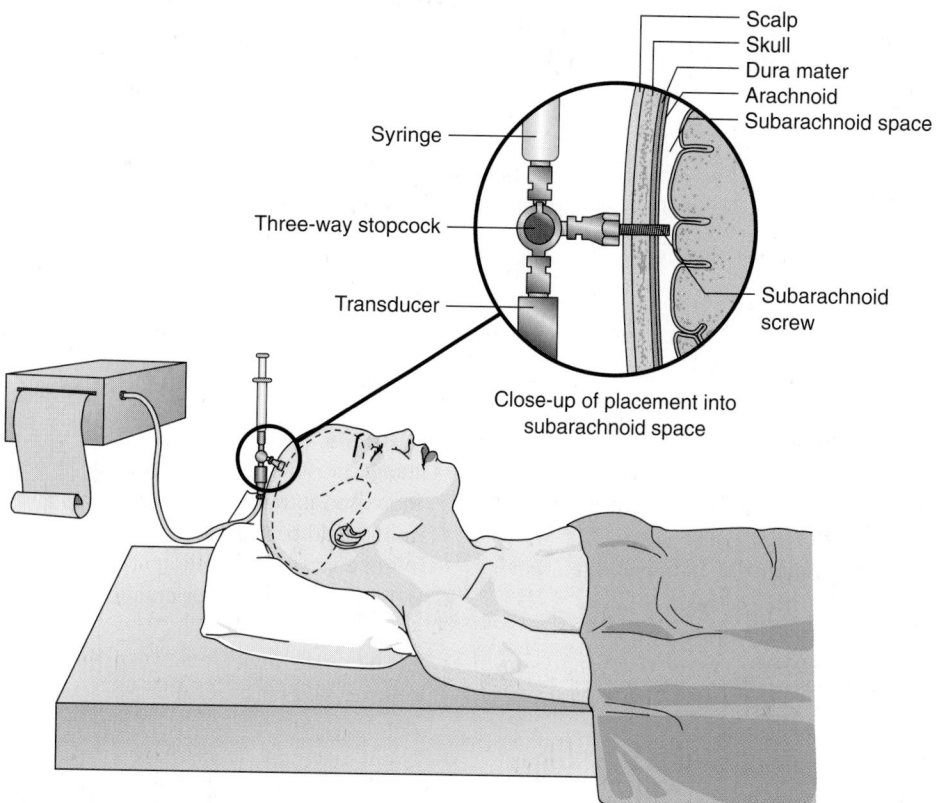

Scalp
Skull
Dura mater
Arachnoid
Subarachnoid space

Syringe

Three-way stopcock

Transducer

Subarachnoid screw

Close-up of placement into subarachnoid space

FIGURE 48.4 Subarachnoid bolt monitor.

Patients with ICP monitors are cared for in an intensive care unit (ICU) and require aggressive nursing care to prevent complications. These patients are often mechanically ventilated and may be pharmacologically paralyzed and sedated. In addition to meeting the patient's physiological needs and preventing complications, provide education and emotional support to the significant others.

Nursing Process for the Patient with an Infectious or Inflammatory Neurological Disorder

Assessment/Data Collection

Collaborate with the registered nurse (RN) to obtain a complete history from the patient, if feasible, and from significant others. Particular attention is paid to exposure to risk factors. The physical assessment must include all body systems because neurological impairment affects the entire person. Following the initial assessment, serial neurological assessments continue to be important to detect and report changes promptly. Pupil response, level of consciousness (LOC), and vital signs are monitored for signs of increased intracranial pressure (Box 48.2 Signs and Symptoms of Increased Intracranial Pressure). Headache is monitored on a pain scale. The Glasgow Coma Scale, presented in Chapter 47, is a valuable tool to monitor level of consciousness.

NURSING DIAGNOSIS, PLANNING, AND IMPLEMENTATION. The patient with increased ICP is usually cared for in an intensive care setting. The LPN/LVN collaborates with the registered nurse in implementing care. For additional interventions for patients with infectious or inflamma-

tory disorders, see Box 48.3 Nursing Care Plan for a Patient with Brain Tumor or Injury.

Pain (headache and nuchal rigidity) related to IICP

EXPECTED OUTCOME: Patient will not exhibit evidence of pain.

- Monitor pain using a 0 to 10 pain scale if the patient is able. *A pain scale is the most accurate way to monitor a patient's pain.*
- If the patient becomes restless, consider pain as a cause. *The patient may not be able to communicate pain sensations.*
- Administer analgesics as ordered. Avoid opioid analgesics. *Opioid analgesics (with the possible*

(Text continued on page 1065)

Box 48.2

Signs and Symptoms of Increased Intracranial Pressure

- Vomiting
- Headache
- Dilated pupil on affected side
- Hemiparesis or hemiplegia
- Decorticate then decerebrate posturing
- Decreasing level of consciousness
- Increasing systolic blood pressure
- Increasing then decreasing pulse rate
- Rising temperature

Box 48.3   NURSING CARE PLAN for a Patient with a Brain Tumor or Injury

Nursing Diagnosis: Disturbed thought processes related to cerebral edema or increased intracranial pressure and cognitive changes with orientation and problem solving

Expected Outcomes Patient will be oriented to person, place, and time, retain memory, and make appropriate decisions to maintain safety.

Evaluation Outcomes Is patient oriented to self, place, and time and able to ask for help appropriately to prevent injury?

Interventions	Rationale	Evaluation
Assess level of consciousness (LOC) using Glasgow Coma Scale. Monitor orientation and reorient as necessary. Observe patient's reaction to simple commands such as "raise your hand." Monitor patient's capabilities as activities increase.	Change in LOC can indicate increased intracranial pressure and should be reported. Giving correct information to patient will assist in orientation. This helps distinguish between reflexes and purposeful movement. Patient may experience dizziness, imbalance, and confusion; the patient will need assistance with mobilization until stable.	Is patient alert and responsive? Is LOC stable? Can patient identify who he/she is, location, and month, year, or season? Is patient able to follow simple commands? Can patient sit up and ambulate to chair without dizziness?

Nursing Diagnosis: Self-care deficit, bathing/hygiene related to mental status changes and inability to perform ADLs independently

Expected Outcomes The patient maintains as much independence with ADLs as possible.

Evaluation Outcomes Is the patient able to participate in self-care at an appropriate level?

Interventions	Rationale	Evaluation
Assess what the patient was able to do prior to admission/injury. Provide all supplies and equipment for hygiene and bath. Encourage the patient to perform activities at own pace. Teach and encourage family to participate with care.	The patient's potential for participation will depend on what he or she was able to do prior to injury. Assembling equipment for the patient reserves energy for performing self-care. The patient may need more time to perform activities. Including the family in the patient's care promotes support and family interaction.	What was the patient able to do? How does that compare with what he or she can do now? Is the patient able to perform the majority of bath and hygiene tasks with appropriate set-up? Does the patient gradually increase performance of self-care in a timely fashion? Is the family involved? Is the patient accepting of their assistance?

Nursing Diagnosis: Pain related to cerebral edema and headache or other signs of discomfort

Expected Outcomes Patient states pain level is acceptable, or demonstrates a decrease in painful behaviors.

Evaluation Outcomes Does patient state pain level is acceptable? Are pain behaviors reduced?

Interventions	Rationale	Evaluation
Assess pain using a scale of 0 to 10, or a faces scale (see Chapter 9). If patient is unable to participate, observe for pain behaviors such as restlessness, grimacing, or moaning. Monitor vital signs.	The patient's self-report is the best measure of the patient's pain. Pulse and blood pressure may be elevated in acute pain.	Is the patient able to rate pain? Is there evidence that pain is present?
Administer appropriate pain medication as ordered.	Nonnarcotic medications are preferred because they do not alter the level of consciousness. If these are not effective, codeine preparations, which have a minimal effect on LOC, may be prescribed.	Does patient state pain has decreased? Is sedation minimized?
Keep head of bed elevated at least 30 degrees.	Elevating the head of the bed helps prevent increased intracranial pressure, which can increase pain.	Does keeping head of bed elevated help prevent pain?
Provide alternative comfort measures such as dim lights, a quiet environment, and positioning for comfort.	Decreasing stimuli in the room by dimming lights and decreasing noise can have a calming effect.	Is patient resting quietly, with no complaints of pain?

Nursing Diagnosis: Sensory-perceptual disturbance (visual, auditory, or tactile) related to brain injury and cranial nerve involvement as evidenced by alterations in sensations

Expected Outcomes Patient will be kept safe from injury related to reduced sensation.

Evaluation Outcomes Is patient safe? Is skin intact?

Interventions	Rationale	Evaluation
Monitor patient's ability to perceive stimuli.	Changes in patient's perceptions must be incorporated into the plan of care.	What can patient feel?
Turn patient and assess skin every 2 hours while in bed; provide moisturizer as needed. Protect bony prominences.	If the patient cannot determine pressure or dryness, the nurse must evaluate and act to prevent skin breakdown.	Is skin intact, pink, warm, dry, and without redness?
Assist the patient out of bed and into a different environment.	This can help prevent sensory deprivation and social isolation.	How does patient respond to being in a chair or wheelchair and taken to sunroom or common area?
Teach the patient to monitor own position and skin, and to direct position changes.	This provides a way for the patient to maintain some control over his body, and to take part in preventing complications.	Is patient able to direct care activities effectively?

(Continued on following page)

Box 48.3　NURSING CARE PLAN for a Patient with a Brain Tumor or Injury *(Continued)*

Nursing Diagnosis: Impaired physical mobility related to motor deficits

Expected Outcome Patient will maintain maximum mobility and be free from complications of immobility.

Evaluation of Outcomes Is patient kept mobile without contractures? Is skin intact?

Interventions	Rationale	Evaluation
Assess degree of mobility limitation.	A good assessment can help determine how much the patient can actively participate in a plan for mobilization.	How much can patient do independently? Is physical/occupational therapy evaluation indicated?
Turn patient every 1 to 2 hours; if postoperative, avoid positioning on the operative site unless specifically permitted by the surgeon.	Turning helps prevent skin and respiratory complications.	Is a turning schedule maintained? Is skin free from redness and breakdown?
Position patient in correct body alignment. High-top tennis shoes, trochanter rolls, and slings can be used to keep the body in alignment.	This keeps the patient in functional position in case function is regained in the future.	Are all joints maintained in correct alignment?
Perform range-of-motion exercises; consult physical therapy as ordered.	ROM helps prevent contractures.	If patient unable to perform active range-of-motion (ROM), is passive ROM provided on a regular schedule?
Consult occupational therapist to assist the patient in learning to perform ADLs.	The patient may be able to participate in self-care with assistive devices.	Do assistive devices help patient mobilize and maintain independence?

Nursing Diagnosis: Risk for injury related to seizures

Expected Outcome Patient will remain free of injury during a seizure.

Evaluation of Outcomes Is safety maintained? Is skin intact, without bruising or discoloration?

Interventions	Rationale	Evaluation
Observe the patient's behavior and time the length of the seizure. When patient is alert following seizure, determine if an aura occurred, and what it was.	Observing the seizure can provide clues for teaching the patient to recognize the warning signs of a future seizure and how to maintain safety.	What did the patient experience? What can be taught to help keep patient safe in the future?
If patient should lose consciousness during the seizure, lay patient on his or her side or turn head to the side.	This helps prevent oral secretions from being aspirated.	Did patient maintain a patent airway without respiratory distress?
Remove objects from patient's surroundings to prevent injury during a seizure. If the patient must have side rails, pad them with blankets or foam. See Table 48.5.	During a tonic-clonic seizure the patient may be harmed by hitting furniture or other objects.	Is patient protected from objects that could cause injury during a seizure?

TABLE 48.3 INTERVENTIONS TO PREVENT INCREASED INTRACRANIAL PRESSURE

Action	Rationale
Keep head of bed elevated 30 degrees unless contraindicated.	Head elevation reduces ICP in some patients.
Avoid flexing the neck; keep head and neck in midline position.	Neck flexion may obstruct venous outflow.
Administer antiemetics and antitussives as necessary to prevent vomiting and cough.	Coughing and vomiting can increase ICP.
Administer stool softeners.	Straining for bowel movement can increase ICP.
Minimize suctioning. If absolutely necessary, oxygenate first and limit suction passes to one or two.	Suctioning can increase ICP.
Avoid hip flexion.	Hip flexion can increase intra-abdominal and thoracic pressure, which can increase ICP.
Prevent unnecessary noise and startling the patient.	Noxious stimuli can increase ICP in some patients.
Space care activities to provide rest between each disturbance.	Clustering care activities may increase ICP.

exception of codeine) are usually avoided because they mask neurological symptoms and make detection of changes difficult.

- Provide a dark, quiet room with few distractions; *avoidance of extra stimuli may help reduce headache.*
- Implement measures to prevent increased intracranial pressure. See Table 48.3 for measures and rationale.

Hyperthermia related to infectious process

- Monitor temperature. *A high temperature can increase risk for seizures.*
- Administer acetaminophen or aspirin as ordered *for fever.*
- Provide a cooling mattress or tepid sponge baths as necessary *to reduce fever. Remember these are uncomfortable for the patient. Comfort can be increased and shivering reduced by cooling the patient gradually and wrapping extremities in bath blankets during cooling mattress therapy.*

EVALUATION. Successful nursing management of a patient with an infectious or inflammatory neurological disorder is evidenced by a patient who is comfortable and with no preventable complications such as pressure ulcers or **contractures.** The absence of complications increases the possibility that the patient with a neurological deficit will benefit from rehabilitation and improve his or her level of functioning.

Patient Education

The nature and focus of teaching depend on the patient's level of consciousness and cognitive status. When appropriate, both the patient and significant others should be included in the education process. If the patient is not able to participate, the significant others become the focus of teaching.

Describing the brain as in control of body functions may help significant others to understand some of the symptoms of neurological disorders. The spinal cord can be compared to a telephone cord, with hundreds of tiny individual wires (nerves) making up the cord. The specific wires affected by disease determine the symptoms the patient experiences.

CRITICAL THINKING

Mr. Chung

■ Mr. Chung is an 18-year-old Asian college student. He comes to the emergency department complaining of headache, stiff neck, and fever. On physical assessment you notice a petechial rash on his legs and torso. The physician diagnoses meningococcal meningitis.

1. What tests are likely to be performed?
2. How patient education should be planned for Mr. Chung?
3. What infection control practices should be instituted?
4. What comfort measures might you offer to Mr. Chung?
5. What concerns do you have about how Mr. Chung contracted his illness?

Suggested answers at end of chapter.

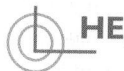 **HEADACHES**

As mentioned throughout this chapter, headache is a common symptom of neurological disorders. However, most headaches are transient events and do not indicate a serious pathological condition. If headaches are recurrent, persistent, or increasing in severity, the patient should undergo a neurological evaluation.

Types of Headaches

Because the causes, signs and symptoms, pathophysiology, and treatment of headaches vary based on the type of headache experienced, these subjects are discussed separately for each type of headache.

Tension or Muscle Contraction Headaches

Persistent contraction of the scalp and facial, cervical, and upper thoracic muscles can cause tension headaches. A cycle of muscle tension, muscle tenderness, and further muscle tension is established. This cycle may or may not be associated with vasodilation of cerebral arteries. Headaches of this type may be associated with premenstrual syndrome or psychosocial stressors such as anxiety, emotional distress, or depression. Symptoms typically develop gradually. Radiation of pain to the crown of the head and base of the skull, with variations in location and intensity, is common. *Pressure, aching, steady,* and *tight* are some of the words patients use to describe the pain of tension headaches.

Care must be taken to thoroughly rule out physical causes before attributing the headache to psychosocial origins. Symptom management may include the use of relaxation techniques, massage of the affected muscles, rest, localized heat application, nonnarcotic analgesics, and appropriate counseling.

Migraine Headaches

A migraine headache is believed to be caused by cerebral vasoconstriction followed by vasodilation. The vasoconstriction may be due to a response triggered by the trigeminal nerve, which stimulates release of substance P, a pain transmitter, into the vessels or by the release of amines such as serotonin, norepinephrine, and epinephrine. A migraine may or may not begin with an aura (visual phenomena, such as a flashing light that precedes an attack). The tendency to develop migraine headaches is often hereditary. Commonly used descriptors of migraine pain include *throbbing, boring, viselike,* and *pounding.* It is usually on one side of the head. Noise and light tend to exacerbate the headache, leading the patient to rest in a dark, quiet environment. Triggers for the headache include specific foods, noise, bright light, alcohol, and stress.

There are two types of migraine headaches: a classic migraine and a common migraine. The classic migraine has a preheadache (**prodromal**) phase in which the patient may experience visual disturbances, difficulty with speaking, and/or numbness or tingling. The headache that follows is often accompanied by nausea and sometimes vomiting, and may last for hours to days. A common migraine does not have the preheadache phase, but the patient experiences an immediate onset of a throbbing headache.

Treatment of migraine may be prophylactic or directed at an acute episode. Prophylactic treatment is usually reserved for those patients experiencing one or more migraine headaches per week. Dietary restrictions may be helpful if precipitating foods or beverages can be identified. Nifedipine (a calcium channel blocker) and propranolol (a beta-adrenergic blocker) are prophylactic treatments that are usually used to control blood pressure. These medications may help prevent the vascular changes that cause the headache. They should be used cautiously because of the potential for lowering blood pressure. Amitriptyline (a tricyclic antidepressant) may also help prevent migraines. Amitriptyline may cause drowsiness, dry mouth, and weight gain. None of these medications should be stopped abruptly after long-term use.

Several types of medications are available to treat the acute migraine headache. Ergot (Cafergot), a vasoconstrictor, is effective only if taken before the vessel walls become edematous, usually within 30 to 60 minutes of headache onset. Sumatriptan (Imitrex) and zolmitriptan (Zomig) are newer medications available for migraine relief. These drugs work at the serotonin receptor sites and have a vasoconstricting action. Sumatriptan is available in both intramuscular and oral forms. The potentially additive nature of multidrug regimens requires careful monitoring.

Cluster Headaches

Vascular disturbance, stress, anxiety, and emotional distress are all proposed causes of cluster headaches. As indicated by the name, these headaches tend to occur in clusters during a time span of several days to weeks. Months or even years may pass between episodes. Alcohol consumption may worsen the episodes.

The patient may state that the headache begins suddenly, typically at the same time of night. *Throbbing* and *excruciating* are often the adjectives used by the patient. The headache tends to be unilateral, affecting the nose, eye, and forehead. A bloodshot, teary appearance of the affected eye is common.

Because of the brief nature of cluster headaches, treatment is difficult. A quiet, dark environment and cold compresses may lessen the intensity of the pain. Nonsteroidal anti-inflammatory drugs (NSAIDs) or tricyclic antidepressants may be prescribed.

Diagnosis

Most headaches are diagnosed based on the patient's history and symptoms. Magnetic resonance imaging (MRI), CT, skull x-ray, arteriogram, electroencephalogram, cranial nerve testing, and lumbar puncture to test CSF may be done to rule out other causes for the headaches.

Nursing Process for the Patient with a Headache

Assessment/Data Collection

The WHAT'S UP? mnemonic is particularly useful in helping the patient provide useful information regarding the headache.

W—Where is the pain? Does it remain in one place or radiate to other areas of the head? Does the headache consistently start in one place?

H—How does the headache feel? Is it throbbing, steady, dull, bandlike, or does it have other qualities?

A—Aggravating or alleviating factors should be assessed. Some aggravating factors include red wine, caffeine, chocolate, and foods containing nitrates or monosodium glutamate (MSG). Other factors include particular stages of the menstrual cycle, emotional stress, and tension. Alleviating factors might include lying down in a dark room, cold compresses, and over-the-counter medications.

T—Timing may be a factor for a patient who experiences headaches just before or during her menstrual period. For other patients, there may be no predictive timing. Also ask how long the headache lasted.

S—Ask the patient to rate the severity on a scale of 0 to 10. Is the severity consistent or does it vary from headache to headache?

U—Are there associated symptoms, such as nausea, vomiting, or bloodshot eyes?

P—Determine the patient's perception of the headache. Does it interfere with the patient's life? If so, how? Has the patient had a previous evaluation of headaches?

Planning, Implementation, and Evaluation

Acute pain (headache) related to lack of knowledge of pain prevention and control techniques

- Assist the patient to identify and reduce or eliminate aggravating factors. This can be accomplished by keeping a headache diary for a time, recording the time of day the headache occurs, foods eaten or other aggravating factors, description of the pain, identification of associated symptoms such as nausea or visual disturbances, and other factors related to headache symptoms. *Identification of triggers can help the patient lessen the frequency and intensity of attacks.*

- Encourage the patient to use alleviating techniques such as biofeedback or stress reduction. *This helps the patient participate in the treatment of the headache and provides a sense of control over his or her illness.*

- Teach the patient to use relaxation exercises and warm, moist compresses. *These interventions may be helpful for tension headaches.*

- Provide a dark room and rest *to reduce stimulation during a migraine headache.*

- Teach the patient about medications, appropriate dosage, expected action, side effects, and consequences of misuse. *The patient will need to understand medication administration for appropriate use at home.*

Evaluation

If interventions have been effective, the patient will understand self-care to prevent and treat headaches, and be able to report a reduction in headache occurrences.

SEIZURE DISORDERS

Seizures/Epilepsy

A seizure is defined as "sudden, abnormal, and excessive electrical discharges from the brain that can change motor or autonomic function, consciousness, or sensation. Seizures can develop at any time during a person's life, and they can occur at any time."[1] A seizure may be a symptom of epilepsy or of other neurological disorders such as a brain tumor or meningitis. Epilepsy is a chronic neurological disorder characterized by recurrent seizure activity.

Pathophysiology

The normal stability of the neuron cell membrane is impaired in individuals with epilepsy. This instability allows for abnormal electrical discharges to occur. These discharges cause the characteristic symptoms seen during a seizure.

Seizures can be classified as partial or generalized. Partial seizures begin on one side of the cerebral cortex. In some cases, the electrical discharge spreads to the other hemisphere and the seizure becomes generalized. Generalized seizures are characterized by involvement of both cerebral hemispheres.

Etiology

Epilepsy may be acquired or idiopathic (unknown cause). Causes of acquired epilepsy include traumatic brain injury and anoxic events. No cause has been identified for idiopathic epilepsy. The most common time for idiopathic epilepsy to begin is before age 20. New-onset seizures after this age are most commonly caused by an underlying neurological disorder.

Signs and Symptoms

Symptoms of seizure activity correlate with the area of the brain where the seizure begins. Some patients experience an aura or sensation that warns the patient that a seizure is about to occur. An aura may be a visual distortion, a noxious odor, or an unusual sound. Patients who experience an aura may have enough time to sit or lie down before the seizure starts, thereby minimizing the chance of injury.

PARTIAL SEIZURES. Repetitive, purposeless behaviors, called automatisms, are the classic symptom of partial seizures. The patient appears to be in a dreamlike state while picking at his or her clothing, chewing, or smacking his or her lips. Patients may be labeled as mentally ill, particularly if automatisms include unacceptable social behaviors such as spitting or fondling themselves. Patients are not aware of their behavior or that it is inappropriate. If the patient does not lose consciousness, the seizure is labeled as simple partial and usually lasts less than 1 minute. Older terms for simple partial seizures include *jacksonian* and *focal motor.* If consciousness is lost, it is called a complex partial seizure or psychomotor seizure, and may last from 2 to 15 minutes.

Partial seizures arising from the parietal lobe may cause paresthesias on the side of the body opposite the seizure focus. Visual disturbances are seen if the occipital lobe is the originating site. Involvement of the motor cortex results in involuntary movements of the opposite side of the body. Typically, movements begin in the arm and hand and may spread to the leg and face.

GENERALIZED SEIZURES. Generalized seizures affect the entire brain. Two types of generalized seizures are absence seizures and tonic-clonic seizures. Absence seizures, sometimes referred to as petit mal seizures, occur most often in children and are manifested by a period of staring that lasts several seconds.

Tonic-clonic seizures are what most people envision when they think of seizures. They are sometimes called grand mal seizures or convulsions. Tonic-clonic seizures follow a typical progression. Aura and loss of consciousness may or may not occur. The tonic phase, lasting 30 to 60 seconds, is characterized by rigidity, causing the patient to fall if not lying down. The pupils are fixed and dilated, the hands and jaws are clenched, and the patient may temporarily stop breathing. The clonic phase is signaled by contraction and relaxation of all muscles in a jerky, rhythmic fashion. The extremities may move forcefully, causing injury if the patient strikes furniture or walls. The patient is often incontinent. Biting the lips or tongue may cause bleeding.

The **postictal** period is the recovery period after a seizure. Following a partial seizure the postictal phase may be no more than a few minutes of disorientation. Patients who experience a generalized seizure may sleep deeply for 30 minutes to several hours. Following this deep sleep, patients may complain of headache, confusion, and fatigue. Patients may realize that they had a seizure but not remember the event itself.

Diagnostic Tests

An EEG is the most useful test for evaluating seizures. An EEG can determine where in the brain the seizures start, the frequency and duration of seizures, and the presence of subclinical (asymptomatic) seizures. Sleep deprivation and flashing light stimulation may be used to evaluate the seizure threshold. See Chapter 47 for more information on EEG.

---

postictal: post—after + ictal—seizure

Therapeutic Interventions

If an underlying cause for the seizure is identified, treatment focuses on correcting the cause. If no cause is found or if the seizures continue despite treatment of concurrent disorders, treatment focuses on the seizure activity.

Numerous anticonvulsant medications are available, each with specific actions, therapeutic ranges, and potential side effects (Table 48.4). Typically, the patient is started on one drug and the dosage is increased until therapeutic levels are attained or side effects become troublesome. If seizures are not controlled on a single drug, another medication is added. Many anticonvulsants require periodic blood tests to monitor serum levels as well as kidney and liver functions. Most of these medications can cause drowsiness, so teach the patient to avoid driving until the effects of the drug are known. Driving is also contraindicated until seizures are under control. If a patient must discontinue an anticonvulsant agent, it should be tapered slowly according to manufacturer directions. Stopping an anticonvulsant abruptly can result in status epilepticus, discussed below. If seizures continue despite anticonvulsant therapy, surgical intervention may be considered.

Surgical Management

The success of surgical intervention for epilepsy depends on identification of an epileptic focus within nonvital brain tissue. The surgeon attempts to resect the area affected to prevent spread of seizure activity. In some cases, seizures may be cured, but in others, the goal is to reduce the frequency or severity of the seizures. If no focus is identified or if it is in a vital area such as the motor cortex or speech center, surgery is not feasible.

TABLE 48.4 ANTICONVULSANT MEDICATIONS

Medication Class/Action	Examples	Route	Side Effects	Nursing Implications
Anticonvulsants Suppress abnormal discharge of neurons, suppress spread of seizure activity from focus to other parts of brain	Phenytoin (Dilantin)	PO, IM, IV	Gingival (gum) hyperplasia, nausea, ataxia, rash; aplastic anemia	Regular dental care essential; therapeutic level is 10–20 μg/mL
	Phenobarbital (Luminal)	PO, IM, IV	Drowsiness, respiratory depression	Monitor vital signs. Therapeutic level 15–40 μg/mL.
	Carbamazepine (Tegretol)	PO	Drowsiness and ataxia, blood disorders	Monitor CBC. Therapeutic level 6–12 μg/mL.
	Valproic acid (Depakote)	PO, IV	GI upset, nausea, vomiting	Therapeutic level 50–100 μg/mL
	Gabapentin (Neurontin)	PO	Drowsiness, dizziness	Blood levels not necessary
	Topiramate (Topamax)	PO	Dizziness, drowsiness, impaired memory, psychomotor slowing, vision changes, weight loss	Blood levels not necessary

The preoperative assessment for epilepsy surgery is an extensive multistage process. Thorough assessment and teaching are essential. To adequately identify seizure foci, the patient is weaned off anticonvulsant therapy. Increasing the frequency of seizures with weaning is anxiety provoking to patients and significant others.

Emergency Care

The prime objective in caring for a patient experiencing a seizure is to prevent injury. Side rails, if used, should be padded to prevent injury if the patient strikes his or her extremities against them. If the patient falls to the floor, move furniture out of the way. Maintain a patent airway and, if possible, turn the patient on his or her side to prevent aspiration if vomiting occurs. Do not force an airway or anything else into the patient's mouth once the seizure has begun. The individual should not be restrained because this may also increase the risk of injury. Observe and document the patient's behavior during the seizure, which part of the body was first involved, progression of the seizure, and the length of time the seizure lasted (see Box 48.4 Patient Perspective). After the seizure, assess the patient for breathing. Suction if necessary and initiate rescue breathing or cardiopulmonary resuscitation (CPR) as indicated.

Status Epilepticus

Status epilepticus is characterized by at least 30 minutes of repetitive seizure activity without a return to consciousness. This is a medical emergency and requires prompt intervention to prevent irreversible neurological damage. Abrupt cessation of anticonvulsant therapy is the usual cause of status epilepticus.

Seizure activity precipitates a significant increase in the brain's need for glucose and oxygen. This metabolic demand is even greater during status epilepticus. Irreversible neuronal damage may occur if cerebral metabolic needs cannot be fulfilled. Adequate oxygenation must be maintained, if necessary, by intubating and mechanically ventilating the patient. These patients are also at significant risk for aspiration.

Intravenous diazepam (Valium) or lorazepam (Ativan) is given to stop the seizures. Because both of these drugs may cause respiratory depression, careful airway management is required. After obtaining serum drug levels, anticonvulsant therapy is adjusted to achieve therapeutic levels.

If seizures remain resistant to treatment, a barbiturate coma may be induced with intravenous pentobarbital. The last line of treatment for status epilepticus is general anesthesia or pharmacological paralysis. Both of these therapies require intubation, mechanical ventilation, and management in an intensive care unit (ICU) setting. Continuous EEG monitoring is used to verify that the seizures have actually stopped. A patient treated with neuromuscular blockade drugs may still be seizing but have no visible manifestations. For more information, visit the Epilepsy Foundation of America at www.efa.org.

Psychosocial Effects

Finances can be a major concern to patients with seizure disorders. Some patients with epilepsy experience hiring discrimination, or they may not qualify for some jobs in which safety is a concern. Remind patients that falsifying information on job applications may be grounds for dismissal. Refusal of health insurance coverage can create financial hardships for patients on long-term medications. Most patients whose seizures are controlled can work and lead productive lives. You can help patients explore options for financial assistance if necessary.

Patients with poorly controlled seizures should not operate motor vehicles. In today's society a driver's license is a sign of adulthood and independence, and patients who cannot drive may experience lowered self-esteem. Job opportunities may be limited for patients who depend on public transportation. Encourage the patient to obtain a state identification card. This can be used in place of a driver's license for identification.

Patients may limit interpersonal relationships out of fear of having a seizure. The involuntary movements, sounds, and possible incontinence that occur with seizures are embarrassing to patients and can be frightening to lay people. Role playing may help the patient determine when and how to confide in others.

Nursing Process for the Patient with Seizures

Assessment/Data Collection

Perform a general neurological assessment of the patient with a history of seizures. Determine the type of seizure

---

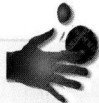

Box 48.4

Patient Perspective

Mrs. Rowley

I have had seizures for 35 years, and as a result of falling during seizures have experienced cuts, bruises, and a broken bone. I usually have an aura that lets me know a seizure is about to occur. This is helpful if I can get myself to a safe place to prevent falling or being injured. When a patient is having a seizure you can best help by using padding such as pillows or blankets for protection, talking calmly, and using gentle touch to prevent injury. You should not sit on or hold down someone during a seizure. I have had the frightening experience of waking up with a nurse sitting on me and holding down my arms. After you have protected the patient, let them come out of the seizure on their own. When the seizure is over, I usually want to sleep because seizures are exhausting and uncomfortable. I will rest better knowing you are watching over me to keep me safe.

manifestations and type of aura if any. Assess the patient's knowledge of the disease and its treatment. It is important to assess whether the patient has the resources to purchase prescribed anticonvulsant medications and whether the medication regimen is adhered to. Drug levels may help determine degree of compliance with therapy.

Nursing Diagnosis, Planning, and Implementation
Risk for injury related to seizure activity

EXPECTED OUTCOME: Patient will remain free from injury.

- Instruct the patient to recognize the aura and to get to safety if it occurs. This may mean lying down away from furniture or other objects. *This helps prevent injury.*
- Institute seizure precautions for the patient admitted to a health-care institution. See Table 48.5 for precautions and interventions *to prevent injury.*
- Encourage all patients to wear medical alert jewelry or other identification *to alert others to the presence of seizure disorder.*
- Assist patients to identify conditions that trigger seizures. Hypoglycemia, hypoxia, and hyponatremia are all potential triggers of hypersensitive neurons. Teach the patient the importance of a consistent schedule of eating and sleeping. *The patient may be able to prevent seizures by avoidance of triggers.*

Risk for ineffective management of therapeutic regimen related to complex regimen and possible lack of resources

EXPECTED OUTCOME: Patient will follow medication regimen as evidenced by therapeutic drug levels and seizure activity controlled.

- Assess patient's ability to obtain and pay for medication. *Sudden discontinuance of a medication can result in status epilepticus.*

TABLE 48.5 INTERVENTIONS FOR SEIZURES

Seizure Precautions
- Pad side rails of hospital bed with commercial pads or bath blankets folded over and pinned in place.
- Keep call light within reach.
- Assist patient when ambulating.
- Keep suction and oral airway at bedside.

Nursing Care During a Seizure
- Stay with patient.
- Do not restrain patient.
- Protect from injury (move nearby objects).
- Loosen tight clothing.
- Turn to side when able to prevent occlusion of airway or aspiration.
- Suction if needed.
- Monitor vital signs when able.
- Be prepared to assist with breathing if necessary.
- Observe and document progression of symptoms.

- Refer patient to a case manager or social worker if necessary *to assist with obtaining resources for medications.*
- Teach the patient about medication action, dose, side effects, schedule, and the importance of not stopping treatment suddenly. *Patients with seizures may have several medications to take several times each day. Patients who understand their regimens are more likely to comply.*
- Teach the patient about the importance of regular blood tests if required. *Therapeutic blood levels help prevent seizures (too low) and toxicity (too high).*

Evaluation
Successful care of a patient with epilepsy is manifested by a decrease in seizures to the lowest possible frequency. Patient verbalization of understanding of needed lifestyle changes is another indication of success. Patients should be able to state measures to prevent injury if a seizure should occur and should verbalize understanding of all medications and their administration schedules. Therapeutic drug levels may be measured to evaluate compliance with the medication regimen.

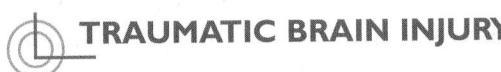
TRAUMATIC BRAIN INJURY

Traumatic brain injury (TBI) is a major cause of death and disability in adults. Young males make up a large proportion of brain injury victims.

Pathophysiology
Traumatic brain injury is a complex phenomenon with results ranging from no detectable effect to persistent vegetative state. Trauma can result in hemorrhage, contusion or laceration of the brain, and damage at the cellular level. In addition to the primary insult, the brain injury may be compounded by cerebral edema, hyperemia, or hydrocephalus.

Etiology
Motor vehicle accidents account for the largest percentage of traumatic brain injuries. Falls, sports-related injuries, and violence are also common causes of traumatic brain injury.

The brain is susceptible to various types of injury and can be classified in several ways. The term *closed head injury* or *nonpenetrating injury* is used when there has been rapid back and forth movement of the brain causing bruising and tearing of brain tissues and vessels, but the skull is intact. An open head injury or penetrating injury refers to a break in the skull. *Acceleration injury* is the term used to describe a moving object hitting a stationary head. An example of this type of injury is a patient who is hit in the head with a baseball bat. A *deceleration injury* occurs when the head is in motion and strikes a stationary surface. This type of injury is seen in patients who trip and fall, hitting their head on furniture or the floor.

A combination of acceleration-deceleration injury occurs when the stationary head is hit by a mobile object and the head then strikes a stationary surface. A soccer player who sustains a blow to the head and then hits the ground with his or her head may sustain an acceleration-deceleration injury.

Rotational injuries have the potential to cause shearing damage to the brain, as well as laceration and contusions. Rotational injuries may be caused by a direct blow to the head or may occur during a motor vehicle accident in which the vehicle is struck from the side. Twisting of the brainstem can damage the reticular activating system, causing loss of consciousness. Movement of the brain within the skull may result in bruising or tearing of brain tissue where it comes in contact with the inside of the skull.

Types of Brain Injury and Signs and Symptoms

Concussion

Cerebral concussion is considered a mild brain injury. If there is a loss of consciousness, it is for 5 minutes or less. Concussion is characterized by headache, dizziness, or nausea and vomiting. The patient may complain of amnesia of events before or after the trauma. On clinical examination there is no skull or dura injury and no abnormality detected on CT or MRI.

Contusion

Cerebral contusion is characterized by bruising of brain tissue, possibly accompanied by hemorrhage. There may be multiple areas of contusion, depending on the causative mechanism. Severe contusions can result in diffuse axonal injury (DAI). The symptoms of a cerebral contusion depend on the area of the brain involved.

Brainstem contusions affect level of consciousness. Decreased level of consciousness may be transient or permanent. Respirations, pupil reaction, eye movement, and motor response to stimuli may also be affected. The autonomic nervous system may be affected by edema or by hypothalamic injury, causing rapid heart rate and respiratory rate, fever, and diaphoresis.

Hematoma

SUBDURAL HEMATOMA. Subdural hematomas are classified as acute or chronic based on the time interval between injury and onset of symptoms. Acute subdural hematoma is characterized by appearance of symptoms within 24 hours following injury. The bleeding is typically venous in nature and accumulates between the dura and arachnoid membranes (Fig. 48.5). Approximately 24% of patients who sustain a severe brain injury develop an acute subdural hematoma. Damage to the brain tissue may cause an altered level of consciousness. Therefore, it can be difficult to recognize a subdural hematoma based only on clinical examination. As the subdural hematoma increases in size, the patient may exhibit one-sided paralysis of extraocular movement, extremity weakness, or dilation of

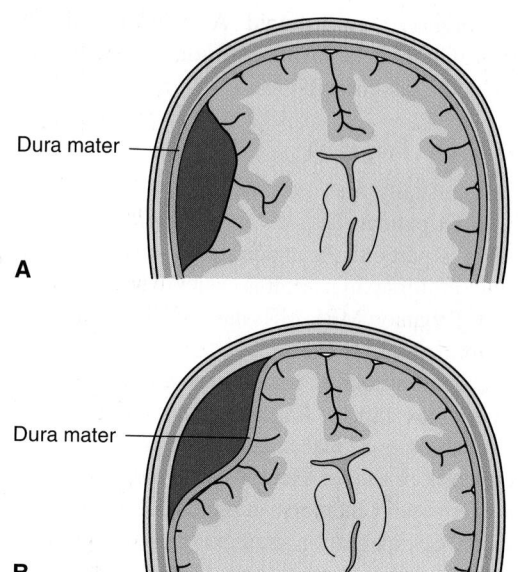

FIGURE 48.5 *(A)* Subdural hematoma is usually venous and forms between the dura and the arachnoid membranes. *(B)* An epidural hematoma is usually from an arterial bleed and forms between the dura mater and the skull.

the pupil. Level of consciousness may deteriorate further as ICP increases.

Older adults and alcoholic individuals are particularly prone to chronic subdural hematomas. Atrophy of the brain, common in these populations, stretches the veins between the brain and the dura. A seemingly minor fall or blow to the head can cause these stretched veins to rupture and bleed. Often there are no other injuries associated with the trauma. Because a chronic subdural hematoma can develop weeks to months after the injury, the patient may not remember an injury occurring.

The patient with a chronic subdural hematoma may be forgetful, lethargic, or irritable or may complain of a headache. If the hematoma persists or increases in size, the patient may develop hemiparesis and pupillary changes. The patient or significant other may not associate the symptoms with a previous injury and therefore may delay seeking medical care.

EPIDURAL HEMATOMA. Approximately 10% of patients with severe brain injuries develop epidural hematomas. This collection of blood between the dura mater and skull is usually arterial in nature and is often associated with skull fracture (see Fig. 48.5.) Arterial bleeding can cause the hematoma to become large very quickly. Patients with epidural hematoma typically exhibit a progressive course of symptoms. The patient loses consciousness directly after the injury; he or she then regains consciousness and is coherent for a brief period. The patient then develops a dilated pupil and paralyzed extraocular muscles on the side of the hematoma and becomes less responsive. If there is no intervention, the patient becomes unresponsive. Seizures or hemiparesis may occur. Once the patient exhibits symptoms, the deterioration may be rapid. Airway management and control of ICP must be instituted immediately. If ICP is not controlled, the patient will die.

Diagnostic Tests

CT scan is usually the first imaging test performed on the brain-injured patient. It is faster and more accessible than MRI. This is particularly important for unstable patients or those with multiple injuries. It is easier to identify skull fractures on CT than on MRI. MRI may be used later to identify damage to the brain tissue.

Neuropsychological testing can be useful in assessing the patient's cognitive function. This information helps direct rehabilitation placement, discharge planning, and return to work or school. Neuropsychological testing identifies problems with memory, judgment, learning, and comprehension. Compensation strategies can be suggested to the patient and significant others based on the results.

Therapeutic Interventions

Surgical Management

Surgical treatment of hematomas is discussed under intracranial surgery later in this chapter.

Medical Management

Medical management of traumatic brain injury involves control of ICP and support of body functions. Brain-injured patients may be partially or completely dependent for maintenance of respiration, nutrition, elimination, movement, and skin integrity.

A variety of techniques are used to control intracranial pressure in the patient with moderate or severe brain injury. The first step is to insert an ICP monitor to allow measurement of the ICP. Refer to the section on increased ICP earlier in this chapter for further information.

If ICP remains elevated despite drainage of cerebrospinal fluid, the next step is use of an osmotic diuretic. The most commonly used drug is intravenous mannitol (Osmitrol). Mannitol utilizes osmosis to pull fluid into the intravascular space and eliminate it via the renal system. Serum osmolarity and electrolytes must be carefully monitored when mannitol is being administered. Some patients experience a rebound increase in ICP after the mannitol wears off.

Mechanical hyperventilation is the next step if the patient is still experiencing increased ICP. Hyperventilation is effective in lowering ICP because it causes vasoconstriction. Vasoconstriction allows less blood into the cranium, thereby lowering ICP. Research has demonstrated, however, that aggressive hyperventilation, particularly within the first 24 hours after injury, may induce ischemia in the already compromised brain. Therefore, hyperventilation is now reserved for increased ICP that does not respond to other treatments.

High-dose barbiturate therapy may be used to induce a therapeutic coma, which reduces the metabolic needs of the brain during the acute phase following injury. These patients

are completely dependent for all their needs and care. They will be mechanically ventilated and cared for in an ICU setting. Vasopressors may be required to maintain blood pressure, and the patient's temperature should be kept as normal as possible.

Complications of Traumatic Brain Injury

Brain Herniation

If interventions to control ICP are unsuccessful, the patient may experience uncontrolled edema or herniation of brain tissue (Fig. 48.6). Herniation is displacement of brain tissue out of its normal anatomical location. This displacement prevents function of the herniated tissue and places pressure on other vital structures, most commonly the brainstem. Herniation usually results in brain death.

Patients who experience brain death may be suitable organ donor candidates. For some significant others, the opportunity to donate their loved one's organs provides some sense of purpose in the death. See Box 48.5 Traumatic Brain Injury Summary.

Diabetes Insipidus

Edema or direct injury affects the posterior portion of the pituitary gland or hypothalamus. Inadequate release of anti-

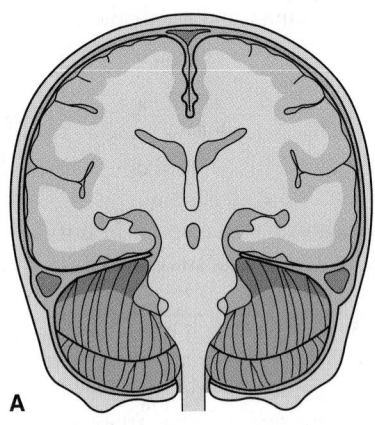

A

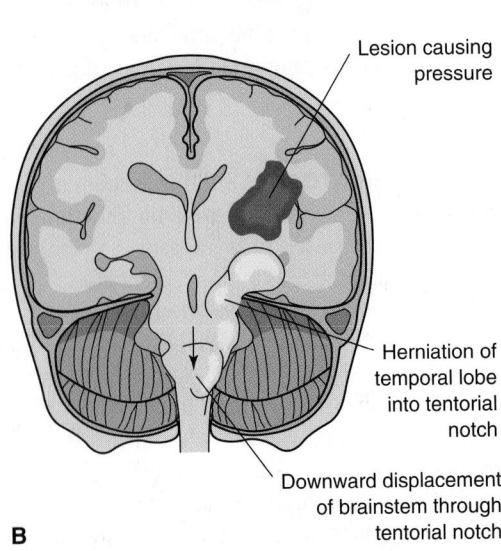

Lesion causing pressure

Herniation of temporal lobe into tentorial notch

Downward displacement of brainstem through tentorial notch

B

FIGURE 48.6 Herniation of the brain. *(A)* Normal brain. *(B)* Herniation of brain tissue into tentorial notch.

Box 48.5

Traumatic Brain Injury Summary

Signs and Symptoms	Loss or decrease in level of consciousness, depending on severity and type of injury Loss of memory before or after the injury Increased ICP Headache, dizziness Nausea and vomiting Unequal pupils Tachycardia, tachypnea Diaphoresis Hemiparesis
Diagnostic Tests	CT scan, MRI Skull x-rays Routine laboratory tests (hemoglobin, electrolytes, coagulation studies, type and crossmatch) Neuropsychological testing
Therapeutic Interventions	Control intracranial pressure Surgical management of hematoma Maintain respiratory function Maintain diet/nutrition Maintain skin integrity Prevent complications Education
Complications	Increased intracranial pressure Diabetes insipidus Acute hydrocephalus Posttraumatic syndrome Cognitive and personality changes
Possible Nursing Diagnoses	Disturbed thought processes related to cerebral edema or increased intracranial pressure Self-care deficit related to increased intracranial pressure Pain related to cerebral edema

diuretic hormone results in polyuria and, if the patient is awake, polydipsia. Fluid replacement and intravenous vasopressin are used to maintain fluid and electrolyte balance.

Acute Hydrocephalus

Cerebral edema can interfere with cerebrospinal fluid circulation, causing **hydrocephalus**. Initial treatment is with an external ventricular drain, followed by a ventriculoperitoneal

shunt if necessary. A shunt drains excess CSF into the peritoneum, where it is reabsorbed into circulation and excreted.

Labile Vital Signs

Direct trauma to or pressure on the brainstem can cause fluctuations in blood pressure, cardiac rhythm, or respiratory pattern. Treatment is aimed at control of intracranial pressure.

Posttraumatic Syndrome

Patients who sustain a concussion may experience ongoing, somewhat vague symptoms. They complain of headache, fatigue, difficulty concentrating, depression, or memory impairment. Symptoms may be severe enough to interfere with work, school, and interpersonal relationships. Neuropsychological testing may provide objective evidence of cognitive dysfunction and establish the need for cognitive rehabilitation. Symptoms may take 3 to 12 months to resolve.

Cognitive and Personality Changes

Alterations in personality and cognition may be the most difficult long-term complication for patients and significant others to adjust to. The patient may have significant short-term memory impairment. This limits his or her ability to learn new information and may interfere with ability to function at work or school. Impaired judgment can make the patient a safety risk to self or others. It also affects social functioning.

Emotional lability, loss of social inhibitions, and personality changes may occur. These consequences of traumatic brain injury have a profound effect on the patient and significant others. Spouses may state, "This is not the person I married." If behavior is violent, bizarre, or profane, children may be unwilling to bring their friends home and may become socially isolated. Young children, in particular, have difficulty understanding why the parent is behaving so differently. Disintegration of relationships is not uncommon following traumatic brain injury.

Neuropsychological testing objectively identifies problems. These deficits can then be addressed with cognitive rehabilitation. Individual and family counseling may be of benefit. Support groups for patients and significant others are often helpful.

Motor and speech impairment are additional possible long-term complications of traumatic brain injury. Intensive rehabilitation provides the best opportunity for maximizing recovery. For more information, visit the Brain Injury Association at www.biausa.org.

Nursing Process for the Patient with Traumatic Brain Injury

Acute care is presented below. Also see Box 48.3 Nursing Care Plan for the Patient with a Brain Tumor or Injury.

Assessment/Data Collection

After stabilization in the emergency department, care of the patient with a traumatic brain injury is in the intensive care setting, where ICP can be carefully monitored. Neurological status is assessed frequently, including Glasgow Coma Scale score, pupil responses, muscle strength, and vital signs.

---

hydrocephalus: hydro—water + cephalus—head

Review Box 48.2 Signs and Symptoms of Increased Intracranial Pressure. Once the patient is stabilized, neurological damage is assessed. Identification of deficits guides nursing care. Assessment of discharge needs should also begin as soon as possible. The patient may require extensive rehabilitation, and early referral may speed transfer to an appropriate facility.

Nursing Diagnosis, Planning, and Implementation

Ineffective cerebral tissue perfusion related to increased ICP

EXPECTED OUTCOME: Changes in cerebral tissue perfusion are recognized and reported promptly.

- Monitor vital signs for widening pulse pressure or falling blood pressure. *These are signs of increased ICP and should be reported promptly.*
- Monitor Glasgow Coma Scale score and report worsening status promptly. *Decreasing level of consciousness (LOC) may indicate increased ICP and may necessitate emergency intervention.*
- Implement measures to prevent increased ICP. See Table 48.3 for interventions and rationale.

Ineffective airway clearance related to reduced cough reflex and decreased level of consciousness

EXPECTED OUTCOME: Patient will maintain a clear airway as evidenced by clear breath sounds and $SaO_2 = 90\%$.

- Monitor airway and breath sounds. *If the patient has excess secretions and is unable to cough effectively, suctioning may be necessary.*
- Limit suction passes to one or two at a time, a maximum of 5 to 10 seconds each time. *Suctioning can increase ICP.*
- Keep head of bed elevated 30 degrees *to reduce risk of aspirating oral secretions.*
- Turn the patient frequently *to help mobilize secretions.*

Risk for ineffective breathing pattern related to pressure on respiratory center

EXPECTED OUTCOME: The patient will maintain oxygenation within normal limits.

- Monitor respiratory rate and depth, ABGs, and SaO_2. Report changes. *If respiratory status is deteriorating, mechanical ventilation may be necessary.*

Evaluation

The plan of care has been successful if the patient shows no unexpected worsening of neurological function and injuries and complications are prevented. The airway is clear. The patient is kept comfortable, and self-care needs are met.

Rehabilitation

Once the patient is stabilized, evaluation for discharge to a rehabilitation facility is completed. The patient must be able to physically tolerate the rehabilitation program, in which the patient is taught to function as independently as possible.

The family must be prepared for changes in the patient's ability to function and possible changes in personality. It may take months to years before the patient reaches his or her maximum potential. In some cases of severe brain damage or continued comatose state, rehabilitation is not feasible and the patient is discharged to home or a long-term facility for custodial care.

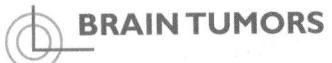

BRAIN TUMORS

Brain tumors are neoplastic growths of the brain or meninges. These tumors may be characterized by vague symptoms such as headache or visual changes or by focal neurological deficits such as hemiparesis or seizures.

Pathophysiology and Etiology

Brain tumors cause symptoms by either compressing or infiltrating brain tissue. Tumors may arise from central nervous system cells or may metastasize from other locations in the body. Primary brain tumors rarely metastasize. If they do metastasize, it is to the spine.

There is no established cause for primary brain tumors. It is unclear what causes the cells to begin reproducing in an uncontrolled fashion. Brain tumors can be classified in several different ways. The traditional distinction of benign and malignant is less helpful when discussing brain tumors. A benign tumor in the brainstem may be fatal, whereas a malignant tumor in the frontal lobe may not. Location of the tumor can be just as important a factor in outcome as the cell type.

Primary tumors are those arising from cells of the central nervous system. Eighty to 90% of brain tumors are primary in nature. Intra-axial tumors are those that arise from the glial cells within the cerebrum, cerebellum, or brainstem. These tumors infiltrate and invade brain tissue. Extra-axial tumors arise from the skull, meninges, pituitary gland, or cranial nerves. These tumors have a compressive effect on the brain.

Approximately 10% to 20% of brain tumors are secondary; that is, they are metastatic from a primary malignancy elsewhere in the body (Fig. 48.7). These tumors commonly spread via the arterial system. If untreated, they cause increased ICP. This may be the cause of the patient's death rather than the primary malignancy.

Signs and Symptoms

The symptoms of a brain tumor are directly related to the location of the tumor in the brain and to the rate of growth. Slow-growing types of tumors such as meningiomas (a tumor arising from the meninges) (Fig. 48.8) can get to be quite large before causing symptoms. Conversely, glioblastoma multiforme or metastatic tumors may abruptly cause seizures or hemiparesis. Other types of tumors include oligodendroglioma, astrocytoma, and acoustic neuroma. The suffix *-oma* refers to tumor. The prefix denotes the type of cell the tumor arises from.

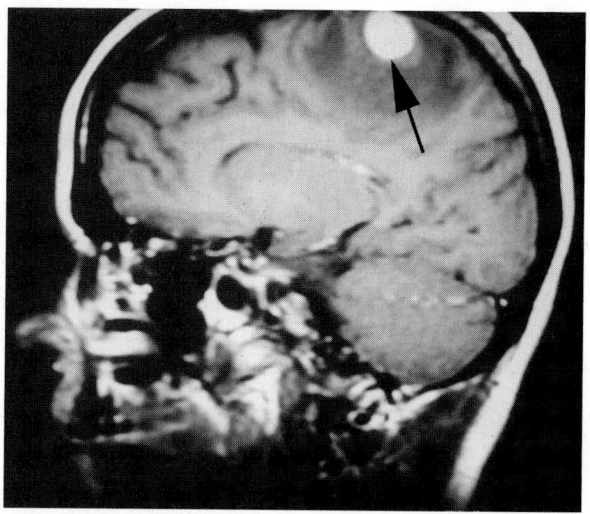

FIGURE 48.7 Metastatic brain tumor. This patient's primary cancer was in the lung.

Symptoms can include seizures, motor and sensory deficits, headaches, and visual disturbances. If the pituitary gland is involved, additional symptoms such as abnormal growth or fluid volume changes are related to changes in hormone secretion.

Diagnostic Tests

MRI gives the clearest images of a brain tumor. Many health-care providers order a CT scan first because it is cheaper. If the tumor appears to be highly vascular or in close proximity to major blood vessels, an angiogram may be performed. It is now possible to do magnetic resonance angiograms, which involve the intravenous administration

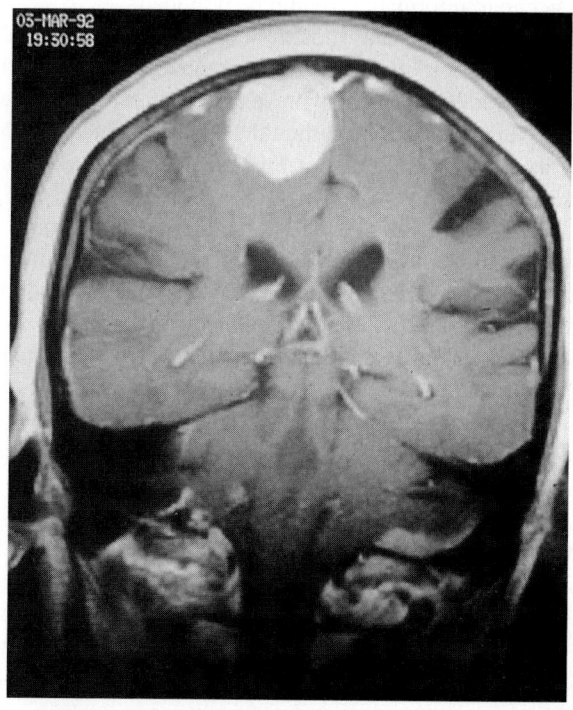

FIGURE 48.8 Meningioma.

of contrast material and is much less invasive than a traditional angiogram. If the tumor is in the region of the pituitary gland, serum hormone levels are evaluated.

Therapeutic Interventions

Surgical treatment involves removal of the tumor or as much of the tumor as possible. Care of the patient undergoing intracranial surgery is discussed later in this chapter.

Medical Treatment

Medical treatment consists of controlling symptoms. Patients who have a seizure are placed on anticonvulsants. If significant cerebral edema is noted on the CT or MRI or if the patient is suffering from headaches or other symptoms, a steroid such as dexamethasone (Decadron) may be prescribed to lessen the edema. Typically, patients do not require narcotics for pain relief.

Radiation Therapy

External beam radiation therapy is standard treatment for many patients with a brain tumor. The therapy is typically given 5 days a week for 6 weeks. Some clinicians use a hyperfractionated schedule, in which the patient has therapy twice a day for less time. Brachytherapy is a means of delivering radiation therapy directly to the tumor. Small catheters are implanted in the tumor and then tiny radioactive particles are inserted into the catheters. The treatment typically takes 3 to 5 days. During this time the patient is confined to a private room and interaction with visitors and staff is kept to a minimum because of radioactivity. This therapy is not appropriate for confused individuals because they may not be able to cooperate with restrictions.

Stereotactic radiosurgery is a technique that utilizes small amounts of radiation directed at the tumor from different angles. A metal frame is affixed to the patient's skull, and the tumor is visualized within the framework on a CT or MRI. A computer plan is generated to direct the radiation. Because multiple small sources are used, the normal brain tissue receives very little radiation while the majority of the radiation accumulates in the tumor.

Chemotherapy

The blood-brain barrier is a protective mechanism that prevents many injurious substances from reaching brain tissue. Unfortunately, it is also effective in preventing most chemotherapeutic agents from reaching the brain. To penetrate the blood-brain barrier, very large doses of chemotherapy may be required. These doses may not be well tolerated by other body systems. New treatments are currently being investigated. Some clinicians place chemotherapeutic substances in the cavity left by surgical resection. Others disrupt the blood-brain barrier with mannitol (an osmotic diuretic) and then deliver intra-arterial chemotherapy under general anesthesia. Gene therapy is also being used in an effort to kill malignant cells.

Complementary Therapies

The rate of success for treatment of brain tumors is not as high as treatment of other neoplasms. Patients may be drawn to nontraditional therapies both as cures and for treatment of symptoms. Encourage patients to look at each option in a rational manner. Some questions they should ask themselves include the following:

- Will this interfere with any of my other treatments or medications?
- What is the cost?
- What are the side effects?
- Is there any objective information (research) available?
- What does my physician think of this?

Additional information on evaluation of complementary therapies is found in Chapter 4.

Acute and Long-Term Complications

It is difficult to distinguish between symptoms of a brain tumor and complications of treatment. Seizures, headaches, memory impairment, cognitive changes, and ataxia may be symptoms of the tumor or the result of surgery or radiation therapy. Patients may experience hemiparesis or aphasia following surgery. If the tumor continues to grow despite treatment, the patient will experience further decline in function. Gradually the patient becomes more lethargic and unresponsive. Once the patient becomes comatose, death occurs within a matter of days, particularly if artificial nutrition and hydration are not administered.

Nursing Process for the Patient with a Brain Tumor

Nursing care of the patient with a brain tumor is similar to the patient with a brain injury, since both experience neurological deficits. See Box 48.3 Nursing Care Plan for Care of the Patient with a Brain Tumor or Injury.

INTRACRANIAL SURGERY

The primary purpose of intracranial surgery is to remove a mass lesion. These types of lesions include hematomas, tumors, arteriovenous malformations, and, occasionally, contused brain tissue. Other indications for surgery include elevation of a depressed skull fracture, removal of a foreign body, débridement of a wound, or resection of a seizure focus. **Craniotomy** refers to any surgical opening in the skull. A burr hole is an opening into the cranium made with a drill. **Craniectomy** is the term used to describe removal of part of the cranial bone. **Cranioplasty** refers to repair of bone or use of a prosthesis to replace bone following surgery.

The goal of intracranial tumor surgery for a tumor is gross total resection of the tumor. This involves removal of all visible tumor, called *debulking*. Even with the use of an operative microscope, there may be viable tumor cells left behind that can give rise to recurrence. If the entire tumor cannot be removed, the surgeon debulks as much as possi-

ble, thereby giving radiation therapy or chemotherapy less of a burden to combat. In some cases, it is not feasible to attempt more than a biopsy of the tumor. Location of the tumor or the patient's age or medical condition may not allow the patient to tolerate a full craniotomy. The biopsy may be done under local or general anesthesia, depending on the patient's condition. The goal of a biopsy is to obtain tissue that allows pathological diagnosis of the tumor. The diagnosis then guides any further treatment.

Intracranial surgery is usually performed under general anesthesia. Occasionally, a procedure requires that the patient be awake and cooperative.

Preoperative Care

Preoperative care of the patient undergoing intracranial surgery is similar to that of patients having other surgeries (see Chapter 11). The patient undergoes a laboratory work-up and anesthesia evaluation. If the patient has cognitive impairments, it is important that a significant other be available to provide information. A thorough baseline neurological assessment should be documented.

Patient education is important preoperatively. The extent of education depends on the patient's ability to absorb new information. This is influenced by the disease process, cognitive functioning, anxiety, and educational level. Significant others are involved as needed. Information about the disease process and surgery are provided by the surgeon. You can play an important role in reinforcing and clarifying the information presented.

Anxiety is also a significant concern before surgery. The patient is anticipating serious surgery, as well as an unknown outcome. Allow time for the patient and significant others to express their fears and ask questions. Honest and accurate information should be provided.

Significant others should be prepared for how the patient will look after surgery. A preoperative visit to the intensive care unit may help prevent some anxiety postoperatively. Significant others should be accompanied on this visit by a knowledgeable nurse who can explain what they are seeing.

Surgery may last 2 hours for a biopsy to 12 hours or longer for more intricate procedures. Patients and significant others should be prepared for the idea that some or all of the patient's hair will be shaved off. Some people prefer to have all their hair shaved rather than just part. The patient should be prepared to see his or her face swollen after surgery, particularly around the eyes. The periorbital region may be bruised. Many patients wish to wear a scarf or scrub cap after the dressing is removed.

Nursing Process for the Postoperative Care of the Patient Having Intracranial Surgery

Acute care of the postoperative patient is presented below. Also see Box 48.3 Nursing Care Plan for the Patient with a Brain Tumor or Injury.

---

craniotomy: crani—skull + otomy

Assessment/Data Collection

After intracranial surgery, plan to assist the RN with frequent neurological assessments in addition to routine postoperative monitoring. Patients should have their neurological status assessed every hour for the first 24 hours or as ordered by the physician. Any deterioration in status should be immediately reported to the RN and physician. Many patients undergo a CT scan within the first 24 hours following surgery to assess cerebral edema.

Nursing Diagnosis, Planning, and Implementation

The primary goal following intracranial surgery is prevention of complications. Initial care will be provided in an intensive care unit, and the LPN works with the RN to provide care. Once the patient is stabilized, goals can change to longer term outcomes such as acceptance of changes in body image and understanding of self-care following discharge. If the patient has severe deficits following surgery, rehabilitation or long-term care may become necessary. A consultation with a social worker can help with planning for this transition. Priority nursing diagnoses include the following.

Risk for ineffective cerebral tissue perfusion related to edema of the operative site

EXPECTED OUTCOME: Patient will have adequate cerebral tissue perfusion as evidenced by stable or improving neurological assessments.

- Monitor neurological status as ordered. Report changes promptly. *Deteriorating status may signify increased ICP.*
- Implement measures to prevent increased ICP. See Table 48.3 for interventions and rationales.
- Position patient with the head of the bed at 30 degrees or higher, unless ordered otherwise, *to promote venous drainage and minimize increases in intracranial pressure.* The exception to this is patients who have had a chronic subdural hematoma removed, who must remain flat. Patients may turn from side to side or lie on their back, but should not lie on the operative side.
- Implement seizure precautions *because the patient is at risk for seizures due to cerebral edema.*
- Use caution to protect the many monitoring systems being used. The patient may have an intracranial monitor in place following surgery *to monitor intracranial pressure.* Some patients may also have central venous pressure catheters or pulmonary artery catheters *to monitor fluid status.* Urinary catheters are used during the immediate postoperative period *to accurately monitor fluid balance.*
- Monitor dressings for drainage. *Drainage that is blood tinged in the center with a yellowish ring around it may be CSF leakage. A suspected CSF leak should be reported to the RN or physician immediately.*

Risk for infection related to surgical procedure

EXPECTED OUTCOME: Patient remains free from infection as evidenced by temperature and white cell count within normal limits and incision sites clean and dry.

- Monitor for rise in temperature, purulence at incision site, and increase in white cell count. *These are signs of infection and should be reported immediately.*
- Use strict aseptic technique for all care of the incision, dressing, and monitoring equipment sites *to reduce risk of infection.*

Body image disturbance related to changes in appearance or function

EXPECTED OUTCOME: Patient will display an accepting attitude toward change in appearance, as evidenced by willingness to look in mirror and/or be seen by others.

- Offer a turban, scarf, or hat if the patient desires *to help conceal a shaved head.*
- Portray an accepting attitude toward the patient. *Patients are likely aware of nurses' nonverbal behavior.*
- Allow the patient to express his or her feelings if desired. *Talking may help the patient work through feelings, but it should not be forced.*

Deficient knowledge related to change in treatment regimen following surgery

EXPECTED OUTCOME: The patient and significant others will verbalize correct information for follow-up care at home. They will state they have the resources to manage care effectively.

- Teach the patient and family or significant other home management, including medication regimen, wound care, and ordered activity restrictions, including driving. Have the patient and significant others verbalize the signs of infection or other possible complications to report. *The patient and family will assume responsibility for care after discharge.*
- Teach patient and family seizure precautions and the importance of taking anticonvulsants as ordered. *The patient will be at risk for seizures following surgery. If seizure-free for 1 year, the physician may discontinue anticonvulsants.*
- Consult social worker or case manager for resources if needed. *The patient may benefit from visiting nurse follow-up. Assistance with obtaining medications can also be provided if necessary.*

Evaluation

Interventions have been effective if infection and other complications have been prevented. The patient might be able to look in the mirror and begin to show evidence of acceptance of changes in body image, although this may not happen until after discharge from the hospital. The patient and significant others should be able to describe appropriate follow-up care.

CRITICAL THINKING

Mr. Evans

■ Mr. Evans is a 24-year-old white male who was involved in a motor vehicle accident. His blood alcohol level was 0.24. Mr. Evans has no preexisting medical problems. Emergency medical services personnel report that Mr. Evans was unconscious on their arrival at the scene and then became alert and combative. His CT scan shows a left-sided epidural hematoma. Mr. Evans is admitted to your unit for observation.

1. What symptoms would you expect to see if Mr. Evans's hematoma increases in size?
2. What emergency preparations should you have ready?
3. What psychosocial assessments should you perform?

Suggested answers at end of chapter.

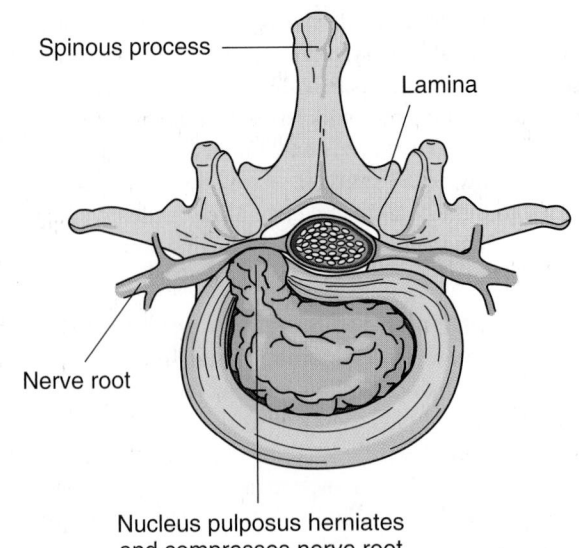

FIGURE 48.9 A herniated disk places pressure on a spinal nerve root.

 SPINAL DISORDERS

Herniated Disks

Herniated intravertebral disks are a common health problem. They are characterized by pain and paresthesias that follow a radicular (nerve path) pattern. It is not uncommon for patients to have more than one herniated disk or to have herniated disks in different areas of the spine.

Pathophysiology

When the disk between two vertebrae herniates, it moves out of its normal anatomical position. In most cases, the annulus fibrosus, the tough outer ring of the disk, tears. This allows escape of the nucleus pulposus, the soft inner portion of the disk. Displacement of the disk compresses one or more nerve roots, causing the characteristic symptoms (Fig. 48.9).

Etiology

In some cases, a specific event can be correlated with a herniated disk. The patient may describe a fall, lifting a heavy object, or a motor vehicle accident. In other instances, the patient cannot identify a triggering incident.

Signs and Symptoms

Cervical disk herniation causes pain and muscle spasm in the neck. The patient may exhibit decreased range of motion secondary to pain. Hand and arm pain is unilateral (one sided) and follows the distribution of the spinal nerve root. Patients often complain of numbness or tingling in the extremity. Asymmetrical weakness and atrophy of specific muscle groups may be detected. If weakness involves the entire extremity, it is unlikely that disk herniation is the etiology. The severity of the pain or paresthesia does not correlate directly with the severity of the nerve compression. However, weakness and atrophy are indicators of significant nerve compression.

Thoracic herniated disks are not common. This portion of the spine is the least mobile; therefore, less stress is exerted on the disks. Patients with herniated thoracic disks may complain of pain in the back. It is uncommon to detect muscular weakness.

A herniated lumbar disk is typically characterized by low back pain, pain radiating down one leg, paresthesias, and weakness. The patient may limp on the affected leg or may have difficulty walking on his or her heels or toes. Muscle spasm is often present. Pain and muscle spasm may limit the patient's range of motion. Depending on the disk affected, the knee or ankle deep tendon reflex may be decreased or absent. A severely herniated L5–S1 disk may affect bowel or bladder continence. This is an emergency situation and should be reported immediately.

The WHAT'S UP? mnemonic can be used to assess symptoms of herniated disks at any level:

W—Where is the pain? Does it radiate into an extremity? In what distribution?

H—How does it feel? Sharp, stabbing, burning?

A—Do certain positions or activities alleviate or aggravate the pain? Holding the affected arm above the head may alleviate cervical pain. Sitting places pressure on disks and aggravates lumbar pain. Lying down may relieve it.

T—Is there a correlation between time and pain? Some patients have more pain at the end of the day. Is the pain constant or intermittent?

S—Ask the patient to rate the severity of the pain on a scale of 0 to 10. Which is the most painful, the spine or the extremity?

U—Ask the patient to identify associated symptoms such as numbness, tingling, or weakness.

P—What is the patient's perception of the pain? Is it interfering with work or other aspects of the patient's life?

Diagnostic Tests

An MRI will detect herniation of a disk and compression or abnormality of the spinal cord. If the patient has previously had surgery in the area of the suspected herniation, the MRI is done with and without contrast to differentiate between scar tissue and a herniated disk.

If the patient cannot tolerate MRI or if the MRI does not provide enough information, a myelogram is done. Refer to Chapter 47 for a description of both tests.

Therapeutic Interventions

Most clinicians and patients prefer to try conservative medical therapy before performing surgery for a herniated disk.

MEDICAL TREATMENT. Rest. In the past, bedrest was advised as part of conservative management. The current recommendation is 1 or 2 days of bedrest, followed by a careful, gradual increase in activity.

Physical Therapy. Physical therapy can be very useful for some patients. A gradually progressive course of exercise strengthens the muscles. This is particularly important in the lumbar spine, where the muscles help stabilize the spine. Techniques such as ultrasound, heat, ice, and deep massage can decrease muscle spasm and allow for increased range of motion. Instructions in proper body mechanics and strategies for avoiding reinjury are important components of physical therapy.

A transcutaneous electrical nerve stimulator (commonly called a TENS unit) is a noninvasive pain-relief technique. Small electrodes are placed on the skin around the area of the pain. The device then transmits a low-voltage electrical current through the skin. The patient feels a tingling or buzzing sensation, which may block the pain impulses. A physical therapist or pain specialist teaches the patient where to place the electrodes and how to operate the unit. The patient decides when to use it and at what settings. This allows the patient to actively participate in his or her care and have some control over the pain level.

Traction. Cervical traction is a noninvasive technique sometimes used by physical therapists for patients with herniated cervical disks. The patient's head is placed in a halterlike device. A series of ropes and pulleys connect the halter to a weight. This gently pulls the head away from the shoulders. The rationale is that this traction slightly separates the vertebral bodies and may allow the disk to return to its proper position. If it is effective in relieving the patient's pain, cervical traction may be done at home on an as-needed basis. Traction is discontinued immediately if it increases the patient's pain. Lumbar traction is not particularly effective because the lumbar paraspinal muscles are very large and strong. The amount of traction needed to overcome the muscular resistance can cause injury.

Medication. Muscle relaxants are often prescribed for patients who are experiencing muscle spasms. These medications decrease pain by decreasing the spasm, helping the patient increase range of motion and activity. Muscle

spasm is actually a protective mechanism. Muscles tighten and become painful, causing the patient to limit movement. This lessens the chance that the disk will be further injured. However, chronic spasm can cause tearing and scarring of the muscles. It is hard to predict which muscle relaxant will be most effective for a given patient. Patients should be warned that drowsiness is a common side effect of many muscle relaxants. They should be cautioned against driving or operating machinery until they determine how well they tolerate the medication. Diazepam is an effective muscle relaxant; however, it has a strong potential for addiction so it is usually used only if muscle spasm cannot be adequately treated with other medications.

Inflammation of the nerve root is caused by compression and irritation from the herniated disk. Nonsteroidal anti-inflammatory drugs (NSAIDs) can be effective in reducing this inflammation, but there is no way of predicting response to a given drug. It may be necessary for the patient to try several nonsteroidal drugs before an effective one is found. Because several of these drugs are now available without prescription, the patient should be cautioned not to use a nonprescription NSAID at the same time as a prescription NSAID. Patients should be instructed to report any stomach upset to the clinician because NSAIDs have the potential to cause gastric bleeding. Occasionally, oral steroids are used on a short-term basis for patients with severe inflammation that does not respond to other treatments. A rapidly tapering dose of steroid over 1 week is often prescribed. Steroids may also cause gastric upset, in addition to elevated serum glucose levels. Instruct patients with diabetes to monitor glucose levels closely and consult a physician if the levels are outside their normal parameters.

Epidural injections are an option for patients who are unable or do not wish to have surgery. A mixture of medications, typically a steroid, long-acting anesthetic, and long-acting pain reliever, is injected into the epidural space. The anesthetic provides immediate relief while the steroid reduces swelling for a longer lasting effect. If relief is obtained, the injection can be repeated every 3 to 4 months.

The use of pain medication is a subject of concern in the treatment of patients with herniated disks. Opioids may be appropriate for short-term use. This includes patients who are trying conservative therapy or those who are not able to have surgery immediately. If surgery is not an option or is not successful, the condition may be a chronic source of pain. In that circumstance, the physician and patient must discuss the potential complications of long-term opioid use, such as constipation, tolerance, and dependence. A referral to a pain clinic for alternative strategies may be appropriate.

SURGICAL MANAGEMENT. Several types of surgery can be done. A **laminectomy** removes one of the laminae, the flat pieces of bone on each side of a vertebra. This may be done to relieve pressure or to gain access for removal of a

---

laminectomy: lamin—posterior portion of the vertebra + ectomy—surgical removal of

herniated disk. A diskectomy removes the entire disk. A spinal fusion uses a bone graft to fuse two vertebrae together if the area is unstable. Surgery may be done through a microscope for less scarring and faster recovery. Most patients are discharged within 24 hours of surgery.

A diskectomy is generally done for a herniated cervical disk. This can be accomplished via an anterior or posterior approach. Most surgeons use the anterior approach for cervical herniations because the muscles in the front of the neck are much smaller and more moveable than those in the back of the neck. Therefore, there is less pain and muscle spasm following surgery. It is also safer than the posterior approach, which involves more maneuvering around the spinal cord.

Most surgeons replace the disk with bone or another material. This prevents collapse of the disk space and creates a spinal fusion. If bone is used, it may be harvested from the patient's iliac crest or donated from a cadaver. Mobility of the spine is lost in the area of a fusion. Spinal fusions may also be done to correct instability of the spine from other causes, such as scoliosis or degenerative disorders.

A posterior approach is used for a herniated lumbar disk. Typically, the vertical incision is 1 to 2 inches long. It is necessary to pull some of the muscle away from the bone, which accounts for some of the postoperative pain that patients experience. A laminectomy is done, and the herniated portion of the disk is resected. The remainder of the disk continues to provide a cushion between the intravertebral bodies. The surgeon removes any free fragments and any disk material that appears unstable.

Percutaneous diskectomy involves insertion of a large needle into the disk under local anesthesia to aspirate herniated disk material. This technique is not used for severely herniated disks. Laser disk surgery may be used to disintegrate the herniated tissue. Laparoscopic techniques may also be used.

Complications After Surgery

HEMORRHAGE. As with any surgery, intraoperative hemorrhage is possible. It is not common in disk surgery. If a postoperative hemorrhage occurs in a patient who has had an anterior cervical diskectomy, the airway may become occluded. The patient is monitored for bleeding from the incision and respiratory distress.

NERVE ROOT DAMAGE. If the nerve root is severed during surgery, the patient has loss of motor and sensory functions in that distribution. This may result in decreased use of the extremity. If the nerve root is damaged or excessive scarring occurs, the patient may experience pain, weakness, or paresthesias. In some cases, physical therapy and NSAIDs may be effective in improving function and lessening pain.

REHERNIATION. Lumbar disks may reherniate. This can occur anywhere from 1 week to several years after the initial surgery. If the reherniation occurs within a few weeks to months after the first surgery, the patient usually undergoes

another microdiskectomy. Reherniation of the cervical disk does not occur because the entire disk is removed.

HERNIATION OF ANOTHER DISK. Fusion of the cervical spine results in loss of movement at that motion segment. This can place increased stress on the disks above and below the fusion. This may increase the risk of another herniated disk, especially if the patient already has degeneration of other disks. The patient should be instructed to maintain an exercise program and to frequently move the spine through range-of-motion exercises.

Nursing Process for the Patient Having Spinal Surgery

Preoperative Care
Routine preoperative care is appropriate for the patient undergoing spinal surgery. In addition to routine teaching, instruct the patient in how to logroll following surgery. This procedure involves keeping the body in alignment and rolling as a unit, without twisting the spine, to prevent injury to the operative site.

Postoperative Care
ASSESSMENT/DATA COLLECTION. In addition to routine postoperative assessment, monitor extremities for changes in circulation, movement, and sensation. Monitor color, warmth, and presence of pulses in the extremities. Assess movement by asking the patient to move the extremities. Assess sensation by gently touching the patient's extremity and asking if feeling is present. Report any changes immediately to the physician because this may indicate nerve or circulatory damage.

Monitor pain frequently. The pain that necessitated surgery should be relieved, but the patient may still have muscular and incisional pain. The patient should be reassured that it will gradually subside. Monitor the surgical dressing and drain (if present) for CSF drainage or bleeding. Any sign of CSF drainage or significant bleeding should be reported to the physician immediately. If bone was taken from a separate donor site, this site must also be monitored. Intake and output are measured to ensure that the patient is able to void. Notify the physician if the patient has difficulty voiding.

NURSING DIAGNOSIS, PLANNING, AND IMPLEMENTATION. Goals of nursing are to keep the patient safe and free from injury or complications and free from pain. Gradual return to normal physical activity is expected. Possible postoperative diagnoses include the following.

Pain related to surgical procedure

EXPECTED OUTCOME: Patient will verbalize an acceptable pain level.

- Monitor pain following surgery using a pain scale. *The patient's self-report is the most reliable method for assessing pain.*
- Administer muscle relaxants, analgesics, and NSAIDs as ordered. If a local anesthetic was injected into the surgical site during surgery, the

patient may not have pain immediately postoperatively. *Medications to relieve pain help the patient to mobilize following surgery, which helps prevent complications.*

- Position the patient in bed in correct body alignment. If ordered, keep the patient flat for 6 to 8 hours. *Correct alignment avoids twisting and injury to the operative site.*
- Place a pillow between the legs when lying on the side *to promote alignment and comfort.*

Risk for impaired urinary elimination related to effects of surgery

EXPECTED OUTCOME: Patient will be able to empty bladder without assistance.

- Monitor urine output for retention. *Patients may have difficulty voiding following lumbar surgery because of anesthesia, immobility, or occasionally because of nerve damage related to surgery.*
- If activity orders allow, assist the patient to get up to urinate (or to stand for men). *This may help the patient urinate.*
- If unable to void, try running warm water over the perineum, or taking a warm bath or shower. *This may stimulate voiding.*
- If difficulty urinating occurs, contact the physician for an order for intermittent catheterization until the problem resolves. *Urinary retention that is not resolved can lead to bladder rupture. Intermittent catheterization is a safe way to empty the bladder.*

Risk for impaired physical mobility related to neuromuscular impairment

EXPECTED OUTCOME: Patient will be able to ambulate and prevent complications of immobility following surgery.

- Assess mobility of affected extremities following surgery. *A reduction in mobility following surgery indicates nerve damage in surgery and should be reported immediately.*
- Assist the patient to logroll to get out of bed and ambulate on the first postoperative day. If spinal fusion has been done, the fused area of the spine will be immobile. *Early mobilization after surgery helps prevent complications.*
- Apply a soft cervical collar to the patient with a cervical laminectomy as ordered *for neck support.*

EVALUATION. The patient is expected to be free of complications and pain, be able to urinate, be able to move all extremities, and return gradually to preillness activity level.

Spinal Stenosis

Spinal stenosis is a condition in which the spinal canal compresses the spinal cord (Fig. 48.10). Arthritis is a major cause of spinal stenosis. The facet joints of the spine become inflamed and enlarged, narrowing the diameter of the spinal canal and compressing the spinal cord. Patients may complain of pain and weakness. Compression of the cervical

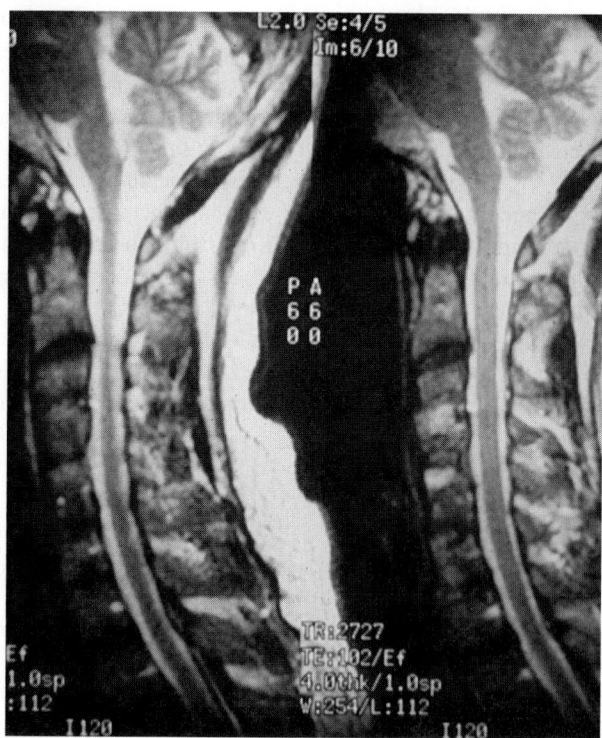

FIGURE 48.10 Stenosis of the cervical spine *(left)*. Compare with normal spinal column *(right)*.

portion of the spinal cord may result in hyperreflexia and weakness of the legs and arms.

A laminectomy may be done to relieve pressure on the spinal cord. The size of the incision depends on the number of vertebrae involved. These patients are often older and may have concurrent illnesses. They may require inpatient rehabilitation before returning home.

SPINAL CORD INJURIES

Injuries to the spinal cord affect people of all ages but take their greatest toll on young people. These injuries are characterized by a decrease or loss of sensory and motor functions below the level of the injury.

Pathophysiology

The spinal cord is made up of nerve fibers that allow communication between the brain and the rest of the body. Damage to the spinal cord results in interference with this communication process. Damage may be caused by bruising, tearing, cutting, edema, or bleeding into the cord. The damage may be caused by external forces or by fragments of fractured bone.

Causes and Types

The causes of spinal cord injury are similar to those of traumatic brain injury. It is not uncommon for a patient to have both a spinal cord injury and traumatic brain injury. Motor vehicle crashes, falls, and sports-related injuries are common causes. Diving into shallow water is often the cause of cervical cord injury. Assaults may cause cord injury if a knife or bullet penetrates the spinal cord.

Spinal cord injuries may be classified by location or by degree of damage to the cord. A complete spinal cord injury means that there is no motor or sensory function below the level of the injury. An incomplete lesion means that there is some function remaining. This does not necessarily mean that the remaining function will be useful to the patient. Some patients find that having areas where sensation is intact may be more painful than useful.

The cervical and lumbar portions of the spine are injured more often than the thoracic or sacral segments. This is because the cervical and lumbar areas are the most mobile portions of the spine.

Signs and Symptoms

Cervical Injuries

Signs and symptoms depend on the level of cord that is damaged (Fig. 48.11). Cervical cord injuries can affect all four extremities, causing paralysis and paresthesias, impaired respiration, and loss of bowel and bladder control. Paralysis of all four extremities is called **quadriplegia;** weakness of all extremities is called **quadriparesis.** If the injury is at C3 or above, the injury is usually fatal because muscles used for breathing are paralyzed. An injury at the fourth or fifth cervical vertebra affects breathing and may necessitate some type of ventilatory support. These patients typically need long-term assistance with activities of daily living.

Thoracic and Lumbar Injuries

Thoracic and lumbar injuries affect the legs, bowel, and bladder. Paralysis of the legs is called **paraplegia;** weakness of the legs is called **paraparesis.** Sacral injuries affect bowel and bladder continence and may affect foot function. Individuals with thoracic, lumbar, and sacral injuries can usually learn to perform activities of daily living independently.

Spinal Shock

Spinal cord injury has a profound effect on the autonomic nervous system. Immediately following injury, the cord below the injury stops functioning completely. This causes a disruption of sympathetic nervous system function, resulting in vasodilation, hypotension, and bradycardia (neurogenic shock or spinal shock). Dilation of the blood vessels allows more blood flow just beneath the skin. This blood cools and is circulated throughout the body, causing hypothermia. The patient is unable to maintain control of body temperature. Keep the patient covered as much as possible but avoid overheating. In addition, all reflexes below the level of the injury are lost, and retention of urine and feces occurs. Spinal shock can last from a week to many weeks in some patients.

---

quadriplegia: quad—four + plegia—paralysis
quadriparesis: quad—four + paresis—partial paralysis
paraplegia: para—beside + plegia—paralysis
paraparesis: para—beside + paresis—partial paralysis

Complications

Infection

Impaired respiratory effort, decreased cough, mechanical ventilation, and immobility all predispose the cervical cord–injured patient to pneumonia. Catheterization, whether indwelling or intermittent, places patients at risk for urinary tract infection.

Deep Vein Thrombosis

Lack of movement in the legs inhibits normal blood circulation. Compression stockings, sequential compression devices, and subcutaneous heparin may be used separately or together to reduce the risk of deep vein thrombosis.

Orthostatic Hypotension

Most spinal cord–injured patients no longer have muscular function in their legs to promote venous return to the heart. They also have impaired vasoconstriction. This leads to pooling of the blood in the legs when the patient moves from a supine to a sitting position. If the movement is sudden, the patient may become dizzy or faint. Gradual elevation of the head, use of elastic stockings, and a reclining wheelchair help lessen this response.

Skin Breakdown

Patients or their caregivers must be diligent about relieving pressure on the skin by position changes and cushioning of bony prominences. Development of pressure ulcers can lead to infection and loss of skin, muscle, or bone. Treatment of pressure ulcers is time consuming and expensive and may interfere with work or school.

SAFETY TIP

Assess and periodically reassess each resident's risk for developing a pressure ulcer (decubitus ulcer) and take action to address any identified risk (2006 National Patient Safety Goals from www.jcaho.org).

Renal Complications

Urinary tract infections are an ongoing concern to spinal cord–injured patients. Both urinary reflux and untreated urinary tract infections can cause permanent damage to the kidneys.

Depression and Substance Abuse

Patients with spinal cord injury have a higher than average incidence of depression and substance abuse. Both these factors can interfere with the patient's ability to care for himself or herself. Individual or family counseling may be helpful. Some rehabilitation centers have support groups for spinal cord–injured patients.

Autonomic Dysreflexia

This life-threatening complication occurs in patients with injuries above the T6 level. The spinal cord injury impairs

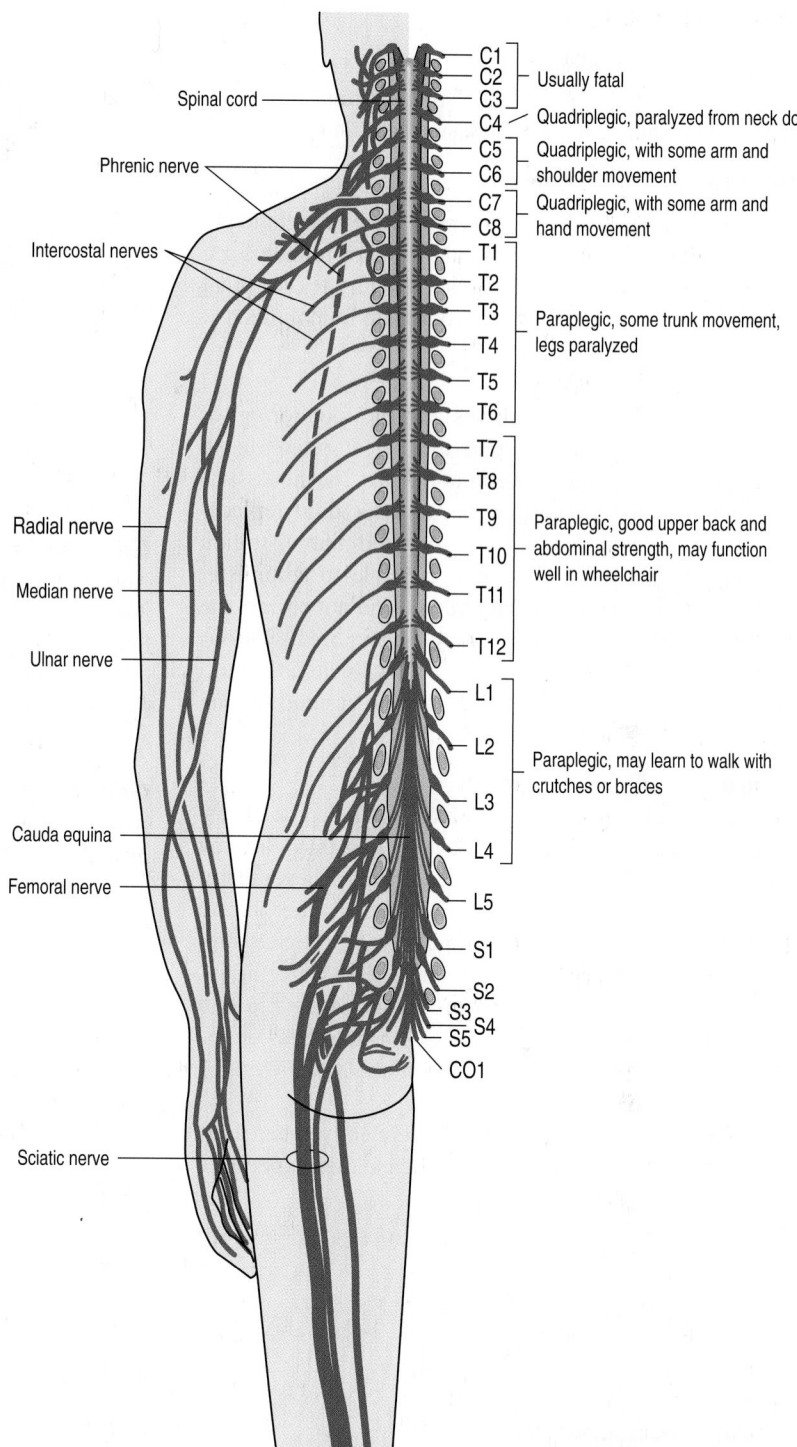

FIGURE 48.11 Spinal cord injury—quadriplegia versus paraplegia. *(Modified from Scanlon, VC, and Sanders, T: Workbook for Essentials of Anatomy and Physiology, ed. 5. F.A. Davis, Philadelphia, 2007, p 163, with permission.)*

the normal equilibrium between the sympathetic and parasympathetic divisions of the autonomic nervous system. Some type of noxious stimuli below the spinal cord injury causes activation of the sympathetic system. This response continues unchecked because the parasympathetic responses cannot descend past the spinal cord injury.

The most common cause of autonomic **dysreflexia** is bladder distention. Other causes include bowel impaction,

urinary tract infection, ingrown toenails, pressure ulcers, pain, and labor. Stimulation of the sympathetic nervous system results in cool, pale skin, gooseflesh, and vasoconstriction below the level of the injury. Blood pressure may rise as high as 300 mm Hg systolic. The parasympathetic response results in vasodilation, causing flushing and diaphoresis above the lesion, and bradycardia as low as 30 beats per minute. The patient complains of a pounding headache and nasal congestion secondary to the dilated blood vessels.

dysreflexia: dys—abnormal + reflexia—reflex activity

Diagnostic Tests

Plain radiographs are done to identify fractures or displacement of vertebrae. A CT scan is also useful for identifying fractures. MRI may demonstrate lesions within the cord.

Therapeutic Interventions

Patients with spinal cord injuries typically are brought to the emergency department. They should be kept immobilized until they are assessed by a physician. If injury to the spinal cord is detected, the patient needs to remain immobilized.

Emergency Management

Emergency management involves careful monitoring of vital signs and airway and keeping the patient immobilized. Intubation and mechanical ventilation may be necessary. Intravenous normal saline may be used for fluid replacement. The physician does not rely on fluid administration alone to correct hypotension. It is possible to administer enough fluid to cause pulmonary edema and not correct the hypotension. Vasoactive drugs may be required. Various medications to reduce the extent of injury, including intravenous methylprednisolone (a steroid), are currently being researched.

Respiratory Management

Patients with injuries above C4–5 have some degree of respiratory impairment. The patient may require a tracheostomy and continuous mechanical ventilation or require a ventilator only at night or when fatigued. Some patients are able to breathe by using a phrenic nerve stimulator. This device, similar to a pacemaker, artificially stimulates the phrenic nerve, causing the diaphragm to move. These patients use a mechanical ventilator at night. This lessens the stress on the phrenic nerve and removes the risk of the system failing while the patient is asleep.

Patients may be breathing independently when they first arrive in the emergency department and then experience respiratory compromise as the spinal cord becomes edematous. Edema can compress the spinal cord above the lesion, leading to symptoms at a higher level. This deterioration is usually temporary. Fatigue of the accessory muscles may also cause respiratory compromise. The intercostal muscles are not normally of major importance in respiration. However, if the diaphragm is paralyzed, the intercostal muscles become very important. As these muscles fatigue, the patient's breathing becomes shallow and rapid. Elective intubation and mechanical ventilation protect the patient from expending huge amounts of energy trying to breathe. Feeling their breathing becoming more labored is terrifying to these patients, and they need to be reassured that it is probably a temporary setback. As the edema recedes and the accessory muscles become stronger, the patient is weaned from the ventilator.

Gastrointestinal Management

Absence of bowel sounds is a common finding on examination. Oral or enteral feedings are not started until bowel function resumes. The metabolic needs of the patients are influenced by the work of breathing and the extent of other injuries. If positioning or paralytic ileus precludes oral or enteral feedings, hyperalimentation is begun.

Genitourinary Management

An indwelling urinary catheter is placed to prevent bladder distention and protect skin integrity until spinal shock resolves. Once it is determined what degree of hand function the patient will have, a bladder management program is devised.

Immobilization

The cervical spine may be immobilized with skeletal traction such as Crutchfield or Gardner-Wells tongs (Fig. 48.12). Some patients have a halo brace, a device that attaches to the skull with four small pins. The skull ring attaches to a rigid plastic vest by four poles (Fig. 48.13).

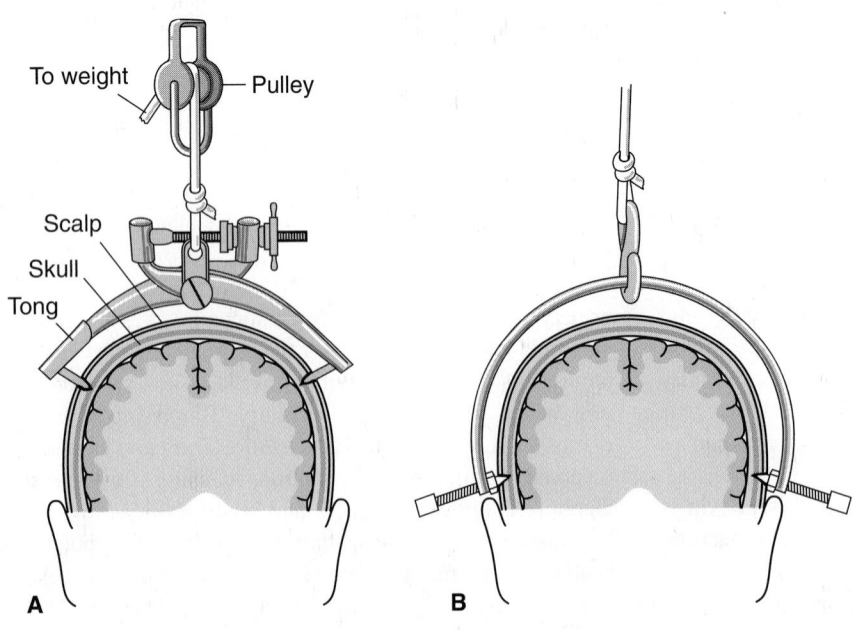

A **B**

FIGURE 48.12 Skeletal traction for cervical injuries. (A) Crutchfield tongs. (B) Gardner-Wells tongs.

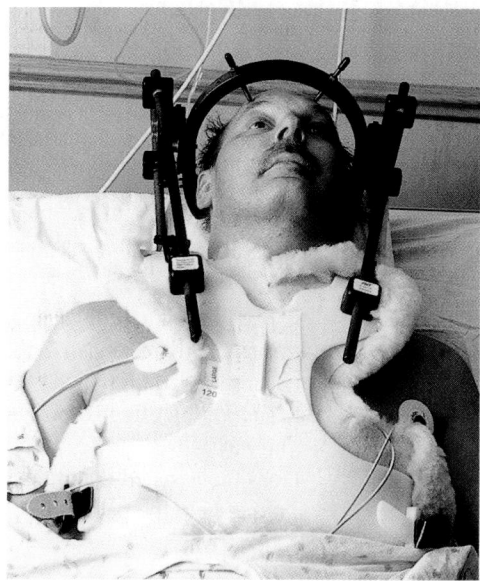

FIGURE 48.13 Halo brace.

This device keeps the head and neck immobile while fusion and healing take place. The advantage over traction is that the patient is not confined to bed.

Surgical Management

The goal of surgery following spinal cord injury is to stabilize the bony elements of the spine and relieve pressure on the spinal cord. Surgery may or may not improve functional outcome.

Stabilization of the spine allows for earlier mobilization of the patient. This decreases the risk of complications from immobility and quickens the transition to a rehabilitation setting. Patients who have been in cervical traction before surgery may be placed in a halo brace postoperatively.

Unstable thoracic and lumbar fractures may also be treated with surgical implantation of rods to stabilize the spine. It is more difficult to stabilize these areas in the postoperative recovery period. Patients may wear a supportive corset, a rigid brace, or occasionally a body cast to supplement the support provided by the internal fixation devices. For more information, visit the Spinal Cord Injury Information Network at http://spinalcord.uab.edu.

Nursing Process for the Care of the Patient with a Spinal Cord Injury

Patients with spinal cord injury need ongoing evaluation of all body systems. Frequent neurological and respiratory assessments are essential. Early assessment of the patient's support systems can help with discharge and rehabilitation planning. Initial goals for the patient include maintenance of safety and prevention of complications. Long-term goals include rehabilitation and maximizing remaining function.

See Box 48.6 Nursing Care Plan for the Patient with a Spinal Cord Injury and Box 48.7 Spinal Cord Injury Summary on page 1093.

NEURODEGENERATIVE DISORDERS AND DISTURBED THOUGHT PROCESSES

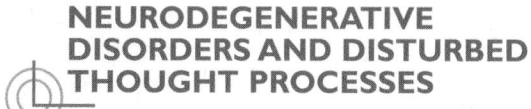

Neurodegenerative is a term that can apply to any nervous system disorder that causes degeneration, or wasting, of the neurons in the nervous system. The following disorders are some of the most common neurodegenerative disorders that

---

neurodegenerative: neuro—nervous system + degenerative—deteriorating

(Text continued on page 1092)

Box 48.6   Nursing Care Plan for the Patient with a Spinal Cord Injury

Nursing Diagnosis: Impaired gas exchange related to respiratory muscle weakness

Expected Outcome Patient will maintain $Sao_2 \geq 90\%$, $Pao_2 \geq 75$ mm Hg, $Paco_2 \leq 45$ mm Hg.

Evaluation of Outcome Are ABGs and Sao_2 within normal limits?

Interventions	Rationale	Evaluation
Monitor respiratory rate, effort, ABGs and Sao_2.	These are indicators of respiratory function. The patient may have difficulty maintaining normal respiration if diaphragm or accessory muscles are weak related to injury.	Are ABGs and Sao_2 within normal limits? Does patient appear distressed?
Notify physician immediately if Sao_2 or Pao_2 drops, or if $Paco_2$ rises.	If patient is unable to maintain blood gases, mechanical ventilation may be necessary.	

(Continued on following page)

Box 48.6 NURSING CARE PLAN for the Patient with a Spinal Cord Injury (Continued)

Nursing Diagnosis: Ineffective airway clearance related to ineffective cough and decreased muscle control

Expected Outcome Patient will maintain a clear airway as evidenced by clear breath sounds and $Sao_2 \geq 90\%$.

Evaluation of Outcome Are breath sounds clear? Is $Sao_2 \geq 90\%$?

Interventions	Rationale	Evaluation
Monitor cough and lung sounds.	Patient may not have adequate muscle strength to cough effectively.	Is patient able to cough up secretions? Is there evidence that secretions are retained?
Suction patient prn if unable to cough effectively.	To keep the airway clear.	Is suctioning effective in clearing airway?
Once the patient is stable, try assisting the patient to cough to clear secretions. Gently push upward and inward on the patient's chest while the patient coughs as strongly as possible.	This may help the patient clear secretions without invasive suctioning. This is similar to the Heimlich maneuver but not as forceful.	Does the assisted cough technique help the patient to clear the airway?
Provide humidified air and oral or enteral fluids.	Humidification helps keep secretions thin and mobile.	Are secretions thin and easily expectorated?

Nursing Diagnosis: Risk for autonomic dysreflexia related to stimuli below the level of injury

Expected Outcome The patient does not demonstrate signs of autonomic dysreflexia as evidenced by stable vital signs. If dysreflexia occurs, it is recognized and corrected promptly.

Evaluation of Outcome Is patient free of signs or are signs recognized and promptly treated?

Interventions	Rationale	Evaluation
Monitor for signs of autonomic dysreflexia: sudden high blood pressure, bradycardia, headache, pale skin below the injury, gooseflesh. Remember that patients with spinal cord injury are typically hypotensive, so a finding of even mild hypertension may represent a dramatic increase from their baseline blood pressure.	Autonomic dysreflexia must be recognized quickly in order to remove cause and prevent complications such as seizures, intracerebral hemorrhage, or death.	Are signs of dysreflexia present?
If you suspect autonomic dysreflexia, immediately take the patient's blood pressure and continue to monitor it every 5 minutes.	Blood pressure must be continually monitored until it is under control, to prevent complications.	Is blood pressure higher than normal for patient? Are emergency interventions warranted?
Place the patient in high-Fowler's position. Remove elastic stockings or any other garment that could prevent blood from pooling in the periphery.	High-Fowler's position utilizes the effect of orthostasis to control blood pressure. Allowing blood to pool in periphery can help reduce blood pressure.	Does position change reduce blood pressure?
Evaluate the indwelling catheter for patency. If it is not patent or a catheter is not in place, obtain an order to insert one immediately. Monitor blood pressure during catheterization.	A full bladder can be the cause of the stimuli causing the dysreflexia.	Is catheter patent? Is bladder full? Does emptying bladder resolve dysreflexia?

Interventions	Rationale	Evaluation
Perform a rectal examination to determine if an impaction is present. Apply anesthetic ointment to the rectum before disimpaction. Simultaneously monitor blood pressure and stop disimpaction if the blood pressure increases.	Fecal impaction can be the stimulus causing the dysreflexia. Anesthetic is used because further rectal stimulation may exacerbate symptoms.	Is impaction present? Does removal resolve dysreflexia?
If bowel or bladder distention is not present, examine the patient for other causative mechanisms. If a cause cannot be identified, or removal of the cause does not relieve hypertension, notify the physician immediately.	If the cause cannot be found and removed, an antihypertensive agent may be ordered.	Are other causes identifiable? Is an antihypertensive agent ordered?
If hypertension is treated with medication, continue to carefully monitor blood pressure.	Blood pressure may decrease rapidly once the cause of the autonomic dysreflexia is corrected.	Is blood pressure stabilized?
Once the acute episode is past, work with patient and significant others to devise a plan to prevent reoccurrence. Teach the patient how to direct caregivers in treating autonomic dysreflexia.	Episodes of dysreflexia can recur.	Do patient and caregivers verbalize understanding of how to prevent and treat future episodes of dysreflexia?

Nursing Diagnosis: Total urinary incontinence related to spinal cord damage and no sensation to void and/or inability to control flow of urine

Expected Outcomes Patient's skin will be dry and free of urine; urine elimination will be controlled.

Evaluation of Outcomes Patient will be continent of urine, free of urinary infection (urine clear, yellow, without burning on urination), and have dry and intact skin.

Interventions	Rationale	Evaluation
Assess patient's ability to control urination.	If patient has some control, a bladder training program may be effective.	Is patient able to sense need to urinate? Is any degree of control present?
Monitor appearance of urine, temperature, and white cell count.	Cloudy urine, and an increase in temperature and white cell count indicate urinary tract infection.	Is urine clear, and temperature and white blood cells within normal limits?
Implement a bladder training program utilizing set times for voiding.	Following a voiding schedule can help reduce incontinence.	Is patient able to avoid incontinence with regular voiding?
Use bladder ultrasound to scan bladder for residual urine.	Incomplete voiding can increase risk for urinary tract infection.	Is patient effectively emptying bladder?
Teach the patient or caregiver self-catheterization as ordered, if bladder training is not effective.	Intermittent self-catheterization is associated with fewer complications than an indwelling catheter.	Is patient able to perform self-catheterization correctly?
Consult with physician re Foley catheter if patient is not a candidate for intermittent self catheterization.	An indwelling catheter can increase risk for infection, but may be necessary as a last resort for some patients.	Is Foley catheter necessary? Are signs of infection avoided?

(Continued on following page)

Box 48.6 NURSING CARE PLAN for the Patient with a Spinal Cord Injury *(Continued)*

Nursing Diagnosis: Constipation related to immobility and nerve damage

Expected Outcome Patient will return to preinjury bowel pattern.

Evaluation of Outcome Does patient pass soft stool at regular intervals?

Interventions	Rationale	Evaluation
Assess previous and current bowel pattern and continence.	Decreased or absent sphincter tone, inability to detect the need to defecate, and immobility put the patient at risk for incontinence and constipation.	What was previous pattern? Is it used to develop goals for patient?
Monitor bowel sounds and abdominal distention.	These monitor bowel function.	Are bowel sounds present? Is abdomen soft?
Institute a bowel management program as soon as oral feedings are resumed. Include a suppository on a scheduled daily or every-other-day basis as ordered.	A management program including stool softeners and routine suppository use can help to restore regular defecation.	Does management program keep bowel movements soft and regular, and maintain continence?
Provide a high-fiber diet with adequate fluid intake.	Fiber and fluids help keep stool soft.	Is patient receiving adequate fiber and fluids?

Nursing Diagnosis: Impaired physical mobility related to hemorrhage, ischemia, and edema of cord as evidenced by paresis or paralysis.

Expected Outcome Patient will maintain maximum mobility and be free from complications of immobility.

Evaluation of Outcomes Is patient kept mobile without contractures? Is skin intact? Can patient complete ADLs with assistance?

Interventions	Rationale	Evaluation
Determine patient's ability to move independently.	Assessment should guide interventions.	What can patient do independently?
Assess patient's ability to feel pressure and pain.	If the patient is unable to feel pain or pressure, it will be even more important to monitor skin and prevent prolonged pressure.	Can patient feel pressure and pain?
Reposition every 2 hours, utilizing supportive devices.	Unrelieved pressure on the skin, especially bony prominences, will result in ischemia and necrosis.	Is skin intact without redness?
Change positions slowly; have patient sit at side of bed before standing (if able) or getting up to chair.	Patients with cervical spine injuries or patients remaining immobile for long periods are prone to orthostatic hypotension.	Does patient become dizzy when getting up?
Perform active or passive range of motion exercises at least once every 8 hours. If patient has arm mobility, teach patient to participate in doing as much ROM as possible.	Range-of-motion exercises maintain mobility and prevent contractures.	Is patient able to perform range-of-motion exercises with minimal difficulty?
Teach patient importance of repositioning self at least every 2 hours.	Patients with some mobility can learn to reposition themselves; this helps prevent total dependence on caregivers.	Does patient demonstrate correct repositioning every 2 hours?
Teach patient to direct own care, if unable to reposition independently.	This allows the patient some control over his or her situation.	Does patient direct own care and prevent complications of immobility?

Nursing Diagnosis: Self-care deficit related to paralysis

Expected Outcome Patient's self-care needs will be met by self or caregivers.

Evaluation of Outcome Are patient's needs met? Does patient verbalize satisfaction with care?

Interventions	Rationale	Evaluation
Determine patient's level of function and ability to perform ADLs.	The patient should be encouraged to be as independent as possible.	What is patient able to do? Is it incorporated into plan of care?
Explain the rationale for nursing activities, and encourage the patient and significant others to participate in hands-on care as much as possible	This will help prepare the patient and significant others to assume responsibility for care at home.	Do patient and significant others verbalize understanding of care? Are they able to demonstrate procedures correctly?
If the patient will not be able to perform self-care, assist him or her to learn to direct care.	This allows the patient some control over his or her care.	Does patient participate by directing care?
Consult with physical and occupational therapy.	Physical and occupational therapy can help the patient learn to adapt to physical limitations; they can provide a wheelchair or other mobility aids.	Is patient adapting to limitations with help?
Discuss discharge to a rehabilitation facility with patient, physician, and discharge planner.	A rehab facility can teach the patient to function independently. Some patients may require long-term care.	Is the patient a candidate for rehabilitation?
Assist patients and caregivers to determine contingency plans. These include what to do in the event of a power failure, fire, or illness of the caregiver.	Planning ahead what to do in an emergency can mean the difference between life and death for an immobile patient.	Do patient and caregivers have a plan to keep the patient safe?
Encourage the patient to establish a relationship with a primary practitioner who is familiar with spinal cord injury.	Spinal cord–injured patients experience the same basic health care needs as noninjured individuals.	Does patient have a primary care practitioner who understands his or her unique needs?

Nursing Diagnosis: Risk for impaired skin integrity related to immobility and possible paresthesias

Expected Outcome Skin will remain intact without redness or breakdown.

Evaluation of Outcomes Is skin intact?

Interventions	Rationale	Evaluation
Monitor skin frequently. When permitted by the physician, turn the patient frequently and assess bony prominences for redness.	The patient who does not have sensation is at increased risk of developing pressure ulcers.	Is the patient turned and repositioned at least every 2 hours? Is skin intact?
Start preventive measures in the emergency department by being sure to remove anything between the patient and the backboard.	Patients have developed pressure ulcers from lying on keys or other objects in their pockets.	Are skin surfaces protected from pressure?
Use a pressure-reducing mattress.	Specialty mattresses or beds can reduce pressure, but do not reduce the need to turn the patient.	Is the patient on an appropriate mattress?

(Continued on following page)

Box 48.6   NURSING CARE PLAN for the Patient with a Spinal Cord Injury *(Continued)*

Interventions	Rationale	Evaluation
If on a self-turning bed, make sure the patient is not sliding as the bed turns. Avoid pulling and friction on skin when repositioning patient in bed.	Sliding can cause friction and shearing damage to the skin.	Is friction damage to skin avoided?
Ensure that the patient's extremities do not get caught in side rails or wheelchair spokes.	The patient may not be aware this is happening, and a pressure ulcer can result.	Are all patient's body parts accounted for and safe?
If a patient is in traction or a halo brace, assess pin sites frequently. Keep the sites clean and dry and report any sign of infection.	Skin sites are at risk for infection and breakdown.	Are pin sites clean and dry?

Nursing Diagnosis: Risk for ineffective role performance related to effects of injury

Expected Outcome Patient will identify new ways to carry out essential roles.

Evaluation of Outcome Is patient able to identify ways to carry out roles?

Interventions	Rationale	Evaluation
Allow the patient to verbalize concerns if he or she wishes.	This may help to clarify potential role problems for the patient, and begin the process of developing a plan.	Is patient able to identify roles he or she has filled in the past that will be difficult to carry out due to injury?
Help patient and family to identify resources.	Interpersonal relationships can be significantly stressed by spinal cord injury. Friends, family, and members of the patient's religious affiliation can provide emotional and physical help.	Does patient have adequate support systems in place to provide help?
Consult a social worker to help the patient gain access to appropriate physical and financial assistance.	Loss of income may be temporary or permanent, and may add to the burden of spinal cord injury. Not all insurance policies cover the extensive inpatient rehabilitation needed by spinal cord–injured patients. Adaptive equipment is expensive and may not be covered by insurance.	Is patient able to access appropriate financial assistance if needed?
Provide information about area support groups.	Individuals who have been through similar experiences can provide support and information for the patient and family.	Is patient willing to contact support groups?

Nursing Diagnosis: Risk for sexual dysfunction related to autonomic nervous system dysfunction

Expected Outcome The patient will state he or she has an acceptable means for sexual expression.

Evaluation of Outcomes Does patient state satisfaction with sexual function?

Interventions	Rationale	Evaluation
If a male patient has an erection during a bath or catheterization, discontinue the procedure and continue at a later time if possible. Maintain a matter-of-fact attitude.	Male patients with quadriplegia may develop an erection during any penile stimulation.	Is patient's dignity maintained during personal care?
Allow patient to voice concerns about sexual function if desired.	Male patients with paraplegia usually have difficulty achieving and maintaining an erection.	Is patient able to voice concerns? Is a consult with a urologist or other specialist needed?
Encourage the patient and partner to explore alternative methods of sexual expression.	Closeness and touching may be a satisfying alternative.	Is patient able to discuss alternative methods with partner?
If a male patient wishes to have children, encourage a consult with a fertility specialist or urologist.	Males with spinal cord injuries do not ejaculate in the normal manner. A specialist may provide some help for conception if desired.	Is patient given information about conception if desired?
Advise female patients who wish to become pregnant to seek an obstetrician familiar with spinal cord injuries	A specialist may be necessary to meet unique needs of these patients.	Is the patient interested in pregnancy? Does she have the information needed related to pregnancy with spinal cord injury?
If the patient does not wish to become pregnant, provide information about contraception. See Table 48.6 for contraception for females with spinal cord injuries.	Spinal cord injury does not impair female fertility.	Does the patient have information and resources to prevent pregnancy if desired?
Encourage partners to verbalize feelings about caregiving activities such as catheterizations and make alternative arrangements for care if possible. Some patients with the financial resources to do so may choose to hire an attendant rather than rely on significant others for personal care.	Performing tasks such as catheterization or bowel care may interfere with feelings of intimacy between partners.	Are patient and partner able to discuss feelings about caregiving activities, and find alternate arrangements if desired?

Nursing Diagnosis: Anxiety related to change in health status as evidenced by behavioral changes such as insomnia, poor eye contact, and irritability

Expected Outcomes The patient will participate in rehabilitation activities. The patient will be able to verbalize fears, concerns, and expectations.

Evaluation of Outcomes Is the patient able to participate in rehabilitation? Does patient verbalize that anxiety is controlled?

Interventions	Rationale	Evaluation
Allow patient to voice feelings of fear and anxiety.	Communication is vital to assess the patient's coping abilities.	Is the patient able to verbalize anxiety?

(Continued on following page)

Box 48.6   NURSING CARE PLAN for the Patient with a Spinal Cord Injury (Continued)

Interventions	Rationale	Evaluation
Provide information about what is happening to the patient physiologically and about procedures.	Understanding of what is happening can help the patient cope with changes.	Does patient verbalize understanding of what is happening? Does information help keep patient less fearful?
Consult a social worker, pastoral care, and/or support groups.	A social worker or pastor can help provide emotional and spiritual support. Discussing rehabilitation with patients and their families who have had similar experiences can provide insight and encouragement.	Does patient state talking with support persons help reduce anxiety?
Encourage the patient to participate in physical and occupational therapy.	Seeing progress toward becoming independent may help reduce anxiety and fear about the future.	Does patient participate in therapies? Is anxiety lessening?

TABLE 48.6 BIRTH CONTROL ISSUES FOR PATIENTS WITH SPINAL CORD INJURY

Method	Comments
Oral contraceptives	Contraindicated because of the risk of deep vein thrombosis
Diaphragm	May be difficult to insert for a patient with poor hand function
Intrauterine device	Patient may not feel IUD move out of position
	Patient may not feel perforation of uterus
Norplant	No contraindications
Condom	No contraindications

cause chronic illness. By the year 2030, it is estimated that 150 million Americans will have one or more chronic conditions. Management of chronic conditions does not focus on the short-term stay in the hospital due to a exacerbation of the disease process, but rather on the long-term goal of facilitating the patient and family to cope with the disease process and maintain the patient's independence for as long as possible. Nursing care involves providing information on management of the illness, education related to prevention and treatment of complications, and guidance to support groups or case managers. As patients decline, many families will come to a time when they can no longer care for their loved one in their homes and must consider care in a long-term facility.

Dementia

Dementia is not a disease, but rather is a symptom of a number of different disorders. According to the National Institute of Neurological Disorders and Stroke, "People with dementia have significantly impaired intellectual functioning that interferes with normal activities and relationships. They also lose their ability to solve problems and maintain emotional control, and they may experience personality changes and behavioral problems, such as agitation, delusions, and hallucinations. While memory loss is a common symptom of dementia, memory loss by itself does not mean that a person has dementia.[2] Some patients may have mild mental status changes that do not interfere significantly with day-to-day functioning. This is sometimes referred to as mild cognitive impairment, or MCI. Patients with MCI are more likely to go on to develop Alzheimer's disease than those without MCI.

Etiology and Pathophysiology

There are many causes of dementia. Huntington's, Parkinson's, and Alzheimer's diseases are discussed later in this chapter. Multiple "ministrokes" (multi-infarct dementia or vascular dementia) is another common cause. Chronic alcoholism, neurological infections, head injuries, and many medications (Box 48.8 Some Medications That Can Cause Disturbed Thought Processes) can also cause changes in mental status leading to dementia. Although aging is associated with more frequent dementia diagnoses, dementia is not a normal part of aging. Pathophysiologies vary depending on the cause. In general, thinking is affected by changes in the brain that result from reduced blood flow or from structural changes related to disease states.

Much research has been done to determine factors related to dementia, and therefore how it can be prevented. Some studies indicate that patients who have more educa-

Box 48.7

Spinal Cord Injury Summary

Signs and Symptoms	Flaccid paralysis and paresthesias (depending on level of the lesion) Loss of reflex activity below the level of the lesion Spinal shock initially Risk for autonomical dysreflexia (injuries above sixth thoracic vertebra)
Diagnostic Tests and Findings	Radiograph CT scan MRI
Therapeutic Interventions	Immobilization Maintenance of airway and respiratory status Bowel and bladder training Nutrition/diet Activity/rehabilitation Prevention of dysreflexia Prevention of skin breakdown Sexual counseling Education
Complications	Infection Deep vein thrombosis Paralysis Orthostatic hypotension Pressure ulcers Depression
Possible Nursing Diagnoses	Impaired physical mobility related to hemiparesis/hemiplegia Total urinary incontinence related to spinal cord damage

Box 48.8

Some Medications That Can Cause Disturbed Thought Processes

- Anticholinergic agents (atropine, some antihistamines)
- Analgesics (meperidine, morphine)
- Cimetidine (Tagamet)
- Central nervous system depressants (sleeping pills, tranquilizers, alcohol)
- Steroids (cortisone, prednisone)

As patients become more forgetful, they may ask the same question repeatedly. They may get lost driving or walking in a familiar neighborhood. They may become disoriented to time, and not be aware of the year. A patient may say that Eisenhower is president, for example, because they remember that as true when they were younger. Later, they may not recognize where they are, and last, they may lose recognition of their own family members.

Later in the course of the dementia, even remote memory may be lost. Patients may forget how to perform simple tasks, such as doing the dishes or making a phone call. They may wander and become lost. Safety is a significant issue with a wandering patient. Patients may develop aphasia and become unable to communicate their needs or follow simple instructions. This can become very frustrating to both the family and nursing caregivers. Behavioral problems may necessitate admission to a long-term care facility. In very late stages, the patient may become totally dependent on caregivers.

Diagnostic Tests

Diagnosis of dementia is twofold: first, dementia must be identified, and then the focus moves to finding the cause of the mental status change. Early diagnosis is essential, since some causes of MCI may be reversible, or early treatment may delay progression. Neuropsychological testing can determine the degree of memory, personality, and behavior changes. The Mini-Mental State Examination is commonly used. The patient should also be tested for depression, since depression can cause mental status changes, but is often easily treated. A review of medications by a knowledgeable nurse, physician, or pharmacist may reveal a medication that can be contributing to the mental changes. MRI, CT scan, positron emission tomographic (PET) scan, and blood tests help diagnose underlying causes.

Therapeutic Interventions

Medical interventions depend on the cause of the dementia. See Table 48.7 for medications that may be used to delay progression of some types of dementia. If medical treatment cannot alter the course of the disease, the focus will shift to delaying progression of symptoms and maintaining patient safety. Excellent nursing care becomes essential for both the

tion, have higher socioeconomic status, and engage in stimulating intellectual and leisure activities are less likely to develop dementia. Some experts believe these individuals develop a sort of "cognitive reserve" that keeps them functioning at a high level, even when changes in their brains on autopsy indicate dementia. People with less education, fewer leisure activities, and less intellectual stimulation are more likely to develop symptoms of Alzheimer's disease.

Signs and Symptoms

Most people have occasional memory lapses. Students may have memory lapses during examinations, but they do not generally have dementia. In patients with dementia, recent memories are usually affected first. Patients may have difficulty recalling whether they ate breakfast, or may accuse a family member of not calling when in reality they called just a few hours earlier. This same patient may easily recall an event or even a phone number from childhood.

TABLE 48.7 MEDICATIONS USED TO TREAT DISTURBED THOUGHT PROCESSES

Medication Class/Action	Examples	Route	Side Effects	Nursing Implications
Cholinesterase Inhibitors Inhibits cholinesterase, to improve function of acetylcholine in CNS	Donepezil (Aricept) Tacrine (Cognex) Rivastigmine (Exelon) Galantamine (Reminyl)	PO	Headache, diarrhea, nausea	Must be taken regularly; patient may need reminders to take, or family member may need to assist. May improve cognitive function but will not alter course of disease.
NMDA Antagonist Reduces binding of glutamate, an excitatory neurotransmitter	Memantine (Namenda)	PO	Dizziness	

patient and family at this point. An important aspect of care in early dementia is determination of the patient's wishes while the patient is still able to make decisions. Decisions related to resuscitation, guardianship, and powers of attorney for health care and finances are essential. Other difficult decisions relate to the patient's continued ability to drive and live alone.

Nursing Process for the Patient with Dementia
See Box 48.9 Nursing Care Plan for the Patient with Disturbed Thought Processes.

Delirium

In comparison to dementia, **delirium** is a mental disturbance that is temporary, and can have either a rapid or gradual onset. It is considered to be a medical emergency, and should be diagnosed and treated promptly. It is characterized with disorganized thinking and difficulty with staying focused, and is seen most commonly in older adults when experiencing an illness. Many times response to medications is the cause (see Box 48.8 Some Medications That Can Cause Disturbed Thought Processes). It may also be the result of anything that is a stressor to the person's body, such as pain, oxygen deficiency, urinary catheters, fluid and electrolyte imbalances, a change in environment, or nutritional deficiency. Often the most effective nursing intervention is to have a family member present to assist with orientation and reassurance. It is also beneficial to have continuity in nursing personnel.

It is essential that delirium not be mistaken for dementia. If an older adult is hospitalized and exhibits confusion, consider that it might be delirium. Correcting electrolyte levels, controlling pain, changing medications, or administering oxygen can be helpful in reversing delirium. See Box 48.9 Nursing Care Plan for the Patient with Disturbed Thought Processes for nursing interventions.

Parkinson's Disease

Parkinson's disease is a chronic degenerative movement disorder that arises in the basal ganglia in the cerebrum. It usually begins in the fourth or fifth decade of life, with symptoms becoming progressively worse as the patient ages. The disease is characterized by tremors, changes in posture and gait, rigidity, and slowness of movements. Approximately 1% of people over 65 have a diagnosis of Parkinson's disease.[3]

Pathophysiology
The substantia nigra is a group of cells located within the basal ganglia, which is situated deep within the brain. These cells are responsible for the production of dopamine, an inhibitory neurotransmitter. Dopamine facilitates the transmission of impulses from one neuron to another. Parkinson's disease is caused by destruction of the cells of the substantia nigra, resulting in decreased dopamine production. Loss of dopamine function results in impairment of semiautomatic movements. Parkinson's disease is sometimes referred to as an extrapyramidal disorder because the extrapyramidal tracts that contain motor neurons are affected.

Acetylcholine, an excitatory neurotransmitter, is secreted normally in individuals with Parkinson's disease. The normal balance of acetylcholine and dopamine is interrupted in these patients, causing a relative excess of acetylcholine, which results in the tremor, muscle rigidity, and **akinesia** (loss of muscle movement) characteristic of Parkinson's disease.

Etiology
The etiology of Parkinson's disease is unknown. It was first described in 1817 by London surgeon James Parkinson. Although scientists now know that the symptoms are caused by death of dopamine-producing cells in the substantia nigra, they do not know what causes the cells to die. There may be a genetic component, especially in younger patients. Certain environmental toxins may also play a role. Parkinson's disease–like symptoms, referred to as parkinsonism, may be associated with use of certain drugs, such as phenothiazines. Parkinsonism was also linked to an outbreak of encephalitis in the 1920s.

---

akinesia: a—not + kinesia—movement

Box 48.9 Nursing Care Plan for the Patient with Disturbed Thought Processes

Nursing Diagnosis: Risk for injury related to impaired memory, thought processes, and judgment

Expected Outcomes Patient will remain free from injury

Evaluation of Outcomes Is patient safe and free from injury? Is environment safe?

Interventions	Rationale	Evaluation
Monitor patient's ability to maintain safety.	As dementia worsens, the patient's needs will change.	Is patient able to make decisions and negotiate the environment safely?
Keep environment simple and familiar; label doors and objects. Keep patient in familiar environment as long as possible.	Change can result in confusion; even a minor change in furniture arrangement can result in falls.	Is patient able to remain in the home with minimum confusion and without injury?
Remove harmful objects (scissors, matches), store medicines in locked cabinet; remove knobs from stoves.	Impaired judgment can make safety a major concern for patients who live at home.	Is the environment safe for the patient?
Make sure patient has eyeglasses and hearing aids if necessary.	Impaired sensory perception can increase confusion and risk of falls.	Is patient able to see and hear effectively?
Use night lights, remove throw rugs, use safety gates on stairs.	These can reduce the risk for falls.	Is environment set up to reduce risk of falling?
Have identification bracelet on patient and sewn into clothes, and locks on doors to prevent leaving. Provide daily walks or exercise.	Patients may wander, making them prone to injury. Exercise can decrease wandering.	Is wandering confined to a monitored area? Is environment set up to allow movement within a safe area?

Nursing Diagnosis: Imbalanced nutrition: less than body requirements related to impaired thought processes and lack of interest or refusal to eat, poor muscle tone, weight loss

Expected Outcome Patient will maintain adequate food intake and weight within normal limits for height.

Evaluation of Outcomes Does patient maintain appropriate weight?

Interventions	Rationale	Evaluation
Monitor intake, weight, and serum albumin.	Loss of weight or serum albumin <3.5 indicates poor nutrition.	Are weight and serum albumin stable and within normal limits?
Develop meal plan to include likes and dislikes, snacks, and protein supplements.	Using the patient's favorite foods will encourage eating.	Is patient consuming majority of meals?
Offer larger meal when patient has the greatest appetite or serve small meals five to six times a day.	A lot of food at one time may feel overwhelming to the patient.	Is patient eating meals that are served?
Offer one food at a time if patient is not successful with a whole plate full.	Too many choices on a plate may feel overwhelming to the patient.	Does patient eat more if one food at a time is offered?
Offer finger foods.	Utensils may be difficult for the patient to use and may discourage eating.	Does patient eat more when finger foods are offered?

Also see Box 48.10 Nutrition Notes (Managing Mealtimes for Patients with Dementia).

(Continued on following page)

Box 48.9   NURSING CARE PLAN **for the Patient with Disturbed Thought Processes** *(Continued)*

Nursing Diagnosis: Disturbed thought processes related to dementia as evidenced by disorientation, inability to concentrate or follow directions.

Expected Outcomes Patient will function at optimal cognitive level.

Evaluation of Outcome Is patient maintaining cognitive function?

Interventions	Rationale	Evaluation
Monitor changes in thought processes.	As cognitive function declines, care plan will need to be revised.	Is patient able to correctly identify objects, remember tasks, speak clearly, identify person, place, and time?
Provide a box of safe, familiar items, such as empty thread spools, or pretty handkerchiefs for women.	Patients often rummage through drawers, closets, or boxes. These patients may not recognize the difference between their own possessions and those of others. Keeping them occupied with a box of safe items may decrease their need to look for things.	Does a box of items keep patient occupied and content?
Place calendars, clocks, personal items, and seasonal decorations in patient's environment.	These provide orientation to the present.	Can patient identify the season or year?
If patient hallucinates or has delusions, do not attempt to correct. Focus instead on the feelings related to the hallucinations, such as "Do you feel frightened?"	Having feelings validated may help develop trust, while not validating the hallucination.	Does patient respond to refocusing on feelings?
Reduce stressors such as fatigue, overstimulation, or pain.	Stress may increase dysfunctional behaviors.	Are stressors eliminated as much as possible? Is patient's behavior calm?
Maintain patient's usual routines as much as possible.	Familiar routines such as sleeping or eating habits are more comfortable for patients. Change can be stressful.	Are routines organized around the patient rather than the staff?
Communicate clearly: make eye contact, speak slowly and directly to the patient, use nonverbal gestures.	Unclear communication can increase confusion and stress.	Do all staff communicate clearly and respectfully with the patient?
Involve family in care planning and implementation.	The family knows the patient's preferences and routines best.	Does family presence help patient stay calm and function at optimum level?
Provide video or audiotapes of patient's family members.	Familiar sounds and pictures may reduce agitation when family is not present.	Do video or audiotapes help calm patient?

Nursing Diagnosis: Caregiver role strain related to demands of caring for patient with declining mental status while balancing other demands

Expected Outcomes Caregiver will have support needed to safely manage care of patient. Caregiver will be able to identify when the patient is too difficult to care for and requires more structured observation.

Evaluation of Outcomes Is caregiver managing demands of caring for patient? Is patient safe? Is additional support or a change in environment for patient indicated?

Interventions	Rationale	Evaluation
Allow caregiver to verbalize concerns related to burden of caring for patient.	An assessment of caregiver concerns and challenges can help the nurse plan appropriate support.	Does the caregiver share concerns? What are the caregiver's current support systems?
Observe for signs of depression or stress in the caregiver.	A stressed or depressed caregiver may have difficulty providing safe care for the patient.	Are signs of stress present? Does patient care appear to be suffering?
Encourage caregiver to identify family and friends that can provide support. If they are involved in a local church or religious organization, encourage caregiver to make his or her needs known.	There are often resources in the family or community that can be accessed without cost, and are able to help if they know the need exists.	Can caregiver identify potential resources to contact?
Refer for assistance with caregiving and/or day care utilizing Alzheimer's support groups and resources.	Formal support systems in the community may be available to help relieve some of the caregiver's burden.	Is caregiver able to obtain support and take some time for him- or herself?
Encourage caregiver to use support systems identified to allow him or her time to care for self; encourage to take care of own health needs, and enjoy some respite time doing something enjoyable on a regular basis.	If the caregiver becomes ill due to the stress of caregiving, he or she will no longer be able to assist the patient.	Does caregiver maintain own physical and emotional health?
Allow the caregiver to grieve over the losses he or she is experiencing: losses in the patient as well as loss of control over his or her own life.	As the disease progresses, the patient gradually loses awareness of the neurological deterioration. Occasional lucid moments can be very difficult for patient and caregiver as they realize what has been lost.	Is the caregiver able to identify feelings of grief, anger, or sorrow?
Discuss progression of the disease process and the possibility of transferring the patient to a nursing home.	The caregiver may feel guilt over not being able to care for the patient, and may need permission to consider nursing home placement.	Is caregiver able to identify when homecare is too demanding, and choose an alternative arrangement?

Signs and Symptoms

The onset of symptoms in patients with Parkinson's disease is usually gradual and subtle. A substantial percentage of the dopamine-producing cells are nonfunctional before the patient becomes symptomatic. Symptoms may be mistakenly attributed to aging or fatigue. In retrospect, patients and their significant others often identify a long period in which symptoms were present but not identified as symptoms of Parkinson's disease.

The primary symptoms of Parkinson's disease are muscular rigidity, **bradykinesia** (slow movement) or akinesia, changes in posture, and tremors. The brain is no longer able to direct the muscles to perform in the usual manner. This lack of communication between the brain and the muscles can have a profound impact on the patient's ability to ambulate safely, perform ADLs and job functions, or enjoy leisure

---

bradykinesia: brady—slow + kinesia—movement

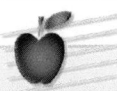

Box 48.10

Nutrition Notes

Managing Mealtimes for Patients with Dementia

Dining rooms should be quiet and have adequate lighting. Occupying the same chair for every meal lends familiarity. Serving one course at a time and providing necessary but not extraneous flatware, large handled if necessary, limits distractions. Dishes with high sides enable the patient to scoop the food onto a spoon or fork. Finger foods that the patient can manage may increase intake with minimal staff assistance.

Patients with dementia must be reminded of the steps involved in self-feeding: putting the food on the spoon, directing it to the mouth, swallowing. Use verbal cues or guide the patient's hand to start the necessary movement. Despite the surroundings, common courtesies model social expectations. Introducing the patient to the other persons at the table, providing a cup rather than a carton for milk, and offering foods separately rather than mixing them all together help maintain a person's dignity.

Quiet music with a slow tempo may relax a patient and help block out environmental noises that might otherwise be startling. It might help relax staff also!

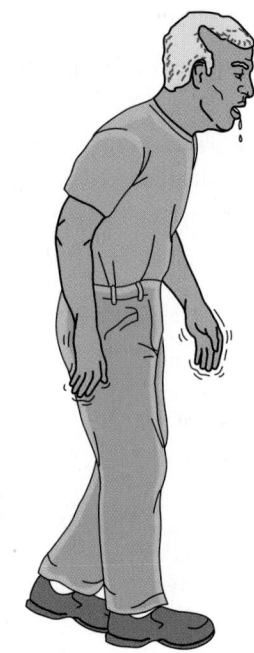

Masklike facial expression
Soft voice
Drooling, dysphagia

Hand tremors at rest

Constipation
Frequent urination

Flexion of knees and hips shifts center of gravity forward

Short, shuffling steps

FIGURE 48.14 Manifestations of Parkinson's disease.

activities. The symptoms may also have a significant negative impact on the patient's self-esteem.

The patient may have difficulty in initiating movement; this may be particularly apparent when the patient attempts to start walking, rise from a sitting position, or begin dressing. Because considerable effort is required to move the rigid muscles, the patient performs voluntary movements very slowly. At times, the patient may experience "freezing" of gait, and be unable to initiate ambulation or negotiate a turn during ambulation.

The extensor muscles are more affected by Parkinson's disease than the flexor muscles. This impaired function of the extensor muscles results in the stooped posture typical of patients with Parkinson's disease (Fig. 48.14). Flexion of the hips, knees, and neck shifts the center of gravity forward. The gait is characterized by shuffling, short steps. This shuffling gait may increase in speed once the patient finally gets walking, and the patient may have difficulty stopping. The patient maintains a broad base when making turns to try to compensate for imbalance. These changes place patients at high risk for falls. Slowness of movement and stiff muscles make it much harder for patients to catch themselves if they start to fall or to relax the muscles to minimize injury.

Tremors typically begin in the hand and then progress to the **ipsilateral** foot. In most patients, the tremor then

moves to the **contralateral** side. Many patients identify one side of the body as being more affected by the tremor than the other. Tremor of the hand has been described as a pill-rolling tremor; the thumb typically moves back and forth across the fingers and looks like the patient is rolling a pill. Tremors typically lessen or disappear during movement and are more noticeable when the extremity is at rest or when trying to hold an object still (this is called a resting tremor). The tremors disappear when the patient is asleep. The inability to hold an object still can make simple acts such as drinking a glass of water or reading a book nearly impossible. The signs and symptoms of Parkinson's disease tend to increase in severity when the patient becomes fatigued.

Another type of tremor, a benign familial (or essential) tremor, may sometimes be mistaken for Parkinson's disease. Treatment is different for each. See Table 48.8 for differen-

---

contralateral: contra—opposite + lateral—side

TABLE 48.8 SYMPTOMS OF PARKINSON'S DISEASE VERSUS ESSENTIAL TREMOR

Disease	Parkinson's Tremor	Benign Familial
Resting tremor	Yes	No
Intention tremor (with movement)	No	Yes
Pill-rolling tremor	Yes	No
Head/voice tremor	No	Yes
Relieved with beta-blocking medication (propranolol)	No	Yes
Relieved with anti-Parkinson's medications	Yes	No

---

ipsilateral: ipsi—same + lateral—side

tiation of these tremors. The secondary symptoms of Parkinson's disease include generalized weakness, muscle fatigue and cramping, and difficulty with fine motor activities. This fine motor dysfunction may make it difficult for the patient to button a shirt or tie shoes. Handwriting typically deteriorates as the disease progresses. A soft, monotone voice and masklike facial expression may make the patient appear to be lacking in emotional responses. It may be necessary to ask patients about their emotional status and help them develop ways of expressing their emotions. The normal blink response is diminished, so the patient and significant others must be educated about eye care to prevent corneal abrasions.

Dysfunction of the autonomic system may be manifested by diaphoresis, constipation, orthostatic hypotension, drooling, dysphagia, seborrhea, and frequent urination. Patients who experience seborrhea and diaphoresis need frequent attention to personal hygiene. Drooling and dysphagia may make the patient reluctant to appear in public. Slowness in initiating walking, balance problems, and frequent urination place the patient at risk for urinary incontinence, which may also increase the patient's reluctance to leave home.

Late in the disease, mental function may become slowed and the patient may develop dementia. This is compounded by the side effects of many anti-Parkinson's drugs. Death is usually from complications of immobility.

Complications

The most typical acute complications of Parkinson's disease are related to the patient's difficulties with mobility and balance. These patients are very prone to falls, which may result in injuries ranging from bruises or fractures to head or spinal cord injuries. Constipation is common because of decreased activity, diminished ability to take in food and fluids, and side effects of anticholinergic medications. Patients are encouraged to increase fiber and fluids in their diet. If constipation is not alleviated by dietary modifications, the patient may need to use stool softeners. The patient should be counseled not to rely on laxatives or enemas.

Muscular rigidity and bradykinesia contribute to joint immobility, which decreases patients' ability to ambulate and care for themselves. Position changes may be painful for patients. A turning sheet and adequate personnel are necessary when turning a patient in bed to prevent stress on the joints. Tremors interfere with ADLs, consume immense amounts of energy, and may prevent the patient from working or performing leisure activities. Swallowing may become so impaired that enteral (tube) feeding is required. Depression is a common complication at any stage of Parkinson's disease and may compromise communication, ability to learn, and performance of ADLs. Patients may require counseling or antidepressants.

Diagnostic Tests

No specific tests are used to diagnose Parkinson's disease. The diagnosis is based on the history given by the patient and a thorough physical examination. An MRI may be done to rule out alternative causes of the patient's symptoms.

Therapeutic Interventions

There is no cure for Parkinson's disease. Treatment is aimed at controlling symptoms and maximizing the patient's functional level. Drugs used to control symptoms are listed in Table 48.9.

Many patients with Parkinson's disease experience fluctuations in motor function related to their drug therapy. This is referred to as the on-off phenomenon. Patients may experience a decreased response to levodopa, or off period, particularly as the dose is wearing off. As the disease progresses, patients may notice that the off periods become less predictable and occur more rapidly. The patient may have a delayed or absent response to the next dose of levodopa, resulting in the patient being stuck in the off stage and being significantly disabled for that period. Fluctuations in motor function may be accompanied by other symptoms, such as pain, diaphoresis, anxiety attacks, hallucinations, or mood swings. These symptoms significantly increase the disability associated with the episodes.

Patients who are taking maximum doses of medication for Parkinson's disease symptoms may benefit from a "drug holiday." During a drug holiday, patients are taken off all drugs for a time, then restarted on lower doses. Hospitalization may be necessary during this time to maintain patient safety.

Surgical Treatment

Pallidotomy is an option for patients whose rigidity, tremor, and bradykinesia are uncontrollable by medical management. During this stereotactic procedure, a destructive lesion is placed in the basal ganglia. The surgery is only performed on one side at a time. The patient remains awake during the surgery to make sure that the lesion is being placed in the appropriate location. These patients need a great deal of education and support before and during the surgery. Some centers have experimented with implanting embryonic stem cells into the brain to develop into dopamine-producing cells, but ethical issues related to use of human embryos have slowed this process. For more information, visit the National Parkinson Foundation at www.parkinson.org.

Nursing Process for the Patient with Parkinson's Disease

ASSESSMENT/DATA COLLECTION. Assess the patient for symptoms of Parkinson's disease and their effect on level of functioning. Observe ability to move, walk, and perform ADLs safely. Determine risk for injury related to immobility or falls. Assess nutritional status and condition of skin. Identify presence of confusion and side effects of medications. Psychosocial assessment includes the patient's and caregiver's responses to the disease, coping strategies, and support systems.

NURSING DIAGNOSIS, PLANNING, AND IMPLEMENTATION. The patient with Parkinson's disease is at risk for many problems. Typical diagnoses are addressed below. Also see Box 48.9 Nursing Care Plan for the Patient with Disturbed Thought Processes.

TABLE 48.9 MEDICATIONS USED TO TREAT PARKINSON'S DISEASE

Medication Class/Action	Examples	Route	Side Effects	Nursing Implications
Anticholinergic Blocks the action of acetylcholine to control tremor and salivation	Trihexyphenidyl (Artane)	PO	Urine retention, dry mouth, constipation, blurred vision, dizziness, confusion	Monitor I&O for urinary retention; teach patient not to discontinue abruptly; implement measures to prevent constipation.
Dopamine Agonist Facilitates release of dopamine	Amantadine (Symmetrel)	PO	Ataxia, hypotension, dizziness, confusion	Use caution with alcohol and other CNS agents.
Dopamine Agonists Convert into dopamine in the brain	Levodopa (L-Dopa)	PO	Nausea, vomiting, dyskinesias	Teach patient to take food shortly after (not before or with) each dose to prevent gastric irritation. May discolor urine and sweat. Teach patient to take ATC to control symptoms.
	Levodopa/carbidopa combination (Sinemet). Carbidopa prevents peripheral breakdown of levodopa so more is available in the CNS.	PO		
Dopamine Agonist Stimulates dopamine receptors in the brain	Pramipexole (Mirapex)	PO	Nausea, dizziness, weakness; may cause sudden excessive sleepiness; constipation, dry mouth	Patients may fall asleep suddenly; caution patient to avoid driving until effects known. Giving with meals may reduce nausea.
Monoamine Oxidase B Inhibitor Blocks metabolism of central dopamine, increasing dopamine in CNS.	Selegiline (Eldepryl, Carbex)	PO	Nausea, dizziness, confusion, insomnia	May slow progression of Parkinson's disease. Administer daily at noon to prevent insomnia. Can cause dangerous interaction with meperidine (Demerol).
COMT Inhibitor Blocks the enzyme COMT to prevent breakdown of levodopa, prolonging levodopa action. For use with Sinemet.	Entacapone (Comtan)	PO	Dyskinesias, hallucinations, nausea, diarrhea, yellow-orange urine, rhabdomyolysis, neuroleptic malignant syndrome	Report elevated temperature, muscular rigidity, altered LOC, elevated CPK.

LOC = level of consciousness; CPK = creatine phosphokinase; COMT = catechol-O-methyltransferase;
ATC = around the clock.
   With all anti–Parkinson's disease agents, teach patient to check with physician before taking over-the-counter medications, especially cold preparations. Teach to rise slowly to prevent orthostasis.

Impaired physical mobility related to muscle stiffness and tremor

EXPECTED OUTCOME: Patient will maintain optimal mobility and ability to ambulate as long as possible.

- Assist patient to plan daily activities based on anticipated response to medications. *Certain times of day may be less troublesome than others.*
- Consult with physical and occupational therapies *to provide assistive devices to help maintain mobility, and provide diversional activities.*
- Provide assistance with range-of-motion exercises *to maintain flexibility of muscles.*
- Teach patients who have difficulty initiating walking to pick up one foot as though attempting to step over something to take the first step. It may also

help to take several steps in place before starting to walk. *This may help overcome freezing of gait.*

Self-care deficit related to reduced mobility

EXPECTED OUTCOME: Patient's self-care needs will be met.

- Encourage the patient to participate in ADLs as much as possible. This helps the patient maintain independence and self-esteem.
- Consult occupational therapist to assist with devices and strategies *for maintaining independence.*
- Instruct the patient or family to provide clothing without buttons or shoes with adherent fasteners *to help maintain independence.*
- Assist the patient and family to make decisions about long-term care. Consult a social worker prn

for assistance. *As the patient ages, so do the significant others who are providing care. The point may be reached at which the caregiver is no longer able to meet the increasing needs of the patient. The decision to place the patient in a skilled nursing facility is extremely difficult and emotional.*

Risk for injury related to reduced mobility and balance

EXPECTED OUTCOME: Patient will remain safe and without injury.

- If the patient is in the hospital or extended care facility, keep the call light within reach at all times. Remind the patient to request assistance with ambulation. *The patient is at risk for injury from falls related to problems with mobility.*
- Maintain bed in the low position, with side rails raised if appropriate (side rails may be prohibited in some institutions). *Maintaining the bed in a low position reduces the risk of injury or fall when getting out of bed. Side rails may increase the risk of injury, and must be used carefully.*
- Use an alarm system that alerts the staff that the patient is getting up *so that staff can assist the patient to get up and ambulate.*
- Avoid use of restraints. *Restraints can increase the risk of injury.*
- Keep environment free from clutter, throw rugs, or other items *that may cause a patient to trip.*
- Provide walkers and other assistive devices *to provide support and prevent falls.*

SAFETY TIP

Implement a fall reduction program and evaluate the effectiveness of the program (2006 National Patient Safety Goals from www.JCAHO.org).

EVALUATION. The care of the patient with Parkinson's disease has been successful if the patient remains as mobile and independent as possible. Self-care needs are met by the patient or others, and the patient should remain safe from injury.

Huntington's Disease

Huntington's disease is a progressive, hereditary, degenerative, incurable neurological disorder. It was first described in 1872 by George Huntington, a general practitioner in New York. The uncontrolled movements associated with Huntington's disease caused some sufferers in the 17th century to be accused of and executed for witchcraft. Many of the cases around the world can be traced back to specific individuals.

Pathophysiology and Etiology

Huntington's disease is inherited in an autosomal dominant manner, which means that each offspring of an affected par-

CRITICAL THINKING

Ms. Simpson

■ Ms. Simpson is a 47-year-old Caucasian woman. She has had Parkinson's disease for the last 5 years, and the symptoms are becoming progressively worse. She is now admitted for a urinary tract infection.

1. What problems do you foresee when caring for Ms. Simpson?
2. What safety measures should you implement?
3. Ms. Simpson is receiving IV fluids of 5% dextrose in 0.45% saline, 1000 mL over 12 hours. The RN on duty is accountable for her IV, but as you are bathing her you notice that the bag is nearly full and it has been hanging for 4 hours. How many milliliters should still be in her IV bag after 4 hours?

Suggested answers at end of chapter.

ent has a 50% chance of inheriting the disorder. It is uncertain what caused the mutation of the gene responsible for Huntington's disease. Structurally the disease is characterized by degeneration of the corpus striatum, caudate nucleus, and other deep nuclei of the brain and portions of the cerebral cortex. This degeneration results in progressive loss of normal movement and intellect.

Signs and Symptoms

Signs and symptoms develop slowly and become progressively more apparent. Cognitive signs may be noticed before movement problems. Patients who are not aware of their hereditary risk for Huntington's disease may be incorrectly diagnosed as being mentally ill or alcoholic.

The patient may display personality changes and inappropriate behavior. The patient may be euphoric or irritable and may rapidly alternate between moods. Paranoia is common, and behavior may become violent as dementia worsens. The patient eventually becomes so demented that he or she is incontinent and totally dependent on others for care. These symptoms are difficult for caregivers, whether family members or professionals, to cope with. They are particularly devastating for offspring, who may or may not know whether they have inherited the disease.

Physical symptoms also develop slowly. Huntington's disease is characterized by involuntary, irregular, jerky, dancelike (choreiform) movements. Initially these symptoms may take the form of mild fidgeting and facial grimacing. In the early stages of the disease, the patient may try to cover the movements by incorporating them into a voluntary movement such as crossing the arms or scratching. The involuntary movements usually start in the arms, face, and neck and progressively involve the remainder of the body. Patients display hesitant speech, eye blinking, irregular trunk movements, abnormal tilt of the head, and constant motion (Fig. 48.15). The gait is wide, and the patient may appear to be dancing. Emotional upset, stress, or trying to perform a

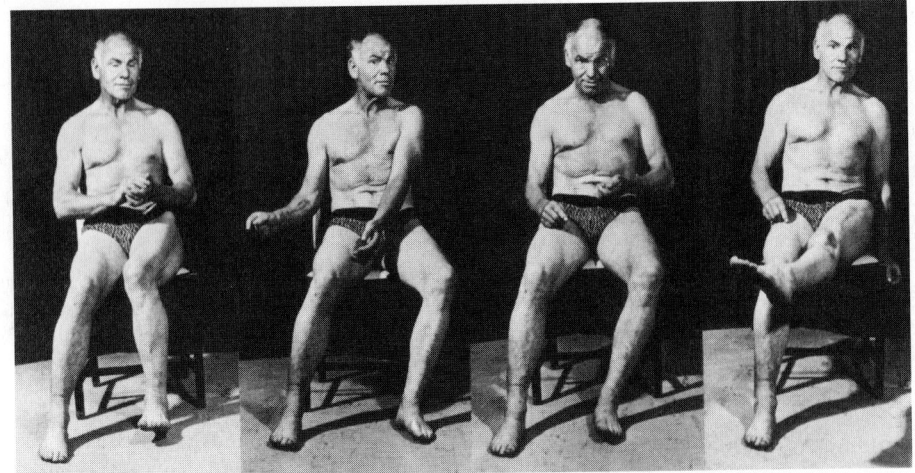

FIGURE 48.15 A 47-year old patient with Huntington's disease. Note constant fidgety movement. *(From Spillane, JD: An Atlas of Clinical Neurology. Oxford University Press, New York, 1968, p 219, with permission.)*

voluntary task can significantly increase the severity and rate of the abnormal movements. The movements typically diminish or disappear during sleep. Dysphagia may significantly impair the patient's nutritional status.

Depression and suicide are common in the earlier stages of the disease, when the patient still has the cognitive ability to carry out a suicidal act. As the disease progresses, the patient becomes more and more dependent. Aspiration resulting in respiratory failure is the primary cause of death. Life span following diagnosis is about 10 to 20 years.

Diagnostic Tests

Huntington's disease has typically been diagnosed based on the clinical examination and a family history of the disease. MRI or CT may be helpful. Genetic testing is available for prenatal use and to determine if an individual has Huntington's disease before he or she becomes symptomatic. This is a significant breakthrough because Huntington's disease does not become symptomatic until patients are in their 30s or 40s, when they may already have children who could be affected (see Box 48.11 Patient Perspective).

Therapeutic Interventions

Because there is no cure, treatment of Huntington's disease focuses on minimizing symptoms and preventing complications. Antipsychotic, antidepressant, and antichoreic drugs may be used to treat both the involuntary movements and behavioral outbursts. Research has been done on the benefits of transplanting fetal nerve tissue in patients with Huntington's disease, but this is limited by ethical debates about using fetal tissue.

Nursing Management

Patients with Huntington's disease are typically cared for on an outpatient basis. When a patient with Huntington's disease is admitted to an inpatient facility, it is important to obtain as much information as possible about that person's response to medication, daily routine, and emotional and cognitive functioning from the caregivers. For example, knowing that a certain patient is intensely afraid of bathtubs but willingly takes showers can prevent unnecessary struggles and outbursts. Providing some objects from home may

make the new environment seem less threatening. The caregivers may relate that the patient has better cognitive functioning at a particular time of day. As the dementia progresses, the patient responds less to attempts at reasoning. Giving directions in a calm but firm tone may help the patient cooperate with activities. The environment should be modified to keep the patient safe. Keep in mind that forceful, involuntary movements of the patient's extremities can happen at any time. These movements should never be misinterpreted as an attempt to harm caregivers.

Difficulty swallowing typically begins toward the middle of the disease course. Patients exhibit trouble swallowing liquids in particular. At this stage, it may still be possible to teach the patient to hold the chin down to the chest while swallowing, which lessens the chance of aspiration. Patients should sit straight upright while eating. Thickening agents may be added to thin liquids to help prevent aspiration. Adaptive devices may prolong the patient's ability to eat independently. Soft foods that are easily manipulated in the mouth are most suitable. These patients may have difficulty taking in adequate calories to maintain a normal body weight, even if a caregiver assists with feeding them. One of the many ethical issues faced by these patients and their significant others is whether artificial feeding should be used, and if so, for how long. Patients and their significant others should be encouraged to discuss end-of-life decisions early in the course of the disease.

See Box 48.9 Nursing Care Plan for the Patient with Disturbed Thought Processes.

Alzheimer's Disease

Alzheimer's disease (also called dementia of the Alzheimer's type [DAT]) is the most common of several types of dementia. Dementia is a progressive loss of mental functioning that interferes with memory, ability to think clearly and learn, and eventually ability to function (see discussion of dementia earlier in this chapter).

Alois Alzheimer, a German neurologist, first described the disease in 1907. He described pathological changes, now referred to as neurofibrillary tangles and neuritic plaques, that he discovered while performing an autopsy on a patient

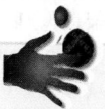

Box 48.11

Patient Perspective

Betty

I was born the second of six children. My mom was diagnosed with Huntington's chorea (an old name for Huntington's disease) after she had all of us. My brother was diagnosed with Huntington's disease at the age of 60. He started out with terrible mood swings and a bad temper, but eventually he had a lot of movement problems, including pronounced facial and tongue movements.

By the time we knew the disease had affected our family, many of us had children and grandchildren of our own. My kids wanted me to be tested. It is a hereditary disease and you have a 50/50 chance of having it if a parent has it. If I had Huntington's, then my kids would have a 50/50 chance of having it. If I tested negative, then they and their children would not be at risk.

I was very nervous and afraid of being tested. When I went for the initial visit at the University of Michigan, they observed my movements, how I walked and talked, and my facial movements. They made me go to a psychologist to see if I could handle the results if they did the blood test that would tell for sure. I understand the suicide rate is kind of high for people with Huntington's. After talking for an hour and a half, they decided I could handle the results.

At my next visit they just drew blood, which was sent out for testing. I had to return to U of M six weeks later for the results. When I went back, I was a nervous wreck. A friend went with me. When the technician came in, she said the doctor would be with me soon. I immediately had bad thoughts. Then when the technician and doctor came back, they were both smiling and had tears in their eyes—I had tested negative. So my friend, the doctor, the technician, and I all hugged and cried.

It is a very hard disease to live with, whether you or another family member has it. My brother has it very bad. Out of my five siblings, four have it for sure, and we think the fifth has it because of mood swings we have observed.

I am the only one of the six who tested clear. I felt very guilty at first that they all had it and I didn't. I'm starting to get over that, but when I see one of them having a bad time with talking, or temper, or movement, the guilt starts to kick in again.

Etiology and Pathophysiology

Many etiologies have been theorized for Alzheimer's disease, including viral or bacterial infection, and autoimmune dysfunction. Markers associated with Alzheimer's disease can be found on several chromosomes. Chromosome 21 in particular has been associated with Alzheimer's disease, and is also the location of the genetic abnormality responsible for Down's syndrome. Patients older than age 40 who have Down's syndrome usually develop Alzheimer's disease. The exact correlation between the two disorders is still being studied.

Although the exact cause of Alzheimer's disease is unknown, the structural changes associated with it have been well documented. An abnormality exists within the protein of the cell membrane of a neuron. As the axon terminals and dendrite branches disintegrate, they collect in neuritic plaques. Within the normal brain is a precise arrangement of filaments and tubules that are responsible for cell integrity. Individuals with Alzheimer's disease develop neurofibrillary tangles instead of the normal orderly arrangement. Instead of remaining a small area of abnormality, these neuritic plaques and neurofibrillary tangles spread via axons to other areas of the brain.

Advancement of neurofibrillary tangles and neuritic plaques typically affect the hippocampus first, resulting in short-term memory dysfunction. As the tangles and plaques spread to the temporal lobe, the memory impairment becomes more severe. It may be at this point that the patient accesses the health-care system. Personality changes and incontinence are inevitable results of Alzheimer's disease. These symptoms can be attributed to the spread of plaques and tangles to the frontal lobes of the brain.

It is believed that the younger the patient is at the time of onset, the faster the neurofibrillary tangles and neuritic plaques spread. Therefore, these patients tend to deteriorate faster, require complete care earlier, and have a shorter life span.

In addition, patients tend to have a deficiency of acetylcholine in the cerebral cortex. Remember that acetylcholine is a neurotransmitter important for nervous system function.

One area of the brain that is left relatively untouched by Alzheimer's is the subcortical area. This structure is responsible for our subconscious urge to survive. The needs for basic requirements such as shelter, food and water, security, and reproduction are controlled by the subcortical area, as are emotional responses to situations. The patient with Alzheimer's disease may experience hunger but no longer know how to meet that basic need. Left to their own devices, these individuals would starve.

Signs and Symptoms

The signs and symptoms of Alzheimer's disease are typically broken down into three stages. The early stage, stage one, lasts from 2 to 4 years and is characterized by increasing forgetfulness. At this stage, the patient may attempt to cope by using lists and reminders. Interest in day-to-day activities, acquaintances, and surroundings tends to diminish. The patient is reluctant to take on tasks because of

with dementia. Alzheimer's disease is a progressively degenerative disease that is inevitably fatal. The incidence of Alzheimer's disease is more common in women than men and doubles for every 5 years a person lives beyond age 65.

uncertainty in how to perform them. If the patient is still working, his or her performance deteriorates and may result in being terminated from the job.

The middle stage, stage two, is the longest in duration, lasting 2 to 12 years. Progressive cognitive deterioration is demonstrated by difficulty doing simple calculations or answering questions. Patients may become irritable, particularly when asked to perform a task that they know they should be able to perform but cannot. It may help the patient to break down the task into manageable steps. Depression is common. Aphasia and the resulting inability to make themselves understood may exacerbate patients' irritability. It is during the middle stage, as cognitive function significantly deteriorates, that the patient becomes more physically active. The normal sleep-wake cycle is disrupted, and the patient tends to wander aimlessly, particularly at night. The patient may become lost in familiar surroundings, which compounds the anxiety that typically develops during this stage. Hallucinations and seizures may occur. Management of day-to-day activities such as feeding a pet or paying bills becomes overwhelming. Personal hygiene deteriorates, as does appropriate social behavior. Patients may make up stories to cover for deficits, saying that possessions they misplaced were stolen. Some patients hoard food or money.

The third stage of Alzheimer's disease is characterized by progression to complete dependency. The patient loses the ability to converse or control bowel or bladder function. Constant supervision is required, if the patient is still mobile, to protect from wandering and avoid injury. Emotional control and ability to recognize significant others are lost. This lack of recognition is particularly devastating for family members. Eventually the patient is unable to move independently, swallow, or express needs. Death usually occurs from complications of immobility.

The duration of the final stage of Alzheimer's disease, characterized by complete dependence, depends in part on the physical stamina and general health of the individual. The healthier the patient, the longer the body will continue to function. Another factor is the decisions that have been made regarding artificial feeding and respiratory support. Few significant others or health-care practitioners advocate intubation and mechanical ventilation for patients with Alzheimer's disease. The issue of enteral (tube) feedings, however, is an emotional one with few easy answers. The use of enteral feedings can prolong the patient's life, despite the absence of cognitive functioning. As with patients suffering from Huntington's disease, every effort should be made to determine the patient's wishes before cognitive impairment makes that impossible. See Table 48.10 for a comparison of the symptoms of Parkinson's, Huntington's, and Alzheimer's diseases.

Diagnostic Tests

The only absolute method of confirming a diagnosis of Alzheimer's disease is by pathological examination at autopsy. In actuality, the disease is diagnosed on the basis of clinical examination, history, and elimination of other possible causes of the symptoms. MRI may reveal the presence of the classic neurofibrillary tangles and neuritic plaques. Positron emission tomography (PET) and single photon emission computed tomography (SPECT) scans show areas of neuronal inactivity. Newer tests are being evaluated that hold promise for better diagnosis.

Therapeutic Interventions

There is no known cure for Alzheimer's disease. Treatment has traditionally focused on minimizing the effects of the disease and maintaining independence as long as possible. Acetylcholinesterase (AChE) inhibitors such as donepezil (Aricept) or rivastigmine (Exelon) are thought to inhibit the breakdown of the neurotransmitter acetylcholine (see Table 48.7). Increased levels of acetylcholine in the brain allow better functioning of the remaining neurons. They appear to be most effective for those patients who exhibit mild to moderate symptoms of Alzheimer's disease. It may take some time to notice any effects of the drugs. Use of AChE inhibitors diminishes the amount of medical care and social service interventions required and delays admission to skilled nursing facilities. This delay in institutionalization can result in significant positive impact on quality of life, as well as thousands of dollars in savings.

A new class of medications, NMDA (N-methyl-D-aspartate) antagonists, may prevent overexcitation of NMDA receptors in the brain and allow more normal function. Memantine (Namenda, Axura) is the only drug currently available in this class. These drugs can be given at any

TABLE 48.10 SYMPTOMS OF PARKINSON'S DISEASE, HUNTINGTON'S DISEASE, AND ALZHEIMER'S DISEASE

Symptom	Parkinson's Disease	Huntington's Disease	Alzheimer's Disease
Tremors	Present	Absent	Absent
Bradykinesia/akinesia	Present	Absent	Absent
Muscle rigidity	Present	Absent	Absent
Memory dysfunction	Late	Late	Early
Cognitive dysfunction	Late	Present	Early
Inability to perform ADLs	Progressive	Progressive	Progressive
Involuntary movements	Absent	Present	Absent
Depression	Present	Present	Present

stage of Alzheimer's disease, and like AChE inhibitors, simply slow the patient's decline.

Antidepressants, antipsychotics, and antianxiety drugs may be used as a last resort to control symptoms of depression and behavioral disturbances, but they do not treat the dementia. Patients should be carefully monitored for drug interactions and side effects. For more information, visit the Alzheimer's Association at www.alz.org.

Nursing Process for the Patient with Alzheimer's Disease

See the earlier discussion of dementia and Box 48.9 Nursing Care Plan for the Patient with Disturbed Thought Processes.

CRITICAL THINKING

Mrs. Johnson

■ Mrs. Johnson has just become a resident at the Valley Bend nursing home. She is diagnosed with Alzheimer's disease and is in the second stage with some signs of stage three disease. When you check on her during the evening, you find her walking around her room, talking to herself. What other signs and symptoms are typical for stage two and stage three Alzheimer's disease? How should you address her behavior?

Home Health Hints

To assess a patient's neurological status at home:
- Note whether the patient's clothes are matched and properly fastened. Is the patient clean and well groomed?
- Observe the patient during bathing, grooming, or dressing to assess motor function and coordination.
- Assess energy level by noting if the patient makes frequent requests to sit or lie down.
- Observe the patient's gait for steadiness.

To help the patient perform ADLs easier at home:
- Ask permission to move furniture and small rugs in order to provide a clear path for ambulation.
- Position frequently used items such as a comb, glass of water, eyeglasses, books, tissues, and phone where they are easily accessible.
- Recommend shoes with Velcro closures.
- Use chairs with armrests—the patient can use the armrests to push against to stand.
- Keep the patient cleaner at meals with a clip-on bib such as those used at the dentist's office. Attach clips from suspenders to a piece of elastic and place around the back of the patient's neck. Attach a clean napkin or washcloth for each meal.

To help the patient with Alzheimer's disease who has perceptual deficits:
- Have things used together the same color (e.g., toothbrush and toothpaste).
- Contrast colors in the environment to help patients function independently—slipper color should be different than the floor, a dark-colored placemat can be used under light dishes, and the first and last steps of a stairway can be painted a contrasting color.
- Use a bath or shower seat, hand-held shower head, and soothing music to help the patient feel safe and oriented to the task while bathing.
- Cover doorknobs with a piece of cloth to keep the patient from wandering away or have a caregiver purchase inexpensive child safety devices that can fit over doorknobs and/or cabinet latches.
- Family members may require respite care and homemaker services. Discuss with the registered nurse or physician about having social services complete a visit to assist the family with access to community resources.

REVIEW QUESTIONS

1. Which of the following problems predisposes someone to develop meningitis?
   a. A sore throat for 3 days
   b. A migraine headache
   c. A muscle injury in the neck
   d. Vision changes

2. A patient with meningitis is experiencing photophobia and a severe headache. Which nursing interventions will be most helpful to relieve symptoms?

   a. Administer antibiotics as ordered, and prepare the patient for a lumbar puncture.
   b. Darken the room and administer analgesics.
   c. Administer acetaminophen as ordered and place a cooling blanket on the patient.
   d. Check level of consciousness with the Glasgow Coma Scale and monitor pulse pressure.

3. Which type of headache is most commonly associated with an aura?

a. Migraine
b. Cluster
c. Tension
d. Muscle contraction

4. A patient makes an appointment to see a primary care practitioner for recurrent severe headaches. Which instruction by the nurse will help gather the best additional data prior to the appointment?
   a. "Try relaxation and warm moist compresses for your headaches."
   b. "Call and come in the next time you have a headache so you can be examined."
   c. "Keep track of how many headaches you have before you come in."
   d. "Keep a diary of your headaches, recording symptoms, timing, and things that trigger them."

5. A patient who has had a generalized tonic-clonic seizure is sound asleep 30 minutes after the seizure. Meals are about to be delivered. Which nursing action is most appropriate?
   a. Wake the patient because nourishment is essential following a seizure.
   b. Wake the patient to do a complete neurological assessment before the meal.
   c. Let the patient sleep during the postictal state, and keep the meal warm.
   d. Do not attempt to wake the patient because of the risk of a repeat seizure.

6. A patient with a history of seizures says he thinks he is about to have a seizure. Place the nurse's interventions in the correct order.
   a. Protect the patient from injury during the seizure.
   b. Document the events of the seizure.
   c. Help the patient lie down in a safe place.
   d. Turn the patient on his or her side to sleep.

7. Which patients should be closely monitored by the nurse for symptoms of increased intracranial pressure? Select all answers that apply.
   a. The patient who has a history of epilepsy.
   b. The patient admitted with a high fever and severe headache.
   c. The patient in the post-anesthesia care unit following craniectomy.
   d. The patient with a brain tumor who is admitted for radiation therapy.
   e. The patient with a history of migraine headaches, admitted for orthopedic surgery.

8. Which of the following actions should the nurse take to help prevent increased ICP in a patient following a traumatic brain injury?

a. Cluster care so the patient can have long periods of rest.
b. Keep the head of the bed elevated at 30 degrees.
c. Suction frequently to keep the airway clear.
d. Do not give anything by mouth.

9. How much function can be expected in a patient with a spinal cord injury at the L2 level?
   a. Quadriplegic from neck down
   b. Quadriplegic with some arm movement
   c. Paraplegic with some trunk movement
   d. Paraplegic, may learn to walk with a brace

10. A patient is admitted following a T4 spinal injury. When taking his morning vital signs, the nurse notes that he appears restless and his blood pressure is elevated. Which of the following actions by the nurse is appropriate?
    a. Recheck his blood pressure in 30 minutes.
    b. No action is necessary. This is an expected finding.
    c. Check for a full bladder.
    d. Encourage him to express his anxiety.

11. The symptoms of Parkinson's disease are caused by depletion of which neurotransmitter?
    a. Dopamine
    b. Acetylcholine
    c. Serotonin
    d. Norepinephrine

12. Which nursing interventions are appropriate for the patient with a neurodegenerative disorder who has difficulty swallowing?
    a. Show the patient how to tuck his or her chin down to the chest during swallowing.
    b. Provide clear to full liquids; avoid solid foods.
    c. Place the patient in semi-Fowler's position for eating.
    d. Provide adaptive eating utensils.

13. A nursing home resident with Alzheimer's disease is sitting in a corner, crying loudly that no one is paying attention to her. Several staff members have tried to find out what's wrong, but the patient won't answer. She just keeps rocking back and forth and crying that no one is paying attention to her. Which approach by the nurse might best help the patient?
    a. Say in a quiet voice, "What is wrong? We can't help you if you don't tell us what's wrong."
    b. Sit quietly by the patient and say, "I'm here; you aren't alone."
    c. Say in a firm voice, "Several staff have asked what you need, now it is time to stop crying."
    d. Ignore the continued crying. Continuing to respond to her will encourage the behavior.

References

1. Gambrell, M, and Flynn, N: Seizures 101. Nursing 2004 34:36–41, 2004.
2. National Institute of Neurological Disorders and Stroke: Dementia Information Page, Updated November 16, 2005.

Accessed http://www.ninds.nih.gov/disorders/dementias/dementia.htm November 29, 2005.
3. National Center for Health Statistics, Data on Parkinson's Disease. Accessed http://www.cdc.gov/nchs/data/factsheets/Parkinsons.pdf, November 17, 2005.

SUGGESTED ANSWERS TO

CRITICAL THINKING

■ *Mr. Chung*

1. Be prepared to assist with a lumbar puncture.
2. You should use short, simple sentences because he may be very anxious or disoriented. Involve his family. Further education can be provided when he is feeling better.
3. Because meningococcal meningitis is contagious, he should be placed in isolation. Gloves, gowns, and masks should be used. Explain the need for these practices to Mr. Chung and his visitors.
4. Comfort measures include tepid baths, a quiet, dark environment, and minimal stimulation. Administer acetaminophen and analgesics as ordered.
5. The health service at his college should be notified of his diagnosis. Close contacts may require prophylactic treatment. If Mr. Chung lives at home rather than at college, his family should be advised to see their family practitioner and begin prophylactic treatment.

■ *Mr. Evans*

1. You might expect to see impaired speech, right-sided weakness, and a rapid decrease in consciousness if Mr. Evans's hematoma is enlarged.
2. Intubation equipment, mannitol, and intravenous access should be ready. He should be given nothing by mouth (NPO) and the results of laboratory tests should be ready in the event of emergency surgery. The location of Mr. Evans's next of kin must be known.
3. Who are Mr. Evans's support people? Was this drinking episode an isolated incident or a chronic problem that should be addressed?

■ *Ms. Simpson*

1. Urinary tract infection is often accompanied by urinary urgency. Ms. Simpson may have difficulty getting to the bathroom quickly and safely.
2. Keep a bedside commode nearby if the bathroom is not close. Assist Ms. Simpson to the bathroom or commode at regular intervals to prevent urgency. Remind her to ask for help if she needs to get up. Make sure that her call light is within reach.
3.

$$\frac{1000 \text{ mL}}{12 \text{ hours}} \Big| \frac{4 \text{ hours}}{} = 333 \text{ mL}$$

After 4 hours: 1000 − 333 mL = 667 mL should remain in the bag. If it is still nearly full, the RN should be notified.

■ *Mrs. Johnson*

Being admitted to a new and unfamiliar facility can increase confusion. Signs of second stage Alzheimer's disease include memory loss, wandering at night, sleeplessness, irritability, loss of way in familiar surroundings, losing possessions and searching for them, and neglect of personal hygiene. During the third stage of the disease, the patient will lose weight, recognize hunger but be unable to eat, be unable to communicate verbally or in writing, lose ability to recognize family, become incontinent of urine and feces, and eventually lose ability to stand and walk. Address Mrs. Johnson by her name and ask her what she needs. Reorient her to where she is and assure her that she is safe and being cared for.

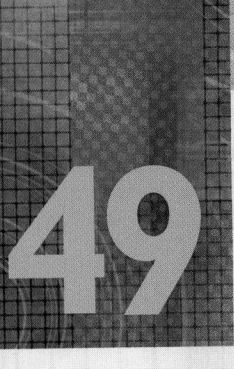

49

Nursing Care of Patients with Cerebrovascular Disorders

WENDY HOCKLEY

KEY TERMS

ataxia (ah-TAK-see-ah)
endarterectomy (end-AR-tur-EK-tuh-mee)
diplopia (dip-LOH-pee-ah)
penumbra (puh–NUM–brah)
thrombolytic (THROM-boh-LIT-ik)
hemiplegia (HEM-ee-PLEE-jee-ah)

QUESTIONS TO GUIDE YOUR READING

1. What are the causes, risk factors, and pathophysiology of transient ischemic attack, stroke, and cerebral aneurysm?

2. What are emergency interventions for transient ischemic attack, stroke, and cerebral aneurysm?

3. What are therapeutic interventions for transient ischemic attack, stroke, and cerebral aneurysm?

4. What outcomes can be expected for a stroke victim?

5. What is appropriate nursing care for a patient with a cerebrovascular disorder?

Cerebrovascular disorders are disorders of the vascular system in the brain. When the vessels are unable to supply blood and oxygen to brain cells, brain tissue dies, causing a cerebrovascular accident (stroke). The most common cerebrovascular disorders include transient ischemic attack (TIA), stroke, and subarachnoid hemorrhage (SAH).

 TRANSIENT ISCHEMIC ATTACK

Transient ischemic attack (TIA) is a temporary impairment of the cerebral circulation causing neurological impairment that lasts less than 24 hours. It is characterized by a sudden, focal (specific area) neurological deficit caused by a brief period of inadequate perfusion of a portion of the brain. The loss of neurological function causes symptoms similar to those of a stroke (see next section). A TIA typically lasts minutes to hours, and the patient will have complete recovery. Symptoms that last longer than 24 hours but do not cause permanent neurological changes are called reversible ischemic neurological deficits (RINDs). If the symptoms do not reverse because an area of the brain is permanently damaged, then the event is considered to be a cerebral vascular accident (CVA), or stroke. Patients who have had a TIA have an increased risk of having a stroke; about 24% to 29% of patients who experience a TIA will have a stroke within 5 years. The risk is highest in the first month after the TIA. A TIA should be evaluated urgently to start appropriate therapy as soon as possible in order to decrease the risk of stroke.[1]

Because TIA is such a significant risk factor for stroke, etiologies, symptoms, diagnostic tests, and therapeutic interventions for TIA are the same as described below for cerebrovascular accident (stroke).

 CEREBROVASCULAR ACCIDENT

Cerebrovascular accident is the infarction (death) of brain tissue caused by the disruption of blood flow to the brain. It is characterized by focal neurological deficits specific to the area of the brain involved that do not fully resolve. The patient does not return to baseline functional level. Although strokes are most common in people over the age of 75, they affect approximately 700,000 people of all ages each year; 500,000 first-time strokes and 200,000 recurrent strokes. On average, every 45 seconds someone in the United States has a stroke, and every 3 minutes someone dies of a stroke. Stroke is our nation's number 3 killer and the leading cause of severe, long-term disability. Some population groups, such as African Americans, American Indians, Alaskan natives, and Mexican Americans, have a higher than average risk. Recent studies indicate that the risk of stroke may be higher in women during pregnancy and the 6 weeks following childbirth.[2]

In order to impress upon practitioners and the community the urgency of treating a stroke quickly, strokes are now being called *brain attacks* in the public setting. This reminds us that, like a heart attack, stroke is an urgent condition that can be treated if medical care is sought immediately. Patients should understand that if they experience any symptoms of a stroke, they should call 911 and go to the hospital immediately by ambulance. If patients receive treatment within 3 hours of symptom onset, they may be able to receive medication that has the potential to fully resolve their deficits.

Pathophysiology

Cerebral function is dependent on oxygen and glucose delivery to neurons of the brain. When blood flow is severely compromised or absent, the oxygen and glucose needed to meet the brain's metabolic needs are not available. The brain has no capability to store oxygen or glucose, so it relies on a constant supply of these nutrients. If the supply of oxygen and glucose is stopped, the brain tissue dies. In contrast to TIA, a brain attack can cause permanent damage if it is not reversed with timely treatment. For a brief period of time following a stroke, there is an area of brain tissue surrounding the damage, called the **penumbra**, which may be revived if the brain is reperfused quickly.

The particular vessel or vessels involved determine the area of the brain affected and therefore the symptoms that result. The duration of ischemia determines whether the symptoms are transient or permanent. A transient ischemic attack may be a warning of an impending stroke.

Etiology

A stroke can be caused by ischemia or hemorrhage. Most strokes present with sudden or rapidly evolving onset of symptoms. Even the best neurological specialist has difficulty making a diagnosis of stroke using clinical examination and history alone. A CT scan or MRI is necessary to make a diagnosis of stroke, and to determine whether the stroke is due to ischemia or hemorrhage. Etiology must be determined before treatment can be initiated.

Ischemic Stroke

An ischemic stroke can be caused by embolism or thrombosis, with resulting decreased perfusion (Fig. 49.1). Although any vessel may be involved, the bifurcation of the common carotid artery into the internal and external branches is the most common location for cerebral atherosclerosis and subsequent occlusion from an embolism or thrombosis.

When arteries are narrowed due to atherosclerotic plaque, they can become occluded (thrombotic stroke). If emboli break away from plaque, they can travel and lodge in narrowed cerebral vessels (embolic stroke). Either case results in ischemia or infarct of the brain cells that are perfused by the affected vessel.

Emboli in the brain may be arterial or cardiac in origin. Patients in atrial fibrillation can have small clots develop in the atria because the blood is not ejected normally, and as a result pools. These clots can be ejected into the circulation and become emboli. Other commonly recognized cardiac

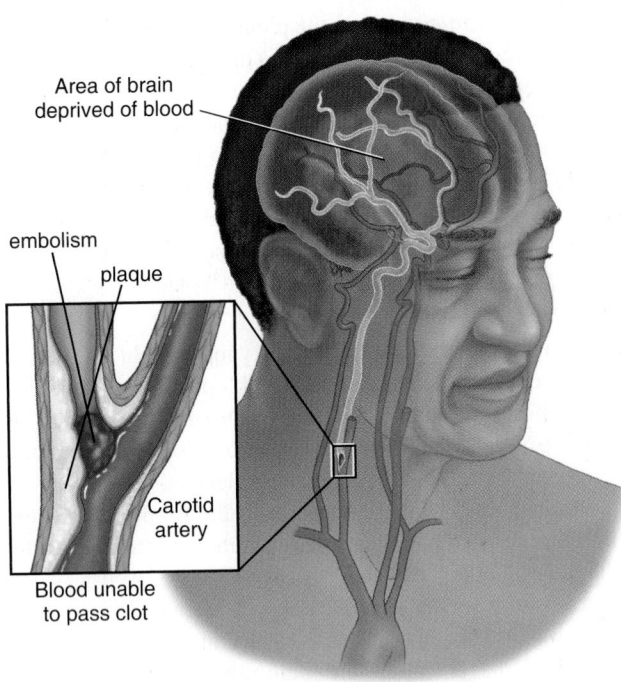

Area of brain
deprived of blood

embolism

plaque

Carotid
artery

Blood unable
to pass clot

FIGURE 49.1 Embolism and thrombosis.

sources for embolism include sinoatrial disorder, recent acute myocardial infarction (AMI), subacute bacterial endocarditis, cardiac tumors, and valve disorders. Most strokes of cardiac origin occur in the first weeks after AMI, but some risk for stroke remains for an indefinite time.

Stroke due to decreased perfusion occurs with severe stenosis of the carotid or basilar arteries, or with stenosis of the small deep arteries of the brain. The smallest, most distal vessels are affected first, before the larger proximal vessels, a process termed "watershed infarction." People with diabetes and hypertension have an increased risk for atherosclerosis and thrombosis.

Decreased perfusion may also occur from vasculitis, an inflammatory condition involving the cerebral blood vessels. Common causes of vasculitis are systemic lupus erythematosus, bacterial or tuberculous meningitis, fungal infection, and herpes zoster arteritis (arterial inflammation).

Hemorrhagic Stroke

Hemorrhagic stroke is caused by the rupture of a cerebral blood vessel. When a cerebral blood vessel ruptures, the brain tissue beyond the vessel does not receive oxygen and nutrients and can die. Additional damage can occur to the brain tissue surrounding the rupture from blood being released in the brain outside of the vascular system. The most common cause of an intracerebral hemorrhage (ICH) is poorly controlled hypertension. Another cause is a ruptured aneurysm. Hemorrhages tend to occur deep within the brain tissue. Subarachnoid hemorrhage (SAH) is caused by rupture of blood vessels on the surface of the brain. This type of infarct has the slowest rate of recovery and the highest probability of leaving the patient with extensive neuro-

logical deficits. A complete discussion of hemorrhagic strokes is presented later in this chapter.

The most common etiology of brain attack in younger patients is illicit drug usage. PCP (phencyclidine), crack, cocaine, amphetamines, and heroin have all been associated with cerebrovascular accident from subarachnoid or intracerebral hemorrhage because these drugs raise the blood pressure and increase pressure within the cerebral vessels.

Risk Factors

Risk factors for ischemic stroke are classified as modifiable or nonmodifiable.

Nonmodifiable risk factors are those things that cannot be altered, such as age, gender, race, prior stroke history, and heredity. Modifiable risk factors are those risks which can be changed by treatment, such as treating high blood pressure, or by lifestyle modification, such as stopping smoking (Box 49.1). Following physician recommendations and medication orders for modifiable risk factors will help individuals reduce stroke risk.

Warning Signs

All patients should be taught to recognize warning signs of a stroke, and to call 911 immediately if they occur. Warning signs include:

- Sudden numbness or weakness of face, arm, or leg, especially on one side of the body
- Sudden confusion, trouble speaking, or understanding
- Sudden trouble seeing in one or both eyes
- Sudden trouble walking, dizziness, loss of balance, or coordination
- Sudden severe headache with no known cause[3]

Box 49.1

Risk Factors for Stroke

Modifiable Risk Factors

- High blood pressure
- Smoking
- Diabetes mellitus
- Atherosclerosis
- Atrial fibrillation
- Other heart disease
- TIAs
- Sickle cell anemia
- High cholesterol
- Obesity
- Excessive alcohol intake
- Certain illegal drugs

Nonmodifiable Risk Factors

- Older age
- Sex (more common in men)
- Heredity
- Prior stroke or heart attack

TIAs = transient ischemic attacks.

Acute Signs and Symptoms

Symptoms are varied and depend on the area of the brain affected. Common symptoms include visual disturbances, language disturbances, weakness or paralysis on one side of the body, and difficulty swallowing (dysphagia). These signs and symptoms are the same for both ischemic and hemorrhagic stroke. In addition, the patient with a hemorrhagic stroke may experience rapid deterioration, drowsiness, and a severe headache, often described as "the worst headache of my life." Symptoms can last a few minutes to a few hours or may persist for an indefinite period of time (Table 49.1)

Language Disturbances

Difficulty with language is frequently associated with a TIA and stroke. *Aphasia* refers to the absence of language; *dysphasia* refers to difficulty with speech and is not as severe as aphasia. The patient may experience trouble selecting correct words, use incomprehensible or nonsense speech, have trouble understanding others' speech, and have trouble writing or reading. Aphasia may be expressive, in which the patient knows what he wants to say but cannot speak or make sense, or receptive, with an inability to understand spoken and/or written words. Global aphasia occurs when both expressive and receptive aphasia are present. Slurred or indistinct speech and abnormal pronunciation of words and articulation because of a motor problem are referred to as dysarthria.

Motor Disturbances

Paralysis, weakness, or numbness can present as clumsiness, heaviness, and facial droop. The onset will be sudden and generally involves one side of the body, the side of the body *opposite* to the damaged area. The deficits may present on both sides of the body if the patient has experienced a brainstem stroke or a vertebrobasilar stroke. The most common paralysis or weakness affects the arm and face together but can present as complete hemiparesis, where the entire one side of the body is flaccid. Another clinical finding that affects mobility is **ataxia**. Ataxia may present as poor balance, a stumbling gait, or staggering. This can be related to damage to the cerebellum, or to poor coordination due to weakness or paralysis on one side of the body. If the muscles of swallowing are affected, dysphagia results.

Visual Disturbances

Visual field disturbances are also a common symptom of a stroke. The visual loss is painless and may involve loss of all or part of the vision in one eye. Patients often describe a "curtain dropping," "fog," "gray-out," or "black-out" of vision. The involved eye is on the *same* side as the diseased artery. Visual field abnormalities include horizontal (top or bottom half of visual field), bitemporal (outside half), homonymous (same side half), or hemianopsia or quadrantic (one-quarter visual loss) defects (Fig. 49.2). When you are assessing the patient, stop talking and keep moving across the room. If the patient does not track you there is a good chance he or she has a deficit in that visual field.

Diagnostic Tests

A new assessment tool is now available to assist community members and emergency medical technicians in identifying stroke symptoms quickly. The Cincinnati Prehospital Stroke Scale (CPSS) was created to facilitate transporting stroke victims to the hospital as soon as possible. Findings in recent studies show that a patient who has one of three positive findings when the CPSS is used has a 72% probability of having an ischemic stroke. If all three findings are positive, the probability increases to 85%.[4]

The CPSS has three components to review:
- Have the patient smile. Look for subtle signs of facial droop or uneven symmetry of the face.
- Ask the patient to hold the arms out straight in front while closing the eyes. Observe the patient's arms closely for any signs of drifting downward. This can be performed with the patient standing or sitting down.
- Ask the patient to repeat a phrase, such as "It is a bright and sunny day in Michigan." Did the patient understand? Did he repeat the phrase exactly? Did he exhibit any slurred speech or difficulty saying words?

If any one of the three tests is positive, the patient should be sent immediately by ambulance to the nearest emergency room or stroke center.

Upon arrival at the emergency department, a computed tomographic (CT) scan will be performed immediately. If the cause of symptoms is a TIA, the CT scan will be negative for stroke since there has been no permanent damage to the brain. However, even an ischemic stroke that causes damage to the brain cells will not be visible on a CT for several days after the event. The purpose of the CT scan is to identify if the symptoms are caused by a hemorrhagic stroke

TABLE 49.1 SYMPTOMS OF STROKE ACCORDING TO ARTERY AFFECTED

	Hemiparesis	Dysphasia	Visual Changes	Altered Level of Consciousness	Ataxia	Dysphagia
Carotid	X	X	X	X		
Middle cerebral	X	X	X	X		
Vertebrobasilar/ cerebellar (brainstem)	Loss on both sides of body	X	X	X	X	X

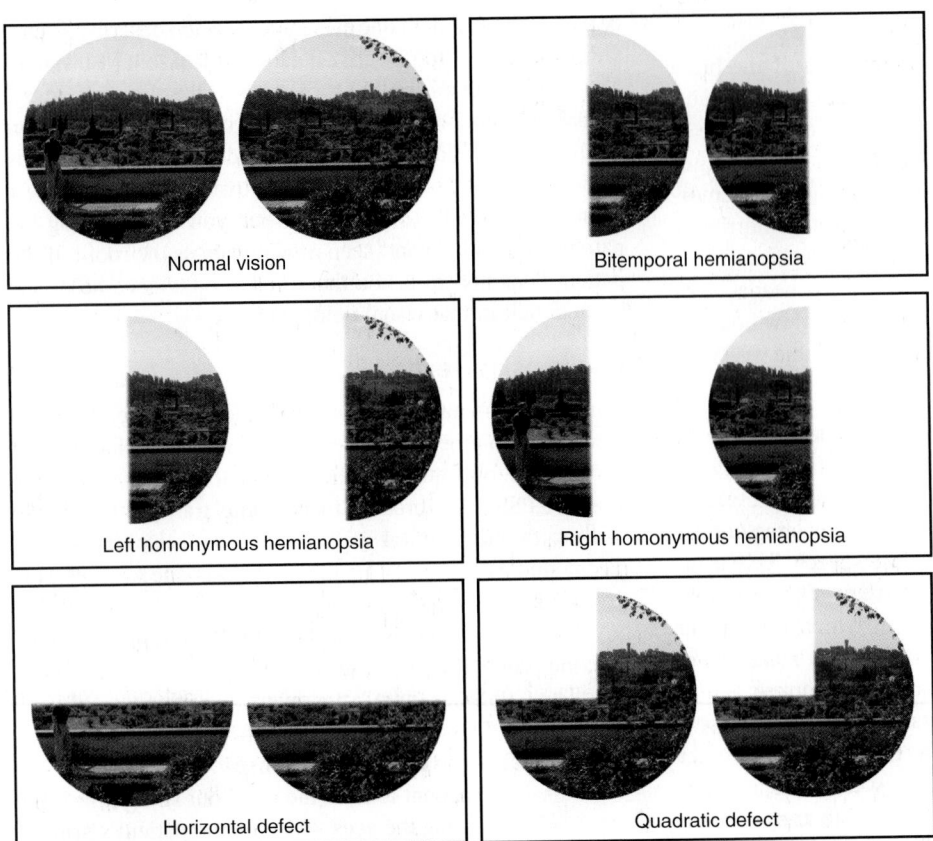

FIGURE 49.2 Visual deficits in stroke.

so the physician can determine the appropriate course of treatment. Hemorrhagic strokes are treated with a different course of care than ischemic strokes. Care for hemorrhagic strokes is discussed later in this chapter.

Patients may have an electrocardiogram (ECG) to determine if atrial fibrillation is present. An echocardiogram may be done to determine the presence of other heart disease that may increase risk of thrombus formation. Other tests that may be performed in the emergency department include complete blood count (CBC), metabolic panel, blood typing, prothrombin time (PT) and international normalized ratio (INR), and serum pregnancy if indicated. Stools and emesis may be checked for blood if possible. The patient will be placed on a cardiac monitor and pulse oximeter. The emergency department (ED) nurse will complete a dysphagia screen before the patient consumes anything.

ED staff may complete the NIH (National Institutes of Health) Stroke Scale to determine the patient's neurological deficit level. This scale is more involved than the Prehospital Scale. See the Stroke Scale at http://www.ninds.nih.gov/doctors/NIH_Stroke_Scale_Booklet.pdf. If the patient has arrived at the ED within 3 hours of the onset of symptoms, the patient will be evaluated for appropriateness for receiving t-PA (tissue plasminogen activator), a **thrombolytic** agent recently approved for use in strokes. If the patient is not a candidate for t-PA, the patient will be further evaluated for appropriate care.

Carotid Doppler testing can determine if stenosis of the carotid arteries exists. This noninvasive test involves bouncing sound waves off the carotid arteries to determine the velocity and turbulence of blood flow. The amount of restricted flow determines if the patient would benefit from a carotid **endarterectomy** to remove the occlusion from the artery. If the patient is symptomatic or the degree of stenosis causes over 70% occlusion of the carotid artery, the patient may be kept at the hospital for surgical intervention.

A cerebral angiogram may be completed to determine the patency of cerebral vessels and the status of any collateral circulation.

Therapeutic Interventions

Initial emergency care is supportive while test results are pending. ABCs (airway, breathing, and circulation) are monitored. Oxygen is administered to maintain oxygen saturation greater than 90%. Vital signs and heart rhythm are monitored. Diagnostic tests are done without delay. When test results verify whether the stroke is hemorrhagic or ischemic, therapeutic interventions are initiated.

Thrombolytic Therapy

Thrombolytic therapy (alteplase or t-PA) is a recent development in the treatment of ischemic brain attack. Other thrombolytic agents that are approved for use in heart attacks

---

thrombolytic: thrombo—clot + lytic—causing breakdown

endarterectomy: endo—inside + arter—artery + ectomy—surgical removal of

are being researched for treatment of strokes. Intracerebral hemorrhage must be ruled out before t-PA therapy is instituted because of the risk of worsening a bleeding vessel. The goal of thrombolytic agents is to actually break down the thrombus causing the occlusion, which can potentially prevent or completely reverse the symptoms of stroke. Plasmin is the enzyme that causes thrombi to break down. Thrombolytic agents accomplish thrombus lysis by causing the conversion of plasminogen to plasmin. Patients treated effectively with t-PA may be able to leave the hospital within 1 or 2 days with no residual effects from the stroke.

Cerebral hemorrhage is a major complication of thrombolytic therapy; therefore, it is only used if the patient meets strict criteria. It is crucial to know when the symptoms began because t-PA can only be given within 3 hours of the stroke occurrence. Assessment for appropriateness of t-PA include asking the patient or the family, "When was the last time you (or your family member saw you) were normal?" This question will determine actual onset time of the TIA or stroke. Asking questions regarding what they were doing at the time of the symptom onset assists in determining the time of onset if there are discrepancies regarding the time. There are other inclusion criteria for administering t-PA including:

- Age greater than 18 years
- NIH Stroke Scale score of 4 or greater

Patients who have a history of intracerebral hemorrhage, recent stroke or serious head trauma, surgery within the past 3 weeks, recent lumbar puncture, GI or urinary bleeding, uncontrolled high blood pressure, or any other risk factors for bleeding cannot have t-PA because of the risk of bleeding.

To be effective, t-PA must be administered within 3 hours of the onset of symptoms. This time frame has clear implications for nurses. Patients with neurological symptoms who are seen in the emergency department must be assessed and stabilized promptly. A CT scan and, if an ischemic cause is suspected, an angiogram are performed quickly. Some people may be surprised to learn that there are treatments available for stroke. Because of time constraints, individuals may be asked to make treatment decisions before other family members are able to arrive. This places a significant burden on people who are already experiencing stress. You can help ease this burden by explaining the time factor, repeating information as needed, and ensuring that the individuals involved have the opportunity to ask questions.

Pharmacological Management

Blood pressure control is vital for the patient. Care is taken not to lower the blood pressure too quickly or too far. If the patient has long-standing hypertension, lowering the blood pressure to a "normal" level may actually cause further ischemia. Current recommendations are to not lower blood pressure more than 10% from baseline at one time. Drugs must be used carefully and blood pressure monitored frequently. If the patient experiences neurological deterioration, the physician may adjust treatment to increase the blood pressure. Some physicians believe that the blood pressure should not be lowered because chronically hypertensive patients require a higher BP to maintain adequate cerebral perfusion.

The patient may receive an antiseizure medication as a prophylactic measure. Sometimes after a hemorrhagic stroke, the patient can experience vasospasm, which could further occlude the arteries and inhibit oxygen and glucose from reaching brain tissue. If this occurs, the patient may be treated with a calcium channel blocker like nimodipine, which relaxes smooth muscles of the vessel wall and reduces the vasospasm. The physician may also order an antifibrinolytic, such as epsilon-aminocaproic acid, to inhibit plasminogen activation. This medication has been reported to reduce the incidence of rebleeding. See Table 49.2 for medications commonly used for cerebrovascular disorders.

Patients suffering from a stroke develop increased intracranial pressure, which further adds to brain damage. Stroke patients are also vulnerable to repeated strokes. Careful serial neurological assessments are needed to promptly detect and report changes.

Postemergent Care

After emergent treatment, medical management focuses on controlling the cause of the transient ischemic attack or stroke. The results of the diagnostic tests assist physicians in determining the course of treatment If there are residual physical deficits, the physician will order physical, occupational, and speech therapist consultations to evaluate the patient's functional status and make recommendations for further treatment. The American Stroke Association recommends that patients who have had a TIA or stroke receive an antiplatelet drug within 24 hours of symptom onset. Antiplatelet drugs include clopidigrel (Plavix), aspirin/dipyridamole (Aggrenox), or aspirin. Decreasing platelet aggregation lessens the likelihood of thrombus formation. Antidysrhythmic medication may be used to control atrial fibrillation. The patient in atrial fibrillation may also receive warfarin (Coumadin) to prevent clot development.

Respiratory compromise may occur related to an increase in intracranial pressure. Patients with stroke are prone to aspiration because of decreased level of consciousness or impaired swallowing ability. Patients should be suctioned as needed to keep the airway clear. If the patient vomits, he or she should be turned to the side to reduce the risk of aspiration. Oral feedings should be initiated carefully and progressed slowly only after the patient is alert and the ability to swallow safely has been determined by an appropriate swallowing evaluation.

LEARNING TIP

Time is brain. This means the faster the patient with a stroke receives treatment, the more brain (and brain function) can be saved.

TABLE 49.2 MEDICATIONS USED IN CEREBROVASCULAR DISORDERS

Medication Class/Action	Examples	Route	Side Effects	Nursing Implicatioins
Thrombolytic agents Lyse existing clots	Tissue plasminogen activator (t-PA)	IV	Intracranial, GI, urinary hemorrhage	Must be administered within 3 hours of symptom onset.
Antiplatelet agents Prevent formation of clots	Aspirin	PO/rectal	Dyspepsia, nausea, vomiting, bleeding	Monitor for bruising, change in LOC, prolonged bleeding time.
	Clopidogrel (Plavix)	PO	Bleeding, abdominal pain, skin rash, edema, headache, backache	
	Aspirin/dipyridamole (Aggrenox)	PO	Headache, dyspepsia, pain, fatigue	
Anticoagulants Prolong time to form clots; prevent new clots	Warfarin (Coumadin)	PO/IV	Hemorrhage, purple toe syndrome, necrosis of skin	Monitor for bruising, change in LOC, prolonged bleeding time.
	Heparin	SC, IV	Hemorrhage, erythema, local irritation, hematoma, ulceration	
Peripheral vasodilators Improve collateral circulation	Cyclandelate (Cyclospasmol)	PO	Flushing, tingling, headache, dizziness, tachycardia	Monitor for therapeutic and nontherapeutic effects of administration (to decrease spasm of cerebral vessels).
	Papaverine (Papacon, Pavabid)	PO, parenteral, IV, IM	Increased heart rate and BP, drowsiness, vertigo, headache	
Statins Reduce cholesterol level	Simvastatin (Zocor), pravastatin (Pravachol), atorvastatin (Lipitor), lovastatin (Mevacor)	PO	Irritability, diarrhea, heartburn, hepatitis, dizziness, headache, muscle aches	Patient should notify prescriber if muscle pain or weakness occur.

BP = blood pressure; LOC = level of consciousness.

Surgical Management of Carotid Stenosis

If tests show carotid stenosis greater than 70%, a carotid endarterectomy may be performed. During this surgical procedure, the carotid artery is opened and the plaque removed. Nursing care focuses on careful neurological assessment for signs of deterioration related to ischemia. The incision is monitored for hematoma development and bleeding. Development of a hematoma can compromise the patient's airway. Bleeding at the suture line, particularly of bright red blood, may indicate failure of the sutures. This emergency situation requires prompt response to prevent massive blood loss. Balloon angioplasty for carotid stenosis is being investigated as a potential treatment in large facilities.

Prevention of Stroke

Incidence of stroke can be lessened by reduction of risk factors (see Box 49.1). Keeping hypertension, cholesterol level, weight, and diabetes controlled can go a long way in preventing strokes. Smoking cessation is essential. Emboli may be prevented with warfarin in individuals at high risk from atrial fibrillation. Aspirin or other antiplatelet agents help prevent abnormal clotting. Carotid endarterectomy can be done in patients with carotid stenosis.

It is important to educate all patients about new treatments for stroke and the potential for reversal of symptoms with the use of the thrombolytic agent t-PA. Patients must be educated about symptoms of stroke and the importance of receiving emergency treatment within 3 hours to maximize the potential for prevention of neurological deficits. *Too often patients ignore early symptoms or delay calling for help. This delay can mean the difference between leading a normal life and permanent disability.*

Long-Term Effects of Stroke

Impaired Motor Function and Sensation

The side of the body opposite the side of the cerebral infarct is affected because nerve fibers cross over as they pass from the brain to the spinal cord (Fig. 49.3). Paralysis on one side of the body is called **hemiplegia** (Fig. 49.4). The affected extremities may be weak or totally paralyzed (flaccid). Depending on the artery affected, the arm may be weaker than the leg or vice versa. These patients are particularly prone to contractures, which cause permanent immobility of a muscle or joint from fibrosis of connective tissue.

hemiplegia: hemi—one side + plegia—paralysis

Mr. Jankowski

■ You are caring for Mr. Jankowski, a 56-year-old man who has been admitted to your orthopedic unit following knee surgery. As you listen to his lungs during your shift assessment, you notice that his lung sounds are diminished. You ask if he is a smoker and find that he has smoked for 40 years. You realize this places Mr. Jankowski at risk for stroke. What further assessment and intervention should you provide?

Suggested answers at end of chapter.

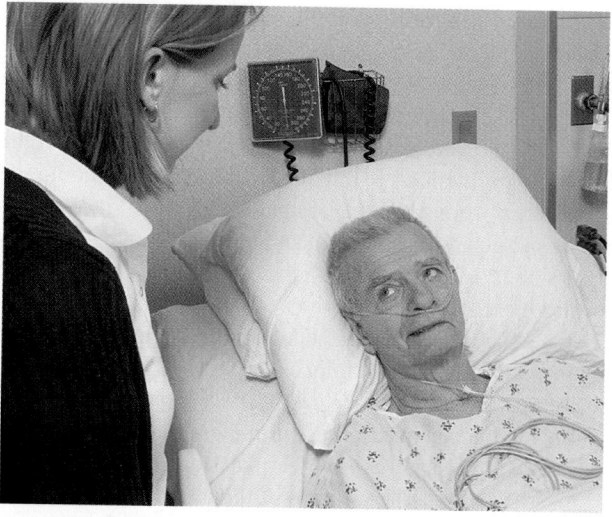

FIGURE 49.4 Note the left-sided weakness in this man's smile as result of a stroke.

Adaptation or assistance with activities of daily living (ADLs) is required. Motor involvement often affects swallowing, control of urination, and bowel function Patients should be mobilized within 24 hours if possible to prevent complications of immobility. Physical, occupational, and speech therapy are provided to maximize functioning and to progress the patient toward a return to baseline functioning.

Sensation changes may prevent the patient from being aware of pressure or injuries on the affected side. Patients must be taught to be aware of these changes and protect the involved limbs.

APHASIA. If the infarct is on the dominant side of the brain, the speech center will probably be affected. Aphasia may be expressive, receptive, or global, as described earlier. Patients may be able to say words but are not able to form coherent

speech, such as the patient who picks up a fork but calls it a comb. A patient with receptive aphasia does not understand what is said. In this situation, it is easy to attempt to speak louder to try to help the patient understand. Remember that it is not the patient's hearing that is affected. You need to be very patient and understanding as the patient tries to communicate with you. Speech therapy can help the patient relearn to communicate. See the Nursing Process section for interventions for the aphasic patient.

Emotional Lability

Emotional lability, or instability, is a common consequence of stroke. Patients may move rapidly from profound sadness to an almost euphoric state and back again. Laughing or crying may have no relationship to the patient's situation at any given moment. Families can be upset by this behavior because they do not understand why a once happy person is now crying all the time or why the patient laughs inappropriately. You can help by explaining that these responses probably do not reflect how the patient is feeling, but rather are caused by the stroke damage.

Impaired Judgment

Patients who have had a stroke, particularly those with right-sided lesions, present safety risks. Patients may have poor understanding of their own limitations and believe that they are capable of performing tasks they did before the stroke. Precautions must be taken to protect the patient from injury.

If the frontal lobes are involved, learned social behaviors may be lost. The patient may undress in public, use profanity, or make inappropriate sexual advances. These behaviors are extremely difficult for significant others to cope with. Education and emotional support of the significant others are essential. Allowing them to talk about their frustration and anger may facilitate coping. Distracting the patient from inappropriate behavior may help. The patient should never be reprimanded or punished because he or she no longer has the cognitive ability to control the behaviors.

Left-side infarct

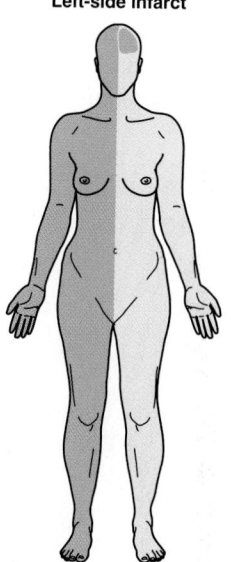

Right-sided weakness or paralysis
Aphasia (in left–brain-dominant clients)
Depression related to disability common

Right-side infarct

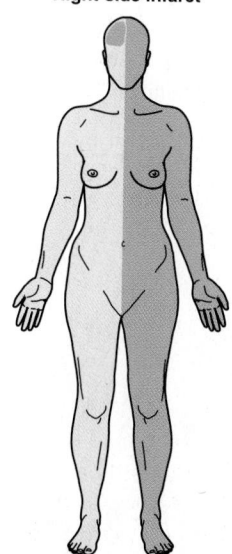

Left-sided weakness or paralysis
Impaired judgment/safety risk
Unilateral neglect more common
Indifferent to disability

FIGURE 49.3 The side opposite the infarct is affected in a stroke.

Unilateral Neglect

The phenomenon of unilateral neglect is seen predominantly in patients who have right hemisphere infarcts. These individuals do not acknowledge the left side of their environment. In severe cases, the patient may forget to dress the left side of the body. Initially these patients should be approached from the right (or unaffected) side. Place essential items such as the call light and telephone on the patient's right side. Position the bed so that the patient's right side is toward the door. Gradually the health team can begin teaching the patient to focus on the left side. This involves teaching the patient to purposefully check where the left limbs are positioned and to look for safety risks. The patient can learn to turn his or her head and scan the environment. Patients may need reminders to turn their plates during meals to recognize the food on the left side of the plate.

Homonymous Hemianopsia

Visual deficits were described earlier. In particular, homonymous hemianopsia can cause the patient to ignore one side of a meal tray or neglect to care for one side of the body. Again, it is important to teach the patient to check the affected side, and to turn his or her plate to recognize food on both sides.

Other Long-Term Effects

The stroke patient may experience other complications after the acute phase of the stroke has passed. These may include pneumonia, deep vein thrombosis, pulmonary embolism, pressure ulcers, malnutrition, and depression. For the homeward bound patient, education for the patient and family regarding prevention and recognition of these complications will assist the patient in a successful recovery. If a patient needs to receive rehabilitation in a skilled nursing facility, prevention of these issues will be a part of the care plan at the facility. For more information, visit the National Stroke Association at www.stroke.org.

NURSING CARE TIP

When preparing a room for a patient with stroke, the caretaker should choose a room in which the patient can have the unaffected side toward the door if at all possible.

CEREBRAL ANEURYSM AND SUBARACHNOID HEMORRHAGE

A cerebral aneurysm is a weakness in the wall of a cerebral artery. It may be congenital, traumatic, or the result of disease. If the aneurysm ruptures, a subarachnoid hemorrhage results. It is unknown what causes the formation of congenital aneurysms or what causes them to rupture. Unruptured aneurysms are typically asymptomatic. The exception to this is a very large aneurysm, which can cause symptoms similar to a brain tumor. Aneurysms often affect young, otherwise healthy adults.

Pathophysiology and Etiology

Aneurysms can occur in any of the cerebral arteries. Eighty percent of cerebral aneurysms occur in the circle of Willis. The most common site is at the bifurcation of an artery. It is theorized that increased turbulence at the bifurcation causes an outpouching of a congenitally weak arterial wall.

Subarachnoid hemorrhage is the collection of blood beneath the arachnoid mater following aneurysm rupture. Rupture of an arteriovenous malformation or head trauma may also result in subarachnoid hemorrhage (Fig. 49.5). The presence of blood outside the blood vessels is very irritating to brain tissue. It is believed that irritation from blood breakdown is the major cause of vasospasm, a common complication of subarachnoid hemorrhage.

It is unclear what causes an aneurysm to rupture at a given time. Some individuals experience a subarachnoid hemorrhage while performing Valsalva's maneuver, engaging in sexual activity, or physically exerting themselves. For other patients, the aneurysm ruptures during a quiet, inactive period. If the aneurysm rupture is associated with a particular activity, the patient may be very frightened of engaging in that activity again. This may have a negative effect on the patient's interpersonal relationships if the associated activity was sexual in nature. The patient's partner may feel guilty or responsible for the hemorrhage. Emotional support and confidentiality regarding associated events help both the patient and significant other.

Signs and Symptoms

Some patients experience a small hemorrhage before diagnosis of subarachnoid hemorrhage. This leakage of blood may cause a mild headache, vomiting, or disorientation. The symptoms may be attributed to a flulike syndrome. Patients may dismiss the symptoms and not seek medical care.

The most common presentation of rupture of an aneurysm is sudden onset of a severe headache. Typically, patients state, "I have never had a headache this bad in my

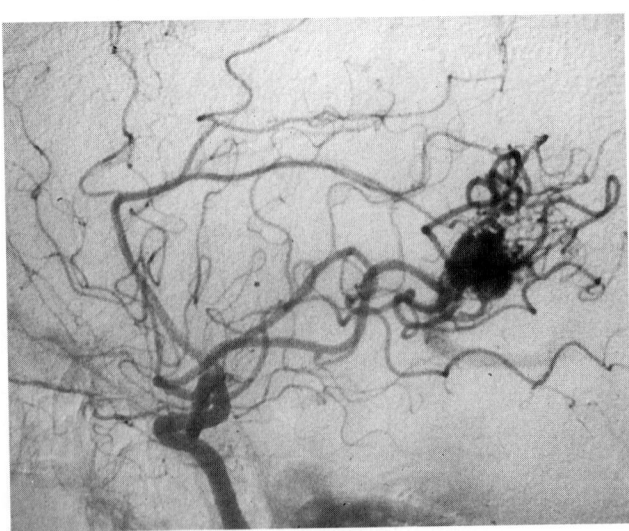

FIGURE 49.5 Arteriovenous malformation. Note tangled vessels.

life." Patients may hold their heads and moan or cry in pain. Sensitivity to light is a common finding. This may make patients reluctant to cooperate with pupil examinations.

Level of consciousness varies based on the severity of the hemorrhage. Patients may be alert and coherent, may lose consciousness immediately, or may gradually become less responsive. The decreased level of consciousness is caused by increased intracranial pressure and impairment of cerebral blood flow. Patients may experience generalized seizures.

Blood in the subarachnoid space causes meningeal irritation. The patient may exhibit nuchal rigidity. The most commonly affected cranial nerves are III and VI. This is manifested as an enlarged pupil or abnormal gaze. Motor dysfunction may involve one or both limbs on the side opposite the hemorrhage.

Diagnostic Tests

Because of the severe nature of the symptoms, patients with subarachnoid hemorrhage almost always come to the emergency department rather than seek care from a primary health-care provider. A CT scan is done to identify the presence and location of a hemorrhage. Precise diagnosis of an aneurysm requires a cerebral angiogram. The contrast material fills the aneurysm if one exists. For a patient with a severe headache and facing a life-threatening illness, this test can be very frightening. If the patient's neurological status does not allow him or her to cooperate, sedation may be required before and during the examination.

Therapeutic Interventions

Patients experiencing a subarachnoid hemorrhage are cared for in an intensive care unit setting. They typically have an arterial line and a central venous pressure monitoring catheter. Blood pressure is carefully monitored because high pressures increase the risk of rerupture of the aneurysm and low pressures may be associated with ischemia. Values outside parameters identified by the physician are reported. Typically, the systolic blood pressure is kept between 120 and 160 mm Hg. Vasoactive drugs may be required to maintain blood pressure within the prescribed parameters.

There is no cure for subarachnoid hemorrhage. Treatment consists of correcting the cause of the hemorrhage if possible. Preventing or managing complications and providing supportive care are important aspects of nursing care.

Surgical Management

Definitive treatment of the aneurysm involves performing a craniotomy and exposing the aneurysm. If the aneurysm has a neck (berry aneurysm), it is identified and clamped with a metal clip (Fig. 49.6). An aneurysm without a neck may be wrapped with a sterile plastic or muslin wrap. This provides stability to the aneurysm walls, lessening the chance of rupture. In some situations, it is possible to clamp the artery on either side of the aneurysm, removing that portion of the vessel, and the aneurysm, from the circulation.

Nonsurgical Management

Nonsurgical intervention may be provided for aneurysms that are inoperable because of size, configuration, or the

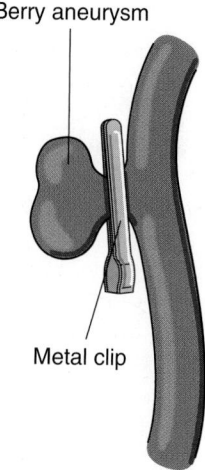

FIGURE 49.6 Surgical management of aneurysms.

patient's medical status. A foreign material such as a tiny metallic coil or fibrin glue may be introduced into the aneurysm. A thrombus develops around the foreign body and, if the treatment is successful, occludes the aneurysm. The goal is to fill the aneurysm enough to prevent blood flowing into it without causing rupture.

Complications

Rebleeding

Recurrent rupture of a cerebral aneurysm carries significant morbidity and mortality rates. Patients are at risk for rebleeding until the aneurysm is surgically repaired. If the aneurysm is wrapped or embolized, there is a risk of rebleeding, but it is much less than if the aneurysm is left untreated.

Hydrocephalus

Blood within the ventricular system interferes with the circulation, and reabsorption of CSF and hydrocephalus may develop. Early in the course of subarachnoid hemorrhage, an external ventricular drain may be used to treat hydrocephalus.

Approximately 25% of patients with subarachnoid hemorrhage require placement of a ventriculoperitoneal shunt to treat hydrocephalus (Fig. 49.7). This surgical procedure involves placement of a ventricular catheter. The catheter is then connected to a valve, which regulates the rate of cerebrospinal fluid drainage. Another catheter connects to the valve and is passed down to the peritoneal cavity. The cerebrospinal fluid drains out of the peritoneal catheter and is absorbed into the peritoneal cavity.

Vasospasm

Vasospasm is responsible for the majority of long-term complications of subarachnoid hemorrhage. Vasospasm is the narrowing of a blood vessel diameter. Although it typically begins in the vessel giving rise to the aneurysm, vasospasm may spread to other vessels. This explains why the ischemia or infarct caused by vasospasm can be so widespread and devastating.

The long-term complications of subarachnoid hemorrhage are similar to those of stroke.

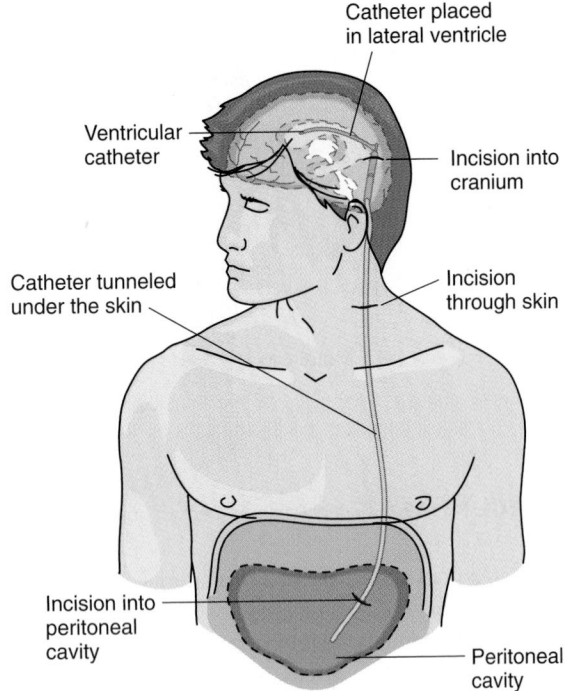

Catheter placed
in lateral ventricle

Ventricular
catheter

Incision into
cranium

Catheter tunneled
under the skin

Incision
through skin

Incision into
peritoneal
cavity

Peritoneal
cavity

FIGURE 49.7 A ventriculoperitoneal shunt drains cerebrospinal fluid into the peritoneal cavity.

Rehabilitation

If the patient is able to tolerate intensive therapy, discharge from the hospital may be to a rehabilitation center. With rehabilitation, most patients can learn to walk, some with a walker or cane. Speech therapy can help the patient learn to communicate. Many patients can learn to take care of themselves. Some may be able to drive again and even have a job.

Nursing Process for the Patient with a Cerebrovascular Disorder

Assessment/Data Collection

Assess the patient for signs and symptoms of decreased cerebral tissue perfusion: decreased level of consciousness, irritability or restlessness, dizziness, syncope, blurred or dimmed vision, **diplopia**, change in visual fields, unequal pupils or a sluggish or absent pupillary reaction to light, paresthesias, motor weakness, paralysis, or seizures. Reassess frequently and report decline. Monitor vital signs and oxygen levels. Monitor laboratory tests: CBC, lipid profile, and INR/PT if on warfarin (Coumadin). Perform a routine respiratory assessment. Monitor lung sounds for adventitious sounds or a change in breath sounds. Assess pain level since pain can impair an effective breathing pattern. Assess swallowing ability before offering oral intake. Promptly report any increase in dyspnea, changes in vital signs or pulse oximetry, or increased white blood cell count or temperature.

---

diplopia: diplo—— double + opia—sight

Mrs. Washington

■ Mrs. Washington is a 68-year-old African American retired office worker. She was admitted to your unit following a right-sided intracerebral hemorrhage. Her daughter states that Mrs. Washington has taken antihypertensive medication for the last 20 years. However, she states that her mother has been "forgetful" lately and that there are five more pills in the medicine bottle than expected. On admission, Mrs. Washington is oriented only to person and has hemiparesis.

1. What may have precipitated Mrs. Washington's stroke?
2. On which side are Mrs. Washington's extremities affected?
3. List two safety concerns and strategies to promote patient safety.
4. List at least two educational needs for Mrs. Washington and her daughter.

Suggested answers at end of chapter.

Nursing Diagnosis, Planning, and Implementation

See Box 49.2 Nursing Care Plan for the Patient with Stroke for nursing diagnoses during acute care. Possible post–acute nursing diagnoses are listed below with outcomes and interventions.

Impaired physical mobility related to decreased motor function

EXPECTED OUTCOMES: Patient will maintain physical mobility as evidenced by maximum physical mobility within limitations of deficits. Patient will not experience complications related to immobility.

- Consult physical and occupational therapists *to assess the patient's abilities and make specific recommendations related to mobility.*
- Maintain the patient in good body alignment *to prevent contractures and promote comfort.*
- Support affected extremities with pillows *to prevent dislocation injuries and promote comfort.*
- Perform range of motion exercises as prescribed by physical therapist *to prevent contractures and atrophy.*
- Follow physical/occupational therapy recommendations for being up in chair or ambulation. *Prolonged bedrest is associated with complications and poor outcomes.*
- If patient is unable to get out of bed, turn and reposition at least every 2 hours to prevent complications *to prevent skin, respiratory, and musculoskeletal complications.*

Box 49.2   Nursing Care Plan for the Patient with Stroke

Nursing Diagnosis: Ineffective cerebral tissue perfusion

Expected Outcomes The patient will experience improved cerebral tissue perfusion as evidenced by:
- Absence of or reduction in dizziness, syncope, visual disturbances
- Improved mental status
- Pupils equal and reactive to light
- Improved motor and sensory function

Evaluation of Outcomes Is patient free of symptoms of decreased perfusion? Are symptoms improving?

Interventions	Rationale	Evaluation
Assess neurological status frequently.	A change in status could indicate decreased perfusion and should be reported immediately.	Is there a change in neurological status since the previous documented assessment?
Assess vital signs q2hr × 4 hours then q4hr × 72 hours.	High or low blood pressure can lead to decreased tissue perfusion and recurrent stroke.	Are vital signs within normal limits? Has there been a change?
Monitor medication for therapeutic and nontherapeutic effects. Monitor coagulation studies if appropriate.	Anticoagulant therapy must be closely monitored to make sure it is at a therapeutic level, and not increasing risk for bleeding.	Are coagulation studies within normal or therapeutic ranges? Are there signs of bleeding?

Nursing Diagnosis: Ineffective airway clearance related to stasis of secretions associated with decreased mobility and poor cough effort; and airway obstruction resulting from tongue falling back in throat

Expected Outcomes Patient will maintain open airway as evidenced by respirations quiet and unlabored, 12–20 per minute, $SaO_2 \geq 90\%$.

Evaluation of Outcomes Are respirations quiet, 12–20 per minute, with SaO_2 90% or greater?

Interventions	Rationale	Evaluation
Monitor lung sounds, cough, and respirations.	Assessment provides the basis for intervention.	Are lung sounds clear? Cough effective? Respirations quiet and easy?
Position the patient to maintain an open airway.	Side lying may keep tongue from obstructing airway.	Is patient positioned to keep airway clear?
Consult with RN or physician about an oral airway if airway is not clear.	An oral airway will keep tongue from obstructing airway if needed.	Is an airway indicated?
Encourage to deep breathe and cough if patient is able.	Coughing and deep breathing will help clear secretions from airway and prevent atelectasis.	Is patient able to deep breathe and cough? Is cough effective?
If cough is ineffective, suction as needed.	Suctioning may be necessary if patient is unable to swallow secretions or cough effectively.	Is suctioning indicated? Is airway clear after suctioning?

(Continued on following page)

Box 49.2   NURSING CARE PLAN **for the Patient with Stroke** (Continued)

Nursing Diagnosis: Risk for injury related to seizure or repeat stroke

Expected Outcomes Patient will remain free from injury.

Evaluation of Outcomes Is patient free from injury? Are problems recognized and reported quickly?

Interventions	Rationale	Evaluation
Monitor neurological status frequently and report changes promptly.	Prompt recognition of a repeat stroke	Are neurological checks WNL? Are changes reported promptly?
Administer anticonvulsant agent as ordered.	The patient is at increased risk for seizures following a stroke.	Is patient seizure-free?
Implement seizure precautions (see Chapter 47).	Precautions help protect patient in event of a seizure.	Are precautions in place?
Assist with transfers and ambulation.	Patient is at risk for falls because of motor and sensory deficits and impaired judgment.	Is patient assisted with mobility? Is patient able to call for help when needed?
Offer toileting on set schedule.	The patient may attempt to get up by her- or himself if no one is available when he or she needs to go to the bathroom.	Is patient toileted often enough to prevent accidents and falls?

WNL = within normal limits.

Imbalanced nutrition, less than requirements related to impaired swallowing and motor deficits

EXPECTED OUTCOME: Patient will maintain adequate nutrition without aspiration as evidenced by stable weight at appropriate level for height.

- Keep patient NPO until swallowing can be evaluated *to prevent aspiration.*
- Perform dysphagia screening. *This quick assessment can identify problems before a complete evaluation can be done.*
  - Observe for facial weakness or inability to completely close mouth.
  - Ask patient to stick out tongue and move it side to side.
  - Observe for drooling.
- If swallowing appears to be intact, have patient swallow a sip of water from a cup before offering other foods or fluids. Observe for coughing, choking, or noisy lung sounds. *These are signs of difficulty swallowing.*
- Request speech pathologist evaluation if indicated *to diagnose specific swallowing problems and make recommendations.*
- Implement measures to prevent aspiration. *Aspiration can lead to pneumonia, which will greatly complicate the patient's recovery.*
  - Stay with patient during meals.
  - Ensure that patient is fully alert before feeding.
  - Have the patient in high-Fowler's position or chair for meals.

- Avoid use of straws.
- Use a thickening agent if swallowing study recommends.
- Place food on unaffected side of mouth.
- Teach the patient to swallow twice after each bite.
- Check the patient's mouth for pocketing of food.
- Have suction equipment available.
- Notify primary care provider if patient is unable to take in adequate oral calories. *A feeding tube may be necessary if patient is unable to take in enough calories to maintain nutrition. Advance directives should be consulted before a feeding tube is placed.*
- Assist with insertion and care of feeding tube if necessary. *If patient is unable to swallow effectively, a feeding tube may be necessary to maintain nutrition.*
- See Box 49.3 Nutrition Notes for additional interventions.

Disturbed sensory perception related to CNS damage

EXPECTED OUTCOME: The patient adapts to sensory-perceptual deficits as evidenced by avoidance of injury to affected areas.

PATIENT CARE TIP

A new stroke patient should never have anything by mouth until a dysphagia screening test has been successfully completed.

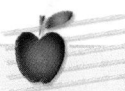

Box 49.3

Nutrition Notes

Feeding Patients with Swallowing Disorders

Suggestions for persons who have difficulty swallowing include the following:
- Eat slowly.
- Avoid distractions while eating.
- Do not talk while eating.
- Sit up straight while eating.
- Use a teaspoon, taking only half a teaspoonful at a time.
- Swallow completely between bites or sips.

Possible nursing interventions to aid a person with a swallowing disorder include the following:
- Remove loose dentures.
- Position the head correctly. A speech therapist can help determine the optimum head position. A hemiplegic patient often benefits from turning the head toward the weak side.
- When spoon feeding a patient with hemiplegia, place the food on the unaffected side of the tongue.
- Consult a dietitian concerning appropriate textures for liquids and solids. A multi-disciplinary assessment may be needed to tailor the diet prescription to the patient's strengths and weaknesses. Foods with mixed textures such as vegetable soup are frequently problematic. Often thicker substances are better managed than liquids. Although infant cereal can be an effective thickener, it may be rejected on a psychological basis in favor of instant potato flakes, unflavored gelatin, or a commercial thickener.

- Assist occupational therapist to assess for visual and/or spatial deficits and decreased sensory perception: heat and cold, position of body parts, pressure. *Identification of specific deficits is the first step in creating a plan of care.*
- Teach patient to scan the environment *to compensate for a visual deficit.*
- Implement plans for skin integrity and mobility *to protect patient from complications related to sensory deficits.*

Risk for impaired skin integrity: irritation or breakdown related to immobility and incontinence

EXPECTED OUTCOME: Skin integrity is maintained as evidenced by no redness or breakdown.
- Assess the skin frequently for redness or breakdown, especially around bony prominences, dependent areas, and perineum. *Any signs of breakdown must be treated immediately to prevent further damage.*
- Thoroughly cleanse and dry perineal area after each episode of incontinence. *Urine and feces can be very irritating to the skin.*

- If incontinence is unavoidable, use a barrier cream such as zinc oxide *to protect skin.*
- Turn and position the client at least every 2 hours, or more often if the client experiences breakdown. *Pressure impairs circulation and increases risk of breakdown.*
- Use a lift sheet to move patient in bed *to avoid damage from friction.*
- Consider the use of a pressure-reducing mattress if patient is not able to be out of bed for long periods. *This helps reduce pressure, but does not eliminate the need to reposition the patient every 2 hours.*
- If breakdown occurs, contact the physician or wound care specialist *for treatment recommendations.*

Incontinence related to loss of voluntary control of elimination

EXPECTED OUTCOME: Episodes of incontinence are avoided, or if unavoidable, they will be cleaned up quickly and skin complications avoided.
- Monitor for incontinence of bowel or bladder *so patient can be cleaned promptly and skin protected.*
- Assess for usual pattern of urinary and bowel elimination. *Keeping the patient on his or her regular prehospitalization pattern may help prevent incontinence.*
- Provide assistance with toileting according to the patient's usual schedule. *The patient who is unable to get up unaided may wait too long for help or try to get up alone and be injured.*
- Respond quickly to requests for assistance with toileting *to avoid accidental incontinence.*

Self-care deficit related to decreased motor function, spatial-perceptual alterations, and fear of injury

EXPECTED OUTCOME: Self-care is accomplished as evidenced by patient's ADL needs being met, and patient becomes increasingly independent.
- Assess patient's ability to perform ADLs. *A good assessment will guide development of a care plan.*
- Work with patient to create a plan for meeting daily physical needs. *The patient will be more likely to participate in a plan if he or she participated in creating it.*
- Encourage highest level of independence possible; facilitate patient's ability to do ADLs. *Providing too much assistance can promote dependence and further loss of mobility.*
- Place objects within reach and within visual field.
- Place food/fluids within patient's visual field.
- Encourage use of assistive devices.
- Assist patient with learning to use nondominant side of body. *If dominant side is affected, the patient may have to use the nondominant side.*
- Provide positive feedback *to help reduce discouragement with slow progress.*
- Provide education for family members and significant others regarding patient's deficits and recovery

plan. *The family can assist the patient with mobility if they understand what needs to be done.*

Impaired verbal communication: dysarthria related to loss of motor function of the muscles of speech articulation, or aphasia or dysphasia related to ischemia of the dominant hemisphere

EXPECTED OUTCOME: *Communication will be effective as evidenced by patient communicating needs and desires effectively, and frustration is avoided.*

- Assess for difficulties in verbal communication (difficulty speaking, articulating or incorrect ordering of words, inability to find or name words and objects). *A good assessment will guide planning of care.*
- Consult speech pathologist for assistance in determining types of aphasia or dysphasia and need for follow-up treatment. *A speech pathologist is specially trained to diagnose and treat communication problems, and can work with nursing staff to develop a plan of care.*
- Implement measures to facilitate communication: *These measures help assure the patient has his or her immediate needs met while learning to adapt to communication impairment.*
  - Answer call light in person.
  - Assess needs frequently.
  - Listen carefully: avoid interrupting patient and allow ample time for communication.

- When patient is tired, ask questions that require short answers.
- Provide and use appropriate aids to communication (picture board, magic slate, pencil and paper). See Figure 49.8.
- Provide education to family members and significant others regarding communication problems and interventions *so they can communicate with patient and participate in care.*
- If the patient is unable to communicate, do not assume that he cannot hear and understand. Every effort should be made to speak to the patient and to keep conversation appropriate when it is within the patient's range of hearing. *The patient may understand exactly what is being said, even if he or she is unable to respond.*
- Contact physician if impairment increases. *This may be a sign of stroke extension.*

Disturbed thought processes related to cerebral ischemia

EXPECTED OUTCOMES: *Patient's thought processes are as clear as possible within limitations of brain damage; patient's safety is maintained; patient feels calm and safe.*

- Assess patient for thought process impairment such as shortened attention span, impaired memory, confusion, slowed or quick and impulsive responses,

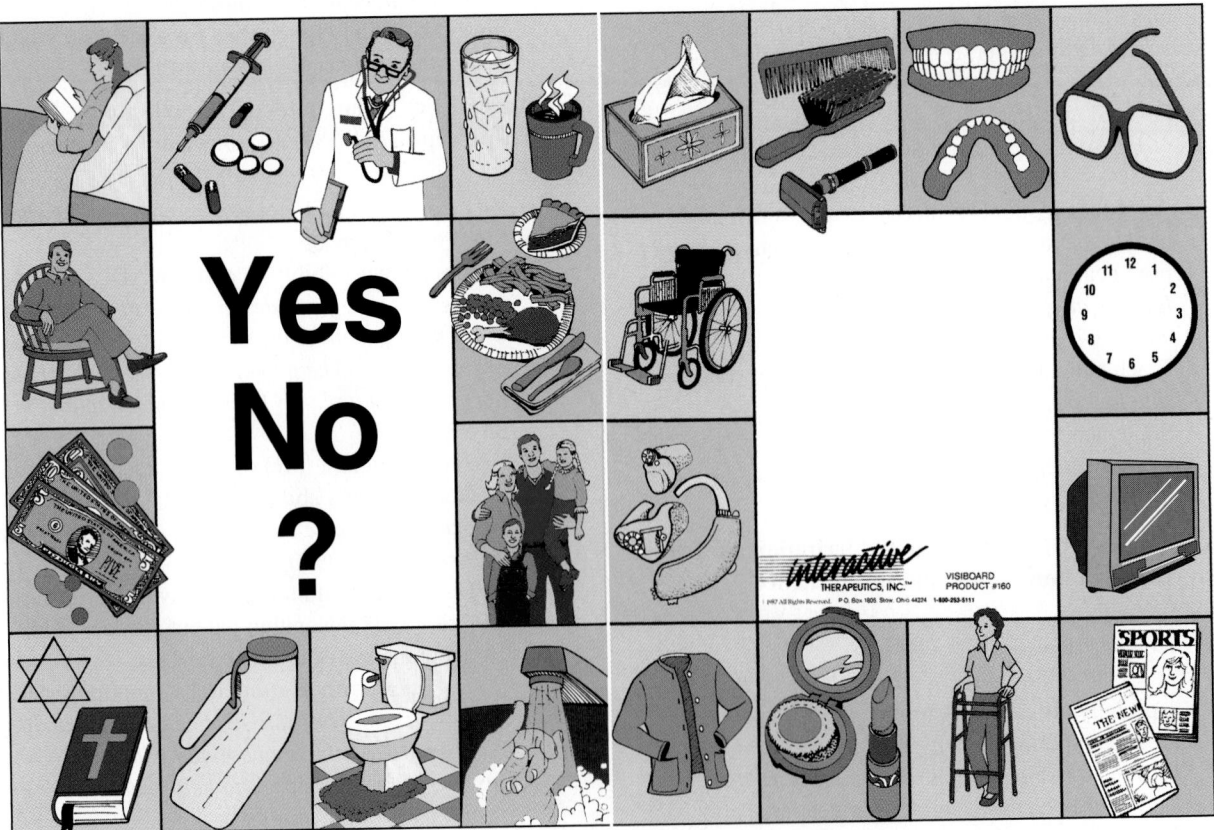

FIGURE 49.8 Picture board.

and aggressive and/or inappropriate responses. *Disturbed thinking can be manifested in a variety of ways (see Chapter 48 for care of patients with disturbed thought processes).*

Deficient knowledge related to diagnosis and treatment

EXPECTED OUTCOME: Patient and family have necessary knowledge to make decisions and assist with care.

- Explain what has happened to the patient. Explain tests, procedures, and care activities. *The patient and significant others are likely to be very frightened of what is happening. Correct information about what a stroke is, tests and procedures, and rationale for care activities help reduce anxiety.*
- Present information in small amounts and as simply as possible. *The patient may have difficulty attending to large amounts of information while acutely ill or if thought processes are disturbed.*
- Orient the patient and family to the ICU or other setting and the constant monitoring provided. *This can help reduce anxiety and reassure the patient and significant others that the patient is receiving competent care.*
- If the patient is to be discharged to home, make sure information is provided related to medications, treatments, and follow-up care. *The patient and family need to know how to provide appropriate care at home.*
- Evaluate the need for home nursing, physical, and occupational therapy, and request appropriate referrals. *The patient will likely need continued therapy after discharge to regain as much function as possible.*

Risk for caregiver role strain related to changes in roles, responsibilities, finances, and intimacy

EXPECTED OUTCOMES: Caregiver is comfortable with role as evidenced by statement that she or he understands how to care for the patient and has the needed resources to do so. Caregiver maintains her or his own health.

- Work with caregiver to assess how the patient's functional level will affect their lives. *Assumption of roles or responsibilities previously fulfilled by the patient may be very stressful to significant others. If the caregiver can anticipate the impact, he or she can plan ahead how to make sure needs are met.*
- Encourage patient and caregiver to identify support systems and make use of community resources. Provide a list of resources. *If support is in place before discharge, they are more likely to use it after the patient goes home.*
- Consult social worker or case manager. *These individuals have access to many resources, and can help the patient and caregiver identify appropriate sources of assistance.*
- Provide support if transfer to a skilled nursing facil-

ity is necessary. *This can be a very difficult decision for a patient and caregiver.*

Evaluation

If interventions have been effective, the patient does not experience increased deficits due to decreased perfusion of brain cells. The patient should recover physical limitations or make a good adjustment to remaining deficits and be independent in ADLs. The patient is able to communicate effectively and has needs and desires understood (see Box 49.4 Stroke Summary).

Box 49.4

Stroke Summary

Signs and Symptoms	Dizziness, syncope, visual disturbances, irritability, restlessness, confusion, decreased level of consciousness, unequal pupils, paresthesias, motor weakness, paralysis, seizures, difficulty swallowing, difficulty understanding language, difficulty speaking
Diagnostic Tests	• CT scan • ECG • Carotid Doppler • Echocardiogram • TEE, angiogram • Laboratory: INR/PT, metabolic panel, CBC, PTT, serum pregnancy (if appropriate), oxygen saturation
Therapeutic Interventions	• Oxygen • Antiplatelet, anticoagulant medication • Physical, occupational, speech therapy • Carotid endarterectomy • Knee-high antiembolism stockings
Complications	Stroke evolves causing more deficits, aspiration pneumonia, skin breakdown, malnutrition
Priority Nursing Diagnoses	Ineffective cerebral tissue perfusion Ineffective airway clearance Risk for injury

CBC = complete blood count; CT = computed tomography; ECG = electrocardiogram; INR/PT = international normalized ratio/prothrombin time; PTT = partial thromboplastin time; TEE = transesophageal echocardiography.

Home Health Hints

- Work with physical therapist, occupational therapist, and speech therapist to assist the patient with rehabilitation.
- Provide assistive devices to aid the patient to function independently.
- Keep home environment clutter-free to prevent falls.
- Offer frequent praise for all achievements.
- Keep regularly used items close by. If the patient is using a walker have him or her tie a small bag to the top to store these items.
- If the patient does not have a portable phone, encourage the purchase of one. Instruct the patient to keep it near at all times in case of an emergency.
- If necessary, assist the patient with obtaining a medical alert device. If the patient falls he or she can access an emergency medical service by pushing a button.

- Assist with obtaining homemaker or respite care for caregivers if necessary.
- Patients on a pureed diet can make their own food at home using a food processor. Baby food can also be purchased to meet swallowing guidelines.
- Patients with one-sided paralysis following a stroke should be instructed to wear clothes that are easy to get on and off. Examples include pants with elastic waists, shoes with elastic laces or slip-on shoes, and pullover shirts without buttons.
- If the patient has difficulty speaking (dysarthria), try using magnetic alphabet letters. Ask questions that require a yes or no answer. The patient can respond with the letter *y* or *n*. You can also help the patient and caregiver develop a communication board of frequently used words and objects.
- Keep bedside commode lids up with patches of Velcro attached to the seat and the frame.

REVIEW QUESTIONS

1. Which of the following are modifiable risk factors for stroke? Choose all answers that are correct.
   a. Heredity
   b. Age
   c. Diabetes
   d. Race
   e. High cholesterol
   f. Obesity

2. What is the most important diagnostic test that is completed immediately on the patient with symptoms of stroke in the emergency department?
   a. Head CT scan
   b. Arteriogram
   c. PT/INR
   d. CPSS

3. How soon after symptom onset must a stroke victim receive thrombolytic treatment?
   a. 1 hour
   b. 2 hours
   c. 3 hours
   d. 4 hours

4. A patient is experiencing receptive aphasia. This means that he has difficulty with which of the following functions?
   a. Swallowing
   b. Forming words
   c. Hearing
   d. Understanding language

5. A nurse is caring for a patient who is recovering from an ischemic stroke. Upon entering his room to pick up his supper tray, the nurse notes that he has only eaten half his meal. What should the nurse do?
   a. Assist him by handing him finger foods and feeding him items that require a utensil.
   b. Remove his tray and do not comment.
   c. Enourage him to eat the rest of his meal.
   d. Turn his plate 180 degrees and observe his response.

6. A nurse is doing an afternoon assessment on a patient transferred to a medical unit from intensive care following a subarachnoid hemorrhage. The patient was alert and oriented during the morning assessment, but complained of being very tired. Now the patient is difficult to arouse. What action should the nurse take?
   a. Let the patient sleep; transferring from ICU can be very strenuous.
   b. Reassess the patient in an hour. If the sleepiness continues, notify the RN.
   c. Call the RN immediately.
   d. Call a code.

References

1. Antonio Culebras, MD, Kase CS, Masdeu JC, et al: Practice guidelines for the use of imaging in transient ischemic attacks and acute stroke-introduction. Stroke 28:1480–1497, 1997.
2. American Heart Association: Heart Disease and Stroke Statistics 2005 Update. Accessed August 4, 2005 at www.americanheart.org.
3. National Institute of Neurological Disorders and Stroke. Brain basics: Preventing stroke. Accessed March 23, 2006 at www.ninds.nih.gov/disorders/stroke/preventing_stroke.htm.
4. Project Brain Save, St. Joseph Mercy Oakland, Michigan. CD Rom printed for education purposes.

SUGGESTED ANSWERS TO

CRITICAL THINKING

■ Mr. Jankowski

Ask Mr. Jankowski about other risk factors for stroke, such as his dietary and alcohol habits. Check his chart for history of diabetes, hypertension, or heart disease. Check his weight and cholesterol levels if drawn. Educate him about risk factors for stroke, and how they can be modified. Consider a dietitian consultation, and provide written information on stroke prevention and smoking cessation. As a nurse, you will be in a position to recognize risks and help patients modify risk factors for many problems before they occur.

■ Mrs. Washington

1. Uncontrolled hypertension, in the presence of a preexisting aneurysm, might have precipitated Mrs. Washington's stroke.
2. Her left extremities are affected.
3. Mrs. Washington is disoriented. Her room should be as close to the nurse's station as possible. Reorient her to her surroundings and condition frequently. Keep side rails up when Mrs. Washington is alone.

   Mrs. Washington also has hemiparesis. Obtain a commode because Mrs. Washington will probably not be able to walk to the bathroom. Place the call light and telephone on her right side. Assist Mrs. Washington with positioning to prevent injury to her affected limbs.
4. If Mrs. Washington will be going back to her home, you should teach Mrs. Washington and her daughter about the relationship of uncontrolled hypertension to intracranial hemorrhage; options for inpatient, outpatient, and in-home therapy; and memory strategies to prevent missed medication doses (e.g., weekly pill box, keeping medications with breakfast food, or an alarm clock or watch).

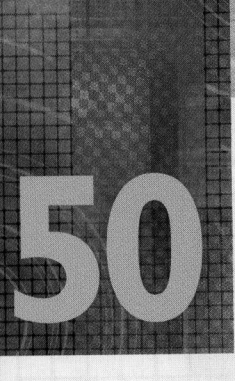

50

Nursing Care of Patients with Peripheral Nervous System Disorders

DEBORAH L. WEAVER

KEY TERMS

amyotrophic (ay-MY-oh-TROH-fik)
anticholinesterase (AN-ti-KOH-lin-ESS-ter-ays)
atrophy (AT-roh-fee)
degeneration (de-jen-er-AY-shun)
demyelination (dee-MY-uh-lin-AY-shun)
exacerbation (egg-sass-ur-BAY-shun)
fasciculation (fah-SIK-yoo-LAY-shun)
neuralgia (new-RAL-jee-ah)
neuropathies (new-RAH-puh-thees)
plasmapheresis (PLAS-mah-fer-EE-sis)
polyneuropathy (PAH-lee-new-RAH-puh-thee)
ptosis (TOH-sis)
remyelination (ree-MY-uh-lin-AY-shun)
sclerosis (skle-ROH-sis)

QUESTIONS TO GUIDE YOUR READING

1. What disorders are caused by disruption of the peripheral nervous system?

2. What are the pathophysiology, major signs and symptoms, and complications of selected peripheral nervous system disorders?

3. What are therapeutic interventions for selected peripheral nervous system disorders?

4. What are the common nursing diagnoses associated with peripheral nervous system disorders?

5. What are priority nursing interventions for patients with peripheral nervous system disorders?

6. How will you know if your nursing care has been effective?

The peripheral nervous system (PNS) consists of all nervous system structures outside the central nervous system (CNS). A variety of disorders affect the PNS. Some of these disorders become chronic and cause **degeneration** of body systems. Some other disorders are of a temporary nature. Two common types of PNS disorders are discussed in this chapter. Neuromuscular disorders compose one group and may include motor or sensory disorders or both. The second group includes cranial nerve disorders. Both types of disorders present a challenge to the nurse caring for the patient and family.

 NEUROMUSCULAR DISORDERS

This group of neurological conditions is chronic and degenerative in nature. Neuromuscular disorders involve a disruption of the transmission of impulses between neurons and the muscles that they stimulate. This breakdown in transmission results in muscle weakness. If the muscles of the respiratory system are affected, deadly complications can develop, including pneumonia and respiratory failure. Common neuromuscular disorders include multiple **sclerosis** (MS), myasthenia gravis (MG), **amyotrophic** lateral sclerosis (ALS), and Guillain-Barré syndrome (GBS). An additional neuropathic disorder, Navajo neuropathy, is discussed in Box 50.1 Cultural Considerations.

Multiple Sclerosis

Pathophysiology

Multiple sclerosis is a chronic progressive degenerative disease that affects the myelin sheath of the neurons in the central nervous system. Myelin is responsible for the smooth transmission of nerve impulses. Muscles contract when nerve impulses stimulate the muscle tissue. If the myelin sheath is damaged (Fig. 50.1), nerve impulses cannot be transmitted to the muscle and contraction of the muscle does not occur. In multiple sclerosis, the myelin sheath begins to break down (degenerate) as a result of the activation of the body's immune system. The nerve becomes inflamed and edematous. Nerve impulses to the muscles slow down. As the disease progresses, sclerosis or scar tissue damages the nerve. Nerve impulses become completely blocked causing permanent loss of muscle function in that area of the body.

Etiology

Damage to the myelin sheath is thought to be from an autoimmune process; however, the disease may be related to viral infections, heredity, and other unknown factors. Some research indicates that there is an inherited tendency to develop MS, and the manifestations of the disease only appear in the presence of environmental triggers. Thus, the cause of MS is not really understood. This disease affects 400,000 persons in the United States and up to 2.5 million people worldwide.[1] Onset of the disease usually occurs between the ages of 20 and 50. Women are affected twice as often as men. The course of the disease is unpredictable, and there are many variations in symptoms, depending on which nerves are affected. Some individuals have mild illness, while others suffer permanent disability or rapid decline and death.

Signs and Symptoms

The patient with MS presents with muscle weakness, tingling sensations, and numbness. Other common symptoms include visual disturbances, usually in one eye at a time; disturbances may be accompanied by pain with eye movement. These symptoms may begin slowly over weeks to months or start suddenly and dramatically. MS affects many systems of

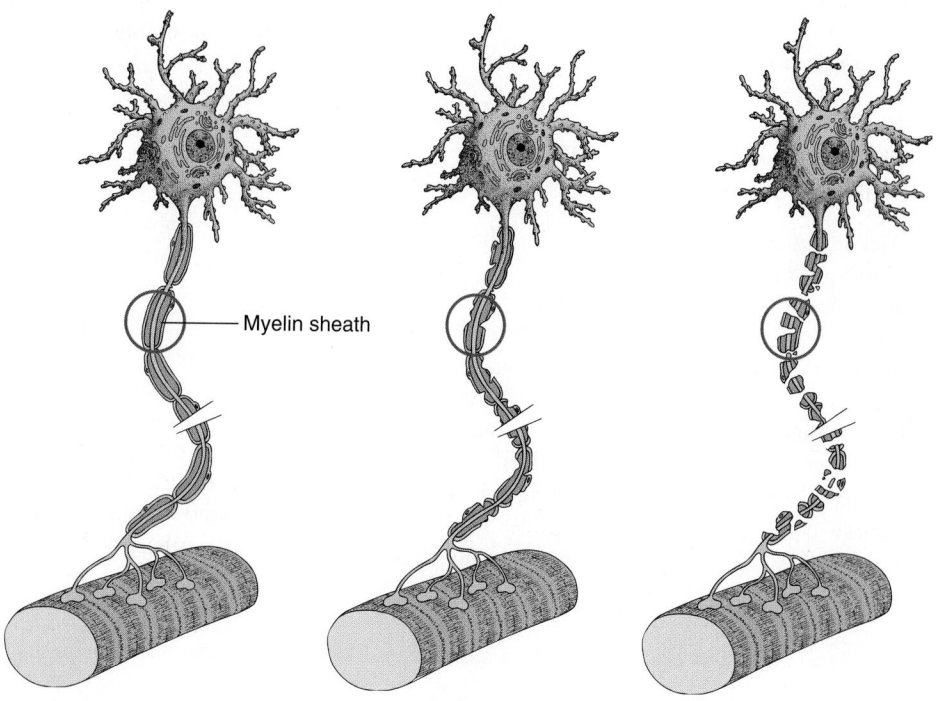

FIGURE 50.1 The myelin sheath breaks down in multiple sclerosis, interrupting transmission of nerve impulses. *(A)* Normal myelin sheath. *(B)* Myelin beginning to break down. *(C)* Total myelin disruption. *(Modified from Scanlon, VC, and Sanders, T: Workbook for Essentials of Anatomy and Physiology, ed. 5. F.A. Davis, Philadelphia, 2007, with permission.)*

Myelin sheath

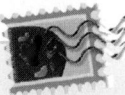

Box 50.1

Cultural Considerations

Navajo neuropathy is unique to the Navajo Indian population. Characteristics include poor weight gain, short stature, sexual infantilism, serious systemic infections, and liver derangement. Manifestations include weakness, hypotonia, areflexia, loss of sensation in the extremities, corneal ulcerations, acral (extremity) mutilation, and painless fractures.[2] Nerve biopsies show a nearly complete absence of myelinated fibers, which is different from other neuropathies, that presents as a gradual demyelination process. Individuals who survive have many complications and are generally ventilator dependent. None has been known to survive past the age of 24.

LEARNING TIP

Myelin facilitates impulse transmission to the muscle. If myelin is interrupted, the impulse cannot get to the muscle efficiently so the muscle response may be sluggish, unpredictable, or absent.

the body (Box 50.2 Problems Associated with Multiple Sclerosis). A variety of factors can trigger the onset of symptoms or aggravate the condition, including extreme heat and cold, fatigue, infection, and physical and emotional stress. Hormonal changes after pregnancy may also cause symptom onset or exacerbations. Periods of **exacerbation** and remission of symptoms lead patients with MS to be uncertain about when the disease will flare up and what system of the body will be affected. Intense fatigue is a common complaint among patients; therefore, immobility can become a problem. Accidents and falls are common because of muscular weakness or numbness of the trunk and extremities. Some people with MS suffer with symptoms such as muscle spasticity, bowel or bladder dysfunction, or paralysis. Difficulty with concentration or forgetfulness can also be problematic. Pneumonia can occur from immobility and from weakness

of the diaphragm and intercostal muscles. Death, often resulting from respiratory infection, typically occurs 20 to 35 years after diagnosis.

Diagnostic Tests

Diagnosis is based on the history and signs and symptoms experienced by the patient. MS cannot be diagnosed by a specific test. Analysis of cerebrospinal fluid (CSF) may show an increase in oligoclonal immunoglobulin G (IgG). Magnetic resonance imaging (MRI) may be helpful in diagnosis because sclerotic plaques can be detected.

Therapeutic Interventions

MS has no cure. Many individuals with MS do well with no medication treatment at all. Interferon therapy with beta-interferons such as Betaseron or Avonex may reduce exacerbations and delay disability. Other treatment is supportive and symptomatic. Steroids such as adrenocorticotropic hormone (ACTH), prednisone, and other corticotropics are given to decrease inflammation and edema of the neuron, which may relieve some symptoms. Immunosuppressant drugs such as azathioprine (Imuran) and cyclophosphamide (Cytoxan) may be given to depress the immune system. Anticonvulsants such as phenytoin (Dilantin) and carbamazepine (Tegretol) help relieve neuropathic pain. Valium (Diazepam), baclofen (Lioresal), and tizanidine (Zanaflex) and physical therapy assist in controlling muscle spasms. Bladder problems are treated with parasympathetic agents such as bethanechol (Urecholine) and oxybutynin (Ditropan). Fatigue may be treated with antidepressants or an antiviral agent such as amantadine (Symmetrel). See Table 50.1 for a summary of medications used to treat PNS disorders.

Rehabilitation after an acute episode includes physical, speech, and occupational therapies. Rehabilitation therapy assists the patient and family in adapting the home environment to the patient's special needs. Instruction in the use of assistive devices (e.g., braces, canes, wheelchairs, splints) by physical and occupational therapists allows the patient increased mobility and independence. Patients who develop speech difficulties benefit from speech therapy. For those individuals who suffer sudden severe attacks or who do not respond to high doses of steroids, plasma exchange or **plasmapheresis** may be used to remove antibodies that may be attacking the myelin from the blood (Table 50.2).

Box 50.2

Problems Associated with Multiple Sclerosis

Weakness/paralysis of limbs, trunk, or head	Impaired hearing
Diplopia (double vision)	Nystagmus
Slurred speech	Ataxia
Spasticity of muscles	Dysarthria
Numbness and tingling	Dysphagia
Patchy blindness (scotomas)	Constipation
Blurred vision	Spastic (uninhibited) bladder
Vertigo	Flaccid (hypotonic) bladder
Tinnitus	Sexual dysfunction
	Anger, depression, euphoria

plasmapheresis: plasma—liquid of blood + pheresis—removal

TABLE 50.1 MEDICATIONS USED TO TREAT PNS DISORDERS

Medication Class/Action	Examples	Route	Side Effects	Nursing Implications
Cholinesterase Inhibitors Increase acetylcholine at synapses	Neostigmine (Prostigmin) Pyridostigmine (Mestinon) Edrophonium chloride (Tensilon, used in diagnosis)	PO PO, IM, IV IM, IV	Cholinergic toxicity (SLUDGE)	Atropine is antidote.
Glucocorticoids Reduce inflammation	Prednisone Prednisolone Prednisolone acetate or sodium phosphate	PO PO IV, IM	Osteoporosis Risk for infection Elevated blood sugar Sodium and water retention Cushing's syndrome	Provide calcium supplement. Avoid crowds and others with infections. Monitor fluid balance. May need to treat blood sugar with insulin while on medication.
Immunosuppressants Suppress immunity and antibody formation	Azathioprine (Imuran) Cyclophosphamide (Cytoxan)	PO, IV PO, IV	Anorexia, hepatotoxicity, nausea, vomiting, anemia, leukopenia, thrombocytopenia, fever, chills	Monitor blood counts. Protect from bleeding and infection. Administer with meals to reduce nausea.
Antispasmodics/Muscle Relaxants Relax muscles, reduce pain	Dantrolene (Dantrium) Baclofen (Lioresal) Diazepam (Valium)	PO, IV PO PO, IM, IV	CNS depression Nausea Constipation Urinary retention Sedation Muscle weakness Diarrhea (dantrolene)	Avoid operating machinery, driving until effects known. Provide measures to prevent constipation (except dantrolene). Monitor for respiratory depression.
Anticonvulsants Treat nerve pain	Phenytoin (Dilantin) Carbamazepine (Tegretol) Gabapentin (Neurontin) Valproic acid (Depakene)	PO PO PO PO	CNS depression Gingival hyperplasia (phenytoin) Ataxia, vertigo Bone marrow suppression GI upset	Teach good oral hygiene with soft bristle brush, floss, and gum massage (phenytoin). Monitor for fall risk. Monitor blood counts.
Glutamate Antagonist Delays progression of ALS	Riluzole (Rilutek)	PO	Decreased strength, diarrhea, nausea, vomiting, abdominal pain, dizziness, vertigo, sedation	Rest, monitor for respiratory depression; administer on empty stomach; avoid large quantities of caffeine; avoid charcoal-broiled foods.

Nursing Care

See Box 50.3 Nursing Care Plan for the Patient with a Progressive Neuromuscular Disorder.

In addition to routine care, instruct the patient to avoid factors that can exacerbate symptoms. This includes avoiding stressful situations as much as possible. Rest, exercise, and a balanced diet are important self-care steps to control symptoms. In addition, avoiding extreme temperature changes, especially heat, as well as avoiding infection and illness, is important. Any infection, especially respiratory, should be reported immediately to a physician. Two sources of information on MS are the National Multiple Sclerosis Society at www.nationalmssociety.org and the Multiple Sclerosis Foundation at www.msfocus.org

Myasthenia Gravis

Pathophysiology

Myasthenia gravis (MG) means "grave muscle weakness," or weakness of the voluntary or skeletal muscles of the body. MG is a disease of the neuromuscular junction (Fig. 50.2).

TABLE 50.2 PLASMAPHERESIS*

Preprocedure Nursing Care	Postprocedure Nursing Care
Teach patient about the procedure and what to expect, including what the machine looks like (similar to but smaller than a dialysis machine), the need for arterial and venous access sites, and the length of the procedure (2 to 5 hours).	Observe the patient for signs of hypovolemia, such as dizziness and hypotension.
The physician may order medications held until after the procedure.	Apply pressure dressings to access sites.
Assess baseline vital signs and weight.	Monitor patient for infection and bruits at the access site.
Assess complete blood cell count (CBC), platelet count, and clotting studies.	Monitor electrolytes and signs of electrolyte loss. Report imbalances, and administer replacement electrolytes as ordered.
Check blood type and crossmatch for replacement blood products.	Compare preprocedure and postprocedure laboratory data, such as CBC, platelet count, and clotting times.

*Plasmapheresis, also known as plasma exchange therapy, is a procedure that removes the plasma component from whole blood and replaces it with fresh plasma. The goal of this therapy is to remove antibodies through exchanging plasma to suppress the immune response and inflammation.

Box 50.3   NURSING CARE PLAN for the Patient with a Progressive Neuromuscular Disorder

Nursing Diagnosis: Ineffective airway clearance related to respiratory muscle weakness, impaired cough and gag reflexes

Expected Outcomes Patient will maintain a patent airway. Patient will be free of signs and symptoms of respiratory distress.

Evaluation of Outcomes Is patient's airway patent? Is patient free of signs and symptoms of respiratory distress?

Interventions	Rationale	Evaluation of Interventions
Monitor respiratory rate and depth, oxygen saturation (SaO_2), and arterial blood gases (as ordered). Report deterioration.	Increasing respiratory distress indicates progressing muscle weakness that may require mechanical ventilation or end-of-life decisions.	Is patient's respiratory rate status stable or is intervention indicated?
Encourage patient to cough and deep breathe every 2 hours.	Effective coughing helps keep airway clear.	Does patient have the strength to cough effectively?
Observe patient for breathlessness while speaking.	Inability to speak without breathlessness indicates declining respiratory function.	Is patient able to finish sentences without needing to take a breath?
Elevate head of bed.	Fowler's position improves lung expansion, decreases work of breathing, improves cough efforts, and decreases risk for aspiration.	Does elevation of head of bed help relieve dyspnea and prevent aspiration?
Evaluate cough, swallow, and gag reflexes frequently. Notify physician if absent.	Frequent evaluation of reflexes is needed to prevent aspiration, respiratory infections, and respiratory failure.	Is patient able to cough effectively? Is gag reflex intact?
Suction secretions as needed, noting color and amount of secretions.	Muscle weakness may result in inability to clear airway.	Does patient require suctioning to clear airway? What color are secretions?

Nursing Diagnosis: Impaired physical mobility related to muscle weakness

Expected Outcomes Patient will identify measures to help maintain mobility. Patient will perform exercises that help maintain current mobility. Patient will maintain optimum mobility and activity level.

Evaluation of Outcomes Can patient identify measures that will help maintain mobility? Does patient perform exercises that help maintain mobility? Is optimum activity level maintained?

Interventions	Rationale	Evaluation of Interventions
Determine current level of mobility.	Provides information to formulate plan of care.	What is patient's present level of mobility?
Identify factors that affect ability to be mobile and active.	Provides opportunity to seek answers for problems.	Is patient able to identify factors that help or hinder mobility?
Encourage patient to perform self-care to maximum ability.	Promotes sense of control and independence for patient.	Does patient perform self-care activities? Is assistance required?
Consult physical therapist (PT) or occupational therapist (OT) to provide assistive devices for walking (canes, braces, walker, wheelchair) and other activities.	Assistive devices decrease fatigue, promote independence, comfort, and safety.	Does patient use assistive devices safely during activities? Do they help keep patient active?
Reposition frequently when patient is immobile.	Prevents skin breakdown and stasis of pulmonary secretions.	Is patient free from complications of immobility?
Provide active/passive range-of-motion (ROM) exercises on a regular basis.	Prevents contractures and disuse atrophy.	Does patient have any contractures or atrophy?
Plan activities with a balance of frequent rest periods.	Rest decreases fatigue.	Is fatigue controlled?
Administer medications as ordered.	Medications may slow progress of disease and reduce symptoms.	Are symptoms controlled?

Nursing Diagnosis: Risk for imbalanced nutrition related to weakness or lack of coordination of muscles for chewing and swallowing

Expected Outcomes Patient will maintain body weight within normal limits for height and frame.

Evaluation of Outcomes Is patient's weight stable and within normal limits (WNL)?

Interventions	Rationale	Evaluation of Interventions
Evaluate cough, swallow, and gag reflexes frequently. Notify physician if absent.	If patient is unable to swallow, a feeding tube may be indicated, depending on patient's wishes.	Does patient eat and drink without aspirating?
Offer soft, easy to chew and swallow foods.	Soft foods require less effort to chew and are less fatiguing.	Is patient able to chew and swallow without excessive fatigue?
Institute swallowing precautions as needed.	Swallowing precautions help prevent aspiration and allow patient to maintain oral intake as long as possible.	Do precautions prevent aspiration?
Request speech therapy and dietitian consultations as indicated.	Speech therapy can help evaluate swallowing and make recommendations. Dietitian can provide appropriate foods.	Are consults indicated? Are recommendations implemented?

(Continued on following page)

Box 50.3   NURSING CARE PLAN for the Patient with a Progressive Neuromuscular Disorder (*Continued*)

Nursing Diagnosis: Impaired verbal communication related to impaired respiratory and muscle function

Expected Outcomes Patient will be able to communicate needs.

Evaluation of Outcomes Does patient indicate that needs are met with a minimum of frustration?

Interventions	Rationale	Evaluation of Interventions
Assess ability to speak and communicate.	Assessment is essential to planning appropriate communication interventions.	Can patient speak or communicate needs?
Request referral to speech therapist for assistance if indicated.	Speech therapist can recommend appropriate alternative communication techniques.	Is speech therapy referral indicated? Is referral completed?
Assess for nonverbal signs of pain or distress, such as restlessness, agitation, grimacing.	Patient may not be able to tell you if he or she is in pain or distress.	Are signs of pain or distress present? Are they attended to?
Use picture board or paper and pencil. Ask questions that require yes or no answer.	These do not require the patient to speak to communicate.	Do alternative methods help patient communicate needs?
Use nonhurried, calm, and caring approach while providing care.	This will help decrease anxiety and provide emotional support to patient and family	Do patient and family appear anxious? Does calm approach help?
Explain all procedures.	Patient can still hear and needs to know what is happening.	Does patient indicate understanding?

Normally, at the neuromuscular junction, the neuron releases the chemical neurotransmitter acetylcholine (ACh), which crosses the synaptic cleft. Receptors on the muscle tissue take up ACh and contraction of the muscle results. In MG, the body's immune system is activated, producing antibodies that attack and destroy ACh receptors at the neuromuscular junction. ACh cannot stimulate muscle contraction because the number of ACh receptors has been reduced, resulting in loss of voluntary muscle strength.

Etiology

Myasthenia gravis is a chronic autoimmune process. No specific cause has been found for MG. However, current thought is that a virus may initiate the disease. Disorders of the thymus gland are often associated with MG. Thymomas or tumors on the thymus gland may account for the malfunction of the immune system that initiates the autoimmune process. All ethnic groups and both genders can develop this disease. Peak age of onset in women is 20 to 30 years. Men are affected more often after age 60. MG occurs slightly more often in women than men.

Signs and Symptoms

MG results in progressive extreme muscle weakness. The hallmark of MG is increased muscle weakness during activity and improvement in muscle strength after rest. Muscles are strongest in the morning, when the person is rested. Activity causes the muscles to fatigue easily, but rest allows the muscles to regain strength. Activities affected by MG include eye and eyelid movements, chewing, swallowing, speaking, and breathing, as well as skeletal muscle function. Patients often present with drooping of the eyelids (**ptosis**). Facial expressions are masklike. After long conversations, the patient's voice may fade. Falls occur because of weakness of the arm and leg muscles. Patients with MG experience periods of exacerbation and remission of symptoms, similar to patients with multiple sclerosis. Exacerbations can be caused by emotional or physical stress, such as pregnancy, menses, illness, trauma, extremes in temperature, electrolyte imbalance, surgery, and drugs that block actions at the neuromuscular junction.

Complications

Major complications associated with MG result from weakness of muscles that assist with swallowing and breathing. Aspiration, respiratory infections, and respiratory failure are the leading causes of death. Sudden onset of muscle weakness in patients with MG resulting from not enough medication is called a myasthenic crisis. Overmedication with

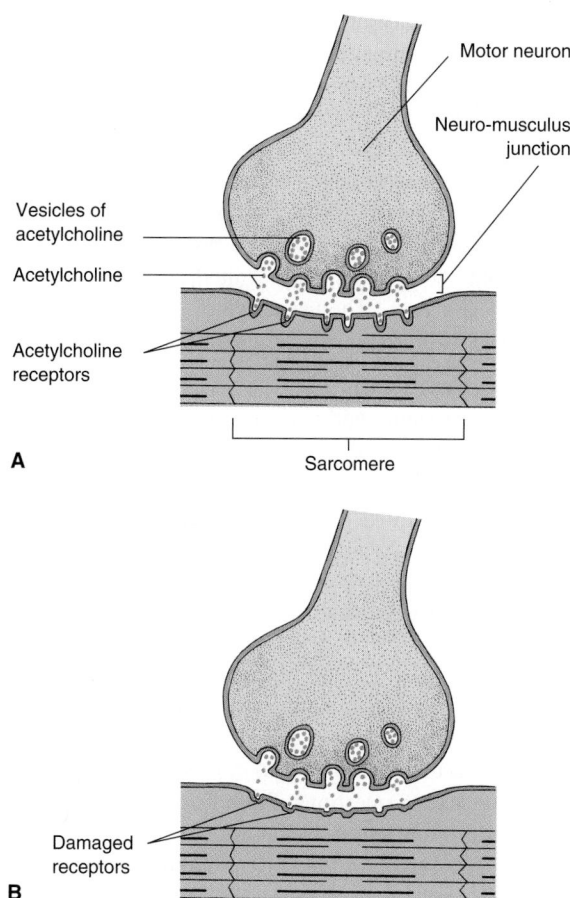

FIGURE 50.2 Myasthenia gravis. (A) Normal neuromuscular junction. (B) Note damaged acetylcholine receptor sites in myasthenia gravis. *(Modified from Scanlon, VC, and Sanders, T: Workbook for Essentials of Anatomy and Physiology, ed. 5. F.A. Davis, Philadelphia, 2007, with permission.)*

 LEARNING TIP

Symptoms of cholinergic crisis can be remembered with the acronym SLUDGE: salivation, lacrimation, urination, diarrhea, gastrointestinal cramping, and emesis. A severe crisis has been described as "liquid pouring out of every body orifice."

anticholinesterase drugs causes a cholinergic crisis (Table 50.3). Both crises require immediate medical attention.

Diagnostic Tests

Diagnosis of myasthenia gravis is based on history of symptoms and physical examination of the patient. A simple test involves the patient looking upward for 2 to 3 minutes. Increased droop of the eyelids (ptosis) occurs if MG is present. After a brief rest, the eyelids can be opened without dif-

anticholinesterase: anti—against + cholinesterase—chemical that breaks down acetylcholine

TABLE 50.3 COMPARISON OF MYASTHENIC CRISIS AND CHOLINERGIC CRISIS

Myasthenic Crisis	Cholinergic Crisis
Cause	***Cause***
Too little medication	Too much medication
Signs and Symptoms	***Signs and Symptoms***
Ptosis	Increasing muscle weakness
Difficulty swallowing	Dyspnea
Difficulty speaking	Salivation
Dyspnea	Nausea or vomiting
Weakness	Abdominal cramping
	Sweating
	Increased bronchial secretions
	Miosis (constriction of pupils)

ficulty. Another test involves an intravenous injection of edrophonium (Tensilon, an anticholinesterase drug). If muscle strength improves dramatically (e.g., the patient can suddenly open the eyes wide), MG is diagnosed. However, improvement is only temporary. An increased number of anti-ACh receptor antibodies in the blood are present in 90% of patients with MG. Electromyography (EMG) may be done to rule out other conditions. Pulmonary function tests may be done to predict or anticipate potential myasthenic crisis leading to respiratory failure.

Therapeutic Interventions

No cure has been found for MG. Treatment is aimed at control of symptoms. Removal of the thymus gland (thymectomy) can decrease production of ACh receptor antibodies and decrease symptoms in most patients. Medications used to treat MG include the anticholinesterase drugs neostigmine (Prostigmin) and pyridostigmine (Mestinon). These drugs improve symptoms of MG by destroying the acetylcholinesterase that breaks down ACh. Remember that ACh causes muscles to contract. If ACh is allowed more time to attach to muscle tissue receptors, the muscle contracts and strength is increased. Steroids such as prednisone and immunosuppressants are used to suppress the body's immune response. Plasmapheresis can be used to remove antibodies from the patient's blood (see Table 50.2).

Nursing Care

See Box 50.3 Nursing Care Plan for the Patient with a Progressive Neuromuscular Disorder.

In addition, schedule anticholinesterase drugs so that peak action occurs at times when increased muscle strength is needed for activities such as meals and physical therapy. Be aware of symptoms and treatment of myasthenic and cholinergic crises, so you can determine what immediate actions need to be taken.

PATIENT EDUCATION. Instruct the patient that nutritious, well-balanced meals provide caloric intake to maintain strength and resistance to infections. Teach the patient to schedule activities such as grocery shopping or errands at times when medication is at peak action, so that muscle strength is increased. Teach methods to conserve energy, such as sitting down to do grooming and housekeeping activities whenever possible. Explain that resting between activities allows time for muscle strength to be restored. Teach the importance of avoidance of persons with infections and exposure to cold to minimize risk for respiratory infections, which can exacerbate symptoms and increase risk for ineffective airway clearance. Teach signs and symptoms of crisis conditions because both crises constitute medical emergencies and require immediate medical attention (see Table 50.3).

There are many medications that should not be used with patients with MG such as D-penicillamine, alpha-interferon, and botulinum toxin. Other medications should be used with caution such as neuromuscular blocking agens, beta blockers, calcium channel blockers, some antibiotics, quinine, quinidine and procainamide. Many of these can exacerbate muscle weakness. Teach the patient to only use medications that are prescribed by the physician. If multiple providers are used, all medications should be checked with the provider who is treating the MG.

Provide information about support groups that can provide encouragement and assistance to patients and their families. More information can be found at the Myasthenia Gravis Foundation of America website www.myasthenia. org.

CRITICAL THINKING

Jamie

■ Jamie is referred to a neurologist with complaints of muscle weakness.

1. What history can help differentiate between MS and MG?
2. What assessment can be done to differentiate between MS and MG?
3. The neurologist prepares to do a Tensilon test and asks you to prepare 2 mg of Tensilon for IV injection. It is supplied as 10 mg per milliliter. How much should you draw up?

Suggested answers at end of chapter.

Amyotrophic Lateral Sclerosis

Pathophysiology and Etiology

Amyotrophic lateral sclerosis (ALS) (also called Lou Gehrig's disease) is a progressive, degenerative condition that affects motor neurons responsible for the control of voluntary muscles. Within the brain and spinal cord, upper and lower motor neurons begin to degenerate and form scar tissue or die, blocking transmission of nerve impulses. Without stimulation, **atrophy** of muscle tissue occurs, and muscle strength and coordination decrease. As the disease progresses, more muscle groups, including muscles controlling breathing and swallowing, become involved. However, the ability to think and reason is not affected.

ALS can occur at any age, but usually does not appear until adulthood. A specific cause has not been discovered, although ALS may have a genetic predisposition in some cases. About 5600 people in the United States are diagnosed with ALS each year.[3] The usual age of onset is between 40 and 70. ALS is more prevalent in men than women.

Signs and Symptoms

Symptoms are vague early in the course of ALS. Primary symptoms include progressive muscle weakness and decreased coordination of arms, legs, and trunk. Atrophy of muscles and twitching (**fasciculations**) also occur. Muscle spasms can cause pain. Difficulty with chewing and swallowing place the patient at a risk for choking and aspiration as the disease progresses. Inappropriate emotional outbursts of laughing and crying may occur. Speech becomes increasingly difficult. Bladder and bowel functions remain intact, yet problems such as constipation, urinary urgency, hesitancy, or frequency may occur. Late in the disease, communication becomes limited to moving and blinking of eyes in response to questions. Pulmonary function becomes severely compromised to the point of requiring mechanical assistance (ventilator) if the patient chooses. Other complications that may occur include extreme malnutrition, falls, pulmonary emboli, and congestive heart failure. ALS eventually leads to death from respiratory complications (atelectasis, respiratory failure, and pneumonia). Death usually occurs 3 to 5 years after diagnosis.

Diagnostic Tests

Diagnosis is made based on clinical symptoms. Additional tests such as CSF analysis, electroencephalogram (EEG), nerve biopsy, or electromyography (EMG) may be done to rule out other conditions. Blood enzymes may be increased as a result of muscle atrophy.

Therapeutic Interventions

Goals of treatment are aimed at improving function as long as possible and emotionally supporting the patient and family through the illness. Baclofen and diazepam may be given to relieve muscle spasticity. Quinine is used for muscle cramps. Riluzole has recently been approved by the Food and Drug Administration (FDA) to help reduce the damage to the motor neurons and may prolong survival by several months. Nonpharmacological measures such as physical therapy, massage, position changes, and diversional activities may be instituted for pain control. Tube feedings via a surgically placed gastrostomy tube help provide adequate nutrition. Prevention of infections, such as pneumonia and urinary tract infection (UTI), is vital. Meticulous skin care

---

atrophy: a—without + trophy—nourishment

minimizes the incidence of pressure ulcers. Rehabilitation therapy, including physical, occupational, and speech therapy, allows the patient to maximize function and control. Therapy may also decrease the occurrence of complications such as aspiration, falls, and contractures.

Individuals with speech problems may benefit from the use of augmentative alternative communication (AAC). A variety of AAC systems are available; most use laptop computers that patients can use to type in words or symbols to generate speech. Medicare now will pay at least a portion of the cost for AAC equipment.

Support groups and counseling provide emotional support for the patient and family. Most patients with ALS die within 3 to 5 years of diagnosis of respiratory failure. Ten percent of patients with ALS survive for 10 or more years.

Nursing Care

See Box 50.3 Nursing Care Plan for the Patient with a Progressive Neuromuscular Disorder.

PATIENT EDUCATION. Reinforce information given by the physician to the patient and family about ALS and its prognosis. Support groups can provide emotional support as the patient and family deal with the reality of eventual death. Rehabilitation using assistive devices and exercises helps prevent complications. Teaching family members how to perform physical therapy and other health-care activities allows the patient to spend as much time as possible at home. Teach the patient to avoid exposure to persons with infections because an infection can be deadly to the patient with a debilitating disease.

LEARNING TIP

A person with ALS has an intact mind—it is the body that is deteriorating.

CRITICAL THINKING

Mr. Miller

■ Mr. Miller has been having difficulty swallowing. He is diagnosed with ALS.
1. What are the priority nursing diagnoses for him?
2. How can the patient and his family be supported in coping with this disease?

Suggested answers at end of chapter.

Guillain-Barré Syndrome

Pathophysiology

Guillain-Barré syndrome (GBS) is also called acute inflammatory **polyneuropathy.** This term is more descriptive of

the actual disease process. GBS is an inflammatory disorder characterized by abrupt onset of symmetrical paresis (weakness) that progresses to paralysis. The myelin sheath of the spinal and cranial nerves is destroyed by a diffuse inflammatory reaction. The peripheral nerves are infiltrated by lymphocytes, which leads to edema and inflammation. Segmental **demyelination** causes axonal atrophy, resulting in slowed or blocked nerve conduction. Typically, the demyelination begins in the most distal nerves and ascends in a symmetrical fashion. **Remyelination,** which is a much slower process, occurs in a descending pattern and is accompanied by a resolution of symptoms.

There are four recognized variants of GBS. The most common form is ascending Guillain-Barré syndrome. It is characterized by progressive weakness and numbness that begins in the legs and ascends up the body. The numbness tends to be mild, but the muscle weakness usually progresses to paralysis. The paralysis may ascend all the way to the cranial nerves or stop anywhere between the legs and head. Deep tendon reflexes are either depressed or absent. In approximately 50% of patients with ascending GBS, respiratory function becomes compromised.

Descending GBS is less common. It affects the cranial nerves that originate in the brainstem first. These patients present with difficulty swallowing and speaking. The weakness progresses downward toward the legs. Respiratory compromise is rapid. Numbness is more problematic in the hands than in the feet, and the reflexes are diminished or absent.

Miller Fisher syndrome, a variant of GBS, is rare. Typically, there is no respiratory compromise or sensory loss. The classic symptoms are profound ataxia, absence of reflexes, and paralysis of the extraocular muscles. Some people believe that the fourth form, pure motor GBS, is actually a milder version of ascending GBS. The symptoms are the same except for the lack of numbness or paresthesias.

Etiology

GBS is believed to be caused by an autoimmune response to some type of viral infection or vaccination, although the exact cause is not known. Usually the viral illness occurs within 2 weeks prior to onset of symptoms. Average age at onset is 30 to 50; men and women are equally affected.

GBS has worldwide distribution, is not seasonal, and affects individuals of all races and ages. Higher rates, however, have been found in people 45 years and older. The incidence of the disease is 50% to 60% higher in Caucasians than in African Americans.

Signs and Symptoms

GBS is divided into three stages. The first stage starts with the onset of symptoms and lasts until the progression of symptoms stops. This stage can last from 24 hours to 3 weeks and is characterized by abrupt and rapid onset of muscle weakness and paralysis, with little or no muscle atrophy. Many patients give a history of a recent viral illness or vaccination, supporting the theory that the cause is autoimmune in nature. The degree of respiratory involvement correlates to the type of GBS and the level of paralysis. Patients with ascending GBS may gradually notice a reduced ability to take deep breaths or carry on conversations and may feel short of breath. These patients are terrified that they will not be able to breathe. Patients with either ascending or descending GBS may require intubation and artificial ventilation.

The autonomic nervous system is often affected by GBS. Patients may experience labile blood pressure, cardiac dysrhythmias, urinary retention, or paralytic ileus. Patient complaints of discomfort range from annoying numbness and cramping to severe pain. The discomfort is exacerbated by the patient's inability to move voluntarily.

The second stage is the plateau stage, when symptoms are most severe but progression has stopped. It may last from 2 to 14 days. Patients may become discouraged if no improvement is evident.

Axonal regeneration and remyelination occur during the recovery phase. This stage lasts from 6 to 24 months. Symptoms slowly improve. Most patients with GBS recover completely within a few months to a year. A few patients experience chronic disability.

Complications

Complications that can occur include respiratory failure, infection, and depression. Fatigue and paralysis of the respiratory muscles lead to insufficient respiratory effort. Some patients with impending respiratory failure attempt to convince the staff that they are not in distress and do not need to be intubated. Discussion of the possible need for intubation early in the patient's illness is important. The decision to intubate in GBS is different than with the other PNS disorders, since GBS patients are expected to recover. Constant monitoring of respiratory parameters and continuous pulse oximetry provide information indicating the need for immediate intervention.

Patients with GBS are prone to pneumonia and UTIs. Maintaining infection control practices and maximizing the patient's nutritional status help decrease the likelihood of infections occurring. Immobility leads to such problems as skin breakdown, pulmonary embolus, deep vein thrombosis, and muscle atrophy. Patients with GBS have little time to adjust to their illness and deterioration. They fear that they will not recover function. Calm, supportive reassurance is important.

Diagnostic Tests

A lumbar puncture is performed to obtain CSF. The CSF analysis shows a normal cell count with an elevated protein level. Electromyographic and nerve conduction velocity tests are done to evaluate nerve function. Pulmonary function testing helps identify impending respiratory problems.

Therapeutic Interventions

During the first stage, patients are partially or completely dependent for all needs. They are often frightened and anxious. Oxygen and mechanical ventilation may be required. Plasmapheresis is used to remove the patient's plasma and replace it with fresh plasma. This procedure is thought to lessen the body's immune response. To be most effective, plasmapheresis should begin 7 to 14 days from the onset of symptoms. Steroid hormones, although used in the past, are not effective and may have a deleterious effect on the individual.

During the plateau phase, patients may become discouraged because they are not getting any better. Emotional support is important during this phase.

Axonal regeneration and remyelination occur during the recovery phase. Intensive rehabilitation helps the patient regain function during this phase.

Nursing Care

See Box 50.3 Nursing Care Plan for the Patient with a Progressive Neuromuscular Disorder.

The goal of therapy is to support body systems until the patient recovers. Monitor vital capacity and ABGs, and promptly report deterioration in respiratory function. Monitor gag, corneal, and swallowing reflexes so protective interventions can be implemented if necessary. Manage pain with administration of narcotics and nonpharmacological methods such as position changes, massage, and diversional activities. Administer tube feedings or parenteral nutrition as ordered to meet nutritional needs if the patient is unable to swallow. Provide a communication board if needed so the patient can indicate needs to staff. Because recovery can be prolonged, diversional activities such as visits from family and friends, listening to music or relaxation tapes, and watching television or videos can help alleviate boredom, loneliness, and depression. As the patient begins to regain function, encourage participation in therapy and point out any returning function to the patient and family.

PATIENT EDUCATION. All procedures should be explained to the patient and family. The patient and family need to understand the reasons for continuous respiratory monitoring. Patients may deny any respiratory difficulty because of a fear of intubation and mechanical ventilation. Informing the patient about the possible need for temporary respiratory support and the measures taken to alleviate discomfort help decrease anxiety and encourage patient cooperation. Information about the disease, treatments, and recovery should be given because recovery may take months or years. Educating family members about how to perform specific patient care activities encourages participation and prepares the patient and family for discharge.

See Table 50.4 for a summary comparison of MS, MG, ALS, and GB.

Postpolio Syndrome

Pathophysiology and Etiology

Postpolio syndrome is a condition that affects survivors of polio 10 to 40 years after they have recovered from infection caused by the poliomyelitis virus. The severity of this syndrome depends on the degree of residual weakness and disability left from the initial illness.

TABLE 50.4 SUMMARY OF PNS DISORDERS

	Multiple Sclerosis (MS)	Myasthenia Gravis (MG)	Amyotrophic Lateral Sclerosis (ALS)	Guillain-Barré Syndrome (GBS)
Signs and Symptoms	Muscle weakness Muscle paralysis Visual disturbances Fatigue	Progressive severe muscle weakness of voluntary muscles Muscles regain strength with rest Masklike face	Progressive muscle weakness Decreased coordination Muscle twitching Muscle spasms Pain Emotional outbursts Difficulty with speech Intact thought processes	3 Stages: 1. Ascending paralysis 2. Plateau 3. Descending resolution Pain, cramping or numbness
Diagnosis	CSF analysis MRI Interferon therapy Steroids Immunosuppressants Plasmapheresis Anticonvulsants Antiviral agents Muscle relaxants Physical therapy	Ptosis test Tensilon test EMG	CSF analysis EEG Nerve biopsy	CSF EMG Nerve conduction velocity
Therapeutic Interventions	Assistive devices for ADLs Speech therapy	Plasmapheresis Thymectomy Anticholinesterase agents Steroids	Antispasmodics/quinine Riluzole (Rilutek) Physical therapy Massage Muscle relaxants Diversional activities Tube feeding Alternative communications devices	Plasmapheresis Ventilation support
Complications	Falls Muscle spasms Bowel and bladder problems, risk for UTI Forgetfulness Extreme fatigue	Aspiration Respiratory infections Respiratory failure Myasthenic crisis or cholinergic crisis	Communication problems Risk for aspiration Pain Respiratory failure	Respiratory infection Respiratory failure Depression Fatigue UTI Complications of immobility
Priority Nursing Diagnoses	Ineffective airway clearance; Impaired physical mobility; Risk for imbalanced nutrition			

CSF = cerebrospinal fluid; EEG = electroencephalography; EMG = electromyography; MRI = magnetic resonance imaging; UTI = urinary tract infection.

Signs and Symptoms

Postpolio syndrome (PPS) involves a further weakening of the muscles that were affected with the first involvement with the poliovirus. Symptoms range from fatigue to progressive muscle weakness leading to atrophy. Sleeping problems, joint pain, scoliosis, and respiratory compromise can occur. Some individuals suffer great debilitation, while others have little problem.

Diagnostic Tests

Observation and history and excluding other problems are most important in diagnosis of this syndrome.

Therapeutic Interventions

No interventions have been found to be effective at this time. Symptoms seem to be best controlled by rest and moderate exercise without pushing the limits of tolerance.

 CRANIAL NERVE DISORDERS

Cranial nerves are the peripheral nerves of the brain. There are 12 pairs of cranial nerves. Areas that the cranial nerves innervate include the head, neck, and special sensory structures. Cranial nerve problems are classified as peripheral **neuropathies.** Disorders may affect the sensory, motor, or both branches of a single nerve. Causes of cranial nerve disorders include tumors, infections, inflammation, trauma, and unknown causes. Two common cranial nerve problems are trigeminal **neuralgia** (tic douloureux) and Bell's palsy.

---

neuropathies: neuro—nerve + pathies—disease
neuralgia: neur—nerve + algia—pain

Trigeminal Neuralgia

Pathophysiology and Etiology

Trigeminal neuralgia (TN), sometimes called tic douloureux, involves the fifth cranial (trigeminal) nerve. This cranial nerve has three branches that include both sensory and motor functions. The branches innervate areas of the face, including the forehead, nose, cheek, gums, and jaw. Trigeminal neuralgia affects only the sensory portion of the nerve. Irritation or chronic compression of the nerve is suspected to initiate onset of symptoms. This condition is seen more often in women and usually begins around age 50 to 60.

Signs and Symptoms

Intense recurring episodes of pain, described as sudden, jabbing, burning, or knifelike, characterize this condition. Episodes of pain begin and end suddenly, lasting a few seconds to minutes. Attacks can occur in clusters up to hundreds of times daily. However, some patients experience only a few attacks per year. Pain is felt in the skin on one side of the face. A slight touch, cold breeze, talking, or chewing can trigger attacks of pain. The areas of the face where pain is triggered are referred to as trigger zones. Areas affected include the lips, upper or lower gums, cheeks, forehead, or side of the nose (Fig. 50.3). Sleep provides a period of relief from the pain. Therefore, persons with trigeminal neuralgia may sleep most of the time to avoid painful attacks. They may also refrain from activities such as talking, face washing, teeth brushing, shaving, and eating to prevent pain. Frequent blinking and tearing of the eye on the affected side also occurs.

Diagnostic Tests

History of symptoms and direct observation of an attack confirm diagnosis. Radiological studies, including computed tomographic (CT) scan and MRI, may be used to rule out other causes of the pain.

Therapeutic Interventions

Initial management includes the use of anticonvulsants such as phenytoin (Dilantin) and carbamazepine (Tegretol)

to reduce transmission of nerve impulses. Baclofen, clonazepam, gabapentin, and valproic acid may also be effective in controlling the symptoms. Most persons experience relief with medications. These drugs cause bone marrow suppression, so routine complete blood counts are necessary. However, medications do not offer a permanent solution because they lose their effectiveness after a period of time. Another treatment option is nerve blocks using local anesthetics. This option offers 8 to 16 months of relief. If medications and nerve blocks do not provide relief, surgical options are available. Surgery is done to identify and remove the cause of irritation and inflammation of the nerve. Radio frequency ablation is used to destroy some of the nerve branches, resulting in anesthesia of the area. Gamma knife radiosurgery is also an option. The gamma knife creates a lesion on the nerve to block the pain signals.

PATIENT EDUCATION POSTPROCEDURE. Many of the above interventions may still apply following nerve block or ablation. If corneal sensation is lost, goggles and sunglasses should be used as needed to protect the affected eye. An eye patch may be needed at night to prevent injury during sleep. Artificial tears may also be needed to prevent corneal damage.

Bell's Palsy

Pathophysiology and Etiology

In Bell's palsy (BP), the facial nerve (cranial nerve VII) becomes inflamed and edematous, causing interruption of nerve impulses. The cause is thought to be nerve trauma from a viral or bacterial infection. There is ongoing research to determine whether this is another autoimmune disorder. Loss of motor control generally occurs on one side of the face; bilateral facial palsy occurs in less than 1% of cases. Contracture of facial muscles may occur if recovery is slow. Men and women are affected equally. Bell's palsy is more common in the third trimester of pregnancy, in individuals with immune disorders such as HIV infection, and individuals with diabetes. It occurs in all ages (including children) and at all times of the year.

Signs and Symptoms

Onset of symptoms may be sudden or may progress over a 2- to 5-day period. The severity of the paralysis usually peaks within several days of onset of symptoms. Pain behind the ear may precede the onset of facial paralysis. Other vague initial symptoms are dry eye or tingling around the lips with progression to the more recognizable symptoms of Bell's palsy. The patient may be unable to close the eyelid, wrinkle the forehead, smile, raise the eyebrow, or close the lips effectively. The mouth is pulled toward the unaffected side (Fig. 50.4). Drooling of saliva occurs, and the affected eye has constant tearing. Sense of taste is lost over the anterior two-thirds of the tongue. Speech difficulties are present. Fifty percent of these patients will have complete recovery in a short period of time. Thirty-five percent will have full recovery in less than 1 year. See Box 50.4 Patient Perspective for Angela's experience with Bell's palsy.

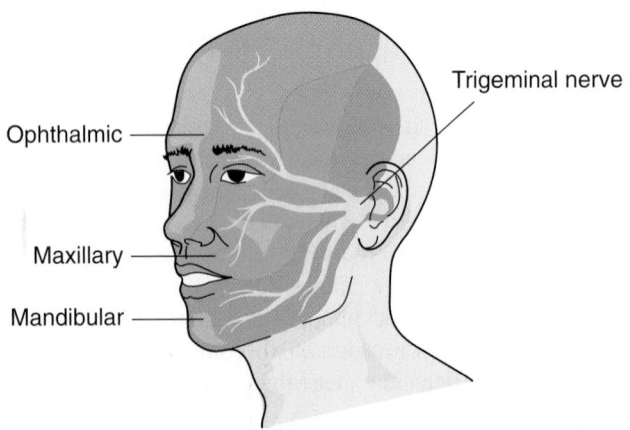

FIGURE 50.3 Areas innervated by the three main branches of the trigeminal nerve (cranial nerve V) are affected in trigeminal neuralgia.

Labels: Trigeminal nerve, Ophthalmic, Maxillary, Mandibular

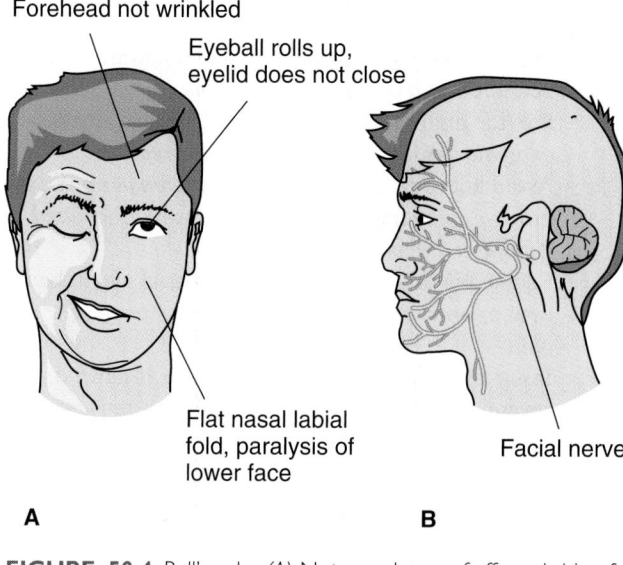

Forehead not wrinkled

Eyeball rolls up, eyelid does not close

Flat nasal labial fold, paralysis of lower face

A

Facial nerve

B

FIGURE 50.4 Bell's palsy. *(A)* Note weakness of affected side of face. *(B)* Distribution of facial nerve.

Diagnostic Tests

History of the onset of symptoms is used to diagnose Bell's palsy. Observation of the patient confirms the diagnosis. An EMG may be done. The possibility of a stroke must be ruled out.

Therapeutic Interventions

Prevention of complications is the goal of treatment. Prednisone may be given over 7 to 10 days to decrease edema. Analgesics are given for pain control. Antiviral medication may be prescribed. Moist heat with gentle massage to the face and ear also eases pain. Use of a facial sling aids in eating and supports facial muscles.

Nursing Process for Cranial Nerve Disorders (Trigeminal Neuralgia and Bell's Palsy)

ASSESSMENT/DATA COLLECTION. Assess attacks using the WHAT'S UP? format, being sure to include factors that trigger pain. Are there sensory or motor problems associated with the pain? Assess the effect of the disorder on the patient's life, including nutritional status, general and oral

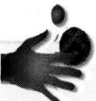

Box 50.4

Patient Perspective

Angela, Bell's Palsy

I woke up that Thursday morning with the same intense pain in my forehead that I had been experiencing for the last week. When I rolled out of bed, I realized that I didn't have morning breath (or so I thought). Knowing that I had not brushed my teeth yet, I proceeded to do so and noticed that I could not taste the toothpaste. The fruit cup I ate for lunch tasted like Clorox. I chomped up and down on each bite, then carefully attempted to swallow. It was like I had been injected with several shots of Novocain. My throat felt like it had closed up, and each swallow took a concentrated effort. Over the course of eating my fruit, I managed to bite my tongue three times.

I was 35 weeks pregnant and on strict bed rest due to pregnancy-induced hypertension and severe edema (which later spiraled into toxemia). We attributed the numbness in my mouth to the edema. I had already swollen up like a balloon and had experienced intense numbness in my extremities since the 12th week of pregnancy. As the afternoon progressed, I grew more and more concerned. I knew something was not quite right. By 5:30 that evening I had lost control of the entire left side of my face. I called my obstetrician and she said to get to the ER because I was either having a stroke or had developed Bell's palsy. The doctor at the ER confirmed that I had Bell's palsy and prescribed Valtrex and prednisone to treat it.

The symptoms of Bell's that I experienced were severe pain in my forehead, not being able to breathe out of the left side of my nose, and difficulty chewing, swallowing, and saying most consonants. I completely lost the ability to smile, blink, close my eye, raise my eyebrow, or use a straw or blow. My eyesight in the left eye blurred, and I could not drive at night due to the intense pain behind my eye triggered by head lights and having to use eye drops every 5 to 20 minutes.

I delivered my baby (after induction, 2 days of labor, 2 hours of pushing, and emergency C-section) 2 weeks after being diagnosed with Bell's palsy. During labor, I continuously asked for my eye drops because the pain in my head was so fierce that it overshadowed the contractions.

After delivery, I was desperate for my face to be "fixed." I tried everything that anyone suggested: herbal supplements, chiropractic, facial massage, laser treatments, facial exercise, shock treatments, a neurologist consultation, and physical therapy. The only thing that has worked for me is time (and lots of it)!

For the first 15 weeks after being diagnosed I wanted to hide from the world. However, here it is 7 months later and I have come to terms with it. I am constantly aware of it, though I have regained a tremendous amount of the muscle control. I still have not shared a "real smile" with my daughter and do not blink my left eye. Covering my mouth when I smile or laugh so others do not see has become almost like a reflex now.

hygiene, behavior, and emotional state. Carefully document all findings.

NURSING DIAGNOSIS, PLANNING, AND IMPLEMENTATION. Acute pain related to inflammation or compression of the nerve

EXPECTED OUTCOME: Patient will state pain is controlled

- Assess pain level and response to interventions prn. *Assessment guides intervention.*
- Administer analgesics as needed for pain. *Analgesics decrease pain and increase comfort.*
- Discuss and implement alternative and complementary pain relief measures *to complement analgesics and increase patient's control over pain.*
  - Biofeedback
  - Diversional activities
- Plan hygiene activities when pain relief is at its peak *to decrease discomfort with activities.*
- Provide alternative communication methods. *Patient may not be able to speak clearly or want to speak due to pain.*
  - Paper and pencil/pen
  - Dry erase board
  - Magnetic letters
  - Communication boards
  - Pain scales for pointing to level of pain
- Teach to chew on opposite side of face *to avoid triggering pain and injury.*
- Encourage use of electric razor rather than blades *to prevent injury of numb areas.*
- Provide the following measures for trigeminal neuralgia *to reduce pain triggers.*
  - Provide soft cloths for facial hygiene using lukewarm water.
  - Avoid touching the patient's face.
  - Provide soft bristle toothbrush for oral care.
  - Teach to protect face from cold or wind.
- Provide the following measures for Bell's palsy *to reduce pain and prevent muscle atrophy.*
  - Provide warm, moist compresses prn.
  - Massage face.
  - Assist with facial exercises several times a day.
  - Provide a facial sling.

Imbalanced nutrition: Less than body requirements related to fear of triggering pain

EXPECTED OUTCOME: Patient will maintain sufficient nutrition as evidenced by stable weight

- Weigh each morning and record *to monitor weight loss or gain.*

- Provide small frequent meals *to provide nutrition without increasing pain.*
- Provide soft, easy-to-chew food at lukewarm temperature *to prevent triggering pain.*
- Provide high-protein and high-calorie diet. *Protein and calories are needed for cellular repair.*
- Avoid hot or cold foods and drinks. *Temperature extremes may trigger pain. If foods are associated with pain, the patient may avoid them.*
- Encourage oral hygiene after each meal and at bedtime *to prevent gum and tooth disease as trigger for pain.*
- Insert feeding tube on unaffected side if nutrition is severely impaired *to provide means for nutrient intake while avoiding painful nerve areas.*

Risk for trauma to eye related to inability to blink, and body image disturbance (Bell's palsy)

EXPECTED OUTCOME: Cornea will remain intact without injury.

- Administer eye drops or eye ointment as ordered by the physician *to protect the eye.*
- Teach the patient to use a patch over the affected eye *to protect the eye.*
- Advise the patient to wear glasses or goggles, especially when outside or in areas with multiple particles in the air *to protect the eyes.*

EVALUATION. Nursing care has been successful if the patient reports that pain is controlled, nutrition is maintained with no inappropriate weight loss, and the eyes are intact and without injury.

LEARNING TIP

Trigeminal neuralgia (cranial nerve V) is a sensory disorder; Bell's palsy (cranial nerve VII) is a motor disorder.

See Table 50.5 for a summary comparison of BP and TN.

Home Health Hints

- If a home-bound patient has difficulty speaking (dysarthria), try using magnetic alphabet letters. Ask questions that require a yes or no answer. The patient can respond with the letter *y* or *n*.
- Keep bedside commode lids up with patches of Velcro attached to the seat and the frame.

TABLE 50.5 SUMMARY OF CRANIAL NERVE DISORDERS

	Trigeminal Neuralgia	Bell's Palsy
Cranial Nerve Involved	5th sensory	7th motor
Signs and Symptoms	Intense pain on one side of face • Sudden onset • Sudden resolution • Jabbing, burning, knifelike Sensitive to temperature and air flow Sensitive to touch Pain exacerbated by talking or chewing Frequent blinking or tearing of the eye on affected side	Loss of motor control, paralysis on one side of face Variable onset of symptoms Facial droop and inability to close affected eye Drooling Loss of taste over anterior one-third of tongue Speech difficulties
Diagnosis	History Observation of attack CT MRI	History EMG
Therapeutic Interventions	Anticonvulsants Antispasmodics Nerve block with local anesthetic Surgical radiofrequency ablation	Prednisone Analgesics Moist heat Gentle massage Facial sling when eating
Complications	Corneal damage Poor nutrition Depression	Corneal damage Poor nutrition Depression

CT = computed tomography; EMG = electomyography; MRI = magnetic resonance imaging.

REVIEW QUESTIONS

1. A patient with TN asks the nurse why she was started on carbamazepine (Tegretol). Which response is best?
   a. "It will help decrease the inflammation in your nervous system."
   b. "It will depress your immune system, which can slow the progression of the disease."
   c. "It can help relieve nerve pain."
   d. "It relaxes the bladder to help control bladder spasms."

2. A patient with ALS asks why he doesn't seem to have enough breath to sing anymore. Which explanation by the nurse is best?
   a. "ALS can damage the nerves to your bronchi and bronchioles, causing constriction and reduced airflow."
   b. "The demyelination of your nerves caused by ALS causes confusion in the impulses to your lungs."
   c. "ALS can affect your vocal cords, making it difficult to form sounds as you speak or sing."
   d. "ALS may be affecting the nerves that go to your respiratory muscles, making them weak."

3. A patient who is newly diagnosed with ALS says to the nurse, "I do not want to be kept alive on machines." Which nursing action is best in response?

   a. Ask the patient if he has advance directives, and provide information about preparing them.
   b. Reassure the patient that he will not need to make decisions about machines for a long time.
   c. Inform the patient that individuals with ALS are not candidates for artificial ventilation.
   d. Explain to the patient that a ventilator will be necessary to keep him breathing as his disease progresses.

4. When caring for a patient admitted with a diagnosis of Guillain-Barré syndrome, which nursing diagnosis should take priority?
   a. Anxiety
   b. Imbalanced nutrition
   c. Impaired gas exchange
   d. Impaired mobility

5. Which nursing interventions are appropriate for the patient with Bell's palsy? Select all that apply.
   a. Administer moisturizing eye drops.
   b. Apply an eye patch.
   c. Avoid touching the patient's face.
   d. Apply warm compresses.
   e. Provide facial massage.
   f. Teach the patient to protect her face from cool breezes.

6. Which meal would be the best choice for a patient with myasthenia gravis?
   a. Baked chicken sandwich, fresh carrots, apple
   b. Meatloaf, mashed potatoes, canned green beans
   c. Steak, baked potato, green salad
   d. Tacos, fresh vegetables, sliced peaches

7. How will the visiting nurse caring for a patient with myasthenia gravis and severe muscle weakness know if interventions have been effective?

a. The patient verbalizes satisfaction with the plan of care.
b. The patient states understanding of the medication regimen.
c. The patient and family state that no further home visits are needed.
d. The patient is able to perform ADLs with SaO_2 remaining at 95%.

References

1. National Multiple Sclerosis Society. Accessed March 26, 2006 at http://www.nationalmssociety.org
2. Singleton, R, Helgerson, SD, Snyder RD, et al: Neuropathy in Navajo children: clinical and epidemiologic features. Neurology 40:363, 1990.
3. ALS Association. Accessed March 26, 2006, at http://www.alsa.org/als/who.cfm

Unit Thirteen Bibliography

1. Amella, EJ: Presentation of illness in older adults. AJN 104:40–51, 2004.
2. American Heart Association www.americanheart.org
3. American Stroke Association www.strokeassociation.org
4. Cunning, S: When the Dx is myasthenia gravis. RN 63:26–31, 2000.
5. Ebersole, P, Hess, P, Touhy, T, and Jett, K: Gerontological Nursing and Healthy Aging, ed. 2. Mosby, St. Louis, 2005.
6. Guillain-Barre Syndrome/Chronic Inflammatory Demyelination Polyneuropathy at www.guillain-barre.com
7. Harvey, J: Countering brain attacks. Nurs Manage 35:27–32, 2004.
8. Kanapaux, W: Alzheimer's researchers target early detection, prevention. Geriatric Times January/February 2004.
9. Lehne, RA: Pharmacology for Nursing Care, ed. 5. Saunders, St. Louis, 2004.
10. Mayo Clinic at http://www.mayoclinic.com
11. National Institute of Neurological Disorders and Stroke. Post-polio syndrome fact sheet, NIH Publication No. 96-4030, accessed November 23, 2005 at http://www.nlm.nih.gov/medlineplus/polioandpostpoliosyndrome.html.
12. Myasthenia Gravis Foundation of America, Inc. (2004). At www.myasthenia.org/information.
13. Naylor, M, Stephens, C, Bowles, KH, and Bixby, MB: Cognitively impaired older adults: from hospital to home. AJN 105:52–61, 2005.
14. Petersen, RJ: MCI as a useful clinical concept. Geriatric Times January/February 2004.
15. Scarmeas, N, and Stern, Y: Does stimulation facilitate cognitive skill maintenance? Geriatric Times January/February 2004.
16. Smith, M, and Buckwalter, K: Behaviors associated with dementia. AJN 105:40–51, 2005.
17. Wasson, K, Tate, H, and Hayes, C: Food refusal and dysphagia in older people with dementia: ethical and practical issues. Int J Palliative Nurs 7:465–471, 2001.
18. Weiner, M: Legal and ethical issues for patients with dementia and their families. Geriatric Times January/February 2004.
19. Wood, T: Talking with technology. Quest, 10 (2) retrieved June 5, 2005 from www.mdausa.org/publications/Quest/q102technology.cfm.
20. Yee, CA: Getting a grip on myasthenia gravis. Nursing 2002 32:, 2002.

SUGGESTED ANSWERS TO

CRITICAL THINKING

■ *Jamie*

1. Muscle weakness caused by myasthenia gravis improves with rest.
2. Have Jamie look up for 2 to 3 minutes. If ptosis occurs, let the patient close her eyes for several minutes. If she can open her eyelids and look up, myasthenia gravis is likely.
3.

$$\frac{2 \text{ mg}}{} \quad \frac{1 \text{ mL}}{10 \text{ mg}} = 0.2 \text{ mL}$$

■ *Mr. Miller*

1. Nursing diagnoses include ineffective airway clearance related to muscle weakness and risk for aspiration related to muscle weakness. If a patient's respiratory system is compromised by a disease, nursing care should be focused on maintaining pulmonary function to preserve life.
2. Compassionate care for the patient and providing information about the disease and its prognosis to the patient and family establish an honest and supportive environment. Support groups provide resources and emotional support.

unit FOURTEEN

UNDERSTANDING THE SENSORY SYSTEM

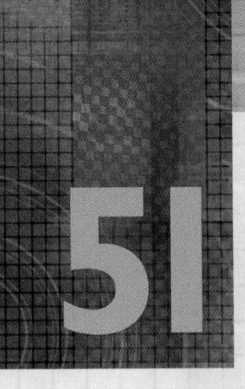

51

Sensory System Function, Assessment, and Therapeutic Measures: Vision and Hearing

DEBRA AUCOIN-RATCLIFF,
LAZETTE V. NOWICKI, AND
JANICE L. BRADFORD

QUESTIONS TO GUIDE YOUR READING

1. What is the normal anatomy of the sensory system?

2. What is the normal function of the sensory system?

3. What data should you collect when caring for a patient with a disorder of the sensory system?

4. What are the diagnostic tests commonly performed to diagnose disorders of the sensory system?

5. What nursing care should you provide for patients undergoing each of the diagnostic tests?

6. What are the common therapeutic measures used for patients with disorders of the sensory system?

Our eyes and ears provide us with a great deal of sensory information. It is difficult to imagine what it would be like not to see or hear the world around us. Nurses have an important role in assessing vision and hearing. Patients depend on health-care personnel to assist them in maintaining these primary senses. To learn more about ways to promote vision and hearing health, visit http://web.health.gov/healthypeople.

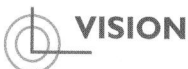

VISION

Normal Anatomy and Physiology of the Eye

The eye contains the receptors for vision and a refracting system that focuses light rays on these photoreceptors in the retina.

External Structures

The eyelids are the protective covers for the front of the eyeball; on the border of each lid are eyelashes that help keep dust out of the eyes. The eyelids are lined with a thin transparent membrane called the conjunctiva, which is also folded over the white of the eye on its anterior surface.

Associated with each eyeball is a lacrimal gland located within the bony socket at the upper, outer corner of the eyeball. Small ducts take tears to the front of the eyeball, and blinking helps spread the tears over the surface. Tears contain lysozyme, an enzyme that inhibits the growth of most bacteria on the surface of the eye. The lacrimal canals at the medial corner of each eye collect tears, which then drain into the lacrimal sac, to the nasolacrimal duct, to the nasal cavities.

Structure of the Eyeball

Most of the eyeball is within the orbit, the bony socket that provides protection from trauma. The six extrinsic muscles that move the eyeball are attached to the orbit and to the outer surface of the eyeball. There are four rectus muscles that move the eyeball side to side or up and down and two oblique muscles that rotate the eye. The cranial nerves that innervate these muscles are the oculomotor, trochlear, and abducens (third, fourth, and sixth cranial nerves, respectively).

The wall of the eyeball has three layers: the outer sclera, the middle choroid, and the inner retina. The sclera is made of fibrous connective tissue that is visible as the white of the eye. The most anterior portion is the transparent cornea (Fig. 51.1), which has no capillaries and is the first part of the eye that refracts light rays.

The choroid layer contains blood vessels and the dark pigment melanin, which prevents glare within the eyeball by absorbing light. The anterior of the choroid is modified into the ciliary body and the iris. The ciliary body has a circular muscle that surrounds the edge of the lens and is connected to the lens by suspensory ligaments. The lens is made of a transparent, elastic protein and, like the cornea, has no capillaries. The shape of the lens is changed by the ciliary muscle, which permits the focusing of light from objects at varying distances.

In front of the lens is the circular iris, which is made of two sets of smooth muscle fibers that change the diameter of the pupil, the central opening. Contraction of the radial fibers is a sympathetic response and dilates the pupil. Contraction of the circular fibers is a parasympathetic response (mediated by the oculomotor nerves) and constricts the pupil. Pupillary constriction is a reflex that protects the retina from intense light or that permits more acute near vision.

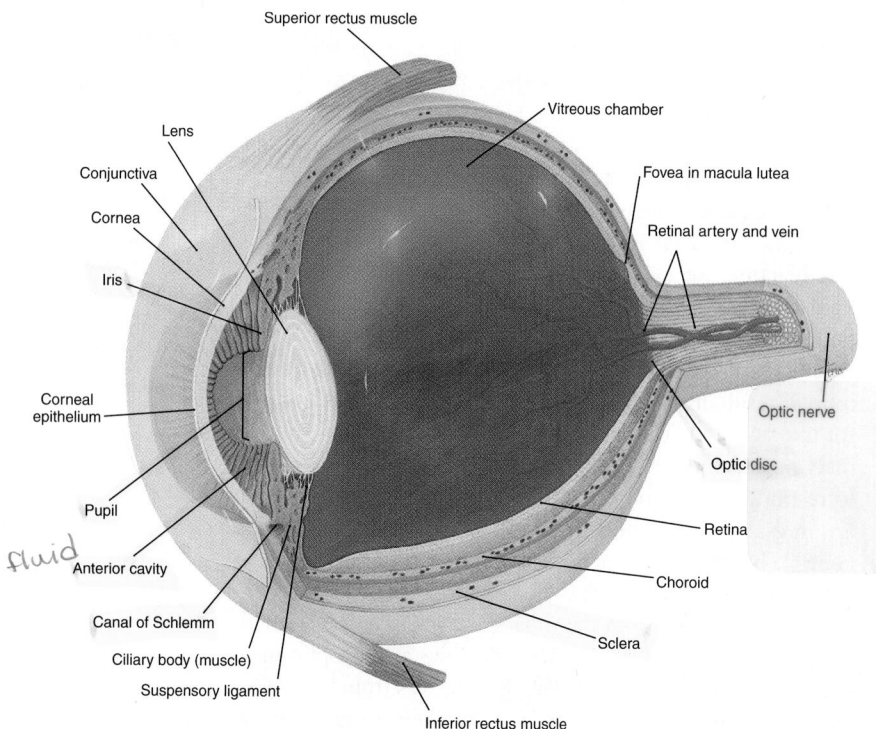

FIGURE 51.1 Internal anatomy of the eye. *(From Scanlon, VC, and Sanders, T: Essentials of Anatomy and Physiology, ed. 5. F.A. Davis, Philadelphia, 2007, with permission.)*

The retina lines the posterior two-thirds of the eyeball and contains the rods and cones, the receptors for vision. Rods detect only the presence of light, whereas cones detect the different wavelengths of light as colors. The fovea centralis is a small depression in the macula lutea of the posterior retina, directly behind the center of the lens, and contains only cones. It is, therefore, the area of most acute color vision. Rods are proportionally more abundant toward the periphery of the retina, and for this reason night vision is best at the sides of the visual field.

Neurons called ganglion cells transmit the impulses generated by the rods and cones. These neurons all converge at the optic disc and pass through the wall of the eyeball as the optic nerve. The optic disc may also be called the blind spot because no rods or cones are present.

Cavities of the Eyeball

There are two cavities divided by the lens within the eye, posterior and anterior. The larger posterior cavity is between the lens and retina and contains vitreous humor. This semisolid substance helps keep the retina in place.

The anterior cavity is between the cornea and the front of the lens and contains aqueous humor, the tissue fluid of the eyeball that nourishes the lens and cornea. Aqueous humor is formed by capillaries in the ciliary body, flows anteriorly through the pupil, and is reabsorbed by the canal of Schlemm (scleral venous sinus) at the junction of the iris and the cornea. The rate of reabsorption normally equals the rate of production.

Physiology of Vision

Vision involves the focusing of light rays on the retina and the transmission of the subsequent nerve impulses to the visual areas of the cerebral cortex.

The refractive structures of the eye are, in order, the cornea, aqueous humor, lens, and vitreous humor. The lens is the only adjustable part of this focusing system. When the eye is focused on a distant object, the ciliary muscle is relaxed and the lens is elongated and thin. When the eye is focused on a near object, the ciliary muscle contracts and forms a smaller circle and the elastic lens recoils and bulges in the middle and has greater refractive power.

When light rays strike the retina, they stimulate chemical reactions in the rods and cones. Receptors contain a light-absorbing molecule called retinal (a derivative of vitamin A) bonded to a protein called an opsin. In the rods, light stimulates the breakdown of rhodopsin into an opsin and retinal; resultant chemical changes generate a nerve impulse for transmission. The cones also contain retinal, and similar reactions take place. The opsins of the cones are specialized to respond to a portion of the visible light spectrum; there are red-absorbing, blue-absorbing, and green-absorbing cones. The chemical reactions within the cones also generate electrical nerve impulses.

The impulses from the rods and cones are transmitted to the ganglion neurons, which converge at the optic disc and become the optic nerve. The optic nerves from both eyes converge at the optic chiasma, just in front of the pituitary gland. Here, the medial fibers of each optic nerve cross to the other side. This crossing permits each visual area to receive impulses from both eyes, which is important for binocular vision.

The visual areas are in the occipital lobes of the cerebral cortex. It is here that the upside-down retinal images are righted and the slightly different pictures from the two eyes are integrated into one image; this is binocular vision, which also provides depth perception.

Aging and the Eye

The most common changes in the aging eye are those in the lens (Fig. 51.2). With age, the lens may become partially or totally opaque. The lens also loses its elasticity with age; most people become farsighted as they get older and by age 40 begin to need corrective lenses. Peripheral vision losses may occur. Depth perception decreases and glare is more difficult to adjust to, which can affect safety. Color vision fades with poorer discrimination of blue, green, and violet colors. Red, yellow, and orange colors are seen best.

Nursing Assessment/Data Collection of the Eye and Visual Status

As with most examinations, nursing assessment of the eye begins with the collection of subjective data, then moves to

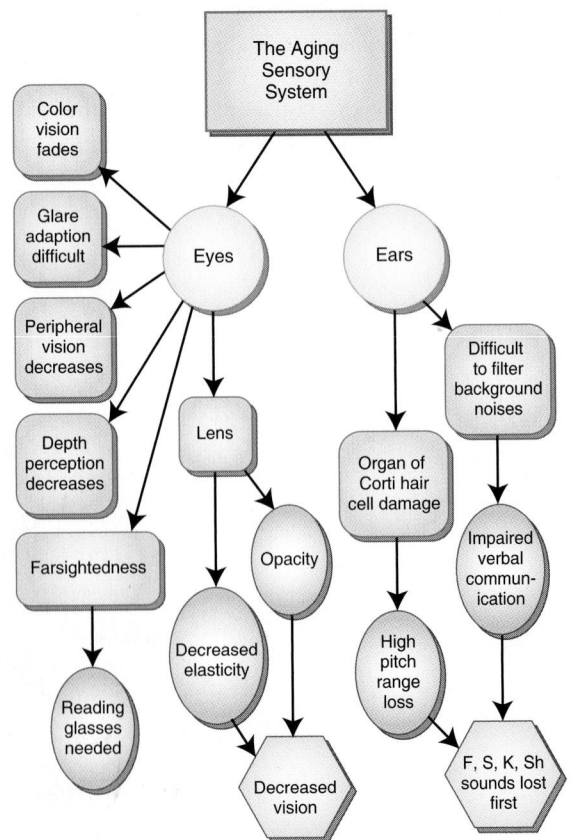

FIGURE 51.2 Legend: Aging and the sensory system. This concept map shows the effects the aging process has on the sensory system.

observation and testing, and finally a more invasive physical examination is performed. Licensed practical nurses/licensed vocational nurses (LPN/LVNs) generally do not conduct invasive examinations on the eye, but rather assist the advanced practitioner in conducting this portion of data collection.

Subjective Data

The nurse interviews patients and collects data about family history that may affect vision, particularly glaucoma, diabetes, blindness, and cataracts. Because many eye disorders are genetically transmitted, this information alerts the nurse to possible alterations in eye health. Patients should be asked about their general health and the presence of diseases such as diabetes and hypertension. The nurse determines the types of medication the patient is taking to assess for any ocular (eye) effects. Last, the nurse asks the patient about any changes in visual acuity or symptoms of abnormality (Table 51.1).

Objective Data

VISUAL ACUITY. Objective data collection begins by checking the patient's visual acuity (Table 51.2). Visual acuity is measured in a variety of ways but usually starts with the use of **Snellen's chart,** E chart, or hand-held visual acuity chart (Rosenbaum's card) to test near and far vision. Snellen's chart is imprinted with alphabetical letters graduating in size from the smallest on the bottom to the largest on the top (Fig. 51.3). The examiner measures 20 feet and marks the distance on the floor. The examiner then asks the patient to cover one eye with a 3 × 5 card or eye cover

and then read out loud an indicated line of letters. The lowest line on the chart that the patient is able to read accurately is used to indicate visual acuity for that eye. Normal vision is 20/20, which means the patient can read at 20 feet what the normal eye can read at 20 feet. Visual impairment occurs at 20/70 and legal blindness at 20/200 or more with correction. An example of findings is the patient who identifies all the letters correctly on the line marked 30; this patient has a visual acuity of 20/30. This means that the patient can see at 20 feet what the average individual can see at 30 feet. The examination is conducted on both eyes separately, then together, and documented as follows: "oculus dexter (OD) [right eye] 20/30, oculus sinister (OS) [left eye] 20/20, oculus uterque (OU) [both eyes] 20/20." In addition to identifying the eye tested, the examiner conducts the examination with and without the patient's corrective lenses, if applicable. When corrective lenses are used, documentation reflects this as "OD 20/100 without correction, OD 20/20 with correction." The E chart is used for patients who are illiterate. The patient is asked to indicate the direction of the E-shaped figure. The hand-held visual acuity chart is used to indicate visual acuity by having the patient hold the card approximately 14 inches from the eyes. The test is conducted and documented in the same way as the Snellen's and E chart examinations.

Visual Fields by Confrontation. The examiner also tests peripheral vision, which is the ability of the eye to see objects peripherally while the eye is fixed or kept in one position. This is also known as testing visual fields by confrontation. To do this, the examiner compares his or her

TABLE 51.1 SUBJECTIVE ASSESSMENT OF THE EYE

Category	Questions to Ask During History Assessment	Rationale/Significance
Family History	Do you have any family members with a history of diabetes? Hypertension? Cataracts? Glaucoma? Blindness? Diabetes mellitus? Do any family members wear glasses or contact lenses? Is their vision corrected with the lens?	Many eye disorders are genetically transmitted.
Patient's General Health	How would you describe your general health? What health problems do you currently have? How are they treated? What health problems have you had in the past? Have you ever had trauma to your eyes? What medications do you take? How often do you have eye examinations? When was the last time you had an eye examination?	Some metabolic disorders are precursors to eye disorders, such as diabetes and hypertension. Assess for ocular effects of systemic medications. Assess preventative practices.
Visual Acuity	Do you wear glasses or contact lenses? Have you had any changes in vision such as difficulty seeing distances, difficulty seeing close up, difficulty seeing at night? Do you see things double? Do you have clouded vision? Do you see halos around lights? Does it look like you are looking through a veil or web? Is there sensitivity to light? Is there pain? Itching? Tearing? Burning? Do you have headaches? If so, what are the precipitating events?	Any of these signs and symptoms could indicate visual disorders/disturbances.

TABLE 51.2 OBJECTIVE ASSESSMENT OF THE EYE

Category	Physical Assessment Findings	Possible Abnormal Findings/Causes
Visual Acuity	Normal vision is 20/20	Hyperopia, myopia, presbyopia, blurred or cloudy vision Possible causes: refractive error, opacity, or disorder of pathway
Visual Fields	Full peripheral fields	Peripheral field loss
Muscle Balance and Eye Movement	Movement in all six cardinal fields of gaze	Nystagmus Inability to move in all six fields can indicate cranial nerve impairment
	Corneal light reflex test—light is at the same place on both pupils	Asymmetry could mean muscle weakness
	Cover test–steady gaze	Drifting eye indicates muscle weakness
Pupillary Reflexes	Pupillary light reflex	Dilated, fixed, or constricted pupils
	Accommodation	Absence of constriction or convergence
External Structures	Inspection and palpation of eyebrows, orbital area, eyelids, palpebral fissure, medial canthus, irises, corneal clarity, anterior chamber	Ptosis (drooping of eyelid) usually indicates nerve dysfunction Opaque whitening of outer rim of cornea can indicate arcus senilis Corneal opaqueness can be from cataract or trauma

own ability to see peripheral objects with that of the patient. This test should be done with an examiner who has normal peripheral vision. The examiner stands 2 feet in front of the patient and instructs the patient to cover one eye. The examiner covers his or her own corresponding eye (e.g., if the patient's right eye is covered, the examiner's left eye is covered). The examiner uses the arm opposite the covered eye, extends it to the space midway between the patient and the examiner, and brings it toward the eye from three directions: superior, inferior, and temporal (middle). The examiner wiggles the finger while moving the arm. The examiner asks the patient to look straight ahead and indicate at what point he or she is able to see the examiner's finger. One eye is tested and then the other. The patient has full visual fields if the point at which the patient sees the finger matches that of the examiner. The examiner documents the results as "visual fields equal to examiner," "full visual fields," or, if abnormal, "visual fields unequal to examiner in. . . ." (identify position, e.g., left superior).

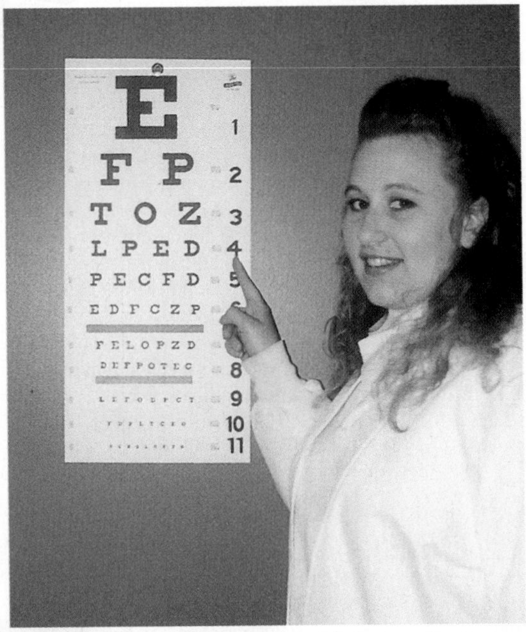

MUSCLE BALANCE AND EYE MOVEMENT. The examiner tests extraocular muscle balance and cranial nerve function by instructing the patient to look straight ahead and follow the examiner's finger movement without moving his or her head. As with the confrontation test, the patient and examiner face each other either standing or sitting. The examiner moves his or her finger in the six cardinal fields of gaze, coming back to the point of origin between each field of gaze (Fig. 51.4). If the patient's eyes are able to follow the examiner's finger in all fields of gaze without nystagmus, the patient is assessed to have adequate extraocular muscle strength and innervation. Nystagmus is an involuntary, cyclical, rapid movement of the eyes in response to vertical, horizontal, or rotary movement.

The corneal light reflex test is used to assess muscle balance. This test is conducted by shining a penlight toward the cornea while the patient is staring at an object straight ahead. The light reflection should be at exactly the same place on both pupils. If the eyes lack symmetry, muscle weakness could be present.

FIGURE 51.3 Using Snellen's chart to assess visual acuity.

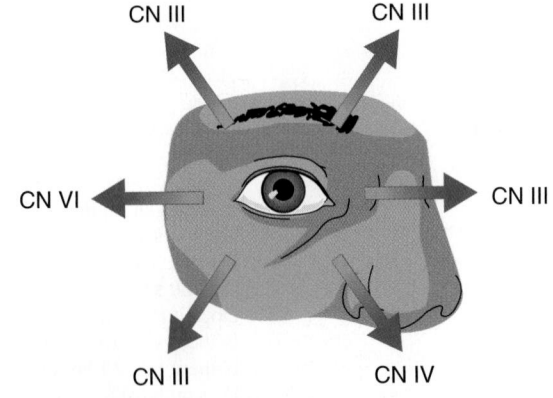

FIGURE 51.4 Six cardinal fields of gaze.

The cover test is used in conjunction with an abnormal corneal light reflex test to evaluate muscle balance. The patient is asked to look straight ahead at a far object. The examiner covers one of the patient's eyes with a 3 × 5 card. The uncovered eye should have a steady gaze; if it moves, there may be muscle weakness. Next, the cover is quickly removed and the action of this eye is observed. If this eye moves to fixate on the light instead of staring straight ahead, it indicates a drifting of the eye when it was covered, which is a sign of muscle weakness. This deviation of the eye away from the visual axis is known as **tropia.** Deviation of the eye toward the nose is known as **esotropia,** movement laterally is known as **exotropia,** and downward deviation is hypotropia.

PUPILLARY REFLEXES. The pupils are observed. They should be round, symmetrical, and reactive to light. To test pupillary response to light, both consensual and direct examinations should be completed. A slightly darkened room works best. The patient is asked to look straight ahead, and the size of the pupil is noted. A penlight is shone toward the pupil from a lateral position, and the movement of the pupil is observed. The pupil should quickly constrict. The size of the pupil is noted when it constricts. This is known as direct response.

To conduct a consensual pupil examination, observe the eye just tested for reaction while shining the penlight into the other eye. The observed pupil should constrict. This is known as **consensual response.** Repeat the procedure for the opposite eye.

The examiner now proceeds to test for **accommodation.** Accommodation is the ability of the pupil to respond to near and far distances. The patient is told to focus on an object far away. The size and shape of the pupils are observed. The examiner continues to observe the pupils as the patient focuses on a near object (the examiner's penlight or finger) held approximately 5 inches from the patient's face. Normally, the patient's eyes turn inward and the pupils constrict. These responses, convergence and constriction, are called accommodation (Box 51.1 Gerontological Issues). Examiners use the acronym PERRLA to indicate pupils equal, round, reactive to light, accommodation. If accommodation is not tested along with the other tests, the examiner may use the acronym PERRL.

INSPECTION AND PALPATION OF EXTERNAL STRUCTURES. The extraocular structures are inspected beginning with the eyebrows. The presence of eyebrows,

---

esotropia: eso—inward + tropia—movement of the eye
exotropia: exo—out + tropia—movement of the eye

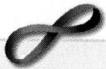

Box 51.1

Gerontological Issues

Age-Related Changes in Vision and Hearing

Vision

Older adults commonly have the following changes in their vision:

- Presbyopia, an inability to focus up close because of decreased elasticity in the ocular lens
- Narrowing of the visual field and more difficulty with peripheral vision
- Decreased pupil size and responsiveness to light
- Difficulty with vision in dimly lit areas or at night (requires more light to see adequately)
- Increased opacity of the lens, which causes sensitivity to glare, blurred vision, and interference with night vision
- Yellowing of the lens, which makes the person less able to differentiate low-tone colors of blues, greens, and violets (yellow, orange, and red hues are more clearly visible)
- Distorted depth perception and difficulty correctly judging the height of curbs and steps
- Decreased lacrimal secretions

Because visual accommodation is decreased with aging, older adults have an increased risk of falling. An older person has difficulty making a visual adjustment when moving from a well-lit room into the evening darkness, for example, or when stepping out of a dark area into the sunlight.

The increased time needed to accommodate to near and far and dark and light is often the reason that older adults do not drive at night. Usually they complain that the light from oncoming traffic blinds them or that their eyes do not focus properly.

One of the most simple and effective ways to improve vision for older adults is to assure that eye glasses are clean.

Hearing

Presbycusis is an age-related change in which progressive hearing loss is caused by loss of hair cells and decreased blood supplying the ear, resulting in a decreased ability to hear high-frequency sounds. Deafness or decreased hearing acuity is one of the main reasons that older adults withdraw from social activities. The loss of high-pitched hearing causes the older adult to hear distracting background noises more clearly than conversation.

Older adults who are deaf may require adaptive equipment in their home for safety. The use of a hearing aid can increase hearing for those who do not have nerve damage deafness. The use of flashing lights instead of buzzers or alarms increases the safety of an older adult who is not able to hear a smoke detector or fire alarm.

symmetry, hair texture, size, and extension of the brow are noted. The examiner inspects and palpates the orbital area for edema, lesions, puffiness, and tenderness. Then the eyelids are inspected for symmetry, presence of eyelashes, eyelash position, tremors, flakiness, redness, and swelling. The patient is asked to open and close the eyelids. When open, the eyelid should cover the iris margin but not the pupil. The distance between the upper and lower eyelid, known as the palpebral fissure, is inspected; it should be equal in both eyes. If the palpebral fissure is nonsymmetrical, observe for ptosis, a drooping of the eyelid, which is commonly seen in stroke patients. Next the medial canthus of the lower lid is gently palpated and observed for exudate. The eyelids are palpated for nodules while the eye is palpated for firmness over the closed eyelid.

The lower eyelid is pulled down, and the patient is asked to look upward. The conjunctiva and sclera are inspected for color, discharge, and pterygium (thickening of the conjunctiva). To inspect the upper eyelid, the upper lid is everted over a cotton-tipped applicator. The patient blinks to return the eyelid to its resting position when the inspection is complete.

The external eyes are inspected for color and symmetry of the irises, clarity of the cornea, and depth and clarity of the anterior chamber. Shining a light obliquely across the cornea assesses the clearness of the cornea. The cornea should be transparent without cloudiness. In individuals older than 40 years of age, there may be bilateral opaque whitening of the outer rim of the cornea known as **arcus senilus.** It is caused from lipid deposits and is considered normal. It does not affect vision. The anterior chamber (the area between the cornea and the iris) of the eye is inspected using oblique light. The anterior chamber should be clear when the light shines on it.

INTERNAL EYE EXAMINATION. Examination of the internal eye is done by the advanced practitioner. The LPN/LVN may be required to explain the procedure to the patient and to assist the practitioner in the examination. To perform the internal eye examination, specialized equipment must be used. It is useful, but not always necessary, to have the pupil dilated for the internal eye examination. Having a dark room allows the pupil to dilate, as does the application of anticholinergic mydriatic eye drops.

The instrument used to examine the internal eye is called an **opthalmoscope.** The opthalmoscope magnifies the structures of the eye, so the examiner can visualize the retina, optic nerve, blood vessels, and macula. The device is handheld and has a light source that is directed into the patient's internal eye. The patient should be instructed to hold the head still with the eyes focused on a distant object. The patient should be notified that the bright light might be uncomfortable. The **ophthalmologist** may examine the eye using a stationary device called a slit-lamp microscope rather than the hand-held ophthalmoscope. The patient is seated and rests the chin on a support. This examination allows the examiner to visualize the internal eye by use of a microscope and light source directed into the eye.

Intraocular Pressure. Estimation of intraocular pressure is measured by using one of several types of tonometer. Often, the procedure is performed with anesthetic drops being instilled. One type of tonometer testing uses a puff of air to make an indentation in the cornea to measure intraocular pressure. Readings above the normal range may indicate glaucoma.

Diagnostic Tests

CULTURE. If there is exudate from any portion of the eye or surrounding structure, a culture may be ordered. Results of the culture determine if anti-infective treatment is necessary.

FLUORESCEIN ANGIOGRAPHY. Fluorescein angiography is a procedure used to monitor, diagnose, and treat eye diseases. The patient is assessed for dye allergies before the procedure. Then the pupil is dilated and fluorescence dye is injected into the patient's venous system. The dye travels to the retinal arteriovenous circulation, and the eye is examined via a slit-lamp microscope. The blood vessels in the eye are extremely visible with the addition of the dye.

ELECTRORETINOGRAPHY. Electoretinography is useful in diagnosing diseases of the rods and cones of the eye. The procedure evaluates differences in the electrical potential between the cornea and retina in response to light wavelengths and intensity. The test is conducted by placing contact lenses with electrodes directly on the eye.

ULTRASONOGRAPHY. Ultrasound is useful as an examination tool when the internal eye cannot be visualized directly because of obstructions such as corneal opacities or bloody vitreous. The eye is anesthetized with instillation of anesthetic drops, and a transducer probe is placed on the eye to perform the ultrasound. Patients should be instructed to keep the eye and head still during the procedure.

RADIOLOGICAL TESTS. Several radiological examinations are used to assess eye health. X-ray films are used to view bone structure and tumors. Computed tomography (CT) and magnetic resonance imaging (MRI) are used to visualize ocular structures and abnormalities of the eye and surrounding tissues.

Therapeutic Interventions

Nurses have an important role in educating individuals, families, and the community about the care of healthy eyes. Nurses often have the opportunity to screen and educate people about the prevention of disease and impairment. To learn more about ways to promote vision health, visit www.lighthouse.org. For resources to help those persons who are blind, visit the American Foundation for the Blind at www.afb.org or the National Federation of the Blind at www.nfb.org.

Regular Eye Examinations

Regular eye examinations should be encouraged. Individuals who are not known to have visual deficits and do not have diseases associated with visual loss such as diabetes should have their eyes examined at regular intervals throughout their life. Screening tests are usually done during an annual physical examination to detect gross visual deficits. Patients who wear corrective lenses or have disease processes that place them at risk for visual loss should have their eyes examined by an eye care provider at least yearly.

Eye care providers include the **ophthalmologist** and **optometrist.** An ophthalmologist is a physician who specializes in the comprehensive care of the eyes and visual system, including diagnosing and treating eye diseases. An optometrist is a health-care provider who specializes in visual examinations, diagnosis, and treatment of visual problems, such as prescribing lenses. The optometrist is not a physician but is identified as a doctor of optometry. An **optician** is a person trained to grind and fit lenses according to prescriptions written by the ophthalmologist or optometrist.

Eye Hygiene

Individuals should be careful to keep debris out of their eyes to prevent scratching of the eye's delicate surfaces. When a foreign object gets into the eye, such as dirt or an eyelash, the individual should be taught not to rub the eye but to allow tears to wash out the object. This can be done by pulling the eyelid down over the eye for a brief time. When wiping the eyes, the nurse should wipe from the inner canthus to the outer canthus.

Nutrition for Eye Health

Adequate nutrition is important not only for the whole body but for the eye as well (Box 51.2 Nutrition Notes). Eye disorders related to inadequate vitamin intake include corneal damage and night blindness from lack of vitamin A and optic neuritis as a result of vitamin B deficiency.

Eye Safety and Prevention of Injury

Many people in the United States suffer eye injuries each year. Common household activities are responsible for the majority of injuries. Activities such as microwave cooking, lawn care, and shooting rubber bands and BB guns all contribute to eye injury. Many of these injuries could be prevented with education and implementation of safety measures (Table 51.3).

Eye Irrigation

It is sometimes necessary to irrigate foreign bodies or chemical substances out of the eye. The nurse prepares the patient by explaining the procedure. Usually an isotonic solution is used to irrigate the eye. The solution is delivered using IV tubing or a Morgan lens. Refer to Box 51.3 (Eye Irrigation) and Figure 51.5.

Medication Administration

A variety of drugs are available for eye application. Most of the drugs are applied as drops, ointments, or irrigations. The nurse must know the usual dosage and strength, desired action, side effects, and contraindications of the medication being administered to prevent harm to the patient. Systemic adverse reactions can occur and medical diseases can be exacerbated from the administration of eye medications. The elderly are especially susceptible to this because they have more chronic diseases, as well as long-term use of ophthalmic agents. These agents can interact with other med-

---

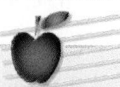

Box 51.2

Nutrition Notes

Interpreting the Role of Antioxidants in Eye Disease

In developing countries, vitamin A deficiency is a leading cause of blindness. In developed countries, antioxidants have been investigated in relation to macular degeneration and cataracts, two conditions that can also lead to severely impaired vision.

Macular Degeneration

High-dose vitamins C and E, beta carotene, and zinc over an average of 6.3 years of follow-up resulted in a 27% reduction in the risk of advanced age-related macular degeneration (ARMD). Such a protocol was recommended to ophthalmologists for certain patients.[1] In addition, observational studies have linked high intakes of foods rich in the carotenoids, lutein, and zeaxanthin, such as spinach, broccoli, and eggs with a 40% reduction in risk of ARMD.[2]

Cataracts

The effect of antioxidants on cataract development is less clear. High doses of vitamins C and E and beta carotene had no apparent effect on cataract development or progression in relatively well-nourished older adults over 6.3 years' time,[3] but a 60% reduction in risk of cataract was found in women who used vitamin C supplements for 10 years or more.[4]

Recommendations

Because there are other risk factors for both eye diseases and because whole foods contain many components besides antioxidant vitamins, many researchers conclude by recommending diets rich in fruits and vegetables to prevent disease and also note that health-conscious individuals who take vitamin supplements often also consume nutrient-dense diets. If a person chooses to take supplements, a multivitamin and multimineral product at Recommended Dietary Allowance levels is advocated rather than separate preparations of individual nutrients.

TABLE 51.3 EYE SAFETY AND INJURY PREVENTION

To Protect From	Use These Eye Safety Measures
Foreign objects	Wear safety goggles. Avoid mowing over rocks or sticks. Always wear safety goggles when using lawn edging yard devices.
Chemical splashes	Use splash shields when working with chemicals such as cleaning solution or body fluids. Close eyes to avoid getting hair spray in them.
Corneal lens abrasions/infections from contact lenses	Follow manufacturer's or eye care professional's directions for length of use and cleaning procedures. Do not overwear lenses.
Ultraviolet light (UV)	Wear UV-protected sunglasses when outdoors. Instruct patients to wear sunglasses with side shields after administration of mydriatics. Wear a hat to shield sun.
Visual deficits in adult with corrective lenses	Update prescription of glasses yearly. Glasses should fit properly, be clean, and be free of scratches.
Eye strain from computer usage	The position of the bottom of the monitor should be 20 degrees below the line of sight and should be positioned 13 to 18 inches from the eyes. The light in the room should prevent glare. Increase the font size on the screen if letters appear too small. If dry eyes are a problem while using a computer, adjust the monitor to a lower level so the eyes do not have to open as wide, which increases evaporation.
Eye injury from sports	Wear protective eye wear with polycarbonate lenses. Wear facemasks or helmets while participating in any high-contact or high-impact sports.

ications the patient is taking. The nurse needs to observe patients for possible reactions.

Chapter 52 discusses specific ophthalmic medications and their uses. To identify the steps in the application of eye medications, see Boxes 51.4 (Administration of Eye Drops) and 51.5 (Administration of Eye Ointments). Whenever eye medications, especially eye drops, are administered, the punctum (tear duct) of the eye should have pressure applied to it by either the nurse wearing gloves or the patient if able for at least 1 minute. This reduces systemic absorption of the medication via the punctum. Some eye medications can have serious cardiac or respiratory effects, and patients have had life-threatening reactions to them. The nurse should educate the patient on the proper instillation of eye medications to reduce these reactions.

 LEARNING TIP

Older patients, when instilling their own eye drops, may not feel the drops go in. Teaching patients to refrigerate the drops, if not contraindicated, for 15 to 30 minutes before instillation helps them feel if the drops go into the eye or on the face.

EYE PATCHING. After treating an injured or infected eye, the physician may order the eye to be patched. The nurse applies ointment or drops if ordered, requests that the patient keep the eyelid shut, and then places a disposable, cotton gauze eye patch over the depression of the eye socket. If the

Box 51.3

Eye Irrigation

1. Explain the procedure to the patient.
2. Wash hands.
3. Gather equipment. For low-volume irrigation, a prefilled squeezable bottle is used. For large-volume irrigation, an intravenous (IV) bag of isotonic solution such as normal saline or lactated Ringer's is used. Attach IV tubing to the bag and flush the line.
4. Apply anesthetic drops, if ordered.
5. Place a basin by the side of the patient's head and pad the area with towels to absorb irrigant.
6. Apply gloves.
7. The eye may be irrigated by holding the distal end of the IV tubing at the inner canthus of the eye, or a Morgan lens may be attached. (See Fig. 51.5.) The lens is placed directly on the anesthetized eye, and the tubing is connected to the IV bag tubing. Proceed with irrigation using a slow, steady stream of irrigant. Generally, use of the lens is more comfortable for patients because the eyelids do not need to be held open.
8. Assess patient's tolerance to the procedure.
9. Remove Morgan lens.
10. Remove gloves. Wash hands.
11. Document assessment, type and amount of irrigant, and patient's tolerance to the procedure.

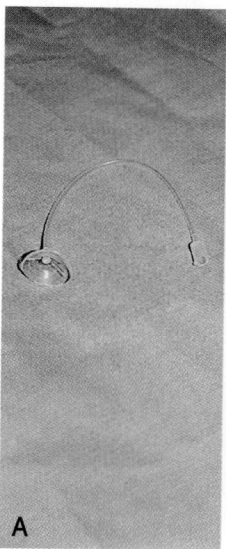
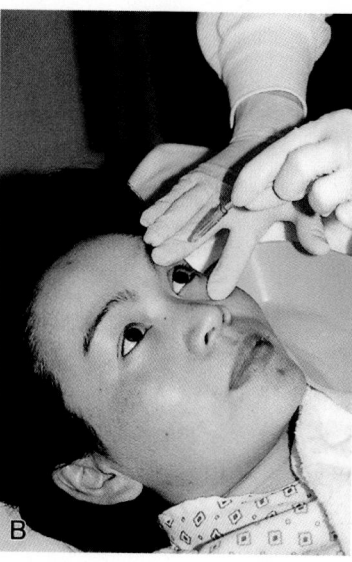

FIGURE 51.5 *(A)* Morgan lens is used for eye irrigation. *(B)* Irrigation of eye.

patient has a deep eye socket, the nurse may need to place two pads over the socket to assist the eyelids to remain closed. The purpose of eye patching is to protect the eye from further damage by keeping the lids closed. Sometimes

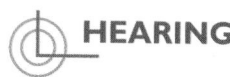

Box 51.4

Administration of Eye Drops

1. Explain procedure to the patient.
2. Check medication for dosage, strength, side effects, contraindications, and expiration date.
3. Wash hands and apply gloves.
4. Instruct patient to tilt head backward and look up toward the ceiling.
5. Gently pull the lower lid down and out. This forms a pocket to catch the eye drop.
6. Approach the patient's eye from the side and instill the prescribed amount of medication into the pocket. Be careful to avoid touching the patient's eye or surrounding structure with the tip of the dropper. It is helpful for the nurse and the patient who is self-administering eye drops to use the forehead as a stabilizing area for the hand administering the drop.
7. Release the lower eyelid.
8. Gently apply pressure with a tissue to the punctum (over the tear duct) for at least 1 minute to prevent the medication from being systemically absorbed. The nurse or patient can do this.
9. Wipe any excess medication off of the eyelids or cheek.
10. Remove gloves. Wash hands.
11. Document medication administration and the patient's tolerance to the procedure.

Box 51.5

Administration of Eye Ointments

1. Explain procedure to the patient.
2. Check medication for dosage, strength, side effects, contraindications, and expiration date.
3. Wash hands and apply gloves.
4. Instruct patient to tilt head backward and look up toward the ceiling.
5. Gently pull the lower lid down. This forms a pocket into which the ointment is placed.
6. Express the ointment directly into the exposed palpebral conjunctiva in the direction of inner to outer canthus. Be careful to avoid touching the patient's eye or surrounding structure with the tip of the ointment tube.
7. Release the lower eyelid over the ointment.
8. Instruct the patient to gently close the eyes.
9. Remove gloves. Wash hands.
10. Instruct the patient that vision may be blurred while the ointment is in the eye.
11. Document medication administration and the patient's tolerance to procedure.

an additional metal shield is placed over the soft pads to protect the eye from external injury. The patch is taped in place and the patient instructed to rest the eyes. The nurse should suggest quiet activities to the patient such as listening to music or an audiotaped book or sleeping. Watching television or reading is not recommended because the patched eye follows the movement of the unpatched eye.

HEARING

Normal Anatomy and Physiology of the Ear

The ear consists of three areas: the outer ear, the middle ear, and the inner ear (Fig. 51.6). The inner ear contains the receptors for the senses of hearing and equilibrium.

Outer Ear
The outer ear consists of the auricle (or pinna) and the ear canal. The auricle is made of cartilage covered with skin. The ear canal is a tunnel into the temporal bone that curves slightly forward and downward. The canal is lined with skin that contains ceruminous glands. Cerumen, or earwax, is the secretion that keeps the eardrum pliable and traps dust.

Middle Ear
The middle ear is an air-filled cavity in the temporal bone. The eardrum (or tympanic membrane) is stretched across the end of the ear canal and vibrates when sound waves strike it. These vibrations are transmitted through the three auditory bones—the malleus, incus, and stapes. The stapes

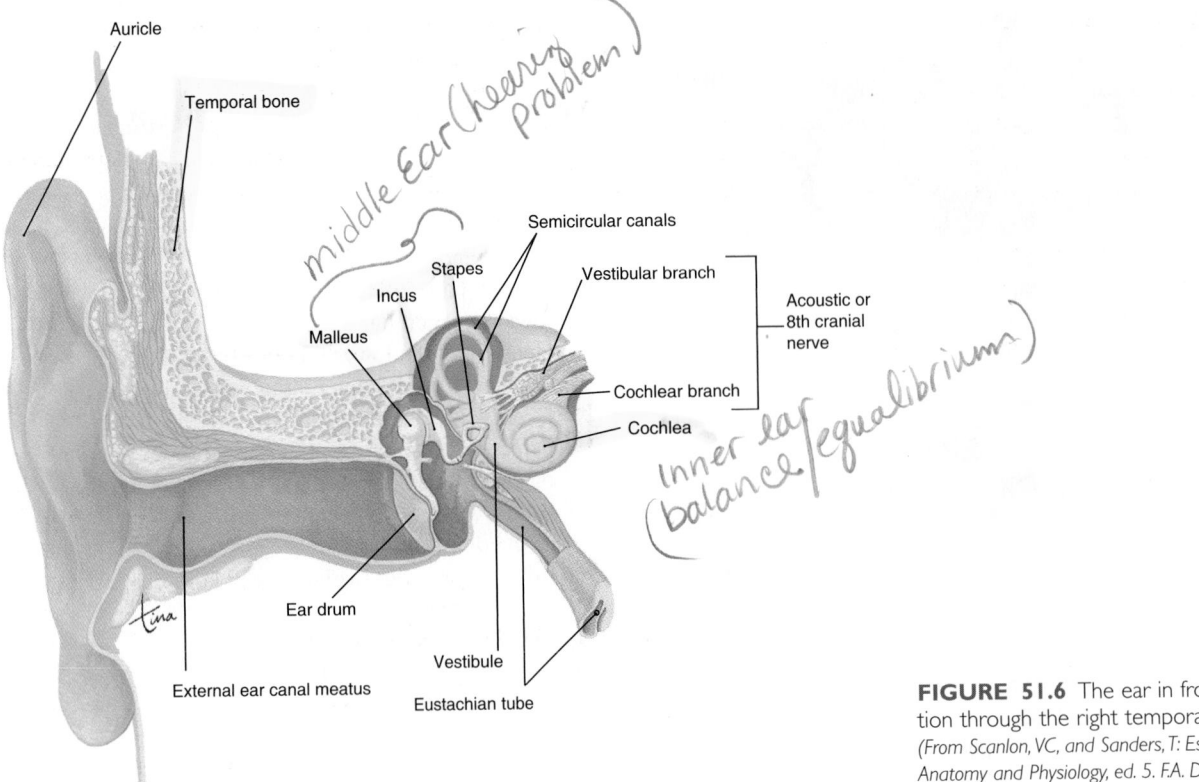

middle Ear (hearing problem)

inner ear (balance/equalibrium)

Auricle

Temporal bone

Semicircular canals

Stapes

Vestibular branch

Incus

Acoustic or 8th cranial nerve

Malleus

Cochlear branch

Cochlea

Ear drum

Vestibule

External ear canal meatus

Eustachian tube

FIGURE 51.6 The ear in frontal section through the right temporal bone. *(From Scanlon, VC, and Sanders, T: Essentials of Anatomy and Physiology, ed. 5. F.A. Davis, Philadelphia, 2007.)*

then transmits vibrations to the fluid-filled inner ear at the oval window.

The eustachian tube (or auditory tube) extends from the middle ear to the nasopharynx and permits air to enter or leave the middle ear cavity. The air pressure in the middle ear must be the same as the external atmospheric pressure for the eardrum to vibrate properly. Swallowing or yawning opens the eustachian tubes and permits equalization of these pressures.

Inner Ear

The inner ear is a cavity in the temporal bone called the bony labyrinth, lined with membrane called the membranous labyrinth. The fluid between bone and membrane is called perilymph, and that within the membrane is called endolymph. These membranous structures are the cochlear ducts, which are concerned with hearing, and the utricle, saccule, and semicircular ducts, which are all concerned with equilibrium.

The cochlea is shaped like a snail shell and is partitioned internally into three fluid-filled canals. The medial canal is the cochlear duct, which contains the receptors for hearing in the organ of Corti (spiral organ). The receptors are called hair cells (their projections are stereocilia), which contain endings of the cochlear branch of the eighth cranial nerve. A membrane called the tectorial membrane hangs over the hair cells.

The process of hearing involves the transmission of vibrations and the generation of nerve impulses. When sound waves enter the ear canal, vibrations are transmitted by the following structures: eardrum, malleus, incus, stapes,

oval window of the inner ear, perilymph and endolymph within the cochlea, and hair cells of the organ of Corti. When the hair cells bend, they generate impulses that are carried by the eighth cranial nerve to the brain. The auditory areas, for both hearing and interpretation, are in the temporal lobes of the cerebral cortex.

The utricle and saccule are membranous sacs between the cochlea and semicircular canals. Each contains a patch of hair cells embedded in a gelatinous structure that contains otoliths, small crystals of calcium carbonate. The hair cells bend in response to the pull of gravity on the otoliths as the position of the head changes. The impulses generated are carried by the vestibular branch of the eighth cranial nerve to the cerebellum, medulla, and pons. The cerebellum sends this information continuously to the cerebral motor cortex. The cerebellum and brainstem use this information to maintain equilibrium at a subconscious level; the cerebrum provides a conscious awareness of the position of the head.

The three semicircular canals are fluid-filled membranous ovals oriented in three planes. At the base of each is an enlarged portion called the ampulla, which contains hair cells (the cristae) that are affected by movement. As the body moves forward, for example, the hair cells at first bend backward. The bending of the hair cells generates impulses carried by the vestibular branch of the eighth cranial nerve to the cerebellum and brainstem; and then impulses continue on to the cerebral motor cortex. These impulses are interpreted as starting or stopping, turning, or changing speeds, and this information is used to maintain equilibrium while a person is moving.

Aging and the Ear

In the ear, cumulative damage to the hair cells in the organ of Corti usually becomes apparent sometime after the age of 60 (see Fig. 51.2). Hair cells that have been damaged by a lifetime of noise cannot be replaced. Sounds in high-pitched ranges are usually those lost first (presbycusis), whereas hearing may still be adequate for lower pitched ranges. The high-pitched sounds *f, s, k,* and *sh* are usually lost first. It becomes more difficult to filter out background noises, so noisy environments make it difficult to hear conversations.

LEARNING TIP

Presbycusis is the loss of hearing high-pitched sounds (pitch = cycles per second; loudness = decibels [dB]). Because the ability to hear pitch is lost rather than loudness, it is not helpful to talk louder to a patient with this type of hearing loss. In fact, talking louder can make it more difficult to discriminate sounds. It is important to know the type of hearing loss a patient has.

Nursing Assessment/Data Collection of the Ear and Hearing Status

A nursing assessment of the ear includes obtaining the patient's health history and performing a physical examination. A complete nursing assessment is conducted on admission. Provide privacy and make the patient as comfortable as possible before beginning the nursing assessment. A quiet environment is helpful for an accurate assessment of hearing. During the initial assessment, observe the patient's behavior and note any information the patient shares.

Subjective Data

To understand the patient's ear disorder, perform a focused health history. Use knowledge of pathophysiology to guide questions in an appropriate and complete manner. Assessment of symptoms includes asking the WHAT'S UP? questions: where it is, how it feels, aggravating and alleviating factors, timing, severity, useful data for associated symptoms, and perception of the problem by the patient.

HEALTH HISTORY. Obtaining the patient's self-appraisal of his or her hearing or related symptoms is completed during the health history. You should also gather information about medications, surgeries, treatments, allergies, and habits. The health history helps in formulating the nursing care plan.

Symptoms and complaints related to the ear include decreased or loss of hearing, **otorrhea** (discharge), **otalgia** (ear pain), itching, fullness, tinnitus (ringing, buzzing, or roaring in the ears), or vertigo (dizziness). If any of these symptoms or complaints is positive, explore the symptoms in more detail using the WHAT'S UP? format. Record all the information accurately and completely.

Other information about the patient's medical history, including previous ear problems and use of **hearing aids** or assistive hearing devices, is obtained. You should also ask about any surgeries, allergies, recent upper respiratory infections, history of infections, injury to the ear, hospitalizations, swimming habits, exposure to pressure changes (flying or diving), medical diseases, and exposure to any loud noises. Positive findings should be assessed using the WHAT'S UP? format and results recorded.

Information about current and past medications should be obtained. Many medications are potentially toxic to the ear and can cause hearing loss or decreased hearing. Pay particular attention to any exposure to medications that are potentially **ototoxic,** such as certain antibiotics or diuretics. (See Chapter 52.) *aminoclyocites*

Family history related to ear disorders includes any hearing problems or hearing loss and family members with Ménière's disease. Significant findings are recorded, including the relationship of the family member with the problem to the patient.

Information about the patient's care of the ears is also gathered. It is important to assess what preventive measures the patient practices and what the patient's learning needs are concerning care and protection of the ears. Determine how the patient cleans the ears, any exposure to loud noises during recreational activities or during work activities, any changes in ability to hear, and any exposure to ototoxic medications. You should determine if the patient has had a hearing evaluation and if there is a history of ear problems. Instruct the patient in ways to care for the ears and maintain ear health (Table 51.4).

Objective Data

Physical data collection of the ear begins by observing the behaviors of the patient. Note how the patient communicates. Observe how the patient talks, noting any slurred speech or words. See Box 51.6 Behaviors Indicating Hearing Loss. Examination of the ear includes inspection, palpation, testing auditory acuity, and, for the advanced practitioner, otoscopic examination (Table 51.5).

INSPECTION AND PALPATION OF THE EXTERNAL EAR. Inspection of the external ear begins with examining the auricle. A penlight or otoscope may be used to improve visualization of the external ear. The external ear should be inspected for size, symmetry, configuration, and angle of attachment. Note any obvious deformities or scars. The skin should be smooth and without breaks, particularly behind the ear in the crevice. The color should be uniform, without signs of inflammation. To inspect the external ear canal, tip the adult patient's head to the side and use a penlight or otoscope to inspect the canal. Note any drainage or cerumen (wax), including the color, odor, and clarity of the drainage.

---

otorrhea: oto—related to the ear + rrhea—to flow
otalgia: ot—related to the ear + algia—signifying pain

ototoxic: oto—related to the ear + toxic—poison

TABLE 51.4 SUBJECTIVE ASSESSMENT OF THE EAR

Category	Questions to Ask During History Assessment	Rationale/Significance
Family History	Has any family member had any hearing problems or loss? Has any family member had Ménière's disease?	This may give information about the patient's current ear problem.
Patient Health History	What medications are you currently taking? Have you had any surgeries or trauma to the ear? Do you have any allergies to food, medications or other substances? Have you had any recent upper respiratory infections? Do you have a history of upper respiratory infections or ear infections? Do you have any discharge from the ear (otorrhea), ear pain (otalgia), itching, fullness, tinnitus or vertigo? Do you have a fever, nausea, or vomiting? Are you exposed to pressure changes such as with flying or diving?	Many medications are ototoxic and can cause hearing loss (see Chapter 52) Recent trauma or surgeries can affect hearing. Can cause nasal congestion leading to middle ear congesion and/or infections. May indicate outer, middle or inner ear infections. May indicate ototoxicity or other ear diseases. Barotrauma may occur due to pressure changes.
Hearing Impairment	Have you noticed any hearing loss? If so, has it been gradual or sudden? Do you have difficulty understanding certain words or entire conversations? Do you have difficulty hearing when there is a lot of background noise? Do you hear better out of one ear versus the other? Have your friends or family commented on your decreased hearing? Do you wear a hearing aid or other assistive device? If so, what is the device and for which ear is it used? How does your hearing loss affect your daily life? Do you feel embarrassed or frustrated because of your hearing loss? How do your friends and family react to your hearing loss? Are you exposed to loud noises, such as with your current or past job, busy traffic, machinery or loud music?	Could indicate hearing loss and further assessment is needed. Patient may already have hearing loss in one or both ears. Hearing loss can cause social isolation. Can cause damage to the ear leading to hearing loss over time.
Self-Care Behaviors	Have you had your hearing checked? If so, when? How do you clean your ears? How do you protect your ears from loud noises?	Provides information about patient's ear self-care and health.

Box 51.6

Behaviors Indicating Hearing Loss

Adults with hearing loss may display any or all of the following behaviors:

- Turns up the volume on the television or radio
- Frequently asks, "What did you say?"
- Leans forward or turns head to one side during conversations to hear better
- Cups hand around ear during conversation
- Complains of people talking softly or mumbling
- Speaks in an unusually quiet or loud voice
- Answers questions inappropriately or not at all
- Has difficulty hearing high-frequency consonants
- Avoids group activities
- Shows loss of sense of humor
- Face looks strained or serious during conversations
- Appears to ignore people or aloof, does not participate
- Is irritable or sensitive in interpersonal relations
- Complains of ringing, buzzing, or roaring noise in the ears

The skin should be smooth and without inflammation, edema, or breaks. There should be no lesions, foreign bodies, erythema, or edema observed within the external ear canal. Inspection of the external ear canal should be completed before obtaining an infrared ear temperature because the presence of cerumen can alter the accuracy of the reading.

Next the auricles are palpated and any tophi, lesions, or masses are noted. Tophi are deposits of uric acid crystals that appear as small, hard nodules in the helix (external ear margin); they may also occur in gout. The auricle should be nontender when it is palpated; tenderness can indicate an external ear infection. A downward protrusion of the helix, called Darwin's tubercle, is a normal finding. The mastoid process should be smooth and hard when palpated. The mastoid process can be of different sizes but should not be tender or swollen.

AUDITORY ACUITY TESTING. Auditory function can be grossly evaluated using three different assessment tests. The whisper voice test is one test to check hearing function in each ear. The patient occludes one ear with a finger, and the nurse stands 1 to 2 feet away on the opposite side. The nurse whispers two-syllable words toward the unoccluded ear. The

TABLE 51.5 OBJECTIVE ASSESSMENT OF THE EAR

Category	Physical Assessment Findings	Possible Abnormal Findings/Causes
Inspection and Palpation of the External Ear	Ears should be symmetrical in size, configuration, and angle of attachment. Skin covering the ear should be intact, smooth, and without edema, erythema, or inflammation. Canal should have minimal or no cerumen. No lesions, tophi, or masses should be palpated. No tenderness of auricle when palpated. No odor detected.	Asymmetrical size and placement could indicate congenital deformities. Discharge, breaks in skin, or inflammation can be caused by trauma, external ear infections, poorly fitting hearing aid or skin disorders. Excessive cerumen may be found. This can alter hearing and cause inaccurate tympanic temperature readings. Excess cerumen may need to be removed. Tophi may be present in the patient with gout. Tenderness could indicate an external ear infection.
Auditory Acuity Testing	Patient able to hear whispered words at 1–2 feet away. Rinne's and Weber's tests normal (see Table 51.7). Able to understand and converse with examiner.	Patient may have indications of conductive or sensorineural hearing loss.
Balance Testing	Patient is able to sit and walk without difficulty. Patient able to complete Romberg's test with minimal swaying.	Difficulty sitting and/or walking; increased swaying or falling with Romberg's test due to balance difficulties. May be due to inner ear infection or disorder.
Otoscopic Examination	Ear canal should be smooth and empty without redness, scaliness, swelling, drainage, excessive cerumen, or foreign objects. Internal otoscope examination is completed by experienced practitioner and should reveal a slightly conical, shiny, smooth, pearly gray eardrum.	Ear canal may be reddened and swollen; drainage may be present; excessive cerumen or foreign object may be present. Caused by infection, improper care, or excessive cerumen production. Eardrum may be dull, bulging or retracted, reddened caused by middle ear infection or blockage.

patient restates the whispered words. The nurse should be by the patient's side to prevent the patient from lip reading. The nurse's voice can be increased from a soft, medium, or loud whisper to a soft, medium, or loud voice. The process is repeated on the other ear. The patient is asked if hearing is better in one ear than in the other ear. The patient should be able to hear a soft whisper equally well in both ears. Findings of one ear hearing better than the other or an inability to hear a soft whisper can be indicative of hearing impairment. Results of the test are documented.

A second acuity test is the **Rinne test.** This test is performed with a tuning fork and is useful for differentiating between conductive and sensorineural hearing loss. To per-

form the test, strike the tuning fork and place it on the patient's mastoid process (Fig. 51.7). Verify that the patient is able to hear the tuning fork and then instruct the patient to say immediately when the sound is no longer heard. When the patient indicates that the sound is not heard, place the vibrating tuning fork 2 inches in front of the ear. (See Fig. 51.7.) Ask the patient if he or she hears the tuning fork and then to indicate when the sound is no longer heard. Normally, air conduction (AC) is heard twice as long as bone conduction (BC). The patient reports this by hearing the tuning fork when placed in front of the ear (AC) after no longer hearing the tuning fork placed on the mastoid process (BC). Normal results are recorded as "AC > BC" (air conduction

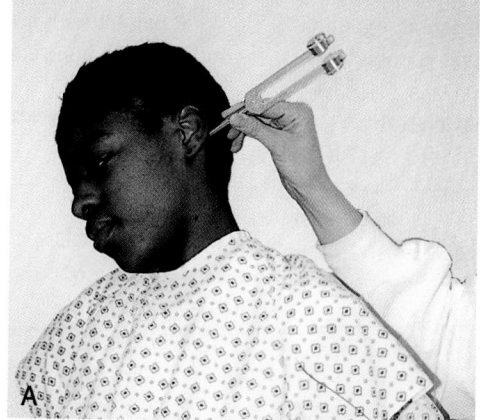
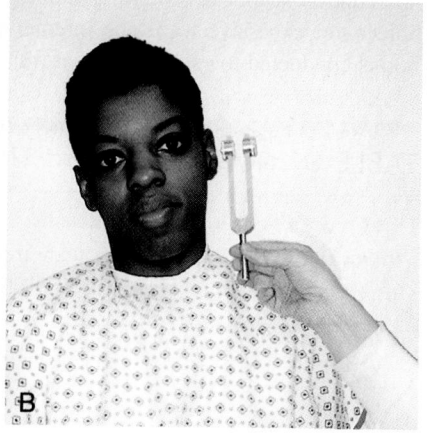

FIGURE 51.7 Rinne test. *(A) Bone conduction. (B) Air conduction.*

is greater than bone conduction). The test is repeated on the other ear and findings recorded. Abnormal findings can indicate conduction or sensorineural problems (Table 51.6).

The **Weber test** is a third test to assess hearing acuity. The Weber test is also performed using a tuning fork. Place the vibrating tuning fork on the center of the patient's forehead or head (Fig. 51.8). Verify that the patient can hear the tuning fork. Then, with a positive answer, ask the patient if he or she hears the sound better in the left ear, better in the right ear, or the same in both ears. It is important to give the patient three choices from which to choose. Normally, the patient hears the sound the same in both ears (see Table 51.6).

BALANCE TESTING. When the patient complains of dizziness, nystagmus, or problems with equilibrium, simple tests can be performed to assess vestibular function. The first test is simply to observe the patient's gait by having the patient walk away from the examiner and then walk back to the examiner. Note the patient's balance, posture, and movement of arms and legs. The patient should be able to walk with an upright position with no difficulties in balance or movement.

Romberg's test, or falling test, is another simple test to assess vestibular function. Instruct the patient to stand with feet together, first with eyes open and then with eyes closed. Normally, the patient has no difficulty maintaining a standing position with only minimal swaying. If the patient has difficulty maintaining balance or loses balance (a positive Romberg's test), it can indicate an inner ear problem. If a fall appears likely, be prepared to support the patient to prevent injury.

OTOSCOPIC EXAMINATION. An otoscope is an instrument consisting of a handle, a light source, a magnifying lens, and an optional speculum for inserting in the ear. Some otoscopes have a pneumatic device for injecting air into the canal to test the eardrum's mobility and integrity. The otoscope is used to visualize the external ear, ear canal, and tympanic membrane. Otoscopic examination is completed to identify specific disorders or infections, remove wax, or remove foreign bodies. Examination of the ear canal should be completed during insertion and removal of the speculum. The ear canal should be smooth and empty. There should be no redness, scaliness, swelling, drainage, nodules, foreign objects, or excessive wax. The internal otoscopic examination is conducted to examine the eardrum and is done by the

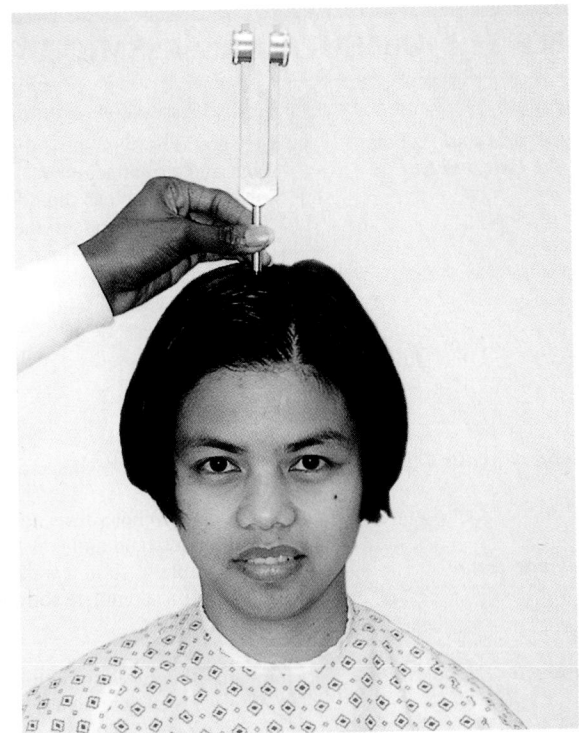

FIGURE 51.8 Weber's test.

experienced practitioner. The eardrum should appear slightly conical, shiny, and smooth and be a pearly gray color.

Diagnostic Tests

AUDIOMETRIC TESTING. Audiometric testing is used as a screening tool to determine the type and degree of hearing loss. An audiologist conducts the hearing tests in a sound-proof booth. The audiometer produces a stimulus that consists of a musical tone, pure tone, or speech. To test air conduction, the patient is placed in the booth, wears earphones, and signals the audiologist when and if the tone is heard. Each ear is tested separately as the patient is exposed to sounds of varying frequency or pitch (hertz) and intensity (decibels). By varying the levels of the sound, a hearing level is established (Table 51.7). The use of earphones measures air conduction, level of speech hearing, and understanding of speech. During bone conduction testing, a vibrator is placed on the mastoid process and the earphones are removed. Testing proceeds as with air conduction.

A patient with normal hearing should have the same air conduction as bone conduction hearing levels. Alterations in

TABLE 51.6 AUDITORY ACUITY TUNING FORK TESTS

Test	Expected Results	Conductive Hearing Loss	Sensorineural Hearing Loss
Rinne Test	Air conduction heard longer than bone conduction	Bone conduction heard longer than air conduction in affected ear	Air conduction heard longer than bone conduction in affected ear (may be less than 2:1 ratio)
Weber Test	Tone heard in center of the head; no lateralization	Sound heard louder in affected ear	Sound heard louder in better ear

TABLE 51.7 COMMON NOISE LEVELS

Human Hearing Threshold	0–25 dB
Quiet room	30–40 dB
Conversational speech	60 dB
Heavy traffic	70 dB
Telephone	70 dB
Alarm clock	80 dB
Vacuum cleaner	80 dB
Unsafe noise levels begin	**90 dB**
Circular saw	100 dB
Rock music	120 dB
Jet planes	120–130 dB
Pain threshold	130 dB
Firearms	140 dB

testing air and bone conduction hearing can provide information about the location and type of hearing loss.

TYMPANOMETRY. Tympanometry is a test used to measure compliance of the tympanic membrane and differentiate problems in the middle ear. Varying amounts of pressure are applied to the tympanic membrane, and the results create a distinctive response recorded on a graph called a tympanogram. The test is useful in determining the amount of negative pressure within the middle ear. The patient is informed that the tympanometry may cause transient vertigo. The patient should report any nausea or dizziness experienced during the test.

CALORIC TEST. The caloric test is used to test the function of the eighth cranial nerve and to assess vestibular reflexes of the inner ear that control balance. The test is performed first on one ear and then the other. Warm (44.5°C [112°F]) or cold (30°C [86° F]) water is instilled into the ear canal. This stimulates the endolymph of the semicircular canals, which stimulates movement of the head. Nystagmus is a normal response. The patient may also experience dizziness. No nystagmus is seen if the patient has a disease of the labyrinth such as Ménière's disease. The test is contraindicated if the patient has a perforated tympanic membrane. Otoscopic examination should be completed before this test to assess for excessive cerumen or perforated tympanic membrane.

ELECTRONYSTAGMOGRAM. The electronystagmogram is used to diagnose the causes of unilateral hearing loss of unknown origin, vertigo, or ringing in the ears. It is similar to the caloric test. The test is usually completed in a darkened room. Five electrodes are taped to the patient's clean face at certain positions around the eye. The electrodes measure nystagmus in response to vestibular stimulation. Measurements are taken at rest, looking at different objects, with eyes open and closed, in different positions, with water of different temperatures, and with air. Usually tranquilizers, alcohol, stimulants, and antivertigo agents are held for 1 to 5 days before the test. The patient should also avoid tobacco and caffeine on the day of the test. The test is contraindicated

in patients who have pacemakers. The patient may experience nausea, vertigo, or weakness following the test.

COMPUTED TOMOGRAPHY. A CT scan produces radiographs similar to those used in conventional radiography. A special scanner system produces cross-sectional images of anatomical structures without superimposing tissues on each other. CT is useful for visualizing the temporal and mastoid bones, the middle and inner ears, and the eustachian tube. The patient should remove hairpins and jewelry from the area of visualization.

MAGNETIC RESONANCE IMAGING. MRI produces cross-sectional images of the human anatomy through exposure to magnetic energy sources without using radiation. It is useful in differentiating between healthy and diseased tissue. The MRI allows the membranous organs, nerve, and blood vessels of the temporal bone to be examined. The test is contraindicated in patients with implanted heart valves, surgical and aneurysm clips, and internal orthopedic screws and rods. The patient should remove dental bridges and appliances, credit cards, keys, hairclips, shoes, belts, jewelry or clothing with metal fasteners, wigs, and hairpieces before entering the magnetic resonance room.

LABORATORY TESTS. Culture. Culture of drainage from the ear canal or surgical incision is important in diagnosis and treatment of acute infections. Identifying the organism responsible for the infection allows the appropriate antibiotic to be used. Often with chronic infections, the culture is less helpful because gram-negative bacilli cover up the original pathogen. Drainage from the external ear is collected using a sterile cotton-tipped or polyester-tipped swab. Samples should be taken to the laboratory immediately.

Pathological Examination. Pathological examination of tissue obtained during surgery is completed to rule out a malignancy and identify any unusual problems. A cholesteatoma (cyst of epithelial cells and cholesterol found in the middle ear) is usually documented by a pathological examination.

Therapeutic Interventions
Medications

The medications most often used to treat ear disorders include anti-infectives, anti-inflammatories, antihistamines, decongestants, cerumenolytics, and diuretics. Anti-infectives can be administered systemically or as a topical solution. Ear medications are generally in a liquid form for ease in administration as drops. Box 51.7 (Administration of Ear Drops) and Figure 51.9 guide the nurse in administering ear drops. Anti-inflammatories, antihistamines, and decongestants are used with acute infections to reduce nasal and middle ear congestion. Cerumenolytics are used to soften cerumen and remove it from the ear canal. Diuretics are used with some inner ear disorders to reduce pressure caused by fluids.

CRITICAL THINKING

Mr. Frank

■ Mr. Frank's wife expressed concern about his changing behavior during the last 6 months. She reports that Mr. Frank no longer enjoys talking to neighbors or visiting with friends in their church group, is irritable, has lost his sense of humor, and does not always answer her questions appropriately.

1. What do you suspect is happening with Mr. Frank?
2. What examination techniques or tests might you use to gather data related to Mr. Frank's signs and symptoms?
3. What would be the expected findings of these tests?
4. What teaching for these symptoms and their affect on Mr. Frank's lifestyle would be helpful?
5. What safety issues should Mr. Frank be taught to address?

Suggested answers at end of chapter.

Ear Health Maintenance

Routine cleaning and care of the ears should be taught to all patients. Patient education should include prevention of trauma, prevention of hearing loss, and early detection of hearing loss. All patients can benefit from this type of education, as found in Table 51.8.

Assistive Devices

Hearing aids are instruments that amplify sounds. (See Chapter 52.) Certain hearing aids may be designed to amplify sounds and attenuate certain portions of the sound signal. A microphone receives the sounds and converts them to electrical signals. These signals are amplified, and a receiver then converts the signal to sound. A small battery serves as the energy source. Digital hearing aids contain computers that provide clearer and crisper sound that is tai-

Box 51.7

Administration of Ear Drops

1. Wash hands.
2. Ensure medication is at room temperature.
3. Position patient sitting up with head tilted toward unaffected side or side lying on unaffected side.
4. Pull auricle down and back on children and pull auricle up and back for adults.
5. Instill prescribed number of drops, being careful not to touch the tip of the dropper to prevent contamination.
6. Have patient remain in position for 2 to 3 minutes.
7. A small cotton plug may be inserted to prevent medication from running out of ear.
8. Wash hands.

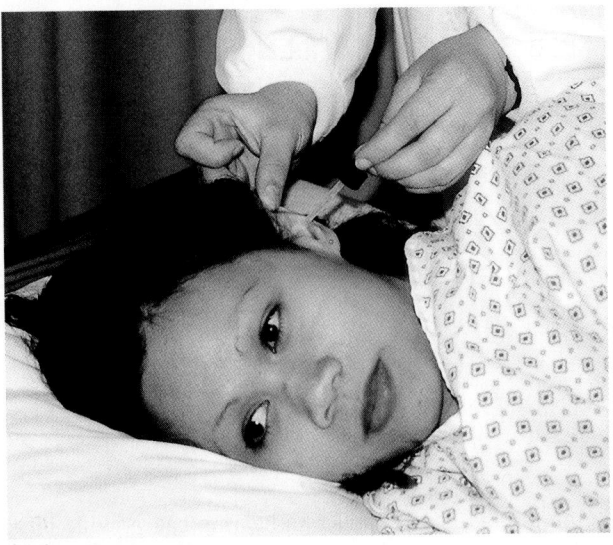

FIGURE 51.9 Ear drop administration.

lored to the person's hearing loss. Digital hearing aids are more expensive than analog hearing aids. There are four types of commonly used hearing aids:

1. The in-the-ear aid fits into the ear. It is small and unobtrusive to the wearer and others.
2. The behind-the-ear, or postauricular, aid is the most common type. This fits behind the ear and is comfortable to wear.
3. The all-in-one eyeglass aid combines eyeglasses with a hearing aid and is the least commonly used type.
4. The body-worn aid has a fitted ear mold inserted into the external ear and is connected to a receiver. The receiver is wired to a transmitter, which is worn around the neck. The wearer is not able to hide the receiver and wires.

To care for a hearing aid, ensure that it is turned off and the battery is removed when it is not in use. This reduces battery expense for the patient, who may be on a fixed income. When turning the hearing aid on, the volume should be turned up just until it squeals and then turned down until the patient indicates it is at the appropriate level for hearing. At least weekly, clean the hearing aid mold portion with either a dry cloth or a damp, soapy cloth and rinse with a damp cloth. A brush may come with the hearing aid for cleaning, or a cotton-tipped swab can be used to clean the small tip that fits into the ear.

Another type of hearing aid is the implantable middle ear hearing device, called the Vibrant Soundbridge (MED-EL, Durham, NC), for those with a sensorineural hearing loss. It provides sound perception by enhancing the normal middle ear hearing function. An audio processor picks up environmental sound and transmits it to the receiver implanted under the skin. The sound is then sent to a tiny floating transducer that directly vibrates the ossicles, which sends the message to the cochlea, as in normal hearing. The hair cells in the cochlea stimulate the auditory nerve, and the brain interprets the message as sound. For more information

TABLE 51.8 PREVENTION OF EAR PROBLEMS

Activity	Patient Education	Rationale
Care of External Ear	Wash external ear with soap and water only.	Keeps external ear clean.
	Do not routinely remove wax from the ear canal.	The ear is generally self-cleaning. Wax is normally removed during showering. Wax serves as a protective mechanism to lubricate and trap foreign material.
Preventing Ear Trauma	Avoid inserting any objects or solutions into the ear. Avoid swimming in polluted areas.	Prevents traumatizing the ear and tympanic membrane or exposing the ear to infection.
	Avoid flying when the ear or upper respiratory system is congested.	Prevents barotrauma due to pressure changes.
Preventing Damage from Noise Pollution	Avoid exposure to excessive occupational noise levels.	Normal speech is 60 dB; heavy traffic is 70 dB. Above 80 dB is uncomfortable. If there is ringing in the ear, damage may be occurring. Occupational noise is the primary cause of hearing loss.
	Avoid other causes of excessive noise such as use of firearms and high-intensity music.	Hearing loss can occur due to exposure to loud noises.
	Use protective earplugs or earmuffs if exposure to noise cannot be avoided.	Protects ears from hearing loss by decreasing exposure to loud noises.
Early Detection of Hearing Loss	Instruct adults to have hearing checked every 2–3 years.	Degenerative changes occur in the ear with aging.
	Monitor for side effects of ototoxic drugs. Instruct patient to report any dizziness, decreased hearing acuity, or tinnitus when taking ototoxic medications.	Prevents side effects of medications from causing hearing loss.
	Caution older patients who use aspirin that it is ototoxic.	Older patients may have hearing loss and not be able to hear the tinnitus.
	Instruct patient to report to physician any prolonged symptoms of ear pain, swelling, drainage, or plugged feeling.	Many medical problems can be prevented with prompt treatment.
	Instruct patient to blow nose with both nostrils open during upper respiratory infections (colds).	Prevents infected secretions from moving up the eustachian tubes into the middle ear.

or to see the Vibrant Soundbridge, visit www.symphonix. com.

A person who is profoundly deaf and has lost all hearing may use a **cochlear implant.** All cochlear implants feature a microelectronic processor for converting the sound into electrical signals, a transmission system to relay signals to the implanted parts, and a long, slender electrode placed in the cochlea to deliver the electrical stimuli directly to the fiber of the auditory nerve. The electrode is surgically placed. Patients commonly have difficulty understanding and learning speech, even with the cochlear implant.

For resources on helping those with hearing impairments, visit the National Association of the Deaf at www. nad.org.

Diet

The patient with an ear problem usually does not have any diet modifications. However, the patient with Ménière's disease may benefit from a lower sodium diet to prevent retention of fluid. Increased fluid may contribute to Ménière's disease symptoms.

Hearing Ear Dogs

Hearing ear dogs are now available to assist those with hearing problems. The dogs are trained to respond to sounds that the person who is hard of hearing cannot hear. Examples include a crying baby, oven timer, and smoke alarm. These dogs provide a valuable service that enriches the lives of those with hearing problems.

REVIEW QUESTIONS

Place the items in correct order. Use all items.

1. In what order does a beam of light pass through the refractive structures in the eye?

   aqueous humor 2

   cornea 1

   lens 3

   vitreous humor 4

2. Which of the following methods can be used to assess visual fields?
   a. Inspection with an ophthalmoscope
   b. Fluorescein angiography
   c. Testing vision with Snellen's chart
   d. Comparing the patient's visual fields with your own

3. Which of the following patient behaviors would the nurse expect to find in a patient's history who has a hearing loss?

   a. Turns volume lower on the television
   b. Is irritable or sensitive in interpersonal relations
   c. Answers questions appropriately
   d. Complains of people talking too loudly

4. The nurse is collecting data during a patient's clinic visit. Which question will best collect data about a patient's preventative ear health?
   a. "What symptoms are you having?"
   b. " Tell me about your ear pain."
   c. "When was your last hearing evaluation?"
   d. "What medications do you take?"

5. Which of the following is the most important nursing intervention during Romberg's test?
   a. Ensure patient safety.
   b. Whisper softly into each ear.
   c. Ensure a quiet environment.
   d. Remove all cerumen from ear canal.

6. Which of the following patient statements indicates that the patient understands ear care teaching?

   a. "I should insert a cotton swab into my ear canal for cleaning."
   b. "I should not get my external ear wet during bathing."
   c. "I should block one nostril when blowing my nose."
   d. "Aspirin can be toxic to the ears."

Multiple response item. Select all that apply.

7. The nurse prepares to provide an eye irrigation to a patient with a methicillin-resistant *S. aureus* (MRSA) infection. Contact precautions are ordered. Which of the following protective items will the nurse need while performing this procedure?
   a. Gloves
   b. Gown
   c. Goggles
   d. Mask
   e. Shoe protectors

8. A patient is taking aspirin. Which of the following findings would indicate to the nurse that the patient is experiencing a toxic effect related to the medication?
   a. Halos around lights
   b. Decreased night vision
   c. Tinnitus
   d. Vertigo

References

1. Age-related Eye Disease Study Research Group: A randomized, placebo-controlled, clinical trial of high-dose supplementation with vitamins C and E, beta-carotene, and zinc for age-related macular degeneration and vision loss. Arch Ophthalmol 119:1417, 2001.
2. Moeller, SM, Jacques, PF, and Blumberg, JB: The potential role of dietary xanthophylls in cataract and age-related macular degeneration. J Am Coll Nutr 19:522S, 2000.
3. Age-related Eye Disease Study Research Group: A randomized, placebo-controlled, clinical trial of high-dose supplementation with vitamins C and E and beta-carotene for age-related cataract and vision loss. Arch Ophthalmol 119: 1439, 2001.
4. Taylor, A, Jacques PF, Chylack LT, et al: Long-term intake of vitamins and carotenoids and odds of early age-related cortical and posterior subcapsular lens opacities. Am J Clin Nutr 75: 540, 2002.

SUGGESTED ANSWERS TO

CRITICAL THINKING

■ Mr. Frank

1. He is exhibiting behaviors of hearing loss.
2. Ear inspection, a whisper voice test, a Rinne test, and a Weber test might be performed.
3. For inspection of ear, cerumen impaction may be found. For a whisper voice test, the whisper is not heard in affected ear. For a Rinne test, bone conduction is heard longer than air conduction in affected ear. For a Weber test, sound is heard louder in affected ear.
4. Explaining to Mr. and Mrs. Frank symptoms of hearing loss will help them understand Mr. Frank's behaviors. Explore with them the effects of these symptoms in daily life to develop plans for coping with the hearing loss until an intervention is implemented.
5. He may not hear telephones or alarms such as smoke or carbon monoxide detectors, so alternatives such as visual alarms could be considered. If he drives, he may not hear car horns or emergency vehicles of which he should be aware to compensate.

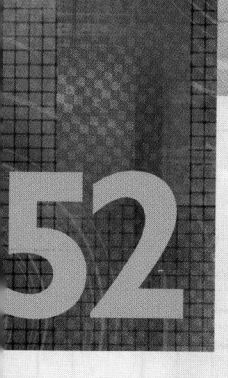

52

Nursing Care of Patients with Sensory Disorders: Vision and Hearing

LAZETTE V. NOWICKI AND
DEBRA AUCOIN-RATCLIFF

KEY TERMS

astigmatism (uh-STIG-mah-TIZM)
blepharitis (BLEF-uh-RIGH-tis)
blindness (BLYND-ness)
carbuncle (KAR-bung-kull)
cataract (KAT-uh-rakt)
chalazion (kah-LAY-zee-on)
conductive hearing loss (kon-DUK-tiv HEER-ing LOSS)
conjunctivitis (kon-JUNK-ti-VIGH-tis)
enucleation (ee-NEW-klee-AY-shun)
external otitis (eks-TER-nuhl oh-TIGH-tis)
furuncle (FYOOR-ung-kull)
glaucoma (glaw-KOH-mah)
hordeolum (hor-DEE-oh-lum)
hyperopia (HIGH-per-OH-pee-ah)
macular (MAK-yoo-lar)
Ménière's disease (ma-NEARS di-ZEEZ)
miotics (my-AH-tiks)
myopia (my-OH-pee-ah)
myringoplasty (mir-IN-goh-PLASS-tee)
myringotomy (MIR-in-GOT-uh-mee)
otosclerosis (OH-toh-skle-ROH-sis)
photophobia (FOH-toh-FOH-bee-ah)
presbycusis (PREZ-by-KYOO-sis)
presbyopia (PREZ-by-OH-pee-ah)
retinopathy (ret-i-NAH-puh-thee)
sensorineural (SEN-suh-ree-NEW-ruhl)
stapedectomy (stuh-puh-DEK-tuh-mee)

QUESTIONS TO GUIDE YOUR READING

1. How would you explain the pathophysiology of each of the disorders of the sensory system?

2. How would you define blindness and the refractive errors of vision?

3. What are the etiologies, signs, and symptoms of sensory disorders?

4. What care would you provide for patients undergoing tests for sensory disorders?

5. What are the therapeutic interventions for each sensory disorder?

6. What medications are contraindicated for patients with acute angle-closure glaucoma?

7. What are three ototoxic drugs?

8. What data should you collect when caring for patients with disorders of the sensory system?

9. What nursing care will you provide for patients with disorders of the eye or ear?

10. What nursing care interventions would you use for the patient with a hearing impairment?

11. How will you know if your nursing interventions for sensory disorders have been effective?

Early detection and treatment of sensory injuries or diseases can reduce their impact. Any disturbance in vision or hearing disrupts a person's role performance, safety, and activities of daily living (ADLs). Treatment for sensory disturbances, such as glasses for refractive errors or hearing aids, can interfere with an individual's self-concept and body image. Nurses play an important role in recognizing symptoms of visual and hearing disorders and in assisting the individual to follow treatment, prevent recurrence, and learn new adaptive skills.

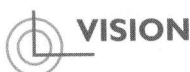 VISION

See Box 52.1 Eye Disorder Summary.

Infections and Inflammation

Infections and inflammation of the eye and surrounding structures can be bacterial or viral in origin. The eye may become aggravated by allergens, chemical substances, or mechanical irritation, leading to infection by microorganisms. Mechanical irritation may be caused by sunburn or bacterial infection. Inflammation results from allergies to environmental substances or by irritation of chemical irritants found in perfumes, make-up, sprays, or plants. Viral agents that cause infection include herpes simplex virus, cytomegalovirus, and human adenovirus. Bacterial agents that infect the eye include *Staphylococcus* and *Strep-*

Box 52.1

Eye Disorder Summary

Signs and Symptoms	Visual disturbances, pain, redness, secretions, itchiness, sensation of pressure in eyes
Diagnostic Tests and Findings	Visual acuity, opthalmoscopic examination of internal and external eye, Amsler grid (identifies visual field disturbances), slit-lamp examination (identifies abnormalities on cornea and sclera), tonometry (identifies intraocular pressure)
Therapeutic Interventions	Medications: reduce IOP, treat infections, anesthetize the eye
Complications	Worsening vision or loss of vision
Possible Nursing Diagnoses	Acute pain Anxiety related to visual-sensory deficit Deficient knowledge

IOP = intraocular pressure.

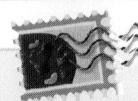

Box 52.2

Cultural Considerations

Vision

Trachoma, a form of conjunctivitis, is a common, chronic disease that affects approximately 600 million people worldwide. It is primarily seen among low-income persons in the Mediterranean, Africa, Brazil, and the Far East. Trachoma is caused by a viral strain of *Chlamydia trachomatis* that is highly contagious. Following the acute conjunctivitis phase, the eyelids shrink as a result of scarring. The shrinking tends to pull the eyelashes inward (entropion), which may scratch the cornea. In addition, granulations form on the inner eyelids. This painful condition may eventually lead to corneal ulceration and blindness. Trachoma is medically treated with topical and oral erythromycin or tetracycline.

---

tococcus. The most common type of acute infection is **conjunctivitis** (Box 52.2 Cultural Considerations).

Conjunctivitis

Conjunctivitis is inflammation of the conjunctiva caused by either a virus or bacteria. Viral conjunctivitis occurs more commonly than bacterial conjunctivitis and is highly contagious. The virus is usually transmitted via contaminated eye secretions on the hand that then touches or rubs an eye, which infects the eye. The virus is hardy and may live on dry surfaces for 2 weeks or more. Viral conjunctivitis lasts 2 to 4 weeks. Bacterial conjunctivitis (commonly called pinkeye) usually is due to staphylococcal or streptococcal bacteria and is also highly contagious. Conjunctivitis can also be caused by the organisms *Haemophilus influenzae, Chlamydia trachomatis,* and *Neisseria gonorrhoeae.* Conjunctivitis is commonly transmitted among children and then among family members. Interestingly, conjunctivitis may also be caused by the use of nonprescription decongestant eye drops containing vasoconstrictors. When the eye drops are discontinued, a pharmacologically induced rebound phenomenon may occur. The eye vessels dilate and may become ischemic. This condition eventually subsides.

The symptoms of conjunctivitis include conjunctival redness and crusting exudate on the lids and in the corners of the eyes. Individuals may complain that their eyes itch and are painful. The eyes may tear excessively in response to the irritation.

Viral conjunctivitis is treated by supportive measures, which seek to keep the patient comfortable until the infection resolves on its own. Treatment includes eyewashes or eye irrigations, which cleanse the conjunctiva and relieve the inflammation and pain. Bacterial conjunctivitis is treated

---

conjunctivitis: conjunctive—joining membrane + itis—inflammation

TABLE 52.1 OPHTHALMIC MEDICATIONS

Medication Class/Action	Examples	Route	Side Effects	Nursing Considerations
Diagnostic Aids				
Fluorescein sodium				
Staining of eye. Lesions of foreign objects pick up bright yellow-orange stain so abnormality can be detected.	Fluorescein (AK-Fluor)	Eye drop	Transient stinging or burning	Stain needs to be irrigated out of eye when examination is complete. Stain is colorfast, so caution should be used when irrigating.
Topical Anesthetics				
Provide local anesthesia to area, making examination painless. Also used to reduce pain of injury.	Tetracaine (Pontocaine)	Eye drop	Rare	Corneal anesthesia is achieved within 1 minute and lasts about 15 minutes. The eye must be protected because the blink reflex is temporarily lost. The lid should be kept closed to keep eye moist when examination and treatment are completed.
Antivascular Endothelial Growth Factor				
Antiangiogenic Inhibits growth of new blood vessels and slows progression of wet ARMD	Pegaptanib (Macugen)	Ophthalmic injection every 6 weeks	Burning, eye pain, redness, light sensitivity, vision loss, cataract, blurred vision, hypertension	Sterile technique must be used during injection by ophthalmologist. Monitor for 1 week after to detect infection early. Retinal detachment is a complication.
Anti-infectives				
Antibiotics				
Combat eye infections of bacterial origin	Erythromycin (AK-Mycin)	Eye drop or PO	Inflammation, burning, stinging, and drug hypersensitivity	Patients must be asked about previous allergic reaction to any ophthalmic or systemic medications.
Antivirals				
Combat eye infections of viral origin	Vidarabine (Vira-A)	Eye drop or PO	Inflammation, burning, stinging, and drug hypersensitivity	To minimize systemic absorption of anti-infectives, apply pressure on tear duct up to 5 minutes after medication is applied.
Antifungals				
Combat eye infections of fungal origin	Natamycin (Natacyn)	Eye drop or PO	Inflammation, burning, stinging, and drug hypersensitivity	Follow instructions for instillation.
Anti-inflammatories				
Reduce inflammation of conjunctiva, cornea, or eyelids due to infection, edema, allergic reaction, cataract surgery or burns				
Steroidal	Dexamethasone (Decadron)	Eye drop or PO	Transient stinging or burning on application.	To minimize systemic absorption of anti-inflammatories, apply pressure on tear duct up to 5 minutes after medication is applied. Long-term use of corticosteroids can contribute to cataract formation.
Nonsteroidal	Ketorolac (Acular)	Eye drop or PO	Transient stinging or burning on application	Use only as prescribed. Solutions preferred for eye infections as ointments can decrease healing.
	Bromfenac (Xibrom)	Eye drop	Headache, abnormal vision, eye pain, pruritus	Reduces ocular inflammation and pain following cataract surgery usually within 2 days of bid treatment.

(Continued on following page)

TABLE 52.1 OPHTHALMIC MEDICATIONS (Continued)

Medication Class/Action	Examples	Route	Side Effects	Nursing Considerations
Lubricants Moisten eyes in healthy and ill persons. Lubricants maintain moisture on eyeball, which contributes to maintenance of the epithelial surface.	Artificial tears (Lacrilube, Tears Plus)	Eye drop or ointment	Rare	Lubricants come in liquid and ointment forms. For patients who have ointments placed in the eye during surgery to prevent eye dryness, inform patients that vision will be distorted in the presence of ophthalmic ointments.
Miotics Lower intraocular pressure by stimulating papillary and ciliary sphincter muscles. This assists in improving blood flow to the retina and flow of aqueous humor.	Pilocarpine (Pilocar) Physostigmine (Isopto Eserine)	Eye drop	Miotic side effects include headache, eye pain, and brow pain. Systemic absorption can cause nausea, vomiting, diarrhea, respiratory attacks in patients with asthma, and respiratory difficulty.	Pilocarpine, a miotic, causes miosis (contraction of the pupil). Expect to see a smaller than normal pupil with little if any reaction to light. Careful administration with gentle pressure on the tear duct for 5 minutes following application will reduce systemic absorption of medications.
Carbonic Anhydrase Inhibitors Used to decrease aqueous humor formation and decrease intraocular pressure. Used primarily for treatment of glaucoma when other miotics have not been successful.	Acetazolaminde (Diamox)	Eye drop	Side effects include lethargy, anorexia, depression, nausea, and vomiting. Do not administer to persons allergic to sulfonamides. Carbonic anhydrase inhibitors may also cause photosensitivity.	Careful administration with gentle pressure on the tear duct for 5 minutes following application will reduce systemic absorption. Instruct patient to wear sunglasses and protect eyes from bright lights if photosensitive. Use of the medication may cause dry eyes and dry oral membranes. Encourage patient to maintain eye and oral hygiene.
Osmotics Used to reduce intraocular pressure in emergency situations such as acute open-angle glaucoma or used preoperatively and postoperatively to decrease vitreous humor volume, thereby reducing intraocular pressure.	Mannitol (Osmitrol)	Eye drop, PO, or IV	Disorientation, especially in elderly, may be caused by change in electrolytes secondary to use of osmotics	Mannitol may result in digitalis toxicity when given concurrently. Monitor for headache, nausea, vomiting, and confusion.
Beta-adrenergic Blockers Used to reduce intraocular pressure by reducing aqueous humor formation and increasing its outflow.	Timolol (Timoptic) Betaxolol (Betoptic)	Eye drop	Drug may cause transient burning and discomfort. There is limited systemic absorption of beta blockers, which may cause headache, dizziness, cardiac irregularities, and bronchospasm.	Careful administration with gentle pressure on the tear duct for 5 minutes following application will reduce systemic absorption. Monitor for bradycardia, heart block, and wheezing.
Mydriatics Used to dilate the pupils for examination or surgical procedures.	Atropine *[handwritten: for days up to 10 days surgery dilate]*	Eye drop	Systemic absorption may cause irregular pulse, confusion, dry mouth, fever. Local side effects include blurred vision and photosensitivity.	If pupils are dilated, they can no longer protect the eye from bright light. Instruct patient to wear dark glasses until the effects of the drug have worn off. Monitor for side effects such as irregular pulse, confusion, dry mouth, and fever. Careful administration with gentle pressure on the tear duct for 5 minutes following application will reduce systemic absorption.
Cycloplegics Paralyzes muscles of accommodation for examination or surgical procedures.	Cyclopentolate	Eye drop	Side effects include tachycardia, dry mouth, and symptoms of atropine toxicity.	Contraindicated in patients with glaucoma because of increase in intraocular pressure with use.

ARMD = age-related macular degeneration.

with antibiotic eye drops or ointments (Table 52.1). Eye drops are generally preferred by adults because they do not impair vision. Ointments are commonly used when the eye is resting (at night) or in children, who may squeeze their eyes shut and cry when ocular medications are applied, thus expelling the medication. With either type of conjunctivitis, hand washing is the best means of preventing the spread of the disease.

Blepharitis

Blepharitis, an inflammation of the eyelid margins, is a chronic inflammatory process. There are two types: seborrheic blepharitis and ulcerative blepharitis. The cause may include staphylococcal infection, seborrhea (dandruff), rosacea (a chronic disease of the skin usually affecting middle-aged and older adults), dry eye, or abnormalities of the meibomian glands and their lipid secretions. Seborrheic blepharitis is characterized by reddened eyelids with scales and flaking at base of the lashes. Ulcerative blepharitis produces crusts at eyelashes, reddened eyes, and inflamed corneas. Eyelids chronically infected with *Staphylococcus* may become thickened and eyelashes may be lost.

Treatment requires a commitment to long-term daily cleansing with cotton-tipped swabs dipped in diluted baby shampoo or sterile eyelid cleanser solutions to prevent infection. If infection occurs, antistaphylococcal antibiotic ointment (bacitracin, erythromycin) is applied to the lid margins one to four times a day after the eyelids have been cleansed. Warm compresses may also be used.

Hordeolum and Chalazion

Another type of eyelid infection is a **hordeolum.** An external hordeolum (sty) is a small staphylococcal abscess in the sebaceous gland at the base of the eyelash (either Zeis's glands or the glands of Moll). Use of cosmetics on the eyes may contribute to hordeolum formation. Styes are small, raised, reddened areas. A second type of abscess, **chalazion** (internal hordeolum), may form in the connective tissue of the eyelids, specifically in the meibomian glands. A chalazion is larger than an external hordeolum. Styes may be tender; however, a chalazion often puts pressure on the cornea, causing more discomfort.

Hordeolums usually form and heal spontaneously within a few days and require no treatment. Chalazions may require surgical incision and drainage (I&D) if they do not drain spontaneously. If either type of abscess persists, administration of oral antibiotics may be prescribed along with application of warm compresses to aid healing.

Keratitis

PATHOPHYSIOLOGY AND ETIOLOGY. Keratitis is inflammation of the cornea and may be acute or chronic and superficial or deep. The depth of keratitis is determined by the layers of the cornea that may be affected. Keratitis may be associated with bacterial conjunctivitis, a viral infection such as herpes simplex, a corneal ulcer, or diseases such as tuberculosis and syphilis. Children may develop keratitis from vitamin A deficiency, allergic reactions, or viral

diseases such as mumps or measles. Herpes simplex keratitis is the most common corneal infection in developed countries, with bacterial and fungal infections being more prevalent throughout the rest of the world. People who wear contact lenses or have dry eyes, practice poor contact lens hygiene, have decreased corneal sensation, or are immunosuppressed are at increased risk of keratitis. Overnight wearing of soft contact lenses increases the risk even more. *Pseudomonas aeruginosa* is the pathogen most commonly associated with infection following the wearing of soft contact lenses overnight. If this infection occurs, the patient may be advised to dispose of the contaminated lenses and be treated with antibiotics.

SIGNS AND SYMPTOMS. The cornea has many pain receptors, so any inflammation of the cornea is painful. This pain increases with movement of the lid over the cornea. Other symptoms of keratitis include decreased vision, **photophobia** (sensitivity to light), tearing, and blepharospasm (spasm of the eyelids). The conjunctiva often appears reddened. In advanced cases, the cornea may appear opaque (cloudy).

DIAGNOSTIC TESTS. Assessment of keratitis or corneal ulcer is made by use of a slit lamp or a hand-held light. The cornea is examined by shining the light source obliquely (diagonally) across the cornea to show opacity in the cornea. Fluorescein stain may also be used to outline the area of involvement. When the stained area is viewed with a blue light, the disruption in the corneal surface shows up clear. If the patient is having pain from blepharospasm (contraction of the orbicularis oculi muscle), the examiner may instill a topical ophthalmic anesthetic such as proparacaine.

THERAPEUTIC INTERVENTIONS. Therapeutic interventions may include topical antibiotics, antiviral medications for herpes simplex, cycloplegic agents (to keep the iris and ciliary body at rest), and warm compresses. If the cornea is severely damaged, corneal transplant may be required. The eye may be patched to decrease the amount of eyelid movement over the cornea during healing.

COMPLICATIONS. Corneal infections are usually serious and are often sight threatening. The corneal tissue may become thin and susceptible to perforation. Untreated, keratitis can cause permanent scarring of the cornea, resulting in permanent loss of vision.

Nursing Process for the Patient with Inflammation and Infection of the Eye

ASSESSMENT/DATA COLLECTION. Gather subjective and objective data (Table 52.2). Objective assessment data includes the condition of the conjunctiva, eyelids, and eyelashes; the presence of exudate, tearing, any visible abscess on the palpebral border, or a palpable abscess in the eyelid; opacity of the cornea; and visual acuity testing comparing unaffected and affected eyes.

---

photophobia: photo—light + phobia—fear of

TABLE 52.2 SUBJECTIVE ASSESSMENT OF EYE INFLAMMATION AND INFECTION CONDITIONS

W	Where is it? What part of the eye is affected? Eyelid, conjunctiva, cornea?
H	How does it feel? Pressure? Itchy? Painful? No pain? Irritated? Spasm?
A	Aggravating and alleviating factors. Is it worse when rubbing eyes or blinking? Is there photosensitivity?
T	Timing. Was there exposure to a pathogen? Previous infection or irritation? How long have symptoms persisted?
S	Severity. Is there visual impairment? Does pain affect ADLs?
U	Useful data for associated symptoms. Is patient infected with lice? Immunosuppression? Do other members of the family or peer group have symptoms? Are decongestant eye drops used? Is there exudate? Are the eyelids stuck together on awakening? Does patient wear contact lenses, soft contact lenses overnight, disposable contact lenses? Does patient have dry eyes? Is patient infected with tuberculosis, syphilis, HIV? What is typical eye hygiene?
P	Perception by the patient of the problem. What does patient think is wrong?

ADLs = activities of daily living; HIV = human immunodeficiency virus.

NURSING DIAGNOSIS, PLANNING, AND IMPLEMENTATION. Acute pain related to inflammation or infection of the eye or surrounding tissues

EXPECTED OUTCOME: *Pain is decreased or absent as evidenced by lower rating on pain scale.*

- Assess the patient for pain. *Use of dark glasses, rubbing the eye, squinting, and avoiding light may be indicators of pain that should be assessed.*
- Administer eye medications as ordered. Eye pain is generally treated with topical anesthetic drops or ointments, antibiotics, anti-inflammatory agents, or analgesics for severe pain.
- Apply warm or cool packs as ordered *to assist in soothing the eye.*
- Patching of the affected eye may help reduce pain *by decreasing the movement of the eye across the eyelid.*
- Explore additional methods of pain reduction, *such as guided imagery, relaxation techniques, music, or distraction.*

Disturbed sensory perception: visual related to altered sensory reception

EXPECTED OUTCOME: *Patient states vision has returned to preillness state.*

- Reading and television should be discouraged *if the patient is to rest the eye.*
- Encourage quiet activity, such as listening to music, radio, or a recorded book, which can be carried out

with the eyes closed *to provide distraction and rest for the eye.*

Risk for injury related to visual impairment

EXPECTED OUTCOME: *Injury does not occur as a result of visual impairment.*

- Assess and plan for visual impairments that may be present *to promote safety.*
- Advise patient with one eye patched that depth perception is altered and not to drive automobile.
- Teach caution when ambulating and reaching for things. *Inflamed eyes often do not focus well and may have exudate, tearing, or ointment present, which can interfere with vision.*

Risk for infection related to poor eye hygiene, use of contact lenses

EXPECTED OUTCOME: *Patient does not develop eye infection.*

- Administer antibiotics as ordered.
- Teach not to wear contact lenses when the eye or surrounding structure is inflamed.
- Teach contact lenses must be sterilized before use after the inflammation resolves *to prevent reinfection of the eye. Soft contact lenses that cannot be sterilized need to be discarded.*

Deficient knowledge related to eye disease process, prevention, and treatment from lack of previous experience

EXPECTED OUTCOMES: *Patient explains disease process, prevention, and treatment measures. Patient demonstrates treatment regimen correctly, such as administration of eye drops.*

- Teach patient prevention, care of the affected eye, medication administration, safety issues *for understanding and compliance with therapeutic plan.*
- Have patient demonstrate the administration of ointments or drops after teaching has occurred *to evaluate understanding.*
- Teach patient and family how to prevent spreading infection *if it is contagious.*
- Teach patient good eye hygiene *to prevent further complications.*

EVALUATION. The interventions have been successful if pain is reduced to an acceptable rating, vision improves or returns to preillness level, injury does not occur as a result of visual impairment, infection does not occur as a result of poor eye hygiene or wearing of contact lenses, patient explains disease process, prevention, or treatment regimen accurately, or prescribed treatment is stated or demonstrated correctly (e.g., administering eye drops or ointments).

Refractive Errors
Pathophysiology and Etiology
Refraction refers to the bending of light rays as they enter the eye. Emmetropia, or normal vision, means that light rays

are bent to focus images precisely on the macula of the retina. *Ametropia* is a term used to describe any refractive error. When an image is not clearly focused on the retina, refractive error is present. Refractive errors account for the largest number of impairments in vision. Ametropia occurs when parallel light rays entering the eye are not refracted to focus on the retina. There are four common ametropic disorders: **myopia, hyperopia, astigmatism,** and **presbyopia.**

HYPEROPIA. Hyperopia, also known as farsightedness, is caused by light rays focusing behind the retina (Fig. 52.1). People who are hyperopic see images that are far away more clearly than images that are close. Physiologically, the globe or eyeball is too short from the front to the back, causing the light rays to focus beyond the retina. Hyperopia is corrected with convex lenses.

MYOPIA. Myopia, commonly referred to as nearsightedness, is caused by light rays focusing in front of the retina. The eyeball is elongated and thus the light rays do not reach the retina. Persons with myopia hold things close to their eyes to see them better. Distance vision is blurred. Myopia is corrected with concave lenses (see Fig. 52.1).

ASTIGMATISM. Astigmatism results from unequal curvatures in the shape of the cornea. When parallel light rays enter the eye, the irregular cornea causes the light rays to be refracted to focus on two different points. This can result in either myopic or hyperopic astigmatism. The person with astigmatism has blurred vision with distortion. The corneal irregularities can be caused by injury, inflammation, corneal surgery, or an inherited autosomal dominant trait.

PRESBYOPIA. Presbyopia is a condition in which the crystalline lenses lose their elasticity, resulting in a decrease in ability to focus on close objects. The loss of elasticity causes light rays to focus beyond the retina, resulting in hyperopia. This condition usually is associated with aging and generally occurs after age 40. If an individual has preexisting hyperopia, the onset of presbyopia may occur earlier than 40 years. Likewise, if an individual has myopia, presbyopia may correct the myopia by projecting the light rays directly on the retina. Because accommodation for close vision is accomplished by lens contraction, people with presbyopia exhibit the inability to see objects at close range. They often compensate for blurred close vision by holding objects to be viewed farther away. Complaints of eyestrain and mild frontal headache are common. These symptoms are relieved with eye rest and corrective lenses.

Signs and Symptoms
Individuals with refractive errors often report difficulty reading or seeing objects. Often the eyestrain that occurs as one attempts to improve visual acuity causes headache. Myopic individuals may hold reading materials close to the eyes. Hyperopic individuals hold reading materials farther away from their eyes.

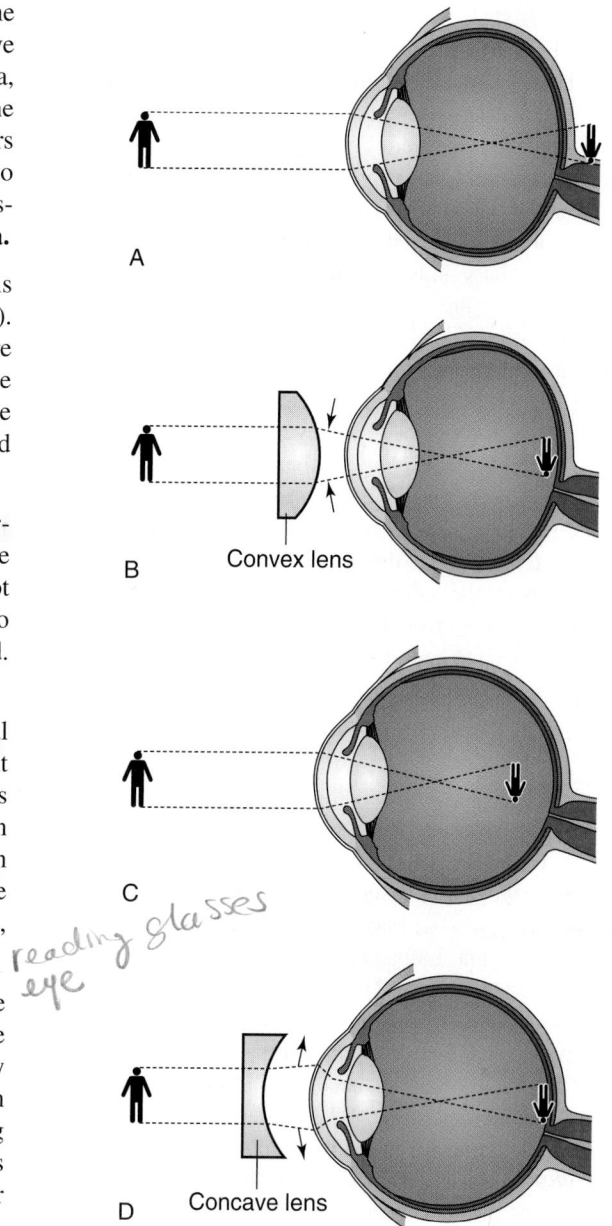

FIGURE 52.1 Refractive disorders. *(A)* Hyperopia (farsighted). The eyeball is too short, causing the image to focus beyond the retina. *(B)* Corrected hyperopia. *(C)* Myopia (nearsighted). A long eyeball causes the image to focus in front of the retina. *(D)* Corrected myopia.

 LEARNING TIP

To remember the type of vision a person has, use this saying: *You are what you say.* For example, if you say you are farsighted, this means that you have clear vision of far away images but difficulty seeing images that are nearer. If you say you are nearsighted, this means that you have clear vision of near images but difficulty seeing images that are farther away.

---

presbyopia: presby—old age + opia—concerning vision

Diagnostic Tests

A refractive error may be roughly estimated by use of Snellen's chart or by determining the individual's vision at different distances and comparing it with that of the examiner. To obtain a more definitive refractive error measurement, a retinoscopic examination is necessary. Before this examination, a cycloplegic drug is often instilled (see Table 52.1). A cycloplegic drug dilates the pupil and temporarily paralyzes the ciliary muscle, thus preventing accommodation. During the examination, an ophthalmologist or optometrist examines the internal and external eye and uses trial lenses via a retinoscope to assess the type of lens best suited to correct the refractive error. If convex-shaped trial lenses correct the focusing power of the eyes, the patient is determined to be hyperopic. If concave-shaped trial lenses correct the focusing power, the patient is said to be myopic. The amount of focusing power needed in the trial lens to correct the visual defect indicates the degree of refractive error. Left and right eyes of the same person may not have the same degree of refractive error. If a cycloplegic agent has been used, patients need to be told that blurred vision will be present and sunglasses need to be worn until the agent wears off. In addition, the patient should be instructed that driving and reading are not possible until the effect of the cycloplegic drug is gone.

Therapeutic Interventions

Refractive errors are commonly treated with corrective lenses; either eyeglasses or contact lenses. The lenses bend the parallel light rays so that they converge on the macular portion of the retina. Incisional radial keratotomy and photorefractive keratectomy (PRK) are surgical procedures used to correct refractive error. With incisional radial keratotomy, surgical incisions are made on the cornea to reshape it. PRK utilizes laser technology to accomplish the same goal of reshaping the cornea (Box 52.3 Laser Treatment). The cornea is made flatter for individuals with myopia and more cone shaped for those with hyperopia.

Complications

Complications of corrective lens use are primarily related to safety. Eyeglasses can be broken. Eyeglass lenses can be made with special polymers that do not break as easily as traditional glass. It is a myth that if corrective lenses are not worn, vision becomes worse. Complications of contact lens use include corneal abrasions, infections, and keratitis. Incisional radial keratotomy and PRK both have surgical risks and may not always be successful.

Blindness

Blindness is described in many terms that are often reflective of the degree of visual impairment an individual has. Generally, blindness is the complete or almost complete absence of the sense of sight. Terms such as *profound blindness, partially sighted,* and *blind* may all have different meanings. Some people consider the terms *blind* and *partially sighted* to be negative and prefer the term *visually impaired* to describe their condition. For information or resources, visit the following sites:

Box 52.3

Laser Treatment

Laser is an acronym for light amplification by stimulated emission of radiation. Lasers are devices that amplify light and produce synchronized light waves. Lasers are based on the principle that atoms, molecules, and ions can be excited by absorption of thermal, electrical, or light energy. After this energy is absorbed, the atoms, molecules, or ions give off a beam of synchronized light waves. By using this extremely intense, highly directional, pure-colored light, lasers can be used for a variety of purposes, such as making incisions, removing tissue, or stopping bleeding.

- American Foundation for the Blind at http://afb.org
- Canadian National Institute for the Blind at www.cnib.ca
- National Federation of the Blind at www.nfb.org

Pathophysiology and Etiology

Few people are born blind. Blindness is caused by a variety of factors, including trauma, complications from various diseases such as hypertension and diabetes, conditions such as **cataract**s and **glaucoma,** and, in children, malnutrition, infectious diseases, and parasitic infestations. Blindness is produced when there is an obstacle to the rays of light on their way to the optic nerve or by disease of the optic nerve or tract of the part of the brain connected with vision. Blindness may be permanent or transient, complete or partial, or may occur only in darkness (night blindness). There are blind people in every age group, but about half the blind people in the United States are older adults.

Signs and Symptoms

Aside from a general loss of vision, patients may describe their visual image as blurred, distorted, or absent in specific areas of the visual field. Objects may appear dark or absent around the peripheral field in glaucoma or retinitis pigmentosa. Retinitis pigmentosa causes this visual disturbance because the pigmented layer of the retina has degenerated. The center of the visual field may appear dark for individuals with diabetic **retinopathy** or **macular** degeneration. Half the visual field may be impaired in patients with hemianopia. This results from a defect in the optic pathways in the brain and is often seen with stroke. Patients may report that the visual field appears blurry or hazy in corneal visual problems, cataracts, diabetic retinopathy, or refractive errors (Fig. 52.2).

Diagnostic Tests

Diagnostic tests are usually done to determine the exact cause of the blindness and may include a visual field exam-

---

retinopathy: retino—having to do with the retina + pathy—illness, disease, or suffering

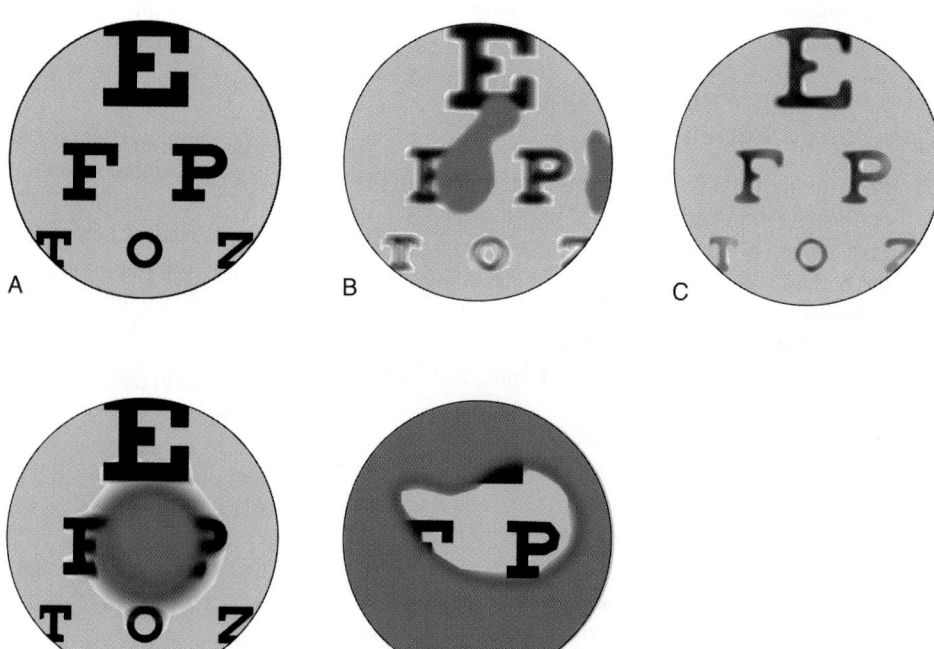

FIGURE 52.2 Visual field abnormalities. *(A)* Normal vision. *(B)* Diabetic retinopathy. *(C)* Cataracts. *(D)* Macular degeneration. *(E)* Advanced glaucoma.

ination, tonometry, and slit-lamp microscope examination. Retinal angiography is used to follow blood flow through the retinal vessels and to detect vascular changes. Ultra-sonography may be used to visualize changes in the posterior eye that cannot be directly examined because of other pathological conditions, such as a cloudy cornea, a bloody vitreous, or an opaque lens.

Therapeutic Interventions

Therapeutic interventions for blindness center on treating the underlying condition and preventing further impairment. Depending on the cause of the blindness, treatment may include medication prescription, surgical intervention, corrective eyewear prescription, and referral to supportive services.

Nursing Process for the Patient with Visual Impairment

ASSESSMENT/DATA COLLECTION. Collection of subjective data for assessment of visual impairment can be made using the WHAT'S UP? format (Table 52.3). Collection of objective data includes observations of the patient. Is there squinting? Rubbing of eyes? Is the patient using compensatory measures—magnifying glass, sitting close to television, using large-print reading materials, avoiding reading, using eyeglasses? Psychosocial data are important because a blind person may be withdrawn or socially isolated, have low self-esteem or poor coping mechanisms, or have poor interpersonal skills as a result of the visual impairment.

NURSING DIAGNOSIS AND PLANNING. Nursing care begins by understanding how to interact with the visually impaired patient (Box 52.4 Interacting with the Visually Impaired Patient). A patient's level of independence must be included in the planning phase. If patients have minimal

visual impairment or have attended rehabilitation, they may be able to function independently. If a patient has recently become visually impaired, he or she may be completely dependent until learning alternative ways of coping with this impairment. Planning focuses on meeting self-care needs, keeping the patient safe from injury, supporting the grieving

TABLE 52.3 SUBJECTIVE ASSESSMENT OF VISUAL DISORDERS

W	Where is it? What part of the visual field is affected? If there is vision, what are the characteristics of what can be seen? Blurry? Hazy? Dark? Halos around lights?
H	How does it feel? Is there associated pain with the visual impairment? Headaches? How does it make the patient feel? Fearful? Anxious? Depressed? Helpless? Hopeless? Accepting?
A	Aggravating and alleviating factors. Is it worse when reading? Is it worse when watching TV? Does it affect the patient only at night? Is vision better at distances or close up?
T	Timing. When did the symptoms start? Do they come and go? Is the impairment progressively getting worse? Was onset sudden?
S	Severity. Does the impairment affect the patient's ADLs? If so, how severely? Does the patient need assistance to cook, dress, bathe, read mail, pay bills, access health care, obtain transportation, maintain household, shop?
U	Useful data for associated symptoms. Does the patient have diabetes, hypertension, a family history of retinitis pigmentosa, a history of eye infection, or eye trauma? Has the patient recently traveled out of the country?
P	Perception of the problem by the patient. What does the patient think is wrong? How severe does the patient perceive the impairment to be?

ADLs = activities of daily living.

Box 52.4

Interacting with the Visually Impaired Patient

- People entering a room and at each contact with the patient should identify themselves.
- Post a sign on the door or over the bed that identifies the patient's visual status so that others can interact appropriately.
- Remember that the individual is not having hearing problems, so use a normal tone of voice and do not yell.
- Ask visually impaired patients what their needs are; do not assume they need help with everything.
- Do not hesitate to use the words *blind* and *see*.
- Talk directly to the impaired patient, not through a companion.
- At mealtime, explain the location of items on the tray by comparing their position to the numbers on a clock (e.g., milk is at 2 o'clock, peas are at 7 o'clock).
- Explain any activity going on in the room or within the patient's auditory range.
- Explain procedures before beginning them. Speak to the patient before touching.
- When walking, allow the patient to grasp assistant's arm and walk a half step behind. Be aware of obstacles on either side when walking.
- When seating a patient, place the patient's hand on the arm of the chair.
- Tell the patient when leaving the room or area so the patient does not continue conversation in an empty room, which may cause embarrassment.
- When orienting the patient to the hospital room, explain the location of items the patient may need, such as the water pitcher, call light, bed controls, urinal, tissues. Attempt to keep these items in the same place at all times.
- If the patient has a seeing eye dog, do not play with the dog, pet it, or feed it without consulting the patient—the dog is working! Make sure the patient's dog is near the bed, on a mat provided especially for the dog, preferably on the side of the bed that is less likely to be used by staff. Instruct staff and visitors about the seeing eye dog.

patients to these resources enhances their ability to maintain independence. Visit the following organizations' websites:

- American Academy of Ophthalmology at www.eye-net.org
- Guide Dogs for the Blind at www.guidedogs.com
- National Association for Visually Handicapped at www.navh.org
- National Eye Institute at www.nei.nih.gov
- Talking books: National Library Service for the Blind and Visually Handicapped at www.loc.gov/nls/index.html

EVALUATION. The outcomes for the visually impaired patient are met if the patient demonstrates the ability to complete activities of daily living with increasing independence, remains free of injury, and demonstrates ability to assess agencies and services for the visually impaired.

Diabetic Retinopathy

Pathophysiology and Etiology

Retinopathy is a disorder in which there are vascular changes in the retinal blood vessels. The most common incidence of retinopathy is found in persons with diabetes. It is estimated that half of the people with diabetes in the United States have at least early signs of retinopathy. The pathological changes that occur with diabetic retinopathy are related to excess glucose, changes in the retinal capillary walls, formation of microaneurysms, and constriction of retinal blood vessels. Three stages of diabetic retinopathy have been identified: background retinopathy, preproliferative retinopathy, and proliferative retinopathy.

Background retinopathy is the earliest stage, in which microaneurysms form on the retinal capillary walls. These microaneurysms may leak blood into the central retina or macula. If the leakage causes edema, the patient may notice a decrease in color discrimination and visual acuity.

The second stage, preproliferative retinopathy, is characterized by swollen and irregularly dilated veins, which results in sluggish or blocked blood flow. Patients generally are not aware of this stage because there are no symptoms.

Proliferative retinopathy, the third stage, is characterized by the formation of new blood vessels growing into the retinal and optic disc area as an attempt to increase the blood supply to the retina. The newly formed blood vessels are fragile and often leak blood into the vitreous and retina. In addition to leaking, the newer vessels may grow into the vitreous, which causes a traction effect, pulling the vitreous away from the retina and subsequently pulling the retina away from the choroid. This condition is called retinal detachment (discussed later).

Signs and Symptoms

Individuals may experience a reduction in central visual acuity or color vision as a result of macular edema (see Fig. 52.2). Many patients with diabetic retinopathy do not have any symptoms until the proliferative stage, at which point vision is lost. Visual loss at the last stage usually cannot be restored.

process, and helping the patient acquire knowledge of agencies, services, and devices that allow maintenance of independence. Families must be included in the planning phase because they need to understand and be supportive of the self-image and role performance changes that may occur (Box 52.5 Nursing Care Plan for the Patient with Visual Loss).

There are organizations whose mission is to enhance the independence of visually impaired persons. Referring

Box 52.5   NURSING CARE PLAN for the Patient with Visual Loss

Nursing Diagnosis: Disturbed sensory perception: visual related to altered sensory reception

Expected Outcomes Patient will attain optimum level of sensory stimulation. Patient will become aware of visual impairment and ways to compensate. Patient will demonstrate ability to perform activities of daily living, with assistance if necessary.

Evaluation of Outcomes Patient perceives maximum visual sensory input. Patient is able to compensate for sensory impairment by using other senses and resources. Patient is able to perform activities of daily living as independently as possible.

Interventions	Rationale	Evaluation
Check visual acuity using a standard Snellen's vision chart. If the individual is unable to read letters, use directional arrows or pictures.	Determines patient's ability to see	Does patient have 20/20 vision? Is there an impairment? If so, how severe is it?
Check visual fields using the cover test or confrontation test.	Identifies deficits in visual fields	Are visual fields of patient equal to examiner's? Is there a deficit? Is it bilateral or unilateral?
Structure environment to compensate for visual loss by adding color and contrast (e.g., chairs and carpeting should be in contrasting colors, bright tape or paint on stairs, medicine bottles color coded with colored dot stickers).	Makes the environment easier to visualize and interpret and assists in depth perception and identifying medications	Does the environment have clearly delineated walkways, sitting areas, and doorways? Are areas with changes in elevation clearly identified using contrasting tape or paint? Is there a way for patient to safely self-administer medications?
Structure environment to compensate for visual loss by use of large-print directional signs and arrows, well-lit areas, nonglare surfaces, consistent placement of objects, traffic areas free of clutter.	Large directional signs assist the individual in maintaining orientation. Shiny floors or areas with bright window glass can impair vision. Traffic areas free of clutter assist in preventing injury.	Can the visually impaired individual identify locations such as bathroom, dining room, and office areas? Is the individual able to ambulate freely without safety hazards?
Provide for optimum care of assistive appliances such as eyeglasses, including maintenance of proper prescription, fit, and cleaning.	Improperly fitting or dirty eyeglasses may impair vision even further. Older adults should have their eyeglass prescription checked yearly.	Do eyeglasses fit properly? Are lenses clean? Is prescription current?
Introduce other assistive devices such as handheld magnifying glasses, tableside magnifiers, television magnifiers, large-print items, and phone dial covers with large numbers, talking watches, alarm clocks, and calculators.	Patients may not be aware of assistive devices, which may help them adapt to visual loss and continue previous activities such as watching TV or reading letters and magazines. Allows people to rely on hearing rather than vision.	Is patient aware of assistive devices that allow participation in previously enjoyed activities such as TV or reading? Is the visually impaired patient able to pay bills? Read mail? Communicate on telephone?

(Continued on following page)

Box 52.5 NURSING CARE PLAN for the Patient with Visual Loss *(Cont'd)*

Interventions	Rationale	Evaluation
Allow patient to verbalize feelings and grieving about visual loss.	Losing a primary sense such as vision can be devastating for patients. Opportunity to ventilate feelings assists in processing the loss.	Is patient able to verbalize feelings about visual impairment and its loss?
Identify coping strategies that have been successful for patient in the past.	By identifying successful coping strategies, the nurse assists patient in dealing with stress or visual loss. A positive approach for nurse to use focuses on individual's capabilities rather than deficits.	Is patient able to identify successful coping strategies and use them to deal with the stress of visual impairment?
Refer to specialized clinician such as ophthalmologist or occupational therapist or to specialized resources such as American Federation for the Blind or Prevent Blindness America.	Specialized clinicians can provide detailed examination and treatment for the disorder. Specialized resource groups have networks in place to assist individuals in coping with loss and assisting with maximizing abilities.	Does patient know who to call for detailed examination and treatment of problems? Does patient know that there are specialized clinicians and resource groups to help with the visual impairment? Does patient know how to access these specialists?

Diagnostic Tests

Diabetic retinopathy, as well as the other retinopathies, can be diagnosed only on examination of the internal eye. The examination is conducted with an ophthalmoscope following dilation of the pupil using a cycloplegic agent. The examination may be enhanced by use of retinoangiography. In the initial stages, vessels may appear swollen and tortuous (twisted).

Therapeutic Interventions

Treatment of diabetic retinopathy focuses on stopping the leakage of blood and fluid into the vitreous and retina. The leaking microaneurysm is sealed by use of laser photocoagulation (see Box 52.3 Laser Treatment). If blood has already leaked into the vitreous, a vitrectomy is performed. During a vitrectomy, the vitreous humor is drained out of the eye chamber and replaced with saline or silicon oil. The replacement fluid is necessary to support the structures of the eyeball until healing can occur. Further treatment may be needed if the patient has sustained retinal detachment.

Complications

Early treatment for diabetic retinopathy is highly successful in preventing further visual loss; however, visual loss cannot be reversed. For this reason, it is very important for patients with diabetes to have a comprehensive eye examination through dilated pupils at least once each year or as directed by their physician. Careful control of diabetes during the first 5 years following diagnosis reduces the occurrence and delays the onset of diabetic retinopathy.

Nursing Process for the Patient with Diabetic Retinopathy

ASSESSMENT/DATA COLLECTION. Nursing assessment for diabetic retinopathy focuses on risk factors associated with the incidence of the disease. The patient may not have any symptoms. If patients with diabetes do have changes in perceptions of visual acuity or color discrimination, they should immediately contact their physician.

NURSING DIAGNOSIS, PLANNING, AND IMPLEMENTATION. The planning phase of the nursing process focuses on prevention of visual loss by early detection and treatment. If the patient has entered phase three and is already visually impaired, the nursing care plan for the visually impaired patient is used. Nursing diagnoses, goals, and interventions for diabetic retinopathy include but are not limited to the following:

Risk for (or actual) ineffective therapeutic regimen management

EXPECTED OUTCOME: Patient will state ability to manage therapeutic regimen.

- Determine if visually impaired patient who is diabetic can monitor blood glucose and draw up and administer the correct amount of insulin. *Specialty devices are available that can be preset to draw up amounts of insulin for the visually impaired patient with diabetes. Family members may have to assist the patient.*

- Teach patient importance of yearly comprehensive eye examinations.

Disturbed sensory perception: visual related to altered sensory reception and transmission

EXPECTED OUTCOME: *Patient will adapt to altered visual perception.*

- Determine patient's abilities and needs to develop plan of action and support needed.
- Assist patient with home and health maintenance as needed.

EVALUATION. Patient goals are met if the patient is able to manage therapeutic regimen and manage visual deficits.

Retinal Detachment

Pathophysiology and Etiology

Retinal detachment is a separation of the retina from the choroid layer of the eye that allows fluid to enter the space between the layers. There are three types of retinal detachment:

1. Rhegmatogenous retinal detachment is caused by a hole or tear in the retina that allows fluid to flow between the two layers. The tears are related to degenerative changes in the retina or vitreous. This type of retinal detachment can also be precipitated by moderate trauma, such as stooping or lifting weights, or by direct trauma to the eye. The incidence of rhegmatogenous detachment increases with age.
2. Nonrhegmatogenous tractional detachment occurs when fibrous tissue in the vitreous humor attaches to the sensory retina and, as it contracts, pulls the retina away from its normal position. It occurs in patients with sickle cell disease or diabetes mellitus.
3. Exudative detachment occurs when fluid or exudate accumulates in the subretinal space and separates the layers. Exudative detachment occurs most often in conditions such as advanced hypertension, preeclampsia, or eclampsia and from intraocular tumors.

Signs and Symptoms

Patients experiencing a retinal detachment report a sudden change in vision. Initially, as the retina is pulled, "flashing lights" are reported, and then "floaters" are seen. The flashing lights are caused by vitreous traction on the retina, and the floaters are caused by the hemorrhage of vitreous fluid or blood. When the retina detaches, the patient describes it as "looking through a veil" or "cobwebs" and finally "like a curtain being lowered over the field of vision," with darkness resulting. There is no pain because the retina does not contain sensory nerves. On visual examination, the patient generally has a loss of peripheral vision when the visual fields are tested and a loss of acuity in the affected eye.

Diagnostic Tests

Indirect ophthalmoscopy is used by the physician to examine the interior of the eye. This examination allows the examiner to visualize the retina, which may be pale, opaque, and in folds with retinal detachment. The examiner is able to diagnose the type of detachment based on this examination. If there are lesions in the eye, the slit-lamp examination allows the examiner to magnify the lesions.

Therapeutic Interventions

Prompt medical treatment must be sought to prevent loss of vision. One of several procedures may be performed to reattach the retina to prevent blindness.

- Laser reattachment involves focusing a laser beam on the detached area of the retina and causing a controlled burn, which reattaches the layers together by forming an adhesion (see Box 52.3 Laser Treatment). This procedure is used when only a small area of the retina is involved.
- Cryosurgery involves the placement of a super-cooled probe on the sclera. The probe causes injury to the tissue, forming an adhesion; a principle similar to the laser procedure.
- Electrodiathermy, the least used procedure, involves placement of an electrode needle into the sclera to allow fluid that has accumulated to drain. The retina later adheres to the choroid layer.
- Scleral buckling is a surgical procedure that involves placing a silicon implant in conjunction with a beltlike device around the sclera to bring the choroid in contact with the retina. Cryosurgery or laser is used before the buckling procedure to seal the tear and form a scar that helps adhere the retina and choroid layers together.
- Pneumatic retinopexy is a procedure that can be conducted in the physician's office and is time consuming for the patient. This procedure involves injecting air or gas into the chamber to hold the retina in place. The patient must be extremely compliant with the treatment regimen, reclining for about 16 hours before the procedure to allow the retina to fall back toward the choroid. Because air rises, the patient must maintain a position that keeps the air bubble against the detached area for up to 8 hours a day for 3 weeks.

Complications

With any of the retinal reattachment procedures there is risk of increased intraocular pressure (IOP) and recurrent detachment. The patient is also at risk for future breaks in the retina.

Nursing Process for the Patient with Retinal Detachment

ASSESSMENT/DATA COLLECTION. Subjective data collected includes patient observation of the loss of peripheral vision, any change in visual acuity, and the presence of floaters, flashing lights, cobwebs, or veil-like visual impairments. There should be an absence of pain. Objective data collected includes the patient's visual acuity, visual fields, ability to perform ADLs, and level of anxiety.

NURSING DIAGNOSIS, PLANNING, IMPLEMENTATION, AND EVALUATION. The nursing process for patients with retinal detachment can be found in the section on nursing process for patients undergoing eye surgery.

CRITICAL THINKING

Mr. Samuel

■ Mr. Samuel, age 65, is working in the yard when a branch strikes his right eye. He sees flashes of light and then a short time later a dark shadow out of the right eye.

1. What should Mr. Samuel do?
2. After having a scleral buckling procedure, Mr. Samuel reports nausea. What action should you take?
3. Compazine 7.5 mg IM prn every 6 hours is ordered. Available is Compazine 2 mL of 5 mg/mL. How many milliliters should you give?

Suggested answers at end of chapter.

Glaucoma

Glaucoma is a group of diseases characterized by abnormal pressure within the eyeball. This pressure causes damage to the cells of the optic nerve, the structure responsible for transmitting visual information from the eye to the brain. The damage is silent, progressive, and irreversible until the end stages, when loss of peripheral vision occurs, followed by reductions in central vision and eventually blindness (see Fig. 52.2). Once glaucoma occurs, the patient will always have it and must follow a treatment regimen to maintain stable intraocular eye pressures.

Pathophysiology

The most common form of glaucoma, called primary, consists of two types: primary open-angle glaucoma (POAG) and acute angle-closure glaucoma (AACG). Secondary glaucoma may be caused by infections, tumors, or injuries. A third form, congenital glaucoma, primarily is due to developmental abnormalities.

AACG occurs in people who have an anatomically narrowed angle at the junction where the iris meets the cornea. When nearby eye structures such as the iris protrude into the anterior chamber, the angle is occluded, which blocks the flow of aqueous fluid. This is considered a medical emergency and results in partial or total blindness if not treated. POAG occurs when the drainage system of the eye, the trabecular meshwork and Schlemm's canal, degenerate and subsequently block the flow of aqueous humor.

give drops that constrict

Etiology and Prevention

The incidence of AACG is highest among Asians, women older than age 45, and nearsighted individuals. The incidence of POAG increases in those older than 40 years of age (older than age 50 for European Americans, older than age 35 for African Americans), in persons with diabetes, and in those with a family history of glaucoma, and is four to five times more prevalent in African Americans than European Americans. Those in high-risk groups should have yearly eye examinations for glaucoma detection.

Signs and Symptoms

An ophthalmic emergency, AACG typically has a unilateral, rapid onset. The patient may complain of severe pain over the affected eye, blurred vision, rainbows around lights, eye redness, a steamy-appearing cornea, photophobia, and tearing. Nausea and vomiting may occur from the increased IOP.

POAG develops bilaterally. The onset is usually gradual and painless, so the patient may not experience noticeable symptoms or after time may experience mild aching in the eyes, headache, halos around lights, or frequent visual changes that are not corrected with eyeglasses.

Diagnostic Tests

Traditionally, tonometry is utilized to detect increased IOP (normal IOP: 12 to 20 mm Hg). Applanation tonometry uses a tiny instrument to apply pressure to the anesthetized cornea. Noncontact tonometry is performed with a tonometer mounted on a slit-lamp microscope using a warm puff of air that flattens an anesthetized area of the cornea to obtain a pressure reading. In contact tonometry, the instrument is placed directly on the anesthetized cornea to measure eye pressure. Tonometry is not adequate to detect glaucoma alone, so three other methods are used. The optic nerve is examined with an ophthalmoscope through dilated pupils, visual field examination looks for loss of peripheral vision, and the angle where the iris meets the cornea is checked. In AACG, IOP may exceed 50 mm Hg. A new glaucoma screening device, the GDx Access (Carl Zeiss Meditec, Dublin, CA), uses infrared laser technology to measure the thickness of the retinal nerve fiber layers to identify damage to the fibers. The advantages of this diagnostic tool are that it catches glaucoma earlier than other tests, which allows greater vision to be saved with treatment, and it is painless.

Therapeutic Interventions

The first-line treatment for glaucoma focuses on opening the aqueous flow by administering cholinergic agents (**miotics**) such as carbachol (Isopto) or pilocarpine (Pilocar) to constrict the pupil. When the pupil is constricted, the iris pulls away from the drainage canal so that the aqueous fluid can flow freely. A second type of medication may be given to slow the production of aqueous fluid. These include carbonic anhydrase inhibitors such as acetazolamide (Diamox), adrenergic agonists such as dipivefrin (Propine), or beta blockers such as timolol (Timoptic). Slowing the aqueous fluid production helps decrease IOP. Additionally, the physician may order steroid eye drops to reduce inflammation. The patient experiencing an acute attack of AACG is given these medications and mannitol, a hyperosmolar agent, to rapidly reduce IOP, as well as analgesics and is ordered to maintain complete bedrest.

Patients with glaucoma are required to administer life-long eye drop medications twice or more daily. In the absence of symptoms, compliance is often an issue. Other factors that contribute to noncompliance include age of the patient, inability to afford the medication, and lack of understanding of the disease process. Patients need to carry medical alert identification indicating they have glaucoma and what their medications are. This can help prevent administration of contraindicated medications in emergency situations.

Certain medications, regardless of their route, are contraindicated in AACG and can result in blindness if given to a patient with AACG. These medications include any anticholinergics such as atropine and antihistamines such as diphenhydramine (Benadryl) or hydroxyzine (Vistaril) because they are mydriatics. Before a medication is given, it should be determined that it is not contraindicated in AACG to prevent blindness from occurring.

LEARNING TIP

1. Mydriatic medications are contraindicated in acute angle-closure glaucoma because they can cause an acute episode of increased IOP by dilating the pupil and pushing the iris back, blocking the outflow of aqueous humor.
2. Miotic medications constrict the pupil and so may be given to patients with acute angle-closure glaucoma.
3. To remember what miotic medications and mydriatic medications do, so that the appropriate medication is given and contraindicated ones are never given, remember the following:
   D = dilate = my**d**riatic = do not
   No D = constricts = miotic = okay to give

Surgical Management

When medication is no longer able to control the flow of aqueous humor, surgical intervention may become necessary. Surgery focuses on creating an area for the aqueous humor to flow freely, thus preventing increased IOP (Fig. 52.3). For AACG, laser peripheral iridotomy or surgical iridectomy is performed. Laser iridotomy is a noninvasive procedure utilizing a laser to remove a portion of the iris, thus allowing aqueous fluid to flow through the area. Prophylactic iridotomy may be performed on the other eye to prevent AACG. POAG is treated with argon laser trabeculoplasty (noninvasive laser beam creates openings in trabecular meshwork), trabeculectomy (part of iris and trabecular meshwork removed), or cyclocryotherapy (cryoprobe destroys part of ciliary body).

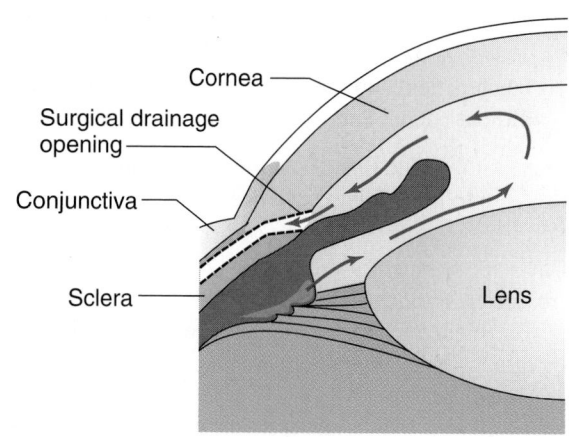

FIGURE 52.3 Flow of aqueous humor after trabeculoplasty (*arrows*).

Nursing Process for the Patient with Glaucoma

ASSESSMENT/DATA COLLECTION. The patient should be assessed for loss of central and peripheral vision, discomfort, understanding of disease and compliance with treatment regimen, and ability to conduct activities of daily living.

NURSING DIAGNOSIS, PLANNING, AND IMPLEMENTATION. The goal of nursing care for the glaucoma patient is to prevent further visual loss and to promote comfort if the patient is experiencing pain with acute glaucoma. The patient who needs surgical intervention has additional goals (see Nursing Process for the Patient Having Eye Surgery).

Pain related to increased intraocular pressure

EXPECTED OUTCOME: *Patient reports pain is relieved.*

- Give analgesics as needed for acute glaucoma *to relieve pain.*

Disturbed sensory perception: visual related to altered sensory reception

EXPECTED OUTCOME: *Patient has no further loss of vision.*

- Interventions that may be implemented if the patient is experiencing severe visual loss or having surgery are in the nursing process sections for impaired vision and the patient having eye surgery, respectively.

Self-care deficit related to decreased vision

EXPECTED OUTCOME: *Patient is able to care for self with assistance if needed.*

- Assist with self-care as needed *to ensure ADLs are met.*

Anxiety related to partial or total visual loss

EXPECTED OUTCOME: *Patient states reduced anxiety.*

- Encourage patient to verbalize concerns about glaucoma *to allow questions to be answered.*

Risk for injury related to decreased vision

EXPECTED OUTCOME: *Patient does not suffer injury as a result of the visual impairment.*

- Refer patient to support services for vision loss *who provide adaptive visual devices*.
- Teach patient and family not to rearrange furniture without patient knowledge *to prevent falls or injury*.

Deficient knowledge related to medical regimen, disease process due to no prior experience

EXPECTED OUTCOME: *Patient demonstrates correct instillation of eye medications and is able to verbalize understanding of condition and treatment.*

- Teach need for having regular eye examinations through dilated pupils *to monitor disease and detect complications*.
- Teach how to administer medications with a return demonstration *to ensure that eye drops are administered properly*.
- Teach the patient to rest his or her hand on the forehead to steady the hand *if the patient has trouble with a steady hand when administering eye drops*.
- Consider large-print labels or audiotaped directions *if the patient is unable to see the label on the eye drop bottle*.
- Consider using large, multicolored dot stickers placed on medication bottle with a corresponding direction card with a matching colored dot *for patients with multiple medications*.
- Advise family members that they are at increased risk of developing glaucoma and should have regular eye examinations *as glaucoma can be hereditary*.

EVALUATION. Interventions are successful if the patient maintains an acceptable level of comfort, has no further loss of vision, is able to care for self with assistance, expresses concerns and anxieties, does not suffer injury as a result of the visual impairment, and is able to verbalize understanding of condition and treatment.

Cataracts

Pathophysiology and Etiology

A cataract is an opacity in the lens of the eye that may cause a loss of visual acuity (see Fig. 52.2). Vision is diminished because the light rays are unable to get to the retina through the clouded lens.

Factors that contribute to cataract development may include age, ultraviolet radiation (sunlight), diabetes, smoking, steroids, nutritional deficiencies, alcohol consumption, intraocular infections, trauma, and congenital defects.

Signs and Symptoms

Cataracts are painless. Symptoms of cataract formation may include halos around lights, difficulty reading fine print or seeing in bright light, increased sensitivity to glare such as when driving at night, double or hazy vision, and decreased color vision.

Diagnostic Tests

Cataract formation is diagnosed through an eye examination. Visual acuity is tested for near and far vision. The direct ophthalmoscope and slit-lamp microscope are used to examine the lens and other internal structures.

Surgical Treatment
help not to fall

The only treatment for cataract formation is surgical removal of the cloudy lens. With the no-stitch cataract operation, there are no postoperative activity restrictions and vision is fine in about 2 days. After the lens is removed, there are several treatment options to correct the visual deficit that occurs when the eye is aphakic (absence of lens) and cannot accommodate or refract light properly. One treatment option is to provide the patient with eyeglasses or contact lenses that help correct the visual deficit. Another option is to replace the lens with a synthetic intraocular lens. For more information, visit the American Society of Cataract and Refractive Surgery at www.ascrs.org.

Complications

Complications of cataract surgery are rare but include inflammation, increased IOP, macular edema, retinal detachment, vitreous loss, hyphema, endophthalmitis, and expulsive hemorrhage.

Nursing Process for the Patient with Cataracts
ASSESSMENT/DATA COLLECTION. The patient is assessed for visual deficits to assist care planning, as well as knowledge needs about the disease process, surgical intervention, postoperative care, and medical regimen. The majority of patients undergoing cataract surgery have same-day surgery and then go home. The home situation, the ability of the patient or family member to follow the medical regimen, and transportation to and from the hospital for the patient are evaluated.

NURSING DIAGNOSES, PLANNING, IMPLEMENTATION, AND EVALUATION. Preoperative and postoperative nursing care is the primary nursing responsibility for the patient with cataracts, which is discussed below.

Nursing Process for the Patient Having Eye Surgery
ASSESSMENT/DATA COLLECTION. Subjective assessment data for patients having eye surgery can be collected using the WHAT'S UP? format (Table 52.4). Objective data may include visual acuity and peripheral field measurements. Visual acuity should be tested with and without corrective lenses. Eye tearing, redness, or swelling is noted.

Nursing Diagnosis, Planning, and Implementation

Risk for injury related to altered visual acuity

EXPECTED OUTCOME: *Patient will remain free of injury.*

- Explain depth perception may be affected by eye surgery, which can result in falls *to help prevent injury*.
- Ambulate with assistance and use clearly marked stairs.
- At home, beverages can be poured and stored in the refrigerator in single-serving glasses *to prevent spills and slippery floors*.

TABLE 52.4 SUBJECTIVE ASSESSMENT FOR PATIENTS HAVING EYE SURGERY

W Where is the visual disturbance? Is it centrally located? Peripherally? Throughout the entire visual field? Unilateral? Bilateral?

H How does it feel? Painful? Is there an absence of pain?

A Aggravating or alleviating factors. Is it worse in bright light or at night? Better when resting eyes or with head of bed elevated?

T Timing. Was there a sudden onset? Gradual onset?

S Severity. Does it affect ADLs? Does it affect close-up work?

U Useful data for associated symptoms. Does the patient suffer from hypertension? Diabetes? Has there been trauma? Vascular disease? What is the level of anxiety? Is the patient older than age 50?

P Perception of the problem by the patient. Will the visual disturbance impair ability to carry out ADLs? Ability to comply with medical regimen? Ability to manage home maintenance?

ADLs = activities of daily living.

Deficient knowledge related to preoperative and postoperative eye care

EXPECTED OUTCOME: Patient will verbalize preoperative and postoperative care directions.

- Teach disease process, surgical intervention, preoperative and postoperative activity restrictions, use of dark glasses to decrease the discomfort of photophobia, use of correct technique for administration of eye medications, reporting for medical follow-up as instructed, and protecting the eye from further injury.
- In some types of cataract surgery, patients may be advised to avoid activities that might increase intraocular pressure, such as vomiting, coughing, sneezing, straining, or bending over or driving a car.
- Patients are told to seek medical treatment if they experience sudden, worsening pain, increase in watery or bloody discharge, or sudden loss of vision, as *these are signs of hemorrhage or problems.*

Anxiety related to visual alteration and surgery

EXPECTED OUTCOME: Patient will have minimal anxiety surrounding the visual alteration, treatment, and recovery.

- Allow patients the opportunity to discuss their feelings about the visual loss, by answering questions honestly, and by explaining any restrictions in activity *to reduce anxiety.*

EVALUATION. The patient goals have been met if the patient is free from injury, the patient verbalizes preoperative and postoperative directions, and anxiety is lessened.

Macular Degeneration

Pathophysiology and Etiology

Age-related macular degeneration (ARMD) is the leading cause of visual impairment in U.S. residents older than age 50. It involves a deterioration in the macula, the area on the retina where light rays converge for the sharp, central vision needed for reading and seeing small objects. The macula is also responsible for color vision (Fig. 52.4). There are two types of ARMD: dry (atrophic) and wet (exudative). In the dry form, photoreceptors in the macula fail to function and are not replaced because of advancing age. This accounts for 70% to 90% of the cases. In the wet form, retinal tissue degenerates, allowing vitreous fluid or blood into the subretinal space. New blood vessels are formed and compromise the macular tissue, causing subretinal edema. Eventually, fibrous scar tissue is formed, severely limiting central vision.

People at risk of developing macular degeneration include those older than age 60, those with a family history of macular degeneration, persons with diabetes, people who smoke, those frequently exposed to ultraviolet light, and Caucasian people.

Signs and Symptoms

Macular degeneration of the dry type is characterized by slow, progressive loss of central and near vision (see Fig. 52.2). Although individuals usually have the condition in both eyes, each eye may be affected in different degrees. Macular degeneration of the wet type has the same loss of central and near vision, but the onset is sudden. The loss can occur in one or both eyes. This visual loss is described as blurred vision, distortion of straight lines, and a dark or empty spot in the central area of vision. For some patients, there may be a decreased ability to distinguish colors.

Diagnostic Tests

Examination of the patient begins with visual acuity for near and far vision and an examination of the internal eye structures with an ophthalmoscope. The examiner uses an Amsler grid (Fig. 52.5) to detect central vision distortion and a color vision test to evaluate color differences. Patients are given an Amsler grid to take home and look at on a regular basis to monitor their vision changes. If any of the grid lines look crooked or disappear, the patient should contact the physician. Intravenous fluorescein (dye) angiography to look at the retina may also be utilized to evaluate blood vessel leakage or abnormalities in the eye.

Therapeutic Interventions

Unfortunately, there is no treatment for the dry type of ARMD. Most patients with the dry type do not lose peripheral vision or become totally blind, but most are classified as legally blind (less than 20/200 vision with correction). Special low-vision lenses can enhance remaining vision.

If the wet type of ARMD is diagnosed early, argon laser photocoagulation can seal the leaking blood vessels, slowing the rate of vision loss. If the patient receives argon laser photocoagulation, there is a small, permanent blind

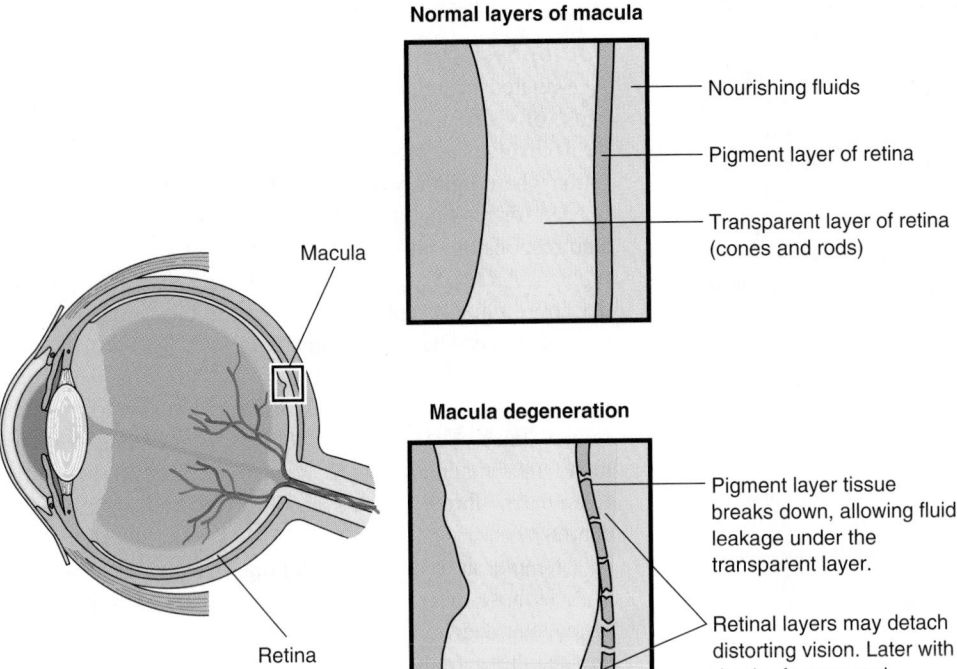

Normal layers of macula

- Nourishing fluids
- Pigment layer of retina
- Transparent layer of retina (cones and rods)

Macula degeneration

- Pigment layer tissue breaks down, allowing fluid leakage under the transparent layer.
- Retinal layers may detach distorting vision. Later with death of cones and rods blind spots occur.

Macula

Retina

FIGURE 52.4 Macular degeneration. The macula is a small area of the retina responsible for central and color vision.

spot at the point of laser contact with the macula. Photodynamic therapy is also available to stop bleeding in blood vessels. New research is exploring treatment options for wet ARMD. New drugs that are antiangiogenic (angiogenic = formation of new blood vessels) to stop the growth of new blood vessels in the eye are becoming available. These drugs inhibit vascular endothelial growth factor (VEGF), which is a protein involved in making new blood vessels and which increases vessel permeability. Examples of these medications are Pegaptanib (Macugen), which is now on the market, and ranibizumab (Lucentis), which is being studied. These medications are injected into the eye by an ophthalmologist. Macugen is most helpful in the early stages of ARMD. It slows the rate of vision loss but does not repair existing damage. Other studies are looking at the use of photodynamic therapy along with this drug to reduce the need for repeated laser treatments.

With either type of ARMD, patients have significant visual loss and need to adapt their patterns of daily living.

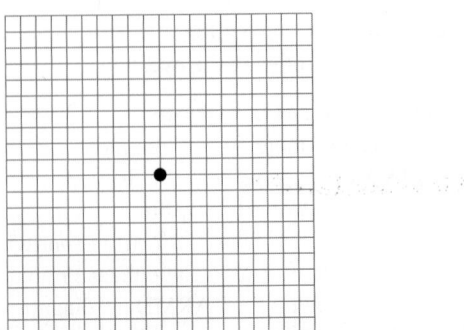

FIGURE 52.5 Amsler grid is used to identify central vision blind spots or distortions.

Research is exploring transplanting retinal pigmented epithelial cells that grow and function normally in an attempt to provide a cure in the future.

Nursing Process for the Patient with Macular Degeneration

See the nursing process section for the visually impaired.

Trauma

Emergencies and trauma of the eye must be assessed immediately so that proper treatment can be initiated. Injuries to the eye include foreign bodies, burns, abrasions, lacerations, and penetrating wounds. Treatment for chemical burns and sudden, painless loss of vision should be initiated within minutes to preserve vision.

Pathophysiology and Etiology

Foreign bodies are the most common cause of corneal injury. Dust particles or propellants may lodge in the conjunctiva or cornea. Patients naturally rub their eyes to dislodge the object, which further irritates the cornea. Burns may occur from chemical, ultraviolet, and direct heat sources. Depending on the agent causing the burn, it may be superficial or deep. Abrasions and lacerations usually occur as a result of something dragging across the eye, such as a fingernail or clothing.

Penetrating wounds are the most serious eye injury. Eye structures may be damaged permanently with complete blindness resulting. A penetrating wound also puts the patient at great risk of infection.

Signs and Symptoms

Foreign bodies produce pain when the eyeball or eyelid moves, causing the foreign body to drag over the opposing surface. Usually the eye tears excessively in an attempt to irrigate the noxious substance out of the eye.

Injuries that irritate or penetrate layers of the cornea range from mild to severe pain. With corneal abrasions, the pain sensation may be delayed for several hours. Other symptoms that may be seen with abrasions, lacerations, and foreign bodies include conjunctival redness, photosensitivity, decreased visual acuity, erythema, and pruritus.

Acute pain and burning are characteristic symptoms of a burn to the eye. Chemical burns must be treated immediately with an eyewash or irrigation to remove the caustic substance from the eye.

Penetrating wounds may result in a variety of symptoms depending on the area of the eye involved and the extent of the damage. If the nerve has been damaged, the patient may have no pain.

Diagnostic Tests

With any eye trauma or injury, visual acuity must be tested. It is important to establish baseline acuity to evaluate effectiveness of treatment, although many patients resist acuity testing because of the discomfort. Testing includes examination by slit-lamp microscope and direct ophthalmoscope. Fluorescein staining is used to evaluate abrasions.

Therapeutic Interventions

Foreign bodies are treated with a normal saline flush to irrigate the object out of the eye or to a point where it can be removed with a swab. Topical antibiotic ointment is prescribed to prevent infection.

Most chemical burns are treated with a 15- to 20-minute irrigation of either tap water at the work site or sterile solution in the health-care facility. Topical antibiotic ointments are usually prescribed. Burns from heat or ultraviolet (UV) radiation are not irrigated.

Abrasions and lacerations are generally treated with anti-infective ointments or drops after cleansing the eye with a normal saline solution.

An eye specialist treats penetrating wounds. At initial injury, both eyes should be covered to prevent ocular movement. If there is a protruding object, it should be stabilized but not removed until the physician can assess the patient. The nature and extent of the penetrating wound determine treatment.

Complications

If the eye cannot be saved via medical treatment, it may be necessary to surgically remove the eye. This procedure is called **enucleation** (entire eyeball removal).

Nursing Process for the Patient with Eye Trauma
ASSESSMENT/DATA COLLECTION AND EMERGENCY INTERVENTION. Foreign Bodies. The eye is inspected for foreign bodies, which may be visible on the eyeball. The lids should be everted to examine the surface. Then the eye is irrigated.

---

enucleation: e—removed from + nuclear—center

Burns. Assessment of the type of burn is done because treatment options vary. Immediate irrigation of the eyes is performed once it has been established that a chemical burn has taken place unless contraindicated for the chemical. Medication and eye patching are applied as indicated.

Abrasions and Lacerations. The eye is assessed for visible lacerations and then cleansed with medication and patching of the eye as indicated.

Penetrating Wounds. The patient is kept calm and relaxed to minimize eye movement and increased IOP. If a protruding object is present, the object is stabilized with tape or other supports.

NURSING DIAGNOSIS, PLANNING, AND IMPLEMENTATION. Acute pain related to inflammatory process and injury

EXPECTED OUTCOME: *Pain level is within an acceptable range for the patient.*
  - Administer analgesics as ordered *to reduce pain.*
  - Assist patient in remaining calm and relaxed *to reduce pain.*

Risk for infection related to eye trauma
EXPECTED OUTCOME: *Patient remains free of infection.*
  - Use sterile technique when irrigating eye, when applying medications, and during examination *to prevent infection.*

Anxiety related to visual-sensory deficit
EXPECTED OUTCOME: *Patient verbalizes a reduction in anxiety.*
  - Encourage the patient to verbalize feelings about visual impairment *to reduce anxiety.*
  - Reassure patient as appropriate.

Deficient knowledge related to medical regimen due to lack of prior experience
EXPECTED OUTCOME: *Patient is able to verbalize care of the eye.*
  - Teach patient about interventions and follow-up care.

EVALUATION. Patient goals have been met if pain level is within an acceptable range for the patient, patient remains free of infection, patient is able to verbalize a reduction in anxiety, and patient is able to verbalize care of the eye.

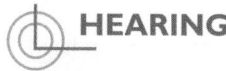 **HEARING**

Hearing Loss

Hearing loss is the most common disability in the United States and can be acquired or congenital. Hearing impairment ranges from difficulty understanding words or hearing certain sounds to total deafness (Box 52.6 Hearing Loss Summary). Hearing impairment can affect communication, social activities, and work activities. Hearing impairment

Box 52.6

Hearing Loss Summary

Signs and Symptoms	Difficulty understanding words or certain sounds, total deafness, changes in social and work activities, turns up volume on TV, asks "What did you say?", complains of people talking softly, speaks in a quiet or loud voice, answers questions inappropriately, avoids group activities, loss of sense of humor, appears aloof, complains of ringing, buzzing or roaring noise in ears
Diagnostic Tests and Findings	Abnormal Rinne's and Weber's tests, audiometric testing indicates hearing loss
Therapeutic Interventions	Ceruminolytics Anti-infectives Anti-inflammatories Assistive devices (hearing aids, implantable middle ear hearing devices, cochlear implants)
Complications	Safety issues related to not hearing; withdrawal from social activities and relationships related to hearing loss
Possible Nursing Diagnoses	Disturbed sensory perception: hearing related to altered sensory reception and transmission Impaired verbal communication related to impaired hearing Impaired social interaction related to impaired hearing and decreased communication skills Disturbed body image related to impaired hearing and use of assistive hearing devices Ineffective coping related to difficult communication Deficient knowledge related to care of hearing aid due to lack of prior experience

can diminish the individual's quality of life. Nurses have a responsibility to communicate with the hearing impaired and provide necessary information regarding health care. For more information on hearing impairment, visit the following sites:

- American Academy of Ear, Nose and Throat athttp://entnet.org
- Canadian Hard of Hearing Association at www.cyberus.ca/~chhanational/english.html
- National Information Center on Deafness at www.galludet.edu/~nicd
- National Institute on Deafness and Other Communication Disorders at www.nidcd.nih.gov
- National Organization for the Deaf at www.nad.org

Conductive Hearing Loss

Conductive hearing loss is any interference with the conduction of sound impulses through the external auditory canal, the eardrum, or the middle ear. The inner ear is not involved in a pure conductive hearing loss. Conductive hearing loss can be caused by anything that interferes with the ability of the sound wave to reach the inner ear. Conductive hearing loss is a mechanical problem. Causes of conductive hearing loss include cerumen, foreign bodies, infection, perforation of the tympanic membrane, trauma, fluid in the middle ear, cysts, tumor, and **otosclerosis.** Many causes of conductive hearing loss, such as infection, foreign bodies, and impacted cerumen, can be corrected. Hearing devices may improve hearing for conditions that cannot be corrected, such as scarred tympanic membrane or otosclerosis. Hearing devices are most effective with conductive hearing loss when no inner ear and nerve damage are present.

Sensorineural Hearing Loss

Sensory hearing loss originates in the cochlea and involves the hair cells and nerve endings. Neural hearing loss originates in the nerve or brainstem. **Sensorineural** hearing loss results from disease or trauma to the sensory or neural components of the inner ear. Some of the causes of nerve deafness are complications of infections (such as measles, mumps, and meningitis), ototoxic drugs (Table 52.5), trauma, noise, neuromas, arteriosclerosis, and the aging process.

Presbycusis is hearing loss caused by the aging process that results from degeneration of the organ of Corti. This degenerative process usually begins in the fifth decade of life. The individual develops an inability to decipher high-frequency sounds (consonants *s, z, t, f,* and *g*). This interferes with the individual's ability to understand what has been said, especially in noisy environments. The aging individual commonly has more difficulty understanding higher pitched female voices than lower pitched male voices.

Other Types of Hearing Loss

Mixed hearing loss occurs when an individual has both conductive and sensorineural hearing loss. This can be caused

---

otosclerosis: oto—ear + sclerosis—hardening

TABLE 52.5 OTOTOXIC DRUGS

Aminoglycosides (Antibiotic)	
Streptomycin	Neomycin
Gentamicin	Netilmicin
Amikacin	Kanamycin
Tobramycin	
Other Antibiotics	
Vancomycin	Minocycline
Erythromycin	
Diuretics	
Furosemide	Hydrochlorothiazide
Bumetanide	
Other Drugs	
Salicylates	Cisplatin
Indomethacin	Methotrexate
Quinidine	

by a combination of any of the disorders previously mentioned. Central hearing loss occurs when the central nervous system cannot interpret normal auditory signals. This condition occurs with such disorders as cerebrovascular accidents and tumors. Functional hearing loss is a hearing loss for which no organic cause or lesion can be found. It is also called psychogenic hearing loss and is precipitated by emotional stress.

Therapeutic Interventions

Medical management consists of improving the patient's hearing. The majority of persons with ear disorders have some degree of hearing loss. With any permanent hearing loss, the use of a hearing aid should always be considered. A hearing aid is designed to amplify sound or attenuate certain portions of the sound signal and amplify other sounds. Various types of hearing aids are available (Fig. 52.6). The in-the-ear aid is a small device that fits in the ear canal. The in-the-ear aid is unobtrusive and may be preferred by the individual. The behind-the-ear aid is worn postauricular.

The all-in-one eyeglass aid is attached to glasses and is positioned behind the ear.

Surgical intervention may be available for patients whose hearing is not improved with hearing aids. Implantable middle ear hearing aids can improve sound perception for patients with moderate-to-severe sensorineural hearing loss. Cochlear implants are surgically placed electrical devices that receive sound and transmit the resulting electrical signal to electrodes implanted in the cochlear of the ear. The signal stimulates the cochlea, allowing the patient to hear. The cochlear implants are able to restore up to half of the patient's hearing.

Nursing Process for the Patient Who Is Hearing Impaired

ASSESSMENT/DATA COLLECTION. Nursing care includes identifying those patients at risk for hearing impairment (Table 52.6). Patients with renal or hepatic disease, using two or more ototoxic drugs, or previously having used ototoxic drugs are at risk for developing hearing impairment. Monitor for signs of vertigo, horizontal nystagmus, nausea, vomiting, and spinning or rocking sensation while sitting still. To collect data for the hearing impaired patient, ask family members, as well as the patient, questions related to the patient's hearing status.

Objective data focus on obtaining a gross screening of hearing function. Assessment should start with engaging in normal conversation with the patient. Observe the patient for any difficulty understanding conversation or interview questions. Clarity of the patient's speech is also determined during the interview. Physical assessment includes the whisper voice, Rinne, and Weber tests. Test results provide an estimate of conductive or sensorineural hearing loss. The patient should be assessed for the underlying cause of the problem to determine if it is an external, middle, or inner ear problem. Examination of the external ear may reveal an external ear problem. The advanced practitioner may examine the ear canal for impacted cerumen or a tympanic mem-

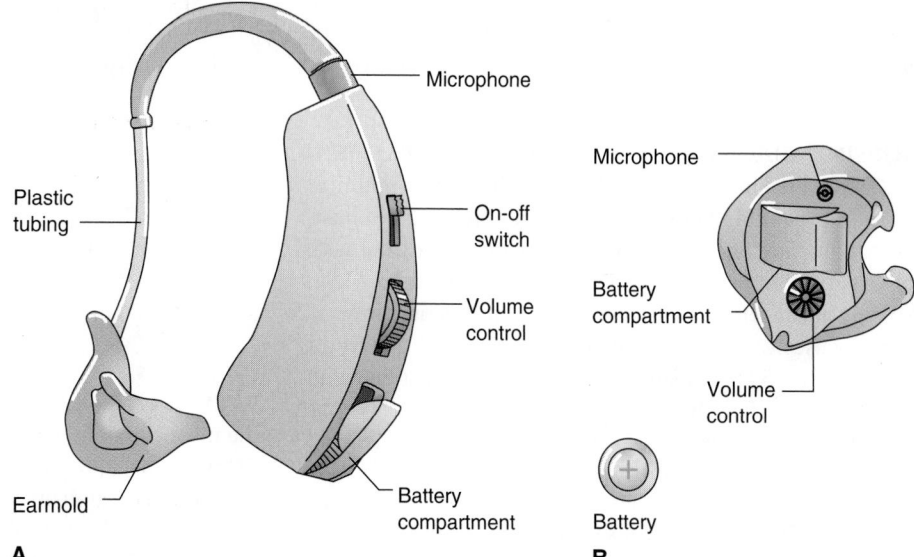

FIGURE 52.6 Hearing aids.
(A) Behind-the-ear hearing aid.
(B) In-the-ear hearing aid.

A

Plastic tubing
Earmold
Microphone
On-off switch
Volume control
Battery compartment

B

Microphone
Battery compartment
Volume control
Battery

TABLE 52.6 SUBJECTIVE ASSESSMENT OF HEARING

W Where is it? Are both ears affected? Is one side worse than the other?

H How does it feel? Are certain words unclear, or entire conversations? Are high-frequency sounds (consonants *s, t, z, f, g,* and female voices) unclear or difficult to understand? Is there any pain associated with the hearing loss? Any tinnitus or vertigo?

A Aggravating and alleviating factors. Is hearing worse in large groups or when there is a lot of background noise? Is hearing improved in a quiet environment or when speaking only to an individual? Is it easier to understand someone when seeing the person's lips move? Does the patient own or use any assistive hearing devices? Are they effective? What type is used?

T Timing. When did the hearing loss start? Was it gradual or sudden? Is the hearing loss associated with any illness or traumatic event? Is it associated with any recent flying? Any history of ototoxic drug use?

S Severity. Does it cause communication impairment? How much? Does it affect ADLs? Does it affect or limit usual social activities? Have family or friends commented on decreased hearing? Does patient avoid communication or social activities because of difficulty hearing? Is patient having difficulties hearing telephone voices, radio, television, or movies?

U Useful data for associated symptoms. Is there any fever, nausea, vomiting, or dizziness? Is there any history of occupational or environmental exposure to loud noises? What are the usual ear self-care habits? Any history of impacted cerumen? Has patient ever had cerumen removed from ears?

P Perception of problem by the patient. What does the patient feel is wrong? Does the patient think that he or she has a hearing problem? How does the patient feel about hearing assistive devices? How does the patient perceive the hearing loss, and how is it influencing the patient's life?

brane problem. Any assistive hearing devices should be noted and inspected for proper functioning. The results of the examination are documented and communicated to other health-team members.

NURSING DIAGNOSIS, PLANNING, AND IMPLEMENTATION. Planning focuses on helping the patient optimize hearing, promoting communication, and promoting adjustment to impaired hearing (Boxes 52.7 Communicating with the Hearing Impaired and 52.8 Care of Hearing Aids). Nursing management for the patient with hearing impairment focuses on enhancing communication and quality of life (see Box 52.9 Nursing Care Plan for the Patient with Hearing Loss). Families should be included in discussions about therapeutic hearing devices and their care, enhancing communication, and limiting isolation.

EVALUATION. The patient's goals are met if the patient communicates effectively, engages in usual social activities,

Box 52.7

Communicating with the Hearing Impaired

1. Get the person's attention before beginning to speak.
2. Face and stand close to the person being spoken to and maintain eye contact.
3. Avoid standing in the glare of bright sunlight or other bright lights.
4. Speak clearly, at a normal rate and volume. Do not shout or overarticulate.
5. Inform the listener of topics to be discussed and when a change of topic occurs. Stick to a topic for a while and avoid quick shifts.
6. Use short sentences and assess for understanding. If the listener does not understand after the message is repeated, rephrase the message. If the listener has difficulty with high-pitched sounds, lower the voice pitch.
7. Allow extra time for the listener to respond and do not rush the listener.
8. Ensure an optimum environment by reducing background noises by turning off television and radio, closing the door, or moving to a quieter area.
9. Encourage nonverbal communication such as touch or gestures as appropriate.
10. If the listener uses a hearing device, ensure that it is operational and in place before beginning to communicate. Give the person time to adjust the hearing device before speaking.
11. Do not smile, chew gum, or cover the mouth when talking.
12. Use active listening with attentive body posture, pleasant facial expressions, and a calm, unhurried manner.
13. Do not avoid conversation with a person who has hearing loss.
14. Use written communication if unable to communicate verbally.

verbalizes acceptance of an assistive hearing device, copes with emotional reaction of hearing impairment, and demonstrates care of hearing aid.

External Ear

Infections

PATHOPHYSIOLOGY AND ETIOLOGY. Infections are the most common disorder of the external ear, with **external otitis** being the most common infection. Exposure to moisture, contamination, or local trauma provides an ideal environment for pathological growth in the external ear, which results in external otitis. It may be caused by bacterial

Box 52.8

Care of Hearing Aids

1. Insert hearing aid while over a soft surface such as a pillow to prevent damage if the hearing aid is dropped during insertion.
2. Remove hearing aid before showering or bathing. Do not immerse in water.
3. Turn the hearing aid off when not in use to conserve battery.
4. Do not expose the hearing aid to extreme heat or cold.
5. Clean the hearing aid daily with a dry, soft cloth. Clean ear mold with small brush or toothpick to keep free of earwax.
6. Turn off the hearing aid and turn the volume down before inserting. Turn hearing aid on and increase volume once it is inserted.
7. Minimize whistling noise by ensuring that the volume is not too high, the aid fits securely, and the aid is free from ear-wax.
8. Check battery or lower the volume if sound is not clear or is intermittent. Buzzing noise may indicate that the battery door is not completely closed.
9. Do not expose the hearing aid to medicinal or hair sprays. Apply sprays before inserting hearing aid.

or fungal pathogens. Staphylococci are the most common causative organisms, but other gram-negative or gram-positive bacteria can cause problems. *Pneumocystis* infections have been seen in patients who have human immunodeficiency virus (HIV). A bacterial or fungal external otitis that occurs when water is left in the ear and washes away protective ear wax often after water exposure or trauma is known as swimmer's ear. External otitis occurs more often in the summer months than in the winter months. However, swimmer's ear can be seen year round in patients who swim indoors.

A localized infection called ear canal **furuncle** or abscess results when a hair follicle becomes infected. A **carbuncle** forms when several hair follicles are involved in forming the abscess. Most furuncles and carbuncles erupt and drain spontaneously. Otomycosis is an infection caused by fungal growth and is typically seen after topical corticosteroid or antibiotic use. Otomycosis occurs more often in hot weather. An infection of the auricle is called perichondritis, which can result in necrosis of cartilage.

SIGNS AND SYMPTOMS. The most common sign of infection of the external ear is pain (Box 52.10 External Ear Disorders Summary). An early indication of infection is pain with gentle pulling on the pinna. The patient may also experience pain when moving the jaw or when the otoscope is inserted into the ear canal. Pruritus (itching) is also a common symptom and can be an early sign of infection. Signs of inflammation are present on the external ear. The ear canal may become swollen or occluded, and as a result hearing may be diminished. Redness, swelling, and drainage can be observed during otoscopic examination. If drainage is present, it usually starts out clear and becomes purulent as the disease progresses. The patient may also be febrile.

DIAGNOSTIC TESTS. Laboratory tests such as a complete blood cell count (CBC) and cultures of discharge may be completed to diagnose infections. The white blood cell (WBC) count may be elevated. Culture and sensitivity tests isolate the specific infective organism, as well as antibiotics to treat the infection. Rinne's and Weber's tests can indicate conductive hearing impairment.

Impacted Cerumen

PATHOPHYSIOLOGY AND ETIOLOGY. Normally, the ear is self-cleaning. However, cerumen (wax) may become impacted, blocking the ear canal. People with large amounts of hair in the ear canal or who work in dusty or dirty areas are prone to cerumen impaction. Improper cleaning can also result in cerumen impaction. The older adult is at risk to develop impacted cerumen. This occurs because the amount of cerumen secreted is decreased and because of increased amounts of keratin. These two factors cause the cerumen to be drier, harder, and more easily impacted. Patients with hearing aids tend to have problems with impacted cerumen. Patients with bony growths secondary to an osteophyte or osteoma are at risk for cerumen impaction.

SIGNS AND SYMPTOMS. The patient may experience hearing loss, a feeling of fullness, or blocked ear if cerumen has become impacted (see Box 52.6 Hearing Loss Summary). Otoscopic examination reveals cerumen blocking the ear canal.

DIAGNOSTIC STUDIES. Audiometric testing reveals conductive hearing loss in the affected ear. Hearing acuity can be decreased by 45 decibels because of an impacted cerumen. Whisper voice, Rinne's, and Weber's tests also indicate conductive hearing loss (see Chapter 51).

Masses

PATHOPHYSIOLOGY AND ETIOLOGY. Benign masses of the external ear are usually cysts resulting from sebaceous glands. Other benign masses are lipomas, warts, keloids, and infectious polyps. Infectious polyps usually arise from the middle ear and enter the external ear through a hole in the tympanic membrane. Actinic keratosis is a precancerous lesion that can be found on the auricle and may be seen in the elderly. Malignant tumors such as basal cell carcinoma on the pinna and squamous cell in the ear canal may develop. These tumors can spread to surrounding tissue and bones if not treated.

SIGNS AND SYMPTOMS. Changes in the appearance of the skin can occur with benign or malignant masses.

Box 52.9   NURSING CARE PLAN for the Patient with Hearing Loss

Nursing Diagnosis: Disturbed sensory perception: hearing related to altered sensory reception and transmission

Expected Outcomes Patient will attain optimum level of sensory stimulation. Patient will become aware of auditory impairment and ways to compensate. Patient will demonstrate ability to perform activities of daily living, with assistance if necessary.

Evaluation of Outcomes Patient perceives maximum auditory sensory input. Patient is able to compensate for sensory impairment by using other senses and resources. Patient is able to perform activities of daily living as independently as possible.

Interventions	Rationale	Evaluation
Begin assessment of hearing by inspecting ear canals for mechanical obstruction. If cerumen is found, the use of a softening product is recommended to assist in wax removal. If canal is clear, continue assessment of hearing by use of a tuning fork, loud ticking clock, or verbal cues to determine auditory ability at various distances.	Hearing loss may occur due to the buildup of cerumen in the auditory canal. Determination of hearing ability assists nurse in developing interventions appropriate to the hearing level of patient.	Is ear canal free of mechanical obstruction? Is patient able to hear verbal input? If not, how severe is the impairment?
Enhance hearing by giving auditory cues in quiet surroundings.	Background noise such as television, radio, or large numbers of people make hearing more difficult.	Are auditory cues being delivered in an environment free of extraneous background noises? Are auditory cues being understood by patient?
Enhance understanding of auditory cues by getting patient's attention before speaking, speak slowly with careful enunciation of words, add hand gestures, speak face to face with impaired person, and adjust pitch downward without increasing volume.	Hearing is enhanced when additional cues assist the impaired individual in understanding the message. Use of hand gestures to point, lip-reading, facial expression, and lower pitch all assist communication.	Are instructions given in step-by-step format with written cues?
Structure environment to compensate for hearing loss by adding visual indicators to telephone ringer, doorbell, smoke detectors, and other emergency sounds.	Assists in communication and safety.	Is patient able to receive input in ways other than auditory?
Provide for optimum care of assistive appliances such as hearing aids by making sure that cerumen has been cleaned from the device, that batteries are charged, and that appliance is placed correctly in ear.	Appliances that are not functioning properly will not assist patient in hearing.	Is patient's hearing aid in place correctly? Is there cerumen blocking sound conduction? Do batteries work?

Interventions	Rationale	Evaluation
Introduce assistive devices such as hearing amplifiers, telephone amplifiers, telephones with extra-loud bells, written communication, and sign language.	Patients may not be aware of assistive devices, which may help them adapt to hearing loss and continue previous activities such as talking on telephone or listening to television.	Is patient aware of assistive devices that will allow him or her to continue to verbally communicate with others? Is patient able to use the devices to compensate for auditory impairment?
Allow patient to verbalize feelings and grieving about hearing loss.	Losing a primary sense such as hearing can be devastating for patients. Opportunity to ventilate feelings assists in processing the loss.	Is patient able to verbalize feelings about the auditory impairment and its loss?
Identify coping strategies that have been successful for patient in the past.	By identifying successful coping strategies, the nurse assists patient in dealing with stress of hearing loss. A positive approach for nurses to use focuses on the individual's capabilities rather than deficits.	Is patient able to identify successful coping strategies and use them to deal with stress of hearing impairment?
Refer to specialized clinician such as audiologist or occupational therapist or to specialized resources such as National Association of the Deaf or American Speech, Language and Hearing Association.	Specialized clinicians can provide detailed examination and treatment for the disorder. Specialized resource groups have networks in place to assist individuals in coping with the loss and assisting them with maximizing abilities.	Does patient know who to call for detailed examination and treatment of problems? Does patient know that there are specialized clinicians and resource groups to help with hearing impairment? Does patient know how to access these specialists?

Usually, impaired conductive or sensorineural hearing loss occurs with masses. Pain is another symptom and is usually described as deep pain radiating inward on the affected side. Ear drainage may be present. As the condition progresses, facial paralysis occurs. Visualization of the mass may be observed during otoscopic examination.

DIAGNOSTIC STUDIES. A biopsy may be obtained to determine if the mass is benign or malignant. Imaging studies are also used to diagnose tumors. Audiometric studies reveal any hearing impairment.

Trauma

PATHOPHYSIOLOGY AND ETIOLOGY. Injuries to the external ear are commonly caused by a blow to the head, automobile accidents, burns, foreign bodies lodged in the ear canal, and cold temperatures. Foreign bodies in the ear canal are common among children, with small toys being the most common object found. Cotton ball pieces and insects are the most common foreign bodies found in adults.

SIGNS AND SYMPTOMS. Lacerations, contusions, hematomas, abrasions, erythema, and blistering are signs seen with thermal or physical trauma. Repeated trauma to the ear can cause swelling, also known as cauliflower ear. This is common among boxers, rugby players, martial artists, and wrestlers. Conductive hearing loss can occur if

the ear canal is partially or totally blocked. Patients who have contusions or hematomas commonly complain of numbness, pain, and paresthesia of the auricle. The patient may or may not have symptoms associated with foreign bodies. These symptoms include decreased hearing, itching, pain, and infection. Examination of the ear canal with a penlight usually reveals the foreign body. Care should be taken during otoscopic examination not to push the foreign body further into the ear canal.

DIAGNOSTIC STUDIES. Imaging studies may be needed to determine the extent of the trauma. Audiometric, whisper voice, Rinne's, and Weber's tests may demonstrate conductive hearing loss.

Complications of External Ear Disorders

Complications can result from delayed treatment, no treatment, or spreading of the external ear disorder. If not treated, infections can spread, causing cellulitis, abscesses, middle ear infection, and septicemia. Metastasis can occur if malignant tumors are not treated. Infection, trauma, and malignant tumors may cause temporary or permanent hearing loss, disfigurement, discoloration, and scarring. Prompt identification and treatment of external ear disorders can prevent many complications.

Box 52.10

External Ear Disorders Summary

Signs and Symptoms	Pain, pruritus, swelling, redness, drainage, lacerations, contusion, hematomas, abrasion, erythema, blistering, hearing loss, foreign body
Diagnostic Tests and Findings	CBC with elevated WBC with infections; audiometric, Rhinne's, Weber's, and whisper voice tests indicate conductive hearing loss with impacted cerumen and trauma; imaging studies to indicate extent of trauma
Therapeutic Interventions	Ceruminolytics to remove ear wax; anti-infectives and anti-inflammatory medications to treat infection; débridement, surgical repair, or application of protective covering with trauma to external ear
Complications	Spread of infection to other parts of the ear, disfigurement, loss of hearing, and scarring
Possible Nursing Diagnoses	Acute pain related to inflammation or trauma Disturbed sensory perception: auditory related to altered sensory reception Risk for injury related to self-cleaning of external ear Deficient knowledge related to care of hearing aid due to lack of prior experience

Therapeutic Interventions for External Ear Disorders

External ear infections are treated with topical antibiotics in the form of drops or ointment. Systemic antibiotics are used for severe infections that are localized or have spread to surrounding tissues. Topical or systemic steroids may be used to treat inflammation. The ear is thoroughly cleaned before starting any topical treatment. If the external ear canal has drainage or is swollen shut, a wick may be inserted. The wick serves to aid in removing drainage or to aid in administering medication into the ear canal. Cerumen may be removed with instillations, a blunt ear curette, or a wire ear curette. Instillation is not used with a history of perfo-

rated tympanic membrane (eardrum). External ear disorders are usually painful, and analgesics are used to control pain.

Débridement, surgical repair, or application of a protective covering may be done when trauma occurs to the external ear. Surgical management consists of incision and drainage of abscesses. Excision of cysts or cutaneous carcinomas may also be required.

Nursing Process for the Patient with External Ear Disorders

ASSESSMENT/DATA COLLECTION. Subjective data are obtained in a patient history. Data include any reports of pain, fullness, previous cerumen impaction, itching, or hearing loss, as well as onset, duration, and severity of symptoms. Additional data include patient's occupation, previous ear problems, use of a hearing aid, and typical ear hygiene. Inspection and palpation are primarily used to obtain objective data. Observe for redness, swelling, drainage, furuncles, carbuncles, lesions, abrasions, lacerations, growths, cerumen, scaliness, or crusting. The patient may report pain when the ear is palpated. Basic hearing acuity tests are conducted to evaluate hearing loss (see Chapter 51).

NURSING DIAGNOSIS, PLANNING, AND IMPLEMENTATION. Possible nursing diagnoses are listed below.

Acute pain related to inflammation or trauma

EXPECTED OUTCOME: *Patient's pain will be decreased or absent as evidenced by a lower rating on the pain scale*

- Assess for nonverbal signs of ear pain *to identify pain.*
- Identify with the patient an optimum analgesic schedule *to promote comfort.*
- Implement nonpharmacological methods such as relaxation, massage, music, guided imagery, or distraction techniques *to relieve pain.*
- Heat may be applied to the area *to promote comfort.*
- Liquid or soft foods may be offered *if the patient experiences pain when chewing.*

Disturbed sensory perception: auditory related to altered sensory reception

EXPECTED OUTCOME: *Patient hearing will return to preillness state.*

- Teach patient how to administer topical antibiotics and anti-inflammatory medications using aseptic technique *to help restore hearing and relieve blockage of the ear canal.*
- Explain to patient if a wick is inserted into the ear canal *to monitor for drainage and report excessive drainage to health-care provider.*
- Explain procedure if health-care provider is to remove cerumen *for patient understanding and to decrease anxiety* (Box 52.11 Removing Cerumen, Fig. 52.7).

Box 52.11

Removing Cerumen

Instillations and irrigations should not be used on any person with a history of perforated tympanic membrane. Commercial ceruminolytics or common products such as baby oil, mineral oil, and virgin olive oil can be used to soften impacted cerumen and aid in the removal of the impacted wax. The patient should instill several drops of the solution at bedtime and then place a cotton plug in the ear to hold the solution in place. Excess oil and drainage are removed in the morning. Earwax is usually softened for 3 to 4 days before an irrigation is attempted. Patients prone to cerumen build-up should be taught how to safely remove earwax. A few drops of half-strength peroxide may be instilled into the ear canal during the day and three drops of glycerine instilled at bedtime. This can be repeated each week to minimize wax build-up.

The ear can be irrigated with an ear irrigation syringe or a Water Pik. The irrigation solution, usually water, should be warmed to body temperature. The patient is draped with a protective plastic drape, and a basin is placed below the ear to catch the irrigating solution. The patient sits with the ear toward the nurse and the head tilted toward the opposite ear. (See Fig. 52.7.) The external ear is pulled upward and backward for the adult. A low-pressure stream of water is directed toward the top of the ear canal. Care is taken not to obstruct the canal with the syringe so that the irrigation solutions can flow back out of the canal. Ensure that only the tip of the syringe is in the ear canal to prevent perforation of the eardrum.

Box 52.12

Ear Care

1. Cleanse the external ear with a wet washcloth. Gently cleanse the helix.
2. Never insert anything into the ear canal, including hairpins, cotton-tipped applicators, matchsticks, safety pins, toothpicks, paper clips, and fingers.
3. An individual with a history of ear infections, perforated tympanic membrane, or swimmer's ear should prevent moisture from entering the ear canal. Avoid swimming in contaminated water. Moisture or water in the ear canal can be prevented by using special earplugs or by using a piece of cotton rolled into a cylinder and covered with petroleum jelly.
4. Avoid home remedies for ear care without consulting a physician.
5. An individual with an upper respiratory infection should gently blow the nose with both nares open to prevent microbes from being forced up the eustachian tubes.

Risk for injury related to self-cleaning of external ear

EXPECTED OUTCOME: *Patient explains or demonstrates prescribed treatment.*

- Instruct patient how to care for ear *to prevent injury.*
- Instruct how to complete prescribed treatment *to ensure completion of treatment.*
- See Box 52.12 (Ear Care) for further instructions on ear care.

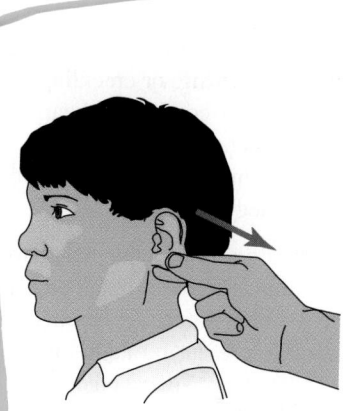

A   Pull ear back and down to straighten ear canal in a child

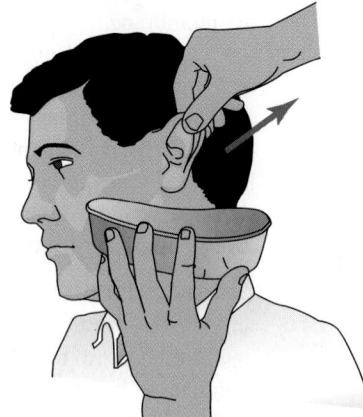

B   Pull ear up and back to straighten ear canal in an adult

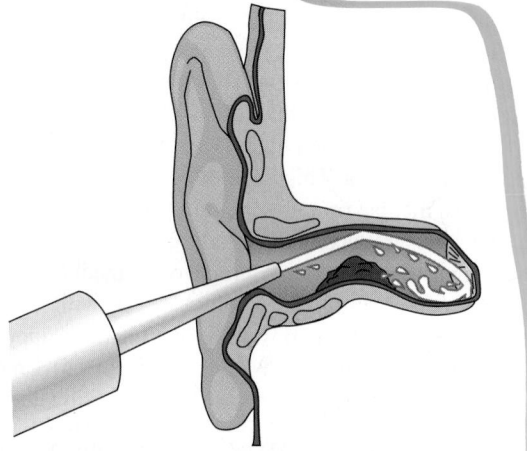

C   Irrigation – Fluid is aimed off top of ear canal wall behind impacted cerumen

FIGURE 52.7 Ear irrigation. *(A)* Child. *(B)* Adult. *(C)* Irrigation.

Deficient knowledge related to lack of information on preventive ear care

EXPECTED OUTCOME: *Patient explains or demonstrates procedures to maintain wellness of the external ear.*

- Instruct patient to keep external ear clean and dry *to prevent problems.*
- Teach patient how to use topical antibiotics, oral antibiotics, and/or anti-inflammatory medications *to promote healing.*
- Teach the patient how to complete the prescribed treatment and maintain ear health (see Box 52.12 Ear Care): include how to administer ear drops or ointments, keep the ear clean and dry, use cotton with petroleum jelly or ear plugs *to avoid getting water in the ears during an infection.*

EVALUATION. The outcomes for the patient are met if patient indicates pain is decreased or absent as evidenced by a lower rating on a pain scale, hearing improves or returns to preillness level, states or demonstrates prescribed treatment (e.g., administering ear drops or ointments), explains or demonstrates measures to maintain wellness of the external ear.

Middle Ear, Tympanic Membrane, and Mastoid Disorders

Infections

PATHOPHYSIOLOGY AND ETIOLOGY. Otitis media is the most common disease of the middle ear. *Otitis media* is a general term for inflammation of the middle ear, mastoid, and eustachian tube. Inflammation of the nasopharynx causes most cases of otitis media. As inflammation occurs, the nasopharyngeal mucosa becomes edematous and discharge is produced. When fluid, pus, or air builds up in the middle ear, the eustachian tube becomes blocked, and this impairs middle ear ventilation.

There are several types of otitis media in which inflammation can occur alone, with infective drainage, or with noninfective drainage. The first type of otitis media is otitis media without effusion. This is an inflammation of the middle ear mucosa without drainage. The second type of otitis media occurs when there is a bacterial infection of the middle ear mucosa. This is called acute otitis media, suppurative otitis media, or purulent otitis media. The infected fluid becomes trapped in the middle ear. If the infection continues longer than 3 months, chronic otitis media results. The third type of otitis media is otitis media with effusion. Other names include serous otitis media, nonsuppurative otitis media, and glue ear. With this type of otitis media, noninfective fluid accumulates within the middle ear.

SIGNS AND SYMPTOMS. Acute otitis media commonly follows an upper respiratory infection. A fever, earache, and feeling of fullness in the affected ear are common symptoms (Box 52.13 Middle Ear Disorers Summary). As purulent drainage forms, there is pain and conductive hearing loss. Nausea and vomiting may also be present. Purulent drainage may be evident in the external ear canal if the tympanic

---

BOX 52.13

Middle Ear Disorders Summary

Signs and Symptoms	Fever, earache, and feeling of fullness in affected ear following upper respiratory infection; nausea, vomiting; mastoid tenderness; otoscopic examination reveals reddened, bulging tympanic membrane; progressive hearing loss; vertigo; disorientation
Diagnostic Tests	Comple blood count Ear cultures Audiometric, Rhinne's, Weber's, and whisper voice tests
Therapeutic Interventions	Antibiotics — infection Analgesics — pain Myringotomy Myringoplasty Stapedectomy — otosclersis hearing aids
Complications	Perforation of tympanic membrane, cholesteatoma, typanosclerosis, mastoiditis, permanent hearing loss
Possible Nursing Diagnoses	Acute pain Fear Deficient knowledge Risk for infection

---

membrane ruptures. Mastoid tenderness indicates that the infection may have spread to the mastoid area. Otoscopic examination reveals a reddened, bulging tympanic membrane.

Symptoms of otitis media with effusion may go undetected in adults because there are no signs of infection. The patient may complain of fullness, bubbling, or crackling in the ear. The patient may have a slight conductive hearing loss or allergies or be a mouth breather. Otoscopic examination can reveal a bulging tympanic membrane with a fluid level, but the eardrum is not reddened.

DIAGNOSTIC STUDIES. Laboratory studies may indicate an elevated WBC count. Ear cultures may be obtained on any drainage to identify the specific infective organism. Conductive hearing loss is usually present on audiometric studies and Rinne's, Weber's, and whisper voice tests. Imaging studies may be done to diagnose infection.

COMPLICATIONS. A perforation may occur with an acute or chronic infection. Build-up of fluid and pressure in the middle ear can cause a spontaneous perforation of the tympanic membrane. The patient usually experiences pain before the rupture and relief of pain after the rupture. The fluid in the middle ear moves through the perforation into the ear canal, relieving the pressure and pain. A tympanic membrane perforation causes hearing loss. The location and size of the perforation determine the extent of hearing loss. Damage to the ossicles can also occur with perforation.

Repeated infections in the middle ear or mastoid can cause a cholesteatoma, which is an epithelial cystlike sac that fills with debris such as degenerated skin and sebaceous material. The cholesteatoma starts in the external ear canal and spreads to the middle ear through a perforation in the tympanic membrane. Damage occurs in the middle ear structures as a result of pressure necrosis. The cholesteatoma causes conductive hearing loss. As the disease progresses, facial paralysis and vertigo may occur.

Tympanosclerosis is another complication of repeated middle ear infections. Tympanosclerosis consists of deposits of collagen and calcium on the tympanic membrane. The condition can slowly progress over time to the area around the middle ear ossicles. These deposits appear as chalky white plaques on the tympanic membrane and contribute to conductive hearing loss.

Mastoiditis can occur if acute otitis media is not treated. The infection spreads to the mastoid area, causing pain. Since the use of antibiotics, acute mastoiditis is relatively uncommon. Chronic mastoiditis is still seen with repeated middle ear infections.

THERAPEUTIC INTERVENTIONS. Bacterial infections are treated with antibiotics. Amoxicillin (Amoxil), penicillin V (Beepen-VK, Veetids), erythromycin (E.E.S.), cefaclor (Ceclor), and cotrimoxazole (Bactrim) are commonly used. Oral analgesics such as aspirin, acetaminophen, or codeine or ear drops are given to control pain.

Surgical intervention includes several techniques. Paracentesis may be performed with a needle and syringe. The tympanic membrane is punctured with the needle, and the fluid is drained from the middle ear. A **myringotomy** may also be performed. During this procedure, an incision is made in the tympanic membrane and fluid is allowed to drain out or is suctioned out of the middle ear. Another technique is laser-assisted myringotomy, which vaporizes the tympanic membrane. Various types of transtympanic tubes may be inserted to keep the incision open. The transtympanic tube keeps the incision in the tympanic membrane open, equalizes pressure, and prevents further fluid formation and build-up. The transtympanic tubes are left in place until the infection is cured. Most tubes spontaneously extrude in 3 to 12 months and rarely have to be removed.

Reconstructive repair of a perforated tympanic membrane is called a **myringoplasty.** One technique involves placing Gelfoam over the perforation. A graft from the temporal muscle behind the ear or tissue from the external ear is then placed over the perforation and Gelfoam. The Gelfoam is absorbed, and the graft repairs the perforation.

A mastoidectomy involves incision, drainage, and surgical removal of the mastoid process if the infection has spread to the mastoid area.

Otosclerosis

PATHOPHYSIOLOGY AND ETIOLOGY. Otosclerosis, or hardening of the ear, results from the formation of new bone along the stapes. With the new bone growth, the stapes becomes immobile and causes conductive hearing loss. The formation of the new bone growth begins in adolescence or early adulthood and progresses slowly. Hearing loss is most apparent after the fourth decade. Otosclerosis is more common in women than in men. The disease usually affects both ears. Although the exact cause of otosclerosis is not known, most patients have a family history of the disease. It is therefore thought to be a hereditary disease.

SIGNS AND SYMPTOMS. The primary symptom of otosclerosis is progressive hearing loss. The patient usually experiences bilateral conductive hearing loss, particularly with soft, low tones. Usually, medical treatment is sought when the hearing loss interferes with the patient's ability to hear conversations. The patient may also experience tinnitus. Otoscopic examination reveals a pinkish orange tympanic membrane because of vascular and bony changes in the middle ear.

DIAGNOSTIC STUDIES. Audiometric testing indicates the type and extent of the hearing loss. Imaging studies indicate the location and the extent of the excessive bone growth. Whisper voice test and normal conversation show decreased hearing. The patient hears best with bone conduction in the Rinne test, whereas lateralization to the most affected ear occurs with the Weber test.

THERAPEUTIC INTERVENTIONS. There is no cure for otosclerosis, but hearing aids may be used to improve hearing for the patient. The hearing aid is most effective for conductive hearing loss when there is no sensorineural involvement.

Although total restoration of hearing is not possible, reconstruction of necrotic ossicles is done to restore some of the patient's hearing. Various methods are used to reposition and replace some or all of the ossicles. Unfortunately, the surgeries are not always successful over the long term. Ossiculoplasty is the reconstruction of the ossicles. Prostheses made of plastic, ceramic, or human bone are used to replace the necrotic ossicles. Total or partial ossicular replacement prosthesis may be used.

Stapedectomy is the treatment of choice for otosclerosis. Either part or all of the stapes is removed and replaced with a prosthesis. The prosthesis is placed between the incus and the oval window. Advances in surgical treatment include the use of lasers for improved visualization, less trauma, and greater precision during surgery. The goal is to restore vibration from the tympanic membrane to the oval window and allow sound transmission. Many patients experience

---

myringoplasty: myringo—tympanic membrane + plasty—surgical repair

stapedectomy: stape(s)—stirrup + ectomy—excision of

improved hearing immediately, others not until swelling subsides. Complications of ossiculoplasty and stapedectomy include extrusion of the prosthesis, infection, hearing loss, dizziness, and facial nerve damage. Some patients may have the surgery repeated if complications develop.

NURSING MANAGEMENT. The operative ear is placed upward when lying in bed. An ear plug may be used to help keep the area aseptic; the proximity of the brain makes this necessary to prevent brain infection. Activity orders may vary. The patient may be dizzy and experience nausea. Antiemetics should be given promptly to prevent vomiting. The patient's safety should be ensured if dizziness occurs. To prevent dislodgment or damage to the prosthesis, patients are instructed not to cough, sneeze, blow their nose, vomit, fly in an airplane, lift heavy objects, or shower. If the patient develops a cold, the physician should be contacted.

CRITICAL THINKING

Mrs. Smith

■ Mrs. Smith is an 83-year-old woman who is scheduled to be discharged from the hospital following a stapedectomy. She lives alone at home and is able to care for herself.

1. How would you communicate with Mrs. Smith to ensure that she understands the discharge instructions?
2. What teaching methods would you use to enhance communication?
3. What ear care instructions would you give her?

Suggested answers at end of chapter.

Trauma

ETIOLOGY AND PHYSIOLOGY. Trauma such as a blasting force, a blunt injury to the side of the head, or sudden changes in atmospheric pressure can cause the tympanic membrane to perforate and middle ear ossicles to fracture. Blast injuries cause injury from the direct pressure on the ear. Blunt injury to the head can cause temporal skull fractures and trauma to both the middle and inner ear. Barotrauma caused by sudden changes in atmospheric pressure in the ears can occur during scuba diving and airplane takeoffs and landings. Pressure changes can occur during normal atmospheric conditions such as nose blowing, heavy lifting, and sneezing. During these rapid changes of pressure, the eustachian tube does not ventilate because of occlusion or dysfunction and a negative pressure develops in the middle ear. The resulting pressure can cause the tympanic membrane to rupture or cause damage to the middle and inner ear.

SIGNS AND SYMPTOMS. Pain and hearing loss are the most common symptoms associated with trauma (see Box 52.12 Ear Care). Other signs and symptoms of barotrauma

TABLE 52.7 SUBJECTIVE ASSESSMENT OF MIDDLE EAR, TYMPANIC MEMBRANE, AND MASTOID DISORDERS

W	Where is it? Are both ears affected? Is it deep within the head?
H	How does it feel? Is there pressure? Fullness? Is it painful—sharp, dull, continuous, intermittent, throbbing, localized? No pain?
A	Aggravating and alleviating factors. Is it worse with change of position? Worse with movement? Is there relief after drainage? Relief with change of position? Relief with heat or analgesics?
T	Timing. When did it start? Has there been any recent upper respiratory infection, airline travel, scuba diving, trauma, or weight lifting? Was it a gradual or sudden onset? How long have symptoms persisted? Has there been a change in symptoms?
S	Severity. Does it cause hearing impairment? How much? Does it affect ADLs?
U	Useful data for associated symptoms. Is there any fever, drainage from the ear canal, nausea, vomiting, dizziness? Is there a family history of otosclerosis? Any previous ear problems or ear surgeries? Any occupational or recreational risk factors, such as scuba diving, weight lifting, or frequent airline travel?
P	Perception by the patient of the problem. What does the patient think is wrong? Has problem occurred before? If so, how was it the same and what was different?

ADLs = activities of daily living.

include fullness of the ears, vertigo, nausea, disorientation, edema of the affected area, and hemorrhage in the external or middle ear. In severe cases of barotrauma when scuba diving, these symptoms can cause drowning or cerebral air embolism from an overly rapid ascent. Otoscopic examination may reveal a retracted, reddened, and edematous tympanic membrane.

DIAGNOSTIC STUDIES. Audiometric studies are completed to determine the hearing loss. Imaging studies may be done to determine the extent of middle and inner ear damage. Conductive or sensorineural hearing loss may be evident, depending on the extent and location of the damage.

Nursing Process for the Patient with Middle Ear, Tympanic Membrane, and Mastoid Disorders

ASSESSMENT/DATA COLLECTION. Assessment of symptoms includes asking the patient for subjective data using the WHAT'S UP? format (Table 52.7).

The external ear should be inspected and palpated to obtain objective data. Pain with palpation is indicative of external ear problems, not middle ear problems. Pain over the mastoid area can indicate a mastoid problem. The middle ear and mastoid cavity cannot be visualized directly. The tympanic membrane is the only middle ear structure that can be directly visualized by the experienced practitioner with an otoscope. Objective assessment should also include vital signs, noting any elevation in temperature. Hearing acuity should be screened by the experienced practitioner using whisper voice, Rinne's, and Weber's tests. Any drainage from the ear should be noted and described.

NURSING DIAGNOSIS, PLANNING, AND IMPLEMENTATION. Risk for infection related to broken skin, pressure necrosis, chronic disease, or surgical procedure

EXPECTED OUTCOME: *Patient exhibits no signs of infection (no drainage from ear, no tenderness over mastoid, negative culture, afebrile).*

- Explain to patient not to blow nose by pinching off nares *to prevent spread of upper respiratory infections up the eustachean tube.*
- Teach patient to never insert anything into ear canal and other ear techniques (see Box 52.12 Ear Care) *to prevent ear damage.*
- Teach patient how to correctly remove cerumen from ear (see Box 52.11 Removing Cerumen).

Acute pain related to fluid accumulation, inflammation, or infection

EXPECTED OUTCOME: *Patient indicates pain is decreased or absent as evidenced by a lower rating on a pain scale.*

- Monitor pain using a pain scale *to determine baseline and need for treatment.*
- Use nonpharmacological measures such as heat, distraction, and relaxation techniques *for pain reduction.*
- Determine optimum analgesic schedule with patient *to maximize pain control.*
- Ensure that the patient knows how to administer ear drops and ear ointment *to help resolve infection and decrease pain.*
- Instruct patient to take all prescribed antibiotics even if symptoms are relieved *to ensure that infection is completely resolved.*

Fear related to hearing loss and lack of information

EXPECTED OUTCOME: *Patient states methods for preventing problems in the middle ear, tympanic membrane, and mastoid process.*

- Teach patient to yawn or perform jaw-thrust maneuver (opening mouth wide and moving jaw) *to equalize ear pressure to maintain ear health.*
- Teach patient to avoid trauma to the ear, loud noise exposure, and environmental or occupational conditions *to prevent damage to the ear.*
- Instruct patient to seek further medical attention if the patient's pain worsens, hearing decreases, or drainage from ear is present.

Deficient knowledge regarding surgery related to lack of exposure to information due to no prior experience

EXPECTED OUTCOME: *Patient states understanding of impending surgery.*

- Ask about patient's knowledge regarding surgery to determine learning needs.
- Include family in teaching sessions to enhance learning and assist with retention of information.
- Provide preoperative instructions and postoperative instructions as needed (Table 52.8).
- Teach patient to avoid getting water in ear to prevent moisture from reaching surgical site.
- Teach patient methods of effective communication (see Box 52.9 Nursing Care Plan for the Patient with Hearing Loss).

EVALUATION. The goals for the patient are met if there is no ear drainage or pain over mastoid; has negative culture and remains afebrile, states that no pain is present or pain is decreased, verbalizes care of ears, methods to prevent further infection; describes signs requiring medical attention, verbalizes rationale and outcome for any upcoming surgery as well as preoperative and postoperative instructions.

Inner Ear

Labyrinthitis

PATHOPHYSIOLOGY AND ETIOLOGY. Labyrinthitis is an inflammation or infection of the inner ear and can be caused by either viral or bacterial pathogens. The bacterium or virus enters the inner ear from the middle ear, meninges, or bloodstream. Serous labyrinthitis is a type of acute labyrinthitis that sometimes follows drug intoxication or overindulgence in alcohol. It can also be caused by an allergy. Diffuse suppurative labyrinthitis occurs when acute or chronic otitis media spreads into the inner ear or after middle ear or mastoid surgery. Destruction of soft tissue structures from the infection can cause permanent hearing loss.

SIGNS AND SYMPTOMS. Vertigo, tinnitus, and sensorineural hearing loss are the most common symptoms. Vertigo, or dizziness, occurs when the vestibular structures are involved. Tinnitus, or ringing in the ear, occurs when the infection is located in the cochlea. Sensorineural hearing loss can be caused by infections in the cochlea or vestibular structures. Nystagmus on the affected side may occur. Other signs and symptoms include pain, fever, ataxia, nausea, vomiting, and beginning nerve deafness.

DIAGNOSTIC TESTS. Laboratory tests such as a CBC may be completed to diagnose infection. Thorough hearing evaluation by an audiologist may reveal mild to complete hearing loss. Rinne's and Weber's tests can indicate conductive or sensorineural hearing loss.

THERAPEUTIC INTERVENTIONS. Antibiotics are used to treat bacterial inner ear infections. Viral infections usually run their course in about 1 week. Mild sedation may help the patient relax. Although there is no specific medicine to relieve dizziness, antihistamines can be used if they prove helpful on an individual basis. Patients may be placed on bedrest.

TABLE 52.8 PREOPERATIVE AND POSTOPERATIVE NURSING INTERVENTIONS FOR THE PATIENT HAVING EAR SURGERY

Preoperative Care

Nursing care for the patient undergoing ear surgery begins as soon as the decision to have surgery is made. The nurse collects data, determines if the patient understands the events, notes the patient's mental readiness, and obtains baseline physiological data.

- Ask understanding of the surgery and whether local or general anesthesia will be used.
- Help alleviate the patient's fear by encouraging the patient to ask questions. Ensure that all questions are answered before the surgery by appropriate person.
- Explain the type of pain, any packing or dressings that may be in place postoperatively, and any other postoperative restrictions that may be needed.
- Establish baseline vital signs and document findings.
- Ensure that the operative permit is signed.
- Determine current medications the patient is taking and document in the patient's record.
- Assess if the patient understands that surgery does not always correct impaired hearing.
- Leave any hearing devices in place as long as possible before the surgery.

Postoperative Care

Postoperatively the nurse is responsible for assessing the patient's physiological status. The nurse is also responsible for ensuring that the patient and family members understand discharge instructions.

- Some degree of pain may be expected, even with minor procedures. Explain how and when to take pain medication when the patient is discharged.
- Monitor postoperative vital signs and return to presurgical baseline.
- Tell patients that if an occlusive dressing is in place, hearing may be decreased until the dressing is removed.
- Instruct patients with tubes to avoid getting water in the ear. A shower cap or ear plugs may be used.
- Instruct the patient to seek medical attention if excessive bleeding or drainage occurs. If a cotton plug is to be left in place, instruct the patient to change it daily.
- Teach the patient, unless contraindicated, to blow the nose very gently one side at a time for the first week after surgery. Instruct the patient to sneeze or cough with the mouth open for 1 week after surgery.
- Avoid airplane flights for 1 week after surgery. For sensations of ear pressure, hold nose, close mouth, and swallow to equalize pressure.
- The patient should avoid strenuous work for several weeks. The patient may return to work in a few days, depending on the type of surgery and the type of work the patient does.
- Tell the patient to take prescribed medication and antibiotics as ordered.
- Have the patient arrange for follow-up appointment by calling physician's office.

NURSING MANAGEMENT. Nursing management includes helping the patient manage symptoms and self-care, and educating the patient about safety issues while on bedrest and sedatives. The patient should avoid turning the head quickly to help alleviate the vertigo. The patient is assisted to cope with anxiety that may be present because of the frustration surrounding hearing loss or loss of work.

Neoplastic Disorders

PATHOPHYSIOLOGY AND ETIOLOGY. Inner ear tumors can be benign or malignant. Acoustic neuroma, a tumor of the eighth cranial nerve, is the most common benign tumor. It is slow growing, occurs at any age, and usually occurs unilaterally. As it spreads, it compresses the nerve and adjacent structures. Malignant tumors arising from the inner ear are rare. Squamous and basal carcinomas arise from the epidermal lining of the inner ear.

SIGNS AND SYMPTOMS. Early symptoms of an acoustic neuroma include progressive unilateral sensorineural hearing loss of high-pitched sounds, unilateral tinnitus, and intermittent vertigo. Headache, pain, and balance disorders may also be present. Symptoms progress as the tumor spreads to other structures. Most malignant tumors grow quickly. The symptoms vary depending on the area of the ear that is involved.

DIAGNOSTIC TESTS. Neurological, audiometric, and vestibular testing are used to diagnose neuroma. Auditory brainstem evoked response (ABR) and electronystagmography (ENG) are completed. Examination of the cerebrospinal fluid shows increased protein. Computed tomography (CT) and magnetic resonance imaging (MRI) are used to determine size and location of the tumor.

THERAPEUTIC INTERVENTIONS. The preferred method of treatment involves surgical removal of the tumor. The labyrinth is destroyed, with a resulting permanent hearing loss. Steroids and radiation may be used to decrease the size of the tumor or for inoperable tumors.

NURSING MANAGEMENT. Nursing management focuses on preparing the patient for surgery and adjusting to the diagnosis and the resulting hearing loss (see Table 52.8).

Ménière's Disease

PATHOPHYSIOLOGY AND ETIOLOGY. Ménière's disease is a balance disorder. Its cause is unknown. With the disease, there is a dilation of the membranous labyrinth resulting from a disturbance in the fluid physiology of the endolymphatic system. The exact etiology is unknown but is thought to stem from hypersecretion, hypoabsorption, deficit membrane permeability, allergy, viral infection, hormonal imbalance, or mental stress. The disease usually develops between 40 and 60 years of age. The symptoms range from vague to severe and debilitating.

SIGNS AND SYMPTOMS. A triad of symptoms of vertigo, hearing loss, and tinnitus characterizes Ménière's disease.

ringing in the ears

Recurring episodic bouts of the incapacitating triad of symptoms and nausea and vomiting occur with Ménière's disease. The attacks may occur suddenly, or the patient may experience warning signs such as headache or fullness in the ears. During an acute episode, the patient experiences vertigo that lasts 2 to 4 hours. The vertigo is usually accompanied by nausea and vomiting, followed by dizziness and unsteadiness. The patient is uncoordinated and has gait changes when walking. Hearing loss is often described as a fluctuating fullness in the ears. Tinnitus is present. Irritability, depression, and withdrawal are common behavioral changes. The vital signs usually remain normal. It takes several weeks for symptoms to resolve, and hearing loss in the affected ear remains. The patient then enters a stage of remission until the next attack. The acute episodes occur two to three times per year. Eventually the patient has complete remission with some degree of permanent hearing loss.

DIAGNOSTIC TESTS. Diagnostic tests include audiometric studies, neurological testing, and radiographs of the internal ear. Audiometric studies identify the type and magnitude of the hearing loss. Neurological testing and radiographic studies are done to rule out other pathological conditions. A caloric stimulation test may demonstrate a difference in eye movement.

THERAPEUTIC INTERVENTIONS. Medical treatment consists of symptomatic treatment for acute attacks and prophylactic treatment between attacks. Tranquilizers and vagal blockers may be needed during acute attacks. Salt-restricted diet, diuretics, antihistamines, and vasodilators are used during prophylactic treatment. The patient should avoid alcohol, caffeine, and tobacco use. The patient may be placed on bedrest during acute attacks. Most patients respond to medical protocol but continue to have acute attacks. Some patients who do not respond to treatment may be placed on low doses of methotrexate. The goals of medical treatment are to preserve hearing and reduce symptoms.

Surgical treatment is used only when medical management has failed. When involvement is unilateral, a labyrinthectomy is performed. This causes complete loss of hearing in that ear. Another surgical intervention establishes a shunt from the inner ear to the subarachnoid space. This procedure helps drain the fluid and prevent future hearing loss. Another surgical treatment is intratympanic gentamicin injection, which is usually done in the physician's office.

NURSING MANAGEMENT. Nursing management focuses on managing the patient's symptoms and providing safety during the acute attacks. Administer medication, monitor fluid and nutritional status, and ensure safety. Because of the unpredictability of Ménière's disease, the nursing care focuses on emotional support for the patient during periods of remission. Provide emotional support and resources to help the patient cope with the unpredictable nature of the disease and the physical impairments associated with the disease.

Nursing Process for the Patient with Inner Ear Disorders

ASSESSMENT/DATA COLLECTION. Assessment of symptoms for the patient with inner ear disorders includes asking the patient for subjective data using the WHAT'S UP? format (Table 52.9).

Objective data include assessment of gross hearing. Whisper voice, Rinne's, and Weber's tests and a physical examination can be performed. The patient should be assessed for any nutritional deficiencies, including dehydration, weight loss, or weight gain. Any musculoskeletal abnormalities, such as unsteady gait, are also noted. The patient's vital signs are taken to determine if symptoms are associated with an infection. Laboratory data and diagnostic data are examined for abnormal findings.

NURSING DIAGNOSIS, PLANNING, AND IMPLEMENTATION. Planning focuses on helping the patient maintain a normal lifestyle, remain free of injuries, cope with the illness or hearing loss, and maintain adequate nutrition and hydration. The major nursing diagnoses and interventions for internal ear disorders may include:

Anxiety related to unpredictability of sudden and severe acute attacks

EXPECTED OUTCOME: Patient states anxiety is decreased.
- Encourage the patient to explore concerns about hearing loss and the unpredictability of acute attacks.
- Assess for signs of anxiety such as fidgeting, restlessness, apprehension, shakiness, and increased heart rate to determine if anxiety is present.

TABLE 52.9 SUBJECTIVE ASSESSMENT OF INNER EAR DISORDERS

W	Where is it? Are both ears affected?
H	How does it feel? Is there pressure? Fullness? Vertigo? Tinnitus? Is it painful—sharp, dull continuous, intermittent, throbbing, localized? No pain?
A	Aggravating and alleviating factors. Is it worse with change of position? Worse with movement? Is there relief with medications? Is the patient taking current medications? Are there any allergies?
T	Timing. When did it start? Was it a gradual or sudden onset? How long have symptoms persisted? Do symptoms progress in a set timing pattern? Do symptoms occur together or separately? Has there been a change in symptoms?
S	Severity. Does it cause hearing impairment? How much? Does it affect ADLs, nutritional intake, work, or leisure?
U	Useful data for associated symptoms. Any fever, nausea, vomiting, or dizziness? Any previous ear problems or ear surgeries? Headache?
P	Perception by the patient of the problem. What does the patient think is wrong? Has patient had this problem before? If so, what was the same and what was different?

- Explore with patient techniques that have and have not worked in the past *to reduce anxiety.*
- Use a calm reassuring approach *to help reduce patient's anxiety.*
- Provide quiet environment and diversional activities *to reduce anxiety.*
- Provide factual information regarding diagnosis and treatment *to reduce anxiety.*

Risk for injury related to impaired equilibrium

EXPECTED OUTCOME: *Patient is not injured from falling due to alterations in equilibrium.*

- Institute fall precautions *to help prevent injury.*
- Ensure that environment is safe and free of obstacles to *prevent falls.* Environmental hazards such as throw rugs, electrical cords in walkways, and poor lighting should be removed by the family.
- Monitor for signs of headache or fullness in the ears *which can indicate oncoming Ménière's disease attack.*
- Instruct patient to avoid sudden movement of the head during periods of vertigo *to prevent increasing symptoms.*
- Instruct patient on correct dosage and administration of medications *to help ensure resolution of symptoms.*
- Instruct patient to avoid use of alcohol, caffeine, and tobacco, *which can increase disruptions of equilibrium.*
- Instruct patient to call for assistance when ambulating *to minimize risk of falling.*
- If indicated, instruct patient to remain on bedrest until symptoms are relieved *to prevent injury.*

Nutrition: less than body requirements related to nausea and vomiting

EXPECTED OUTCOME: *Patient experiences adequate nutrition and hydration with relief of nausea and vomiting.*

- Monitor for signs of nausea, vomiting, and inadequate hydration *to determine baseline information.*
- Instruct patient to use deep breathing and voluntary swallowing *to suppress the vomiting reflex.*
- Instruct patient to eat slowly.
- Medicate as ordered *to relieve symptoms and prevent episodes of nausea and vomiting.*
- Institute salt-restricted diet, if ordered, and instruct patient on low- and high-sodium foods.

EVALUATION. The goals for the patient are met if signs of anxiety are decreased, patient remains free from injury, patient maintains weight within normal range with no signs of dehydration.

CRITICAL THINKING

■ Mrs. Belmont is a 48-year-old woman diagnosed with Ménière's disease. She is currently in a state of remission. She states she is fearful that the next attack will occur during her daughter's upcoming wedding.
1. What information would you ask Mrs. Belmont about her attacks?
2. What instructions can you provide her regarding treatment during her attacks?
3. How will you handle Mrs. Belmont's fears about future attacks?

Suggested answers at end of chapter.

REVIEW QUESTIONS

1. A patient is diagnosed with otosclerosis and asks the nurse what this disease is. Which of the following is the most appropriate response by the nurse?
   a. "Infection of the external ear most commonly caused by moisture or contamination."
   b. "Hardening of the stapes due to new bone growth."
   c. "Inflammation of the inner ear caused by pathogens."
   d. "Tumor of the eighth cranial nerve."

2. A patient is diagnosed with a refractive error and asks the nurse what this means. What would be the appropriate explanation by the nurse?
   a. "You will lose your vision and become blind."
   b. "You will need corrective lenses in order to see clearly."
   c. "The pressure in your eyes is higher than normal."
   d. "Your vision is 20/20."

3. A patient comes to the health clinic for a suspected ear infection. Which of the following data collection findings does the nurse expect with an external ear infection?
   a. Pain
   b. Fullness in ears
   c. Fever
   d. Dizziness

4. A patient has been prepped for an internal eye examination. Anesthetic drops as well as a mydriatic drug have been administered. Which of the following should the patient be taught for eye safety?
   a. "Wear sunglasses outdoors."
   b. "Rub your eye hourly to increase blood circulation."
   c. "You may reapply contact lenses when eye exam is completed."
   d. "Flush your eye with water to remove the eye drops."

5. A nurse is working on a postoperative unit for eye surgery. In planning interventions for an eye surgery patient, the nurse understands that which of the following patients needs specific positioning orders postoperatively to prevent complications?
   a. 19-year-old after removal of congenital cataract
   b. 30-year-old woman after scleral buckling
   c. 52-year-old man after trabeculectomy
   d. 82-year-old man after corneal transplant

Multiple response item. Select all that apply.
6. Which of the following medications should the nurse question before giving to prevent serious eye complications for a patient who has a history of acute angle-closure glaucoma?
   a. Morphine
   b. Cefazolin (Kefzol)
   c. Atropine
   d. Ranitidine (Zantac)
   e. Hydroxyzine (Vistaril)
   f. Warfarin (Coumadin)

7. Which of the following medications can cause hearing loss?
   a. Furosemide (Lasix)
   b. Acetaminophen (Tylenol)
   c. Warfarin (Coumadin)
   d. Penicillin (Pen-Vee K)

8. Which of the following symptoms would the nurse expect to be in the patient's history who has macular degeneration?
   a. Loss of peripheral vision
   b. Sudden darkness
   c. Dull ache in the eyes
   d. Loss of central vision

9. The nurse is contributing to the plan of care for a patient with Ménière's disease. Which of the following is the primary goal for a patient with Ménière's disease that the nurse should recommend be included in the plan of care?
   a. Prevent dehydration
   b. Decrease pain
   c. Prevent injury
   d. Preserve hearing

10. The nurse is caring for a patient with presbycusis. Which of the following techniques would be most important for the nurse to use to increase communication with this patient?
    a. Talk in a very loud voice.
    b. Lower voice pitch.
    c. Do not smile or chew gum when talking to the patient.
    d. Allow extra time for patient to respond.

11. A patient with acute angle-closure glaucoma reports use of the following medications. Using which of these medications indicates to the nurse that further instruction is needed.
    a. Acetaminophen
    b. Cefazolin (Kefzol)
    c. Ranitidine(Zantac)
    d. Diphenhydramine(Benadryl)

Unit Fourteen Bibliography

1. Age, hearing loss and hearing aids. Harvard Health Lett 26, 2000.
2. Age-Related Eye Disease Research Group: A randomized, placebo-controlled, clinical trial of high-dose supplementation with vitamins C and E, beta carotene, and zinc for age-related cataract and vision loss. AREDS Report No. 9. Arch Ophthalmol 119:1439–1452, 2001.
3. Cober, MP, and Johnson, CE: Otitis media: review of the 2004 Treatment Guidelines (CE) (November). Ann Pharmacother 39(11):1879–1887, 2005.
4. Cohen, HS, and Kimball, KT: Decreased ataxia and improved balance after vestibular rehabilitation. Otolaryngol Head Neck Surg 130:418–25, 2004.
5. Crews, JE, and Campbell, VA: Vision impairment and hearing loss among community-dwelling older Americans: implications for health and functioning. Am J Public Health 94:823–829, 2004.
6. Dalton, DS, Cruickshanks, KJ, Klein, BE, et al: The impact of hearing loss on quality of life in older adults. Gerontologist 43:661–668, 2003.
7. Eichenbaum, J: Vitamins for cataracts and macular degeneration. J Ophthal Nurs Technol 15:2, 1996.
8. Epstein, S: What you should know about ototoxic medications. Self Help for Hard of Hearing People Journal available online at http://www.pub.utdallas.edu/dybala/theaudpa/blah/shhh/ototoxic.htm.
9. Gragoudas, ES, Adamis, AP, Cunningham, ET Jr, et al, for the VEGF Inhibition Study in Ocular Neovascularization Clinical Trial Group.
10. Henney, JE: New hearing implant approved. JAMA 284:1640, 2000.
11. Kilpatrick, JK, Sismanis, A, Spencer, R, et al: Low-dose methotrexate management of patients with bilateral Meniere's disease. Ear Nose Throat J 79:82, 2000.
12. Lassig, AA, Zwolan, TA, and Telian, SA: Cochlear implant failures and revision. Otol Neurotol 26:624–634, 2005.
13. Lin, MY, Gutierrez, PR, Stone, KL, et al: Study of Osteoporotic Fractures Research Group. Vision impairment and combined vision and hearing impairment predict cognitive and functional decline in older women. J Am Geriatr Soc 52:1996–2002, 2004.
14. Lyle, BJ, Mayes-Perlman, J, Klien, BEK, et al: Antioxidant intake and risk of incident age-related nuclear cataracts in the Beaver Dam Eye Study. Am J Epidemiol 149:801, 1999.
15. McConnell, E: Communicating with a hearing-impaired patient. Nursing 28:32, 1998.

16. McCord, H, and McVeigh, G: Eat your spinach, save your eyesight. Prevention 52:60, 2000.
17. McHugh, M, and Schaller, P: Ergonomic nursing workstation design to prevent cumulative trauma disorders. Computers Nurs 15:5, 1997.
18. Moeller, SM, Jacques, PF, and Blumberg, JB: The potential role of dietary xanthophylls in cataract and age-related macular degeneration. J Am Coll Nutr 19:522S, 2000.
19. New treatment may help stem vision loss from macular degeneration. Tufts University Health & Nutrition Letter 18:3, 2000.
20. Gragoudas, ES, Adamis, AP, Cunningham, ET, Pegaptanib for neovascular age-related macular degeneration. N Engl J Med 351:2805–2816, 2004.
21. Reiley, JS, Deutsch, ES, and Cook, S: Laser-assisted myringotomy for otitis media: a feasibility study with short-term follow-up. Ear Nose Throat J 79:650, 2000.
22. Smith, W, Mitchell, P, Webb, K et al: Dietary antioxidants and age-related maculopathy: The Blue Mountains Eye Study. Ophthalmology 106:761, 1999.
23. Taylor, A, et al: Long-term intake of vitamins and carotenoids and odds of early age-related cortical and posterior subcapsular lens opacities. Am J Clin Nutr 75: 540, 2002.
24. Wallhagen, MI, Strawbridge, WJ, Shema, SJ, Kaplan, GA: Impact of self-assessed hearing loss on a spouse: a longitudinal analysis of couples. J Gerontol B Psychol Sci Soc Sci 59:S190–S196, 2004.

SUGGESTED ANSWERS TO

CRITICAL THINKING

■ *Mr. Samuel*

1. Mr. Samuel should seek assistance, patch both eyes, and have someone take him to receive medical treatment immediately.
2. Ensure that an antiemetic is ordered postoperatively on the patient's return to the unit. When Mr. Samuel reports nausea, the antiemetic should be given promptly.
3. Did you recognize that the concentration is 5 mg/1 mL, and the volume of the vial is 2 mL? The concentration is what is needed to calculate the dose.

$$\frac{7.5 \text{ mL}}{} \quad \frac{1 \text{ mL}}{5 \text{ mL}} = 1.5 \text{ mL}$$

■ *Mrs. Smith*

1. Gain her attention, face and stand in her visual field, avoid glare, speak clearly, inform her of topics to be discussed, assess for understanding, allow extra time, reduce background noises, use nonverbal communication, and do not cover your mouth when talking.
2. Use active listening. Use written communication to enhance spoken words. Use demonstration and return demonstration. Allow questions. Do not hurry. Provide information in short segments. Reassess understanding at each session.

3. Place the operative ear upward when lying in bed. Use ear plug as ordered. Do not cough, sneeze, blow nose, vomit, fly in an airplane, lift heavy objects, or shower. If a cold develops, call the physician. If dizzy, be careful when up.

■ *Mrs. Belmont*

1. You would ask Mrs. Belmont about specific signs she may have prior to attacks, such as headache or fullness in the ears. You should also ask her specifically what symptoms she has during attacks. Common symptoms include the triad of vertigo, hearing loss, and tinnitus. She may also have nausea, vomiting, and unsteady gait.
2. Discuss treatment that Mrs. Belmont has used with previous attacks. Ask her which treatments seemed to help. Common treatments you can recommend include taking recommended medication such as tranquilizers and vagal blockers; instruct her to maintain adequate fluid and nutritional intake during attacks; ambulate with assistance; limit salt in diet; avoid alcohol, caffeine, and tobacco use.
3. Discuss with Mrs. Belmont prophylactic treatment such as salt-restricted diet, diuretics, antihistamines, and vasodilators. Discuss the normal progress of the disease. Provide emotional support and discuss methods to help her cope with the disease, such as counseling and relaxation techniques.

unit FIFTEEN

UNDERSTANDING THE INTEGUMENTARY SYSTEM

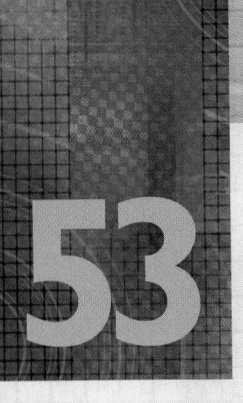

53

Integumentary Function, Assessment, and Therapeutic Measures

RITA BOLEK TROFINO,
MARTY KOHN, AND
JANICE L. BRADFORD

KEY TERMS

alopecia (AL-oh-PEE-she-ah)
ecchymosis (ek-uh-MOH-sis)
erythema (ER-i-THEE-mah)
petechiae (pe-TEE-kee-eye)
turgor (TER-ger)

QUESTIONS TO GUIDE YOUR READING

1. What is the normal anatomy of the integumentary system?

2. What is the normal function of the integumentary system?

3. What are the effects of aging on the integumentary system?

4. What data should you collect when caring for a patient with a disorder of the integumentary system?

5. What laboratory and diagnostic tests are commonly performed to diagnose integumentary disorders?

6. What common therapeutic measures are used for patients with integumentary disorders?

REVIEW OF NORMAL ANATOMY AND PHYSIOLOGY

The skin, its accessory structures, and the subcutaneous tissue make up the integumentary system, the covering of the body that separates the living internal environment from the external environment. The skin itself is considered an organ and consists of two layers, the outer epidermis and the inner dermis (Fig. 53.1).

Epidermis

The epidermis is made of stratified squamous epithelial tissue and is avascular—meaning that it has no capillaries within it. Its nourishment comes from the dermis beneath it. The epidermis is thickest on the palms of the hands and soles of the feet. The innermost layer of the epidermis is called the stratum germinativum, and it is here that mitosis takes place to produce new epidermal cells. The rate of mitosis is fairly constant, but it may be increased by chronic pressure on the skin, as in callus formation. The new cells produce the protein keratin. As they are pushed to the surface of the skin, they die and become the stratum corneum, the outermost of the epidermal layers.

The stratum corneum consists of many layers of dead cells; all that remains is their keratin. An unbroken stratum corneum is an effective barrier against pathogens and most chemicals, although even microscopic breaks are sufficient to permit their entry. Keratin is relatively waterproof, so it prevents the loss of water and therefore dehydration, and also prevents the entry of excess water by way of the body surface. As dead cells are worn off the surface of the skin (which contributes to the removal of pathogens), they are continuously replaced by cells from within. Loss of large portions of the stratum corneum, as with extensive third-degree burns, greatly increases the risk for infection and dehydration.

Melanocytes are cells in the lower epidermis that produce the protein melanin; the amount of melanin is a genetic characteristic and gives color to skin and hair. When the skin is exposed to ultraviolet (UV) rays from the sun or artificial lighting, production of melanin increases and it is incorporated into the epidermal cells before they die, making the cells darker. Melanin is a pigment barrier to prevent further exposure of living cells in the stratum germinativum to UV rays. Ultraviolet rays are mutagenic; that is, they are capable of damaging the DNA within cells and causing mutations that may result in malignancy.

Also in the epidermis are Langerhans' cells, a type of macrophage that presents foreign antigens to helper T cells. This is the first step in the destruction of pathogens that have penetrated the epidermis.

Dermis

The dermis consists of two layers: the outer papillary region is made of mainly adipose tissue with fine elastin contribution, and the inner reticular region is of dense irregular

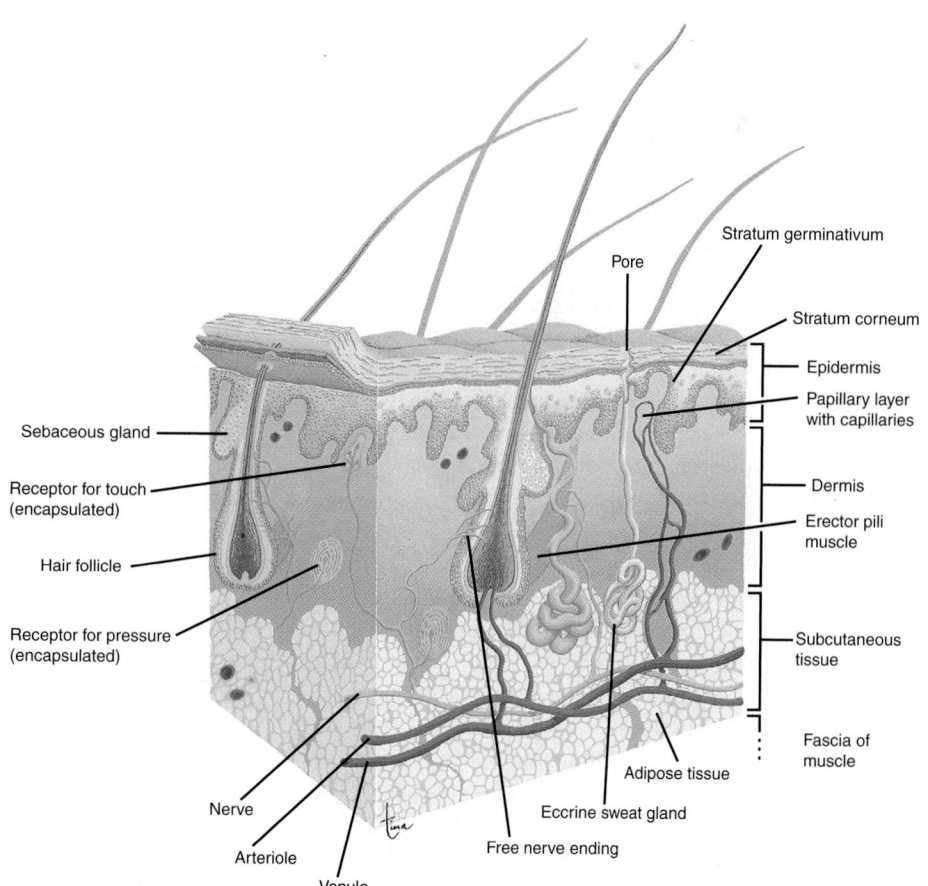

FIGURE 53.1 Structure of the skin and subcutaneous tissue. *(Modified from Scanlon, VC, and Sanders, T: Essentials of Anatomy and Physiology, ed. 5. F.A. Davis, Philadelphia, with permission.)*

Sebaceous gland

Receptor for touch (encapsulated)

Hair follicle

Receptor for pressure (encapsulated)

Nerve

Arteriole

Venule

Free nerve ending

Eccrine sweat gland

Adipose tissue

Pore

Stratum germinativum

Stratum corneum

Epidermis

Papillary layer with capillaries

Dermis

Erector pili muscle

Subcutaneous tissue

Fascia of muscle

connective tissue. This reticular region contains cells called fibroblasts, a large contribution of collagen, and some coarse elastic fibers. Fibroblasts produce the protein fibers collagen and elastin. Collagen fibers form the strength of the dermis; elastin fibers are capable of recoil and make the dermis somewhat elastic. Within the dermis are the hair and nail follicles, glands, nerve endings, and blood vessels. The capillaries in the papillary layer of the dermis are important to nourish the stratum germinativum, which has no capillaries of its own.

Hair

Hair develops in epidermal structures called follicles. At the base of the hair root in its follicle is the matrix, a group of cells that undergo mitosis to produce the hair shaft. The cells quickly die after producing keratin and incorporating melanin. Human hair with significant functions includes the eyelashes and eyebrows, which keep dust and sweat out of the eyes, and nostril hair, which filters air entering the nasal cavities. Hair on the head provides thermal insulation.

Nails

Nail follicles are found at the ends of the fingers and toes, and growth of nails is similar to growth of hair. Mitosis in the nail root is a continuous process to produce new cells, which contain keratin. As these cells die, they form the visible nail. Nails protect the ends of the digits from mechanical injury and are useful for picking up small objects.

Receptors

The sensory receptors in the dermis are those for the cutaneous senses. Free nerve endings are the receptors for heat, cold, and pain; encapsulated nerve endings are specific for touch and pressure. The sensitivity of an area of skin is determined by the number of receptors present.

Sebaceous Glands

Most ducts of sebaceous glands open into hair follicles; a few open directly onto the skin surface. Their secretion is sebum, a lipid substance that inhibits the growth of some bacteria and prevents drying of skin and hair. Skin that is dry tends to crack or fissure more easily, and even these small breaks in the epidermis are potential portals of entry for pathogens.

Sudoriferous (Sweat) Glands

Sudoriferous glands are also known as sweat glands. There are two kinds of sudoriferous glands: apocrine and eccrine. Apocrine glands are really modified scent glands and are most numerous in the axillae and genital area; they are activated by stress and emotions.

Eccrine glands are found throughout the dermis but are most numerous on the face, palms, and soles. They are activated by high temperatures or by exercise and secrete sweat onto the skin surface. The sweat is evaporated by excess body heat, which is a very effective cooling mechanism, although it does have the potential to lead to dehydration if water is not replaced by drinking.

Modified sweat glands called ceruminous glands are found in the dermis of the ear canals. Their secretion is called cerumen or earwax. Cerumen prevents drying of the outer surface of the eardrum. Excess cerumen, however, may become impacted against the eardrum, prevent it from vibrating properly, and diminish the hearing acuity.

Blood Vessels

The blood vessels in the dermis serve the usual function of tissue nourishment, but the arterioles are also involved in the maintenance of body temperature. Blood carries the heat produced by active organs and distributes it throughout the body. In a warm environment, dilation of blood vessels in the dermis increases blood flow and loss of heat to air or clothing. Constriction of blood vessels in a cold environment decreases blood flow to the skin and conserves body heat.

Stressful situations also bring about vasoconstriction in the dermis, which allows blood to circulate to more vital organs, such as the heart, liver, brain, or muscles.

Other functions of the skin are the formation of vitamin D from cholesterol when the skin is exposed to the UV rays of the sun and the excretion of small amounts of urea and sodium chloride in sweat.

Subcutaneous Tissue

The subcutaneous tissue, between the dermis and the muscles, is made of areolar and adipose connective tissues. Although an unbroken stratum corneum is an excellent barrier to pathogens, even small breaks provide portals of entry. In the subcutaneous tissue are numerous white blood cells that destroy any pathogens that have entered by way of broken skin. Subcutaneous adipose tissue cushions some bones and provides some insulation from cold, but its most important function is energy storage. Excess nutrients are changed to triglyceride and stored as potential energy for times when food intake may decrease.

Aging and the Integumentary System

The effects of age on the integumentary system are often quite visible (Fig. 53.2).

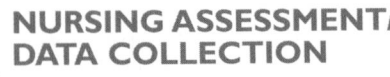

NURSING ASSESSMENT/ DATA COLLECTION

Health History

Skin problems are a fairly common complaint for the patient entering the health system. Many factors can influence the integumentary system. A skin problem may be the only complaint the patient has, or it may be a manifestation of an underlying systemic condition or psychological stress. Most important, the skin can visibly communicate the patient's health. Therefore, the questions that are posed to the patient are important in determining if the skin problem is a disease entity of its own or a sign of a more systemic

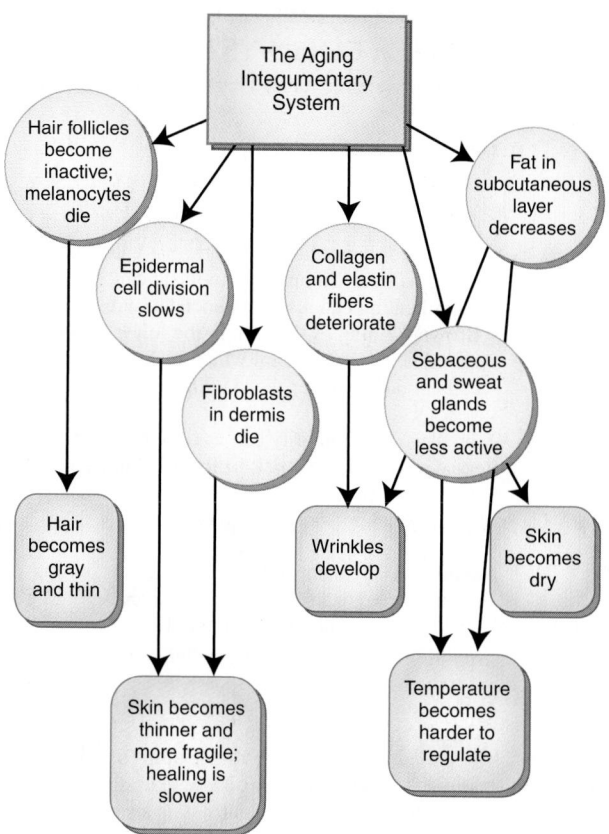

FIGURE 53.2 Aging and the integumentary system.

disorder. Table 53.1 provides examples of general questions that can be asked of the patient to elicit information.

If further assessment of a particular problem area is necessary, the WHAT'S UP? line of questioning can be used. For example, if the patient has a rash, you can respond with the following questions:

Where is it? Is that the only area where you have a rash?

How does it feel? Does it itch? Burn? Hurt?

Aggravating and alleviating factors. Does scratching aggravate it? Does anything else aggravate it, such as soaps and detergents? What relieves it? How have you treated it in the past?

Timing. How long have you had this problem? Does it recur?

Severity. How bad is the discomfort on a scale of 0 to 10, with 0 being comfortable and 10 being unable to touch the area?

Useful other data. Do you have other symptoms besides the rash, such as itching, discharge, tingling, or loss of sensation?

Patient's perception. What do you think is causing your rash?

Physical Assessment

Assessment of the skin involves not only the entire skin area, but also the hair, nails, scalp, and mucous membranes. The main techniques utilized in physical assessment of the skin are inspection and palpation. Ensure that the patient is disrobed but adequately draped in a well-lighted and warm environment. Use a hand-held magnifying glass or penlight to see small details and further illuminate the area.

Normally the skin is intact, with no abrasions, and is smooth, dry, well hydrated, and warm. Skin **turgor** is firm and elastic. The skin surface is flexible and soft. Skin color ranges from light to ruddy pink or olive in white-skinned patients and light brown to deep brown in dark-skinned patients.

You need to be aware of normal developmental changes when performing an assessment. The skin of the neonate is very thin and friable (easily broken). During adolescence, the skin becomes thicker, with active sebaceous, eccrine, and apocrine glands. Body hair also changes during adolescence as a result of hormonal influences. In older patients, the skin loses some of its elasticity and moisture. There is decreased activity of sebaceous and sweat glands. The older patient's skin is thinner, more fragile, and more wrinkled.

Inspection

Inspect each area of the skin, including nails, hair, scalp, and mucous membranes, for color, moisture, lesions, edema, intactness, vascular markings, turgor, and cleanliness. This examination should be done in an orderly sequence, such as hair, scalp, nails, buccal mucosa, and then the general skin surface from head to toe.

COLOR. Skin color can be influenced by many factors, including the temperature of the patient, oxygenation, blood flow, exposure to UV rays, and positioning. Because skin color can differ genetically from very light to very dark, skin assessment can be difficult for the novice practitioner.

Commonly noted alterations can include pallor, **erythema** (redness), jaundice, cyanosis, and brown color. Pallor is a paleness or decrease in color and can be caused by vasoconstriction, decreased blood flow, or decreased hemoglobin levels from anemia. Pallor is best assessed on the face, conjunctivae, nailbeds, and lips. Erythema, or red discoloration, may indicate circulatory changes and can be caused by vasodilation or increased blood flow to the skin from fever or inflammation. Erythema is best assessed on the face or in an area of trauma.

Jaundice, a yellow-orange discoloration, may occur as a result of liver disease. The best place to inspect for jaundice is in the sclera of the eye. Cyanosis, or bluish discoloration, may indicate a cardiac, pulmonary, or perfusion problem. The best places to inspect for cyanosis are the lips, nailbeds, conjunctivae, and palms. People of Mediterranean descent normally have a bluish tone to their lips; this is not cyanosis.

A brown color may be caused by increased melanin production and can indicate chronic exposure to sunlight or pregnancy. This is best assessed on areas exposed to the sun; changes in pregnancy can be seen on the face, areolae, and nipples. A brownish color may also be the result of chronic peripheral vascular disease, especially noted on the lower extremities.

TABLE 53.1 SUBJECTIVE ASSESSMENT OF THE INTEGUMENTARY SYSTEM

Catagory	Questions to Ask During History Assessment	Rationale
History	Do you (or does anyone in your family) have a history of dryness, rashes, itching, skin diseases, psoriasis, eczema, dermatitis, asthma, hay fever, hives, or allergies?	These conditions may be hereditary.
Risk Factors	Have you noticed any changes in your skin, such as a sore that does not heal, rashes, lumps, or a change in an existing mole?	• Sores that do not heal or moles that change color along with any lumps may indicate cancer. • Slow healing can also be associated with diabetes. • Brown staining of the skin in the lower legs is called hemosiderin stain which is due to red blood cells breaking under the skin in a condition called venous stasis.
	Have you had any recent trauma to your skin? Do you have a tendency to sunburn easily? Do you use sunblock? Do you go to tanning salons or utilize sun lamps or tanning pills?	A break in skin integrity can lead to infection. Repeat sunburns are a risk factor for skin cancer. These are risk factors for skin cancer.
Hair	Do you wear a wig or hairpiece? Have you noticed a change in the growth or loss of your hair?	Adequate assessment of the scalp requires permission for removal of a wig or hairpiece. Hair loss can result from systemic illness or treatment or sometimes from infections or hair care products.
Nails	Have you experienced recent trauma or changes in your nails? Do you wear artificial nails?	Nail changes may be caused by circulatory problems. Artificial nails may mask changes.
Medications	What medications do you take every day (prescription or nonprescription)? What is the dosage and frequency? What medications did you take most recently? When did you take your last dose?	The patient may be taking medication for a skin disorder. Many medications cause skin reactions, from hives and photosensitivity to serious inflammatory conditions. This might help pinpoint the cause of a new reaction.
Exposures	What is your occupation? How often to you bathe or shower? What kind of soap do you use? What recreational activities to you participate in? Do you or any members of your immediate family or your coworkers have recent skin complaints? Have you traveled recently? Is there anything in your current environment, at home or work, that may be causing any skin problems (e.g., animals, plants, chemicals, infections, new carpeting, or new soaps or detergents)? Is there anything that touches your skin that causes a rash?	Occupational exposures can lead to skin problems. Some soap may cause allergic reactions. Skin disorders can be caused by gym equipment that was not cleaned properly. Poison ivy may result from jogging in wooded areas. Some skin disorders are contagious. This could help to pinpoint causes of suspicious skin changes. Various environmental factors can be causes of contact dermatitis; release of some chemicals can cause skin disorders. This may help pinpoint causes of contact dermatitis.

LESIONS. A lesion is any change or injury to tissue. Assessment of skin lesions helps determine the cause of a skin disorder. Lesions are described as primary or secondary. Primary lesions are the initial reaction to a disease process. Secondary lesions are the changes that take place in the primary lesion because of trauma, scratching, infection, or various stages of a disease. Lesions are further described according to type and appearance in Figure 53.3.

When assessing and documenting skin lesions, note the color or colors of the lesion, the size (usually in centimeters), location, distribution, and configuration. *Configuration* refers to the pattern of the lesions; shown in Figure 53.4. Also note any exudate, including amount, color, and odor,

and any accompanying symptoms. Gently stretching the skin over the rash area makes it stand out more for further assessment.

In general, healthy patients with naturally dark skin have a reddish undertone, with pinkish buccal mucosa, tongue, nails, and lips. If a dark-skinned patient is pale, the mucous membranes have an ash-gray color, lips and nailbeds appear paler than usual, and the skin appears yellow-brown to ash gray. Erythema presents as a purplish gray color. Cyanosis presents as a gray cast to the skin. The nailbeds, palms, and soles may have a bluish cast. Jaundice can be noted in the oral mucosa (particularly the hard palate) and in the sclera closest to the cornea.

PRIMARY LESIONS

Macule:
Flat, nonpalpable change in skin color, with different sizes, shapes, color; usually smaller than 1 cm (e.g., rubella, scarlet fever freckles)
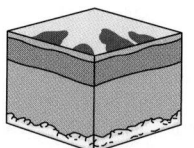

Papule:
Palpable solid raised lesion that is less than 1 cm in diameter due to superficial thickening in the epidermis (e.g., ringworm, rosea, wart, mole)
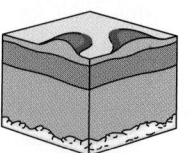

Nodule:
Solid elevated lesion that is larger and deeper than a papule (e.g., fibroma, intradermal nevi)
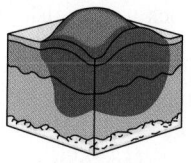

Vesicle:
A small, blister-like raised area of the skin that contains serous fluid, up to 1 cm in diameter (e.g., poison ivy, shingles, chickenpox)
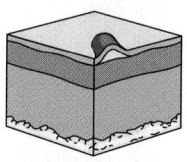

Bulla:
A fluid-filled vesicle or blister larger than 1 cm (e.g., burns, contact dermatitis)
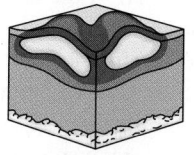

Pustule:
Small elevation of skin or vesicle or bulla that contains lymph or pus (e.g., impetigo, scabies, acne)
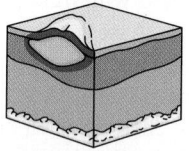

Wheal:
Round, transient elevation of the skin caused by dermal edema and surrounding capillary dilatation; white in center and red in periphery (e.g., hives, insect bites)
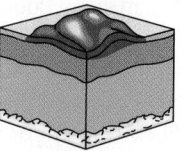

Plaque:
A patch or solid, raised lesion on the skin or mucous membrane that is greater than 1 cm in diameter (e.g., psoriasis)
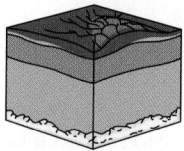

Cyst:
A closed sac or pouch which consists of semisolid, solid, or liquid material (e.g., sebaceous cyst)
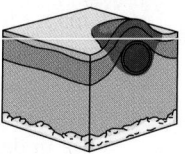

SECONDARY LESIONS

Scale:
Dry exfoliation of dead epidermis that may develop as a result of inflammatory changes (e.g., very dry skin, cradle cap, psoriasis)
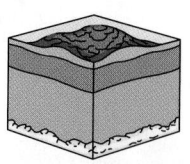

Crust:
A scab formed by dry serum, pus, or blood (e.g., infected dermatitis, impetigo)
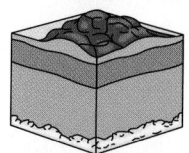

Excoriation:
Traumatized abrasions of the epidermis or linear scratch marks (e.g., scabies, dermatitis, burns)
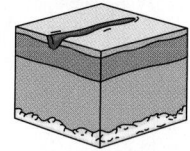

Fissure:
A slit or cracklike sore that extends into dermis usually due to continuous inflammation and drying (e.g., athlete's foot, anal fissure)
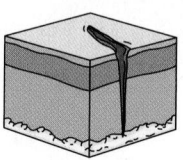

Ulcer:
An open sore or lesion that extends to the dermis (e.g., pressure sores)
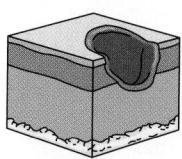

Lichenification:
Thickening and hardening of skin from continued irritation such as intense scratching looks like surface of mass
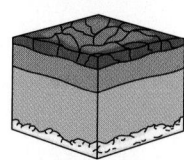

Scar:
A mark left in the skin due to fibrotic changes following healing of a wound or sore or surgical incision
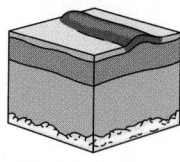

FIGURE 53.3 Description of skin lesions.

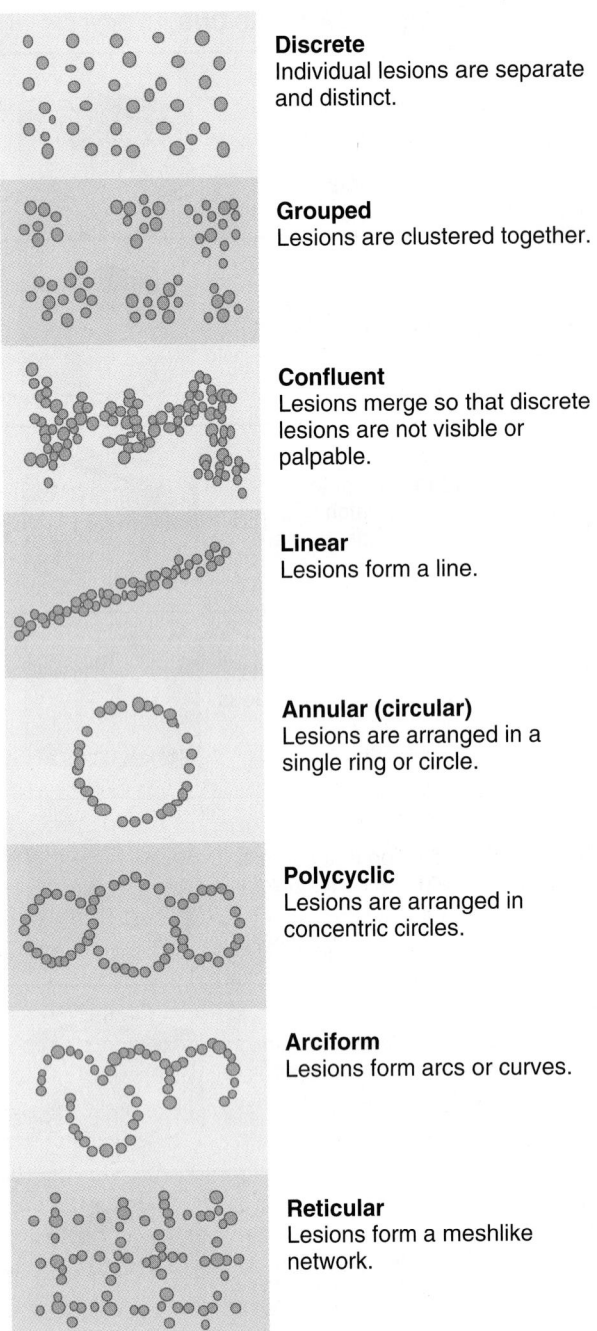

Discrete
Individual lesions are separate and distinct.

Grouped
Lesions are clustered together.

Confluent
Lesions merge so that discrete lesions are not visible or palpable.

Linear
Lesions form a line.

Annular (circular)
Lesions are arranged in a single ring or circle.

Polycyclic
Lesions are arranged in concentric circles.

Arciform
Lesions form arcs or curves.

Reticular
Lesions form a meshlike network.

FIGURE 53.4 To assess configuration, observe the relationship of the lesions to each other. Then characterize the configuration by one of the patterns illustrated in the chart.

MOISTURE/DRYNESS. Assessment of moisture provides clues to the patient's level of hydration. Observe the skin for dryness, moisture, scales, and flakes. Moisture may be found in skin fold areas. The skin should normally be smooth and dry. Flaking and scaling of the skin indicate dry skin.

EDEMA. Edema occurs because of a build-up of fluid in the tissues. Edema can cause the skin to become stretched, dry, and shiny. Assess and document the location, distribution, and color of edematous areas. If edema is unilateral, compare it with the opposite side of the body. Measure

edematous extremities to track improvement or worsening of the condition. Dependent edema is edema that occurs in the part of the body that is at the lowest point, typically noted in the feet and ankles or in the sacrum if the patient is lying down.

VASCULAR MARKINGS. Vascular markings can be classified as normal and abnormal. Two common abnormal vascular changes are **petechiae** and **ecchymosis** (see Figures 28.1 and 28.5). Petechiae are reddish purple hemorrhagic spots that are smaller than 0.5 mm in diameter. In the darker skinned patient, petechiae are usually not visible on the skin but can be visualized in the conjunctivae and oral mucosa. Ecchymosis is a bruise in which the color changes from blue-black to greenish brown or yellow over time.

GENERAL INTEGRITY AND CLEANLINESS. Assess the integrity of the skin. Elderly patients have thin, fragile skin that is easily broken or torn. Be sure to check between toes and skin folds and under a pendulous abdomen or breasts. Check over bony prominences for signs of pressure. Note general cleanliness and odors.

Palpation

Palpation is used in conjunction with inspection. Use the dorsum (back) of the hand to palpate temperature because this part of the hand is most sensitive to changes in temperature. Use the fingertips to gently palpate over the skin to determine size, contour (flat, raised, depressed), and consistency (soft or indurated) of lesions. If the lesion is moist or draining, wear gloves to protect against the spread of infectious organisms. Note the degree of pain or discomfort associated with light palpation of lesions.

Assess turgor and texture of the skin. Skin turgor is a measure of the amount of skin elasticity. To assess for turgor, the skin on the back of the forearm or over the sternum is pinched between the thumb and forefinger and then released. Normally, the skin lifts easily and then quickly returns to its normal state. Poor skin turgor is indicated by "tenting" of the skin, with more gradual return to its normal state. Poor skin turgor may indicate dehydration. Normal aging of skin produces some loss of skin elasticity; the preferred place to check skin turgor in the elderly is over the sternum.

If edema is suspected, palpate those areas to assess for tenderness, mobility, and consistency. When pressure from your fingers leaves an indentation, this is called pitting edema. Pitting edema is classified by its depth. Press the edematous area (against bone, if possible) with your thumb for 5 seconds and then release. One way to measure edema is to measure depth of the pitting in millimeters. For example:

1+ edema = 2-mm depth, or trace edema
2+ edema = 4-mm depth of indentation, or a small
       amount
3+ = 6-mm depth, moderate edema
4+ = 8-mm depth, indentation lasts 2 to 3 minutes,
       very edematous

ecchymosis: ec—out + cchymos—juice + is—condition

Inspect and/or palpate over the entire body for hair color, quantity, thickness, and texture. Note any areas of **alopecia** (hair loss). Determine any recent changes in color and growth pattern. Note cleanliness, itching, redness, scaling, flakes, and tenderness. If lesions or lice are suspected, use disposable gloves to avoid spread of infection.

Terminal hair is the hair on the scalp, eyebrows, axillae, and pubic areas and on the face and chest of males. Vellus hairs are the soft, tiny hairs covering the body. Normally, body hair has a uniform distribution. Note male or female pubic hair distribution. Scalp hair can normally be thick, thin, coarse, smooth, shiny, curly, or straight. Describe scalp hair distribution and cleanliness.

Nails can reflect the patient's general health. Assess fingers and nails for color, shape, texture, thickness, and abnormalities. Normally, the nails appear pink, smooth, hard, and slightly convex (160-degree angle), with a firm base. The nails of elderly patients may have a yellowish gray color, thickening, and ridges. Brown or black pigmentation between the nail and nail base is normal in dark-skinned patients. Abnormal findings include clubbing, which may indicate hypoxia, and spoon nails (concave nails, also called koilonychia), which may be associated with anemia. Thick nails may indicate fungal infection. Palpate for nail consistency and observe for redness, swelling, or tenderness around the nail area. See Table 53.2 for other nail abnormalities.

Describe any abnormal skin conditions in detail. Include findings such as color of lesion, pain, swelling, redness, location, size, drainage (including amount, color, and odor), and eruption patterns. If equipment is available, an excellent way to supplement documentation is by photographing the area; serial photographs can be mounted in the chart to document healing progression. See Box 53.1 Gerontological Issues for assessment and care specific to the elderly.

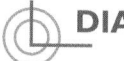 DIAGNOSTIC TESTS

Laboratory Tests

Cultures

Skin cultures are done to determine the presence of fungi, bacteria, and viruses. When a fungal infection is suspected, gently scrape scales from the lesion into a Petri dish or other indicated container. The specimen is then treated with a 10% potassium hydroxide (KOH) solution to make fungi more

NURSING CARE TIP

When scraping scales for culture position the patient so that the skin lesion is vertical. Place the slide against the skin below the lesion. Be sure to wear gloves when collecting specimens, and wash your hands before and after.

prominent. The specimen can remain at room temperature until sent to the laboratory.

If a viral culture is ordered, the fluid is expressed (gently squeezed) from an intact vesicle, collected with a sterile cotton swab, and placed in a special viral culture tube. If the lesion has crusts, they are removed or punctured before swabbing. The viral culture tube must be kept in ice and sent to the laboratory as soon as possible.

Bacterial cultures may be collected with a sterile swab or wound culture kit. See Box 53.2 (Steps in Culturing a Wound) for specific instructions.

Skin Biopsy

A skin biopsy is indicated for deeper infections, to establish an accurate diagnosis, or for the evaluation of current treatment. A biopsy is an excision of a small piece of tissue for microscopic assessment. Three common types of skin biopsies are punch, shave, and incisional.

A punch biopsy uses a small round cutting instrument, called a punch, to cut a cylinder-shaped plug of tissue for a full-thickness specimen. An incisional biopsy is performed with a scalpel to make a deep incision and almost always requires sutures for closure. A shave biopsy removes just the area that has risen above the rest of the skin.

For all biopsies, explain the procedure, assist in preparing a sterile field, calm and comfort the patient during the procedure, and assist in dressing the site following the procedure. The most uncomfortable part of the procedure is usually the injection of the local anesthetic agent. Explaining the procedure and calming the patient can make the procedure less traumatic.

Other Diagnostic Tests

Wood's Light Examination

Wood's light examination is the use of ultraviolet rays to detect fluorescent materials in the skin and hair present in certain diseases such as tinea capitis (ringworm). This

TABLE 53.2 ABNORMALITIES OF THE NAILS

Physical Assessment Finding	Description	Possible Causes
Beau's lines	Transverse depressions in the nails	Systemic illnesses or nail injury
Splinter hemorrhages	Red or brown streaks in the nailbed	Minor trauma, subacute bacterial endocarditis, or trichinosis
Paronychia	Inflammation of the skin at the base of the nail	Local infection or trauma

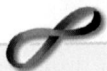

Box 53.1

Gerontological Issues

In acute care settings, priorities are determined by medical diagnoses and often center around cardiovascular, respiratory, nutrition, comfort, or other immediate concerns. The feet may be forgotten in the rush to care for the patient and plan a timely discharge.

Feet are also viewed by some as dirty; washing the feet may be seen as a lowly job. It may be assumed that people take care of their own feet. However, many older people are unable to bend down or bring the feet up high enough to see or care for them.

For these reasons it is especially important for the nurse to assess and care for the feet, both in institutional settings and at home. General guidelines for assessment include the following:

- Inspect feet for redness or pressure ulcers over bony prominences.
- Inspect feet for dryness or cracking.
- Inspect between toes for cracking, wounds, or excess moisture.
- Inspect and palpate for callouses.
- Palpate dorsalis pedis and posterior tibial pulses for circulatory status.
- Assess patient's sensation using a wisp of cotton, monofilament, or light touch.

Hints to promote healthy feet:

- Soak the patient's feet briefly in warm water and wash using a gentle soap. Test the water to be sure it is not too warm, especially for the patient with reduced sensation.
- Thoroughly dry the feet, including between the toes. Water left to evaporate can cause drying and cracking.
- Use a pumice stone to help remove dry dead skin over heels or calluses. Work gently, rubbing the stone in one direction only and removing only a small amount of dead skin at any one time.
- Use a cream or lotion that does not contain alcohol to moisturize the feet. Do not apply between toes. Apply it with a gentle massage while moving the patient's feet through range-of-motion exercises. To prevent falls, never apply lotion before the patient steps into the tub or shower.
- Use gauze or a commercially made pad to decrease pressure and friction in areas between toes that cross or other areas where breakdown is likely.
- Encourage the patient to wear cotton or dry weave socks that allow feet to stay dry with perspiration. Encourage wearing shoes or hard soled-slippers to avoid injury to the feet and prevent falls.
- Take extra care to assess and care for feet in patients with diabetes because of their increased risk for injury and slow healing.

Box 53.2

Steps in Culturing a Wound

1. Use sterile saline to remove excess drainage and debris from the wound. Purulent material may have different bacteria than those actually causing the infection.
2. Using a sterile calcium alginate swab in a rotating motion, swab wound and wound edges 10 times in a diagonal pattern across the entire surface of the wound.
3. Do not swab over eschar.

examination is performed with a hand-held black light in a darkened room.

Skin Testing

Patch and scratch tests are performed when allergic contact dermatitis is suspected. These are usually done by a dermatologist on uninvolved skin, such as the upper back or arms. Any hair in the area must first be shaved.

For the scratch test, the skin is superficially scratched or pricked with an allergen for an immediate reaction. If a reaction such as a wheal occurs, the test is positive for that allergen. Resuscitation equipment should be in the immediate vicinity in the event of a severe allergic (anaphylactic) reaction.

With the patch test, a delayed hypersensitivity reaction develops in 48 to 96 hours. The allergens are applied under occlusive tape patches. For this test, the skin should be free of oils to promote patch adhesion, so cleanse the skin first with alcohol. The test site must remain dry and free from moisture. The patch is removed in 2 days. Any reaction is noted, with a final reading in 2 to 5 days.

THERAPEUTIC MEASURES

Open Wet Dressings

Wet compresses may be ordered for acute, weeping, crusted, inflammatory, or ulcerated lesions. The purpose of wet dressings is to decrease inflammation, cleanse and dry the wound, and continue drainage of infected areas. They may be ordered either sterile or clean, depending on the risk for infection. The solutions commonly consist of room temperature to cool tap water or normal saline, aluminum acetate solution (Burow's solution), or magnesium sulfate. The dressing is saturated with the solution before it is applied. Wet dressings are usually applied every 3 to 4 hours for 15 to 30 minutes.

Wet dressings should not be prescribed for more than 72 hours because the skin may become too dry or macerated. If cool compresses are used, they should be reapplied every 5 to 10 minutes because they become too warm from body heat. If warm compresses are used, monitor the skin closely to prevent burns.

NURSING CARE TIP

To prevent chilling, no more than one-third of the body should be treated at one time. Keep the patient warm during wet dressing treatment.

Balneotherapy

Balneotherapy (therapeutic bath) is useful in applying medications to large areas of the skin, as well as for débridement, or removing old crusts; for removing old medications; and to relieve itching and inflammation. The temperature of the water should be kept at a comfortable level, avoiding hot baths. The bath should last for 15 to 30 minutes, while maintaining its warmth. Fill the tub half full. Keep the room warm to minimize changes in temperature. Advise the patient to wear loose clothing after the bath.

NURSING CARE TIP

A bath mat should be used for treatment baths because some may make the tub slippery.

Water and saline are utilized for weeping, oozing, and erythematous lesions. Colloidal baths (such as oatmeal or Aveeno) are utilized for widely distributed skin lesions, for drying, and for relief of itching. Medicated tar baths, such as Almar-Tar or Bainetar, are used for chronic eczema problems and psoriasis. Any loose skin crusts can be removed after the bath. The room should be well ventilated because tars are volatile.

To increase hydration after the bath, a lubricating agent is applied to damp skin if emollient action is prescribed. Bath oils, such as Alpha-Keri, Avenol, and Lubath, are used for lubrication and to relieve itching.

Topical Medications

Many types of topical medications are used to treat skin conditions. These include lotions, ointments and creams, powders, gels, pastes, and intralesional therapy. Systemic medications may also be given for more serious conditions.

Lotions tend to cool the skin through water evaporation. They may also have a protective effect and may be antipruritic (treat itching). Lotions are usually applied with cotton gauze, gloves, or a soft brush.

Ointments and creams have a varied base (greasy, nongreasy, or penetrating), depending on the drug applied. These medications can protect the skin, provide lubrication, and prevent water loss. They are used for localized or chronic skin conditions. Ointments and creams can cause some reduction in blood flow to the skin. They are applied with a gloved hand or wooden tongue depressor.

Powders usually have a zinc oxide, talc, or cornstarch base. They act as a hygroscopic agent to absorb moisture and reduce friction. Powders are usually applied with a

NURSING CARE TIP

Avoid applying too much powder in skin fold areas. Dermatitis can occur with too much powder in these areas. Products with a cornstarch base can provide a good medium for growth of microorganisms.

shaker top. Powders are avoided around patients with respiratory disease or tracheostomies.

Gels, or semisolid emulsions, become liquid with topical application. They are usually greaseless and do not stain. Many topical steroids are prescribed in this manner.

Pastes are semisolid substances comprised of ointments and powders. They are used for inflammatory disorders. Mineral oil can facilitate removal of pastes.

Topical corticosteroids are used to reduce or relieve pain and itching by decreasing inflammation. Steroids should be used sparingly and according to package directions. Overuse of topical steroids can cause thinning of the skin. Caution is needed when used on the face to prevent glaucoma, cataracts, and perioral dermatitis.

Intralesional therapy has an anti-inflammatory action. This procedure utilizes a tuberculin syringe, most often of a sterile suspension of a corticosteroid, injected just below the lesion. Local atrophy may occur if the injection is made into subcutaneous tissue. Common conditions that are treated with this therapy include psoriasis and keloids.

CRITICAL THINKING

Mr. Evans

■ Mr. Evans comes to the doctor's office with atrophic skin (thin, shiny, pink, with visible vessels) at the area of psoriasis where he is applying his corticosteroid ointment. He states that he has been applying a thick layer of ointment four times a day.

1. What might be the cause of this condition?
2. What should you include when you document his skin condition?

Suggested answers at end of chapter.

Dressings

Dressings may be used to enhance absorption of topical medications, promote retention of moisture, prevent evaporation of medication, and reduce pain and itching. Occlusive dressings (for sealing the wound) are commonly used for skin disorders. An airtight plastic film is applied directly over the topical agent. Corticosteroids are also available as a special plastic surgical tape and can be cut to size. See Box 53.3 Nursing Care Plan for the Patient with an Occlusive Dressing. Proper application of a plastic wrap dressing

Box 53.3 NURSING CARE PLAN **for the Patient with an Occlusive Dressing**

Nursing Diagnosis: Impaired skin integrity related to open lesions

Expected Outcome Improved skin integrity as evidenced by reduction in size of lesion

Evaluation of Outcome Is there a decrease in wound size?

Interventions	Rationale	Evaluation
Assess areas of lesions for changes three times a day or as ordered.	Areas of redness, swelling, pain, and drainage may indicate infection.	Are lesions free of redness, swelling, pain, and drainage?
Assess lesions for presence or absence of dead tissue and exudates.	Appearance indicates areas of healing and infection.	Are lesions free of exudates and dead tissue?
Cleanse wound as prescribed (see text for specific bathing instructions). Lightly pat dry.	Cleansing helps provide a healthy granulation area for healing.	Is wound clean and free of debris, crusts, and exudate?
Apply prescribed topical agent (see text for specifics) to moist skin. Apply sparingly or as directed.	Various agents have specific properties (control bacterial growth, prevent itching, have a protective effect, provide lubrication, relieve pain, or decrease inflammation).	Does area exhibit signs of healing (e.g., decrease in size and numbers of lesions, free from infection, less itching)?
Apply plastic film, cut to size. Cover with an appropriate dressing to seal edges.	Film enhances absorption of medication and helps retain moisture.	Is the topical agent adherent to the skin?
Remove dressing for 12 out of 24 hours.	Continued use may cause skin atrophy, folliculitis, erythema, and systemic absorption of medication.	Are there signs of healthy granulation tissue? Is skin pink? Are there less open areas? Is dressing removed for at least 12 hours?

Nursing Diagnosis: Disturbed body image related to presence of lesion or wound

Expected Outcomes Patient verbalizes acceptance of condition. Patient is willing to participate in care of lesion or wound.

Evaluation of Outcomes Does patient verbalize acceptance of condition? Does patient participate in care of lesions?

Interventions	Rationale	Evaluation
Assess patient's feelings regarding condition.	Assessment provides a baseline for care. If patient denies condition, he or she may not comply with care.	Does patient state willingness to follow care instructions?
Care for patient with an accepting attitude.	Patient will be aware of nuances in nurse's behavior.	Does patient allow nurse to partake in care of lesion or wound?
Allow opportunities for patient to verbalize concerns about condition.	Verbalizations allow patient to begin to accept and problem solve.	Does patient verbalize feelings appropriately?
Provide referrals to support groups and counselors as appropriate.	Patient may benefit from talking to others with similar condition or to another professional for objective evaluation.	Is patient receptive to appropriate referrals?
Assist patient in concealing lesion or wound in a safe and appropriate manner.	Long sleeves and long pants may help conceal lesions, protect lesions, and prevent further skin damage.	Is patient accepting of appearance of lesions? Are lesions or wounds visible?

Nursing Diagnosis: Bathing/hygiene self-care deficit, related to presence of lesions or wound and discomfort

Expected Outcomes Patient verbalizes importance of good hygiene. Patient is willing to participate in bathing/hygiene.

Evaluation of Outcomes Does patient verbalize importance of good hygiene? Is patient clean?

Interventions	Rationale	Evaluation
Assess patient's level of hygiene.	Provides a baseline for care.	Is patient's level of hygiene at an acceptable level?
Instruct patient in appropriate bathing/hygiene: • Avoid strong detergents and soaps; utilize gentle emollient soaps or prescribed soaps. • Gently stroke areas of lesions. • Pat dry; no friction. • Maintain a little moisture on skin. • Maintain comfortable environmental temperature. • Have temperature of bath at a comfortable level to patient, but not too hot.	Patient needs to be able to properly cleanse lesions to prevent infection. Avoidance of friction and strong soaps prevents further trauma to skin. Patient will not shiver in comfortable temperatures.	Is patient able to verbalize understanding, as well as demonstrate good bathing techniques? Are lesions free of infection?

includes washing the area, lightly patting it dry, applying the medication to moist skin, covering the medicated area with plastic wrap, and covering with a dressing to seal the edges. Wet dressings and ointments should only be applied to affected areas, *not* to healthy intact skin, because this can cause maceration of good skin. Plastic wrap dressings should be used for no more than 10 to 12 hours a day.

NURSING CARE TIP

Continued use of occlusive dressings can cause skin atrophy, folliculitis, maceration, erythema, and systemic absorption of the medication. To prevent some of these complications, the dressing is removed for 12 out of every 24 hours.

Other dressings commonly used with topical treatments for skin conditions include gauze or cotton cloth held in place with small, stretchable tubular material (e.g., Surgi-

tube, tube gauze) for fingers, toes, and extremities; disposable polyethylene gloves sealed at the wrist; cotton socks or plastic bags for the feet; cotton cloth held in place with tubular material for the extremities; disposable diapers or cotton diapers for the groin and perineal areas; cotton cloth held in place with dress shields for the axillae; cotton or light flannel pajamas for the trunk; a shower cap for the scalp; and a face mask made from gauze and stretchable dressings with holes cut out for eyes, nose, mouth, and ears. The patient's primary care provider should specify the type of dressing and particular materials needed for this dressing.

A variety of other types of dressing materials are available for wound and skin care. Transparent dressings (e.g., Op-Site, Tegaderm) can be used over skin tears or intravenous insertion sites. Hydrocolloid dressings (e.g., Duoderm, Tegasorb thin) can help protect areas exposed to pressure and treat pressure ulcers in early stages. Gels, pastes, and granules can be used to fill in deep wounds to promote granulation and aid healing. See Chapter 54 for additional dressings used specifically for pressure ulcers.

REVIEW QUESTIONS

1. Which of the following is the protein in epidermal cells that makes the skin relatively waterproof?
   a. Collagen
   b. Keratin
   c. Melanin
   d. Elastin

Multiple response item. Select all that apply.
2. What are functions of subcutaneous tissue?
   a. It nourishes the dermis.
   b. It cushions bony prominences.
   c. It lubricates the epidermis.
   d. It provides insulation.
   e. It stores energy.

3. Older adults have fewer fibroblasts, and epidermal division slows. How do these changes affect nursing care?
   a. The nurse should take care to protect fragile skin.
   b. The nurse should provide blankets to keep the patient warm.
   c. The nurse should apply lubricating lotions to prevent drying.
   d. The nurse should massage the skin to enhance circulation.

4. Which skin lesion is typically seen in chickenpox?
   a. Macule
   b. Papule
   c. Vesicle
   d. Wheal

5. What equipment is most important to have readily available when a patient is undergoing skin testing for allergies?
   a. Resuscitation equipment
   b. Flashlight
   c. Measuring device
   d. Alcohol and cotton swabs

6. Why should wet dressings be applied only to one-third of the body at one time?
   a. So the rest of the body can be observed for reaction to the dressing
   b. To prevent chilling the patient
   c. To prevent absorption of too much water, causing fluid overload
   d. To enable the patient to be more mobile

SUGGESTED ANSWERS TO

CRITICAL THINKING

■ *Mr. Evans*

1. He may be sensitive or allergic to the medication. Most likely, he is applying too much too often. This ointment is applied as a thin layer, and usually only twice daily.

2. Note the size (usually in centimeters), location, color, distribution, and configuration of lesions. Describe exactly what you see, avoiding judgments about what you think it is. Document any teaching you provided related to how his medication should be applied.

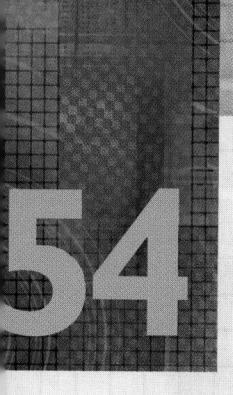

Nursing Care of Patients with Skin Disorders

MARTY KOHN AND
RITA BOLEK TROFINO

KEY TERMS

blanching (BLANCH-ing)
cellulitis (sell-yoo-LYE-tis)
comedo (KOH-me-doh)
dermatitis (DER-mah-TIGH-tis)
dermatophytosis (DER-mah-toh-fye-TOH-sis)
eschar (ESS-kar)
lichenified (lye-KEN-i-fyed)
onychomycosis (ON-i-koh-my-KOH-sis)
pediculosis (pe-DIK-yoo-LOH-sis)
pemphigus (PEM-fi-gus)
pruritus (proo-RYE-tus)
psoriasis (suh-RYE-ah-sis)
purulent (PURE-u-lent)
pyoderma (PYE-oh-DER-mah)
seborrhea (SEB-oh-REE-ah)

QUESTIONS TO GUIDE YOUR READING

1. How would you explain the pathophysiology of each of the skin disorders listed in this chapter?

2. What are the etiologies, signs, and symptoms of each of the skin disorders?

3. What are current therapeutic interventions for each of the skin disorders?

4. What data should you collect when caring for patients with disorders of the integumentary system?

5. What nursing care will you provide for patients with each of the covered skin disorders?

6. How will you know if your nursing interventions have been effective?

Skin disorders cover a wide array of diseases and conditions. These disorders can be generalized or localized, acute, chronic, or traumatic. This chapter discusses common skin disorders encountered by nurses. An excellent resource on skin disorders, with photographs, is at www.nsc.gov.sg/commskin/skin.html. The American Academy of Dermatology can be accessed at www.aad.org.

PRESSURE ULCERS

Pathophysiology and Etiology

Pressure ulcers are often referred to by patients with old terms such as *bedsores, decubitus ulcers,* or *pressure sores.* Essentially a pressure ulcer is a lesion caused by prolonged pressure against the skin. This may occur from spending a prolonged period in one position, causing the weight of the body to compress the capillaries against a bed or chair, especially over bony prominences. Pressure ulcers are the result of tissue anoxia and begin to develop within 20 to 40 minutes of unrelieved pressure on the skin. Other causes include pressure from a tight splint or cast, traction, or other device. Those at risk are immobile patients, those with decreased circulation, and those with impaired sensory perception or neurological function.

Mechanical forces (pressure, friction, and shear) lead to the formation of pressure ulcers. The pressure level that closes capillaries in healthy people is 25 to 32 mm Hg. When pressure applied to the skin is greater than the pressure in the capillary bed, it can impair cellular metabolism. It decreases the blood supply to the tissues and eventually causes tissue ischemia. This reduction in blood flow causes **blanching** of the skin. The longer the pressure lasts, the greater the risk of skin breakdown and the development of a pressure ulcer.

Friction is the rubbing of the skin surface with an external mechanical force. Also referred to as "sheet burns," this can happen when the patient is dragged or pulled across bed linens instead of being lifted.

Shearing occurs when the patient slides down in bed when the head of the bed is raised, or when being pulled or repositioned without being lifted off the sheets. With shearing, the skin and subcutaneous tissue remain stationary and the fat, muscle, and bone shift in the direction of body movement. As a result, there is damage deep within the tissues.

Any patient experiencing prolonged pressure is at risk for a pressure ulcer. Elderly patients have increased risk because of normal aging changes of the skin. Because thin patients have little padding when pressure is present, they have the greatest pressure applied to their capillaries. Obesity also is a contributing factor because adipose tissue is poorly vascularized and is therefore more likely to develop ischemic changes. Impaired peripheral circulation also makes the skin more susceptible to ischemic damage.

Prevention

There are many interventions for the prevention of pressure ulcers. Assess and document the condition of the skin daily, so all are aware of developing problems. Gently cleanse the skin daily with tepid water and mild soap to prevent drying. To reduce friction, pat the skin dry rather than rubbing it dry. After bathing, daily lifelong lubrication of the skin with moisturizers is important to prevent dryness. Thoroughly dry skin-to-skin surfaces, such as under the breasts, skin folds (especially in the groin and abdominal folds), and between the toes, to prevent prolonged exposure to moisture. If incontinence is a problem, clean the skin promptly with tepid water and mild soap, pat dry, and apply a moisture barrier to prevent breakdown. Avoid massaging bony prominences or reddened skin areas; research has shown that blood vessels are damaged by massage when ischemia is present or when they lie over a bone.

Teach patients to shift their weight every 15 minutes if possible when lying or sitting. When the patient is immobile, the highest possible level of mobility should be maintained; frequent active or passive range-of-motion exercises should be performed, as well as turning according to a written repositioning schedule. If patients are on bedrest, turn and reposition them at least every 2 hours, but preferably more often because ischemia development begins after 20 to 40 minutes of pressure. The head of the bed should not be elevated more than 30 degrees to reduce pressure on the coccyx, and to reduce friction and shear damage from sliding down in the bed. When positioning patients on their side, place them at a 30-degree angle or less and not directly on the trochanter because this area is especially sensitive to pressure and can quickly break down. If patients are placed on the trochanter, they usually become restless and squirm around to get off the trochanter. If the patient is seated in a chair, repositioning every hour is important. A mobility program specific to the patient must be developed.

The patient's heels should not rest on the bed surface. They should be elevated off the bed with pillows placed lengthwise under the calf or with heel elevators. Take care so pressure is not applied on the calf from the pillows. Be sure to also protect the patient's elbows, sacrum, scapulae, ears, and occipital area from pressure.

Donut-shaped cushions should never be used. They create a circle of pressure that cuts off the circulation to the surrounding tissue, promoting ischemia rather than preventing it. Pad skin contact surfaces, especially bony prominences, so they do not press against each other. (For example, place a small pillow between the knees when the patient is in a side-lying position.) Provide an appropriate pressure-relieving or pressure-reducing mattress and chair cushion for immobile patients. To avoid friction, use a sheet to lift and move patients; provide an overbed trapeze to assist patients to move themselves. Prevent malnutrition and dehydration by ensuring an adequate intake of protein, calories, and fluid; provide 2500 mL of fluid each day if not contraindicated by other medical problems. See

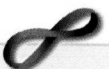

Box 54.1

Gerontological Issues

Interventions to Prevent Skin Breakdown

- Avoid the use of soap and water on dry skin areas. Use a moisture barrier cream or ointment on dry skin areas *before* bathing to protect the skin from the drying effects of water.
- Clean and dry areas between toes.
- Use perineal cleansing products to cleanse urine and feces residue from the perineum and anal areas. These products are specially designed to break down and facilitate the complete removal of urine and feces without irritating the skin.
- Use moisturizing creams that have no alcohol or perfume, which can irritate the skin.
- Avoid areas of skin pressure, especially over bony areas, by assisting the older adult to change positions on a regular schedule.
- Assess skin for areas of redness. If redness occurs, the positioning schedule should be more frequent.
- Keep fingernails short.
- Use pillows and pads to help maintain alignment with position changes. Use specialized mattresses and chair cushions designed to decrease pressure. Keep the patient's heels off the bed with pillows under the calves for support and to prevent pressure.
- Encourage the older adult to be out of bed and active throughout the day. Remember to assess skin and reposition frequently even when out of bed, because areas of pressure occur whether the patient is in or out of bed.
- Remind the patient to change position or shift weight frequently while sitting in a chair to avoid prolonged pressure.
- Provide a high-protein vitamin-rich diet if not contraindicated.

Box 54.1 Gerontological Issues for additional preventive measures.

An important aspect of prevention is identification of patients at risk for pressure ulcer development. Most institutions have adopted assessment tools such as the Braden or Norton scales to assess patients for physical condition, mental status, activity, mobility, and incontinence to determine the risk for pressure ulcers. Advanced age, low diastolic blood pressure, elevated body temperature, and inadequate current intake of protein are all risk factors associated with the development of pressure ulcers. See Table 54.1 for the Braden instrument.

Signs and Symptoms

The most common sites for pressure ulcers are the sacrum, heels, elbows, lateral malleoli, greater trochanters, ischial

LEARNING TIP

Pressure ulcers may be described according to a three-color system.
- Black wounds indicate necrosis.
- Yellow wounds have exudate and are infected.
- Red wounds are pink or red and are in the healing stage.

tuberosities, base of the skull, scapulae, and ears. Most patients experience pain at the ulcer site. A report of pain requires continual assessment, documentation, and treatment.

A wound may contain a mixture of black, yellow, and red colors. Necrotic wounds are the worst because they contain dead tissue. Beefy red wounds are desired because they are healing wounds. It is important to consider treating the worst color present first or healing will be delayed. For example, if a wound is both yellow and black, the dead tissue must be removed first before the infection can be effectively treated. This color system is a helpful system for patients and families to use to describe wounds to the home care nurse because colors are easily recognized and understood by most people.

Complications

Wound infection is a common complication. New ulcers can also appear, and the present ulcer can progress to a deeper wound. Some wounds take a prolonged time to heal or never heal.

Diagnostic Tests

All pressure ulcers are considered to be colonized with bacteria. This means that bacteria are present, but the wound is not necessarily infected. In most cases, adequate cleansing and debridement can prevent bacterial colonization from advancing to clinical infection. Swab cultures and culture and sensitivity tests may be done to identify the causative organism in suspected infection sites. (See Chapter 53 for instructions for obtaining a culture.) Results need to be interpreted to distinguish between true wound infection and bacterial colonization. If the wound is healing by secondary intention, it becomes colonized by bacterial flora on the skin and from the environment. If, however, the wound is extensive, bacterial growth may exceed the local tissue defenses and a true wound infection results.

If the wound does not demonstrate signs of healing or if an ischemic ulcer is suspected, noninvasive and invasive arterial blood supply studies are recommended. Wound biopsies may be performed for large, extensive wounds.

Therapeutic Interventions

Treatment varies according to the size, depth, and stage of the pressure ulcer, as well as special needs of the patient and

(Text continued on page 1218)

TABLE 54.1 BRADEN SCALE FOR PREDICTING PRESSURE SORE RISK

Patient's Name _____   Evaluator's Name _____   Date of Assessment _____

SENSORY PERCEPTION ability to respond meaningfully to pressure-related discomfort	**1. Completely Limited** Unresponsive (does not moan, flinch, or grasp) to painful stimuli, due to diminished level of consciousness or sedation. OR Limited ability to feel pain over most of body	**2. Very Limited** Responds only to painful stimuli. Cannot communicate discomfort except by moaning or restlessness OR Has a sensory impairment which limits the ability to feel pain or discomfort over 1/2 of body	**3. Slightly Limited** Responds to verbal commands, but cannot always communicate discomfort or the need to be turned OR Has some sensory impairment which limits ability to feel pain or discomfort in 1 or 2 extremities	**4. No Impairment** Responds to verbal commands. Has no sensory deficit which would limit ability to feel or voice pain or discomfort.
MOISTURE degree to which skin is exposed to moisture	**1. Constantly Moist** Skin is kept moist almost constantly by perspiration, urine, etc. Dampness is detected every time patient is moved or turned.	**2. Very Moist** Skin is often, but not always moist. Linen must be changed at least once a shift.	**3. Occasionally Moist** Skin is occasionally moist, requiring an extra linen change approximately once a day.	**4. Rarely Moist** Skin is usually dry, linen only requires changing at routine intervals.
ACTIVITY degree of physical activity	**1. Bedfast** Confined to bed	**2. Chairfast** Ability to walk severely limited or nonexistent. Cannot bear own weight and/or must be assisted into chair or wheelchair.	**3. Walks Occasionally** Walks occasionally during day, but for very short distances, with or without assistance. Spends majority of each shift in bed or chair.	**4. Walks Frequently** Walks outside room at least twice a day and inside room at least once every two hours during waking hours
MOBILITY ability to change and control body position	**1. Completely Immobile** Does not make even slight changes in body or extremity position without assistance	**2. Very Limited** Makes occasional slight changes in body or extremity position but unable to make frequent or significant changes independently	**3. Slightly Limited** Makes frequent though slight changes in body or extremity position independently	**4. No Limitation** Makes major and frequent changes in position without assistance
NUTRITION usual food intake pattern	**1. Very Poor** Never eats a complete meal. Rarely eats more than 1/3 of any food offered. Eats 2 servings or less of protein (meat or dairy products) per day. Takes fluids poorly. Does not take a liquid dietary supplement OR Is NPO and/or maintained on clear liquids or IVs for more than 5 days	**2. Probably Inadequate** Rarely eats a complete meal and generally eats only about 1/2 of any food offered. Protein intake includes only 3 servings of meat or dairy products per day. Occasionally will take a dietary supplement. OR Receives less than optimum amount of liquid diet or tube feeding	**3. Adequate** Eats over half of most meals. Eats a total of 4 servings of protein (meat, dairy products) per day. Occasionally will refuse a meal, but will usually take a supplement when offered. OR Is on a tube feeding or TPN regimen which probably meets most of nutritional needs	**4. Excellent** Eats most of every meal. Never refuses a meal. Usually eats a total of 4 or more servings of meat and dairy products. Occasionally eats between meals. Does not require supplementation.
FRICTION & SHEAR	**1. Problem** Requires moderate to maximum assistance in moving. Complete lifting without sliding against sheets is impossible. Frequently slides down in bed or chair, requiring frequent repositioning with maximum assistance. Spasticity, contractures, or agitation leads to almost constant friction .	**2. Potential Problem** Moves feebly or requires minimum assistance. During a move skin probably slides to some extent against sheets, chair, restraints, or other devices. Maintains relatively good position in chair or bed most of the time but occasionally slides down.	**3. No Apparent Problem** Moves in bed and in chair independently and has sufficient muscle strength to lift up completely during move. Maintains good position in bed or chair.	

Total Score _____

MANAGE MOISTURE

USE COMMERCIAL MOISTURE BARRIER
USE ABSORBANT PADS OR DIAPERS THAT
WICK & HOLD MOISTURE
ADDRESS CAUSE IF POSSIBLE
OFFER BEDPAN/URINAL AND GLASS OF
WATER IN CONJUNCTION WITH TURNING
SCHEDULES

MANAGE NUTRITION

INCREASE PROTEIN INTAKE
INCREASE CALORIE INTAKE TO SPARE
PROTEINS
SUPPLEMENT WITH MULTIVITAMIN
(SHOULD HAVE VIT A, C, & E)
ACT QUICKLY TO ALLEVIATE DEFICITS
CONSULT DIETITIAN

MANAGE FRICTION & SHEAR

ELEVATE HOB NO MORE THAN 30°
USE TRAPEZE WHEN INDICATED
USE LIFT SHEET TO MOVE PATIENT
PROTECT ELBOWS & HEELS IF BEING
EXPOSED TO FRICTION

OTHER GENERAL CARE ISSUES

NO MASSAGE OF REDDENED BONY
PROMINENCES
NO DONUT TYPE DEVICES
MAINTAIN GOOD HYDRATION
AVOID DRYING THE SKIN

AT RISK (15–18)*

FREQUENT TURNING
MAXIMAL REMOBILIZATION
PROTECT HEELS
MANAGE MOISTURE, NUTRITION,
AND FRICTION AND SHEAR
PRESSURE-REDUCTION SUPPORT SURFACE IF
BED- OR CHAIRBOUND
*If other major risk factors are present
(advanced age, fever, poor dietary intake of protein, diastolic
pressure below 60, hemodynamic instability)
advance to next level of risk.

MODERATE RISK (13–14)*

TURNING SCHEDULE
USE FOAM WEDGES FOR 30° LATERAL
POSITIONING
PRESSURE-REDUCTION SUPPORT SURFACE
MAXIMAL REMOBILIZATION
PROTECT HEELS
MANAGE MOISTURE, NUTRITION,
AND FRICTION AND SHEAR
*If other major risk factors present,
advance to next level of risk.

HIGH RISK (10–12)

INCREASE FREQUENCY OF TURNING
SUPPLEMENT WITH SMALL SHIFTS
PRESSURE REDUCTION SUPPORT SURFACE
USE FOAM WEDGES FOR 30° LATERAL
POSITIONING
MAXIMAL REMOBILIZATION
PROTECT HEELS
MANAGE MOISTURE, NUTRITION,
AND FRICTION AND SHEAR

VERY HIGH RISK (9 or below)

ALL OF THE ABOVE
+
USE PRESSURE-RELIEVING SURFACE IF
PATIENT HAS INTRACTABLE PAIN
OR
SEVERE PAIN EXACERBATED BY TURNING
OR
ADDITIONAL RISK FACTORS
*Low air loss beds do not substitute for turning schedules.

health-care provider preference. All pressure must be removed from the affected area for healing to occur. Cleanliness must be maintained. Basic treatment includes debridement, cleansing, and dressing of the wound to provide a moist and healing environment.

LEARNING TIP

The epidermis skates on moisture, so the wound must be kept moist to heal.

Debridement

Debridement is the removal of dead or nonviable tissue from a wound to help clean up the wound and facilitate formation of granulation tissue. It may be done surgically or nonsurgically. Nonsurgical debridement includes mechanical, enzymatic, and autolytic methods. Surgical debridement is used only if the patient has sepsis or **cellulitis,** or to remove extensive **eschar.** Eschar is a black or brown hard scab or dry crust that forms from necrotic tissue. It may hide the true depth of the wound and must be removed for the wound to heal.

MECHANICAL DEBRIDEMENT. Scissors and forceps can be used for mechanical debridement to selectively debride nonviable tissue. Dextranomer beads, another method of mechanical debridement, may also be sprinkled over the wound to absorb exudate and all other products of tissue breakdown, as well as surface bacteria. Whirlpool baths and wet-to-dry saline gauze dressings may also be used for mechanical debridement. For wet-to-dry dressings, the wet gauze is placed directly on the wound (avoiding surrounding healthy tissue) and allowed to dry completely. The drying process causes the gauze to adhere to the wound; when it is pulled off, tissue is pulled off with it. This results in nonselective debridement because viable tissue may also be removed in this process. These methods are painful, so the patient should be premedicated for pain and assessed frequently.

ENZYMATIC DEBRIDEMENT. Enzymatic debridement involves the application of a topical debriding agent. These agents vary as to application methods, so careful reading of instructions is necessary. Most of these debriding agents are proteolytic enzymes that selectively digest necrotic tissue. Be careful to keep them off of healthy tissue.

AUTOLYTIC DEBRIDEMENT. Autolytic debridement is the use of a synthetic dressing or moisture-retentive dressing over the ulcer. The eschar is then self-digested via the action of the enzymes that are present in the fluid environment of the wound. This method is not used for infected wounds.

SURGICAL DEBRIDEMENT. Surgical debridement is the removal of devitalized tissue, slough, or thick, adherent

eschar, utilizing a scalpel, scissors, or other sharp instrument. Slough is a loose yellow to tan stringy necrotic tissue. Slough, like eschar, can be tightly adhered to the wound bed.

Depending on the amount of debridement to be done, this may be performed in the operating room, a treatment room, or the patient's room. Following surgical debridement, grafting may be required to close the wound. This becomes necessary if it is a full-thickness ulcer, if there is loss of joint function, or for cosmetic purposes. For procedures performed without anesthesia, be sure to premedicate the patient. Continually monitor for pain during the procedure, especially if there is a donor site for grafting.

Wound Cleansing

The ulcer should be thoroughly cleansed via whirlpool, hand-held shower head, or irrigating system with a pressure between 4 and 15 pounds per square inch (psi), such as a 30-mL syringe with an 18-gauge needle. Pressure less than 4 psi does not adequately cleanse the wound, and greater than 15 psi may damage tissue. If an irrigating system is used, 250 mL of normal saline (or sometimes tap water for home wound care) should be used to thoroughly cleanse the wound. If the wound is red, gentle irrigation with a needle-less 30- to 60-mL syringe should be used to prevent trauma and bleeding. When bleeding occurs, wound healing has been impaired. However, if the wound has been diagnosed as being infected, pressure flushing with a 30- to 60-mL syringe and an 18-gauge needle is needed to help remove bacteria.

LEARNING TIP

Dilution is the solution to wound pollution!

Once the wound is cleansed and debrided, apply a dressing. Wounds heal more rapidly in a moist environment, with minimal bacterial colonization and a healing temperature. This takes 12 hours to occur after the wound is covered with an occlusive dressing. If a dressing is frequently removed, the wound may not reach its healing temperature and healing may be impaired. When possible, the dressing should be left in place for extended periods. Infected wounds are not covered with occlusive dressings; draining wounds may require frequent dressing changes.

Wound Dressings

Dressings vary according to size, location, depth, stage of ulcer, and preference of the ordering practitioner. Commonly used dressing materials include hydrogel dressings, polyurethane films, hydrocolloid wafers, biological dressings, alginates, and cotton gauze. These materials promote an optimum healing environment. Hypoallergenic tape should be used to secure dressings if tape is necessary. Protective paste may be applied to protect nonaffected tissue from topical agents. In all cases, pressure should be kept off the wound. No treatment will be effective if pressure continues to damage the tissue.

---

cellulitis: cellu—cell + itis—inflammation

eschar: eschara—scab

Negative Pressure Wound Therapy

Negative pressure wound therapy (NPWT) is a relatively new development that is proving effective for healing of large open pressure ulcers (Fig. 54.1). In NPWT, a wound is packed loosely with a sterile sponge, then covered with an occlusive dressing. A vacuum source is placed in the wound and gentle negative pressure is applied. The negative pressure allows excess drainage and infectious material to be removed, which reduces pressure on delicate new tissue. With small vessels decompressed, circulation is increased, and healing is accelerated. NPWT also maintains a moist environment for optimal healing.

Nursing Process for the Patient with a Pressure Ulcer

Assessment/Data Collection

Provide an ongoing assessment of the status of the pressure ulcer, as well as underlying causes and barriers to healing. Monitor for risk factors such as prolonged immobility, incontinence, and inadequate nutrition and hydration.

Use transparency film or a disposable ruler to measure the diameter of the ulcer in centimeters. Imagine a clock superimposed over the wound with 12 o'clock at the head and 6 o'clock at the feet. Measure in centimeters from 12 to 6 o'clock, and from 9 to 3 o'clock. Depth can be measured with a cotton-tipped applicator. Also, gently probe a cotton-tipped applicator under the skin edges to detect tunneling and measure lateral tissue destruction.

There are several different staging systems for pressure sores based on the depth of tissue destroyed. In general, the staging systems are categorized from stage I to stage IV (Fig. 54.2).

- Stage I: The skin is still intact, but the area is red and does not blanch. There may also be warmth, hardness, and discoloration of the skin. Be aware that even though the skin is intact, there may be deeper tissue damage that is difficult to observe.
- Stage II: There is a break in the skin, with partial-thickness skin loss of epidermis, dermis, or both.

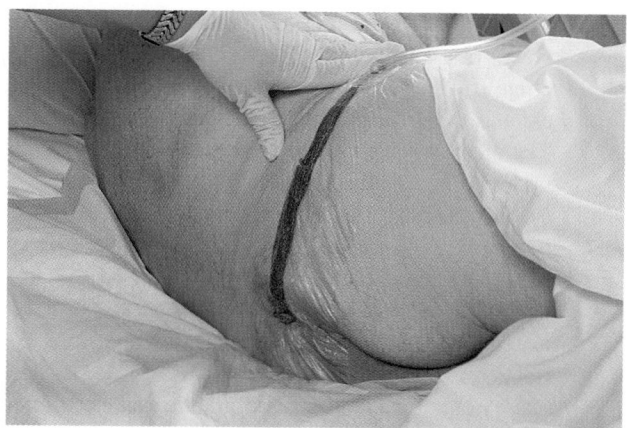

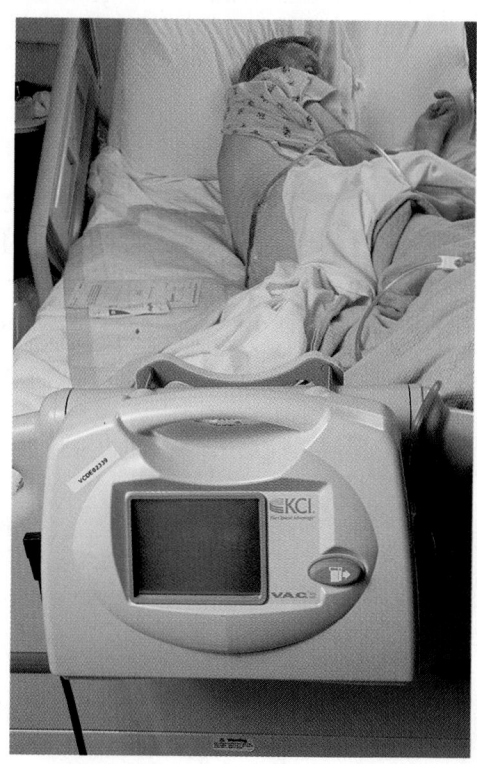

FIGURE 54.1 Wound vac therapy.

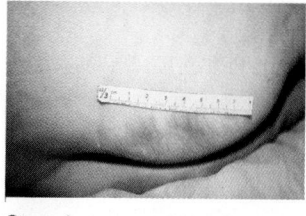
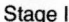
Stage I

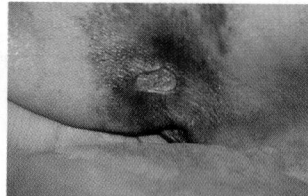
Stage II

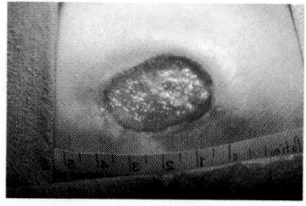
Stage III

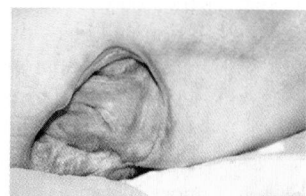
Stage IV

FIGURE 54.2 Staging criteria for pressure ulcers. Stage I. Nonblanchable erythema of intact skin indicates potential for ulceration. Stage II. Partial-thickness loss involving both epidermis and dermis. Ulcer is still superficial and appears as a blister, abrasion, or very shallow crater. Stage III. Full-thickness loss involving subcutaneous tissue. Ulcer may extend to but not through fascia. A deep crater that may undermine adjacent tissues. Stage IV. Full-thickness loss with extensive involvement of muscles, bone, or supporting structures. This deep ulcer may involve undermining and sinus tracts of adjacent tissues. *(From Dillon PM: Nursing Health Assessment, 2nd ed. F.A. Davis, Philadelphia, 2007, with permission.)*

The ulcer may appear as an abrasion, a shallow crater, or a blister.

- Stage III: There is full-thickness skin loss, which extends to the subcutaneous tissue, but not fascia. The ulcer looks like a deep crater and may have undermining of adjacent tissue. If a wound has eschar you cannot determine depth until the eschar is removed.
- Stage IV: There is full-thickness skin loss with damage to the muscle, bone, or support structures such as tendons. There may be undermining and sinus tracts (tunneling).

Assess wound exudate. Two common types of wound exudate are serosanguineous and **purulent.** Serosanguineous exudate is fluid consisting of serum and blood. It is blood-tinged, amber-colored fluid. Purulent fluid is a fluid that contains pus. It can vary in color and have different odors, which are suggestive of different wound colonizations. Creamy yellow pus may indicate *Staphylococcus.* Beige pus that has a fishy odor may suggest *Proteus.* Green-blue pus with a fruity odor may indicate *Pseudomonas.* Brown pus with a fecal odor may suggest *Bacteroides.*

Gently palpate the wound with a gloved hand to assess the texture of granulations. Granulation tissue has a budding appearance from the development of tiny new capillaries. If the granulations are healthy, they have a slightly spongy texture.

Document all findings carefully in the medical record, so all health team members can monitor progress of healing. Many institutions have specific forms for drawing pictures of the locations and sizes of wounds. There may be a special instant camera to document progress. Follow policy at the institution where you work.

NURSING DIAGNOSIS, PLANNING, IMPLEMENTATION, AND EVALUATION. See Box 54.2 Nursing Care Plan for the Patient with a Pressure Ulcer.

---

purulent: purulentus—pus

Box 54.2 NURSING CARE PLAN for the Patient with a Pressure Ulcer

Nursing Diagnosis: Impaired skin integrity related to pressure on skin surface

Expected Outcomes Skin integrity is improved as evidenced by decrease in wound size, no development of additional pressure ulcers.

Evaluation of Outcomes Is there a decrease in wound size? Are there any new pressure ulcers?

Interventions	Rationale	Evaluation
Assess status of pressure ulcer according to stage, color, exudate, texture, size, and depth.	Provides baseline data on which care is based	What stage is ulcer? Are there any other outstanding characteristics?
Assess cause of pressure (e.g., immobility, friction, shearing).	Allows for correction and also prevents further trauma	What is the cause of this ulcer?
Cleanse wound gently with warm water; rinse; pat dry gently with gauze. Do not rub the area.	Reduces number of bacteria. Drying prevents maceration of skin. Gentle handling prevents further trauma.	Is wound clean and dry?
Debride wound as prescribed (method depends on patient's condition and goals of care).	Debridement removes drainage and wound debris. Permits granulation of tissue.	Does wound look clean and free of debris?
Dress wound appropriately for prescribed topical agent. Make sure it stays intact with movement and that edges do not roll, causing more pressure.	Protects underlying wound and helps promote healing	Is dressing applied appropriately?
Position patient off the ulcer.	Prevents further pressure and trauma on ulcer	Is patient positioned off the ulcer?
If a leg ulcer, provide for frequent rest periods with leg elevated; if immobile, reposition every 2 hours.	Prevents further tissue breakdown	Is leg elevated? Is patient repositioned every 2 hours?

Nursing Diagnosis: Risk for infection related to open wound

Expected Outcomes Patient will not experience wound infection or systemic sepsis. (Total elimination of bacteria is impossible due to nature of the condition.)

Evaluation of Outcomes Is patient free from signs and symptoms of further infection? Is patient free from systemic infection?

Interventions	Rationale	Evaluation
Assess ulcer at every dressing change or at least every 24 hours. Look for areas of tenderness, swelling, redness, and heat; and drainage.	Allows for early recognition of infection and response to treatment	Are signs of infection present?
Monitor temperature at least every 12 hours.	Elevated body temperature is one sign of infection.	Is patient afebrile?
Provide meticulous wound care (see Impaired Skin Integrity).	Helps decrease the level of contamination and prevent infection	Is wound showing signs of healing without purulent drainage?
Use thorough handwashing techniques. Use sterile technique for dressing changes.	Prevents cross-contamination	Does nurse take proper wound precautions?

Nursing Diagnosis: Pain related to ulcer and treatments

Expected Outcomes Patient will be as comfortable and as pain-free as possible as evidenced by statement of increased comfort, statement of decreased pain, and ability to sleep at night.

Evaluation of Outcomes Does patient express comfort? Does patient express a decrease in pain? Is patient able to sleep?

Interventions	Rationale	Evaluation
Assess level of pain with pain scale, and by observing facial expressions and positioning of body.	Monitors level of pain and response to therapy	At what level is pain? Is it better or worse with treatment?
Offer analgesics as prescribed. Request order for topical analgesics as needed with dressing changes and cleaning of the wound.	Analgesics help relieve pain.	Do analgesics relieve pain?
Decrease anxiety with relaxation techniques (e.g., distraction, music).	Relaxation can lessen pain intensity.	Is patient less anxious? Does patient verbalize less pain?
Maintain a comfortable environment: provide for privacy; position in good alignment and comfortably; and maintain a comfortable room temperature.	Relaxes patient and lessens intensity of discomfort	Does patient express an increase in comfort?

NURSING CARE TIP

Many institutions now have nurses who have been specially trained in wound care. Consult one of these nurses for expert wound assessment and treatment recommendations.

CRITICAL THINKING

Mr. Russ

■ Mr. Russ is an 84-year-old man who was admitted from home to the medical surgical unit after a fall that fractured his femur. He has a history of type 2 diabetes. He had an open reduction and internal fixation of his femur and is now in a brace. He is 6 ft tall and weighs 160 pounds. His appetite is poor; his wife states he has lost 15 lb in the last 3 months. He is occasionally incontinent of urine. What preventive measures can be taken to prevent skin breakdown in this patient?

Suggested answers at end of chapter.

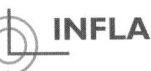 **INFLAMMATORY SKIN DISORDERS**

Dermatitis

Pathophysiology and Etiology

Dermatitis is inflammation of the skin and is characterized by itching, redness, and skin lesions, with varying borders and distribution patterns. Dermatitis can be caused by exposure to allergens or irritants, by heredity, or by emotional stress. Many times the cause is not known; in this case, the terms *eczema* or *nonspecific eczematous dermatitis* may be used. The terms *eczema* and *dermatitis* are sometimes used interchangeably. There are three common types of dermatitis: contact dermatitis, atopic dermatitis, and seborrheic dermatitis. All types tend to be chronic and respond well to treatment, but are prone to recur. See Table 54.2 for common types of dermatitis.

Prevention

The patient should prevent irritation to the skin by avoiding irritants, allergens, excessive heat and dryness, and by controlling perspiration. Baths should be short, and water

dermatitis: derma—skin + itis—inflammation

TABLE 54.2 COMMON TYPES OF DERMATITIS

Type	Description
Contact	Acute or chronic condition; caused by contact with irritant or allergen
Irritant contact	Caused by direct contact with an irritating substance, such as soap, detergent, strong medication, astringent, cosmetic, or industrial chemical
Allergic contact	From contact with an allergen, such as perfume, tanning lotion, medication, hair dye, poison ivy, poison oak; contact results in cell-mediated immune response
Atopic	Chronic inherited condition; may be associated with respiratory allergies or asthma; can vary between bright red maculas, papules, oozing, **lichenified,** and hyperpigmented areas
Seborrheic	Chronic, inflammatory disease usually accompanied by scaling, itching, and inflammation; **seborrhea** is excessive production of sebaceous secretions; found in areas with abundant sebaceous glands (scalp, face, axilla., genitocrural areas) and where there are folds of skin; can appear as dry, moist, or greasy scales, yellow or pink-yellow crusts, redness, and dry flakiness; can be associated with emotional stress; genetic predisposition may exist

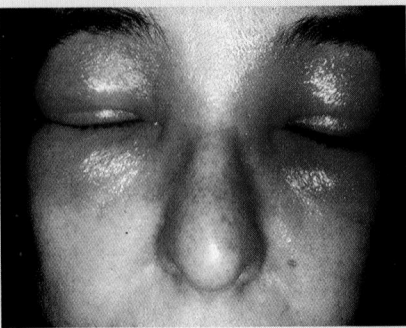

Contact dermatitis caused by nail polish

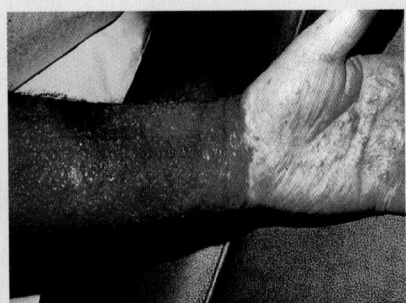

Contact dermatitis caused by topical anesthetic

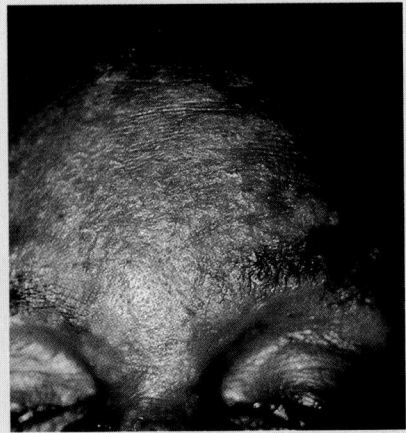

Seborreic dermatitis

lichenified: leichen—scaly growth + facere—to make
seborrhea: sebum—tallow + rhoia—flow

should be tepid. Deodorant soaps should be avoided; mild superfatted soaps are recommended instead. Dry skin is lubricated with creams, oils, or ointments as appropriate. Itching and scratching are prevented as much as possible.

Signs and Symptoms

Itching and rashes or lesions are the main clinical manifestations of dermatitis. The lesions vary depending on the type and location of dermatitis. Rashes and lesions may present as dry, flaky scales, yellow crusts, redness, fissures, macules, papules, and vesicles. (These are described in Chapter 53.) Scratching can make any of these lesions worse.

NURSING CARE TIP

Itching and scratching can occur during sleep, causing the rash to worsen. Have the patient wear cotton gloves at night.

Complications

The lesion or rash worsens with continued irritation, exposure to offending agents, or scratching. Infections of the skin are common and may be due to the many open areas and breaks in the skin, as well as the patient's reluctance to properly wash the affected area because of pain from the lesions. Some infections can also become systemic.

Diagnostic Tests

Diagnosis is usually based on history, symptoms, and clinical findings. If infection is suspected, cultures of the lesions may be ordered to identify the infecting agent.

Therapeutic Interventions

Treatment varies according to symptoms. Basic treatment objectives are to control itching, alleviate discomfort and pain, decrease inflammation, control or prevent crust formation and oozing, prevent infection, prevent further damage to the skin, and heal the skin as much as possible.

Itching (**pruritus**) and discomfort can be somewhat relieved by antihistamines, analgesics, and antipruritic medications as ordered. Colloidal oatmeal preparations added to baths may also help.

Steroids such as hydrocortisone or methylprednisolone may be used to suppress inflammation. They can be administered as a topical, intralesional, or systemic agent. The specific type and vehicle used depends on the type of lesion, the body area involved, and the extent of the lesion. Topical administration is preferred if possible because systemic steroids can cause serious systemic side effects, including adrenal suppression.

Tub baths and wet dressings help control oozing and prevent further crust formation. These interventions serve to loosen exudates, scales, and other wound debris, providing a clean area for topical application of medication. Skin is protected by lightly patting dry, avoiding friction,

avoiding hot water, and using a sunscreen agent when outdoors.

Nursing Process for the Patient with Dermatitis

ASSESSMENT/DATA COLLECTION. You can use the WHAT'S UP? format to assess the rash, as described in Chapter 53. Also refer to Chapter 53, Table 53.1 for specific questions to ask. Observe the rash or lesions for character, distribution, description, skin tenderness, signs of scratching, and other associated problems.

NURSING DIAGNOSIS, PLANNING, AND IMPLEMENTATION. Impaired skin integrity related to rash, lesions, and scratching

EXPECTED OUTCOME: Skin integrity will improve as evidenced by reduction in lesions; no signs or symptoms of infection.

- Monitor skin condition regularly *to determine if treatment is working.*
- Cleanse the area as ordered by the physician, taking care not to further irritate the skin *to keep area clean and prevent infection.*
- Provide cool moist compresses, dressings, or tepid tub baths *to help relieve inflammation and itching, debride lesions, and soften crusts and scales.*
- Pat the skin dry rather than rubbing *to prevent further trauma.*
- Apply topical agents as ordered *to help suppress inflammation.*
- Provide skin care at bedtime *to help promote comfortable sleep. Many antihistamines also have a sedative effect.*
- Encourage patient to eat a high-protein diet *to promote healing and replace lost protein. If lesions are generalized, protein can be lost through oozing of serum.*
- Encourage use of gloves or mitts, especially at night, *to help prevent scratching.*
- Advise the patient to keep fingernails short *to prevent scratching.*
- Teach the patient that application of slight pressure with a clean cloth *may help relieve itching.*
- Teach relaxation exercises *to help the patient cope with distressing symptoms.*

Disturbed body image related to visible rash or lesions

EXPECTED OUTCOME: The patient will have improved body image as evidenced by a statement of acceptance of the condition and ability to socialize with others.

- Allow patients to verbalize concerns only if they wish to do so. *Talking about concerns may help patient to begin to work through feelings about body image, but should not be forced.*
- Refer to a support group, if available, *to receive support from others in similar circumstances.*
- Display an accepting attitude while caring for skin lesions. *The patient will be quick to pick up*

---

pruritus: prur—itch + itis—condition

your reaction to the lesions, especially if it is negative.

- Encourage the patient to participate in skin care *to allow more control over the situation.*
- Encourage the patient to wear long sleeves or other appropriate covering if the patient desires *to make the lesions less noticeable and the patient more comfortable.*

Deficient knowledge related to disease and treatment

EXPECTED OUTCOME: The patient will verbalize understanding of the condition and demonstrate ability to perform self-care measures.

- Assess patient's baseline knowledge of condition and treatment. *Teaching should build on baseline understanding.*
- Instruct the patient in application of topical agents and dressings. *Overuse of medications can further traumatize skin, so application of a very thin layer is advised.*
- Instruct the patient in how to recognize changes, improvement, or flare-ups of the disorder and what symptoms to report to the health care provider. *Because most skin conditions are cared for at home, it is important for the patient to have the skills needed to monitor the condition and carry out treatment appropriately.*
- Advise the patient to avoid overexposure to sun and to use sunscreen agents when outdoors *to prevent skin damage.*
- Encourage use of a humidifier in the home *to help maintain hydration of skin and control itching during dry weather, especially in winter.*
- Teach the patient measures to prevent future flare-ups if possible. *Flare-ups may be avoided if the patient understands what triggers them.*

PATIENT CARE TIP

When applying topical medications, more is not better!

EVALUATION. If medical and nursing care have been effective, the lesions will be controlled or in remission, the patient will state that itching and other discomforts are controlled, the patient will be able to socialize without undue difficulty, and the patient will be able to describe and demonstrate self-care measures.

Psoriasis

Pathophysiology and Etiology

Psoriasis is a chronic inflammatory skin disorder in which the epidermal cells proliferate abnormally fast. Usually, epi-

---

psoriasis: psor—itch + iasis—inflammation

dermal cells take about 27 days to shed. With psoriasis, the cells shed every 4 to 5 days. The abnormal keratin forms loosely adherent scales with dermal inflammation.

Psoriasis is characterized by exacerbations and remissions. The cause is not known; however, often there may be a family history. The average age at onset is 27 years, although it can begin at any age. The condition can be severe if the onset is in childhood. Many factors can influence the suppression and outbreak of lesions, but this varies from individual to individual. Sun and humidity may suppress lesions. Aggravating factors include streptococcal pharyngitis, emotional upset, stress, hormonal changes, cold weather, skin trauma, and certain drugs (e.g., antimalarials, lithium, beta blockers).

Prevention

Because the exact etiology is not known, measures to prevent exacerbation of symptoms are specific to the patient's circumstances. General preventive measures include avoidance of upper respiratory infections, especially streptococcal infections; avoidance of or coping with emotional stress; avoidance of skin trauma, including sunburns; and avoidance of medications that may precipitate a flare-up.

Signs and Symptoms

Signs and symptoms vary according to the patient and the particular type of psoriasis. Lesions are red papules that join to form plaques with distinct borders (Fig. 54.3). Silvery scales develop on untreated lesions. Areas most often affected are the elbows and knees, scalp, umbilicus, and genitals. Other signs and symptoms include nail involvement, intergluteal pinking (involvement in the gluteal fold), itching, and dry or brittle hair.

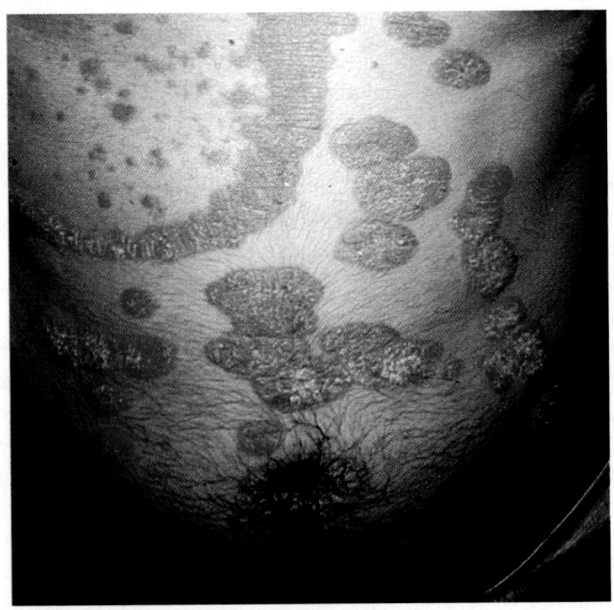

FIGURE 54.3 Psoriasis. Note bright red scaly plaque with silvery scale. *(From Goldsmith, LA, Lazarus, GS, and Tharp, MD: Adult and Pediatric Dermatology. F.A. Davis, Philadelphia, 1997, p 258, with permission.)*

Complications

Because of the nature of the disease, with its lesions and itching, secondary infections can occur. Psoriatic arthritis may develop after the psoriasis has developed, with nail changes and destructive arthritis of large joints, the spine, and interphalangeal joints. If the psoriasis becomes severe and widespread, fever, chills, increased cardiac output, and benign lymphadenopathy can result.

Diagnostic Tests

Testing depends on the severity of the psoriasis. Normally, this disease is diagnosed by physical assessment alone. Diagnostic tests may be performed to rule out concurrent disease or secondary infections.

Therapeutic Interventions

Treatment varies according to the type and extent of the disease, as well as physical preference. Psoriasis is a chronic disease with remissions and exacerbations. Basic treatment objectives are to decrease the rapid epidermal proliferation, inflammation, and itching and scaling. Usually, the patient is instructed to bathe daily in a tub, using a soft brush to assist in the removal of scales.

Topical therapy includes corticosteroids, salicylic acid, keratolytics, coal tar, anthralin, ultraviolet (UV) light, and, in severe cases, antimetabolite chemotherapeutic agents. Topical corticosteroids may be used for their anti-inflammatory effect. Occlusive dressings are commonly used to enhance penetration of medications. (See Chapter 53.) Keratolytic ointments or gels enhance the effects of salicylic acid to loosen or remove scales.

Tar preparations are usually prescribed along with the corticosteroids for conditions that warrant it. The tar acts as an antimitotic, slowing the epidermal cell division. Occlusive dressings are not used with tars. Anthralin is a substance extracted from coal tar. It also suppresses mitotic activity. The anthralin may be mixed with salicylic acid in a stiff paste. The patient must be closely observed because the anthralin is a strong irritant and can cause chemical burns. It is usually applied for no longer than 2 hours. Both coal tar and anthralin are commonly used in combination with UV light and are usually administered in inpatient settings or specialized outpatient clinics.

Topical preparations for the scalp are used in shampoo form. Teach the patient to read package instructions; these preparations generally need to be left in the hair for a period of time to work.

Ultraviolet light may be designated as UVB, shorter wavelength, or UVA, longer wavelength. UVA is from an artificial source, such as special mercury vapor lamps. The amount of exposure depends on the patient's condition, pigmentation, and susceptibility to burning. The patient must wear eye guards during treatments. Oral psoralen tablets (a photosensitizing agent) followed by exposure to UVA is called PUVA therapy. PUVA therapy temporarily inhibits DNA synthesis, which is antimitotic. Because psoralen is a photosensitizing agent, the patient must not only wear dark glasses during the treatment period, but also for the entire day after a treatment. The long-term safety of PUVA therapy is still unknown. Possible side effects include increased skin carcinomas, premature skin aging, and actinic keratosis (premalignant lesions of the skin). The patient should be observed closely for redness, tenderness, edema, and eye changes. Therefore, initial and follow-up eye examinations, skin biopsies, urinalysis, and blood tests may be ordered.

Retinoids are oral agents such as acitretin (Soriatane) that promote skin cell differentiation and inhibit malignancies from forming in the skin. They may be used in combination with UV therapy.

Antimebolites, usually used for cancer chemotherapy, are reserved for the most severe cases. Methotrexate is the most common agent given. Because of its hepatotoxicity, it is contraindicated in patients with liver disease, alcoholism, renal disease, and bone marrow suppression. Before therapy, a liver biopsy and routine laboratory tests are completed.

CRITICAL THINKING

Mrs. Long

■ Mrs. Long arrives at the health clinic to complain that the prescribed shampoo she is using for her scalp is not working. She states that she washes her hair thoroughly with the medicated shampoo and immediately rinses completely. She wants to know why her scalp shows no signs of improvement. What should you tell her?

Suggested answers at end of chapter.

Nursing Care

Nursing care for the patient with psoriasis is the same as nursing care for the patient with dermatitis. The only addition is to encourage frequent periods of rest to enhance the antimitotic effects of the therapeutic agents.

 INFECTIOUS SKIN DISORDERS

A variety of infections can affect the skin. The most common disorders are discussed in this section. See Table 54.3 for a summary of additional skin infections.

Herpes Simplex

Pathophysiology and Etiology

Herpes simplex virus (HSV) infection is a common viral infection that tends to recur repeatedly. There are two types of herpes simplex: that caused by type I virus (HSV-I), which occurs above the waist and causes a fever blister or cold sore (Fig. 54.4), and that caused by type II virus (HSV-II), which occurs below the waist and causes genital herpes. See Chapter 44 for information on genital herpes.

TABLE 54.3 INFECTIOUS SKIN DISORDERS

Type	Description	Complications	Treatment/Nursing Care
Impetigo Contagiosa	Common contagious, infectious, inflammatory skin disorders usually caused by *Streptococcus* or *Staphylococcus aureus*; sources of infection include swimming pools, pets, dirty fingernails, beauty and barber shops, and contaminated clothing, towels, sheets; may occur secondary to scrapes, cuts, insect bites, burns, dermatitis, poison ivy Primary skin infection can appear on exposed areas of the body (extremities, hands, face, neck) or skin-fold areas (axillae). Rash appears as oozing, thin-roofed vesicle that rapidly grows and develops a honey-colored crust; crusts are easily removed, and new crusts appear; lesions heal in 1 to 2 weeks if allowed to dry.	Glomerulonephritis resulting from a particular strain of streptococcus infection Lesions may spread from one skin area to another. Lesions may persist if not permitted to dry. Secondary **pyoderma,** or acute inflammatory purulent dermatitis, may occur if lesions are unresponsive to treatment.	Systemic antibiotics are administered as prescribed. Topical antibiotics are used after crust removal. Gentle washing with a mild soap, or soaking with warm, moist compresses, aids in crust removal, removes debris, and provides a clean bed for topical therapy. Appropriate antipyretics are prescribed as necessary. Keep fingernails short and clean. Glove or mitt hands as necessary to prevent scratching. Patient must remain home until all lesions are healed. Teach proper disposal or washing of any material that comes in contact with lesions. Good hygiene must be practiced to prevent skin-to-skin or person-to-person spread. Observe client for 6 to 7 weeks for signs/ symptoms of glomerulonephritis.
Furuncles and Carbuncles	A furuncle is a small, tender boil that occurs deep in one or more hair follicles and spreads to surrounding dermis; may be single or multiple; usually caused by *Staphylococcus*; usually occurs on body areas prone to excessive perspiration, friction, and irritation (e.g., buttocks, axillae); can recur; the boil eventually comes to a soft yellow, black, or white head; there is localized pain, tenderness, and surrounding cellulitis; lymphadenopathy may be present.	Furuncles may progress to carbuncles.	Prevent trauma; avoid squeezing or irritation.

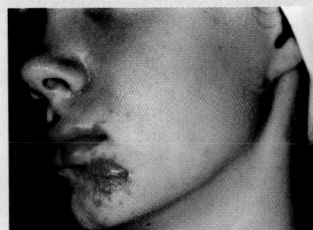

Impetigo on the face.

---

pyoderma: pyo—pus + derma—skin

Type	Description	Complications	Treatment/Nursing Care
Furuncles and Carbuncles *(cont'd)*	A carbuncle is an extension of a furuncle; an abscess of skin and subcutaneous tissue; deeper than furuncle; caused by *Staphylococcus*; usually appears where skin is thick, fibrous, and inelastic (e.g., back of neck, upper back, and buttocks); associated symptoms may include fevers, pain, leukocytosis, prostration. Both tend to occur in debilitated clients, and more often in diabetics. Occasionally, scarring may occur. 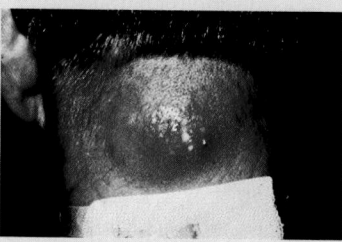	Carbuncles may progress to infection of bloodstream. Further spread of infection can occur to self and others.	Cleanse surrounding skin with antibacterial soap, followed by application of antibacterial ointment. Surgical incision and drainage may be performed. Cover draining lesion with dressing. Follow standard precautions. Double bag all soiled dressings and dispose of properly. Systemic antibiotic therapy (based on sensitivity studies) is instituted for carbuncles or spreading furuncles. Analgesia and antipyretics are ordered as necessary. Bedrest is advised with carbuncles or furuncles on perineal or anal regions. Cover mattress and pillows with plastic and wipe daily with a disinfectant. Wash all linens, towels, and clothing after each use. Properly discard razor blades after each use. Strict hand washing is maintained to prevent cross-contamination.

The primary infection occurs through direct contact, respiratory droplet, or fluid exposure from another infected person. Following the initial infection, the virus lies dormant in nerve ganglia near the spinal column, where the immune system cannot destroy it. The patient is asymptomatic at this time.

Recurrence of symptomatic infection can happen spontaneously or be triggered by fever, sunburn, stress, illness, menses, fatigue, or injury. The secondary lesion may appear isolated or as groups of small vesicles or pustules on an erythematous base. Crusts eventually form, and the lesions heal in about 1 week. The lesions are contagious for 2 to 4 days before dry crusts form.

Prevention

Avoidance of contact with a known infected lesion during the blistering phase can prevent the primary lesions. Patients should also be taught to avoid sharing contaminated items such as toothbrushes, lipsticks, and drinking glasses. This disease can recur spontaneously. Avoidance of stressors, such as sunburn, injury, and fatigue, may delay a recurrence. The use of sunscreens, especially on the lips, may be helpful.

Signs and Symptoms

Some patients may have a prodromal phase of burning or tingling at the site for a few hours before eruption. The area becomes erythematous and swollen. Vesicles and pustules erupt in 1 to 2 days. There may also be redness with no blistering. Lesions can burn, itch, and be painful. The attacks vary in frequency but diminish with age. The patient is contagious until scabs are formed.

Complications

If herpes simplex is present in the vagina at childbirth, the newborn may be infected (meningoencephalitis or a panvisceral infection may occur). If the person touches the affected area and then rubs the eyes, the eyes can become severely infected. Secondary bacterial infection of lesions can occur. Rarely, herpes encephalitis can occur. This is deadly if not treated promptly.

Diagnostic Tests

Cultures of the lesions provide a definitive diagnosis. Most lesions are diagnosed on the basis of history, signs, and symptoms.

Therapeutic Interventions

There is no complete cure for herpes simplex. Recurrences will happen. Topical acyclovir (Zovirax) ointment is the drug of choice for primary lesions, to suppress the multiplication of vesicles. It does not benefit secondary lesions. Oral

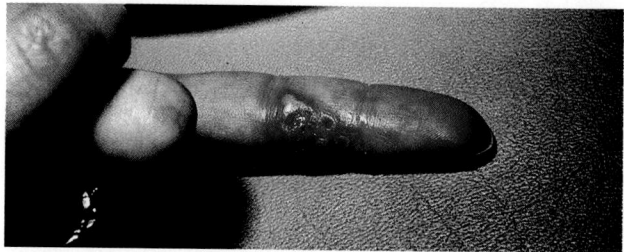

FIGURE 54.4 Herpes simplex. *(From Goldsmith, LA, Lazarus, GS, and Tharp, MD: Adult and Pediatric Dermatology. F.A. Davis, Philadelphia, 1997, p 306, with permission.)*

acyclovir may be recommended for severe or frequent attacks (six or more attacks per year) or for patients who are immunosuppressed. Various lotions, creams, and ointments may be prescribed to accelerate drying and healing of lesions (e.g., camphor, phenol, alcohol). Antibiotics may be indicated for secondary infections.

Herpes Zoster (Shingles)

Pathophysiology and Etiology

Herpes zoster, or shingles, is an acute inflammatory and infectious disorder that produces a painful vesicular eruption on bright red edematous plaques along the distribution of nerves from one or more posterior ganglia. This eruption follows the course of the cutaneous sensory nerve and is almost always unilateral (one sided) (Fig. 54.5).

Herpes zoster is caused by the varicella zoster virus. This virus appears to be identical to the one that causes chickenpox. It is thought that herpes zoster is a reactivation of this latent varicella virus. The incubation period is 7 to 21 days. The vesicles appear in 3 to 4 days. Eruption usually occurs posteriorly and progresses anteriorly and peripherally along the dermatome. The total duration of the disease can vary from 10 days to 5 weeks.

This disease occurs most commonly in the elderly or in those who have a diminished resistance, such as the patient with acquired immunodeficiency syndrome (AIDS), the patient on immunosuppressant agents, or the patient with a malignancy or injury to the spine or a cranial nerve.

Prevention

Avoidance of the person with this disease during the contagious phase (a few days before eruption until vesicles dry or scab) is the best prevention.

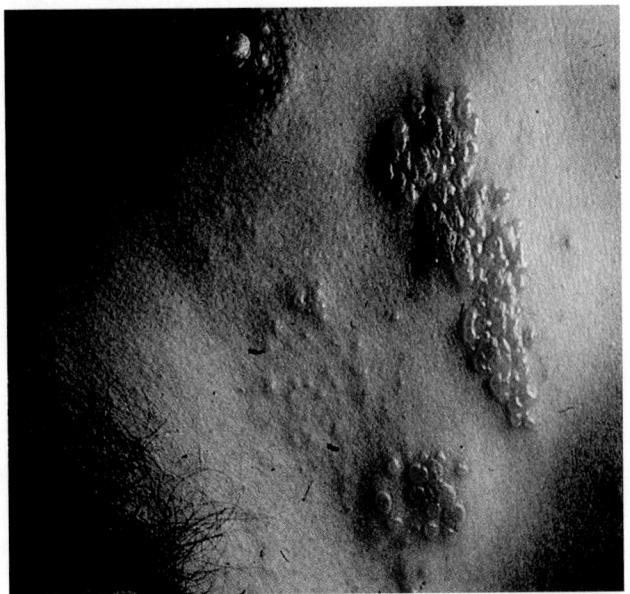

FIGURE 54.5 Herpes zoster (shingles). *(From Goldsmith, LA, Lazarus, GS, and Tharp, MD: Adult and Pediatric Dermatology. F.A. Davis, Philadelphia, 1997, p 307, with permission.)*

Signs and Symptoms

In addition to the vesicles and plaques, there may be irritation, itching, fever, malaise, and, depending on the location of lesions, visceral involvement. Lesions may be very painful; the likelihood of pain increases with age.

Complications

Postherpetic neuralgia, persistent dermatomal pain, and hyperesthesia are common in the elderly and can last for weeks to months after the lesions have healed. The incidence and severity of these complications increase with age.

Ophthalmic herpes zoster affects the fifth cranial nerve and can be a serious complication. Consultation with an ophthalmologist is imperative because this complication can affect eyesight. Other complications can occur with facial and acoustic nerve involvement, including hearing loss, tinnitus, facial paralysis, and vertigo. Full-thickness skin necrosis and scarring can occur if lesions do not heal properly; systemic infection can occur from scratching, causing the virus to enter the bloodstream.

Diagnostic Tests

Diagnosis is usually confirmed by the clinical picture of the patient and associated signs and symptoms. Cultures may be ordered if secondary bacterial infections are suspected.

Therapeutic Interventions

Treatment is aimed at controlling the outbreak, reducing pain and discomfort, and preventing complications. Acyclovir, either intravenous (IV), oral, or topical, may be prescribed in the early stages of the initial infection, for a severe outbreak, and if the patient is immunosuppressed or debilitated. Acyclovir does not cure, but it may help control the initial outbreak. Analgesics are prescribed for pain and discomfort. Corticosteroids may be administered to prevent postherpetic neuralgia and reduce pain but are not used for ocular involvement. Topical steroids should not be applied if a secondary infection is present because they suppress the immune system. Antihistamines are administered to control itching. Antibiotics are prescribed for secondary bacterial infections.

Fungal Infections

Pathophysiology and Etiology

Dermatophytosis, or a fungal infection of the skin, occurs when there is an impairment of the skin integrity in a warm, moist environment. This infection occurs through direct contact with infected humans, animals, or objects. *Tinea* is the term used to describe fungal skin infections; the name used after tinea indicates the body area affected. For example, tinea capitis is a fungal infection of the scalp. Common fungal infections and treatments are described in Table 54.4.

---

dermatophytosis: derma—skin + phyton—plant + osis—condition

TABLE 54.4 FUNGAL INFECTIONS

Type	Description	Treatment/Nursing Care
Tinea Pedis (Athlete's Foot)	Common fungal infection, most frequently seen in those with warm, moist, sweaty feet; occlusive shoes; or friction/trauma to the feet Three types: chronic plantar scaling, acute vesicular, and interdigital Chronic plantar scaling will have slight redness and mild to severe scaling; fold lines on sole appear to have white powder because of scaling; there may be toenail involvement; itching is usually not present. Acute vesicular appears as a sudden eruption of small, painful, itchy vesicles; may also accompany chronic plantar scaling.	Chronic plantar scaling may be treated with kerolytics and topical antifungal agents; these agents help in relieving symptoms and improve appearance; they are not curative. Acute vesicular is treated with soaks or baths two or three times a day for 2 to 3 days to dry up blisters; astringent paint is applied to debrided areas; topical corticosteroids help relieve itching. Interdigital may be treated with combined antifungal and antibacterial therapies or antifungals alone; soak feet twice daily and dry well. Teach patient prevention measures: keep feet dry; dry carefully between toes; apply foot powder to absorb perspiration; wear cotton socks to absorb perspiration; if weather permits, use perforated shoes or sandals; avoid plastic or rubber-soled shoes; wear water shoes in public showers and near swimming pools. Apply topical agents properly: apply thin layer; treat for time specified, even after apparent clearing.
Tinea Capitis (Ringworm of Scalp)	Contagious; commonly causes hair loss in children Appears as scattered round, red, scaly patches; small papules or pustules may be evident at edges of patches; hair is brittle at site, breaks off, and temporary areas of baldness result; may be mild itching; kerion inflammation may occur after weeks 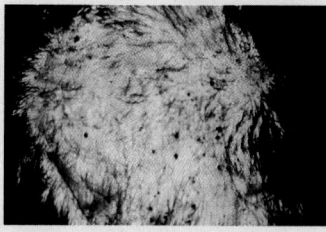 Tinea capitis.	Teach prevention measures: never share combs, brushes, pillowcases, or headgear. Systemic antifungals are prescribed because of high relapse rate with topical agents; review side effects with patient. Oral corticosteroids are indicated for kerion inflammation to help prevent alopecia; review side effects with client. Instruct family on contagious aspect of disease; assess other family members and pets for organism.
Tinea Corporis (Tinea Circinata, Ringworm of Body)	Erythematous macule that progresses to rings of vesicles or scale with a clear center that appears alone or in clusters; usually occurs on exposed areas of body; can be moderately to intensely itchy Infected pet is common source of infection.	Teach prevention measures: keep skin areas, especially folds, dry; use clean towel and wash cloth daily; wear cotton clothing, especially on hot, humid days. Topical antifungals are prescribed for small, localized lesions. Oral antifungals are indicated for severe, widespread, resistant, or follicular cases. Topical corticosteroids are prescribed for itching. Teach patient prevention measures: avoid heat, moisture, and friction.
Tinea Cruris (Ringworm of Groin, Jock Itch)	May extend to inner thighs and buttocks area; may occur with tinea pedis; often in obese people who are athletic Lesion first appears as a small red scaly patch and then progresses to a sharply demarcated plaque with elevated scaly or vesicular borders; itching can range from absent to severe.	Topical antifungals are prescribed; apply in a thin layer to rash and a few centimeters beyond border.

(Continued on following page)

TABLE 54.4 FUNGAL INFECTIONS *(Continued)*

Type	Description	Treatment/Nursing Care
Tinea Cruris (Ringworm of Groin, Jock Itch) (cont'd)	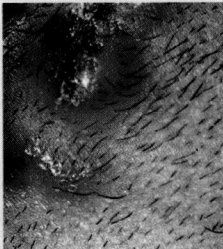 Tinea cruris.	Oral antifungals may be indicated for widespread cases or those resistant to topical therapy. Topical corticosteroids may be prescribed for itching.
Tinea Unguium (Ringworm of Nails)	Also called **onychomycosis** Chronic fungal infection of nails, usually the toenails; a lifelong disease There is yellow thickening of nail plate; it is friable and lusterless; eventually crumbly debris accumulates under free edge of the nail and causes nail plate to become separated; over time, the nail may become thickened, painful, and destroyed. 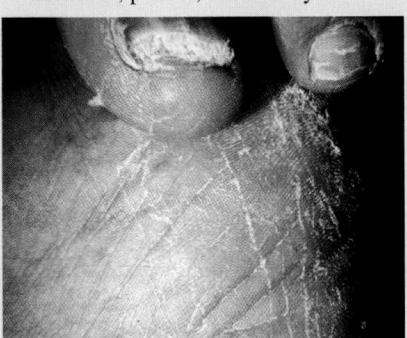 Onychomycosis (tinea unguium).	Systemic antifungals are rarely given for toenail involvement, but may be prescribed for fingernail involvement (review side effects). Topical antifungals are usually ineffective. Nail may have to be surgically removed (nail avulsion). Explain high relapse rate to patient. Keep nails neatly trimmed and buffed flat; gently scrape out any nail debris.

onychomycosis: onyx—nail + myc—fungus + osis—condition

Cellulitis

Pathophysiology and Etiology
Cellulitis is inflammation of the skin and subcutaneous tissue resulting from a generalized infection, usually with *Staphylococcus* or *Streptococcus* bacteria. It can occur as a result of skin trauma or a secondary bacterial infection of an open wound, such as a pressure sore, or it may be unrelated to skin trauma. It most often occurs in the extremities, especially the lower legs.

Prevention
Good hygiene and prevention of cross-contamination are important. If there is an open wound, preventing infection and promoting healing are critical.

Signs and Symptoms
The initial sign of cellulitis is a localized area of inflammation that may become more generalized if not treated properly. Common clinical manifestations include warmth, redness, localized edema, pain, tenderness, fever, and lymphadenopathy. It may be seen in any areas of an open wound, with skin trauma, and in the lower legs. The infection can worsen rapidly if not treated properly.

Diagnostic Tests
Culture and sensitivity testing of any pustules or drainage is necessary to identify the infecting organism. Blood cultures may also be indicated to rule out bacteremia.

Therapeutic Interventions
Topical and systemic antibiotics are prescribed according to culture and sensitivity test results. Debridement of nonviable tissue is necessary if there is an open wound. Systemic antibiotics are indicated if fever and lymphadenopathy are present. Warm, moist compresses may be ordered, although there is no evidence that this is useful in treating pain or infection.

Acne Vulgaris

Pathophysiology and Etiology

Acne vulgaris is a common skin disorder of the sebaceous glands and their hair follicles that usually occurs on the face, chest, upper back, and shoulders. The etiology is multifocal. The most common cause is hormonal changes during puberty.

The sebaceous glands are under endocrine control, especially the androgens. Stimulation of androgens (e.g., during adolescence or the menstrual cycle) in turn stimulates the sebaceous glands to increase sebum production. This, along with gradual obstruction of the pilosebaceous ducts with accumulated debris, ruptures the sebaceous glands, which causes an inflammatory reaction that may lead to papules, pustules, nodules, and cysts. Acne occurs when the ducts through which this sebum flows become plugged.

Other factors that influence the occurrence and severity of acne include a hereditary tendency, stress, and external irritants such as strong soaps or cosmetics. It is not related to diet, chocolate, sexual activity, or uncleanliness.

Prevention

Acne vulgaris occurs regardless of interventions; however, certain interventions can lessen the severity or prevent complications. Avoidance of "picking" pimples prevents further inflammation and scarring. The patient should avoid excessive washing, irritants, and abrasives.

Signs and Symptoms

The initial lesions are called comedones. Closed comedones, or whiteheads, are small white papules with tiny follicular openings. These may eventually become open **comedones,** or blackheads. The color is not caused by dirt but by lipids and melanin pigment. Scarring occurs as a result of significant skin inflammation; picking can worsen inflammation and lead to further scarring. The resulting inflammation can lead to papules, pustules, nodules (Fig. 54.6), cysts, or abscesses.

Therapeutic Interventions

Medical treatment helps prevent new lesions and helps control current lesions. Effective topical agents include benzoyl peroxide (Desquam-X; Benzagel), which is an antibacterial agent that may help prevent pore plugging; antibiotics (erythromycin, tetracycline) to kill bacteria in follicles; and vitamin A acid (Retin-A, tretinoin) to loosen pore plugs and prevent occurrence of new comedones. Topical agents may be used alone or in combination. It may take 3 to 6 weeks before improvement is seen.

All topical agents should be applied with clean hands to acne-prone areas, not just where the acne occurs. They must be applied to dry skin. Medications should not be applied near eyes, nasolabial folds, or the corners of the mouth because of the potential for irritation. If the patient is ordered a combination of topical agents, unless contraindicated, the tretinoin is used at night and the others in the morning or afternoon. Tretinoin can be neutralized if mixed directly with other agents. The patient must be careful with

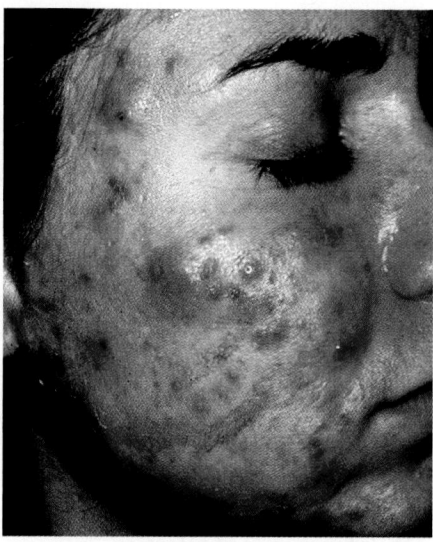

FIGURE 54.6 Acne vulgaris. *(From Goldsmith, LA, Lazarus, GS, and Tharp, MD: Adult and Pediatric Dermatology. F.A. Davis, Philadelphia, 1997, p 351, with permission.)*

sun or sunlamp exposure while using tretinoin. Also, remind the patient that it may be necessary to continue treatment even after the skin clears.

Systemic antibiotics (long term, low dose) and isotretinoin (Accutane) are usually reserved for severe cases of acne; the patient must be closely monitored for side effects. Estrogen therapy (oral contraceptives) may also be prescribed for young women; however, the risks often outweigh the benefits. Women should be aware that some antibiotics reduce the effectiveness of oral contraceptives. Systemic corticosteroids may occasionally be prescribed for severe nodular acne, but they are associated with severe side effects.

Other medical treatments include comedone extraction, intralesional injections of corticosteroids, cryosurgery (freezing with liquid nitrogen), mild peeling (UV light, carbon dioxide, liquid nitrogen, mild acid), dermabrasion (deep chemical peel), excision of scars, and injection of fibrin or collagen below the scars. These treatments depend on the severity, age, condition, and physician and patient preference.

NURSING CARE TIP

Topical benzoyl peroxide may bleach colored fabrics. Have the patient wear a white cotton T-shirt under clothing if benzoyl peroxide is used on the back, and use an old or white pillowcase at night.

Nursing Process for the Patient with a Skin Infection

Assessment/Data Collection

Subjective assessment of a skin infection can begin with the WHAT'S UP? acronym. Determine **W**here the skin infection is located; **H**ow it feels (does it itch, burn, hurt?); what **A**ggravates and **A**lleviates the symptoms; the **T**iming, or how long it has been present; how **S**evere it is; and **U**seful other data, such as whether there is swelling, drainage, or fever. The **P**atient's **P**erception is important because he or she may have information about the source or cause of the infection.

Objective assessment includes observing the affected area and describing the infection in terms of type and configuration of lesions, color, size, and presence of drainage. Also observe for swelling, and check for elevated temperature. If the patient has cellulitis of an extremity, measure and document the circumference of the extremity daily and prn.

Assess the patient's understanding of the cause of the infection, and of infection control measures.

NURSING DIAGNOSIS, PLANNING, AND IMPLEMENTATION. Risk for spread of infection

EXPECTED OUTCOME: The infected area will not spread to other areas on patient or to other individuals.

- Monitor and document size and location of infected area daily and prn. *Careful monitoring can identify improvement or new spread of infection.*
- Monitor temperature every 8 hours and prn. *An increasing temperature can indicate worsening or systemic infection.*
- Monitor for signs and symptoms of systemic spread of infection. *Systemic infection must be reported and treated promptly to prevent complications, including sepsis.*
- Use standard precautions, including careful hand washing, when providing patient care *to prevent transmission to yourself or to others.*
- Implement appropriate isolation precautions for patients with a contagious infection. Contact precautions are usually sufficient, although airborne precautions may be necessary if immunocompromised individuals are present. *Isolation reduces spread of infection.*
- Instruct the patient on wound care, appropriate hand washing, and disposal of soiled dressings. *The patient must follow precautions to protect self and others.*
- Instruct patient on use of prescribed anti-infective agent, including the importance of taking it exactly as directed *to prevent development of a resistant infection.*
- For the patient with acne:
  - Advise the patient to keep hands away from the face and especially not to touch or squeeze pimples. Keep hair clean and off the face. *These measures help prevent spread and secondary infection.*

Acute pain

EXPECTED OUTCOME: Patient will state that pain is controlled at an acceptable level.

- Monitor pain (if present) using a pain scale. *Assessment provides a basis for nursing intervention.*
- Administer analgesics as ordered, especially prior to dressing changes or treatments. *Analgesics relieve pain and help prevent pain during dressing changes.*
- For the patient with shingles:
  - Apply cool, moist compresses to painful or itching lesions *to help cleanse and dry lesions and reduce itching.*
  - Apply firm dressings such as wraps, stockings, or a snug T-shirt *to reduce pain from postherpetic neuralgia.*
- For the patient with cellulitis:
  - Elevate affected extremity as ordered *to reduce swelling and increase comfort.*

Evaluation

If interventions have been effective, the skin lesions will improve, and will not spread to new areas or to others. The patient will state that pain is manageable.

PARASITIC SKIN DISORDERS

Pediculosis

Pathophysiology and Etiology

Pediculosis is an infestation by lice. There are three basic types: pediculosis capitis (head lice), pediculosis corporis (body lice), and pediculosis pubis (pubic, or crab, lice). Generally, the lice bite the skin and feed on human blood, leaving their eggs and excrement, which can cause intense itching. The lice are oval and are approximately 2 mm in length.

In pediculosis capitis, the female louse lays eggs (nits) close to the scalp, where the nits become firmly attached to hair shafts. The most common areas of infestation are the back of the scalp and behind the ears. The nits are about 1 to 3 mm in length and appear silvery white and glistening. Transmission is by direct contact or contact with infested objects, such as combs, brushes, wigs, hats, and bedding. It is most common in children and people with long hair.

Pediculosis corporis is caused by body lice that lay eggs in the seams of clothing and then pierce the skin. Areas of the skin usually involved are the neck, trunk, and thighs.

Pediculosis pubis is caused by crab lice. It is generally localized in the genital region, but it can also be seen on hairs of the chest, axillae, eyelashes, and beard. The lice are about 2 mm in length and have a crablike appearance. It is chiefly transmitted through sexual contact or to a lesser degree by infested bed linen.

Prevention

Prevention involves avoidance of contact with an infected person or object. Brushes, combs, hats, and other personal items should not be shared. Good personal hygiene and routine clothes washing are other preventive measures; however, even someone with meticulous hygiene can develop this infection if there is contact with the organism.

Signs and Symptoms

Pediculosis capitis can result in no itching or intense itching and scratching, especially at the back of the head. Nits may be noticeably attached to hair. A papular rash may be seen.

Pediculosis corporis may appear as minute hemorrhagic points. Excoriations may be noted on the back, shoulders, abdomen, and extremities. It may also cause intense itching.

Pediculosis pubis results in mild to severe itching, especially at night. Black or reddish brown dots (lice excreta) may be noted at the base of hairs or in underclothing. Gray-blue macules may also be noted on the trunk, thighs, and axillae; this is the result of the insects' saliva mixing with bilirubin.

Complications

Secondary bacterial infections can occur with pediculosis capitis, resulting in impetigo, furuncles, pustules, crusts, and matted hair. Secondary lesions that can occur with pediculosis corporis include parallel linear scratches, hyperemia, eczema, and hyperpigmentation. Most important, body lice may be vectors for rickettsial disease. Complications with pediculosis pubis include dermatitis and the coexistence of other sexually transmitted diseases.

Diagnostic Tests

Diagnosis is through history and physical assessment. The patient may also be tested for other sexually transmitted diseases if pediculosis pubis is present.

Therapeutic Interventions

Medical treatment is aimed at killing the parasites and mechanically removing nits. Pediculicides containing pyrethrins or permethrin are the most commonly recommended compounds. These agents should kill the lice and nits, although some lice develop pesticide resistance, making mechanical removal necessary. Permethrin (Nix) remains active for about a week, killing the adult lice immediately and the nits when they hatch days later. Pyrethrins (RID, A-200 Pyrinate) must be reapplied in 1 week to kill newly hatched lice.

Complications are treated, as appropriate, with antipruritics, topical corticosteroids, and systemic antibiotics. Physostigmine ophthalmic ointment is applied to affected eyebrows and eyelashes. Other medications should not be applied to eyebrows or eyelashes.

Patient Education

Reassure the patient and family that head lice can happen to anyone, and this is not a sign of uncleanliness. Lice infestations are treated on an outpatient basis, so patient education is important. Package instructions should be followed for correct usage of all medications.

Instruct the patient to bathe with soap and water and to disinfect combs and brushes in hot, medicated soapy water. A fine-toothed comb dipped in vinegar can be used to remove nits from hairy areas. Nits can be removed from eyebrows and eyelashes with a cotton-tipped applicator after treatment. Clothing, linens, and towels should be laundered in hot water and detergent; unwashable clothing should be dry-cleaned or sealed in a plastic bag for 10 days. Treatment should be started immediately to prevent rapid spread. Family members and close contacts (sexual contact with pediculosis pubis) should be examined for infestation and should put on clean clothing.

Shampoos and lotions kill nits, but they do not remove them. To loosen nits from the scalp, the hair may be soaked in a solution of equal parts vinegar and water and a shower cap worn for 15 minutes. The hair is then combed with a fine-toothed comb and thoroughly rinsed or shampooed to mechanically remove the nits. Children may return to school after adequate medical treatment, even if dead nits are still present.

NURSING CARE TIP

It is not possible to dry clean or wash all infected items, such as mattresses and upholstered furniture. Adult lice can live away from humans for only 3 to 4 days. Therefore, simply vacuum the upholstered furniture. The lice die in 3 to 4 days without human contact.

Scabies

Pathophysiology and Etiology

Scabies is a contagious skin disease caused by the mite *Sarcoptes scabiei*. It is results from intimate or prolonged skin contact or prolonged contact with infected clothing, bedding, or animals (e.g., dogs, cats, other small animals). The parasite burrows into the superficial layer of the skin (Fig. 54.7). These burrows appear as short, wavy, brownish black lines. The patient is asymptomatic while the organism multiplies, but it is most contagious at this time. Symptoms do not occur for almost 4 weeks from time of contact.

Prevention

All persons (and animals) in intimate contact with an infected patient should be treated at the same time to eliminate the mites. The mites survive less than 24 hours without human contact. Therefore, bed linen, clothes, and towels should be washed, but furnishings need not be cleaned. Clean clothing and linens should be applied.

Signs and Symptoms

The major complaints are itching and rash. Itching can be intense, especially at night. The itching occurs 1 month after infestation and may persist for days to weeks after treatment. The rash may appear as small, scattered erythematous papules, concentrated in finger webs, axillae, wrist folds, umbilicus, groin, and genitals. Male patients may exhibit excoriated papules on the penis and groin area.

Complications

Hypersensitivity reactions to the mite can result in crusted lesions, vesicles, pustules, excoriations, and bacterial superinfections.

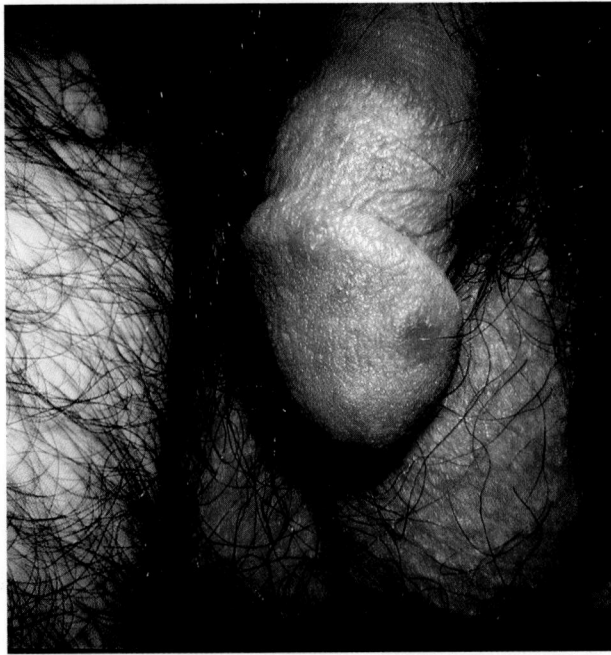

FIGURE 54.7 Scabies. *(From Goldsmith, LA, Lazarus, GS, and Tharp, MD: Adult and Pediatric Dermatology. F.A. Davis, Philadelphia. 1997, p 295, with permission.)*

Diagnostic Tests

Diagnosis is confirmed by a superficial shaving of a lesion and microscopic evaluation for adult mites, eggs, or feces.

Therapeutic Interventions

Topical scabicides are used for chemical disinfection. Usually, the cream or lotion is applied in a thin layer to the entire body from neck to feet (including genitals, umbilicus, and skin-fold areas), is left on overnight (8 to 12 hours), and is washed off in the morning; however, package instructions should be referred to for each medication. One or two applications are usually curative, depending on the agent prescribed. Antipruritics and corticosteroids may be prescribed for itching.

Patient Education

A warm soapy bath or shower removes scales and skin debris. Advise the patient to apply the topical medication as ordered; not to repeatedly use scabicides because they can increase itching and cause further skin irritation; to follow medication directions; to treat family members and close contacts simultaneously to eliminate mites; to wear clean clothing; and to use clean linens. Remind the patient that itching may continue for up to 2 weeks after treatment, until the allergic reaction subsides. (Dead mites remain in the epidermis until exfoliated.)

NURSING CARE TIP

Animals infested with scabies should be treated by a veterinarian, so they won't infect humans.

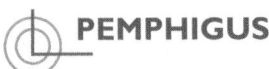
PEMPHIGUS

Pathophysiology and Etiology

Pemphigus is an acute or chronic serious skin disease characterized by the appearance of bullae (large fluid-filled blisters) of various sizes on otherwise normal skin and mucous membranes. The etiology is unknown, but it is believed to be an autoimmune disorder. Sun exposure, genetic predisposition, and certain foods and drugs (e.g., penicillamine, captopril, and enalapril) may trigger the disorder. It usually occurs in patients from middle to older age.

The autoimmune response that occurs in pemphigus causes a patient's own antibodies to attack the skin and mucous membranes, and destroy the protein "glue" that holds the cells together. The result is skin that separates from itself, causing the characteristic blisters.

Signs and Symptoms

Successive crops of bullae suddenly appear on skin or mucous membranes. The bullae are fragile and flaccid. They enlarge, rupture, and form painful, raw, eroded, partial-thickness wounds that bleed, ooze, and form crusts. Pemphigus usually originates in the oral mucosa and then spreads to the trunk. Large areas of the body become involved.

Besides the appearance of the blisters, the patient experiences pain, burning, and itching. The lesions have a foul smell. Involvement of the oral mucosa can interfere with chewing, swallowing, and talking. The patient is in constant misery.

Complications

The major complication is a secondary bacterial infection. There is a high morbidity and mortality rate associated with this disease.

Diagnostic Tests

A positive Nikolsky's sign is a characteristic finding. This occurs when there is sloughing or blistering of normal skin when minimal pressure is applied. A biopsy of a blister reveals acantholysis, or separation of epidermal cells from one another.

Therapeutic Intervention

Treatment is aimed at controlling the disease, healing the skin, and preventing complications. Corticosteroids in large doses and cytotoxic agents are prescribed to control the disease and bring about remission. Medicated mouthwashes may be prescribed for mouth lesions. Analgesics and antipruritics are prescribed according to the patient's specific signs and symptoms. Because of fluid, blood, and protein losses through the partial-thickness injury, a high-protein, high-calorie diet is recommended along with appropriate fluid replacement therapy.

---

pemphigus: pemphix—blister

Nursing Care

Monitor fluid balance with regular intake and output, body weight, and blood pressure measurement. Encourage the patient to maintain adequate fluid intake. Offer cool drinks often to lessen discomfort.

Tepid wet dressings or baths help lessen secondary infection, cleanse the area, decrease odor, and increase comfort. Potassium permanganate baths may decrease infection and clean and deodorize the area. Always thoroughly dissolve potassium permanganate crystals in a small container before adding to tub water. Undissolved crystals may further damage and burn the skin. Dry the patient thoroughly after the bath. Do not use tape on the patient because this may cause further blistering. Talcum powder may be indicated to keep the skin from sticking to linens and bedclothes.

Teach the patient to maintain meticulous oral hygiene. Explain the effects and side effects of medications. Teach the importance of avoiding sun exposure or other triggers. Provide appropriate psychosocial support because of the length of illness, the chronic nature of the condition, and the physical appearance of lesions.

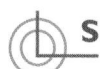 SKIN LESIONS

Skin lesions can be either benign (noncancerous) or malignant. Benign lesions are described in Table 54.5. Malignant lesions are discussed next. See also Box 54.3 Cultural Considerations.

Malignant Skin Lesions

Pathophysiology and Etiology

The most common skin malignancies include basal cell carcinoma, squamous cell carcinoma, and malignant melanoma. The major cause of skin malignancies is overexposure to ultraviolet rays, most commonly sunlight. Other factors include being fair skinned and blue eyed, genetic tendencies, history of x-ray therapy, exposure to certain chemical agents (e.g., arsenic, paraffin, coal tar), burn scars, chronic osteomyelitis, and immunosuppressive therapy.

Basal cell carcinoma arises from the basal cell layer of the epidermis. It is the most common type of skin cancer. This tumor is mainly seen on sun-exposed areas of the body. The lesion appears as a small pearly or translucent papule with a rolled, waxy edge, depressed center, telangiectasia (lesion formed by dilation of vessels), crusting, and ulceration (Fig. 54.8). Metastasis is rare, although it may be locally invasive.

Squamous cell carcinoma arises from the epidermis. This tumor can occur on sun-exposed areas of the skin and mucous membranes and is mainly seen on the lower lip, neck, tongue, head, and dorsa of the hands. It can occur on normal skin or on a preexisting lesion (actinic keratosis). The lesion appears as a single, crusted, scaled, eroded papule, nodule, or plaque (Fig. 54.9). A neglected lesion appears more rough, scaly, and darker colored. The lesion is fragile and prone to oozing and bleeding. This is a truly invasive car-

Box 54.3

Cultural Considerations

Some African American men have facial hair that is kinky, curls back on itself, and penetrates the skin, which can result in pustules and small keloids. Many use depilatories or electric razors to prevent nicking the skin, which can also cause keloids.

Darker skinned people have an increased incidence of birthmarks and Mongolian spots compared with lighter skinned people, Mongolian spots disappear over time. The nurse must be cautious to not mistake these spots for bruising indicating injury or abuse.

Darker skinned people have a tendency toward an overgrowth of connective tissue components concerned with the protection against infection and repair after injury. Keloid formation is one example of this tendency toward overgrowth of connective tissue. Lymphoma and systemic lupus erythematosus may occur due to this overgrowth of connective tissue.

For people with light skin, such as Germans, Polish, and Irish, prolonged exposure to the sun may increase the incidence of skin cancer. The nurse needs to teach patients to protect themselves from sun exposure to reduce their risk of skin cancer. Nevi (freckles and skin discolorations) occur more often in lighter skinned individuals. They are most common in European Americans, followed by Asians, and then darker skinned African Americans.

cinoma. Metastasis is related to histological type, depth of invasion, and size of the lesion.

Malignant melanoma, as the name implies, is a malignant growth of pigment cells (melanocytes) (Fig. 54.10). It is highly metastatic, with a higher mortality rate than basal or squamous cell carcinoma. This tumor can occur anywhere on the body, and about half arise from pre-existing nevi or moles. There are three general types: lentigo maligna, superficial spreading, and nodular.

Lentigo maligna melanoma appears as a slow-growing dark macule on exposed skin surfaces (especially the face) of elderly patients (Fig. 54.11) The lesion has irregular borders and brown, tan, and black coloring. Prognosis is good if treated in the early stage.

Superficial spreading melanoma is the most common melanoma. It can occur anywhere on the body and is usually seen in middle-aged persons. The lesion appears as a slightly elevated plaque with an irregular border. The coloring of the lesion varies in combinations of black, brown, and pink. The fragile surface may bleed or ooze. Eventually the plaque develops into a nodule. The cure rate is excellent when it is in the plaque phase; prognosis is poor with the nodular phase.

(Text continued on page 1238)

TABLE 54.5 BENIGN SKIN LESIONS

Type	Description	Treatment
Cyst	A saclike growth with a definite wall that may contain liquid, semifluid, or solid material An epidermal cyst is a saclike growth of the upper portion of a hair follicle. It is due to blockage of the pilosebaceous follicle. It is a soft hemispherical nodule, usually with an overlying comedo, that is usually seen on the face, neck, or upper trunk. It is usually symptomatic. A pilar cyst, or sebaceous cyst, is a saclike growth of the middle portion of the hair follicle that contains hair and cuticlelike material. It is a hard, hemispherical nodule without a surmounted pore that is usually seen on the scalp. 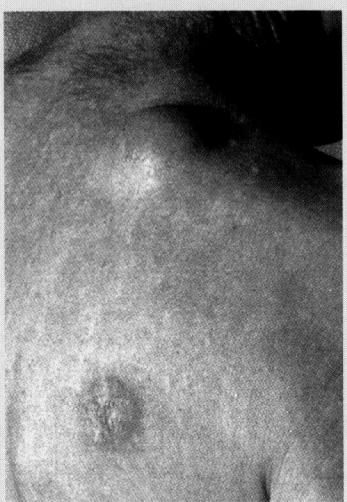 Epidermoid cyst.	Treatments include surgical excision, intralesional steroid therapy, low-dose radiation, and pressure garments worn over the area, or a combination of these therapies. If bothersome, it may be surgically excised. If excision is done, the entire cyst wall is removed to prevent recurrence.
Seborrheic Keratosis	A benign skin lesion that is pigmented light tan to dark brown patches. The plaques or papules have a "stuck on" appearance caused by the proliferation of epidermal cells and keratin piled on the skin surface. Cause is unknown, but it tends to occur in middle-aged to older patients, most commonly on the trunk, scalp, face, and extremities. 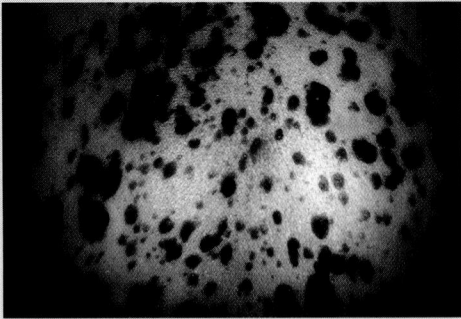 Seborrheic keratosis.	Treatment is cosmetic only, or if lesion becomes irritated from friction. Liquid nitrogen cryotherapy or light curettage is performed if necessary for removal.
Keloid	A benign growth of fibrous tissue (scar formation) at the site of trauma or surgical incision; occurs in various sizes. Growth of tissue is out of proportion to what is needed for normal healing. The benign wartlike lesion or nodule extends beyond the original injury and occurs mainly in middle-aged and elderly clients and darker skinned patients.	Treatment varies, is not always successful, and is difficult; a larger scar may ensue.

Type	Description	Treatment

Pigmented Nevus

A benign, flesh-colored to dark brown macule or papule located randomly over the entire skin surface of the body. Can be inherited or acquired and occurs mostly in light-skinned patients. Usually begin to appear between 1 to 4 years of age, increasing in number into adulthood. Some contain a few hairs. There are many variations.

Rate of transformation to a malignant melanoma is higher in congenital moles and larger lesions. Clinical signs to observe for in differentiating between a mole and a melanoma include change in color or size; inflammation of surrounding skin; irregular borders; spreading borders; variegated colors, especially a bluish pigmentation; bleeding; and oozing, crusting, and itching. Usually nevi larger than 1 cm should be carefully examined.

Treatment is indicated for any of the previously listed indications of melanoma, unsightly nevi (cosmetic), repeated irritation (rubbing from belt, bra), trauma, large moles, and client report of a change in the mole.

Surgical removal can include excision (preferred) or surgical shave. All excised moles should be examined histologically.

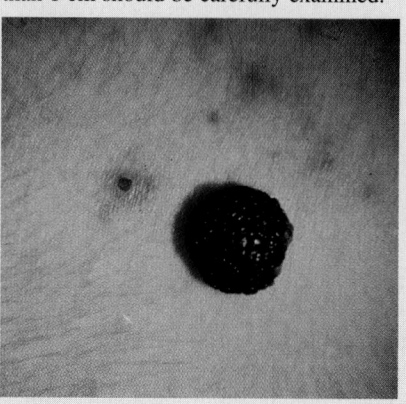

Dermal mole.

Wart

Small, common, benign growth of the skin resulting from the hypertrophy of the papillae and epidermis

Caused by a virus

Common warts, often seen on hands and fingers, appear as raised, flesh-colored papules that have a rough surface. These warts may crack, fissure, bleed, and be painful to lateral pinching and direct, firm pressure.

Plantar warts occur on the sole of the foot. They may appear granular, pitted, or protuberant, with a callous of surrounding normal skin.

Incubation period can be several weeks to months. Virus is spread by direct contact into areas of broken skin or to other nails by nail cuticle biting.

If no pain or discomfort, no treatment may be indicated.

Patient should be cautioned not to spread lesions by picking or biting them.

Treatment is indicated for symptomatic warts and for cosmetic purposes. General treatments include kerolytic agents (e.g., salicylic acid plasters) to soften and reduce keratin; cryotherapy (liquid nitrogen); and light electrodesiccation and curettage (requires local anesthesia).

Treatment of choice is usually cryotherapy because local anesthesia is not necessary and it leaves little scarring.

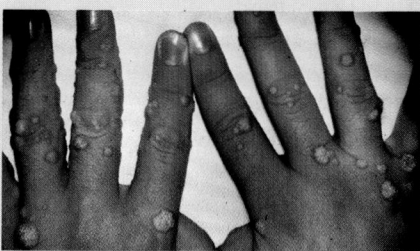

Warts.

(Continued on following page)

TABLE 54.5 BENIGN SKIN LESIONS *(Continued)*

Type	Description	Treatment
Hemangioma (Angioma)	Benign vascular tumor of dilated blood vessels that can have varied clinical manifestations Nevus flammeus involves mature capillaries on the face and neck. It is a congenital neoplasm that appears as a pink-red to bluish purple macular patch. Port-wine stains or port-wine angiomas appear as violet-red macular patches, usually singular lesions, growing proportionately as the child grows. These lesions can persist indefinitely. Cherry hemangiomas are commonly seen in the elderly patient. They appear as small round papules that can vary in color from red to purple.	Nevus flammeus is usually treated for cosmetic reasons. Port-wine stains, if large enough, may require surgical excision with skin grafting. Laser therapy may also be used. Noninvasive treatment is the use of cosmetics to camouflage the affected area. Treatment for cherry hemangiomas is usually not prescribed, except for cosmetic purposes.

Nodular melanoma occurs suddenly as a spherical papule or nodule on the skin or in a mole. Coloration is blue-black, blue-gray, or reddish blue color that may have a rim of inflammation. The lesion is fragile and bleeds easily. Metastasis occurs rapidly. This type of melanoma has the least favorable prognosis. Early diagnosis and treatment is imperative.

Prevention

Most types of skin cancer can be prevented by limiting or avoiding direct exposure to ultraviolet rays (sun, tanning booths). If exposure to the sun is necessary, exposure should be avoided during its highest intensity (10 a.m. to 2 p.m.). The patient should use a protective sunscreen with sun protection factor (SPF) of 15 or more. The patient should also wear sun-protective clothing, such as hats and long sleeves. The patient should seek medical advice if there is a change in color, size, shape, sensation, or character of a lesion or mole.

Diagnostic Tests

A preliminary diagnosis can be based on the appearance of the lesion. A definitive diagnosis is made by biopsy. Other tests are performed based on the results of the pathological examination.

Therapeutic Interventions

Medical treatment depends on the type, thickness, and location of the lesion; the stage of the disease; and the age and general health of the patient. Generally, lesions are surgically excised with a 1- to 2-cm margin. Regional node dissection varies; it may be advised if the nodes in the area drain to one group. Grafting may be necessary for closure or repair. Chemotherapy may be used for metastasis. Radiation therapy may be used as adjunct treatment, or may be recommended for patients with a deeply invasive tumor or those who are poor surgical risks. Other therapies that also may be used include cryosurgery and curettage and electrodessication.

Nursing Care

Perform a complete skin assessment. Palpate lesions to determine texture, size, and firmness. Document size, location, color, surface characteristics, pain, discomfort, itching, and bleeding. Note when the patient first discovered the lesion.

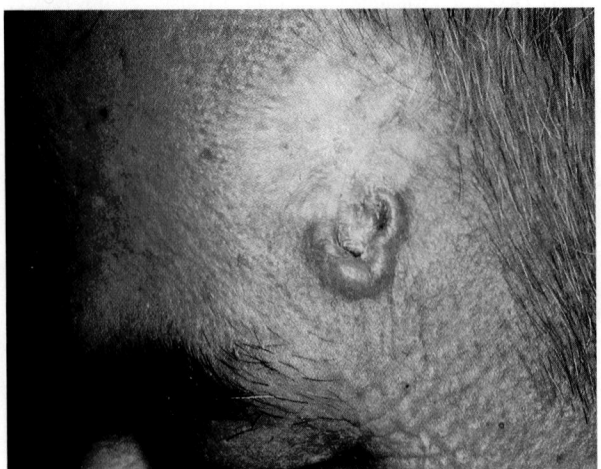

FIGURE 54.8 Basal cell carcinoma. Note pearly, flesh-colored papule with depressed center and rolled edge. *From Goldsmith, LA, Lazarus, GS, and Tharp, MD: Adult and Pediatric Dermatology. F.A. Davis, Philadelphia, 1997, p 158, with permission.)*

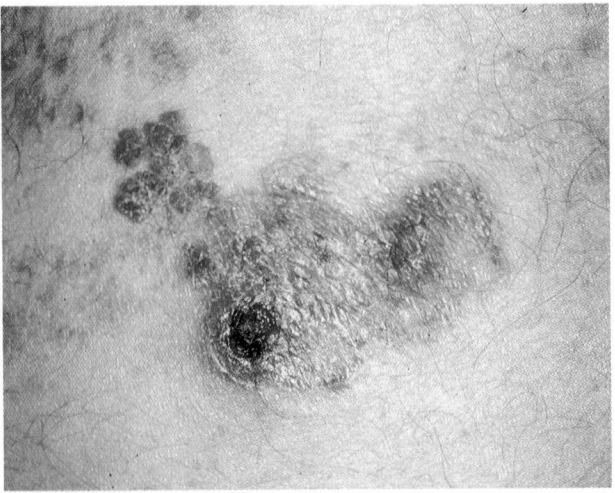

FIGURE 54.9 Squamous cell carcinoma. Surface is fragile and bleeds easily. *(From Goldsmith, LA, Lazarus, GS, and Tharp, MD: Adult and Pediatric Dermatology. F.A. Davis, Philadelphia. 1997, p 237, with permission.)*

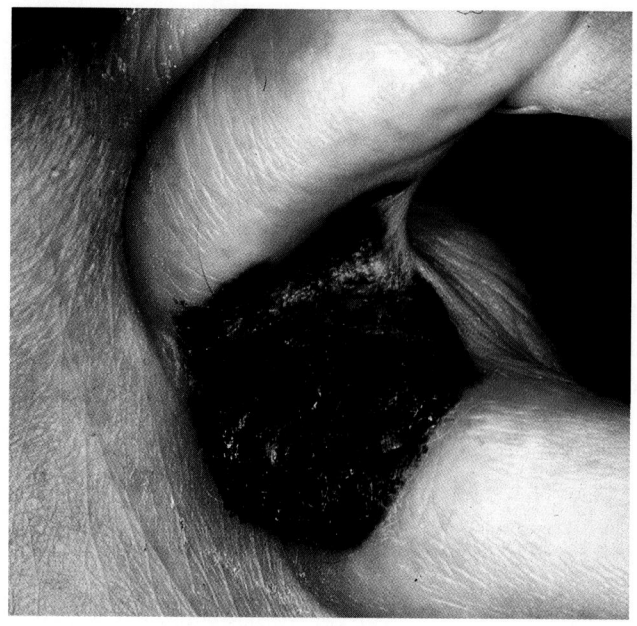

FIGURE 54.10 Malignant melanoma. *(From Goldsmith, LA, Lazarus, GS, and Tharp, MD: Adult and Pediatric Dermatology. F.A. Davis, Philadelphia. 1997, p 137, with permission.)*

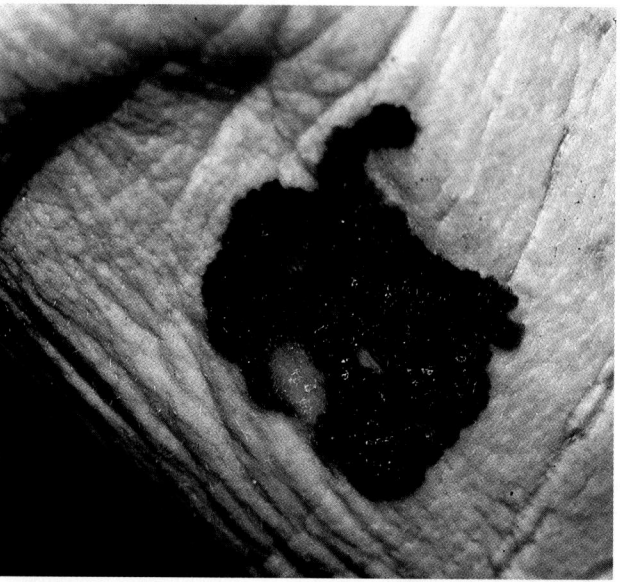

FIGURE 54.11 Lentigo maligna. *(From Goldsmith, LA, Lazarus, GS, and Tharp, MD: Adult and Pediatric Dermatology. F.A. Davis, Philadelphia. 1997, p 55, with permission.)*

Nursing care of the patient with cancer is documented in Chapter 10. Specific nursing care related to cryosurgery includes preparing the patient for the procedure. Minor discomfort can be expected with little or no local anesthesia. Expect swelling, local tenderness, and hemorrhagic blister formation 1 to 2 days after the procedure. After the procedure, the area is cleansed as ordered and prescribed ointments are applied.

Specific nursing care for curettage and electrodesiccation includes preparing the patient for the procedure. After local anesthesia, a dermal curette is used to scrape away the lesion, followed by electrodesiccation of the remaining wound; the wound heals by secondary intention, usually with minimal scarring. After the procedure the wound is cleansed and dressed as prescribed.

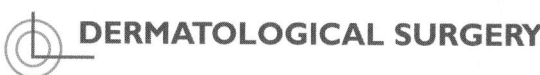 **DERMATOLOGICAL SURGERY**

Plastic or reconstructive surgery is performed to correct certain defects, scars, and malformations, as well as to restore function or prevent further loss of function. This type of surgery is usually an elective procedure; it may be prescribed by the physician or it may be the wish of the patient in hopes of improving his or her body image. Common types of plastic surgical procedures are listed in Table 54.6. Care of the surgical patient is covered in Chapter 11.

TABLE 54.6 COMMON PLASTIC SURGICAL PROCEDURES

Operation	Description	Purpose	Possible Complications	Postoperative Nursing Care Considerations
Rhinoplasty (Nose)	Removal of excessive nasal cartilage, tissue, or bone; reshaping of nose	Correct congenital or acquired septal defects; improve cosmetic shape of nose	Hemorrhage, hematoma; temporary ecchymosis and edema; infection, septal perforation	Monitor dressing and packing for bright-red bleeding; monitor vital signs and level of consciousness; maintain semi-Fowler's position to minimize edema.
Blepharoplasty (Eyelid)	Incisions on upper and lower lids with excision of fat and skin and primary closure	Removal of bags under eyes and wrinkles and bulges	Corneal injury; hematoma; ectropion; rarely visual loss and wound infection	Eye dressings; antibiotic ointment around eyes and lids; discoloration and swelling usually subsides in about 10 days; maintain semi-Fowler's position to minimize edema.

(Continued on following page)

TABLE 54.6 COMMON PLASTIC SURGICAL PROCEDURES *(Continued)*

Operation	Description	Purpose	Possible Complications	Postoperative Nursing Care Considerations
Rhytidoplasty (Face)	Incision anterior to ear with removal of excessive skin and tissue; the subcutaneous tissue and fascia are folded and stretched	Removal of excessive wrinkling or sagging skin	Hemorrhage; hematoma, ecchymosis, and edema (temporary); wound infection, facial nerve damage	Surgical improvement lasts from 5 to10 years; apply antibiotic ointment to suture line; maintain semi-Fowler's position to minimize edema.
Otoplasty (Ear)	Incision of ear for correction of defect	Correct congenital defects; correct deformities; improve cosmetic shape of ear	Hemorrhage; hematoma; edema; wound infection	Ear dressing for about 1 week; protect ear at times of sleep for about 3 weeks.

Home Health Hints

- A wound-measuring device that will not be misplaced is your hand. Measure your hand, such as the nailbed of a particular finger or the space between joints. Use these as a guide to determine wound measurements.
- Sanitary pads make great cushions for bony prominences. You can also place them in a cotton sock for better molding.
- A hand-held shower head is useful in debriding some leg ulcers. Do not use it if it is too painful.
- To relieve pruritus (itchy skin), oatmeal baths are sometimes prescribed. An inexpensive way to do this is to place a half cup of quick-cooking oatmeal in a cotton sock. Put it under the faucet as you fill the tub and ring out the sock.
- Instruct patients to prevent red, dried, cracked skin on hands by wearing gloves outside in the cold or windy weather to prevent chapping, avoiding overheating the house, using a humidifier to keep the air moist, applying hand lotion two or three times a day and after each hand washing, using soaps with added oil and avoiding those with deodorants, using sunscreen with an SPF factor of at least 15, and stopping smoking (smoking reduces blood flow to the skin).
- If necessary, a specialty bed or mattress can be obtained to use in a patient's home.
- Instruct patients who are confined to a wheelchair to rise up briefly, using their armrests, and shift weight every 15 minutes to prevent pressure ulcers.
- Instruct patients with dressings to keep them clean and dry. Unless the patient or caregiver has been instructed on how to perform the dressing change, inform him or her to contact the home care agency if the dressing falls off.
- A patient can wear a cast shoe over a dressing on his or her foot. This will help protect the dressing and provide additional support for the patient while ambulating.
- Surgi-net, or a similar stretchy cover, can be used to cover dressings for patients with tape sensitivities. They are also good for additional support to prevent a dressing from falling off.

REVIEW QUESTIONS

1. Psoriasis is an inflammatory skin disorder that is characterized by which underlying pathology?
   a. Epidermal proliferation
   b. Excessive subcutaneous fat
   c. Herpes infection
   d. Excessive melanin production

2. Which of the following is the most common etiology of malignant skin lesions?
   a. Fair skin, blue eyes, red hair
   b. Genetic predisposition
   c. Overexposure to ultraviolet rays
   d. Numerous moles on body

3. Which of the following actions by the nurse is appropriate when caring for the patient with dermatitis?
   a. Bathe in hot oatmeal baths.
   b. Dry vigorously to prevent moisture build-up.
   c. Apply gloves to hands at night.
   d. Apply a thick layer of the prescribed topical agent.

4. A patient develops several wounds on his sacrum and buttocks in spite of being turned and repositioned regularly. Which factors may have contributed to his skin breakdown? Choose all that apply.
   a. He supplements his regular diet with protein shakes.
   b. He commonly slides down in his chair.
   c. Staff use a lift sheet to move him in bed.
   d. Once repositioned, he often rolls back to his favorite position.
   e. He is often diaphoretic.

5. Which instruction should the nurse provide to the patient being treated for scabies?
   a. "Dry-clean all linens, towels, and clothes."
   b. "Wash linens, towels, and clothes."
   c. "Discard infested mattresses."
   d. "Remove infested pets from the home."

6. A patient with impetigo contagiosa wants to know when he will no longer be contagious. Which response by the nurse is correct?
   a. One week after treatment is started
   b. After spread of lesions has stopped
   c. After all the lesions crust over
   d. When all lesions are healed

SUGGESTED ANSWERS TO

CRITICAL THINKING

■ *Mr. Russ*
- The nurse should assess the patient's mobility and bed surface. A specialty pressure-relieving bed should be ordered for the patient.
- Change patient's position at least every 2 hours if not more frequently. Keep patient's heels off of the bed at all times by propping them on pillows.
- Request a dietary consult as the body cannot meet the increased healing demands if there is an albumin deficiency. Patients will need increased protein if they do not have renal failure. They also need fats, carbohydrates, vitamins, and minerals for wound healing. A dietitian can help determine the amounts of calories and types of foods for the best healing.

- If the patient is able to sit up in a chair, he will need the proper chair cushion to prevent skin breakdown. There are Roho chair cushions which provide pressure relief for patients while they are sitting.
- If the patient is wearing a brace or a splint that must be removed, examine the underlying tissue for pressure areas. Braces and splints must be padded to avoid skin breakdown.

■ *Mrs. Long*
You should ask Mrs. Long if she read the package instructions. She would find that for medicated scalp shampoos to work properly, they must remain on the scalp for several minutes. Package instructions should be carefully checked for each product because they vary from product to product.

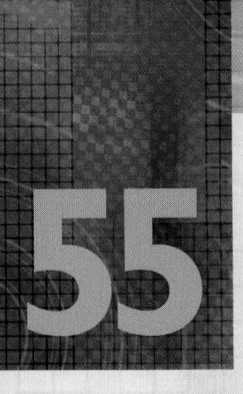

Nursing Care of Patients with Burns

RITA BOLEK TROFINO

QUESTIONS TO GUIDE YOUR READING

1. How would you explain the pathophysiology of burns?

2. What are current therapeutic interventions for burns?

3. What data should you collect when caring for patients with burns?

4. What nursing care will you provide for patients with burns?

5. How will you know if your nursing interventions have been effective?

Many people are hospitalized each year for burns. Burns affect not only the skin but every major body system. Smoke inhalation and wound infections complicate care of the patient who has been burned.

PATHOPHYSIOLOGY AND SIGNS AND SYMPTOMS

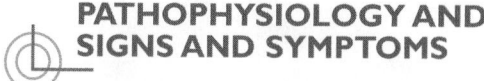

Burns are wounds caused by an energy transfer from a heat source to the body, heating the tissue enough to cause damage. Locally, the heat denatures cellular protein and interrupts the blood supply. The three zones of tissue damage that occur with burns are described in Figure 55.1.

The amount of skin damage is related to (1) the temperature of the burning agent, (2) the burning agent, (3) the duration of exposure, (4) the conductivity of tissue, and (5) the thickness of the involved dermal structures. Alterations in normal skin functioning resulting from a major burn injury include loss of protective functions, impaired ability to regulate temperature, increased risk for infection, changes in sensory function, loss of fluids, impaired skin regeneration, and impaired secretory and excretory functions.

Systemic Responses

The alterations in the functional capacity of the skin affect virtually all major body systems.

Fluid Balance

Following a major burn, increased capillary permeability leads to the leakage of plasma and proteins into the tissue,

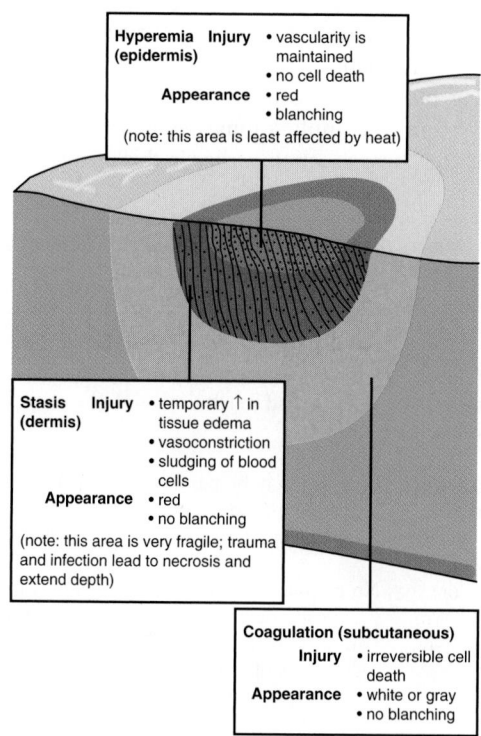

FIGURE 55.1 Three zones of tissue damage. *(Modified from Ruppert, SD, Kernick, JG, and Dolan, JT: Dolan's Critical Care Nursing. F.A. Davis, Philadelphia, 1996, p 942, with permission.)*

resulting in the formation of edema and loss of intravascular volume. There is also water loss by evaporation through burn tissue that can be 4 to 15 times normal. Increased metabolism leads to further water loss through the respiratory system.

Cardiac

Cardiac function is affected. There is an initial decrease in cardiac output, which is further compromised by the circulating plasma volume loss. Severe hematological changes resulting from tissue damage and vascular changes occur in patients with major burns. Plasma moves into the interstitial space because of increased capillary permeability. In the first 48 hours after a burn, fluid shifts lead to hypovolemia and, if untreated, hypovolemic shock. Loss of intravascular fluid causes an increase in hematocrit, and there is red blood cell destruction. The intense heat decreases platelet function and half-life. Leukocyte and platelet aggregation may progress to thrombosis.

Metabolic

Metabolic demands are very high in patients with burns. A high metabolic rate proportional to the severity of the burn is usually maintained until wound closure. This hypermetabolism is further compromised by associated injuries, surgical interventions, and the stress response. Severe catabolism also begins early and is associated with a negative nitrogen balance, weight loss, and decreased wound healing. Elevated catecholamine (epinephrine, norepinephrine) levels are triggered by the stress response. This, along with elevated glucagon levels, can stimulate hyperglycemia.

Gastrointestinal

A few of the gastrointestinal problems that can develop with a major burn include gastric dilation, peptic ulcers, and paralytic ileus. Most of these problems occur in response to fluid shifting, dehydration, opioid analgesics, immobility, depressed gastric motility, and the stress response.

Renal

Acute renal insufficiency can occur as a result of hypovolemia and decreased cardiac output. Fluid loss and inadequate fluid replacement can lead to decreased renal blood flow and glomerular filtration rate. With an electrical burn injury, renal damage can occur from direct electrical current or the formation of myoglobin casts (because of the muscle destruction), which can cause acute renal tubular necrosis.

Pulmonary

Pulmonary effects are mostly related to smoke inhalation. However, hyperventilation may occur and is usually proportional to the severity of the burn. There is increased oxygen consumption resulting from the hypermetabolic state, fear, anxiety, and pain.

Immune

With the skin destroyed, the body loses its first line of defense against infection. Major burns also cause a depression of the immunoglobulins IgA, IgG, and IgM.

Classification of Burn Injuries

The severity of a burn injury is influenced by the depth of destruction, percentage of injury, cause of the burn, age of the patient, concomitant injuries, medical history (e.g., heart disease, diabetes), and location of the burn wound. Table 55.1 describes classification of burn depth (Figs. 55.2, 55.3, and 55.4).

CRITICAL THINKING

Mr. Weinberg

■ Mr. Weinberg is admitted to hospital with superficial and deep partial thickness burns. His wife asks how long it will take for the burns to heal. What should you tell her?

Suggested answers at end of chapter.

The size of a burn wound is estimated based on parts of the body affected. A common method is the Rule of Nines. This method divides the body into segments whose areas are either 9% or multiples of 9% of the total body surface, with the perineum being counted as 1% (Fig. 55.5). This formula is easy, but it is not as accurate in assessing children. A more accurate method uses a table with a relative anatomical scale or diagram that estimates total burned area by ages and by smaller anatomical areas of the body.

LEARNING TIP

For a quick estimation of percentage of burn injury, using the Rule of Nines on an adult burn patient, the palm of your hand is about 1%.

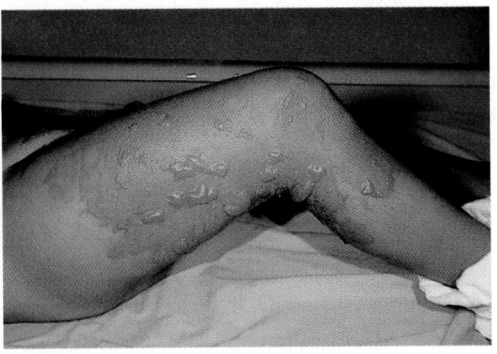

FIGURE 55.2 Partial-thickness burn. *(From Trofino, RB: Nursing Care of the Burn-Injured Patient. F.A. Davis, Philadelphia, 1991, plate 1, with permission.)*

 ETIOLOGY

Burn injuries have many causes. The most common causes include flame, contact, chemical, electrical, and radiation (Table 55.2).

 COMPLICATIONS

A major complication that can occur with a flame burn in an enclosed space is inhalation injury. Infection is another common complication with a major burn. The incidence of infection increases with the size of the burn wound because the first line of defense against microorganisms is the skin.

Neurovascular compromise can also occur with a major burn. Eschar formation creates pressure and contributes to decreasing blood flow to areas distal to the burned area. Other systemic complications were reviewed in the Systemic Responses section earlier in this chapter.

TABLE 55.1 CLASSIFICATION OF BURN DEPTH

Classification	Formerly	Areas Involved	Appearance	Sensitivity	Healing Time
Partial-thickness (superficial)	1st degree to 2nd degree	Epidermis Papillae of dermis	Bright red to pink. Blanches to touch. Serum-filled blisters. Glistening, moist.	Sensitive to air, temperature, and touch	7–10 days
Partial-thickness (deep)	2nd degree	Epidermis, 1/2 to 7/8 of dermis	Blisters may be present. Pink to light red to white. Soft and pliable. Blanching present.	Pressure may be painful from exposed nerve endings.	14–21 days. May need grafting to decrease scarring.
Full-thickness	3rd degree to 4th degree	Epidermis Dermis Tissue Muscle Bone	Snowy white, gray, or brown. Texture is firm and leathery. Inelastic.	No pain as nerve endings are destroyed, unless surrounded by areas of partial-thickness burns	Needs grafting to complete healing

Source: Trofino, RB: Nursing management of the patient with burns. In Ruppert, SD, Kernick, JG, and Dolan, JT (eds): Dolan's Critical Care Nursing. F.A. Davis, Philadelphia, 1996, p 943.

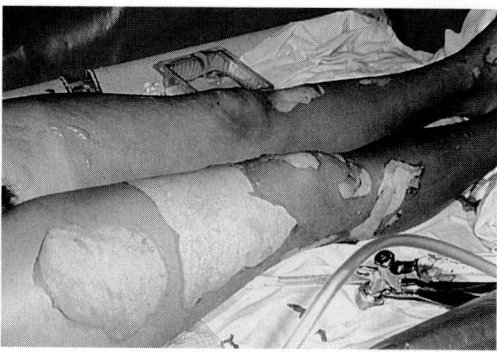

FIGURE 55.3 Partial-thickness burn. *(From Trofino, RB: Nursing Care of the Burn-Injured Patient. F.A. Davis, Philadelphia, 1991, plate 2, with permission.)*

CRITICAL THINKING

Mrs. Rivera

■ Mrs. Rivera is admitted to the emergency room after sustaining injuries from a house fire. Both arms and hands are burned, she has a right leg fracture and a possible neck fracture, her lips are swollen, her face is sooty, and she is spitting up grayish, blackish sputum.
1. What is your priority concern with all of these injuries?
2. An IV is ordered at 1 L over 6 hours. How many milliliters per hour should be set on the controller?

DIAGNOSTIC TESTS

Burns are diagnosed through clinical manifestations. Various diagnostic tests are performed for systemic reactions, infection, and other complications. Common tests for systemic reactions include complete blood cell count (CBC) and differential, blood urea nitrogen (BUN), serum glucose and electrolytes, arterial blood gases, serum protein and albumin, urine cultures, urinalysis, clotting studies, cervical spine series, electrocardiogram, wound cultures, and, if

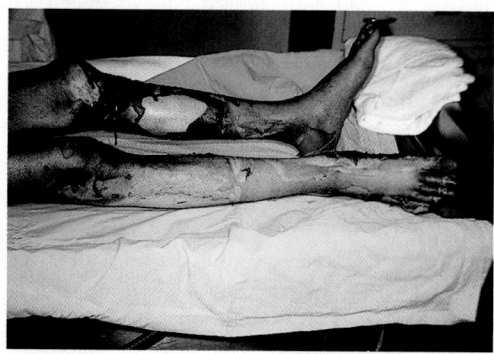

FIGURE 55.4 Full-thickness burn. *(From Trofino, RB: Nursing Care of the Burn-Injured Patient. F.A. Davis, Philadelphia, 1991, plate 3, with permission.)*

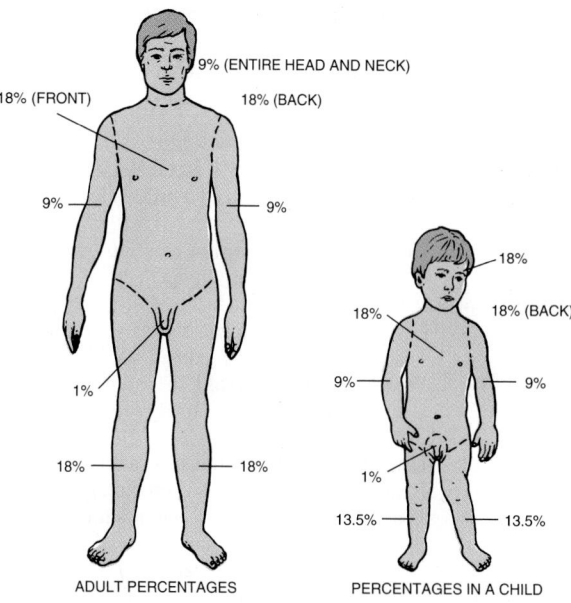

9% (ENTIRE HEAD AND NECK)
18% (FRONT)   18% (BACK)
9%   9%
1%
18%   18%

ADULT PERCENTAGES

18%
18%   18% (BACK)
9%   9%
1%
13.5%   13.5%

PERCENTAGES IN A CHILD

RULE OF NINES

FIGURE 55.5 Estimation of extent of burn injury. (From Venes, D [ed]: Taber's Cyclopedic Medical Dictionary, ed. 19. F.A. Davis, Philadelphia, 2001. Beth Anne Willert, MS, Dictionary Illustrator, with permission.)

there is a suspected inhalation injury, arterial blood gases, bronchoscopy, and carboxyhemoglobin levels.

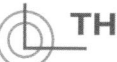 THERAPEUTIC INTERVENTIONS

Therapeutic interventions vary according to the severity of the burn and the stage the patient is in. Treatment is managed over three overlapping stages (Table 55.3).

Emergent Stage

At the time of injury, the burning process must be stopped. The clothes are removed, and the wound is cooled with tepid water and covered with clean sheets to decrease shivering and contamination. The burn wound itself takes a lower priority to the ABCs (airway, breathing, circulation) of trauma resuscitation. The patient should be stabilized in terms of fractures, hemorrhage, spine immobilization, and other injuries. Inhalation injury is suspected if the patient sustained a burn from a fire in an enclosed space or was exposed to smoldering materials, if the face and neck were burned, if there are vocal changes, and if the patient is coughing up carbon particles. Intravenous fluids are given to prevent and treat hypovolemic shock. The patient is treated for pain with appropriate IV opioid analgesics. Patient-controlled analgesia (PCA) is very effective.

An accurate history of the injury is obtained to determine severity, probable complications, and any associated trauma. The patient's medical history is also obtained. Admission to the facility and burn care treatment are explained to the patient and family.

TABLE 55.2 COMMON CAUSES OF BURNS

Flame	House fire is a common cause.
	Usually associated with an inhalation injury.
	Flash injury occurs from a sudden ignition or explosion.
Contact	Hot tar, hot metals, or hot grease produce a full-thickness injury on contact.
Scald	A burn from hot liquid.
	Common in children less than 5 years and adults older than 65 years.
	With an immersion scald, there are usually no splash marks; usually involves lower regions of body.
Chemical	Usually occurs in an industrial setting.
	Extent and depth of injury are directly proportional to concentration and quantity of agent, duration of contact, and chemical activity and penetrability of agent.
Electrical	One of the most serious types of burn injury; can be full thickness with possible loss of limbs, as well as cause internal injuries.
	Entry wound is usually ischemic, charred, and depressed.
	Exit wound may have an explosive appearance.
	Extent of injury depends on voltage, resistance of body, type of current, amperage, pathway of current, and duration of contact.
	Bones offer greatest resistance to the current; can have much damage.
	Tissue fluid, blood, and nerves offer least resistance; therefore, the current travels this path.
Radiation	Can occur in an industrial setting, due to treatment of diseases, or from ultraviolet light (sun or tanning salons).
	Severity depends on type of radiation, duration of exposure, depth of penetration, distance from source, and absorbed dose.

NURSING CARE TIP

Interview all involved family members to determine the cause of the injury, as well as past and current medical history. The patient may not be able to verbalize current medical conditions, current medications, and so forth. Getting a full description of the cause of the injury may lead to the detection of other injuries that may not be readily visible.

Acute Stage

If the patient is in a facility with a special burn unit, multidisciplinary care from a burn team is provided during the acute stage. Management goals include wound closure with no infection, minimum scarring, maximum function, maintenance of comfort as much as possible, adequate nutritional support, and maintenance of fluid, electrolyte, and acid-base

TABLE 55.3 STAGES OF BURN CARE

Stage	Duration
I (Emergent)	From onset of injury to completion of fluid resuscitation
II (Acute)	From start of diuresis to near completion of wound closure
III (Rehabilitation)	From wound closure to return of optimal level of physical and psychosocial function

Source: Trofino, RB: Nursing management of the patient with burns. In Ruppert, SD, Kernick, JG, and Dolan, JT (eds): Dolan's Critical Care Nursing. F.A. Davis, Philadelphia, 1996, p 948.

balance. The patient continues to be medicated for pain as needed, especially before painful treatments. Nutritional support is maintained via a small Silastic nasogastric feeding tube (Box 55.1 Nutrition Notes).

The wound is cleansed and debrided daily to promote healing, prevent infection, and provide a clean bed for grafting. Wound cleansing is achieved by tubbing with a

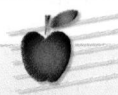

Box 55.1

Nutrition Notes

Burns

The body's response to severe stress, whether caused by trauma, sepsis, or burns, occurs in three stages: ebb (hypometabolic), flow (hypermetabolic), and anabolic (recovery), each driven by hormonal changes that affect the storage, breakdown, and utilization of various nutrients. In addition, a person does not necessarily progress linearly through the stages but may regress several times, although a burned patient may be hypermetabolic for several weeks. Consequently, multiple means are used to monitor a patient's status and a team effort is required to frequently revise nutrient prescriptions to avoid both underfeeding and overfeeding (also a cause of complications).

The first concern is replacement of fluid that is lost through the burned area, which may receive 10 times the blood flow to normal skin, and provision of sufficient fluid to excrete waste products of metabolism. The next concern is meeting the patient's energy needs since a major burn is the most severe stress a person can sustain, doubling caloric needs if greater than 50% of the body surface is affected. If nutrients are not available from external sources, the body breaks down muscle tissue for this energy requirement. As in other conditions, tube feeding (often into the small intestine rather than the stomach) is preferred to intravenous nutrition if the patient can tolerate it. The patient's condition and ability to utilize the nutrients dictates the mode of nutrition implemented.

Hubbard tank, showering using a shower trolley or shower chair, and bedside care.

Debridement, or the removal of nonviable tissue (eschar), can be mechanical, chemical, surgical, or a combination of these methods. Mechanical debridement can involve the use of scissors and forceps to manually excise loose nonviable tissue, or the use of wet-to-moist or wet-to-dry fine mesh gauze. Chemical debridement involves the use of a proteolytic enzymatic debriding agent that digests necrotic tissue. Surgical debridement is the excision of full-thickness and deep partial-thickness burns. This method is followed by an application of a skin graft.

If the patient has a circumferential burn (one that surrounds an extremity or area), an increase in tissue pressure secondary to tissue edema occurs. The burn then acts like a tourniquet, impeding arterial and venous flow. Common sites for these burns are the extremities, trunk, and chest. If this occurs on the chest and trunk, respiratory insufficiency can occur as a result of restricted chest expansion. An **escharotomy** is immediately necessary to relieve this pressure. An escharotomy is a linear excision through the eschar to the superficial fat that allows for expansion of the skin and return of blood flow (Fig. 55.6).

NURSING CARE TIP
Remember to provide adequate padding of the bed with an escharotomy, as there can be copious amounts of drainage. Provide for appropriate disposal of the drainage.

Once the area is cleaned, the burn dressing and topical treatment are prescribed. The type of dressing and topical agent chosen are dependent on the area involved, extent and depth of injury, and physician preference. Several common topical agents are listed in Table 55.4.

Dressings may be open, closed, biological, synthetic, or a combination. The open method is the use of a topical agent without any dressing. The closed method involves the

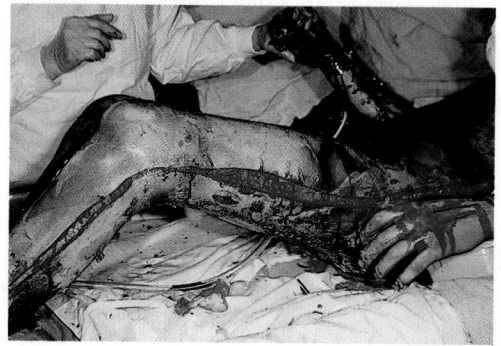

FIGURE 55.6 Escharotomy. *(From Trofino, RB: Nursing Care of the Burn-Injured Patient. F.A. Davis, Philadelphia, 1991, plate 16, with permission.)*

escharotomy: eschara—scab + otomy—incision

use of an occlusive dressing over the wound. General principles for dressings include the following:

1. Limit the bulk of the dressing to facilitate range of motion.
2. Never wrap skin-to-skin surfaces (e.g., wrap fingers or toes separately; place a donut gauze dressing around the ear).
3. Base dressings on the size of wounds, absorption, protection, and type of debridement.
4. Wrap extremities distal to proximal to promote venous return.
5. Elevate affected extremities.

Biological dressing refers to tissue from living or deceased humans (cadaver skin), deceased animals (e.g., pigskin), or cellular dressings that may use animal tissue, human tissue, and synthetics. Biological dressings assist with wound healing and stimulate **epithelialization.** These dressings may be used as donor site dressings, to manage a partial-thickness burn, and to cover the clean, excised wound before autografting. Some of the cellular wound dressings have varied layers that form a matrix onto which the patient's own cells migrate over a few weeks and form a new dermis. A very thin layer of the person's own skin is then grafted onto this new dermis.

Synthetic dressings are used in the management of partial-thickness burns and donor sites. These dressings are more readily available, less costly, and easier to store than biological dressings. They are made from a variety of materials and come in many different sizes and shapes. Most of these dressings contain no antimicrobial agents.

Biological and synthetic dressings are used as temporary wound coverings over clean partial- and full-thickness injuries. They act as skin substitutes to help maintain the wound surface until healing occurs, a donor site becomes available, or the wound is ready for autografting.

Skin Grafts
An autograft is a skin graft from the patient's unburned skin to be placed on the clean excised burn. The two common types of autografts are the split-thickness skin graft (STSG), which includes the epidermis and part of the dermis, and the full-thickness skin graft (FTSG), which includes the epidermis and entire dermal layer.

An STSG (0.006 to 0.016 inch) may be applied as a sheet graft or a meshed graft. A sheet graft is used for cosmetic effect, such as for a face, neck, upper chest, breast, or hand burn. It is placed on the area as a full sheet. A meshed graft is passed through a mesher that produces tiny splits in the skin, similar to a fishnet, with openings in the shape of diamonds (Fig. 55.7), to permit the skin to expand one and a half to nine times its original size. The meshing allows for coverage of a large burn area with a small piece of skin by stretching it and securing it with sutures or staples. A mesh graft is especially useful when there are extensive burns

epithelialization: epi—over + thele—nipple + ization—condition

TABLE 55.4 COMMON TOPICAL ANTIBIOTIC AGENTS

Medication Class/Action	Examples	Route	Side Effects	Nursing Implications
Broad-spectrum Antibiotics	Silver sulfadiazine 1% cream	Topical	Intermediate penetration of eschar; leukopenia.	Buttered on in thick layer, covered with light dressings once or twice a day.
	Mafenide acetate (Sulfamylon)	Topical	Pain on application. Pulmonary toxicity. Metabolic acidosis. Inhibits wound healing. Hypersensitivity.	Buttered on. Open exposure method. Applied three to four times daily.
	Silver nitrate solution 0.5%	Topical	Poor penetration of eschar. Ineffective on established wound infections. Can cause an electrolyte imbalance. Discoloration of wound and environment makes assessment difficult.	Wet dressings. Change bid. Resoak every 2 hours.
	Bacitracin	Topical	Poor penetration of eschar. Not effective in reducing sepsis in large burns. Occasional allergic sensitivity.	Buttered on. Reapply every 4–6 hours.
	Gentamicin	Topical	Ototoxic, nephrotoxic. Pain on application.	Apply gently three to four times daily.
	Nitrofurazone	Topical	Painful application. May lead to overgrowth of fungus and *Pseudomonas*.	Apply thin layer directly to wounds or impregnate into gauze. Change dressings twice daily.

resulting in few available donor sites. Graft "take," or vascularization, is complete in about 3 to 5 days.

Full-thickness skin grafts (0.035 to 0.040 inch) can be sheet grafts or pedicle flaps. FTSGs are used over areas of muscle mass, soft tissue loss, hands, feet, and eyelids. They are not used for extensive wounds because the donor sites usually require an STSG for closure, or closure from the wound edges. A pedicle graft or flap includes the skin flap and subcutaneous tissue that is attached by its pedicle to a blood supply (artery and vein); it is then attached to the area in need of grafting. Once the distal part of the graft takes, it remains in place and the flap is divided, with the remainder returning to the original site. Pedicle flaps are not as popular as free skin flaps because they require more than one sur-

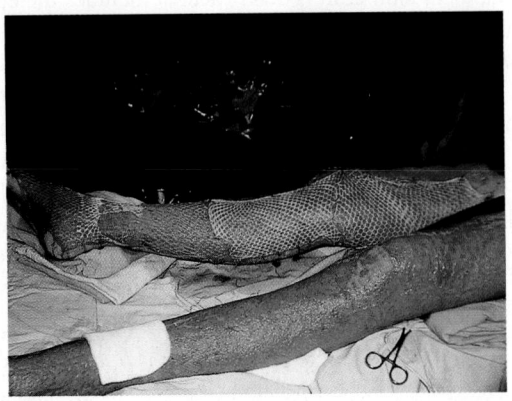

FIGURE 55.7 Meshed graft. *(From Trofino, RB: Nursing Care of the Burn-Injured Patient. F.A. Davis, Philadelphia, 1991, plate 17, with permission.)*

gery and take longer for the graft site and donor site to heal. Table 55.5 provides a comparison of split-thickness and full-thickness grafts.

Donor sites are considered a partial-thickness wound. Donor sites usually heal in 10 to 14 days, but this is dependent on thickness and method of grafting and the general health of the patient. Treatment for the donor site varies with the individual patient, the area of the body, and physician preference. Considerations for care include promoting comfort and preventing trauma and infection. Use of semiocclusive, transparent dressings such as Op-Site or Tegaderm allow a moist healing environment and are associated with reduced risk of infection. The donor site is very painful. Appropriate pain medications are provided, along with nonpharmacological measures (e.g., back rub, distraction).

With any type of graft, the patient must keep the graft site immobilized until the graft takes to prevent movement or slippage of the grafted skin. Dressings may be bulky to assist in immobilization. These dressings must not be disturbed. The involved area requires frequent circulatory checks (color, warmth, sensation, pulses, and capillary refill). Any involved extremities must be elevated to maintain circulation. Table 55.6 describes factors affecting graft viability. A graft has been successful if there is good adherence of the graft to the wound with no evidence of necrosis or infection.

Rehabilitation Phase

The therapy started during the acute phase continues in the rehabilitation phase. There is wound closure, and the goal is

TABLE 55.5 COMPARISON OF SPLIT-THICKNESS AND FULL-THICKNESS SKIN GRAFTS

	Split-Thickness	Full-Thickness
Layers	Epidermis Partial layer of dermis	Epidermis Entire dermal layer
Advantages	Donor site may be reused Healing of donor site is more rapid, results in good "take"	Allows more elasticity over joints Can reconstruct cosmetic defects Soft, pliable Gives full appearance Provides good color-match Less hyperpigmentation May allow hair growth
Disadvantages	Prone to chronic breakdown Likely to hypertrophy More likely to contract	Donor site takes longer to heal Requires split-thickness graft to heal or closure from wound edges

Source: Konop, D: General local treatment. In Trofino, RB (ed): Nursing Care of the Burn-Injured Patient. F.A. Davis, Philadelphia, 1991, p 61.

to return the patient to an optimum level of physical and psychosocial function. This may take months to years to accomplish, depending on the extent of the injury. Reconstructive surgery can be ongoing for many years.

Two things to keep in mind when caring for the patient with a major burn are that (1) the most comfortable position (flexion) is the position of contracture, and (2) the burn wound will shorten until it meets an opposing force. To

TABLE 55.6 FACTORS AFFECTING GRAFT VIABILITY

Factors Inhibiting Graft "Take"	Factors Promoting Graft "Take"
Infection	Adequate hemostasis
Necrotic skin (tissue)	Anatomical location of graft
Anatomic location of graft	Smooth contour
Perineum	Nonjoint areas
Axillae	Graft secured well
Buttocks	Immobilization of graft area
Poor-quality donor skin	Good nutritional status
Poor nutritional status	
Bleeding	
Mechanical trauma	
Shock	

Source: Konop, D: General local treatment. In Trofino, RB (ed): Nursing Care of the Burn-Injured Patient. F.A. Davis, Philadelphia, 1991, p 62.

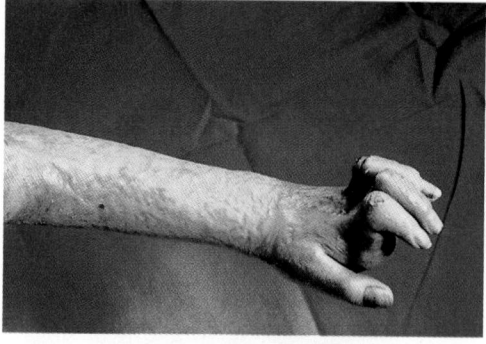

FIGURE 55.8 Burn deformity: contracture. *(From Trofino, RB: Nursing Care of the Burn-Injured Patient. F.A. Davis, Philadelphia, 1991, plate 36, with permission.)*

avoid contractures (Fig. 55.8), a specific exercise program is begun 24 to 48 hours after injury, along with the use of splinting devices to maintain proper positioning and stretching. Hypertrophic scarring, or a proliferation of scar tissue, can be minimized or prevented through the use of a pressure garment (Fig. 55.9).

The burn affects the patient's psychosocial status in many ways. The magnitude of these effects are related to the age of the patient, location of the burn (e.g., face, hands), recovery from injury, cause of the injury (especially if related to negligence or a deliberate act), and ability to continue at preburn level of normal daily activities. The patient may experience a disruption of role function and general health and coping ability. Treatment involves the patient and significant others. Support groups, counselors, and psychiatrists should be utilized appropriately.

CRITICAL THINKING

Mrs. Potter

■ Mrs. Potter is recovering from partial-thickness burns and skin grafts. She mentions that she and her family will be going on a much needed vacation to the shore. What concerns do you have?

NURSING PROCESS FOR A BURNED PATIENT

Assessment/Data Collection

A major burn is painful and frightening to the patient and frightening to the family. Elicit information from the patient, family, and rescuers. If the injury occurred in an enclosed space with flames or smoldering materials, inhalation injury is suspected. If an electrical injury has occurred, ask about voltage, duration of contact, host susceptibility (wet or dry skin), entry and exit sites, and associated falls. With

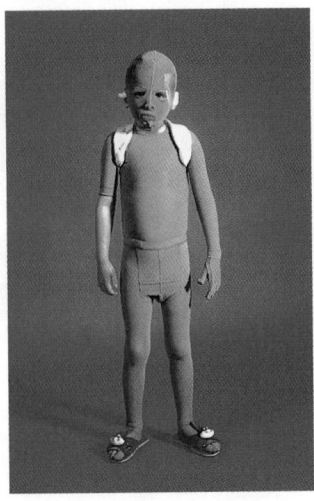

FIGURE 55.9 Full-body pressure garment. *(From Trofino, RB: Nursing Care of the Burn-Injured Patient. F.A. Davis, Philadelphia, 1991, plate 39, with permission.)*

chemical burns, determine type of agent and duration of exposure.

General information to assess in all burns (in addition to normally assessed data, such as medical history, allergies, and current medications) include extent, depth, type and location of the burn; duration of contact with the burning agent; amount and location of pain; and associated injuries. Determine the immediate first aid treatment provided at the scene. Elicit psychosocial information: other people injured, additional losses (home, pets), whether the patient was at fault, and how this injury affects the patient's role function.

Nursing Diagnosis, Planning, Implementation, and Evaluation

See Box 55.2 Nursing Care Plan for the Patient with a Burn Injury and Box 55.3 Burn Summary on page 1255. For more information on burns, go to the American Burn Association website at www.ameriburn.org.

Box 55.2   Nursing Care Plan for the Patient with a Burn Injury

Nursing Diagnosis: Impaired gas exchange related to upper airway edema, carbon monoxide poisoning, edema of alveolar capillary membranes

Expected Outcomes Gas exchange will be improved as evidenced by patent airway, CO level less than 10%, clear lung sounds, Pao_2 80–100 mm Hg, $Paco_2$ 35–45 mm Hg, responsiveness and awareness.

Evaluation of Outcomes Are blood levels improved: CO, Pao_2, $Paco_2$? Do the lungs sound clear on auscultation? Is patient aware of surroundings? Are there no signs of respiratory distress (e.g., retractions, nasal flaring, use of accessory muscles)?

Interventions	Rationale	Evaluation
Assess respiratory status: auscultate breath sounds every 15 minutes or as necessary; note any adventitious breath sounds; observe for chest excursion: monitor ability to cough.	Detects changes in pulmonary function to alter therapy.	What is patient's respiratory status? Are any adventitious lung sounds noted?
Monitor arterial blood gases and CO level.	Assesses level of oxygenation. Helps guide oxygen therapy.	What are the patient's blood gas levels? Are they abnormal?
Monitor for nasal flaring, retractions, wheezing, and stridor.	Stridor may signal upper airway involvement; nasal flaring, retractions, and wheezing may indicate lower airway involvement.	Does patient exhibit nasal flaring, retractions, wheezing, and stridor?
Administer humidified 100% oxygen by tight-fitting face mask for the breathing patient.	Provides oxygen for adequate gas exchange.	Is oxygen administered appropriately? Are blood gases improving?
Elevate head of bed (if no cervical spine injuries or no history of multiple trauma).	Decreases swelling of face and neck.	Is head of bed elevated? Is there any change in facial or neck swelling?
Provide appropriate pulmonary care: turn, cough, deep breathe every 2–4 hours. Provide incentive spirometer every 2–4 hours, suction frequently as needed.	Mobilizes secretions and promotes lung expansion.	Is patient on scheduled activities for vigorous pulmonary care?

Interventions	Rationale	Evaluation
Obtain sputum cultures. Note amount, color, and consistency of pulmonary secretions.	Carbonaceous sputum is diagnostic for smoke inhalation injury. Infection changes color, amount, and consistency of sputum. Culture and sensitivity (C&S) assists in selection of appropriate antibiotic.	Is patient coughing up any sputum? Has character of sputum been documented?
Administer bronchodilators and antibiotics as prescribed.	Bronchodilators decrease bronchospasms and edema; antibiotics fight infection.	Are medications given appropriately?

Nursing Diagnosis: Impaired skin integrity related to thermal injury

Expected Outcomes Skin integrity is improved as evidenced by healing of burned areas with no infection present, healing of burning process.

Evaluation of Outcomes Is burned area healed? Is it free from infection? Did burning process stop?

Interventions	Rationale	Evaluation
Assess burning process. If heat is felt on wound, cool with tepid tap water or sterile water.	Depth of injury increases with length of exposure to burning agent.	Is heat felt over wounds?
Assist registered nurse (RN) or physician to assess the burn area for extent (percentage) and depth (partial thickness, full thickness) of injury.	Provides basis for triage of care. Important also for calculating resuscitation fluid therapy.	What is the estimation of percentage of burn injury? What is depth of injury?
Remove clothing and jewelry.	These items can retain heat and thermal agent, therefore increasing depth of injury. Jewelry can be constrictive when edema develops.	Are clothing and jewelry removed?
Do not apply ice.	Ice causes vasoconstriction, further increasing wound damage. Ice also causes a decrease in core body temperature, which may promote shock.	Is water tepid? Has use of ice been avoided?
Cover patient with clean sheet or blanket.	Prevents excessive heat loss. Decreases pain from air exposure. Protects patient from environmental contamination.	Is patient covered?
Obtain history of burning agent.	Provides information related to depth, duration of contact, and resistance of tissues. If fire scenario, provides clues to possible inhalation injury.	What caused this thermal injury? How long was patient in contact with agent?
Initiate immediate copious tepid water lavage for 20 minutes for all chemical burns, along with simultaneous removal of contaminated clothing. (Do not neutralize chemical because this takes too much time and resulting reaction may generate heat and cause further skin injury.)	Dilution and removal of chemical agent halts burning process. Lavage dissipates heat.	Has lavage been initiated? Were there any injuries to health-care workers?

(Continued on following page)

BOX 55.2 Nursing Care Plan for the Patient with a Burn Injury (Cont'd)

Interventions	Rationale	Evaluation
Brush off dry chemicals before lavage.	To prevent further burn damage due to reaction of dry chemical with water.	
Use heavy rubber gloves or thick gauze for removal of clothing.	Gloves and gauze are necessary to protect health care workers from injury.	
Cleanse wound via tubbing or showers.	Promotes healing and helps decrease infection.	Is burn wound clean and free of wound debris?
Assist RN or physician with debriding wound via surgical, chemical, or mechanical means. Apply topical agent as prescribed.	Promotes healing and healthy granulation bed. Most agents prevent infection and promote healing.	Is there any eschar? Is wound free of wound debris? Is agent applied as directed?
Apply dressing as prescribed.	Dressing types vary and are influenced by area, extent, and depth of injury, as well as by topical agent used. Dressing protects burn area and promotes healing.	Is dressing applied appropriately?
• Do not wrap skin surface to skin surface (e.g., wrap fingers and toes separately; donut bandage around ears).	Wrapping separately prevents webbing and contractures.	
• Limit bulk of dressings.	Mobility is enhanced with less bulky dressing.	
Wrap extremities distal to proximal.	Circulation is increased when extremities are wrapped distal to proximal.	Is wrapping done correctly? Is edema of distal extremity avoided?

Nursing Diagnosis: Deficient fluid volume related to evaporative losses from wound, capillary leak, and decreased fluid intake

Expected Outcomes Patient will maintain adequate circulating volume as evidenced by urine output of 50 mL/hr (in the adult), blood pressure within normal limits, heart rate between 60 and 100 beats per minute (adult), and stabilized body weight.

Evaluation of Outcomes Is urine output maintained at least at 50 mL/hr? Are the blood pressure and heart rate within normal limits? Is patient's weight stable?

Interventions	Rationale	Evaluation
Obtain admission weight and monitor weight daily.	Helps measure fluid loss or gain.	Is patient's weight documented? Is it stable?
Record intake and output (I&O) hourly.	Serves as guide for fluid loss and replacement.	What is patient's I&O?
Assess for signs and symptoms of hypovolemia (hypotension, tachycardia, tachypnea, extreme thirst, restlessness, disorientation).	Fluid volume loss is multifocal (e.g., through increased capillary permeability, insensible loss).	Does patient exhibit any signs or symptoms of hypovolemia?
Monitor electrolytes, complete blood count (CBC).	Serves as guide for electrolyte replacement and blood product replacement.	What are patient's lab values? Are they within normal limits?

Interventions	Rationale	Evaluation
Administer IV fluids as ordered via large bore IV catheter.	Fluid replacement begins immediately. Large vessels are needed for rapid delivery of fluids.	Is patient's fluid replacement adequate? Is catheter patent?
Insert indwelling urinary catheter.	Fluid replacement is titrated based on urine output.	Is catheter patent?
Monitor urine for amount, specific gravity, and hemochromogens.	Specific gravity can predict volume replacement; hemochromogens can cause renal tubular damage.	What are patient's urine values?
Administer osmotic diuretics as ordered; monitor response to therapy.	Decreased urinary output can be caused by decreased renal flow (due to myoglobin in urine).	What is urinary output? Has it changed due to therapy?
Assess gastrointestinal function for absence of bowel sounds. Maintain nasogastric tube.	Splanchnic constriction due to hypovolemia can cause a paralytic ileus.	Are patient's bowel sounds normal? Is nasogastric tube patent?

Nursing Diagnosis: Pain related to burns or graft donor sites

Expected Outcomes Patient will experience pain control as evidenced by verbalizations of pain tolerance, nonverbal cues: less thrashing; able to rest or sleep; body positioning.

Evaluation of Outcomes Does patient verbalize pain control? How many hours of rest/sleep does patient have in 24 hours? Does patient state she or he feels rested?

Interventions	Rationale	Evaluation
Assess level of pain: nature, location, intensity, and duration at various times (during procedures, at rest). Rate pain on visual analog scale.	Provides baseline to monitor response to therapy.	Is patient's individual response to pain documented?
Observe for varied responses to pain: increase in blood pressure, pulse, respiration; increased restlessness and irritability; increased muscle tension; facial grimaces; guarding.	Responses to pain are variable. These parameters change in response to pain.	What are patient's responses to pain? Do responses change with treatment?
Acknowledge presence of pain. Explain causes of pain.	Encourages trust and understanding.	Is patient more trusting of the treatments?
Administer narcotics IV. Utilize patient controlled analgesia (PCA) as appropriate.	IV administration is necessary due to edema and poor tissue perfusion. Narcotics are necessary for severe burn pain. PCA allows patient more control.	Is patient being medicated for pain appropriately?
Offer diversional activities (e.g., music, TV, books, games, relaxation techniques).	Helps patient focus on something other than pain.	Does patient utilize diversional activities? Do they help?
Properly position patient.	Increases comfort.	Is patient positioned as comfortably as possible?
Elevate burned extremities.	Elevation decreases edema and pain.	Are extremities elevated?
Maintain comfortable environment (e.g., bed cradle; comfortable environmental temperature, 86–91.4°F [30–33°C]; quiet environment).	Pressure from bed linens may cause discomfort; with loss of integument, body cannot self-regulate temperature.	Does patient verbalize comfort of environment?

(Continued on following page)

Box 55.2   Nursing Care Plan for the Patient with a Burn Injury *(Cont'd)*

Nursing Diagnosis: Ineffective peripheral tissue perfusion related to circumferential burns, blood loss, decreased cardiac output

Expected Outcomes Patient will maintain adequate tissue perfusion as evidenced by presence of peripheral pulses; minimal edema; intact sensation and motion; and warm extremities.

Evaluation of Outcomes Are peripheral pulses present? Are extremities warm, with adequate sensation, motion, and circulation? Is edema decreased?

Interventions	Rationale	Evaluation
Elevate burned extremity above level of the heart.	Enhances venous return and decreases edema formation.	Are all burned extremities elevated above heart level? Is edema decreasing?
Assess pulses on burned extremities every 15 minutes.	Assesses need for escharotomy.	Are pulses present and documented?
Use Doppler as necessary. Assess capillary refill, sensation, color, swelling, and motion.	Assesses peripheral perfusion.	Is the extremity warm, with adequate color, sensation, motion, and capillary refill?
Assess for numbness, tingling, and increased pain in burned extremity.	Can be indicative of increased pressure from edema.	Does patient complain of numbness, tingling, or pain?
Measure circumference of burned extremities.	Monitors edema formation.	Is there evidence of edema? Is it getting better or worse?
Apply burn dressing loosely.	Prevents constriction and allows for expansion as edema forms.	Is dressing too tight?
Assist with muscle compartment pressures.	Helps determine need for escharotomy (if pressure greater than 25 mm Hg).	What is patient's pressure?
Assist with escharotomy as necessary.	If indicated, removal of eschar allows for edema expansion and permits peripheral perfusion.	Does patient require an escharotomy? Is edema relieved?

Nursing Diagnosis: Risk for sepsis related to wound infection

Expected Outcomes Patient will not develop a wound infection or sepsis.

Evaluation of Outcomes Is there healthy granulation tissue on unhealed areas with less than 10^5 colonies of bacteria on wound culture? Are donor sites free of infection? Have skin grafts taken? Is there absence of clinical manifestation of infection (temperature 98.6°F [37°C]; normal white blood cell [WBC] count)?

Interventions	Rationale	Evaluation
Use sterile technique with wound care.	The unhealed burn wound is a culture medium for bacterial growth.	Is sterile technique used for all wound care?
Maintain protective isolation with good hand-washing technique.	Prevents spread of bacteria from patient to patient or nurse to patient.	Do all persons in contact with patient maintain proper precautions?
Administer immunosupportive medications as prescribed: tetanus and gamma globulin.	Immunoglobulins are depressed at time of severe burn injury.	Does patient require these medications?

Interventions	Rationale	Evaluation
Perform wound care as prescribed, which may include the following: inspect and debride wounds daily; culture wound three times a week or at sign of infection; shave hair at least 1 inch around burn areas (excluding eyebrows); inspect invasive line sites for inflammation (especially if line is through a burn area).	Provides quick identification of bacterial wound invasion and decreases incidence of infection. Presence of hair increases medium for bacterial growth.	What does wound look like? Is it debrided? What are culture results? Is there any hair near burn or line sites?
Continually assess for and report signs and symptoms of sepsis: temperature elevation; change in sensorium; changes in vital signs and bowel sounds; decreased output; positive blood/wound cultures.	The burn patient is at risk for sepsis until wound is healed.	Does patient exhibit any signs or symptoms of sepsis?
Administer systemic antibiotics and topical agents as prescribed.	Antibiotics prevent or treat infection.	Does patient require systemic antibiotics? Are they working? Are topical agents applied appropriately? Is wound healing?

Box 55.3

Burn Summary

Signs and Symptoms	Pain
	Superficial partial thickness—pink to red skin, blisters
	Deep partial thickness—pink to light red or white skin, blisters, blanching
	Full thickness—white, gray, or brown color, firm and leathery
Diagnostic Tests	Wound cultures
	Complete blood count, blood urea nitrogen, glucose, electrolytes, urine studies
Therapeutic Interventions	IV fluid replacement
	Antibiotic/antimicrobial agents
	Analgesics
Complications	Shock
	Wound infection
Priority Nursing Diagnoses	Impaired skin integrity related to thermal injury
	Deficient fluid volume related to evaporative losses from wound, capillary leak, and decreased fluid intake
	Pain related to burns or graft donor sites
	Risk for sepsis related to wound infection

REVIEW QUESTIONS

1. A patient is brought to the emergency department following a house fire, with burns over 36% of his body. The areas are blistered and pinkish white, and very painful when pressure is applied. Which type of burn does he have?
   a. Superficial partial thickness
   b. Deep partial thickness
   c. Full thickness

2. Which of the following actions is appropriate initial treatment of a chemical burn?
   a. Lavage with water.
   b. Neutralize the chemical.
   c. Apply the prescribed topical agent.
   d. Wrap the patient in sterile sheets.

3. A patient is admitted to the emergency department with flame burns to her entire chest, abdomen, back, and upper extremities. Using the Rule of Nines, what is the approximate percentage of burns?
   a. 36%
   b. 45%
   c. 54%
   d. 64%

Multiple response item. Select all that apply.

4. What nursing interventions are appropriate for a patient with a circumferential burn to an extremity?
   a. Apply compression bandages starting at the distal end of the extremity.
   b. Administer analgesics if numbness or tingling occur.
   c. Check neurovascular status hourly.
   d. Assist with escharotomy if indicated.
   e. Elevate the extremity.

5. How will the nurse know if interventions for impaired gas exchange related to smoke inhalation have been effective?
   a. $Paco_2$ is >45 mm Hg
   b. Sao_2 is <90%
   c. pH is 7.34
   d. Pao_2 is 88 mm Hg

Unit Fifteen Bibliography

1. American Burn Association: Burn Incidence Fact Sheet, 2002.
2. Baranoski, S, and Ayello, E: Wound Care Essentials. Lippincott Williams & Wilkins Philadelphia, 2003.
3. Bergstrom, N, Allman, RM, Alvarez, OM, et al: Treatment of pressure ulcers. Clinical Practice Guideline, No. 15. AHCPR Publication No. 95-0652. US Department of Health and Human Services, Public Health Service, Agency for Health Care Policy and Research, Rockville, MD, December 1994.
4. Doctor, JN, Patterson, DR, Mann, R, et al: Health outcome for burn survivors. J Burn Care Rehab 18:490, 1997.
5. Drago, DA: Kitchen scalds and thermal burns in children five years and younger. Pediatrics 115:10, 2005.
6. Dumiel-Peeters, I: Preventing pressure ulcers with massage? AJN 105:31–33, 2005.
7. Fraser, S: Scorched! How to handle different types of burns. Curr Health 31:28, 2005.
8. Gaskin, FC: Detection of cyanosis in the person with dark skin. J Natl Black Nurses Assoc 1:52, 1986.
9. Goldsmith, LA, Lazarus, GS, and Tharp, MD: Adult and Pediatric Dermatology: A Color Guide to Diagnosis and Treatment. F.A. Davis, Philadelphia, 1997.
10. Hall, B: Wound care for burn patients in acute rehabilitation settings. Rehab Nurs 3:114, 2005.
11. Harris, CL, and Fraser, C: Malnutrition in the institutionalized elderly: The effects of wound healing. Ostomy Wound Manage 50:54–63, 2004.
12. Herndon, DN, and Tompkins, RG: Support of the metabolic response to burn injury. Lancet 363:1895, 2004.
13. Hess, CT: Care tips for chronic wounds: pressure ulcers. Adv Skin Wound Care 17:477–479, 2004.
14. Krasner, DL, Rodeheaver, GT, and Sibbald, RS: Chronic Wound Care: A Clinical Source Book for Healthcare Professionals. HMP Communications, Wayne, PA, 2001.
15. Lyder, CH, and Van Rijswijk, L: Pressure ulcer prevention and care. Ostomy Wound Manage Suppl April:2–6, 2005.
16. Ratliff, C: WOCN evidenced based pressure ulcer guideline. Adv Skin Wound Care 18:204–08, 2005.
17. Reeves, JR, and Maibach, H: Clinical Dermatology Illustrated, ed. 3. F.A. Davis, Philadelphia, 1998.
18. Selvaggi, G, Monstrey, S, Van Landuyt, K, et al. Rehabilitation of burn injured patients following lightning and electrical trauma. NeuroRehabilitation 1:35, 2005.
19. Torte, SJ, and Hanifin, JM: Current management and therapy of atopic dermatitis. J Am Acad Dermatol 44: 13–15, 2001.
20. Trofino, RBT: Nursing Care of the Burn-Injured Patient. F.A. Davis, Philadelphia, 1991.

SUGGESTED ANSWERS TO

CRITICAL THINKING

■ *Mr. Weinberg*

In general, superficial partial-thickness burns usually heal in 7–10 days. Deep partial thickness burns may take up to 3 weeks. All of this depends upon the location of the injury, the health of the patient, and if he or she remains infection free.

■ *Mrs. Rivera*

Mrs. Rivera has an inhalation injury. This takes precedence over the burn and other injuries.

1.

$$\frac{1\ L}{6\ hours} \cdot \frac{1000\ mL}{1\ L} = 167\ mL/hour$$

■ *Mrs. Potter*

The burned and graft areas will be sensitive to sunlight for up to 1 year. These areas should be covered, and she needs to use sunscreen anytime she is out in the sun. Her physician should offer guidance as to whether any exposure is safe, and if so, what type of sunscreen agent is recommended.

unit SIXTEEN

UNDERSTANDING MENTAL HEALTH CARE

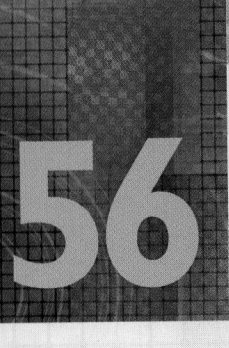

56

Mental Health Function, Assessment, and Therapeutic Measures

MARINA MARTINEZ-KRATZ

KEY TERMS

adaptation (ad-dap-TAY-shun)
affect (AF-feckt)
anxiety (ang-ZIGH-uh-tee)
behavior management (be-HAYV-yer MAN-ij-ment)
cognitive (KOG-ni-tiv)
coping (KOH-ping)
electroconvulsive therapy (ee-LEK-troh kun-VUL-siv THER-uh-pee)
imagery (IM-ij-ree)
insight (IN-sight)
mental health (MEN-tuhl HELLTH)
mental illness (MEN-tuhl ILL-ness)
milieu (meel-YOO)
orientation (OR-ee-en-TAY-shun)
psychoanalysis (SIGH-koh-uh-NAL-i-sis)
psychopharmacology (SIGH-koh-FAR-meh-KAHL-uh-jee)
psychotherapy (SIGH-koh-THER-uh-pee)
stress (STRESS)
stressor (STRESS-er)

QUESTIONS TO GUIDE YOUR READING

1. What are definitions of mental health and mental illness?

2. What are the components of a mental health status assessment?

3. What is the DSM-IV-TR, and what are other methods for diagnosing mental illness?

4. How can you identify common ego defense mechanisms?

5. What is a therapeutic milieu?

6. What are the methods for psychoanalysis, behavior management, cognitive behavioral therapy, humanistic/person-centered therapy, counseling, electroconvulsive therapy, group therapy, and relaxation therapy?

7. What is the LPN/LVN's role in mental health nursing?

REVIEW OF ANATOMY AND PHYSIOLOGY

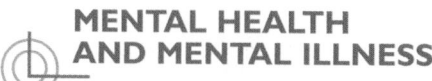

Although there is much debate about the cause(s) of mental illness, it is important to review and understand the anatomy and physiology of the brain and central nervous system (CNS). The brain is involved in thinking, decision making, speaking, emotion, memory, motor and sensory activity, and basic functions such as temperature regulation and breathing, to name a few. In mental health, it is important to distinguish between a neurological disorder (delirium, Parkinson's) and a mental disorder (schizophrenia). Sometimes a patient has both a mental disorder and a neurological or other physical disorder. Refer to Chapter 47 to review the nerves, structure of neurons, synapses, neurotransmitters, and the autonomic nervous system, as well as the structure and function of the brain. Also see Table 56.1 for the possible roles of CNS neurotransmitters in mental illness.

MENTAL HEALTH AND MENTAL ILLNESS

There are differing opinions within the mental health community as to what **mental health** and **mental illness** are. *Mental health* has been defined in many ways. These definitions include the ability to do the following:

- Be flexible
- Be successful
- Form close relationships
- Make appropriate judgments
- Solve problems
- Cope with daily **stress**
- Have a positive sense of self

Mental illness is defined as experiencing the following:

- Impaired ability to think
- Impaired ability to feel
- Impaired ability to make sound judgments
- Impaired ability to adapt
- Difficulty or inability in coping with reality
- Difficulty or inability to form strong personal relationships

It is important to remember that mental health and mental illness exist on a continuum. It is natural for emotions to ebb and flow from day-to-day in response to the degree of stress that is experienced. People who remain mentally healthy are able to keep their stress in perspective. Others are not able to do so, and over time they may develop physical or emotional illnesses as a result of the constant stress in their life.

Visualize the seesaw that children play on. Mental health and mental illness are like a seesaw. When children of approximately equal weight get on each end of the seesaw, they can balance each other and keep the seesaw even. Mentally healthy people keep themselves in a state of emotional balance. Sometimes one child weighs just a little more

than the other and the seesaw tips just a little to one side. Mentally healthy people can cope with this fluctuation. Sometimes another child gets on or one child greatly outweighs the other, and the seesaw gets out of balance completely; one end goes way up while the other goes way down, and it stays there until someone alters the balance. Ultimately it must be the patient who finds his or her own balance. When a person's moods are way down or way up, he is not in emotional homeostasis.

Etiologies

The discussion surrounding the etiologies of mental illness continues to revolve around the "nature versus nurture" or "organic versus inorganic or functional" arguments. The connections between physical and emotional health are so closely intertwined that it is sometimes hard to decide if emotional causes trigger physical responses or vice versa. It is important to have a basic understanding of both the nature and nurture schools of thought on the causes of alterations in mental health.

Explanations of mental illness in this unit include concepts from the psychoanalytic (or psychological) and the psychobiological (or biological) theories. When pertinent, other theories (e.g., behavioral, environmental) are also presented. Most mental illnesses have no identifiable cause. Some etiological theories have stronger positive correlations to illnesses than others. When it is appropriate, this unit gives the most current or most widely accepted view of an etiology.

Social and Cultural Environments

Many professionals in the field of psychology believe that social and cultural environments have a great influence on the way people develop and process life experiences. Some psychoanalysts believe that some cultural traditions and beliefs cause disturbances in personal relationships, which can lead to forms of emotional disturbances. It is part of the nurse's role to take time to learn about the traits that are common among people and those traits that are different. It is important to have an understanding of people's customs and beliefs to avoid unrealistic expectations of patients. See Box 56.1 Cultural Considerations for more detailed information about culture and mental health issues.

Spirituality and Religion

Spirituality and religion are extremely important to some patients and unimportant to others. A person's success in recuperating from physical or emotional illness may be deeply tied to her or his spirituality. It is necessary to be comfortable talking to the patient about spiritual needs while being careful not to impose personal values on the patient. If you are not comfortable in these situations, you should offer to call the spiritual or religious leader of the patient's choice.

It is important to keep the lines of communication open. People learn by sharing with each other. It is much

(Text continued on page 1264)

TABLE 56.1 NEUROTRANSMITTERS IN THE CNS

Neurotransmitter	Location/Function	Possible Implications for Mental Illness
I. Cholinergics		
A. Acetylcholine	ANS: Sympathetic and parasympathetic presy-naptic nerve terminals; parasympathetic post-synaptic nerve terminals CNS: Cerebral cortex, hippocampus, limbic structures, and basal ganglia Functions: Sleep, arousal, pain perception, movement, memory	Increased levels: Depression Decreased levels: Alzheimer's disease, Huntington's disease, Parkinson's disease
II. Monoamines		
A. Norepinephrine	ANS: Sympathetic postsynaptic nerve terminals CNS: Thalamus, hypothalamus, limbic system, hippocampus, cerebellum, cerebral cortex Functions: Mood, cognition, perception, loco-motion, cardiovascular functioning, and sleep and arousal	Decreased levels: Depression Increased levels: Mania, anxiety states, schizophrenia
B. Dopamine	Frontal cortex, limbic system, basal ganglia, thalamus, posterior pituitary, and spinal cord Functions: Movement and coordination, emo-tions, voluntary judgment, release of pro-lactin	Decreased levels: Parkinson's disease and depression Increased levels: Mania and schizophrenia
C. Serotonin	Hypothalamus, thalamus, limbic system, cere-bral cortex, cerebellum, spinal cord Functions: Sleep and arousal, libido, appetite, mood, aggression, pain perception, coordi-nation, judgment	Decreased levels: Depression Increased levels: Anxiety states
D. Histamine	Hypothalamus	Decreased levels: Depression
III. Amino Acids		
A. Gamma-amino-butyric acid (GABA)	Hypothalamus, hippocampus, cortex, cerebel-lum, basal ganglia, spinal cord, retina Functions: Slowdown of body activity	Decreased levels: Huntington's disease, anxiety disorders, schizophrenia, and various forms of epilepsy
B. Glycine	Spinal cord and brain stem Functions: Recurrent inhibition of motor neurons	Toxic levels: "glycine encephalopathy," decreased levels are correlated with spastic motor movement
C. Glutamate and aspartate	Pyramidal cells of the cortex, cerebellum, and the primary sensory afferent systems; hippocampus, thalamus, hypothalamus, spinal cord Functions: Relay of sensory information and in the regulation of various motor and spinal reflexes	Increased levels: Huntington's disease, temporal lobe epilepsy, spinal cere-bellar degeneration
IV. Neuropeptides		
A. Endorphins and enkephalins	Hypothalamus, thalamus, limbic structures, midbrain, and brain stem; enkephalins are also found in the gastrointestinal tract Functions: Modulation of pain and reduced peristalsis (enkephalins)	Modulation of dopamine activity by opi-oid peptides may indicate some link to the symptoms of schizophrenia
B. Substance P	Hypothalamus, limbic structures, midbrain, brain stem, thalamus, basal ganglia, and spinal cord; also found in gastrointestinal tract and salivary glands Function: Regulation of pain	Decreased levels: Huntington's disease and Alzheimer's disease Increased levels: Depression
C. Somatostatin	Cerebral cortex, hippocampus, thalamus, basal ganglia, brain stem, and spinal cord Function: Inhibits release of norepinephrine; stimulates release of serotonin, dopamine, and acetylcholine	Decreased levels: Alzheimer's disease Increased levels: Huntington's disease

ANS = autonomic nervous system; CNS = central nervous system.
Source: Townsend MC: Psychiatric Mental Health Nursing: Concepts of Care in Evidence-Based Practice, 5th Edition. FA Davis, Philadelphia, 2004, pp 60–61.

Box 56.1

Cultural Considerations

Among many Haitians, some African Americans, and some other groups, conjuring (practicing magic) and root doctors are believed to know more about mental illness than Western-educated physicians. Some depressive and obsessive behaviors are viewed as culture-bound syndromes. These behaviors are expected of some Haitians, and those affected fulfill some expected roles in the society. Some of these illnesses are viewed as having no cure. Thus, the nurse may need to include folk healers when working with African Americans and patients of Haitian descent.

Smoking, alcoholism, and deaths from suicide or violence are prevalent problems in the American culture. Violent deaths account for high mortality rates among adolescents and young adults of African American, Cuban, Mexican American, and Puerto Rican origin. Programs targeting these populations should be personalized to include adolescents and their families. Given their strong family values, an important approach is to begin early in church groups or family settings.

Hispanic individuals may require lower doses of antidepressants and experience greater side effects than other Caucasians. Thus, careful observations need to be undertaken when observing for side effects of medications in patients of Mexican heritage.

Asian patients require lower dosages and have side effects at lower dosages than Caucasians for a variety of psychoactive drugs (e.g., lithium, haloperidol) even when matched with body weight. Asians commonly believe that Western drugs are too strong for them and take less than prescribed. Most Asians are more sensitive to alcohol, resulting in facial flushing, palpitations, and tachycardia.

Mental illness among the Navajo is perceived as resulting from placing a curse on an individual. In these instances, a healer who deals with dreams or a crystal gazer is consulted. Individuals may wear turquoise to ward off evil; however, an individual who wears too much turquoise is sometimes thought to be an evil person and someone to avoid. In some tribes, mental illness may mean that the affected person has special powers. Additionally, many Native Americans metabolize alcohol at a faster rate than European Americans, resulting in them having a higher tolerance for alcohol.

Newer immigrants from Ireland have a higher incidence of mental illness than the rest of the population. Undocumented Irish immigrants in the United States report more stressors and mental health problems than their legal counterparts. Because many Irish people have difficulty expressing emotions, health-care providers may need to encourage Irish Americans to express their concerns.

Mental illness is strongly stigmatized among Iranians and is thought to be genetic. Should a family member have mental illness, it is likely to be called a "neurological disorder" so as not to stigmatize the family, which may result in daughters having a lesser chance of marrying. Psychotherapeutic help may be avoided because of stigma or because it is perceived as irrelevant. People prefer a medicine that might cure them. There is a tendency to pay more attention to somatic symptoms when under emotional stress; Iranians consider psychopharmacology most effective, and have a high rate of compliance.

Because of the stigma attached to seeking professional psychiatric help, many Hindus do not access the health-care system. Instead, family and friends seem to be the best help, and a general belief is that time is the best healer. Physical and mental illnesses are considered God's will, or karma, and are associated with a fatalistic attitude.

Among Greeks, mental illness is accompanied by social stigma for the afflicted individual, as well as the relatives. The shame originates in the notion that mental illness is hereditary, and afflicted individuals are viewed as having lifelong conditions that pollute the bloodline.

Because of social stigma attached to mental illness and retardation, Arabs may keep their family from public view. However, when Arab patients suffer from mental distress, they generally seek medical care. They are likely to have complaints such as abdominal pain, lassitude, anorexia, or shortness of breath. Arabs have an increased tendency to experience elevated blood levels and adverse affects when customary dosages of antidepressants are prescribed. Patients often expect and insist on somatic treatment, at least vitamins and tonics.

African Americans may be at a greater risk for being misdiagnosed with a psychiatric disorder than Caucasians. African Americans with psychiatric disorders are more likely to have hallucinations, delusions, somatization, and hostility, even when controlled for socioeconomic class. Maintaining direct eye contact with some African Americans may be misinterpreted as aggressive behavior. Thus, nurses must take these nonverbal behaviors into consideration when working with the patient with an emotional or mental concern. Additionally, African Americans are more susceptible to toxic side effects with tricyclic antidepressants.

better to ask a person about something (to clarify or explore what was said) than to make an assumption about it. For more information about mental health and illness, visit the National Institute of Mental Health at www.nimh.nih.gov, the American Psychiatric Association at www.psych.org, the American Psychiatric Nurses Association (www.apna.org), or the International Society of Psychiatric Mental Health Nurses (www.ispn-psych.org).

NURSING ASSESSMENT/ DATA COLLECTION

During the data collection/assessment part of the nursing process, the mental status examination is performed. This is a series of questions and activities that evaluate eight areas:
- Appearance and behavior
- Level of awareness and reality **orientation**
- Thinking/content of thought
- Memory, speech, and ability to communicate
- Mood and **affect**
- Judgment
- Perception

There are a number of different tools of varying names, lengths, and formats used to assess the patient's mental capabilities. See Table 56.2 for a sample mental status examination.

After data have been collected, the licensed practical nurse/licensed vocational nurse (LPN/LVN) collaborates with the registered nurse (RN) to develop nursing diagnoses. Box 56.2 Nursing Diagnoses Commonly Used for Patients with Mental Health Problems.

DIAGNOSTIC TESTS

Physicians use a variety of diagnostic criteria to diagnose mental illness. It is important to rule out physical illness as a cause of symptoms. The physician may choose to refer the patient to a psychiatrist or other mental health professional for further testing and diagnosis.

The diagnostic tool that is used most widely by psychiatrists and other mental health professionals is the *Diagnostic and Statistical Manual of Mental Disorders IV-Text Revision*, or DSM-IV-TR. The DSM-IV-TR groups illnesses into categories of clinical disorders. This is a complex diagnostic tool. Although as an LPN you will not be responsible to complete the assessment, you can contribute valuable information.

There are also batteries of psychological tests that can be administered and interpreted by psychiatrists or psychologists. Age, hand tremors, vision, language barriers, educational background, and the interpretation of the psychiatrist, the psychologist, or the advanced practice nurse are some factors that can influence the results of these tests.

Distinguishing Physical Versus Mental Disorders

There are many physical disorders that can mimic mental disorders, therefore tests may be performed to either confirm or rule out a diagnosis of a mental illness:
- Laboratory tests to rule out problems such as electrolyte imbalances, hypothyroidism, infections, dehydration, drug toxicity, or pregnancy.

TABLE 56.2 SAMPLE MENTAL STATUS EXAMINATION

Area of Assessment	Type of Assessment	Normal Parameters	Alterations from Normal
Appearance and Behavior	Observations about dress, hygiene, posture, and appearance and about the patient's actions and reactions to health-care personnel.	Clean, combed hair. Clothing intact and appropriate to weather or situation. Teeth/dentures in good repair. Posture erect. Cooperates with health-care personnel.	Displays either unusual apathy or concern about appearance. Displays uncooperative, hostile, or suspicious behaviors toward health-care personnel.
Level of Awareness and Orientation	Subjective and objective assessment of the patient's degree of alertness (wakefulness) and the degree of the patient's knowledge of self.	Awareness is measured on a continuum that ranges from unconsciousness to mania. "Normal alertness" is the desired behavior. Facilities may provide a standard format for this assessment, but observations can be documented as well if the patient is not able to stay awake for even short intervals or if the patient is overly active and has difficulty staying in one place. Orientation is assessed by asking the patient questions relating to person, place, and time, such as, "Who is this sitting next to you?" "Where are you right now?" Or "What year is it?"	Outcome is not considered within accepted normal limits if the patient is difficult to arouse and keep awake or if the patient has difficulty feeling calm. Abnormal results of orientation are the patient's inability to correctly answer orientation questions or inability to answer commonly known questions, such as "Who is the president?"

Area of Assessment	Type of Assessment	Normal Parameters	Alterations from Normal
Thinking/Content of Thought	Subjective assessment of what the patient is thinking and the process the patient uses in his or her thinking.	Formal testing may be done by the psychologist or psychiatrist to determine the patient's general thought content and pattern. Nurses may contribute to the assessment of thought by documenting statements the patient makes regarding daily care and routines.	Abnormal behaviors include flight of ideas, loose associations, phobias, delusions, and obsessions.
Memory	Subjective assessment of the mind's ability to recall recent and remote (long-term) information.	Recent memory: Recall of events that are immediately past or within 2 weeks before the assessment, such as a recent news event. One measurement technique is to verbally list five items. After 1 minute, can the patient recall four or five of those items? Continue with the assessment, and at 5 minutes the patient should be able to recall three or four of the items. Remote memory: Recall of events of the past beyond 2 weeks before assessment. Patients may be asked where they were born, where they went to grade school, etc.	Inability to accurately perform recent or remote (long-term) recall exercises within parameters. May indicate symptom of delirium or dementia.
Speech and Ability to Communicate	Objective and subjective assessment of how the patient uses verbal and nonverbal communication.	Patient can coherently produce words appropriate to age, education, and life experience. Rate of speech reflects other psychomotor activity (e.g., faster if the patient is agitated). Volume is not too soft or too loud. Stuttering, repetition of words, and words that the patient makes up (neologisms) are also assessed.	Limited speech production. Rate of speech is inconsistent with other psychomotor activity. Volume is not appropriate to situation (speaks louder or softer than appropriate). Presence of stuttering, word repetition, or neologisms may indicate physical or psychological illness.
Mood and Affect	Subjective and objective assessment of the patient's stated feelings and emotions. Affect measures the outward expression of those feelings.	Mood is the stated emotional condition of the patient and should fluctuate to reflect situations as they occur. Facial expression, body language (affect) should match (be congruent with) the stated mood. Affect should change to fluctuate with the changes in mood.	Mood and affect do not match (e.g., facial expression does not appear sad while the patient is expressing sad feelings).
Judgment	Subjective assessment of a patient's ability to make appropriate decisions about his or her situation or to understand concepts.	Give the patient a proverb or situation to solve, such as "You can't teach an old dog new tricks." The patient should be able to give some sort of acceptable interpretation, such as "Old habits are hard to break" or "It is hard to learn something new." Another example is to ask the patient what he or she would do if a small child was lost in a store. An appropriate response might be "Call the manager" or "Try to calm the child."	Patient cannot interpret the sayings in some acceptable manner. Patient cannot complete problem-solving questions appropriately. The patient might answer very literally, "Dogs can't learn anything when they get old" or might say, "I would go through the child's pockets looking for phone numbers."
Perception	Assess the way a person experiences reality. Observe the patient's statements about his or her environment and the behaviors expressed in association with those statements. Document exactly what you see and hear.	All five senses are monitored for the patient's perception of reality. The patient's insight into his or her condition is also assessed.	Presence of hallucinations and illusions may occur with schizophrenia. Patient unable to state understanding of the origin of the illness; associated behaviors inappropriate.

Box 56.2

Nursing Diagnoses Commonly Used for Patients with Mental Health Problems

Disturbed thought processes
Ineffective role performance
Anxiety (mild to panic)
Disturbed body image
Dysfunctional grieving
Impaired religiosity
Impaired social interaction
Ineffective coping
Defensive coping
Disturbed personal identity
Powerlessness
Fear
Posttrauma syndrome
Risk for violence (toward self or others)
Risk for injury
Risk for suicide
Self-mutilation
Self-care deficit
Low self-esteem (chronic or situational)
Disturbed sensory perception
Sexual dysfunction
Disturbed sleep pattern
Social isolation

- Computed tomographic (CT) scans or magnetic resonance imaging (MRI) to rule out tumors, lesions, or other physical problems.
- Positron emission tomographic (PET) scans to identify how the parts of the brain are functioning by showing chemical activity or metabolism.

COPING AND EGO DEFENSE MECHANISMS

"Oh, just learn to cope with it." "Get a grip." "Don't make a mountain out of a molehill." These are pieces of advice that people may have heard or given at some point. But what do they mean? What is **coping**? Coping is the way one adapts psychologically, physically, and behaviorally to a **stressor**. Individuals have different methods of coping or dealing with their stressors. Culture, religion, individual belief systems, experience, and personal choice influence an individual's responses to stress. It is not the value of a behavior that we assess as nurses; it is the desired outcome that is important. What is an effective coping skill? Is it healthy? Does it work? How do we as nurses observe and measure it?

Effective Coping Skills

Effective coping skills offer healthy choices for dealing with stressors. Hospitalization is stressful for patients and families. Many things are unknown and unfamiliar. The patient may not understand the illness or the implications of the treatment plan. It is common for patients to use coping mechanisms during hospitalization. The process of effective coping is sometimes called **adaptation.** Allowing the patient to practice new coping techniques will give him or her confidence and will decrease the stress that can accompany change.

Often the dividing line between effective and ineffective coping is the frequency of its use. For instance, mild **anxiety** can be positive. Generally, when there is a little anxiety, people are more alert and ready to respond. The *fight-or-flight mechanism* can actually help one adapt to a new situation. However, too much anxiety begins to cloud the consciousness and interfere with the ability to make appropriate choices and to recall the new adaptive tools one has learned. One of the most helpful roles you can perform is to listen to the patient's thoughts and feelings about the stressor, assist him or her to identify precipitating factors and patterns to the patient's stress, encourage the patient to problem solve, and provide assistance to develop alternative solutions.

CRITICAL THINKING

Joe

■ Joe is noted wailing loudly and continuously after the death of his wife. It is disturbing the other patients on the wing, and one of the nurses comments, "He is a real nut case. Get him out of here."

What is an appropriate response to this nurse and patient? How would you document his behavior?

Suggested answers at end of chapter.

Ineffective Coping Skills

Sometimes coping is ineffective. When conscious techniques are not successful, individuals may unconsciously fall into habits that give the illusion of coping. These habits are called *ego defense mechanisms* (or coping or mental mechanisms). Ego defense mechanisms act as mental pressure valves. The purpose of ego defense mechanisms is to reduce

CRITICAL THINKING

Mrs. Beison

■ Mrs. Beison, a 44-year-old mother of three teenagers, is diagnosed with breast cancer. She is refusing treatment because she does not believe she has cancer. She says if anything is really wrong, her vitamins will take care of it.

What coping mechanism is Mrs. Beison using? Is it effective or ineffective? Why? How can you help?

Suggested answers at end of chapter.

or eliminate anxiety. They give the impression that they are helping alleviate the stress level. When used in very small doses, ego defense mechanisms can be helpful. When they are overused, or are the only means used to deal with anxiety, they can become ineffective and unhealthy. People are not born with these coping behaviors; they are learned as responses to stress. Many times they develop by the age of 10 years old. They may appear to be conscious, but they are, for the most part, unconscious mechanisms. Some commonly used ego defense mechanisms are listed in Table 56.3.

TABLE 56.3 EGO DEFENSE MECHANISMS

Mechanism	Description	Examples
Denial	Usually the first defense learned and used. Unconscious refusal to see reality. Not conscious lying.	The alcoholic states, "I can quit any time I want to."
Repression (Stuffing)	An unconscious "burying" or "forgetting" mechanism. Excludes or withholds from consciousness events or situations that are unbearable.	A step deeper than "denial." A patient may "forget" about an appointment he or she does not want to keep.
Rationalization	Using a logical-sounding excuse to cover up true thoughts and feelings. The most frequently used defense mechanism.	1. "I did not make a medication error; I followed the doctor's order." 2. "I failed the test because the teacher wrote bad questions."
Compensation	Making up for something perceived as an inadequacy by developing some other desirable trait.	1. The small boy who wants to be a basketball center instead becomes an honor roll student. 2. The physically unattractive person who wants to model instead becomes a famous designer.
Reaction Formation (Overcompensation)	Similar to compensation, except the person usually develops the exact opposite trait.	1. The small boy who wants to be a basketball center becomes a political voice to decrease the emphasis on sports in the elementary grades. 2. The physically unattractive person who wants to be a model speaks out for eliminating beauty pageants.
Regression	Emotionally returning to an earlier time in life when patient experienced far less stress. Commonly seen in patients while hospitalized. NOTE: Everyone will not go back to the same developmental age. This is highly individualized.	1. Children who are toilet trained beginning to wet themselves. 2. Adults who may start crying and have a "temper tantrum."
Projection (Scapegoating)	Blaming others. A mental or verbal "finger-pointing" at another for patient's own problem. **Memory tool:** Think of a projector at the movie theater. It "points" the images of the film onto the screen just as a person using this defense mechanism "points" blame on another person or situation.	1. "I didn't get the promotion because you don't like me." 2. "I'm overweight because you make me nervous."
Displacement (Transference)	The "kick-the-dog syndrome." Transferring anger and hostility to another person or object that is perceived to be less powerful than oneself.	Parent loses job without notice; goes home and verbally abuses spouse, who unjustly punishes child, who slaps the dog.
Restitution (Undoing)	Make amends for a behavior one thinks is unacceptable. Makes an attempt at reducing guilt.	1. Giving a treat to a child who is being punished for a wrongdoing. 2. The person who sees someone lose a wallet with a large amount of cash does not return the wallet, but puts extra in the collection plate at the next church service.
Conversion Reaction	Anxiety is channeled into physical symptoms. NOTE: Often the symptoms disappear soon after the threat is over.	Nausea develops the night before a major exam, causing the person to miss the exam. Nausea may disappear soon after the scheduled test is finished.
Avoidance	Unconsciously staying away from events or situations that might open feelings of aggression or anxiety.	"I can't go to the class reunion tonight. I'm just so tired, I have to sleep."

THERAPEUTIC MEASURES

People who experience alterations in their mental health have special treatment needs. When emotional health is threatened, many other daily activities can be altered as well. **Cognitive** ability (the ability to think rationally and to process those thoughts) can be impaired. Emotional responses can be decreased or even absent in some conditions. This can be extremely frightening and can lead to a worsening of the mental disorder or even the development of another disorder. This section will provide an overview of selected therapies to help patients deal with alterations in mental health.

Therapeutic Communication

Many people take communication for granted. In the mental health setting, communication is a tool used to relate therapeutically with patients. It is important to keep in mind what message we want to communicate to patients. Therapeutic communication is accomplished through the deliberate use of verbal and nonverbal techniques. Other areas to consider when communicating are the patient's personal values, attitudes, beliefs, culture, religion, social status, gender, and age or developmental level.

Verbal therapeutic communication techniques can help facilitate an interpersonal interaction. For instance, if you ask a patient to explain something to you in more detail, you are using the therapeutic communication technique of exploring. Verbal communication is also influenced by the tone, pitch, speed, and volume of speech. Some commonly used therapeutic communication techniques are listed in Table 56.4.

Components of *nonverbal communication* include physical appearance, dress, body movement and posture, touch, facial expression, and eye contact. It is believed that most communication takes place nonverbally so it is possible that while you are saying one thing to a patient, your body language could be saying something else.

There are also barriers to effective communication which are commonly called *communication blocks*. A nurse who tells a patient "Don't worry, everything will be all right" has just given the patient false reassurance. This barrier communicates to the patient that his concerns are not being taken seriously. Some commonly encountered communication blocks are listed in Table 56.5.

TABLE 56.4 THERAPEUTIC COMMUNICATION TECHNIQUES

Technique	Description	Examples
Encouraging Descriptions of Perceptions	Asking the patient what he or she is seeing or hearing	"Tell me what the voices are saying to you."
Encouraging Comparison	Asking the patient to compare similarities or differences	"How is this medication working for you compared to the last time you used it?"
Exploring	Looking deeper into a subject, idea, or experience	"Tell me more about the last time you were depressed."
Focusing	Concentrating on a single idea or event	"Tell me more about how your divorce made you feel."
Formulating a Plan of Action	Assisting the patient to come up with a plan to cope with stress	"When this happens in the future how could you handle it more constructively?"
Giving Broad Openings	Allowing the patient to steer the interaction	"What would you like to work on today?"
Giving Recognition	Acknowledging or showing awareness	"I see you went to your therapy group today."
Making Observations	Verbalizing what is observed	"I notice you seemed upset after your visit."
Offering Self	Extending one's presence	"I am available to talk whenever you would like."
Offering General Leads	Giving the patient encouragement to continue	"I see... ." "Go on... ."
Placing Event in Time or Sequence	Clarification of events in time	"Was this before or after your first hospitalization?"
Presenting Reality	Defining reality in simple terms	"The voices may seem real to you, but they are a symptom of your illness."
Restating	Repeating the main idea of what the patient has verbalized	"It sounds as if you are feeling frustrated."
Reflecting	Statements, questions, or feelings are referred back to the patient	"What do you think you should do?"
Seeking Clarification	Searching for understanding of what was said	"Tell me if this is what you meant when you said..."
Verbalizing the Implied	Putting into words what the patient has implied or said indirectly	"You must be feeling very sad right now."
Using Silence	Gives both the nurse and the patient a chance to collect their thoughts and organize what they are going to say	

TABLE 56.5 COMMUNICATION BLOCKS

Mechanism	Description	Examples
Agreeing/Disagreeing	Implies that the patient's ideas or feelings are somehow right or wrong	"That is right on target. I agree 100%."
Asking "Why Questions"	Asking why implies that the patient knows the reason for their behavior and feelings.	"Why were you feeling so angry?"
Changing the Subject	Changing the subject takes control of the conversation away from the patient.	Patient: "I am feeling so hopeless." Nurse: "Did you go to group therapy today?"
Giving Advice	Telling the patient what to do implies that the nurse knows what is best.	"I think you should… ."
Giving Approval or Disapproval	Passes judgment on the patient's ideas or opinions	"That's right."
Giving False Reassurance	Devalues the patient's feelings	"Everything will be all right."
Self-focusing Behavior	The nurse focuses on his or her own feelings at the expense of the patient's.	"That happened to me once…let me tell you about it."
Double-bind Messages	When the nonverbal message doesn't match the verbal message	"I am listening." As the nurse fidgets in her chair, doesn't make eye contact, and then coughs.

Milieu

One area over which you can have some control is the therapeutic environment. In the mental health setting, this therapeutic environment is called the **milieu** or therapeutic milieu. It is believed that environment has an effect on behavior. Milieu therapy is the systematic management of the social environment as a treatment modality.

A *therapeutic milieu* is an environment that provides containment, support, structure, involvement, and validation during the patient's stay. The goals of milieu therapy are resocialization, ego development, and prevention of regression. Resocialization occurs when patients help govern the running of the unit and attend regular meetings to set rules and assign tasks. Ego development is fostered with structured activities that are provided to assist the patient to learn coping and social skills. Regression is prevented when patients help with washing dishes or other small jobs that foster independence. Common milieu interventions include role modeling, positive reinforcement, a schedule of events, consistent expectations and rules for behavior, and unit meetings. Milieu therapy is more difficult in this era of managed care because of shorter hospital stays.

Psychopharmacology

Psychopharmacology is the use of medications to treat psychological disorders. Since the introduction of the phenothiazine class of drugs in the 1950s (e.g., chlorpromazine), the number of medications available for treating mental health disorders has increased greatly, with newer medications having fewer side effects. The reason for using medications is twofold: first, the medications manage the symptoms, helping the patient feel more comfortable emotionally. Second, the patient is generally more receptive and

able to focus on other types of therapy if medications are effective. More information on psychoactive drugs is provided in Chapter 57.

Psychotherapies

Psychotherapy is the term used to describe the form of treatment chosen by the psychologist, psychiatrist, social worker, or advanced practice psychiatric nurse. The goals of psychotherapy include the following:

- Reduce the patient's emotional discomfort
- Increase the level of the patient's social functioning
- Increase the ability of the patient to behave or perform in a manner appropriate to the situation

Several specific types of therapy that are typically used are described next.

Psychoanalysis

Psychoanalysis was developed from Sigmund Freud's psychoanalytic theory. Freud believed that anxiety was the primary motivation for behavior and therefore all behavior had meaning. Psychoanalytic therapy consists of clarifying the meaning of events, feelings, and behavior and thereby gaining **insight** into them. The role of the patient is to provide the psychoanalyst with clues to the unconscious source of problems and to try to develop with insights into behavior. The role of the therapist is to uncover these unconscious experiences and interpret their meanings to the patient. Some believe that psychoanalysis will lose popularity as we gain a better understanding of the role of the brain, neurotransmitters, and genetics in mental health.

Behavior Management

Behavior management (also called behavior modification) is a treatment method that stems from the studies of behavioral theorists such as Skinner and Pavlov. It is a common

---

psychopharmacology: psycho—soul or mind + pharmaco—drug or medicine + ology—study of

psychoanalysis: psycho—soul or mind + analysis—dissolving

treatment modality used in long-term care facilities, with children and adolescents, and with individuals who have a low level of cognitive functioning.

According to behavior management theory, all behavior is learned, so it can be unlearned. The belief is that behavior can be changed by either positive or negative reinforcement. *Positive reinforcement* is the act of rewarding the patient with something pleasant when the desired behavior has been performed. For instance, if a patient has the habit of using foul language in an attempt to have a need met, the desired behavior change might be to come to a staff member and ask quietly for what he or she needs. If this patient loves to be outside but is not allowed out except at supervised times, then a suitable positive reinforcement for her might be to allow 15 more minutes outdoors when she remembers to come ask for her needs quietly.

Negative reinforcement is the act of responding to the undesired behavior by taking away a privilege or adding a responsibility. Negative reinforcement can be misinterpreted as punishment. Parents who "ground" their children for unacceptable behavior are using negative reinforcement; requiring the child to perform extra household tasks for a stated period is reinforcing the fact that the behavior has consequences. The child may not repeat the undesired behavior after negative reinforcement has been used. It is necessary to be very careful when performing behavior management with patients to avoid violating the Patient's Bill of Rights. A signed consent from the patient is advised when using this form of therapy.

The patient must understand the consequences of the behavior to be changed and the purpose for the type of consequence that is chosen. If the person is not capable of understanding the situation or is not able to remember the consequences because of some other problem, behavior management could be considered a questionable alternative to other kinds of treatment.

Cognitive Behavioral Therapy

Cognitive behavioral therapists believe that people teach themselves to be ill because of the way they "think" about their situations. Cognitive behavioral therapy stresses ways of rethinking situations. The therapist confronts the patient with certain distortions of thinking and then works out ways of thinking about them differently.

Feeling sad about an unpleasant experience (such as the death of a loved one) is acceptable and normal, but long-term depression about the death is an extreme emotion and therefore considered to be unhealthy. In this situation, the patient might be helped to see the death as a sad loss. Behavioral techniques are also used more often with phobias or panic disorders, in which fear may interfere with reasoning.

Cognitive therapies are gaining in popularity because they are usually significantly more short term than psychoanalysis and therefore less costly to the patient. It is

commonly performed in groups. The patients are given "homework" that is specific to their needs. Patients practice their assignments between sessions.

Person-Centered/Humanistic Therapy

Abraham Maslow and Carl Rogers are two theorists who are often credited with the concept of person-centered or humanistic therapy. In this form of treatment, caregivers focus on the whole person and work in the "present." It is not important in humanistic treatment to understand the cause of the problem or what happened in the person's past; what is important is the here and now. With this therapy, the patient learns to see himself or herself as a person who has value and who is respected by others.

Nursing is very strongly centered in person-centered principles. Three qualities are essential for caregivers: empathy, which is the ability to identify with the patient's feelings without actually experiencing them with the patient; unconditional positive regard (respect); and genuineness or honesty. Although you may not be an active participant in the actual therapy sessions with patients, it is important to maintain these three qualities in all therapeutic relationships.

Counseling

Counseling is the provision of help or guidance by a healthcare professional. The area of counseling is licensed and regulated differently not only state by state but sometimes municipality by municipality. Nurses prepared at an LPN/LVN level or at an RN level can, in some areas and with special advanced education, practice some forms of counseling.

You may be asked or expected to accompany patients to counseling sessions or even to facilitate a group discussion. Remember that these are confidential sessions, even if they are group oriented. Patients are there to work; others are there by invitation for special reasons.

Group Therapy

Groups are formed for many reasons; they can be ongoing or short term, depending on the needs of the patients or the type of disorder. Group therapy is a cost-effective means of providing treatment. For example, Alcoholics Anonymous (AA) and similar 12-step self-help groups are well-established, ongoing groups formed around treatment of a specific problem. Family counseling sessions may occur with individual therapists with a specialty in the problem area for that family. Marriage counseling may be done in a group with other couples. Many times, peer counselors are used.

Therapists and counselors are tools, or facilitators, in the therapeutic process. They do not heal the patient; the patient heals himself or herself. Patients must take the suggestions given by the therapist, try them, and see what works for them. You can help by reinforcing the good work patients do in learning to stay mentally healthy and develop more effective life skills.

Electroconvulsive Therapy

Electroconvulsive therapy (ECT) is a form of treatment that is used for severely depressed patients who are not responding to psychotropic medications. It uses electric shock to produce a convulsion (seizure). Most mental health professionals believe ECT stimulates an increase in the circulating levels of the neurotransmitters serotonin, norepinephrine, and dopamine in the brain. In essence, ECT impacts neurotransmitter activity much like antidepressants do. ECT may be frightening to patients; it is important for the nurse to provide education and information to the patient and family. Many changes have been made in this form of therapy since the 1940s, and ECT is currently a safe and effective treatment for severe depression.

Procedure

ECT often takes place in the recovery room of an operating suite, where there is ready access to emergency equipment. Informed consent is required and should be obtained by the physician. About 30 minutes before the procedure, the patient is given a medication to dry secretions and counteract stimulation of the vagus nerve, which can cause bradycardia and syncope. Patients are given a short-acting anesthetic before the treatment and a smooth muscle relaxant to minimize injury. Before giving the muscle relaxant, a blood pressure cuff is placed on one of the patient's lower limbs and inflated. This is to ensure that the seizure activity can be visually monitored in this limb. Blood pressure and pulse are carefully monitored before and after the treatment. The patient is oxygenated with pure oxygen during and after the seizure until spontaneous respirations return. During treatment, an electrical stimulus is delivered to the brain via unilateral or bilateral electrodes. The amount of electrical energy used is individualized to the patient. The tonic-clonic (grand mal) seizure must last at least 30 seconds to be effective. The seizure activity is monitored with an electroencephalogram (EEG) and also in the cuffed limb.

Side Effects

Side effects of ECT can be unpleasant, but are usually temporary. The patient may feel confused and forgetful immediately after the treatment. This can be from a combination of the ECT itself and the medication that was used before the treatment. If there has been a strong seizure, the patient may have some muscle soreness.

Electroconvulsive therapy is not used indiscriminately. It is used when other therapies have not been helpful, and it is usually reserved for severe or long-term depression and certain types of schizophrenia (Box 56.3 Patient Perspective).

Nursing Responsibilities

The nurse's responsibilities include careful monitoring of vital signs and accurate documentation relating to the

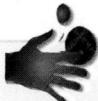

Box 56.3

Patient Perspective

My mom is now 83 and has had a total of 35 electroconvulsive therapy (ECT) treatments in her lifetime. If you met her, you'd never know; you'd find her delightful. She's a sweet little plump German lady with a big heart. I am a nurse, and when I tell fellow nurses about my mom, they often ask me why I didn't get her on antidepressants. I want to scream, "How dumb do you think I am?!" Of course Mom is on antidepressants. But at intervals they don't work and she sinks into severe depression. My choice then is to help her have ECT or let her stay depressed and miserable and put her in a nursing home. And she would soon die because when she is depressed she refuses to move, doesn't sleep, and is horribly miserable.

The first time my mom was scheduled for ECT, one of the nurses in our local community hospital told her to refuse it, that no one should have to go through that. It was a cruel thing to do. My mom doesn't do well in counseling—she doesn't believe in it. In her mind you don't talk about your "dirty linen." My mom was in an abusive relationship with my father for 47 years, and she hid all the problems away and doesn't talk about them to this day. I'm so grateful to have my mom doing okay and grateful that ECT treatments exist. With ECT my mother is doing well and enjoying life. Without treatment she would be gone. Please understand that there are times when ECT treatments are the best thing for severely depressed people, when other treatments have been ineffective.

patient's subjective and objective responses to the treatment. The patient should receive nothing by mouth (NPO) for at least 4 hours before a treatment. Remind the patient to empty his or her bladder and to remove dentures, contact lenses, hair pins, and other items on the body. Stay with the patient until he or she is oriented and able to care for himself or herself. Oral medications and food should be withheld until the gag reflex returns. Ensuring that the person is kept safe after therapy is a major concern.

Relaxation Therapy

A variety of relaxation techniques can be taught to help patients manage their responses to stress. Relaxation exercises such as deep, rhythmic breathing can increase oxygenation and provide distraction from stressors. Breathing exercises may be coupled with progressive muscle relaxation exercises. For this technique, patients are taught to start at the head and neck and systematically tense and then relax muscle groups as they progress toward the lower extremities. Soft music may enhance the patient's ability to fully relax.

Imagery is the use of the imagination to promote relaxation. For this technique, the patient is taught to imagine a pleasurable experience from his or her past, such as lying on a beach or soaking in a warm bath. Use of all senses is encouraged—for a beach image, the patient might see a beach, feel the warm sun, smell salt air, and hear waves crashing against the shore. The patient might also be taught to visualize being successful in a problem situation.

Relaxation techniques may be used individually, but they are often used in combination with each other or with other therapies for maximum effect.

Home Health Hints

Assess the safety of the home and patient for:
- Risk of falls (especially if the patient is experiencing orthostatic hypotension from medications)
- Suicide ideation, plan, and means
- Ability to access medications, missed doses, or overdoses
- Need for additional services for activities of daily living (ADLs), such as housekeeping, medication assistance, or safety rails

REVIEW QUESTIONS

1. When assessing mental health, which patient behavior would cause the nurse to be concerned or ask further questions?
   a. Patient is always happy and smiling.
   b. Patient can verbalize emotions.
   c. Patient is able to cope with bad news.
   d. Patient maintains some close, personal relationships.

Multiple response item. Select all that apply.
2. Which of the following assessments are important parts of a mental health assessment?
   a. Orientation to reality
   b. Mobility
   c. Ability to communicate clearly
   d. Heart sounds
   e. Memory

3. A patient being evaluated for depression asks why he has to have his blood drawn. Which response by the nurse is best?
   a. "Your physical illnesses must be under control before your depression can be treated effectively."
   b. "The clinician needs to rule out physical causes for your symptoms."
   c. "Most mental health disorders can be identified with blood tests."
   d. "If your lab work is out of balance, then correcting the imbalance will reverse your depression."

4. A person who always sounds like he or she is making excuses is displaying which ego defense mechanism?
   a. Denial
   b. Fantasy
   c. Rationalization
   d. Transference

5. Which of the following best defines a therapeutic milieu?
   a. An environment that is able to provide for all the patient's physical and emotional needs
   b. An environment that is locked and supervised
   c. An environment that is structured to decrease stress and encourage learning new behavior
   d. An environment designed to be homelike for persons who are institutionalized for life

6. What is the primary reason a patient may be placed on psychopharmacology?
   a. It can provide a cure for mental illness and substance abuse.
   b. It is used only when necessary to control violent behavior.
   c. It is used to alter the pain receptors in the brain.
   d. It can decrease symptoms and facilitate other therapies.

7. Which of the following is one of the major skills a chemically dependent person and family can learn during treatment?
   a. Honest communication
   b. Avoidance of difficult topics
   c. Denial
   d. Scapegoating

8. A patient shares some very traumatic life experiences with the LPN. What is the best response by the LPN?
   a. Assure the patient that the staff will not allow such experiences to happen to the patient again.
   b. Ask probing questions about the patient's emotional responses to the experiences.
   c. Encourage the patient to forget the experiences and move on with life.
   d. Listen attentively to the patient and show empathy.

SUGGESTED ANSWERS TO

CRITICAL THINKING

■ Joe

Different people cope in different ways. This may be a healthy way to cope in this man's culture. Gently guide the grieving husband to a room where he can express his emotions without disturbing others. Ask if he would like you to contact someone to come in to support him. Document objectively: "Patient's husband weeping loudly; guided to consultation room for privacy."

■ Mrs. Beison

Mrs. Beison is using denial to cope with her cancer diagnosis. Although at times denial can be an effective coping mechanism, if Mrs. Beison continues to deny her disease and refuse treatment, her life will be in danger. You can help Mrs. Beison verbalize her fears about cancer and cancer treatment and can provide accurate information to help her make wise choices. If necessary, a psychiatric evaluation can be requested.

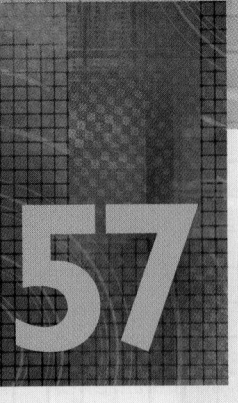

57

Nursing Care of Patients with Mental Health Disorders

MARINA MARTINEZ-KRATZ

KEY TERMS

abuse (uh-BYOOS)
addiction (ah-DIK-shun)
anhedonia (AN-he-DOH-nee-uh)
alogia (ah-LOH-jee-uh)
avolition (A-voh-LISH-un)
bipolar (bye-POH-ler)
codependence (KO-de-PEN-dense)
compulsion (kum-PUHL-shun)
conversion disorder (kon-VER-zhun dis-OR-der)
delirium tremens (dee-LIR-ee-uhm TREE-menz)
delusions (dee-LOO-zhuns)
dependence (dee-PEN-dens)
displacement (dis-PLAYSS-ment)
dysfunctional (dis-FUNCK-shun-uhl)
eustress (YOO-stress)
hallucinations (hah-LOO-si-NAY-shuns)
illusions (i-LOO-zhuns)
mania (MAY-nee-ah)
obsession (ob-SESH-un)
phobia (FOH-bee-ah)
psychosomatic (SIGH-koh-soh-MAT-ik)
somatoform (soh-MAT-oh-form)
tolerance (TALL-ler-ens)
withdrawal (with-DRAW-ul)

QUESTIONS TO GUIDE YOUR READING

1. What are etiologic theories for mental health disorders?

2. What are the signs and symptoms of common mental health disorders?

3. What therapeutic management can be used for each of the disorders?

4. What are nursing interventions to help patients with mental health disorders?

5. What is the role of the LPN/LVN in care of patients with mental health disorders?

6. What are the classifications, actions, side effects, and nursing considerations for selected classifications of psychoactive medications?

MENTAL HEALTH DISORDERS

Anxiety Disorders

Stress is everywhere in our society. Stress produces anxiety. Most often, stress is associated with negative situations, but the good things that happen to us, such as weddings and job promotions, also produce stress. The stress from positive experiences is called **eustress.** Eustress can produce just as much anxiety as the negative stressors. A stressor is any person or situation that produces an anxiety response. Stress and stressors are different for each person; therefore, it is important to ask patients what their personal stress producers are.

Anxiety is the uncomfortable feeling of dread that occurs in response to extreme or prolonged periods of stress. It is commonly ranked as mild, moderate, severe, or panic. It is believed that a mild amount of anxiety is a normal part of being human and that mild anxiety is necessary to change and develop new ways of coping with stress.

Anxiety may also be influenced by one's culture. It may be acceptable for some people to acknowledge and discuss stress, but others may believe that one does not discuss personal problems with others. This cultural behavior can be a challenge for the nurse during an assessment.

Anxiety is usually referred to as either *free-floating anxiety* or signal anxiety. Free-floating anxiety is described as a general feeling of impending doom. The person cannot pinpoint the cause but might say something like "I just know something bad is going to happen if I go on vacation." *Signal anxiety,* on the other hand, is an uncomfortable response to a known stressor ("Finals are only a week away and I've got that nausea again.") Both types of anxiety are involved in the various anxiety disorders.

Etiological Theories

Psychoanalytical theorists believe that anxiety is a conflict between the id (the "all for me" part of the personality) and the superego (the conscience), which was repressed in early development but emerges again in adulthood.

Biological theory looks at anxiety differently. One biological theory points to the sympathoadrenal (fight-or-flight) responses to stress to explain signs and symptoms of anxiety, and observes that the blood vessels constrict because epinephrine and norepinephrine have been released, causing blood pressure to rise. Another biological theory implicates a lack of the neurotransmitter gamma-aminobutyric acid (GABA) in the etiology of anxiety. GABA is an inhibitory neurotransmitter which prevents postsynaptic excitation. If the body adapts to the stress, hormone levels adjust and body functions return to a homeostatic state. If the body does not adapt to the stress, the immune system is challenged and risk for physical illness increases.

You may observe psychological responses to medical-surgical illness. It is important to recognize the relationship between physical and emotional responses to stress. Some examples of medical conditions and the effects of the body's adaptation response to stress are shown in Table 57.1.

Differential Diagnosis

Because there are so many symptoms associated with anxiety disorders, it is important for people to have a complete physical examination before diagnosing an anxiety disorder, as some medical disorders, such as hyperthyroidism, may mimic anxiety. More than one condition may occur at the same time.

Types of Anxiety Disorders

PHOBIA. Phobias are the most common of the anxiety disorders. There are more than 700 documented phobias. *Simple phobias* are defined as irrational fears of specific objects or situations such as snakes or bridges. *Social phobias* are characterized by a persistent fear of behaving or performing in a way that will be humiliating or embarrassing to the individual, such as public speaking, eating in front of others, or using public restrooms. The person is very aware of the fear and even the fact that it is irrational, but is unable to gain control over the stressor and the fear continues.

The psychoanalytical view implies that it really is not the object that is the source of the fear, but rather the fear is a result of a defense mechanism called **displacement.** For example, the person with a phobia of snakes may have seen a frightening movie in which someone died from a snake bite. The stated object of the phobia would be interpreted as a symbol for the underlying cause of the fear.

PANIC DISORDER. Panic is a state of extreme fear that cannot be controlled. It is also referred to as panic attack, and lay people may not consider it to be a serious disorder.

Panic episodes are recurrent and occur unpredictably. Patients may present themselves at the emergency room because they believe they are having a heart attack or other significant physical illness. Patients must exhibit several episodes within a specified time frame to be given the diagnosis of panic disorder. Some of the symptoms associated with panic disorder include the following:
- Fear (usually of dying, losing control of self, or "going crazy")
- Feelings of impending doom
- Dissociation (feeling that it is happening to someone else or not happening at all)
- Nausea
- Diaphoresis
- Chest pain
- Palpitations
- Shaking

GENERALIZED ANXIETY DISORDER. In generalized anxiety disorder (GAD), the anxiety itself (also referred to as excessive worry or severe stress) is the expressed symptom. These patients worry about everything. Symptoms that may be present in GAD include the following:
- Restlessness or feeling "on edge"
- Shaking

---

eustress: eu—normal or good + stress

TABLE 57.1 ADAPTATION RESPONSES TO STRESS

Stress-Related Medical Condition	Body's Adaptation to the Stress	Outcome of Stress on the Body
Lowered Immunity	Interferes with effectiveness of the body's antibodies; possibly related to interactions among the hypothalamus, pituitary gland, adrenal glands, and immune system	Increased susceptibility to colds and other viruses and illnesses
Burnout	Associated with stress-related depression	Emotional detachment
Migraine, Cluster, and Tension Headaches	Tightening skeletal muscles, dilating of cranial arteries	Nausea, vomiting, tight feeling in or around head and shoulders, tinnitus, inability to tolerate light, weakness of a limb
Stress (Peptic) Ulcers	Stress contributes to the formation of ulcers by stimulating the vagus nerve and ultimately leading to hypersecretion of hydrochloric acid	Nausea, vomiting, gastrointestinal bleeding, perforation of intestinal walls
Hypertension	Role of stress not positively known; thought to contribute to hypertension by negatively interacting with the kidneys, autonomic nervous system, and endocrine system	Resistance to blood flow through the cardiovascular system, causing pressure on the arteries; can lead to stroke, heart attack, and kidney failure
Coronary Artery Disease	Stressor increases the amount of epinephrine and norepinephrine	Coronary vessels dilate, pulse and respirations increase
Cancer	Stress lowers immune response	Lowered immunity may allow for overcolonization of opportunistic cancer cells
Asthma	Autonomic nervous system stimulates mucus, increases blood flow, and constricts airways; may be associated with other stress-related conditions such as allergy and viral infection	Wheezing, coughing, dyspnea, apprehension; may lead to respiratory infections, respiratory failure, or pneumothorax

- Palpitations
- Dry mouth
- Nausea, vomiting
- Easy frightening
- Hot flashes
- Chills
- Muscle aches
- Hypervigilance (excessive attention to stimuli)
- Polyuria
- Difficulty swallowing

OBSESSIVE-COMPULSIVE DISORDER. Obsessive-compulsive disorder (OCD) is a different type of anxiety disorder. It consists of two parts: the **obsession** (repetitive thought, urge, or emotion) and the **compulsion** (repetitive act that may appear purposeful). An example of obsessive-compulsive disorder is the need to check that the doors are locked numerous times before one is able to sleep or leave the house. This need to repetitively check the locks may prevent the person from sleeping or leaving the house at all. Some individuals wash their hands compulsively to the point of having raw and bleeding hands. Behaviors become very ritualistic. The person with OCD is unable to stop the thought or the action. Performing the action (such as checking the locks or hand washing) is the mechanism that reduces the anxiety. Although you should not interfere with the repetitive acts, OCD patients can be helped by cognitive-behavioral therapy, medications (such as fluoxetine), and therapeutic interventions.

CRITICAL THINKING

Tommy

■ Tommy has come to your clinic with numerous cracks on his hands. They are bleeding and very sore. Tommy tells you that he has to wash his hands all the time. His mother says he washes for 2 to 3 hours at a time and he will not stop when she tells him to. The doctor has diagnosed Tommy with obsessive-compulsive disorder and has explained the illness to Tommy and his mother. When the doctor leaves the room, Tommy's mother begins to cry. "What did he just say? What am I supposed to do? What did I do wrong that Tommy got this illness?" How do you respond?

Suggested answers at end of chapter.

POSTTRAUMATIC STRESS DISORDER. Posttraumatic stress disorder (PTSD) develops in response to some unexpected emotional or physical trauma when there is the *real threat of death or harm* and the patient is helpless to do anything about it. People who have fought in wars, who have been raped, or who have survived violent storms or violent acts (such as terrorist acts) are examples of those who are susceptible to suffering from this disorder.

A condition that is associated with PTSD is *survivor guilt*, which is the feeling of guilt expressed by those who have survived a tragedy. A survivor of an airline crash may say, "Why me? Why did I make it? I should have died too!" This is especially true if a loved one died in the crash.

Symptoms may appear immediately or may not appear until years later. A key symptom of PTSD is *flashbacks* in which the person may relive the traumatic event as if it were happening at that moment. Sounds and smells associated with the trauma may trigger the flashback.

Signs and symptoms of PTSD include the following:

- Flashbacks
- Social withdrawal
- Feelings of low self-esteem
- Changes in relationships with significant others
- Difficulty forming new relationships
- Hypervigilance
- Irritability and outbursts of anger seemingly for no obvious reason
- Depression
- Chemical dependency

Therapeutic Interventions for Patients with Anxiety Disorders

Treatment is individualized for the patient and may include one or more of the following: psychopharmacology, individual psychotherapy, group therapy, systematic desensitization, hypnosis, imagery, relaxation exercises, and biofeedback.

Psychopharmacology usually involves the antianxiety classification of medications. The benzodiazepines, such as diazepam (Valium) and alprazolam (Xanax), are commonly used and are effective in most cases. Benzodiazepines are used for short-term treatment because of the strong potential for chemical dependency. Individuals who need longer term therapy for anxiety or who have chemical dependency issues can be safely and effectively treated with buspirone (Buspar); clonazepam (Klonopin), the SSRIs paroxetine (Paxil), or sertraline (Zoloft); the antihistamine hydroxyzine hydrochloride (Atarax); or the antihypertensive clonidine (Catapres). See Table 57.2 for a review of medications.

In *systematic desensitization*, the patient is gradually exposed to the object (rating the fear on a scale from 1 to 10) that causes the anxiety. *Hypnosis* places the patient in a subconscious state, then helps the patient recall events that may be producing anxiety so they can be dealt with. Other therapies were discussed in Chapter 56.

Nursing Process for the Patient with Anxiety

ASSESSMENT/DATA COLLECTION. Assess the patient's anxiety level. Ask about triggers of anxiety and coping mechanisms that have been successful or unsuccessful in the past. Observe for physical symptoms such as changes in vital signs, diaphoresis, or tremor. Assess for the presence of suicidal thoughts and observe for suicidal behavior. It is important to identify anxiety and intervene at the lower levels, before escalation to severe and panic anxiety levels.

NURSING DIAGNOSIS, PLANNING, AND IMPLEMENTATION. Anxiety

EXPECTED OUTCOMES: *The patient will identify precipitants and patterns for anxiety and demonstrate techniques to*

control anxiety. The patient will verbalize that anxiety is controlled.

- Assist the patient to identify precipitants and patterns to anxiety. *Recognition of patterns can help guide care and allow the patient to initiate measures to stop anxiety from progressing.*
- Maintain a calm milieu and manner. *A chaotic environment can increase the patient's anxiety. Anxiety is contagious and may be transmitted from staff to patient.*
- Maintain open communication. Encourage the patient to verbalize thoughts and feelings. Observe nonverbal communication. *Honesty in dealing with patients helps them learn to trust others and enhances their self-esteem.*
- Encourage the patient to use positive self-talk such as "I can do this. Anxiety can't kill me." *This helps the patient replace negative anxious thoughts with positive statements to decrease anxiety.*
- Report and document any changes in behavior. Positive or negative alterations in the way a patient responds to the nursing staff, to the treatment plan, or to other people and situations should be reported. *Any change can be significant to the patient's care.*
- Encourage activities, but avoid placing the patient in a competitive situation. *Activities that are enjoyable and nonstressful provide diversion and give staff an opportunity to provide positive feedback about the progress the patient is making.*
- Encourage problem solving and assist to develop alternative solutions. Assist to identify what has worked in the past. *This can help the patient focus on strategies that were effective in the past, and eliminate those that are not effective.*
- Stay with patients during severe or panic levels of anxiety. *Feelings of being abandoned can increase anxiety. The nurse's presence will also provide safety for the patient.*
- Implement suicide precautions if indicated. *The patient may need to be protected from self-harm until treatment is effective.*
- Assess your own level of anxiety. *An anxious nurse may make the patient more anxious.*

EVALUATION. Is the patient able to implement strategies to control anxiety? Does the client recognize triggers of anxiety? Does the patient state he or she feels less anxious?

See Box 57.1 Anxiety Summary.

Mood Disorders

Mood disorders (also called affective disorders) are disorders in which the major symptom is extreme changes in mood (emotions) and affect (the outward expression of the mood). Moods involving both highs and lows are bipolar disorders, where as low moods without any highs, are described as depressive disorders. Mood disorders are

(Text continued on page 1280)

TABLE 57.2 MEDICATIONS USED FOR ALTERATIONS IN MENTAL HEALTH

Medication Class/Action	Examples	Route	Side Effects	Nursing Implications
Typical Antipsychotics Block dopamine receptors (*used less frequently because of serious side effects*)	Chlorpromazine (Thorazine) Haloperidol (Haldol) Fluphenazine (Prolixin)	PO, IM PO, IM, long-acting IM PO, IM, long-acting IM	Extrapyramidal side effects (EPSEs): parkinsonism, akathisia, dystonia, tardive dyskinesia, photosensitivity, orthostatic hypotension, gynecomastia, neuroleptic malignant syndrome	Monitor for EPSEs. Use sunscreen when outside, do not use/take with alcohol or other CNS depressants, avoid use during first trimester of pregnancy, have patient rise slowly to prevent dizziness.
Atypical Antipsychotics Block dopamine and serotonin receptors	Clozapine (Clozaril) Risperidone (Risperdal) Olanzapine (Zyprexa)	PO PO, IM, long-acting IM PO, fast-dissolving tablets	Agranulocytosis (Clozaril), weight gain, type 2 diabetes, dose-related EPSE (Risperdal). Lowers seizure threshold.	Monitor CBC (Clozaril), monitor weight gain and onset of type 2 diabetes.
Selective Serotonin Reuptake Inhibitor (SSRI) Antidepressants Block the reuptake of serotonin at the presynaptic receptor.	Fluoxetine (Prozac, Prozac Weekly) Sertraline (Zoloft) Paroxetine (Paxil) Escitalopram (Lexapro)	PO, weekly dosing form available PO PO	Excitation, nausea and vomiting, decreased libido, anorexia, weight loss	Allow time for side effects to subside; do not administer after 3 p.m. to prevent excitation from affecting sleep; teach patient that it will take 2–4 weeks for therapeutic effects to occur, and possibly longer with Prozac.
Tricyclic Antidepressants Partially block the reuptake of serotonin and norepinephrine at the presynaptic receptor (*used less frequently because of side effects*)	Amitriptyline (Elavil) Amoxapine (Asendin) Nortriptyline (Pamelor) Imipramine (Tofranil)	PO PO PO PO	Anticholinergic effects, sedation, weight gain, orthostatic hypotension, tachycardia	Decreases effects of antihypertensives, lowers seizure threshold, will affect oral contraceptives. Teach patient that it will take 2–4 weeks for therapeutic effects to occur.
Selective Serotonin Norepinephrine Reuptake Inhibitor (SNRI)	Venlafaxine (Effexor, Effexor XR)	PO	Anxiety, abnormal dreams, dizziness, nervousness	Monitor blood pressure for systolic hypertension
Monoamine Oxidase Inhibitor (MAOI) Antidepressants Block the action of monoamine oxidase	Phenelzine (Nardil) Tranylcypromine (Parnate) Isocarboxazid (Marplan)	PO PO PO	Anticholinergic effects, orthostatic hypotension, will interact with foods containing tyramine and cause hypertensive crisis, headache.	Teach about tyramine-free diet. Interacts with many prescribed and over-the-counter medications. Serious fatal reactions with SSRI or SNRI. Teach patient not to stop taking abruptly.

Medication Class/Action	Examples	Route	Side Effects	Nursing Implications
Benzodiazepines *Antianxiety* Potentiate effects of GABA, which causes a calming effect	Alprazolam (Xanax)	PO	Sedation, hangover effect, ataxia, confusion, dizziness, anticholinergic effects	Short-term use only; addictive, do not use in pregnancy, caution in the elderly, do not operate heavy machinery, do not abruptly stop taking.
	Diazepam (Valium)	PO		
	Lorazepam (Ativan)	PO, IM		
Buspar *Antianxiety* Unknown action	Buspirone (BuSpar)	PO	Headaches, dizziness, GI upset, lightheadedness	Teach patient that it will take 3–6 weeks to work; non–habit forming, little sedating effect.
Anticonvulsant Mood Stabilizers Antikindling effect, affect GABA receptors	Carbamazepine (Tegretol)	PO	Dizziness, drowsiness, blurred vision, nausea, headache, weight gain, blood dyscrasias	Use cautiously with MAOIs, elderly, liver, renal, or cardiac disease, and pregnancy.
	Clonazepam (Klonopin)	PO	Nausea, vomiting, ataxia, dizziness, drowsiness	Do not use in pregnancy, caution in elderly, caution in patients with liver or renal disease.
	Lamotrigine (Lamictal)	PO	Headache, dizziness, ataxia, nausea, vomiting, photosensitivity, rash, Stevens-Johnson syndrome	Caution patient to use sunscreen and to report any signs of rash immediately. Avoid with breastfeeding.
	Valproic acid (Depakote)	PO	Nausea, headache, menstrual disturbances, weight gain, hair loss, lethargy, tremors	Caution with hepatic toxicity, monitor for signs of bleeding, do not use in pregnancy, loading dose may be ordered for acute mania.
Lithium *Antimanic* Decreases postsynaptic receptor sensitivity	Lithium carbonate (Eskalith)	PO	Thirst, nausea and vomiting, weight gain, tremors, skin rash (acne), hair loss, hypothyroidism	Narrow therapeutic range increases risk for toxicity; monitor blood levels; do not use in cardiac or renal disease, do not use with diuretics, do not use in pregnancy.
Antiparkinsonian Agents Restore the natural balance of acetylcholine and dopamine in the CNS	Benztropine (Cogentin)	PO, IM	Anticholinergic effects, nausea, GI upset, sedation, dizziness, orthostatic hypotension	Caution with hypersensitivity, glaucoma, history of urinary retention.
	Trihexyphenidyl (Artane)	PO, IM		
	Diphenhydramine (Benadryl)	PO, IM		

CNS = central nervous system; GABA = gamma-aminobutyric acid; GI = gastrointestinal.

Box 57.1

Anxiety Summary

Signs and Symptoms	• Phobia: Irrational fear of object or situation • Panic disorder: Extreme fear, feelings of impending doom, palpitations • Generalized anxiety disorder: Worry, restlessness, palpitations • Obsessive-compulsive disorder: Uncontrollable repetitive thoughts, urges, or actions
Diagnosis	History of symptoms; physical causes for symptoms must be ruled out first
Therapeutic Interventions	Antianxiety medication, selective serotonin reuptake inhibitors, systematic desensitization, psychotherapy, relaxation exercises
Nursing Diagnosis	Anxiety

diagnosed when symptoms begin to interfere with normal day-to-day functioning. People of all age groups and all ethnic and socioeconomic groups can develop mood disorders.

Etiological Theories

Psychoanalytical theory indicates that people who have suffered loss in their lives are at risk for developing depression. This has been supported by recent research. Depression is also associated with unresolved anger and has been explained as "anger turned inward." In other words, people who cannot or do not deal appropriately with situations that anger them may repress the anger (turn it inside) and become depressed.

Cognitive theorists believe that the way people perceive events and situations may lead to depression. Instead of thinking about failing an examination as being unfortunate and disappointing, some people with tendencies toward depression may exaggerate the emotion and turn the situation into something much deeper, such as thoughts of "I'm stupid" or "I'll never get anywhere."

Biological theories offer genetic links and neurotransmitter dysfunctions as two etiologies. Serotonin, norepinephrine, and dopamine have an effect on mood; if these neurotransmitters are elevated, mood is elevated, and if they are low, mood is low. Biological theorists also believe that there is a connection between these neurotransmitters and female hormones.

Differential Diagnosis

Symptoms of depression may occur in conjunction with other disorders, such as schizophrenia or drug side effects or overuse. Heart failure, nutritional deficiencies, drug toxicity, thyroid disease, fluid and electrolyte imbalances, infections, and diabetes can be associated with depression. Depression related to grief is considered a normal reaction unless it is prolonged (unresolved grief).

Types of Mood Disorders

MAJOR (UNIPOLAR) DEPRESSION. Major depression is an episodic condition, and symptoms interfere with the individual's usual social or occupational functioning. Depressed individuals view the world through "gray tinted glasses." The *Diagnostic and Statistical Manual of Mental Disorders IV-Text Revision* (DSM-IV-TR) specifies that symptoms of major depression include either a depressed mood or **anhedonia** (the loss of pleasure in things that are usually pleasurable) along with at least five of the following symptoms:

• Significant weight loss or gain
• Increase or decrease in appetite
• Sleep pattern disturbances—insomnia or hypersomnia
• Increased fatigue
• Increased agitation or psychomotor retardation
• Diminished libido
• Anergia
• Social withdrawal
• Decreased ability to think, remember, or concentrate
• Feelings of guilt or hopelessness
• Indecisiveness
• Suicidal ideation

BIPOLAR DISORDER. Approximately 2 million people in the United States suffer from **bipolar** disorder. Bipolar disorder (formerly called manic depressive illness) is a mood disorder in which patients experience both **mania** (extreme elation or agitation) and extreme depression. Bipolar disorder is more severe than major depression. Affected individuals stay depressed longer, relapse more frequently, display more depressive symptoms, have more **delusions** and **hallucinations**, commit suicide more often, require more hospitalizations, and overall experience more incapacitation.

Individuals can cycle slowly (over weeks or months or even years), or they can be "rapid cyclers" who can change moods several times in an hour.

Common signs of depression were covered in the preceding section. Common signs of mania include the following:

• Excessive high (euphoric) moods
• Increased energy, activity, restlessness
• Decreased need for sleep
• Grandiosity (unrealistic belief in one's abilities or powers)

---

anhedonia: an—not + hedonia—pleasure

- Extreme irritability and distractibility
- Uncharacteristically poor judgment
- Pressured and rapid speech
- Flight of ideas or subjective experience that one's thoughts are racing
- Increase in goal-directed behavior
- Excessive involvement in pleasurable activities that have a high potential for unpleasant consequences, such as sex, substance abuse, or shopping sprees
- Obnoxious, provocative, or intrusive behavior

Therapeutic Interventions for Patients with Mood Disorders

Approximately 80% of people with major depression respond to treatment. Bipolar disorder is more difficult to treat. Some common medical treatments for *all* mood disorders include the following:

- Antidepressants
- Mood stabilizers
- Psychotherapy
- Electroconvulsive therapy

Lithium was once the drug of choice for the treatment of bipolar disorder. Lithium is an antimanic medication with a very narrow therapeutic range (toxic drug levels can easily develop). Lithium levels must be drawn regularly to assess that serum levels are in the therapeutic range. Antidepressants should be used carefully as they may induce a manic episode. See Table 57.2 for a summary of medications. Also see Box 57.2 Nutrition Notes.

Mood stabilizers like the anticonvulsants valproic acid (Depakote) and lamotrigine (Lamictal) are now more commonly used to treat bipolar disorder. Atypical antipsychotics are also commonly used in conjunction with the mood stabilizer when the patient is in the acute manic state.

Psychotherapy for the patient and family may be helpful for any type of mood disorder. It can help the patient understand the illness and learn problem solving and other new adaptive coping behaviors. For young children, play therapy is the most common and effective form of therapy. Electroconvulsive therapy is an option for individuals with

SAFETY TIP

When you do your nursing assessment, be sure to ask about herbal supplements the patient may use in addition to prescription and over-the-counter medications. Many people take St. John's wort, an over-the-counter herbal supplement, for depression. While it may be effective for some people with mild depression, it can interact with many prescribed medications that influence serotonin levels. If combined with prescription antidepressants, it can cause an excess of serotonin, resulting in agitation, confusion, diarrhea, muscle spasms, and even death.

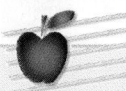

Box 57.2
Nutrition Notes

Anticipating Food-Drug Interactions in Patients with Mental Health Disorders

Monoamine Oxidase Inhibitors. Some antidepressant drugs (e.g., isocarboxazid, phenelzine, tranylcypromine) are monoamine oxidase inhibitors (MAOIs). These drugs counteract depression by preventing the breakdown of dopamine and tyramine, an intermediate product in the conversion of tyrosine to epinephrine. The increased concentration of these chemicals in the central nervous system elevates the patient's mood.

When a patient taking an MAOI consumes foods high in tyramine, the drug prevents the normal breakdown of tyramine, leading to excessive epinephrine. Hypertension results, sometimes severe enough to cause intracranial hemorrhage. Some other drugs (e.g., furazolidone, isoniazid, linezolid, procarbazine, selegiline) produce similar reactions with tyramine-containing foods.

All food groups except breads and cereals have some items with sufficient tyramine to cause problems for patients taking MAOIs. Examples of common foods to be avoided are bananas, aged cheese, yogurt, bologna, salami, pepperoni, summer sausage, chocolate, beer, and wine.

Lithium Carbonate. Lithium carbonate, used to treat bipolar disorder, is absorbed, distributed, and excreted alongside sodium. Fluctuations in sodium intake affect the metabolism of lithium. Thus, decreased sodium intake with decreased fluid intake may lead to retention of lithium and overmedication. Increased sodium intake from food or medications and increased fluid intake may hasten excretion of lithium, resulting in worsening signs and symptoms of mania.

rapid-cycling bipolar disorder or major depression that is not responsive to conventional treatment on page 1284.

Nursing Process for the Patient with a Mood Disorder

See Box 57.3 Nursing Care Plan for the Patient with Depression. Also see Box 57.4 Depression Summary on page 1284.

Somatoform/Psychosomatic Disorders

The **somatoform** (or **psychosomatic**) disorders are conditions in which physical symptoms occur with no known organic cause. It is believed that the physical symptoms are an expression of psychological pain or distress. Because the patient is not able to control the symptoms, they are considered to be caused by some unconscious mechanism.

---

psychosomatic: psych(e)—soul or mind + somatic—body

CRITICAL THINKING

Mr. Zenz

■ Mr. Zenz is the manager of a busy office/clinic. His usual behavior is rather sullen and he comes across as "quiet" or "sad" to various members of the staff. He is in his 40s, married, with three children ages 4, 5, and 7. He speaks of them proudly but always comments that they "take after their mother." His management style in the office is to let people do their jobs; he rarely interferes, although his door is always open and staff members are told they are welcome any time. Recently, however, staff members are noticing a change in Mr. Zenz. He moves quickly, speaks quickly, and has set grandiose goals for the staff. He frequently says he has called the president of the company to tell him of his new ideas. He says he has not slept in several days and he feels terrific. He has changed his wardrobe and has begun pointing out specific performance issues to staff. He jokes with staff. Staff is made aware that he has "bipolar disorder" and has quit taking his medications. His wife has asked for the staff's help. Remember: He is your boss. How do you respond to Mrs. Zenz? How do you approach him?

Suggested answers at end of chapter.

Etiological Theories

Psychoanalytical theorists believe that the somatoform disorders are rooted in unconscious mechanisms that develop to deny, repress, and displace anxiety. Biological research suggests the possibility of a genetic predisposition to somatic difficulties.

Types of Somatoform Disorders

There are five separate illnesses within the category of somatoform disorders and two additional illnesses that are closely related. These include **conversion disorder,** hypochondriasis, dysmorphophobia/body dysmorphic disorder, somatization disorder, and somatoform pain disorder. Discussion of all these disorders is beyond the scope of this book. This chapter gives a brief explanation of conversion disorder.

CONVERSION DISORDER. Conversion disorder is an illness that emerges from overuse of the conversion reaction defense mechanism. (See Table 56.2 in Chapter 56.) In conversion disorder there is a loss or decrease in physical functioning that seems to have a neurological connection. Paralysis and blindness are the two most common examples of this disorder. Age of onset is usually adolescence and young adulthood, but it can occur later in life as well.

The symptoms, although not caused by organic disease, are very real to the patient. It should not be conveyed to the patient that you think the person is "faking" the illness; this is not true. Patients are truly experiencing the symptoms.

It is believed that the symptom is allowing the person to avoid some situation that is unacceptable to him or her. The symptom helps the patient relieve the anxiety. This is called primary gain. Secondary gain results from the extra benefits one may acquire as a result of staying ill, such as extra emotional support, sympathy, love, or financial benefits.

Box 57.3   NURSING CARE PLAN **for the Patient with Depression**

Nursing Diagnosis: Risk for suicide

Expected Outcome The patient will not harm him/herself.

Evaluation of Outcome Did the patient remain free from self-harm during hospitalization?

Interventions	Rationale	Evaluation
Ask patient directly about suicidal ideations each shift.	Ongoing assessment of suicidal risk is essential to patient safety.	Is the patient verbalizing warning signs of suicide?
Create a safe environment for the patient.	Patient safety is a nursing priority.	Are means of harming self kept from patient?
Initiate suicide precautions according to agency protocol.	The patient must be protected until risk is reduced.	Is increased surveillance of patient implemented and communicated to all staff?
Encourage the patient to seek out nursing staff when experiencing suicidal thoughts.	Active listening and therapeutic communication by staff provide the patient with empathy and alternatives to acting on suicidal thoughts.	Does the patient seek out nursing staff when experiencing suicidal thoughts?

Nursing Diagnosis: Ineffective coping

Expected Outcomes The patient will cope effectively as evidenced by (1) verbalizing the ability to cope and asking for help when needed; (2) demonstrating new effective coping strategies.

Evaluation of Outcomes Does the patient exhibit increased ability to problem solve?

Interventions	Rationale	Evaluation
Use therapeutic communication and encourage the patient to verbalize feelings.	Verbalization of feelings in a supportive environment may assist patient to work through issues.	Does the patient verbalize feelings to nursing staff?
Assist the patient to describe stressors and coping mechanisms used.	Reviewing successful coping strategies can strengthen effective coping and diminish ineffective methods.	Is the patient able to identify stressors and related coping strategies in used in the past?
Help the patient set realistic goals and identify his or her skills and knowledge.	Providing validation of actual stress and available coping resources and strategies aids in positive adaptation to stress.	Does the patient set realistic goals?
Encourage the patient to make choices and participate in care.	Active involvement in care increases the possibility of positive adjustment.	Is the patient actively involved in care?

Nursing Diagnosis: Powerlessness

Expected Outcomes The patient will reduce feelings of powerlessness as evidenced by (1) verbal expression of having control over life, situation, or care; (2) participation in care or decision making when opportunities are provided.

Evaluation of Outcomes Does patient identify feelings of powerlessness? Does patient identify factors that are controllable and actively participate in care?

Interventions	Rationale	Evaluation
Assess for factors contributing to powerlessness.	Correct identification of actual or perceived problems is essential to providing appropriate support.	Has there been correct identification of factors contributing to powerlessness?
Help the patient to identify factors not under his or her control.	Identifying factors within the patient's control encourages the patient to take some control over the situation.	Is the patient able to identify what is controllable and what is not controllable in his or her life?
Encourage the ventilation of feelings.	Sharing feelings can lead to the realization that similar feelings are experienced by others and reduce powerlessness.	Is the patient sharing feelings with nursing staff and in therapeutic groups?
Encourage the patient to actively participate in care with goal-directed activities.	Goal-directed behavior increases self-efficacy and empowerment.	Does the patient set realistic goals daily and achieve them daily?

Therapeutic Interventions for Patients with Somatoform Disorders

Because of the physical symptoms, hospitalized patients are usually admitted to a medical unit rather than a psychiatric unit. True physiological causes for symptoms must be ruled out. Treatment is individualized for the patient. Hypnosis and relaxation techniques are used with many patients. Methods of stress management are taught. Behavior management may be effective for some patients. Patients may resist accepting the fact that their problem is psychological or emotional in nature and may feel insulted and become resistant to treatment.

Box 57.4

Depression Summary

Signs and Symptoms	• Unipolar: depressed mood, weight changes, anhedonia, sleep disturbance, social withdrawal • Bipolar: Signs and symptoms of depression cycling with euphoria; delusions, hallucinations
Diagnosis	History; physiological causes must be ruled out
Therapeutic Interventions	Antidepressant medication, mood stabilizers (anticonvulsants), psychotherapy, electroconvulsive therapy
Nursing Diagnosis	Ineffective coping, powerlessness, risk for suicide

Medications are used sparingly. When they are ordered for a patient, the classifications of choice are usually antidepressants, antianxiety agents, or both.

Nursing Management for Patients with Somatoform Disorders

Nursing management for somatoform disorders includes the following:

• *Skillful communication.* Honesty and gaining trust encourage the patient to verbalize thoughts and feelings about the physical and emotional aspects of this disorder. An example of a way to be honest about the situation would be to reinforce what the physician has said to the patient, such as, "Ms. Parks, your doctor can find no physical or life-threatening conditions at this time. We will continue to observe and examine you. We will make every attempt to help you improve." Sometimes the practitioner helps the patient find a healthy behavior to substitute for the symptom.

• *Therapy.* Keeping the patient focused on other topics than the symptoms may help in the recovery. Spend time with the patient other than when they have physical complaints.

• *Support.* When caring for the patient with a somatoform disorder, you must pay attention to the person but must not reinforce the symptoms. Use a matter of fact approach and don't imply that the symptoms are not real. A thorough head-to-toe assessment should always be done. Observe and record frequency of complaints. Provide explanations and support during diagnostic tests. The patient will see your concern for his or her health, but you will not

be focusing on the area of dysfunction or reinforcing the problem. All findings should be documented objectively.

Schizophrenia

Schizophrenia is becoming more widely viewed as a group of illnesses rather than a single condition. Onset is often during adolescence or young adulthood. The National Institute of Mental Health estimates that nearly 3 million persons in the United States will develop schizophrenia during the course of their lives.

The term *schizophrenia* (which means "split mind") was first used by a Swiss psychiatrist, Eugene Bleuler.[1] Schizophrenia is a serious brain disorder of thought and association and is characterized by an inability to distinguish between what is real and what is not, hallucinations, delusions, and limited socialization. People who have schizophrenia may not be able to differentiate between what is "theirs" and what is "everybody else's" in relation to social functioning. Poor self-esteem may be an issue. It is difficult for them to focus on one topic for any length of time. Schizophrenia is not the same thing as multiple personality disorder.

Schizophrenia has an insidious onset. This means that it develops over time, and symptoms may go unnoticed for a time prior to diagnosis. There are four phases of schizophrenia:

1. *Schizoid Personality.* Individuals in this phase are perceived as being indifferent, cold, and aloof. They are often described as loners and don't seem to enjoy close relationships with others. In an adolescent, these behaviors may be dismissed as normal for age. Not all individuals with schizoid personality go on to develop schizophrenia.

2. *Prodromal Phase.* Individuals continue to be socially withdrawn and begin to exhibit behavior that is peculiar or eccentric. Role functioning is impaired, personal hygiene is neglected, and disturbances are evident in communication, ideation, and perception.

3. *Schizophrenia.* This is the third and active phase of the disorder. Psychotic symptoms are prominent and include delusions, hallucinations, and impairment in work, social relations, and self-care.

4. *Residual Phase.* Symptoms are similar to the prodromal phase with flat affect and impairment in role functioning.

Positive and Negative Symptoms

Positive symptoms of schizophrenia can be thought of as those symptoms that reflect an "excess" or distortion of normal functioning. Positive symptoms include hallucinations, delusions, disorganized thinking, and disorganized behavior. **Delusions** are fixed, false beliefs that cannot be changed by logic or factual proof. Typically, patients exhibit delusions of grandeur, persecution, or guilt. **Hallucinations** are false sensory perceptions. They can affect any of the five senses; auditory and visual delusions are most common. For example, a person might see a person that no one else sees, or hear voices that no one else hears. In contrast, **illusions** are mistaken perceptions of reality. For example, a person may see a glowing sunset and think the horizon is on fire. Both the typical and atypical antipsychotic medications work well on the positive symptoms of schizophrenia.

Negative symptoms of schizophrenia can be thought of as a loss of normal functioning. Negative symptoms include affective blunting or flattening, **alogia**, **avolition**, apathy, anhedonia, and social isolation. It is thought that these are the most debilitating symptoms of schizophrenia because they keep the individual from living a normal life. These symptoms respond to atypical antipsychotic medications, but not the typical antipsychotic agents.

Pathophysiology and Etiology

There are psychoanalytical and biological theories of the causes of schizophrenia. The causes of schizophrenia are highly debated on both sides of the nature-versus-nurture theories.

The psychoanalytical, or nurture, theories refer to the anal stage of Freudian theory. The inability to meet the challenge of oral gratification leaves people in the adolescent and young adult years unable to handle their developing sexuality, according to Freud. Lack of nurturing mother-child relationships can also lead to personalities that are cool or indifferent in their relationships. Freud would also attribute the disruption of effective communication to failure to attain oral gratification.

The role of genetics in schizophrenia (psychobiological, or nature, theory) has been examined in twins studies, family studies, and adoption studies for more than 75 years. Studies of identical twins show that if one twin has schizophrenia, the other has about a 50% chance of developing it also. In fraternal twins that percentage drops to about 10%. It is believed that the more genes twins or family members have in common, the greater the probability of the second twin developing schizophrenia.

Other studies have examined the relationship of dopamine and schizophrenia. Patients with schizophrenia generally have elevated amounts of dopamine or a brain that overreacts to the amount of dopamine that is present. Today, schizophrenia is primarily thought of as a series of brain disorders characterized by brain abnormalities and excessive dopamine transmission.

Types of Schizophrenia

There are several categories of schizophrenia. This chapter discusses only the most common: paranoid schizophrenia. Paranoid schizophrenia is defined as schizophrenia in which the person exhibits unusual suspiciousness and fear. They may also be hostile and aggressive in their behavior.

Patients with paranoid schizophrenia tend to have delusions of persecution or grandeur. Patients experiencing persecutory delusions state that they feel tormented and followed by people. Patients often integrate people around them into their delusions. They may feel that nursing staff, relatives, or the announcer on the radio or television is trying to harm them. In delusions of grandeur, patients may state that they are God or the President of the United States.

Hallucinations often accompany delusions. The hallucinations can affect any of the five senses but are most commonly auditory followed by visual. Patients with paranoid schizophrenia talk about hearing "voices." These voices are frightening and derogatory to the patient and are responsible for many of the actions performed by people with paranoid schizophrenia. Patients experience increased fear, anxiety, and suicidal ideation as a result of the voices. You may see or hear patients arguing with what at first appears to be themselves. Actually the patient is arguing with the voices. Describing the voices is difficult, but imagine that you are in a room with six televisions on different stations at the same time. This example comes close to what some patients have described as the voices.

Therapeutic Interventions for the Patient with Schizophrenia

Medications, social skills training, and individual and family psychotherapy are indicated for patients with schizophrenia. Among the classifications of medications that may be prescribed for certain patients are the typical and atypical antipsychotics, which block dopamine action in the brain. There are different dopamine tracts in the brain, and the typical antipsychotics have a greater effect on the motor function tract, resulting in extrapyramidal symptoms such as parkinsonism (see medications in Table 57.2). Anticholinergic medications such as benztropine (Cogentin) or trihexyphenidyl (Artane) are used to combat the extrapyramidal side effects of the typical antipsychotics by helping return balance between dopamine, acetylcholine, and other neurotransmitters. Newer, atypical antipsychotic medications such as clozapine (Clozaril) and risperidone (Risperdal) have fewer extrapyramidal side effects, and are effective in treating both the positive and negative symptoms of schizophrenia.

Psychotherapy may include individual, group, and family therapy. Electroconvulsive therapy (ECT) is used in some severe cases or in cases that are difficult to treat; ECT is usually not used until other methods of therapy have been exhausted. Referral of the patient and family to organizations such as the National Alliance on Mental Illness (NAMI) provides helpful education and support (www. nami.org).

Nursing Process for the Patient with Schizophrenia

ASSESSMENT/DATA COLLECTION. Observe the patient with schizophrenia for positive and negative symptoms, including hallucinations, delusions, or illusions. Observe interactions with others. Monitor for response to medications, including side effects. Determine the individual's ability to function and manage own activities of daily living (ADLs).

---

alogia: a—not + logia—(able to) speak
avolition: a—not + volition—energy or initiative to do something

NURSING DIAGNOSIS, PLANNING, AND IMPLEMEN-TATION. Disturbed thought processes

EXPECTED OUTCOME: Patient will be oriented to person, place, and time; be able to manage medications, perform ADLs, and function in a community.

- Develop trust. Be honest and consistent in all areas of the patient's treatment plan. *Trust is essential to a therapeutic relationship.*
- Allow the patient to verbalize thoughts and feelings when appropriate to the time and place. *Verbalizing feelings can help the patient clarify concerns and feel supported.*
- Whenever possible, maintain consistent staff assignments *to ensure the best possible continuity of care and to promote the development of a trusting relationship.*
- Never whisper or laugh when the patient cannot hear the whole conversation. Face the patient when having a conversation. *Whispering or turning away may be interpreted as rejection; secretive behaviors can reinforce paranoia and suspiciousness.*
- Avoid placing the patient in situations of competition or embarrassment. *These situations can be threatening to the patient.*
- Never reinforce hallucinations, delusions, or illusions. Orient to reality as needed. *The patient needs to know what is real and what is not.*
- Use distraction to deal with the hallucinations. Assist to connect the delusions and hallucinations to times of increased anxiety. (See Table 57.3.) *This models strategies for the patient to use during times of anxiety.*
- Provide a calm and therapeutic milieu *to help reduce anxiety.*
- Provide written instructions and information boards *to help promote reality and self-responsible behavior.*

- Monitor medication use and initiate mouth checks as needed. *Patients may have difficulty maintaining a medication schedule or choose to not take medications as ordered due to paranoia.*
- Keep communication simple. Be brief and clear with all directions. State what is acceptable, giving the rationale and consequences at the same time. State information in positive rather than negative terms: "Eat your food calmly" rather than "Do not throw your food!" *Patients are more likely to process and respond to simple, direct communication.*
- Use touch cautiously. *Perceptions and distortions of reality may cause patients to misconstrue touch.*

EVALUATION. Is the patient alert and oriented? Is he or she able to manage medications, or is there a plan in place to make sure medications are administered? Is the patient able to manage ADLs and live in a community?

See Box 57.5 Schizophrenia Summary.

Substance Abuse Disorders

Alcoholism and chemical dependency are serious conditions. People start using alcohol and drugs for many reasons, but often it is to feel accepted by a peer group or to feel comfortable and reduce anxiety in a social situation. People mistake the temporary high as a stimulant. In reality, alcohol is a depressant. Any chemical can be potentially dangerous.

It is important to understand the following terms and their definitions:

- **Addiction**—the repeated compulsive use of a substance that continues in spite of negative consequences (physical, social, legal).
- **Tolerance**—increased amounts of a substance are needed over time to achieve the same effect as obtained previously with smaller amounts.
- Physical **withdrawal** syndrome—the physiological response to the abrupt stopping or reduction in a

TABLE 57.3 SUGGESTED INTERVENTIONS FOR PATIENTS WITH SCHIZOPHRENIA WHO ARE HALLUCINATING

Suggested Action	Rationale
1. "Mr. R., I don't see any snakes. It is time for lunch. I will walk to the dining room with you."	1. Lets the patient know you heard him, but brings him immediately into the reality of time of day and need to go to the dining room.
2. "I see a crack in the wall, Mr. R. It is harmless; you are safe. Susan is here to take you down to occupational therapy now."	2. This is in response to a probable illusion. It lets the patient know that you see something. It validates his fear, but it tells him what you see and then moves him into the here and now.
3. "I know that your thoughts seem very real to you, Ms. C., but they do not seem logical to me. I would like for you to come to your room and get dressed now, please."	3. Again, you are validating the patient's concern without exploring and focusing on the delusion.
4. "Ms. C, it appears to me that you are listening to someone. Are you hearing voices other than mine?"	4. This is a method of validating your impression of what you see. This is as far as you will go into exploring what she may be hearing.
5. "Thank you, Ms. C. I want to help you focus away from the other voices. I am real; they are not. Please come with me to the reading room."	5. Responds to her in the present and reinforces her response to you. Attempts to redirect her thinking.

Box 57.5

Schizophrenia Summary

Signs and Symptoms	• Disorganized speech and behavior • Ineffective thinking and decision making • Trouble functioning at school and work; self-care deficits • Positive symptoms: hallucinations, delusions • Negative symptoms: apathy, flat affect, anhedonia
Diagnosis	History; psychiatric evaluation
Therapeutic Interventions	Antipsychotic medications, anticholinergic agents to control side effects, psychotherapy; family education and therapy
Nursing Diagnosis	Disturbed thought processes

CRITICAL THINKING

Anne

■ While preparing to invite Anne, a patient receiving chemotherapy on your oncology unit, to a movie in the day room, you observe her standing in the corner of her room trembling. You ask her what's wrong and she responds that she's talking to the woman in the wall. Your first instinct is to giggle, but you ask her, "What woman?" She tells you that you wouldn't understand and says, "You helped put her there and you told me that it is my job to be sure she can't get out." You report this to the charge nurse, who calls the doctor. Tests are run, and it is determined that Anne is not experiencing side effects from the chemotherapy. Further work-up delivers the diagnosis of paranoid-type schizophrenia for Anne. What responses are appropriate for the situation above? What special needs might Anne now experience relating to her chemotherapy, if any? How will you get Anne to the movie or to participate in other care activities?

Suggested answers at end of chapter.

substance used (usually) for a long time. Withdrawal symptoms are specific to the substance used.

The general definitions of substance **abuse** and substance dependence apply to any substance. Substance **dependence** is a condition in which a person has several

(usually three) of the following symptoms for a single 12-month period. The patient:

• Needs more of the substance and at more frequent intervals to achieve the same "high," or desired effect of the substance.
• Spends significant time obtaining the substance.
• Gives up important social or professional functions to use the substance.
• Has tried at least once to quit but still obsesses about the substance.
• Experiences difficulty with job, family, or social activities because of use or withdrawal symptoms.
• Uses the substance regardless of the problems it causes.
• Uses the substance to avoid withdrawal symptoms.

Substance abuse is a maladaptive pattern of substance use leading to clinically significant impairment or distress manifested by one or more of the following within a 12-month period:

• Inability to fulfill major role obligations at work, school, or home
• Recurrent legal or interpersonal problems
• Continued use despite social and interpersonal problems
• Participation in physically hazardous situations while impaired, such as driving

Nurses need to be informed about chemical dependency for several reasons. First, many medical-surgical patients are chemically dependent. This affects their healing and the effect of their medications. Second, as part of the human experience, your chance of being in a close personal relationship with a person who is chemically dependent is great. Third, and perhaps most importantly, you are part of a profession whose members are statistically high users and abusers of drugs and alcohol (Box 57.6 Ethical Considerations). Studies indicate that anywhere from 5% to 20% of nurses in the United States will be chemically impaired at some point in their lifetime.

Substance abuse is not a one-person illness; it affects personal and professional relationships with people who are associated with the user. The term **dysfunctional** is often used to refer to the relationships within an alcoholic family or work environment. Dishonesty and inability to discuss the situation are strong components of the disease. Many times, people who live or work in the dysfunctional group begin to cover up for the user's behaviors and lack of responsibility. Family members or significant others may take sides, begin to be dishonest with each other, and erode the bond within that group. Eventually this leads to a condition called **codependence,** which can be as serious as the use and abuse of the substance. Codependent members of a family group begin to lose their own sense of identity and purpose and exist solely for the abuser. Their actions take away the opportunity for the user to take responsibility for his or her own actions. This is called *enabling*.

dysfunctional: dys—bad or difficult + functional—performance

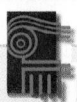

Box 57.6

Ethical Considerations

Whistle Blowing

Ellen and Julie are LPNs who work on a busy medical unit in a large hospital. They were close friends in nursing school and have been working the night shift together for 3 years. Recently, Ellen went through a difficult and painful divorce, and Julie has noticed that Ellen's personality has changed. Ellen, usually serious and almost compulsive in the completion of her work, has taken on a very lackadaisical attitude and often calls in sick. She also displays hostility toward the hospital administration and seems very irritated when corrected. Julie has observed Ellen taking increasingly large doses of pain medication and fears her friend is losing control.

One evening, Ellen arrives at work with glassy eyes and slurred speech. She asks Julie to watch her patients for her while she "takes a little nap." Julie asks Ellen if she is abusing her pain medication, and after some initial denial, Ellen admits that she has been taking increasingly large doses of medication and alcohol to continue functioning from day to day. Ellen pleads with Julie not to tell anyone else about the problem. Because of their friendship, Julie consents to cover for Ellen this night.

The next night, Ellen again comes to work with obvious signs of intoxication. She again asks Julie to cover for her, swearing that this would be the absolute last time it would happen. Ellen falls asleep while listening to the taped report for the change of shifts. What should Julie do?

Etiological Theories

Why do some people become addicted or dependent and others do not? Can it be the chemical, or is it the person? Some theorists believe in the existence of an addictive personality, which may begin to explain addictions to food, sex, and gambling, as well as alcohol, chemicals, and other dependencies.

Psychoanalytical theorists believe that people who develop addictions to alcohol or other substances are people who failed to successfully pass through the "oral" stage of development.

Biological theories include numerous studies that imply that there is some sort of genetic metabolic disorder. Many of these studies were done on twins born to an alcoholic parent or parents and who were separated from the parents at birth or shortly after birth. The number of twins who were born of alcoholic parents but raised by nonalcoholic adoptive or foster parents and yet developed alcoholism was consistently elevated.

Cognitive-behavioral theorists suggest the way in which a person perceives being high may influence the act of becoming high. It can be a very innocent beginning:

obtaining relief from the medications given by the doctor can, according to cognitive theory, leave people perceiving that the drugs offer a miracle cure. It becomes appealing to want that kind of relief again, and very soon a pattern is formed and other substances may be added.

Differential Diagnosis

Commonly, the alcoholic patient is admitted to the medical unit with primary medical diagnoses including dehydration, hyperemesis, or respiratory infection. Nursing assessment, patient need for frequent pain medication, or symptoms of withdrawal may lead you or the physician to pursue the possibility of chemical dependency. Laboratory tests can rule out physiological problems; drug levels of alcohol or drugs can also be measured. A patient who is uncommonly anxious for early discharge should also be further assessed.

Types

ALCOHOL ABUSE AND DEPENDENCE. Use and abuse of alcohol is present in all walks of life, in all economic levels, and in both genders. Sometimes a very fine line exists between a person who is a social drinker and a person who has an abuse condition. One factor used to make that differentiation is the degree of need or compulsion to drink. There is a high incidence of alcohol use and abuse among the elderly, teenagers, and even younger children. Alcoholism either directly or indirectly decreases a person's life expectancy by an average of 10 to 12 years.

Denial is a common ego defense mechanism used by people who are substance abusers. The alcohol-dependent person often uses statements such as "I can quit anytime I want to" or "I just need a little bump to loosen me up."

Characteristics of dependence were described earlier. In addition, the alcoholic patients may experience:

- Binges usually lasting 2 days or more
- Blackouts (unable to recall what happened during period of drinking)
- Vomiting and dehydration
- Disorientation
- Increased vulnerability to infections, accidents, and other injuries

Sometimes patients who are actively using drugs or alcohol when admitted to an inpatient setting, or who are cut off from their alcohol abruptly, experience a condition called **delirium tremens** (DTs). In DTs, hyperexcitability in the sensory activity of the individual can cause visual hallucinations, tremors, and possibly tonic-clonic seizures. Elevated blood pressure and pulse and cardiac dysrhythmias may also occur. Symptoms of withdrawal begin within 4 to 12 hours after the patient has stopped drinking and will peak in 24 to 48 hours. Hospitalization is necessary to maintain the patient's safety.

Therapeutic Interventions for Alcohol Abuse and Dependence. Treatment for and recovery from alcohol dependency and abuse is a slow process. With very few exceptions, an alcoholic who is recovering cannot ever have another drink, or he or she will risk the chance of returning to previous abusive patterns. Some treatment options are described below. Several forms of treatment may be used together.

Support Groups. A common and effective treatment for alcoholism is involvement in Alcoholics Anonymous (AA). AA is a 12-step program that offers support through others who have stopped drinking. For more information on AA, go to http://www.alcoholics-anonymous.org. Another program for women only is Women for Sobriety (www.womenforsobriety.org).

Cognitive Behavioral Therapy. Cognitive behavioral therapy (CBT) is used as an adjunct therapy for control of substance abuse. CBT advocates believe that with homework and practice, a person can learn to think differently about the event that led to the drinking. When the person changes the belief system about the activating event and the drinking, the consequences of drinking will be less powerful.

Psychotherapy. Psychotherapy provides one-on-one therapy. Because addiction affects an entire family, family therapy is important in reinstating honesty in communications. A commitment to stop drinking is required and therapy will only help with some of the issues resulting from years of drinking.

Medications. Medications are used cautiously because of risk for abuse. It is not always wise to substitute another chemical for alcohol. If, however, the anxiety level prohibits participation in therapy, or if a depressive disorder accompanies the abuse, medications may be prescribed. Antidepressant or nonaddictive antianxiety drugs are most often prescribed.

Disulfiram (Antabuse) is a medication that is sometimes prescribed as a deterrent to using alcohol. Disulfiram should never be administered without full informed consent of the patient. If the patient taking disulfiram ingests alcohol, a severe reaction causes chest pain, nausea, vomiting, confusion, and other symptoms. Persons taking disulfiram can also be adversely affected if they use products that contain alcohol, such as cologne, mouthwash, aftershave, or cough syrup. The effects of disulfiram last 2 to 3 weeks after the last dose.

Acamprosate (Campral) is a new drug that works on neurotransmitters to alter functions of other brain chemicals that have been affected by long-term drinking. Naltrexone (ReVia) may decrease alcohol cravings and impulsive behavior. Use of benzodiazepines (Valium, Ativan) can help prevent symptoms of DTs during acute withdrawal, but are not used long term because of risk for dependence.

Hospitalization. Therapy may range from in-house hospitalizations of 2 weeks or more to step down to halfway houses to eventual independence, usually attending AA meetings. It is common for patients to seek treatment multiple times. This should not be interpreted as a weakness in the individual or the treatment program. It is only a sign that the person is learning more about the disorder and the need to help him- or herself. People with all kinds of chronic disease experiences relapse at times.

Nursing Process for the Patient with Alcohol Abuse and Dependence

Assessment/Data Collection. A common screening tool to determine if a patient has a drinking problem is the CAGE questionnaire[2]:

- Have you ever felt you should *Cut down* on your drinking?
- Have people *Annoyed* you by criticizing your drinking?
- Have you ever felt bad or *Guilty* about your drinking?
- Have you ever had a drink first thing in the morning (as an "*Eye opener*") to steady your nerves or get rid of a hangover?

A yes answer to two or more questions suggests a drinking problem.

Alcohol can also have many physiological effects on a patient. See Chapter 32 for assessment of patients with liver disorders.

Nursing Diagnosis, Planning, and Implementation. Nursing diagnoses include ineffective denial and ineffective coping.

EXPECTED OUTCOMES: *The patient will accept responsibility for her or his behavior, verbalize acceptance of the relationship between substance abuse and personal problems, and will identify effects of alcohol on the body.*

- Expect sobriety. *This establishes sobriety as the norm.*
- Identify recent behavior while under the influence. *Patients need to see the relationship between their substance use and their personal problems.*
- Teach about the physical impact of drugs and alcohol on the body. *Many patients lack correct information about the effects of substance abuse on the body.*
- Be honest. You need to be in touch with your own thoughts and feelings about addictions. *Effective communication is essential for a therapeutic relationship.*
- Provide group support such as a 12-step program. Many chemical dependency units provide group support meetings. *Peer support is an effective treatment that is often more acceptable to patients.*
- Confront the patient immediately if projection, rationalization, or denial behaviors are noted. *Projection, rationalization, and denial are ego defense mechanisms that discourage the patient from accepting responsibility for behavior.*
- Use positive reinforcement. *Positive reinforcement for successes is important when helping a person with an addiction. Every step is a big one in this field; every step taken is a new one.*
- Provide a safe environment. *Patients who are chemically addicted may become suicidal or display other bizarre behavior, especially during DTs. A patient under the influence of alcohol or another chemical may have poor impulse control or judg-*

ment. *Maintaining a safe milieu and calm demeanor will help the patient through this difficult time.*

- Remain alert to the possibility that the patient may be using a substance even in the hospital. Express suspicions honestly and nonjudgmentally to the patient. Report and document all findings and behaviors that may be potential safety issues for the patient. *The fact that a patient is hospitalized does not guarantee that he or she does not have access to the chemical or even use it in your presence. Unfortunately, family members or friends sometimes smuggle drugs or alcohol in to the patient.*
- Practice "tough love." "Doing for" patients may be tempting, but it is not in the patient's best interest most of the time. Praise and validate the patient's attempts at self-responsible behavior and use therapeutic communication skills to constructively confront behaviors that are inconsistent with the plan of care. *This encourages patients to be responsible for their own healing.*

Evaluation. Does the patient verbalize acceptance of responsibility for own behavior? Does the patient understand the relationship between personal problems and substance abuse? Does the patient understand the effects of substance abuse on their body?

For additional information, go to the National Institute for Alcohol Abuse and Alcoholism at http://www.niaaa.nih.gov/.

DRUG ABUSE AND DEPENDENCE. Many substances other than alcohol can be addictive to humans. Caffeine and nicotine are two that are very readily available. Coffee, tea, soda, and cigarettes are everywhere in our society and yet are very addicting. Many experts believe that the single most difficult addiction to overcome is the addiction to nicotine. Illegal substances, such as marijuana, cocaine, crack, and PCP, and prescription medications for pain and mental health treatment are also potentially addictive. Methamphetamine (meth) is becoming a growing substance use/abuse problem affecting families and society.

It is also popular among the youth in the United States to use inhalants such as lighter fluid, paint, paint thinners, and gasoline to get high. The term for this is *huffing*. These are highly toxic substances, potentially lethal, and usually available in the house or garage.

Signs and Symptoms of Drug Abuse and Dependence. The signs and symptoms of drug abuse and dependence can be very similar to those of alcohol abuse. Additional signs of drug abuse include the following:

- Red, watery eyes
- Runny nose
- Hostile behavior
- Paranoia
- Needle tracks on arms or legs

Therapeutic Interventions for Patients with Drug Abuse and Dependence. These include:

- Narcotics Anonymous
- Group therapy

- Psychotherapy
- Methadone programs

Methadone acts as a sort of "step down" for people addicted to certain opiate drugs. Methadone can be legally prescribed and dispensed. It, too, is potentially addicting, and its critics believe it is only a substitute for heroin. It is typically given once a day. Psychotherapy is also provided for patients in methadone programs.

SAFETY TIP

To help prevent misuse of prescription medications:

Implement a process for obtaining and documenting a complete list of the client's current medications upon the client's entry to the organization and with the involvement of the client. This process includes a comparison of the medications the organization provides to those on the list.

A complete list of the client's medications is communicated to the next provider of service when a client is referred or transferred to another setting, service, practitioner, or level of care within or outside the organization. (2006 National Patient Safety Goals from www.jcaho.org.)

Nursing Interventions for Patients with Drug Abuse and Dependence. Nursing care for people who are drug dependent is essentially the same as for those who are alcohol dependent. It is important to remember that nurses and doctors cannot "fix" the patient who is chemically dependent. The desire to be chemically free must come from the individual who is addicted.

Caring for patients with mental health disorders is challenging and rewarding. You will learn that there are very few absolutes in the area of mental health nursing. There are many guidelines about the illnesses, but caring for the patients who have the illnesses is as individualized as the patients themselves. It is also important to remember to care for the whole person. The mind and body work together, so be sure to take care of the physical, emotional, cognitive, and behavioral parts of patients.

See Box 57.7 Substance Abuse Summary.

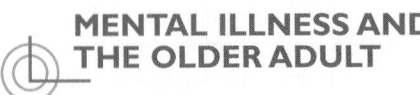

MENTAL ILLNESS AND THE OLDER ADULT

It is not uncommon for older adults to be admitted to the hospital for "change in mental status." It is important to distinguish between physical and mental disorders in these circumstances. Some disorders that affect older adults' mental status are below.

- *Dementia* is an impairment of mental functioning that interferes with daily activities and relationships.

Box 57.7

Substance Abuse Summary

Signs and Symptoms	• Inability to fulfill obligations at work, school, or home • Recurrent legal or interpersonal problems • Continued use despite social and interpersonal problems • Participation in physically hazardous situations while impaired
Diagnosis	History, liver function studies, serum drug or alcohol levels; evaluate for other coexisting disorders (bipolar disorder)
Therapeutic Interventions	12-step programs; cognitive behavioral therapy; psychotherapy; disulfiram (Antabuse), acamprosate (Campral), naltrexone (ReVia); benzodiazepines for acute withdrawal
Nursing Diagnosis	Ineffective denial, ineffective coping

Causes of dementia include Alzheimer's disease, vascular dementia, Huntington's disease, and others.
• *Delirium* is an acute change in mental status needing immediate evaluation and treatment. This is often due to a physiological condition such as an infection, and can be reversed if recognized and the underlying condition corrected. Read more about dementia and delirium in Chapter 48.
• *Pseudodementia* is a condition in which the patient appears to have dementia but is really depressed. Treating the depression can help reverse the mental status changes.

Depression in the elderly should not be viewed as a normal part of aging; it should be diagnosed and treated. Older adults may be dealing with physical and mental decline, loss of function, isolation, and loss of a marriage partner and friends, and may express their depression through bodily complaints such as pain. If not evaluated and treated, depression may lead to suicide. (See Box 57.8 Suicide and the Older Adult). Be sure to review Chapter 14 Nursing Care of Older Adult Patients.

CRITICAL THINKING

Maria

■ You are a school nurse in your local high school. You notice that Maria, a 17-year-old student, is behaving oddly. She has always been rather loud and even has been referred to as "obnoxious" by several of her peers. Lately you have observed her sitting alone, as if waiting for someone, but when you approach her, she barely greets you and then moves away. What are your concerns about Maria? What are some of the possibilities that might be affecting her? How can you approach her more effectively the next time you see her?

Suggested answers at end of chapter.

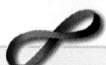

Box 57.8

Gerontological Issues

Suicide and the Older Adult

Older adults are not immune to suicidal thoughts. White males over the age of 75 have an especially high suicide rate.

Comments by any older adult referring to hopelessness or desire to die must be explored to assess suicide risk. The following comments could be a reflection of suicide potential in an older adult who is depressed:
• "Living is harder than dying could ever be."
• "I am a used-up old man who is a burden for everyone."
• "I am useless. I can't do anything anymore."
• "I don't know why God won't take me."

To adequately assess suicide potential, the nurse must ask questions that establish whether the older adult has done the following:

• Thought about ending his or her life
• Attempted to end his or her life in the past
• Developed a plan to end his or her life
• Set the plan into action (i.e., bought a gun, has a full bottle of pills in the bed stand)

Any older adult who has a plan to end his or her life and has the ability or resources to do so must be immediately referred for psychological evaluation. Never leave a person with suicidal thoughts alone.

Crisis Intervention for an Older Adult Who Is Suicidal

• Remove any items that the older adult could use to inflict an injury or end his or her life, such as razors, jewelry with pins or sharp points, and mirrors.

(Continued on following page)

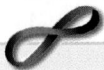

Box 57.8 (Continued)

Gerontological Issues

- Make arrangements for direct supervision and observation that are reliable, considering personnel and family resources. Often, hospital admission is the most appropriate intervention for a person at a very high risk for suicide.
- Help the older adult talk about the crisis or life event that has devastated his or her desire to live. For example, encourage reminiscence about the patient's spouse, or allow the older person to express the frustration of being unable to physically meet the daily demands of life.
- Develop a "do no harm" or suicide contract with the older adult. Outline a short-term, structured plan to keep the older adult safe. Focus on decreasing social

isolation by requiring personal social contacts (e.g., stay at daughter's home for a weekend; go to the senior center for lunch; call a specific person who is willing and wants to listen to feelings and concerns; exercise; take a walk outside; volunteer services at a nursing home, hospital, or school).

Older adults often need assistance to develop or enhance skills required to cope with life events. Self-care and personal independence in care choices need to be encouraged. Developing an understanding and a manner of avoiding personal thinking patterns and behaviors that increase depression are important skills to learn as part of managing depression.

Home Health Hints

- Help patients and families identify pharmacies that will deliver medications.
- Set up medications using a system the patient can easily follow.
- Maintain communication with and act as a liaison between the psychiatrist and medical physician.

- Assist the patient and family to identify community resources such as support groups and respite care.
- Assess family members for evidence of caregiver role strain.
- Provide education for family/caregivers related to the patient's illness, medications, and symptom management.

ETHICAL CONSIDERATIONS DISCUSSION

The substance-abusing health professional is one of the most common situations nurses may encounter during their careers. It is estimated that about 40,000 nurses who work in the United States are alcoholics, and drug addiction among nurses is reported to be 30 to 100 times greater than among the general population. Nurses have easy access to drugs in most work settings. Other factors that contribute to the increased drug abuse among nurses include job stress, short staffing, double shifts, unrealistic expectations, frustration and anxiety, personal problems, and lack of autonomy in practice.

The drug-abusing nurse's colleagues may experience professional and emotional conflicts. Underlying the ethical dilemma is the right of the patient to safe and competent treatment versus the nurse's right to **self-determination**. However, the nurse does not have a totally unrestricted right to self-determination. This right has limits when it comes to endangering others, especially the patients assigned to this nurse for their care and safety. Although the National Association

for Practical Nurse Education and Services (NAP-NES) Code does not directly address any obligation to protect the public from practitioners who are unsafe, various elements that are related include faithfulness and responsibility with a general admonition to protect patients.

In this particular situation, Julie does have an obligation to do something about Ellen's drug problem. Covering for Ellen will not solve the problem. Julie should document Ellen's behavior and inform her supervisor. If the institution hierarchy does not take any action, Julie should submit the report to the state board of nursing. Some states have programs where health professionals can be helped without fear of losing their jobs or licenses, as long as they comply with treatment.

To allow Ellen to practice while under the influence of drugs puts Julie in a very serious legal position. If Ellen were to do something wrong and harm a patient and Julie knew that Ellen was under the influence of drugs, Julie could be held legally liable.

REVIEW QUESTIONS

1. A patient believes his poor relationship with his mother when he was young is the primary cause of his schizophrenia. Which theory explains this belief?
   a. Psychoanalytic theory
   b. Genetic theory
   c. Biological theory
   d. Cognitive theory

2. A patient suddenly and dramatically experiences a loss of vision. The onset of blindness doesn't seem to bother the patient. This person is most likely experiencing which of the following?
   a. Posttraumatic stress disorder
   b. Schizophrenia
   c. Conversion disorder
   d. Dissociative disorder

3. If an extrapyramidal side effect such as dystonia occurs in the patient on antipsychotic medication, which of the following interventions might help?
   a. Administer anticholinergic agents as ordered.
   b. Discontinue the antipsychotic agent immediately.
   c. Administer prn antianxiety agents as ordered.
   d. Encourage progressive muscle relaxation and imagery.

4. A patient who is a veteran of the Gulf War hears the hospital fire alarm go off during a drill and cries, "There are people hiding behind the pillars! They have guns! Be careful!" What action should the nurse take first?
   a. Tell the patient that his behavior is inappropriate and that he is frightening the other patients.
   b. Administer a prn antipsychotic medication as ordered.
   c. Ask him if he is afraid of the guns.
   d. Stay with the patient while calmly reorienting him.

5. A patient is being treated on the mental health unit for a somatoform disorder. The patient approaches the nurse and says she feels dizzy, weak, and her heart is racing. Her nursing care plan includes interventions of imagery exercises and prn alprazolam (Xanax) for identified symptoms of anxiety. What should the nurse do first?
   a. Instruct the patient to sit and breathe deeply.
   b. Give the patient the prescribed prn Xanax.
   c. Measure the patient's vital signs.
   d. Instruct the patient in an imagery exercise.

References

1. Bleuler, E: Dementia Praecox (Emil Kraepelin) or the Group of Schizophrenias. International Press, New York, 1911, p 26.
2. Ewing, JA: Detecting alcoholism: The CAGE questionnaire. JAMA 252:1905–1907, 1984.

Unit Sixteen Bibliography

1. Ackley, BJ, and Ladwig, GB: Nursing Diagnosis Handbook: A Guide to Planning Care, ed. 7. Mosby, St. Louis, 2006.
2. Alcohol, Drug Abuse and Mental Health Administration. DHHS pub. No. (ADM) 90–1609, Bethesda, MD, 1990.
3. American Psychiatric Association: Diagnostic and Statistical Manual of Mental Disorders, ed. 4, text revision. Washington DC, 2000.
4. Arnold, E, and Boggs, KA: Interpersonal Relationships: Professional Communication Skills for Nurses. Saunders, St. Louis, 2003.
5. Bauer, J: RN news watch: Complementary therapies. Can St. John's wort really alleviate depression? RN 64:20, 2001.
6. Bleuler, E: Dementia Praecox (Emil Kraepelin) or the Group of Schizophrenias. International Press, New York, 1911, p 26.
7. Helpful Facts About Depressive Illness. DHHS-NIH pub. no. 94-3875, Bethesda, MD, 1994.
8. Pedersen, DD: PsychNotes: Clinical Pocket Companion. F.A. Davis, Philadelphia, 2005.
9. Purnell, L, and Paulanka, B (eds): Transcultural Health Care: A Culturally Competent Approach, ed. 2. F.A. Davis, Philadelphia, 2003.
10. Sloan, A, and Vernarec, E: Impaired nurses: Reclaiming careers. RN 64:58–63, 2001.
11. Townsend, MC: Psychiatric Mental Health Nursing: Concepts of Care, ed. 5. F.A. Davis, Philadelphia, 2006.
12. Townsend, MC: Nursing Diagnoses in Psychiatric Nursing: Care Plans and Psychotropic Medications, ed. 6. F.A. Davis, Philadelphia, 2004.
13. Weitzel, CA: Could you spot this psych emergency? RN 63:35–40, 2000.

CRITICAL THINKING

■ Tommy

You can reassure Tommy's mother that his OCD is not her fault. Tommy can learn to control his illness with medications and therapy. The family must be part of the therapy, for both Tommy's sake and the family's sake. Positive communication between Tommy and his family is encouraged. Tommy's mother can also be encouraged to attend a support group herself.

■ Mr. Zenz

It is important to be supportive of Mrs. Zenz while maintaining Mr. Zenz's confidentiality and privacy. Encouraging Mrs. Zenz to talk to Mr. Zenz's physician is appropriate. Showing empathy with statements such as, "It must be confusing and difficult to watch your husband change moods so quickly" are good tools to use. It may be a bit more challenging to approach him as your boss. You may certainly ask him if you can speak frankly and share specific observations. You may share your concern, such as "Mr. Zenz, you are a wonderful boss, but I am frightened when you become loud and boisterous." This may help him to reflect. Chances are, however, that if he is in manic stage, he will not hear your concern. It may require delicate talking to the next in the corporate chain of command. This is a tough one. Good luck!

■ Anne

Appropriate communication skills include being positive, reassuring, and not reinforcing the hallucinations. "I don't see or hear a woman, Anne. It is time for the movie. I'd like you to come with me for a while at least" is an example of an appropriate verbal interaction. Reinforcing expectations is also appropriate. "Anne, part of your care plan includes attending one major activity per day. This is the last opportunity for you to meet your care plan objective for today" is also acceptable. At all times, nurses need to be aware of drug interactions. Anne will most likely be medicated for her schizophrenia and those medications may interact unfavorably with her chemotherapy. Good nursing data collection skills are essential.

■ Maria

A number of options may explain Maria's behavior, including depression, drug use, schizophrenia, anorexia, or bulimia. Next time you see Maria you might try constructively confronting her behavior by saying something like, "Maria, you used to be much more outgoing. We always were friendly and now you leave when I'm near. That change in you concerns me. I'm here if you want to talk." Or, "Maria, I see your behavior is changing. You are loud one moment and very quiet the next. That is unusual for you. What is happening?"

North American Nursing Diagnosis Association (NANDA) Nursing Diagnoses

Activity Intolerance [specify level]
Activity Intolerance, risk for
Adjustment, impaired
Airway Clearance, ineffective
Allergy Response, latex
Allergy Response, risk for latex
Anxiety [specify level]
Anxiety, death
Aspiration, risk for
Attachment, risk for impaired parent/infant/child
Autonomic Dysreflexia
Autonomic Dysreflexia, risk for

Body Image, disturbed
Body Temperature, risk for imbalanced
Bowel Incontinence
Breastfeeding, effective
Breastfeeding, ineffective
Breastfeeding, interrupted
Breathing Pattern, ineffective

Cardiac Output, decreased
Caregiver Role Strain
Caregiver Role Strain, risk for
Communication, impaired verbal
Communication, readiness for enhanced
Conflict, decisional (specify)
Conflict, parental role
Confusion, acute
Confusion, chronic
Constipation
Constipation, perceived
Constipation, risk for
Coping, compromised family
Coping, defensive
Coping, disabled family
Coping, ineffective
Coping, ineffective community
Coping, readiness for enhanced
Coping, readiness for enhanced community
Coping, readiness for enhanced family

Death Syndrome, risk for sudden infant
Denial, ineffective
Dentition, impaired
Development, risk for delayed
Diarrhea
Disuse Syndrome, risk for
Diversional Activity, deficient

Energy Field, disturbed
Environmental Interpretation Syndrome, impaired

Failure to Thrive, adult
Falls, risk for

Family Processes: alcoholism, dysfunctional
Family Processes, interrupted
Family Processes, readiness for enhanced
Fatigue
Fear [specify focus]
Fluid Balance, readiness for enhanced
Fluid Volume, deficient [hyper/hypotonic]
Fluid Volume, deficient [isotonic]
Fluid Volume, excess
Fluid Volume, risk for deficient
Fluid Volume, risk for imbalanced

Gas Exchange, impaired
Grieving, anticipatory
Grieving, dysfunctional
Grieving, risk for dysfunctional
Growth, risk for disproportionate
Growth and Development, delayed

Health Maintenance, ineffective
Health-Seeking Behaviors (specify)
Home Maintenance, impaired
Hopelessness
Hyperthermia
Hypothermia

Identity: disturbed, personal
Infant Behavior, disorganized
Infant Behavior, readiness for enhanced organized
Infant Behavior, risk for disorganized
Infant Feeding Pattern, ineffective
Infection, risk for
Injury, risk for
Injury, risk for perioperative positioning
Intracranial Adaptive Capacity, decreased

Knowledge, deficient [Learning Need] (specify)
Knowledge (specify), readiness for enhanced

Lifestyle, sedentary
Loneliness, risk for

Memory, impaired
Mobility, impaired bed
Mobility, impaired physical
Mobility, impaired wheelchair

Nausea
Neglect, unilateral
Noncompliance [Ineffective Adherence] [specify]
Nutrition: less than body requirements, imbalanced

Nutrition: more than body requirements, imbalanced
Nutrition: more than body requirements, risk for imbalanced
Nutrition, readiness for enhanced

Oral Mucous Membrane, impaired

Pain, acute
Pain, chronic
Parenting, impaired
Parenting, readiness for enhanced
Parenting, risk for impaired
Peripheral Neurovascular Dysfunction, risk for
Poisoning, risk for
Post-Trauma Syndrome [specify stage]
Post-Trauma Syndrome, risk for
Powerlessness [specify level]
Powerlessness, risk for
Protection, ineffective

Rape-Trauma Syndrome
Rape-Trauma Syndrome: compound reaction
Rape-Trauma Syndrome: silent reaction
Religiosity, impaired
Religiosity, readiness for enhanced
Religiosity, risk for impaired
Relocation Stress Syndrome
Relocation Stress Syndrome, risk for
Role Performance, ineffective

Self-Care Deficit: bathing/hygiene
Self-Care Deficit: dressing/grooming
Self-Care Deficit: feeding
Self-Care Deficit: toileting
Self-Concept, readiness for enhanced
Self-Esteem, chronic low
Self-Esteem, situational low
Self-Esteem, risk for situational low
Self-Mutilation
Self-Mutilation, risk for
Sensory Perception, disturbed (specify: visual, auditory, kinesthetic, gustatory, tactile, olfactory)
Sexual Dysfunction
Sexuality Pattern, ineffective
Skin Integrity, impaired
Skin Integrity, risk for impaired
Sleep, readiness for enhanced
Sleep Deprivation
Sleep Pattern, disturbed
Social Interaction, impaired
Social Isolation
Sorrow, chronic
Spiritual Distress

Spiritual Distress, risk for
Spiritual Well-Being, readiness for
  enhanced
Suffocation, risk for
Suicide, risk for
Surgical Recovery, delayed
Swallowing, impaired

Therapeutic Regimen Management, effective
Therapeutic Regimen Management, ineffective
Therapeutic Regimen Management, ineffective community
Therapeutic Regimen Management, ineffective family

Therapeutic Regimen Management, readi-
  ness for enhanced
Thermoregulation, ineffective
Thought Processes, disturbed
Tissue Integrity, impaired
Tissue Perfusion, ineffective (specify
  type: renal, cerebral, cardiopulmonary,
  gastrointestinal, peripheral)
Transfer Ability, impaired
Trauma, risk for

Urinary Elimination, impaired
Urinary Elimination, readiness for
  enhanced
Urinary Incontinence, functional
Urinary Incontinence, reflex

Urinary Incontinence, risk for urge
Urinary Incontinence, stress
Urinary Incontinence, total
Urinary Incontinence, urge
Urinary Retention [acute/chronic]

Ventilation, impaired spontaneous
Ventilatory Weaning Response,
  dysfunctional
Violence, [actual/] risk for other-
  directed
Violence, [actual/] risk for self-directed

Walking, impaired
Wandering [specify sporadic or continu-
  ous]

Normal Adult Reference Laboratory Values

BLOOD, PLASMA, OR SERUM VALUES

Determination	Reference Range	
	Conventional	SI
Aldolase	Less than 7.4 U/L	
Ammonia	12–55 μmol/L	12–55 μmol/L
Amylase	30–110 units/mL	
Atrial natriuretic peptide	20–77 pg/mL	20–77 ng/L

	BNP	Pro-BNP (N-Terminal)
Male	<100 pg/mL	60 pg/mL
Female	<100 pg/mL	12–150 pg/mL

Determination	Conventional	SI
Bilirubin (total)	0.3–1.2 mg/dL	5–21 μmol/L
Calcium	8.2–10.2 mg/dL	2.05–2.55 mmol/L
Carbon dioxide content	23–29 mEq/L	23–29 mmol/L
Chloride	97–107 mEq/L	97–107 mmol/L
Creatine kinase (CK)	Female: 26–140 U/L	
	Male: 38–174 U/L	
CK isoenzymes		
CK-BB	Absent	
CK-MB	4%–6%	
CK-MM	94%–96%	
CK-MB by immunoassay	10 ng/mL	
Creatinine		
Male	0.6–1.2 mg/dL	53–106 μmol/L
Female	0.5–1.1 mg/dL	44–97 μmol/L
d-Dimer	*Semiquantitative:* No fragments detected. *Quantitative:* <250 ng/mL	
Erythrocyte sedimentation rate (ESR)	(Westergren method)	
Male	<50 years, <15 mm/hr; >50 years, <20 mm/hr	
Women	<50 years, <20 mm/hr; >50 years, <30 mm/hr	
Glucose	Fasting: 70–100 mg/dL	3.9–5.5 mmol/L
Iron		
Male	65–175 μg/dL	11.6–31.3 μmol/L
Female	50–170 μg/dL	9–30.4 μmol/L
Iron-binding capacity	250–350 μg/dL	45–63 μmol/L
Lactic dehydrogenase	90–176 U/L	
Lipase	0–160 U/L	
Lipids (desirable)		
Cholesterol	<200 mg/dL	<5.18 mmol/L
Low-density lipoprotein	Less than 100 mg/dL	<2.59 mmol/L
High-density lipoprotein	Greater than 60 mg/dL	>1.56 mmol/L
Triglycerides	Less than 150 mg/dL	<1.70 mmol/L
Magnesium	1.6–2.6 mg/dL	0.62–0.91 mmol/L
Myoglobin	0–85 ng/mL	
Osmolality	275–295 mOsm/kg	275–295 mmol/kg
Oxygen saturation (arterial)	95–100%	
P_{CO_2}	35–45 mm Hg	4.66–5.98 kPa
pH	7.35–7.45	Same
P_{O_2}	80–95 mm Hg	10.6–12.6 kPa

(Continued on following page)

BLOOD, PLASMA, OR SERUM VALUES *(Continued)*

Determination	Reference Range	
	Conventional	SI
Phosphatase (prostatic acid)	<2.5 ng/mL	
Phosphatase (alkaline)		
Male	35–142 U/L	
Female	25–125 U/L	
Phosphorus (blood)	2.5–4.5 mg/dL	0.8–1.4 mmol/L
Potassium	3.5–5.0 mEq/L	3.5–5.0 mmol/L
Protein: Total	6.0–8.0 g/dL	60–80 g/L
Albumin	3.4–4.8 g/dL	34–48 g/L
Sodium	135–145 mEq/L	135–145 mmol/L
Transaminase, aspartate aminotransferase (AST)		
Male	15–40 U/L	
Female	13–35 U/L	
Transaminase, alanine aminotransferase (ALT)		
Male	10–40 U/L	
Female	7–35 U/L	
Troponin I	<0.35 ng/mL	
Troponin T	<0.20 µg/L	
Urea nitrogen (BUN)	8–21 mg/dL	2.9–7.5 mmol/L
Uric acid		
Male	4.4–7.6 mg/dL	0.26–0.45 mmol/L
Female	2.3–6.6 mg/dL	0.14–0.39 mmol/L

URINALYSIS

Reference Value:

Dipstick pH	5.0–9.0
Protein	<20 mg/dL
Glucose	Negative
Ketones	Negative
Hemoglobin	Negative
Bilirubin	Negative
Urobilinogen	Up to 1 mg/dL
Nitrite	Negative
Leukocyte esterase	Negative
Microscopic examination	
Red blood cells	Less than 5/hpf
White blood cells	Less than 5/hpf
Renal cells	None seen
Transitional cells	None seen
Squamous cells	Rare; usually no clinical significance
Casts	Rare hyaline; otherwise, none seen
Crystals in acid urine	Uric acid, calcium oxalate, amorphous urates
Crystals in alkaline urine	Triple phosphate, calcium phosphate, ammonium biurate, calcium carbonate, amorphous phosphates
Bacteria, yeast, parasites	None seen

HEMATOLOGICAL VALUES

Determination	Reference Range	
	Conventional	SI
Coagulation screening tests:		
Bleeding time (template)	2.5–10 minutes	
Prothrombin time	11–13.5 seconds	
International Normalized Ratio (INR) = Less than 2.0 for patients not receiving anticoagulation therapy; 2.0 to 3.0 for patients receiving treatment for venous thrombosis, pulmonary embolism, and valvular heart disease; 2.5 to 3.5 for patients with mechanical heart valves and/or receiving treatment for recurrent systemic embolism.		
Partial thromboplastin time (activated)	25–38 sec	25–38 sec
Complete blood count (CBC)		
Hematocrit		
Male	43–49	0.43–0.49
Female	38–44	0.38–0.44
Hemoglobin		
Male	13.2–17.3 g/dL	132–173 mmol/L
Female	11.7–15.5 g/dL	117–155 mmol/L
White blood cell count and differential		

White Blood Cell Count and Differential	SI Units	Neutrophils	Lymphocytes	Monocytes	Eosinophils	Basophils
	WBC $\times$ 10^3/mm^3 or cells/mL	Total (Absolute) and %	Bands (Absolute) and %	Segments (Absolute) and %	(Absolute) and %	(Absolute) and %
Adult	4.5–11.0	(1.8–7.7) 59%	(0–0.7) 3.0%	(1.8–7.0) 56%	(1.0–4.8) 34%	(0–0.8) 4.0%

Erythrocyte count		
Male	4.71–5.14 million cells/mm^3	4.71–5.14 $\times$ 10^{12} cells/L
Female	4.20–4.87 million cells/mm^3	4.20–4.87 $\times$ 10^{12} cells/L

Red Blood Cell Indices	MCV (fl)	MCH (pg/cell)	MCHC (g/dL)	RDW
MCV = mean corpuscular volume; MCH = mean corpuscular hemoglobin; MCHC = mean corpuscular hemoglobin concentration; RDW = RBC distribution width index.				
Male	85–95	28–32	33–35	11.6–14.8
Female	85–95	28–32	33–35	11.6–14.8

Platelet count	150–450 $\times$ 10^3/μL/mm^3	181–521 $\times$ 10^9/L

THERAPEUTIC DRUG LEVELS

Determination	Reference Range	
	Conventional	SI
Carbamazepine	4.0–12.0 mg/mL	17–51 μmol/L
Digoxin	0.5–2.0 ng/mL	0.6–2.6 nmol/L
Ethanol	0 mg/dL	0 mmol/L
Lithium	0.6–1.4 mEq/L	0.6–1.4 mmol/L
Phenobarbital	15–40 μg/mL	65–172 μmol/L
Phenytoin (Dilantin)	10–20 μg/mL	40–79 μmol/L
Salicylate	15–20 mg/dL	1.1–1.4 mmol/L

MISCELLANEOUS VALUES

	Reference Range	
Determination	Conventional	SI
Carcinoembryonic antigen (CEA)	0–2.5 ng/mL	0–2.5 μg/L
Gastrin	25–90 pg/mL	25–90 ng/L
Immunologic tests:		
Alpha-1-antitrypsin	126–226 mg/dL	1.26–2.26 g/L
Antinuclear antibodies	Negative at a 1:8 dilution of serum	

Reference range values may differ from one institution to another. Most data from VanLeeuwen, A, Kranpitz, T, Smith, L: Davis's Comprehensive Handbook of Laboratory and Diagnostic Tests with Nursing Implications, 2/E. FA Davis: Philadelphia, 2005.

Answers to Review Questions

Chapter 1: 1. b 2. d 3. a 4. d 5. c 6. c, a, d, e, b, 7. a 8. d 9. c
Chapter 2: 1. b; 2. c; 3. b; 4. a; 5. d; 6. c; 7. a; 8. a; 9. c; 10. d; 11. b
Chapter 3: 1. b; 2. d; 3. a; 4. c; 5. a
Chapter 4: 1. c; 2. c; 3. d; 4. a, c, e; 5. b
Chapter 5: 1. a,e; 2. b; 3. d; 4. c; 5. a; 6. a; 7. d; 8. b, c, d; 9. b; 10. a
Chapter 6: 1. b; 2. a, b, c, e, f; 3. a; 4. b, e, f, a, c, h, i, d, g; 5. c; 6. b; 7. d; 8. c; 9. 33 gtts/min; 10. 83 mL/hour
Chapter 7: 1. e, b, c, a, f, d; 2. c; 3. b; 4. c; 5. a; 6. d; 7. c
Chapter 8: 1. c; 2. a; 3. d; 4. b; 5. b; 6. d; 7. c; 8. b, c, a
Chapter 9: 1. b; 2. d; 3. c; 4. a; 5. b; 6. c; 7. a, c, d; 8. c; 9. d; 10. b; 11. d; 12. 0.7
Chapter 10: 1. b; 2. a, e, f; 3. a; 4. d; 5. d; 6. c; 7. c; 8. a
Chapter 11: 1. a, c, d; 2. a; 3. d, e, f; 4. b; 5. a, e, f; 6. b; 7. a; 8. d; 9. Assisting patient with recovery process.
Chapter 12: 1. b, c, d, e; 2. a; 3. b; 4. c; 5. a; 6. d; 7. d; 8. c; 9. c 10. 1.25 mL
Chapter 13: 1. d; 2. b; 3. b; 4. a; 5. b, c, f
Chapter 14: 1. c; 2. d; 3. b; 4. b; 5. c; 6. a, c, d, e
Chapter 15: 1. d; 2. a, b, c, d; 3. d; 4. b; 5. a; 6. d
Chapter 16: 1. c; 2. d; 3. a; 4. d; 5. b; 6. a, b, f; 7. c; 8. c; 9. a
Chapter 17: 1. d; 2. a; 3. a; 4. c; 5. b; 6. 8 mL
Chapter 18: 1. a, d, f, g, h; 2. b; 3. c, d, e, g; 4. c; 5. a; 6. d; 7. a, e; 8. b; 9. c
Chapter 19: 1. d; 2. b, c, a; 3. c; 4. b, c, e, f; 5. a, b, e; 6. c; 7. a; 8; 15 mL
Chapter 20: 1. a; 2. c; 3. b; 4. d; 5. b; 6. c; 7. d; 8. a; 9. b; 10. d; 11. a, d, e; 12. b; 13. c
Chapter 21: 1. d; 2. a; 3. b; 4. d, e, f; 5. c; 6. b; 7. b; 8. b; 9. c
Chapter 22: 1. a; 2. d; 3. b; 4. a, d, e, 5. a
Chapter 23: 1. b; 2. a; 3. b; 4. c; 5. c; 6. 325 mg
Chapter 24: 1. b; 2. a; 3. b; 4. d; 5. c; 6. a; 7. a, e
Chapter 25: 1. b; 2. a; 3. c; 4. c; 5. b 6. b 7. 2 tablets
Chapter 26: 1. b; 2. a; 3. a; 4. c; 5. a 6. 454 mg/dose
Chapter 27: 1. b; 2. c; 3. b; 4. c; 5. b; 6. a; 7. a, c, and d; 8. d
Chapter 28: 1. b; 2. c; 3. d; 4. a; 5. d; 6. a; 7. a, d, f; 8. 1,715; 9. a; 10. d
Chapter 29: 1. a; 2. c; 3. d; 4. b; 5. d; 6. c, e, b, a, d; 7. b
Chapter 30: 1. b; 2. a; 3. d; 4. d; 5. a, b, e; 6. a
Chapter 31: 1. c; 2. b; 3. d; 4. c; 5. c; 6. a; 7. b; 8. a
Chapter 32: 1. b; 2. a; 3. b; 4. d; 5. b; 6. b; 7. b, c, d; 8. c; 9. b
Chapter 33: 1. b; 2. c; 3. d; 4. c; 5. c; 6. d; 7. c; 8. b; 9. 25 drops per minute
Chapter 34: 1. a; 2. b; 3. a, b, d, e, f; 4. a; 5. d; 6. c 7. a, b, d, e; 8. a; 9. a; 10. a; 11. b
Chapter 35: 1. b; 2. a; 3. b; 4. d; 5. d; 6. a; 7. c; 8. a; 9. b, c and e; 10. 0.25
Chapter 36: 1. c; 2. b; 3. d; 4. b, d 5. d; 6. c; 7. 912 mL
Chapter 37: 1. a, e; 2. b; 3. a; 4. b; 5. a; 6. b; 7. d; 8. a 9. c; 10. d; 11. 4 tablets
Chapter 38: 1. a, e; 2. d; 3. c; 4. a; 5. b
Chapter 39: 1. c; 2. c; 3. b, e, f; 4. a; 5. d; 6. a; 7. a
Chapter 40: 1. a; 2. b; 3. 126; 4. d; 5. a; 6. c; 7. d; 8. c, f, d, e, b, a 9. a; 10. a; 11. b
Chapter 41: 1. c; 2. d; 3. d; 4. b, c, d, e; 5. b; 6. c
Chapter 42: 1. c; 2. c; 3. d; 4. a; 5. b; 6. c; 7. b; 8. 240; 9. a
Chapter 43: 1. c; 2. c; 3. a; 4. b; 5. b; 6. a; 7. a, d; 8. d
Chapter 44: 1. a; 2. a, b, c, d, e, f; 3. c; 4. d; 5. c; 6. a;
Chapter 45: 1. b; 2. c, e; f; 3. d; 4. a; 5. b;
Chapter 46: 1. b; 2. b; 3. a, e; 4. c; 5. a; 6. c; 7. a; 8. b; 9. b; 10. c; 11. d; 12. d; 13. 0.5 mL
Chapter 47: 1. b; 2. a; 3. b; 4. b, c, d; 5. d; 6. b; 7. c
Chapter 48: 1. a; 2. b; 3. a; 4. d; 5. c; 6. c, a, d, b; 7. b, c, d; 8. b; 9. d; 10. c; 11. a; 12. a; 13. b
Chapter 49: 1. c, e, f; 2. a; 3. c; 4. d; 5. d; 6. c
Chapter 50: 1. c; 2. d; 3. a; 4. c; 5. a, b, d, e; 6. b; 7. d
Chapter 51: 1. cornea, aqueous humor, lens, and vitreous humor; 2. d; 3. b; 4. c; 5. a; 6. d; 7. a, b, c; 8. c;
Chapter 52: 1. b; 2. b; 3. a; 4. a; 5. b; 6. c, e; 7. a; 8. d; 9. c; 10. b; 11. d
Chapter 53: 1. b; 2. b, d, e; 3. a; 4. c; 5. a; 6. b
Chapter 54: 1. a; 2. c; 3. c; 4. b, d, e; 5. b; 6. d
Chapter 55: 1. b; 2. a; 3. c; 4. c, d, e; 5. d
Chapter 56: 1. a; 2. a, c, e; 3. b; 4. c; 5. c; 6. d; 7. a; 8. d
Chapter 57: 1. a; 2. c; 3. a; 4. d; 5. c

Medical Abbreviations

ABG	arterial blood gas	lb.	pound
ac	before a meal	lmp	last menstrual period
AD	advance directive	mEq	milliequivalent
ad lib	freely; as desired	mg	milligram
ALT	alanine aminotransferase	mL	milliliter
AM	morning	mm	millimeter
A-P	anterior-posterior	MRI	magnetic resonance imaging
AST	aspartate aminotransferase	MS	mitral stenosis; multiple sclerosis
AV	atrioventricular	mEq	microequivalent
bid	twice a day	mg	microgram
BM	bowel movement	npo	nothing by mouth
BP	blood pressure	NSAID	nonsteroidal anti-inflammatory drug
BUN	blood urea nitrogen	NSR	normal sinus rhythm
c̄	with	OB	obstetrics
cap	a capsule	O.C.	oral contraceptive
CBC	complete blood count	O.D.	right eye
cc	cubic centimeter	O.S.	left eye
cm	centimeter	O.U.	both eyes
CNS	central nervous system	oz	ounce
CSF	cerebrospinal fluid	p̄	after
CV	cardiovascular	pc	after meals
D & C	dilatation and curettage	P_{CO_2}	carbon dioxide pressure
dc	discontinue	PERRLA	pupils equal, regular, react to light and accommodation
dL	deciliter		
DNR	do not resuscitate	pH	hydrogen ion concentration
DOA	dead on arrival	PM	afternoon/evening
dr	dram	PMI	point of maximal impulse
Dx	diagnosis	post	posterior
ECF	extracellular fluid	pr	through the rectum
ECG	electrocardiogram	prn	as needed
ECT	electroconvulsive therapy	qhr	every hour
EEG	electroencephalogram	q2hr	every 2 hours
EMG	electromyogram	q3hr	every 3 hours
EMS	emergency medical service	qid	four times a day
ENT	ear, nose, and throat	qs	as much as is needed
EOM	extraocular muscles	RBC	red blood cell; red blood count
ER	Emergency Room	s̄	without
ESR	erythrocyte sedimentation rate	SA	sinoatrial
F	Fahrenheit	SC, sc,	subcutaneous(ly)
g, gm	gram	SOB	shortness of breath
GERD	gastroesophageal reflux disease	s.o.s	if necessary
GI	gastrointestinal	sq	subcutaneous(ly)
gr	grain	stat.	immediately
Gtt, gtt	drops	STD	sexually transmitted disease
GYN	gynecology	T	temperature
h, hr	hour	tab	medicated tablet
hgb	hemoglobin	temp	temperature
hor som, hs	bedtime	tid	three times a day
IM	intramuscular	top	topically
IUD	intrauterine device	URI	upper respiratory infection
IV	intravenous	USP	United States Pharmacopeia
IVP	intravenous pyelogram	UTI	urinary tract infection
J	joule	WBC	white blood cell; white blood count
kg	kilogram	WF/BF	white female/black female
KUB	kidney, ureter, and bladder	WM/BM	white male/black male
L	liter	wt.	weight

Adapted from Thomas, CL: Taber's Cyclopedic Medical Dictionary, ed. 20. F.A. Davis, Philadelphia, 2005, p. 2463.

Prefixes, Suffixes, and Combining Forms

a-, an-. Without; away from; not.
ab-, abs-. From; away from; absent.
abdomin-, abdomino-. Abdomen.
-ad. Toward; in the direction of.
aden-, adeno-. Gland.
adip-, adipo-. Fat.
-aemia. Blood.
aer-, aero-. Air.
-algesia, -algia. Suffering; pain.
andro-. Man; male; masculine
angi-, angio-. Blood or lymph vessels.
aniso-. Unequal; asymmetrical; dissimilar.
ankyl-, ankylo-. Crooked; bent; fusion or growing together of parts.
ante-. Before.
antero-. Anterior; front; before.
ant-, anti-. Against.
arteri-, arterio-. Artery.
arthr-, arthro-. Joint.
-ase. Enzyme.
-asis, esis, -iasis, -isis, -sis. Condition; pathological state.
aut-, auto-. Self.
axo-. Axis; axon.
bacteri-, bacterio-. Bacteria; bacterium.
bi-, bis-. Two; double; twice.
bili-. Bile.
bio-. Life.
blast-, -blast. Germ; bud; embryonic state of development.
blephar-, blepharo-. Eyelid.
brady-. Slow.
bronch-, bronchi-, broncho-. Airway.
cardi-, cardio-. Heart.
cat-, cata-, cath-, kat-, kata-. Down; downward; destructive; against; according to.
cent-. Hundred.
cephal-, cephalo-. Head.
cervic-, cervice-. Head; the neck of an organ.
chrom-, chromo-. Color.
-cide. Causing death.
contra-. Against; opposite.
crani-, cranio-. Skull; cranium.
cry-, cryo-. Cold.
cyan-, cyano-. Blue.
cyst-, cysto-, -cyst. Cyst; urinary bladder.
cyt-, cyto-, -cyte. Cell.
derm-, derma-, dermato-, dermo-. Skin.
di-. Double; twice; two; apart from.
dors-, dorsi-, dorso-. Back.
-dynia. Pain.
dys-. Difficult; bad; painful.
ec-, ecto-. Out; on the outside.
-ectomy. Excision.
ef-, es-, ex-, exo-. Out.
electr-, electro-. Electricity.
-emesis. Vomiting.
-emia. Blood.

en-. In; into.
end-, endo-. Within.
ent-, ento-. Within; inside.
enter-, entero-. Intestine.
ep-, epi-. Upon; over; at; in additon to; after.
erythr-, erythro-. Red.
eury-. Broad.
ex-. Out; away from; completely.
exo-. Out; outside of; without.
extra-. Outside of; in addition; beyond.
-facient. Causing; making happen.
-ferous. Producing.
ferri-, ferro-. Iron.
fluo-. Flow.
fore-. Before; in front of.
-form. Form.
-fuge. To expel; to drive away; fleeing.
gaster-, gastero-, gastr-, gastro-. Stomach.
gen-. Producing; forming.
-gen, -gene, -genesis, -genetic, -genic. Producing; forming.
glosso-. Tongue.
gluc-, gluco-, glyc-, glyco-. Sugar; glycerol or similar substance.
gyn-, gyne-, gyneco-, gyno-. Woman; female.
hem-, hema-, hemato-, hemo-. Blood.
hemi-. Half.
hepat-, hepato-. Liver.
heter-, hetero-. Other; different.
histo-. Tissue.
homo-. Same; likeness.
hydra-, hydro, hydr-. Water.
hyp-, hyph-, hypo-. Less than; below; under.
hyper-. Above; excessive; beyond.
hyster-, hystero-. Uterus.
-ia. Condition, esp. an abnormal state.
-iasis. SEE: *-asis.*
-iatric. Medicine; medical profession; physicians.
in-. In; inside; within; intensive action; negative.
infra-. Below; under; beneath; inferior to; after.
inter-. Between; in the midst.
intra-, intro-. Within; in; into.
ipsi-. Same.
irid-, irido-. Iris.
-ism. Condition; theory.
iso-. Equal.
-itis. Inflammation of.
kera-, kerato-. Horny substance; cornea.
kolp-, kolpo, colp-, colpo-. Vagina.
kypho-. Humped.
leuk-, leuko-. White; colorless; rel. to a leukocyte.

lip-, lipo-. Fat.
-lite, -lith, lith-, litho-. Stone; calculus.
-logia,-logy. Science of; study of.
lumbo-. Loins.
-lysis. 1. Setting free; disintegration. 2. In medicine, reduction of; relief from.
macr-, macro-. Large; long.
mal-. Ill; bad; poor.
med-, medi-, medio-. Middle.
mega-, megal-, megalo-. Large; of great size.
-megalia, -megaly. Enlargement of a body part.
melan-, melano-. Black.
mening-, meningo-. Meninges.
-meter. Measure.
metr-, metra-, metro-. Uterus.
micr-, micro-. Small.
mon-, mono-. Single; one.
muc-, muci-, muco-, myxa-, myxo-. Mucus.
multi-. Many; much.
musculo-, my-, myo-. Muscle.
my-, myo-. SEE *musculo-.*
myel-, myelo-. Spinal cord; bone marrow.
naso-. Nose.
necr-, necro-. Death; necrosis.
neo-. New; recent.
nephr-, nephra-, nephro-. Kidney.
neur-, neuri-, neuro-. Nerve; nervous system.
non-. No.
normo-. Normal; usual.
oculo-. Eye.
-ode, -oid. Form; shape; resemblance.
-odynia, odyno-. Pain.
olig-, oligo-. Few; small.
-ology. Science of; study of.
-oma. Tumor.
onco-. Tumor; swelling; mass.
oo-, ovi-, ovo-. Egg; ovum.
oophor-, oophoro-, oophoron-. Ovary.
ophthalm-, ophthalmo-. Eye.
-opia. Vision.
optico-, opto-. Eye; vision.
orchi-, orchid-, orchido-. Testicle.
orth-, ortho-. Straight; correct; normal; in proper order.
os-. Mouth; bone.
-osis. Condition; status, process; abnormal increase.
oste-, osteo-. Bone.
ostomosis, -ostomy, -stomosis, -stomy. A created mouth or outlet.
ot-, oto-. Ear.
-otomy. Cutting.
-ous. 1. Possessing; full of; 2. Pertaining to.
pan-. All; entire.

para-, -para. 1. Prefix: near; alongside of; departure from normal. 2. Suffix: Bearing offspring.

path-, patho-, -path, -pathic, -pathy. Disease; suffering.

ped-, pedi-, pedo-. Foot.

-penia. Decrease from normal; deficiency.

peri-. Around; about.

perineo-. Perineum.

phaco-. Lens of the eye.

phag-, phago-. Eating; ingestion; devouring.

-phil, -philia, -philic. Love for; tendency toward; craving for.

phlebo-. Vein.

-phobia. Abnormal fear or aversion.

photo-. Light.

phren-, phreno-, -phrenia. Mind; diaphragm.

-phylaxis. Protection.

-plasia. Growth; cellular proliferation.

plasm-, -plasm. 1. Prefix: Living substance or tissue. 2. Suffix: To mold.

-plastic. Molded; indicates restoration of lost or badly formed features.

-plegia. Paralysis; stroke.

pneo-. Breath; breathing.

pneum-, pneuma-, pneumato-. Air; gas; respiration.

-poiesis, -poietic. Production; formation.

poly-. Much; many.

post-. After.

pre-. Before; in front of.

presby-. Old age.

pro-. Before; in behalf of.

proct-, procto-. Anus; rectum.

pseud-, pseudo-. False.

psych-, psycho-. Mind; mental processes.

pulmo-. Lung.

py-, pyo-. Pus.

pyro-. Heat; fire.

ren-, reno-. kidneys.

retro-. Backward; back; behind.

rheo-, -(r)rhea. Current; stream; to flow; to discharge.

rhino-. Nose.

-(r)rhage, -(r)rhagia. Rupture; profuse fluid discharge.

-(r)rhaphy. A suturing or stitching.

salping-, salpingo-. Auditory tube; fallopian tube.

sclero-. Hard; relating to the sclera.

-scopy. Examination.

semi-. Half.

sero-. Serum.

somat-, somato-. Body.

sperma-, spermat-, spermato-. Sperm; spermatozoa.

steno-. Narrow; short.

-stomosis, -stomy. SEE: *-ostomosis.*

sub-. Under; beneath; in small quantity; less than normal.

super-. Above; beyond; superior.

supra-. Above; beyond; on top.

tachy-. Swift; rapid.

tel-, tele-. 1. End. 2. Distant; far.

tendo-, teno-. Tendon.

thorac-, thoraci-, thoraco-. Chest; chest wall.

thrombo-. Blood clot; thrombus.

thyro-. Thyroid gland; oblong; shield.

-tomy. Cutting operation; excision.

top-, topo-. Place; locale.

tox-, toxi-, toxico-, toxo-, -toxic. Toxin; poison; toxic.

tracheo-. Trachea; windpipe.

trans-. Across; over; beyond; through.

-tropin. Stimulation of a target organ by a substance, esp. a hormone.

tympano-. Eardrum; tympanum.

ultra-. Beyond; excess.

-uria. Urine.

uter-, utero-. Uterus.

vaso-. Vessel (e. g., blood vessel).

veno-. Vein.

ventro-, ventr-, ventri-. Abdomen; anterior surface of the body.

vertebro-. Vertebra; vertebrae.

vesico-. Bladder; vesicle.

Adapted from Thomas, CL: Taber's Cyclopedic Medical Dictionary, ed. 19. F.A. Davis, Philadelphia, 2001, pp 2465–2469.

Ablation: (uh-BLAY-shun) Removal of part, pathway, or function by surgery, chemical electrocautery, or radiofrequency.

Abrasion: (a-BRAY-zhun) A scraping away of skin or mucous membrane as a result of injury or by mechanical means.

Abuse: (uh-BYOOS) Misuse; excessive or improper use. May refer to substances or individuals.

Accommodation: (uh-KOM-uh-DAY-shun) A reflex action of the eye for focusing.

Acidosis: (ass-i-DOH-sis) An actual or relative increase in the acidity of blood caused by an accumulation of acid or a loss of base.

Acquired immunodeficiency syndrome (AIDS): (uh-KWHY-erd IM-yoo-noh-de-FISH-en-see SIN-drohm) Suppression or deficiency of the cellular immune response, acquired by exposure to human immunodeficiency virus (HIV).

Active immunity: (AK-tiv im-YOO-ni-tee) Acquired immunity attributable to the presence of antibodies or of immune lymphoid cells formed in response to antigenic stimulus.

Activities of daily living (ADLs): (ack-TIV-i-tees of DAY-lee LIV-ing) Those activities and behaviors that are performed in the care and maintenance of self (e.g., bathing, dressing, eating).

Acupuncture: (ak-yoo-PUNGK-chur) Technique using needles inserted at specific points to create anesthesia or treat certain conditions.

Acute coronary syndromes: (a-KEWT KOR-un-na-ree sin-DROMES) Group of conditions, including unstable angina, non-Q wave myocardial infarction, and ST segment elevation myocardial infarction, caused by a lack of oxygen to the heart muscle.

Acute pulmonary hypertension: (ah-KEWT PULL-muh-NAIR-ee HIGH-per-TEN-shun) Sudden obstruction of the pulmonary artery causes excessive buildup of pressure in the pulmonary arteries.

Adaptation: (ad-dap-TAY-shun) Adjustment to changes in internal or external conditions or circumstances; coping.

Addiction: (uh-DIK-shun) Psychological dependence characterized by drug seeking and craving for an opioid or other substance for effects other than the intended purpose of the substance.

Adjunct: (ADD-junkt) An addition to the principal procedure or course of therapy.

Adjuvant: (ad-JOO-vant) Something that assists something else, such as a second form of treatment added to treat a disease.

Administrative laws: (ad-MIN-i-STRAY-tiv LAWZ) Establish the licensing authority of the state to create, license, and regulate the practice of nursing.

Adnexa: (ad-NECK-sah) Appendages or accessory organs.

Advance Medical Directive: (ad-VANS MED-ik-uhl dur-EK-tiv) A set of documents (Living Will and Durable Medical Power of Attorney) that explain a person's end-of-life wishes and direct care when the patient is no longer able to do so.

Adventitious: (ad-ven-TI-shus) Abnormal or extra; often refers to extra breath sounds, such as wheezes or crackles.

Advocate: (ADD-voh-kut) Someone who makes sure a person's wishes are adhered to; someone who represents the best interests of the patient.

Aerobic: (air-O-bick) Living only in the presence of oxygen.

Affect: (AF-feckt) Emotional tone.

Afterload: (AFF-ter-lohd) The forces impeding the blood flow out of the heart (vascular pressure, aortic compliance, blood mass, and viscosity).

Agenesis: (ay-JEN-uh-sis) Failure of an organ or part to develop or grow.

Agonist: (AG-un-ist) A type of opioid that binds to opioid receptors in the central nervous system to relieve pain.

Akinesia: (a-ki-NEE-zee-ah) Absence or loss of the power of voluntary movement.

Alkalosis: (al-ka-LOH-sis) An actual or relative decrease in the acidity of blood caused by loss of acid or accumulation of base.

Allopathic: (AL-oh-PATH-ik) Method of treating disease with remedies that produce effects different from those caused by the disease.

Alopecia: (AL-oh-PEE-she-ah) The loss of hair from the body and the scalp.

Amenorrhea: (ay-MEN-uh-REE-ah) The absence or suppression of menstruation. Amenorrhea is normal before puberty, after menopause, and during pregnancy and lactation.

Amputation: (am-pew-TAY-shun) The removal of a limb or other appendage or outgrowth of the body.

Anaerobic: (AN-air-ROH-bik) Able to live without oxygen.

Analgesic: (AN-uhl-JEE-zik) A drug that relieves pain.

Anaphylactic shock: (AN-uh-fi-LAK-tik) Systemic reaction that produces life-threatening changes in the circulation and bronchioles.

Anaphylaxis: (AN-uh-fi-LAK-sis) A sudden severe allergic reaction.

Anastomose: (uh-NAS-tuh-MOS) To surgically connect two parts.

Anemia: (uh-NEE-mee-yah) A condition in which there is reduced delivery of oxygen to the tissues as a result of reduced numbers of red cells or hemoglobin.

Anergy: (AN-er-jee) Diminished ability of the immune system to react to an antigen.

Anesthesia: (AN-es-THEE-zee-uh) Lack of feeling or sensation; artificially induced loss of ability to feel pain.

Anesthesiologist: (an-es-THEE-zee-uhl-la-just) A physician who specializes in anesthesiology.

Aneurysm: (AN-yur-izm) A sac formed by the localized dilation of the wall of an artery, a vein, or the heart.

Angina pectoris: (an-JIGH-nah PEK-tuh-riss) Severe pain and pressure in the chest caused by insufficient supply of blood and oxygenation to the heart.

Angioedema: (AN-gee-o-eh-DEE-ma) A localized edematous reaction of the deep dermis or subcutaneous or submucosal tissues appearing as giant wheals.

Anion: (AN-eye-on) Electrolyte that carries a negative electrical charge.

Anisocoria: (an-i-soh-KOH-ree-ah) Inequality in size of the pupils of the eyes.

Ankylosing spondylitis: (ANG-ki-LOH-sing SPON-da-LIGHT-is) Inflammatory disease of the spine causing stiffness and pain.

Annuloplasty: (AN-yoo-loh-PLAS-tee) Repair of a cardiac valve.

Anorexia: (AN-oh-REK-see-ah) Absence or loss of appetite for food. Seen in depression, with illness, and as a side effect of some medications.

Anorexia nervosa: (AN-oh-REK-see-ah ner-VOH-sah) Refusal to maintain body weight over a minimal normal weight for age and height.

Antagonist: (an-TAG-on-ist) Medication used to counteract the effects of an opioid (e.g., naloxone).

Anteflexion: (AN-tee-FLECK-shun) The abnormal bending forward of part of an organ.

Anteversion: (AN-tee-VER-zhun) A tipping forward of an organ as a whole, without bending.

Anthrax (AN-thrax) A disease caused by the spore-forming bacterium *Bacillus anthracis* that has three clinical forms in humans: inhalational, cutaneous, and gastrointestinal. It can be used as a biological weapon.

Antibodies: (AN-ti-baw-dees) An immunoglobin molecule having a specific amino acid sequence that gives each antibody the ability to adhere to and interact only with the antigen that induced the synthesis.

Anticholinesterase: (AN-ti-KOH-lin-ESS-ter-ays) A substance that breaks down acetylcholinesterase.

Antidiuretic: (AN-ti-DYE-yoo-RET-ik) Lessening urine excretion.

Antigen: (AN-tih-jen) A protein marker on the surface of cells that identifies the type of cell.

Antitussive: (an-tee-TUSS-iv) An agent that prevents or relieves cough.

Anuria: (an-YOO-ree-ah) Complete suppression of urine formation by the kidney.

Anxiety: (ang-ZIGH-uh-tee) The uncomfortable feeling of apprehension or dread that occurs in response to a known or unknown threat.

Aphasia: (ah-FAY-zee-ah) Defect or loss of the power of expression by speech, writing, or signs, or of comprehension of spoken or written language, caused by disease or injury of the brain centers, such as stroke syndrome.

Aphthous stomatitis: (AF-thus STOH-mah-TIGH-tis) Small, white, painful ulcers (also known as canker sores) that appear on the inner cheeks, lips, gums, tongue, palate, and pharynx. They tend to recur.

Apnea: (ap-NEE-ah) Temporary absence of breathing.

Appendicitis: (uh-PEN-di-SIGH-tis) Inflammation of the vermiform appendix.

Arcus senilus: (AR-kus se-NILL-us) A benign white or gray opaque ring in the corneal margin of the eye.

Arrhythmia: (uh-RITH-mee-yah) Irregular rhythm, especially heart-beat.

Arteriosclerosis: (ar-TIR-ee-oh-skle-ROH-sis) Term applied to a number of pathological conditions in which there is gradual thickening, hardening, and loss of elasticity of the walls of the arteries.

Arthritis: (are-THRYE-tis) Inflammation of a joint.

Arthrocentesis: (ar-THROW-sen-tee-sis) Puncture of a joint space with a needle to remove fluid accumulated in the joint.

Arthroplasty: (AR-throw-PLAS-te) Repair of a joint. Also called joint replacement.

Arthroscopy: (are-THROSS-scop-ee) Examination of the interior of a joint with an arthroscope.

Articular: (ar-TIK-yoo-lar) Pertaining to a joint.

Artificial feeding: (ART-ih-FISH-uhl FEE-ding) Feeding via a tube into the stomach or intestine when a person is unable to take oral nutrition.

Artificial hydration: (ART-ih-FISH-uhl hy-DRAY-shun) Administration of water via intravenous or gastric tube when a person is unable to take oral fluids.

Ascites: (a-SIGH-teez) Abnormal accumulation of fluid in the peritoneal cavity.

Asepsis: (ah-SEP-sis) A condition free from germs, infection, and any form of life.

Aseptic: (ah-SEP-tik) Free of pathogenic organisms; asepsis.

Asphyxia: (as-FIX-ee-a) A condition in which there is a deficiency of oxygen in the blood and an increase in carbon dioxide in the blood and tissues.

Aspiration: (ASS-pi-RAY-shun) Accidental drawing in of foreign substances into the throat or lungs during inspiration.

Assessment: (ah-SESS-ment) An appraisal or evaluation of a patient's condition.

Asterixis: (AS-ter-ICK-sis) Hand flapping tremor and involuntary movements of tongue and feet; may be present in hepatic encephalopathy.

Astigmatism: (uh-STIG-mah-TIZM) An error of refraction in which a ray of light is not sharply focused on the retina but is spread over a more or less diffuse area.

Ataxia: (ah-TAK-see-ah) Failure of muscular coordination; irregularity of muscular action.

Atelectasis: (AT-e-LEK-tah-sis) Collapsed or airless condition of the lung or portion of lung, caused by obstruction or hypoventilation.

Atheroma: (ATH-er-OMA) Fatty deterioration or thickening of the walls of the larger arteries occurring in atherosclerosis.

Atherosclerosis: (ATH-er-oh-skle-ROH-sis) A form of arteriosclerosis characterized by accumulation of plaque, blood, and blood products lining the wall of the artery, causing partial or complete blockage of an artery.

Atrial depolarization: (AY-tree-uhl DE-poh-lahr-i-ZAY-shun) Electrical activation of the atria.

Atrial systole: (AY-tree-uhl SIS-tuh-lee) The contraction of the atria.

Atrioventricular node: (AY-tree-oh-ven-TRICK-yoo-lar NOHD) Located in lower right atrium; receives an impulse from the sinoatrial (SA) node and relays it to the ventricles.

Atrophy: (AT-ruh-fee) Without nourishment; wasting.

Atypical: (ay-TIP-i-kuhl) Deviating from normal.

Augmentation: (AWG-men-TAY-shun) The act or process of increasing in size, quantity, degree or severity.

Auscultation: (AWS-kul-TAY-shun) Process of listening for sounds within the body, usually sounds of thoracic or abdominal viscera, to detect an abnormality.

Autoimmune: (AW-toh-im-YOON) A condition in which the body does not recognize itself and the immune system attacks normal cells.

Ayurvedic: (AY-YUR-VAY-dik) An ancient Hindu system of medicine that improves health by harmonizing mind and body.

Azotemia: (AY-zoh-TEE-me-ah) An increase in nitrogenous bodies in the blood, especially urea, as measured by the serum blood urea nitrogen (BUN) level.

Bacteria: (back-TEER-e-ah) One-celled organisms that can reproduce but need a host for food and supportive environment. Bacteria can be harmless, normal flora, or disease-producing pathogens.

Balanitis: (BAL-uh-NIGH-tis) Inflammation of the skin covering the glans penis.

Bariatric: (BAR-ry-AT-rick) Branch of medicine that deals with the prevention, control, and treatment of obesity.

Basal cell secretion test: (BAY-zuhl SELL see-KREE-shun TEST) Part of a gastric analysis; measures the amount of gastric acid produced in 1 hour.

Behavior management: (be-HAYV-yer MAN-ij-ment) Treatment method that uses positive and negative reinforcement to alter behavior.

Belief: (bee-LEEF) Something accepted as true. Does not have to be proven.

Beneficence: (buh-NEF-i-sens) To provide good care; to do good for patients. One of the oldest requirements for health care providers.

Benign: (bee-NINE) Not progressive; for example, a tumor that is not cancerous.

Beta-hemolytic streptococci: (BAY-tuh-HEE-moh-LIT-ick STREP-toh-KOCK-sigh) Gram-positive bacteria that, when grown on blood-agar plates, completely hemolyze the blood and produce a clear zone around the bacteria colony. Group A beta-hemolytic streptococci cause disease in humans.

Bigeminy: (bye-JEM-i-nee) Occurring every second beat, as in bigeminal premature ventricular contractions.

Bilateral salpingo-oophorectomy: (by-LAT-er-uhl sal-PINJ-oh-ah-fuh-RECK-tuh-mee) Surgical removal of both fallopian tubes and ovaries.

Bimanual: (by-MAN-yoo-uhl) With both hands.

Biofeedback: (BYE-oh-FEED-bak) A form of therapy that uses provision of visual or auditory evidence to a person of the status of an autonomic body function such as heart rate, blood pressure, or respiratory rate.

Biopsy: (BY-ahp-see) A sample of tissue removed for examination.

Bioterrorism (BYE-oh-TER-oh-RIZ-um) Biological agent use or threat of use with a pathological organism for terrorist purposes.

Bipolar: (bye-POH-ler) Having two poles or pertaining to both poles. Bipolar disorder is characterized by episodes of manic and depressive behavior.

Blanch: (BLANCH) To lose color.

Bleb: (BLEB) An irregularly shaped elevation of the skin, such as a blister. May also occur in lung tissue.

Blepharitis: (BLEF-uh-RIGH-tis) Inflammation of the glands and lash follicles along the margin of the eyelids.

Blindness: (BLYND-ness) Lack or loss of ability to see.

Bolus: (BOH-lus) A dose of intravenous medication injected all at once.

Bone: (BOWN) The hard, rigid form of connective tissue constituting most of the skeleton of vertebrates, composed chiefly of calcium salts.

Botulism (BOTCH-u-liz-um) A paralytic illness caused by a potent neurotoxin produced by *Clostridium botulinum,* an anaerobic, spore-forming bacterium. It can be used as a biological weapon.

Bowel sounds: (BOW'L SOWNDS) Gurgling and clicking sounds heard over the abdomen caused by air and fluid movement from peristaltic action. Normal bowel sounds occur every 5 to 15 seconds at a rate of 5 to 35 sounds per minute. Absent—no bowel sounds heard after 5 minutes of listening in each quadrant. Hyperactive—bowel sounds that are frequent, high-pitched, and loud. Hypoactive—bowel sounds that occur at a rate of one every minute or longer.

Bradycardia: (BRAY-dee-KAR-dee-yah) A slow heartbeat characterized by a pulse rate below 60 beats per minute.

Bradykinesia: (BRAY-dee-kin-EE-zee-ah) Abnormal slowness of movement; sluggishness.

Breakthrough pain: (BRAYK-throo) Pain that occurs while medicated with long-acting analgesics.

Bronchiectasis: (BRONG-key-EK-tah-sis) Chronic dilation of a bronchus or bronchi, usually associated with secondary infection and excessive sputum production.

Bronchitis: (brong-KIGH-tis) Inflammation of the mucous membrane

of the bronchial airways; may be viral or bacterial.

Bronchodilator: (BRONG-koh-DYE-lay-ter) A drug that expands the bronchial tubes by relaxing bronchial smooth muscle.

Bronchospasm: (BRONG-koh-spazm) Spasm of the bronchial smooth muscle resulting in narrowing of the airways; associated with asthma and bronchitis.

Bruit: (BROUT) A humming heard when auscultating a blood vessel that is caused by turbulent blood flow through the vessel.

Bulimia nervosa: (buh-LEE-mee-ah ner-VOH-sah) Recurrent episodes of binge eating and self-induced vomiting.

Bulla: (BUHL-ah) A large blister or skin lesion filled with fluid. May also occur in lung tissue.)

Bundle of His: (BUN-duhl of HISS) A bundle of fibers of the impulse-conducting system of the heart. Originates in the atrioventricular (AV) node.

Bursae: (BURR-sah) A small fluid-filled sac or saclike cavity situated in tissues such as joints where friction would otherwise occur.

Calculi: (KAL-kyoo-lye) An abnormal concentration, usually composed of mineral salts, occurring within the body, chiefly in the hollow organs or their passages. Also called stones, as in kidney stones and gallstones.

Cancer: (KAN-sir) A general name for over 100 diseases in which abnormal cells grow out of control; a malignant tumor.

Cannula: (KAN-yoo-lah) A flexible tube that can be inserted into the body guided by a stiff, pointed rod. For example, an intravenous cannula is guided by a metal needle.

Capillary permeability: (KAP-i-lar-ee PER-me-a-BILL-i-tee) The ability of substances to diffuse through capillary walls into tissue spaces.

Capillary refill: (KAP-i-lar-ee RE-fill) The amount of time required for color to return to the nailbed after having been compressed; normally 3 seconds or less. Indicator of peripheral circulation.

Caput medusae: (KAP-ut mi-DOO-see) Dilated veins around the umbilicus, associated with cirrhosis of the liver.

Carbuncle: (KAR-bung-kull) A necrotizing infection of skin and subcutaneous tissue composed of a cluster of boils.

Carcinoembryonic antigens (CEA): (KAR-sin-oh-EM-bree-ah-nik AN-ti-jens) A class of antigens normally present in fetal cells; CEA level is elevated in many cancers and is measured to guide cancer treatment.

Carcinogen: (kar-SIN-oh-jen) Specific agent known to promote the cancer process.

Cardiac output: (KAR-dee-yak OWT-put) A measure of the pumping ability of the heart; amount of blood pumped by the heart per minute.

Cardiac tamponade: (KAR-dee-yak TAM-pon-AID) The life-threatening compression of the heart by the fluid accumulating in the pericardial sac surrounding the heart.

Cardiogenic shock: (KAR-dee-o-JEN-ick SHOCK) Occurs when the heart muscle is unhealthy and contractility is impaired.

Cardiomegaly: (KAR-dee-oh-MEG-ah-lee) Enlargement of the heart.

Cardiomyopathy: (KAR-dee-oh-my-AH-pah-thee) A group of diseases that affect the myocardium's (heart muscle's) structure or function.

Cardioplegia: (KAR-dee-oh-PLEE-jee-ah) Arrest of myocardial contraction, as by use of chemical compounds or cold temperatures in cardiac surgery.

Cardioversion: (KAR-dee-oh-VER-zhun) An elective procedure in which a synchronized shock is delivered to attempt to restore the heart to a normal sinus rhythm.

Cataract: (KAT-uh-rakt) Opacity of the lens of the eye.

Cation: (KAT-eye-on) Electrolyte that carries a positive electrical charge.

Ceiling effect: (SEE-ling e-FEKT) The dose of medication at which the maximum therapeutic effect is achieved. Increasing the dose beyond the therapeutic dose will not result in increased relief and may result in undesirable side effects.

Cell-mediated immunity: (SELL ME-dee-ay-ted im-YOO-ni-tee) Production of lymphocytes by thymus in response to antigen exposure.

Cellulitis: (sell-yoo-LYE-tis) Inflammation of cellular or connective tissue.

Cerebrovascular: (SER-ee-broh-VAS-kyoo-lur) Pertaining to the blood vessels of the cerebrum or brain.

Chalazion: (kah-LAY-zee-on) A small eyelid mass resulting from chronic inflammation of a meibomian gland.

Chancre: (SHANK-er) A hard, syphilitic primary ulcer, the first sign of syphilis, appearing approximately 2 to 3 weeks after infection.

Chemotherapy: (KEE-moh-THER-uh-pee) The treatment of disease with medication; often refers to cancer therapy.

Chiropractic: (ky-RUH-prak-tik) Treatment modality that uses manual adjustment of the vertebral column and extremities to remove interference with nerve function.

Cholecystitis: (KOH-lee-sis-TIGH-tis) Inflammation of the gallbladder.

Choledocholithiasis: (koh-LED-oh-koh-li-THIGH-ah-sis) Gallstones in the common bile duct.

Choledochoscopy: (KOH-LED-oh-KOS-koh-pee) An endoscopic test of the gallbladder and common bile duct.

Cholelithiasis: (KOH-lee-li-THIGH ah-sis) Gallstones in the gallbladder.

Chorea: (kaw-REE-ah) A nervous condition marked by involuntary muscular twitching of the limbs or facial muscles.

Chronic illness: (KRAH-nick ILL-ness) An illness that is long-lasting or recurring, which usually interferes with a person's ability to perform activities of daily living. Medical care and hospitalization are often required on an ongoing basis.

Circumcise: (SIR-kuhm-size) Surgical removal of the foreskin covering the head of the penis.

Cirrhosis: (si-ROH-sis) Chronic disease of the liver, associated with fat infiltration and development of fibrotic tissue.

Civil law: (SIV-il LAW) Provides the rules by which individuals seek to protect their personal and property rights.

Claudication: (KLAW-di-KAY-shun) Severe pain in the calf muscle from inadequate blood supply.

Clubbing: (KLUB-ing) A condition in which the ends of the fingers and toes appear bulbous and shiny, most often the result of lung disease.

Cochlear implant: (KOK-lee-er IM-plant) A device consisting of a microphone, signal processor, external transmitter, and implanted receiver to aid hearing.

Code of ethics: (KOHD of ETH-icks) A traditional compilation of ideal behaviors of a professional group.

Codependence: (KO-de-PEN-dense) A situation in which the significant others in a family group begin to lose their own sense of identity and purpose and exist solely for the abuser.

Cognitive: (KAHG-ni-tiv). The ability to think rationally and to process thoughts.

Colectomy: (koh-LEK-tuh-me) Excision of the colon or a portion of it.

Colic: (KAH-lick) Spasm of a hollow organ or duct, causing pain.

Colitis: (koh-LYE-tis) Inflammation of the colon.

Collateral circulation: (koh-LA-ter-al SIR-kew-LAY-shun) Small branches off of larger blood vessels that will increase in size and capacity next to a main blood vessel that is obstructed.

Colonization: (COLLIN-i-ZAY-shun) The presence of pathogenic microbes in the body, without development of a symptomatic infection

Colonoscopy: (KOH-lun-AHS-kuh-pee) Examination of the upper portion of the rectum with a colonoscope.

Colostomy: (koh-LAH-stuh-me) An artificial opening (stoma) created in the large intestine and brought to the surface of the abdomen for evacuating the bowels.

Colporrhaphy: (kohl-POOR-ah-fee) Surgical repair of the vagina.

Colposcopy: (kul-POS-koh-pee) Examination of the vulva, vagina, and cervix by means of a magnifying lens and a bright light.

Comedone: (KOH-me-doh) Skin lesion that occurs in acne vulgaris (closed form: whitehead; open form: blackhead).

Commissurotomy: (KOM-i-shur-AHT-oh-mee) Surgical incision of any commissure as in cardiac valves to increase the size of the orifice.

Compliance: (kom-PLIGH-ens) The ability to alter size or shape in response to an outside force; the ability of the lungs to distend.

Compulsion: (kum-PUHL-shun) A recurrent, unwanted, and distressing urge to perform an act.

Conductive hearing loss: (kon-DUK-tiv HEER-ing LOSS) Impaired transmission of sound waves through the external ear canal to the bones of the middle ear.

Condylomata acuminata: (KON-di-LOH-ma-tah ah-KYOOM-in-AH-tah) Warts in the genital region caused by the human papillomavirus (HPV); a contagious sexually transmitted disease.

Condylomatous: (KON-di-LOH-ma-tus) Pertaining to a condyloma.

Confidentiality: (KON-fi-den-she-AL-i-tee) Maintaining privacy of patient information. Patient and patient's care can be discussed only in the professional setting.

Congestive heart failure: (kon-JESS-tive HART FAIL-yur) Results from inability of heart to pump sufficient amounts of blood because of impaired pumping function and sodium and water retention. Congestion refers to the buildup of fluid that ranges from mild to life-threatening (pulmonary edema). With left-sided heart failure, the fluid buildup occurs in the lungs and if severe, immediate treatment is required or death can occur. With right-sided heart failure, the fluid buildup is seen systemically (lower legs/feet, sacral area in bedridden persons, jugular veins, liver, spleen).

Conization: (KOH-ni-ZAY-shun) The removal of a cone of tissue, as in partial excision of the cervix uteri.

Conjunctivitis: (kon-JUNK-ti-VIGH-tis) Inflammation of the conjunctiva of the eye.

Consensual response: (kon-SEN-shoo-uhl ree-SPONS) Reaction of both pupils when one eye is exposed to greater intensity of light than the other.

Constipation: (KON-sti-PAY-shun) A condition of sluggish or difficult bowel action/evacuation.

Contraceptive: (KON-truh-SEP-tiv) Any process, device, or method that prevents conception.

Contracture: (kon-TRACK-chur) Abnormal accumulation of fibrosis connective tissue in skin, muscle, or joint capsule that prevents normal mobility at that site.

Contralateral: (KON-truh-LAT-er-uhl) Originating in or affecting the opposite side of the body.

Conversion disorder: (kon-VER-zhun dis-OR-der) An illness that emerges from overuse of the conversion reaction defense mechanism, in which there is impaired physical functioning that appears to be neurological, but no organic disease can be identified.

Coping: (KOH-ping) The process of contending with the stresses of daily life in an effort to overcome or work through them.

Coronary artery disease: (KOR-uh-na-ree AR-tuh-ree di-ZEEZ) Narrowing of the coronary arteries sufficient to prevent adequate blood supply to the myocardium.

Cor pulmonale: (KOR PUL-mah-NAH-lee) Hypertrophy or failure of the right ventricle from disorders of the chest wall, lungs, and pulmonary vessels, as with increased pulmonary pressure caused by chronic obstructive pulmonary disease (COPD).

Craniectomy: (KRAY-nee-EK-tuh-me) Excision of a segment of the skull.

Cranioplasty: (KRAY-nee-oh-plas-tee) Any plastic repair operation on the skull.

Craniotomy: (KRAY-nee-AHT-oh-mee) Any incision through the cranium.

Crepitation: (crep-i-TAY-shun) A dry, crackling sound or sensation, such as that produced by the grating of the ends of a fractured bone.

Crepitus: (KREP-i-tuss) Crepitation.

Criminal law: (KRIM-i-nuhl LAW) Regulates behaviors for citizens within a country.

Critical thinking: (KRIT-i-kuhl THING-king) Use of knowledge and skills to make the best decisions possible in client care situations.

Cryotherapy: (KRY-oh-THER-uh-pee) The therapeutic use of cold.

Cryptorchidism: (kript-OR-ki-dizm) A birth condition in which one or both of the testicles have not descended into the scrotum.

Culdocentesis: (KUL-doh-sen-TEE-sis) The procedure for obtaining material from the posterior vaginal cul-de-sac by aspiration or surgical incision through the vaginal wall, performed for therapeutic or diagnostic reasons.

Culdoscopy: (kul-DOS-koh-pee) Direct visual examination of the female viscera through an endoscope introduced into the pelvic cavity through the posterior vaginal fornix.

Culdotomy: (KUL-DOT-uh-mee) Incision or needle puncture of the cul-de-sac of Douglas through the vagina.

Cultural awareness: (KUL-chur-uhl a-WARE-ness) Being aware of history and ancestry and having an appreciation of and attention to the crafts, arts, music, foods, and clothing of various cultures.

Cultural competence: (KUL-chur-uhl KOM-pe-tens) Having an awareness of one's own culture and not letting it have an undue influence over another person's culture. Having the knowledge and skills about a culture that are required to provide care.

Cultural diversity: (KUL-chur-uhl di-VER-si-tee) Representing two or more cultures; the differences among cultures. For example, the United States includes people from many different countries.

Cultural sensitivity: (KUL-chur-uhl SEN-si-TIV-i-tee) Being aware of and sensitive to cultural differences. Avoiding behavior or language that may be offensive to another person's cultural beliefs.

Culture: (KUL-chur) The socially transmitted behavior patterns, beliefs, values, customs, arts, and all other characteristics of people that guide their worldview.

Curet: (kyoo-RET) A loop, ring, or spoon-shaped instrument, attached to a handle and having sharp or blunt edges; used to scrape tissue from a surface.

Custom: (KUS-tum) A custom is the usual way of acting in a given circumstance or something that an individual or group does out of habit. For example, many people eat turkey on Thanksgiving.

Cyanosis: (SIGH-uh-NOH-sis) Slightly bluish, grayish, or dark purple discoloration of the skin caused by the presence of abnormal amounts of reduced hemoglobin in the blood.

Cystic: (SIS-tik) Pertaining to cysts or the urinary bladder.

Cystitis: (sis-TIGH-tis) Inflammation of the urinary bladder.

Cystocele: (SIS-toh-seel) A bladder hernia that protrudes into the vagina.

Cystoscopy: (sis-TAHS-koh-pee) A diagnostic procedure using an instrument (cystoscope) via the urethra to view the bladder.

Cytomegalovirus: (sigh-TOW-meg-ul-low-vigh-rus) Species-specific herpesvirus; usually harmless to those with functional immune systems. May cause fatal pneumonia in those who are immunocompromised. Affects retina and may cause blindness in those with acquired immunodeficiency syndrome.

Cytotoxic: (SIGH-toh-TOCK-sick) Destructive to cells.

Data, objective: SEE objective data.

Data, subjective: SEE subjective data.

Data: (DAY-tuh) A group of facts or statistics.

Debridement: (day-breed-MAHNT) The removal of foreign material and contaminated and devitalized tissues from or adjacent to a traumatic or infected area until surrounding healthy tissue is exposed.

Decerebrate: (dee-SER-e-brayt) Posture of an individual with absence of cerebral function.

Decorticate: (dee-KOR-ti-kayt) Posture of an individual with a lesion at or above the upper brain stem.

Defibrillation: (dee-FIB-ri-lay-shun) Use of an electrical device that applies countershock to the heart through electrodes placed on the chest wall to stop fibrillation of the heart.

Degeneration: (de-jen-er-AY-shun) Deterioration.

Dehiscence: (dee-HISS-ents) A splitting open (i.e., rupture) of an incision.

Dehydration: (DEE-high-DRAY-shun) A condition resulting from excessive loss of body fluid that occurs when fluid output exceeds intake.

Delirium tremens: (dee-LIR-ee-uhm TREE-menz) An acute alcohol withdrawal syndrome marked by acute, transient disturbance of consciousness.

Delusions: (dee-LOO-zhuns) False beliefs that are firmly maintained in spite of incontrovertible proof to the contrary.

Dementia: (dee-MEN-cha) A broad term that refers to cognitive deficit, including memory impairment.

Demyelination: (dee-MY-uh-lin-AY-shun) Loss of myelin from neurons.

Deontology: (DA-on-TOL-o-gee) The study of moral obligations and commitments, including medical ethics.

Dependence: (di-PEN-dens) A state of reliance on something. Psychological craving for a drug that may or may not be accompanied by a physiological need.

Depression: (dee-PRESS-shun) A mental disorder marked by altered mood with loss of interest.

Dermatitis: (DER-mah-TIGH-tis) Inflammation of the skin.

Dermatophytosis: (DER-mah-toh-fye-TOH-sis) A fungal infection of the skin.

Dermoid: (DER-moyd) Resembling the skin.

Developmental stage: (DEE-vell-up-MEN-tal STAYJ) An age-defined period with specific psychological tasks that need to be accomplished to maintain ego as proposed by Erik Erikson, a psychoanalyst.

Diabetes mellitus: (DYE-ah-BEE-tis mel-LYE-tus) A chronic disease characterized by impaired production or use of insulin and high blood glucose levels.

Diarrhea: (DYE-uh-REE-ah) Passage of fluid or unformed stools.

Diastolic blood pressure: (dye-ah-STAH-lik BLUHD PRE-shure) The amount of pressure exerted on the wall of the arteries when the ventricles are at rest. The bottom number in a blood pressure reading.

Diffusion: (di-FEW-zhun) The tendency of molecules of a substance (gaseous, liquid, or solid) to move from a region of high concentration to one of lower concentration.

Dilation and curettage: (DIL-AY-shun and kyoor-e-TAHZH) A surgical procedure that expands the cervical canal of the uterus (dilation) so that the surface lining of the uterine wall can be scraped (curettage).

Diplopia: (dip-LOH-pee-ah) Double vision.

Displacement: (dis-PLAYSS-ment) Transference of emotion from the original idea with which it was associated to a different idea, allowing the client to avoid acknowledging the original source.

Disseminated intravascular coagulation: (dis-SEM-i-NAY-ted IN-trah-VAS-kyoo-lar koh-AG-yoo-LAY-shun) A pathological form of coagulation that is diffuse (widespread) rather than localized, as would be the case in normal coagulation. Clotting factors are consumed to such an extent that generalized bleeding may occur.

Distributive justice: (dis-TRIB-yoo-tiv JUS-tiss) The right of individuals to be treated equally regardless of race, sex, marital status, sexual preference, medical diagnosis, social standing, economic level, or religious belief.

Distributive shock: (dis-TRIB-yoo-tiv) Excessive dilation of the venules and arterioles, leading to decreased distribution of blood, resulting in shock.

Diverticulitis: (DYE-ver-tik-yoo-LYE-tis) Inflammation of a diverticulum (a sac or pouch in the walls of a canal or organ, usually the colon), especially inflammation involving diverticula of the colon.

Diverticulosis: (DYE-ver-tik-yoo-LOH-sis) The presence of diverticula in the absence of inflammation.

Do Not Resuscitate: (DOO not re-SUSS-i-TATE) An order not to do CPR at the end of life.

Dormant: (DOOR-mant) Condition of greatly reduced metabolic activity permitting long-term survival and possible reactivation of bacterial endospores, protozoan cysts, larval stages of worm parasites, and viruses.

Dressler's syndrome: (DRESS-lers SIN-drohm) Postmyocardial infarction syndrome; pericarditis.

Durable Medical Power of Attorney: (DUR-uh-buhl POW-ur uv uh-TUR-nee) Person legally designated to speak for a patient when the patient is no longer able to speak for himself or herself.

Dysarthria: (dis-AR-three-ah) Imperfect articulation of speech caused by disturbances of muscular control resulting from central or peripheral nervous system damage.

Dysfunctional: (dis-FUNCK-shun-uhl) Family or work environment that does not function effectively, sometimes because of other problems of members.

Dysmenorrhea: (DIS-men-oh-REE-ah) Pain in association with menstruation.

Dyspareunia: (DIS-puh-ROO-nee-ah) Occurrence of pain in the labia, vagina, or pelvis during or after sexual intercourse.

Dysphagia: (dis-FAYJ-ee-ah) Inability to swallow or difficulty swallowing.

Dysplasia: (dis-PLAY-zee-ah) Abnormal development of tissue.

Dyspnea: (DISP-nee-ah) Subjective sense of labored breathing that occurs because of insufficient oxygenation.

Dysreflexia: (DIS-re-FLEK-see-ah) State in which an individual with a spinal cord injury at or above T6 experiences an uninhibited sympathetic response to a noxious stumulus.

Dysrhythmia: (dis-RITH-mee-yah) Abnormal, disordered, or disturbed cardiac rhythm.

Dysuria: (dis-YOO-ree-ah) Difficult or painful urination.

Ecchymoses: (ECK-uh-MOH-sis) A bruise of varying size, the color of which may be blue-black, changing to greenish yellow or yellow with time.

Ectasia: (ek-TAY-zee-ah) Replacement of normal tissue with fibrous tissue.

Ectopic: (eck-TOP-ick) Ectopic hormones are secreted from sites other than the gland where they would normally be found.

Edema: (uh-DEE-muh) Collection of excess fluid in body tissues.

Ejaculation: (ee-JAK-yoo-LAY-shun) The release of semen from the male urethra.

Electrocardiogram: (ee-LECK-troh-KAR-dee-oh-GRAM) A recording of the electrical activity of the heart.

Electrocautery: (ee-LECK-troh-CAW-tur-ee) Cauterization using platinum wires heated to red or white heat by an electric current, either direct or alternating.

Electrocoagulated: (ee-LECK-troh-coh-AG-yoo-LAY-ted) Coagulation of tissue by means of a high-frequency electric current.

Electroconvulsive therapy (ECT): (ee-LEK-troh-kun-VUL-siv THER-uh-pee) A type of somatic therapy in which an electric current is used to produce convulsions to treat such conditions as depression.

Electroencephalogram: (ee-LEK-troh-en-SEFF-uh-loh-gram) A record produced by electroencephalography; tracing of the electrical impulses of the brain.

Electrolyte: (ee-LEK-troh-lite) A substance that when dissolved in water can conduct electricity.

Electroretinography: (ee-LEK-troh-RET-in-AHG-ruh-fee) Measurement of the electrical response of the retina to light stimulation.

Emboli: (EM-boh-li) Solid, liquid, or gaseous masses of undissolved matter traveling with the fluid current in a blood or lymphatic vessel.

Embolism: (EM-buh-lizm) Foreign substance or blood clot that travels through the circulatory system until it obstructs a vessel.

Empathy: (EM-puh-thee) Objective awareness of and insight into the feelings, emotions, and behavior of another person.

Emphysema: (EM-fi-SEE-mah) Distention of interstitial tissue by gas or air; chronic pulmonary disease marked by terminal bronchiole and alveolar destruction and air trapping.

Empyema: (EM-pigh-EE-mah) Pus in a body cavity, especially the pleural space.

Encephalitis: (EN-seff-uh-LYE-tis) Inflammation of the brain.

Encephalopathy: (en-SEFF-uh-LAHP-ah-thee) Dysfunction of the brain.

Endarterectomy: (end-AR-tur-ECK-tuh-mee) Excision of thickened atheromatous areas of the innermost coat of an artery.

Endogenous: (en-DAH-jen-us) Produced or originating from within a cell or organism.

Endometritis: (EN-doh-me-TRY-tis) Inflammation of the endometrium of the uterus.

Endorphins: (en-DOR-fins) Naturally occurring opioids in the body, many times more potent than analgesic medications.

Endoscope: (EN-doh-skohp) A device consisting of a tube and optical system for observing the inside of a hollow organ or cavity. Can be flexible or rigid.

Enkephalins: (en-KEF-e-lins) One type of endorphin.

Enteritis: (en-ter-EYE-tis) Inflammation of the intestines, particularly of the mucosa and submucosa of the small intestine.

Enucleation: (ee-NEW-klee-AY-shun) Removal of an organ or other mass intact from its supporting tissues, as of the eyeball from the orbit.

Epidemiological: (EP-i-DEE-me-ah-LAHJ-i-kuhl) The study of the distribution and determinants of health-related states and events in populations and the application of this study to the control of health problems.

Epididymitis: (EP-i-DID-i-MY-tis) Inflammation or infection of the epididymis.

Epidural: (EP-i-DUHR-uhl) Situated on or outside the dura mater.

Epinephrine: (EP-i-NEFF-rin) A hormone secreted by the adrenal medulla in response to stimulation of the sympathetic nervous system.

Epispadias: (EP-i-SPAY-dee-ahz) A congenital male defect in which the opening of the urethra is on the dorsum of the penis, instead of the tip.

Epistaxis: (EP-iss-TAX-iss) Nosebleed.

Epithelialization: (ep-i-THEE-lee-al-eye-ZAY-shun) The growth of skin over a wound.

Equianalgesic: (EE-kwee-AN-uhl-JEE-zik) Drugs having equal pain killing effect. The same degree of pain relief may require different doses when different medications are given or medications are given by different routes.

Erectile dysfunction: (e-RECK-tile dis-FUNCK-shun) Inability to have an erection sufficient for sexual intercourse.

Erection: (e-REK-shun) Enlargement and hardening of the penis caused by engorgement of blood.

Erythema: (ER-i-THEE-mah) Diffuse redness over the skin.

Eschar: (ESS-kar) Hard scab or dry crust that results from necrotic tissue.

Escharotomy: (ess-kar-AHT-oh-mee) Removal of a slough or scab formed on the skin and underlying tissue of severely burned skin.

Esophagogastroduodenoscopy: (e-SOFF-ah-go-GAS-troh-doo-AH-den-AHS-kuh-pee) An endoscopic procedure that allows the physician to view the esophagus, stomach, and duodenum.

Esophagoscopy: (ee-soff-ah-GAHS-kuh-pee) Examination of the esophagus using an endoscope.

Esotropia: (ESS-oh-TROH-pee-ah) Strabismus in which there is deviation of the visual axis of one eye toward that of the other eye, resulting in diplopia. Also called cross-eyed.

Essential hypertension: (e-SEN-shul HIGH-per-TEN-shun) Chronic elevation of blood pressure resulting from an unknown cause.

Ethical: (ETH-i-kuhl) Describes behavior guided by a system of moral principles or standards.

Ethnic: (ETH-nick) Pertaining to a religious, racial, national, or cultural group. For example, individuals may identify with the Jewish, Catholic, or Islamic religions.

Ethnocentrism: (ETH-noh-SEN-trizm) The tendency to think that one's own ways of thinking, believing, and acting are the only right ways. People who are different are seen as strange or bizarre. An example is one who believes that his or her religious beliefs are the only right beliefs and other religions are wrong.

Eustress: (YOO-stress) Stress from positive experiences.

Euthyroid: (yoo-THY-royd) Normal thyroid function.

Evaluation: (e-VAL-yoo-AY-shun) The judgment of anything.

Evisceration: (E-VIS-sir-a-shun) Extrusion of viscera outside the body, especially through a surgical excision.

Exacerbation: (egg-sass-sir-BAY-shun) Aggravation of symptoms.

Exophthalmos: (ECKS-off-THAL-mus) Abnormal protrusion of the eyeball.

Exotropia: (EKS-oh-TROH-pee-ah) Abnormal turning outward of one or both eyes; divergent strabismus.

Expectorant: (ek-SPEK-tuh-rant) Agent that promotes removal of pulmonary secretions.

Expectorate: (eck-SPECK-tuh-RAYT) The act or process of coughing up materials from the air passageways leading to the lungs.

External otitis: (eks-TER-nuhl oh-TIGH-tis) Inflammation of the external ear.

Extracardiac: (EX-trah-KAR-dee-ack) Outside the heart.

Extracellular: (EX-trah-SELL-yoo-ler) Outside the cell.

Extracorporeal shock wave lithotripsy (ESWL): (ECKS-trah-koar-POR-ee-uhl SHAHK WAYV LITH-oh-TRIP-see) Noninvasive treatment using shock waves to break up gallstones or kidney stones.

Extravasation: (eks-TRA-vah-ZAY-shun) The escape of fluids into surrounding tissue.

Extrinsic factors: (eks-TRIN-sik FAK-ters) External variables.

Exudate: (EKS-yoo-dayt) Accumulated fluid in a cavity; oozing of pus or serum; often the result of inflammation.

Fasciculation: (fah-SIK-yoo-LAY-shun) Twitching.

Fasciotomy: (fash-e-OTT-oh-me) Incision of fascia.

Feminist: (FEM-un-nist) A person who advocates for women the same rights as men.

Fetor hepaticus: (FEE-tor he-PAT-i-kus) Foul breath associated with liver disease.

Fibrocystic: (FIGH-broh-SIS-tik) Consisting of fibrocysts, which are fibrous tumors that have undergone cystic degeneration or accumulated fluid.

Fidelity: (fi-DEL-i-tee) The obligation to be faithful to commitments made to self and others.

Filtration: (fill-TRAY-shun) The process of removing particles from a solution by allowing the liquid portion to pass through a membrane or other partial barrier.

Fissure: (FISH-er) A narrow slit or cleft, especially one of the deeper or more constant furrows separating the gyri of the brain.

Fistula: (FIST-yoo-lah) Any abnormal, tubelike passage within body tissue, usually between two internal organs, or leading from an internal organ to the body surface.

Flaccid: (FLA-sid) Weak, lax, soft muscles.

Flail chest: (FLAY-ul chesst) Condition of the chest wall caused by two or more fractures on each affected rib resulting in a segment of rib that is not attached on either end; the flail portion moves paradoxically in with inspiration and out with expiration.

Flora: (FLOOR-a) Microbial life adapted for living in a specific environment such as the intestines, skin, or urinary tract.

Fluoroscope: (FLAW-or-oh-skohp) A device consisting of a fluorescent screen suitably mounted, either separately or in conjunction with an x-ray tube, by means of which the shadows of objects interposed between the tube and the screen are made visible.

Fluoroscopy: (fluh-RAHS-kuh-pee) The use of a fluoroscope for medical diagnosis or for testing various materials by roentgen rays.

Full-thickness burn: (FUL-THICK-ness BERN) Burn in which all of the epithelializing elements and those lining the sweat glands, hair follicles, and sebaceous glands are destroyed.

Fungi: (FUNG-guy) A general term for a group of eukaryotic organisms (e.g., mushrooms, yeasts, molds).

Furuncle: (FYOOR-ung-kull) An acute circumscribed inflammation of the subcutaneous layers of the skin or of a gland or hair follicle.

Gastrectomy: (gas-TREK-tuh-mee) Any surgery that involves partial or total removal of the stomach.

Gastric acid stimulation test: (GAS-trik ASS-id STIM-yoo-LAY-shun TEST) A test that measures the amount of gastric acid for 1 hour after subcutaneous injection of a drug that stimulates gastric acid secretion.

Gastric analysis: (GAS-trik ah-NAL-i-sis) A test performed to measure secretions of hydrochloric acid and pepsin in the stomach.

Gastric lavage: (GAS-trik la-VAHJ) Washing out of the stomach; used to empty the stomach when the contents are irritating.

Gastritis: (gas-TRY-tis) Acute—The inflammation of the stomach mucosa; also known as heartburn or indigestion. Chronic—Gastritis that is recurrent; classified as type A (asymptomatic) or type B (symptomatic).

Gastroduodenostomy: (GAS-troh-DOO-oh-den-AHS-toh-mee) Excision of the pylorus of the stomach with anastomosis of the upper portion of the stomach to the duodenum.

Gastroepiploic: (GAS-troh-EP-i-PLOH-ick) Pertaining to the stomach and greater omentum.

Gastrojejunostomy: (GAS-troh-JAY-joo-NAHS-toh-mee) Subtotal excision of the stomach with closure of the proximal end of the duodenum and side-to-side anastomosis of the jejunum to the remaining portion of the stomach.

Gastroparesis: (GAS-troh-puh-REE-sis) Paralysis of the stomach, resulting in poor emptying.

Gastroplasty: (GAS-troh-PLAS-tee) Plastic surgery of the stomach. Used to decrease the size of the stomach to treat morbid obesity.

Gastroscopy: (gas-TRAHS-kuh-pee) Examination of the stomach and abdominal cavity by use of a gastroscope.

Gastrostomy: (gas-TRAHS-toh-mee) Surgical creation of a gastric fistula through the abdominal wall.

Gavage: (gah-VAZH) Feeding with a stomach tube or with a tube passed through the nares, pharynx, and esophagus into the stomach. The food is in liquid or semiliquid form at room temperature.

Generalization: (JEN-er-al-i-ZAY-shun) An assumption about a group or an individual item or person that leads to seeking additional information to determine if the generalization fits the individual. Whereas generalizations are true for the group, they may not be true for the individual.

Glaucoma: (glaw-KOH-mah) A group of eye diseases characterized by increased intraocular pressure.

Glomerulonephritis: (gloh-MER-yoo-loh-ne-FRY-tis) A form of nephritis in which the lesions involve primarily the glomeruli.

Glossitis: (glah-SIGH-tis) An inflammation of the tongue.

Glycosuria: (GLY-kos-YOO-ree-ah) Abnormal amount of glucose in the urine, often associated with diabetes mellitus.

Goitrogens: (GOY-troh-jenz) Foods or medications that cause a goiter.

Gravida: (GRAV-id-ah): Number of times a woman has been pregnant.

Gummas: (GUM-ahs) A soft granulomatous tumor of the tissues characteristic of the tertiary stage of syphilis.

Gynecomastia: (JIN-e-koh-MASS-tee-ah) Excessive breast tissue on a male.

Hallucinations: (huh-LOO-si-NAY-shuns) False perceptions having no relation to reality and not accounted for by any exterior stimuli.

Hand hygiene (hand HY-jeen) Cleansing of the hands with hand washing as defined by the Centers for Disease Control and Prevention (CDC) or an alcohol-based hand sanitizer solution

Health: (HELLTH) A condition in which all functions of the body and mind are normally active.

Hearing aid: (HEER-ing AYD) An instrument to amplify sounds for those with hearing loss.

Heatstroke: (HEET-strohk) An acute and dangerous reaction to heat exposure, characterized by high body temperature, usually higher than 105°F (40.5°C).

Helicobacter pylori: (HEH-lick-co-back-tur PIE-lori) Bacterium that causes some peptic ulcers.

Hemarthrosis: (HEEM-ar-THROH-sis) Bleeding into a joint.

Hematochezia: (HEM-uh-toh-KEE-zee-uh) Blood in the feces.

Hematoma: (HEE-muh-TOH-mah) A localized collection of extravasated blood, usually clotted, in an organ, space, or tissue.

Hematuria: (HEM-uh-TYOOR-ee-ah) Blood in the urine.

Hemiparesis: (hem-ee-puh-REE-sis) Weakness affecting one side of the body.

Hemipelvectomy: (hem-ee-pell-VEC-toe-me) The surgical removal of half of the pelvis and the leg.

Hemiplegia: (hem-ee-PLEE-jee-ah) Paralysis of only one side of the body.

Hemodialysis: (HEE-moh-dye-AL-i-sis) A method for replacing the function of the kidneys by circulating blood through tubes made of semipermeable membranes.

Hemolysis: (he-MAHL-e-sis) The destruction of the membrane of red blood cells with the liberation of hemoglobin, which diffuses into the surrounding fluid.

Hemophilia: (HEE-moh-FILL-ee-ah) A hereditary blood disease marked by greatly prolonged coagulation time, with consequent failure of the blood to clot and abnormal bleeding.

Hemoptysis: (hee-MOP-ti-sis) Coughing up of blood from the respiratory tract.

Hemorrhoids: (HEM-uh-royds) A mass of dilated, tortuous veins in the anorectum involving the venous plexuses of that area.

Hemothorax: (HEE-moh-THAW-raks) Blood in the pleural space; may be associated with trauma, tuberculosis, or pneumonia.

Hepatitis: (HEP-uh-TIGH-tis) Inflammation of the liver, most often viral.

Hepatomegaly: (HEP-uh-toh-MEG-ah-lee) Enlargement of the liver.

Hepatorenal syndrome: (hep-PAT-oh-REE-nuhl SIN-drohm) A deadly kidney failure that sometimes accompanies liver disease.

Hepatosplenomegaly: (he-PA-toh-SPLE-noh-MEG-ah-lee) Enlargement of the liver and spleen.

Hernia: (HER-nee-uh) The protrusion or projection of an organ or a part of an organ through the wall of the cavity that normally contains it.

Herpetic: (her-PET-ick) Pertaining to herpes.

Hiatal hernia: (high-AY-tuhl HER-nee-ah) A condition in which part of the stomach protrudes through and above the diaphragm.

High-density lipoprotein (HDL): (HIGH DEN-si-tee LIP-oh-PROH-teen) Plasma lipids bound to albumin consisting of lipoproteins. It has been found that those with high levels of HDL have less chance of having coronary artery disease.

Histamine: (HISS-ta-mean) A substance produced in the body that increases gastric secretion, increases capillary permeability, and contracts the bronchial smooth muscle. Plays a role in allergic reaction.

Homans' sign: (HOH-manz SIGHN) An assessment for venous thrombosis in which calf pain with dorsiflexion occurs if thrombosis is present.

Homeopathy: (HO-mee-AH-pa-thee) System of medicine based on the theory that "like cures like," and uses tiny doses of a substance that create the symptoms of disease.

Homeostasis: (HOH-mee-oh-STAY-sis) Maintaining a constant balance, especially whenever a change occurs.

Hopelessness: (HOHP-less-ness) Subjective state in which a person sees limited or unavailable alternatives; lacking energy.

Hordeolum: (hor-DEE-oh-lum) Sty.

Hospice: (HOS-pis) A service provided to patients and their families in the last 6 months of life to manage pain and provide emotional support.

Host: (HOE-st) The organism from which a parasite obtains its nourishment.

Human immunodeficiency virus (HIV): (HYOO-man im-YOO-noh-dee-FISH-en-see VIGH-rus) A retrovirus that causes acquired immunodeficiency syndrome (AIDS).

Humoral: (HYOO-mohr-uhl) Pertaining to body fluids or substances contained in them.

Hydrocele: (HIGH-droh-seel) A collection of fluid in the scrotal sack.

Hydrocephalus: (HIGH-droh-SEF-uh-luhs) A condition caused by enlargement of the cranium caused by abnormal accumulation of cerebrospinal fluid within the cerebral ventricular system.

Hydronephrosis: (HIGH-droh-ne-FROH-sis) Abnormal dilation of kidneys caused by obstruction of urine flow.

Hydrostatic: (HIGH-droh-STAT-ik) Pertaining to the pressure of liquids in equilibrium and to the pressure exerted by liquids.

Hypercalcemia: (HIGH-per-kal-SEE-mee-ah) An excessive amount of calcium in the blood.

Hyperglycemia: (HIGH-per-gligh-SEE-mee-ah) Excess glucose in the blood.

Hyperkalemia: (HIGH-per-kuh-LEE-mee-ah) An excessive amount of potassium in the blood.

Hyperlipidemia: (HIGH-per-LIP-i-DEE-mee-ah) Excessive quantity of fat in the blood.

Hypermagnesemia: (HIGH-per-MAG-nuh-ZEE-mee-ah) Excess magnesium in the blood.

Hypernatremia: (HIGH-per-nuh-TREE-mee-ah) Excess sodium in the blood.

Hyperopia: (HIGH-per-OH-pee-ah) Farsightedness.

Hyperplasia: (HIGH-per-PLAY-zee-ah) Excessive increase in the number of normal cells.

Hypertension: (HIGH-per-TEN-shun) Abnormally elevated blood pressure.

Hypertensive emergency: (HIGH-per-TEN-siv) Systolic blood pressure above 180 mm Hg and diastolic blood pressure above 120 to 130 mm Hg.

Hypertonic: (HIGH-per-TAHN-ik) Exerts greater osmotic pressure than blood.

Hypertrophy: (high-PER-truh-fee) An increase in the size of an organ or structure, or of the body, owing to growth rather than tumor formation.

Hyperuricemia: (HIGH-per-yoor-a-SEE-me-ah) An excess of uric acid or urates in the blood.

Hyperventilation: (HIGH-per-VEN-ti-LAY-shun) Increased ventilation that results in a lowered carbon dioxide (CO_2) level (hypocapnia).

Hypervolemia: (HIGH-per-voh-LEE-mee-ah) An abnormal increase in the volume of circulating blood.

Hypocalcemia: (HIGH-poh-kal-SEE-mee-ah) Reduced amount of calcium in the blood.

Hypoglycemia: (HIGH-poh-gligh-SEE-mee-ah) Below-normal amount of glucose in the blood.

Hypokalemia: (HIGH-poh-kuh-LEE-mee-ah) Reduced amount of potassium in the blood.

Hypomagnesemia: (HIGH-poh-MAG-nuh-ZEE-mee-ah) Reduced amount of magnesium in the blood.

Hyponatremia: (HIGH-poh-nuh-TREE-mee-ah) Reduced amount of sodium in the blood.

Hypophysectomy: (HIGH-pah-fi-SECK-tuh-mee) Surgical removal of the pituitary gland.

Hypoplasia: (HIGH-poh-PLAY-zee-ah) Underdevelopment of a tissue organ or body.

Hypospadias: (HIGH-poh-SPAY-dee-ahz) A congenital male defect in which the opening of the urethra is on the underside of the penis, instead of the tip.

Hypostatic: (HIGH-poh-STA-tik) Hypostatic pneumonia occurs from congestion in the lungs associated with lack of activity.

Hypotension: (HIGH-poh-TEN-shun) Abnormally low blood pressure below 90 mm Hg systolic.

Hypothermia: (HIGH-poh-THER-mee-ah) Body temperature below 95° F (35° C).

Hypotonic: (HIGH-poh-TAHN-ik) Pertaining to defective muscular tone or tension; having a lower concentration of solute than intracellular or extracellular fluid.

Hypovolemia: (HIGH-poh-voh-LEE-mee-ah) The most common form of dehydration resulting from the loss of fluid from the body; results in decreased blood volume.

Hypovolemic shock: (HIGH-poh-voh-LEEM-ick SHAHK) Shock that occurs when blood or plasma is lost in such quantities that the remaining blood cannot fill the circulatory system despite constriction of the blood vessels.

Hypovolemic: (HIGH-poh-voh-LEEM-ick) Low volume of blood in the circulatory system.

Hypoxemia: (HIGH-pock-SEE-mee-ah) Deficient oxygenation of the blood.

Hypoxia: (high-POCK-see-ah) Diminished availability of oxygen to the body tissues.

Hysterectomy: (HISS-tuh-RECK-tuh-mee) Surgical removal of the uterus through the abdominal wall or vagina.

Hysterosalpingogram: (HIS-tur-oh-SAL-pinj-oh-gram) Radiograph of the uterus and fallopian tubes.

Hysteroscopy: (HIS-tur-AHS-koh-pee) Endoscopic direct visual examination of the canal of the uterine cervix and the cavity of the uterus.

Hysterotomy: (HISS-tuh-RAH-tuh-mee) Incision of the uterus.

Icterus: (ICK-ter-us) Yellowing of the skin and the sclera of the eye.

Idiopathic thrombocytopenic purpura: (ID-ee-oh-PATH-ik THROM-boh-SIGH-toh-PEE-nik PUR-pew-rah) The total number of circulating platelets is greatly diminished, even though platelet production in the bone marrow is normal, resulting in slowed blood clotting.

Ileostomy: (ILL-ee-AH-stuh-me) An artificial opening (stoma) created in the small intestine (ileum) and brought to the surface of the abdomen for the purpose of evacuating feces.

Illness: (ILL-ness) The state of being sick.

Illusions: (i-LOO-zhuns) Mistaken perceptions of reality.

Imagery: (IM-ij-ree) The use of the imagination to promote relaxation.

Immunocompromised: (IM-yoo-noh-KAHM-prah-mized) Having an immune system that is not capable of reacting to a pathogen or tissue damage.

Impaction: (im-PAK-shun) An immovable accumulation of feces in the bowels.

Imperforate: (im-PER-foh-rate) Without an opening.

In situ: (in-SIT-yoo) Localized, not invading surrounding tissue.

In vitro fertilization: (in VEE-troh FER-ti-li-ZAY-shun) Fertilization in a test tube.

Induction: (in-DUCK-shun) The process or act of causing to occur, as in anesthesia induction.

Induration: (IN-dyoo-RAY-shun) Area of hardened tissue.

Infective endocarditis: (in-FECK-tive EN-doh-kar-DYE-tis) Inflammation of the heart lining caused by microorganisms.

Inspection: (in-SPEK-shun) Use of observation skills to systematically gather data that can be seen.

Insufficiency: (IN-suh-FISH-en-see) The condition of being inadequate for a given purpose, such as heart valves that do not close properly.

Insufflation: (in-suff-LAY-shun) Used to inflate the abdomen during laparoscopic or endoscopic procedures to enhance visualization of structures.

Intermittent claudication: (IN-ter-MIT-ent KLAW-di-KAY-shun) A symptom associated with arterial occlusive disease. It refers to pain in the calf of a lower extremity, usually brought on by activity or exercise, and ceases with rest.

International normalized ratio: (IN-ter-NASH-uh-nul NOR-muh-lized RAY-she-oh) The World Health Organization's standardization for reporting the prothrombin time assay test when the thromboplastin reagent developed by the first International Reference Preparation is used. The reagent was developed to prevent variability in prothrombin time testing results and provide uniformity in monitoring therapeutic levels for coagulation during oral anticoagulation therapy.

Interstitial: (IN-ter-STISH-uhl) Fluid between tissues.

Intervention: (in-ter-VEN-shun) One or more actions taken in order to modify an effect.

Intracellular: (IN-trah-SELL-yoo-ler) Fluids located within the blood cell.

Intracranial: (IN-trah-KRAY-nee-uhl) Within the cranium or skull.

Intraoperative: (IN-trah-AHP-er-uh-tiv) Occurring during a surgical procedure.

Intravascular: (IN-trah-VAS-kyoo-lar) Fluids located within the blood vessels.

Intravenous: (IN-trah-VEE-nus) Within or into a vein.

Intrinsic factors: (in-TRIN-sik FAK-ters) Internal variables.

Intussusception: (IN-tuh-suh-SEP-shun) The slipping of one part of an intestine into another adjacent to it.

Ipsilateral: (IP-si-LAT-er-uhl) On the same side; affecting the same side of the body.

Ischemia: (iss-KEY-me-ah) Condition of inadequate blood supply.

Isoelectric line: (EYE-so-e-LEK-trick LINE) The period when the electrical tracing is at zero and is neither positive nor negative.

Isolated systolic hypertension: (EYE-suh-lay-ted sis-TAH-lik high-per-TEN-shun) The systolic pressure is 160 mm Hg or more, but the diastolic pressure is lower than 95 mm Hg.

Isotonic: (EYE-so-TAHN-ik) A fluid that has the same osmolarity as the blood.

Jaundice: (JAWN-diss) Yellowing of the skin and the sclera of the eye.

Joint: (JOYNT) An articulation. The point of juncture between two bones.

Kaposi's sarcoma: (ka-POE-sees sar-CO-mah) A vascular malignancy that is often first apparent in the skin or mucous membranes but may involve the viscera.

Ketoacidosis: (KEE-toh-ass-i-DOH-sis) A condition in which fat breakdown produces ketones, which cause an acidic state in the body; may be associated with weight loss or diabetes mellitus.

Kussmaul's: (KOOS-mahlz) Term describing deep respirations of an individual with ketoacidosis.

Laceration: (la-sir-A-shun) A wound or irregular tear of the flesh.

Lactic acid: (LAK-tik ASS-id) By-product of anaerobic metabolism.

Laminectomy: (LAM-i-NEK-toh-mee) The excision of a vertebral posterior arch, usually to remove a lesion or herniated disk.

Laparoscopy: (LAP-uh-roh-SKOP-ee) Exploration of the abdomen with an endoscope.

Laparotomy: (LAP-uh-RAH-tuh-mee) The surgical opening of the abdomen; an abdominal operation.

Laryngeal edema: (lah-RIN-jee-uhl uh-DEE-muh) Sudden swelling of the larynx occurring with severe allergic reactions.

Laryngectomy: (lar-in-JEK-tah-mee) Surgical removal of the larynx.

Laryngitis: (lare-in-JIGH-tiss) Inflammation of the larynx.

Laser ablation: (LAY-zer uh-BLAY-shun) Therapeutic destruction of a growth or part of a growth by laser treatment.

Lavage: (lah-VAZH) Washing out of a cavity.

Law: (LAW) The further formalization of moral considerations.

Leiomyoma: (LYE-oh-my-OH-ma) A myoma consisting principally of smooth muscle tissue.

Leukemia: (loo-KEE-mee-ah) A malignancy of the blood-forming cells in the bone marrow.

Leukocytosis: (LOO-koh-sigh-TOH-sis) An increase in the number of leukocytes in the blood, generally caused by presence of infection and usually transient.

Leukopenia: (LOO-koh-PEE-nee-yah) Abnormal decrease of white blood cells, usually below 5000/mm^3.

Liability: (LYE-uh-BIL-i-tee) The level of responsibility that society places on individuals for their actions.

Libido: (li-BEE-doh) Sexual drive, conscious or unconscious.

Lichenified: (lye-KEN-i-fyed) Thickened or hardened from continued irritation.

Limitation of liability: (lim-i-TAY-shun OF LYE-uh-BIL-i-tee) Steps that health care professionals can take to limit their liability.

Living Will: (LIV-ing WIL) A document instructing health-care workers about a patient's preferences when he or she is no longer able to communicate. Implementation of Living Wills varies by state.

Lobectomy: (loh-BEK-tuh-mee) Surgical removal of a lobe of any organ or gland.

Lower gastrointestinal series (lower GI): (LOH-er GAS-troh-in-TES-ti-nuhl SEER-ees) The use of barium sulfate as an enema to facilitate x-ray and fluoroscopic examination of the colon.

Lymphadenopathy: (lim-FAD-e-NAH-puh-thee) Any disorder of the lymph nodes.

Lymphangitis: (lim-FAN-je-EYE-tis) Inflammation of lymphatic channels or vessels.

Lymphedema: (LIMPF-uh-DEE-mah) An abnormal accumulation of tissue fluid (potential lymph) in the interstitial space.

Lymphocytes: (LIM-foh-sites) Cells present in the blood and lymphatic tissue that provide the main means of immunity for the body; white blood cells.

Lymphoma: (lim-FOH-mah) A usually malignant lymphoid neoplasm.

Macular degeneration: (MACK-you-lar dee-JEN-uh-RAY-shun) Age-related breakdown of the macular area of the retina of the eye.

Malignant: (muh-LIG-nunt) Growing, resisting treatment; used to describe a tumor of cancerous cells.

Malpractice: (mal-PRAK-tiss) A breach of duty arising out of the relationship that exists between the patient and the health care worker.

Mammography: (mah-MOG-rah-fee) Use of radiography of the breast to diagnose breast cancer.

Mammoplasty: (MAM-oh-PLAS-tee) Plastic surgery of the breast.

Mania: (MAY-nee-ah) Mental disorder characterized by excessive excitement.

Marsupialization: (mar-SOO-pee-al-i-ZAY-shun) Process of raising the borders of an evacuated tumor sac to the edges of the abdominal wound and stitching them there to form a pouch.

Mastalgia: (mass-TAL-jee-ah) Pain in the breast.

Mastectomy: (mass-TECK-tuh-mee) Excision of the breast.

Mastitis: (mass-TIGH-tis) Inflammation of the breast.

Mastopexy: (MAS-toh-PEKS-ee) Correction of a pendulous breast by surgical fixation and plastic surgery.

Mediastinum: (ME-dee-ah-STYE-num) A septum or cavity between two principal portions of an organ.

Megacolon: (MEG-ah-KOH-lun) Extremely dilated colon.

Melena: (muh-LEE-nah) Black, tarry feces caused by action of intestinal secretions on free blood.

Menarche: (me-NAR-kee) The initial menstrual period, normally occurring between the ninth and seventeenth year.

Ménière's disease: (ma-NEARS di-ZEEZ) A recurrent and usually progressive group of symptoms including progressive deafness, ringing in the ears, dizziness, and a sensation of fullness or pressure in the ears.

Meningitis: (men-in-JIGH-tis) Inflammation of the membranes of the spinal cord and brain.

Menopause: (MEN-oh-pawz) The period that marks the permanent cessation of menstrual activity, usually occurring between the ages of 35 and 58.

Mental health: (MEN-tuhl HELLTH) State of being adjusted to life; able to be flexible, successful, maintain close relationships, solve problems, make appropriate judgments, and cope with daily stresses.

Mental illness: (MEN-tuhl ILL-ness) Any illness that affects the mind or behavior.

Metastasis: (muh-TASS-tuh-sis) Movement of bacteria or body cells (especially cancer cells) from one part of the body to another.

Milieu: (me-LYU) Environment.

Miotic: (my-AH-tik) An agent that causes the pupil to contract.

Morality: (muh-RAL-i-tee) A social barometer that dictates what is good or bad in a society.

Morbidity: (more-BID-it-ee) State of being diseased.

Mortality: (more-TAL-it-ee) Condition of being mortal; number of deaths in a population.

Mucolytic: (MYOO-koh-LIT-ik) Agent that liquefies sputum.

Mucopurulent cervicitis: (MYOO-koh-PYOOR-uh-lent SIR-vi-SIGH-tis) Inflammation of the cervix producing mucus and purulent discharge.

Mucositis: (MYOO-koh-SIGH-tis) Inflammation of a mucous membrane.

Multifocal: (MUHL-tee-FOH-kuhl) Many foci (areas) or sites.

Murmur: (MUR-mur) An abnormal sound heard on auscultation of the heart and adjacent large blood vessels.

Muscle: (MUSS-uhl) A bundle of long slender cells or fibers that have the power to contract and hence to produce movement.

Myalgia: (my-AL-jee-ah) Muscle pain or tenderness.

Myectomy: (my-ECK-tuh-mee) Surgical removal of a hypertrophied muscle.

Myelogram: (MY-e-loh-gram) The film produced by radiography of the spinal cord after injection of a contrast medium into the subarachnoid space.

Myocardial infarction: (MY-oh-KAR-dee-yuhl in-FARK-shun) Death of cells of an area of the heart muscle, myocardium, as a result of oxygen deprivation, which in turn is caused by obstruction of the blood supply. Commonly referred to as a heart attack.

Myocarditis: (MY-oh-kar-DYE-tis) The inflammatory process that causes nodules to form in the myocardial tissue;

the nodules become scar tissue over time. Inflammation of the heart muscle.

Myocardium: (MY-oh-KAR-dee-um) Heart muscle.

Myomectomy: (my-oh-MECK-tuh-mee) Removal of a portion of muscle or muscular tissue.

Myopia: (my-OH-pee-ah) The error of refraction in which rays of light entering the eye parallel to the optic axis are brought to a focus in front of the retina; nearsightedness.

Myringoplasty: (mir-IN-goh-PLASS-tee) Surgical reconstruction of the tympanic membrane.

Myringotomy: (MIR-in-GOT-uh-mee) Incision of the tympanic membrane, usually performed to relieve pressure and allow for drainage of either serous or purulent fluid in the middle ear behind the tympanic membrane.

Myxedema: (MICK-suh-DEE-mah) Condition resulting from hypofunction of the thyroid gland.

Nasoseptoplasty: (NAY-zoh-SEP-toh-plass-tee) Surgical correction of the nasal septum.

Naturopathy: (NAY-chur-AH-pa-thee) System of medicine that uses natural therapies such as nutrition, herbs, hydrotherapy, counseling, physical medicine, and homeopathy to treat disease, promote healing, and prevent illness.

Negligence: (NEG-li-jense) An unintentional tort.

Neoplasm: (NEE-oh-PLAZ-uhm) New abnormal tissue growth, as in a tumor.

Nephrectomy: (ne-FREK-tuh-mee) Surgical removal of a kidney.

Nephrogenic: (NEFF-roh-JEN-ick) Caused by the kidneys.

Nephrolithotomy: (NEFF-roh-li-THOT-uh-mee) Incision of a kidney for removal of kidney stones.

Nephropathy: (ne-FROP-uh-thee) Any disease of the kidney.

Nephrosclerosis: (NEFF-roh-skle-ROH-sis) Hardening of the kidney associated with hypertension and disease of the renal arterioles.

Nephrostomy: (ne-FRAHS-toh-mee) Creation of a permanent opening into the renal pelvis.

Nephrotoxin: (NEFF-roh-TOCK-sin) A toxin having a specific destructive effect on kidney tissue.

Neuralgia: (new-RAL-jee-ah) Nerve pain.

Neurogenic: (NEW-roh-JEN-ik) Originating in the nervous system.

Neuropathic pain: (NEW-roh-PATH-ik PAYN) Pain resulting from peripheral nerve injury.

Neuropathy: (new-RAH-puh-thee) A general term denoting functional disturbances and pathologic changes in the peripheral nervous system.

Neutrophils: (NEW-troh-fils) Granular leukocytes (white blood cells) having a nucleus with three to five lobes connected by threads of chromatin and cytoplasm containing very fine granules.

Nociceptive: (NOH-see-SEP-tiv) Pain sensitive.

Nocturia: (nock-TYOO-ree-ah) Excessive urination at night.

Nodal or junctional rhythm: (NOHD-uhl or JUNGK-shun-uhl RITH-uhm) A cardiac rhythm with its origin at the atrioventricular (AV) node.

Nonmaleficence: (NON-muh-LEF-i-sens) The requirement that health care providers do no harm to their patients, either intentionally or unintentionally.

Norepinephrine: (NOR-ep-i-NEFF-rin) A hormone produced by the adrenal medulla, similar in chemical and pharmacological properties to epinephrine, but chiefly a vasoconstrictor with little effect on cardiac output.

Normotensive: (nor-moh-TEN-siv) Normal blood pressure.

Nosocomial infection: (no-zoh-KOH-mee-uhl in-FECK-shun) Infection acquired in a health care agency.

Nuchal rigidity: (NEW-kuhl re-JID-i-tee) Rigidity of the nape, or back, of the neck.

Nursing diagnosis: (NER-sing DYE-ag-NOH-sis) A standardized label placed on a patient's problem to make it understandable to all nurses.

Nursing process: (NER-sing PRAH-sess) An orderly, logical approach to administering nursing care so that the patient's needs for such care are met comprehensively and effectively.

Nystagmus: (nis-TAG-muss) Involuntary, rapid, rhythmic eye movement.

Obesity: (oh-BEE-si-tee) Abnormal amount of fat on the body from 20% to 30% over average weight for age, sex, and height.

Objective data: (ob-JEK-tiv DAY-tuh) Factual data obtained through physical assessment and diagnostic tests; objective data are observable or knowable through the five senses.

Obsession: (ub-SESH-un) Repetitive thought, urge, or emotion.

Obstipation: (OB-sti-PAY-shun) Intractable constipation.

Obstructive shock: (ub-STRUCK-tive SHAHK) Shock caused by indirect pump failure.

Occult blood test: (ah-KULT BLUHD TEST) A chemical test or microscopic examination for blood, especially in feces, that is not apparent on visual inspection.

Oligura: (AWH-li-GYOO-ree-ah) Diminished urination.

Oncology: (on-CAW-luh-jee) The study of cancer and cancer treatment.

Oncovirus: (ON-koh-VIGH-russ) Viruses linked to cancer in humans.

Onychomycosis: (ON-i-koh-my-KOH-sis) Disease of the nails caused by fungus.

Ophthalmia neonatorum: (ahf-THAL-mee-ah NEE-oh-nuh-TOR-uhm) Conjunctivitis in the newborn resulting from exposure to infectious or chemical agents.

Ophthalmologist: (AHF-thal-MAH-luh-jist) A physician who specializes in the treatment of disorders of the eye.

Ophthalmoscope: (ahf-THAL-muh-skohp) An instrument used for examining the interior of the eye, especially the retina.

Opioid: (OHP-ee-OYD) A narcotic drug with morphine-like effects. True opioids are derived from opium.

Optician: (ahp-TISH-uhn) One who specializes in filling prescriptions for corrective lenses for eyeglasses and contact lenses.

Optimum level of functioning: (OP-teh-mum LEV-uhl of FUNK-shun-ing) Highest level of patient activity considering the patient's condition.

Optometrist: (ahp-TOM-uh-trist) A doctor of optometry who diagnoses and treats conditions and diseases of the eye per state laws.

Orchiectomy: (or-ki-EK-toh-mee) Removal of one or both testicles; a treatment for prostate cancer.

Orchitis: (or-KIGH-tis) Inflammation of a testis.

Orgasm: (OR-gazm) Pleasurable physical release sensation related to physical, sexual, and psychological stimulation.

Orientation: (OR-ee-en-TAY-shun) The ability to comprehend and to adjust oneself in an environment with regard to time, location, and identity of persons.

Orthopnea: (or-THOP-knee-a) Labored breathing that occurs when lying flat; relieved when sitting up; associated with left ventricular heart failure.

Osmolality: (ahs-moh-LAL-i-tee) Osmotic concentration; ionic concentration of the dissolved substances per unit of solvent.

Osmosis: (ahs-MOH-sis) The passage of solvent through a semipermeable membrane that separates solutions of different concentrations.

Osteomyelitis: (AHS-tee-oh-my-LIGHT-tis) Inflammation of bone, especially the marrow, caused by a pathogenic organism.

Osteopathy: (AHS-tee-ah-PATH-ee) System of medicine emphasizing the inter-relationship of the body's nerves, muscles, bones, and organs; involves treating the whole person, and stresses the importance of diet, exercise, and fitness, with a focus on prevention.

Osteoporosis: (AHS-tee-oh-por-OH-sis) A condition in which there is a reduction in the mass of bone per unit volume.

Osteosarcoma: (AHS-tee-oh-sar-KOH-mah) A malignant sarcoma of a bone.

Otalgia: (oh-TAL-jee-ah) Pain in the ear.

Otorrhea: (OH-toh-REE-ah) Inflammation of the ear with purulent discharge.

Otosclerosis: (OH-toh-skle-ROH-sis) A condition characterized by chronic, progressive deafness, especially for low tones.

Ototoxic: (OH-toh-TOK-sik) Having a detrimental effect on the eighth cranial nerve or the organs of hearing.

Pain: (PAYN) An unpleasant sensory and emotional experience associated with actual or potential tissue damage, or described in terms of such damage. Is whatever the patient says it is whenever the patient says it occurs.

Palliation: (pal-ee-AY-shun) The relief of symptoms without cure.

Palpation: (pal-PAY-shun) Use of the fingers or hands to feel something.

Pancreatectomy: (PAN-kree-uh-TECK-tuh-mee) Removal of all or part of the pancreas.

Pancreatitis: (PAN-kree-uh-TIGH-tis) Inflammation of the pancreas.

Pancytopenia: (PAN-sigh-toh-PEE-nee-ah) Abnormal depression of all the cellular elements of the blood.

Panhysterectomy: (PAN-hiss-tuh-RECK-tuh-mee) Excision of the entire uterus, including the cervix uteri.

Panmyelosis: (PAN-my-e-LOH-sis) Increased level of all bone marrow components, red blood cells, white blood cells, and platelets.

Para: (PAR-ah) Number of deliveries a woman has had from pregnancies after 20 weeks gestation.

Paradoxical respirations: (PAR-uh-DOK-si-kuhl RES-pi-RAY-shuns) Chest movement on respiration that is opposite to that expected.

Paranoia: (PAR-uh-NOY-uh) Behavior that is marked by delusions of persecution or delusional jealousy.

Paraparesis: (PAR-ah-pah-REE-sis) Partial paralysis of the lower extremities.

Paraphimosis: (PAR-uh-figh-MOH-sis) Uncircumcised foreskin that has swollen and stuck behind the head of the penis.

Paraplegia: (PAR-ah-PLEE-jah) Paralysis of the lower body, including both legs, resulting from a spinal cord lesion.

Paresis: (puh-REE-sis) Weakness; incomplete paralysis.

Paresthesia: (PAR-es-THEE-zee-ah) A heightened sensation, such as burning, prickling, or tingling.

Paroxysmal nocturnal dyspnea: (PEAR-ox-IS-mall knock-TURN-al DISP-knee-a) Sudden attacks of shortness of breath that usually occur during sleep. Person wakes gasping for breath and sits up to relieve symptoms; associated with left ventricular heart failure.

Partial-thickness burn: (PAR-shul THICK-ness BERN) Burn in which the epithelializing elements remain intact.

Passive immunity: (PASS-iv im-YOO-ni-tee) Reinforcement of the immune system with immune serum for such conditions as tetanus, diptheria, and venomous snake bite.

Paternalism: (puh-TER-nuhl-izm) A unilateral and sometimes unreasonable decision by health care providers that implies they know what is best, regardless of the patient's wishes.

Pathogen: (PATH-o-jen) A microorganism or substance capable of producing a disease.

Pathological fracture: (PATH-uh-LAH-jik-uhl FRAHK-chur) Fracture resulting from weakening of the bone structure by pathological processes such as neoplasia or osteomalacia.

Patient-controlled analgesia (PCA): (PAY-shent kon-TROHLD an-uhl-JEE-zee-ah) An apparatus that delivers an intravenous analgesic to relieve pain, which is controlled by the patient.

Pedicle: (PED-i-kuhl) The stem that attaches a new growth.

Pediculosis: (pe-DIK-yoo-LOH-sis) Infestation with lice.

Pemphigus: (PEM-fi-gus) Acute or chronic serious skin disease characterized by the appearance of bullae (blisters) of various sizes on normal skin and mucous membranes.

Penumbra: (puh-NUM-bra) An area of brain tissue surrounding damage from a stroke that may be revived if the brain is reperfused quickly.

Peptic ulcer disease: (PEP-tick UL-sir di-ZEEZ) A condition in which the lining of the esophagus, stomach, or duodenum is eroded.

Perception: (per-SEP-shun) A unique impression of events by an individual. These impressions are strongly influenced by personality, cultural orientation, attitudes, and life experiences.

Percussion: (per-KUSH-un) A tapping technique used by physicians and advanced practice nurses to determine the consistency of underlying tissues.

Percutaneous: (PER-kyoo-TAY-nee-us) Through the skin; may refer to an injection, a medication application, or a biopsy.

Perfusion: (per-FEW-zhun) Supplying an organ or tissue with blood.

Pericardial effusion: (PER-ee-KAR-dee-uhl ee-FYOO-zhun) A buildup of fluid in the pericardial space.

Pericardial friction rub: (PER-ee-KAR-dee-uhl FRICK-shun RUB) Friction sound heard over the fourth left intercostal space near the sternum; a classic sign of pericarditis.

Pericardial tamponade: (PER-ee-KAR-dee-uhl TAM-pon-AID) Compression of the heart by an abnormal filling of the pericardial sac with blood.

Pericardiectomy: (PER-ee-kar-dee-ECK-tuh-mee) Excision of part or all of the pericardium.

Pericardiocentesis: (PER-ee-KAR-dee-oh-sen-TEE-sis) Surgical perforation of the pericardium.

Pericardiotomy: (PER-ee-KAR-dee-AH-tah-mee) Incision of the pericardium.

Pericarditis: (PER-ee-kar-DYE-tis) Inflammation of the pericardium.

Perimenopausal: (PER-ee-MEN-oh-PAWS-uhl) The phase before the onset of menopause, during which the cycle of a woman with regular menses changes, perhaps abruptly, to a pattern of irregular cycles and increased periods of amenorrhea.

Perinatal: (PAIR-ee-NAY-tuhl) Concerning the period beginning after the 28th week of pregnancy and ending 28 days after birth.

Perioperative: (PER-ee-AHP-er-uh-tiv) Occurring in the period immediately before, during, and after surgery.

Peripheral arterial disease: (puh-RIFF-uh-ruhl ar-TIR-ee-uhl di-ZEEZ) Disease of the peripheral arteries that interferes with adequate flow of blood.

Peripheral parenteral nutrition: (puh-RIFF-uh-ruhl par-EN-te-ruhl new-TRISH-un) Nutrition by intravenous injection.

Peripheral vascular resistance: (puh-RIFF-uh-ruhl VAS-kyoo-lar ree-ZIS-tense) Opposition to blood flow through the vessels.

Peristalsis: (paris-TALL-sis) Progressive, wave-like movement that occurs involuntarily in hollow tubes of the body such as the alimentary (digestive) canal; causes contents of tube to be moved onward.

Peristomal: (PER-i-STOH-muhl) Area around a stoma.

Peritoneal dialysis: (PER-i-toh-NEE-uhl dye-AL-i-sis) The employment of the peritoneum surrounding the abdominal cavity as a dializing membrane for the purpose of removing waste products or toxins accumulated as a result of renal failure.

Peritonitis: (per-i-toh-NIGH-tis) Inflammation of the peritoneum.

Personal protective equipment (PUR-sun-al proh-TEK-tiv i-KWIP-mant) Items worn to protect oneself and one's patients from direct transmission of organisms that includes gloves, surgical masks, goggles, gowns, and shoe booties based on the task to be performed and the type of isolation precautions in use.

Petechiae: (pe-TEE-kee-ee, puh-TEE-kee-eye) Small, purplish, hemorrhagic spots on the skin that appear in certain illnesses and bleeding disorders.

Phagocytosis: (fay-go-sigh-TOH-sis) Ingestion and digestion of bacteria and particles by phagocytes, cells that have the ability to ingest and destroy particulate substances such as bacteria, protozoa, and cell debris.

Pharyngitis: (fair-in-JIGH-tiss) Inflammation of the mucous membranes and lymph tissues of the pharynx, usually caused by infection.

Pheochromocytoma: (FEE-oh-KROH-moh-sigh-TOH-mah) Rare tumor of the adrenal system that secretes catecholamines.

Phimosis: (figh-MOH-sis) Uncircumcised foreskin that cannot be moved down from the head of the penis.

Phlebitis: (fla-BYE-tis) Inflammation of a vein; may be due to irritating IV fluids or thrombosis.

Phlebotomy: (fle-BAH-tuh-mee) Entry into a vein for the removal or withdrawal of blood.

Phobia: (FOH-bee-ah) A persistent, irrational, intense fear of a specific object, activity, or situation.

Photophobia: (FOH-toh-FOH-bee-ah) Abnormal visual intolerance to light.

Physical dependence: (FIZ-ik-uhl dee-PEN-dens) A pharmacologic phenomenon characterized by signs and symptoms of withdrawal when medication is withdrawn.

Phytoestrogens: (FI-toh-ES-troh-jens) Naturally occurring plant sterols that have an estrogenlike effect.

Plague: (PLAYG) A severe febrile illness caused by the gram-negative coccobacillus *Yersinia pestis* that is usually transmitted by the bite of an infectious flea. It can also be used as a biological weapon in which primary pneumonic plague would likely occur.

Plaque: (PLAK) A deposit of fatty material on the lining of an artery.

Plasmapheresis: (PLAS-mah-fer-EE-sis) Removal of blood to separate cells from plasma.

Pleurodesis: (PLOO-roh-DEE-sis) Creation of adhesions between the parietal and visceral pleura to treat recurrent pneumothorax.

***Pneumocystis carinii* pneumonia:** (new-mo-SIS-tis ca-RIN-ee-eye new-MOH-nee-ya) An acute pneumonia caused by *Pneumocystis carinii*, a fungus. It occurs in immunodeficient adults and is a defining opportunistic infection of AIDS.

Pneumonectomy: (NEW-moh-NEK-tuh-mee) Surgical removal of all or part of a lung.

Pneumothorax: (NEW-moh-THAW-raks) Air in the pleural space.

Poikilothermy: (POY-ki-loh-THER-mee) The absence of sufficient arterial blood flow, causing the extremity to become the temperature of the environment.

Point of maximal impulse: (POYNT of MAKS-i-muhl IM-puls) The area of the chest where the greatest force can be felt with the palm of the hand when the heart contracts or beats. Usually at the fourth to fifth intercostal space in the midclavicular line.

Polycythemia: (PAH-lee-sigh-THEE-mee-ah) Excessive red cells in the blood.

Polydipsia: (PAH-lee-DIP-see-ah) Excessive thirst.

Polymyositis: (PAH-lee-my-oh-SIGH-tis) A rare, inflammatory disease of the skeletal muscle tissue characterized by symmetric weakness of proximal muscles of the limbs, neck, and pharynx.

Polyneuropathy: (PAH-lee-new-RAH-puh-thee) A disease involving multiple nerves.

Polyphagia: (PAH-lee-FAY-jee-ah) Excessive eating.

Polyuria: (PAH-lee-YOOR-ee-ah) Excessive urination.

Portal hypertension: (POR-tuhl HIGH-per-TEN-shun) Persistent blood pressure elevation in the portal circulation of the abdomen.

Postcoital: (post-KOH-i-tal) Following sexual intercourse.

Postictal: (pohst-IK-tuhl) Occurring after a sudden attack, such as an epileptic seizure.

Postmortem Care: (post-MOR-tum KARE) Care after death.

Postoperative: (post-AHP-er-uh-tiv) Following a surgical operation.

Postprandial: (POST-PRAN-dee-uhl) After a meal.

Powerlessness: (POW-er-less-nes) Perceived lack of control over a situation.

Preload: (PREE-lohd) End-diastolic stretch of cardiac muscle fibers; equals end-diastolic volume.

Preoperative: (pre-AHP-er-uh-tiv) Preceding an operation.

Preprandial: (PREE-PRAN-dee-uhl) Before a meal.

Presbycusis: (PRESS-by-KYOO-sis) Progressive, bilaterally symmetrical perceptive hearing loss occurring with age; usually occurs after age 50 and is caused by structural changes in the organs of hearing.

Presbyopia: (PREZ-by-OH-pee-ah) Diminution of accommodation of the lens of the eye occurring normally with

aging, and usually resulting in hyperopia, or farsightedness.

Pressure ulcer: (PRESS-sure ULL-sir) An open sore or lesion of the skin that develops because of prolonged pressure against an area.

Priapism: (PRY-uh-pizm) Erection that lasts too long.

Primary hypertension: (PRY-mare-ee HIGH-per-TEN-shun) Abnormally elevated blood pressure of unknown cause. Also called essential hypertension.

Proctitis: (prock-TIGH-tis) Inflammation of the rectum and anus.

Proctosigmoidoscopy: (PROK-toh-SIG-moy-DAHS-kuh-pee) Visual examination of the rectum and sigmoid colon by use of a sigmoidoscope.

Prodrome: (PROH-drohm) A symptom indicating the onset of a disease.

Prostaglandins: (PRAHS-tah-GLAND-ins) Chemical neurotransmitters usually associated with pain at the site of an injury, periphery.

Prostatectomy: (PRAHS-tuh-TEK-tuh-mee) Removal of the prostate gland.

Prostatitis: (PRAHS-tuh-TIGH-tis) Inflammation or infection of the prostate gland.

Protozoa: (pro-tow-ZOH-ah) Single-celled parasitic organisms that can move and live mainly in the soil.

Pruritus: (proo-RYE-tis) Severe itching.

Pseudoaddiction: (soo-doh-ad-DICK-shun) Syndrome in which behaviors similar to addiction appear as a result of inadequate pain control and patients fear not receiving adequate pain medications and pain relief.

Psoriasis: (suh-RYE-ah-sis) Chronic inflammatory skin disorder in which epidermal cells proliferate abnormally fast.

Psychoanalysis: (SIGH-koh-uh-NAL-i-sis) Form of therapy based on the theories of Sigmund Freud, regarding the dynamics of the unconscious.

Psychogenic: (SIGH-koh-JEN-ick) Of mental origin.

Psychological dependence: (SY-ko-LAW-ick-al dee-PEN-dens) Obsession of obtaining drugs for use other than medicinal; addiction.

Psychopharmacology: (SIGH-koh-FAR-meh-KAHL-uh-jee) The study of the action of drugs on psychological functions and mental states.

Psychosomatic: (SIGH-koh-soh-MAT-ik) Having bodily symptoms of psychological, emotional, or mental origin; illness traceable to an emotional cause.

Psychotherapy: (SIGH-koh-THER-uh-pee) A method of treating disease (especially mental illness) by mental rather than pharmacological means.

Ptosis: (TOH-sis) Drooping of eyelid.

Puerperal: (pyoo-ER-per-uhl) Concerning the puerperium, or period of 42 days after childbirth.

Pulmonary edema: (PULL-muh-NAIR-ee uh-DEE-muh) Acute heart failure in which there is severe fluid congestion in the alveoli of the lungs; life-threatening.

Pulse deficit: (PULS DEF-i-sit) A condition in which the number of pulse beats counted at the radial artery is less than those counted in the same period of time at the apical heart rate.

Purpura: (PUR-pur-uh) Hemorrhage into the skin, mucous membranes, internal organs, and other tissues.

Purulent: (PURE-u-lent) Fluid that contains pus.

Pyelogram: (PIE-loh-GRAM) A diagnostic procedure involving x-ray of the kidneys; may be done after injection of a dye into the bloodstream or directly into the kidneys.

Pyelonephritis: (PYE-e-loh-ne-FRY-tis) Inflammation of the kidney and renal pelvis.

Pyoderma: (PYE-oh-DER-mah) Any acute, inflammatory, purulent bacterial dermatitis.

Quadriparesis: (kwod-ri-par-E-sis) Weakness involving all four limbs caused by spinal cord injury.

Quadriplegia: (KWA-dri-PLEE-jah) Paralysis of all four limbs caused by spinal cord injury.

Radiation therapy: (RAY-dee-AY-shun THER-uh-pee) Cancer treatment with ionizing radiation.

Range of motion (ROM): (RANJE of MOH-shun) The range of movement of a body joint.

Raynaud's disease: (ra-NOHZ di-ZEEZ) A primary or idiopathic vasospastic disorder characterized by bilateral and symmetrical pallor and cyanosis of the fingers.

Reality orientation: (ree-AL-i-tee OR-ee-en-TAY-shun) A process to orient a person to facts such as names, dates, and time, through the use of verbal and nonverbal repeating messages.

Rectocele: (RECK-toh-seel) Protrusion or herniation of the posterior vaginal wall with the anterior wall of the rectum through the vagina.

Regurgitation: (ree-GUR-ji-TAY-shun) A backward flowing, as in the backflow of blood through a defective heart valve.

Remyelination: (ree-MY-uh-lin-AY-shun) Replacement of myelin or neurons.

Replantation: (re-plan-TAY-shun) The replacement of an organ or other structure, such as a digit, limb, or tooth, to the site from which it was previously lost or removed.

Reservoir: (REZ-er-VWAR) A person, animal, arthropod, plant, soil, or substance in which an infectious agent normally lives and multiplies, on which it depends for survival.

Respiratory excursion: (RES-pi-rah-TOR-ee eks-KUR-zhun) Downward movement of the diaphragm with inspiration.

Respite care: (RES-pit CARE) Short-term, intermittent care for the chronically ill; provides rest for the family members or caregivers from the stress of sustained caregiving.

Respondeat superior: (ress-POND-ee-et sue-PEER-ee-or) An institution that employs a worker may be liable for the acts or omissions of its employees.

Retinopathy: (RET-i-NAH-puh-thee) Disease of the retina of the eye.

Retroflexion: (RET-roh-FLECK-shun) A bending or flexing backward.

Retrograde cholangiopancreatography: (RET-roh-grayd koh-LAN-jee-oh-PAN-kree-ah-TOG-rah-fee) An endoscopic procedure that permits the physician to visualize the liver, gallbladder, and pancreas using an endoscope, dye, and x-ray examinations.

Retrograde: (RET-roh-grayd) Moving backward; degenerating from a better to a worse state.

Retroversion: (RET-roh-VER-zhun) A turning, or a state of being turned back; the tipping of an entire organ.

Rheumatic carditis: (roo-MAT-ick kar-DYE-tis) Serious complication of rheumatic fever in which all layers of the heart become inflamed.

Rheumatic fever: (roo-MAT-ick FEE-ver) A hypersensitivity reaction to antigens of group A beta-hemolytic streptococci.

Rhinitis: (rye-NIGH-tis) Inflammation of the nasal mucosa, usually associated with congestion, itching, sneezing, and nasal discharge.

Rhinoplasty: (RYE-noh-plass-tee) Plastic surgery of the nose.

Rickettsia: (ra-KET-see-ah) A genus of bacteria of the tribe Rickettsiae that multiply only in host cells.

Rinne test: (RIN-nee TEST) A test of hearing made with tuning forks.

Romberg's test: (RAHM-bergs TEST) A test to determine if a person has the ability to maintain body balance when the eyes are shut and the feet are close together.

Roux-en-Y: (roo-ehn-Y) Gastric bypass surgery. A small stomach pouch the size of a thumb is created with staples, then a Y-shaped section of the small intestine is attached to the pouch to allow food to bypass the lower stomach and duodenum.

Rule of nines: (ROOL of NINES) A formula for estimating percentage of body surface area, particularly helpful in judging the portion of skin that has been burned.

Sacral radiculopathy: (SAY-krul ra-DICK-yoo-LAH-puh-thee) Pathology of sacral nerve roots.

Salpingitis: (SAL-pin-JIGH-tis) Inflammation of a fallopian tube.

Salpingoscopy: (SAL-ping-AHS-koh-pee) Endoscopic visualization of the fallopian tubes.

Scleroderma: (SKLER-ah-DER-ma) A chronic manifestation of progressive systemic sclerosis in which the skin is taut, firm, and edematous, limiting movement.

Sclerosis: (skle-ROH-sis) A hardening or induration of an organ or tissue, especially from excessive growth of fibrous tissue.

Seborrhea: (SEB-oh-REE-ah) Disease of the sebaceous glands marked by increase in the amount and often alteration of the quality of sebaceous secretions.

Secondary hypertension: (SEK-un-DAR-ee HIGH-per-TEN-shun) High blood pressure that is a symptom of a specific cause, such as a kidney abnormality.

Semipermeable: (SEM-ee-PER-mee-uh-buhl) Partly permeable; said of a membrane that will allow fluids but not the dissolved substance to pass through it.

Sensorineural: (SEN-soh-ree-NEW-ruhl) Hearing loss caused by impairment of a sensory nerve.

Sensory deprivation: (SEN-suh-ree DEP-ri-VAY-shun) No or minimal stimulation of the senses that creates the potential for maladaptive coping.

Sensory overload: (SEN-suh-ree OH-ver-lohd) Excessive stimulation of the senses that creates the potential for maladaptive coping.

Sepsis: (SEP-sis) Systematic infection caused by microorganisms in the bloodstream.

Serologic: (SEAR-uh-LAJ-ick) Study of substances present in blood serum.

Serosanguineous: (SEER-oh-SANG-gwin-ee-us) Fluid consisting of serum and blood.

Serotonin: (SER-ah-TOH-nin) A chemical neurotransmitter important in sleep-wake cycles. Reduced serotonin levels are associated with depression.

Shock: (SHAHK) A clinical syndrome in which the peripheral blood flow is inadequate to return sufficient blood to the heart for normal function, particularly transport of oxygen to all organs and tissues.

Sinoatrial node: (SIGH-noh-AY-tree-al NOHD) Node at the junction of the superior vena cava and right atrium, regarded as the starting point of the heartbeat.

Sinusitis: (SINE-u-SIGH-tiss)

Inflammation of the sinuses; may be due to viral or bacterial infection, or to allergies.

Smallpox: (small-POX) A disease characterized by high fever and a rash caused by variola virus, an orthopoxvirus unique to humans that has a 30% fatality rate.

Snellen's chart: (SNEL-ens CHART) A chart imprinted with lines of black letters graduating in size from smallest on the bottom to largest on top; used for testing visual acuity.

Somatoform: (soh-MAT-uh-form) Denoting psychogenic symptoms resembling those of physical disease; psychosomatic.

Spider angioma: (SPY-der an-jee-OH-mah) Thin reddish-purple vein lines close to the skin surface.

Spirituality: (SPIHR-it-u-AL-it-tee) Sense of connectedness with all of life and the universe.

Splenectomy: (sple-NEK-tuh-mee) Excision of the spleen.

Splenomegaly: (SPLEE-noh-MEG-ah-lee) Enlargement of the spleen.

Standard of best interest: (STAND-erd OF BEST IN-ter-est) A type of decision made about patients' health care when they are unable to make an informed decision about their own care.

Standard precautions: (STAN-derd pre-KAW-shuns) Guidelines recommended by the Centers for Disease Control and Prevention to reduce the risk of the spread of infection.

Stapedectomy: (stay-pee-DEK-toh-mee) Excision of the stapes in order to improve hearing, especially in cases of otosclerosis.

Staphylococcus: (STAFF-il-oh-KOCK-uss) A genus of gram-positive bacteria; they are constantly present on the skin and in the upper respiratory tract and are the most common cause of localized suppurating infections.

Status asthmaticus: (STAT-us az-MAT-i-kus) Prolonged period of unrelieved asthma symptoms.

Steatorrhea: (STEE-ah-toh-REE-ah) Fat in the stools; may be associated with pancreatic disease.

Stenosis: (ste-NOH-sis) The constriction or narrowing of a passage or orifice, such as a cardiac valve.

Stent: (STENT) Any mold or device used to hold tissue in place or to provide a support, graft, or anastomosis while healing is taking place.

Stereotype: (STER-ee-oh-TIGHP) An opinion or belief about an individual or group that may not be true.

Sternotomy: (stir-NAH-tuh-mee) The operation of cutting through the sternum.

Stoma: (STOH-mah) A mouth, small opening, or pore.

Stomatitis: (STOH-mah-TIGH-tis) Inflammation of the mouth.

Stress: (STRESS) The physical (gravity, mechanical, pathogenic, injury) and psychological (fear, anxiety, crisis, joy) forces that are experienced by individuals.

Stressor: (STRESS-er) Any person or situation that produces an anxiety response.

Striae: (STRIGH-ee) A line or band of elevated or depressed tissue; may differ in color or texture from surrounding tissue.

Subarachnoid: (SUB-uh-RAK-noyd) Below or under the arachnoid membrane and the pia mater of the covering of the brain and spinal cord.

Subdural: (sub-DUHR-uhl) Beneath the dura mater.

Subjective data: (sub-JEK-tiv DAY-tuh) Information that is provided verbally by the patient.

Suffering: (SUFF-er-ing) A state of severe distress associated with events that threaten the intactness of the person. Emotional pain associated with real or potential tissue damage.

Summons: (SUM-muns) A notice of suit.

Suprapubic: (SOO-pruh-PEW-bik) Bone of the groin (or region) located above the pubic arch.

Surgeon: (SURGE-on) A medical practitioner who specializes in surgery.

Synovitis: (sin-oh-VIGH-tis) Inflammation of the synovial membrane that may be the result of an aseptic wound, a subcutaneous injury, irritation, or exposure to cold and dampness.

Systolic blood pressure: (sis-TAL-ik BLUHD PRESS-ur) Maximal pressure exerted on the arteries during contraction of the left ventricle of the heart. The top number of a blood pressure reading.

Tachycardia: (TAK-ee-KAR-dee-yah) An abnormal rapidity of heart action, usually defined as a heart rate greater than 100 beats per minute in adults.

Tachydysrhythmia: (TACK-ee-dis-RITH-mee-yah) An abnormal heart rhythm with rate greater than 100 beats per minute in an adult.

Tachypnea: (TAK-ip-NEE-ah) Abnormally rapid respiratory rate.

Tamponade: (TAM-pon-AYD) Compression of a part.

Tension pneumothorax: (TEN-shun NEW-moh-THOR-raks) Abnormal accumulation of air with buildup of pressure in the pleural space.

Teratoma: (ter-uh-TOH-muh) A congenital tumor containing one or more of the three primary embryonic germ layers.

Terminal illness: (TERM-in-al ILL-ness) An illness that will probably cause death in 6 months or less.

Tetanus: (TET-nus) A highly fatal disease caused by the bacillus *Clostridium tetani* and characterized by muscle spasm and convulsions.

Tetany: (TET-uh-nee) Muscle spasms, numbness, and tingling caused by changes in pH and low serum calcium.

Thoracentesis: (THOR-uh-sen-TEE-sis) Insertion of a large-bore needle into the pleural space to remove fluid.

Thoracotomy: (THAW-rah-KAH-tah-mee) Surgical incision into the chest wall.

Thrill: (THRILL) Abnormal vessel that has a bulging or narrowed wall; a vibration is felt.

Thrombi: (THROM-bye) Blood clots.

Thrombocytopenia: (THROM-boh-SIGH-toh-PEE-nee-uh) Abnormal decrease in the number of blood platelets.

Thrombolytic: (throm-bo-LIT-ik) Agent that dissolves or splits up a thrombus, an aggregation of blood factors.

Thrombophlebitis: (THROM-boh-fle-BYE-tis) The formation of a clot and inflammation within a vein.

Thrombosis: (throm-BOH-sis) Formation, development, or presence of a thrombus, an aggregation of blood factors.

Tidaling: (TIGH-dah-ling) Rise and fall; may refer to water in water-seal chamber of a chest drainage system.

Titration: (tigh-TRAY-shun) Adjustment of medication up or down to meet patient needs.

Tolerance: (TALL-er-ens) The response of the body to medication that requires increased medication administration to achieve the same effect. Often refers to opioids.

Torts: (TORTS) Lawsuits involving civil wrongs.

Toxemia: (tock-SEE-me-ah) Spread of poisonous products of bacteria throughout the body.

Tracheostomy: (TRAY-key-AHS-tuh-me) A surgical opening in the neck into the trachea to provide an airway when the trachea is obstructed.

Tracheotomy: (TRAY-key-AH-tuh-me) An opening in the neck into the trachea.

Traditions: (tra-DISH-uns) Practices and customs handed down through the generations, often by word of mouth.

Transcellular: (trans-SELL-yoo-lar) Across cell membranes.

Transdermal: (trans-DER-mal) Entering through the dermis, or skin, as in administration of a drug applied to the skin in ointment or patch form.

Transillumination: (TRANS-i-loo-mi-NAY-shun) The passage of strong light through a body structure to permit inspection of an observer on the opposite side.

Transjugular intrahepatic portosystemic shunt (TIPS): (TRANZ-jug-yoo-lar intra-hep-PAT-ik POR-toh-sis-TEM-ik SHUNT) Shunt that sidetracks venous blood around the liver to the vena cava for treatment of ascites.

Transmyocardial (TRANS-my-o-KAR-dee-yah) Across all layers of the heart.

Trauma: (TRAW-mah) Physical injury caused by an external force.

Trendelenburg's position: (tren-DELL-en-bergz POH-si-shun) A position in which the patient's head is low and the body and legs are on an elevated and inclined plane.

Triage: (TREE-ahj) To sort.

Trigeminy: (try-JEM-i-nee) Occurring every third beat, as in trigeminal premature ventricular contractions.

Tropia: (TROH-pee-ah) A manifest deviation of an eye from the normal position when both eyes are open and uncovered.

T-tube: (TEE-toob) A T-shaped tube in the bile duct that allows drainage of bile following gallbladder surgery.

Tumor: (TOO-mur) An abnormal growth of cells or tissues; tumors may be benign or malignant.

Turbid: (TER-bid) Cloudy.

Turgor: (TER-ger) The resistance of the skin to being grasped between the fingers. Dehydration causes poor skin turgor.

Unifocal: (YOO-ni-FOH-kuhl) Coming or originating from one site or focus.

Upper gastrointestinal series (upper GI, UGI): (UH-per GAS-troh-in-TES-ti-nuhl SEER-ees) X-ray and fluoroscopic examinations of the stomach and duodenum after the ingestion of a contrast medium.

Uremia: (yoo-REE-mee-ah) An excess in the blood of urea, creatinine, and other nitrogenous end products of protein and amino acid metabolism.

Urethritis: (YOO-ree-THRIGH-tis) Inflammation of the urethra.

Urethroplasty: (yoo-REE-throh-PLAS-tee) Plastic repair of the urethra.

Urinary incontinence: (YOOR-i-NAR-ee in-KON-ti-nents) Inability to control urine excretion creating accidental urinary leakage.

Urodynamic: (YOO-roh-dye-NAM-ik) The study of the holding or storage of urine in the bladder, the facility with which it empties, and the rate of movement of urine out of the bladder during urination.

Urosepsis: (YOO-roh-SEP-sis) Septicemia resulting from urinary tract infection.

Urticaria: (UR-ti-CARE-ee-ah) Hives signifying an allergic reaction.

Utilitarian: (yoo-TILL-I-TAR-I-en) Consequences or outcomes of a dilemma are the most important element.

Vaginosis: (VAJ-i-NOH-sis) Inflammation of the vagina caused by *Gardnerella vaginalis*.

Values: (VAL-use) Ideals or concepts that give meaning to an individual's life.

Valvotomy: (val-VAH-tuh-mee) Cutting through a valve.

Valvuloplasty: (VAL-vyoo-loh-PLAS-tee) Plastic or restorative surgery on a valve, especially a cardiac valve.

Varices: (VAR-i-seez) Dilated veins.

Varicocele: (VAR-i-koh-seel) Varicose veins of the scrotum; can lead to infertility.

Varicose veins: (VAR-i-kohs VAINS) Swollen, distended, and knotted veins, usually in the subcutaneous tissue of the leg.

Vasculitis: (VAS-kue-LIGH-tis) Inflammation of a vessel.

Vasectomy: (va-SEK-tuh-mee) Surgically cutting and sealing the vas deferens to prevent sperm from getting outside the body. Used as a birth control method for men.

Vector: (VECK-tur) Living organism that transmits disease.

Venous stasis ulcers: (VEE-nus STAY-sis UL-sers) Poorly healing ulcers that result from inadequate venous drainage.

Ventricular diastole: (ven-TRICK-yoo-lar dye-AS-tuh-lee) The period of relaxation of the two ventricles.

Ventricular escape rhythm: (ven-TRICK-yoo-lar es-KAYP RITH-uhm) The naturally occurring rhythm of the ventricles when the rest of the cardiac conduction system fails.

Ventricular repolarization: (ven-TRICK-yoo-lar RE-pol-lahr-i-ZAY-shun) Reestablishment of the polarized state of the muscle after contraction.

Ventricular systole: (ven-TRICK-yoo-lar SIS-tuh-lee) The contraction of the two ventricles.

Ventricular tachycardia: (ven-TRICK-yoo-lar TACK-ee-KAR-dee-yah) A series of at least three beats arising from a ventricular focus at a rate greater than 100 beats per minute.

Verrucous: (ve-ROO-kus) Wartlike, with raised portions.

Vertebrae: (VER-te-bray) Any of the 33 bony segments of the spinal column: 7 cervical, 12 thoracic, 5 lumbar, 5 sacral, and 4 coccygeal vertebrae.

Vesicant: (VESS-i-kant) Agent that causes blistering of tissue.

Vesicular: (ve-SICK-yoo-ler) Pertaining to vesicles or small blisters.

Virulence: (VEER-you-lence) The power of an organism to cause disease.

Virus: (VIGH-rus) The smallest organism identified by use of electron microscopy; intracellular parasites that may cause disease.

Viscosity: (vis-KAH-si-tee) Thickness, as of the blood.

Volvulus: (VOL-view-lus) A twisting of the bowel on itself, causing obstruction.

Vulvovaginitis: (VUL-voh-VAJ-I-NIGH-tis) Inflammation of the vulva and vagina.

Weber test: (VAY-ber TEST) A test for unilateral deafness.

Welfare rights: (WELL-fare RIGHTS) Also called legal rights; rights that are based on a legal entitlement to some good or benefit.

White blood cells: (WIGHT BLUHD SELLS) Leukocytes; the body's primary defense against infection.

Withdrawal: (with-DRAW-ul) Symptoms caused by cessation of administration of a drug, especially a narcotic or alcohol, to which the individual has become either physiologically or psychologically addicted.

Worldview: (WERLD-vyoo) The way individuals look on the world to form values and beliefs about life and the world around them.

Xerostomia: (ZEE-roh-STOH-mee-ah) Dry mouth caused by reduction in secretions.

Index

Note: Page numbers in *italics* indicate figures. Page numbers followed by t indicate tables and by b indicate boxes.